Goodman and Gilman's

Manual of Pharmacology and Therapeutics

second edition

Editors

Randa Hilal-Dandan, PhD
Lecturer in Pharmacology
University of California, San Diego
La Jolla, California

Laurence L. Brunton, PhD
Professor of Pharmacology and Medicine
University of California, San Diego
La Jolla, California

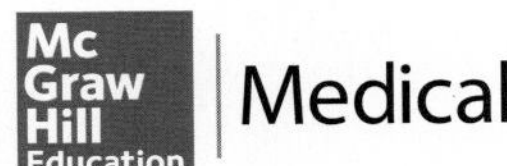

New York Chicago San Francisco Lisbon London Mad
New Delhi San Juan Seoul Singapore Sydney Toronto

Goodman and Gilman's Manual of Pharmacology and Therapeutics
Second Edition

1 2 3 4 5 6 7 8 9 0 CTP/CTP 18 17 16 15 14 13

ISBN 978-0-07-176917-4
MHID 0-07-176917-X

ISE ISBN 978-0-07-179288-2
ISE MHID 0-07-179288-0

This book was set in Times New Roman PS by Thomson Digital.
The editors were James F. Shanahan and Christie Naglieri.
The production supervisor was Richard Ruzycka.
The illustration manager was Armen Ovsepyan.
Project management was provided by Saloni Narang, Thomson Digital.
The designer was Janice Bielawa; the cover designer was Thomas De Pierro.
China Translation & Printing Services, Ltd. was printer and binder.

This book is printed on acid-free paper.

Library of Congress Cataloging-in-Publication Data

Hilal-Dandan, Randa.
Goodman and Gilman's manual of pharmacology and therapeutics. — 2nd ed. / Randa Hilal-Dandan, Laurence L. Brunton.
p. ; cm.
Manual of pharmacology and therapeutics
Rev. ed. of: the Goodman and Gilman's manual of pharmacological therapeutics / [edited] by Laurence L. Brunton ... [et al.]. 2007.
Companion v. to: Goodman & Gilman's the pharmacological basis of therapeutics. 12th ed. 2011.
Includes index.
ISBN 978-0-07-176917-4 (alk. paper) — ISBN 0-07-176917-X
I. Brunton, Laurence L. II. Goodman, Louis S. (Louis Sanford), 1906-2000. III. Goodman and Gilman's manual of pharmacological therapeutics. IV. Goodman & Gilman's the pharmacological basis of therapeutics. V. Title. VI. Title: Manual of pharmacology and therapeutics.
[DNLM: 1. Pharmacological Phenomena—Handbooks. 2. Drug Therapy—Handbooks. QV 39]
615'.7—dc23

2012048756

Contents

Section IV

Inflammation, Immunomodulation, and Hematopoiesis 561

Section V

Hormones and Hormone Antagonists 669

Section VI

Drugs Affecting Gastrointestinal Function 789

Section VII

Chemotherapy of Microbial Diseases 829

Section VIII

Chemotherapy of Neoplastic Diseases 1015

Section IX

Special Systems Pharmacology 1091

Preface to the Second Edition

This *Manual* derives from the 12th edition of *Goodman & Gilman's* The Pharmacological Basis of Therapeutics. The parent text covers not just principles and mechanisms of action but also details of clinical use and recent basic research that supports therapeutic applications and points the way toward new therapies; as a consequence of this thoroughness, the book is large and not in the fashion of the shorter texts preferred by students of this era. To make core material from G&G more accessible, we have abridged the 12th edition of the parent text, trying to present the essentials of mechanism and clinical use while omitting research data, references, and the pharmacokinetic data of Appendix II, all of which can be found at the G&G website on *AccessMedicine.com* and *AccessPharmacy.com*, along with regular therapeutic updates and mechanistic animations. We have also generally omitted the structures of therapeutics agents, which are readily available on the book's website and on PubChem (*pubchem.ncbi.nlm.nih.gov/*). This Manual of Pharmacology and Therapeutics is organized identically to the parent text, using many of the same figures and tables; a number of figures have been improved or added anew for this edition.

Some realizations gained from editing the 12th edition and this volume stand out:

- The invention of new classes of drugs has slowed to a trickle.
- Therapeutics has barely begun to capitalize on the information from the Human Genome Project.
- The development of resistance to antimicrobial agents, mainly through their overuse and misuse in agriculture and medicine, threatens to return us to the pre-antibiotic era.

We have the ingenuity to correct these shortcomings if we can muster the will and the research support to do so.

We thank the contributors and editors of the 12th edition of G&G, Saloni Narang of Thomson Digital, Christie Naglieri and James Shanahan of McGraw-Hill, and a long line of contributors and editors who have worked on *Goodman & Gilman* over 12 editions. It is a tribute to Louis Goodman and Alfred Gilman that their book is alive and vigorous 72 years after the publication of the first edition.

Randa Hilal-Dandan
Laurence Brunton
San Diego, California
St. Patrick's Day, 2013

In Memoriam

Desmond R.H. Gourley (1922–2012)

Steven E. Mayer (1929–2010)

Section I General Principles

chapter 1 Drug Invention and the Pharmaceutical Industry

The first edition of *Goodman & Gilman* helped to organize the field of pharmacology, giving it intellectual validity and an academic identity. That edition began: "The subject of pharmacology is a broad one and embraces the knowledge of the source, physical and chemical properties, compounding, physiological actions, absorption, fate, and excretion, and therapeutic uses of drugs. A *drug* may be broadly defined as any chemical agent that affects living protoplasm, and few substances would escape inclusion by this definition." This *General Principles* section provides the underpinnings for these definitions by exploring the processes of drug invention, followed by the basic properties of the interactions between the drug and biological systems: *pharmacodynamics*, *pharmacokinetics* (including drug transport and metabolism), and *pharmacogenomics*. Subsequent sections deal with the use of drugs as therapeutic agents in human subjects.

Use of the term *invention* to describe the process by which a new drug is identified and brought to medical practice, rather than the more conventional term *discovery,* is intentional. The term *invention* emphasizes the process by which drugs are sculpted and brought into being based on experimentation and optimization of many independent properties; there is little serendipity.

FROM EARLY EXPERIENCES WITH PLANTS TO MODERN CHEMISTRY

The human fascination—and sometimes infatuation—with chemicals that alter biological function is ancient and results from long experience with and dependence on plants. Many plants produce harmful compounds for defense that animals have learned to avoid and humans to exploit.

Examples are described in earlier editions of this text: the appreciation of coffee (caffeine) by the prior of an Arabian convent who noted the behavior of goats that gamboled and frisked through the night after eating the berries of the coffee plant; the use of mushrooms and the deadly nightshade plant by professional poisoners; of belladonna ("beautiful lady") to dilate pupils; of the Chinese herb ma huang (containing ephedrine) as a circulatory stimulant; of curare by South American Indians to paralyze and kill animals hunted for food; and of poppy juice (opium) containing morphine (from the Greek Morpheus, the god of dreams) for pain relief and control of dysentery. Morphine, of course, has well-known addicting properties, mimicked in some ways by other problematic ("recreational") natural products—nicotine, cocaine, and ethanol.

Although terrestrial and marine organisms remain valuable sources of compounds with pharmacological activities, drug invention became more allied with synthetic organic chemistry as that discipline flourished over the past 150 years, beginning in the dye industry. Dyes are colored compounds with selective affinity for biological tissues. Study of these interactions stimulated Paul Ehrlich to postulate the existence of chemical receptors in tissues that interacted with and "fixed" the dyes. Similarly, Ehrlich thought that unique receptors on microorganisms or parasites might react specifically with certain dyes and that such selectivity could spare normal tissue. Ehrlich's work culminated in the invention of arsphenamine in 1907, which was patented as "salvarsan," suggestive of the hope that the chemical would be the salvation of humankind. This and other organic arsenicals were invaluable for the chemotherapy of syphilis until the discovery of penicillin. Through the work of Gerhard Domagk, another dye, prontosil (the first clinically useful sulfonamide), was shown to be dramatically effective in treating streptococcal infections, launching the era of antimicrobial chemotherapy. The collaboration of pharmacology with chemistry on the one hand, and with clinical medicine on the other, has been a major contributor to the effective treatment of disease, especially since the middle of the 20th century.

SMALL MOLECULES ARE THE TRADITION

With the exception of a few naturally occurring hormones (e.g., insulin), most drugs were small organic molecules (typically <500 Da) until recombinant DNA technology permitted synthesis of proteins by various organisms (bacteria, yeast) and mammalian cells. The usual approach to invention of a small-molecule drug is to screen a collection of chemicals ("library") for compounds with the desired features. An alternative is to synthesize and focus on close chemical relatives of a substance known to participate in a biological reaction of interest (e.g., congeners of a specific enzyme substrate chosen to be possible inhibitors of the enzymatic reaction), a particularly important strategy in the discovery of anticancer drugs.

Drug discovery in the past often resulted from serendipitous observations of the effects of plant extracts or individual chemicals on animals or humans; today's approach relies on high-throughput screening of libraries containing hundreds of thousands or even millions of compounds for their capacity to interact with a specific molecular target or elicit a specific biological response. Ideally, the target molecules are of human origin, obtained by transcription and translation of the cloned human gene. The potential drugs that are identified in the screen ("hits") are thus known to react with the human protein and not just with its relative (ortholog) obtained from mouse or another species.

Among the variables considered in screening are the "drugability" of the target and the stringency of the screen in terms of the concentrations of compounds that are tested. "Drugability" refers to the ease with which the function of a target can be altered in the desired fashion by a small organic molecule. If the protein target has a well-defined binding site for a small molecule (e.g., a catalytic or allosteric site), chances are excellent that hits will be obtained. If the goal is to employ a small molecule to mimic or disrupt the interaction between 2 proteins, the challenge is much greater.

FROM HITS TO LEADS

Initial hits in a screen are rarely marketable drugs, often having modest affinity for the target, and lacking the desired specificity and pharmacological properties. Medicinal chemists synthesize derivatives of the hits, thereby defining the structure–activity relationship and optimizing parameters such as affinity for the target, agonist/antagonist activity, permeability across cell membranes, absorption and distribution in the body, metabolism, and unwanted effects.

This approach was driven largely by instinct and trial and error in the past; modern drug development frequently takes advantage of determination of a high-resolution structure of the putative drug bound to its target. X-ray crystallography offers the most detailed structural information if the target protein can be crystallized with the lead drug bound to it. Using techniques of molecular modeling and computational chemistry, the structure provides the chemist with information about substitutions likely to improve the "fit" of the drug with the target and thus enhance the affinity of the drug for its target. Nuclear magnetic resonance (NMR) studies of the drug-receptor complex also can provide useful information, with the advantage that the complex need not be crystallized.

The holy grail of this approach to drug invention is to achieve success entirely through computation. Imagine a database containing detailed chemical information about millions of chemicals and a second database containing detailed structural information about all human proteins. The computational approach is to "roll" all the chemicals over the protein of interest to find those with high-affinity interactions. The dream gets bolder if we acquire the ability to roll the chemicals that bind to the target of interest over all other human proteins to discard compounds that have unwanted interactions. Finally, we also will want to predict the structural and functional consequences of a drug binding to its target (a huge challenge), as well as all relevant pharmacokinetic properties of the molecules of interest. Indeed, computational approaches have suggested new uses for old drugs and offered explanations for recent failures of drugs in the later stages of clinical development (e.g., torcetrapib; see below).

LARGE MOLECULES ARE INCREASINGLY IMPORTANT

Protein therapeutics were uncommon before the advent of recombinant DNA technology. Insulin was introduced into clinical medicine for the treatment of diabetes following the experiments of Banting and Best in 1921. Insulins purified from porcine or bovine pancreas are active in humans, although antibodies to the foreign proteins are occasionally problematic. Growth hormone, used to treat pituitary dwarfism, exhibits more stringent species specificity: only the human hormone could be used after purification from pituitary glands harvested during autopsy, and such use had its dangers. Some patients who received the human hormone developed

Creutzfeldt-Jakob disease (the human equivalent of mad cow disease), a fatal degenerative neurological disease caused by prion proteins that contaminated the drug preparation. Thanks to gene cloning and the production of large quantities of proteins by expressing the cloned gene in bacteria or eukaryotic cells, protein therapeutics now use highly purified preparations of human (or humanized) proteins. Rare proteins can be produced in quantity, and immunological reactions are minimized. Proteins can be designed, customized, and optimized using genetic engineering techniques. Other types of macromolecules may also be used therapeutically. For example, antisense oligonucleotides are used to block gene transcription or translation, as are small interfering RNAs (siRNAs).

Proteins used therapeutically include hormones, growth factors (e.g., erythropoietin, granulocyte-colony stimulating factor), cytokines, and a number of monoclonal antibodies used in the treatment of cancer and autoimmune diseases. Murine monoclonal antibodies can be "humanized" (by substituting human for mouse amino acid sequences). Alternatively, mice have been engineered by replacement of critical mouse genes with their human equivalents, such that they make completely human antibodies. Protein therapeutics are administered parenterally, and their receptors or targets must be accessible extracellularly.

TARGETS OF DRUG ACTION

Early drugs came from observation of the effects of plants after their ingestion by animals, with no knowledge of the drug's mechanism and site of action. Although this approach is still useful (e.g., in screening for the capacity of natural products to kill microorganisms or malignant cells), modern drug invention usually takes the opposite approach—starting with a statement (or hypothesis) that a certain protein or pathway plays a critical role in the pathogenesis of a certain disease, and that altering the protein's activity would therefore be effective against that disease. Crucial questions arise:

- Can one find a drug that will have the desired effect against its target?
- Does modulation of the target protein affect the course of disease?
- Does this project make sense economically?

The effort expended to find the desired drug will be determined by the degree of confidence in the answers to the latter 2 questions.

IS THE TARGET DRUGABLE?

The drugability of a target with a low-molecular-weight organic molecule relies on the presence of a binding site for the drug that exhibits considerable affinity and selectivity.

If the target is an enzyme or a receptor for a small ligand, one is encouraged. If the target is related to another protein that is known to have, for example, a binding site for a regulatory ligand, one is hopeful. However, if the known ligands are large peptides or proteins with an extensive set of contacts with their receptor, the challenge is much greater. If the goal is to disrupt interactions between 2 proteins, it may be necessary to find a "hot spot" that is crucial for the protein-protein interaction, and such a region may not be detected. Accessibility of the drug to its target also is critical. Extracellular targets are intrinsically easier to approach and, in general, only extracellular targets are accessible to macromolecular drugs.

HAS THE TARGET BEEN VALIDATED?

This question is obviously a critical one. A negative answer, frequently obtained only retrospectively, is a common cause of failure in drug invention.

Biological systems frequently contain redundant elements, or can alter expression of drug-regulated elements to compensate for the effect of the drug. In general, the more important the function, the greater the complexity of the system. For example, many mechanisms control feeding and appetite, and drugs to control obesity have been notoriously difficult to find. The discovery of the hormone leptin, which suppresses appetite, was based on mutations in mice that cause loss of either leptin or its receptor; either kind of mutation results in enormous obesity in both mice and people. Leptin thus appeared to be a marvelous opportunity to treat obesity. However, obese individuals have high circulating concentrations of leptin and appear quite insensitive to its action.

Modern techniques of molecular biology offer powerful tools for validation of potential drug targets, to the extent that the biology of model systems resembles human biology. Genes can be inserted, disrupted, and altered in mice. One can thereby create models of disease in animals or mimic the effects of long-term disruption or activation of a given biological process. If, for example, disruption of the gene encoding a specific enzyme or receptor has a beneficial effect in a valid murine model of a human disease, one may believe that the potential drug target has been validated. Mutations in humans also can provide extraordinarily valuable information. For example, loss-of-function mutations in the *PCSK9* gene (encoding proprotein convertase subtilisin/kexin type 9) greatly lower concentrations of LDL cholesterol in plasma and reduce the risk of myocardial infarction. Based on these findings, many drug companies are actively seeking inhibitors of *PCSK9* function.

IS THIS DRUG INVENTION EFFORT ECONOMICALLY VIABLE?

Drug invention and development is expensive (see below), and economic realities influence the direction of pharmaceutical research.

For example, investor-owned companies generally cannot afford to develop products for rare diseases or for diseases that are common only in economically underdeveloped parts of the world. Funds to invent drugs targeting rare diseases or diseases primarily affecting developing countries (especially parasitic diseases) usually come from taxpayers or very wealthy philanthropists.

ADDITIONAL PRECLINICAL RESEARCH

Following the path just described can yield a potential drug molecule that interacts with a validated target and alters its function in the desired fashion. Now one must consider all aspects of the molecule in question—its affinity and selectivity for interaction with the target, its pharmacokinetic properties (absorption, distribution, metabolism, excretion: ADME), issues of its large-scale synthesis or purification, its pharmaceutical properties (stability, solubility, questions of formulation), and its safety. One hopes to correct, to the extent possible, any obvious deficiencies by modification of the molecule itself or by changes in the way the molecule is presented for use.

Before being administered to people, potential drugs are tested for general toxicity by monitoring the activity of various systems in 2 species of animals for extended periods of time. Compounds also are evaluated for carcinogenicity, genotoxicity, and reproductive toxicity. Animals are used for much of this testing. Usually 1 rodent (usually mouse) and 1 nonrodent (often rabbit) species are used. In vitro and ex vivo assays are used when possible, both to spare animals and to minimize cost. If an unwanted effect is observed, an obvious question is whether it is mechanism-based (i.e., caused by interaction of the drug with its intended target) or caused by an off-target effect of the drug, which might be minimized by further optimization of the molecule.

Before the drug candidate can be administered to human subjects in a clinical trial, the sponsor must file an IND (Investigational New Drug) application, a request to the U.S. Food and Drug Administration (FDA; *see* the next section) for permission to administer the drug to human test subjects. The IND describes the rationale and preliminary evidence for efficacy in experimental systems, as well as pharmacology, toxicology, chemistry, manufacturing, and so forth. It also describes the plan for investigating the drug in human subjects. The FDA has 30 days to review the application, by which time the agency may disapprove the application, ask for more data, or allow initial clinical testing to proceed.

CLINICAL TRIALS

ROLE OF THE FDA

The FDA is a regulatory agency within the U.S. Department of Health and Human Services.

The FDA is responsible for protecting the public health by assuring the safety, efficacy, and security of human and veterinary drugs, biological products, medical devices, our nation's food supply, cosmetics, and products that emit radiation. The FDA is also responsible for advancing the public health by helping to speed innovations that make medicines and foods more effective, safer, and more affordable; and helping the public get the accurate, science-based information they need to use medicines and foods to improve their health. One of the FDA's responsibilities is to protect the public from harmful medications. The 1962 Kefauver-Harris Amendments to the Food, Drug, and Cosmetic Act established the requirement for proof of efficacy as well of documentation of relative safety in terms of the risk-to-benefit ratio for the disease entity to be treated (the more serious the disease, the greater the acceptable risk).

The FDA faces an enormous challenge, especially in view of the widely held belief that its mission cannot possibly be accomplished with the available resources. Moreover, harm from drugs that cause unanticipated adverse effects is not the only risk of an imperfect system; harm also occurs when the approval process delays the marketing of a new drug with important beneficial effects.

THE CONDUCT OF CLINICAL TRIALS

Clinical trials of drugs are designed to acquire information about the pharmacokinetic and pharmacodynamic properties of a candidate drug in humans. Efficacy must be proven and an adequate margin of safety established for a drug to be approved for sale in the U.S.

The U.S. National Institutes of Health notes 7 ethical requirements that must be met before a clinical trial can begin: social value, scientific validity, fair and objective selection of subjects, informed consent, favorable ratio of risks to benefits, approval and oversight by an independent review board (IRB), and respect for human subjects.

FDA-regulated clinical trials typically are conducted in 4 phases. The first 3 are designed to establish safety and efficacy, while phase IV postmarketing trials delineate additional information regarding new indications, risks, and optimal doses and schedules. Table 1–1 and Figure 1–1 summarize the important features of each phase of clinical trials; note the attrition at each successive stage over a relatively long and costly process. When initial phase III trials are complete, the sponsor (usually a pharmaceutical company) applies to the FDA for approval to market the drug; this application is called either a *New Drug Application* (NDA) or a *Biologics License Application* (BLA). These applications contain comprehensive information, including individual case-report forms from the hundreds or thousands of individuals who have received the drug during its phase III testing. Applications are reviewed by teams of specialists, and the FDA may call on the help of panels of external experts in complex cases.

Under the provisions of the Prescription Drug User Fee Act (PDUFA; enacted initially in 1992 and renewed in 2007), pharmaceutical companies now provide a significant portion of the FDA budget via user fees, a legislative effort to expedite the drug approval review process. PDUFA also broadened the FDA's drug safety program and increased resources for review of television drug advertising. A 1-year review time is considered standard, and 6 months is the target if the drug candidate is granted priority status because of its importance in filling an unmet need. Unfortunately, these targets are not always met.

Before a drug is approved for marketing, the company and the FDA must agree on the content of the "label" (package insert)—the official prescribing information. This label describes the approved indications for use of the drug and clinical pharmacological information including dosage, adverse reactions, and special warnings

Table 1–1

Typical Characteristics of the Various Phases of the Clinical Trials Required for Marketing of New Drugs

PHASE I First in Human	PHASE II First in Patient	PHASE III Multi-Site Trial	PHASE IV Post-Marketing Surveillance
10-100 participants	50-500 participants	A few hundred to a few thousand participants	Many thousands of participants
Usually healthy volunteers; occasionally patients with advanced or rare disease	Patient-subjects receiving experimental drug	Patient-subjects receiving experimental drug	Patients in treatment with approved drug
Open label	Randomized and controlled (can be placebo-controlled); may be blinded	Randomized and controlled (can be placebo-controlled) or uncontrolled; may be blinded	Open label
Safety and tolerability	Efficacy and dose ranging	Confirm efficacy in larger population	Adverse events, compliance, drug-drug interactions
Months to 1 year	1-2 years	3-5 years	No fixed duration
U.S. $10 million	U.S. $20 million	U.S. $50-100 million	—
Success rate: 50%	Success rate: 30%	Success rate: 25-50%	—

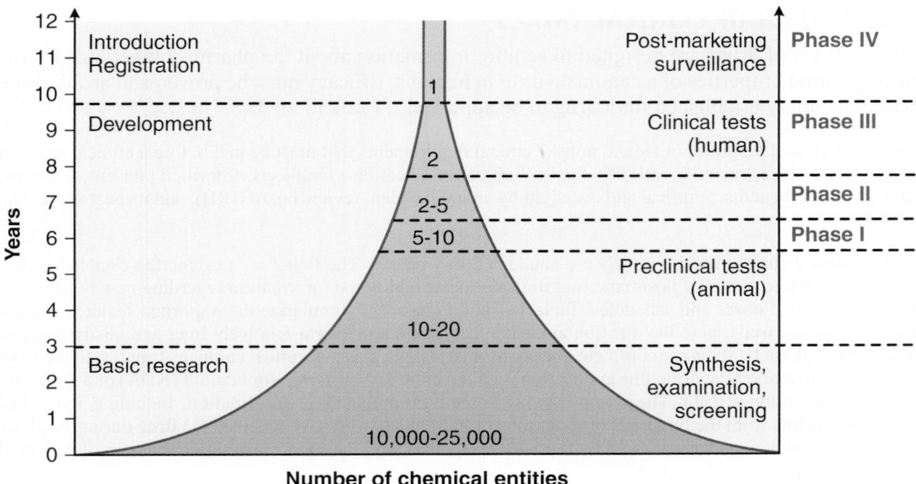

Figure 1–1 *The phases, time lines, and attrition that characterize the invention of new drugs. See* also Table 1–1.

and precautions (sometimes posted in a "black box"). Promotional materials used by pharmaceutical companies cannot deviate from information contained in the package insert. Importantly, the physician is not bound by the package insert; a physician in the U.S. *may* legally prescribe a drug for any purpose that she or he deems reasonable. However, third-party payers (insurance companies, Medicare, and so on) generally will not reimburse a patient for the cost of a drug used for an "off-label" indication unless the new use is supported by one of several compendia such as the U.S. Pharmacopeia. Furthermore, a physician may be vulnerable to litigation if untoward effects result from an unapproved use of a drug.

DETERMINING "SAFE" AND "EFFECTIVE"

Demonstrating efficacy to the FDA requires performing "adequate and well-controlled investigations," generally interpreted to mean 2 replicate clinical trials that are usually, but not always, randomized, double-blind, and placebo-controlled.

Is a placebo the proper control? The World Medical Association's *Declaration of Helsinki* (2000) discourages use of placebo controls when an alternative treatment is available for comparison. What must be measured in the trials? In a straightforward trial, a readily quantifiable parameter (a secondary or surrogate end point), thought to be predictive of relevant clinical outcomes, is measured in matched drug- and placebo-treated groups. Examples of surrogate end points include LDL cholesterol as a predictor of myocardial infarction, bone mineral density as a predictor of fractures, or hemoglobin A_{1c} as a predictor of the complications of diabetes mellitus. More stringent trials would require demonstration of reduction of the incidence of myocardial infarction in patients taking a candidate drug in comparison with those taking an HMG-CoA reductase inhibitor (statin) or other LDL cholesterol-lowering agent, or reduction in the incidence of fractures in comparison with those taking a bisphosphonate. Use of surrogate end points significantly reduces cost and time required to complete trials, but there are many mitigating factors, including the significance of the surrogate end point to the disease that the candidate drug is intended to treat.

Some of the difficulties are well illustrated by recent experiences with ezetimibe, a drug that inhibits absorption of cholesterol from the GI tract and lowers LDL cholesterol concentrations in plasma, especially when used in combination with a statin. Lowering of LDL cholesterol was assumed to be an appropriate surrogate end point for the effectiveness of ezetimibe to reduce myocardial infarction and stroke. Surprisingly, the ENHANCE trial demonstrated that the combination of ezetimibe and a statin did not reduce intima-media thickness of carotid arteries (a more direct measure of subendothelial cholesterol accumulation) compared with the statin alone, despite the fact that the drug combination lowered LDL cholesterol concentrations substantially more than did either drug alone. Critics of ENHANCE argue that the patients in the study had familial hypercholesterolemia, had been treated with statins for years, and did not have carotid artery thickening at the initiation of the study. Should ezetimibe have been approved? Must we return to measurement of true clinical end points (e.g., myocardial infarction) before approval of drugs that lower cholesterol by novel mechanisms? The costs involved in such extensive and expensive trials must be borne somehow (see below). Such a study (IMPROVE-IT) is now in progress.

The drug torcetrapib provides a related example in the same therapeutic area. Torcetrapib elevates HDL cholesterol (the "good cholesterol"), and higher levels of HDL cholesterol are statistically associated with (are a surrogate end point for) a lower incidence of myocardial infarction. Surprisingly, clinical administration of torcetrapib caused a significant *increase* in mortality from cardiovascular events, ending a development path of 15 years and $800 million. In this case, approval of the drug based on this secondary end point would have been a mistake.

No drug is totally safe; all drugs produce unwanted effects in at least some people at some dose. Many unwanted and serious effects of drugs occur so infrequently, perhaps only once in several thousand patients, that they go undetected in the relatively small populations (a few thousand) in the standard phase III clinical trial (*see* Table 1–1).

To detect and verify that such events are in fact drug-related would require administration of the drug to tens or hundreds of thousands of people during clinical trials, adding enormous expense and time to drug development and delaying access to potentially beneficial therapies. In general, the true spectrum and incidence of untoward effects becomes known only after a drug is released to the broader market and used by a large number of people (phase IV, postmarketing surveillance). Drug development costs and drug prices could be reduced substantially if the public were willing to accept more risk. This would require changing the way we think about a pharmaceutical company's liability for damages from an unwanted effect of a drug that was not detected in clinical trials deemed adequate by the FDA.

While the concept is obvious, many lose sight of the fact that extremely severe unwanted effects of a drug, including death, may be deemed acceptable if its therapeutic effect is sufficiently unique and valuable. Such dilemmas are not simple and can become issues for great debate.

Several strategies exist to detect adverse reactions after marketing of a drug. Formal approaches for estimation of the magnitude of an adverse drug response include the follow-up or "cohort" study of patients who are receiving a particular drug; the "case-control" study, where the frequency of drug use in cases of adverse responses is compared to controls; and meta-analysis of pre- and post-marketing studies. Additional approaches also must be used. Spontaneous reporting of adverse reactions has proven to be an effective way to generate an early signal that a drug may be causing an adverse event. Recently, considerable effort has gone into improving the reporting system in the U.S., called *MedWatch* (*see* Appendix I). The primary sources for the reports are responsible, alert physicians; other useful sources are nurses, pharmacists, and students in these disciplines. In addition, hospital-based pharmacy and therapeutics committees and quality assurance committees frequently are charged with monitoring adverse drug reactions in hospitalized patients. The simple forms for reporting may be obtained 24 h a day, 7 days a week by calling 800-FDA-1088; alternatively, adverse reactions can be reported directly using the Internet (www.fda.gov/medwatch). Health professionals also may contact the pharmaceutical manufacturer, who is legally obligated to file reports with the FDA.

PUBLIC POLICY CONSIDERATIONS AND CRITICISMS OF THE PHARMACEUTICAL INDUSTRY

Drugs can save lives, prolong lives, and improve the quality of people's lives. However, in a free-market economy, access to drugs is not equitable. Not surprisingly, there is tension between those who treat drugs as entitlements and those who view drugs as high-tech products of a capitalistic society. Supporters of the entitlement position argue that a constitutional right to life should guarantee access to drugs and other healthcare, and they are critical of pharmaceutical companies and others who profit from the business of making and selling drugs. Free-marketers point out that, without a profit motive, it would be difficult to generate the resources and innovation required for new drug development. Given the public interest in the pharmaceutical industry, drug development is both a scientific process and a political one in which attitudes can change quickly. Little more than a decade ago Merck was named as America's most admired company by *Fortune* magazine 7 years in a row—a record that still stands. In the 2011 survey, no pharmaceutical company ranked in the top 10 most admired companies in the U.S.

Critics of the pharmaceutical industry frequently begin from the position that people (and animals) need to be protected from greedy and unscrupulous companies and scientists. In the absence of a government-controlled drug development enterprise, our current system relies predominantly on investor-owned pharmaceutical companies that, like other companies, have a profit motive and an obligation to shareholders. The price of prescription drugs causes great consternation among consumers, especially as many health insurers seek to control costs by choosing not to cover certain "brand-name" products. Further, a few drugs (especially for treatment of cancer) have been introduced to the market in recent years at prices that greatly exceeded the costs of development, manufacture, and marketing of the product. Many of these products were discovered in government laboratories or in university laboratories supported by federal grants. The U.S. is the only large country that places no controls on drug prices and where price plays no role in the drug approval process.

Many U.S. drugs cost much more in the U.S. than overseas; thus, U.S. consumers subsidize drug costs for the rest of the world, and they are irritated by that fact.

The drug development process is long, expensive, and risky (*see* Figure 1–1 and Table 1–1). Consequently, drugs must be priced to recover the substantial costs of invention and development, and to fund the marketing efforts needed to introduce new products to physicians and patients. Nevertheless, as U.S. healthcare spending continues to rise at an alarming pace, prescription drugs account for only ~10% of total healthcare expenditures, and a significant fraction of this drug cost is for low-priced nonproprietary medicines. Although the increase in prices is significant in certain classes of drugs (e.g., anticancer agents), the total price of prescription drugs is growing at a slower rate than other healthcare costs. Even drastic reductions in drug prices that would severely limit new drug invention would not lower the overall healthcare budget by more than a few percent.

Are profit margins excessive among the major pharmaceutical companies? There is no objective answer to this question. Pragmatic answers come from the markets and from company survival statistics. The costs to bring products to market are enormous; the success rate is low (accounting for much of the cost); effective patent protection is only about a decade (*see* "Intellectual Property and Patents"), requiring every company to completely reinvent itself on a roughly 10-year cycle; regulation is stringent; product liability is great; competition is fierce; with mergers and acquisitions, the number of companies in the pharmaceutical world is shrinking.

WHO PAYS?

The cost of prescription drugs is borne by consumers ("out-of-pocket"), private insurers, and public insurance programs such as Medicare, Medicaid, and the State Children's Health Insurance Program (SCHIP). Recent initiatives by major retailers and mail-order pharmacies run by private insurers to offer consumer incentives for purchase of generic drugs have helped to contain the portion of household expenses spent on pharmaceuticals; however, more than one-third of total retail drug costs in the U.S. are paid with public funds—tax dollars.

Healthcare in the U.S. is more expensive than everywhere else, but it is not, on average, demonstrably better than everywhere else. Forty-five million Americans are uninsured and seek routine medical care in emergency rooms. Solutions to these real problems must recognize both the need for effective ways to incentivize innovation and to permit, recognize, and reward compassionate medical care.

INTELLECTUAL PROPERTY AND PATENTS

Drug invention produces intellectual property eligible for patent protection, protection that is important for innovation. The U.S. patent protection system provides protection for only 20 years from the time the patent is filed. During this period, the patent owner has exclusive rights to market and sell the drug. When the patent expires, equivalent (*generic*) products can come on the market; a generic product must be therapeutically equivalent to the original, contain equal amounts of the same active chemical ingredient, and achieve equal concentrations in blood when administered by the same routes. These generic preparations are sold much more cheaply than the original drug, and without the huge development costs borne by the original patent holder.

The long time course of drug development, usually >10 years (*see* Figure 1–1), reduces the time during which patent protection functions as intended. The Drug Price Competition and Patent Term Restoration Act of 1984 (the "Hatch-Waxman Act") permits a patent holder to apply for extension of a patent term to compensate for delays in marketing caused by FDA approval processes; nonetheless, the average new drug brought to market now enjoys only ~10-12 years of patent protection. Some argue that patent protection for drugs should be shortened, so that earlier generic competition will lower healthcare costs. The counterargument is that new drugs would have to bear higher prices to provide adequate compensation to companies during a shorter period of protected time. If that is true, lengthening patent protection would actually permit lower prices. Recall that patent protection is worth little if a superior competitive product is invented and brought to market.

The Bayh-Dole Act (35 U.S.C. § 200) of 1980 created strong incentives for scientists at academic medical centers to approach drug invention with an entrepreneurial spirit. The Act transferred intellectual property rights to the researchers and their respective institutions in order to encourage partnerships with industry that would bring new products to market for the public's benefit. This encouragement of public-private research collaborations has given rise to concerns about conflicts of interest by scientists and universities.

DRUG PROMOTION

In an ideal world, physicians would learn all they need to know about drugs from the medical literature, and good drugs would thereby sell themselves. Instead, we have print advertising and visits from salespeople directed at physicians, and extensive direct-to-consumer advertising aimed at the public (in print, on the radio, and especially on television). There are roughly 100,000 pharmaceutical sales representatives in the U.S. who target ~10 times that number of physicians. It has been noted that college cheerleading squads are attractive sources for recruitment of this sales force. The amount spent on promotion of drugs approximates or perhaps even exceeds that spent on research and development. Pharmaceutical companies have been especially vulnerable to criticism for some of their marketing practices.

Promotional materials used by pharmaceutical companies cannot deviate from information contained in the package insert. In addition, there must be an acceptable balance between presentation of therapeutic claims for a product and discussion of unwanted effects. Nevertheless, direct-to-consumer advertising of drugs remains controversial and is permitted only in the U.S. and New Zealand. Physicians frequently succumb with misgivings to patients' advertising-driven requests for specific medications. The counterargument is that patients are educated by such marketing efforts and in many cases will then seek medical care, especially for conditions that they may have been denying (e.g., depression). The major criticism of drug marketing involves some of the unsavory approaches used to influence physician behavior. Gifts of value (e.g., sports tickets) are now forbidden, but dinners where drug-prescribing information is presented are widespread. Large numbers of physicians are paid as "consultants" to make presentations in such settings. The acceptance of any gift, no matter how small, from a drug company by a physician, is now forbidden at many academic medical centers and by law in several states. The board of directors of the Pharmaceutical Research and Manufacturers of America has adopted an enhanced code on relationships with U.S. healthcare professionals that prohibits the distribution of noneducational items, prohibits company sales representatives from providing restaurant meals to healthcare professionals, and requires companies to ensure that their representatives are trained about laws and regulations that govern interactions with healthcare professionals.

EXPLOITATION OR "MEDICAL IMPERIALISM"

There is concern about the degree to which U.S. and European patent protection laws have restricted access to potentially lifesaving drugs in developing countries. Because development of new drugs is so expensive, private-sector investment in pharmaceutical innovation naturally has focused on products that will have lucrative markets in wealthy countries such as the U.S., which combines patent protection with a free-market economy. To lower costs, companies increasingly test their experimental drugs outside the U.S. and the E.U., in countries such as China, India, and Mexico, where there is less regulation and easier access to large numbers of patients. If the drug is successful in obtaining marketing approval, consumers in these countries often cannot afford the drugs.

Some ethicists have argued that this practice violates the justice principle articulated in the Belmont Report (1979), which states that "research should not unduly involve persons from groups unlikely to be among the beneficiaries of subsequent applications of the research." Conversely, the conduct of trials in developing nations also frequently brings needed medical attention to underserved populations.

PRODUCT LIABILITY

Product liability laws are intended to protect consumers from defective products. Pharmaceutical companies can be sued for faulty design or manufacturing, deceptive promotional practices, violation of regulatory requirements, or failure to warn consumers of known risks. So-called "failure to warn" claims can be made against drug makers even when the product is approved by the FDA. With greater frequency, courts are finding companies that market prescription drugs directly to consumers responsible when these advertisements fail to provide an adequate warning of potential adverse effects.

Although injured patients are entitled to pursue legal remedies, the negative effects of product liability lawsuits against pharmaceutical companies may be considerable. First, fear of liability may cause pharmaceutical companies to be overly cautious about testing, delaying access to the drug. Second, the cost of drugs increases for consumers when pharmaceutical companies increase the length and number of trials they perform to identify even the smallest risks, and when regulatory agencies increase the number or intensity of regulatory reviews. Third, excessive liability costs create disincentives for development of *orphan drugs*, pharmaceuticals that benefit a small number of patients. Should pharmaceutical companies be liable for failure to warn when all of the rules were followed and the product was approved by the FDA but the unwanted effect was not detected because of its rarity or another confounding factor? The only way to find "all" of the unwanted effects that a drug may have is to market it—to conduct a phase IV "clinical trial" or observational study. This basic friction between risk to patients and the financial risk of drug development does not seem likely to be resolved except on a case-by-case basis.

The U.S. Supreme Court added further fuel to these fiery issues in 2009 in the case *Wyeth v. Levine*. A patient (Levine) suffered gangrene of an arm following inadvertent arterial administration of the drug promethazine. The healthcare provider had intended to administer the drug by so-called intravenous push. The FDA-approved label for the drug *warned against* but did not prohibit administration by intravenous push. The state courts and then the U.S. Supreme Court held both the healthcare provider *and the company* liable for damages. FDA approval of the label apparently neither protects a company from liability nor prevents individual states from imposing regulations more stringent than those required by the federal government.

"ME TOO" VERSUS TRUE INNOVATION: THE PACE OF NEW DRUG DEVELOPMENT

"Me-too drug" is a term used to describe a pharmaceutical that is usually structurally similar to a drug already on the market. Other names used are *derivative medications*, *molecular modifications*, and *follow-up drugs*. In some cases, a me-too drug is a different molecule developed deliberately by a competitor company to take market share from the company with existing drugs on the market. When the market for a class of drugs is especially large, several companies can share the market and make a profit. Other me-too drugs result coincidentally from numerous companies developing products simultaneously without knowing which drugs will be approved for sale.

Some me-too drugs are only slightly altered formulations of a company's own drug, packaged and promoted as if it really offers something new. An example of this type of me-too is the heartburn medication esomeprazole, marketed by the same company that makes omeprazole. Omeprazole is a mixture of 2 stereoisomers; esomeprazole contains only 1 of the isomers and is eliminated less rapidly. Development of esomeprazole created a new period of market exclusivity, although generic versions of omeprazole are marketed, as are branded congeners of omeprazole/esomeprazole.

There are valid criticisms of me-too drugs. First, an excessive emphasis on profit may stifle true innovation. Of the 487 drugs approved by the FDA between 1998 and 2003, only 67 (14%) were considered by the FDA to be new molecular entities. Second, some me-too drugs are more expensive than the older versions they seek to replace, increasing the costs of healthcare without corresponding benefit to patients. Nevertheless, for some patients, me-too drugs may have better efficacy or fewer side effects or promote compliance with the treatment regimen. For example, the me-too that can be taken once a day rather than more frequently is convenient and promotes compliance. Some me-too drugs add great value from a business and medical point of view. Atorvastatin was the seventh statin to be introduced to market; it subsequently became the best-selling drug in the world. Now that nonproprietary versions of simvastatin are available, sales of atorvastatin are declining.

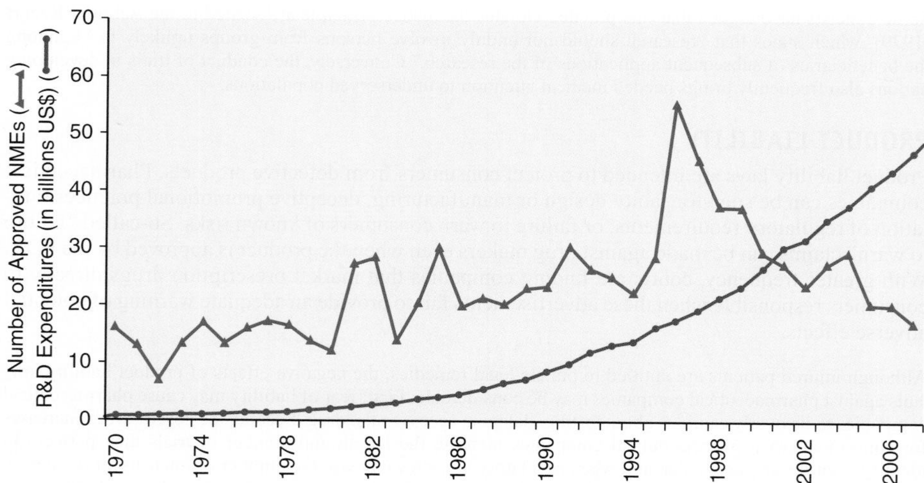

Figure 1–2 *The cost of drug invention is rising dramatically while productivity is declining.* The peak in the mid-1990s was caused by the advent of PDUFA (see text), which facilitated elimination of a backlog.

Billions of dollars might be saved, likely with little loss of benefit, if nonproprietary simvastatin were substituted for proprietary atorvastatin, with appropriate adjustment of dosages.

Critics argue that pharmaceutical companies are not innovative and do not take risks and, further, that medical progress is actually slowed by their excessive concentration on me-too products. Figure 1–2 summarizes a few of the facts behind this and other arguments. Clearly, smaller numbers of new molecular entities reached FDA approval over the past decade, despite the industry's enormous investment in research and development. This disconnect has occurred at a time when combinatorial chemistry was blooming, the human genome was being sequenced, highly automated techniques of screening were being developed, and new techniques of molecular biology and genetics were offering novel insights into the pathophysiology of human disease. Despite their innovations and successes (e.g., insulin, growth hormone, erythropoietin, and monoclonal antibodies to extracellular targets), the biotechnology companies have not, on balance, been more efficient at drug invention or discovery than the traditional major pharmaceutical companies.

The trends evident in Figure 1–2 must be reversed. The current path will not sustain today's companies as they face a major wave of patent expirations over the next several years. There are arguments, some almost counterintuitive, that development of much more targeted, individualized drugs, based on a new generation of molecular diagnostic techniques and improved understanding of disease in individual patients, could improve both medical care and the survival of pharmaceutical companies. Finally, many of the advances in genetics and molecular biology are still new, particularly when measured in the time frame required for drug development. One can hope that modern molecular medicine will sustain the development of more efficacious and more specific pharmacological treatments for an ever wider spectrum of human diseases.

For a complete Bibliographical Listing see Goodman & Gilman's ***The Pharmacological Basis of Therapeutics***, 12th ed., or Goodman & Gilman Online at www.AccessMedicine.com.

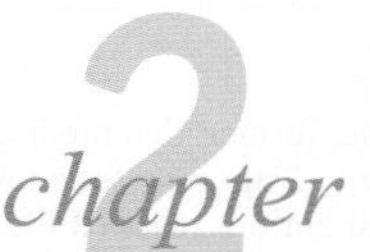

chapter 2 Pharmacokinetics: The Dynamics of Drug Absorption, Distribution, Metabolism, and Elimination

The absorption, distribution, metabolism (biotransformation), and elimination of drugs (ADME) are the processes of *pharmacokinetics* (Figure 2–1). Understanding and employing pharmacokinetic principles can increase the probability of therapeutic success and reduce the occurrence of adverse drug effects in the body.

PHYSICOCHEMICAL FACTORS IN TRANSFER OF DRUGS ACROSS MEMBRANES

The absorption, distribution, metabolism, excretion, and action of a drug involve its passage across cell membranes. Mechanisms by which drugs cross membranes and the physicochemical properties of molecules and membranes that influence this transfer are critical to understanding the disposition of drugs in the human body. The characteristics of a drug that predict its movement and availability at sites of action are its molecular size and structural features, degree of ionization, relative lipid solubility of its ionized and nonionized forms, and its binding to serum and tissue proteins. Although barriers to drug movement may be a single layer of cells (e.g., intestinal epithelium) or several layers of cells and associated extracellular protein (e.g., skin), the plasma membrane represents the common barrier to drug distribution.

The plasma membrane consists of a bilayer of amphipathic lipids with their hydrocarbon chains oriented inward to the center of the bilayer to form a continuous hydrophobic phase, with their hydrophilic heads oriented outward. Individual lipid molecules in the bilayer vary according to the particular membrane and can move laterally and organize themselves with cholesterol (e.g., sphingolipids), endowing the membrane with fluidity, flexibility, organization, high electrical resistance, and relative impermeability to highly polar molecules. Membrane proteins embedded in the bilayer serve as structural anchors, receptors, ion channels, or transporters to transduce electrical or chemical signaling pathways and provide selective targets for drug actions. Membranes are highly ordered and compartmented. Membrane proteins may be associated with caveolin and sequestered within caveolae, excluded from caveolae, or be organized in signaling domains rich in cholesterol and sphingolipid not containing caveolin or other scaffolding proteins (i.e., lipid rafts). Cell membranes are

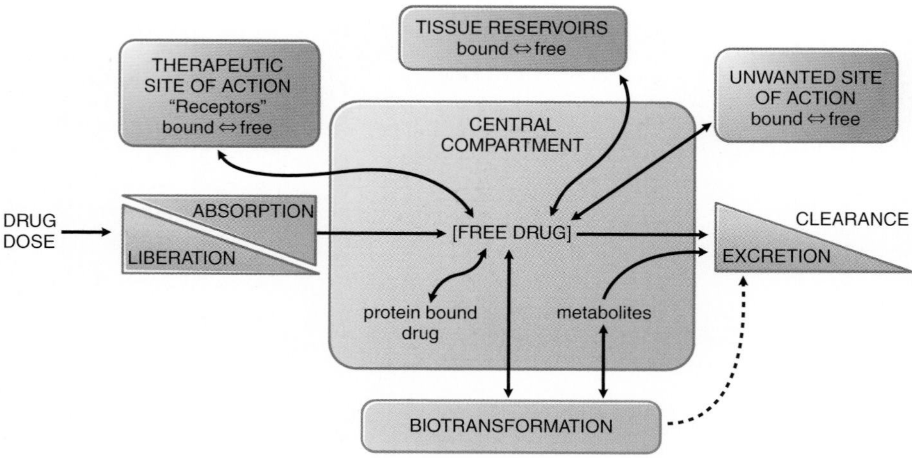

Figure 2–1 *The interrelationship of the absorption, distribution, binding, metabolism, and excretion of a drug and its concentration at its sites of action.* Possible distribution and binding of metabolites in relation to their potential actions at receptors are not depicted.

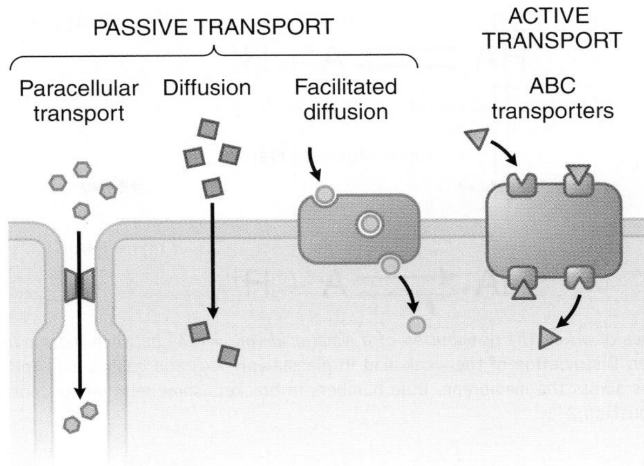

Figure 2–2 *The variety of ways drugs move across cellular barriers in their passage throughout the body.* See details in Figure 5–4.

relatively permeable to water either by diffusion or by flow resulting from hydrostatic or osmotic differences across the membrane, and bulk flow of water can carry with it small drug molecules (<200 Da). Paracellular passage through intercellular gaps is sufficiently large that transfer across capillary endothelium is generally limited by blood flow (Figure 2–2). Capillaries of the central nervous system (CNS) and a variety of epithelial tissues have tight junctions. Bulk-flow transfer is limited when the molecular mass of the solute exceeds 100-200 Da. Accordingly, most large lipophilic drugs must pass through the cell membrane itself (*see* Figure 2–2) by passive and active processes.

PASSIVE MEMBRANE TRANSPORT. In passive transport, the drug molecule usually penetrates by diffusion along a concentration gradient by virtue of its solubility in the lipid bilayer. Such transfer is directly proportional to the magnitude of the concentration gradient across the membrane, to the lipid-water partition coefficient of the drug, and to the membrane surface area exposed to the drug. At steady state, the concentration of the unbound drug is the same on both sides of the membrane if the drug is a nonelectrolyte. For ionic compounds, the steady-state concentrations depend on the electrochemical gradient for the ion and on differences in pH across the membrane, which will influence the state of ionization of the molecule disparately on either side of the membrane and can effectively trap drug on one side of the membrane.

WEAK ELECTROLYTES AND THE INFLUENCE OF pH. Many drugs are weak acids or bases that are present in solution as both the lipid-soluble and diffusible nonionized form, and the relatively lipid-insoluble nondiffusible ionized species. The transmembrane distribution of a weak electrolyte is influenced by its pK_a and the pH gradient across the membrane. The pK_a is the pH at which half the drug (weak acid or base electrolyte) is in its ionized form. The ratio of nonionized to ionized drug at any pH may be calculated from the Henderson-Hasselbalch equation:

$$\log \frac{[\text{protonated form}]}{[\text{unprotonated form}]} = pK_a - pH \qquad \text{(Equation 2–1)}$$

Equation 2–1 relates the pH of the medium around the drug and the drug's acid dissociation constant (pK_a) to the ratio of the protonated (HA or BH^+) and unprotonated (A^- or B) forms, where $HA \leftrightarrow A^- + H^+$ ($K_a = [A^-][H^+]/[HA]$) describes the dissociation of an acid, and $BH^+ \leftrightarrow B + H^+$ ($K_a = [B][H^+]/[BH^+]$) describes the dissociation of the protonated form of a base. At steady state, an acidic drug will accumulate on the more basic side of the membrane and a basic drug on the more acidic side. This phenomenon, known as *ion trapping*, is an important process in drug distribution (Figure 2–3).

CARRIER-MEDIATED MEMBRANE TRANSPORT. *Active transport* and *facilitated diffusion* are carrier-mediated processes. Pharmacologically important transporters may mediate either drug uptake or efflux and often facilitate vectorial transport across polarized cells. An important efflux transporter is the P-glycoprotein encoded

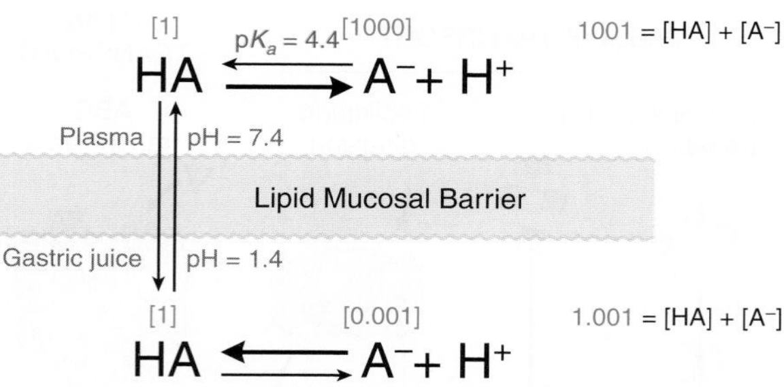

Figure 2–3 *Influence of pH on the distribution of a weak acid (pK_a = 4.4) between plasma and gastric juice separated by a lipid barrier.* Dissociation of the weak acid in plasma (pH 7.4) and gastric acid (pH 1.4). The uncharged form, HA, equilibrates across the membrane. Blue numbers in brackets show relative concentrations of HA and A^-, as calculated from Equation 2–1.

by the multidrug resistance-1 (*MDR1*) gene (*see* Table 5–4). P-glycoprotein localized in the enterocyte limits the absorption of some orally administered drugs because it exports compounds into the lumen of the GI tract subsequent to their absorption. The P-glycoprotein also can confer resistance to some cancer chemotherapeutic agents (*see* Chapters 60–63). Transporters and their roles in drug action are presented in detail in Chapter 5.

DRUG ABSORPTION, BIOAVAILABILITY, AND ROUTES OF ADMINISTRATION

Absorption is the movement of a drug from its site of administration into the central compartment (*see* Figure 2–1). For solid dosage forms, absorption first requires dissolution of the tablet or capsule, thus liberating the drug. The clinician is concerned primarily with bioavailability rather than absorption. *Bioavailability* describes the fractional extent to which a dose of drug reaches its site of action or a biological fluid from which the drug has access to its site of action.

For example, a drug given orally must be absorbed first from the GI tract, but net absorption may be limited by the characteristics of the dosage form, the drug's physicochemical properties, by intestinal metabolism, and by export into the intestinal lumen. The absorbed drug then passes through the liver, where metabolism and biliary excretion may occur before the drug enters the systemic circulation. Accordingly, a fraction of the administered and absorbed dose of drug will be inactivated or diverted in the intestine and liver before it can reach the general circulation and be distributed to its sites of action. If the metabolic or excretory capacity of the liver and the intestine for the drug is large, bioavailability will be reduced substantially (*first-pass effect*). This decrease in availability is a function of the anatomical site from which absorption takes place; other anatomical, physiological, and pathological factors can influence bioavailability (described later), and the choice of the route of drug administration must be based on an understanding of these conditions.

ORAL (ENTERAL) VERSUS PARENTERAL ADMINISTRATION. Some characteristics of the major routes employed for systemic drug effect are compared in Table 2–1.

Oral ingestion is the most common method of drug administration. It also is the safest, most convenient, and most economical. Its disadvantages include limited absorption of some drugs because of their physical characteristics (e.g., low water solubility or poor membrane permeability), emesis as a result of irritation to the GI mucosa, destruction of some drugs by digestive enzymes or low gastric pH, irregularities in absorption or propulsion in the presence of food or other drugs, and the need for cooperation on the part of the patient. In addition, drugs in the GI tract may be metabolized by the enzymes of the intestinal flora, mucosa, or liver before they gain access to the general circulation.

Parenteral injection of drugs has distinct advantages over oral administration. In some instances, parenteral administration is essential for the drug to be delivered in its active form, as in the case of monoclonal antibodies. Availability usually is more rapid, extensive, and predictable when a drug is given by injection; the effective dose can be delivered more accurately. In emergency therapy and when a patient is unconscious, uncooperative, or unable to retain anything given by mouth, parenteral therapy may be necessary. Parenteral administration also has its disadvantages: asepsis must be maintained, especially when drugs are given over time (e.g., intravenous or intrathecal administration); pain may accompany the injection; and it is sometimes difficult for patients to perform the injections themselves if self-medication is necessary.

ORAL ADMINISTRATION. Absorption from the GI tract is governed by factors such as surface area for absorption, blood flow to the site of absorption, the physical state of the drug (solution, suspension, or solid dosage

Table 2–1

Some Characteristics of Common Routes of Drug Administration[a]

ROUTE	ABSORPTION PATTERN	SPECIAL UTILITY	LIMITATIONS AND PRECAUTIONS
Intravenous	Absorption circumvented Potentially immediate effects Suitable for large volumes, irritating substances, or complex mixtures	Valuable for emergency use Permits titration of dosage Usually required for high MW drugs (peptides, proteins)	Increased risk of adverse effects Must inject solutions *slowly* as a rule Not suitable for oily solutions or poorly soluble substances
Subcutaneous	Prompt from aqueous solution Slow and sustained from repository preparations	Suitable for some poorly soluble suspensions and slow-release implants	Not suitable for large volumes Possible pain or necrosis from irritants
Intramuscular	Prompt from aqueous solution Slow and sustained from repository preparations	Suitable for moderate volumes, oily vehicles, and some irritants Appropriate for self-administration (e.g., insulin)	Precluded during anticoagulant therapy May interfere with interpretation of certain diagnostic tests (e.g., creatine kinase)
Oral ingestion	Variable, depends on many factors (see text)	Most convenient and economical; usually more safe	Requires patient compliance Bioavailability potentially erratic and incomplete

[a]See text for discussion and for other routes.

form), its water solubility, and the drug's concentration at the site of absorption. For drugs given in solid form, the rate of dissolution may limit their absorption. Because most drug absorption from the GI tract occurs by passive diffusion, absorption is favored when the drug is in the nonionized, more lipophilic form. Based on the pH-partition concept (Figure 2–3), one would predict that drugs that are weak acids would be better absorbed from the stomach (pH 1-2) than from the upper intestine (pH 3-6), and vice versa for weak bases. However the epithelium of the stomach is lined with a thick mucus layer, and its surface area is small; by contrast, the villi of the upper intestine provide an extremely large surface area (~200 m^2). Accordingly, the rate of absorption of a drug from the intestine will be greater than that from the stomach even if the drug is predominantly ionized in the intestine and largely nonionized in the stomach. Thus, any factor that accelerates gastric emptying will generally increase the rate of drug absorption, whereas any factor that delays gastric emptying is expected to have the opposite effect. Gastric emptying rate is influenced by numerous factors, including the caloric content of food; volume, osmolality, temperature, and pH of ingested fluid; diurnal and interindividual variation; metabolic state (rest or exercise); and the ambient temperature. Gastric emptying is influenced in women by the effects of estrogen (i.e., compared to men, it is slower for premenopausal women and those taking estrogen replacement therapy).

Drugs that are destroyed by gastric secretions and low pH or that cause gastric irritation sometimes are administered in dosage forms with an enteric coating that prevents dissolution in the acidic gastric contents. Enteric coatings are useful for drugs such as aspirin, which can cause gastric irritation, and for presenting a drug such as mesalamine to sites of action in the ileum and colon (*see* Figure 47–4).

Controlled-Release Preparations. The rate of absorption of a drug administered as a tablet or other solid oral dosage form is partly dependent on its rate of dissolution in GI fluids. This is the basis for *controlled-release, extended-release, sustained-release,* and *prolonged-action* pharmaceutical preparations that are designed to produce slow, uniform absorption of the drug for 8 h or longer. Potential advantages of such preparations are reduction in the frequency of administration compared with conventional dosage forms (often with improved compliance by the patient), maintenance of a therapeutic effect overnight, and decreased incidence and/or intensity of undesired effects (by dampening of the peaks in drug concentration) and nontherapeutic blood levels of the drug (by elimination of troughs in concentration) that often occur after administration of immediate-release dosage forms. Controlled-release dosage forms are most appropriate for drugs with short half-lives ($t_{1/2}$ <4 h) or in selected patient groups such as those receiving antiepileptics.

Sublingual Administration. Venous drainage from the mouth is to the superior vena cava, bypassing the portal circulation and thereby protecting the drug from rapid intestinal and hepatic first-pass metabolism. For example, nitroglycerin (*see* Chapter 27) is effective when retained sublingually because it is nonionic and has very high lipid solubility.

TRANSDERMAL ABSORPTION. Absorption of drugs able to penetrate the intact skin is dependent on the surface area over which they are applied and their lipid solubility (*see* Chapter 65). Systemic absorption of drugs occurs much more readily through abraded, burned, or denuded skin. Toxic effects result from absorption through the skin of highly lipid-soluble substances (e.g., a lipid-soluble insecticide in an organic solvent). Absorption through the skin can be enhanced by suspending the drug in an oily vehicle and rubbing the resulting preparation into the skin. Hydration of the skin with an occlusive dressing may be used to facilitate absorption. Controlled-release topical patches have become increasingly available, including nicotine for tobacco-smoking withdrawal, scopolamine for motion sickness, nitroglycerin for angina pectoris, testosterone and estrogen for replacement therapy, various estrogens and progestins for birth control, and fentanyl for pain relief.

RECTAL ADMINISTRATION. Approximately 50% of the drug that is absorbed from the rectum will bypass the liver; thus reducing hepatic first-pass metabolism. However, rectal absorption can be irregular and incomplete, and certain drugs can cause irritation of the rectal mucosa.

PARENTERAL INJECTION. The major routes of parenteral administration are intravenous, subcutaneous, and intramuscular. Absorption from subcutaneous and intramuscular sites occurs by simple diffusion along the gradient from drug depot to plasma. The rate is limited by the area of the absorbing capillary membranes and by the solubility of the substance in the interstitial fluid. Relatively large aqueous channels in the endothelial membrane account for the indiscriminate diffusion of molecules regardless of their lipid solubility. Larger molecules, such as proteins, slowly gain access to the circulation by way of lymphatic channels. Drugs administered into the systemic circulation by any route, excluding the intraarterial route, are subject to possible first-pass elimination in the lung prior to distribution to the rest of the body. The lungs also serve as a filter for particulate matter that may be given intravenously and provide a route of elimination for volatile substances.

Intravenous. Factors limiting absorption are circumvented by intravenous injection of drugs in aqueous solution because bioavailability is complete and rapid. Also, drug delivery is controlled and achieved with an accuracy and immediacy not possible by any other procedure. Certain irritating solutions can be given only in this manner because the drug, when injected slowly, is greatly diluted by the blood.

There are advantages and disadvantages to intravenous administration. Unfavorable reactions can occur because high concentrations of drug may be attained rapidly in plasma and tissues. There are therapeutic circumstances where it is advisable to administer a drug by bolus injection (e.g., tissue plasminogen activator) and other circumstances where slower administration of drug is advisable (e.g., antibiotics). Intravenous administration of drugs warrants close monitoring of the patient's response; once the drug is injected, there is often no retreat. Repeated intravenous injections depend on the ability to maintain a patent vein. Drugs in an oily vehicle, those that precipitate blood constituents or hemolyze erythrocytes, and drug combinations that cause precipitates to form must not be given by this route.

Subcutaneous. Injection into a subcutaneous site can be done only with drugs that are not irritating to tissue; otherwise, severe pain, necrosis, and tissue sloughing may occur. The rate of absorption following subcutaneous injection of a drug often is sufficiently constant and slow to provide a sustained effect. Moreover, altering the period over which a drug is absorbed may be varied intentionally, as is accomplished with insulin for injection using particle size, protein complexation, and pH. The incorporation of a vasoconstrictor agent in a solution of a drug to be injected subcutaneously also retards absorption. Absorption of drugs implanted under the skin in a solid pellet form occurs slowly over a period of weeks or months; some hormones (e.g., contraceptives) are administered effectively in this manner.

Intramuscular. Drugs in aqueous solution are absorbed rapidly after intramuscular injection depending on the rate of blood flow to the injection site. This may be modulated to some extent by local heating, massage, or exercise. Generally, the rate of absorption following injection of an aqueous preparation into the deltoid or vastus lateralis is faster than when the injection is made into the gluteus maximus. The rate is particularly slower for females after injection into the gluteus maximus. This has been attributed to the different distribution of subcutaneous fat in males and females and because fat is relatively poorly perfused. Slow, constant absorption from the intramuscular site results if the drug is injected in solution in oil or suspended in various other repository (depot) vehicles.

Intraarterial. Occasionally, a drug is injected directly into an artery to localize its effect in a particular tissue or organ, such as in the treatment of liver tumors and head and neck cancers. Diagnostic agents sometimes are administered by this route (e.g., technetium-labeled human serum albumin).

Intrathecal. The blood-brain barrier and the blood-cerebrospinal fluid (CSF) barrier often preclude or slow the entrance of drugs into the CNS. Therefore, when local and rapid effects of drugs on the meninges or cerebrospinal axis are desired, drugs sometimes are injected directly into the spinal subarachnoid space. Brain tumors also may be treated by direct intraventricular drug administration.

PULMONARY ABSORPTION. Gaseous and volatile drugs may be inhaled and absorbed through the pulmonary epithelium and mucous membranes of the respiratory tract. Access to the circulation is rapid by this route because the lung's surface area is large. In addition, solutions of drugs can be atomized and the fine droplets in air (aerosol) inhaled. Advantages are the almost instantaneous absorption of a drug into the blood, avoidance of hepatic first-pass loss, and in the case of pulmonary disease, local application of the drug at the desired site of action (*see* Chapters 19 and 36).

TOPICAL APPLICATION

Mucous Membranes. Drugs are applied to the mucous membranes of the conjunctiva, nasopharynx, oropharynx, vagina, colon, urethra, and urinary bladder primarily for their local effects.

Eye. Topically applied ophthalmic drugs are used primarily for their local effects (*see* Chapter 64).

BIOEQUIVALENCE

Drug products are considered to be pharmaceutical equivalents if they contain the same active ingredients and are identical in strength or concentration, dosage form, and route of administration. Two pharmaceutically equivalent drug products are considered to be *bioequivalent* when the rates and extents of bioavailability of the active ingredient in the 2 products are not significantly different under suitable test conditions. However, brand name and generic forms of the same drug are not always legally equivalent; law suits that have succeeded against the makers of brand name drugs have failed against the producers of the equivalent generic forms (*see* recent cases involving Phenergan and generic promethazine). Generic versus brand name prescribing is further discussed in connection with drug nomenclature and the choice of drug name in writing prescription orders (*see* Appendix I).

DISTRIBUTION OF DRUGS

Following absorption or systemic administration into the bloodstream, a drug distributes into interstitial and intracellular fluids depending on the particular physicochemical properties of the individual drug. Cardiac output, regional blood flow, capillary permeability, and tissue volume determine the rate of delivery and potential amount of drug distributed into tissues. Initially, liver, kidney, brain, and other well-perfused organs receive most of the drug; delivery to muscle, most viscera, skin, and fat is slower. This second distribution phase may require minutes to several hours before the concentration of drug in tissue is in equilibrium with that in blood. The second phase also involves a far larger fraction of body mass (e.g., muscle) than does the initial phase and generally accounts for most of the extravascularly distributed drug. With exceptions such as the brain, diffusion of drug into the interstitial fluid occurs rapidly because of the highly permeable nature of the capillary endothelial membrane. Thus, tissue distribution is determined by the partitioning of drug between blood and the particular tissue.

PLASMA PROTEINS. Many drugs circulate in the bloodstream bound to plasma proteins. Albumin is a major carrier for acidic drugs; α_1-acid glycoprotein binds basic drugs. Nonspecific binding to other plasma proteins generally occurs to a much smaller extent. The binding is usually reversible. In addition, certain drugs may bind to proteins that function as specific hormone carrier proteins, such as the binding of estrogen or testosterone to sex hormone–binding globulin or the binding of thyroid hormone to thyroxin-binding globulin.

The fraction of total drug in plasma that is bound is determined by the drug concentration, the affinity of binding sites for the drug, and the number of binding sites. For most drugs, the therapeutic range of plasma concentrations is limited; thus, the extent of binding and the unbound fraction are relatively constant. The extent of plasma protein binding also may be affected by disease-related factors (e.g., hypoalbuminemia). Conditions resulting in the acute-phase reaction response (e.g., cancer, arthritis, myocardial infarction, Crohn disease) lead to elevated levels of α_1-acid glycoprotein and enhanced binding of basic drugs. Changes in protein binding caused by disease states and drug-drug interactions are clinically relevant mainly for a small subset of so-called high-clearance drugs of narrow therapeutic index that are administered intravenously, such as lidocaine. When changes in plasma protein binding occur in patients, unbound drug rapidly equilibrates throughout the body and only a transient significant change in unbound plasma concentration will occur. Only drugs that show an almost instantaneous relationship between free plasma concentration and effect (e.g., anti-arrhythmics) will show a measureable effect. Thus, unbound plasma drug concentrations will exhibit significant changes only when either drug input or clearance of unbound drug occurs, as a consequence of metabolism or active transport. A more common problem resulting from competition of drugs for plasma protein-binding sites is misinterpretation of measured concentrations of drugs in plasma because most assays do not distinguish free drug from bound drug.

Binding of a drug to plasma proteins limits its concentration in tissues and at its site of action because only unbound drug is in equilibrium across membranes. Accordingly, after distribution equilibrium is achieved, the concentration of active, unbound drug in intracellular water is the same as that in plasma except when carrier-mediated transport is involved. Binding of a drug to plasma protein also limits the drug's glomerular filtration. Drug transport and metabolism also are limited by binding to plasma proteins, except when these are especially efficient, and drug clearance, calculated on the basis of unbound drug, exceeds organ plasma flow.

TISSUE BINDING. Many drugs accumulate in tissues at higher concentrations than those in the extracellular fluids and blood. Tissue binding of drugs usually occurs with cellular constituents such as proteins, phospholipids, or nuclear proteins and generally is reversible. A large fraction of drug in the body may be bound in this fashion and serve as a reservoir that prolongs drug action in that same tissue or at a distant site reached through the circulation. Such tissue binding and accumulation also can produce local toxicity.

FAT AS A RESERVOIR. Many lipid-soluble drugs are stored by physical solution in the neutral fat. In obese persons, the fat content of the body may be as high as 50%, and even in lean individuals, fat constitutes 10% of body weight; hence, fat may serve as a reservoir for lipid-soluble drugs. Fat is a rather stable reservoir because it has a relatively low blood flow.

BONE. The tetracycline antibiotics (and other divalent metal-ion chelating agents) and heavy metals may accumulate in bone by adsorption onto the bone crystal surface and eventual incorporation into the crystal lattice. Bone can become a reservoir for the slow release of toxic agents such as lead or radium; their effects thus can persist long after exposure has ceased. Local destruction of the bone medulla also may lead to reduced blood flow and prolongation of the reservoir effect because the toxic agent becomes sealed off from the circulation; this may further enhance the direct local damage to the bone. A vicious cycle results, whereby the greater the exposure to the toxic agent, the slower is its rate of elimination. The adsorption of drug onto the bone crystal surface and incorporation into the crystal lattice have therapeutic advantages for the treatment of osteoporosis.

REDISTRIBUTION. Termination of drug effect after withdrawal of a drug usually is by metabolism and excretion but also may result from redistribution of the drug from its site of action into other tissues or sites. Redistribution is a factor in terminating drug effect primarily when a highly lipid-soluble drug that acts on the brain or cardiovascular system is administered rapidly by intravenous injection or inhalation, such as intravenous anesthetic thiopental, a highly lipid-soluble drug. Because blood flow to the brain is so high, thiopental reaches its maximal concentration in brain within a minute of its intravenous injection. After injection is concluded, the plasma and brain concentrations decrease as thiopental redistributes to other tissues, such as muscle. The concentration of the drug in brain follows that of the plasma because there is little binding of the drug to brain constituents. Thus, both the onset and termination of thiopental anesthesia are rapid and both are related directly to the concentration of drug in the brain.

CNS AND CEREBROSPINAL FLUID. The brain capillary endothelial cells have continuous tight junctions; therefore, drug penetration into the brain depends on transcellular rather than paracellular transport. The unique characteristics of brain capillary endothelial cells and pericapillary glial cells constitute the blood-brain barrier. At the choroid plexus, a similar blood-CSF barrier is present, formed by epithelial cells that are joined by tight junctions. The lipid solubility of the nonionized and unbound species of a drug is therefore an important determinant of its uptake by the brain; the more lipophilic a drug, the more likely it is to cross the blood-brain barrier. Pharmaceutical chemists have used this fact to regulate the extent to which drugs penetrate into the CNS (e.g., compare first- and second-generation antihistamines; *see* Chapter 32). In general, the blood-brain barrier's function is well maintained; however, meningeal and encephalic inflammation increase local permeability. Drugs may also be imported to and exported from the CNS by specific transporters (*see* Chapter 5).

PLACENTAL TRANSFER OF DRUGS. The transfer of drugs across the placenta is of critical importance because drugs may cause anomalies in the developing fetus. Lipid solubility, extent of plasma binding, and degree of ionization of weak acids and bases are important general determinants in drug transfer across the placenta. The fetal plasma is slightly more acidic than that of the mother (pH 7.0-7.2 versus 7.4), so that ion trapping of basic drugs occurs. The view that the placenta is an absolute barrier to drugs is inaccurate, in part because a number of influx transporters are also present. The fetus is to some extent exposed to all drugs taken by the mother.

EXCRETION OF DRUGS

Drugs are eliminated from the body either unchanged or as metabolites. Excretory organs, the lung excluded, eliminate polar compounds more efficiently than substances with high lipid solubility. Lipid-soluble drugs thus are not readily eliminated until they are metabolized to more polar compounds. The kidney is the most important organ for excreting drugs and their metabolites. Renal excretion of unchanged drug is a major route of elimination for 25-30% of drugs administered to humans. Substances excreted in the feces are principally unabsorbed orally ingested drugs or drug metabolites excreted either in the bile or secreted directly into the intestinal tract and not reabsorbed. Excretion of drugs in breast milk is important not because of the amounts eliminated, but because the excreted drugs may affect the nursing infant. Excretion from the lung is important mainly for the elimination of anesthetic gases (*see* Chapter 19).

RENAL EXCRETION. Excretion of drugs and metabolites in the urine involves 3 distinct processes: glomerular filtration, active tubular secretion, and passive tubular reabsorption. Changes in overall renal function generally affect all 3 processes to a similar extent. In neonates, renal function is low compared with body mass but matures rapidly within the first few months after birth. During adulthood, there is a slow decline in renal function, ~1% per year, so that in elderly patients a substantial degree of functional impairment may be present.

The amount of drug entering the tubular lumen by filtration depends on the glomerular filtration rate and the extent of plasma binding of the drug; only unbound drug is filtered. In the proximal renal tubule, active, carrier-mediated tubular secretion also may add drug to the tubular fluid (*see* Chapter 5). Membrane transporters, mainly located in the distal renal tubule, also are responsible for any active reabsorption of drug from the tubular lumen back into the systemic circulation; however, in the proximal and distal tubules, the nonionized forms of weak acids and bases undergo net passive reabsorption. The concentration gradient for back diffusion is created by the reabsorption of water with Na^+ and other inorganic ions. Because the tubular cells are less permeable to the ionized forms of weak electrolytes, passive reabsorption of these substances depends on the pH. When the tubular urine is made more alkaline, weak acids are largely ionized and thus are excreted more rapidly and to a greater extent; conversely, acidification of the urine will reduce fractional ionization and excretion of weak acids. Alkalinization and acidification of the urine have the opposite effects on the excretion of weak bases. In the treatment of drug poisoning, the excretion of some drugs can be hastened by appropriate alkalinization or acidification of the urine.

BILIARY AND FECAL EXCRETION. Transporters present in the canalicular membrane of the hepatocyte (*see* Chapter 5) actively secrete drugs and metabolites into bile. P-gp and BCRP (breast cancer resistance protein, or ABCG2) transport a plethora of amphipathic lipid-soluble drugs, whereas MRP2 is mainly involved in the secretion of conjugated metabolites of drugs (e.g., glutathione conjugates, glucuronides, and some sulfates). Ultimately, drugs and metabolites present in bile are released into the GI tract during the digestive process. Subsequently, drugs and metabolites can be reabsorbed into the body from the intestine, which, in the case of conjugated metabolites, such as glucuronides, may require their enzymatic hydrolysis by the intestinal microflora. Such *enterohepatic recycling*, if extensive, may prolong significantly the presence of a drug (or toxin) and its effects within the body prior to elimination by other pathways. For this reason, drugs may be given orally to bind substances excreted in the bile.

EXCRETION BY OTHER ROUTES. Excretion of drugs into sweat, saliva, and tears is quantitatively unimportant. Elimination by these routes depends mainly on diffusion of the nonionized lipid-soluble form of drugs through the epithelial cells of the glands and on the pH. The same principles apply to excretion of drugs in breast milk. Because milk is more acidic than plasma, basic compounds may be slightly concentrated in this fluid; conversely, the concentration of acidic compounds in the milk is lower than in plasma. Nonelectrolytes (e.g., ethanol and urea) readily enter breast milk and reach the same concentration as in plasma, independent of the pH of the milk. Thus, the administration of drugs to breast-feeding women carries the general caution that the suckling infant will be exposed to some extent to the medication and/or its metabolites. In certain cases, such as treatment with the β-blocker atenolol, the infant may be exposed to significant amounts of drug. Although excretion into hair and skin is quantitatively unimportant, sensitive methods of detection of drugs in these tissues have forensic significance.

METABOLISM OF DRUGS

The majority of therapeutic agents are lipophilic compounds filtered through the glomerulus and reabsorbed into the systemic circulation during passage through the renal tubules. The metabolism of drugs and other xenobiotics into more hydrophilic metabolites is essential for their elimination from the body, as well as for termination of their biological and pharmacological activity. In general, biotransformation reactions generate more polar, inactive metabolites that are readily excreted from the body. However, in some cases, metabolites with potent biological activity or toxic properties are generated. Many of the enzyme systems that transform drugs to inactive metabolites also generate biologically active metabolites of endogenous compounds, as in steroid biosynthesis.

The enzyme systems involved in the biotransformation of drugs are localized primarily in the liver. Other organs with significant drug metabolizing capacity include the GI tract, kidneys, and lungs. *Prodrugs* are pharmacologically inactive compounds designed to maximize the amount of the active species that reaches its site of action. Inactive prodrugs are converted rapidly to biologically active metabolites often by the hydrolysis of an ester or amide linkage (*see* Chapter 6 for details of drug metabolism).

CLINICAL PHARMACOKINETICS

Clinical pharmacokinetics rely on a relationship between the pharmacological effects of a drug and an accessible concentration of the drug (e.g., in blood or plasma). In most cases, the concentration of drug at its sites of action will be related to the concentration of drug in the systemic circulation (*see* Figure 2–1). The pharmacological effect that results may be the clinical effect desired, or an adverse or toxic effect. The 4 most important parameters governing drug disposition are *bioavailability*, the fraction of drug absorbed as such into the systemic circulation; *volume of distribution,* a measure of the apparent space in the body available to contain the drug based on how much is given versus what is found in the systemic circulation; *clearance,* a measure of the body's efficiency in eliminating drug from the systemic circulation; and *elimination* $t_{1/2}$, a measure of the rate of removal of drug from the systemic circulation.

For some drugs, no clear or simple relationship has been found between pharmacological effect and concentration in plasma, whereas for other drugs, routine measurement of drug concentration is impractical as part of therapeutic monitoring.

CLEARANCE

Clearance is the most important concept to consider when designing a rational regimen for long-term drug administration. The clinician usually wants to maintain steady-state concentrations of a drug within a *therapeutic window* or range associated with therapeutic efficacy and a minimum of toxicity for a given agent. Assuming complete bioavailability, the steady-state concentration of drug in the body will be achieved when the rate of drug elimination equals the rate of drug administration (Equation 2–2). Thus:

$$\text{Dosing rate} = CL \cdot C_{ss} \qquad \text{(Equation 2–2)}$$

where CL is clearance of drug from the systemic circulation and C_{ss} is the steady-state concentration of drug. If the desired steady-state concentration of drug in plasma or blood is known, the rate of clearance of drug by the patient will dictate the rate at which the drug should be administered.

Metabolizing enzymes and transporters usually are not saturated, and thus the absolute rate of elimination of the drug is essentially a linear function of its concentration in plasma (first-order kinetics), where a constant fraction of drug in the body is eliminated per unit of time. If mechanisms for elimination of a given drug become saturated, the kinetics approach zero order (the case for ethanol), in which a constant amount of drug is eliminated per unit of time. With first-order kinetics, clearance (CL) will vary with the concentration of drug, often according to Equation 2–3:

$$CL = v_m/(K_m + C) \qquad \text{(Equation 2–3)}$$

where K_m represents the concentration at which half the maximal rate of elimination is reached (in units of mass/volume) and v_m is equal to the maximal rate of elimination (in units of mass/time). Thus, clearance is derived in units of volume/time. This equation is analogous to the Michaelis-Menten equation for enzyme kinetics.

Clearance of a drug is its rate of elimination by all routes normalized to the concentration of drug C in some biological fluid where measurement can be made:

$$CL = \text{rate of elimination}/C \qquad \text{(Equation 2–4)}$$

Thus, when clearance is constant, the rate of drug elimination is directly proportional to drug concentration. Clearance indicates the volume of biological fluid such as blood or plasma from which drug would have to be completely removed to account for the clearance per unit of body weight (e.g., mL/min per kg). Clearance can be defined further as blood clearance (CL_b), plasma clearance (CL_p), or clearance based on the concentration of unbound drug (CL_u), depending on the measurement made (C_b, C_p, or C_u). Clearance of drug by several organs is additive. Elimination of drug from the systemic circulation may occur as a result of processes that occur in the kidney, liver, and other organs. Division of the rate of elimination by each organ by a concentration of drug (e.g., plasma concentration) will yield the respective clearance by that organ. Added together, these separate clearances will equal systemic clearance:

$$CL_{renal} + CL_{hepatic} + CL_{other} = CL \qquad \text{(Equation 2–5)}$$

Systemic clearance may be determined at steady state by using Equation 2–2. For a single dose of a drug with complete bioavailability and first-order kinetics of elimination, systemic clearance may be determined from mass balance and the integration of Equation 2–4 over time:

$$CL = \text{Dose}/AUC \qquad \text{(Equation 2–6)}$$

AUC is the total area under the curve that describes the measured concentration of drug in the systemic circulation as a function of time (from zero to infinity), as in Figure 2–6.

Examples. The plasma clearance for the antibiotic cephalexin is 4.3 mL/min/kg, with 90% of the drug excreted unchanged in the urine. For a 70-kg man, the clearance from plasma would be 301 mL/min, with renal clearance accounting for 90% of this elimination. In other words, the kidney is able to excrete cephalexin at a rate such that the drug is completely removed (cleared) from ~270 mL of plasma every minute (renal clearance = 90% of total clearance). Because clearance usually is assumed to remain constant in a medically stable patient (e.g., no acute decline in kidney function), the rate of elimination of cephalexin will depend on the concentration of drug in the plasma (*see* Equation 2–4).

The β adrenergic receptor antagonist propranolol is cleared from the blood at a rate of 16 mL/min/kg (or 1120 mL/min in a 70-kg man), almost exclusively by the liver. Thus, the liver is able to remove the amount of propranolol contained in 1120 mL of blood in 1 min. Even though the liver is the dominant organ for elimination, the plasma clearance of some drugs exceeds the rate of blood flow to this organ. Often this is so because the drug partitions readily into red blood cells (RBCs) and the rate of drug delivered to the eliminating organ is considerably higher than expected from measurement of its concentration in plasma. The parent text has a more extended presentation of clearance in Chapter 2 and Appendix II.

HEPATIC CLEARANCE. For a drug that is removed efficiently from the blood by hepatic processes (metabolism and/or excretion of drug into the bile), the concentration of drug in the blood leaving the liver will be low, the extraction ratio will approach unity, and the clearance of the drug from blood will become limited by hepatic blood flow. Drugs that are cleared efficiently by the liver (e.g., drugs with systemic clearances >6 mL/min/kg, such as diltiazem, imipramine, lidocaine, morphine, and propranolol) are restricted in their rate of elimination not by intrahepatic processes but by the rate at which they can be transported in the blood to the liver.

RENAL CLEARANCE. Renal clearance of a drug results in its appearance in the urine. The rate of filtration of a drug depends on the volume of fluid that is filtered in the glomerulus and the unbound concentration of drug in plasma, because drug bound to protein is not filtered. The rate of secretion of drug by the kidney will depend on the drug's intrinsic clearance by the transporters involved in active secretion as affected by the drug's binding to plasma proteins, the degree of saturation of these transporters, and the rate of delivery of the drug to the secretory site. In addition, processes involved in drug reabsorption from the tubular fluid must be considered. These factors are altered in renal disease.

DISTRIBUTION

VOLUME OF DISTRIBUTION. The volume of distribution (V) relates the amount of drug in the body to the concentration of drug (C) in the blood or plasma depending on the fluid measured. This volume does not necessarily refer to an identifiable physiological volume but rather to the fluid volume that would be required to contain all of the drug in the body at the same concentration measured in the blood or plasma:

$$\text{Amount of drug in body}/V = C \quad \text{or} \quad V = \text{amount of drug in body}/C \qquad \text{(Equation 2–7)}$$

A drug's volume of distribution therefore reflects the extent to which it is present in extravascular tissues and not in the plasma. View V as an imaginary volume, because for many drugs V exceeds the known volume of any and all body compartments. For example, the value of V for the highly lipophilic antimalarial chloroquine is some 15,000 L, yet the plasma volume of a typical 70-kg man is 3 L, blood volume is ~5.5 L, extracellular fluid volume outside the plasma is 12 L, and the volume of total-body water is ~42 L.

Many drugs exhibit volumes of distribution far in excess of these values. For example, if 500 μg of the cardiac glycoside digoxin were in the body of a 70-kg subject, a plasma concentration of ~0.75 ng/mL would be observed. Dividing the amount of drug in the body by the plasma concentration yields a volume of distribution for digoxin of ~667 L, or a value ~15 times greater than the total-body volume of a 70-kg man. In fact, digoxin distributes preferentially to muscle and adipose tissue and to its specific receptors (Na^+, K^+-ATPase), leaving a very small amount of drug in the plasma to be measured. For drugs that are bound extensively to plasma proteins but are not bound to tissue components, the volume of distribution will approach that of the plasma volume because drug bound to plasma protein is measurable in the assay of most drugs. In contrast, certain drugs have high volumes of distribution even though most of the drug in the circulation is bound to albumin because these drugs are also sequestered elsewhere.

The volume of distribution may vary widely depending on the relative degrees of binding to high-affinity receptor sites, plasma and tissue proteins, the partition coefficient of the drug in fat, and accumulation in poorly perfused tissues. The volume of distribution for a given drug can differ according to patient's age, gender, body composition, and presence of disease. Total-body water of infants younger than 1 year of age, for example, is 75% to 80% of body weight, whereas that of adult males is 60% and that of females is 55%.

The volume of distribution defined in Equation 2–7 considers the body as a single homogeneous compartment. In this one-compartment model, all drug administration occurs directly into the central compartment, and distribution of drug is instantaneous throughout the volume (V). Clearance of drug from this compartment occurs in a first-order fashion, as defined in Equation 2–4; that is, the amount of drug eliminated per unit of time depends on the amount (concentration) of drug in the body compartment. Figure 2–4A and Equation 2–8 describe the decline of plasma concentration with time for a drug introduced into this central compartment:

$$C = [\text{dose}/V][e^{-kt}] \qquad \text{(Equation 2–8)}$$

where k is the rate constant for elimination that reflects the fraction of drug removed from the compartment per unit of time. This rate constant is inversely related to the $t_{1/2}$ of the drug [$kt_{1/2} = \ln 2 = 0.693$]. The idealized one-compartment model does not describe the entire time course of the plasma concentration. That is, certain tissue reservoirs can be distinguished from the central compartment, and the drug concentration appears to decay in a manner that can be described by multiple exponential terms (Figure 2–4B).

RATE OF DISTRIBUTION. In many cases, groups of tissues with similar perfusion-to-partition ratios all equilibrate at essentially the same rate such that only one apparent phase of distribution is seen (rapid initial decrease in concentration of intravenously injected drug, as in Figure 2–4B). It is as though the drug starts in a

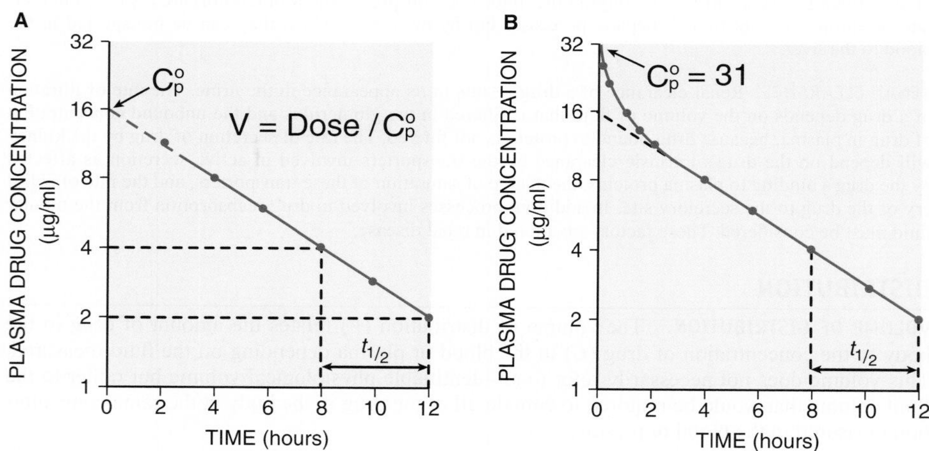

Figure 2–4 *Plasma concentration-time curves following intravenous administration of a drug (500 mg) to a 70-kg patient.* **A.** Drug concentrations are measured in plasma at 2-hour intervals following drug administration. The semilogarithmic plot of plasma concentration (C_p) versus time suggests that the drug is eliminated from a single compartment by a first-order process (*see* Equation 2–8) with a $t_{1/2}$ of 4 h ($k = 0.693/t_{1/2} = 0.173$ hr^{-1}). The volume of distribution (V) may be determined from the value of C_p obtained by extrapolation to 0-time. Volume of distribution (*see* Equation 2–7) for the one-compartment model is 31.3 L, or 0.45 L/kg ($V = \text{dose}/C_p^o$). The clearance for this drug is 90 mL/min; for a one-compartment model, $CL = kV$. **B.** Sampling before 2 h indicates that in fact the drug follows multiexponential kinetics. The terminal disposition $t_{1/2}$ is 4 h, clearance is 84 mL/min (*see* Equation 2–6), V_{area} is 29 L (*see* Equation 2–8), and V_{ss} is 26.8 L. The initial or "central" distribution volume for the drug ($V = \text{dose}/C_p^o$) is 16.1 L. The example indicates that multicompartment kinetics may be overlooked when sampling at early times is neglected. In this particular case, there is only a 10% error in the estimate of clearance when the multicompartment characteristics are ignored. For many drugs, multicompartment kinetics may be observed for significant periods of time, and failure to consider the distribution phase can lead to significant errors in estimates of clearance and in predictions of the appropriate dosage. Also, the difference between the "central" distribution volume and other terms reflecting wider distribution is important in deciding a loading dose strategy.

"central" volume (*see* Figure 2–1), which consists of plasma and tissue reservoirs that are in rapid equilibrium, and distributes to a "final" volume, at which point concentrations in plasma decrease in a log-linear fashion with a rate constant of k (*see* Figure 2–4B). The multicompartment model of drug disposition can be viewed as though the blood and highly perfused lean organs such as heart, brain, liver, lung, and kidneys cluster as a single central compartment, whereas more slowly perfused tissues such as muscle, skin, fat, and bone behave as the final compartment (the tissue compartment).

STEADY STATE. Equation 2–2 (dosing rate = $CL \cdot C_{ss}$) indicates that a steady-state concentration eventually will be achieved when a drug is administered at a constant rate. At this point, drug elimination (the product of clearance and concentration; Equation 2–4) will equal the rate of drug availability. This concept also extends to regular intermittent dosage (e.g., 250 mg of drug every 8 h). During each interdose interval, the concentration of drug rises with absorption and falls by elimination. At steady state, the entire cycle is repeated identically in each interval (Figure 2–5). Equation 2–2 still applies for intermittent dosing, but it now describes the average steady-state drug concentration ($\bar{C}_{ss}$) during an interdose interval, where F is fractional bioavailability of the dose and T is dosage interval (time). By substitution of infusion rate for $F \cdot \text{dose}/T$, the formula is equivalent to Equation 2–2 and provides the concentration maintained at steady state during continuous intravenous infusion.

HALF-LIFE. The $t_{1/2}$ is the time it takes for the plasma concentration to be reduced by 50%. For a one-compartment model (Figure 2–4A), $t_{1/2}$ may be determined readily by inspection and used to make decisions about drug dosage. However, as indicated in Figure 2–4B, drug concentrations in plasma often follow a multiexponential pattern of decline, reflecting the changing amount of drug in the body. When using pharmacokinetics to calculate drug dosing in disease, note in Equation 2–9 that $t_{1/2}$ changes as a function of both clearance and volume of distribution:

$$t_{1/2} \cong 0.693 \cdot V_{ss}/CL \qquad \text{(Equation 2–9)}$$

This $t_{1/2}$ reflects the decline of systemic drug concentrations during a dosing interval at steady-state as depicted in Figure 2–5.

Clearance is the measure of the body's ability to eliminate a drug; thus, as clearance decreases, owing to a disease process, for example, $t_{1/2}$ would be expected to increase as long as the volume of distribution remains unchanged. For example, the $t_{1/2}$ of diazepam increases with increasing age; however, it is not clearance that changes as a function of age but rather the volume of distribution. Similarly, changes in protein binding of a drug may affect its clearance as well as its volume of distribution, leading to unpredictable changes in $t_{1/2}$ as a

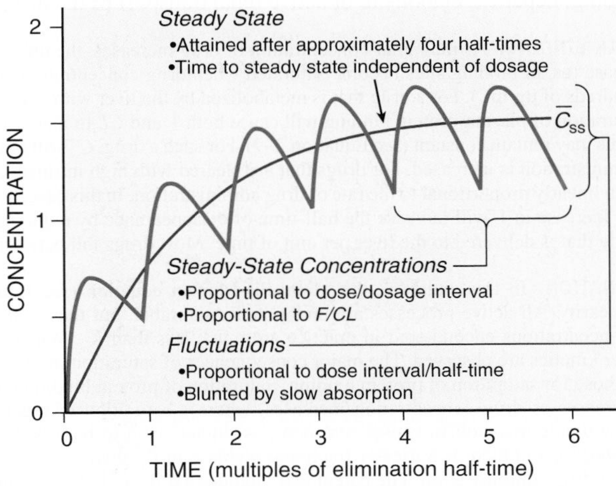

Figure 2–5 *Fundamental pharmacokinetic relationships for repeated administration of drugs.* The red line is the pattern of drug accumulation during repeated administration of a drug at intervals equal to its elimination half-time when drug absorption is 10 times as rapid as elimination. As the rate of absorption increases, the concentration maxima approach 2 and the minima approach 1 during the steady state. The blue line depicts the pattern during administration of equivalent dosage by continuous intravenous infusion. Curves are based on the one-compartment model. Average drug concentration at steady state ($\bar{C}_{ss}$) is given by Equation 2–10, where dosing rate is dose per time interval (T), F is fractional bioavailability, and CL is clearance. Substituting infusion rate for $F \cdot \text{dose}/T$ provides the concentration maintained at steady state during continuous intravenous infusion.

function of disease. The $t_{1/2}$ defined in Equation 2–9 provides an approximation of the time required to reach steady state after a dosage regimen is initiated or changed (e.g., 4 half-lives to reach ~94% of a new steady state) and a means to estimate the appropriate dosing interval.

EXTENT AND RATE OF ABSORPTION

BIOAVAILABILITY. It is important to distinguish between the rate and extent of drug absorption and the amount of drug that ultimately reaches the systemic circulation. This depends not only on the administered dose but also on the fraction of the dose (F) that is absorbed and escapes any first-pass elimination. This fraction is the drug's *bioavailability*.

When drugs are administered by a route that is subject to first-pass loss, the equations presented previously that contain the terms *dose* or *dosing rate* (*see* Equations 2–2, 2–6, and 2–8) also must include the bioavailability term F such that the available dose or dosing rate is used. For example, Equation 2–2 is modified to Equation 2–10:

$$F \cdot \text{dosing rate} = CL \cdot C_{ss} \qquad \text{(Equation 2–10)}$$

where the value of F is between 0 and 1. The value of F varies widely for drugs administered by mouth, and successful therapy can still be achieved for some drugs with F values as low as 0.03 (e.g., etidronate and aliskiren).

RATE OF ABSORPTION. Although the rate of drug absorption does not, in general, influence the average steady-state concentration of the drug in plasma, it may still influence drug therapy. If a drug is absorbed rapidly (e.g., a dose given as an intravenous bolus) and has a small "central" volume, the concentration of drug initially will be high. It will then fall as the drug is distributed to its "final" (larger) volume (*see* Figure 2–4B). If the same drug is absorbed more slowly (e.g., by slow infusion), a significant amount of the drug will be distributed while it is being administered, and peak concentrations will be lower and will occur later. Controlled-release oral preparations are designed to provide a slow and sustained rate of absorption in order to produce smaller fluctuations in the plasma concentration-time profile during the dosage interval compared with more immediate-release formulations. Because the beneficial, nontoxic effects of drugs are based on knowledge of an ideal or desired plasma concentration range, maintaining that range while avoiding large swings between peak and trough concentrations can improve therapeutic outcome.

NONLINEAR PHARMACOKINETICS

Nonlinearity in pharmacokinetics (i.e., changes in such parameters as clearance, volume of distribution, and $t_{1/2}$ as a function of dose or concentration of drug) is usually caused by saturation of either protein binding, hepatic metabolism, or active renal transport of the drug.

SATURABLE PROTEIN BINDING. As the molar concentration of drug increases, the unbound fraction eventually also must increase (as all binding sites become saturated when drug concentrations in plasma are in the range of tens to hundreds of μg/mL). For a drug that is metabolized by the liver with a low intrinsic clearance-extraction ratio, saturation of plasma-protein binding will cause both V and CL to increase as drug concentrations increase; $t_{1/2}$ thus may remain constant (*see* Equation 2–9). For such a drug, C_{ss} will not increase linearly as the rate of drug administration is increased. For drugs that are cleared with high intrinsic clearance-extraction ratios, C_{ss} can remain linearly proportional to the rate of drug administration. In this case, hepatic clearance will not change, and the increase in V will increase the half-time of disappearance by reducing the fraction of the total drug in the body that is delivered to the liver per unit of time. Most drugs fall between these 2 extremes.

SATURABLE ELIMINATION. In this situation, the Michaelis-Menten equation (*see* Equation 2–3) usually describes the nonlinearity. All active processes are undoubtedly saturable, but they will appear to be linear if values of drug concentrations encountered in practice are much less than K_m. When drug concentrations exceed K_m, nonlinear kinetics are observed. The major consequences of saturation of metabolism or transport are the opposite of those for saturation of protein binding. Saturation of protein binding will lead to increased CL because CL increases as drug concentration increases, whereas saturation of metabolism or transport may decrease CL. Saturable metabolism causes oral first-pass metabolism to be less than expected (higher *fractional bioavailability*), and there is a greater fractional increase in C_{ss} than the corresponding fractional increase in the rate of drug administration. The parent text includes a more detailed treatment.

DESIGN AND OPTIMIZATION OF DOSAGE REGIMENS

The intensity of a drug's effect is related to its concentration above a minimum effective concentration, whereas the duration of the drug's effect reflects the length of time the drug level is above this value (Figure 2–6). These considerations, in general, apply to both desired and undesired (adverse) drug effects; as a result, a *therapeutic window* exists that reflects a concentration range that provides efficacy without unacceptable toxicity.

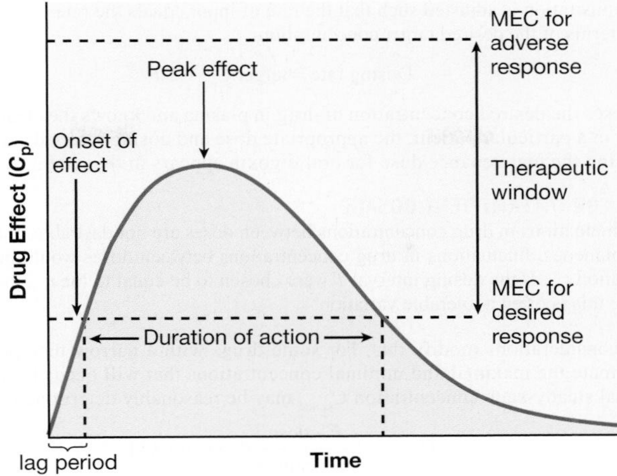

Figure 2–6 *Temporal characteristics of drug effect and relationship to the therapeutic window (e.g., single dose, oral administration).* A lag period is present before the plasma drug concentration (C_p) exceeds the minimum effective concentration (MEC) for the desired effect. Following onset of the response, the intensity of the effect increases as the drug continues to be absorbed and distributed. This reaches a peak, after which drug elimination results in a decline in C_p and in the effect's intensity. Effect disappears when the drug concentration falls below the MEC. The duration of a drug's action is determined by the time period over which concentrations exceed the MEC. An MEC exists for each adverse response, and if the drug concentration exceeds this, toxicity will result. The therapeutic goal is to obtain and maintain concentrations within the therapeutic window for the desired response with a minimum of toxicity. Drug response below the MEC for the desired effect will be subtherapeutic; above the MEC for an adverse effect, the probability of toxicity will increase. Increasing or decreasing drug dosage shifts the response curve up or down the intensity scale and is used to modulate the drug's effect. Increasing the dose also prolongs a drug's duration of action but at the risk of increasing the likelihood of adverse effects. Unless the drug is nontoxic (e.g., penicillins), increasing the dose is not a useful strategy for extending the duration of action. Instead, another dose of drug should be given, timed to maintain concentrations within the therapeutic window. The area under the blood concentration-time curve (area under the curve, or AUC, shaded in red) can be used to calculate the clearance (*see* Equation 2–6) for first-order elimination. The AUC is also used as a measure of bioavailability (defined as 100% for an intravenously administered drug). Bioavailability will be less than 100% for orally administered drugs, due mainly to incomplete absorption and first-pass metabolism and elimination.

Similar considerations apply after multiple dosing associated with long-term therapy, and they determine the amount and frequency of drug administration to achieve an optimal therapeutic effect. In general, the lower limit of a drug's therapeutic range is approximately equal to the drug concentration that produces about half the greatest possible therapeutic effect, and the upper limit of the therapeutic range is such that no more than 5-10% of patients will experience a toxic effect. For some drugs, this may mean that the upper limit of the range is no more than twice the lower limit. Of course, these figures can be highly variable, and some patients may benefit greatly from drug concentrations that exceed the therapeutic range, whereas others may suffer significant toxicity at much lower values (e.g., with digoxin).

For a limited number of drugs, some effect of the drug is easily measured (e.g., blood pressure, blood glucose) and can be used to optimize dosage using a trial-and-error approach. Even in an ideal case, certain quantitative issues arise, such as how often to change dosage and by how much. These usually can be settled with simple rules of thumb based on the principles discussed (e.g., change dosage by no more than 50% and no more often than every 3-4 half-lives). Alternatively, some drugs have very little dose-related toxicity, and maximum efficacy usually is desired. In such cases, doses well in excess of the average required will ensure efficacy (if this is possible) and prolong drug action. Such a "maximal dose" strategy typically is used for penicillins. For many drugs, however, the effects are difficult to measure (or the drug is given for prophylaxis), toxicity and lack of efficacy are both potential dangers, or the therapeutic index is narrow. In these circumstances, doses must be titrated carefully, and drug dosage is limited by toxicity rather than efficacy.

MAINTENANCE DOSE

In most clinical situations, drugs are administered in a series of repetitive doses or as a continuous infusion to maintain a steady-state concentration of drug associated with the therapeutic window. Calculation of the appropriate maintenance dosage is a primary goal. To maintain the chosen steady-state or target concentration, the rate of drug administration is adjusted such that the rate of input equals the rate of loss. This relationship is expressed here in terms of the desired target concentration:

$$\text{Dosing rate} = \text{target } C_p \cdot CL/F \qquad \text{(Equation 2–11)}$$

If the clinician chooses the desired concentration of drug in plasma and knows the clearance and bioavailability for that drug in a particular patient, the appropriate dose and dosing interval can be calculated. An example of calculating the maintenance dose for oral digoxin appears in the parent text.

DOSING INTERVAL FOR INTERMITTENT DOSAGE

In general, marked fluctuations in drug concentrations between doses are not desirable. If absorption and distribution were instantaneous, fluctuations in drug concentrations between doses would be governed entirely by the drug's elimination $t_{1/2}$. If the dosing interval T were chosen to be equal to the $t_{1/2}$, then the total fluctuation would be 2-fold; this is often a tolerable variation.

Pharmacodynamic considerations modify this. For some drugs with a narrow therapeutic range, it may be important to estimate the maximal and minimal concentrations that will occur for a particular dosing interval. The minimal steady-state concentration $C_{ss,min}$ may be reasonably determined as:

$$C_{ss,\,min} = \frac{F \cdot \text{dose}/V_{ss}}{1 - \exp(-kT)} \cdot \exp(-kT) \qquad \text{(Equation 2–12)}$$

where k equals 0.693 divided by the clinically relevant plasma $t_{1/2,}$ and T is the dosing interval. The term $\exp(-kT)$ is, in fact, the fraction of the last dose (corrected for bioavailability) that remains in the body at the end of a dosing interval. The parent text gives examples employing Equation 2–12.

LOADING DOSE

The *loading dose* is one or a series of doses that may be given at the onset of therapy with the aim of achieving the target concentration rapidly. The appropriate magnitude for the loading dose is:

$$\text{Loading dose} = \text{target } C_p \cdot V_{ss}/F \qquad \text{(Equation 2–13)}$$

A loading dose may be desirable if the time required to attain steady state by the administration of drug at a constant rate (4 elimination $t_{1/2}$ values) is long relative to the temporal demands of the condition being treated as is the case for treatment of arrhythmias and cardiac failure. The use of a loading dose also has significant disadvantages. First, the particularly sensitive individual may be exposed abruptly to a toxic concentration of a drug that may take a long time to decrease (i.e., long $t_{1/2}$). Loading doses tend to be large, and they are often given parenterally and rapidly; this can be particularly dangerous if toxic effects occur as a result of actions of the drug at sites that are in rapid equilibrium with plasma. It is therefore usually advisable to divide the loading dose into a number of smaller fractional doses that are administered over a period of time. Alternatively, the loading dose should be administered as a continuous intravenous infusion over a period of time using computerized infusion pumps. See the parent text for sample calculations.

THERAPEUTIC DRUG MONITORING

The major use of measured concentrations of drugs (at steady state) is to refine the estimate of CL/F for the patient being treated, using Equation 2–10 as rearranged:

$$CL/F\text{ (patient)} = \text{dosing rate}/C_{ss}\text{(measured)} \qquad \text{(Equation 2–14)}$$

The new estimate of CL/F can be used in Equation 2–11 to adjust the maintenance dose to achieve the desired target concentration. See the parent text for a fuller presentation of details, precautions, and pitfalls associated with therapeutic drug monitoring.

For a complete Bibliographical Listing see Goodman & Gilman's ***The Pharmacological Basis of Therapeutics***, 12th ed., or Goodman & Gilman Online at www.AccessMedicine.com.

Pharmacodynamics: Molecular Mechanisms of Drug Action

Pharmacodynamic Concepts

Pharmacodynamics is the study of the biochemical and physiological effects of drugs and their mechanisms of action. The effects of most drugs result from their interaction with macromolecular components of the organism. The term drug *receptor* or drug *target* denotes the cellular macromolecule or macromolecular complex with which the drug interacts to elicit a cellular response. Drugs commonly alter the rate or magnitude of an intrinsic cellular response rather than create new responses. Drug receptors are often located on the surface of cells, but may also be located in specific intracellular compartments such as the nucleus.

Many drugs also interact with *acceptors* (e.g., serum albumin) within the body. Acceptors are entities that do not directly cause any change in biochemical or physiological response. However, interactions of drugs with acceptors can alter the pharmacokinetics of a drug's actions.

PHYSIOLOGICAL RECEPTORS

Many drug receptors are proteins that normally serve as receptors for endogenous regulatory ligands. These drug targets are termed *physiological receptors*. Drugs that bind to physiological receptors and mimic the regulatory effects of the endogenous signaling compounds are termed *agonists*. If the drug binds to the same *recognition site* as the endogenous agonist, the drug is said to be a *primary agonist*. *Allosteric* (or *allotopic*) agonists bind to a different region on the receptor referred to as an allosteric or allotopic site. Drugs that block or reduce the action of an agonist are termed *antagonists*. Antagonism generally results from competition with an agonist for the same or overlapping site on the receptor (a *syntopic* interaction), but can also occur by interacting with other sites on the receptor (allosteric antagonism), by combining with the agonist (chemical antagonism), or by functional antagonism by indirectly inhibiting the cellular or physiological effects of the agonist. Agents that are only partly as effective as agonists are termed *partial agonists*. Many receptors exhibit some constitutive activity in the absence of a regulatory ligand; drugs that stabilize such receptors in an inactive conformation are termed *inverse agonists* (Figure 3–1). In the presence of a full agonist, partial and inverse agonists will behave as competitive antagonists.

SPECIFICITY OF DRUG RESPONSES

The strength of the reversible interaction between a drug and its receptor, as measured by the *dissociation constant*, is defined as the affinity of one for the other. Both the affinity of a drug for its receptor and its *intrinsic activity* are determined by its chemical structure. The chemical structure of a drug also contributes to the drug's *specificity*. A drug that interacts with a single type of receptor that is expressed on only a limited number of differentiated cells will exhibit high specificity. Conversely, drugs acting on a receptor expressed ubiquitously throughout the body will exhibit widespread effects.

Many clinically important drugs exhibit a broad (low) specificity because they interact with multiple receptors in different tissues. Such broad specificity might enhance the clinical utility of a drug, but also contribute to a spectrum of adverse side effects because of off-target interactions. One example of a drug that interacts with multiple receptors is amiodarone, an agent used to treat cardiac arrhythmias. Amiodarone also has a number of serious toxicities, some of which are caused by the drug's structural similarity to thyroid hormone and its ability to interact with nuclear thyroid receptors. Amiodarone's salutary effects and toxicities may also be mediated through interactions with receptors that are poorly characterized or unknown. Some drugs are administered as racemic mixtures of stereoisomers. The stereoisomers can exhibit different pharmacodynamic as well as pharmacokinetic properties. For example, the anti-arrhythmic drug sotalol is prescribed as a racemic mixture; the D- and L-enantiomers are equipotent as K^+ channel blockers, but the L-enantiomer is a much more

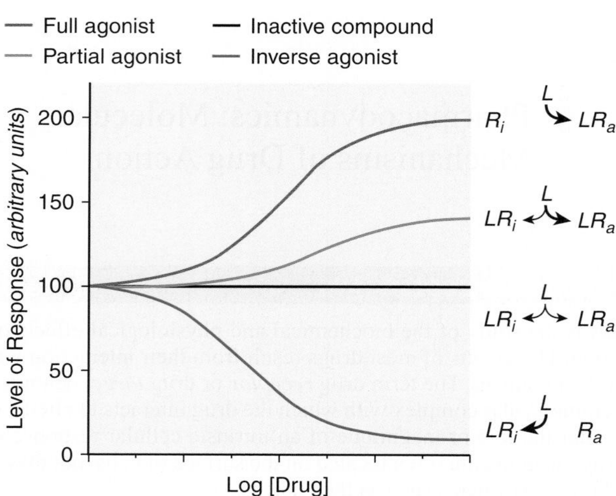

Figure 3–1 *Regulation of the activity of a receptor with conformation-selective drugs.* The ordinate is the activity of the receptor produced by R_a, the active receptor conformation (e.g., stimulation of adenylyl cyclase by a β adrenergic receptor). If a drug *L* selectively binds to R_a, it will produce a maximal response. If *L* has equal affinity for R_i and R_a, it will not perturb the equilibrium between them and will have no effect on net activity; *L* would appear as an inactive compound. If the drug selectively binds to R_i, then the net amount of R_a will be diminished. If *L* can bind to receptor in an active conformation R_a but also bind to inactive receptor R_i with lower affinity, the drug will produce a partial response; *L* will be a partial agonist. If there is sufficient R_a to produce an elevated basal response in the absence of ligand (agonist-independent constitutive activity), then activity will be inhibited; *L* will then be an inverse agonist. Inverse agonists selectively bind to the inactive form of the receptor and shift the conformational equilibrium toward the inactive state. In systems that are not constitutively active, inverse agonists will behave like competitive antagonists, which helps explain why the properties of inverse agonists and the number of such agents previously described as competitive antagonists were only recently appreciated. Receptors that have constitutive activity and are sensitive to inverse agonists include benzodiazepine, histamine, opioid, cannabinoid, dopamine, bradykinin, and adenosine receptors.

potent β adrenergic antagonist (*see* Chapter 29). A drug may have multiple mechanisms of action that depend on receptor specificity, the tissue-specific expression of the receptor(s), drug access to target tissues, drug concentration in different tissues, pharmacogenetics, and interactions with other drugs.

Chronic administration of a drug may cause a *downregulation* of receptors or *desensitization* of response that can require dose adjustments to maintain adequate therapy. Chronic administration of nitrovasodilators to treat angina results in the rapid development of complete tolerance, a process known as *tachyphylaxis*. Drug resistance may also develop because of pharmacokinetic mechanisms (i.e., the drug is metabolized more rapidly with chronic exposure), the development of mechanisms that prevent the drug from reaching its receptor (i.e., increased expression of the multidrug resistance transporter in drug-resistant cancer cells; *see* Chapter 5), or the clonal expansion of cancer cells containing drug-resistant mutations in the drug receptor.

Some drug effects do not occur by means of macromolecular receptors; aluminum and magnesium hydroxides [$Al(OH)_3$ and $Mg(OH)_2$] reduce gastric acid chemically, neutralizing H^+ with OH^- and raising gastric pH. Mannitol acts osmotically to cause changes in the distribution of water to promote diuresis, catharsis, expansion of circulating volume in the vascular compartment, or reduction of cerebral edema (*see* Chapter 25). Anti-infective drugs such as antibiotics, antivirals, and antiparasitics target receptors or cell processes that are critical for the growth or survival of the infective agent but are nonessential or lacking in the host organism. Resistance to antibiotics, antivirals, and other drugs can result through a variety of mechanisms including mutation of the target receptor, increased expression of enzymes that degrade or increase efflux of the drug from the infective agent, and development of alternative biochemical pathways that circumvent the drug's effects on the infective agent.

STRUCTURE-ACTIVITY RELATIONSHIPS AND DRUG DESIGN

The receptors responsible for the clinical effects of many drugs have yet to be identified. Conversely, sequencing of the entire human genome has identified novel genes related by sequence to known receptors, for which endogenous and exogenous ligands are unknown; these are called *orphan receptors*.

Both the affinity of a drug for its receptor and its intrinsic activity are determined by its chemical structure. This relationship frequently is quite stringent. Relatively minor modifications in the drug molecule may result in major changes in its pharmacological properties based on altered affinity for 1 or more receptors. Exploitation of structure-activity relationships has frequently led to the synthesis of valuable therapeutic agents. Because changes in molecular configuration need not alter all actions and effects of a drug equally, it is sometimes possible to develop a congener with a more favorable ratio of therapeutic to adverse effects, enhanced selectivity among different cells or tissues, or more acceptable secondary characteristics than those of the parent drug. Therapeutically useful antagonists of hormones or neurotransmitters have been developed by chemical modification of the structure of the physiological agonist.

With information about the molecular structures and pharmacological activities of a relatively large group of congeners, it is possible to use computer analysis to identify the chemical properties (i.e., the pharmacophore) required for optimal action at the receptor: size, shape, position, and orientation of charged groups or hydrogen bond donors, and so on. Advances in molecular modeling of organic compounds and the methods for drug target (receptor) discovery and biochemical measurement of the primary actions of drugs at their receptors have enriched the quantitation of structure-activity relationships and its use in drug design. Such information increasingly is allowing the optimization or design of chemicals that can bind to a receptor with improved affinity, selectivity, or regulatory effect. Similar structure-based approaches also are used to improve pharmacokinetic properties of drugs, particularly if knowledge of their metabolism is known. Knowledge of the structures of receptors and of drug-receptor complexes, determined at atomic resolution by X-ray crystallography, is even more helpful in the design of ligands and in understanding the molecular basis of drug resistance and circumventing it. Emerging technology in the field of pharmacogenetics (*see* Chapter 7) is improving our understanding of the nature of and variation in receptors.

QUANTITATIVE ASPECTS OF DRUG INTERACTIONS WITH RECEPTORS

Receptor occupancy theory assumes that response emanates from a receptor occupied by a drug, a concept that has its basis in the law of mass action. The *dose-response curve* depicts the observed effect of a drug as a function of its concentration in the receptor compartment. Figure 3–2 shows a typical dose-response curve.

Some drugs cause low-dose stimulation and high-dose inhibition of response. These U-shaped relationships for some receptor systems are said to display *hormesis*. Several drug-receptor systems can display this property (e.g., prostaglandins, endothelin, and purinergic and serotonergic agonists), which may be at the root of some drug toxicities.

AFFINITY, EFFICACY, AND POTENCY. In general, the drug-receptor interaction is characterized by (1) binding of drug to receptor and (2) generation of a response in a biological system, as illustrated in Equation 3–1 where the drug or ligand is denoted as *L* and the inactive receptor as *R*.

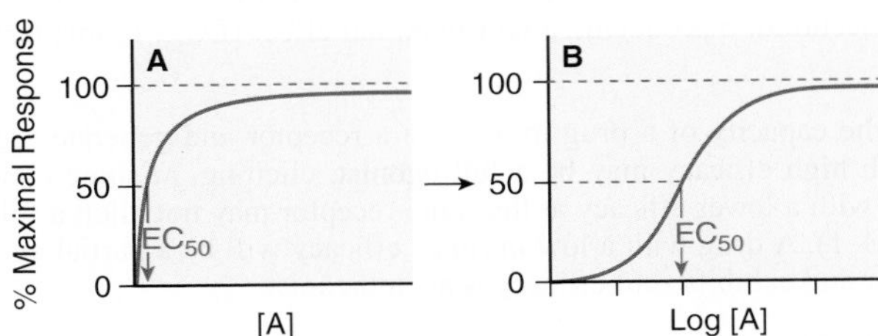

Figure 3–2 *Graded responses (y axis as a percentage of maximal response) expressed as a function of the concentration of drug A present at the receptor.* The hyperbolic shape of the curve in panel **A** becomes sigmoid when plotted semi-logarithmically, as in panel **B**. The concentration of drug that produces 50% of the maximal response quantifies drug activity and is referred to as the EC_{50} (effective concentration for 50% response). The range of concentrations needed to fully depict the dose-response relationship (~3 log_{10} [10] units) is too wide to be useful in the linear format of Figure 3–2A; thus, most dose-response curves use log [Drug] on the *x* axis, as in Figure 3–2B. Dose-response curves presented in this way are sigmoidal in shape and have 3 properties: threshold, slope, and maximal asymptote. These 3 parameters quantitate the activity of the drug.

The first reaction, the reversible formation of the ligand-receptor complex *LR*, is governed by the chemical property of *affinity*.

$$L + R \underset{k_{-1}}{\overset{k_{+1}}{\rightleftharpoons}} LR \underset{k_{-2}}{\overset{k_{+2}}{\rightleftharpoons}} LR^* \qquad \text{(Equation 3–1)}$$

*LR** is produced in proportion to [LR] and leads to a response. This simple relationship illustrates the reliance of the affinity of the ligand (*L*) with receptor (*R*) on both the forward or *association rate* (k_{+1}) and the reverse or *dissociation rate* (k_{-1}). At any given time, the concentration of ligand-receptor complex [LR] is equal to the product of $k_{+1}[L][R]$, the rate of formation of the bimolecular complex *LR*, minus the product k_{-1}[LR], the rate dissociation of *LR* into *L* and *R*. At equilibrium (i.e., when $\delta[\text{LR}]/\delta t = 0$), $k_{+1}[\text{L}][\text{R}] = k_{-1}[\text{LR}]$. The *equilibrium dissociation constant* (K_D) is then described by ratio of the *off* and *on* rate constants (k_{-1}/k_{+1}).

Thus, at equilibrium,

$$K_D = \frac{[\text{L}][\text{R}]}{[\text{LR}]} = \frac{k_{-1}}{k_{+1}} \qquad \text{(Equation 3–2)}$$

The *affinity constant* or *equilibrium association constant* (K_A) is the reciprocal of the equilibrium dissociation constant (i.e., $K_A = 1/K_D$); thus, a high-affinity drug has a low K_D and will bind a greater number of a particular receptor at a low concentration than a low-affinity drug. As a practical matter, the affinity of a drug is influenced most often by changes in its off-rate (k_{-1}) rather than its on-rate (k_{+1}).

Equation 3–2 permits us to write an expression of the fractional occupancy (*f*) of receptors by agonist:

$$f = \frac{[\text{ligand-receptor complexes}]}{[\text{total receptors}]} = \frac{[\text{LR}]}{[\text{R}] + [\text{LR}]} \qquad \text{(Equation 3–3)}$$

This can be expressed in terms of K_A (or K_D) and [L]:

$$f = \frac{K_A[\text{L}]}{1 + K_A[\text{L}]} = \frac{[\text{L}]}{[\text{L}] + K_D} \qquad \text{(Equation 3–4)}$$

From this relationship, it follows that when the concentration of drug equals the K_D (or $1/K_A$), $f = 0.5$, that is, the drug will occupy 50% of the receptors. This relationship describes only receptor occupancy, not the eventual response that may be amplified by the cell. Many signaling systems reach a full biological response with only a fraction of receptors occupied.

Potency is defined by example in Figure 3–3. Basically, when 2 drugs produce equivalent responses, the drug whose dose-response curve (plotted as in Figure 3–3A) lies to the left of the other (i.e., the concentration producing a half-maximal effect [EC_{50}] is smaller) is said to be the more potent.

Efficacy reflects the capacity of a drug to activate a receptor and generate a cellular response. Thus, a drug with high efficacy may be a full agonist, eliciting, at some concentration, a full response. A drug with a lower efficacy at the same receptor may not elicit a full response at any dose (*see* Figure 3–1). A drug with a low intrinsic efficacy will be a partial agonist. A drug that binds to a receptor and exhibits zero efficacy is an antagonist.

QUANTIFYING AGONISM. When the relative potency of 2 agonists of equal efficacy is measured in the same biological system, and downstream signaling events are the same for both drugs, the comparison yields a relative measure of the affinity and efficacy of the 2 agonists (*see* Figure 3–3). We often describe agonist response by determining the *half-maximally effective concentration* (EC_{50}) for producing a given effect. We can also compare maximal asymptotes in systems where the agonists do not produce maximal response (Figure 3–3B). The advantage of using maxima is that this property depends solely on efficacy, whereas drug *potency* is a mixed function of both affinity and efficacy.

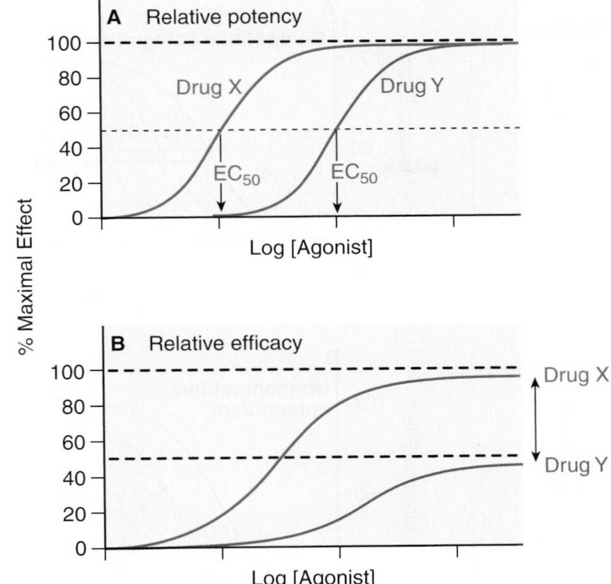

Figure 3–3 *Two ways of quantifying agonism.* **A.** The relative potency of 2 agonists (Drug X, *red line;* Drug Y, *purple line*) obtained in the same tissue is a function of their relative affinities and intrinsic efficacies. The EC_{50} of Drug X occurs at a concentration that is one-tenth the EC_{50} of Drug Y. Thus, Drug X is more potent than Drug Y. **B.** In systems where the 2 drugs do not both produce the maximal response characteristic of the tissue, the observed maximal response is a nonlinear function of their relative intrinsic efficacies. Drug X is more efficacious than Drug Y; their asymptotic fractional responses are 100% (Drug X) and 50% (Drug Y).

QUANTIFYING ANTAGONISM. Characteristic patterns of antagonism are associated with certain mechanisms of blockade of receptors. One is straightforward *competitive antagonism*, whereby a drug with affinity for a receptor but lacking intrinsic efficacy competes with the agonist for the primary binding site on the receptor. The characteristic pattern of such antagonism is the concentration-dependent production of a parallel shift to the right of the agonist dose-response curve with no change in the maximal response (Figure 3–4A). The magnitude of the rightward shift of the curve depends on the concentration of the antagonist and its affinity for the receptor. A competitive antagonist will reduce the response to zero.

A *partial agonist* similarly can compete with a "full" agonist for binding to the receptor. However, increasing concentrations of a partial agonist will inhibit response to a finite level characteristic of the drug's intrinsic efficacy. Partial agonists may be used therapeutically to buffer a response by inhibiting excessive receptor stimulation without totally abolishing receptor stimulation.

An antagonist may dissociate so slowly from the receptor that its action is exceedingly prolonged. In the presence of a slowly dissociating antagonist, the maximal response to the agonist will be depressed at some antagonist concentrations (Figure 3–4B). Operationally, this is referred to as *noncompetitive antagonism,* although the molecular mechanism of action cannot be inferred unequivocally from the effect. An *irreversible antagonist* competing for the same binding site as the agonist can produce the pattern of antagonism shown in Figure 3–4B. Noncompetitive antagonism can be produced by an *allosteric* or *allotopic antagonist*, which binds to a site on the receptor distinct from that of the primary agonist, thereby changing the affinity of the receptor for the agonist. In the case of an allosteric antagonist, the affinity of the receptor for the agonist is decreased by the antagonist (Figure 3–4C). In contrast, a drug binding at an allosteric site could potentiate the effects of primary agonists (Figure 3–4D); such a drug would be referred to as an *allosteric agonist* or *co-agonist*.

The affinity of a competitive antagonist (K_i) for its receptor can be determined in radioligand binding assays or by measuring the functional response of a system to a drug in the presence of the antagonist. Concentration curves are run with the agonist alone and with the agonist plus an effective concentration of the antagonist (*see* Figure 3–4A). As more antagonist (I) is added, a higher concentration of the agonist (A) is needed to

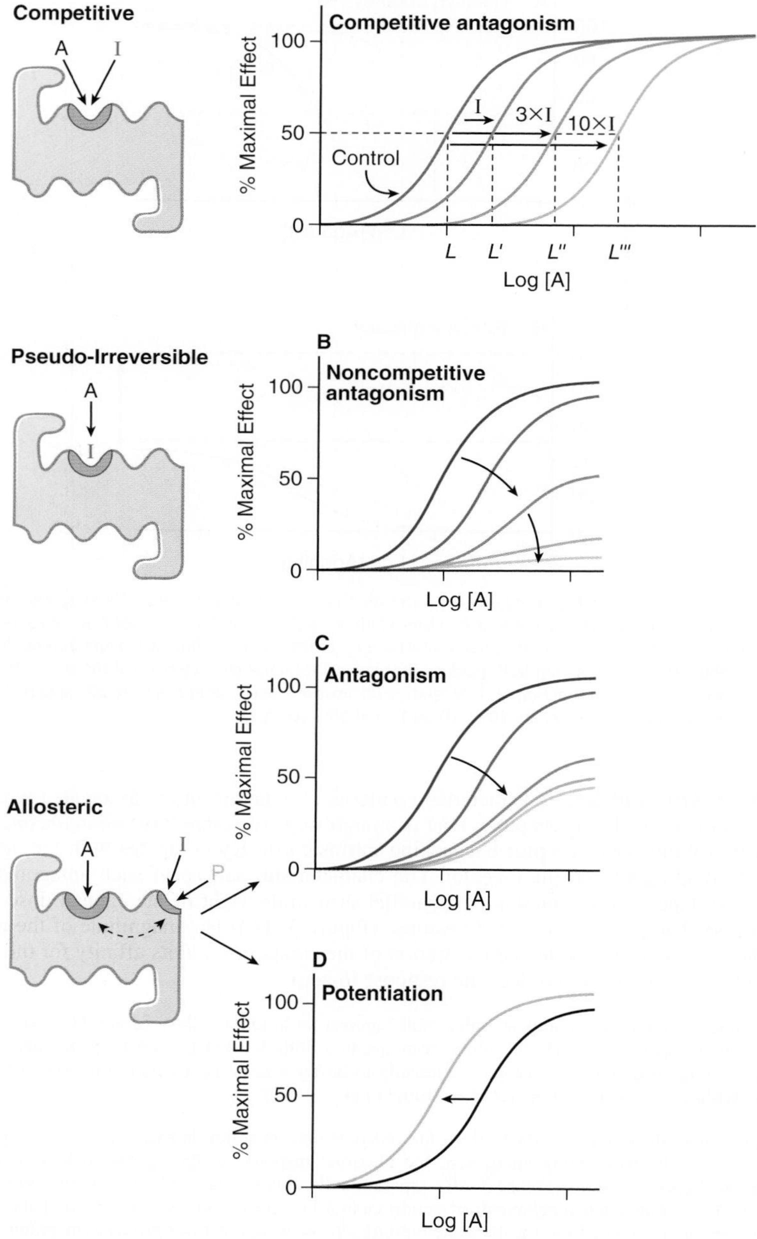

Figure 3–4 *Mechanisms of receptor antagonism.* **A.** Competitive antagonism occurs when the agonist A and antagonist I compete for the same binding site on the receptor. Response curves for the agonist are shifted to the right in a concentration-related manner by the antagonist such that the EC_{50} for the agonist increases (e.g., *L* versus *L′*, *L″*, and *L‴*) with the concentration of the antagonist. **B.** If the antagonist binds to the same site as the agonist but does so irreversibly or pseudo-irreversibly (slow dissociation but no covalent bond), it causes a shift of the dose-response curve to the right, with further depression of the maximal response. Allosteric effects occur when an allosteric ligand I or P binds to a different site on the receptor to either inhibit (I) the response (see panel **C**) or potentiate (P) the response (see panel **D**). This effect is saturable; inhibition or potentiation reaches a limiting value when the allosteric site is fully occupied.

produce an equivalent response (the half-maximal or 50%, response is a convenient and accurately determined level of response). The extent of the rightward shift of the concentration-dependence curve is a measure of the affinity of the inhibitor, and a higher-affinity inhibitor will cause a greater rightward shift than a lower-affinity inhibitor at the same inhibitor concentration. Using Equations 3–3 and 3–4, one may write mathematical expressions of *fractional occupancy* (f) of the receptor by agonist for the agonist alone (control) and agonist in the presence of inhibitor.

For the agonist drug (L) alone,

$$f_{\text{control}} = \frac{[L]}{[L] + K_D} \quad \text{(Equation 3–5)}$$

For the case of agonist plus antagonist (I),

$$f_{+I} = \frac{[L]}{[L] + K_D\left(1 + \frac{I}{K_i}\right)} \quad \text{(Equation 3–6)}$$

Assuming that equal responses result from equal fractional receptor occupancies in both the absence and presence of antagonist, one can set the fractional occupancies equal at agonist concentrations (L and L') that generate equivalent responses in Figure 3–4A. Thus,

$$\frac{L}{L + K_D} = \frac{L'}{L' + K_D\left(1 + \frac{[I]}{K_i}\right)} \quad \text{(Equation 3–7)}$$

Simplifying, one gets:

$$\frac{L'}{L} - 1 = \frac{[I]}{K_i} \quad \text{(Equation 3–8)}$$

where all values are known except K_i. Thus, one can determine the K_i for a reversible, competitive antagonist without knowing the K_D for the agonist and without needing to define the precise relationship between receptor and response.

PHARMACODYNAMIC VARIABILITY: INDIVIDUAL AND POPULATION PHARMACODYNAMICS

Individuals vary in the magnitude of their response to the same concentration of a single drug, and a given individual may not always respond in the same way to the same drug concentration. Drug responsiveness may change because of disease or because of previous drug administration. Receptors are dynamic, and their concentration and function may be up- or downregulated by endogenous and exogenous factors.

Data on the correlation of drug levels with efficacy and toxicity must be interpreted in the context of the pharmacodynamic variability in the population (e.g., genetics, age, disease, and the presence of coadministered drugs). The variability in pharmacodynamic response in the population may be analyzed by constructing a quantal concentration-effect curve (Figure 3–5A). The dose of a drug required to produce a specified effect in 50% of the population is the *median effective dose* (ED_{50}; *see* Figure 3–5A). In preclinical studies of drugs, the *median lethal dose* (LD_{50}) is determined in experimental animals (Figure 3–5B). The LD_{50}/ED_{50} ratio is an indication of the *therapeutic index*, which is a statement of how selective the drug is in producing its desired effects versus its adverse effects. A similar term, the *therapeutic window,* is the range of steady-state concentrations of drug that provides therapeutic efficacy with minimal toxicity (Figures 2–6 and 3–6). In clinical studies, the dose, or preferably the concentration, of a drug required to produce toxic effects can be compared with the concentration required for therapeutic effects in the population to evaluate the *clinical therapeutic index*. The concentration or dose of drug required to produce a therapeutic effect in most of the population usually will overlap the concentration required to produce toxicity in some of the population, even though the drug's therapeutic index in an individual patient may be large. Thus, a *population therapeutic window* expresses a range of concentrations at which the likelihood of efficacy is high and the probability of adverse effects is low (*see* Figure 3–6); it does not guarantee efficacy or safety. *Therefore, use of the population therapeutic window to adjust dosage of a drug should be complemented by monitoring appropriate clinical and surrogate markers for drug effect(s).*

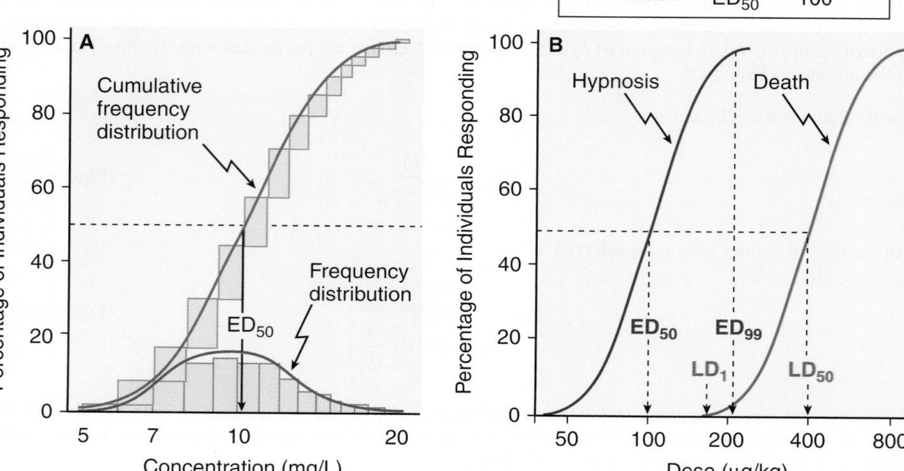

Figure 3–5 *Frequency distribution curves and quantal concentration-effect and dose-effect curves.* **A.** *Frequency distribution curves.* An experiment was performed on 100 subjects, and the effective plasma concentration that produced a quantal response was determined for each individual. The number of subjects who required each dose was plotted, giving a log-normal frequency distribution (*purple bars*). The normal frequency distribution, when summated, yields the cumulative frequency distribution—a sigmoidal curve that is a quantal concentration-effect curve (red bars, red line). **B.** *Quantal dose-effect curves.* Animals were injected with varying doses of a drug and the responses were determined and plotted. The calculation of the therapeutic index, the ratio of the LD_{50} to the ED_{50}, is an indication of how selective a drug is in producing its desired effects relative to its toxicity. See text for additional explanation.

FACTORS MODIFYING DRUG ACTION. Numerous factors contribute to the wide patient-to-patient variability in the dose required for optimal therapy observed with many drugs (Figure 3–7). The effects of these factors on variability of drug pharmacokinetics are described more thoroughly in Chapters 2, 5, 6, and 7.

COMBINATION THERAPY. Marked alterations in the effects of some drugs can result from coadministration with other agents, including prescription and nonprescription drugs, as well as supplements and nutraceuticals. Such interactions can cause toxicity, or inhibit the drug effect and the therapeutic benefit. Drug

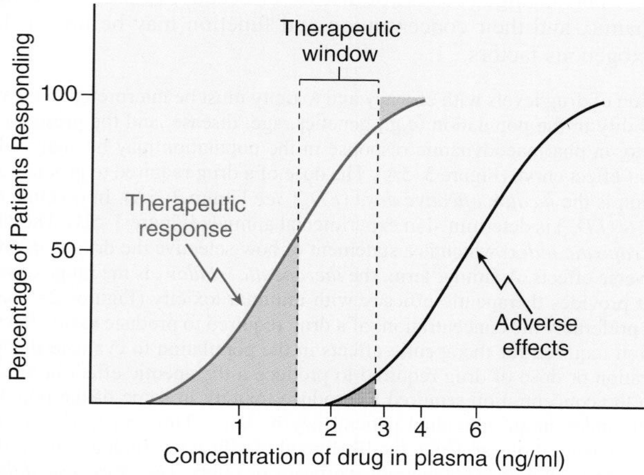

Figure 3–6 *Relation of the therapeutic window of drug concentrations to therapeutic and adverse effects in the population.* The ordinate is linear; the abscissa is logarithmic.

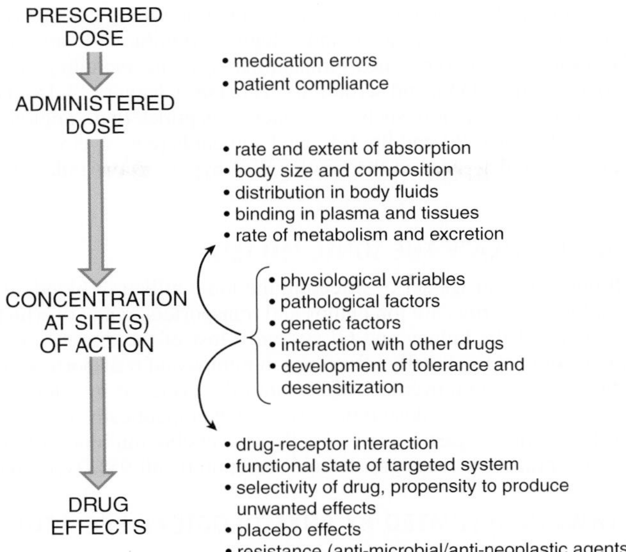

Figure 3–7 *Factors influencing the response to a prescribed drug dose.*

interactions always should be considered when unexpected responses to drugs occur. Understanding the mechanisms of drug interactions provides a framework for preventing them. Drug interactions may be pharmacokinetic (the delivery of a drug to its site of action is altered by a second drug) or pharmacodynamic (the response of the drug target is modified by a second drug). Examples of pharmacokinetic interactions that can enhance or diminish the delivery of drug to its site of action are provided in Chapter 2. In a patient with multiple comorbidities requiring a variety of medications, it may be difficult to identify adverse effects due to medication interactions, and to determine whether these are pharmacokinetic, pharmacodynamic, or some combination of interactions.

Combination therapy constitutes optimal treatment for many conditions, including heart failure (*see* Chapter 28), hypertension (*see* Chapter 27), and cancer (*see* Chapters 60-63). However, some drug combinations produce pharmacodynamic interactions that result in adverse effects. For example, nitrovasodilators produce relaxation of vascular smooth muscle (vasodilation) via NO-dependent elevation of cyclic GMP in vascular smooth muscle. The pharmacologic effects of sildenafil, tadalafil, and vardenafil result from inhibition of the type 5 cyclic nucleotide phosphodiesterase (PDE5) that hydrolyzes cyclic GMP to 5′GMP in the vasculature. Thus, coadministration of an NO donor (e.g., nitroglycerin) with a PDE5 inhibitor can cause potentially catastrophic hypotension. The oral anticoagulant warfarin has a narrow margin between therapeutic inhibition of clot formation and bleeding complications and is subject to numerous important pharmacokinetic and pharmacodynamic drug interactions. Alterations in dietary vitamin K intake may significantly affect the pharmacodynamics of warfarin and mandate altered dosing; antibiotics that alter the intestinal flora reduce the bacterial synthesis of vitamin K, thereby enhancing the effect of warfarin; concurrent administration of nonsteroidal anti-inflammatory drugs (NSAIDs) with warfarin increases the risk of GI bleeding almost 4-fold compared with warfarin alone. By inhibiting platelet aggregation, aspirin increases the incidence of bleeding in warfarin-treated patients.

Most drugs are evaluated in young and middle-aged adults, and data on their use in children and the elderly are sparse. At the extremes of age, drug pharmacokinetics and pharmacodynamics can be altered, possibly requiring substantial alteration in the dose or dosing regimen to safely produce the desired clinical effect.

Mechanisms of Drug Action

RECEPTORS THAT AFFECT CONCENTRATIONS OF ENDOGENOUS LIGANDS

A large number of drugs act by altering the synthesis, storage, release, transport, or metabolism of endogenous ligands such as neurotransmitters, hormones, and other intercellular mediators. For example, some of the drugs acting on adrenergic neurotransmission (*see* Chapters 8 and 12) include α-methyltyrosine [inhibits synthesis of norepinephrine (NE)], cocaine (blocks NE reuptake), amphetamine (promotes NE release), and selegiline (inhibits NE breakdown by MAO). There are similar examples for other neurotransmitter systems including acetylcholine (*see* Chapters 8 and 10), dopamine (DA), and serotonin (5HT) (*see* Chapters 13-15). Drugs that affect the synthesis of circulating mediators such as vasoactive peptides (e.g., angiotensin-converting enzyme inhibitors; *see* Chapter 26) and lipid-derived autocoids (e.g., cyclooxygenase inhibitors; *see* Chapter 33) are also widely used in the treatment of hypertension, inflammation, and myocardial ischemia.

RECEPTORS THAT REGULATE THE IONIC MILIEU

A relatively small number of drugs act by affecting the ionic milieu of blood, urine, and the GI tract. The receptors for these drugs are ion pumps and transporters, many of which are expressed only in specialized cells of the kidney and GI system. Most of the diuretics (e.g., furosemide, chlorothiazide, amiloride) act by directly affecting ion pumps and transporters in epithelial cells of the nephron that increase the movement of Na^+ into the urine, or by altering the expression of ion pumps in these cells (e.g., aldosterone). Another therapeutically important target is the H^+,K^+-ATPase (proton pump) of gastric parietal cells. Irreversible inhibition of this proton pump by drugs such as esomeprazole reduces gastric acid secretion by 80-95% (*see* Chapter 45).

CELLULAR PATHWAYS ACTIVATED BY PHYSIOLOGICAL RECEPTORS

SIGNAL TRANSDUCTION PATHWAYS. Physiological receptors have 2 major functions, ligand binding and message propagation (i.e., signaling). These functions imply the existence of at least 2 functional domains within the receptor: a *ligand-binding domain* and an *effector domain*.

The regulatory actions of a receptor may be exerted directly on its cellular target(s), on *effector protein(s),* or may be conveyed by intermediary cellular signaling molecules called *transducers*. The receptor, its cellular target, and any intermediary molecules are referred to as a *receptor-effector system* or *signal transduction pathway*. Frequently, the proximal cellular effector protein is not the ultimate physiological target but rather is an enzyme, ion channel, or transport protein that creates, moves, or degrades a small molecule (e.g., a cyclic nucleotide, inositol trisphosphate, or NO) or ion (e.g., Ca^{2+}) termed a *second messenger*. Second messengers can diffuse in the proximity of their synthesis or release and convey information to a variety of targets, which may integrate multiple signals. Even though these second messengers originally were thought of as freely diffusible molecules within the cell, imaging studies show that their diffusion and intracellular actions are constrained by compartmentation—selective localization of receptor-transducer-effector-signal termination complexes—established by protein-lipid and protein-protein interactions. All cells express multiple forms of proteins designed to localize signaling pathways by protein-protein interactions; these proteins are termed *scaffolds* or *anchoring proteins*.

Receptors and their associated effector and transducer proteins also act as integrators of information as they coordinate signals from multiple ligands with each other and with the differentiated activity of the target cell. For example, signal transduction systems regulated by changes in cyclic AMP (cAMP) and intracellular Ca^{2+} are integrated in many excitable tissues. In cardiac myocytes, an increase in cellular cAMP caused by activation of β adrenergic receptors enhances cardiac contractility by augmenting the rate and amount of Ca^{2+} delivered to the contractile apparatus; thus, cAMP and Ca^{2+} are positive contractile signals in cardiac myocytes. By contrast, cAMP and Ca^{2+} produce opposing effects on the contractility of smooth muscle cells: as usual, Ca^{2+} is a contractile signal, however, activation of β adrenergic receptors on these cells activates the cAMP-PKA pathway, which leads to relaxation through the phosphorylation of proteins that mediate Ca^{2+} signaling, such as myosin light chain kinase and ion channels that hyperpolarize the cell membrane.

Another important property of physiological receptors is their capacity to significantly amplify a physiological signal. Neurotransmitters, hormones, and other extracellular ligands are often present at the ligand-binding domain of a receptor in very low concentrations (nM to μM levels). However, the effector domain or the signal transduction pathway often contains enzymes and enzyme cascades that catalytically amplify the intended signal. These signaling systems are excellent targets for drugs.

STRUCTURAL AND FUNCTIONAL FAMILIES OF PHYSIOLOGICAL RECEPTORS

Receptors for physiological regulatory molecules can be assigned to functional families that share common molecular structures and biochemical mechanisms. Table 3–1 outlines 6 major families of receptors with examples of their physiological ligands, signal transduction systems, and drugs that affect these systems.

Table 3–1

Physiological Receptors

STRUCTURAL FAMILY	FUNCTIONAL FAMILY	PHYSIOLOGICAL LIGANDS	EFFECTORS AND TRANSDUCERS	EXAMPLE DRUGS
	β Adrenergic receptors	NE, Epi, DA	G_s; AC	Dobutamine, propranolol
GPCR	Muscarinic cholinergic receptors	ACh	G_i and G_q; AC, ion channels, PLC	Atropine
	Eicosanoid receptors	Prostaglandins, leukotrienes, thromboxanes	G_s, G_i and G_q proteins	Misoprostol, montelukast
	Thrombin receptors (PAR)	Receptor peptide	$G_{12/13}$, GEFs	(in development)
Ion channels	Ligand-gated	ACh (M_2), GABA, 5HT	Na^+, Ca^{2+}, K^+, Cl^-	Nicotine, gabapentin
	Voltage-gated	None (activated by membrane depolarization)	Na^+, Ca^{2+}, K^+, other ions	Lidocaine, verapamil
Transmembrane enzymes	Receptor tyrosine kinases	Insulin, PDGF, EGF VEGF, growth factors	Proteins with PTB and SH2 domains	Herceptin, imatinib
	Membrane-bound GC	Natriuretic peptides	Cyclic GMP	Neseritide
Transmembrane, non-enzymes	Cytokine receptors	Interleukins and other cytokines	Jak/STAT, soluble tyrosine kinases	
	Toll-like receptors	LPS, bacterial products	MyD88, IARKs, NF-κB	
Nuclear receptors	Steroid receptors	Estrogen, testosterone	Co-activators	Estrogens, androgens, cortisol
	Thyroid hormone receptors	Thyroid hormone		Thyroid hormone
	PPARγ	Eicosanoids, oxidized LDL	RXR	Thiazolidinediones
Intracellular enzymes	Soluble GC	NO, Ca^{2+}	Cyclic GMP	Nitrovasodilators

AC, adenylyl cyclase; GC, guanylyl cyclase; LDL, low density lipoprotein; PAR, protease-activated receptor; PLC, phospholipase C; PPAR, peroxisome proliferator-activated receptor; PTB and SH2, phosphotyrosine binding domains; RXR, retinoid X receptor.

G PROTEIN–COUPLED RECEPTORS (GPCRs)

GPCRs span the plasma membrane as a bundle of 7 α-helices (Figure 3–8). Among the ligands for GPCRs are neurotransmitters such as ACh, biogenic amines such as NE, all eicosanoids and other lipid-signaling molecules, peptide hormones, opioids, amino acids such as GABA, and many other peptide and protein ligands. GPCRs are important regulators of nerve activity in the CNS and are the receptors for the neurotransmitters of the peripheral autonomic nervous system. Because of their number and physiological importance, GPCRs are the targets for many drugs.

GPCR Subtypes. There are multiple receptor subtypes within families of receptors. Ligand-binding studies initially identified receptor subtypes; molecular cloning has greatly accelerated the discovery and definition of additional receptor subtypes; their expression as recombinant proteins has facilitated the discovery of

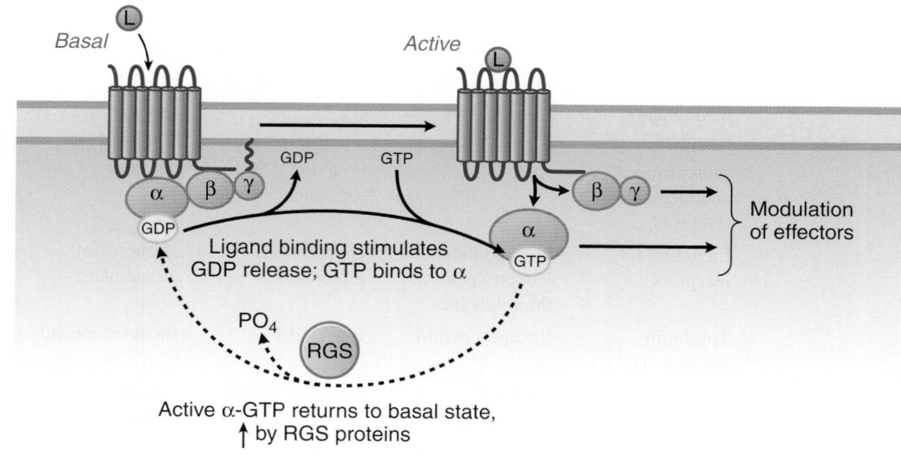

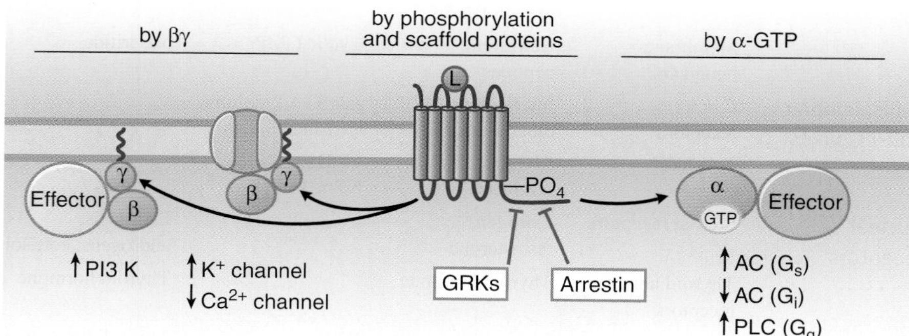

Figure 3–8 *Stimulation of a G–protein coupled receptor by ligand, the activation of the G protein, and stimulation of selected effectors.* In the absence of ligand, the receptor and G protein heterotrimer form a complex in the membrane with the Gα subunit bound to GDP. Following binding of ligand, the receptor and G protein α subunit undergo a conformational change leading to release of GDP, binding of GTP, and dissociation of the complex. The activated GTP-bound Gα subunit and the freed βγ dimer bind to and regulate effectors. The system is returned to the basal state by hydrolysis of the GTP on the α subunit; a reaction that is markedly enhanced by the regulators of G protein signaling (RGS) proteins. Prolonged stimulation of the receptor can lead to downregulation of the receptor. This event is initiated by G protein receptor kinases (GRKs) that phosphorylate the C terminal tail of the receptor, leading to recruitment of proteins termed arrestins; arrestins bind to the receptor on the internal surface, displacing G proteins and inhibiting signaling. Detailed descriptions of these signaling pathways are given throughout the text in relation to the therapeutic actions of drugs affecting these pathways.

subtype-selective drugs. The distinction between classes and subtypes of receptors, however, is often arbitrary or historical. The α_1, α_2, and β adrenergic receptors differ from each other both in ligand selectivity and in coupling to G proteins (G_q, G_i, and G_s, respectively), yet α and β are considered receptor classes and α_1 and α_2 are considered subtypes. Pharmacological differences among receptor subtypes are exploited therapeutically through the development and use of receptor-selective drugs. For example, β_2 adrenergic agonists such as terbutaline are used for bronchodilation in the treatment of asthma in the hope of minimizing cardiac side effects caused by stimulation of the β_1 adrenergic receptor (*see* Chapter 12). Conversely, the use of β_1-selective antagonists minimizes the chance of bronchoconstriction in patients being treated for hypertension or angina (*see* Chapters 12 and 27).

Receptor Dimerization. GPCRs undergo both homo- and heterodimerization and possibly oligomerization. Dimerization of receptors may regulate the affinity and specificity of the complex for G proteins and the sensitivity of the receptor to phosphorylation by receptor kinases and the binding of arrestin, events important in termination of the action of agonists and removal of receptors from the cell surface. Dimerization also may permit binding of receptors to other regulatory proteins such as transcription factors.

G PROTEINS. GPCRs couple to a family of heterotrimeric GTP-binding regulatory proteins termed *G proteins*. G proteins are signal transducers that convey the information from the agonist-bound receptor to 1 or more effector proteins. G protein–regulated effectors include enzymes such as adenylyl cyclase, phospholipase C, cyclic GMP phosphodiesterase (PDE6), and membrane ion channels selective for Ca^{2+} and K^+ (*see* Table 3–1 and Figure 3–8).

The G protein heterotrimer consists of a guanine nucleotide-binding α subunit, which confers specific recognition to both receptors and effectors, and an associated dimer of β and γ subunits that helps confer membrane localization of the G protein heterotrimer by prenylation of the γ subunit. In the basal state of the receptor-heterotrimer complex, the α subunit contains bound GDP and the α-GDP:βγ complex is bound to the unliganded receptor (*see* Figure 3–8). The α subunits fall into 4 families (G_s, G_i, G_q, and $G_{12/13}$) which are responsible for coupling GPCRs to relatively distinct effectors. The G_s α subunit uniformly activates adenylyl cyclase; the G_i α subunit inhibits certain isoforms of adenylyl cyclase; the G_q α subunit activates all forms of phospholipase C-β (PLCβ); and the $G_{12/13}$ α subunits couple to guanine nucleotide exchange factors (GEFs), such as p115RhoGEF for the small GTP-binding proteins Rho and Rac. The signaling specificity of the large number of possible βγ combinations is not yet clear; nonetheless, it is known that K^+ channels, Ca^{2+} channels, and PI-3 kinase (PI3K) are some of the effectors of free βγ dimer. Figure 3–8 and its legend summarize the basic activation/inactivation scheme for GPCR-linked systems.

SECOND MESSENGER SYSTEMS

CYCLIC AMP. Cyclic AMP is synthesized by adenylyl cyclase; stimulation is mediated by the G_s α subunit, inhibition by the G_i α subunit. There are 9 membrane-bound isoforms of adenylyl cyclase (AC) and 1 soluble isoform found in mammals. Cyclic AMP generated by adenylyl cyclases has 3 major targets in most cells, the cyclic AMP dependent protein kinase (PKA), cAMP-regulated guanine nucleotide exchange factors termed EPACs (exchange factors directly activated by cAMP), and via PKA phosphorylation, a transcription factor termed CREB (cAMP response element binding protein). In cells with specialized functions, cAMP can have additional targets such as cyclic nucleotide-gated ion channels, cyclic nucleotide-regulated phosphodiesterases (PDEs), and several ABC transporters (MRP4 and MRP5) (*see* Chapter 7).

PKA. The PKA holoenzyme consists of 2 catalytic (C) subunits reversibly bound to a regulatory (R) subunit dimer to form a heterotetramer complex (R_2C_2). When AC is activated and cAMP concentrations are increased, 4 cyclic AMP molecules bind to the R_2C_2 complex, 2 to each R subunit, causing a conformational change in the R subunits that lowers their affinity for the C subunits, causing their activation. The active C subunits phosphorylate serine and threonine residues on specific protein substrates. There are multiple isoforms of PKA; molecular cloning has revealed α and β isoforms of both the regulatory subunits (RI and RII), as well as 3 C subunit isoforms Cα, Cβ, and Cγ. The R subunits exhibit different subcellular localization and binding affinities for cAMP, giving rise to PKA holoenzymes with different thresholds for activation. PKA function also is modulated by subcellular localization mediated by A-kinase anchoring proteins (AKAPs).

PKG. Stimulation of receptors that raise intracellular cyclic GMP concentrations (*see* Figure 3–11) leads to the activation of the cyclic GMP-dependent protein kinase G (PKG) that phosphorylates some of the same substrates as PKA and some that are PKG-specific. Unlike the heterotetramer (R_2C_2) structure of the PKA holoenzyme, the catalytic domain and cyclic nucleotide-binding domains of PKG are expressed as a single polypeptide, which dimerizes to form the PKG holoenzyme.

PKG exists in 2 homologous forms, PKG-I and PKG-II. PKG-I has an acetylated N terminus, is associated with the cytoplasm, and has 2 isoforms (Iα and Iβ) that arise from alternate splicing. PKG-II has a myristylated N terminus, is membrane-associated, and can be localized by PKG-anchoring proteins in a manner analogous to that known for PKA, although the docking domains of PKA and PKG are very different structurally. Pharmacologically important effects of elevated cyclic GMP include modulation of platelet activation and relaxation of smooth muscle. Receptors linked to cGMP synthesis are covered below in a separate section.

PDES. Cyclic nucleotide PDEs form another family of important signaling proteins whose activities are regulated via the rate of gene transcription as well as by second messengers (cyclic nucleotides or Ca^{2+}) and interactions with other signaling proteins such as β arrestin and protein kinases. PDEs hydrolyze the cyclic 3′,5′-phosphodiester bond in cAMP and cGMP, thereby terminating their action.The enzymes comprise a superfamily with >50 different PDE proteins. The substrate specificities of the different PDEs include those specific for cAMP hydrolysis, cGMP hydrolysis, and some that hydrolyze both cyclic nucleotides. PDEs (mainly PDE3 forms) are drug targets for treatment of diseases such as asthma, cardiovascular diseases such as heart failure, atherosclerotic coronary and peripheral arterial disease, and neurological disorders. PDE5 inhibitors (e.g., sildenafil) are used in treating chronic obstructive pulmonary disease and erectile dysfunction.

G_q-PLC-DAG/IP_3-CA^{2+} PATHWAY. Calcium is an important messenger in all cells and can regulate diverse responses including gene expression, contraction, secretion, metabolism, and electrical activity. Ca^{2+} can enter the cell through Ca^{2+} channels in the plasma membrane (see "Ion Channels," below) or be released by hormones or growth factors from intracellular stores. In keeping with its role as a signal, the basal Ca^{2+} level in cells is maintained in the 100 nM range by membrane Ca^{2+} pumps that extrude Ca^{2+} to the extracellular space and a sarcoplasmic reticulum (SR) Ca^{2+}-ATPase (SERCA) in the membrane of the endoplasmic reticulum (ER) that accumulates Ca^{2+} into its storage site in the ER/SR.

Hormones and growth factors release Ca^{2+} from its intracellular storage site, the ER, via a signaling pathway that begins with activation of phospholipase C (PLC) at the plasma membrane, of which there are 2 primary forms, PLCβ and PLCγ. GPCRs that couple to G_q or G_i activate PLCβ by activating the G protein α subunit (*see* Figure 3–8) and releasing the βγ dimer. Both the active, G_q-GTP bound α subunit and the βγ dimer can activate certain isoforms of PLCβ. PLCγ isoforms are activated by tyrosine phosphorylation, including phosphorylation by receptor and nonreceptor tyrosine kinases.

PLCs are cytosolic enzymes that translocate to the plasma membrane upon receptor stimulation. When activated, they hydrolyze a minor membrane phospholipid, phosphatidylinositol-4, 5-bisphosphate, to generate 2 intracellular signals, inositol-1,4,5-trisphosphate (IP_3) and the lipid, diacylglycerol (DAG). DAG directly activates members of the protein kinase C (PKC) family. IP_3 diffuses to the ER where it activates the IP_3 receptor in the ER membrane causing release of stored Ca^{2+} from the ER. Release of Ca^{2+} from these intracellular stores raises Ca^{2+} levels in the cytoplasm manyfold within seconds and activates calmodulin-sensitive enzymes such as cyclic AMP PDE and a family of Ca^{2+}/calmodulin-sensitive protein kinases (e.g., phosphorylase kinase, myosin light chain kinase, and CaM kinases II and IV). Depending on the cell's differentiated function, the Ca^{2+}/calmodulin kinases and PKC may regulate the bulk of the downstream events in the activated cells.

ION CHANNELS

Changes in the flux of ions across the plasma membrane are critical regulatory events in both excitable and nonexcitable cells. To establish the electrochemical gradients required to maintain a membrane potential, all cells express ion transporters for Na^+, K^+, Ca^{2+}, and Cl^-. For example, the Na^+,K^+-ATPase expends cellular ATP to pump Na^+ out of the cell and K^+ into the cell. The electrochemical gradients thus established are used by excitable tissues such as nerve and muscle to generate and transmit electrical impulses, by nonexcitable cells to trigger biochemical and secretory events, and by all cells to support a variety of secondary symport and antiport processes (*see* Chapter 5). Because of their roles as regulators of cell function, these proteins are important drug targets. The diverse ion channel family can be divided into subfamilies based on the mechanisms that open the channels, their architecture, and the ions they conduct. They can also be classified as voltage-activated, ligand-activated, store-activated, stretch-activated, and temperature-activated channels.

VOLTAGE-GATED CHANNELS. Humans express multiple isoforms of voltage-gated channels for Na^+, K^+, Ca^{2+}, and Cl^- ions. In nerve and muscle cells, voltage-gated Na^+ channels are responsible for the generation of robust action potentials that depolarize the membrane from its resting potential of –70 mV up to a potential of +20 mV within a few msec. These Na^+ channels are composed of 3 subunits, a pore-forming α subunit and 2 regulatory β subunits (Figure 3–9A). The voltage-activated Na^+ channels in pain neurons are targets for local anesthetics such as lidocaine and tetracaine, which block the pore, inhibit depolarization, and thus block the sensation of pain. They are also the targets of the naturally occurring marine toxins, tetrodotoxin and saxitoxin (*see* Chapter 20). Voltage-activated Na^+ channels are also important targets of many drugs used to treat cardiac arrhythmias (*see* Chapter 29).

Voltage-gated Ca^{2+} channels have a similar architecture to voltage-gated Na^+ channels with a large α subunit (4 domains of 5 membrane-spanning helices) and 3 regulatory subunits (the β, δ, and γ subunits). Ca^{2+} channels can be responsible for initiating an action potential (as in the pacemaker cells of the heart), but are more commonly responsible for modifying the shape and duration of an action potential initiated by fast voltage-gated Na^+ channels. These channels initiate the influx of Ca^{2+} that stimulates the release of neurotransmitters in the central, enteric, and autonomic nervous systems, and that control heart rate and impulse conduction in cardiac tissue (*see* Chapters 8, 14, and 27). The L-type voltage-gated Ca^{2+} channels are subject to additional regulation via phosphorylation by PKA. Voltage-gated Ca^{2+} channels expressed in smooth muscle regulate vascular tone; the intracellular concentration of Ca^{2+} is critical to regulating the phosphorylation state of the contractile apparatus via the activity of the Ca^{2+}/calmodulin-sensitive myosin light chain kinase. Ca^{2+} channel

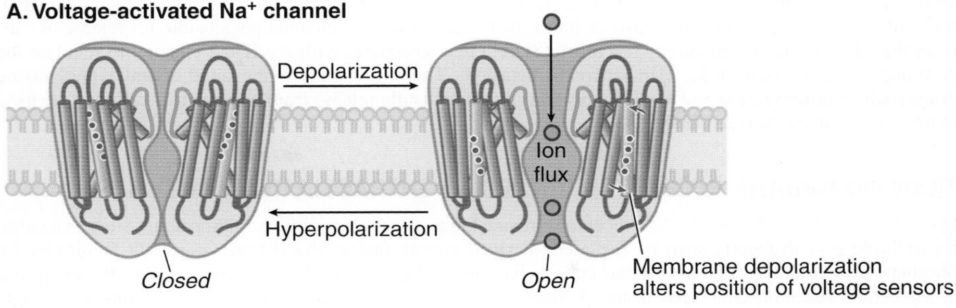

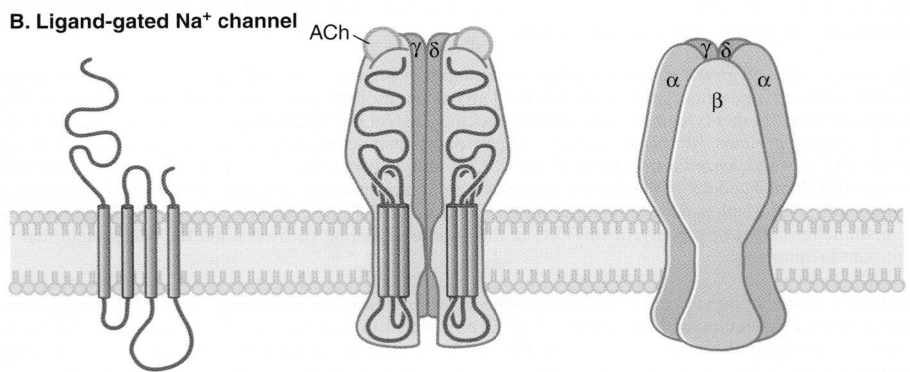

Figure 3–9 *Two types of ion channels regulated by receptors and drugs.* **A.** Diagram of a voltage-activated Na^+ channel with the pore in the open and closed state. The pore-forming P loops are shown in blue, angled into the pore to form the selectivity filter. The S4 helices forming the voltage sensor are shown in orange, with the positively charged amino acids displayed as red dots. **B.** Ligand-gated nicotinic acetylcholine receptor expressed in the skeletal muscle neuromuscular junction. The pore is made up of 5 subunits, each with a large extracellular domain and 4 transmembrane helices (1 of these subunits is shown at the left of panel B). The helix that lines the pore is shown in blue. The receptor is composed of 2 α subunits, and β, γ, and δ subunits. See text for discussion of other ligand-gated ion channels. Detailed descriptions of specific channels are given throughout the text in relation to the therapeutic actions of drugs affecting these channels (see especially Chapters 11, 14, and 20). (Adapted with permission from Purves D, Augustine GJ, Fitzpatrick D, Hall WC, LaMantia AS, McNamara JO, and White LE, eds. *Neuroscience*, 4th ed. Sunderland, MA: Sinauer Associates, Inc., 2008.)

antagonists such as nifedipine, diltiazem, and verapamil are effective vasodilators and are widely used to treat angina, cardiac arrhythmias, and hypertension.

Voltage-gated K^+ channels are the most numerous and structurally diverse members of the voltage-gated channel family and include the voltage-gated K_v channels, the inwardly rectifying K^+ channel, and the tandem or 2-pore domain "leak" K^+ channels. The inwardly rectifying channels and the 2-pore channels are voltage insensitive, regulated by G proteins and H^+ ions, and greatly stimulated by general anesthetics. Increasing K^+ conductance through these channels drives the membrane potential more negative (closer to the equilibrium potential for K^+); thus, these channels are important in regulating resting membrane potential and restoring the resting membrane at –70 to –90 mV following depolarization.

LIGAND-GATED CHANNELS. Channels activated by the binding of a ligand to a specific site in the channel protein have a diverse architecture and set of ligands. Major ligand-gated channels in the nervous system are those that respond to excitatory neurotransmitters such as acetylcholine (Figure 3–9B) or glutamate (or agonists such as AMPA and NMDA) and inhibitory neurotransmitters such as glycine or γ-aminobutyric acid (GABA). Activation of these channels is responsible for the majority of synaptic transmission by neurons both in the CNS and in the periphery (*see* Chapters 8, 11, and 14). In addition, there are a variety of more specialized ion channels that are activated by intracellular small molecules, and are structurally distinct from conventional ligand-gated ion channels. These include ion channels that are formally members of the K_v family, such as the hyperpolarization and cyclic nucleotide-gated (HCN) channel expressed in the heart (*see* Chapter 29), and the cyclic nucleotide-gated (CNG) channels important for vision (*see* Chapter 64). The intracellular small molecule category of ion channels also includes the IP_3-sensitive Ca^{2+} channel responsible for release of Ca^{2+} from the ER and the sulfonylurea "receptor" (SUR1) that associates with the $K_{ir}6.2$ channel to regulate the ATP-dependent K^+ channel (K_{ATP}) in pancreatic beta cells. The K_{ATP} channel is the target of oral hypoglycemic drugs such as sulfonylureas and meglitinides that stimulate insulin release from pancreatic β cells and are used to treat type 2 diabetes (*see* Chapter 43).

TRANSMEMBRANE RECEPTORS LINKED TO INTRACELLULAR ENZYMES

RECEPTOR TYROSINE KINASES. The receptor tyrosine kinases include receptors for hormones such as insulin, for multiple growth factors such EGF, platelet-derived growth factor (PDGF), nerve growth factor (NGF), fibroblast growth factor (FGF), vascular endothelial growth factor (VEGF), and ephrins. With the exception of the insulin receptor, which has α and β chains (*see* Chapter 43), these macromolecules consist of single polypeptide chains with large, cysteine-rich extracellular domains, short transmembrane domains, and an intracellular region containing 1 or 2 protein tyrosine kinase domains. Activation of growth factor receptors leads to cell survival, cell proliferation, and differentiation. Activation of the ephrin receptors leads to neuronal angiogenesis, axonal migration, and guidance.

The inactive state of growth factor receptors is monomeric; binding of ligand induces dimerization of the receptor and cross-phosphorylation of the kinase domains on multiple tyrosine residues (Figure 3–10A). The phosphorylation of other tyrosine residues forms docking sites for the SH2 domains contained in a large number of signaling proteins. Molecules recruited to phosphotyrosine-containing proteins by their SH2 domains include PLCγ, which raises intracellular levels of Ca^{2+} and activates PKC. The α and β isoforms of PI3K contain SH2 domains, dock at the phosphorylated receptor, are activated, and increase the level of phosphatidylinositol 3,4,5 trisphosphate (PIP_3) and protein kinase B (PKB, also known as Akt). PKB can regulate the mammalian target of rapamycin (mTOR) in the various signaling pathways and the bad protein that is important in apoptosis.

In addition to recruiting enzymes, phosphotyrosine-presenting proteins can interact with SH2 domain-containing adaptor molecules without activity (e.g., Grb2), which in turn attract guanine nucleotide exchange factors (GEFs) such as Sos that can activate the small GTP-binding protein, Ras. The small GTP-binding proteins Ras and Rho belong to a large family of small monomeric GTPases. All of the small GTPases are activated by GEFs that are regulated by a variety of mechanisms and inhibited by GTPase-activating proteins (GAPs). Activation of members of the Ras family leads in turn to activation of a protein kinase cascade termed the mitogen-activated protein kinase (MAP kinase or MAPK) pathway. Activation of the MAPK pathway is one of the major routes used by growth factor receptors to signal to the nucleus and stimulate cell growth.

JAK-STAT RECEPTOR PATHWAY. Cells express a family of receptors for cytokines such as γ-interferon and hormones like growth hormone and prolactin, which signal to the nucleus by a more direct manner than the receptor tyrosine kinases. These receptors have no intrinsic enzymatic activity, rather the intracellular domain binds a separate, intracellular tryosine kinase termed a Janus kinase (JAK). Upon dimerization induced by ligand binding, JAKs phosphorylate other proteins termed *signal transducers and activators of transcription* (STATs), which translocate to the nucleus and regulate transcription (Figure 3–10B). The entire pathway is termed the JAK-STAT pathway. There are 4 JAKs and 5 STATs in mammals that, depending on the cell type and signal, combine differently to activate gene transcription.

RECEPTOR SERINE-THREONINE KINASES. Protein ligands such as TGF-β activate a family of receptors that are analogous to the receptor tyrosine kinases except that they have a serine/threonine kinase domain in the cytoplasmic region of the protein. There are 2 isoforms of the monomeric receptor protein, type I (7 forms) and type II (5 forms). In the basal state, these proteins exist as monomers; upon binding an agonist ligand, they dimerize, leading to phosphorylation of the kinase domain of the type I monomer, which activates the receptor. The activated receptor then phosphorylates a gene regulatory protein termed a *Smad*. Once phosphorylated by the activated receptor on a serine residue, Smad dissociates from the receptor, migrates to the nucleus, associates with transcription factors, and regulates genes leading to morphogenesis and transformation. There are also inhibitory Smads (the Smad6 or Smad7 isoforms) that compete with the phosphorylated Smads to terminate signaling.

TOLL-LIKE RECEPTORS. Signaling related to the innate immune system is carried out by a family of >10 single membrane-spanning receptors termed *Toll-like receptors* (TLR), which are highly expressed in hematopoietic cells. In a single polypeptide chain, these receptors contain a large extracellular ligand-binding domain, a short membrane-spanning domain, and a cytoplasmic region termed the TIR domain that lacks intrinsic enzymatic activity. Ligands for TLR are comprised of a multitude of pathogen products including lipids, peptidoglycans, lipopeptides, and viruses. Activation of these receptors produces an inflammatory response to the pathogenic microorganisms.

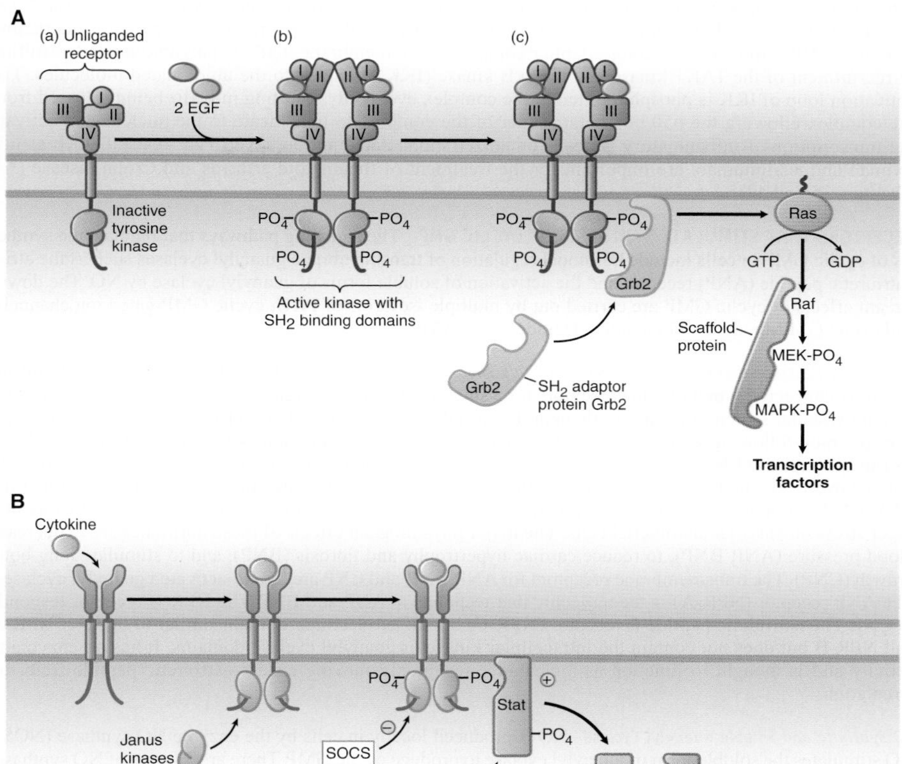

Figure 3–10 *Mechanism of activation of a receptor tyrosine kinase and a cytokine receptor.* **A.** Activation of the EGF receptor. The extracellular structure of the unliganded receptor (a) contains 4 domains (I-IV), which rearrange significantly upon binding 2 EGF molecules. (b). The conformational changes lead to activation of the cytoplasmic tyrosine kinase domains and tyrosine phosphorylation of intracellular regions to form SH2 binding sites. (c). The adapter molecule Grb2 binds to the phosphorylated tyrosine residues and activates the Ras-MAP kinase cascade. **B.** Activation of a cytokine receptor. Binding of the cytokine causes dimerization of the receptor and recruits the Janus kinases (JAKs) to the cytoplasmic tails of the receptor. JAKs transphosphorylate and lead to the phosphorylation of the signal transducers and activators of transcription (STATs). The phosphorylated STATS translocate to the nucleus and regulate transcription. There are proteins termed suppressors of cytokine signaling (SOCS) that inhibit the JAK-STAT pathway.

The first step in activation of TLR by ligands is dimerization, which in turn causes signaling proteins to bind to the receptor to form a signaling complex. Ligand-induced dimerization recruits a series of adaptor proteins including Mal and the myeloid differentiation protein 88 (MyD88) to the intracellular TIR domain, which in turn recruit the interleukin-associated kinases termed IRAKs. The IRAKs autophosphorylate in the complex and subsequently form a more stable complex with MyD88. The phosphorylation event also recruits TRAF6 to the complex, which facilitates interaction with a ubiquitin ligase that attaches a polyubiquitin molecule to TRAF6. This complex can now interact with the protein kinase TAK1 and the adaptor TAB1. TAK1 is a member of the MAP kinase family, which activates the NF-κB kinases; phosphorylation of the NF-κB transcription factors causes their translocation to the nucleus and transcriptional activation of a variety of inflammatory genes.

TNF-α RECEPTORS. The mechanism of action of tumor necrosis factor α (TNF-α) signaling to the NF-κB transcription factors is very similar to that used by Toll-like receptors in that the intracellular domain of the receptor has no enzymatic activity. The TNF-α receptor is another single membrane-spanning receptor with an extracellular ligand-binding domain, a transmembrane domain, and a cytoplasmic domain termed the *death domain*. TNF-α binds a complex composed of TNF-receptor 1 and TNF-receptor 2. On trimerization, the death domains bind the adaptor protein TRADD, which recruits the receptor interacting protein 1 (RIP1) to form a receptor-adapto r complex at the membrane. RIP1 is polyubiquinated, resulting in recruitment of the TAK1 kinase and the IκB kinase (IKK) complex to the ubiquinated molecules. The activation loop of IKK is phosphorylated in the complex eventually resulting in IκBα being released from the complex allowing the p50/p65 heterodimer of the complex to translocate to the nucleus and activate the transcription of inflammatory genes. Humanized monoclonal antibodies to TNF-α itself, such as infliximab and adalimumab, are important for the treatment of rheumatoid arthritis and Crohn disease (*see* Chapters 35 and 47).

RECEPTORS THAT STIMULATE SYNTHESIS OF CYCLIC GMP. The signaling pathways that regulate the synthesis of cyclic GMP in cells include hormonal regulation of transmembrane guanylyl cyclases such as the atrial natriuretic peptide (ANP) receptor and the activation of soluble forms of guanylyl cyclase by NO. The downstream effects of cyclic GMP are carried out by multiple isoforms of PKG, cyclic GMP-gated ion channels, and cyclic GMP-modulated PDEs that degrade cyclic AMP.

Natriuretic Peptide Receptors: Ligand-Activated Guanylyl Cyclases. The class of membrane receptors with intrinsic enzymatic activity includes the receptors for 3 small peptide ligands released from cells in cardiac tissues and the vascular system, the natriuretic peptides: atrial natriuretic peptide (ANP), released from atrial storage granules following expansion of intravascular volume or stimulation with pressor hormones; brain natriuretic peptide (BNP), synthesized and released in large amounts from ventricular tissue in response to volume overload; and C-type natriuretic peptide (CNP), synthesized in the brain and endothelial cells. Like BNP, CNP is not stored in granules; rather, its synthesis and release are increased by growth factors and sheer stress on vascular endothelial cells. The major physiological effects of these hormones are to decrease blood pressure (ANP, BNP), to reduce cardiac hypertrophy and fibrosis (BNP), and to stimulate long bone growth (CNP). The transmembrane receptors for ANP, BNP, and CNP are ligand-activated guanylyl cyclases. The ANP receptor (NPR-A) is the molecule that responds to ANP and BNP. The NPR-B receptor responds to CNP. The natriuretic peptide C receptor (NPR-C) has an extracellular domain similar to those of NPR-A and NPR-B but does not contain the intracellular kinase or guanylyl cyclase domains. It has no enzymatic activity and is thought to function as a clearance receptor, removing excess natriuretic peptide from the circulation.

NO Synthase and Soluble Guanylyl Cyclase. NO is produced locally in cells by the enzyme NO synthase (NOS). NO stimulates the soluble form of guanylyl cyclase to produce cyclic GMP. There are 3 forms of NO synthase, neuronal NOS (nNOS or NOS1), endothelial NOS (eNOS or NOS3), and inducible NOS (iNOS or NOS2). All 3 forms of this enzyme are widely expressed but are especially important in the cardiovascular system, where they are found in myocytes, vascular smooth muscle cells, endothelial cells, hematopoietic cells, and platelets. Elevated cell Ca^{2+}, acting via calmodulin, markedly activates nNOS and eNOS; the inducible form is less sensitive to Ca^{2+} but synthesis of iNOS protein in cells can be induced >1000-fold by inflammatory stimuli such as endotoxin, TNF-α, interleukin-1β, and interferon-γ.

NOS produces NO by catalyzing the oxidation of the guanido nitrogen of L-arginine, producing L-citrulline and NO. NO activates the soluble guanylyl cyclase (sGC), a heterodimer that contains a protoporphyrin-IX heme domain. NO binds to this domain at low nM concentrations and produces a 200- to 400-fold increase in the V_{max} of guanylyl cyclase, leading to an elevation of cellular cyclic GMP. The cellular effects of cyclic GMP on the vascular system are mediated by a number of mechanisms, but especially by PKG. In vascular smooth muscle, activation of PKG leads to vasodilation by:

- Inhibiting IP_3-mediated Ca^{2+} release from intracellular stores
- Phosphorylating voltage-gated Ca^{2+} channels to inhibit Ca^{2+} influx
- Phosphorylating phospholamban, a modulator of the sarcoplasmic Ca^{2+} pump, leading to a more rapid reuptake of Ca^{2+} into intracellular stores
- Phosphorylating and opening the Ca^{2+}-activated K^+ channel leading to hyperpolarization of the cell membrane, which closes L-type Ca^{2+} channels and reduces the flux of Ca^{2+} into the cell.

NUCLEAR HORMONE RECEPTORS AND TRANSCRIPTION FACTORS

Nuclear hormone receptors comprise a superfamily of 48 receptors that respond to a diverse set of ligands. The receptor proteins are transcription factors able to regulate the expression of genes controlling numerous physiological processes such as reproduction, development, and metabolism. Members of the family include receptors for circulating steroid hormones such as androgens, estrogens, glucocorticoids, thyroid hormone, and vitamin D. Other members of the family are receptors for a diverse group of fatty acids, bile acids, lipids, and lipid metabolites.

Examples include the retinoic acid receptor (RXR); the liver X receptor (LXR—the ligand is 22-OH cholesterol); the farnesoid X receptor (FXR—the ligand is chenodeoxycholic acid); and the peroxisome

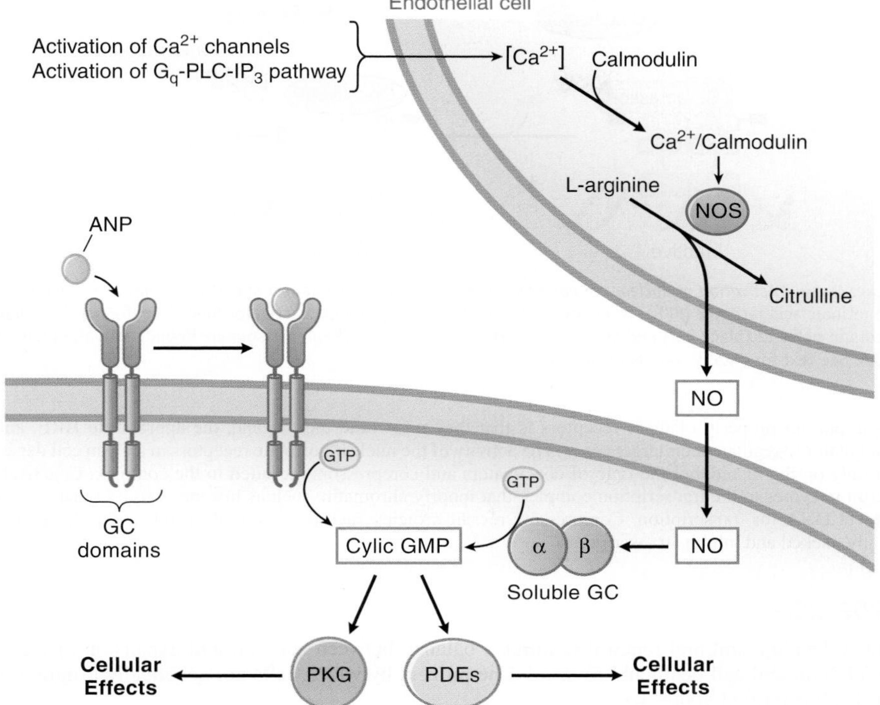

Figure 3–11 *Cyclic GMP signaling pathways.* Formation of cyclic GMP is regulated by cell surface receptors with intrinsic guanylyl cyclase (GC) activity and by soluble forms of GC. The cell surface receptors respond to natriuretic peptides such as atrial natriuretic peptide (ANP) with an increase in cyclic GMP. Soluble GC responds to nitric oxide (NO) generated from L-arginine by NO synthase (NOS). Cellular effects of cyclic GMP are carried out by PKG and cyclic GMP-regulated phosphodiesterases (PDEs). In this diagram, NO is produced by a Ca^{2+}/calmodulin-dependent NOS in an adjacent endothelial cell. Detailed descriptions of these signaling pathways are given throughout the text in relation to the therapeutic actions of drugs affecting these pathways.

proliferator-activated receptors (PPARs α, β, and γ; 15 deoxy prostaglandin J2 is a possible ligand for PPARγ; the cholesterol-lowering fibrates bind to and regulate PPARγ). In the inactive state, receptors for steroids such as glucocorticoids reside in the cytoplasm and translocate to the nucleus upon binding ligand. Other members of the family such as the LXR and FXR receptors reside in the nucleus and are activated by changes in the concentration of hydrophobic lipid molecules.

Nuclear hormone receptors contain 4 major domains in a single polypeptide chain. The N-terminal domain can contain an activation region (AF-1) essential for transcriptional regulation followed by a very conserved region with 2 zinc fingers that bind to DNA (the *DNA-binding domain*). The N-terminal activation region (AF-1) is subject to regulation by phosphorylation and other mechanisms that stimulate or inhibit transcription. The C terminal half of the molecule contains a *hinge region* (which can be involved in binding DNA), the domain responsible for binding the hormone or ligand (the *ligand-binding domain* or LBD), and specific sets of amino acid residues for binding coactivators and corepressors in a second activation region (AF-2). The LBD is formed from a bundle of 12 helices; ligand binding induces a major conformational change in helix 12 that affects the binding of the coregulatory proteins essential for activation of the receptor-DNA complex (Figure 3–12).

When bound to DNA, most of the nuclear hormone receptors act as dimers—some as homodimers, others as heterodimers. Steroid hormone receptors such as the glucocorticoid receptor are commonly homodimers, whereas those for lipids are heterodimers with the RXR receptor. The receptor dimers bind to repetitive DNA sequences, either direct repeat sequences or an inverted repeat termed hormone response elements (HRE) that are specific for each type of receptor. The hormone response elements in DNA are found upstream of the regulated genes or in some cases within the regulated genes. An agonist-bound nuclear hormone receptor often activates a large number of genes to carry out a program of cellular differentiation or metabolic regulation.

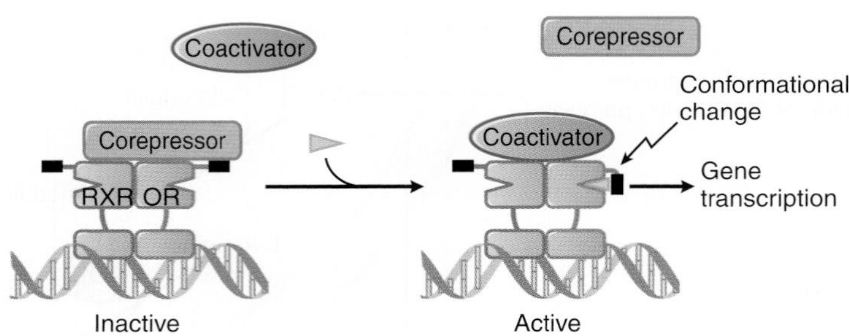

Figure 3–12 *Activation of nuclear hormone receptors.* A nuclear hormone receptor (OR) is shown in complex with the retinoic acid receptor (RXR). When an agonist (yellow triangle) and coactivator bind, a conformational change occurs in helix 12 (black bar) and gene transcription is stimulated. If corepressors are bound, activation does not occur. See text for details; *see* also Figure 6–13.

An important property of these receptors is that they must bind their ligand, the appropriate HRE, and a coregulator to regulate their target genes. The activity of the nuclear hormone receptors in a given cell depends not only on the ligand, but the ratio of coactivators and corepressors recruited to the complex. Coactivators recruit enzymes to the transcription complex that modify chromatin, such as histone acetylase that serves to unravel DNA for transcription. Corepressors recruit proteins such as histone deacetylase that keeps DNA tightly packed and inhibits transcription.

APOPTOSIS

Organ development and renewal requires a balance between survival and expansion of the cell population, and cell death and removal. The process by which cells are genetically programmed for death is termed *apoptosis*.

Apoptosis is a highly regulated program of biochemical reactions that leads to cell rounding, shrinking of the cytoplasm, condensation of the nucleus and nuclear material, and changes in the cell membrane that eventually lead to presentation of phosphatidylserine on the outer surface of the cell. Phosphatidylserine is recognized as a sign of apoptosis by macrophages, which engulf and phagocytize the dying cell. During this process, the membrane of the apoptotic cell remains intact and the cell does not release its cytoplasm or nuclear material. Thus, unlike necrotic cell death, the apoptotic process does not initiate an inflammatory response. Alterations in apoptotic pathways are implicated in a variety of diseases such as cancer, and neurodegenerative and autoimmune diseases.

Two major signaling pathways induce apoptosis. Apoptosis can be initiated by external signals that have features in common with those used by ligands such as TNF-α or by an internal pathway activated by DNA damage, improperly folded proteins, or withdrawal of cell survival factors (Figure 3–13). The apoptotic program is carried out by a large family of cysteine proteases termed *caspases*. The caspases are highly specific cytoplasmic proteases that are inactive in normal cells but become activated by apoptotic signals.

The external apoptosis signaling pathway can be activated by ligands such as TNF, Fas (also called Apo-1), or the TNF-related apoptosis-inducing ligand (TRAIL). The receptors for Fas and TRAIL are transmembrane receptors with no enzymatic activity, similar to the organization of the TNF receptor described above. Upon binding TNF, Fas ligand, or TRAIL, these receptors form a receptor dimer, undergo a conformational change, and recruit adapter proteins to the death domain. The adaptor proteins then recruit the receptor-interacting protein kinase (RIP1) and caspase 8 to form a complex that results in the activation of caspase 8. Activation of caspase 8 leads to the activation of caspase 3, which initiates the apoptotic program. The final steps of apoptosis are carried out by caspase 6 and 7, leading to degradation of enzymes, structural proteins, and DNA fragmentation characteristic of cell death (*see* Figure 3–13).

The internal apoptosis pathway can be activated by signals such as DNA damage leading to increased transcription of the p53 gene and involves damage to the mitochondria by pro-apoptotic members of the Bcl-2 family of proteins. This family includes proapoptotic members such as Bax, Bak, and Bad, which induce damage at the mitochondrial membrane. There are also anti-apoptotic Bcl-2 members, such as Bcl-2, Bcl-X, and Bcl-W, which serve to inhibit mitochondrial damage and are negative regulators of the system. When DNA damage occurs, p53 transcription is activated and holds the cell at a cell cycle checkpoint until the damage is repaired. If the damage cannot be repaired, apoptosis is initiated through the pro-apoptotic Bcl-2

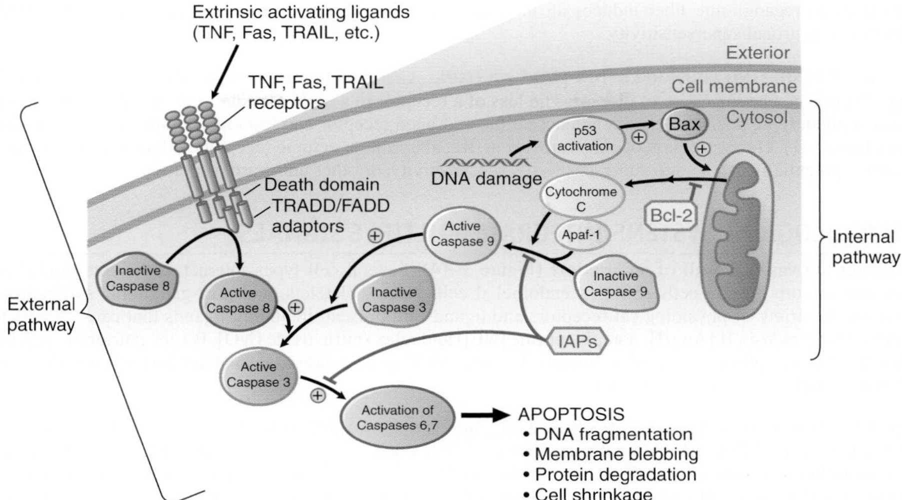

Figure 3–13 *Two pathways leading to apoptosis.* Apoptosis can be initiated by external ligands such as TNF, Fas, or TNF-related apoptosis-inducing ligand (TRAIL) at specific transmembrane receptors (left half of figure). Activation leads to trimerization of the receptor, and binding of adaptor molecules such as TRADD, to the intracellular death domain. The adaptors recruit caspase 8, activate it leading to cleavage and activation of the effector caspase, caspase 3, which activates the caspase pathway, leading to apoptosis. Apoptosis can also be initiated by an intrinsic pathway regulated by Bcl-2 family members such as Bax and Bcl-2. Bax is activated by DNA damage or malformed proteins via p53 (right half of figure). Activation of this pathway leads to release of cytochrome c from the mitochondria, formation of a complex with Apaf-1 and caspase 9. Caspase 9 is activated in the complex and initiates apoptosis thru activation of caspase 3. Either the extrinsic or the intrinsic pathway can overwhelm the inhibitors of apoptosis proteins (IAPs) that otherwise keep apoptosis in check.

members such as Bax. Bax is activated, translocates to the mitochondria, overcomes the anti-apoptotic proteins, and induces the release of cytochrome c and a protein termed the *second mitochondria-derived activator of caspase* (SMAC). SMAC binds to and inactivates the inhibitors of apoptosis proteins (IAPs) that normally prevent caspase activation. Cytochrome C combines in the cytosol with another protein, apoptotic activating protease factor -1 (Apaf-1), and with caspase 9. This complex leads to activation of caspase 9 and ultimately to the activation of caspase 3. Once activated, caspase 3 activates the same downstream pathways as the external pathway described above, leading to the cleavage of proteins, cytoskeletal elements, DNA repair proteins, with subsequent DNA condensation and membrane blebbing that eventually lead to cell death and engulfment by macrophages (*see* Figure 3–13).

RECEPTOR DESENSITIZATION AND REGULATION OF RECEPTORS

Receptors are almost always subject to feedback regulation by their own signaling outputs. Continued stimulation of cells with agonists generally results in a state of *desensitization* (also referred to as *adaptation, refractoriness,* or *downregulation*) such that the effect that follows continued or subsequent exposure to the same concentration of drug is diminished. This phenomenon, called *tachyphylaxis,* occurs rapidly and is important therapeutically; an example is attenuated response to the repeated use of β adrenergic receptor agonists as bronchodilators for the treatment of asthma (*see* Chapters 12 and 36).

Desensitization can result from temporary inaccessibility of the receptor to agonist or from fewer receptors being synthesized (e.g., downregulation of receptor number). Phosphorylation of GPCR receptors by specific GPCR kinases (GRKs) plays a key role in triggering rapid desensitization. Phosphorylation of agonist-occupied GPCRs by GRKs facilitates the binding of cytosolic proteins termed *arrestins* to the receptor, resulting in the uncoupling of G protein from the receptor. The β arrestins recruit proteins, such as PDE4, that limit cyclic AMP signaling, and clathrin and β2-adaptin, that promote sequestration of receptor from the membrane (*internalization*), thereby providing a scaffold that permits additional signaling steps.

Conversely, *supersensitivity* to agonists also frequently follows chronic reduction of receptor stimulation. Such situations can result, e.g., following withdrawal from prolonged receptor blockade (e.g., the long-term administration of β adrenergic receptor antagonists such as metoprolol) or in the case where chronic denervation of a preganglionic fiber induces an increase in neurotransmitter release per pulse, indicating post-ganglionic neuronal supersensitivity.

DISEASES RESULTING FROM RECEPTOR MALFUNCTION. Alteration in receptors and their immediate signaling effectors can be the cause of disease. The loss of a receptor in a highly specialized signaling system may cause a phenotypic disorder (e.g., deficiency of the androgen receptor and testicular feminization syndrome; *see* Chapter 41). The expression of constitutively active, aberrant, or ectopic receptors, effectors, and coupling proteins potentially can lead to supersensitivity, subsensitivity, or other untoward responses.

PHYSIOLOGICAL SYSTEMS INTEGRATE MULTIPLE SIGNALS

Consider the vascular wall of an arteriole (Figure 3–14). Several cell types interact at this site, including vascular smooth muscle cells (SMCs), endothelial cells (ECs), platelets, and post-ganglionic sympathetic neurons. A variety of physiological receptors and ligands are present, including ligands that cause SMCs to contract (angiotensin II [AngII], norepinephrine [NE]) and relax (nitric oxide [NO], B-type natriuretic peptide [BNP], and epinephrine), as well as ligands that alter SMC gene expression (platelet-derived growth factor [PDGF], AngII, NE, and eicosanoids).

AngII has both acute and chronic effects on SMC. Interaction of AngII with AT_1 receptors (AT_1R) mobilizes stored Ca^{2+} via G_q-PLC-IP_3-Ca^{2+} pathway. The Ca^{2+} binds and activates calmodulin and its target protein, myosin light-chain kinase (MLCK). The activation of MLCK results in the phosphorylation of myosin, leading to smooth muscle cell contraction. Activation of the sympathetic nervous system also regulates SMC tone through release of NE from post-ganglionic sympathetic neurons. NE binds α_1 adrenergic receptors that also activate the G_q-PLC-IP_3-Ca^{2+} pathway, resulting in SMC contraction, an effect that is additive to that of AngII.

The contraction of SMCs is opposed by mediators that promote relaxation, including NO, BNP, and catecholamines acting at β_2 receptors. NO is formed in ECs by eNOS when the G_q-PLC-IP_3-Ca^{2+} pathway is activated, and by iNOS when that isoform is induced. The NO formed in ECs diffuses into SMCs, and activates the soluble form of guanylyl cyclase (sGC), which catalyzes the formation of cyclic GMP, which leads to activation of PKG and phosphorylation of proteins in SMCs that reduce intracellular concentrations of Ca^{2+} and thereby promote relaxation. Intracellular concentrations of cyclic GMP are also increased by activation of the transmembrane BNP receptor (BNP-R), whose guanylyl cyclase activity is increased when BNP binds.

As a consequence of the variety of pathways that affect arteriolar tone, a patient with hypertension may be treated with 1 or several drugs that alter signaling through these pathways. Drugs commonly used to treat hypertension include β_1 antagonists to reduce secretion of renin (the rate-limiting first step in AngII synthesis),

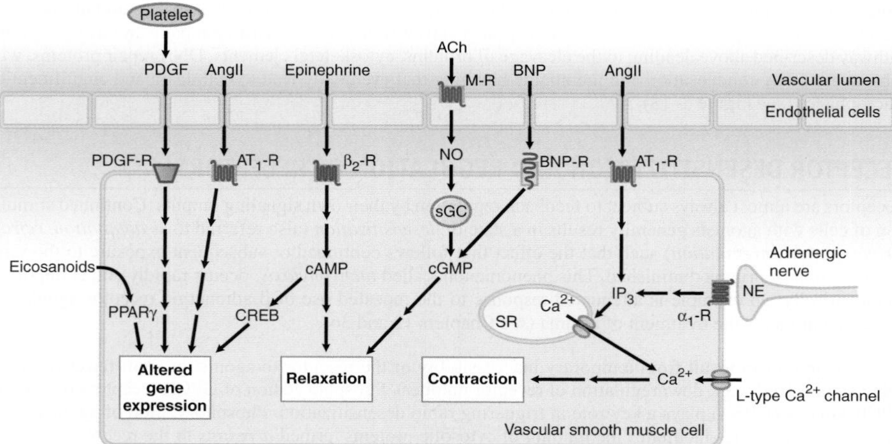

Figure 3–14 *Interaction of multiple signaling systems regulating vascular smooth muscle cells.* See text for explanation of signaling and contractile pathways and abbreviations.

a direct renin inhibitor (aliskiren) to block the rate-limiting step in AngII production, angiotensin-converting enzyme (ACE) inhibitors (e.g., enalapril) to reduce the concentrations of circulating AngII, AT_1 receptor blockers (e.g., losartan) to block AngII binding to AT_1Rs on SMCs, α_1 adrenergic blockers to block NE binding to SMCs, sodium nitroprusside to increase the quantities of NO produced, or a Ca^{2+} channel blocker (e.g., nifedipine) to block Ca^{2+} entry into SMCs. β_1 antagonists would also block the baroreceptor reflex increase in heart rate and blood pressure elicited by a drop in blood pressure induced by the therapy. ACE inhibitors also inhibit the degradation of a vasodilating peptide, bradykinin (*see* Chapter 26). Thus, the choices and mechanisms are complex, and the appropriate therapy in a given patient depends on many considerations, including the diagnosed causes of hypertension in the patient, possible side effects of the drug, efficacy in a given patient, and cost.

For a complete Bibliographical Listing see Goodman & Gilman's ***The Pharmacological Basis of Therapeutics***, 12th ed., or Goodman & Gilman Online at www.AccessMedicine.com.

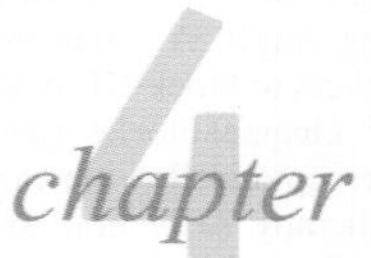

Drug Toxicity and Poisoning

Pharmacology intersects with *toxicology* when the physiological response to a drug is an *adverse effect*. A *poison* is any substance, including any drug, that has the capacity to harm a living organism. *Poisoning* generally implies that damaging physiological effects result from exposure to pharmaceuticals, illicit drugs, or chemicals.

DOSE-RESPONSE

There is a graded dose-response relationship in an *individual* and a quantal dose-response relationship in the *population* (*see* Chapters 2 and 3). Graded doses of a drug given to an individual usually result in a greater magnitude of response as the dose increases. In a quantal dose-response relationship, the percentage of the population affected increases as the dose is raised; the relationship is quantal in that the effect is judged to be either present or absent in a given individual. This quantal dose-response phenomenon is used to determine the *median lethal dose* (LD_{50}) of drugs, as defined in Figure 4–1.

One can also determine a quantal dose-response curve for the therapeutic effect of a drug to generate a median effective dose (ED_{50}), the concentration of drug at which 50% of the population will have the desired response, and a quantal dose-response curve for lethality by the same agent. These 2 curves can be used to generate a *therapeutic index* (TI), which quantifies the relative safety of a drug:

$$\text{TI} = LD_{50}/ED_{50}$$

Clearly, the higher the ratio, the safer the drug.

Values of TI vary widely, from 1-2 to >100. Drugs with a low TI must be administered with caution (e.g., cardiac glycoside digitalis and cancer chemotherapeutic agents). Agents with very high TI (e.g., penicillin) are extremely safe in the absence of a known allergic response in a given patient. Note that use

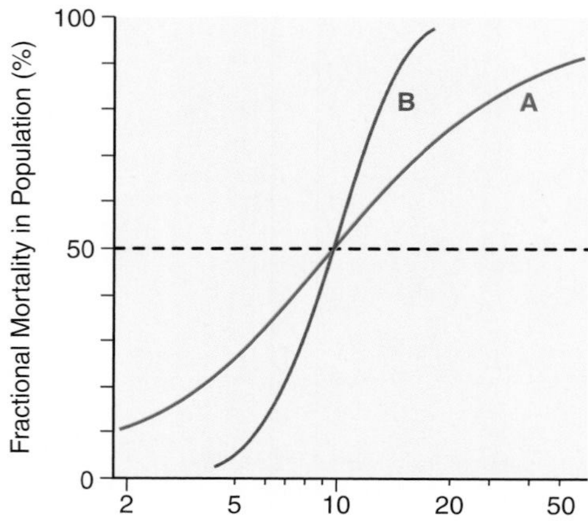

Figure 4–1 *Dose-response relationships*. The LD_{50} of a compound is determined experimentally, usually by administration of the chemical to mice or rats (orally or intraperitoneally). The midpoint of the curve representing percent of population responding (response here is death) versus dose (log scale) represents the LD_{50}, or the dose of drug that is lethal in 50% of the population. The LD_{50} values for both compounds are the same (~10 mg/kg); however, the slopes of the dose-response curves are quite different. Thus, at a dose equal to one-half the LD_{50} (5 mg/kg), less than 5% of the animals exposed to compound **B** would die, but 30% of the animals given compound **A** would die.

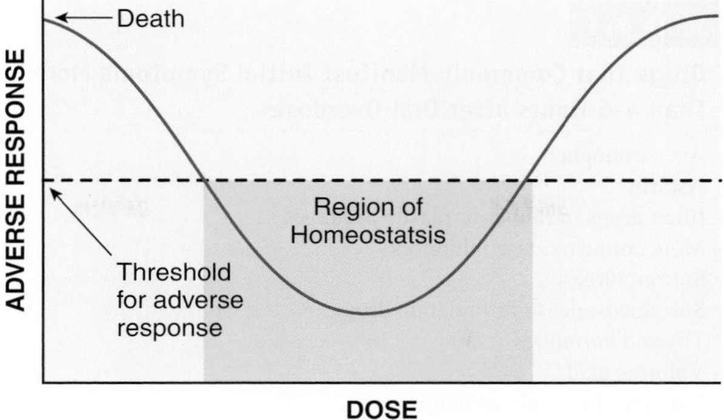

Figure 4–2 *U-Shaped dose-response curve for essential metals and vitamins.* Vitamins and essential metals are essential for life and their lack can cause adverse responses (plotted on the vertical axis), as can their excess, giving rise to a U-shaped dose-dependence curve.

of median doses fails to consider that the slopes of the dose-response curves for therapeutic and lethal (toxic) effects may differ (Figure 4–1). As an alternative the ED_{99} for the therapeutic effect can be compared to the LD_1 for lethality (toxic effect), to yield a *margin of safety*.

$$\text{Margin of Safety} = LD_1/ED_{99}$$

These quantal dose-response relationships are typical sigmoidal dose-response curves. However, not all dose-response curves follow this shape. *U-shaped dose-response curves* can be observed for essential metals and vitamins (Figure 4–2). At low dose, adverse effects are observed since there is a deficiency of these nutrients to maintain homeostasis. As dose increases, homeostasis is achieved, and the bottom of the U-shaped dose-response curve is reached. As dose increases to surpass the amount required to maintain homeostasis, overdose toxicity can ensue. Thus, adverse effects are seen at both low and high dose.

PHARMACOKINETICS VERSUS TOXICOKINETICS

Absorption, distribution, metabolism, and elimination (ADME; *see* Chapters 2, 5, and 6) may differ significantly after poisoning, and these differences can profoundly alter treatment decisions and prognosis. The pharmacokinetics of a drug under circumstances that produce toxicity or excessive exposure are referred to as *toxicokinetics*. Ingesting larger than therapeutic doses of a pharmaceutical may prolong its absorption, alter its protein binding and apparent volume of distribution, and change its metabolic fate. When confronted with a potential poisoning, 2 questions should be foremost in the clinician's mind:

- *How long will an asymptomatic patient need to be monitored (drug absorption and dynamics)?*
- *How long will it take an intoxicated patient to get better (drug elimination and dynamics)?*

DRUG ABSORPTION. Aspirin poisoning is a leading cause of overdose morbidity and mortality as reported to U.S. poison control centers. In therapeutic dosing, aspirin reaches peak plasma concentrations in ~1 h. However, aspirin overdose may cause spasm of the pyloric valve, delaying entry of the drug into the small intestine. Aspirin, especially enteric-coated forms, may coalesce into bezoars, reducing the effective surface area for absorption. Peak plasma salicylate concentrations from aspirin overdose may not be reached for 4-35 h after ingestion.

DRUG ELIMINATION. After therapeutic dosing, valproic acid has an elimination $t_{1/2}$ of ~14 h. Valproic acid poisoning may lead to coma. In predicting the duration of coma, it is important to consider that, after overdose, first-order metabolic processes appear to become saturated and the apparent elimination $t_{1/2}$ may exceed 30-45 h. Table 4–1 lists some pharmaceuticals notorious for their predilection to have initial symptoms develop *after* a typical 4-6 h emergency medical observation period.

TYPES OF THERAPEUTIC DRUG TOXICITY

In therapeutics, a drug typically produces numerous effects, but usually only 1 is sought as the primary goal of treatment; most of the other effects are undesirable effects for that therapeutic indication (Figure 4–3). *Side effects* of drugs usually are bothersome but not deleterious. Other undesirable effects may be characterized as toxic effects.

Table 4–1

Drugs That Commonly Manifest Initial Symptoms More Than 4-6 Hours after Oral Overdose[a]

Acetaminophen
Aspirin
Illicit drugs in rubber or plastic packages
Monoamine oxidase inhibitors
Sulfonylureas
Sustained-release formulation drugs
Thyroid hormones
Valproic acid
Warfarin-like anticoagulants

[a]Drugs co-ingested with agents having anticholinergic activity, manifest by diminished GI motility, may also exhibit delayed onset of action.

DOSE-DEPENDENT REACTIONS. Toxic effects of drugs may be classified as *pharmacological, pathological, or genotoxic*. Typically, the incidence and seriousness of the toxicity is proportionately related to the concentration of the drug in the body and to the duration of the exposure.

Pharmacological Toxicity. The CNS depression produced by barbiturates is largely predictable in a dose-dependent fashion. The progression of clinical effects goes from anxiolysis to sedation to somnolence to coma. Similarly, the degree of hypotension produced by nifedipine is related to the dose of the drug administered. Tardive dyskinesia (*see* Chapter 16), an extrapyramidal motor disorder associated with use of antipsychotic medications, seems to be dependent on duration of exposure. Pharmacological toxicity can also occur when the correct dose is given: there is phototoxicity associated with exposure to sunlight in patients treated with tetracyclines, sulfonamides, chlorpromazine, and nalidixic acid.

Pathological Toxicity. Acetaminophen is metabolized to nontoxic glucuronide and sulfate conjugates, and to a highly reactive metabolite *N*-acetyl-*p*-benzoquinoneimine (NAPQI) via CYP isoforms. At therapeutic dose, NAPQI binds to nucleophilic glutathione; but, in overdose, glutathione depletion may lead to the pathological finding of hepatic necrosis (Figure 4–4).

Genotoxic Effects. Ionizing radiation and many environmental chemicals are known to injure DNA, and may lead to mutagenic or carcinogenic toxicities. Many of the cancer chemotherapeutic agents (*see* Chapters 60-63) may be genotoxic (*see* Chapters 6 and 7).

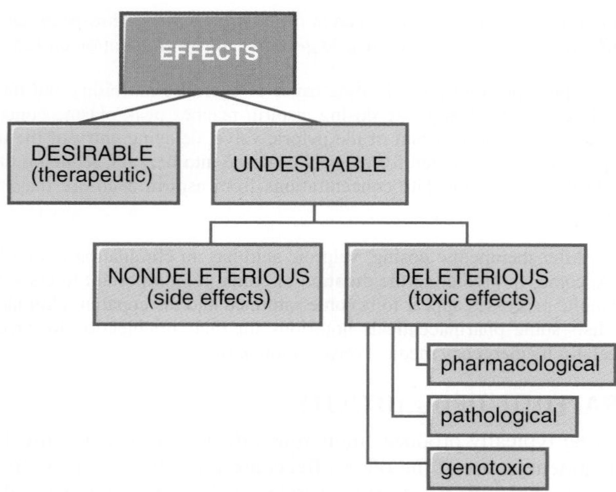

Figure 4–3 *Spectrum of the effects of pharmaceuticals.*

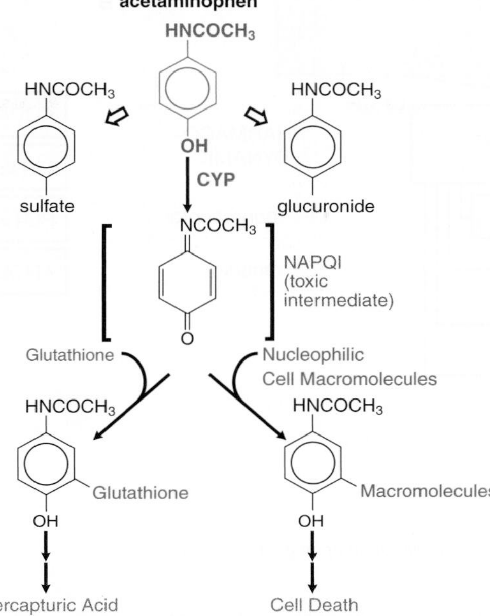

Figure 4–4 *Pathways of acetaminophen metabolism and toxicity.* The toxic intermediate NAPQI is *N*-acetyl-*p*-benzoquinoneimine.

ALLERGIC REACTIONS. An *allergy* is an adverse reaction, mediated by the immune system, that results from previous sensitization to a particular chemical or to 1 that is structurally similar. Allergic responses have been divided into 4 general categories based on the mechanism of immunological involvement.

TYPE I: ANAPHYLACTIC REACTIONS. Anaphylaxis is mediated by IgE antibodies. The Fc portion of IgE can bind to receptors on mast cells and basophils. If the Fab portion of the antibody molecule then binds an antigen, various mediators (e.g., histamine, leukotrienes, and prostaglandins) are released and cause vasodilation, edema, and an inflammatory response. The main targets of this type of reaction are the GI tract (food allergies), the skin (urticaria and atopic dermatitis), the respiratory system (rhinitis and asthma), and the vasculature (anaphylactic shock). These responses tend to occur quickly after challenge with an antigen to which the individual has been sensitized and are termed *immediate hypersensitivity reactions*.

TYPE II: CYTOLYTIC REACTIONS. Type II allergies are mediated by both IgG and IgM antibodies and usually are attributed to their capacity to activate the complement system. The major target tissues for cytolytic reactions are the cells in the circulatory system. Examples of type II allergic responses include penicillin-induced hemolytic anemia, quinidine-induced thrombocytopenic purpura, and sulfonamide-induced granulocytopenia. These autoimmune reactions to drugs usually subside within several months after removal of the offending agent.

TYPE III: ARTHUS REACTIONS. Type III allergic reactions are mediated predominantly by IgG; the mechanism involves the generation of antigen-antibody complexes that subsequently fix complement. The complexes are deposited in the vascular endothelium, where a destructive inflammatory response called *serum sickness* occurs. The clinical symptoms of serum sickness include urticarial skin eruptions, arthralgia or arthritis, lymphadenopathy, and fever. Several drugs, including commonly used antibiotics, can induce serum sickness-like reactions. These reactions usually last 6-12 days and then subside after the offending agent is eliminated.

TYPE IV: DELAYED HYPERSENSITIVITY REACTIONS. These reactions are mediated by sensitized T-lymphocytes and macrophages. When sensitized cells come in contact with antigen, an inflammatory reaction is generated by the production of lymphokines and the subsequent influx of neutrophils and macrophages. An example of type IV or delayed hypersensitivity is the contact dermatitis caused by poison ivy.

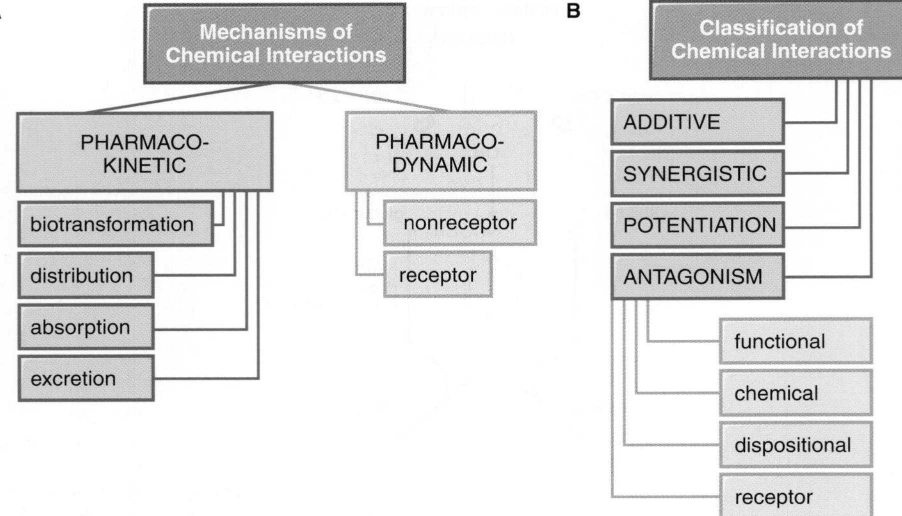

Figure 4–5 *Mechanisms and classification of drug interactions.*

IDIOSYNCRATIC REACTIONS; PHARMACOGENETIC CONTRIBUTIONS. *Idiosyncrasy* is an abnormal reactivity to a chemical that is peculiar to a given individual; the idiosyncratic response may be extreme sensitivity to low doses or extreme insensitivity to high doses of drugs.

Many interindividual differences in drug responses have a *pharmacogenetic basis* (*see* Chapter 7). Some black males (~10%) develop a serious hemolytic anemia when they receive primaquine as an antimalarial therapy, due to a genetic deficiency of erythrocyte glucose-6-phosphate dehydrogenase. Variability in the anticoagulant response to warfarin is due to polymorphisms in CYP2C9 and VKORC1 (vitamin K epoxide reductase complex 1) (*see* Figure 30–6 and Table 30–2).

DRUG–DRUG INTERACTIONS. Patients are commonly treated with more than 1 drug, may also be using over-the-counter (OTC) medications, vitamins, and other "natural" supplements, and may have unusual diets; all of these factors can contribute to interactions of drugs, a failure of therapy, and toxicity. Figure 4–5 summarizes the mechanisms and types of interactions.

INTERACTION OF ABSORPTION. A drug may cause either an increase or a decrease in the absorption of another drug from the intestinal lumen. Ranitidine, an antagonist of histamine H_2 receptors, raises gastrointestinal pH and may increase the absorption of basic drugs such as triazolam. Conversely, the bile-acid sequestrant cholestyramine leads to significantly reduced serum concentrations of propranolol.

INTERACTION OF PROTEIN BINDING. Many drugs, such as aspirin, barbiturates, phenytoin, sulfonamides, valproic acid, and warfarin, are highly protein-bound in the plasma, and it is the free (unbound) drug that produces the clinical effects. These drugs may have enhanced toxicity in overdose if protein binding sites become saturated, in physiological states that lead to hypoalbuminemia, or when displaced from plasma proteins by other drugs.

INTERACTION OF METABOLISM. A drug can frequently influence the metabolism of 1 or several other drugs (*see* Chapter 6), especially when hepatic CYPs are involved. Acetaminophen is partially transformed by CYP2E1 to the toxic metabolite NAPQI (*see* Figure 4–4). Intake of ethanol, a potent inducer of CYP2E1, may lead to increased susceptibility to acetaminophen poisoning after overdose.

INTERACTION OF RECEPTOR BINDING. Buprenorphine is an opioid with partial agonist and antagonist receptor activities, commonly used to treat opioid addiction. The drug binds opioid receptors with high affinity, and can prevent euphoria from concomitant use of narcotic drugs of abuse.

INTERACTION OF THERAPEUTIC ACTION. Aspirin is an inhibitor of platelet aggregation and heparin is an anticoagulant; given together they may increase risk for bleeding. Sulfonylureas cause hypoglycemia by stimulating pancreatic insulin release, whereas biguanide drugs (metformin) lead to decreased hepatic glucose production, and these drugs can be used together to control diabetic hyperglycemia.

Such drug interactions are *additive* when the combined effect of 2 drugs equals the sum of the effect of each agent given alone and *synergistic* when the combined effect exceeds the sum of the effects of each drug given alone. *Potentiation* describes the creation of a toxic effect from 1 drug due to the presence of another drug. *Antagonism* is the interference of 1 drug with the action of another. *Functional* or *physiological* antagonism occurs when 2 chemicals produce opposite effects on the same physiological function. *Chemical* antagonism, or *inactivation*, is a reaction between 2 chemicals to neutralize their effects, such as is seen with chelation therapy. *Dispositional* antagonism is the alteration of the disposition of a substance (its absorption, biotransformation, distribution, or excretion) so that less of the agent reaches the target organ or its persistence in the target organ is reduced. *Receptor* antagonism is the blockade of the effect of 1 drug by another drug that competes at the receptor site.

DESCRIPTIVE TOXICITY TESTING IN ANIMALS

Two main principles or assumptions underlie all descriptive toxicity tests performed in animals.

First, those effects of chemicals produced in laboratory animals, when properly qualified, apply to human toxicity. When calculated on the basis of dose per unit of body surface, toxic effects in human beings usually are encountered in the same range of concentrations as those in experimental animals. On the basis of body weight, human beings generally are more vulnerable than experimental animals.

Second, exposure of experimental animals to toxic agents in high doses is a necessary and valid method to discover possible hazards to human beings who are exposed to much lower doses. This principle is based on the quantal dose-response concept. As a matter of practicality, the number of animals used in experiments on toxic materials usually will be small compared with the size of human populations potentially at risk. For example, 0.01% incidence of a serious toxic effect (such as cancer) represents 25,000 people in a population of 250 million. Such an incidence is unacceptably high. Yet, detecting an incidence of 0.01% experimentally probably would require a minimum of 30,000 animals. To estimate risk at low dosage, large doses must be given to relatively small groups. *The validity of the necessary extrapolation is clearly a crucial question.*

The parent text, 12th edition, briefly discusses the rationale, design, size, and duration of such toxicity studies.

SAFETY PHARMACOLOGY AND CLINICAL TRIALS

Fewer than one-third of the drugs tested in clinical trials reach the marketplace. U.S. federal law and ethical considerations require that the study of new drugs in humans be conducted in accordance with stringent guidelines.

Once a drug is judged ready to be studied in humans, a **Notice of Claimed Investigational Exemption for a New Drug (IND)** must be filed with the FDA. The IND includes: (1) information on the composition and source of the drug; (2) chemical and manufacturing information; (3) all data from animal studies; (4) proposed clinical plans and protocols; (5) the names and credentials of physicians who will conduct the clinical trials; and (6) a compilation of the key data relevant to study the drug in man made available to investigators and their institutional review boards (IRBs).

It often requires 4-6 years of clinical testing to accumulate and analyze all required data. Testing in humans is begun after sufficient acute and subacute animal toxicity studies have been completed. Chronic safety testing in animals, including carcinogenicity studies, is usually done concurrently with clinical trials. In each of the 3 formal phases of clinical trials, volunteers or patients must be informed of the investigational status of the drug as well as the possible risks and must be allowed to decline or to consent to participate and receive the drug. These regulations are based on the ethical principles set forth in the Declaration of Helsinki. In addition, an interdisciplinary IRB at the facility where the clinical drug trial will be conducted must review and approve the scientific and ethical plans for testing in humans.

The prescribed phases, time lines, and costs for developing a new drug are presented in Table 1–1 and Figure 1–1.

EPIDEMIOLOGY OF ADVERSE DRUG RESPONSES AND PHARMACEUTICAL POISONING

Poisoning can occur in many ways following both therapeutic and nontherapeutic drug or chemical exposures (Table 4–2). In U.S., it is estimated that ~2 million hospitalized patients have serious adverse drug reactions each year, and ~100,000 suffer fatal adverse drug reactions. Use of good principles of prescribing, as described in Appendix I and Table 4–6, can aid in avoiding such adverse outcomes.

Table 4–2

Potential Scenarios for Poisoning

Therapeutic drug toxicity
Exploratory exposure by young children
Environmental exposure
Occupational exposure
Recreational abuse
Medication error
Prescribing error
Dispensing error
Administration error
Purposeful administration for self-harm
Purposeful administration to harm another

Table 4–3

Top Agents in Drug-Related Deaths

Cocaine
Opioids
Benzodiazepines
Alcohol
Antidepressants

U.S. DHSS. https://dawninfo.samhsa.gov/default.asp.

Some toxicities of pharmaceuticals can be predicted based on their known pharmacological mechanism; however, it is often not until the postmarketing period that the therapeutic toxicity profile of a drug becomes fully appreciated. The Adverse Event Reporting System of the FDA relies on 2 signals to detect rarer adverse drug events. *First*, the FDA requires drug manufacturers to perform postmarketing surveillance of prescription drugs and nonprescription products. *Second*, the FDA operates a voluntary reporting system (MedWatch, at http://www.fda.gov/Safety/MedWatch/default.htm) available to both health professionals and consumers. Hospitals may also support adverse drug event committees to investigate potential adverse drug events. Unfortunately, any national dataset will significantly underestimate the morbidity and mortality attributable to adverse drug events because of underreporting and because it is difficult to estimate the denominator of total patient exposures for each event reported once a drug is available on the open market.

Therapeutic drug toxicity is only a subset of poisoning, as noted in Table 4–2. Misuse and abuse of both prescription and illicit drugs is a major public health problem. The incidence of unintentional, non-iatrogenic poisoning is bimodal, primarily affecting exploratory young children, ages 1-5 years, and the elderly. *Intentional* overdose with pharmaceuticals is most common in adolescence and through adulthood. The top 5 drugs involved in drug-related deaths reported in 2005 are presented in Table 4–3. The substances most frequently involved in human exposures and fatalities are presented in Tables 4–4 and 4–5.

PREVENTION OF POISONING

REDUCTION OF MEDICATION ERRORS. Over the past decade considerable attention has been given to the reduction of medication errors and adverse drug events. Medication errors can occur in any part of the medication prescribing or use process, whereas adverse drug events (ADEs) are injuries related to the use or nonuse of medications. It is believed that medication errors are 50-100

Table 4–4

Substances Most Frequently Involved in Human Poisoning

SUBSTANCE	%
Analgesics	12.5
Personal care products	9.1
Cleaning substances	8.7
Sedatives/hypnotics/antipsychotics	6.2
Foreign bodies	5.1
Topical preparations	4.5
Cold and cough medications	4.5
Antidepressants	4.0

Data from Bronstein et al., Clin Toxicol, 2008;46:927–1057.

Table 4–5

Poisons Associated with the Largest Number of Human Fatalities

Sedatives/hypnotics/antipsychotics
Acetaminophen
Opioids
Antidepressants
Cardiovascular drugs
Stimulants and street drugs
Alcohols

Data from Bronstein et al., Clin Toxicol, 2008;46:927–1057.

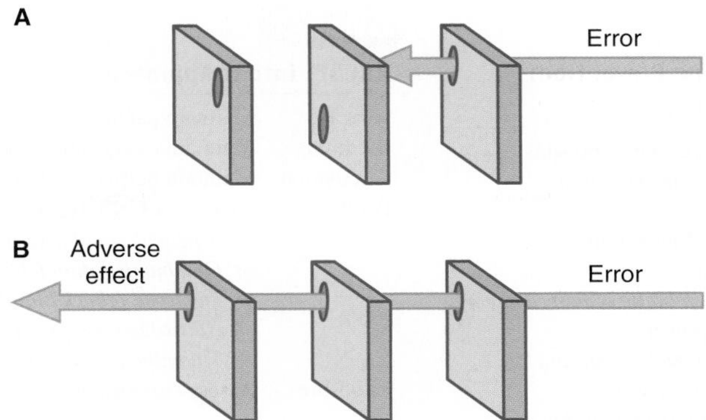

Figure 4–6 *The "Swiss cheese" model of medication error.* Several checkpoints typically exist to identify and prevent an adverse drug event, and that adverse event can only occur if holes in several systems align. **A.** One systematic error does not lead to an adverse event, because it is prevented by another check in the system. **B.** Several systematic errors align to allow an adverse event to occur. (Adapted from Reason J, *Br Med J,* 2000;320:768–770.)

times more common than ADEs. The "5 Rights" of safe medication administration attempt to help practitioners avoid medication errors:

Right drug, right patient, right dose, right route, right time.

In practice, accomplishing a reduction in medication errors involves scrutiny of the systems involved in prescribing, documenting, transcribing, dispensing, administering, and monitoring a therapy, as presented in Appendix I. Good medication use practices have mandatory and redundant checkpoints (Figure 4–6), such as having a pharmacist, a doctor, and a nurse all review and confirm that an ordered dose of a medication is appropriate for a patient prior to the drug's administration. Several practical strategies have can help to reduce medication errors within healthcare settings (Table 4–6).

POISONING PREVENTION IN THE HOME. Table 4–2 demonstrates that there are several contexts into which poisoning prevention can be directed. Depression and suicidal ideation need to be identified and treated. Exposure to hazards in the home, outdoor, and work environments need to be reduced to reasonably achievable levels.

Table 4–6

Best Practice Recommendations to Reduce Medication Administration Errors[a]

Short Term

- Maintain unit-dose distribution systems for non-emergency medications
- Have pharmacies prepare intravenous solutions
- Remove inherently dangerous medications (e.g., concentrated KCl) from patient care areas
- Develop special procedures for high-risk drugs
- Improve drug-related clinical information resources
- Improve medication administration education for clinicians
- Educate patients about the safe and accurate use of medications
- Improve access of bedside clinicians to pharmacists

Long Term

Implement technology-based safeguards:

- Computerized order entry
- Computerized dose and allergy checking
- Computerized medication tracking
- Use of bar codes or electronic readers for medication preparation and administration

[a]*See Mass. Hosp. Assoc., http://macoalition.org/documents/Best_Practice_Medication_Errors.pdf.*

Table 4–7

Passive Poisoning Prevention: Strategies and Examples

Reduce manufacture/sale of poisons
Withdrawal of phenformin from U.S. market
Decrease amount of poison in a consumer product
Limiting of pills in bottle of baby aspirin
Prevent access to poison
Use of child-resistant packaging
Change product formulation
Removing ethanol from mouthwash

Table 4–8

ABCDE: Initial Approach for Acute Poisoning

Airway	Maintain patency
Breathing	Maintain oxygenation and ventilation
Circulation	Maintain perfusion of vital organs
Disability	Assess for CNS dysfunction *For neurological disability, consider:* • *O_2 administration (check pulse oximetry)* • *Dextrose (check blood glucose)* • *Naloxone (consider empiric trial)* • *Thiamine (for adults receiving dextrose)*
Exposure	Assess "toxidrome" (*see* Table 4–9)

Poisoning prevention strategies may be categorized as being *passive*, requiring no behavior change on the part of the individual, or *active*, requiring sustained adaptation to be successful. Passive prevention strategies are the most effective (Table 4–7). The incidence of poisoning in children has decreased dramatically over the past 4 decades. This favorable trend is largely due to improved safety packaging of drugs, drain cleaners, turpentine, and other household chemicals; improved medical training and care; and increased public awareness of potential poisons.

PRINCIPLES OF TREATMENT OF POISONING

When toxicity is expected or occurs, the priorities of poisoning treatment are to:

- *Maintain vital physiological functions from impairment*
- *Keep the concentration of poison in tissues as low as possible by preventing absorption and enhancing elimination*
- *Combat the toxicological effects of the poison at the effector sites*

INITIAL STABILIZATION OF THE POISONED PATIENT. The "ABC" mnemonic of emergency care applies to the treatment of acute poisoning (Table 4–8). In severe cases, endotracheal intubation, mechanical ventilation, pharmacological blood pressure support, and/or extracorporeal circulatory support may be necessary and appropriate.

IDENTIFICATION OF CLINICAL PATTERNS OF TOXICITY. A medical history may allow for the creation of a list of available medications or chemicals that might be implicated in a poisoning event. Often, an observation of physical symptoms and signs may be the only additional clues to a poisoning diagnosis. Groups of physical signs and symptoms associated with specific poisoning syndromes are known as *toxidromes* (Table 4–9).

The urine drug toxicology test is an immunoassay designed to detect common drugs of abuse such as amphetamines, barbiturates, benzodiazepines, cannabis, cocaine, and opiates. Acute poisoning with these substances can usually be determined on clinical grounds, and the results of these assays are infrequently available fast enough to guide stabilization. Additionally, detection of drugs or their metabolites on a urine immunoassay does not mean that the detected drug is responsible for the currently observed poisoning illness. When ingestion of acetaminophen or aspirin cannot clearly be excluded via the exposure history, serum quantification of these drugs is recommended. An ECG may be useful at detecting heart blocks, Na^+ channel blockade, or K^+ channel blockade associated with specific medication classes (Table 4–10). Further laboratory analysis should be tailored to the individual poisoning circumstance.

DECONTAMINATION OF THE POISONED PATIENT. Poisoning exposures may be by inhalation, by dermal or mucosal absorption, by injection, or by ingestion. The first step in preventing absorption of poison is to stop any ongoing exposure. If necessary, eyes and skin should be washed copiously. GI decontamination prevents or reduces absorption of a substance after it has been ingested. The strategies for GI decontamination are *gastric emptying, adsorption of poison, and catharsis*. Minimal indications for considering GI decontamination include: (1) the poison must be potentially dangerous; (2) the poison must still be unabsorbed in the stomach or intestine, so it must be soon after ingestion; and (3) the procedure must be able to be performed safely and with proper technique. Gastric emptying is rarely recommended anymore, but the administration

Table 4–9

Common Toxidromes

DRUG CLASS	EXAMPLE(S)	MENTAL STATUS	HR	BP	RR	T	PUPIL SIZE	OTHER
Sympathomimetic	Cocaine Amphetamine	Agitation	↑	↑		↑	↑	Tremor, diaphoresis
Anticholinergic	Diphenhydramine *Belladonna atropa*	Delirium	↑	↑		↑	↑	Ileus, flushing
Cholinergic	Organophosphates	Somnolence, coma			↑		↓	SLUDGE[a], fasciculation
Opioid	Heroin Oxycodone	Somnolence, coma	↓		↓		↓	
Sedative-hypnotic	Benzodiazepines Barbiturates	Somnolence, coma		↓	↓			
Salicylate	Aspirin	Confusion	↑		↑	↑		Diaphoresis, vomiting
Ca^{2+} channel blocker	Verapamil		↓	↓				

HR, heart rate; BP, blood pressure; RR, respiratory rate; T, temperature.
[a]SLUDGE, muscarinic effects of Salivation, Lacrimation, Urination, Defecation, Gastric cramping, and Emesis.

of activated charcoal and the performance of whole bowel irrigation remain therapeutic options. Gastric emptying reduces drug absorption by ~1/3 under optimal conditions.

Based upon review of existing evidence, the American Academy of Pediatrics no longer recommends syrup of ipecac as part of its childhood injury prevention program, and the American Academy of Clinical Toxicology dissuades routine use of gastric emptying in the poisoned patient.

ADSORPTION. Adsorption of a poison refers to the binding of a poison to the surface of another substance so that the poison is less available for absorption into the body. Fuller's earth has been suggested as an adsorbent for paraquat, Prussian blue binds thallium and cesium, and sodium polystyrene can adsorb lithium. The most common adsorbent used in the treatment of acute drug overdose is activated charcoal.

Table 4–10

Differential Poisoning Diagnosis (Partial Listing) for Electrocardiographic Manifestations of Toxicity

BRADYCARDIA/HEART BLOCK	QRS INTERVAL PROLONGATION	QT_C INTERVAL PROLONGATION
Cholinergic agents Physostigmine Neostigmine Organophosphates, carbamates *Sympatholytic agents* β receptor antagonists Clonidine Opioids *Other* Digoxin Ca^{2+} channel blockers Lithium	Anti-arrhythmia drugs Bupropion Chloroquine Diphenhydramine Lamotrigine Phenothiazines Propranolol Tricyclic antidepressants	(See Arizona Center for Education and Research on Therapeutics website, http://www.azcert.org/medical-pros/drug-lists/drug-lists.cfm)

ACTIVATED CHARCOAL. Charcoal is created through controlled pyrolysis of organic matter, and is *activated* through steam or chemical treatment that increases its internal pore structure and adsorptive surface capacity. The surface of activated charcoal contains carbon moieties that are capable of binding poisons. The recommended dose is typically 0.5-2 g/kg of body weight, up to a maximum tolerated dose of ~75-100 g. As a rough estimate, 10 g of activated charcoal is expected to bind ~1 g of drug. Alcohols, corrosives, hydrocarbons, and metals are not well adsorbed by charcoal. Complications of activated charcoal therapy include vomiting, constipation, pulmonary aspiration, and death. Nasogastric administration of charcoal increases the incidence of vomiting, and may increase the risk for pulmonary aspiration. Charcoal should not be given to patients with suspected GI perforation, or to patients who may be candidates for endoscopy.

WHOLE BOWEL IRRIGATION. Whole bowel irrigation (WBI) involves the enteral administration of large amounts of a high molecular weight, iso-osmotic polyethylene glycol electrolyte solution with the goal of passing poison by the rectum before it can be absorbed. Potential candidates for WBI include: (1) "body-packers" with intestinal packets of illicit drugs; (2) patients with iron overdose; (3) patients who have ingested patch pharmaceuticals; and (4) patients with overdoses of sustained-release or bezoar-forming drugs. Polyethylene glycol electrolyte solution is typically administered at a rate of 25 to 40 mL/kg/h until the rectal effluent is clear and no more drug is being passed. To achieve these high administration rates, a nasogastric tube may be used. WBI is contraindicated in the presence of bowel obstruction or perforation, and may be complicated by abdominal distention or pulmonary aspiration.

CATHARTICS. The 2 most common categories of simple cathartics are the magnesium salts, such as magnesium citrate and magnesium sulfate, and the nondigestible carbohydrates, such as sorbitol. The use of simple cathartics has been abandoned as a GI decontamination strategy.

Gastric Lavage. The procedure for gastric lavage involves passing an orogastric tube into the stomach with the patient in the left-lateral decubitus position with head lower than feet. After withdrawing stomach contents, 10 to 15 mL/kg (up to 250 mL) of saline lavage fluid is administered and withdrawn. This process continues until the lavage fluid returns clear. Complications of the procedure include mechanical trauma to the stomach or esophagus, pulmonary aspiration of stomach contents, and vagus nerve stimulation.

Syrup of Ipecac. The alkaloids cephaeline and emetine within syrup of ipecac act as emetics because of both a local irritant effect on the enteric tract and a central effect on the chemoreceptor trigger zone in the area postrema of the medulla. Ipecac is given orally at a dose of 15 mL for children up to 12 years, and 30 mL for older children and adults. Administration of ipecac is typically followed by a drink of water, and reliably produces emesis in 15-30 min. Contraindications for syrup of ipecac administration include existing or impending CNS depression, ingestion of a corrosive or hydrocarbon drug (due to the emergence of chemical pneumonia), or presence of a medical condition that might be exacerbated by vomiting.

ENHANCING THE ELIMINATION OF POISONS. Once absorbed, the deleterious toxicodynamic effects of some drugs may be reduced by methods that hasten their elimination from the body, as described below.

MANIPULATING URINARY pH: URINARY ALKALINIZATION. Drugs subject to renal clearance are excreted into the urine by glomerular filtration and active tubular secretion; nonionized compounds may be reabsorbed far more rapidly than ionized polar molecules (*see* Chapter 2). Weakly acidic drugs are susceptible to "ion-trapping" in the urine. Aspirin is a weak acid with a $pK_a = 3.0$. As the pH of the urine increases, more salicylate is in its ionized form at equilibrium, and more salicylic acid is diffused into the tubular lumen of the kidney. Urinary alkalinization is also believed to speed clearance of phenobarbital, chlorpropamide, methotrexate, and chlorophenoxy herbicides. The American Academy of Clinical Toxicologists recommends urine alkalinization as first-line treatment only for moderately severe salicylate poisoning that does not meet criteria for hemodialysis. To achieve alkalinization of the urine, 100-150 mEq of sodium bicarbonate in 1 L of D5W is infused intravenously at twice the maintenance fluid requirements and then titrated to effect. Hypokalemia should be treated since it will hamper efforts to alkalinize the urine due to H^+-K^+ exchange in the kidney. Urine alkalinization is contraindicated in renal failure, or if fluid administration may worsen pulmonary edema or congestive heart failure. Acetazolamide is not used to alkalinize urine as it promotes acidemia.

MULTIPLE-DOSE ACTIVATED CHARCOAL. Activated charcoal adsorbs drug to its surface and promotes enteral elimination. Multiple doses of activated charcoal can speed elimination of absorbed drug by 2 mechanisms. Charcoal may interrupt enterohepatic circulation of hepatically metabolized drug excreted in the bile, and charcoal may create a diffusion gradient across the GI mucosa and promote movement of drug from the bloodstream onto the charcoal in the intestinal lumen. Activated charcoal may be administered in multiple doses, 12.5 g/h every 1, 2, or 4 h (smaller doses may be used for children). Charcoal enhances the clearance of many drugs of low molecular weight, small volume of distribution, and long elimination $t_{1/2}$. Multiple-dose activated charcoal is believed to have the most potential utility in overdoses of carbamazepine, dapsone, phenobarbital, quinine, theophylline, and yellow oleander.

Table 4–11

Some Common Antidotes and Their Indications

ANTIDOTE	POISONING INDICATION(S)
Acetylcysteine	Acetaminophen
Atropine sulfate	Organophosporus and carbamate pesticides
Benztropine	Drug-induced dystonia
Bicarbonate, sodium	Na^+ channel blocking drugs
Bromocriptine	Neuroleptic malignant syndrome
Calcium gluconate or chloride	Ca^{2+} channel blocking drugs, Fluoride
Carnitine	Valproate hyperammonemia
Crotalidae polyvalent immune Fab	North American rattlesnake bite
Dantrolene	Malignant hyperthermia
Deferoxamine	Iron
Digoxin immune Fab	Cardiac glycosides
Diphenhydramine	Drug-induced dystonia
Dimercaprol (BAL)	Lead, mercury, arsenic
EDTA, $CaNa_2$	Lead
Ethanol	Methanol, ethylene glycol
Fomepizole	Methanol, ethylene glycol
Flumazenil	Benzodiazepines
Glucagon hydrochloride	β adrenergic antagonists
Hydroxocobalamin hydrochloride	Cyanide
Insulin (high dose)	Ca^{2+} channel blockers
Leucovorin calcium	Methotrexate
Methylene blue	Methemoglobinemia
Naloxone hydrochloride	Opioids
Octreotide acetate	Sulfonylurea-induced hypoglycemia
Oxygen, hyperbaric	Carbon monoxide
Penicillamine	Lead, mercury, copper
Physostigmine salicylate	Anticholinergic syndrome
Pralidoxime chloride (2-PAM)	Organophosphorus pesticides
Pyridoxine hydrochloride	Isoniazid seizures
Succimer (DMSA)	Lead, mercury, arsenic
Thiosulfate, sodium	Cyanide
Vitamin K_1 (phytonadione)	Coumarin, indanedione

EXTRACORPOREAL DRUG REMOVAL. The ideal drug amenable to removal by hemodialysis has a low molecular weight, a low volume of distribution, high solubility in water, and minimal protein binding. Hemoperfusion involves passing blood through a cartridge containing adsorbent particles. The most common poisonings for which hemodialysis is sometimes used include salicylate, methanol, ethylene glycol, lithium, carbamazepine, and valproic acid.

ANTIDOTAL THERAPIES. Antidotal therapy involves antagonism or chemical inactivation of an absorbed poison. Among the most common specific antidotes used are *N*-acetyl-*L*-cysteine for acetaminophen poisoning, opioid antagonists for opioid overdose, and chelating agents for poisoning from certain metal ions. A list of antidotes used is presented in Table 4–11.

The pharmacodynamics of a poison can be altered by competition at a receptor, as in the antagonism provided by naloxone therapy in the setting of heroin overdose. A physiological antidote may use a different cellular mechanism to overcome the effects of a poison, as in the use of glucagon to circumvent a blocked β adrenergic receptor and increase cellular cyclic AMP in the setting of propranolol overdose. Antivenoms and chelating agents bind and directly inactivate poisons. The biotransformation of a drug can also be altered by an antidote; for example, fomepizole will inhibit alcohol dehydrogenase and stop the formation of toxic acid metabolites from ethylene glycol and methanol. Many drugs used in the supportive care of a poisoned patient (anticonvulsants, vasoconstricting agents, etc.) may be considered nonspecific functional antidotes.

The mainstay of therapy for poisoning is good support of the airway, breathing, circulation, and vital metabolic processes of the poisoned patient until the poison is eliminated from the body.

IMPORTANT RESOURCES FOR INFORMATION RELATED TO DRUG TOXICITY AND POISONING

Additional information on poisoning from drugs and chemicals can be found in many dedicated books of toxicology. A popular computer database for information on toxic substances is POISINDEX (Micromedex, Inc., Denver, CO). The National Library of Medicine offers information on toxicology and environmental health (http://sis.nlm.nih.gov/enviro.html), including a link to ToxNet (http://toxnet.nlm.nih.gov/). Regional poison control centers are a resource for valuable poisoning information and may be contacted within the U.S. through a national PoisonHelp hotline: 1-800-222-1222.

For a complete Bibliographical Listing see Goodman & Gilman's ***The Pharmacological Basis of Therapeutics***, 12th ed., or Goodman & Gilman Online at www.AccessMedicine.com.

Membrane Transporters and Drug Response

Transporters are membrane proteins that are present in all organisms. These proteins control the influx of essential nutrients and ions and the efflux of cellular waste, environmental toxins, drugs, and other xenobiotics (Figure 5–1), consistent with their critical roles in cellular homeostasis, ~2000 genes in the human genome, ~7% of the total number of genes, code for transporters or transporter-related proteins. The functions of membrane transporters may be facilitated (equilibrative, not requiring energy) or active (requiring energy). In considering the transport of drugs, pharmacologists generally focus on transporters from 2 major superfamilies, ABC (*A*TP *b*inding *c*assette) and SLC (*so*lute *c*arrier) transporters.

Most ABC proteins are primary active transporters, which rely on ATP hydrolysis to actively pump their substrates across membranes. Among the best recognized transporters in the ABC superfamily are P-glycoprotein (Pgp, encoded by *ABCB1*, also termed *MDR1*) and the cystic fibrosis transmembrane regulator (CFTR, encoded by *ABCC7*). The *SLC* superfamily includes genes that encode facilitated transporters and ion-coupled secondary active transporters. Forty-eight SLC families with ~315 transporters have been identified in the human genome. Many SLC transporters serve as drug targets or in drug absorption and disposition. Widely recognized SLC transporters include the serotonin transporter, SERT, and the dopamine transporter, DAT, both targets for antidepressant medications.

MEMBRANE TRANSPORTERS IN THERAPEUTIC DRUG RESPONSES

PHARMACOKINETICS. Transporters important in pharmacokinetics generally are located in intestinal, renal, and hepatic epithelia, where they function in the selective absorption and elimination of endogenous substances and xenobiotics, including drugs. Transporters work in concert with drug-metabolizing enzymes to eliminate drugs and their metabolites (Figure 5–2). In addition,

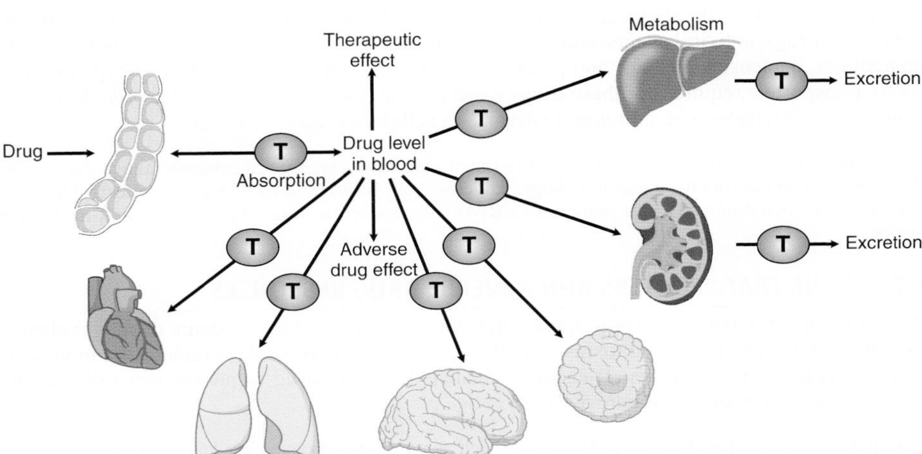

Figure 5–1 *Membrane transporters in pharmacokinetic pathways.* Membrane transporters (T) play roles in pharmacokinetic pathways (drug absorption, distribution, metabolism, and excretion), thereby setting systemic drug levels. Drug levels often drive therapeutic and adverse drug effects.

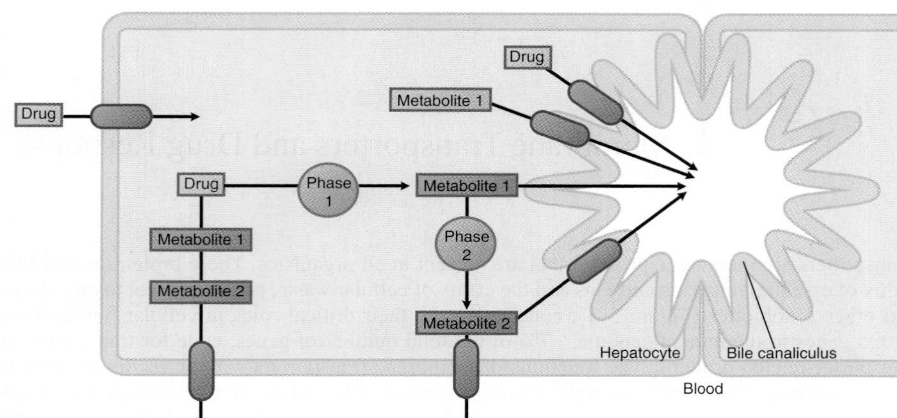

Figure 5–2 *Hepatic drug transporters.* Membrane transporters (*red ovals with arrows*) work in concert with phase 1 and phase 2 drug-metabolizing enzymes in the hepatocyte to mediate the uptake and efflux of drugs and their metabolites.

transporters in various cell types mediate tissue-specific drug distribution (drug targeting). Conversely, transporters also may serve as protective barriers to particular organs and cell types. For example, P-glycoprotein in the blood-brain barrier protects the central nervous system (CNS) from a variety of structurally diverse drugs through its efflux mechanisms.

PHARMACODYNAMICS: TRANSPORTERS AS DRUG TARGETS. Membrane transporters are the targets of many clinically used drugs. SERT (*SLC6A4*) is a target for a major class of antidepressant drugs, the selective serotonin reuptake inhibitors (SSRIs). Other neurotransmitter reuptake transporters serve as drug targets for the tricyclic antidepressants, various amphetamines (including amphetamine-like drugs used in the treatment of attention deficit disorder in children), and anticonvulsants.

These transporters also may be involved in the pathogenesis of neuropsychiatric disorders, including Alzheimer and Parkinson diseases. Transporters that are nonneuronal also may be potential drug targets, e.g., cholesterol transporters in cardiovascular disease, nucleoside transporters in cancers, glucose transporters in metabolic syndromes, and Na^+-H^+ antiporters in hypertension.

DRUG RESISTANCE. Membrane transporters play critical roles in the development of resistance to anticancer drugs, antiviral agents, and anticonvulsants. *Decreased uptake of drugs*, such as folate antagonists, nucleoside analogs, and platinum complexes, is mediated by reduced expression of influx transporters required for these drugs to access the tumor. *Enhanced efflux of hydrophobic drugs* is one mechanism of antitumor resistance in cellular assays of resistance.

For example, P-glycoprotein is overexpressed in tumor cells after exposure to cytotoxic anticancer agents. P-glycoprotein pumps out the anticancer drugs, rendering cells resistant to their cytotoxic effects. The overexpression of multidrug resistance protein 4 (MRP4) is associated with resistance to antiviral nucleoside analogs.

MEMBRANE TRANSPORTERS AND ADVERSE DRUG RESPONSES

As controllers of import and export, transporters ultimately control the exposure of cells to chemical carcinogens, environmental toxins, and drugs. Thus, transporters play crucial roles in the cellular toxicities of these agents. Transporter-mediated adverse drug responses generally can be classified into 3 categories (Figure 5–3).

Transporters expressed in the liver and kidney, as well as metabolic enzymes, are key determinants of drug exposure in the circulating blood, thereby affecting exposure, and hence toxicity, in all organs (Figure 5–3, *top panel*). For example, after oral administration of an HMG-CoA reductase inhibitor (e.g., pravastatin), the efficient first-pass hepatic uptake of the drug by the *organic anion-transporting polypeptide* OATP1B1 maximizes the effects of such drugs on hepatic HMG-CoA reductase. Uptake by OATP1B1 also minimizes the

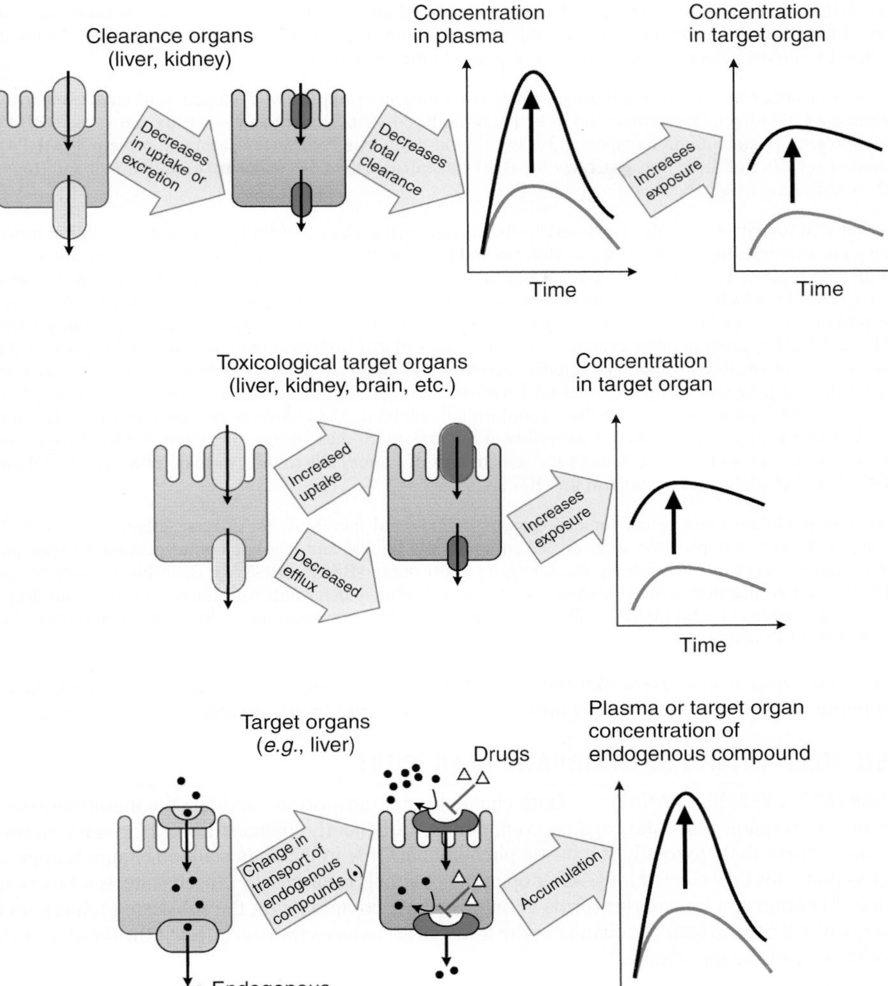

Figure 5–3 *Major mechanisms by which transporters mediate adverse drug responses.* Three cases are given. The *left panel* of each case provides a representation of the mechanism; the *right panel* shows the resulting effect on drug levels. (*Top panel*) Increase in the plasma concentrations of drug due to a decrease in the uptake and/or secretion in clearance organs (e.g., liver and kidney). (*Middle panel*) Increase in the concentration of drug in toxicological target organs due to the enhanced uptake or reduced efflux. (*Bottom panel*) Increase in the plasma concentration of an endogenous compound (e.g., a bile acid) due to a drug's inhibiting the influx of the endogenous compound in its eliminating or target organ. The diagram also may represent an increase in the concentration of the endogenous compound in the target organ owing to drug-inhibited efflux of the endogenous compound.

escape of these drugs into the systemic circulation, where they can cause adverse responses such as skeletal muscle myopathy.

Transporters expressed in tissues that may be targets for drug toxicity (e.g., brain) or in barriers to such tissues (e.g., the blood-brain barrier [BBB]) can tightly control local drug concentrations and thus control the exposure of these tissues to the drug (Figure 5–3, *middle panel*). For example, endothelial cells in the BBB are linked by tight junctions, and some efflux transporters are expressed on the blood-facing (luminal) side, thereby restricting the penetration of compounds into the brain. The interactions of loperamide and quinidine are a good example of transporter control of drug exposure at this site. Loperamide is a peripheral opioid used in the treatment of diarrhea and is a substrate of P-glycoprotein. Inhibition of P-glycoprotein-mediated efflux in the BBB would cause an increase in the concentration of loperamide in the CNS and potentiate adverse effects. Indeed, coadministration of loperamide and the potent P-glycoprotein inhibitor quinidine results in significant respiratory depression, an adverse response to the loperamide.

The case of oseltamivir (the antiviral drug TAMIFLU) provides an example that dysfunction of an active barrier may cause a CNS effect. Oseltamivir and its active form, Ro64-0802, undergo active efflux across the BBB by P-glycoprotein, organic anion transporter 3 (OAT3), and multidrug resistance-associated protein 4 (MRP4). Decreased activities of these transporters at the BBB can enhance the CNS exposure to oseltamivir and Ro64-0802, contributing to an adverse effect on the CNS.

Drug-induced toxicity sometimes is caused by the concentrative tissue distribution mediated by influx transporters. For example, biguanides (e.g., metformin and phenformin), used for the treatment of type 2 diabetes mellitus, can produce lactic acidosis, a lethal side effect. Biguanides are substrates of the organic cation transporter 1 (OCT1), which is highly expressed in the liver. OCT1-mediated hepatic uptake of biguanides plays an important role in lactic acidosis. The organic anion transporter 1 (OAT1) and organic cation transporters (OCT1 and OCT2) provide other examples of transporter-related toxicity. OAT1 is expressed mainly in the kidney and is responsible for the renal tubular secretion of anionic compounds. Substrates of OAT1, such as cephaloridine (a β-lactam antibiotic), and adefovir and cidofovir (antiviral drugs), reportedly cause nephrotoxicity. In vitro experiments suggest that cephaloridine, adefovir, and cidofovir are substrates of OAT1 and that OAT1-expressing cells are more susceptible to the toxicity of these drugs than control cells. Exogenous expression of OCT1 and OCT2 enhances the sensitivities of tumor cells to the cytotoxic effect of oxaliplatin for OCT1, and cisplatin and oxaliplatin for OCT2.

Drugs may modulate transporters for endogenous ligands and thereby exert adverse effects (Figure 5–3, *bottom panel*). For example, bile acids are taken up mainly by *N*a$^+$-*t*aurocholate *c*otransporting *p*olypeptide (NTCP) and excreted into the bile by the *b*ile *s*alt *e*xport *p*ump (BSEP, *ABCB11*). Bilirubin is taken up by OATP1B1 and conjugated with glucuronic acid, and bilirubin glucuronide is excreted by the *m*ultidrug-*r*esistance-associated *p*rotein (MRP2, *ABCC2*). Inhibition of these transporters by drugs may cause cholestasis or hyperbilirubinemia.

Uptake and efflux transporters determine the plasma and tissue concentrations of endogenous compounds and xenobiotics, thereby influencing the systemic or site-specific toxicity of drugs.

BASIC MECHANISMS OF MEMBRANE TRANSPORT

TRANSPORTERS VERSUS CHANNELS. Both channels and transporters facilitate the membrane permeation of inorganic ions and organic compounds. In general, channels have 2 primary states, open and closed, that are totally stochastic phenomena. Only in the open state do channels appear to act as pores for the selected ions. After opening, channels return to the closed state as a function of time. In contrast, a transporter forms an intermediate complex with the substrate (solute), and subsequently a conformational change in the transporter induces translocation of the substrates to the other side of the membrane.

The turnover rate constants of typical channels are 10^6 to 10^8 s^{-1}; those of transporters are, at most, 10^1 to 10^3 s^{-1}. Because a particular transporter forms intermediate complexes with specific compounds (referred to as *substrates*), transporter-mediated membrane transport is characterized by saturability and inhibition by substrate analogs, as described in "Kinetics of Transport."

The basic mechanisms involved in solute transport across biological membranes include passive diffusion, facilitated diffusion, and active transport. Active transport can be further subdivided into primary and secondary active transport. These mechanisms are depicted in Figure 5–4.

PASSIVE DIFFUSION. Simple diffusion of a solute across the plasma membrane consists of 3 processes: partition from the aqueous to the lipid phase, diffusion across the lipid bilayer, and repartition into the aqueous phase on the opposite side. Diffusion of any solute (including drugs) occurs down an electrochemical potential gradient of the solute.

FACILITATED DIFFUSION. Diffusion of ions and organic compounds across the plasma membrane may be facilitated by a membrane transporter. Facilitated diffusion is a form of transporter-mediated membrane transport that does not require energy input. Just as in passive diffusion, the transport of ionized and nonionized compounds across the plasma membrane occurs down their electrochemical potential gradient. Therefore, steady state will be achieved when the electrochemical potentials of the compound on both sides of the membrane become equal.

ACTIVE TRANSPORT. Active transport is the form of membrane transport that requires the input of energy. It is the transport of solutes against their electrochemical gradients, leading to the concentration of solutes on

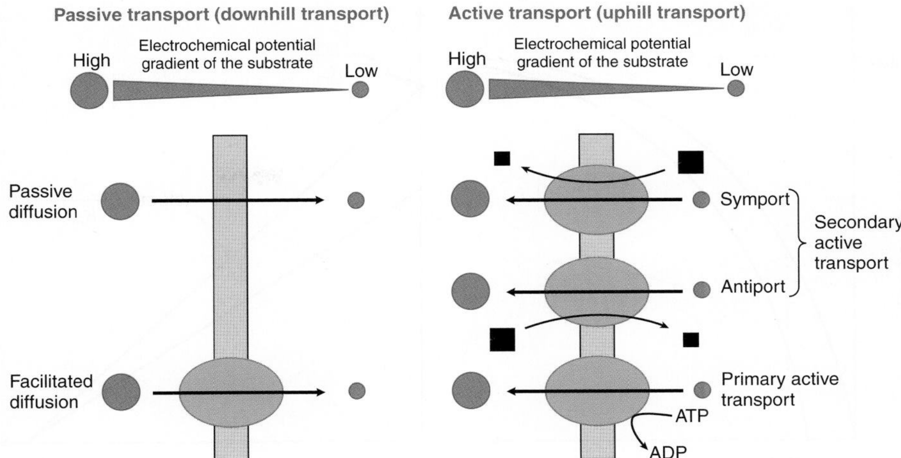

Figure 5–4 *Classification of membrane transport mechanisms. Red circles* depict the substrate. Size of the circles is proportional to the concentration of the substrate. *Arrows* show the direction of flux. *Black squares* represent the ion that supplies the driving force for transport (size is proportional to the concentration of the ion). *Blue ovals* depict transport proteins.

1 side of the plasma membrane and the creation of potential energy in the electrochemical gradient formed. Active transport plays an important role in the uptake and efflux of drugs and other solutes. Depending on the driving force, active transport can be subdivided into primary and secondary active transport (*see* Figure 5–4).

Primary Active Transport. Membrane transport that directly couples with ATP hydrolysis is called *primary active transport*. ABC transporters are examples of primary active transporters. In mammalian cells, ABC transporters mediate the unidirectional efflux of solutes across biological membranes.

Secondary Active Transport. In secondary active transport, the transport across a biological membrane of 1 solute S_1 against its concentration gradient is energetically driven by the transport of another solute S_2 in accordance with its concentration gradient. For example, an inwardly directed Na^+ concentration gradient across the plasma membrane is created by Na^+, K^+-ATPase. Under these conditions, inward movement of Na^+ produces the energy to drive the movement of a substrate S_1 against its concentration gradient by a secondary active transporter, as in Na^+/Ca^{2+} exchange. Depending on the transport direction of the solute, secondary active transporters are classified as either symporters or antiporters. *Symporters*, also termed *cotransporters*, transport S_2 and S_1 in the same direction, whereas *antiporters*, also termed *exchangers*, move their substrates in opposite directions (*see* Figure 5–4).

KINETICS OF TRANSPORT

The flux of a substrate (rate of transport) across a biological membrane *via* transporter-mediated processes is characterized by saturability. The relationship between the flux v and substrate concentration C in a transporter-mediated process is given by the Michaelis-Menten equation:

$$v = \frac{V_{max} C}{K_m + C} \qquad \text{(Equation 5–1)}$$

where V_{max} is the maximum transport rate and is proportional to the density of transporters on the plasma membrane, and K_m is the Michaelis constant, which represents the substrate concentration at which the flux is half the V_{max} value. K_m is an approximation of the dissociation constant of the substrate from the intermediate complex.

The K_m and V_{max} values can be determined by examining the flux at different substrate concentrations. The Eadie-Hofstee plot provides a graphical method for determining the V_{max} and K_m values (Figure 5–5).

$$\frac{v}{C} = \frac{V_{max}}{K_m} - \frac{C}{K_m} \qquad \text{(Equation 5–2)}$$

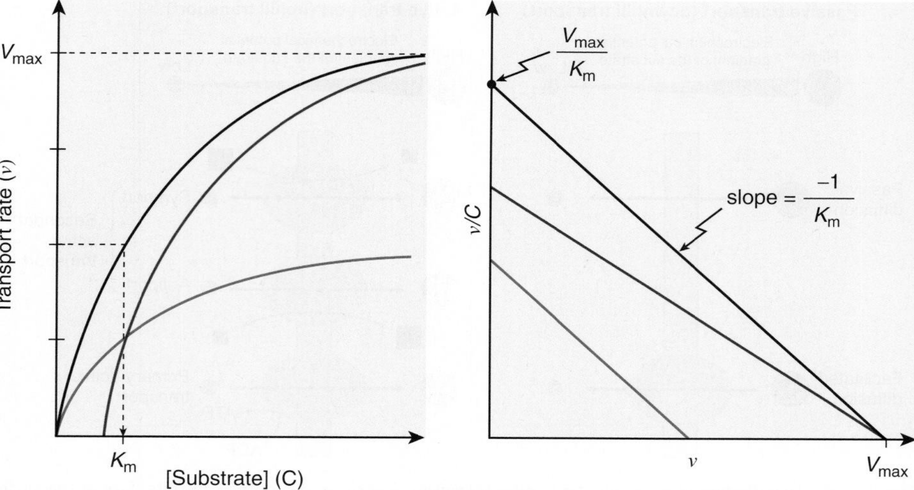

Figure 5–5 *Eadie-Hofstee plot of transport data.* The black lines show the hyperbolic concentration-dependence curve (v vs C, left panel) and the Eadie-Hofstee transformation of the transport data (v/C vs v, right panel) for a simple transport system. The blue lines depict transport in the presence of a competitive inhibitor (surmountable inhibition; achieves same V_{max}). The red lines depict the system in the presence of a noncompetitive inhibitor that reduces the number of transporting sites by half but leaves the K_m of the functional sites unchanged. Involvement of multiple transporters with different K_m values gives an Eadie-Hofstee plot that is curved. Algebraically, the Eadie-Hofstee plot of kinetic data is equivalent to the Scatchard plot of equilibrium binding data.

Transporter-mediated membrane transport of a substrate is also characterized by inhibition by other compounds. The manner of inhibition can be categorized as 1 of 3 types: *competitive*, *noncompetitive*, and *uncompetitive*. *Competitive* inhibition occurs when substrates and inhibitors share a common binding site on the transporter, resulting in an increase in the apparent K_m value in the presence of inhibitor. The flux of a substrate in the presence of a competitive inhibitor is

$$v = \frac{V_{max} C}{K_m(1 + I/K_i) + C} \qquad \text{(Equation 5–3)}$$

where I is the concentration of inhibitor, and K_i is the inhibition constant.

Noncompetitive inhibition assumes that the inhibitor has an allosteric effect on the transporter, does not inhibit the formation of an intermediate complex of substrate and transporter, but does inhibit the subsequent translocation process.

$$v = \frac{V_{max}/(1 + I/K_i) \cdot C}{K_m + C} \qquad \text{(Equation 5–4)}$$

Uncompetitive inhibition assumes that inhibitors can form a complex only with an intermediate complex of the substrate and transporter and inhibit subsequent translocation.

$$v = \frac{V_{max}/(1 + I/K_i) \cdot C}{K_m/(1 + I/K_i) + C} \qquad \text{(Equation 5–5)}$$

VECTORIAL TRANSPORT

Asymmetrical transport across a monolayer of polarized cells, such as the epithelial and endothelial cells of brain capillaries, is called *vectorial transport* (Figure 5–6). Vectorial transport is important for the absorption of nutrients and bile acids in the intestine. Vectorial transport plays a major role in hepatobiliary and urinary excretion of drugs from the blood to the lumen and in the intestinal absorption of drugs. In addition, efflux of drugs from the brain via brain endothelial cells and brain choroid plexus epithelial cells involves vectorial transport. The ABC transporters mediate only unidirectional efflux, whereas SLC transporters mediate either drug uptake or efflux. For lipophilic compounds that have sufficient membrane permeability, ABC transporters

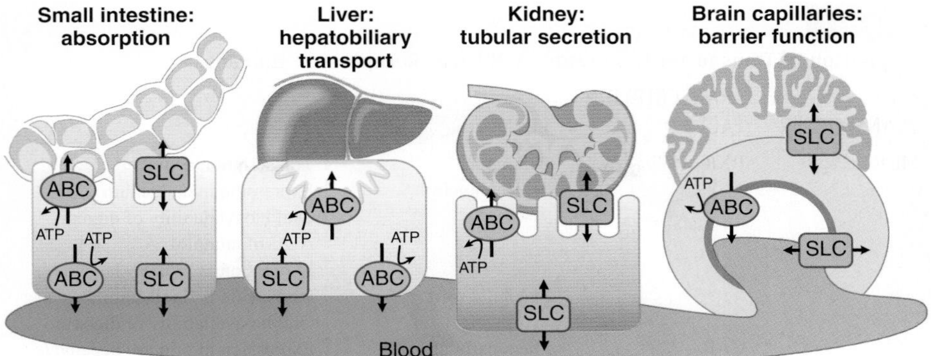

Figure 5–6 *Transepithelial and transendothelial flux.* Transepithelial or transendothelial flux of drugs requires distinct transporters at the 2 surfaces of the epithelial or endothelial barriers. These are depicted diagrammatically for transport across the small intestine (absorption), the kidney and liver (elimination), and the brain capillaries that comprise the blood-brain barrier.

alone are able to achieve vectorial transport without the help of influx transporters. For relatively hydrophilic organic anions and cations, coordinated uptake and efflux transporters in the polarized plasma membranes are necessary to achieve the vectorial movement of solutes across an epithelium. Common substrates of coordinated transporters are transferred efficiently across the epithelial barrier.

In the liver, a number of transporters with different substrate specificities are localized on the sinusoidal membrane (facing blood). These transporters are involved in the uptake of bile acids, amphipathic organic anions, and hydrophilic organic cations into the hepatocytes. Similarly, ABC transporters on the canalicular membrane (facing bile) export such compounds into the bile. Multiple combinations of uptake (OATP1B1, OATP1B3, OATP2B1) and efflux transporters (MDR1, MRP2, and BCRP) are involved in the efficient transcellular transport of a wide variety of compounds in the liver by using a model cell system called "doubly transfected cells," which express both uptake and efflux transporter on each side. In many cases, overlapping substrate specificities between the uptake transporters (OATP family) and efflux transporters (MRP family) make the vectorial transport of organic anions highly efficient. Similar transport systems also are present in the intestine, renal tubules, and endothelial cells of the brain capillaries (*see* Figure 5–6).

REGULATION OF TRANSPORTER EXPRESSION. Transporter expression can be regulated transcriptionally in response to drug treatment and pathophysiological conditions, resulting in induction or down-regulation of transporter mRNAs. Recent studies have described important roles of type II nuclear receptors, which form heterodimers with the 9-cis-retinoic acid receptor (RXR), in regulating drug-metabolizing enzymes and transporters (*see* Table 6–4 and Figure 6–8). Table 5–1 summarizes the effects of drug activation of type II nuclear receptors on expression of transporters.

DNA methylation is one mechanism underlying the epigenetic control of gene expression. Reportedly, the tissue-selective expression of transporters is achieved by DNA methylation (silencing in the transporter-negative tissues) as well as by transactivation in the transporter-positive tissues. Transporters subjected to epigenetic control include OAT3, URAT1, OCT2, Oatp1b2, Ntcp, and PEPT2 in the SLC families; and MDR1, BCRP, BSEP, and ABCG5/ABCG8.

TRANSPORTER STRUCTURE AND MECHANISM

Predictions of secondary structure of membrane transport proteins based on hydropathy analysis indicate that membrane transporters in the SLC and ABC superfamilies are multi-membrane-spanning proteins. ABC transporters have nucleotide-binding domains (NBDs) on the cytoplasmic side that may be thought of as the motor domains with conserved motifs (e.g., Walker-A motif, ABC signature motif) that participate in binding and hydrolysis of ATP. Crystal structures of ABC transporters show 2 NBDs in contact with each other. The ABC transport mechanism appears to involve binding of ATP to the NBDs, which triggers one conformation of the transporter; dissociation of the hydrolysis products of ATP results in a conformation open toward the opposite side of the membrane. In the case of drug extrusion, when ATP binds, the transporters open to the outside, releasing their substrates to the extracellular media; when the hydrolysis products dissociate, the transporter returns to the inward-facing conformation, permitting the binding of ATP and transportable substrate. Chapter 5 of the 12th edition of the parent text provides additional details.

Table 5–1

Regulation of Transporter Expression by Nuclear Receptors in Humans

TRANSPORTER	TRANSCRIPTION FACTOR	LIGAND	EFFECT
MDR1 (P-gp)	PXR	Rifampin (rifampicin)	↑ Transcription activity ↑ Expression in duodenum ↓ Oral bioavailability of digoxin ↓ AUC of talinolol ↑ Expression in primary hepatocye
		St John's wort	↑ Expression in duodenum ↓ Oral bioavailability of digoxin
	CAR	Phenobarbital	↑ Expression in primary hepatocye
MRP2	PXR	Rifampin	↑ Expression in duodenum
		Rifampin/hyperforin	↑ Expression in primary hepatocye
	FXR	GW4064/ chenodeoxycholate	↑ Expression in HepG2-FXR
	CAR	Phenobarbital	↑ Expression in hepatocye
BCRP	PXR CAR	Rifampin Phenobarbital	↑ Expression in primary hepatocyte
MRP3	PXR	Rifampin	↑ Expression in hepatocye
OATP1B1	SHP1	Cholic acid	Indirect effect on HNF1α expression
	PXR	Rifampin	↑ Expression in hepatocye
OATP1B3	FXR	Chenodeoxycholate	↑ Expression in Hepatoma cells
BSEP	FXR	Chenodeoxycholate	↑ Transcription activity
OSTα/β	FXR	Chenodeoxycholate/ GW4064	↑ Transcription activity
	FXR	Chenodeoxycholate	↑ Expression in ileal biopsies

See 12th edition of parent text for details and for examples from other mammals.

TRANSPORTER SUPERFAMILIES IN THE HUMAN GENOME

SLC TRANSPORTERS. The solute carrier (SLC) superfamily includes 48 families and represents ~315 genes in the human genome, some of which are associated with certain genetic diseases (Table 5–2). Transporters in the SLC superfamily transport diverse ionic and nonionic endogenous compounds and xenobiotics. SLC superfamily transporters may be facilitated transporters or secondary active symporters or antiporters.

ABC SUPERFAMILY. The 7 groups of ABC transporters are essential for many cellular processes, and mutations in at least 13 of the genes for ABC transporters cause or contribute to human genetic disorders (Table 5–3). In addition to conferring multidrug resistance, an important pharmacological aspect of these transporters is xenobiotic export from healthy tissues. In particular, MDR1/ABCB1, MRP2/ABCC2, and BCRP/ABCG2 have been shown to be involved in overall drug disposition.

The ABC superfamily includes 49 genes, each containing 1 or 2 conserved ABC regions. The ABC region is a core catalytic domain of ATP hydrolysis and contains Walker A and B sequences and an intervening ABC transporter-specific signature C sequence. The ABC regions of these proteins bind and hydrolyze ATP, and the proteins use the energy for uphill transport of their substrates across the membrane. Although some ABC superfamily transporters contain only a single ABC motif, they form homodimers (BCRP/ABCG2) or heterodimers (ABCG5 and ABCG8) that exhibit a transport function. ABC transporters (e.g., MsbA) in prokaryotes are involved in the import of essential compounds that cannot be obtained by passive diffusion (sugars, vitamins, metals, etc.). Most ABC genes in eukaryotes transport compounds from the cytoplasm to the outside or into an intracellular compartment (endoplasmic reticulum, mitochondria, peroxisomes).

Table 5–2

The Human Solute Carrier Superfamily

GENE	FAMILY	SELECTED DRUG SUBSTRATES	EXAMPLES OF LINKED HUMAN DISEASES
SLC1	Low-K_m glu/neutral aa T		ALS
SLC2	Facilitative GLUT		
SLC3	Heavy subunits, heteromeric aa Ts	Melphalan	Classic cystinuria I
SLC4	Bicarbonate T		Hemolytic anemia, blindness–auditory impairment
SLC5	Na^+ glucose co-T	Dapagliflozin	Gluc–gal malabsorption
SLC6	Na^+/Cl^--dependent neurotransmitter T	Paraoxetine, fluoxetine	X-linked creatine deficit
SLC7	Cationic aa T	Melphalan	Lysinuric protein intolerance
SLC8	Na^+/Ca^{2+} Exch	di-CH_3-arg	
SLC9	Na^+/H^+ Exch	Thiazide diuretics	Secretory diarrhea
SLC10	Na^+ bile salt co-T	Benzothiazepines	Bile salt malabsorp
SLC11	H^+ coupled metal ion T		Hereditary hemochromatosis
SLC12	Electroneutral cation–Cl^- co-T		Gitelman's syndrome
SLC13	Na^+–SO_4^-/COO^- co-T	SO_4^-/cys conjugates	
SLC14	Urea T		Kidd antigen blood group
SLC15	H^+–oligopeptide co-T	Valacyclovir	
SLC16	Monocarboxylate T	Salicylate, T_3/T_4 atorvastatin	Muscle weakness
SLC17	Vesicular glu T		Sialate storage disease
SLC18	Vesicular amine T	Reserpine	Myasthenic syndromes
SLC19	Folate/thiamine T	Methotrexate	Thiamine-responsive anemia
SLC20	Type III Na^+–PO_4^- co-T		
SLC21	Organic anion T	Pravastatin	
SLC22	Organic ion T	Pravastatin, metformin	Carnitine deficit
SLC23	Na^+-dependent ascorbate T	Vitamin C	
SLC24	$Na^+/(Ca^{2+}$-$K^+)$ Exch		
SLC25	Mitochondrial carrier		Senger's syndrome
SLC26	Multifunctional anion Exch	Salicylate, ciprofloxacin	Cl^--losing diarrhea
SLC27	Fatty acid T		
SLC28	Na^+-coupled nucleoside T	Gemcitabine, cladribine	
SLC29	Facilitative nucleoside T	Dipyridamole, gemcitabine	
SLC30	Zn efflux		
SLC31	Cu T	Cisplatin	
SLC32	Vesicular inhibitory aa T	Vigabatrin	
SLC33	Acetyl-CoA T		
SLC34	Type II Na^+–PO_4^-/ co-T		Hypophosphatemic rickets
SLC35	Nucleoside-sugar T		Leukocyte adhesion deficiency II
SLC36	H^+-coupled aa T	D-Serine, cycloserine	
SLC37	Sugar-phosphate/PO_4^- Exch		Glycogen storage disease
SLC38	Na^+-coupled neutral aa T		
SLC39	Metal ion T		Acrodermatitis enteropathica
SLC40	Basolateral Fe T		Hemochromatosis IV
SLC41	MgtE-like Mg^{2+} T		
SLC42	Rh ammonium T		Rh-null regulator
SLC43	Na^+-independent L-like aa T		

aa, amino acid; ALS, amytrophic lateral sclerosis; Exch, exchanger; T, Transporter.

Table 5–3

The ATP Binding Cassette (ABC) Superfamily in the Human Genome and Linked Genetic Diseases

GENE	FAMILY	NUMBER OF MEMBERS	EXAMPLES OF LINKED HUMAN DISEASES
ABCA	ABC A	12	Tangier disease (defect in cholesterol transport; ABCA1), Stargardt syndrome (defect in retinal metabolism; ABCA4)
ABCB	ABC B	11	Bare lymphocyte syndrome type 1 (defect in antigen-presenting; ABCB3 and ABCB4), progressive familial intrahepatic cholestasis type 3 (defect in biliary lipid secretion; MDR3/ABCB4), X-linked sideroblastic anemia with ataxia (a possible defect in iron homeostasis in mitochondria; ABCB7), progressive familial intrahepatic cholestasis type 2 (defect in biliary bile acid excretion; BSEP/ABCB11)
ABCC	ABC C	13	Dubin–Johnson syndrome (defect in biliary bilirubin glucuronide excretion; MRP2/ABCC2), pseudoxanthoma (unknown mechanism; ABCC6), cystic fibrosis (defect in Cl^- channel regulation; ABCC7), persistent hyperinsulinemic hypoglycemia of infancy (defect in inwardly rectifying K^+ conductance regulation in pancreatic B cells; SUR1)
ABCD	ABC D	4	Adrenoleukodystrophy (a possible defect in peroxisomal transport or catabolism of very long-chain fatty acids; ABCD1)
ABCE	ABC E	1	
ABCF	ABC F	3	
ABCG	ABC G	5	Sitosterolemia (defect in biliary and intestinal excretion of plant sterols; ABCG5 and ABCG8)

PROPERTIES OF ABC TRANSPORTERS RELATED TO DRUG ACTION

The tissue distribution of drug-related ABC transporters in humans is summarized in Table 5–4 together with information about typical substrates.

TISSUE DISTRIBUTION OF DRUG-RELATED ABC TRANSPORTERS. MDR1 (*ABCB1*), MRP2 (*ABCC2*), and BCRP (*ABCG2*) are all expressed in the apical side of the intestinal epithelia, where they serve to pump out xenobiotics, including many orally administered drugs. MRP3 (*ABCC3*) is expressed in the basal side of the epithelial cells.

Key to the vectorial excretion of drugs into urine or bile, ABC transporters are expressed in the polarized tissues of kidney and liver: MDR1, MRP2, and MRP4 (*ABCC4*) on the brush-border membrane of renal epithelia; MDR1, MRP2, and BCRP on the bile canalicular membrane of hepatocytes; and MRP3 and MRP4 on the sinusoidal membrane of hepatocytes. Some ABC transporters are expressed specifically on the blood side of the endothelial or epithelial cells that form barriers to the free entrance of toxic compounds into tissues: the BBB (MDR1 and MRP4 on the luminal side of brain capillary endothelial cells), the blood-cerebrospinal fluid (CSF) barrier (MRP1 and MRP4 on the basolateral blood side of choroid plexus epithelia), the blood-testis barrier (MRP1 on the basolateral membrane of mouse Sertoli cells and MDR1 in several types of human testicular cells), and the blood-placenta barrier (MDR1, MRP2, and BCRP on the luminal maternal side and MRP1 on the antiluminal fetal side of placental trophoblasts).

MRP/ABCC FAMILY. The substrates of transporters in the MRP/ABCC family are mostly organic anions. Both MRP1 and MRP2 accept glutathione and glucuronide conjugates, sulfated conjugates of bile salts, and nonconjugated organic anions of an amphipathic nature (at least 1 negative charge and some degree of hydrophobicity). They also transport neutral or cationic anticancer drugs, such as vinca alkaloids and anthracyclines, possibly by means of a cotransport or symport mechanism with reduced glutathione. MRP3

Table 5–4

ABC Transporters Involved in Drug Absorption, Distribution, and Excretion Processes

NAME	SUBSTRATES
MDR1 (ABCB1)	**Characteristics:** Bulky neutral or cationic compounds (many xenobiotics) etoposide, doxorubicin, vincristine; diltiazem, verapamil; indinavir, ritonavir; erythromycin, ketoconazole; testosterone, progesterone; cyclosporine, tacrolimus; digoxin, quinidine, fexofenadine, loperamide
MRP1 (ABCC1)	**Characteristics:** Negatively charged amphiphiles vincristine (with GSH), methotrexate; GSH conjugate of LTC_4, ethacrynic acid; glucuronide of estradiol, bilirubin; estrone-3-sulfate; saquinavir; grepafloxacin; folate, GSH, GS-SG
MRP2 (ABCC2)	**Characteristics:** Negatively charged amphiphiles methotrexate, vincristine; GSH conjugates of LTC_4, ethacrynic acid; glucuronides of estradiol, bilirubin; taurolithocholate sulfate; statins, AngII receptor antagonists, temocaprilat; indinavir, ritonavir; GSH, GS-SG
MRP3 (ABCC3)	**Characteristics:** Negatively charged amphiphile etoposide, methotrexate; GSH conjugates of LTC_4, PGJ_2; glucuronides of estradiol, etoposide, morphine, acetaminophen, hymecromone, harmol; sulfate conjugates of bile salts; glycocholate, taurocholate; folate, leucovorin
MRP4 (ABCC4)	**Characteristics:** Nucleotide analogs 6-mercaptopurine, methotrexate; estradiol glucuronide; dehydroepiandrosterone sulfate; cyclic AMP/GMP; furosemide, trichlormethiazide; adefovir, tenofovir; cefazolin, ceftizoxime; folate, leucovorin, taurocholate (with GSH)
MRP5 (ABCC5)	**Characteristics:** Nucleotide analogs 6-mercaptopurine; cyclic AMP/GMP; adefovir
MRP6 (ABCC6)	doxorubicin*, etoposide*; GSH conjugate of LTC_4; BQ-123 (cyclic peptide)
BCRP (MXR) (ABCG2)	methotrexate, mitoxantrone, camptothecins, SN-38, topotecan, imatinib; glucuronides of 4-methylumbelliferone, estradiol; sulfate conjugates of dehydroepiandrosterone, estrone; nitrofurantoin, fluoroquinolones; pitavastatin, rosuvastatin; cholesterol, estradiol, dantrolene, prazosin, sulfasalazine
MDR3 (ABCB4)	**Characteristics:** Phospholipids
BSEP (ABCB11)	**Characteristics:** Bile salts
ABCG5, G8	**Characteristics:** Plant sterols

**indicates substrates and cytotoxic drugs with increased resistance (cytotoxicity with increased resistance is usually caused by the decreased accumulation of the drugs). Although MDR3 (ABCB4), BSEP (ABCB11), ABCG5 and ABCG8 are not directly involved in drug disposition, their inhibition will lead to unfavorable side effects.*

also has a substrate specificity that is similar to that of MRP2 but with a lower transport affinity for glutathione conjugates compared with MRP1 and MRP2. MRP3 is expressed on the sinusoidal side of hepatocytes and is induced under cholestatic conditions. MRP3 functions to return toxic bile salts and bilirubin glucuronides into the blood circulation. MRP4 accepts negatively charged molecules, including cytotoxic compounds (e.g., 6-mercaptopurine and methotrexate), cyclic nucleotides, antiviral drugs (e.g., adefovir and tenofovir), diuretics (e.g., furosemide and trichlormethiazide), and cephalosporins (e.g., ceftizoxime and cefazolin). Glutathione enables MRP4 to accept taurocholate and leukotriene B_4. MRP5 has a narrower substrate specificity and accepts nucleotide analog and clinically important anti–human immunodeficiency virus (HIV) drugs. No substrates have been identified that explain the mechanism of the MRP6-associated disease, pseudoxanthoma.

BCRP/ABCG2. BCRP accepts both neutral and negatively charged molecules, including cytotoxic compounds (e.g., topotecan, flavopiridol, and methotrexate), sulfated conjugates of therapeutic drugs and hormones (e.g., estrogen sulfate), antibiotics (e.g., nitrofurantoin and fluoroquinolones), statins (e.g., pitavastatin and rosuvastatin), and toxic compounds found in normal food [phytoestrogens, 2-amino-1-methyl-6-phenylimidazo[4,5-*b*]pyridine (PhIP) and pheophorbide A, a chlorophyll catabolite].

ABC TRANSPORTERS IN DRUG ABSORPTION AND ELIMINATION. With respect to clinical medicine, MDR1 is the most important ABC transporter yet identified. The systemic exposure to orally administered digoxin is decreased by coadministration of rifampin (an MDR1 inducer) and is negatively correlated with the MDR1 protein expression in the human intestine. MDR1 is also expressed on the brush-border membrane of renal epithelia, and its function can be monitored using digoxin (>70% excreted in the urine). MDR1 inhibitors (e.g., quinidine, verapamil, valspodar, spironolactone, clarithromycin, and ritonavir) all markedly reduce renal excretion of digoxin. Drugs with narrow therapeutic windows (e.g., digoxin, cyclosporine, tacrolimus) should be used with great care if MDR1-based drug-drug interactions are likely.

In the intestine, MRP3 can mediate the intestinal absorption in conjunction with uptake transporters. MRP3 mediates sinusoidal efflux in the liver, decreasing the efficacy of the biliary excretion from the blood, and excretion of intracellularly formed metabolites, particularly, glucuronide conjugates. Thus, dysfunction of MRP3 results in a shortening of the elimination $t_{1/2}$. MRP4 substrates also can be transported by OAT1 and OAT3 on the basolateral membrane of the epithelial cells in the kidney. The rate-limiting process in renal tubular secretion is likely the uptake process at the basolateral surface. Dysfunction of MRP4 enhances the renal concentration, but has limited impact on the blood concentration.

GENETIC VARIATION IN MEMBRANE TRANSPORTERS: IMPLICATIONS FOR CLINICAL DRUG RESPONSE

There are inherited defects in SLC transporters (*see* Table 5–2) and ABC transporters (*see* Table 5–3). Polymorphisms in membrane transporters play a role in drug response and are yielding new insights in pharmacogenetics (*see* Chapter 7).

Clinical studies have focused on a limited number of transporters, relating genetic variation in membrane transporters to drug disposition and response. For example, 2 common single-nucleotide polymorphisms (SNPs) in *SLCO1B1* (OATP1B1) have been associated with elevated plasma levels of pravastatin, a widely used drug for the treatment of hypercholesterolemia. Recent studies using genome-wide association methods have determined that genetic variants in SLCO1B1 (OATP1B1) predispose patients to risk for muscle toxicity associated with use of simvastatin. Other studies indicate that genetic variants in transporters in the SLC22A family associate with variation in renal clearance and response to various drugs including the antidiabetic drug, metformin.

TRANSPORTERS INVOLVED IN PHARMACOKINETICS

Drug transporters play a prominent role in pharmacokinetics (*see* Figure 5–1 and Table 5–4). Transporters in the liver and kidney have important roles in removal of drugs from the blood and hence in metabolism and excretion.

HEPATIC TRANSPORTERS

Hepatic uptake of organic anions (e.g., drugs, leukotrienes, and bilirubin), cations, and bile salts is mediated by SLC-type transporters in the basolateral (sinusoidal) membrane of hepatocytes: OATPs (SLCO) and OATs (SLC22), OCTs (SLC22), and NTCP (SLC10A1), respectively. These transporters mediate uptake by either facilitated or secondary active mechanisms.

ABC transporters such as MRP2, MDR1, BCRP, BSEP, and MDR2 in the bile canalicular membrane of hepatocytes mediate the efflux (excretion) of drugs and their metabolites, bile salts, and phospholipids against a steep concentration gradient from liver to bile. This primary active transport is driven by ATP hydrolysis.

Vectorial transport of drugs from the circulating blood to the bile using an uptake transporter (OATP family) and an efflux transporter (MRP2) is important for determining drug exposure in the circulating blood and liver. Moreover, there are many other uptake and efflux transporters in the liver (Figures 5–7 and 5–8).

The following examples illustrate the importance of vectorial transport in determining drug exposure in the circulating blood and liver and the role of transporters in drug-drug interactions.

HMG-CoA REDUCTASE INHIBITORS. Statins are cholesterol-lowering agents that reversibly inhibit HMG-CoA reductase, which catalyzes a rate-limiting step in cholesterol biosynthesis (*see* Chapter 31). Most of the statins in the acid form are substrates of uptake transporters, so they are taken up efficiently by the liver and

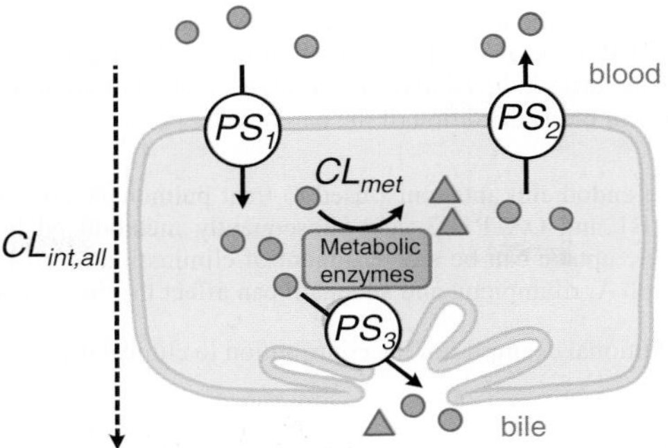

Figure 5–7 *Hepatic uptake, backflux into blood, metabolism, and efflux into bile.* The *red circles* represent parent drugs; the *green triangles* represent drug metabolites. PS, permeability surface product; CL_{met}, metabolic clearance; CL_{int}, intrinsic clearance.

undergo enterohepatic circulation (*see* Figures 5–5 and 5–8). In this process, hepatic uptake transporters such as OATP1B1 and efflux transporters such as MRP2 act cooperatively to produce vectorial trans-cellular transport of bisubstrates in the liver. The efficient first-pass hepatic uptake of these statins by OATP1B1 helps them to exert their pharmacological effect and also minimizes the systemic drug distribution, thereby minimizing adverse effects in smooth muscle. Recent studies indicate that the genetic polymorphism of OATP1B1 also affects the function of this transporter.

GEMFIBROZIL. The cholesterol-lowering agent gemfibrozil, a PPARa activator, can enhance toxicity (myopathy) to several statins by a mechanism that involves transport. Gemfibrozil inhibits the uptake of the active hydroxy forms of statins into hepatocytes by OATP1B1, resulting in an increase in the plasma concentration of the statin.

IRINOTECAN (CPT-11). Irinotecan hydrochloride (CPT-11) is a potent anticancer drug, but late-onset gastrointestinal toxic effects, such as severe diarrhea, make it difficult to use CPT-11 safely. After intravenous administration, CPT-11 is converted to SN-38, an active metabolite, by carboxylesterase. SN-38 is subsequently

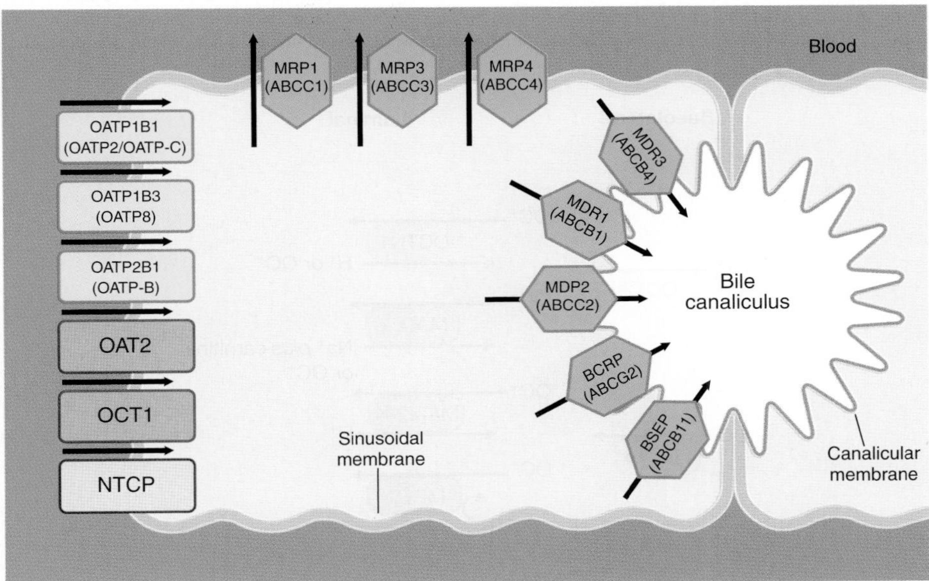

Figure 5–8 *Transporters in the hepatocyte that function in the uptake and efflux of drugs across the sinusoidal membrane and efflux of drugs into the bile across the canalicular membrane.* See text for details of the transporters pictured.

conjugated with glucuronic acid in the liver. SN-38 and SN-38 glucuronide are then excreted into the bile by MRP2. The inhibition of MRP2-mediated biliary excretion of SN-38 and its glucuronide by coadministration of probenecid reduces the drug-induced diarrhea, at least in rats. For additional details, *see* Figures 6–5 and 6–6; *see* also Figure 6–7 in the 12th edition of the parent text.

BOSENTAN. Bosentan is an endothelin antagonist used to treat pulmonary arterial hypertension. It is taken up in the liver by OATP1B1 and OATP1B3, and subsequently metabolized by CYP2C9 and CYP3A4. Transporter-mediated hepatic uptake can be a determinant of elimination of bosentan, and the inhibition of hepatic uptake by cyclosporin A, rifampicin, and sildenafil can affect its pharmacokinetics.

The parent text contains additional examples of the contribution to clinical drug use of vectorial transport and its genetic variability.

RENAL TRANSPORTERS

ORGANIC CATION TRANSPORT. Structurally diverse organic cations are secreted in the proximal tubule. A primary function of organic cation secretion is ridding the body of xenobiotics, including many positively charged drugs and their metabolites (e.g., cimetidine, ranitidine, metformin, procainamide, and *N*-acetylprocainamide) and toxins from the environment (e.g., nicotine). Organic cations that are secreted by the kidney may be either hydrophobic or hydrophilic. Hydrophilic organic drug cations generally have molecular weights < 400 daltons; a current model for their secretion in the proximal tubule of the nephron is shown in Figure 5–9, involving the transporters described below.

For the transepithelial flux of a compound (e.g., secretion), the compound must traverse 2 membranes sequentially, the basolateral membrane facing the blood side and the apical membrane facing the tubular lumen. Organic cations appear to cross the basolateral membrane in human proximal tubule by 2 distinct transporters in the SLC family 22 (SCL22): OCT2 (*SLC22A2*) and OCT3 (*SLC22A3*). Organic cations are transported across this membrane down an electrochemical gradient.

Transport of organic cations from cell to tubular lumen across the apical membrane occurs through an electroneutral proton–organic cation exchange. The recent discovery of a new transporter family, SLC47A, *m*ultidrug *a*nd *t*oxin *e*xtrusion family (MATEs), has provided the molecular identities of the previously characterized electroneutral proton–organic cation antiport mechanism. Transporters in the MATE family, assigned to the apical membrane of the proximal tubule, appear to play a key role in moving hydrophilic organic cations from tubule cell to lumen. In addition, *novel organic cation transporters* (OCTNs), located on the apical membrane, appear to contribute to organic cation flux across the proximal tubule. In humans, these include OCTN1 (*SLC22A4*) and OCTN2 (*SLC22A5*). These bifunctional transporters are involved not only in organic cation

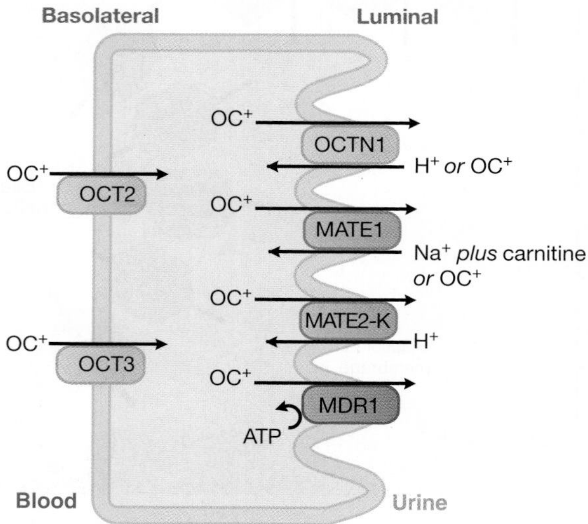

Figure 5–9 *Organic cation secretory transporters in the proximal tubule.* OC+, organic cation. See text for details of the transporters pictured.

secretion but also in carnitine reabsorption. In the reuptake mode, the transporters function as Na^+ cotransporters, relying on the inwardly driven Na^+ gradient created by Na^+,K^+-ATPase to move carnitine from tubular lumen to cell. In the secretory mode, the transporters appear to function as proton–organic cation exchangers. That is, protons move from tubular lumen to cell interior in exchange for organic cations, which move from cytosol to tubular lumen. The inwardly directed proton gradient (from tubular lumen to cytosol) is maintained by transporters in the SLC9 family, which are Na^+/H^+ exchangers (NHEs, antiporters). Of the 2 steps involved in secretory transport, transport across the luminal membrane appears to be rate-limiting.

OCT2 *(SLC22A2)*. Human, mouse, and rat orthologs of OCT2 are expressed in abundance in human kidney and to some extent in neuronal tissue such as choroid plexus. In the kidney, OCT2 is localized to the proximal tubule and to distal tubules and collecting ducts. In the proximal tubule, OCT2 is restricted to the basolateral membrane. OCT2-mediated transport of model organic cations MPP^+ and TEA is electrogenic, and both OCT2 and OCT1 can support organic cation–organic cation exchange. OCT2 generally accepts a wide array of monovalent organic cations with molecular weights < 400 daltons. OCT2 is also present in neuronal tissues; however, monoamine neurotransmitters have low affinities for OCT2.

OCT3 *(SLC22A3)*. OCT3 is located in tandem with OCT1 and OCT2 on chromosome 6. Tissue distribution studies suggest that human OCT3 is expressed in liver, kidney, intestine, and placenta, although it appears to be expressed in considerably less abundance than OCT2 in the kidney. Like OCT1 and OCT2, OCT3 appears to support electrogenic potential-sensitive organic cation transport. OCT3 may play only a limited role in renal drug elimination.

OCTN1 *(SLC22A4)*. OCTN1 seems to operate as an organic cation–proton exchanger. OCTN1-mediated influx of model organic cations is enhanced at alkaline pH, whereas efflux is increased by an inwardly directed proton gradient. OCTN1 contains a nucleotide-binding sequence motif, and transport of its substrates appears to be stimulated by cellular ATP. OCTN1 also can function as an organic cation–organic cation exchanger. OCTN1 functions as a bidirectional pH- and ATP-dependent transporter at the apical membrane in renal tubular epithelial cells.

OCTN2 *(SLC22A5)*. OCTN2 is a bifunctional transporter, it functions as both a Na^+-dependent carnitine transporter and a Na^+-independent organic cation transporter. OCTN2 transport of organic cations is sensitive to pH, suggesting that OCTN2 may function as an organic cation exchanger. The transport of *L*-carnitine by OCTN2 is a Na^+-dependent electrogenic process, and mutations in OCTN2 appear to be the cause of primary systemic carnitine deficiency.

MATE1 AND MATE2-K (*SLC47A1* AND *SLC47A2*). Multidrug and toxin extrusion family members MATE1 and MATE2-K interact with structurally diverse hydrophilic organic cations including the antidiabetic drug metformin, the H_2 antagonist cimetidine, and the anticancer drug, topotecan. In addition to cationic compounds, the transporters also recognize some anions, including the antiviral agents acyclovir and ganciclovir. The zwitterions cephalexin and cephradine are specific substrates of MATE1. The herbicide paraquat, a bisquaternary ammonium compound, which is nephrotoxic in humans, is a potent substrate of MATE1. Both MATE1 and MATE2-K have been localized to the apical membrane of the proximal tubule. MATE1, but not MATE2-K, is also expressed on the canalicular membrane of the hepatocyte. These transporters appear to be the long-searched-for organic cation–proton antiporters on the apical membrane of the proximal tubule, that is, an oppositely directed proton gradient can drive the movement of organic cations via MATE1 or MATE2-K. The antibiotics, levofloxacin and ciprofloxacin, though potent inhibitors, are not translocated by either MATE1 or MATE2-K.

Polymorphisms of OCTs. OCT1 exhibits the greatest number of amino acid polymorphisms, followed by OCT2 and then OCT3. Recent studies suggest that genetic variants of OCT1 and OCT2 are associated with alterations in the renal elimination and response to the anti-diabetic drug, metformin.

ORGANIC ANION TRANSPORT. The primary function of organic anion secretion appears to be the removal from the body of xenobiotics, including many weakly acidic drugs (e.g., pravastatin, captopril, *p*-aminohippurate [PAH], and penicillins) and toxins (e.g., ochratoxin). Organic anion transporters move both hydrophobic and hydrophilic anions but also may interact with cations and neutral compounds. A current model for the transepithelial flux of organic anions in the proximal tubule is shown in Figure 5–10.

OAT1 *(SLC22A6)*. Mammalian isoforms of OAT1 are expressed primarily in the kidney, with some expression in brain and skeletal muscle. OAT1 generally transports small-molecular-weight organic anions that may be endogenous (e.g., PGE_2 and urate) or ingested drugs and toxins.

OAT2 *(SLC22A7)*. OAT2 is present in both kidney and liver. In the kidney, the transporter is localized to the basolateral membrane of the proximal tubule, and appears to function as a transporter for nucleotides, particularly guanine nucleotides such as cyclic GMP.

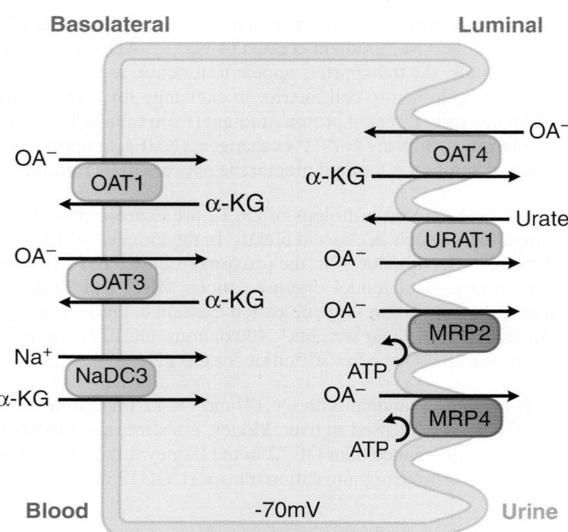

Figure 5–10 *Organic anion secretory transporters in the proximal tubule.* Two primary transporters on the basolateral membrane mediate the flux of organic anions from interstitial fluid to tubule cell: OAT1 (*SLC22A6*) and OAT3 (*SLC22A8*). Hydrophilic organic anions are transported across the basolateral membrane against an electrochemical gradient in exchange with intracellular α-ketoglutarate, which moves down its concentration gradient from cytosol to blood. The outwardly directed gradient of α-ketoglutarate is maintained at least in part by a basolateral Na^+-dicarboxylate uptake transporter (NaDC3). The Na^+ gradient that drives NaDC3 is maintained by Na^+,K^+-ATPase. OA, organic anion; α-KG, α-ketoglutarate.

OAT3 *(SLC22A8)*. OAT3 transports a wide variety of organic anions, including model compounds, PAH and estrone sulfate, as well as many drug products (e.g., pravastatin, cimetidine, 6-mercaptopurine, and methotrexate).

OAT4 *(SLC22A9)*. In humans, OAT4 is expressed in placenta and kidney (on the luminal membrane of the proximal tubule). Organic anion transport by OAT4 can be stimulated by transgradients of α-ketoglutarate, suggesting that OAT4 may be involved in the reabsorption of organic anions from tubular lumen into cell.

OTHER ANION TRANSPORTERS. URAT1 (*SLC22A12*) is a kidney-specific transporter confined to the apical membrane of the proximal tubule. URAT1 is primarily responsible for urate reabsorption, mediating electroneutral urate transport that can be trans-stimulated by Cl^-gradients. NPT1 (*SLC17A1*) is expressed on the luminal membrane of the proximal tubule as well as in the brain. NPT1 transports PAH, probenecid, and penicillin G. It appears to be part of the system involved in organic anion efflux from tubule cell to lumen.

MRP2 (*ABCC2*) is considered to be the primary transporter involved in efflux of many drug conjugates such as glutathione conjugates across the canalicular membrane of the hepatocyte. However, MRP2 is also found on the apical membrane of the proximal tubule, where it is thought to play a role in the efflux of organic anions into the tubular lumen. In general, MRP2 transports larger, bulkier compounds than do most of the organic anion transporters in the SLC22 family. MRP4 (*ABCC4*), localized on the apical membrane of the proximal tubule, transports a wide array of conjugated anions, including glucuronide and glutathione conjugates. MRP4 appears to interact with drugs, including methotrexate, cyclic nucleotide analogs, and antiviral nucleoside analogs.

Polymorphisms of OATs. Polymorphisms in OAT1 and OAT3 have been identified in ethnically diverse human populations.

TRANSPORTERS AND PHARMACODYNAMICS: DRUG ACTION IN THE BRAIN

Neurotransmitters are packaged in vesicles in presynpatic neurons, released in the synapse by fusion of the vesicles with the plasma membrane, and, excepting acetylcholine, are then taken back into the presynpatic neurons or postsynaptic cells (*see* Chapter 8). Transporters involved in the neuronal reuptake of the neurotransmitters and the regulation of their levels in the synaptic cleft belong to 2 major superfamilies, SLC1 and SLC6. Transporters in both families play roles in reuptake of γ-aminobutyric acid (GABA), glutamate, and the monoamine neurotransmitters norepinephrine (NE), serotonin (5HT), and dopamine (DA). These transporters may serve as pharmacologic targets for neuropsychiatric drugs. SLC6 family members localized in the brain and involved in the reuptake of neurotransmitters into presynaptic neurons include the NE transporter (NET, *SLC6A2*), the DA transporter (DAT, *SLC6A3*), the serotonin transporter (SERT, *SLC6A4*), and several GABA reuptake transporters (GAT1, GAT2, and GAT3).

SLC6 family members depend on the Na^+ gradient to actively transport their substrates into cells. Cl^- is also required, although to a variable extent depending on the family member. Through reuptake mechanisms, the neurotransmitter transporters in the SLC6A family regulate the concentrations and dwell times of neurotransmitters in the synaptic cleft; the extent of transmitter uptake also influences subsequent vesicular storage of transmitters. Many of these transporters are present in other tissues (e.g., kidney and platelets) and may serve other roles. Further, the transporters can function in the reverse direction. That is, the transporters can export neurotransmitters in a Na^+-independent fashion.

SLC6A1 (GAT1), _SLC6A11_ (GAT3), AND _SLC6A13_ (GAT2). GAT1 is the most important GABA transporter in the brain, expressed in GABAergic neurons and found largely on presynaptic neurons. GAT1 is found in abundance in the neocortex, cerebellum, basal ganglia, brainstem, spinal cord, retina, and olfactory bulb. GAT3 is found only in the brain, largely in glial cells. GAT2 is found in peripheral tissues, including the kidney and liver, and within the CNS in the choroid plexus and meninges. Physiologically, GAT1 appears to be responsible for regulating the interaction of GABA at receptors. The presence of GAT2 in the choroid plexus and its absence in presynaptic neurons suggest that this transporter may play a primary role in maintaining the homeostasis of GABA in the CSF. GAT1 is the target of the antiepileptic drug tiagabine, which presumably acts to increase GABA levels in the synaptic cleft of GABAergic neurons by inhibiting the reuptake of GABA. GAT3 is the target for the nipecotic acid derivatives that are anticonvulsants.

SLC6A2 (NET). NET is found in central and peripheral nervous tissues as well as in adrenal chromaffin tissue. NET colocalizes with neuronal markers, consistent with a role in reuptake of monoamine neurotransmitters. The transporter functions in the Na^+-dependent reuptake of NE and DA. NET limits the synaptic dwell time of NE and terminate its actions, salvaging NE for subsequent repackaging. NET participates in the regulation of many neurological functions, including memory and mood. NET serves as a drug target for the antidepressant desipramine, other tricyclic antidepressants, and cocaine. Orthostatic intolerance, a rare familial disorder characterized by an abnormal blood pressure and heart rate response to changes in posture, has been associated with a mutation in NET.

SLC6A3 (DAT). DAT is located primarily in the brain in dopaminergic neurons. The primary function of DAT is the reuptake of DA, terminating its actions. Although present on presynaptic neurons at the neurosynaptic junction, DAT is also present in abundance along the neurons, away from the synaptic cleft, suggesting that DAT may play a role in clearance of excess DA in the vicinity of neurons. Physiologically, DAT is involved in functions attributed to the dopaminergic system, including mood, behavior, reward, and cognition. Drugs that interact with DAT include cocaine and its analogs, amphetamines, and the neurotoxin MPTP.

SLC6A4 (SERT). SERT plays a role in the reuptake and clearance of serotonin in the brain. Like the other SLC6A family members, SERT transports its substrates in a Na^+-dependent fashion and is dependent on Cl^- and possibly on the countertransport of K^+. Substrates of SERT include 5HT, various tryptamine derivatives, and neurotoxins such as 3,4-methylenedioxymethamphetamine (MDMA; ecstasy) and fenfluramine. SERT is the specific target of the selective serotonin reuptake inhibitor antidepressants (e.g., fluoxetine and paroxetine) and 1 of several targets of tricyclic antidepressants (e.g., amitriptyline). Genetic variants of SERT have been associated with an array of behavioral and neurological disorders. The precise mechanism by which a reduced activity of SERT, caused by either a genetic variant or an antidepressant, ultimately affects behavior, including depression, is not known.

BLOOD-BRAIN BARRIER AND BLOOD-CEREBROSPINAL FLUID BARRIER

Drugs acting in the CNS have to cross the BBB or blood-CSF barrier, which are formed by brain capillary endothelial cells and epithelial cells of the choroid plexus, respectively. These are not static anatomical barriers but dynamic ones in which efflux transporters play a role. P-glycoprotein extrudes its substrate drugs on the luminal membrane of the brain capillary endothelial cells into the blood, thereby, limiting the brain penetration. Thus, recognition by P-glycoprotein as a substrate is a major disadvantage for drugs used to treat CNS diseases. Other transporters involved in the efflux of organic anions from the CNS are being identified in the BBB and the blood-CSF barrier and include the members of OATP1A4 and OATP1A5 and OAT3 families. They mediate the uptake of organic compounds such as β-lactam antibiotics, statins, *p*-aminohippurate, H_2 receptor antagonists, and bile acids on the plasma membrane facing the brain-CSF. Further clarification of influx and efflux transporters in the barriers will enable delivery of CNS drugs efficiently into the brain while avoiding undesirable CNS side effects.

For a complete Bibliographical Listing see Goodman & Gilman's ***The Pharmacological Basis of Therapeutics***, 12th ed., or Goodman & Gilman Online at www.AccessMedicine.com.

Drug Metabolism

COPING WITH EXPOSURE TO XENOBIOTICS

Substances foreign to the body, or *xenobiotics*, are metabolized by the same enzymatic pathways and transport systems that are used for normal metabolism of dietary constituents. Drugs are considered xenobiotics and most are extensively metabolized in humans. The capacity to metabolize xenobiotics has made development of drugs very time consuming and costly due in large part to:

- *Interindividual variations in the capacity of humans to metabolize drugs*
- *Drug-drug interactions*
- *Metabolic activation of chemicals to toxic and carcinogenic derivatives*
- *Species differences in expression of enzymes that metabolize drugs, thereby limiting the use of animal models to predict effects in humans*

Most xenobiotics are subjected to 1 or multiple enzymatic pathways that constitute *phase 1 oxidation* and *phase 2 conjugation*. Metabolism serves to convert these hydrophobic chemicals into more hydrophilic derivatives that can easily be eliminated from the body through the urine or the bile.

Many drugs are hydrophobic, a property that allows entry through the lipid bilayers into cells where the agents can interact with their target receptors or proteins. This property of hydrophobicity renders drugs difficult to eliminate, because in the absence of metabolism, they accumulate in fat and cellular phospholipid bilayers in cells. The xenobiotic-metabolizing enzymes convert drugs and other xenobiotics into derivatives that are more hydrophilic and thus easily eliminated through excretion into the aqueous compartments of the tissues.

Drug metabolism that leads to elimination also plays a major role in diminishing the biological activity of a drug. For example, *(S)-phenytoin*, an anticonvulsant used in the treatment of epilepsy, is virtually insoluble in water. Metabolism by the phase 1 cytochromes P450 (CYPs) followed by phase 2 uridine diphosphate-glucuronosyltransferases (UGTs) produces a metabolite that is highly water soluble and readily eliminated from the body (Figure 6–1). Metabolism also terminates the biological activity of the drug.

Paradoxically, these drug metabolizing enzymes can also convert certain chemicals to highly reactive, toxic, and carcinogenic metabolites or *carcinogens*. Depending on the structure of the chemical substrate, xenobiotic-metabolizing enzymes can produce electrophilic metabolites that react with nucleophilic cellular macromolecules such as DNA, RNA, and protein. Reaction of these electrophiles with DNA can sometimes result in cancer through the mutation of genes, such as oncogenes or tumor suppressor genes. This potential for carcinogenic activity makes testing the safety of drug candidates of vital importance, particularly for drugs that will be used chronically.

THE PHASES OF DRUG METABOLISM

Xenobiotic metabolizing enzymes are grouped into those that carry out: *phase 1 reactions*, which include oxidation, reduction, or hydrolytic reactions; and the *phase 2 reactions*, in which enzymes catalyze the conjugation of the substrate (the phase 1 product) with a second molecule (Table 6–1). *Oxidation by phase 1 enzymes adds or exposes a functional group, permitting the products of phase 1 metabolism to serve as substrates for the phase 2 conjugating or synthetic enzymes.* While many phase 1 reactions result in the biological inactivation of the drug, phase 2 reactions produce a metabolite with improved water solubility, thereby facilitating drug elimination. The example of phase 1 and phase 2 metabolism of phenytoin is shown in Figure 6–1.

The *phase 1 enzymes* lead to the introduction of functional groups such as –OH, –COOH, –SH, –O–, or NH_2. *The phase 1 oxidation reactions* are carried out by CYPs, flavin-containing monooxygenases (FMOs), and epoxide hydrolases (EHs).

CYPs and FMOs comprise superfamilies of enzymes containing multiple genes. The addition of functional groups does little to increase the water solubility of the drug, but can dramatically alter the biological properties of the drug. Reactions carried out by phase 1 enzymes usually lead to the inactivation of a drug. However,

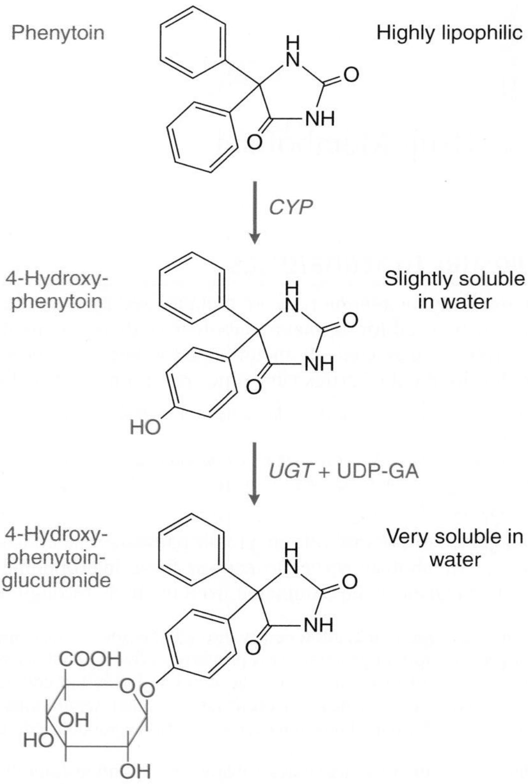

Phenytoin — Highly lipophilic

CYP

4-Hydroxy-phenytoin — Slightly soluble in water

UGT + UDP-GA

4-Hydroxy-phenytoin-glucuronide — Very soluble in water

COOH O O OH HO OH

Figure 6–1 *Metabolism of phenytoin by phase 1 cytochrome P450 (CYP) and phase 2 uridine diphosphate-glucuronosyltransferase (UGT).* CYP facilitates 4-hydroxylation of phenytoin. The hydroxy group serves as a substrate for UGT that conjugates a molecule of glucuronic acid (in green) using UDP-glucuronic acid (UDP-GA) as a cofactor. This converts a very hydrophobic molecule to a larger hydrophilic derivative that is eliminated via the bile.

Table 6–1

Xenobiotic Metabolizing Enzymes

ENZYMES	REACTIONS
Phase 1 "oxygenases"	
Cytochrome P450s (P450 or CYP)	C and O oxidation, dealkylation, others
Flavin-containing monooxygenases (FMO)	N, S, and P oxidation
Epoxide hydrolases (mEH, sEH)	Hydrolysis of epoxides
Phase 2 "transferases"	
Sulfotransferases (SULT)	Addition of sulfate
UDP-glucuronosyltransferases (UGT)	Addition of glucuronic acid
Glutathione-S-transferases (GST)	Addition of glutathione
N-acetyltransferases (NAT)	Addition of acetyl group
Methyltransferases (MT)	Addition of methyl group
Other enzymes	
Alcohol dehydrogenases	Reduction of alcohols
Aldehyde dehydrogenases	Reduction of aldehydes
NADPH-quinone oxidoreductase (NQO)	Reduction of quinones

mEH and sEH are microsomal and soluble epoxide hydrolase. UDP, uridine diphosphate; NADPH, reduced nicotinamide adenine dinucleotide phosphate.

in certain instances, metabolism, usually the hydrolysis of an ester or amide linkage, results in bioactivation of a drug. Inactive drugs that undergo metabolism to an active drug are called *prodrugs*. For example, the antitumor drug cyclophosphamide, is bioactivated to a cell-killing electrophilic derivative (*see* Chapter 61); clofibrate, used to reduce triglyceride levels, is converted in the cell from an ester to an active acidic metabolite.

Phase 2 enzymes facilitate the elimination of drugs and the inactivation of electrophilic and potentially toxic metabolites produced by oxidation. *Phase 2 enzymes* include several superfamilies of conjugating enzymes, such as the glutathione-S-transferases (GSTs), UDP-glucuronosyltransferases (UGTs), sulfotransferases (SULTs), *N*-acetyltransferases (NATs), and methyltransferases (MTs). These conjugation reactions usually require the substrate to have oxygen (hydroxyl or epoxide groups), nitrogen, or sulfur atoms that serve as acceptor sites for a hydrophilic moiety, such as glutathione, glucuronic acid, sulfate, or an acetyl group.

In the case of the UGTs, glucuronic acid is delivered to the functional group, forming a glucuronide metabolite that is more water soluble and is targeted for excretion either in the urine or bile. When the substrate is a drug, these reactions usually convert the original drug to a form that is not able to bind to its target receptor, thus attenuating the biological response to the drug.

SITES OF DRUG METABOLISM

Xenobiotic metabolizing enzymes are found in most tissues in the body, with the highest levels located in the GI tract (liver, small and large intestines). The liver is the major "metabolic clearing house" for both endogenous chemicals (e.g., cholesterol, steroid hormones, fatty acids, and proteins) and xenobiotics. The small intestine plays a crucial role in drug metabolism because drugs that are orally administered are absorbed by the gut and taken to the liver through the portal vein. The xenobiotic-metabolizing enzymes located in the epithelial cells of the GI tract are responsible for the initial metabolic processing of most oral medications. The absorbed drug then enters the portal circulation for its first pass through the liver, where it can undergo significant metabolism. A portion of active drug escapes metabolism in the GI tract and liver and enters the systemic circulation; subsequent passes through the liver result in more metabolism of the parent drug until the agent is eliminated. Thus, drugs that are poorly metabolized remain in the body for longer periods of time (have longer elimination half-lives). Other organs that contain significant xenobiotic-metabolizing enzymes include tissues of the nasal mucosa and lung, which play important roles in the metabolism of drugs that are administered as aerosols.

At the cellular level, the phase 1 CYPs, FMOs, and EHs, and some phase 2 conjugating enzymes, notably the UGTs, are all located in the endoplasmic reticulum of the cell (Figure 6–2). Once subjected to oxidation, drugs can be directly conjugated by the UGTs (in the lumen of the endoplasmic reticulum) or by the cytosolic transferases such as GST and SULT. The metabolites can then be transported out of the cell into the bloodstream. Hepatocytes, which constitute > 90% of the cells in the liver, carry out most drug metabolism and produce conjugated substrates that can also be transported through the bile canalicular membrane into the bile, from which they are eliminated into the gut (*see* Chapter 5).

PHASE 1 REACTIONS

CYPs: THE CYTOCHROME P450 SUPERFAMILY

The CYPs are a superfamily of enzymes, all of which contain a molecule of heme that is noncovalently bound to the polypeptide chain (*see* Figure 6–2). The heme iron binds oxygen in the CYP active site, where oxidation of the substrates occurs. The H^+ is supplied through the enzyme NADPH-cytochrome P450 oxidoreductase and its cofactor NADPH. Metabolism of a substrate by a CYP consumes 1 molecule of O_2 and produces an oxidized substrate and a molecule of water. Depending on the nature of the substrate, the reaction is "uncoupled," consuming more O_2 than substrate metabolized and producing what is called activated oxygen or O_2^-. The O_2^- is usually converted to water by the enzyme superoxide dismutase. Elevated O_2^-, a *reactive oxygen species* (ROS), can give rise to oxidative stress that is detrimental to cells and associated with diseases.

Among the diverse reactions carried out by mammalian CYPs are *N*-dealkylation, *O*-dealkylation, aromatic hydroxylation, *N*-oxidation, *S*-oxidation, deamination, and dehalogenation (Table 6–2). CYPs are involved in the metabolism of dietary and xenobiotic chemicals, in the synthesis of endogenous compounds (e.g., steroids; fatty acid-derived signaling molecules, such as epoxyeicosatrienoic acids), and in the production of bile acids from cholesterol. In contrast to the drug-metabolizing CYPs, the CYPs that catalyze steroid and bile acid synthesis have very specific substrate preferences. For example, the CYP that produces estrogen from

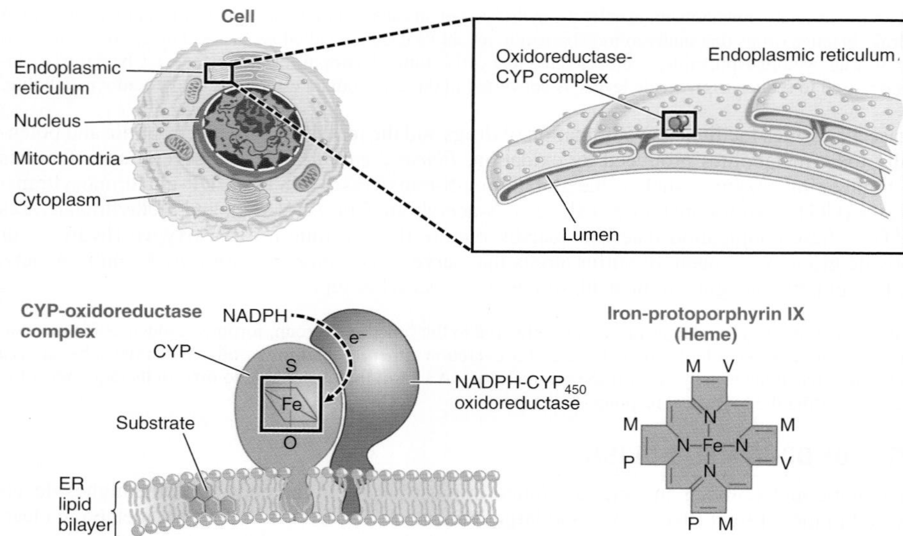

Figure 6–2 *Location of CYPs in the cell.* The figure shows increasingly microscopic levels of detail, sequentially expanding the areas within the *black boxes*. CYPs are embedded in the phospholipid bilayer of the endoplasmic reticulum (ER). Most of the enzyme is located on the cytosolic surface of the ER. A second enzyme, NADPH-cytochrome P_{450} oxidoreductase, transfers electrons to the CYP where it can, in the presence of O_2, oxidize xenobiotic substrates, many of which are hydrophobic and dissolved in the ER. A single NADPH-CYP oxidoreductase species transfers electrons to all CYP isoforms in the ER. Each CYP contains a molecule of iron-protoporphyrin IX that functions to bind and activate O_2. Substituents on the porphyrin ring are methyl (M), propionyl (P), and vinyl (V) groups.

testosterone, CYP19 or aromatase, can metabolize only testosterone or androstenedione and does not metabolize xenobiotics. Specific inhibitors for aromatase, such as *anastrozole*, have been developed for use in the treatment of estrogen-dependent tumors (*see* Chapters 40 and 60-63). CYPs involved in bile acid production have strict substrate requirements and do not participate in xenobiotic or drug metabolism.

The CYPs that carry out xenobiotic metabolism can metabolize structurally diverse chemicals. This is due both to multiple forms of CYPs, to the capacity of a single CYP to metabolize many structurally distinct chemicals, to significant overlapping substrate specificity amongst CYPs, and to the capacity of CYPs to metabolize a single compound at different positions on the molecule. Indeed, CYPs are promiscuous in their capacity to bind and metabolize multiple substrates (*see* Table 6–2). This property sacrifices metabolic turnover rates; CYPs metabolize substrates at a fraction of the rate of more typical enzymes involved in intermediary metabolism and mitochondrial electron transfer. As a result, drugs have, in general, half-lives in the range of 2-30 h, while endogenous compounds have half-lives of the order of seconds or minutes (e.g., dopamine and insulin).

The extensive overlapping substrate specificities by the CYPs is one of the underlying reasons for the predominance of drug-drug interactions. When 2 coadministered drugs are both metabolized by a single CYP, they compete for binding to the enzyme's active site. This can result in the inhibition of metabolism of 1 or both of the drugs, leading to elevated plasma levels. If there is a narrow therapeutic index for the drugs, the elevated serum levels may elicit unwanted toxicities. Drug-drug interactions are among the leading causes of adverse drug reactions (ADRs).

THE NAMING OF CYPs. Genome sequencing has revealed the existence of 57 putatively functional genes and 58 pseudogenes in humans. These genes are grouped, based on amino acid sequence similarity, into a superfamily composed of families and subfamilies with increasing sequence similarity. CYPs are named with the root CYP followed by a number designating the family, a letter denoting the subfamily, and another number designating the CYP form. Thus, *CYP3A4* is family 3, subfamily A, and gene number 4.

A DOZEN CYPs SUFFICE FOR METABOLISM OF MOST DRUGS. In humans, 12 CYPs (CYP1A1, 1A2, 1B1, 2A6, 2B6, 2C8, 2C9, 2C19, 2D6, 2E1, 3A4, and 3A5) are known to be important for metabolism of xenobiotics. The

Table 6–2

Major Reactions Involved in Drug Metabolism

	REACTION	EXAMPLES
I. Oxidative Reactions		
N-Dealkylation	$RNHCH_3 \rightarrow RNH_2 + CH_2O$	Imipramine, diazepam, codeine, erythromycin, morphine, tamoxifen, theophylline, caffeine
O-Dealkylation	$ROCH_3 \rightarrow ROH + CH_2O$	Codeine, indomethacin, dextromethorphan
Aliphatic hydroxylation	$RCH_2CH_3 \rightarrow RCHOHCH_3$	Tolbutamide, ibuprofen, phenobarbital, meprobamate, cyclosporine, midazolam
Aromatic hydroxylation	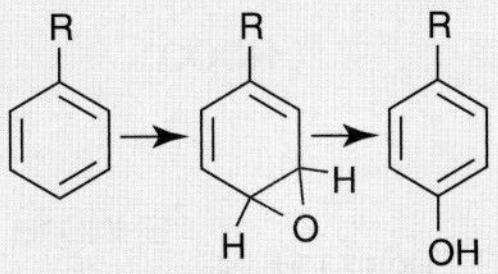 R–benzene → R–arene epoxide (H, O, H) → R–phenol (OH)	Phenytoin, phenobarbital, propanolol, ethinyl estradiol, amphetamine, warfarin
N-Oxidation	$RNH_2 \rightarrow RNHOH$ 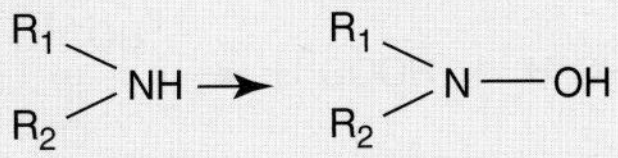 $R_1R_2NH \rightarrow R_1R_2N{-}OH$	Chlorpheniramine, dapsone, meperidine
S-Oxidation	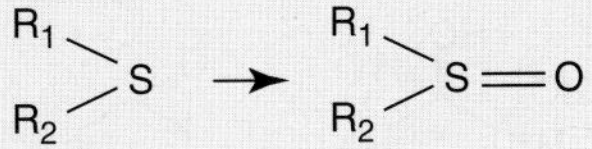 $R_1R_2S \rightarrow R_1R_2S{=}O$	Cimetidine, chlorpromazine, thioridazine, omeprazole
Deamination	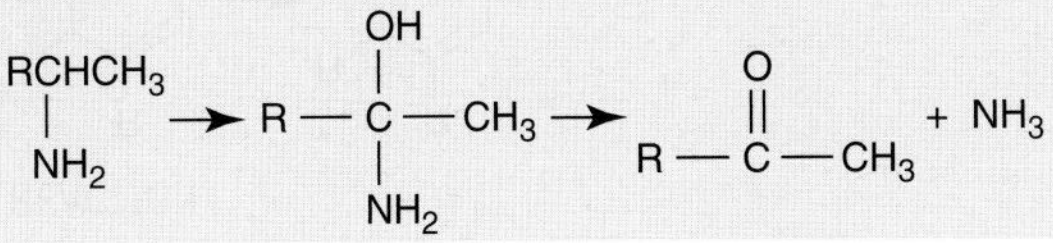 $RCH(NH_2)CH_3 \rightarrow R{-}C(OH)(NH_2){-}CH_3 \rightarrow R{-}C({=}O){-}CH_3 + NH_3$	Diazepam, amphetamine

(*continued*)

Table 6–2

Major Reactions Involved in Drug Metabolism (*Continued*)

	REACTION	EXAMPLES
II. Hydrolysis Reactions	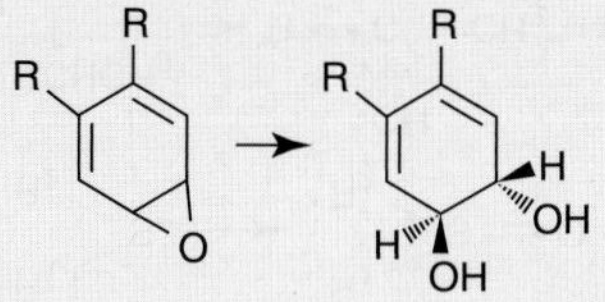 R, R, O → R, R, H, OH, H, OH	Carbamazepine (*see* Figure 6–4)
	R_1COR_2 (C=O) → $R_1COOH + R_2OH$	Procaine, aspirin, clofibrate, meperidine, enalapril, cocaine
	R_1CNHR_2 (C=O) → $R_1COOH + R_2NH_2$	Lidocaine, procainamide, indomethacin
III. Conjugation Reactions		
Glucuronidation	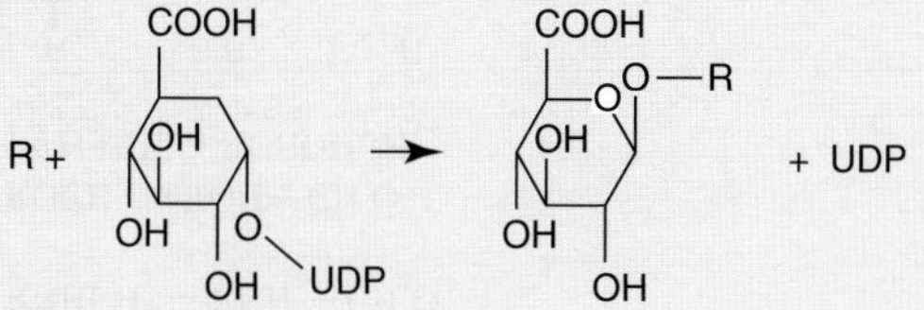 R + COOH, OH, OH, OH, O–UDP → COOH, O–R, OH, OH, OH + UDP	Acetaminophen, morphine, oxazepam, lorazepam
Sulfation	PAPS + ROH → $R{-}O{-}SO_2{-}OH$ + PAP	Acetaminophen, steroids, methyldopa
Acetylation	$CoAS{-}CO{-}CH_3 + RNH_2 \rightarrow RNH{-}CO{-}CH_3$ + CoA-SH	Sulfonamides, isoniazid, dapsone, clonazepam
Methylation	RO-, RS-, RN- + AdoMet → $RO{-}CH_3$ + AdoHomCys	L-Dopa, methyldopa, mercaptopurine, captopril
Glutathionylation	GSH + R →R-GSH	Adriamycin, fosfomycin, busulfan

PAPS, 3′-phosphoadenosine-5′ phosphosulfate; PAP 3′-phosphoadenosine-5′-phosphate.

liver contains the greatest abundance of xenobiotic-metabolizing CYPs, thus ensuring efficient first-pass metabolism of drugs. CYPs are also expressed throughout the GI tract, and in lower amounts in lung, kidney, and even in the CNS. The most active CYPs for drug metabolism are those in the CYP2C, 2D, and 3A subfamilies. CYP3A4, the most abundantly expressed in liver, is involved in the metabolism of over 50% of clinically used drugs (Figure 6–3A). The CYP1A, 1B, 2A, 2B, and 2E subfamilies are not significantly involved in the metabolism of therapeutic drugs, but they do catalyze the metabolic activation of many protoxins and procarcinogens.

CYPs AND DRUG-DRUG INTERACTIONS. Differences in the rate of metabolism of a drug can be caused by drug interactions. Most commonly, an interaction occurs when 2 drugs (e.g., a statin and a macrolide antibiotic or antifungal agent) are metabolized by the same enzyme and affect each other's metabolism. Thus, it is important to determine the identity of the CYP that metabolizes a particular drug and to avoid coadministering drugs that are metabolized by the same enzyme. Some drugs can also inhibit CYPs independently of being substrates for a CYP.

For example, the common antifungal agent, ketoconazole (NIZORAL), is a potent inhibitor of *CYP3A4* and other CYPs, and coadministration of ketoconazole with an anti-HIV viral protease inhibitor reduces the clearance of the protease inhibitor and increases its plasma concentration and the risk of toxicity. For most drugs, information found on the package insert lists the CYP that metabolizes the drug and determines the potential for drug interactions.

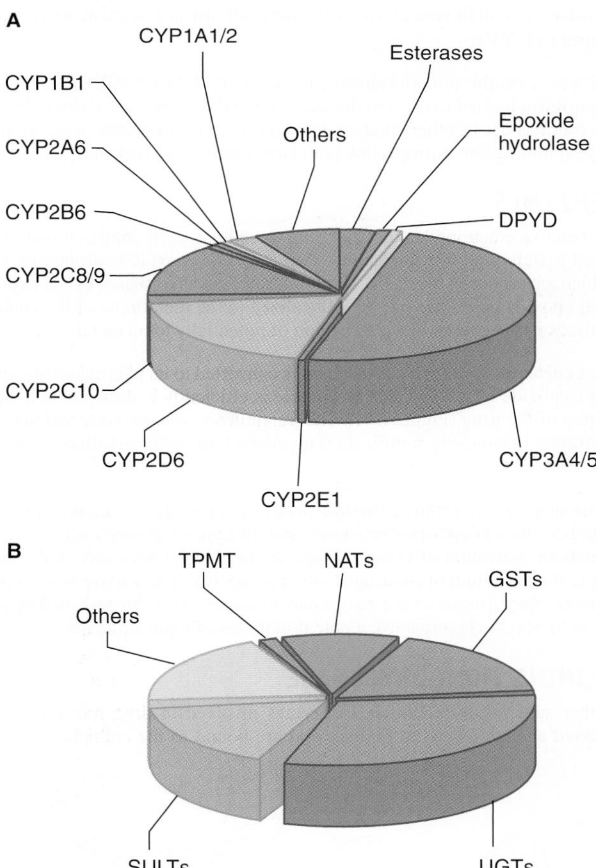

Figure 6–3 *The fraction of clinically used drugs metabolized by the major phase 1 and phase 2 enzymes.* The relative size of each pie section represents the estimated percentage of drugs metabolized by the major phase 1 (panel **A**) and phase 2 (panel **B**) enzymes, based on studies in the literature. In some cases, more than a single enzyme is responsible for metabolism of a single drug. CYP, cytochrome P450; DPYD, dihydropyrimidine dehydrogenase; GST, glutathione-S-transferase; NAT, *N*-acetyltransferase; SULT, sulfotransferase, TPMT, thiopurine methyltransferase; UGT, UDP-glucuronosyltransferase.

Some drugs are CYP inducers that can increase not only their own rates of metabolism, but also induce metabolism of other coadministered drugs (*see* below and Figure 6–8).

For example, steroid hormones and herbal products such as St. John's wort can increase hepatic levels of *CYP3A4*, thereby increasing the metabolism of many orally administered drugs. Indeed, St. John's wort can induce hepatic metabolism of the steroid components of birth control pills, rendering the standard dose ineffective in preventing pregnancy.

Drug metabolism can also be influenced by diet.

Components found in grapefruit juice (e.g., naringin, furanocoumarins) are potent inhibitors of *CYP3A4*, and thus grapefruit juice can increase the bioavailability of certain drugs that are substrates for *CYP3A4*. Terfenadine, a once popular antihistamine, was removed from the market because its metabolism was inhibited *by CYP3A4* substrates such as erythromycin and grapefruit juice. Terfenadine was actually a prodrug that required oxidation by *CYP3A4* to its active metabolite, and at high doses the parent compound caused the potentially fatal arrhythmia, torsades de pointes. Thus, as a result of *CYP3A4* inhibition by a coadministered agent, plasma levels of the parent drug could become dangerously elevated, causing ventricular tachycardia in some individuals; this led to terfenadine's withdrawal from the market. Subsequently, the metabolite was developed as a drug, fexofenadine, which retains the therapeutic properties of the parent compound but avoids the step involving *CYP3A4.*

In addition, interindividual differences in drug metabolism are significantly influenced by heritable polymorphisms in CYPs.

Several human CYP genes exhibit polymorphisms, including *CYP2A6, CYP2C9, CYP2C19*, and *CYP2D6*. The *CYP2D6* polymorphism has led to the withdrawal of several clinically used drugs (e.g., debrisoquine and perhexiline) and the cautious use of others that are known *CYP2D6* substrates (e.g., encainide and flecainide [anti-arrhythmics], desipramine and nortriptyline [antidepressants], and codeine).

HYDROLYTIC ENZYMES

Epoxides are highly reactive electrophiles that can bind to cellular nucleophiles found in protein, RNA, and DNA, resulting in cell toxicity and transformation. Two forms of epoxide hydrolase carry out hydrolysis of epoxides, most of which are produced by CYPs. The soluble epoxide hydrolase (EH) is expressed in the cytosol while the microsomal epoxide hydrolase (mEH) is localized to the membrane of the endoplasmic reticulum. Thus, epoxide hydrolases participate in the deactivation of potentially toxic metabolites generated by CYPs.

The antiepileptic drug *carbamazepine* is a prodrug that is converted to its pharmacologically active derivative, carbamazepine-10, 11-epoxide by a CYP. This metabolite is efficiently hydrolyzed to a dihydrodiol by mEH, resulting in inactivation of the drug (Figure 6–4). The tranquilizer *valnoctamide* and anticonvulsant *valproic acid* inhibit mEH, resulting in clinically significant drug interactions with carbamazepine by causing elevation of the active derivative.

The carboxylesterases superfamily catalyze the hydrolysis of ester- and amide-containing chemicals. These enzymes are found in both the endoplasmic reticulum and the cytosol of many cell types and are involved in detoxification or metabolic activation of various drugs, environmental toxicants, and carcinogens. Carboxylesterases also catalyze the activation of prodrugs to their respective free acids. For example, the prodrug and cancer chemotherapeutic agent irinotecan is a camptothecin analog that is bioactivated by plasma and intracellular carboxylesterases to SN-38 (Figure 6–5), a potent inhibitor of topoisomerase 1.

FLAVIN-CONTAINING MONOOXYGENASE

The FMOs are another superfamily of phase 1 enzymes involved in drug metabolism. Similar to CYPs, the FMOs are expressed at high levels in the liver and are bound to the endoplasmic reticulum. There are

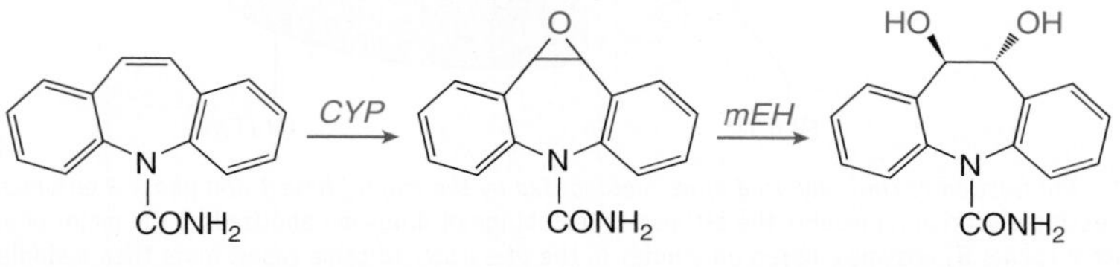

Figure 6–4 *Metabolism of carbamazepine by CYP and microsomal epoxide hydrolase (mEH).* Carbamazepine is oxidized to the pharmacologically active metabolite carbamazepine-10, 11-epoxide by CYP. The epoxide is converted to a transdihydrodiol by mEH. This metabolite is biologically inactive and can be conjugated by phase 2 enzymes.

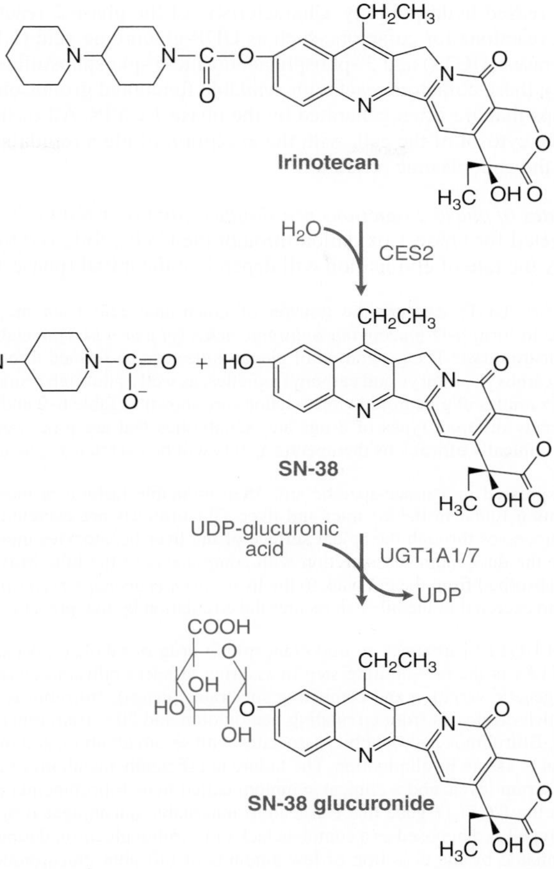

Figure 6–5 *Metabolism of irinotecan (CPT-11).* The prodrug CPT-11 is initially metabolized by a serum esterase (CES2) to the topoisomerase inhibitor SN-38, which is the active camptothecin analog that slows tumor growth. SN-38 is then subject to glucuronidation, which results in loss of biological activity and facilitates elimination of the SN-38 in the bile.

6 families of FMOs, with FMO3 being the most abundant in liver. A genetic deficiency in this enzyme causes the *fish-odor syndrome* due to a lack of metabolism of trimethylamine *N*-oxide (TMAO) to trimethylamine (TMA). FMOs are considered minor contributors to drug metabolism and they almost always produce benign metabolites. FMOs are not induced by any of the xenobiotic receptors (see below) or easily inhibited; thus, in contrast to CYPs, FMOs are less involved in drug-drug interactions. In fact, this has been demonstrated by comparing the pathways of metabolism of 2 drugs used in the control of gastric motility, itopride, and cisapride. Itopride is metabolized by FMO3 while cisapride is metabolized by *CYP3A4*; thus, itopride is less likely to be involved in drug-drug interactions than is cisapride. *CYP3A4* participates in drug-drug interactions through induction and inhibition of metabolism, whereas FMO3 is not induced or inhibited by any clinically used drugs. FMOs could be of importance in the development of new drugs. A candidate drug could be designed by introducing a site for FMO oxidation with the knowledge that favorable metabolism and pharmacokinetic properties could be accurately predicted.

CONJUGATING ENZYMES (PHASE 2 REACTIONS)

The phase 2 conjugating enzymes, synthetic in nature, catalyze reactions that normally terminate the biological activity of drugs, although for drugs like morphine and minoxidil, glucuronide and sulfate conjugates, respectively, are more pharmacologically active than the parent. The contributions of different phase 2 reactions to drug metabolism are shown in Figure 6–3B. Two of the phase 2 reactions, glucuronidation and sulfation, result in the formation of metabolites with a significantly increased hydrophilicity. Characteristic of the phase 2 reactions is the dependency on the catalytic reactions for cofactors, such as UDP-glucuronic acid (UDP-GA) for UDP-glucuronosyltransferases (UGTs) and 3′-phosphoadenosine-5′-phosphosulfate (PAPS) for sulfotransferases (SULTs); these cofactors react with available functional groups on the substrates, reactive functional groups that are often generated by the phase 1 CYPs. All of the phase 2 reactions are carried out in the cytosol of the cell, with the exception of glucuronidation, which occurs on the luminal side of the endoplasmic reticulum.

The catalytic rates of phase 2 reactions are significantly faster than the rates of the CYPs. Thus, if a drug is targeted for phase 1 oxidation through the CYPs, followed by a phase 2 conjugation reaction, usually the rate of elimination will depend on the initial (phase 1) oxidation reaction.

GLUCURONIDATION. UGTs catalyze the transfer of glucuronic acid from the cofactor UDP-glucuronic acid to a substrate to form β-D-glucopyranosiduronic acids (*glucuronides*), metabolites that are sensitive to cleavage by β-glucuronidase. The generation of glucuronides can be formed through alcoholic and phenolic hydroxyl groups, carboxyl, sulfuryl, and carbonyl moieties, as well as through primary, secondary, and tertiary amine linkages. Examples of glucuronidation reactions are shown in Table 6–2 and Figure 6–5. The structural diversity in the many different types of drugs and xenobiotics that are processed through glucuronidation assures that most clinically efficacious therapeutic agents will be excreted as glucuronides.

The UGTs are expressed in a tissue-specific and often inducible fashion in most human tissues, with the highest concentration found in the GI tract and liver. Glucuronides are excreted into the urine or through active transport processes through the apical surface of the liver hepatocytes into the bile ducts where they are transported to the duodenum for excretion with components of the bile. Most of the bile acids that are conjugated are reabsorbed from the gut back to the liver via *enterohepatic recirculation*; many drugs that are glucuronidated and excreted in the bile can reenter the circulation by this process.

The expression of UGT1A1 assumes an important role in drug metabolism, because the glucuronidation of bilirubin by UGT1A1 is the rate-limiting step in assuring efficient bilirubin clearance, and this rate can be affected by both genetic variation and competing substrates (drugs). Bilirubin is the breakdown product of heme, 80% of which originates from circulating hemoglobin and 20% from other heme-containing proteins such as the CYPs. Bilirubin is hydrophobic, associates with serum albumin, and must be metabolized further by glucuronidation to assure its elimination. The failure to efficiently metabolize bilirubin by glucuronidation leads to elevated serum levels and a clinical symptom called hyperbilirubinemia or jaundice. There are >50 genetic lesions in the *UGT1A1* gene that can lead to inheritable unconjugated hyperbilirubinemia. Crigler-Najjar syndrome type I is diagnosed as a complete lack of bilirubin glucuronidation; Crigler-Najjar syndrome type II is differentiated by the detection of low amounts of bilirubin glucuronides in duodenal secretions. These rare syndromes result from genetic polymorphisms in the *UGT1A1* gene, resulting in abolished or highly diminished levels of functional protein.

Gilbert syndrome is a generally benign condition present in up to 10% of the population; it is diagnosed clinically because circulating bilirubin levels are 60-70% higher than those seen in normal subjects. The most common genetic polymorphism associated with Gilbert syndrome is a mutation in the *UGT1A1* gene promoter, which leads to reduced expression levels of UGT1A1. Subjects diagnosed with Gilbert syndrome may be predisposed to adverse drug reactions (ADRs) (Table 6–3) that result from a reduced capacity of UGT1A1 to metabolize drugs. If a drug undergoes selective metabolism by UGT1A1, competition for drug

Table 6–3

Drug Toxicity and Gilbert's Syndrome

PROBLEM	FEATURE
Gilbert's syndrome	UGT1A1*28 (main variant in Caucasians)
Established toxicity reactions	Irinotecan, atazanavir
UGT1A1 substrates (potential risk?)	Gemfibrozil[a], ezetimibe
	Simvastatin, atorvastatin, cerivastatin[a]
	Ethinylestradiol, buprenorphine, fulvestrant
	Ibuprofen, ketoprofen

[a]A severe drug reaction owing to the inhibition of glucuronidation (UGT1A1) and CYP2C8 and CYP2C9 when both drugs were combined led to the withdrawal of cerivastatin. Reproduced with permission from Strassburg CP. Pharmacogenetics of Gilbert's syndrome. Pharmacogenomics, 2008, 9:703–715.

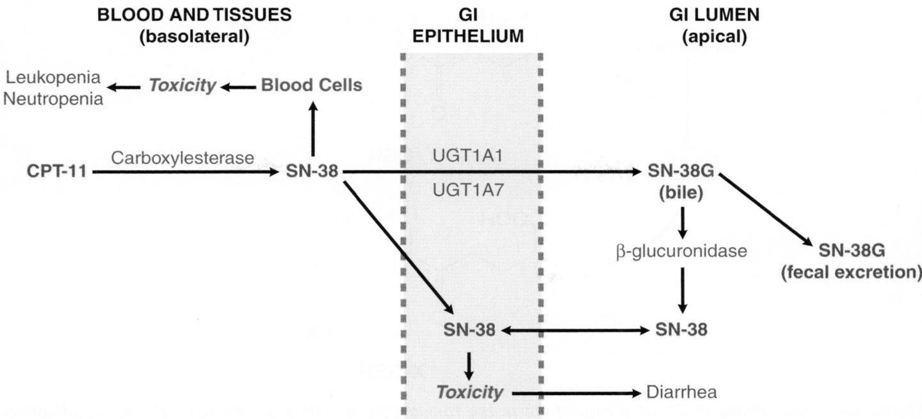

Figure 6–6 *Cellular* targets *of SN-38 in the blood and intestinal tissues.* Excessive accumulation of SN-38 can lead to bone marrow toxicities such as leukopenia and neutropenia, as well as damage to the intestinal epithelium. These toxicities are pronounced in individuals that have reduced capacity to form the SN-38 glucuronide, such as patients with Gilbert syndrome. Note the different body compartments and cell types involved. (Modified with permission from Tukey RH *et al.* Pharmacogenetics of human UDP-glucuronosyltransferases and irinotecan toxicity. *Mol Pharmacol,* 2002;62:446–450. Copyright © 2002 The American Society for Pharmacology and Experimental Therapeutics.)

metabolism with bilirubin glucuronidation will exist, resulting in pronounced hyperbilirubinemia as well as reduced clearance of the metabolized drug. Gilbert syndrome also alters patient responses to irinotecan (CPT-11). Irinotecan, a prodrug used in chemotherapy of solid tumors (*see* Chapter 61), is metabolized to its active form, SN-38, by serum carboxylesterases (*see* Figure 6–5). SN-38, a potent topoisomerase inhibitor, is inactivated by UGT1A1 and excreted in the bile (Figure 6–6). Once in the lumen of the intestine, the SN-38 glucuronide undergoes cleavage by bacterial β-glucuronidase and reenters the circulation through intestinal absorption. Elevated levels of SN-38 in the blood lead to bone marrow toxicities characterized by leukopenia and neutropenia, as well as damage to the intestinal epithelial cells (*see* Figure 6–6), resulting in acute and life-threatening diarrhea. Patients with Gilbert syndrome who are receiving irinotecan therapy are predisposed to the hematological and GI toxicities resulting from elevated serum levels of SN-38.

SULFATION. The sulfotransferases (SULTs) are cytosolic and conjugate sulfate derived from 3′-phosphoadenosine-5′-phosphosulfate (PAPS) to the hydroxyl and, less frequently, amine groups of aromatic and aliphatic compounds. In humans, significant fractions of circulating catecholamines, estrogens, iodothyronines, and DHEA exist in the sulfated form. In humans, 13 SULT isoforms have been identified and classified into 4 families [SULT1 (8 members), SULT2 (3 members), SULT4 (1 member), and SULT6 (1 member) families]. SULTs play an important role in normal human homeostasis. For example, SULT2B1b is a predominant form expressed in skin, carrying out the catalysis of cholesterol. Cholesterol sulfate is an essential metabolite in regulating keratinocyte differentiation and skin development. SULT2A1 is very highly expressed in the fetal adrenal gland, where it produces the large quantities of dehydroepiandrosterone sulfate that are required for placental estrogen biosynthesis during the second half of pregnancy. SULT1A3 is highly selective for catecholamines; SULT1E1 sulfates estrogens.

Members SULT1 family are the major forms involved in xenobiotic metabolism, with SULT1A1 being the most important in the liver. It displays extensive diversity in its capacity to catalyze the sulfation of a wide variety of structurally heterogeneous xenobiotics with high affinity. SULT1B1 is similar to SULT1A1, but it is much more abundant in the intestine than the liver. Three SULT1C isoforms exist in humans, but little is known about their substrate specificity. SULT1C enzymes are expressed abundantly in human fetal tissues and decline in abundance in adults. SULT1E catalyzes the sulfation of steroids, and is localized in liver, as well as in hormone-responsive tissues such as the testis, breast, adrenal gland, and placenta. In the upper GI tract, SULT1A3 and SULT1B1 are particularly abundant. Drug metabolism through sulfation often leads to the generation of chemically reactive metabolites, where the sulfate is electron withdrawing and may be heterolytically cleaved, leading to the formation of an electrophilic cation. Examples of the generation by sulfation of a carcinogenic or toxic response in mutagenicity assays have been documented with chemicals derived from the environment or from food mutagens generated from well-cooked meat. Thus, it is important to understand whether genetic linkages can be made by associating known human SULT polymorphisms to cancers related to environmental sources.

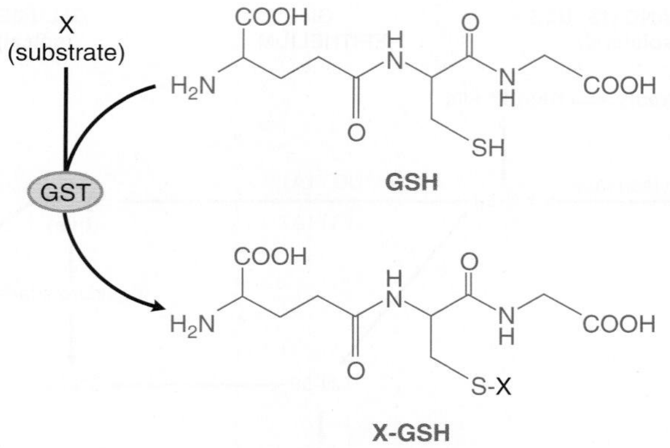

Figure 6–7 *Glutathione (GSH) as a cosubstrate in the conjugation of a drug or xenobiotic (X) by glutathione-S-transferase (GST).*

GLUTATHIONE CONJUGATION. The glutathione-S-transferases (GSTs) catalyze the transfer of glutathione to reactive electrophiles, a function that protects cellular macromolecules from interacting with electrophiles that contain electrophilic heteroatoms (-O, -N, and -S). The cosubstrate in the reaction is the tripeptide glutathione, which is synthesized from γ-glutamic acid, cysteine, and glycine (Figure 6–7). Glutathione exists in the cell as oxidized (GSSG) or reduced (GSH) forms, and the ratio of GSH:GSSG is critical in maintaining a cellular environment in the reduced state. In addition to affecting xenobiotic conjugation with GSH, a severe reduction in GSH content can predispose cells to oxidative damage, a state that has been linked to a number of human health issues.

The formation of glutathione conjugates generates a thioether linkage with drug or xenobiotic to the cysteine moiety of the tripeptide. Because the concentration of glutathione in cells is usually very high, typically in the 10 mM range, many drugs and xenobiotics can react nonenzymatically with glutathione. However, the GSTs have been found to occupy up to 10% of the total cellular protein concentration, a property that assures efficient conjugation of glutathione to reactive electrophiles. More than 20 human GSTs have been identified and divided into 2 subfamilies: the cytosolic and the microsomal forms. The cytosolic forms have more importance in the metabolism of drugs and xenobiotics, whereas the microsomal GSTs are important in the endogenous metabolism of leukotrienes and prostaglandins. The high concentration of GSTs also provides the cells with a sink of cytosolic protein that sequesters compounds that are not substrates for glutathione conjugation. The cytosolic pool of GSTs binds steroids, bile acids, bilirubin, cellular hormones, and environmental toxicants, in addition to complexing with other cellular proteins.

The high concentrations of GSH in the cell and the plenitude of GSTs mean that few reactive molecules escape detoxification. However, there is always concern that some reactive intermediates will escape detoxification, and by nature of their electrophilicity, will cause toxicity. The potential for such an occurrence is heightened if GSH is depleted or if a specific form of GST is polymorphic. Reactive therapeutic agents that require large doses for clinical efficacy have the greatest potential to lower cellular GSH levels. Acetaminophen, which is normally metabolized by glucuronidation and sulfation, is also a substrate for oxidative metabolism by CYP2E1 and CYP3A4, which generate the toxic metabolite *N*-acetyl-*p*-benzoquinone imine (NAPQI) that, under normal dosing, is readily neutralized through conjugation with GSH. An overdose of acetaminophen can deplete cellular GSH levels, thereby increasing the potential for NAPQI to interact with other cellular components resulting in toxicity and cell death (*see* Figure 4–4).

The GSTs are polymorphic, and several of the polymorphic forms express a null phenotype; thus, individuals polymorphic at these loci are predisposed to toxicities by agents that are selective substrates for these GSTs. For example, the mutant GSTM1*0 allele is observed in 50% of the Caucasian population and has been linked genetically to human malignancies of the lung, colon, and bladder. Null activity in the GSTT1 gene has been associated with adverse side effects and toxicity in cancer chemotherapy with cytostatic drugs; the toxicities result from insufficient clearance of the drugs by GSH conjugation. Expression of the null genotype can be as high as 60% in Chinese and Korean populations. GST polymorphisms may influence efficacies and severity of adverse side effects of drugs. GSTs activities in cancerous tissues have been linked to the development of drug resistance toward chemotherapeutic agents. *See* Figures 6–10 and 6–11 in the 12th edition of the parent text for more on this subject.

***N*-ACETYLATION.** The cytosolic *N*-acetyltransferases (NATs) are responsible for the metabolism of drugs and environmental agents that contain an aromatic amine or hydrazine group. The addition of the acetyl group from the cofactor acetyl-coenzyme A often leads to a metabolite that is less water soluble because the potential ionizable amine is neutralized by the covalent addition of the acetyl group. There are 2 functional NAT genes in humans, *NAT1* and *NAT2*. NATs are among the most polymorphic of all the human xenobiotic drug-metabolizing enzymes. More than 25 allelic variants of *NAT1* and *NAT2* have been characterized, and in individuals in whom acetylation of drugs is compromised, homozygous genotypes for at least 2 variant alleles are required to predispose a patient to lowered drug metabolism. The frequency of the slow acetylation patterns are attributed mostly to the polymorphism in the *NAT2* gene. The characterization of an acetylator phenotype in humans was one of the first hereditary traits identified, and was responsible for the development of the field of pharmacogenetics (*see* Chapter 7). Following the discovery that isonicotinic acid hydrazide (isoniazid, INH) could be used in the cure of tuberculosis, a significant proportion of the patients (5-15%) experienced toxicities. Individuals suffering from the toxic effects of the drug excreted the largest amount of unchanged drug and the least amount of acetylated isoniazid. Pharmacogenetic studies led to the classification of "rapid" and "slow" acetylators, with the "slow" phenotype being associated with toxicity. Characterization of *N*-acetyltransferase revealed polymorphisms that correspond to the "slow" acetylator phenotype. *See* Figures 56–3 and 56–4 for details of isoniazid metabolism and NAT2 polymorphisms.

Drug substrates of NATs and their toxicities are listed in Table 6–4. If a drug is known to be metabolized through acetylation, determining an individual's phenotype can be important in maximizing outcome in subsequent therapy. Several drugs, such as the sulfonamides, that are targets for acetylation have been implicated in idiosyncratic hypersensitivity reactions; in such instances, an appreciation of a patient's acetylating phenotype is particularly important. Sulfonamides are transformed into hydroxylamines that interact with cellular proteins, generating haptens that can elicit autoimmune responses. Individuals who are slow acetylators are predisposed to drug-induced autoimmune disorders.

Tissue-specific expression patterns of NAT1 and NAT2 have a significant impact on drug metabolism and the potential for toxicity. NAT1 is expressed in most tissues, whereas NAT2 is found predominantly in the liver and GI tract. Both NAT1 and NAT2 can form *N*-hydroxy–acetylated metabolites from bicyclic aromatic hydrocarbons, a reaction that leads to the nonenzymatic release of the acetyl group and the generation of highly reactive nitrenium ions. Thus, *N*-hydroxy acetylation is thought to activate certain environmental toxicants. In contrast, direct *N*-acetylation of bicyclic aromatic amines is stable and leads to detoxification.

Table 6–4

Indications and Unwanted Side Effects of Drug Metabolized by *N*-Acetyltransferases

DRUG	INDICATION	MAJOR SIDE EFFECTS
Acebutolol	Arrhythmias, hypertension	Drowsiness, weakness, insomnia
Amantadine	Influenza A, parkinsonism	Appetite loss, dizziness, headache, nightmares
Aminobenzoic acid	Skin disorders, sunscreens	Stomach upset, contact sensitization
Aminoglutethimide	Adrenal cortex carcinoma, breast cancer	Clumsiness, nausea, dizziness, agranulocytosis
Aminosalicylic acid	Ulcerative colitis	Allergic fever, itching, leukopenia
Amonafide	Prostate cancer	Myelosuppression
Amrinone	Advanced heart failure	Thrombocytopenia, arrhythmias
Benzocaine	Local anesthesia	Dermatitis, itching, rash, methemoglobinemia
Caffeine	Neonatal respiratory distress syndrome	Dizziness, insomnia, tachycardia
Clonazepam	Epilepsy	Ataxia, dizziness, slurred speech
Dapsone	Dermatitis, leprosy, AIDS-related complex	Nausea, vomiting, hyperexcitability, methemoglobinemia, dermatitis
Dipyrone, metamizole	Analgesic	Agranulocytosis
Hydralazine	Hypertension	Hypotension, tachycardia, flush, headache
Isoniazid	Tuberculosis	Peripheral neuritis, hepatotoxicity
Nitrazepam	Insomnia	Dizziness, somnolence
Phenelzine	Depression	CNS excitation, insomnia, orthostatic hypotension, hepatotoxicity
Procainamide	Ventricular tachyarrhythmia	Hypotension, systemic lupus erythematosus
Sulfonamides	Antibacterial agents	Hypersensitivity, hemolytic anemia, fever, lupus-like syndromes

For details, see Meisel P. Arylamine N-acetyltransferases and drug response. Pharmacogenomics, 2002;3:349–366.

Individuals who are NAT2 fast acetylators are able to efficiently metabolize and detoxify bicyclic aromatic amines through liver-dependent acetylation. Slow acetylators (NAT2 deficient) accumulate bicyclic aromatic amines, which are metabolized by CYPs to *N*-OH metabolites that are eliminated in the urine. In bladder epithelium, NAT1 is highly expressed and can catalyze the *N*-hydroxy acetylation of bicyclic aromatic amines and the formation of the mutagenic nitrenium ion, especially in NAT2-deficient subjects. Slow acetylators are predisposed to bladder cancer if exposed environmentally to bicyclic aromatic amines.

METHYLATION. In humans, drugs and xenobiotics can undergo O-, N-, and S-methylation. Methyltransferases (MTs) are identified by substrate and methyl conjugate. Humans express 3 *N*-methyltransferases, 1 catechol-*O*-methyltransferase (COMT), 1 phenol-*O*-methyltransferase (POMT), 1 thiopurine *S*-methyltransferase (TPMT), and 1 thiol methyltransferase (TMT). These MTs use *S*-adenosyl-methionine (SAM; AdoMet) as the methyl donor. With the exception of a signature sequence that is conserved among the MTs, there is limited conservation in sequence, indicating that each MT has evolved to display a unique catalytic function. Although all MTs generate methylated products, the substrate specificity is high.

Nicotinamide *N*-methyltransferase (NNMT) methylates serotonin and tryptophan and pyridine-containing compounds (e.g., nicotinamide and nicotine). Phenylethanolamine *N*-methyltransferase (PNMT) methylates norepinephrine to epinephrine; the histamine *N*-methyltransferase (HNMT) metabolizes drugs containing an imidazole ring (e.g., histamine). COMT methylates neurotransmitters containing a catechol moiety (e.g., dopamine and norepinephrine, methyldopa and drugs of abuse such as ecstasy).

Clinically, the most important MT may be thiopurine *S*-methyltransferase (TPMT), which catalyzes the S-methylation of aromatic and heterocyclic sulfhydryl compounds, including azathioprine (AZA), 6-mercaptopurine (6-MP), and thioguanine. AZA and 6-MP are used for inflammatory bowel disease (*see* Chapter 47) and autoimmune disorders such as systemic lupus erythematosus and rheumatoid arthritis. Thioguanine is used in the treatment of acute myeloid leukemia, and 6-MP is used for the treatment of childhood acute lymphoblastic leukemia (*see* Chapters 61-63). Because TPMT is responsible for the detoxification of 6-MP, a genetic deficiency in TPMT can result in severe toxicities in patients taking these drugs. The toxic side effects arise when a lack of 6-MP methylation by TPMT causes a buildup of 6-MP, resulting in the generation of toxic levels of 6-thioguanine nucleotides (*see* Figure 47–5). Tests for TPMT activity have made it possible to identify individuals who may be predisposed to the toxic side effects of 6-MP therapy.

XENOBIOTIC METABOLISM, EFFICACY, AND ADVERSE RESPONSES

Metabolism of drugs normally results in the inactivation of their therapeutic effectiveness and facilitates their elimination. The extent of metabolism can determine the efficacy and toxicity of a drug by controlling its biological $t_{1/2}$. Among the most serious considerations in the clinical use of drugs are adverse drug responses (ADRs). If a drug is metabolized too quickly, it rapidly loses its therapeutic efficacy. A drug that is metabolized too slowly can accumulate in the bloodstream; the plasma clearance of the drug is decreased and the pharmacokinetic parameter AUC (area under the plasma concentration-time curve; *see* Figure 2–6) is elevated. An increase in AUC often results when specific xenobiotic-metabolizing enzymes are inhibited by diet or drug interactions.

For example, the consumption of grapefruit juice (which contains CYP3A4 inhibitors naringin and furanocoumarins) can inhibit intestinal CYP3A4, blocking the metabolism and altering the oral bioavailability of many classes of drugs, including, immunosuppressants, antidepressants, antihistamines, statins, and certain antihypertensives. Phenotypic changes in drug metabolism are also observed in individuals that are genetically predisposed to adverse drug reactions because of pharmacogenetic differences in the expression of xenobiotic-metabolizing enzymes (*see* Chapter 7). See, for example, the discussion of Gilbert syndrome, above (*see* Figures 6–5 and 6–6).

Nearly every class of therapeutic agent has been reported to initiate an ADR. In the U.S., the annual costs of ADRs have been estimated at >100,000 deaths and $100 billion. About 56% of drugs that are associated with adverse responses are subjected to metabolism by CYPs and UGTs. Because many of the CYPs and UGTs are subject to induction as well as inhibition by drugs, dietary factors, and other environmental agents, these enzymes play an important role in most ADRs. Thus, before a new drug application (NDA) is filed with the FDA, the route of metabolism and the enzymes involved in the metabolism must be known.

Xenobiotics can influence the extent of drug metabolism by activating transcription and expression of genes encoding drug-metabolizing enzymes. Thus, a drug may induce its own metabolism. One potential consequence of this is a decrease in plasma drug concentration over the course of treatment, resulting in loss of efficacy. Many ligands and receptors participate in this way to induce drug metabolism (Table 6–5). A particular receptor, when activated by a ligand, can induce the transcription of a battery of target genes, including CYPs and drug transporters,

Table 6–5

Nuclear Receptors and Ligands That Induce Drug Metabolism

RECEPTOR	LIGANDS
Aryl hydrocarbon receptor (AHR)	Omeprazole
Constitutive androstane receptor (CAR)	Phenobarbital
Pregnane X receptor (PXR)	Rifampin
Farnesoid X receptor (FXR)	Bile acids
Vitamin D receptor	Vitamin D
Peroxisome proliferator activated receptor (PPAR)	Fibrates
Retinoic acid receptor (RAR)	*all-trans*-Retinoic acid
Retinoid X receptor (RXR)	9-*cis*-Retinoic acid

leading to drug interactions. The aryl hydrocarbon receptor (AHR) is a member of a superfamily of transcription factors. The AHR induces expression of genes encoding CYP1A1, CYP1A2, and CYP1B1, which metabolically activate chemical carcinogens, including environmental contaminants and carcinogens derived from food. Many of these substances are inert unless metabolized by CYPs. Induction of these CYPs by a drug could potentially result in an increase in the toxicity and carcinogenicity of procarcinogens.

For example, omeprazole, a proton pump inhibitor used to treat gastric and duodenal ulcers (*see* Chapter 45), is a ligand for the AHR and can induce CYP1A1 and CYP1A2, possibly activating toxins/carcinogens as well as drug-drug interactions in patients receiving agents that are substrates for either of these CYPs.

Another important induction mechanism is caused by type 2 nuclear receptors that are in the same superfamily as the steroid hormone receptors. Figure 6–8 shows the scheme by which a drug may interact with nuclear receptors to induce its own metabolism. Many of these receptors were originally termed "orphan receptors," because they had no known endogenous ligands. The type 2 nuclear receptors of most importance to drug metabolism and drug therapy include the pregnane

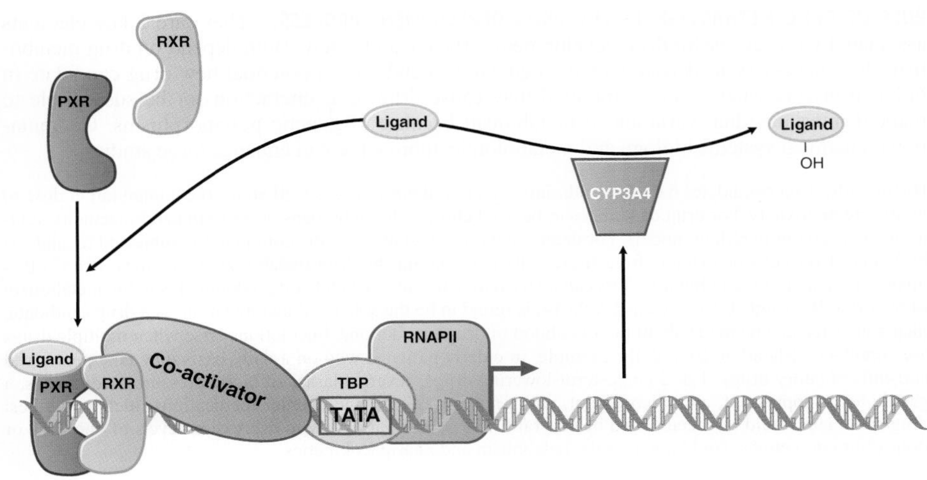

Figure 6–8 *Induction of drug metabolism by nuclear receptor–mediated signal transduction.* When a drug such as atorvastatin (the Ligand) enters the cell, it can bind to a nuclear receptor such as the pregnane X receptor (PXR). PXR then forms a complex with the retinoid X receptor (RXR), binds to DNA upstream of target genes, recruits coactivator (which binds to the TATA box binding protein, TBP), and activates transcription by RNA polymerase II (RNAP II). Among PXR target genes are CYP3A4, which can metabolize the atorvastatin and decrease its cellular concentration. Thus, atorvastatin induces its own metabolism. Atorvastatin undergoes both *ortho* and *para* hydroxylation.

X receptor (PXR), constitutive androstane receptor (CAR), and the peroxisome proliferator activated receptors (PPARs).

PXR is activated by a number of drugs including, antibiotics (rifampicin and troleandomycin), Ca^{2+} channel blockers (nifedipine), statins (mevastatin), antidiabetic drugs (troglitazone), HIV protease inhibitors (ritonavir), and anticancer drugs (paclitaxel). Hyperforin, a component of St. John's wort, an over-the-counter herbal remedy used for depression, also activates PXR. This activation is thought to be the basis for the increase in failure of oral contraceptives in individuals taking St. John's wort: Activated PXR induces CYP3A4, which can metabolize steroids found in oral contraceptives. PXR also induces the expression of genes encoding certain drug transporters and phase 2 enzymes including SULTs and UGTs. Thus, PXR facilitates the metabolism and elimination of xenobiotics, including drugs, with notable consequences.

The nuclear receptor CAR was discovered based on its ability to activate genes in the absence of ligand. Steroids such as *androstenol*, the antifungal agent *clotrimazol*e, and the antiemetic *meclizine* are inverse agonists that inhibit gene activation by CAR, while the pesticide 1,4-bis[2-(3,5-dichloropyridyloxy)]benzene, the steroid 5-β-pregnane-3,20-dione, are agonists that activate gene expression when bound to CAR. Genes induced by CAR include those encoding several CYPs (*CYP2B6, CYP2C9*, and *CYP3A4*), phase 2 enzymes (including GSTs, UGTs, and SULTs), and drug and endobiotic transporters. *CYP3A4* is induced by both PXR and CAR and thus its level is highly influenced by a number of drugs and other xenobiotics. There are species differences in the ligand specificities of these receptors. For example, *rifampin* activates human PXR, but not mouse or rat PXR, while *meclizine* activates mouse CAR, but inhibits gene induction by human CAR. These findings further underscore that data from rodent model systems do not always reflect the response of humans to drugs.

Members of a receptor family do not always show similar activities toward xenobiotics. One peroxisome proliferator activated receptor, PPARα, is the target for the fibrate class of hyperlipidemic drugs (e.g., *gemfibrozil* and *fenofibrate*). Activation of PPARα results in induction of genes encoding fatty acid metabolizing enzymes (result: ↓serum triglycerides) and of CYP4 enzymes that oxidize fatty acids and compounds with fatty acid side chains, such as leukotriene and arachidonic acid analogs. Another family member, PPARγ, is the target for the thiazolidinedione class of agents for type 2 diabetes (e.g., rosiglitazone and pioglitazone); PPARγ does not induce xenobiotic metabolism.

The UGT genes, especially *UGT1A1*, are inducible via a host of transcriptional activation pathways, including AHR, Nrf2 (a transcriptional regulator of cytoprotective genes that is induced by an antioxidant response), PXR, CAR, and PPARα. Because the UGTs are abundant in the GI track and liver, regulation of the UGTs by drug-induced activation of these receptors could affect the pharmacokinetic parameters of many orally administered therapeutics.

ROLE OF DRUG METABOLISM IN THE DRUG DEVELOPMENT PROCESS. There are 2 key elements associated with successful drug development: efficacy and safety. Both depend on drug metabolism. It is necessary to determine which enzymes metabolize a potential new drug candidate in order to predict whether the compound may cause drug-drug interactions or be susceptible to marked interindividual variation in metabolism because of genetic polymorphisms. Computational chemical systems biology and metabolomic approaches can enhance these studies.

Historically, drug candidates have been administered to rodents at doses well above the human target dose to predict acute toxicity. For drug candidates to be used chronically in humans, long-term carcinogenicity studies are carried out in rodent models. For determination of metabolism, the compound is subjected to analysis by human liver cells or extracts from these cells that contain the drug-metabolizing enzymes. If a CYP is involved, a panel of recombinant CYPs can be used to determine which CYP predominates in the metabolism of the drug. If a single CYP, such as CYP3A4, is found to be the sole CYP that metabolizes a drug candidate, then a decision can be made about the likelihood of drug interactions. Interactions arise when multiple drugs are simultaneously administered, for example, in elderly patients, who on a daily basis may take prescribed anti-inflammatory drugs, 1 or 2 cholesterol-lowering drugs, several classes of blood pressure medications, a gastric acid suppressant, an anticoagulant, and a number of over-the-counter medications. Ideally, the best drug candidate would be metabolized by several CYPs so that variability in expression levels of one CYP or drug-drug interactions would not alter its metabolism and pharmacokinetics.

Similar studies can be carried out with phase 2 enzymes and drug transporters. In addition to the use of recombinant human xenobiotic-metabolizing enzymes in predicting drug metabolism, human receptor-based (PXR and CAR) systems or cell lines expressing these receptors are used to determine whether a particular drug candidate could be a ligand or activator of PXR, CAR, or PPARα. For example, a drug that activates PXR may result in rapid clearance of other drugs that are CYP3A4 substrates, thus decreasing their bioavailability and efficacy.

Traditional toxicity studies in animals can be a bottleneck in the drug development process of lead compound optimization. A new technology of high-throughput screening for biomarkers of toxicity is being adopted for drug development using *metabolomics*, the systematic identification and quantification of all metabolites in a given organism or biological sample. Analytical platforms such as ^{1}H-NMR and liquid or gas chromatography coupled to mass spectrometry, in conjunction with chemometric and multivariate data analysis, allow the simultaneous determination and comparison of thousands of chemicals in biological fluids such as serum and urine, as well as the chemical constituents of cells and tissues. Metabolomics can be used to find biomarkers for drug efficacy and toxicity that can be of value in clinical trails to identify responders and nonresponders.

For a complete Bibliographical Listing see Goodman & Gilman's ***The Pharmacological Basis of Therapeutics***, 12th ed., or Goodman & Gilman Online at www.AccessMedicine.com.

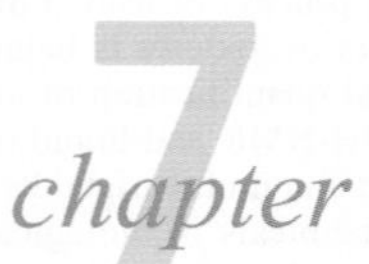

Pharmacogenetics

Pharmacogenetics is the study of the genetic basis for variation in drug response. In this broadest sense, pharmacogenetics encompasses *pharmacogenomics*, which employs tools for surveying the entire genome to assess multigenic determinants of drug response. Individuals differ from each other approximately every 300-1000 nucleotides, with an estimated total of 10 million *single nucleotide polymorphisms* (SNPs; single base pair substitutions found at frequencies ≥1% in a population) and thousands of copy number variations in the genome. Identifying which of these variants or combinations of variants have functional consequence for drug effects is the task of modern pharmacogenetics.

IMPORTANCE OF PHARMACOGENETICS TO VARIABILITY IN DRUG RESPONSE

Drug response is considered to be a gene-by-environment phenotype. An individual's response to a drug depends on the complex interplay between environmental factors (e.g., diet, age, infections, drugs, exercise level, occupation, exposure to toxins, tobacco, and alcohol use) and genetic factors (e.g., gender, variants of drug transporters, and drug metabolizing enzymes expressed). Variation in drug response therefore may be explained by variation in environmental and genetic factors, alone or in combination.

Drug metabolism is highly heritable, with genetic factors accounting for most of the variation in metabolic rates for many drugs.

Comparison of intra-twin vs inter-pair variability suggests that ~75-85% of the variability in pharmacokinetic half-lives for drugs that are eliminated by metabolism is heritable. Extended kindreds may be used to estimate heritability. Inter- vs. intra-family variability and relationships among members of a kindred are used to estimate heritability. Using this approach with lymphoblastoid cells, cytotoxicity from chemotherapeutic agents was shown to be heritable, with ~20-70% of the variability in sensitivity to 5-fluorouracil, cisplatin, docetaxel, and other anticancer agents estimated as inherited.

For "monogenic" phenotypic traits, it is often possible to predict phenotype based on genotype. Several genetic polymorphisms of drug metabolizing enzymes result in monogenic traits. Based on a retrospective study, 49% of adverse drug reactions were associated with drugs that are substrates for polymorphic drug metabolizing enzymes, a proportion larger than estimated for all drugs (22%) or for top-selling drugs (7%). Prospective genotype determinations may result in the ability to prevent adverse drug reactions. Defining multigenic contributors to drug response will be much more challenging. For some multigenic phenotypes, such as response to antihypertensives, the large numbers of candidate genes will necessitate a large patient sample size to produce the statistical power required to solve the "multigene" problem.

GENOMIC BASIS OF PHARMACOGENETICS

PHENOTYPE-DRIVEN TERMINOLOGY

A trait (e.g., CYP2D6 "poor metabolism") is deemed *autosomal recessive* if the responsible gene is located on an autosome (i.e., it is not sex-linked) and a distinct phenotype is evident only with nonfunctional alleles on both the maternal and paternal chromosomes. An autosomal recessive trait does not appear in heterozygotes. A trait is deemed *codominant* if heterozygotes exhibit a phenotype that is intermediate to that of homozygotes for the common allele and homozygotes for the variant allele. With the advances in molecular characterization of polymorphisms and a genotype-to-phenotype approach, many polymorphic traits (e.g., CYP2C19 metabolism of drugs such as mephenytoin and omeprazole) are now recognized to exhibit some degree of codominance. Two major factors complicate the historical designation of recessive, codominant, and dominant traits. *First*, even within a single gene, a vast array of polymorphisms (promoter, coding, noncoding, completely inactivating, or modestly modifying) are possible. Each polymorphism may produce a different effect on gene function and therefore differentially affect a measured trait. *Second*, most traits (pharmacogenetic and otherwise) are multigenic, not monogenic. Thus, even if the designations of recessive, codominant, and dominant are informative for a given gene, their utility in describing the genetic variability that underlies variability in drug response phenotype is diminished, because variability is likely to be multigenic.

TYPES OF GENETIC VARIANTS

A *polymorphism* is a variation in the DNA sequence that is present at an allele frequency of 1% or greater in a population. Two major types of sequence variation have been associated with variation in human phenotype: *single nucleotide polymorphisms* (SNPs) and *insertions/deletions* (indels). In comparison to base pair substitutions, indels are much less frequent in the genome and are of particularly low frequency in coding regions of genes. Single base pair substitutions that are present at frequencies ≥ 1% in a population are termed SNPs and are present in the human genome at ~1 SNP every few hundred to a thousand base pairs.

SNPs in the coding region are termed *cSNPs* (coding SNPs), and are further classified as *nonsynonymous* (or *missense*) or *synonymous* (or *sense*). Coding nonsynonymous SNPs result in a nucleotide substitution that changes the amino acid codon (e.g., proline [CCG] to glutamine [CAG]), which could change protein structure, stability, substrate affinities, or introduce a stop codon. Coding synonymous SNPs do not change the amino acid codon, but may have functional consequences (transcript stability, splicing). Typically, substitutions of the third base pair, termed the *wobble position*, in a 3 base pair codon, such as the G to A substitution in proline (CCG → CCA), do not alter the encoded amino acid. Base pair substitutions that lead to a stop codon are termed *nonsense* mutations. In addition, ~10% of SNPs can have more than 2 possible alleles (e.g., a C can be replaced by either an A or G), so that the same polymorphic site can be associated with amino acid substitutions in some alleles but not others.

Synonymous polymorphisms have sometimes been found to contribute directly to a phenotypic trait. One of the most notable examples is a polymorphism in ABCB1, which encodes P-glycoprotein, an efflux pump that interacts with many clinically used drugs. The synonymous polymorphism, C3435T, is associated with various phenotypes and results in a change from a preferred codon for isoleucine to a less preferred codon. Presumably, the less preferred codon is translated at a slower rate, which apparently changes the folding of the protein, its insertion into the membrane, and its interaction with drugs.

Noncoding SNPs may be in promoters, introns, or other regulatory regions that may affect transcription factor binding, enhancers, transcript stability, or splicing. Polymorphisms in noncoding regions of genes may occur in the 3′ and 5′ untranslated regions, in promoter or enhancer regions, in intronic regions, or in large regions between genes, intergenic regions (for nomenclature guide, *see* Figure 7–1). Noncoding SNPs in promoters or enhancers may alter *cis*- or *trans*-acting elements that regulate gene transcription or transcript stability. Noncoding SNPs in introns or exons may create alternative exon splicing sites, and the altered transcript may have fewer or more exons, or shorter or larger exons, than the wild-type transcript. Introduction or deletion of exonic sequence can cause a frame shift in the translated protein and thereby change protein structure or function, or result in an early stop codon, which makes an unstable or nonfunctional protein. Because 95% of the genome is intergenic, most polymorphisms are unlikely to directly affect the encoded transcript or protein. However, intergenic polymorphisms may have biological consequences by affecting DNA tertiary structure, interaction with chromatin and topoisomerases, or DNA replication. Thus, intergenic polymorphisms cannot be assumed to be without pharmacogenetic importance.

The second major type of polymorphism is indels. SNP indels can have any of the same effects as SNP substitutions: short repeats in the promoter (which can affect transcript amount), or insertions/deletions that add

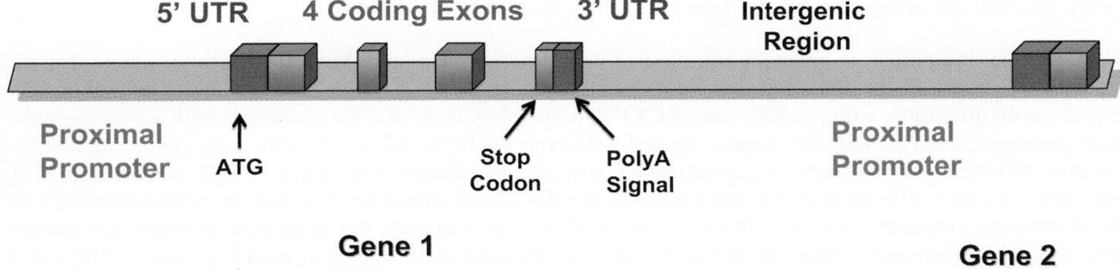

Figure 7–1 *Nomenclature of genomic regions.*

or subtract amino acids. A remarkable diversity of indels is tolerated as germline polymorphisms. A common glutathione-S-transferase M1 (*GSTM1*) polymorphism is caused by a 50-kilobase (kb) germline deletion, and the null allele has a population frequency of 0.3-0.5. Biochemical studies indicate that livers from homozygous null individuals have only ~50% of the glutathione conjugating capacity of those with at least 1 copy of the *GSTM1* gene. The number of TA repeats in the *UGT1A1* promoter affects the quantitative expression of this crucial glucuronosyltransferase in liver; 6 or 7 repeats constitute the most common alleles.

Some deletion and duplication polymorphisms can be seen as a special case of *copy number variations* (CNVs). Copy number variations involve large segments of genomic DNA that may involve gene duplications (stably transmitted inherited germline gene replication that causes increased protein expression and activity), gene deletions that result in the complete lack of protein production, or inversions of genes that may disrupt gene function. CNVs range in size from 1 kb to many megabases. CNVs appear to occur in ~10% of the human genome and in 1 study accounted for ~18% of the detected genetic variation in expression of around 15,000 genes in lymphoblastoid cell lines. There are notable examples of CNVs in pharmacogenetics; gene duplications of CYP2D6 are associated with an ultra-rapid metabolizer phenotype.

A *haplotype*, which is defined as a series of alleles found at a linked locus on a chromosome, specifies the DNA sequence variation in a gene or a gene region on 1 chromosome. For example, consider 2 SNPs in *ABCB1*, which encodes for the multidrug resistance protein, P-glycoprotein. One SNP is a T-to-A base pair substitution at position 3421 and the other is a C-to-T change at position 3435. Possible haplotypes would be $T_{3421}C_{3435}$, $T_{3421}T_{3435}$, $A_{3421}C_{3435}$, and $A_{3421}T_{3435}$. For any gene, individuals will have 2 haplotypes, 1 maternal and 1 paternal in origin. A haplotype represents the constellation of variants that occur together for the gene on each chromosome. In some cases, this constellation of variants, rather than the individual variant or allele, may be functionally important. In others, however, a single mutation may be functionally important regardless of other linked variants within the haplotype(s).

Two terms describe the relationship of genotypes at 2 loci: *linkage equilibrium* and *linkage disequilibrium*. Linkage equilibrium occurs when the genotype present at 1 locus is independent of the genotype at the second locus. Linkage disequilibrium occurs when the genotypes at the 2 loci are not independent of one another. In complete linkage disequilibrium, genotypes at 2 loci always occur together. Patterns of linkage disequilibrium are population specific and as recombination occurs linkage disequilibrium between 2 alleles will decay and linkage equilibrium will result.

ETHNIC DIVERSITY. Polymorphisms differ in their frequencies within human populations and have been classified as either cosmopolitan or population (or race and ethnic) specific. *Cosmopolitan polymorphisms* are those polymorphisms present in all ethnic groups, although frequencies may differ among ethnic groups. Likely to have arisen before migrations of humans from Africa, cosmopolitan polymorphisms are generally older than population-specific polymorphisms. The presence of ethnic and *race-specific polymorphisms* is consistent with geographical isolation of human populations. These polymorphisms probably arose in isolated populations and then reached a certain frequency because they are advantageous (positive selection) or, more likely, neutral to a population. African Americans have the highest number of population-specific polymorphisms in comparison to European Americans, Mexican Americans, and Asian Americans.

PHARMACOGENETIC STUDY DESIGN CONSIDERATIONS

PHARMACOGENETIC TRAITS

A *pharmacogenetic trait* is any measurable or discernible trait associated with a drug. Thus, enzyme activity, drug or metabolite levels in plasma or urine, blood pressure or lipid lowering produced by a drug, and drug-induced gene expression patterns are examples of pharmacogenetic traits. Directly measuring a trait (e.g., enzyme activity) has the advantage that the net effect of the contributions of all genes that influence the trait is reflected in the phenotypic measure. However, it has the disadvantage that it is also reflective of nongenetic influences (e.g., diet, drug interactions, diurnal, or hormonal fluctuation) and thus, may be "unstable."

For CYP2D6, if a patient is given an oral dose of dextromethorphan, and the urinary ratio of parent drug to metabolite is assessed, the phenotype is reflective of the genotype for CYP2D6. However, if dextromethorphan is given with quinidine, a potent inhibitor of CYP2D6, the phenotype may be consistent with a poor metabolizer genotype, even though the subject carries wild-type CYP2D6 alleles. In this case, quinidine administration results in a *drug-induced haploinsufficiency*, and the assignment of a CYP2D6 poor metabolizer phenotype would not be accurate for that subject in the absence of quinidine. If a phenotypic measure, such as the erythromycin breath test (for CYP3A), is not stable within a subject, this is an indication that the phenotype is highly influenced by nongenetic factors, and may indicate a multigenic or weakly penetrant effect of a monogenic trait. *Most pharmacogenetic traits are multigenic rather than monogenic* (Figure 7–2), and considerable effort is being made to identify the important polymorphisms that influence variability in drug response.

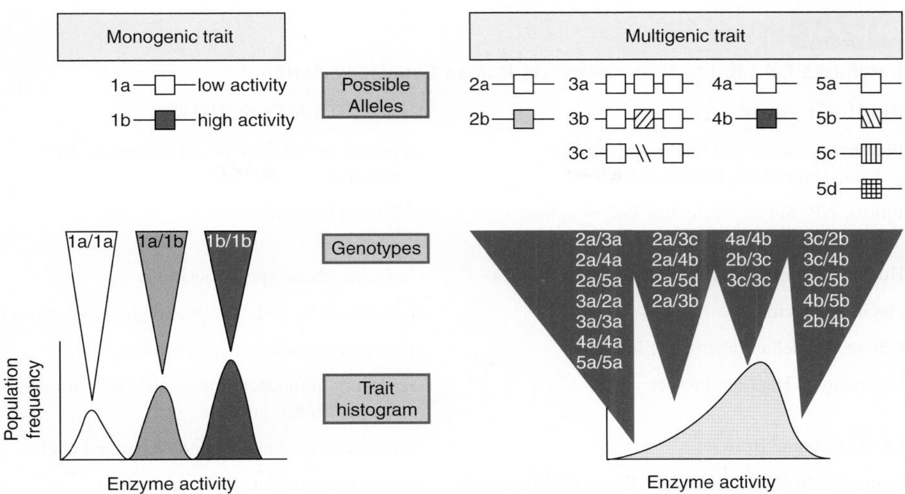

Figure 7–2 *Monogenic versus multigenic pharmacogenetic traits.* Possible alleles for a monogenic trait (*upper left*), in which a single gene has a low-activity (1a) and a high-activity (1b) allele. The population frequency distribution of a monogenic trait (*bottom left*), here depicted as enzyme activity, may exhibit a trimodal frequency distribution among low activity (homozygosity for 1a), intermediate activity (heterozygote for 1a and 1b), and high activity (homozygosity for 1b). This is contrasted with multigenic traits (e.g., an activity influenced by up to 4 different genes, genes 2 through 5), each of which has 2, 3, or 4 alleles (a through d). The population histogram for activity is unimodal-skewed, with no distinct differences among the genotypic groups. Multiple combinations of alleles coding for low activity and high activity at several of the genes can translate into low-, medium-, and high-activity phenotypes.

GENETIC TESTING. Most genotyping methods use constitutional or germline DNA, that is, DNA extracted from any somatic, diploid cells, usually white blood cells or buccal cells. DNA is extremely stable if appropriately extracted and stored and DNA sequence is generally invariant throughout an individual's lifetime. Because genotyping tests are directed at specific known polymorphic sites, and because not all known functional polymorphisms are likely to be known for any particular gene, it is critical to understand the methodology for interrogating the polymorphic sites. One method to assess the reliability of any specific genotype determination in a group of individuals is to assess whether the relative number of homozygotes to heterozygotes is consistent with the overall allele frequency at each polymorphic site. *Hardy-Weinberg* equilibrium is maintained when mating within a population is random and there is no natural selection effect on the variant. Such assumptions are described mathematically when the proportions of the population that are observed to be homozygous for the variant genotype (q^2), homozygous for the wild-type genotype (p^2), and heterozygous ($2*p*q$) are not significantly different from that predicted from the overall allele frequencies (p = frequency of wild-type allele; q = frequency of variant allele) in the population. Proportions of the observed 3 genotypes must add up to 1.

CANDIDATE GENE VERSUS GENOME-WIDE APPROACHES

After genes in drug response pathways are identified, the next step in the design of a candidate gene association pharmacogenetic study is to identify the genetic polymorphisms that are likely to contribute to the therapeutic and/or adverse responses to the drug. There are several databases that contain information on polymorphisms and mutations in human genes (Table 7–1); these databases allow the investigator to search by gene for reported polymorphisms. Some of the databases, such as the Pharmacogenetics and Pharmacogenomics Knowledge Base (PharmGKB), include phenotypic as well as genotypic data.

In candidate gene association studies, specific genes are prioritized as playing a role in response or adverse response to a drug, it is important to select polymorphisms in those genes for association studies. For this purpose, there are 2 categories of polymorphisms. The first are polymorphisms that do not, in and of themselves, cause altered function or expression level of the encoded protein (e.g., an enzyme that metabolizes the drug or the drug receptor). Rather, these polymorphisms are linked to the variant allele(s) that produces the altered function. The second type of polymorphism is the causative polymorphism, which directly precipitates the phenotype. For example, a causative SNP may change an amino acid residue at a site that is highly

Table 7–1

Databases Containing Information on Human Genetic Variation

DATABASE NAME	DESCRIPTION OF CONTENTS
Pharmacogenetics and Pharmacogenomics Knowledge Base (PharmGKB)	Genotype and phenotype data related to drug response
EntrezSNP (Single Nucleotide Polymorphism) (dbSNP)	SNPs and frequencies
Human Genome Variation Database (HGVbase)	Genotype/phenotype associations
HuGE Navigator	Annotations for genotype/phenotype associations
Online Mendelian Inheritance in Man	Human genes and genetic disorders
International HapMap Project	Genotypes, frequency/linkage data for variants in ethnic/racial groups
UCSC Genome Browser	Sequence of the human genome; variant alleles
Genomics Institute of Novartis Research Foundation	Gene expression data for human genes
The Broad Institute Software	Software tools for the analysis of genetic studies

conserved throughout evolution. This substitution may result in a protein that is nonfunctional or has reduced function. If biological information indicates that a particular polymorphism alters function, e.g., in cellular assays of nonsynonymous variants, this polymorphism is an excellent candidate to use in an association study. When causative SNPs are unknown, tag SNPs can be typed to represent important, relatively common blocks of variation within a gene. Once a tag SNP is found to associate with a drug response phenotype, the causative variant or variants, which may be in linkage with the tag SNP, should be identified. Because the causative variant may be an unknown variant, sequencing the gene may be necessary to identify potential causative variants. These additional causative variants may be uncovered by further deep resequencing of the gene.

GENOME-WIDE AND ALTERNATIVE LARGE-SCALE APPROACHES. A potential drawback of the candidate gene approach is that the wrong genes may be studied. Genome-wide approaches, using gene expression arrays, genome-wide scans, or proteomics, can complement and feed into the candidate gene approach by providing a relatively unbiased survey of the genome to identify previously unrecognized candidate genes. For example, RNA, DNA, or protein from patients who have unacceptable toxicity from a drug can be compared with identical material from identically treated patients who did not have such toxicity. Differences in gene expression, DNA polymorphisms, or relative amounts of proteins can be ascertained using computational tools, to identify genes, genomic regions, or proteins that can be further assessed for germline polymorphisms differentiating the phenotype. Gene expression and proteomic approaches have the advantage that the abundance of signal may itself directly reflect some of the relevant genetic variation; however, both types of expression are highly influenced by choice of tissue type, which may not be available from the relevant tissue; for example, it may not be feasible to obtain biopsies of brain tissue for studies on CNS toxicity. DNA has the advantage that it is readily available and independent of tissue type, but the vast majority of genomic variation is not in genes, and the large number of polymorphisms presents the danger of *type I error* (finding differences in genome-wide surveys that are false positives). Current research challenges include prioritizing among the many possible differentiating variations in genome-wide surveys of RNA, DNA, and protein to focus on those that hold the most promise for future pharmacogenomic utility.

FUNCTIONAL STUDIES OF POLYMORPHISMS

For most polymorphisms, functional information is not available. Therefore, to select polymorphisms that are likely to be causative, it is important to predict whether a polymorphism may result in a change in expression level of a protein or a change in protein function, stability, or subcellular localization. One way to gain an understanding of the functional effects of various types of genomic variations is to survey the mutations that have been associated with human Mendelian disease. The greatest numbers of DNA variations associated with Mendelian diseases or traits are *missense* and *nonsense mutations*, followed by *deletions*.

Functional genomics studies of numerous variants in membrane transporters suggest that the variants that alter function are likely to change an evolutionarily conserved amino acid residue and to be at low allele frequencies. These data indicate that SNPs that alter evolutionarily conserved residues are most deleterious.

For example, substitution of a charged amino acid (Arg) for a nonpolar, uncharged amino acid (Cys) is more likely to affect function than substitution of residues that are more chemically similar (e.g., Arg to Lys). The data also suggest that rare SNPs, at least in the coding region, are likely to alter function.

Among the first pharmacogenetic examples to be discovered was glucose-6-phosphate dehydrogenase (G6PD) deficiency, an X-linked monogenic trait that results in severe hemolytic anemia in individuals after ingestion of fava beans or various drugs, including many antimalarial agents. G6PD is normally present in red blood cells and helps to regulate levels of glutathione (GSH), an antioxidant. Antimalarials such as primaquine increase red blood cell fragility in individuals with G6PD deficiency, leading to profound hemolytic anemia. The severity of the deficiency syndrome varies among individuals and is related to the amino acid variant in G6PD. The severe form of G6PD deficiency is associated with changes at residues that are highly conserved across evolutionary history. Collectively, studies of Mendelian traits and polymorphisms suggest that nonsynonymous SNPs that alter residues that are highly conserved among species and those that result in more radical changes in the nature of the amino acid are likely to be the best candidates for causing functional changes. *The information in Table 7–2 can be used as a guide for prioritizing polymorphisms in candidate gene association studies.*

Table 7–2

Predicted Functional Effect and Relative Risk That a Variant Will Alter Function of SNP Types in the Human Genome

TYPE OF VARIANT	LOCATION	FREQUENCY IN GENOME	PREDICTED RELATIVE RISK OF PHENOTYPE	FUNCTIONAL EFFECT
Nonsense	Coding region	Very low	Very high	Stop codon
Nonsynonymous Evolutionarily conserved	Coding region	Low	High	Substitution of AA conserved across evolution
Nonsynonymous Evolutionarily unconserved	Coding region	Low	Low to moderate	Substitution of AA not conserved across evolution
Nonsynonymous Radical chemical change	Coding region	Low	Moderate to high	Substitution of AA chemically dissimilar to original
Nonsynonymous Low to moderate chemical change	Coding region	Low	Low to high	Substitution of AA chemically similar to original
Insertion/deletion	Coding/noncoding region	Low	Low to high	Coding region: can cause frameshift
Synonymous	Coding region	Medium	Low	Can affect mRNA stability or splicing
Regulatory region	Promoter, 5′ UTR, 3′ UTR	Medium	Low to High	Can affect mRNA transcript level by changing rate of transcription or transcript stability
Intron/exon boundary	Within 8 bp of intron	Low	High	May affect splicing
Intronic	Deep within intron	Medium	Unknown	May affect mRNA transcript levels via enhancer mechanism
Intergenic	Noncoding region between genes	High	Unknown	

AA, amino acid.

Adapted by permission from Macmillan Publishers Ltd: Tabor HK, Risch NJ, Myers RM. Candidate-gene approaches for studying complex genetic traits: Practical considerations. Nat Rev Genet, 2002;3:391–397. Copyright 2002.

With the increasing number of SNPs that have been identified, it is clear that computational methods are needed to predict the functional consequences of SNPs. To this end, predictive algorithms have been developed to identify potentially deleterious amino acid substitutions. These methods can be classified into 2 groups. The first group relies on sequence comparisons alone to identify and score substitutions according to their degree of conservation across multiple species; different scoring matrices have been used (e.g., BLOSUM62, SIFT, and PolyPhen). The second group of methods relies on mapping of SNPs onto protein structures, in addition to sequence comparisons. For example, rules have been developed that classify SNPs in terms of their impact on folding and stability of the native protein structure as well as shapes of its binding sites.

Functional activity of amino acid variants for many proteins can be studied in cellular assays. An initial step in characterizing the function of a non-synonymous variant is to isolate the variant gene or construct the variant by site-directed mutagenesis, express it in cells, and compare its functional activity to that of the reference or most common form of the protein. For many proteins, including enzymes, transporters, and receptors, the mechanisms by which amino acid substitutions alter function have been characterized in kinetic studies. Figure 7–3 shows simulated curves depicting the rate of metabolism of a substrate by 2 amino acid variants of an enzyme and the most common genetic form of the enzyme.

In contrast to the studies with SNPs in coding regions, we know much less about noncoding region SNPs. SNPs identified in genome-wide association studies as being associated with clinical phenotypes including drug response phenotypes have largely been in noncoding regions, either intergenic or intronic regions, of the genome. An example of profound functional effect of a noncoding SNP is provided by CYP3A5; a common noncoding intronic SNP in CYP3A5 accounts for its polymorphic expression in humans. The SNP accounting for variation in CYP3A5 protein creates an alternative splice site, resulting in a transcript with a larger exon 3 but also the introduction of an early stop codon (Figure 7–4).

PHARMACOGENETIC PHENOTYPES

Candidate genes for therapeutic and adverse response can be divided into 3 categories: *pharmacokinetic*, *receptor/target*, and *disease modifying*.

PHARMACOKINETIC ALTERATIONS. Germline variability in genes that encode determinants of the pharmacokinetics of a drug, in particular metabolizing enzymes and transporters, affect drug concentrations, and are therefore major determinants of therapeutic and adverse drug response (Table 7–3). Multiple enzymes and transporters may be involved in the pharmacokinetics of a single drug. Several polymorphisms in drug metabolizing enzymes were discovered as monogenic phenotypic trait variations.

For example, a very large number of medications (estimated at 15-25% of all medicines in use) have been shown to be substrates for CYP2D6 (*see* Table 7–3 and Figure 6–3A). Phenotypic consequences of the

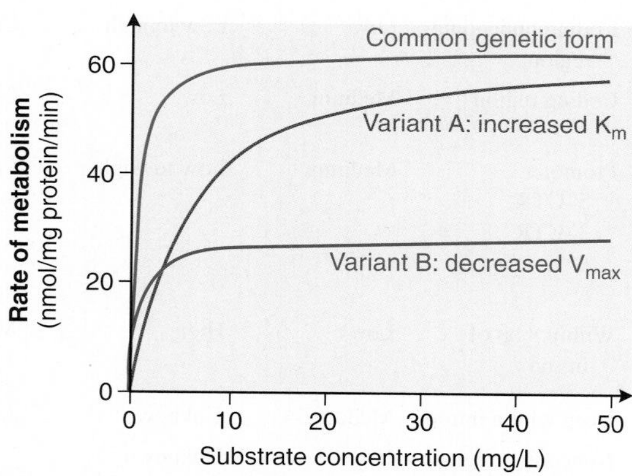

Figure 7–3 *Concentration-dependence curves showing the rate of metabolism of a hypothetical substrate by the common genetic form of an enzyme and 2 nonsynonymous variants.* Variant A exhibits an increased K_m and likely reflects a change in the substrate binding site of the protein by the substituted amino acid. Variant B exhibits a change in the maximum rate of metabolism (V_{max}) of the substrate. This may be due to reduced expression level of the enzyme.

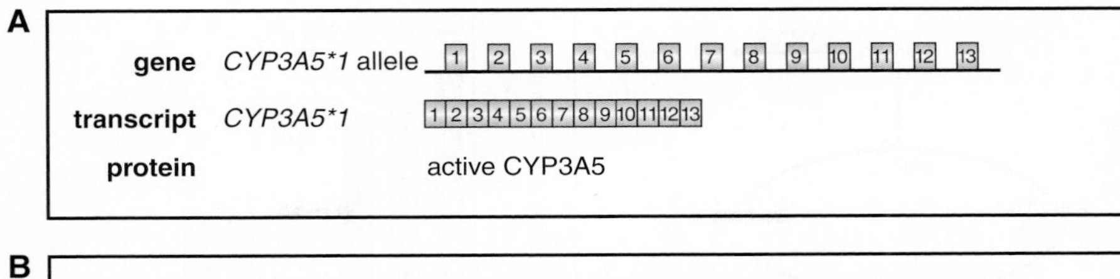

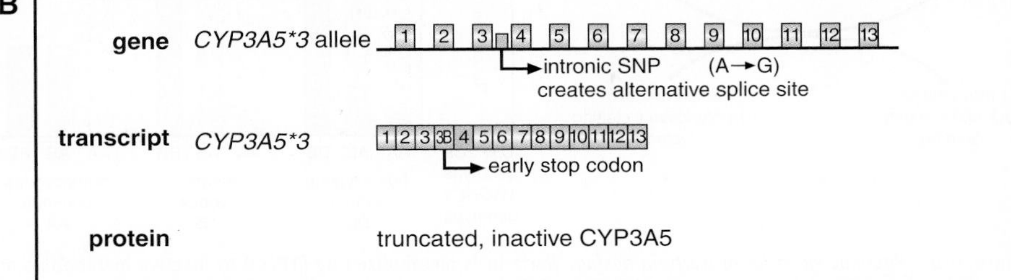

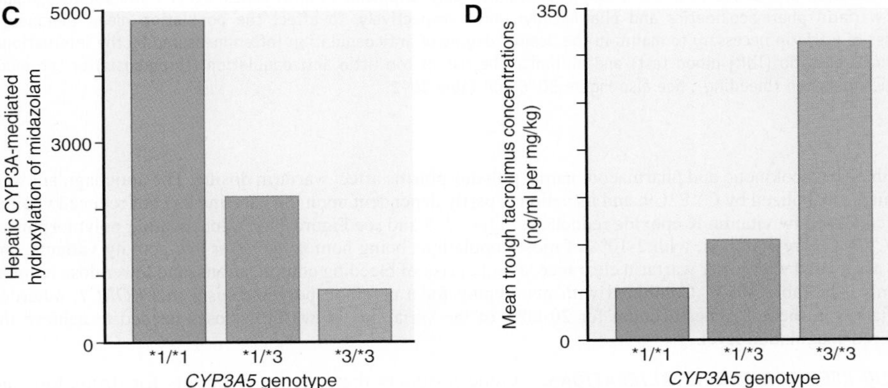

Figure 7–4 *An intronic SNP can affect splicing and account for polymorphic expression of CYP3A5.* A common polymorphism (A > G) in intron 3 of CYP3A5 defines the genotypes associated with the wild-type CYP3A5*1 allele, or the variant nonfunctional CYP3A5*3 allele. This intronic SNP creates an alternative splice site that results in the production of an alternative CYP3A5 transcript carrying an additional intron 3B (panel **B**), with an early stop codon and truncated CYP3A5 protein. The wild-type gene (more common in African than Caucasian or Asian populations) results in production of active CYP3A5 protein (panel **A**); the *3 variant results in a truncated and inactive protein. Thus, metabolism of CYP3A5 substrates is diminished in vitro (panel **C**) and blood concentrations of such medications are higher in vivo (panel **D**) for those with the *3 than the *1 allele.

deficient CYP2D6 phenotype include increased risk of toxicity of antidepressants or antipsychotics (catabolized by the enzyme), lack of analgesic effects of codeine (anabolized by the enzyme), and lack of activation of tamoxifen, leading to a greater risk of relapse or recurrence in breast cancer. Conversely, the ultrarapid phenotype is associated with extremely rapid clearance and thus inefficacy of antidepressants.

A promoter region variant in the enzyme UGT1A1, UGT1A1*28, which has an additional TA in comparison to the more common form of the gene, has been associated with a reduced transcription rate of *UGT1A1* and lower glucuronidation activity of the enzyme. This reduced activity has been associated with higher levels of the active metabolite SN38 of the cancer chemotherapeutic agent *irinotecan* (*see* Chapter 6), which is associated with the increased risk of toxicity (*see* Figures 6–5 and 6–6). CYP2C19, historically termed mephenytoin hydroxylase, displays penetrant pharmacogenetic variability, with just a few SNPs accounting for the majority of the deficient, poor metabolizer phenotype. The deficient phenotype is much more common in Chinese and Japanese populations. Several proton pump inhibitors, including omeprazole and lansoprazole, are inactivated by CYP2C19. Thus, the deficient patients have higher exposure to active parent drug, a greater pharmacodynamic effect (higher gastric pH), and a higher probability of ulcer cure than heterozygotes or homozygous wild-type individuals.

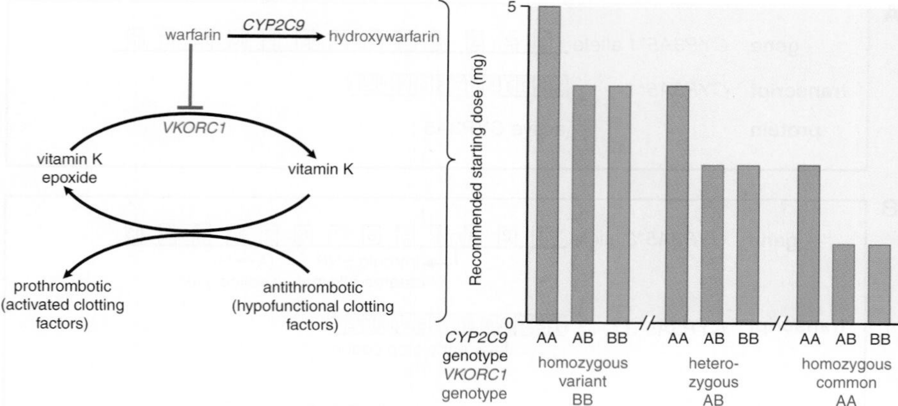

Figure 7–5 *Pharmacogenetics of warfarin dosing.* Warfarin is metabolized by *CYP2C9* to inactive metabolites and exerts its anticoagulant effect partly via inhibition of *VKORC1* (vitamin K epoxide hydrolase), an enzyme necessary for reduction of inactive to active vitamin K. Common polymorphisms in both genes, *CYP2C9* and *VKORC1*, impact on warfarin pharmacokinetics and pharmacodynamics, respectively, to affect the population mean therapeutic doses of warfarin necessary to maintain the desired degree of anticoagulation (often measured by the international normalized ratio [INR] blood test) and minimize the risk of too little anticoagulation (thrombosis) or too much anticoagulation (bleeding). See also Figure 30–6 and Table 30–2.

Both pharmacokinetic and pharmacodynamic polymorphisms affect warfarin dosing. The anticoagulant warfarin is catabolized by CYP2C9, and its action is partly dependent upon the baseline level of reduced vitamin K (catalyzed by vitamin K epoxide reductase; Figure 7–5 and *see* Figure 30–6). Inactivating polymorphisms in *CYP2C9* are common, with 2-10% of most populations being homozygous for low-activity variants, and are associated with lower warfarin clearance, a higher risk of bleeding complications, and lower dose requirements (*see* Table 30–2). Combined with genotyping for a common polymorphism in *VKORC1*, inherited variation in these 2 genes account for 20-60% of the variability in warfarin doses needed to achieve the desired coagulation level.

DRUG RECEPTOR/TARGET ALTERATIONS. Gene products that are direct targets for drugs have an important role in pharmacogenetics. Highly penetrant variants with profound functional consequences in some genes may cause disease phenotypes that confer negative selective pressure; more subtle variations in the same genes can be maintained in the population without causing disease, but nonetheless causing variation in drug response.

For example, complete inactivation by means of rare point mutations in methylenetetrahydrofolate reductase (MTHFR) causes severe mental retardation, cardiovascular disease, and a shortened lifespan. Conversely, the 677C→T SNP causes an amino acid substitution that is maintained in the population at a high frequency (frequency in most white populations = 0.4) and is associated with modestly lower MTHFR activity (~30% less than the 677C allele) and modest but significantly elevated plasma homocysteine concentrations (~25% higher). This polymorphism does not alter drug pharmacokinetics, but does appear to modulate pharmacodynamics by predisposing to GI toxicity to the antifolate drug methotrexate in stem cell transplant recipients.

FACTORS MODIFYING METHOTREXATE ACTION. The methotrexate pathway involves metabolism, transport, drug modifier, and drug target polymorphisms. Methotrexate is a substrate for transporters and anabolizing enzymes that affect its intracellular pharmacokinetics and that are subject to common polymorphisms. Several of the direct targets (dihydrofolate reductase, purine transformylases, and thymidylate synthase [TYMS]) are also subject to common polymorphisms. A polymorphic indel in *TYMS* (2 vs. 3 repeats of a 28-base pair repeat in the enhancer) affects the amount of enzyme expression in both normal and tumor cells. The *TYMS* polymorphism can affect both toxicity and efficacy of anticancer agents (e.g., fluorouracil and methotrexate) that target TYMS. Thus, the genetic contribution to variability in the pharmacokinetics and pharmacodynamics of methotrexate cannot be understood without assessing genotypes at a number of different loci.

OTHER EXAMPLES OF DRUG TARGET POLYMORPHISMS. Many drug target polymorphisms have been shown to predict responsiveness to drugs (Table 7–3). Serotonin receptor polymorphisms predict not only the responsiveness to antidepressants, but also the overall risk of depression. β Adrenergic receptor polymorphisms have been linked to asthma responsiveness, renal function following angiotensin-converting enzyme (ACE) inhibitors, and heart rate following β blockers. Polymorphisms in HMG-CoA reductase have been linked to the degree of lipid lowering following statins (*see* Chapter 31), and to the degree of positive effects on high-density lipoproteins among women on estrogen replacement therapy. Ion channel polymorphisms have been linked to a risk of cardiac arrhythmias in the presence and absence of drug triggers.

POLYMORPHISM-MODIFYING DISEASES. Some genes may be involved in an underlying disease being treated, but do not directly interact with the drug. Modifier polymorphisms are important for the de novo risk of some events and for the risk of drug-induced events.

For example, the *MTHFR* polymorphism is linked to homocysteinemia, which in turn affects thrombosis risk. The risk of a drug-induced thrombosis is dependent not only on the use of prothrombotic drugs, but on environmental and genetic predisposition to thrombosis, which may be affected by germline polymorphisms in *MTHFR*, factor V, and prothrombin. These polymorphisms do not directly act on the pharmacokinetics or pharmacodynamics of prothrombotic drugs, such as glucocorticoids, estrogens, and asparaginase, but may modify the risk of the phenotypic event (thrombosis) in the presence of the drug. Likewise, polymorphisms in ion channels (e.g., *HERG*, KvLQT1, Mink, and *MiRP1*) may affect the overall risk of cardiac dysrhythmias, risk that may be accentuated by a drug that can prolong the QT interval in some circumstances (e.g., macrolide antibiotics, antihistamines).

CANCER AS A SPECIAL CASE. Cancer pharmacogenetics have an unusual aspect in that tumors exhibit somatically acquired mutations in addition to the underlying germline variation of the host. Thus, the efficacy of some anticancer drugs depends on the genetics of both the host and the tumor.

For example, non-small-cell lung cancer is treated with an inhibitor of epidermal growth factor receptor (EGFR), gefitinib. Patients whose tumors have activating mutations in the tyrosine kinase domain of *EGFR* appear to respond better to gefitinib than those without the mutations. Breast cancer patients with expression of the Her2 antigen (as an acquired genetic changes) are more likely to benefit from the antibody trastuzumab than are those who are negative for Her2 expression, and this results in a common tailoring of anticancer therapy in patients with breast cancer based on tumor genetics. Some genetic alterations affects both tumor and host: the presence of 2 instead of 3 copies of a *TYMS* enhancer repeat polymorphism increases the risk of host toxicity but also increases the chance of tumor susceptibility to thymidylate synthase inhibitors.

PHARMACOGENETICS IN CLINICAL PRACTICE

Three major types of evidence should accumulate to implicate a polymorphism in clinical care:

1. *Screens of tissues from multiple humans linking the polymorphism to a trait*
2. *Complementary preclinical functional studies indicating that the polymorphism is plausibly linked with the phenotype*
3. *Multiple supportive clinical phenotype/genotype association studies*

Most drug dosing relies on a population "average" dose of drug. Adjusting dosages for variables such as renal or liver dysfunction is often accepted in drug dosing. Even though there are many examples of significant effects of polymorphisms on drug disposition (e.g., *see* Table 7–3), there is much more hesitation from clinicians to adjust doses based on genetic testing than on indirect clinical measures of renal and liver function. The frequency of functionally important polymorphisms means that complexity of dosing will be likely to increase substantially in the postgenomic era. Even if every drug has only 1 important polymorphism to consider when dosing, the scale of complexity could be large. The potential utility of pharmacogenetics to optimize drug therapy is great. With continued incorporation of pharmacogenetics into clinical trials, the important genes and polymorphisms will be identified, and data will demonstrate whether dosage individualization can improve outcomes and decrease short- and long-term adverse effects.

There are useful resources that permit clinicians to access information on pharmacogenetics, (*see* Table 7–1). Passage of laws to prevent genetic discrimination may assuage concerns that genetic data placed in medical records could penalize those with "unfavorable" genotypes.

Table 7–3

Examples of Genetic Polymorphisms Influencing Drug Response

GENE PRODUCT *(GENE)*	DRUGS[a]	RESPONSES AFFECTED
Drug Metabolism and Transport		
CYP2C9	Tolbutamide, warfarin,[a] phenytoin, nonsteroidal anti-inflammatory	Anticoagulant effect of warfarin
CYP2C19	Mephenytoin, omeprazole, voriconazole[a], hexobarbital, mephobarbital, propranolol, proguanil, phenytoin, clopidogrel	Peptic ulcer response to omeprazole; cardiovascular events after clopidogrel
CYP2D6	β blockers, antidepressants, antipsychotics, codeine, debrisoquine, atomoxetine[a], dextromethorphan, encainide, flecainide, fluoxetine, guanoxan, *N*-propylajmaline, perhexiline, phenacetin, phenformin, propafenone, sparteine, tamoxifen	Tardive dyskinesia from antipsychotics, narcotic side effects, codeine efficacy, imipramine dose requirement, β blocker effect; breast cancer recurrence after tamoxifen
CYP3A4/3A5/3A7	Macrolides, cyclosporine, tacrolimus, Ca^{2+} channel blockers, midazolam, terfenadine, lidocaine, dapsone, quinidine, triazolam, etoposide, teniposide, lovastatin, alfentanil, tamoxifen, steroids	Efficacy of immunosuppressive effects of tacrolimus
Dihydropyrimidine dehydrogenase	Fluorouracil, capecitabine[a]	5-Fluorouracil toxicity
N-acetyltransferase *(NAT2)*	Isoniazid, hydralazine, sulfonamides, amonafide, procainamide, dapsone, caffeine	Hypersensitivity to sulfonamides, amonafide toxicity, hydralazine-induced lupus, isoniazid neurotoxicity
Glutathione transferases *(GSTM1, GSTT1, GSTP1)*	Several anticancer agents	Decreased response in breast cancer, more toxicity and worse response in acute myelogenous leukemia
Thiopurine methyltransferase *(TPMT)*	Mercaptopurine[a], thioguanine[a], azathioprine[a]	Thiopurine toxicity and efficacy, risk of second cancers
UDP-glucuronosyl-transferase *(UGT1A1)*	Irinotecan[a], bilirubin	Irinotecan toxicity
P-glycoprotein *(ABCB1)*	Natural product anticancer drugs, HIV protease inhibitors, digoxin	Decreased CD4 response in HIV-infected patients, decreased digoxin AUC, drug resistance in epilepsy
UGT2B7	Morphine	Morphine plasma levels
Organic anion transporter *(SLC01B1)*	Statins, methotrexate, ACE inhibitors	Statin plasma levels, myopathy; methotrexate plasma levels, mucositis
COMT	Levodopa	Enhanced drug effect
Organic cation transporter *(SLC22A1, OCT1)*	Metformin	Pharmacologic effect and pharmacokinetics
Organic cation transporter *(SLC22A2, OCT2)*	Metformin	Renal clearance
Novel organic cation transporter *(SLC22A4, OCTN1)*	Gabapentin	Renal clearance
CYP2B6	Cyclophosphamide	Ovarian failure

(continued)

Table 7–3

Examples of Genetic Polymorphisms Influencing Drug Response (*Continued*)

GENE PRODUCT *(GENE)*	DRUGS[a]	RESPONSES AFFECTED
Targets and Receptors		
Angiotensin-converting enzyme (ACE)	ACE inhibitors (e.g., enalapril)	Renoprotective effects, hypotension, left ventricular mass reduction, cough
Thymidylate synthase	5-Fluorouracil	Colorectal cancer response
Chemokine receptor 5 (CCR5)	Antiretrovirals, interferon	Antiviral response
β_2 Adrenergic receptor *(ADBR2)*	β_2 Antagonists (e.g., albuterol, terbutaline)	Bronchodilation, susceptibility to agonist-induced desensitization, cardiovascular effects (e.g., increased heart rate, cardiac index, peripheral vasodilation)
β_1 Adrenergic receptor *(ADBR1)*	β_1 Antagonists	Blood pressure and heart rate after β_1 antagonists
5-Lipoxygenase (ALOX5)	Leukotriene receptor antagonists	Asthma response
Dopamine receptors (D_2, D_3, D_4)	Antipsychotics (e.g., haloperidol, clozapine, thioridazine, nemonapride)	Antipsychotic response (D_2, D_3, D_4), antipsychotic-induced tardive dyskinesia (D_3) and acute akathisia (D_3), hyperprolactinemia in females (D_2)
Estrogen receptor α	Estrogen hormone replacement therapy	High-density lipoprotein cholesterol
Serotonin transporter (5-HTT)	Antidepressants (e.g., clomipramine, fluoxetine, paroxetine, fluvoxamine)	Clozapine effects, 5-HT neurotransmission, antidepressant response
Serotonin receptor (5-HT_{2A})	Antipsychotics	Clozapine antipsychotic response, tardive dyskinesia, paroxetine antidepression response, drug discrimination
HMG-CoA reductase	Pravastatin	Reduction in serum cholesterol
Vitamin K oxidoreductase (VKORC1)	Warfarin[a]	Anticoagulant effect, bleeding risk
Corticotropin releasing hormone receptor (CRHR1)	Glucocorticoids	Bronchodilation, osteopenia
Ryanodine receptor (RYR1)	General anesthetics	Malignant hyperthermia
Modifiers		
Adducin	Diuretics	Myocardial infarction or strokes, blood pressure
Apolipoprotein E	Statins (e.g., simvastatin), tacrine	Lipid-lowering; clinical improvement in Alzheimer's disease
Human leukocyte antigen	Abacavir, carbamazepine, phenytoin	Hypersensitivity reactions
G6PD deficiency	Rasburicase[a], dapsone[a]	Methemoglobinemia
Cholesteryl ester transfer protein	Statins (e.g., pravastatin)	Slowing atherosclerosis progression

(*continued*)

Table 7–3

Examples of Genetic Polymorphisms Influencing Drug Response (*Continued*)

GENE PRODUCT *(GENE)*	DRUGS[a]	RESPONSES AFFECTED
Ion channels *(HERG, KvLQT1, Mink, MiRP1)*	Erythromycin, cisapride, clarithromycin, quinidine	Increased risk of drug-induced *torsades de pointes,* increased QT interval
Methylguanine-methyltransferase	DNA methylating agents	Response of glioma to chemotherapy
Parkin	Levodopa	Parkinson disease response
MTHFR	Methotrexate	GI toxicity
Prothrombin, factor V	Oral contraceptives	Venous thrombosis risk
Stromelysin-1	Statins (e.g., pravastatin)	Reduction in cardiovascular events and in repeat angioplasty
Inosine triphosphatase (ITPA)	Azathioprine, mercaptopurine	Myelosuppression
Vitamin D receptor	Estrogen	Bone mineral density

[a]*Information on genetics-based dosing, adverse events, or testing added to FDA-approved drug label (Grossman I. Routine pharmacogenetic testing in clinical practice: Dream or reality? Pharmacogenomics, 2007, 8:1449–1459).*

For a complete Bibliographical Listing see Goodman & Gilman's ***The Pharmacological Basis of Therapeutics***, 12th ed., or Goodman & Gilman Online at www.AccessMedicine.com.

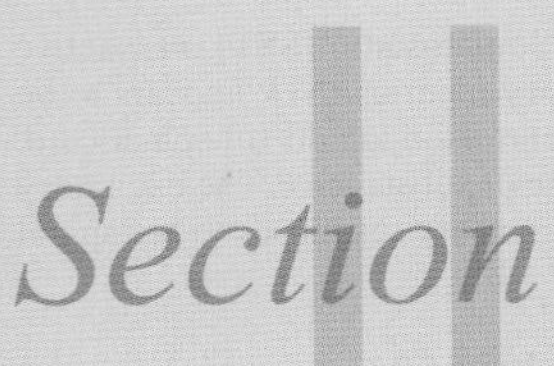

Section II Neuropharmacology

chapter 8 Neurotransmission: The Autonomic and Somatic Motor Nervous Systems

ANATOMY AND GENERAL FUNCTIONS

The autonomic nervous system (ANS; a.k.a. the *visceral, vegetative,* or *involuntary nervous system*) regulates autonomic functions that occur without conscious control. In the periphery, it consists of nerves, ganglia, and plexuses that innervate the heart, blood vessels, glands, other visceral organs, and smooth muscle in various tissues.

DIFFERENCES BETWEEN AUTONOMIC AND SOMATIC NERVES

- The *efferent nerves* of the ANS supply all innervated structures of the body except skeletal muscle, which is served by *somatic nerves*.
- The most distal synaptic junctions in the autonomic reflex arc occur in *ganglia* that are entirely *outside the cerebrospinal axis*. Somatic nerves contain no peripheral *ganglia*, and the synapses are located entirely *within the cerebrospinal axis*.
- Many autonomic nerves form extensive peripheral plexuses; such networks are absent from the somatic system.
- Postganglionic autonomic nerves generally are *nonmyelinated*; motor nerves to skeletal muscles are *myelinated*.
- When the spinal efferent nerves are interrupted, smooth muscles and glands generally retain some level of spontaneous activity, whereas the *denervated* skeletal muscles are paralyzed.

VISCERAL AFFERENT FIBERS. The afferent fibers from visceral structures are the first link in the reflex arcs of the autonomic system. With certain exceptions, such as local axon reflexes, most visceral reflexes are mediated through the central nervous system (CNS).

Information on the status of the visceral organs is transmitted to the CNS through 2 main sensory systems: *the cranial nerve (parasympathetic) visceral sensory* system and *the spinal (sympathetic) visceral afferent* system. The cranial visceral sensory system carries mainly *mechanoreceptor* and *chemosensory information*, whereas the afferents of the spinal visceral system principally convey sensations related to *temperature* and *tissue injury* of mechanical, chemical, or thermal origin.

Cranial visceral sensory information enters the CNS by 4 cranial nerves: the trigeminal (V), facial (VII), glossopharyngeal (IX), and vagus (X) nerves. These 4 cranial nerves transmit visceral sensory information from the internal face and head (V); tongue (taste, VII); hard palate and upper part of the oropharynx (IX); and carotid body, lower part of the oropharynx, larynx, trachea, esophagus, and thoracic and abdominal organs (X), with the exception of the pelvic viscera. The pelvic viscera are innervated by nerves from the second through fourth sacral spinal segments. The visceral afferents from these 4 cranial nerves terminate topographically in the *solitary tract nucleus*.

Sensory afferents from visceral organs also enter the CNS from the spinal nerves and convey information concerned with temperature as well as nociceptive visceral inputs related to mechanical, chemical, and thermal stimulation. Those concerned with muscle chemosensation may arise at all spinal levels, whereas sympathetic visceral sensory afferents generally arise at the thoracic levels where sympathetic preganglionic neurons are found. The neurotransmitters that mediate transmission from sensory fibers have not been characterized unequivocally. Substance P and calcitonin gene-related peptide (CGRP), are leading candidates for neurotransmitters that communicate nociceptive stimuli from the periphery. Somatostatin (SST), vasoactive intestinal polypeptide (VIP), and cholecystokinin (CCK), also occur in sensory neurons. ATP appears to be a neurotransmitter in certain sensory neurons. Enkephalins, present in interneurons in the dorsal spinal cord, have antinociceptive effects both pre- and postsynaptically to inhibit the release of substance P. The excitatory amino acids glutamate and aspartate also play major roles in transmission of sensory responses to the spinal cord. These transmitters and their signaling pathways are reviewed in Chapter 14.

DIVISIONS OF THE PERIPHERAL AUTONOMIC SYSTEM. The ANS consists of 2 large divisions: the *sympathetic* and the *parasympathetic* (Figure 8–1).

The neurotransmitter of all preganglionic autonomic fibers, most postganglionic parasympathetic fibers, and a few postganglionic sympathetic fibers is *acetylcholine* (ACh). Some postganglionic parasympathetic nerves use *nitric oxide* (NO) and are referred to as *nitrergic*. The majority of the postganglionic sympathetic fibers are *adrenergic,* in which the transmitter is *norepinephrine* (NE, noradrenaline). The terms *cholinergic* and *adrenergic* describe neurons that liberate ACh or NE, respectively. Substance P and glutamate may also mediate many afferent impulses.

SYMPATHETIC NERVOUS SYSTEM. The cells that give rise to the preganglionic fibers of this division lie mainly in the intermediolateral columns of the spinal cord and extend from the first thoracic to the second or third lumbar segment. The axons from these cells are carried in the anterior (ventral) nerve roots and synapse, with neurons lying in sympathetic ganglia outside the cerebrospinal axis. Sympathetic ganglia are found in 3 locations: paravertebral, prevertebral, and terminal.

The 22 pairs of paravertebral sympathetic ganglia form the lateral chains on either side of the vertebral column. The ganglia are connected to each other by nerve trunks and to the spinal nerves by *rami communicantes*. The white rami carry the preganglionic myelinated fibers that exit the spinal cord by the anterior spinal roots. The gray rami carry postganglionic fibers back to the spinal nerves for distribution to sweat glands and pilomotor muscles and to blood vessels of skeletal muscle and skin. The prevertebral ganglia lie in the abdomen and the pelvis near the ventral surface of the bony vertebral column and consist mainly of the celiac (solar), superior mesenteric, aorticorenal, and inferior mesenteric ganglia. The terminal ganglia are few in number, lie near the organs they innervate, and include ganglia connected with the urinary bladder and rectum and the cervical ganglia in the region of the neck. In addition, small intermediate ganglia lie outside the conventional vertebral chain, especially in the thoracolumbar region. They are variable in number and location but usually are in close proximity to the communicating rami and the anterior spinal nerve roots.

Preganglionic fibers from the spinal cord may synapse with the neurons of more than 1 sympathetic ganglion. Their principal ganglia of termination need not correspond to the original level from which the preganglionic fiber exits the spinal cord. Many of the preganglionic fibers from the fifth to the last thoracic segment pass through the paravertebral ganglia to form the splanchnic nerves. Most of the splanchnic nerve fibers do not synapse until they reach the celiac ganglion; others directly innervate the adrenal medulla (*see* below).

Postganglionic fibers arising from sympathetic ganglia innervate visceral structures of the thorax, abdomen, head, and neck. The trunk and the limbs are supplied by the sympathetic fibers in spinal nerves. The prevertebral ganglia contain cell bodies whose axons innervate the glands and smooth muscles of the abdominal and the pelvic viscera. Many of the upper thoracic sympathetic fibers from the vertebral ganglia form terminal plexuses, such as the cardiac, esophageal, and pulmonary plexuses. The sympathetic distribution to the head and the neck (vasomotor, pupillodilator, secretory, and pilomotor) is by means of the cervical sympathetic chain and its 3 ganglia. All postganglionic fibers in this chain arise from cell bodies located in these 3 ganglia; all preganglionic fibers arise from the upper thoracic segments of the spinal cord, there being no sympathetic fibers that leave the CNS above the first thoracic level.

Pharmacologically, the chromaffin cells of the adrenal medulla resemble a collection of postganglionic sympathetic nerve cells. Typical preganglionic fibers that release ACh innervate these chromaffin cells, stimulating the release of epinephrine (EPI, adrenaline), in distinction to the NE released by postganglionic sympathetic fibers.

PARASYMPATHETIC NERVOUS SYSTEM. The parasympathetic nervous system consists of preganglionic fibers that originate in the CNS and their postganglionic connections. The regions of central origin are the midbrain, the medulla oblongata, and the sacral part of the spinal cord. The midbrain, or tectal, outflow consists of fibers arising from the Edinger-Westphal nucleus of the third cranial nerve and going to the ciliary ganglion in the orbit. The medullary outflow consists of the parasympathetic components of the VII, IX, and X cranial nerves.

The fibers in the VII (facial) cranial nerve form the chorda tympani, which innervates the ganglia lying on the submaxillary and sublingual glands. They also form the greater superficial petrosal nerve, which innervates

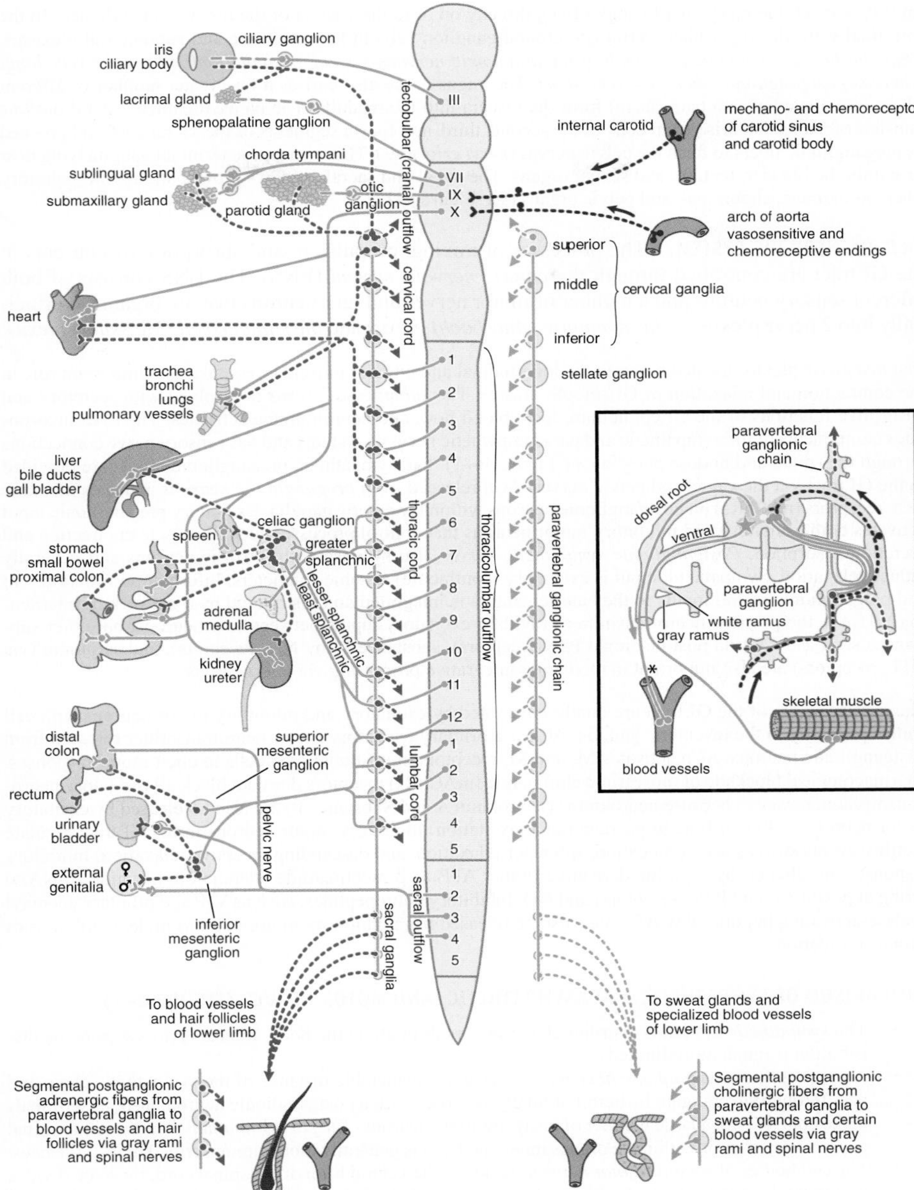

Figure 8–1 *The autonomic nervous system. Yellow*, cholinergic; *red*, adrenergic; *dotted blue*, visceral afferent; *solid lines*, preganglionic; *broken lines*, postganglionic. The *rectangle* at right shows the finer details of the ramifications of adrenergic fibers at any 1 segment of the spinal cord, the path of the visceral afferent nerves, the cholinergic nature of somatic motor nerves to skeletal muscle, and the presumed cholinergic nature of the vasodilator fibers in the dorsal roots of the spinal nerves. The asterisk (*) indicates that it is not known whether these vasodilator fibers are motor or sensory or where their cell bodies are situated.

the sphenopalatine ganglion. The autonomic components of the IX (glossopharyngeal) cranial nerve innervate the otic ganglia. Postganglionic parasympathetic fibers from these ganglia supply the sphincter of the iris (pupillary constrictor muscle), the ciliary muscle, the salivary and lacrimal glands, and the mucous glands of the nose, mouth, and pharynx. These fibers also include vasodilator nerves to these same organs. The X (vagus) cranial nerve arises in the medulla and contains preganglionic fibers, most of which do not synapse until they reach the many small ganglia lying directly on or in the viscera of the thorax and abdomen. In the intestinal wall, the vagal fibers terminate around ganglion cells in the myenteric and submucosal plexuses. *Thus, in the parasympathetic branch of the autonomic nervous system, preganglionic fibers are very long, whereas postganglionic fibers are very short.* The vagus nerve also carries a far greater number of afferent fibers (but apparently no pain fibers) from the viscera into the medulla. The parasympathetic sacral outflow consists of axons that arise from cells in the second, third, and fourth segments of the sacral cord and proceed as preganglionic fibers to form the pelvic nerves (*nervi erigentes*). They synapse in terminal ganglia lying near or within the bladder, rectum, and sexual organs. The vagal and sacral outflows provide motor and secretory fibers to thoracic, abdominal, and pelvic organs (*see* Figure 8–1).

ENTERIC NERVOUS SYSTEM. The processes of mixing, propulsion, and absorption of nutrients in the GI tract are controlled through the *enteric nervous system* (ENS). The ENS consists of both afferent sensory neurons and a number of motor nerves and interneurons that are organized principally into 2 nerve plexuses: *the myenteric (Auerbach) plexus* and *the submucosal (Meissner) plexus*.

The myenteric plexus, located between the longitudinal and circular muscle layers, plays an important role in the contraction and relaxation of GI smooth muscle. The *submucosal plexus* is involved with secretory and absorptive functions of the GI epithelium, local blood flow, and neuroimmune activities. The ENS incorporates components of the sympathetic and parasympathetic nervous systems and has sensory nerve connections through the spinal and nodose ganglia (*see* Figure 46–1). Parasympathetic preganglionic inputs are provided to the GI tract via the vagus and pelvic nerves. ACh released from *preganglionic neurons* activates nicotinic ACh receptors (nAChRs) on postganglionic neurons within the enteric ganglia. Excitatory preganglionic input activates both excitatory and inhibitory motor neurons that control processes such as muscle contraction and secretion/absorption. *Postganglionic sympathetic nerves* also synapse with intrinsic neurons and generally induce relaxation. Sympathetic input is excitatory (contractile) at some sphincters. Information from afferent and preganglionic neural inputs to the enteric ganglia is integrated and distributed by a network of interneurons. ACh is the primary neurotransmitter providing excitatory inputs between interneurons, but other substances such as ATP (via postjunctional P2X receptors), substance P (by NK_3 receptors), and serotonin (via $5HT_3$ receptors) are also important in mediating integrative processing via interneurons.

The muscle layers of the GI tract are dually innervated by excitatory and inhibitory motor neurons with cell bodies primarily in the myenteric ganglia. ACh is a primary excitatory motor neurotransmitter released from postganglionic neurons. ACh activates M_2 and M_3 receptors in postjunctional cells to elicit motor responses. Pharmacological blockade of muscarinic cholinergic (mAChRs) receptors does not block all excitatory neurotransmission, however, because neurokinins (neurokinin A and Substance P) are also coreleased by excitatory motor neurons and contribute to postjunctional excitation. Inhibitory motor neurons in the GI tract regulate motility events such as accommodation, sphincter relaxation, and descending receptive relaxation. Inhibitory responses are elicited by a purine derivative (either ATP or β-nicotinamide adenine dinucleotide (β-NAD) acting at postjunctional $P2Y_1$ receptors) and NO. Inhibitory neuropeptides, such as VIP and pituitary adenylyl cyclase-activating peptide (PACAP), may also be released from inhibitory motor neurons under conditions of strong stimulation.

COMPARISON OF SYMPATHETIC, PARASYMPATHETIC, AND MOTOR NERVES (FIGURE 8–2)

- The *sympathetic* system is distributed to effectors throughout the body, whereas *parasympathetic* distribution is much more limited.
- A *preganglionic sympathetic fiber* may traverse a considerable distance of the sympathetic chain and pass through several ganglia before it finally synapses with a postganglionic neuron; also, its terminals make contact with a large number of postganglionic neurons. *The parasympathetic system* has terminal ganglia very near or within the organs innervated and is generally more circumscribed in its influences.
- The cell bodies of *somatic motor neurons* reside in the ventral horn of the spinal cord; the axon divides into many branches, each of which innervates a single muscle fiber, so more than 100 muscle fibers may be supplied by 1 motor neuron to form a motor unit. At each neuromuscular junction, the axonal terminal loses its myelin sheath and forms a terminal arborization that lies in apposition to a specialized surface of the muscle membrane, termed the *motor end plate* (*see* Figure 11–3).

RESPONSES OF EFFECTOR ORGANS TO AUTONOMIC NERVE IMPULSES. In most instances, the sympathetic and parasympathetic neurotransmitters can be viewed as physiological or functional antagonists (Table 8–1).

Most viscera are innervated by both divisions of the autonomic nervous system, and their activities on specific structures may be either discrete and independent or integrated and interdependent. For example, the effects of sympathetic and parasympathetic stimulation of the heart and the iris show a pattern of functional antagonism in controlling heart rate and pupillary aperture, respectively, whereas their actions on male sexual organs are complementary and are integrated to promote sexual function.

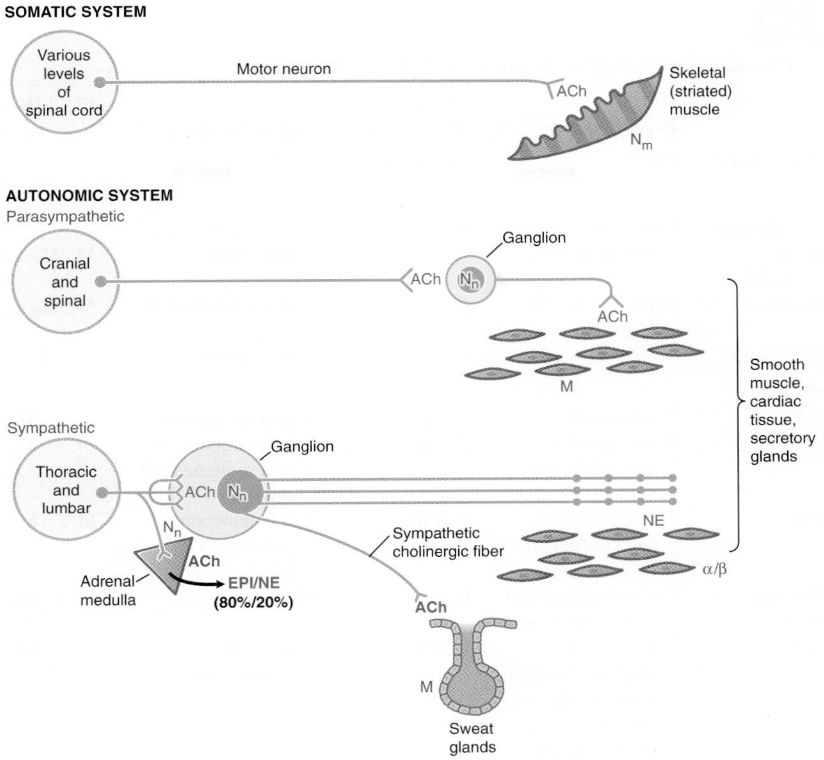

Figure 8–2 *Wiring diagram for somatic motor nerves and the efferent nerves of the autonomic nervous system.* The principal neurotransmitters, acetylcholine (ACh) and norepinephrine (NE), are shown in *red*. The receptors for these transmitters, nicotinic (N) and muscarinic (M) cholinergic receptors, α and β adrenergic receptors, are shown in *green*.

- Somatic nerves innervate skeletal muscle directly at a specialized synaptic junction, the motor end plate, where ACh activates N_m receptors.
- Autonomic nerves innervate smooth muscles, cardiac tissue and glands. Both parasympathetic and sympathetic systems have ganglia, where ACh is released by the preganglionic fibers; ACh acts on N_n receptors on the postganglionic nerves. ACh is also the neurotransmitter at cells of the adrenal medulla, where it acts on N_n receptors to cause release of EPI and NE into the circulation.
- ACh is the dominant neurotransmitter released by postganglionic parasympathetic nerves and acts on muscarinic receptors. The ganglia in the parasympathetic system are near or within the organ being innervated with generally a one-to-one relationship between pre- and post-ganglionic fibers.
- NE is the principal neurotransmitter of postganglionic sympathetic nerves, acting on α- or β-adrenergic receptors. Autonomic nerves form a diffuse pattern with multiple synaptic sites. In the sympathetic system the ganglia are generally far from the effector cells (e.g., within the sympathetic chain ganglia). Preganglionic sympathetic fibers may make contact with a large number of postganglionic fibers.

GENERAL FUNCTIONS OF THE AUTONOMIC NERVOUS SYSTEM. The ANS is the primary regulator of the constancy of the internal environment of the organism.

The sympathetic system and its associated adrenal medulla are not essential to life in a controlled environment, but the lack of sympathoadrenal functions becomes evident under circumstances of stress. In the absence of the sympathetic system: body temperature cannot be regulated when environmental temperature varies; the concentration of glucose in blood does not rise in response to urgent need; compensatory vascular responses to hemorrhage, oxygen deprivation, excitement, and exercise are lacking; and resistance to fatigue is lessened. Sympathetic components of instinctive reactions to the external environment are lost; and other serious deficiencies in the protective forces of the body are discernible. The sympathetic system normally is continuously active, the degree of activity varying from moment to moment and from organ to organ, adjusting to a constantly changing environment. The sympathoadrenal system can discharge as a unit. Heart rate is accelerated;

Table 8–1

Responses of Effector Organs to Autonomic Nerve Impulses

ORGAN SYSTEM	SYMPATHETIC EFFECT[a]	ADRENERGIC RECEPTOR SUBTYPE[b]	PARASYMPATHETIC EFFECT[a]	CHOLINERGIC RECEPTOR SUBTYPE[b]
Eye				
Radial muscle, iris	Contraction (mydriasis)++	α_1		
Sphincter muscle, iris			Contraction (miosis)+++	M_3, M_2
Ciliary muscle	Relaxation for far vision+	β_2	Contraction for near vision+++	M_3, M_2
Lacrimal glands	Secretion+	α	Secretion+++	M_3, M_2
Heart[c]				
SA node	↑ in heart rate++	$\beta_1 > \beta_2$	↓ in heart rate+++	$M_2 >> M_3$
Atria	↑ in contractility and conduction velocity++	$\beta_1 > \beta_2$	↓ in contractility++ and shortened AP duration	$M_2 >> M_3$
AV node	↑ in automaticity and conduction velocity++	$\beta_1 > \beta_2$	↓ in conduction velocity; AV block+++	$M_2 >> M_3$
His-Purkinje system	↑ in automaticity and conduction velocity	$\beta_1 > \beta_2$	Little effect	$M_2 >> M_3$
Ventricle	↑ in contractility, conduction velocity, automaticity, and rate of idioventricular pacemakers+++	$\beta_1 > \beta_2$	Slight ↓ in contractility	$M_2 >> M_3$
Blood Vessels				
Arteries and arterioles[d]				
Coronary	Constriction+; dilation[e]++	$\alpha_1, \alpha_2; \beta_2$	No innervation[h]	—
Skin and mucosa	Constriction+++	α_1, α_2	No innervation[h]	—
Skeletal muscle	Constriction; dilatione[e,f]++	α_1, β_2	Dilation[h] (?)	—
Cerebral	Constriction (slight)	α_1	No innervation[h]	—
Pulmonary	Constriction+; dilation	$\alpha_1; \beta_2$	No innervation[h]	—
Abdominal viscera	Constriction+++; dilation+	$\alpha_1; \beta_2$	No innervation[h]	—
Salivary glands	Constriction+++	α_1, α_2	Dilation[h]++	M_3
Renal	Constriction++; dilation++	$\alpha_1\ \alpha_2; \beta_1, \beta_2$	No innervation[h]	
Veins[d]	Constriction; dilation	$\alpha_1, \alpha_2; \beta_2$		
Endothelium	—	—	↑ NO synthase[h]	M_3
Lung				
Tracheal and bronchial smooth muscle	Relaxation	β_2	Contraction	$M_2 = M_3$
Bronchial glands	↓ secretion, ↑ secretion	α_1 β_2	Stimulation	M_2, M_3

(*continued*)

Table 8–1

Responses of Effector Organs to Autonomic Nerve Impulses (*Continued*)

ORGAN SYSTEM	SYMPATHETIC EFFECT[a]	ADRENERGIC RECEPTOR SUBTYPE[b]	PARASYMPATHETIC EFFECT[a]	CHOLINERGIC RECEPTOR SUBTYPE[b]
Stomach				
Motility and tone	↓ (usually)[i]+	α_1, α_2, β_1, β_2	↑[i]+++	$M_2 = M_3$
Sphincters	Contraction (usually)+	α_1	Relaxation (usually)+	M_3, M_2
Secretion	Inhibition	α_2	Stimulation++	M_3, M_2
Intestine				
Motility and tone	Decrease[h]+	α_1, α_2, β_1, β_2	↑[i]+++	M_3, M_2
Sphincters	Contraction+	α_1	Relaxation (usually)+	M_3, M_2
Secretion	↓	α_2	↑++	M_3, M_2
Gallbladder and Ducts Kidney	Relaxation+	β_2	Contraction+	M
Renin secretion	↓+; ↑++	α_1; β_1	No innervation	—
Urinary Bladder				
Detrusor	Relaxation+	β_2	Contraction+++	$M_3 > M_2$
Trigone and sphincter	Contraction++	α_1	Relaxation++	$M_3 > M_2$
Ureter				
Motility and tone	↑	α_1	↑ (?)	M
Uterus	Pregnant contraction;	α_1		
	Relaxation	β_2	Variable[j]	M
	Nonpregnant relaxation	β_2		
Sex Organs, Male Skin	Ejaculation+++	α_1	Erection+++	M_3
Pilomotor muscles	Contraction++	α_1	—	
Sweat glands	Localized	α_1	—	
	secretion[k]++	—	Generalized secretion+++	M_3, M_2
Spleen Capsule	Contraction+++	α_1	—	—
	Relaxation+	β_2	—	
Adrenal Medulla	—		Secretion of epinephrine and norepinephrine	N $(\alpha_3)_2(\beta_4)_3$; M (secondarily)
Skeletal Muscle	Increased contractility; glycogenolysis; K^+ uptake	β_2	—	—
Liver	Glycogenolysis and gluconeogenesis+++	α_1 β_2	—	—
Pancreas				
Acini	↓ secretion+	α	Secretion++	M_3, M_2
Islets (β cells)	↓ secretion+++	α_2	—	
	↑ secretion+	β_2		
Fat Cells[l]	Lipolysis+++; thermogenesis	α_1, β_1, β_2, β_3	—	—
Salivary Glands	Inhibition of lipolysis	α_2		
	K+ and water secretion+	α_1	K+ and water secretion+++	M_3, M_2

(*continued*)

Table 8–1

Responses of Effector Organs to Autonomic Nerve Impulses (*Continued*)

ORGAN SYSTEM	SYMPATHETIC EFFECT[a]	ADRENERGIC RECEPTOR SUBTYPE[b]	PARASYMPATHETIC EFFECT[a]	CHOLINERGIC RECEPTOR SUBTYPE[b]
Nasopharyngeal Glands	—		Secretion++	M_3, M_2
Pineal Glands	Melatonin synthesis	β	—	
Posterior Pituitary	ADH secretion	β_1	—	
Autonomic Nerve Endings				
Sympathetic terminal				
Autoreceptor	Inhibition of NE release	$\alpha_{2A} > \alpha_{2C}(\alpha_{2B})$		
Heteroreceptor	—		Inhibition of NE release	M_2, M_4
Parasympathetic terminal				
Autoreceptor	—	—	Inhibition of ACh release	M_2, M_4
Heteroreceptor	Inhibition ACh release	$\alpha_{2A} > \alpha_{2C}$	—	—

[a]*Responses are designated + to +++ to provide an approximate indication of the importance of sympathetic and parasympathetic nerve activity in the control of the various organs and functions listed.*

[b]*Adrenergic receptors: α_1, α_2 and subtypes thereof; β_1, β_2, β_3. Cholinergic receptors: nicotinic (N); muscarinic (M), with subtypes 1-4. The receptor subtypes are described more fully in Chapters 9 and 12 and in Tables 8–2, 8–3, 8–6 and 8–7. When a designation of subtype is not provided, the nature of the subtype has not been determined, unequivocally. Only the principal receptor subtypes are shown. Transmitters other than ACh and NE contribute to many of the responses.*

[c]*In the human heart, the ration of β_1 to β_2 is about 3:2 in atria and 4:1 in ventricles. While M_2 receptors predominate, M_3 receptors are also present.*

[d]*The predominant α_1 receptor subtype in most blood vessels (both arteries and veins) is α_{1A}, although other α_1 subtypes are present in specific blood vessels. The α_{1D} is the predominant subtype in the aorta.*

[e]*Dilation predominates in situ owing to metabolic autoregulatory mechanisms.*

[f]*Over the usual concentration range of physiologically released circulating epinephrine, the β receptor response (vasodilation) predominates in blood vessels of skeletal muscle and liver; β receptor response (vasoconstriction) in blood vessels of other abdominal viscera. The renal and mesenteric vessels also contain specific dopaminergic receptors whose activation causes dilation.*

[g]*Sympathetic cholinergic neurons cause vasodilation in skeletal muscle beds, but this is not involved in most physiological responses.*

[h]*The endothelium of most blood vessels releases NO, which causes vasodilation in response to muscarinic stimuli. However, unlike the receptors innervated by sympathetic cholinergic fibers in skeletal muscle blood vessels, these muscarinic receptors are not innervated and respond only to exogenously added muscarinic agonists in the circulation.*

[i]*While adrenergic fibers terminate at inhibitory β receptors on smooth muscle fibers and at inhibitory β receptors on parasympathetic (cholinergic) excitatory ganglion cells of the myenteric plexus, the primary inhibitory response is mediated via enteric neurons through NO, P2Y receptors, and peptide receptors.*

[j]*Uterine responses depend on stages of menstrual cycle, amount of circulating estrogen and progesterone, and other factors.*

[k]*Palms of hands and some other sites ("adrenergic sweating").*

[l]*There is significant variation among species in the receptor types that mediate certain metabolic responses. All three β adrenergic receptors have been found in human fat cells. Activation of β_3 receptors produces a vigorous thermogenic response as well as lipolysis. The significance is unclear. Activation of β receptors also inhibits leptin release from adipose tissue.*

blood pressure rises; blood flow is shifted from the skin and splanchnic region to the skeletal muscles; blood glucose rises; the bronchioles and pupils dilate; and the organism is better prepared for "fight or flight." Many of these effects result primarily from or are reinforced by the actions of epinephrine secreted by the adrenal medulla.

The parasympathetic system is organized mainly for discrete and localized discharge. Although it is concerned primarily with conservation of energy and maintenance of organ function during periods of minimal activity, its elimination is not compatible with life. The parasympathetic system slows the heart rate, lowers the blood pressure, stimulates GI movements and secretions, aids absorption of nutrients, protects the retina from excessive light, and empties the urinary bladder and rectum.

NEUROTRANSMISSION

Nerve impulses elicit responses in smooth, cardiac, and skeletal muscles, exocrine glands, and postsynaptic neurons by liberating specific chemical neurotransmitters. Neurohumoral transmission relates to the transmission of impulses from postganglionic autonomic fibers to effector cells. Evidence supporting this concept includes:

- Demonstration of the presence of a physiologically active transmitter and its biosynthetic enzymes at appropriate sites
- Recovery of the transmitter from the perfusate of an innervated structure during periods of nerve stimulation but not (or in greatly reduced amounts) in the absence of stimulation
- Demonstration that the putative transmitter is capable of producing responses identical to responses to nerve stimulation
- Demonstration that the responses to nerve stimulation and to the administered transmitter candidate are modified in the same manner by various drugs, usually competitive antagonists

While these criteria are applicable for most neurotransmitters, including NE and ACh, there are now exceptions to these general rules. For example, NO has been found to be a neurotransmitter; however, NO is not stored in neurons and released by exocytosis. Rather, it is synthesized when needed and readily diffuses across membranes. Synaptic transmission in many instances may be mediated by the release of more than 1 neurotransmitter.

STEPS INVOLVED IN NEUROTRANSMISSION

The sequence of events involved in neurotransmission is of particular importance because pharmacologically active agents modulate the individual steps.

AXONAL CONDUCTION. At rest, the interior of the typical mammalian axon is ~70 mV negative to the exterior. In response to depolarization to a threshold level, an action potential is initiated at a local region of the membrane. The action potential consists of 2 phases. Following depolarization that induces an open conformation of the channel, *the initial phase* is caused by a rapid increase in the permeability and inward movement of Na^+ through voltage-sensitive Na^+ channels, and a rapid depolarization from the resting potential continues to a positive overshoot. *The second phase* results from the rapid inactivation of the Na^+ channel and the delayed opening of a K^+ channel, which permits outward movement of K^+ to terminate the depolarization.

The transmembrane ionic currents produce local circuit currents such that adjacent resting channels in the axon are activated, and excitation of an adjacent portion of the axonal membrane occurs, leading to propagation of the action potential without decrement along the axon. The region that has undergone depolarization remains momentarily in a refractory state.

The puffer fish poison, *tetrodotoxin*, and a close congener found in some shellfish, *saxitoxin*, selectively block axonal conduction by blocking the voltage-sensitive Na^+ channel and preventing the increase in Na^+ permeability associated with the rising phase of the action potential. In contrast, *batrachotoxin*, an extremely potent steroidal alkaloid secreted by a South American frog, produces paralysis through a selective increase in permeability of the Na^+ channel, which induces a persistent depolarization. Scorpion toxins are peptides that also cause persistent depolarization by inhibiting the inactivation process. Na^+ and Ca^{2+} channels are discussed in more detail in Chapters 11, 14, and 20.

JUNCTIONAL TRANSMISSION. The arrival of the action potential at the axonal terminals initiates events that trigger transmission of an excitatory or inhibitory impulse across the synapse or neuroeffector junction. These events, summarized by Figure 8–3, are:

1. *Release of the transmitter*. The nonpeptide (small molecule) neurotransmitters are largely synthesized in the region of the axonal terminals and stored there in synaptic vesicles. An action potential causes the synchronous release of several hundred quanta of neurotransmitter. The influx of Ca^{2+}, is a critical

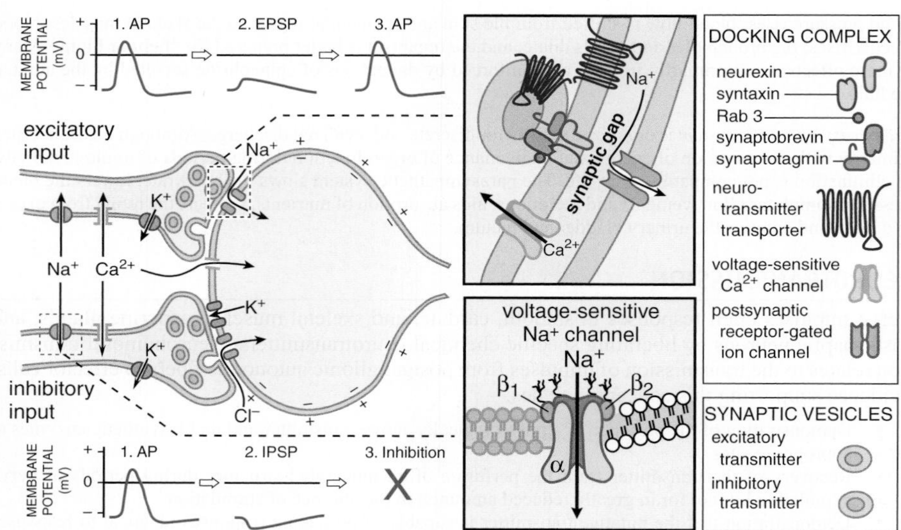

Figure 8–3 *Excitatory and inhibitory neurotransmission.*

1. The nerve action potential (AP) consists of a transient self-propagated reversal of charge on the axonal membrane. The internal potential E_i goes from a negative value, through zero potential, to a slightly positive value primarily through increases in Na^+ permeability and then returns to resting values by an increase in K^+ permeability. When the AP arrives at the presynaptic terminal, it initiates release of the excitatory or inhibitory transmitter. Depolarization at the nerve ending and entry of Ca^{2+} initiate docking and then fusion of the synaptic vesicle with the membrane of the nerve ending.
2. Combination of the excitatory transmitter with postsynaptic receptors produces a localized depolarization, the excitatory postsynaptic potential (EPSP), through an increase in permeability to cations, most notably Na^+. An inhibitory transmitter causes a selective increase in permeability to K^+ or Cl^-, resulting in a localized hyperpolarization, the inhibitory postsynaptic potential (IPSP).
3. The EPSP initiates a conducted AP in the postsynaptic neuron; this can be prevented, however, by the hyperpolarization induced by a concurrent IPSP. The transmitter is dissipated by enzymatic destruction, by reuptake into the presynaptic terminal or adjacent glial cells, or by diffusion. Depolarization of the postsynaptic membrane can permit Ca^{2+} entry if voltage-gated Ca^{2+} channels are present.

step; Ca^{2+} enters the axonal cytoplasm and promotes fusion between the axoplasmic membrane and those vesicles in proximity to it. The contents of the vesicles, are discharged to the exterior by a process termed *exocytosis*.

Receptors on soma, dendrites, and axons of neurons, respond to neurotransmitters or modulators released. *Soma–dendritic receptors*; when activated, they primarily modify functions of the soma–dendritic region such as protein synthesis and generation of action potentials. *Presynaptic receptors*; when activated, they modify functions of the terminal region such as synthesis and release of transmitters. Two main classes of presynaptic receptors have been identified on most neurons: *Heteroreceptors* are presynaptic receptors that respond to neurotransmitters, neuromodulators, or neuro-hormones released from adjacent neurons or cells. *Autoreceptors* are receptors located on or close to axon terminals of a neuron through which the neuron's own transmitter can modify transmitter synthesis and release (*see* Figures 8–3, 8–4, and 8–6).

2. *Combination of the transmitter with postjunctional receptors and production of the postjunctional potential.* The transmitter diffuses across the synaptic or junctional cleft and combines with specialized receptors on the postjunctional membrane; this often results in a localized increase in the ionic permeability, or conductance, of the membrane. With certain exceptions, 1 of 3 types of permeability change can occur:

   - A generalized increase in the permeability to cations (notably Na^+ but occasionally Ca^{2+}), resulting in a localized depolarization of the membrane, that is, an excitatory postsynaptic potential (EPSP)
   - A selective increase in permeability to anions, usually Cl^-, resulting in stabilization or actual hyperpolarization of the membrane, which constitutes an inhibitory postsynaptic potential (IPSP)
   - An increased permeability to K^+. Because the K^+ gradient is directed out of the cell, hyperpolarization and stabilization of the membrane potential occur (an IPSP)

Electric potential changes associated with the EPSP and IPSP at most sites are the results of passive fluxes of ions down their concentration gradients. The changes in channel permeability that cause these potential changes are specifically regulated by the specialized postjunctional receptors for the neurotransmitter that initiates the response (*see* Figures 8–4, 8–6, and 11–4; and Chapter 14). *High-conductance ligand-gated ion channels* usually permit passage of Na^+ or Cl^-; K^+ and Ca^{2+} are involved less frequently. The ligand-gated channels belong to a superfamily of ionotropic receptor proteins that includes the nicotinic, glutamate, and certain serotonin ($5HT_3$) and purine receptors, which conduct primarily Na^+, cause depolarization, and are excitatory; and GABA acid and glycine receptors, which conduct Cl^-, cause hyperpolarization, and are inhibitory. Neurotransmitters also can modulate the permeability of K^+ and Ca^{2+} channels indirectly. In these cases, the receptor and channel are separate proteins, and information is conveyed between them by G proteins (*see* Chapter 3).

3. *Initiation of postjunctional activity*. If an EPSP exceeds a certain threshold value, it initiates a propagated action potential in a postsynaptic neuron or a muscle action potential in skeletal or cardiac muscle by activating voltage-sensitive channels in the immediate vicinity. In certain smooth muscle types in which propagated impulses are minimal, an EPSP may increase the rate of spontaneous depolarization, cause Ca^{2+} release, and enhance muscle tone; in gland cells, the EPSP initiates secretion through Ca^{2+} mobilization. An IPSP, which is found in neurons and smooth muscle will tend to oppose excitatory potentials simultaneously initiated by other neuronal sources. Whether a propagated impulse or other response ensues depends on the summation of all the potentials.
4. *Destruction or dissipation of the transmitter*. At cholinergic synapses, which are involved in rapid neurotransmission, high and localized concentrations of acetylcholinesterase (AChE) rapidly hydrolyze the ACh. When AChE activity is inhibited, removal of the transmitter is accomplished principally by diffusion. Under these circumstances, the effects of released ACh are potentiated and prolonged (*see* Chapter 10).

   Rapid termination of NE occurs by a combination of simple diffusion and reuptake by the axonal terminals of the released NE. Termination of the action of amino acid transmitters is by active transport into neurons and surrounding glia. Peptide neurotransmitters are hydrolyzed by various peptidases and dissipated by diffusion.
5. *Nonelectrogenic functions*. The activity and turnover of enzymes involved in the synthesis and inactivation of neurotransmitters, the density of presynaptic and postsynaptic receptors, and other characteristics of synapses are controlled by trophic actions of neurotransmitters or other trophic factors released by the neuron or target cells.

CHOLINERGIC TRANSMISSION

The neurochemical events that underlie cholinergic neurotransmission are summarized in Figure 8–4.

SYNTHESIS AND STORAGE OF ACh. Two enzymes, choline acetyltransferase and AChE, are involved in ACh synthesis and degradation, respectively.

Choline Acetyltransferase. *Choline acetyltransferase* catalyzes the final step in the synthesis of ACh—the acetylation of choline with acetyl coenzyme A (CoA). Choline acetyltransferase is synthesized within the perikaryon and then is transported along the length of the axon to its terminal. Axonal terminals contain a large number of mitochondria, where acetyl CoA is synthesized. Choline is taken up from the extracellular fluid into the axoplasm by active transport. The final step in the synthesis occurs within the cytoplasm, following which most of the ACh is sequestered within synaptic vesicles.

Choline and Choline Transport. Choline availability is rate limiting to the synthesis of ACh and is provided from the diet as there is little *de novo* synthesis. Choline is taken up from the extracellular space by 2 transport systems: a ubiquitous low affinity, *Na^+-independent transport* system that is inhibited by *hemicholinium-3* with a K_i of ~50 μM, and high affinity *Na^+- and Cl^--dependent choline transport* system that is also sensitive to inhibition by *hemicholinium-3* (K_i = 10-100 nM). This second transport system is found predominantly in cholinergic neurons. ACh is released from cholinergic neurons is hydrolyzed by *acetylcholine esterase* (*AChE*) to acetate and choline. Choline is recycled after reuptake into the nerve terminal and reused for ACh synthesis.

Storage of ACh. ACh is transported into synaptic vesicles by vesicular ACh transporter (VAChT) using the potential energy of a proton electrochemical gradient. The process is inhibited by the noncompetitive and reversible inhibitor *vesamicol*, which does not affect the vesicular ATPase.

RELEASE OF ACh. Exocytotic release of ACh and cotransmitters (e.g., ATP, VIP, NO) occurs upon depolarization of the nerve terminals. Depolarization of the terminals allows the entry of Ca^{2+} through voltage-gated Ca^{2+} channels and promotes fusion of the vesicular membrane with the plasma membrane, allowing exocytosis to occur.

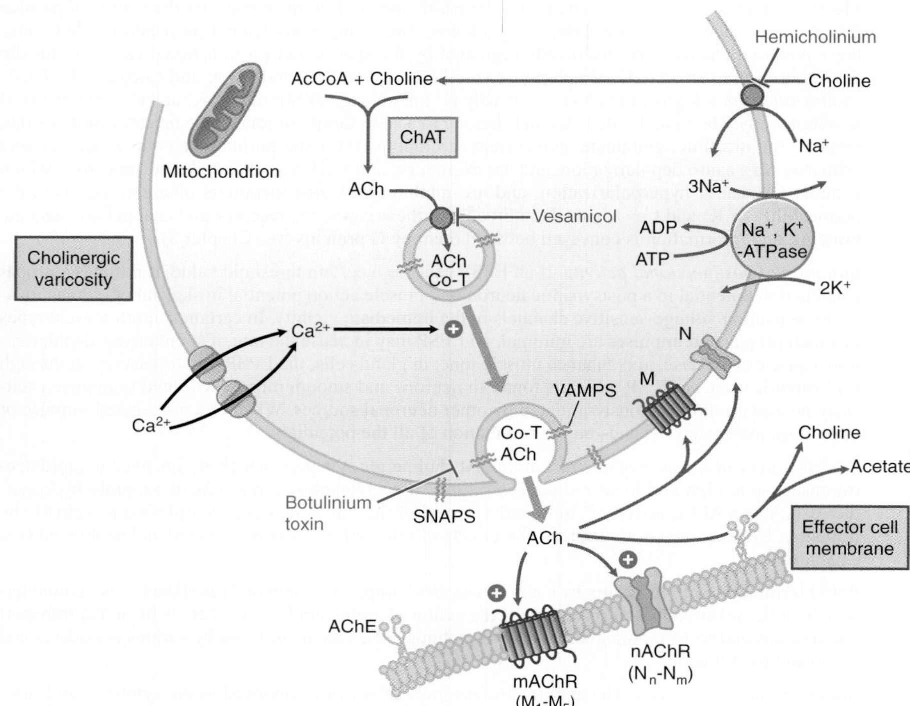

Figure 8–4 *A cholinergic neuroeffector junction.* The synthesis of ACh in the depends on the uptake of choline via a sodium-dependent carrier that can be blocked by hemicholinium. Choline and the acetyl moiety of acetyl coenzyme A, derived from mitochondria, form ACh, a process catalyzed by the enzyme choline acetyl transferase (ChAT). ACh is transported into the storage vesicle by another carrier that can be inhibited by vesamicol. ACh is stored in vesicles along with other potential cotransmitters (Co-T) such as ATP and VIP at certain neuroeffector junctions. Release of ACh and the Co-T occurs on depolarization of the varicosity, which allows the entry of Ca^{2+} through voltage-dependent Ca^{2+} channels. Elevated $[Ca^{2+}]_{in}$ promotes fusion of the vesicular membrane with the cell membrane, and exocytosis of the transmitters occurs. This fusion process involves the interaction of specialized proteins associated with the vesicular membrane (vesicle-associated membrane proteins [VAMPs]) and the membrane of the varicosity (synaptosome-associated proteins [SNAPs]). The exocytotic release of ACh can be blocked by botulinum toxin. Once released, ACh can interact with the muscarinic receptors (M), which are GPCRs, or nicotinic receptors (N), which are ligand-gated ion channels, to produce the characteristic response of the effector. ACh also can act on presynaptic mAChRs or nAChRs to modify its own release. The action of ACh is terminated by metabolism to choline and acetate by acetylcholinesterase (AChE), which is associated with synaptic membranes.

ACh is stored in vesicles located close to presynaptic membranes. A multiprotein complex appears to attach the vesicle to the plasma membrane close to other signaling elements. Various synaptic proteins, including the plasma membrane protein syntaxin and synaptosomal protein 25 kDa (SNAP-25), and the vesicular membrane protein, synaptobrevin, form a complex designated as SNAP regulators (SNARES). SNARE proteins are involved in transmitter release which is blocked by botulinum neurotoxins.

ACETYLCHOLINESTERASE. At the neuromuscular junction, immediate removal is required to prevent lateral diffusion and activation of adjacent receptors. The time required for hydrolysis of ACh at the neuromuscular junction is less than a millisecond.

AChE is found in cholinergic neurons and is highly concentrated at the postsynaptic end plate of the neuromuscular junction. *Butyrylcholinesterase* (BuChE) is virtually absent in neuronal elements of the central and peripheral nervous systems. BuChE is synthesized primarily in the liver and is found in liver and plasma; its likely physiological function is the hydrolysis of ingested esters from plant sources. AChE and BuChE typically are distinguished by the relative rates of ACh and butyrylcholine hydrolysis and by effects of selective inhibitors (*see* Chapter 10).

CHARACTERISTICS OF CHOLINERGIC TRANSMISSION AT VARIOUS SITES

Skeletal Muscle. At the neuromuscular junction (*see* Figure 8–2), ACh stimulates the nicotinic receptor's intrinsic channel, which opens for ~1 ms, admitting ~50,000 Na^+ ions. The channel-opening process is the basis for the localized depolarizing end-plate potential (EPP) within the end plate, which triggers the muscle AP and leads to contraction.

Autonomic Effector Cells. Stimulation or inhibition of autonomic effector cells occurs on activation of mAChRs. In contrast to skeletal muscle and neurons, smooth muscle and the cardiac conduction system exhibit intrinsic activity (both electrical and mechanical) that is modulated but not initiated by nerve impulses.

In the heart, spontaneous depolarizations normally arise from the SA node. In the cardiac conduction system, particularly in the SA and AV nodes, stimulation of the cholinergic innervation or the direct application of ACh causes inhibition, associated with hyperpolarization of the membrane and a marked decrease in the rate of depolarization. These effects are due, at least in part, to a selective increase in permeability to K^+.

Autonomic Ganglia. The primary pathway of cholinergic transmission in autonomic ganglia is similar to that at the neuromuscular junction of skeletal muscle. The initial depolarization is the result of activation of nAChRs, which are ligand-gated cation channels with properties similar to those found at the neuromuscular junction. Several secondary transmitters or modulators either enhance or diminish the sensitivity of the postganglionic cell to ACh (*see* Chapter 11).

Prejunctional Sites. ACh release is subject to complex regulation by mediators, including ACh itself acting on M_2 and M_4 *autoreceptors*, and activation of *heteroreceptors* (e.g., NE acting on α_{2A} and α_{2C} adrenergic receptors) or substances produced locally in tissues (e.g., NO). ACh-mediated inhibition of ACh release following activation of M_2 and M_4 autoreceptors is a physiological negative-feedback control mechanism. At some neuroeffector junctions (e.g., the myenteric plexus in the GI tract or the cardiac SA node), sympathetic and parasympathetic nerve terminals often lie juxtaposed to each other. There, opposing effects of NE and ACh result not only from the opposite effects of the 2 transmitters on the smooth muscle or cardiac cells but also from the inhibition of ACh release by NE or inhibition of NE release by ACh acting on heteroreceptors on parasympathetic or sympathetic terminals.

Extraneuronal Sites. All elements of the cholinergic system are functionally expressed independently of cholinergic innervation in numerous non-neuronal cells. These *non-neuronal cholinergic* systems can both modify and control phenotypic cell functions such as proliferation, differentiation, formation of physical barriers, migration, and ion and water movements.

CHOLINERGIC RECEPTORS AND SIGNAL TRANSDUCTION

Acetylcholine elicits responses similar to those of either nicotine or muscarine depending on the pharmacological preparation. The physiological receptors for ACh are classified as having a "nicotine action" (*nicotinic*) or a "muscarine action" (*muscarinic*). *Tubocurarine* and *atropine* block nicotinic and muscarinic effects of ACh, respectively.

Nicotinic receptors are ligand-gated ion channels whose activation always causes a rapid (millisecond) increase in cellular permeability to Na^+ and Ca^{2+}, depolarization, and excitation. *Muscarinic receptors* are G protein-coupled receptors (GPCRs). Responses to muscarinic agonists are slower; they may be either excitatory or inhibitory, and they are not necessarily linked to changes in ion permeability.

SUBTYPES OF NICOTINIC ACETYLCHOLINE RECEPTORS (TABLE 8–2). The *nicotinic ACh receptors* (nAChRs) exist at the skeletal neuromuscular junction, autonomic ganglia, adrenal medulla, the CNS and in nonneuronal tissues. The nAChRs are composed of 5 homologous subunits organized around a central pore (*see* Chapter 11). In general the nAChRs are further divided into 2 groups:

1. *Muscle type* (N_m), found in vertebrate skeletal muscle, where they mediate transmission at the neuromuscular junction (NMJ)
2. *Neuronal type* (N_n), found mainly throughout the peripheral nervous system, central nervous system, and also nonneuronal tissues

Neuronal nAChRs are widely distributed in the CNS and are found at presynaptic, perisynaptic, and postsynaptic sites. At pre- and perisynaptic sites, nAChRs appear to act as autoreceptors or heteoreceptors to regulate the release of several neurotransmitters (ACh, DA, NE, glutamate, and 5HT) at several diverse sites throughout the brain.

SUBTYPES OF MUSCARINIC RECEPTORS (TABLE 8–3). Five distinct subtypes of muscarinic ACh receptors (mAChRs) have been identified, each produced by a different gene. Like the different forms of nicotinic receptors, these variants have distinct anatomic locations in the periphery and CNS and differing chemical specificities (*see* Table 8–3 and Chapter 9).

Table 8–2

Characteristics of Subtypes of Nicotinic Acetylcholine Receptors (nAChRs)

RECEPTOR (Primary Receptor Subtype)[a]	MAIN SYNAPTIC LOCATION	MEMBRANE RESPONSE	MOLECULAR MECHANISM	AGONISTS	ANTAGONISTS
Skeletal Muscle (N_m) $(\alpha_1)_2\beta_1\varepsilon\delta$ adult $(\alpha_1)_2\ \beta_1\gamma\delta$ fetal	Skeletal neuromuscular junction (postjunctional)	Excitatory; end-plate depolarization; skeletal muscle contraction	Increased cation permeability (Na^+; K^+)	ACh Nicotine Succinylcholine	Atracurium Vecuronium *d*-Tubocurarine Pancuronium α-Conotoxin α-Bungarotoxin
Peripheral Neuronal (N_n) $(\alpha_3)_2(\beta_4)_3$	Autonomic ganglia; adrenal medulla	Excitatory; depolarization; firing of postganglion neuron; depolarization and secretion of catecholamines	Increased cation permeability (Na^+; K^+)	ACh Nicotine Epibatidine Dimethylphenyl-piperazinium	Trimethaphan Mecamylamine
Central Neuronal (CNS) $(\alpha_4)_2(\beta_4)_3$(α-btox-insensitive)	CNS; pre- and postjunctional	Pre- and post-synaptic excitation Prejunctional control of transmitter release	Increased cation permeability (Na^+; K^+)	Cytosine, epibatidine Anatoxin A	Mecamylamine Dihydro-β-erythrodine Erysodine Lophotoxin
$(\alpha_7)_5$ (α-btox-sensitive)	CNS; Pre- and post-synaptic	Pre- and post-synaptic excitation Prejunctional control of transmitter release	Increased permeability (Ca^{2+})	Anatoxin A	Methyllycaconitine α-Bungarotoxin α-Conotoxin ImI

[a] *Nine α (α_2-α_{10}) and three β (β_2-β_4) subunits have been identified and cloned in human brain, which combine in various conformations to form individual receptor subtypes. The structure of individual receptors and the subtype composition are incompletely understood. Only a finite number of naturally occurring functional nAChR constructs have been identified. α-btox, β-bungarotoxin.*

Table 8–3

Characteristics of Muscarinic Acetylcholine Receptor Subtypes (mAChRs)

RECEPTOR	CELLULAR AND TISSUE LOCATION[a]	CELLULAR RESPONSE[b]	FUNCTIONAL RESPONSE[c]	DISEASE RELEVANCE
M_1	CNS; Most abundant in cerebral cortex, hippocampus, striatum, and thalamus Autonomic ganglia Glands (gastric and salivary) Enteric nerves	Couples by $G_{q/11}$ to activate PLC-IP_3/DAG-Ca^{2+}-PKC pathway Depolarization and excitation (↑ sEPSP) Activation of PLD_2, PLA_2; ↑AA	Increased cognitive function (learning and memory) Increased seizure activity Decrease in dopamine release and locomotion Increase in depolarization of autonomic ganglia Increase in secretions	Alzheimer disease Cognitive dysfunction Schizophrenia
M_2	Widely expressed in CNS, hind brain, thalamus, cerebral cortex, hippocampus, striatum, heart, smooth muscle, autonomic nerve terminals	Couples by G_i/G_o (PTX-sensitive) Inhibition of AC, ↓ cAMP Activation of inwardly rectifying K^+ channels Inhibition of voltage-gated Ca^{2+} channels Hyperpolarization and inhibition	***Heart:*** SA node: slowed spontaneous depolarization; hyperpolarization, ↓ HR AV node: decrease in conduction velocity Atrium: ↓ refractory period, ↓ contraction Ventricle: slight ↓ contraction ***Smooth muscle:*** ↑ Contraction ***Peripheral nerves:*** Neural inhibition *via* autoreceptors and heteroreceptor ↓ Ganglionic transmission. ***CNS:*** Neural inhibition ↑ Tremors; hypothermia; analgesia	Alzheimer's disease Cognitive dysfunction Pain
M_3	Widely expressed in CNS (< than other mAChRs), cerebral cortex, hippocampus Abundant in smooth muscle and glands Heart	Couples by $G_{q/11}$ to activate PLC-IP_3/DAG-Ca^{2+}-PKC pathway Depolarization and excitation (↑ sEPSP) Activation of PLD_2, PLA_2; ↑ AA	*Smooth muscle* ↑ contraction (predominant in some, *e.g.*, bladder) *Glands:* ↑ secretion (predominant in salivary gland) Increases food intake, body weight fat deposits Inhibition of DA release Synthesis of NO	Chronic obstructive pulmonary disease (COPD) Urinary incontinence Irritable bowel disease

(continued)

Table 8–3

Characteristics of Muscarinic Acetylcholine Receptor Subtypes (mAChRs) (*Continued*)

RECEPTOR	CELLULAR AND TISSUE LOCATION[a]	CELLULAR RESPONSE[b]	FUNCTIONAL RESPONSE[c]	DISEASE RELEVANCE
M_4	Preferentially expressed in CNS, particularly forebrain, also striatum, cerebral cortex, hippocampus	Couples by G_i/G_0 (PTX-sensitive) Inhibition of AC, ↓ cAMP Activation of inwardly rectifying K^+ channels Inhibition of voltage-gated Ca^{2+} channels Hyperpolarization and inhibition	Autoreceptor- and heteroreceptor-mediated inhibition of transmitter release in CNS and periphery Analgesia; cataleptic activity Facilitation of DA release	Parkinson disease Schizophrenia Neuropathic pain
M_5	Substantia nigra Expressed in low levels in CNS and periphery Predominant mAchR in neurons in VTA and substantia nigra	Couples by $G_{q/11}$ to activate PLC-IP_3/DAG-Ca^{2+}-PKC pathway Depolarization and excitation (↑ sEPSP) Activation of PLD_2, PLA_2; ↑ AA	Mediator of dilation in cerebral arteries and arterioles (?) Facilitates DA release Augmentation of drug-seeking behavior and reward (e.g., opiates, cocaine)	Drug dependence Parkinson disease Schizophrenia

PLC, phospholipase C; IP_3, inositol-l,4,5-triphosphate; DAG, diacylglycerol; PLD_2, phospholipase D; AA, arachidonic acid; PLA, phospholipase A; AC, adenylyl cyclase; DA, dopamine; cAMP, cyclic AMP; SA node, sinoatrial node; AV node, atrioventricular node; HR, heart rate; PTX, pertussis toxin; VTA, ventral tegmentum area.

[a]*Most organs, tissues, and cells express multiple mAChRs.*

[b]*M_1 M_3, and M_5 mAChRs appear to couple to the same G proteins and signal through similar pathways. Likewise, M_2 and M_4 mAChRs couple through similar G proteins and signal through similar pathways.*

[c]*Despite the fact that in many tissues, organs, and cells multiple subtypes of mAChRs coexist, one subtype may predominate in producing a particular function; in others, there may be equal predominance.*

The functions of mAChRs are mediated by interactions with G proteins. The M_1, M_3, and M_5 subtypes couple through $G_{q/11}$ to stimulate the PLC-IP_3/DAG-Ca^{2+} pathway, leading to activation of PKC and Ca^{2+}-sensitive enzymes. Activation of M_1, M_3, and M_5 receptors can also cause the activation of phospholipase A_2, leading to the release of arachidonic acid and consequent eicosanoid synthesis; these effects of M_1, M_3, and M_5 mAChRs are generally secondary to elevation of intracellular Ca^{2+}. Stimulated M_2 and M_4 cholinergic receptors couple to G_i and G_o, with a resulting inhibition of adenylyl cyclase, leading to a decrease in cellular cyclic AMP, activation of inwardly rectifying K^+ channels, and inhibition of voltage-gated Ca^{2+} channels. The functional consequences of these effects are hyperpolarization and inhibition of excitable membranes. In the myocardium, inhibition of adenylyl cyclase and activation of K^+ conductances account for the negative inotropic and chronotropic effects of ACh.

ADRENERGIC TRANSMISSION

Norepinephrine (NE) is the principal transmitter of most sympathetic postganglionic fibers and of certain tracts in the CNS; dopamine (DA) is the predominant transmitter of the mammalian extrapyramidal system and of several mesocortical and mesolimbic neuronal pathways; and epinephrine (EPI) is the major hormone of the adrenal medulla. Collectively, these 3 amines are called *catecholamines*.

SYNTHESIS OF CATECHOLAMINES. The steps in the synthesis of catecholamines and the characteristics of the enzymes involved are shown in Figure 8–5 and Table 8–4.

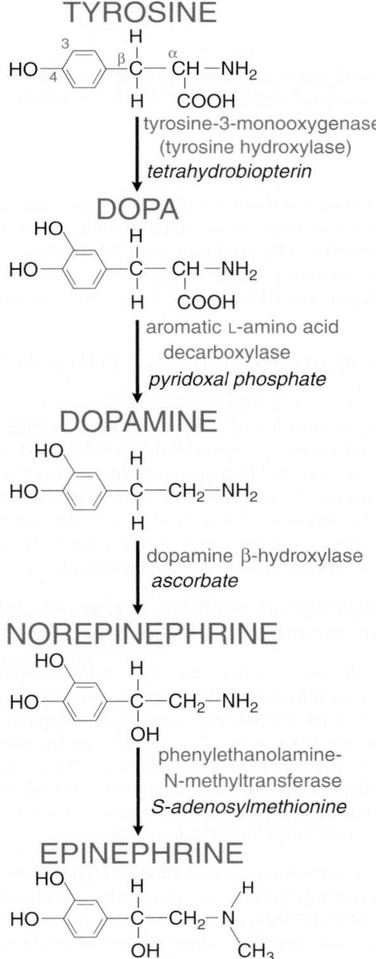

Figure 8–5 *Biosynthesis of catecholamines.* The enzymes involved are shown in *red;* essential cofactors in italics. The final step occurs only in the adrenal medulla and in a few epinephrine-containing neuronal pathways in the brainstem.

Table 8–4

Enzymes for Synthesis of Catecholamines

ENZYME	OCCURRENCE	SUBCELLULAR DISTRIBUTION	COFACTORS	SUBSTRATE SPECIFICITY	COMMENTS
TH	Widespread	Cytoplasm	BH_4, O_2, Fe^{2+}	Specific for L-tyrosine	Rate limiting step. Inhibition can deplete NE
AAADC	Widespread	Cytoplasm	Pyridoxal PO_4	Nonspecific	Inhibition does not alter tissue NE and EPI appreciably
DβH	Widespread	Synaptic vesicles	Ascorbate, O_2 (DβH contains Cu)	Nonspecific	Inhibition can ↓ NE and EPI levels
PNMT	Largely in adrenal gland	Cytoplasm	SAM (CH_3 donor)	Nonspecific	Inhibition can ↓ adrenal EPI/NE; regulated by glucocorticoids

TH, tyrosine hydroxylase; AAADC, aromatic amino acid decarboxylase; DβH, dopamine β hydroxylase; PNMT, phenylethanolamine N-methyltransferase; SAM, S-adenosyl methionine; BH_4, tetrahydrobiopterin.

Table 8–4 summarizes the characteristics of these synthetic enzymes. These enzymes are not completely specific; consequently, other endogenous substances, as well as certain drugs, are also substrates. For example, 5-hydroxytryptamine (5HT, serotonin) can be produced from 5-hydroxy-*L*-tryptophan by aromatic *L*-amino acid decarboxylase (or dopa decarboxylase). Dopa decarboxylase also converts dopa into DA (*see* Chapter 13) and methyldopa to α-methyldopamine, which in turn is converted by dopamine β-hydroxylase (DβH) to methylnorepinephrine.

The hydroxylation of tyrosine by *tyrosine hydroxylase* (TH) is the rate-limiting step in the biosynthesis of catecholamines.

This enzyme is activated following stimulation of sympathetic nerves or the adrenal medulla. The enzyme is a substrate for PKA, PKC, and CaM kinase; phosphorylation is associated with increased hydroxylase activity. In addition, there is a delayed increase in TH gene expression after nerve stimulation. These mechanisms serve to maintain the content of catecholamines in response to increased transmitter release. TH also is subject to feedback inhibition by catechol compounds. TH deficiency has been reported in humans and is characterized by generalized rigidity, hypokinesia, and low cerebrospinal fluid (CSF) levels of NE and DA metabolites homovanillic acid (HVA) and 3-methoxy-4-hydroxyphenylethylene glycol.

The main features of the mechanisms of synthesis, storage, and release of catecholamines and their modifications by drugs are summarized in Figure 8–6.

In the case of adrenergic neurons, the enzymes that participate in the formation of NE are synthesized in the cell bodies of the neurons and then are transported along the axons to their terminals. In the course of synthesis, the hydroxylation of tyrosine to dopa and the decarboxylation of dopa to DA take place in the cytoplasm. DA then is actively transported into the DβH-containing storage vesicles, where it is converted to NE by DβH in sympathetic nerves (about 90%); the remainder is metabolized. DA is converted by MAO to an aldehyde intermediate DOPAL, and then mainly converted to 3,4-dihydroxyphenyl acetic acid (DOPAC) by aldehyde dehydrogenase and to a minor extent 3,4-dihydroxyphenylethanol (DOPET) by aldehyde reductase. DOPAC is further converted to HVA by O-methylation in nonneuronal sites.

The *adrenal medulla* has 2 distinct catecholamine-containing cell types: those with NE and those with primarily EPI. The latter cell population contains the enzyme phenylethanolamine-*N*-methyltransferase (PNMT). In these cells, the NE formed in the granules leaves these structures and is methylated in the cytoplasm to EPI. Epinephrine then reenters the chromaffin granules, where it is stored until released. EPI accounts for ~80% of the catecholamines of the adrenal medulla and NE ~20%. The level of *glucocorticoids*, secreted by the adrenal cortex, is a major factor that controls the rate of synthesis of EPI and the amount available for release from the adrenal medulla. The intra-adrenal portal vascular system carries the corticosteroids directly to the adrenal

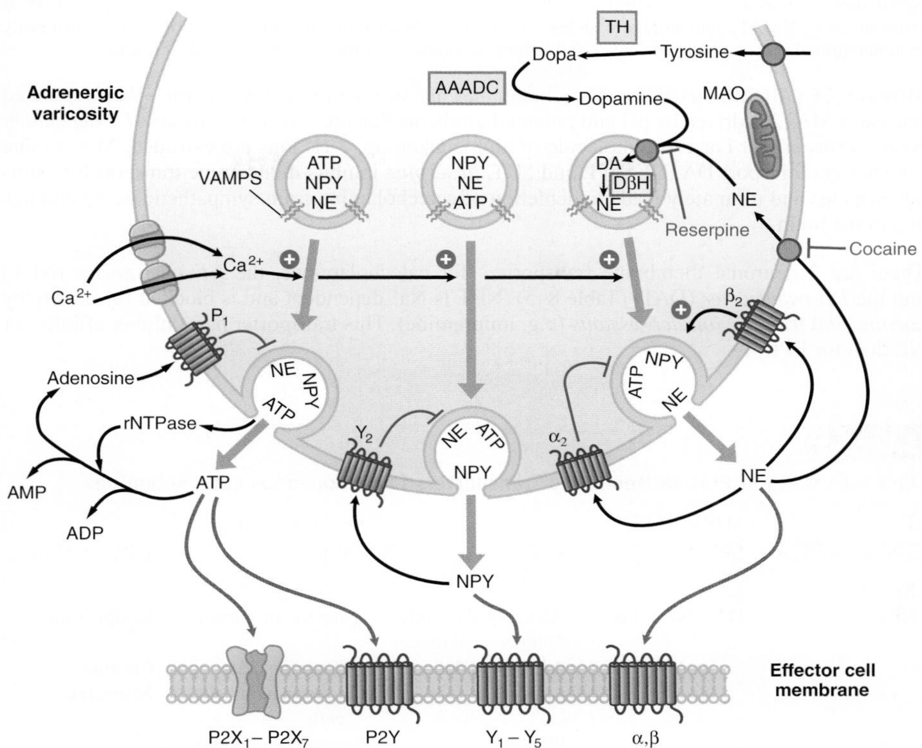

Figure 8–6 *An adrenergic neuroeffector junction.* Tyrosine is transported into the varicosity and converted to dopa by tyrosine hydroxylase (TH); aromatic L-amino acid decarboxylase (AAADC) converts dopa to dopamine (DA). Dopamine is taken up into the vesicles of the varicosity by a transporter, VMAT2, that can be blocked by reserpine. Cytoplasmic NE also can be taken up by this transporter. DA is converted to NE within the vesicle by dopamine-β-hydroxylase (DβH). NE is stored in vesicles along with other cotransmitters, NPY and ATP, depending on the particular neuroeffector junction. Release of the transmitters occurs upon depolarization of the varicosity, which allows entry of Ca^{2+} through voltage-dependent Ca^{2+} channels. Elevated levels of Ca^{2+} promote the fusion of the vesicular membrane with the membrane of the varicosity, with subsequent exocytosis of transmitters, as described in the legend to Figure 8–4. NE, NPY, and ATP may be stored in the same or different vesicles and co-released. Once in the synapse, NE can interact with α and β adrenergic receptors to produce the characteristic response of the effector. The adrenergic receptors are GPCRs. α and β Receptors also can be located presynaptically where NE can either diminish (α_2), or facilitate (β) its own release and that of the cotransmitters. The principal mechanism by which NE is cleared from the synapse is via a cocaine-sensitive neuronal uptake transporter, NET. Once transported into the cytosol, NE can be re-stored in the vesicle or metabolized by monoamine oxidase (MAO). NPY produces its effects by activating NPY receptors, of which there are at least 5 types (Y_I through Y_5), all GPCRs. NPY can modify its own release and that of the other transmitters via presynaptic receptors of the Y_2 type; NPY is removed from the synapse by metabolic breakdown by peptidases. ATP produces its effects by activating P2X receptors or P2Y receptors (*see* Table 14–8). ATP can act prejunctionally to modify its own release *via* receptors for ATP or *via* its metabolic breakdown to adenosine that acts on P1 (adenosine) receptors. ATP is cleared from the synapse primarily by releasable nucleotidases (rNTPase) and by cell-fixed ectonucleotidases.

medullary chromaffin cells, where they induce the synthesis of PNMT. The activities of both TH and DβH also are increased in the adrenal medulla when the secretion of glucocorticoids is stimulated.

In addition to de novo synthesis, NE stores in the terminal portions of the adrenergic fibers are also replenished by reuptake and re-storage of NE following its release. At least 2 distinct carrier-mediated transport systems are involved:

1. One across the axonal membrane from the extracellular fluid to the cytosol (*the NE transporter [NET]*, previously called *uptake 1*)
2. The other from the cytosol into the storage vesicles (*the vesicular monoamine transporter [VMAT2]*)

Sympathetic nerves as a whole remove ~87% of released NE by NET. More than 70% of recaptured NE is sequestered by VMAT2 into storage vesicles. In contrast, clearance of circulating catecholamines is primarily by nonneuronal mechanisms, with liver and kidney accounting for more than 60% of the clearance.

STORAGE OF CATECHOLAMINES. Catecholamines are stored in vesicles, ensuring their regulated release. VMAT2 is driven by pH and potential gradients that are established by an *ATP-dependent proton translocase*. For every molecule of amine taken up, 2 H^+ ions are extruded. Monoamine transporters transport DA, NE, EPI, and 5HT. *Reserpine* inhibits monoamine transport into storage vesicles and ultimately leads to depletion of catecholamine from sympathetic nerve endings and in the brain.

There are 2 neuronal membrane transporters for catecholamines, the *NE transporter* (NET) and the *DA transporter* (DAT) (Table 8–5). NET is Na^+-dependent and is blocked selectively by *cocaine* and *tricyclic antidepressants* (e.g. imipramine). This transporter has a higher affinity for NE than for EPI.

Table 8–5

Characteristics of Plasma Membrane Transporters for Endogenous Catecholamines

TYPE OF TRANSPORTER	SUBSTRATE SPECIFICITY	TISSUE	REGION/CELL TYPE	INHIBITORS
Neuronal				
NET	DA > NE > Epi	All sympathetically innervated tissue	Sympathetic nerves	Desipramine
		Adrenal medulla	Chromaffin cells	Cocaine
		Liver	Capillary endothelial cells	Nisoxetine
		Placenta	Syncytiotrophoblast	
DAT	DA > NE > Epi	Kidney	Endothelium	Cocaine
		Stomach	Parietal and endothelial cells	Imazindol
		Pancreas	Pancreatic duct	
Nonneuronal				
OCT1	DA > Epi >> NE	Liver	Hepatocytes	Isocyanines
		Intestine	Epithelial cells	Corticosterone
		Kidney (not human)	Distal tubule	
OCT2	DA >> NE > Epi	Kidney	Medullary proximal and distal tubules	Isocyanines
		Brain	Glial cells of DA-rich regions, some non-adrenergic neurons	Corticosterone
ENT (OCT 3)	Epi >> NE > DA	Liver	Hepatocytes	Isocyanines
		Brain	Glial cells, others	Corticosterone
		Heart	Myocytes	*O*-methyl-isoproterenol
		Blood vessels	Endothelial cells	
		Kidney	Cortex, proximal and distal tubules	
		Placenta	Syncytiotrophoblasts (basal membrane)	
		Retina	Photoreceptors, ganglion amacrine cells	

NET, norepinephrine transporter, originally known as uptake 1; DAT, dopamine transporter; ENT (OCT3), extraneuronal transporter, originally known as uptake 2; OCT 1, OCT 2, organic cation transporters; Epi, epinephrine; NE, norepinephrine; DA, dopamine.

Indirectly acting sympathomimetic drugs (e.g., ephedrine and tyramine) produce some of their effects by displacing and releasing NE from the nerve terminals to the effector cells. These agents are substrates for NET. As a result of their transport across the neuronal membrane and release into the axoplasm, they make NET available at the inner surface of the membrane for the outward transport of NE ("facilitated exchange diffusion"). These amines also mobilize NE stored in the vesicles by competing for the vesicular uptake process (VMAT2).

Three *extraneuronal transporters* (ENTs) handle a range of endogenous and exogenous substrates (*see* Table 8–5). The ENT (or uptake-2 and OCT3), is an organic cation transporter that exhibits lower affinity for catecholamines, compared to NET, and favors EPI over NE and DA. Other members of this family are the organic cation transporters OCT1 and OCT2 (*see* Chapter 5).

RELEASE OF CATECHOLAMINES. Details of excitation-secretion coupling in sympathetic neurons and adrenal medulla are not completely known, The triggering event is the entry of Ca^{2+}, which results in the exocytosis of the granular contents, including EPI, ATP, some neuroactive peptides or their precursors, chromogranins, and DβH.

PREJUNCTIONAL REGULATION OF NOREPINEPHRINE RELEASE. Following their release from sympathetic terminals, the 3 sympathetic cotransmitters—*NE, neuropeptide Y (NPY), and ATP*—can feed back on *prejunctional receptors* to inhibit the release of each other. The α_{2A} and α_{2C} adrenergic receptors are the principal prejunctional receptors that inhibit sympathetic neurotransmitter release, whereas the α_{2B} adrenergic receptors also may inhibit transmitter release at selected sites. NPY, acting on Y_2 receptors, and ATP-derived adenosine, acting on P1 receptors, also can inhibit sympathetic neurotransmitter release. Numerous heteroreceptors on sympathetic nerve varicosities also inhibit the release of sympathetic neurotransmitters; these include: M_2 and M_4 muscarinic, 5HT, PG E_2, histamine, enkephalin, and DA receptors. Enhancement of sympathetic neurotransmitter release can be produced by activation of β_2 adrenergic receptors, angiotensin AT_2 receptors, and nAChRs.

TERMINATION OF THE ACTIONS OF CATECHOLAMINES. The actions of NE and EPI are terminated by:

- Reuptake *into nerve terminals* by NET
- *Dilution by diffusion* out of junctional cleft and *extraneuronal uptake* by ENT, OCT1, and OCT2

METABOLISM OF CATECHOLAMINES. Following uptake, catecholamines are either metabolized by *monoamine oxidase* (MAO) and *catechol-O-methyltransferase* (COMT). MAO metabolizes transmitter that is released within the nerve terminal. COMT, particularly in the liver, plays a major role in the metabolism of endogenous circulating and administered catecholamines. MAO and COMT can act sequentially in conjunction with aldehyde reductase, aldehyde dehydrogenase, and alcohol dehydrogenase to produce a variety of intermediates en route to vanillylmandelic acid, which is secreted into the urine (Figure 8–7).

The 2 enzymes have different subcellular localizations: MAO is associated chiefly with the outer surface of mitochondria; COMT is largely cytoplasmic. Both MAO and COMT are distributed widely throughout the body, however, little or no COMT is found in sympathetic neurons. The physiological substrates for COMT include L-dopa, all 3 endogenous catecholamines (DA, NE, and EPI), their hydroxylated metabolites, catecholestrogens, ascorbic acid, and dihydroxyindolic intermediates of melanin. Two different isozymes of MAO (MAO-A and MAO-B) occur in widely varying proportions in different cells in the CNS and in peripheral tissues. In the brain, MAO-A is located in all regions containing catecholamines. MAO-B, on the other hand, is found primarily in regions that are known to synthesize and store 5HT. MAO inhibitors are useful in the treatment of Parkinson disease and mental depression (*see* Chapters 15 and 22). Inhibitors of MAO (e.g., *pargyline* and *nialamide*) can cause an increase in the concentration of NE, DA, and 5HT in the brain and other tissues.

Adrenal medullary chromaffin cells contain both MAO and COMT; the COMT is mainly present as the membrane-bound form of the enzyme in contrast to the form found in the cytoplasm of extra-neuronal tissue.

CLASSIFICATION OF ADRENERGIC RECEPTORS. Adrenergic receptors are broadly classified as either α or β, with subtypes within each group (Table 8–6). The original subclassification was based on the rank order of potency of agonists:

- Epinephrine ≥ norepinephrine >> isoproterenol for α adrenergic receptors
- Isoproterenol > epinephrine ≥ norepinephrine for β adrenergic receptors

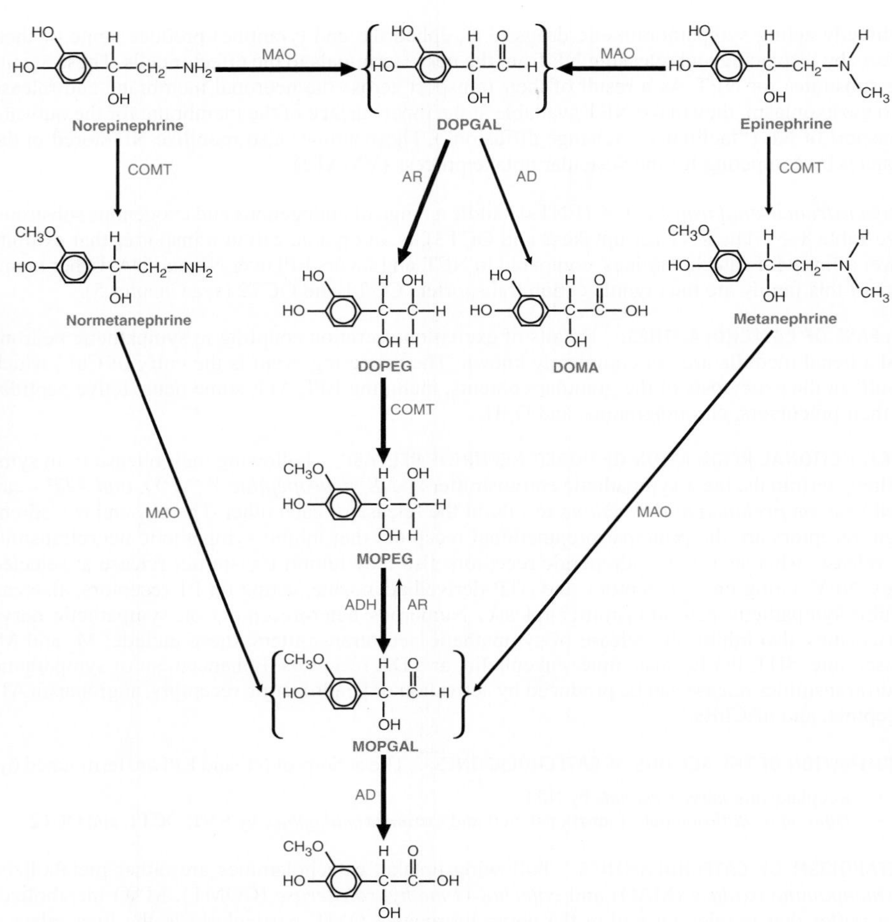

Figure 8–7 *Metabolism of catecholamines.* NE and EPI are first oxidatively deaminated to a short-lived intermediate (DOPGAL) by monoamine oxidase (MAO). DOPGAL then undergoes further metabolism to more stable alcohol or acid deaminated metabolites. Aldehyde dehydrogenase (AD) metabolizes DOPGAL to 3,4-dihydroxymandelic acid (DOMA) while aldehyde reductase (AR) metabolizes DOPGAL to 3,4-dihydroxyphenyl glycol (DOPEG). Under normal circumstances DOMA is a minor metabolite with DOPEG being the major metabolite produced from NE and EPI. Once DOPEG leaves the major sites of its formation (sympathetic nerves; adrenal medulla), it is converted to 3-methoxy, 4-hydroxyphenylglycol (MOPEG) by catechol-*O*-methyl transferase (COMT). MOPEG is then converted to the unstable aldehyde (MOPGAL) by alcohol dehydrogenase (ADH) and finally to vanillylmandelic acid (VMA) by aldehyde dehydrogenase. VMA is the major end product. Another route for the formation of VMA is conversion of NE or EPI into normetanephrine or metanephrine by COMT either in the adrenal medulla or extraneuronal sites, with subsequent metabolism to MOPGAL and thence to VMA. Catecholamines are also metabolized by *sulfotransferases*.

MOLECULAR BASIS OF ADRENERGIC RECEPTOR FUNCTION. All adrenergic receptors are GPCRs that link to heterotrimeric G proteins. Each major type shows preference for a particular class of G proteins, that is, α_1 to G_q, α_2 to G_i, and β to G_s (*see* Table 8–6). The responses that follow activation result from G protein–mediated effects on the generation of second messengers and on the activity of ion channels, as discussed in Chapter 3. The pathways overlap broadly with those discussed for muscarinic ACh receptors.

α ADRENERGIC RECEPTORS. The α_1 receptors (α_{1A}, α_{1B}, and α_{1D}) and the α_2 receptors (α_{2A}, α_{2B}, and α_{2C}) are heptahelical proteins that couple differentially to a variety of G proteins to regulate smooth muscle contraction, secretory pathways, and cell growth (*see* Table 8–6).

Table 8–6

Characteristics for Adrenergic Receptor Subtypes[a]

	G-PROTEIN COUPLING	PRINCIPLE EFFECTORS	TISSUE LOCALIZATION	DOMINANT EFFECTS[b]
α_{1A}	$G\alpha_q$ ($\alpha_{11}/\alpha_{14}/\alpha_{16}$)	↑ PLC, ↑ PLA_2 ↑ Ca^{2+} channels ↑ Na^+/H^+ exchanger Modulation of K^+ channels ↑ MAPK Signaling	Heart, Lung Liver Smooth muscle Blood vessels Vas deferens Prostate Cerebellum Cortex Hippocampus	• Dominant receptor for contraction of vascular smooth muscle • Promotes cardiac growth and structure • Vasoconstriction of large resistant arterioles in skeletal muscle
α_{1B}	$G\alpha_q$ ($\alpha_{11}/\alpha_{14}/\alpha_{16}$)	↑ PLC, ↑ PLA_2 ↑ Ca^{2+} channels ↑ Na^+/H^+ exchanger Modulation of K^+ channels ↑ MAPK Signaling	Kidney, Lung Spleen Blood vessels Cortex Brainstem	• Most abundant subtype in heart • Promotes cardiac growth and structure
α_{1D}	$G\alpha_q$ ($\alpha_{11}/\alpha_{14}/\alpha_{16}$)	↑ PLC, ↑ PLA_2 ↑ Ca^{2+} channels ↑ Na^+/H^+ exchanger Modulation of K^+ channels ↑ MAPK Signaling	Platelets, Aorta Coronary artery Prostate Cortex Hippocampus	• Dominant receptor for vasoconstriction in aorta and coronaries
α_{2A}	$G\alpha_i$ $G\alpha_o$ ($\alpha_{o1},/\alpha_{o2}$)	↓ AC-cAMP-PKA pathway	Platelets Sympathetic neurons Autonomic ganglia Pancreas Coronary/ CNS vessels Locus ceruleus Brainstem, Spinal cord	• Dominant inhibitory receptor on sympathetic neurons • Vasoconstriction of precapillary vessels in skeletal muscle
α_{2B}	$G\alpha_i$ Family $G\alpha_o$ Family ($\alpha_{o1},/\alpha_{o2}$)	↓ AC-cAMP-PKA pathway	Liver, Kidney Blood vessels Coronary/ CNS vessels Diencephalon Pancreas, Platelets	• Dominant mediator of α_2 vasoconstriction
α_{2C}	$G\alpha_i$ ($\alpha_{11}/\alpha_{12}/\alpha_{13}$) $G\alpha_o$ (α_{o1}/α_{o2})	↓ AC-cAMP-PKA pathway	Basal ganglia Cortex, Cerebellum Hippocampus	• Dominant receptor modulating DA neurotransmission • Dominant receptor inhibiting hormone release from adrenal medulla
β_1	$G\alpha_s$	↑ AC-cAMP-PKA pathway ↑ L type Ca^{2+} channels	Heart, Kidney Adipocytes Skeletal muscle Olfactory nucleus Cortex, Brain stem Cerebellar nuclei Spinal cord	• Dominant mediator of positive inotropic and chronotropic effects in heart

(continued)

Table 8–6

Characteristics for Adrenergic Receptor Subtypes[a] (*Continued*)

	G-PROTEIN COUPLING	PRINCIPLE EFFECTORS	TISSUE LOCALIZATION	DOMINANT EFFECTS[b]
β_2[c]	$G\alpha_s$	↑ AC-cAMP-PKA pathway ↑ Ca^{2+} channels	Heart, Lung Blood vessels Bronchial and GI smooth muscle Kidney Skeletal muscle Olfactory bulb Cortex Hippocampus	• Smooth muscle relaxation • Skeletal muscle hypertrophy
β_3[c,d]	$G\alpha_s$	↑ AC-cAMP-PKA pathway ↑ Ca^{2+} channels	Adipose tissue GI tract, Heart	• Metabolic effects

AC, adenylyl cyclase; Epi, epinephrine; NE, norepinephrine; Iso, isoproterenol; GI, gastrointestinal; GU, genitourinary.

[a]*At least 3 subtypes each of α_1 and α_2 adrenergic receptors are known, but distinctions in their mechanisms of action have not been clearly defined.*

[b]*In some species (e.g., rat), metabolic responses in the liver are mediated by α_1 adrenergic receptors, whereas in others (e.g., dog) β_2 adrenergic receptors are predominantly involved. Both types of receptors appear to contribute to responses in human beings.*

[c]*β Receptor coupling to cell signaling can be more complex. In addition to coupling to G_s to stimulate AC, β_2 receptors can activate signaling via a GRK/β-arrestin pathway. β_2 and β_3 receptors can couple to both G_s and G_i in a manner that may reflect agonist stereochemistry. See also Chapter 12.*

[d]*Metabolic responses in tissues with atypical pharmacological characteristics (e.g., adipocytes) may be mediated by β_3 receptors. Most β receptor antagonists (including propranolol) do not block these responses.*

***α_1* ADRENERGIC RECEPTORS.** Stimulation of α_1 receptors activates the G_q-PLCβ-IP_3/DAG-Ca^{2+} pathway and results in the activation of PKC and other Ca^{2+} and calmodulin sensitive pathways such as CaM kinases, with sequelae depending on cell differentiation (e.g., contraction of vascular smooth muscle, activation of eNOS in vascular endothelium) (*see* Chapter 3). Activation of α_1 receptor subtypes also stimulates several phospholipases (PLA_2, PLD).

PKC phosphorylates many substrates, including membrane proteins such as channels, pumps, and ion-exchange proteins (e.g., Ca^{2+}-transport ATPase). α_1 Receptor stimulation of PLA_2 leads to the release of free arachidonate, which is then metabolized by cyclooxygenase (yielding prostaglandins) and lipoxygenase (yielding leukotrienes) (*see* Chapter 33); PLD hydrolyzes phosphatidylcholine to yield phosphatidic acid. In most smooth muscles, the increased concentration of intracellular Ca^{2+} causes contraction (*see* Chapter 3 and Figure 3–14). In contrast, the increased concentration of intracellular Ca^{2+} that result from stimulation of α_1 receptors in GI smooth muscle causes hyperpolarization and relaxation by activation of Ca^{2+}-dependent K^+ channels. α_1 Receptors activate MAPKs, PI3K, and others to affect cell growth and proliferation.

***α_2* ADRENERGIC RECEPTORS.** *α_2 Adrenergic receptors* (α_{2A}, α_{2B}, and α_{2C}) couple to a variety of effectors, generally inhibiting adenylyl cyclase (reducing signaling via the cyclic AMP-PKA pathway) and activating G protein–gated K^+ channels (resulting in membrane hyperpolarization).

Activation of α_{2A} receptors inhibits NE release from sympathetic nerve endings and suppresses sympathetic outflow from the brain, leading to hypotension. In the CNS, α_{2A} receptors, probably produce the antinociceptive effects, sedation, hypothermia, hypotension, and behavioral actions of α_2 agonists. The α_{2B} receptor is the main receptor mediating α_2-induced vasoconstriction, whereas the α_{2C} receptor is the predominant receptor inhibiting the release of catecholamines from the adrenal medulla and modulating dopamine neurotransmission in the brain.

β ADRENERGIC RECEPTORS. β Receptors regulate numerous functions, including heart rate and contractility, smooth muscle relaxation, and multiple metabolic events in numerous tissues including adipose and hepatic cells and skeletal muscle (*see* Table 8–1). All 3 of the β receptor subtypes

(β_1, β_2, and β_3) couple to G_s and activate adenylyl cyclase (*see* Table 8–6). However, recent data suggest possible differences in downstream signals and events activated by the 3 β receptors.

β_1, β_2, and β_3 receptors can differ in their intracellular signaling pathways and subcellular location. Stimulation of β_2 receptors cause a transient increase in heart rate that is followed by a prolonged decrease. Following pretreatment with pertussis toxin, which prevents activation of G_i, the negative chronotropic effect of β_2 activation is abolished. It is thought that these specific signaling properties of β receptor subtypes are linked to subtype-selective association with intracellular scaffolding and signaling proteins. β_2 receptors normally are confined to caveolae in cardiac myocyte membranes; the importance of compartmentation of components of the cyclic AMP pathway are discussed in Chapter 3.

REFRACTORINESS TO CATECHOLAMINES. Exposure of catecholamine-sensitive cells and tissues to adrenergic agonists causes a progressive diminution in their capacity to respond to such agents. This phenomenon, variously termed *refractoriness, desensitization,* or *tachyphylaxis* (*see* Chapter 3). Multiple mechanisms are involved in desensitization, including receptor phosphorylation by both G-protein receptor kinases (GRKs) and by signaling kinases such as PKA and PKC, receptor sequestration and endocytosis, interaction with scaffold proteins, and activation of specific cyclic nucleotide phosphodiesterases. The β_2 receptor system is the best studied in this regard.

PHARMACOLOGICAL CONSIDERATIONS

Each step involved in neurotransmission (*see* Figures 8–3, 8–4, and 8–6) represents a potential point of therapeutic intervention. This is depicted in the diagrams of the cholinergic and adrenergic terminals and their postjunctional sites (*see* Figures 8–4 and 8–6). Drugs that affect processes involved in each step of transmission at cholinergic and adrenergic junctions are summarized in Table 8–7.

OTHER AUTONOMIC NEUROTRANSMITTERS

Most neurons in both the central and peripheral nervous systems contain more than 1 putative neurotransmitter (*see* Chapter 14). Although the parasympathetic and sympathetic components of the autonomic nervous system and the actions of ACh and NE still provides the essential framework for studying autonomic function, a host of other chemical messengers such as purines, eicosanoids, NO, and peptides modulate or mediate responses that follow stimulation of the ANS.

ATP. ATP is a cotransmitter with NE. The sympathetic nerves store ATP and NE in the same synaptic vesicles, and the 2 cotransmitters are released together. ATP and NE may also be released from separate subsets of vesicles and be subject to differential regulation. There is also evidence that ATP may be a cotransmitter with ACh in certain post-ganglionic parasympathetic nerves.

NPY. NPY peptides are distributed widely in the central and peripheral nervous systems. NPY is colocalized and coreleased with NE and ATP in most sympathetic nerves in the peripheral nervous system, especially those innervating blood vessels. Thus, NPY, together with NE and ATP, is likely a third sympathetic cotransmitter. The functions of NPY include (1) direct postjunctional contractile effects; (2) potentiation of the contractile effects of the other sympathetic cotransmitters; and (3) inhibitory modulation of the nerve stimulation–induced release of all 3 sympathetic cotransmitters.

VIP AND ACh. VIP and ACh coexist in peripheral autonomic neurons, possibly in separate populations of storage vesicles. There is evidence for their cotransmission in the regulation of salivation.

NONADRENERGIC, NONCHOLINERGIC (NANC) TRANSMISSION BY PURINES. There is evidence for the existence of NANC transmission in the ANS and of purinergic neurotransmission in the GI tract, genitourinary tract, and certain blood vessels. Indeed, ATP has fulfilled all the criteria for a neurotransmitter. Adenosine, generated from the released ATP by ectoenzymes and releasable nucleotidases acts as a modulator by causing feedback inhibition of release of the transmitter. Purinergic receptors are classified as adenosine *(P1)* receptors and ATP *(P2X and P2Y)* receptors. Adenosine receptors and P2Y receptors mediate their responses via G proteins, whereas the P2X receptors are a subfamily of ligand-gated ion channels (*see* Figure 14–8). Methylxanthines (e.g., caffeine and theophylline) preferentially block adenosine receptors (*see* Chapter 36).

MODULATION OF VASCULAR RESPONSES BY ENDOTHELIUM-DERIVED FACTORS; NO. An intact endothelium is necessary to achieve vascular relaxation in response to physiological ligands with G_q-linked receptors on endothelial cells and to exogenous ACh. In response to a variety of vasoactive agents and physical stimuli, endothelial cells produce and release a vasodilator called endothelium-derived relaxing factor (EDRF), now

Table 8–7

Representative Agents Acting at Peripheral Cholinergic and Adrenergic Neuroeffector Junctions

MECHANISM OF ACTION	SYSTEM	AGENTS	EFFECT
1. Interference with synthesis of transmitter	Cholinergic	ChAT inhibitors	Minimal depletion of ACh
	Adrenergic	α-Methyltyrosine (inhibition of TH)	Depletion of NE
2. Metabolic transformation endogenous transmitter pathway	Adrenergic	Methyldopa	Displacement of NE by α-methyl-NE, an α_2 agonist that reduces sympathetic outflow from CNS (similar to clonidine)
3. Blockade of transport system at nerve terminal membrane	Cholinergic	Hemicholinium	Block of choline uptake with consequent depletion of ACh
	Adrenergic	Cocaine, imipramine	Accumulation of NE at receptors
4. Blockade of transport system of storage vesicle	Cholinergic	Vesamicol	Block of ACh storage
	Adrenergic	Reserpine	Depletion of NE from storage vesicles; chemical sympathectomy
5. Promotion of exocytosis or displacement of transmitter from storage sites	Cholinergic	Latrotoxins	Cholinomimetic followed by anticholinergic
	Adrenergic	Amphetamine, tyramine	Sympathomimetic
6. Prevention of release of transmitter	Cholinergic	Botulinum toxin	Anti-cholinergic
	Adrenergic	Bretylium, guanadrel	Anti-adrenergic
7. Mimicry of transmitter at postjunctional sites	Cholinergic		
	Muscarinic[a]	Methacholine, bethanechol	Cholinomimetic
	Nicotinic[b]	Nicotine, epibatidine, cytisine	Cholinomimetic
	Adrenergic		
	α_1	Phenylephrine	Selective α_1 agonist
	α_2	Clonidine	Sympathomimetic (periphery); reduced sympathetic outflow (CNS)
	α_1, α_2	Oxymetazoline	Nonselective α agonist
	β_1	Dobutamine	Selective cardiac stimulation (some α_1 activation)
	β_2	Terbutaline, albuterol metaproterenol	Selective β_2 receptor agonist (selective inhibition of smooth muscle contraction)
	β_1, β_2	Isoproterenol	Nonselective β agonist

(*continued*)

Table 8–7

Representative Agents Acting at Peripheral Cholinergic and Adrenergic Neuroeffector Junctions (*Continued*)

MECHANISM OF ACTION	SYSTEM	AGENTS	EFFECT
8. Blockade of postsynaptic receptor	Cholinergic		
	Muscarinic[a]	Atropine	Muscarinic blockade
	Nicotinic (N_m)[b]	*d*-tubucurarine, atracurium	Neuromuscular blockade
	Nicotinic (N_n)[b]	Trimethaphan	Ganglionic blockade
	Adrenergic		
	α_1, α_2	Phenoxybenzamine	Nonselective α receptor blockade (irreversible)
	α_1, α_2	Phentolamine	Nonselective α receptor blockade (reversible)
	α_1	Prazosin, terazosin, doxasozin	Selective α_1 receptor blockade (reversible)
	α_2	Yohimbine	Selective α_2 receptor blockade
	β_1, β_2	Propranolol	Nonselective β blockade
	β_1	Metoprolol, atenolol	Selective β_1 receptor blockade (cardiomyocytes; renal j-g cells)
	β_2	—	Selective β_2 receptor blockade (smooth muscle)
9. Inhibition of enzymatic breakdown of transmitter	Cholinergic	AChE inhibitors Edrophonium, neostigmine, pyridostigmine	Cholinomimetic (muscarinic sites)
			Depolarization blockade (nicotinic sites)
	Adrenergic	Nonselective MAO inhibitors Pargyline, nialamide	Little direct effect on NE or sympathetic response; potentiation of tyramine
		Selective MAO-B inhibitor Selegeline	Adjunct in Parkinson disease
		Peripheral COMT inhibitor Entacapone	
		COMT inhibitor Tolcapone	Adjunct in Parkinson disease

ACh, acetylcholine; AChE, acetylcholine esterase; ChAT, choline acetyl transferase; COMT, catechol-O-methyl transferase; MAO, monoamine oxidase; NE, norepinephrine; j-g cells, renin-secreting cells in the juxta-glomerular complex of the kidney; TH, tyrosine hydroxylase.

[a]*At least five subtypes of muscarinic receptors exist. Agonists show little selectivity for subtypes whereas several antagonists show partial subtype selectivity (see Table 8–3).*

[b]*Two subtypes of muscle acetylcholine nicotinic receptors and several subtypes of neuronal receptors have been identified (see Table 8–2).*

known to be NO. Less commonly, an endothelium-derived hyperpolarizing factor (EDHF) and endothelium-derived contracting factor (EDCF) are released. NO production contributes to vascular tone and thus can modulate the influence of α- and β-agonists and antagonists thereon. *See* Figure 3–14 for more information on the multiple signaling systems that can influence vascular tone.

For a complete Bibliographical Listing see Goodman & Gilman's ***The Pharmacological Basis of Therapeutics***, 12th ed., or Goodman & Gilman Online at www.AccessMedicine.com.

Muscarinic Receptor Agonists and Antagonists

ACETYLCHOLINE AND ITS MUSCARINIC RECEPTOR TARGET

Muscarinic acetylcholine receptors in the peripheral nervous system occur primarily on autonomic effector cells innervated by postganglionic parasympathetic nerves. Muscarinic receptors are also present in autonomic ganglia and on some cells (e.g., vascular endothelial cells) that, paradoxically, receive little or no cholinergic innervation. Within the CNS, the hippocampus, cortex, and thalamus have high densities of muscarinic receptors. Acetylcholine (ACh), the naturally occurring neurotransmitter for these receptors, has virtually no systemic therapeutic applications because its actions are diffuse, and its hydrolysis, catalyzed by both acetylcholinesterase (AChE) and plasma butyrylcholinesterase, is rapid. Muscarinic agonists mimic the effects of ACh at these sites and are longer-acting congeners of ACh or natural alkaloids.

Cholinergic synapses are found at:

- Autonomic effector sites innervated by postganglionic parasympathetic nerves (or, in the sweat glands, by postganglionic sympathetic nerves)
- Sympathetic and parasympathetic ganglia and the adrenal medulla, innervated by preganglionic autonomic nerves
- Motor end plates on skeletal muscle, innervated by somatic motor nerves
- Certain synapses in the CNS, where ACh can have either pre- or postsynaptic actions

The actions of ACh and related drugs at autonomic effector sites are termed *muscarinic*, based on the observation that the alkaloid muscarine acts selectively at those sites and produces the same qualitative effects as ACh (*see* Table 8–1). Muscarinic receptors are present in autonomic ganglia and the adrenal medulla but primarily function to modulate the nicotinic actions of ACh at these sites (*see* Chapter 11). In the CNS, muscarinic receptors are widely distributed and mediate many important responses. The actions of ACh and its congeners at muscarinic receptors can be blocked competitively by atropine.

PROPERTIES AND SUBTYPES OF MUSCARINIC RECEPTORS

Muscarinic receptors comprise 5 distinct gene products, designated as M_1 through M_5 (*see* Table 8–3). Muscarinic receptors are GPCRs that in turn couple to various cellular effectors. Selectivity is not absolute but, in general, stimulation of M_1, M_3, and M_5 receptors activates the G_q-PLC-IP_3/DAG-Ca^{2+} pathway, resulting in a variety of Ca^{2+}-mediated responses. By contrast, M_2 and M_4 muscarinic receptors couple to the pertussis toxin–sensitive G proteins, G_i and G_o, to inhibit adenylyl cyclase and regulate specific ion channels.

The 5 muscarinic receptor subtypes are widely distributed in both the CNS and peripheral tissues; most cells express at least 2 subtypes (*see* Table 8–3). The M_2 receptor is the predominant subtype in the cholinergic control of the heart, whereas the M_3 receptor is the predominant subtype in the cholinergic control of smooth muscle, secretory glands, and the eye. The M_1 receptor has an important role in the modulation of nicotinic cholinergic transmission in ganglia.

PHARMACOLOGICAL EFFECTS OF ACETYLCHOLINE

CARDIOVASCULAR SYSTEM. ACh has 4 primary effects on the cardiovascular system:

- Vasodilation
- Decrease heart rate (negative chronotropic effect)
- Decrease the conduction velocity in the atrioventricular (AV) node (negative dromotropic effect)
- Decrease in the force of cardiac contraction (negative inotropic effect)

The negative inotropic effect is less significant in the ventricles than in the atria. Some of these responses can be obscured by baroreceptor and other reflexes that dampen the direct responses to ACh. Although ACh rarely is given systemically, its cardiac actions are important because the cardiac effects of cardiac glycosides, antiarrhythmic agents, and many other drugs are at least partly due to changes in parasympathetic (vagal) stimulation of the heart; in addition, afferent stimulation of the viscera during surgical interventions can reflexly increase the vagal stimulation of the heart.

The intravenous injection of a small dose of ACh produces a transient fall in blood pressure owing to generalized vasodilation (mediated by vascular endothelial NO), which is usually accompanied by reflex tachycardia. A considerably larger dose is required to see direct effects of ACh on the heart, such as eliciting bradycardia or AV nodal conduction block. The generalized vasodilation produced by exogenously administered ACh is due to the stimulation of muscarinic receptors, primarily of the M_3 subtype, located on vascular endothelial cells despite the apparent lack of cholinergic innervation. Occupation of the receptors by agonist activates the G_q-PLC-IP_3 pathway, leading to Ca^{2+}-calmodulin–dependent activation of endothelial NO synthase and production of NO, which diffuses to adjacent vascular smooth muscle cells and causes them to relax (*see* Chapters 3 and 8). If the endothelium is damaged, as occurs under various pathophysiological conditions, ACh acts predominantly on M_3 receptors located on vascular smooth muscle cells, causing vasoconstriction.

ACh affects cardiac function *directly* and also *indirectly* through inhibition of the adrenergic stimulation of the heart. Cardiac effects of ACh are mediated primarily by M_2 muscarinic receptors, which couple to G_i/G_o. The *direct* effects include:

- Increase in the ACh-activated K^+ current ($I_{K\text{-}ACh}$) due to activation of K-ACh channels
- Decrease in the L-type Ca^{2+} current ($I_{Ca\text{-}L}$) due to inhibition of L-type Ca^{2+} channels
- Decrease in the cardiac pacemaker current (I_f) due to inhibition of HCN (pacemaker) channels

The *indirect* effects include:

- G_i-mediated decrease in cyclic AMP, which opposes and counteracts the β_1 receptor/G_s–mediated increase in cyclic AMP
- Inhibition of the release of NE from sympathetic nerve terminals

The inhibition of NE release is mediated by presynaptic M_2 and M_3 receptors, which are stimulated by ACh released from adjacent parasympathetic postganglionic nerve terminals. Presynaptic M_2 receptors also inhibit ACh release from parasympathetic postganglionic nerve terminals in the human heart.

ACh slows the heart rate primarily by decreasing the rate of spontaneous depolarization of the *SA node* (*see* Chapter 29); attainment of the threshold potential and the succeeding events in the cardiac cycle are therefore delayed. In the *atria,* ACh causes hyperpolarization and a decreased action potential duration by increasing IK-ACh. ACh also inhibits cyclic AMP formation and NE release, decreasing atrial contractility. The rate of impulse conduction is either unaffected or may increase in response to ACh; the increase probably is due to the activation of additional Na^+ channels in response to ACh-induced hyperpolarization. In contrast, in the *AV node* (which has Ca^{2+} channel-dependent action potentials; *see* Chapter 29), ACh slows conduction and increases the refractory period by inhibiting $I_{Ca\text{-}L}$; the decrement in AV conduction is responsible for the complete heart block that may be observed when large quantities of cholinergic agonists are administered systemically.

Cholinergic (vagal) innervation of the His-Purkinje system and ventricular myocardium is sparse and the effects of ACh are smaller than those observed in the atria and nodal tissues. In the ventricles, ACh, whether released by vagal stimulation or applied directly, has a small negative inotropic effect; this inhibition is most apparent when there is concomitant adrenergic stimulation or underlying sympathetic tone. Automaticity of Purkinje fibers is suppressed, and the threshold for ventricular fibrillation is increased.

RESPIRATORY TRACT. The parasympathetic nervous system plays a major role in regulating bronchomotor tone. The effects of ACh on the respiratory system include not only bronchoconstriction but also increased tracheobronchial secretion and stimulation of the chemoreceptors of the carotid and aortic bodies. These effects are mediated primarily by M_3 muscarinic receptors.

URINARY TRACT. Parasympathetic sacral innervation causes detrusor muscle contraction, increased voiding pressure, and ureteral peristalsis. M_2 receptors appear most prevalent in the bladder; M_3 receptor mediates detrusor muscle contraction.

GI TRACT. Stimulation of vagal input to the GI tract increases tone, amplitude of contractions, and secretory activity of the stomach and intestine. The muscarinic receptors of the M_2 subtype are most prevalent, but M_3 muscarinic receptors are primarily responsible for mediating the cholinergic control of GI motility.

SECRETORY AND OCULAR EFFECTS. ACh stimulates secretion from glands that receive parasympathetic or sympathetic cholinergic innervation, including the lacrimal, nasopharyngeal, salivary, and sweat glands. These effects are mediated primarily by M_3 muscarinic receptors; M_1 receptors also contribute significantly to the cholinergic stimulation of salivary secretion. When instilled into the eye, ACh produces miosis by contracting the pupillary sphincter muscle and accommodation for near vision by contracting the ciliary muscle (*see* Chapter 64); both effects are mediated primarily by M_3 muscarinic receptors.

CNS EFFECTS. All 5 muscarinic receptor subtypes are found in the brain, and studies suggest that muscarinic receptor-regulated pathways may have an important role in cognitive function, motor control, appetite regulation, nociception, and other processes. Elevation of ACh with AChE inhibitors is used in treating some of the cognitive symptoms of Alzheimer disease (*see* Table 22–2).

MUSCARINIC RECEPTOR AGONISTS

Muscarinic cholinergic receptor agonists can be divided into 2 groups:

- Choline esters, including ACh and several synthetic esters
- Naturally occurring cholinomimetic alkaloids (particularly *pilocarpine*, *muscarine*, and *arecoline*) and their synthetic congeners

Of several hundred synthetic choline derivatives investigated, only methacholine, carbachol, and bethanechol have had clinical applications, along with a few natural alkaloids (Figure 9–1; Table 9–1).

Methacholine (acetyl-β-methylcholine), the β-methyl analog of ACh, is a synthetic choline ester that differs from ACh chiefly in its greater duration of action (the added methyl group increases its resistance to hydrolysis by cholinesterases) and its predominantly muscarinic selectivity. *Carbachol* and *bethanechol* are unsubstituted carbamoyl esters that are completely resistant to hydrolysis by cholinesterases; their $t_{1/2}$ are thus sufficiently long that they become distributed to areas of low blood flow. Carbachol retains substantial nicotinic activity, particularly on autonomic ganglia. Bethanechol has mainly muscarinic actions, with prominent effects on motility of the GI tract and urinary bladder. The major natural alkaloid muscarinic agonists are *muscarine, pilocarpine*, and *arecoline*. Muscarine acts almost exclusively at muscarinic receptor sites and is of toxicological significance (see below). Pilocarpine has a dominant muscarinic action but is a partial rather than a full agonist; the sweat glands are particularly sensitive to pilocarpine. Arecoline acts at nicotinic receptors. Although these naturally occurring alkaloids are of great value as pharmacological tools, present clinical use is restricted largely to the employment of pilocarpine as a sialagogue and miotic agent (*see* Chapter 64).

ABSORPTION, DISTRIBUTION, AND ELIMINATION. Muscarine and the choline esters are quaternary amines (*see* Figure 9–1), hence they are poorly absorbed following oral administration and have a limited ability to cross the blood-brain barrier. The choline esters are short-acting agents due to rapid elimination by the kidneys. Muscarine can still, however, be toxic when ingested and can even have CNS effects. Pilocarpine and arecoline, being tertiary amines, are readily absorbed and can cross the blood-brain barrier. Pilocarpine clearance is decreased in patients with hepatic impairment. The natural alkaloids are primarily eliminated by the kidneys; excretion of the tertiary amines can be accelerated by acidification of the urine.

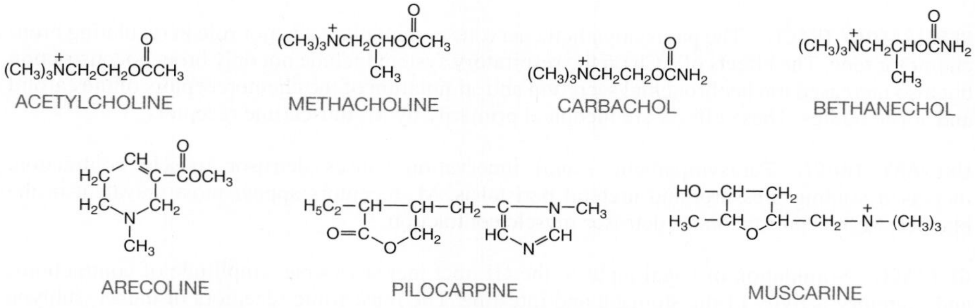

$(CH_3)_3\overset{+}{N}CH_2CH_2OC(=O)CH_3$
ACETYLCHOLINE

$(CH_3)_3\overset{+}{N}CH_2CH(CH_3)OC(=O)CH_3$
METHACHOLINE

$(CH_3)_3\overset{+}{N}CH_2CH_2OC(=O)NH_2$
CARBACHOL

$(CH_3)_3\overset{+}{N}CH_2CH(CH_3)OC(=O)NH_2$
BETHANECHOL

ARECOLINE

PILOCARPINE

MUSCARINE

Figure 9–1 *Structural formulas of acetylcholine, choline esters, and natural alkaloids that stimulate muscarinic receptors.*

Table 9–1

Some Pharmacological Properties of Choline Esters and Natural Alkaloids

MUSCARINIC AGONIST	HYDROLYSIS BY AChE	MUSCARINIC ACTIVITY: *CV*	*GI*	*Urinary Bladder*	*Eye (topical)*	*Antagonism by Atropine*	NICOTINIC ACTIVITY
Acetylcholine	+++	++	++	++	+	+++	++
Methacholine	+	+++	++	++	+	+++	+
Carbachol	−	+	+++	+++	++	+	+++
Bethanechol	−	±	+++	+++	++	+++	−
Muscarine	−	++	+++	+++	++	+++	−
Pilocarpine	−	+	+++	+++	++	+++	−

THERAPEUTIC USES OF MUSCARINIC RECEPTOR AGONISTS

Muscarinic agonists are currently used in the treatment of urinary bladder disorders and xerostomia and in the diagnosis of bronchial hyper-reactivity. They are also used in ophthalmology as miotic agents and for the treatment of glaucoma. There is growing interest in the role of muscarinic receptors in cognition and the potential utility of M_1 agonists in treating the cognitive impairment associated with Alzheimer disease.

ACETYLCHOLINE. ACh (MIOCHOL-E) is used topically for the induction of miosis during ophthalmologic surgery; it is instilled into the eye as a 1% solution (*see* Chapter 64).

METHACHOLINE. Methacholine (PROVOCHOLINE) is administered by inhalation for the diagnosis of bronchial airway hyperreactivity in patients who do not have clinically apparent asthma. Contraindications to methacholine testing include severe airflow limitation, recent myocardial infarction or stroke, uncontrolled hypertension, or pregnancy. The response to methacholine also may be exaggerated or prolonged in patients taking β adrenergic receptor antagonists. Methacholine is available as a powder that is diluted with 0.9% NaCl and administered via a nebulizer.

BETHANECHOL. Bethanechol (URECHOLINE, others) primarily affects the urinary and GI tracts. In the urinary tract, bethanechol has utility in treating urinary retention and inadequate emptying of the bladder as in postoperative urinary retention. When used chronically, 10-50 mg of the drug is given orally 3 to 4 times daily, administered on an empty stomach (i.e., 1 h before or 2 h after a meal) to minimize nausea and vomiting. In the GI tract, bethanechol stimulates peristalsis, increases motility, and increases resting lower esophageal sphincter pressure. Bethanechol formerly was used to treat postoperative abdominal distention, gastric atony, gastroparesis, adynamic ileus, and gastroesophageal reflux; more efficacious therapies for these disorders are now available (*see* Chapters 45 and 46).

CARBACHOL. Carbachol (MIOSTAT, ISOPTO CARBACHOL, others) is used topically in ophthalmology for the treatment of glaucoma and the induction of miosis during surgery; it is instilled into the eye as a 0.01-3% solution (*see* Chapter 64).

PILOCARPINE. Pilocarpine hydrochloride (SALAGEN, others) is used for the treatment of xerostomia that follows head and neck radiation treatments or that is associated with Sjögren syndrome, an autoimmune disorder occurring primarily in women in whom secretions, particularly salivary and lacrimal, are compromised. Side effects typify cholinergic stimulation. The usual dose is 5-10 mg 3 times daily; the dose should be lowered in patients with hepatic impairment. Pilocarpine (ISOPTO CARPINE, others) is used topically in ophthalmology for the treatment of glaucoma and as a miotic agent; it is instilled in the eye as a 0.5-6% solution and also can be delivered via an ocular insert (*see* Chapter 64).

CEVIMELINE. Cevimeline (EVOXAC), a quinuclidine derivative of ACh, is a muscarinic agonist with a high affinity for M_3 muscarinic receptors on lacrimal and salivary gland epithelia. Cevimeline has a long-lasting sialogogic action and may have fewer side effects than pilocarpine. The usual dose is 30 mg 3 times daily.

CONTRAINDICATIONS, PRECAUTIONS, AND ADVERSE EFFECTS

Contraindications to the use of muscarinic agonists include asthma, chronic obstructive pulmonary disease, urinary or GI tract obstruction, acid-peptic disease, cardiovascular disease, hypotension, and hyperthyroidism (muscarinic agonists may precipitate atrial fibrillation in hyperthyroid patients). Common adverse effects include diaphoresis; diarrhea, abdominal cramps, nausea/vomiting, and other GI side effects; a sensation of tightness in the urinary bladder; difficulty in visual accommodation; and hypotension. The adverse effects are of limited concern with topical administration for ophthalmic use.

TOXICOLOGY

Poisoning from the ingestion of plants containing pilocarpine, muscarine, or arecoline is characterized chiefly by exaggeration of their various parasympathomimetic effects and resembles that produced by consumption of mushrooms of the genus *Inocybe*. Treatment consists of the parenteral administration of atropine in doses sufficient to cross the blood-brain barrier and measures to support the respiratory and cardiovascular systems.

MUSHROOM POISONING (MYCETISM). High concentrations of muscarine are present in various species of *Inocybe* and *Clitocybe*. The symptoms of intoxication attributable to muscarine develop within 30-60 min of ingestion; they include salivation, lacrimation, nausea, vomiting, headache, visual disturbances, abdominal colic, diarrhea, bronchospasm, bradycardia, hypotension, and shock. Treatment with atropine (1-2 mg intramuscularly every 30 min) effectively blocks these effects.

Other mushroom species produce toxins unrelated to ACh. Intoxication by *Amanita* species arises from the neurologic and hallucinogenic properties of muscimol (a $GABA_A$ agonist), ibotenic acid, and other isoxazole derivatives that stimulate excitatory and inhibitory amino acid receptors. Mushrooms from *Psilocybe* and *Panaeolus* species contain hallucinogens [psilocybin (a $5HT_{2A}$ pro-agonist) and related derivatives of tryptamine]. *Gyromitra* species (false morels) produce GI disorders and a delayed hepatotoxicity. The most serious mycetism is produced by *Amanita phalloides*, other *Amanita* species, *Lepiota*, and *Galerina* species. These species account for > 90% of all fatal cases. Ingestion of as little as 50 g of *A. phalloides* (deadly nightcap) can be fatal. The principal toxins are the amatoxins (α- and β-amanitin), a group of cyclic octapeptides that inhibit RNA polymerase II and thereby block mRNA synthesis. Initial symptoms, which often are unnoticed or when present are due to other toxins, include diarrhea and abdominal cramps. A symptom-free period lasting up to 24 h is followed by hepatic and renal malfunction. Death occurs in 4-7 days from renal and hepatic failure. Treatment is largely supportive.

Because the severity of toxicity and treatment strategies for mushroom poisoning depend on the species ingested, seek their identification. Regional poison control centers in the U.S. maintain up-to-date information on the incidence of poisoning in the region and treatment procedures.

MUSCARINIC RECEPTOR ANTAGONISTS

Muscarinic antagonists prevent the effects of ACh by blocking its binding to muscarinic receptors on effector cells. In general, muscarinic antagonists cause little blockade of nicotinic receptors. However, the quaternary ammonium antagonists generally exhibit a greater degree of nicotinic blocking activity and therefore are more likely to interfere with ganglionic or neuromuscular transmission. An important consideration in the therapeutic use of muscarinic antagonists is the fact that physiological functions in different organs vary in their sensitivity to muscarinic receptor blockade (Table 9–2).

Table 9–2

Effects of Atropine in Relation to Dose

DOSE (mg)	EFFECTS
0.5	Slight cardiac slowing; some dryness of mouth; inhibition of sweating
1	Definite dryness of mouth; thirst; acceleration of heart, sometimes preceded by slowing; mild dilation of pupils
2	Rapid heart rate; palpitation; marked dryness of mouth; dilated pupils; some blurring of near vision
5	Above symptoms marked; difficulty in speaking and swallowing; restlessness and fatigue; headache; dry, hot skin; difficulty in micturition; reduced intestinal peristalsis
≥10	Above symptoms more marked; pulse rapid and weak; iris practically obliterated; vision very blurred; skin flushed, hot, dry, and scarlet; ataxia, restlessness, and excitement; hallucinations and delirium; coma

The clinical picture of a high (toxic) dose of atropine may be remembered by an old mnemonic device that summarizes the symptoms: Red as a beet, Dry as a bone, Blind as a bat, Hot as firestone, and Mad as a hatter.

The muscarinic receptor antagonists include:

- The naturally occurring alkaloids, atropine and scopolamine
- Semisynthetic derivatives of these alkaloids, which primarily differ from the parent compounds in their disposition in the body or their duration of action
- Synthetic derivatives, some of which show selectivity for subtypes of muscarinic receptors

Noteworthy agents among the latter 2 categories are homatropine and tropicamide, which have a shorter duration of action than atropine, and methscopolamine, ipratropium, and tiotropium, which are quaternized and do not cross the blood-brain barrier or readily cross membranes. The synthetic derivatives possessing some degree of receptor selectivity include pirenzepine, which shows selectivity for M_1 receptors; and darifenacin and solifenacin, which show selectivity for M_3 receptors.

Small doses of atropine depress salivary and bronchial secretion and sweating. Much larger doses are required to inhibit gastric motility and secretion, which are associated with unwanted side effects. This hierarchy of relative sensitivities is not a consequence of differences in the affinity of atropine for the muscarinic receptors at these sites; atropine lacks selectivity toward different muscarinic receptor subtypes. More likely determinants include the degree to which the functions of various end organs are regulated by parasympathetic tone, the "spareness" of receptors and signaling mechanisms, the involvement of intramural neurons and reflexes.

Most clinically available muscarinic antagonists are nonselective and their actions differ little from those of atropine. No subtype-selective antagonist, including pirenzepine, is completely selective. In fact, the clinical efficacy of some agents may arise from a balance of antagonistic actions on 2 or more receptor subtypes. Atropine and related compounds compete with ACh and other muscarinic agonists for a common binding site on the muscarinic receptor. Because antagonism by atropine is competitive, it can be overcome if the concentration of ACh at muscarinic receptors of the effector organ is increased sufficiently.

PHARMACOLOGICAL EFFECTS OF MUSCARINIC ANTAGONISTS

The pharmacological effects of atropine provide a good background for understanding the therapeutic uses of the various muscarinic antagonists. The effects of other muscarinic antagonists will be mentioned only when they differ significantly from those of atropine. Table 9–2 summarizes the major pharmacological effects of increasing doses of atropine.

CARDIOVASCULAR SYSTEM

Heart. Although the dominant response is tachycardia, the heart rate often decreases transiently with average clinical doses (0.4-0.6 mg). The slowing is modest (4-8 beats per minute) and is usually absent after rapid intravenous injection. Larger doses of atropine cause progressive tachycardia by blocking M_2 receptors on the SA nodal pacemaker cells, thereby antagonizing parasympathetic (vagal) tone to the heart. The resting heart rate is increased by ~35-40 beats per minute in young men given 2 mg of atropine intramuscularly. The maximal heart rate (e.g., in response to exercise) is not altered by atropine. The influence of atropine is most noticeable in healthy young adults, in whom vagal tone is considerable. In infancy and old age, even large doses of atropine may fail to accelerate the heart. Atropine often produces cardiac arrhythmias, but without significant cardiovascular symptoms.

Atropine can abolish many types of reflex vagal cardiac slowing or asystole, such as from inhalation of irritant vapors, stimulation of the carotid sinus, pressure on the eyeballs, peritoneal stimulation, or injection of contrast dye during cardiac catheterization. Atropine also prevents or abruptly abolishes bradycardia or asystole caused by choline esters, acetylcholinesterase inhibitors, or other parasympathomimetic drugs, as well as cardiac arrest from electrical stimulation of the vagus. The removal of vagal tone to the heart by atropine also may facilitate AV conduction.

Circulation. Atropine, alone, has little effect on blood pressure, since most vessels lack significant cholinergic innervation. However, in clinical doses, atropine completely counteracts the peripheral vasodilation and sharp fall in blood pressure caused by choline esters. In toxic and occasionally in therapeutic doses, atropine can dilate cutaneous blood vessels, especially those in the blush area (atropine flush). This may be a compensatory reaction permitting the radiation of heat to offset the atropine-induced rise in temperature that can accompany inhibition of sweating.

RESPIRATORY SYSTEM. Atropine inhibits the secretions of the nose, mouth, pharynx, and bronchi, and thus dries the mucous membranes of the respiratory tract. Atropine can inhibit the bronchoconstriction caused by histamine, bradykinin, and the eicosanoids, which presumably reflects the participation of reflex parasympathetic (vagal) activity in the bronchoconstriction elicited by these agents. The ability to block the indirect bronchoconstrictive effects of these mediators forms the basis for the use of muscarinic receptor antagonists, along with β adrenergic receptor agonists, in the treatment of asthma and COPD (*see* Chapter 36).

EYE. Muscarinic receptor antagonists block the cholinergic responses of the pupillary sphincter muscle of the iris and the ciliary muscle controlling lens curvature (*see* Chapter 64). Thus, they dilate the pupil (*mydriasis*) and paralyze accommodation (cycloplegia). Locally applied atropine produces ocular effects of considerable duration; accommodation and pupillary reflexes may not fully recover for 7-12 days. Other muscarinic receptor antagonists with shorter durations of action are therefore preferred as mydriatics in ophthalmologic practice (*see* Chapter 64). Muscarinic receptor antagonists administered systemically have little effect on intraocular pressure except in patients predisposed to angle-closure glaucoma, in whom the pressure may occasionally rise dangerously.

GI TRACT. Muscarinic receptor antagonists are used as antispasmodic agents for GI disorders and in the treatment of peptic ulcer disease. Although atropine can completely abolish the effects of ACh (and other parasympathomimetic drugs) on GI motility and secretion, it inhibits only incompletely the GI responses to vagal stimulation. This difference can be attributed to the fact that preganglionic vagal fibers innervating the GI tract synapse not only with postganglionic cholinergic fibers, but also with a network of noncholinergic intramural neurons. In addition, vagal stimulation of gastrin secretion is mediated by gastrin-releasing peptide (GRP), not ACh. The gastric parietal cell secretes acid in response to at least 3 agonists: gastrin, histamine, and ACh; furthermore, stimulation of muscarinic receptors on enterochromaffin-like cells will cause histamine release. Atropine inhibits the component of acid secretion that results from muscarinic stimulation of enterochromaffin cells and parietal cells (*see* Figure 45–1).

Secretions. Salivary secretion is particularly sensitive to inhibition by muscarinic receptor antagonists, which can completely abolish the copious, watery secretion induced by parasympathetic stimulation. The mouth becomes dry, and swallowing and talking may become difficult. *Gastric secretion* during the cephalic and fasting phases is also reduced markedly by muscarinic receptor antagonists. In contrast, the intestinal phase of gastric secretion is only partially inhibited. Although muscarinic antagonists can reduce gastric secretion, the doses required also affect salivary secretion, ocular accommodation, micturition, and GI motility (*see* Table 9–2). Thus, histamine H_2 receptor antagonists and proton pump inhibitors have replaced muscarinic antagonists as inhibitors of acid secretion (*see* Chapter 45).

Motility. The parasympathetic nerves enhance both tone and motility and relax sphincters, thereby favoring the passage of gastrointestinal contents. Muscarinic antagonists produce prolonged inhibitory effects on the motor activity of the stomach, duodenum, jejunum, ileum, and colon, characterized by a reduction in tone, amplitude and frequency of peristaltic contractions. Relatively large doses are needed to produce such inhibition. This probably can be explained by the ability of the enteric nervous system to regulate motility independently of parasympathetic control (*see* Chapter 8 and Figure 46–1).

OTHER SMOOTH MUSCLE

Urinary Tract. Muscarinic antagonists decrease the normal tone and amplitude of contractions of the ureter and bladder, and often eliminate drug-induced enhancement of ureteral tone. However, this inhibition cannot be achieved in the absence of inhibition of salivation and lacrimation and blurring of vision (*see* Table 9–2).

Biliary Tract. Atropine exerts a mild antispasmodic action on the gallbladder and bile ducts in humans. However, this effect usually is not sufficient to overcome or prevent the marked spasm and increase in biliary duct pressure induced by opioids, for which nitrates (*see* Chapter 27) are more effective.

SWEAT GLANDS AND TEMPERATURE. Small doses of atropine inhibit the activity of sweat glands innervated by sympathetic cholinergic fibers, and the skin becomes hot and dry. Sweating may be depressed enough to raise the body temperature, but only notably so after large doses or at high environmental temperatures.

CNS. Atropine has minimal effects on the CNS at therapeutic doses, although mild stimulation of the parasympathetic medullary centers may occur. With toxic doses of atropine, central excitation becomes more prominent, leading to restlessness, irritability, disorientation, hallucinations, or delirium. With still larger doses, stimulation is followed by depression, leading to circulatory collapse and respiratory failure after a period of paralysis and coma. In contrast to atropine, scopolamine has prominent central effects at low therapeutic doses; atropine therefore is preferred over scopolamine for many purposes. The basis for this difference is probably the greater permeation of scopolamine across the blood-brain barrier. Specifically, scopolamine in therapeutic doses normally causes CNS depression manifest as drowsiness, amnesia, fatigue, and dreamless sleep, with a reduction in REM sleep. Scopolamine is effective in preventing motion sickness.

Muscarinic receptor antagonists have long been used in the treatment of Parkinson disease. These agents can be effective adjuncts to treatment with levodopa (*see* Chapter 22). Muscarinic receptor antagonists also are used to treat the extrapyramidal symptoms that commonly occur as side effects of conventional antipsychotic drug therapy (*see* Chapter 16). Certain antipsychotic drugs are relatively potent muscarinic receptor antagonists and, perhaps for this reason, cause fewer extrapyramidal side effects.

IPRATROPIUM AND TIOTROPIUM. The quaternary ammonium compounds ipratropium and tiotropium are used exclusively for their effects on the respiratory tract. When inhaled, their action is confined almost completely to the mouth and airways. Dry mouth is the only frequently reported side effect, as the absorption of these drugs from the lungs or the GI tract is very inefficient. Ipratropium appears to block all subtypes of muscarinic receptors and accordingly also antagonizes the inhibition of ACh release by presynaptic M_2 receptors on parasympathetic postganglionic nerve terminals in the lung; the resulting increase in ACh release may counteract its blockade of M_3 receptor-mediated bronchoconstriction. In contrast, tiotropium shows some selectivity for M_1 and M_3 receptors; its lower affinity for M_2 receptors minimizes its presynaptic effect to enhance ACh release.

ABSORPTION, DISTRIBUTION, AND ELIMINATION. The belladonna alkaloids and the *tertiary* synthetic and semisynthetic derivatives are absorbed rapidly from the GI tract. They also enter the circulation when applied locally to the mucosal surfaces of the body. Absorption from intact skin is limited, although efficient absorption does occur in the postauricular region for some agents, allowing delivery by transdermal patch. Systemic absorption of inhaled or orally ingested *quaternary* muscarinic receptor antagonists is limited even from the conjunctiva of the eye. Quaternary agents do not cross the blood-brain barrier. Atropine has a $t_{1/2}$ of ~4 h; hepatic metabolism accounts for the elimination of about half of a dose; the remainder is excreted unchanged in the urine.

Ipratropium is administered as an aerosol or solution for inhalation whereas tiotropium is administered as a dry powder. As with most drugs administered by inhalation, ~90% of the dose is swallowed. Most of the swallowed drug appears in the feces. Maximal responses develop over 30-90 min, with tiotropium having the slower onset. The effects of ipratropium last for 4-6 h, while tiotropium's effects persist for 24 h.

THERAPEUTIC USES OF MUSCARINIC RECEPTOR ANTAGONISTS

Muscarinic receptor antagonists have been used in the treatment of a wide variety of clinical conditions, predominantly to inhibit effects of parasympathetic activity in the respiratory tract, urinary tract, GI tract, eye, and heart. Their CNS effects have resulted in their use in the treatment of Parkinson disease, the management of extrapyramidal side effects of antipsychotic drugs, and the prevention of motion sickness.

RESPIRATORY TRACT. Ipratropium (ATROVENT, others) and tiotropium (SPIRIVA) are important agents in the treatment of chronic obstructive pulmonary disease. These agents often are used with inhaled long-acting β_2 adrenergic receptor agonists. Ipratropium is administered 4 times daily via a metered-dose inhaler or nebulizer; tiotropium is administered once daily via a dry powder inhaler (*see* Chapter 36). Ipratropium also is used in nasal inhalers for the treatment of the rhinorrhea associated with the common cold or with allergic or nonallergic perennial rhinitis.

GENITOURINARY TRACT. Overactive urinary bladder can be successfully treated with muscarinic receptor antagonists. Muscarinic antagonists can be used to treat enuresis in children, particularly when a progressive increase in bladder capacity is the objective, and to reduce urinary frequency and increase bladder capacity in spastic paraplegia. The muscarinic receptor antagonists indicated for overactive bladder are oxybutynin (DITROPAN, others), tolterodine (DETROL), trospium chloride (SANCTURA), darifenacin (ENABLEX), solifenacin (VESICARE), and fesoterodine (TOVIAZ); available preparations and dosages are summarized in Table 9–3. The most important adverse reactions are consequences of muscarinic receptor blockade and include xerostomia, blurred vision, and GI side effects such as constipation and dyspepsia. CNS-related antimuscarinic effects, including drowsiness, dizziness, and confusion, can occur and are particularly problematic in elderly patients.

GI TRACT. Although muscarinic receptor antagonists can reduce gastric motility and the secretion of gastric acid, antisecretory doses produce pronounced side effects (*see* Table 9–2). As a consequence, patient compliance in the long-term management of symptoms of acid-peptic disease with these drugs is poor. Pirenzepine, a tricyclic drug similar in structure to imipramine, has selectivity for M_1 over M_2 and M_3 receptors. However, pirenzepine's affinities for M_1 and M_4 receptors are comparable, so it does not possess total M_1 selectivity. Telenzepine, an analog of pirenzepine, has higher potency and similar selectivity for M_1 muscarinic receptors. Both drugs are used in the treatment of acid-peptic disease in Europe, Japan, and Canada, but not currently in the U.S. At therapeutic doses of pirenzepine, the incidence of xerostomia, blurred vision, and central muscarinic disturbances is relatively low. Central effects are not seen because of the drug's limited penetration into the CNS. H_2 receptor antagonists and proton pump inhibitors generally are the current drugs of choice to reduce gastric acid secretion (*see* Chapter 45).

The belladonna alkaloids (atropine, hyoscyamine sulfate [ANASPAZ, others], and scopolamine) alone or in combination with sedatives (phenobarbital [DONNATAL, others]) or anti-anxiety agents (chlordiazepoxide [LIBRAX]) have been used in a variety of conditions known to involve irritable bowel and increased tone (spasticity) or motility of the GI. Glycopyrrolate (ROBINUL, others), a muscarinic antagonist structurally unrelated

Table 9–3

Muscarinic Receptor Antagonists Used in the Treatment of Overactive Urinary Bladder

NONPROPRIETARY NAME	$t_{1/2}$ (hours)	PREPARATIONS[a]	DAILY DOSE (adult)
Oxybutynin	2–5	IR ER Transdermal patch Topical gel	10–20 mg[b] 5–30 mg[b] 3.9 mg 100 mg
Tolterodine	2–9.6[c] 6.9–18[c]	IR ER	2–4 mg[b,d] 4 mg[b,d]
Trospium chloride	20 35	IR ER	20–40 mg[e] 60 mg[e]
Solifenacin	55	IR	5–10 mg[b]
Darifenacin	13–19	ER	7.5–15 mg[f]
Fesoterodine	7	ER	4–8 mg

[a]Preparations are designated as follows: IR, immediate-release tablet; ER, extended-release tablet or capsule.
[b]Doses may need to be reduced in patients taking drugs that inhibit CYP3A4.
[c]Longer times in indicated ranges are seen in poor metabolizers.
[d]Doses should be reduced in patients with significant renal or hepatic impairment.
[e]Doses should be reduced in patients with significant renal impairment; dosage adjustments also may be needed in patients with hepatic impairment.
[f]Doses may need to be reduced in patients taking drugs that inhibit CYPs 3A4 or 2D6.

to the belladonna alkaloids, also is used to reduce GI tone and motility; as a quaternary amine, it is less likely to cause adverse CNS effects. The belladonna alkaloids and synthetic substitutes are very effective in reducing excessive salivation, such as drug-induced salivation and that associated with heavy-metal poisoning and Parkinson disease. A subtherapeutic dose of atropine is included with diphenoxylate in antidiarrheal LOMOTIL to discourage overuse.

Dicyclomine hydrochloride (BENTYL, others) is a weak muscarinic receptor antagonist that also has nonspecific direct spasmolytic effects on smooth muscle of the GI tract. It is occasionally used in the treatment of diarrhea-predominant irritable bowel syndrome.

EYE. Effects limited to the eye are obtained by topical administration of muscarinic receptor antagonists to produce mydriasis and cycloplegia. Cycloplegia is not attainable without mydriasis and requires higher concentrations or more prolonged application of a given agent. Homatropine hydrobromide (ISOPTO HOMATROPINE, others), a semisynthetic derivative of atropine, cyclopentolate hydrochloride (CYCLOGYL, others), and tropicamide (MYDRIACYL, others) are agents used in ophthalmological practice. These agents are preferred to topical atropine or scopolamine because of their shorter duration of action (*see* Chapter 64).

CARDIOVASCULAR SYSTEM. The cardiovascular effects of muscarinic receptor antagonists are of limited clinical utility. Atropine may be considered in the initial treatment of patients with acute myocardial infarction in whom excessive vagal tone causes sinus bradycardia or AV nodal block. Dosing must be judicious; doses that are too low can cause a paradoxical bradycardia (described earlier), while excessive doses will cause tachycardia that may extend the infarct by increasing the demand for oxygen. Atropine may reduce the degree of AV block when increased vagal tone is a major factor in the conduction defect, such as the second-degree AV block that can be produced by digitalis.

CNS. Scopolamine is the most effective prophylactic agent for short (4-6 h) exposures to severe motion, and probably for exposures of up to several days. All agents used to combat motion sickness should be given prophylactically. A transdermal preparation of scopolamine (TRANSDERM SCOP), used for the prevention of motion sickness, is applied to the postauricular mastoid region, an area where transdermal absorption of the drug is especially efficient, resulting in the delivery of ~0.5 mg of scopolamine over 72 h. Dry mouth is common, drowsiness is not infrequent, and blurred vision occurs in some individuals. Mydriasis and cycloplegia can occur. Rare but severe psychotic episodes have been reported. Centrally acting muscarinic antagonists are efficacious in preventing extrapyramidal side effects such as dystonias or parkinsonian symptoms in patients treated with antipsychotic drugs (*see* Chapter 16). The muscarinic antagonists used for Parkinson disease and drug-induced extrapyramidal symptoms include benztropine mesylate (COGENTIN, others), trihexyphenidyl hydrochloride (ARTANE, others), and biperiden; all are tertiary amines that readily gain access to the CNS.

USES IN ANESTHESIA. Atropine commonly is given to block responses to vagal reflexes induced by surgical manipulation of visceral organs. Atropine or glycopyrrolate is used with neostigmine to block its parasympathomimetic effects when the latter agent is used to reverse skeletal muscle relaxation after surgery (*see* Chapter 11). Serious cardiac arrhythmias have occasionally occurred.

ANTICHOLINESTERASE POISONING. The use of atropine in large doses for the treatment of poisoning by anticholinesterase organophosphorus insecticides is discussed in Chapter 10. Atropine also may be used to antagonize the parasympathomimetic effects of pyridostigmine or other anticholinesterases administered in the treatment of myasthenia gravis. It is most useful early in therapy, before tolerance to muscarinic side effects of anticholinesterases have developed.

OTHER THERAPEUTIC USES OF MUSCARINIC ANTAGONISTS. Methscopolamine bromide (PAMINE) is a quaternary ammonium derivative of scopolamine is primarily used in combination products for the temporary relief of symptoms of allergic rhinitis, sinusitis, and the common cold.

CONTRAINDICATIONS AND ADVERSE EFFECTS

Most contraindications, precautions, and adverse effects of muscarinic antagonists are predictable consequences of muscarinic receptor blockade: xerostomia, constipation, blurred vision, dyspepsia, and cognitive impairment. Important contraindications to the use of muscarinic antagonists include urinary tract obstruction, GI obstruction, and uncontrolled (or susceptibility to attacks of) angle-closure glaucoma.

TOXICOLOGY OF DRUGS WITH ANTIMUSCARINIC PROPERTIES

The deliberate or accidental ingestion of natural belladonna alkaloids is a major cause of poisonings. Many histamine H_1 receptor antagonists, phenothiazines, and tricyclic antidepressants also block muscarinic receptors and, in sufficient dosage, produce syndromes that include features of atropine intoxication.

Among the tricyclic antidepressants, protriptyline and amitriptyline are the most potent muscarinic receptor antagonists, with an affinity for the receptor that is ~ one-tenth of that reported for atropine. Since these drugs are administered in therapeutic doses considerably higher than the effective dose of atropine, antimuscarinic effects are often observed clinically (*see* Chapter 15) and overdose with suicidal intent is a danger in the population using antidepressants. Fortunately, most of the newer antidepressants and SSRIs have more limited anticholinergic properties. The newer antipsychotic drugs, classified as "atypical" and characterized by their low propensity for inducing extrapyramidal side effects, also include agents that are potent muscarinic receptor antagonists (e.g., clozapine and olanzapine). A paradoxical side effect of clozapine is increased salivation and drooling, possibly the result of partial agonist properties of this drug.

Infants and young children are especially susceptible to the toxic effects of muscarinic antagonists. Indeed, cases of intoxication in children have resulted from conjunctival instillation for ophthalmic refraction and other ocular effects. Systemic absorption occurs either from the nasal mucosa after the drug has traversed the nasolacrimal duct or from the GI tract if the drug is swallowed. Poisoning with diphenoxylate-atropine (LOMOTIL, others), used to treat diarrhea, has been extensively reported in the pediatric literature. Transdermal preparations of scopolamine used for motion sickness have been noted to cause toxic psychoses, especially in children and in the elderly. Jimson weed contains a variety of belladonna alkaloids; serious intoxication can result from ingestion and smoking of the plant.

Table 9–2 shows the oral doses of atropine causing undesirable responses or symptoms of overdosage. These symptoms are predictable results of blockade of parasympathetic innervation. In cases of full-blown atropine poisoning, the syndrome may last 48 h or longer. Intravenous injection of the anticholinesterase agent physostigmine may be used for confirmation. Depression and circulatory collapse are evident only in cases of severe intoxication; the blood pressure declines, convulsions may ensue, respiration becomes inadequate, and death due to respiratory failure may follow. If marked excitement is present and more specific treatment is not available, a benzodiazepine is the most suitable agent for sedation and for control of convulsions. Phenothiazines or agents with antimuscarinic activity should not be used, because their antimuscarinic action is likely to intensify toxicity. Support of respiration and control of hyperthermia may be necessary.

For a complete Bibliographical Listing see Goodman & Gilman's ***The Pharmacological Basis of Therapeutics***, 12th ed., or Goodman & Gilman Online at www.AccessMedicine.com.

Anticholinesterase Agents

Acetylcholinesterase (AChE) terminates the action of acetylcholine (ACh) at the junctions of the various cholinergic nerve endings with their effector organs or postsynaptic sites (*see* Chapter 8). Drugs that inhibit AChE are called anticholinesterase (anti-ChE) agents. They cause ACh to accumulate in the vicinity of cholinergic nerve terminals and thus are potentially capable of producing effects equivalent to excessive stimulation of cholinergic receptors throughout the central and peripheral nervous systems. The anti-ChE agents have received extensive application as toxic agents, in the form of agricultural insecticides, pesticides, and potential chemical warfare "nerve gases." Nevertheless, some compounds of this class are used therapeutically for the treatment of Alzheimer disease.

History. Physostigmine, also called *eserine,* is an alkaloid obtained from the Calabar or ordeal bean, the dried, ripe seed of *Physostigma venenosum,* a West African perennial. The Calabar bean once was used by native tribes of West Africa as an "ordeal poison" in trials for witchcraft, in which guilt was judged by death from the poison, innocence by survival after ingestion of a bean. The recent suggestion that we apply this test to politicians was narrowly rejected on humanitarian grounds.

Prior to World War II, only the "reversible" anti-ChE agents were generally known, of which physostigmine is the prototype. Shortly before and during World War II, a new class of highly toxic chemicals, the organophosphates, was developed, first as agricultural insecticides and later as potential chemical warfare agents. The extreme toxicity of these compounds is due to their "irreversible" inactivation of AChE, which results in prolonged enzyme inhibition. Because the pharmacological actions of both the reversible and irreversible anti-ChE agents are qualitatively similar, they are discussed here as a group.

STRUCTURE OF ACETYLCHOLINESTERASE. AChE exists in 2 general molecular classes: simple homomeric oligomers of catalytic subunits and heteromeric associations of catalytic subunits with structural subunits. The homomeric forms are found as soluble species in the cell, presumably destined for export or for association with the outer membrane of the cell, typically through an attached glycophospholipid. One heteromeric form, largely found in neuronal synapses, is a tetramer of catalytic subunits disulfide-linked to a 20-kDa lipid-linked subunit and localized to the outer surface of the cell membrane. The other heteromeric form consists of tetramers of catalytic subunits, disulfide linked to each of 3 strands of a collagen-like structural subunit. This molecular species, whose molecular mass approaches 10^6 Da, is associated with the basal lamina of junctional areas of skeletal muscle. A separate, structurally related gene encodes butyrylcholinesterase, which is synthesized in the liver and is primarily found in plasma.

The active center of mammalian AChE is at the base of a 2 nm gorge, at the bottom of which lie the catalytic triad (Ser203, His447, and Glu334), an acyl pocket, and a choline subsite; a "peripheral" site lies at the mouth of the gorge. The interactions of ligands with AChE can be usefully considered by examining their interactions with these domains (*see* Figure 10–1). The catalytic mechanism resembles that of other hydrolases; the serine hydroxyl group is rendered highly nucleophilic through a charge-relay system involving the carboxylate anion from glutamate, the imidazole of histidine, and the hydroxyl of serine (Figure 10–1A). During enzymatic attack of ACh, an ester with trigonal geometry, a tetrahedral intermediate between enzyme and substrate is formed (*see* Figure 10–1A) that collapses to an acetyl enzyme conjugate with the concomitant release of choline. The acetyl enzyme is very labile to hydrolysis, which results in the formation of acetate and active enzyme. AChE is one of the most efficient enzymes known: 1 molecule of AChE can hydrolyze 6×10^5 ACh molecules/min; this yields a turnover time of 100 μsec.

MECHANISM OF ACTION OF AChE INHIBITORS. Anti-ChE agents are divided into 3 classes whose interactions with AChE are depicted Figure 10–1: *noncovalent "reversible' inhibitors," carbamoylating inhibitors, and organophosphate inhibitors.*

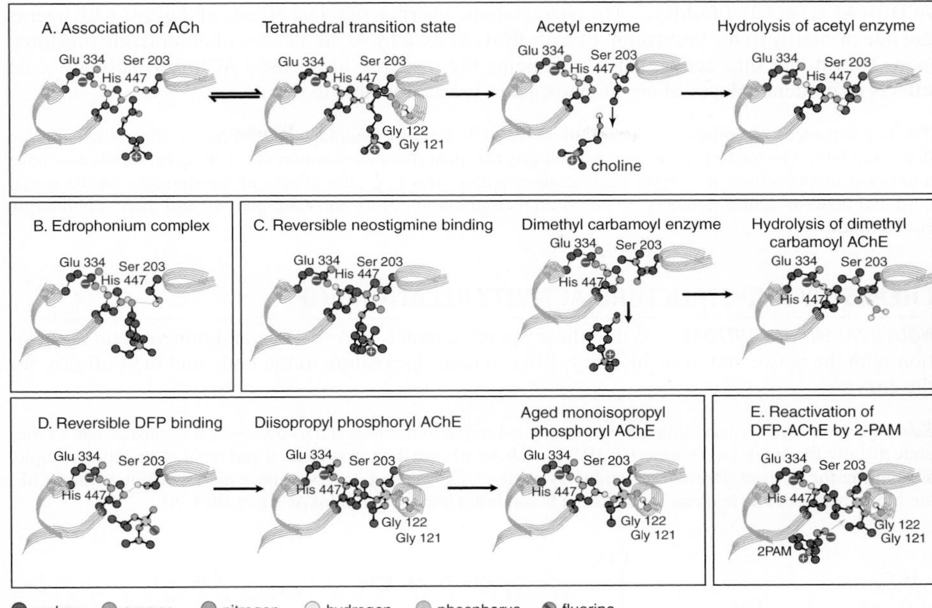

Figure 10–1 *Steps involved in the hydrolysis of acetylcholine by acetylcholinesterase and in the inhibition and reactivation of the enzyme.* Only the 3 residues of the catalytic triad are depicted. The associations and reactions shown are: **A.** Acetylcholine (ACh) catalysis: binding of ACh, formation of a tetrahedral transition state, formation of the acetyl enzyme with liberation of choline, rapid hydrolysis of the acetyl enzyme with return to the original state. **B.** Reversible binding and inhibition by edrophonium. **C.** Neostigmine reaction with and inhibition of AChE: reversible binding of neostigmine, formation of the dimethyl carbamoyl enzyme, slow hydrolysis of the dimethyl carbamoyl enzyme. **D.** Diisopropyl fluorophosphate (DFP) reaction and inhibition of AChE: reversible binding of DFP, formation of the diisopropyl phosphoryl enzyme, formation of the aged monoisopropyl phosphoryl enzyme. Hydrolysis of the diisopropyl enzyme is very slow (not shown). The aged monoisopropyl phosphoryl enzyme is virtually resistant to hydrolysis and reactivation. The tetrahedral transition state of ACh hydrolysis resembles the conjugates formed by the tetrahedral phosphate inhibitors and accounts for their potency. Amide bond hydrogens from Gly121 and Gly122 stabilize the carbonyl and phosphoryl oxygens. **E.** Reactivation of the diisopropyl phosphoryl enzyme by pralidoxime (2-PAM). 2-PAM attack of the phosphorus on the phosphorylated enzyme will form a phospho-oxime with regeneration of active enzyme.

- ***Reversible inhibitors***, such as *edrophonium* and *tacrine*, bind to the choline subsite (Figure 10–1B). Additional reversible inhibitors include *donepezil, propidium*, and the peptidic snake toxin *fasciculin.*
- ***Carbamoylating inhibitors*** with a carbamoyl ester linkage, such as *physostigmine* and *neostigmine*, are hydrolyzed by AChE, generating the carbamoylated enzyme (Figure 10–1C). In contrast to the acetyl enzyme, methylcarbamoyl AChE and dimethylcarbamoyl AChE are far more stable (the $t_{1/2}$ for hydrolysis of the dimethylcarbamoyl enzyme is 15-30 min). Sequestration of the enzyme in its carbamoylated form thus precludes the enzyme-catalyzed hydrolysis of ACh for extended periods of time. When administered systemically, the duration of inhibition is 3-4 h.
- ***Organophosphate inhibitors***, such as *diisopropyl fluorophosphate* (DFP), form very stable conjugates with AChE, with the active center serine phosphorylated or phosphonylated (Figure 10–1D). If the alkyl groups in the phosphorylated enzyme are ethyl or methyl, spontaneous regeneration of active enzyme requires several hours. Secondary (as in DFP) or tertiary alkyl groups further enhance the stability of the phosphorylated enzyme, and significant regeneration of active enzyme usually is not observed. The stability of the phosphorylated enzyme is *strengthened* through "*aging*," which results from the loss of 1 of the alkyl groups.

Thus, the terms *reversible* and *irreversible* as applied to the carbamoyl ester and organophosphate anti-ChE agents, respectively, reflect only quantitative differences in rates of decarbamoylation or dephosphorylation of the conjugated enzyme. Both chemical classes react covalently with the active center serine in essentially the same manner as does ACh.

ACTION AT EFFECTOR ORGANS. The characteristic pharmacological effects of the anti-ChE agents are due primarily to the prevention of hydrolysis of ACh by AChE at sites of cholinergic transmission. Transmitter thus accumulates, enhancing the response to released ACh. Virtually all acute effects of moderate doses of organophosphates are attributable to this action.

The consequences of enhanced concentrations of ACh at motor endplates are unique to these sites and are discussed later. The tertiary amine and particularly the quaternary ammonium anti-ChE compounds may have additional direct actions at certain cholinergic receptor sites (e.g., the effects of neostigmine on the spinal cord and neuromuscular junction are based on a combination of its anti-ChE activity and direct cholinergic stimulation).

CHEMISTRY AND STRUCTURE-ACTIVITY RELATIONSHIPS

NONCOVALENT INHIBITORS. While these agents interact by reversible and noncovalent association with the active site in AChE, they differ in their disposition in the body and their affinity for the enzyme.

Edrophonium, a quaternary drug whose activity is limited to peripheral nervous system synapses, has a moderate affinity for AChE (*see* Figure 10–1B). Its volume of distribution is limited and renal elimination is rapid, accounting for its short duration of action. By contrast, *tacrine* and *donepezil* have higher affinities for AChE, are more hydrophobic, and readily cross the blood-brain barrier to inhibit AChE in the CNS.

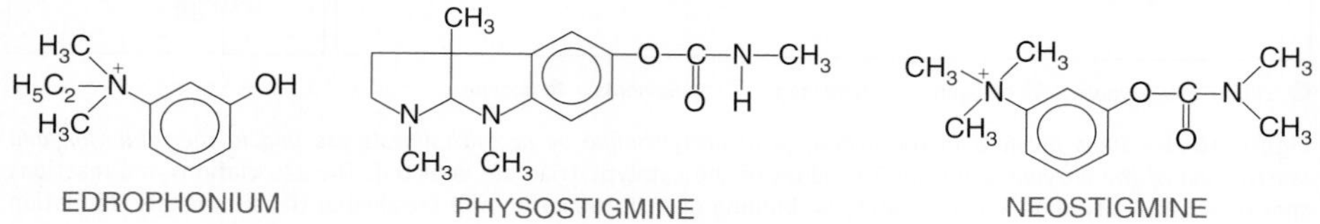

EDROPHONIUM PHYSOSTIGMINE NEOSTIGMINE

"REVERSIBLE" CARBAMATE INHIBITORS. Drugs of this class that are of therapeutic interest include physostigmine, neostigmine, and rivastigmine. Their interaction with AChE is depicted in Figure 10–1C.

The essential moiety of the physostigmine molecule is the methyl carbamate of an amine-substituted phenol. An increase in anti-ChE potency and duration of action can result from the linking of 2 quaternary ammonium moieties. An example is the miotic agent demecarium, which consists of 2 neostigmine molecules connected by a series of 10 methylene groups. The second quaternary group confers additional stability to the interaction. Carbamoylating inhibitors with high lipid solubilities (e.g., rivastigmine), which readily cross the blood-brain barrier and have longer durations of action, are approved or in clinical trial for the treatment of Alzheimer disease (*see* Chapter 22).

The carbamate insecticides carbaryl (SEVIN), propoxur (BAYGON), and aldicarb (TEMIK), which are used extensively as garden insecticides, inhibit ChE in a fashion identical with other carbamoylating inhibitors. The symptoms of poisoning closely resemble those of the organophosphates.

ORGANOPHOSPHORUS COMPOUNDS. The general formula for this class of ChE inhibitors is shown at the top of Table 10–1. The group includes DFP, soman, malathion, and echothiophate.

DFP produces virtually irreversible inactivation of AChE and other esterases by diisopropylphosphorylation followed by "aging" (conversion to the monoisopropylphosphoryl AChE (*see* Figure 10–1D). Its high lipid solubility, low molecular weight, and volatility facilitate inhalation, transdermal absorption, and penetration into the CNS. The "*nerve gases*"—*tabun, sarin,* and *soman*—are among the most potent synthetic toxins known; they are lethal to laboratory animals in nanogram doses. Insidious employment of these agents has occurred in warfare and terrorism attacks. *Because of their low volatility and stability in aqueous solution, parathion* and *methylparathion* were widely used as insecticides; however, acute and chronic toxicity has limited their use. These compounds are inactive in inhibiting AChE in vitro; paraoxon is the active metabolite produced in vivo via a substitution of phosphoryl oxygen for sulfur carried out by hepatic CYPs. This reaction also occurs in the insect, typically with more efficiency than in mammals and many other animals. Other insecticides possessing the phosphorothioate structure have been widely employed, including *diazinon* (SPECTRACIDE, others) and *chlorpyrifos* (DURSBAN, LORSBAN). Both of these agents have been placed under restricted use because of evidence of chronic toxicity in the newborn animal. They have been banned since 2005.

Table 10–1

Representative Organophosphorus Compounds

General formula R_1 O (S) / P / R_2 X

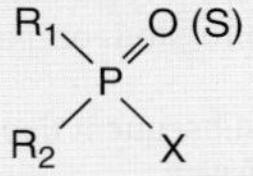

Group **A,** X = halogen, cyanide, or thiocyanate leaving group; group **B,** X = alkylthio, arylthio, alkoxy, or aryloxy leaving group; group **C,** thionophosphorus or thio-thionophosphorus compounds; group **D,** quaternary ammonium leaving group. R_1 can be an alkyl (phosphonates), alkoxy (phosphorates) or an alkylamino (phosphoramidates) group.

GROUP	STRUCTURAL FORMULA	COMMON, CHEMICAL, AND OTHER NAMES	COMMENTS
A	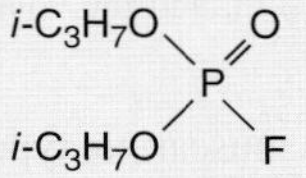 i-C_3H_7O O P i-C_3H_7O F	DFP; Isoflurophate; diisopropyl fluorophosphate	Potent, irreversible inactivator
	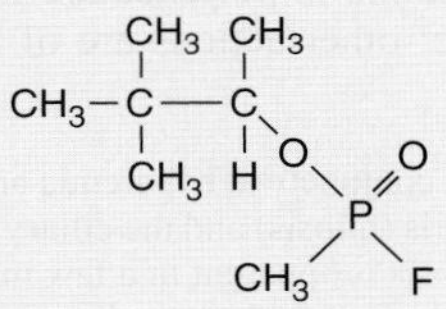 CH_3 CH_3 CH_3—C—C CH_3 H O O P CH_3 F	Soman (GD) Pinacolyl methylphosphonofluoridate	Extremely toxic "nerve gas"; greatest potential for irreversible action/rapid aging
B	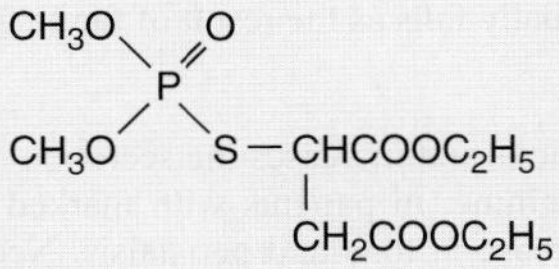 CH_3O O P CH_3O S−$CHCOOC_2H_5$ $CH_2COOC_2H_5$	Malaoxon *O,O*-Dimethyl S-(1,2-dicarboxyethyl)-phosphorothioate	Active metabolite of malathion
C	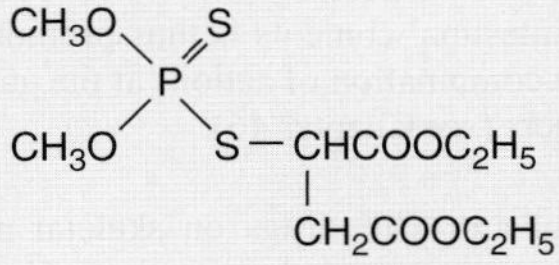 CH_3O S P CH_3O S−$CHCOOC_2H_5$ $CH_2COOC_2H_5$	Malathion *O,O*-Dimethyl S-(1,2-dicarbethoxyethyl) phosphorodithioate	Widely employed insecticide; safer than parathion or other agents due to rapid detoxification by higher organisms
D	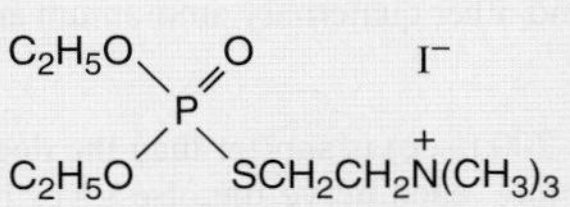 C_2H_5O O I^- P C_2H_5O $SCH_2CH_2\overset{+}{N}(CH_3)_3$	Echothiophate (PHOSPHOLINE IODIDE), MI-217 Diethoxyphosphinylthiocholine iodide	Extremely potent choline derivative; administered locally in treatment of glaucoma; relatively stable in water

Malathion (CHEMATHION, MALA-SPRAY) also requires replacement of a sulfur atom with oxygen in vivo, conferring resistance in mammalian species. This insecticide can be detoxified by hydrolysis of the carboxyl ester linkage by plasma carboxylesterases, and plasma carboxylesterase activity dictates species resistance to malathion. The detoxification reaction is much more rapid in mammals and birds than in insects. Malathion has been employed in aerial spraying of relatively populous areas for control of citrus orchard-destructive Mediterranean fruit flies and mosquitoes that harbor and transmit viruses harmful to human beings (e.g., West Nile encephalitis virus). Evidence of acute toxicity from malathion arises only with suicide attempts or deliberate poisoning. The lethal dose in mammals is ~1 g/kg. Exposure to the skin results in a small fraction (<10%) of systemic absorption. Malathion is used topically in the treatment of pediculosis (lice) infestations.

Of the quaternary organophosphate AChE inhibitors (*see* Table 10–1, group D), only *echothiophate* is useful clinically and it is limited to ophthalmic administration. Being positively charged, it is not volatile and does not readily penetrate the skin.

Anti-ChE agents potentially can produce all the following effects:

- Stimulation of muscarinic receptor responses at autonomic effector organs
- Stimulation, followed by depression or paralysis, of all autonomic ganglia and skeletal muscle (nicotinic actions)
- Stimulation, with occasional subsequent depression, of cholinergic receptor sites in the CNS

In general, compounds containing a quaternary ammonium group do not penetrate cell membranes readily; hence, anti-ChE agents in this category are absorbed poorly from the GI tract or across the skin and are excluded from the CNS by the blood-brain barrier after moderate doses. However, such compounds act preferentially at the neuromuscular junctions of skeletal muscle, exerting their action both as anti-ChE agents and as direct agonists. They have comparatively less effect at autonomic effector sites and ganglia.

By contrast, the more lipid-soluble agents are well absorbed after oral administration, have ubiquitous effects at both peripheral and central cholinergic sites, and may be sequestered in lipids for long periods of time. Lipid-soluble organophosphorus agents also are well absorbed through the skin, and the volatile agents are transferred readily across the alveolar membrane.

The actions of anti-ChE agents where the receptors are largely of the muscarinic type are blocked by atropine. The sites of action of anti-ChE agents of therapeutic importance are the CNS, eye, intestine, and the neuromuscular junction of skeletal muscle; other actions are of toxicological consequence.

EYE. When applied locally to the conjunctiva, anti-ChE agents cause conjunctival hyperemia and constriction of the pupillary sphincter muscle around the pupillary margin of the iris (miosis) and the ciliary muscle (block of accommodation reflex with resultant focusing to near vision). Miosis is apparent in a few minutes and can last several hours to days. The block of accommodation is more transient and generally disappears before termination of miosis. Intraocular pressure, when elevated, usually falls as the result of facilitation of outflow of the aqueous humor (*see* Chapter 64).

GI TRACT. In humans, neostigmine enhances gastric contractions and increases the secretion of gastric acid. The lower portion of the esophagus is stimulated by neostigmine; in patients with marked achalasia and dilation of the esophagus, the drug can cause a salutary increase in tone and peristalsis. Neostigmine also augments motor activity of the small and large bowel; the colon is particularly stimulated. Propulsive waves are increased in amplitude and frequency, and movement of intestinal contents is thus promoted. The effect of anti-ChE agents on intestinal motility probably represents a combination of actions at the ganglion cells of the myenteric (Auerbach) plexus and at the smooth muscle fibers (*see* Chapter 46).

NEUROMUSCULAR JUNCTION. Most of the effects of potent anti-ChE drugs on skeletal muscle can be explained adequately on the basis of their inhibition of AChE at neuromuscular junctions. However, there is good evidence for an accessory direct action of neostigmine and other quaternary ammonium anti-ChE agents on skeletal muscle.

The lifetime of free ACh within the nerve-muscle synapse (~200 μsec) is shorter than the decay of the endplate potential or the refractory period of the muscle. Therefore, each nerve impulse gives rise to a single wave of depolarization on the muscle fiber. After inhibition of AChE, the residence time of ACh in the synapse increases, allowing for lateral diffusion and interaction of the transmitter with multiple receptors. This successive stimulation of neighboring receptors site in the endplate results in a prolongation of the decay time of the endplate potential. Consequently, asynchronous excitation and fasciculations of muscle fibers occur. With sufficient inhibition of AChE, depolarization of the endplate predominates, and depolarization blockade ensues (*see* Chapter 11). When ACh persists in the synapse, it also may depolarize the axon terminal, resulting in antidromic firing of the motoneuron; this effect contributes to fasciculations that involve the entire motor unit.

The anti-ChE agents will reverse the antagonism caused by competitive neuromuscular blocking agents. Neostigmine is not effective against the skeletal muscle paralysis caused by succinylcholine; this agent also produces neuromuscular blockade by depolarization, and depolarization will be enhanced by neostigmine.

ACTIONS AT OTHER SITES. Secretory glands that are innervated by postganglionic cholinergic fibers include the bronchial, lacrimal, sweat, salivary, gastric (antral G cells and parietal cells), intestinal, and pancreatic acinar glands. Low doses of anti-ChE agents augment secretory responses to nerve stimulation, and higher doses actually produce an increase in the resting rate of secretion. Anti-ChE agents increase contraction of smooth muscle fibers of bronchioles and ureters, and ureters may show increased peristaltic activity.

The cardiovascular actions of anti-ChE agents are complex; they reflect both ganglionic and postganglionic effects of accumulated ACh on the heart and blood vessels and actions in the CNS. The predominant effect on the heart from the peripheral action of accumulated ACh is bradycardia, resulting in a fall in cardiac output. Higher doses usually cause a fall in blood pressure, often as a consequence of effects of anti-ChE agents on the medullary vasomotor centers of the CNS.

Anti-ChE agents augment vagal influences on the heart, thereby shortening the effective refractory period of atrial muscle fibers and increasing the refractory period and conduction time at the SA and AV nodes. At the ganglionic level, accumulating ACh initially is excitatory on nicotinic receptors, but at higher concentrations, ganglionic blockade ensues as a result of persistent depolarization. The excitatory action on the parasympathetic ganglion cells can reinforce the diminished cardiac output, whereas enhanced cardiac function would result from the action of ACh on sympathetic ganglion cells. ACh also elicits excitation followed by inhibition at the central medullary vasomotor and cardiac centers. These effects are complicated by the hypoxemia resulting from the bronchoconstrictor and secretory actions of increased ACh on the respiratory system; hypoxemia, in turn, can reinforce both sympathetic tone and ACh-induced discharge of epinephrine from the adrenal medulla. Hence, it is not surprising that an increase in heart rate is seen with severe ChE inhibitor poisoning. Hypoxemia is a major factor in the CNS depression after large doses of anti-ChE agents. The CNS-stimulant effects are antagonized by larger doses of atropine, although not as completely as are the muscarinic effects at peripheral autonomic effector sites.

ADME. Physostigmine is absorbed readily from the GI tract, subcutaneous tissues, and mucous membranes. The conjunctival instillation of solutions of the drug may result in systemic effects if measures (e.g., pressure on the inner canthus) are not taken to prevent absorption from the nasal mucosa. Parenterally administered physostigmine is largely destroyed within 2-3 h by plasma esterases; renal excretion plays only a minor role in its elimination. Neostigmine and pyridostigmine are absorbed poorly after oral administration; the effective parenteral dose of neostigmine is 0.5-2 mg whereas the equivalent oral dose may be 15-30 mg or more. Neostigmine and pyridostigmine are destroyed by plasma esterases, and the quaternary aromatic alcohols and parent compounds are excreted in the urine; the half-lives of these drugs are 1-2 h.

Organophosphate anti-ChE agents with the highest risk of toxicity are highly lipid-soluble liquids; many have high vapor pressures. The less volatile agents that are commonly used as agricultural insecticides (e.g., diazinon, malathion) generally are dispersed as aerosols or as dusts adsorbed to an inert, finely particulate material. Consequently, the compounds are absorbed rapidly through the skin and mucous membranes following contact with moisture, by the lungs after inhalation, and by the GI tract after ingestion.

Following their absorption, most organophosphates are hydrolyzed by plasma and liver esterases; the hydrolysis products are excreted in the urine. *Plasma and liver esterases are responsible for hydrolysis to the corresponding phosphoric and phosphonic acids. However, the CYPs are responsible for converting the inactive phosphorothioates containing a phosphorus-sulfur (thiono) bond to phosphorates with a phosphorus-oxygen bond, resulting in their activation.* These enzymes also play a role in the inactivation of certain organophosphorus agents, and allelic differences are known to affect rates of metabolism. Plasma and hepatic carboxylesterases (aliesterases) and plasma butyrylcholinesterase are inhibited irreversibly by organophosphates; their scavenging capacity for organophosphates affords partial protection against inhibition of AChE in the nervous system. The carboxylesterases also catalyze hydrolysis of malathion and other organophosphates that contain carboxyl-ester linkages, rendering them less active or inactive. Since carboxylesterases are inhibited by organophosphates, toxicity from simultaneous exposure to 2 organophosphorus insecticides can be synergistic.

TOXICOLOGY

The toxicological aspects of the anti-ChE agents are of practical importance to clinicians. In addition to cases of accidental intoxication from the use and manufacture of organophosphorus compounds as agricultural insecticides, these agents have been used frequently for homicidal and suicidal purposes. Organophosphates account for as many as 80% of pesticide-related hospital admissions. Pesticide toxicity is a widespread global problem associated with >200,000 deaths a year; most poisonings occur in Southeast Asia. Occupational exposure occurs most commonly by the dermal and pulmonary routes, while oral ingestion is most common in cases of nonoccupational poisoning.

ACUTE INTOXICATION. The effects of acute intoxication by anti-ChE agents are manifested by muscarinic and nicotinic signs and symptoms, and, except for compounds of extremely low lipid solubility, by signs referable to the CNS. The broad spectrum of effects of acute AChE inhibition on the CNS includes confusion, ataxia, slurred speech, loss of reflexes, Cheyne-Stokes respiration, generalized convulsions, coma, and central respiratory paralysis. Actions on the vasomotor and other cardiovascular centers in the medulla oblongata lead to hypotension.

Systemic effects appear within minutes after inhalation of vapors or aerosols. The onset of symptoms is delayed after GI and percutaneous absorption. The duration of toxic symptoms is determined largely by the properties of the compound: its lipid solubility, whether it must be activated to form the oxon, the stability of the organophosphate-AChE bond, and whether "aging" of the phosphorylated enzyme has occurred.

After local exposure to vapors or aerosols or after their inhalation, ocular and respiratory effects generally appear first. Ocular manifestations include marked miosis, ocular pain, conjunctival congestion, diminished vision, ciliary spasm, and brow ache. With acute systemic absorption, miosis may not be evident due to sympathetic discharge in response to hypotension. In addition to rhinorrhea and hyperemia of the upper respiratory tract, respiratory responses consist of tightness in the chest and wheezing respiration, caused by the combination of bronchoconstriction and increased bronchial secretion. GI symptoms occur earliest after ingestion and include anorexia, nausea and vomiting, abdominal cramps, and diarrhea.

With percutaneous absorption of liquid, localized sweating and muscle fasciculations in the immediate vicinity are generally the earliest symptoms. Severe intoxication is manifested by extreme salivation, involuntary defecation and urination, sweating, lacrimation, penile erection, bradycardia, and hypotension.

Nicotinic actions at the neuromuscular junctions of skeletal muscle usually consist of generalized weakness, involuntary twitchings, scattered fasciculations, and eventually severe weakness and paralysis. The most serious consequence is paralysis of the respiratory muscles. The time of death after a single acute exposure may range from <5 min to nearly 24 h, depending on the dose, route, agent, and other factors. The cause of death primarily is respiratory failure, usually accompanied by a secondary cardiovascular component. Delayed symptoms appearing after 1-4 days and marked by persistent low blood ChE and severe muscle weakness are termed the *intermediate syndrome*. Delayed neurotoxicity also may be evident after severe intoxication.

DIAGNOSIS AND TREATMENT. In cases of mild or chronic intoxication, determination of the ChE activities in erythrocytes and plasma generally will establish the diagnosis. Although these values vary considerably in the normal population, they usually are depressed well below the normal range before symptoms are evident. *Atropine* in sufficient dosage effectively antagonizes the actions at muscarinic receptor sites, including increased tracheobronchial and salivary secretion, bronchoconstriction, bradycardia, and to a moderate extent, peripheral ganglionic and central actions.

Atropine should be given in doses sufficient to cross the blood-brain barrier. Following an initial injection of 2-4 mg, given intravenously if possible, otherwise intramuscularly, 2 mg should be given every 5-10 min until muscarinic symptoms disappear, if they reappear, or until signs of atropine toxicity appear. More than 200 mg may be required on the first day. A mild degree of atropine block then should be maintained for as long as symptoms are evident. The AChE reactivators can be of great benefit in the therapy of anti-ChE intoxication, but their use is supplemental to the administration of atropine.

Atropine is ineffective against the peripheral neuromuscular compromise caused by moderate or severe intoxication with an organophosphorus anti-ChE agent; the condition can be reversed by *pralidoxime (2-PAM)*, a cholinesterase reactivator.

The recommended adult dose of pralidoxime is 1-2 g, infused intravenously over ≥5 min. If weakness is not relieved or if it recurs after 20-60 min, the dose should be repeated. Early treatment is very important to assure that the oxime reaches the phosphorylated AChE while the latter still can be reactivated. With severe toxicities from the lipid-soluble agents, it is necessary to continue treatment with atropine and pralidoxime for a week or longer.

General supportive measures also are important, including:

- Termination of exposure, by removal of the patient or application of a gas mask; removal of contaminated clothing; copious washing of contaminated skin or mucous membranes with water; gastric lavage, if indicated
- Maintenance of a patent airway, including endobronchial aspiration
- Artificial respiration; administration of O_2, if required
- Alleviation of persistent convulsions with diazepam (5-10 mg, intravenously)
- Treatment of shock

CHOLINESTERASE REACTIVATORS. The phosphorylated esteratic site of AChE undergoes hydrolytic regeneration at a slow or negligible rate, but nucleophilic agents, such as hydroxylamine (NH_2OH), hydroxamic acids (RCONH—OH), and oximes (RCH=NOH), reactivate the enzyme more rapidly than does spontaneous hydrolysis. Reactivation with pralidoxime occurs at a million times the rate of that with hydroxylamine. The oxime is oriented proximally to exert a nucleophilic attack on the phosphorus, forming a phosphoryloxime and regenerating the enzyme (Figure 10–1E). Several *bis*-quaternary oximes are more potent as reactivators for insecticide and nerve gas poisoning (e.g., HI-6, used in Europe as an antidote).

The reactivating action of oximes in vivo is most marked at the skeletal neuromuscular junction. Following a dose of an organophosphorus compound that produces total blockade of transmission, the intravenous injection of an oxime can restore the response to stimulation of the motor nerve within a few minutes. Antidotal effects are less striking at autonomic effector sites, and the quaternary ammonium group restricts entry into the CNS. Although high doses or accumulation of oximes can inhibit AChE and cause neuromuscular blockade, oximes should be given until one can be assured of clearance of the offending organophosphate. Many organophosphates partition into lipid and are released slowly as the active entity. Current antidotal therapy for organophosphate exposure resulting from warfare or terrorism includes parenteral atropine, an oxime (2-PAM or HI-6), and a benzodiazepine as an anticonvulsant. The oximes and their metabolites are readily eliminated by the kidney.

THERAPEUTIC USES

AVAILABLE AGENTS

Physostigmine salicylate (ANTILIRIUM) is available for injection. Physostigmine sulfate ophthalmic ointment and physostigmine salicylate ophthalmic solution also are available. Pyridostigmine bromide is available for oral (MESTINON) or parenteral (REGONOL, MESTINON) use. Neostigmine bromide (PROSTIGMIN) is available for oral use. Neostigmine methylsulfate (PROSTIGMIN) is marketed for parenteral injection. Ambenonium chloride (MYTELASE) is available for oral use. *Tacrine* (COGNEX), donepezil (ARICEPT), rivastigmine (EXELON), and galantamine (REMINYL) have been approved for the treatment of Alzheimer disease. Pralidoxime chloride (PROTOPAM CHLORIDE) is the only AChE reactivator currently available in the U.S. and can be obtained in a parenteral formulation. HI-6 is available in several European and Near Eastern countries.

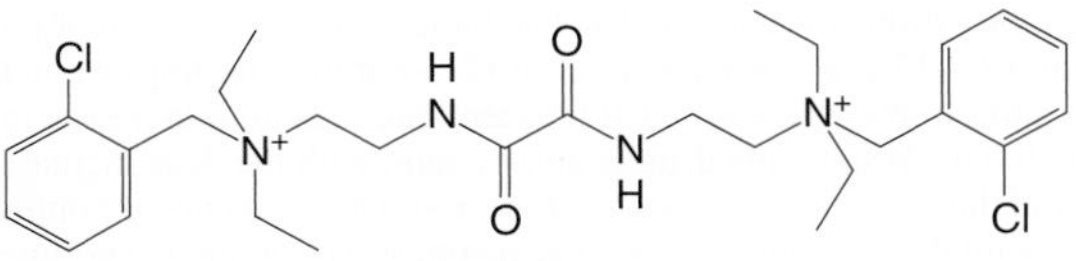

Cl N+ H N O O N H N+ Cl

AMBENONIUM

CH_3 N+ CH=NOH

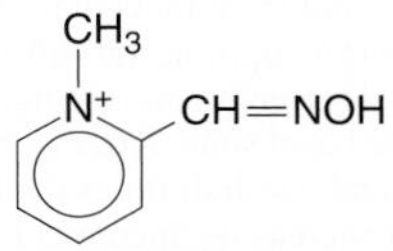

PRALIDOXIME (2-PAM)

USES. Current use of anti-AChE agents is limited to 4 conditions in the periphery:

- Atony of the smooth muscle of the intestinal tract and urinary bladder
- Glaucoma
- Myasthenia gravis
- Reversal of the paralysis of competitive neuromuscular blocking drugs

and 1 in the CNS:

- Treatment of dementia symptoms of Alzheimer disease

PARALYTIC ILEUS AND ATONY OF THE URINARY BLADDER. Neostigmine generally is preferred among the anti-ChE agents in the treatment of these conditions. Directly acting muscarinic agonists (*see* Chapter 9) are employed for the same purposes. The usual subcutaneous dose of neostigmine methylsulfate for postoperative paralytic ileus is 0.5 mg, given as needed. Peristaltic activity commences 10-30 min after parenteral administration, whereas 2-4 h are required after oral administration of neostigmine bromide (15-30 mg). It may be necessary to assist evacuation with a small low enema or gas with a rectal tube. A similar dose of neostigmine is used for the treatment of atony of the detrusor muscle of the urinary bladder. Neostigmine should not be used when the intestine or urinary bladder is obstructed, when peritonitis is present, when the viability of the bowel is doubtful, or when bowel dysfunction results from inflammatory bowel disease.

GLAUCOMA AND OTHER OPHTHALMOLOGIC INDICATIONS. *See* Chapter 64.

MYASTHENIA GRAVIS. Myasthenia gravis is a neuromuscular disease characterized by weakness and marked fatigability of skeletal muscle; exacerbations and partial remissions occur frequently. The defect in myasthenia gravis is in synaptic transmission at the neuromuscular junction such that mechanical responses to nerve stimulation are not well sustained. Myasthenia gravis is caused by an autoimmune response primarily to the ACh receptor at the postjunctional endplate. Antireceptor antibodies are detectable in sera of 90% of patients with the disease. Immune complexes along with marked ultrastructural abnormalities appear in the synaptic cleft and enhance receptor degradation through complement-mediated lysis in the endplate. In ~10% of patients presenting with a myasthenic syndrome, muscle weakness has a congenital rather than an autoimmune basis, with mutations in the ACh receptor that affect ligand-binding and channel-opening kinetics, or mutations in the form of AChE that contains the collagen-like tail unit. Administration of anti-ChE agents does not result in subjective improvement in most congenital myasthenic patients.

Diagnosis. Although the diagnosis of autoimmune myasthenia gravis usually can be made from the history, signs, and symptoms, its differentiation from certain neurasthenic, infectious, endocrine, congenital, neoplastic, and degenerative neuromuscular diseases can be challenging. Myasthenia gravis is the only condition in which muscular weakness can be improved dramatically by anti-ChE medication. The edrophonium test for evaluation of possible myasthenia gravis is performed by rapid intravenous injection of 2 mg of edrophonium chloride, followed 45 sec later by an additional 8 mg if the first dose is without effect; a positive response consists of brief improvement in strength, unaccompanied by lingual fasciculation (which generally occurs in nonmyasthenic patients).

An excessive dose of an anti-ChE drug results in a *cholinergic crisis*, a condition characterized by weakness resulting from generalized depolarization of the motor endplate; other features result from overstimulation of muscarinic receptors. The weakness resulting from depolarization blockade may resemble *myasthenic weakness*, which is manifest when anti-ChE medication is insufficient. The distinction is of obvious practical importance, because the former is treated by withholding, and the latter by administering, the anti-ChE agent. When the edrophonium test is performed cautiously (limiting the dose to 2 mg and with facilities for respiratory resuscitation available) a further decrease in strength indicates *cholinergic crisis*, while improvement signifies *myasthenic weakness*. Atropine sulfate, 0.4-0.6 mg or more intravenously, should be given immediately if a severe muscarinic reaction ensues. Detection of antireceptor antibodies in muscle biopsies or plasma is now widely employed to establish the diagnosis.

Treatment. Pyridostigmine, neostigmine, and ambenonium are the standard anti-ChE drugs used in the symptomatic treatment of myasthenia gravis. All can increase the response of myasthenic muscle to repetitive nerve impulses, primarily by the preservation of endogenous ACh.The optimal single oral dose of an anti-ChE agent can be determined empirically. Baseline recordings are made for grip strength, vital capacity, and a number of signs and symptoms that reflect the strength of various muscle groups. The patient then is given an oral dose of pyridostigmine (30-60 mg), neostigmine (7.5-15 mg), or ambenonium (2.5-5 mg). The improvement in muscle strength and changes in other signs and symptoms are noted at frequent intervals until there is a return to the basal state. After an hour or longer in the basal state, the drug is given again, with the dose increased to one and one-half times the initial amount, and the same observations are repeated. This sequence is continued, with increasing increments of one-half the initial dose, until an optimal response is obtained. The interval between oral doses required to maintain muscle strength usually is 2-4 h for neostigmine, 3-6 h for pyridostigmine, or 3-8 h for ambenonium. However, the dose required may vary from day to day; physical or emotional stress, intercurrent infections, and menstruation usually necessitate an increase in the frequency or size of the dose. Unpredictable exacerbations and remissions of the myasthenic state may require adjustment of dosage.

Pyridostigmine is available in sustained-release tablets containing a total of 180 mg, of which 60 mg is released immediately and 120 mg over several hours; this preparation is of value in maintaining patients for 6–8-h periods, but should be limited to use at bedtime. Muscarinic cardiovascular and GI side effects of anti-ChE agents generally can be controlled by atropine or other anticholinergic drugs (*see* Chapter 9). However, these anticholinergic drugs mask many side effects of an excessive dose of an anti-ChE agent. In most patients, tolerance develops eventually to the muscarinic effects.

Several drugs, including curariform agents and certain antibiotics and general anesthetics, interfere with neuromuscular transmission (*see* Chapter 11); their administration to patients with myasthenia gravis requires proper adjustment of anti-ChE dosage and other precautions. Other therapeutic measures are essential elements in the management of this disease. Glucocorticoids promote clinical improvement in a high percentage of patients. Initiation of steroid treatment augments muscle weakness; however, as the patient improves with continued administration of steroids, doses of anti-ChE drugs can be reduced. Immunosuppressive agents such as azathioprine and cyclosporine have been beneficial in more advanced cases (*see* Chapter 35).

ALZHEIMER DISEASE. A deficiency of intact cholinergic neurons, particularly those extending from subcortical areas such as the nucleus basalis of Meynert, has been observed in patients with progressive dementia of the Alzheimer type (*see* Chapter 22). Using a rationale similar to that in other CNS degenerative diseases, therapy for enhancing concentrations of cholinergic neurotransmitters in the CNS has been used in mild to moderate Alzheimer disease. Long-acting and hydrophobic ChE inhibitors are the only inhibitors with well-documented, albeit limited, efficacy.

Donepezil may improve cognition and global clinical function and delay symptomatic progression of the disease. Side effects are largely attributable to excessive cholinergic stimulation, with nausea, diarrhea, and vomiting being most frequently reported. The drug is well tolerated in single daily doses. Usually, 5-mg doses are administered at night; if this dose is well tolerated, the dose can be increased to 10 mg daily. Rivastigmine, a long-acting carbamoylating inhibitor, has efficacy, tolerability, and side effects similar to those of donepezil. Galantamine has a side-effect profile similar to those of donepezil and rivastigmine. These 3 cholinesterase inhibitors, which have good affinity, sufficient hydrophobicity to cross the blood-brain barrier, and prolonged durations of action constitute current modes of therapy, along with an excitatory amino acid transmitter mimic, memantine.

INTOXICATION BY ANTICHOLINERGIC DRUGS. In addition to atropine and other muscarinic agents, many other drugs, such as the phenothiazines, antihistamines, and tricyclic antidepressants, have central and peripheral anticholinergic activity. The effectiveness of physostigmine in reversing the anticholinergic effects of these agents has been clearly documented (Physostigmine, a tertiary amine, crosses the blood-brain barrier, in contrast to the quaternary anti-AChE drugs). However, other toxic effects of the tricyclic antidepressants and phenothiazines (*see* Chapters 15 and 16), such as intraventricular conduction deficits and ventricular arrhythmias, are not reversed by physostigmine. In addition, physostigmine may precipitate seizures; hence, its usually small potential benefit must be weighed against this risk. The initial intravenous or intramuscular dose of physostigmine is 2 mg, with additional doses given as necessary.

For a complete Bibliographical Listing see Goodman & Gilman's ***The Pharmacological Basis of Therapeutics***, 12th ed., or Goodman & Gilman Online at www.AccessMedicine.com.

11 chapter Agents Acting at the Neuromuscular Junction and Autonomic Ganglia

The nicotinic acetylcholine (ACh) receptor mediates neurotransmission postsynaptically at the neuromuscular junction and peripheral autonomic ganglia; in the CNS, it largely controls release of neurotransmitters from presynaptic sites. The receptor is called the *nicotinic acetylcholine receptor* because both the alkaloid nicotine and the neurotransmitter ACh can stimulate the receptor. Distinct subtypes of nicotinic receptors exist at the neuromuscular junction and the ganglia.

THE NICOTINIC ACETYLCHOLINE RECEPTOR

The binding of ACh to the nicotinic ACh receptor initiates an endplate potential (EPP) in muscle or an excitatory postsynaptic potential (EPSP) in peripheral ganglia (*see* Chapter 8). The nicotinic receptor is the prototype for other pentameric ligand-gated ion channels, which include the receptors for the inhibitory amino acids (γ-aminobutyric acid [GABA] and glycine; *see* Chapter 14) and serotonin (the $5HT_3$ receptor) (Figure 11–1).

NICOTINIC RECEPTOR STRUCTURE. Nicotinic receptors of vertebrate skeletal muscle (N_m) are pentamers composed of 4 distinct subunits (α, β, γ, and δ) in the stoichiometric ratio of 2:1:1:1. In mature, innervated muscle endplates, the γ subunit is replaced by ε, a closely related subunit. The individual subunits are ~40% identical in their amino acid sequences. The 5 subunits of the nicotinic acetylcholine receptor are arranged around a pseudo-axis of symmetry to circumscribe a channel. Agonist-binding sites occur at the subunit interfaces; in muscle, only 2 of the 5 subunit interfaces, αγ and αδ, bind ligands (Figure 11–2). Both of the subunits forming the subunit interface contribute to ligand specificity.

Neuronal nicotinic (N_n) receptors found in ganglia and the CNS also exist as pentamers of 1 or more types of subunits. Subunit types α2 through α10 and β2 through β4 are found in neuronal tissues (*see* Figure 11–2). Although not all permutations of α and β subunits lead to functional receptors, the diversity in subunit composition is large and exceeds the capacity of ligands to distinguish subtypes on the basis of their selectivity.

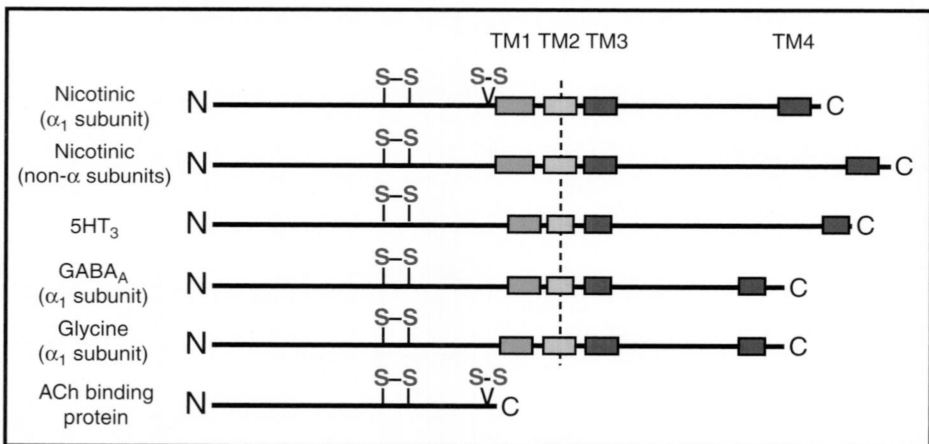

Figure 11–1 *Subunit organization of pentameric ligand-gated ion channels and the ACh binding protein.* For each receptor, the amino terminal region of ~210 amino acids is found at the extracellular surface. It is then followed by 4 hydrophobic regions that span the membrane (TM1-TM4), leaving the small carboxyl terminus on the extracellular surface. The TM2 region is α-helical, and TM2 regions from each subunit of the pentameric receptor line the internal pore of the receptor. Two disulfide loops at positions 128-142 and 192-193 are found in the α-subunit of the nicotinic receptor. The 128-142 motif is conserved in the family of pentameric receptors; the vicinal cysteines at 192-193 occur only in α-subunits of the nicotinic receptor and in the ACh binding protein.

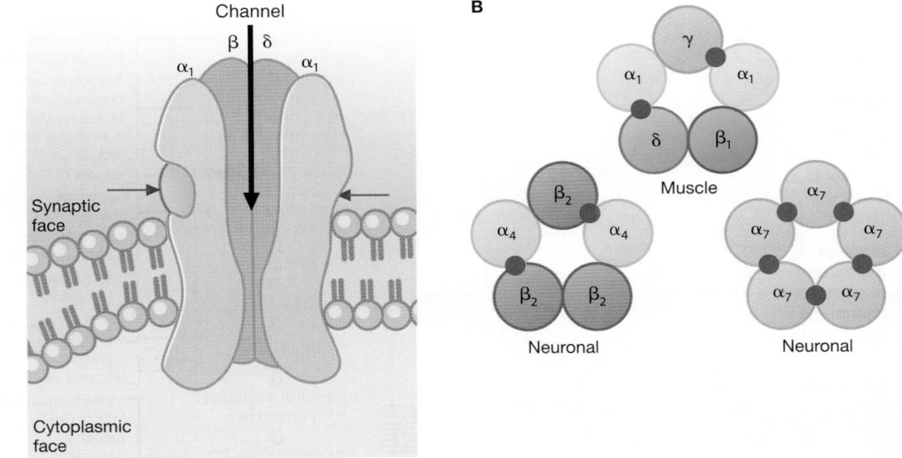

Figure 11–2 *Subunit arrangement and molecular structure of the nicotinic acetylcholine receptor.* **A.** Longitudinal view of receptor schematic with the γ subunit removed. The remaining subunits, 2 copies of α, 1 of β, and 1 of δ, are shown to surround an internal channel with an outer vestibule and its constriction located deep in the membrane bilayer region. Spans of α-helices with slightly bowed structures form the perimeter of the channel and come from the TM2 region of the linear sequence (Figure 11–1). ACh binding sites, indicated by *red arrows*, occur at the $\alpha\gamma$ and $\alpha\delta$ (not visible) interfaces. **B.** Nicotinic receptor subunit arrangement, with examples of subunit assembly. Agonist binding sites (*red circles*) occur at α subunit-containing interfaces. A total of 17 functional receptor isoforms have been observed in vivo, with different ligand specificity, relative Ca^{2+}/Na^{+} permeability, and physiological function as determined by their subunit composition. The only isoform found at the neuromuscular junction is that shown here. There are 16 neuronal receptor isoforms found at autonomic ganglia and in the CNS, homo- and hetero-pentamers of α (α2-α10) and β (β2-β4) subunits.

NEUROMUSCULAR BLOCKING AGENTS

Modern-day neuromuscular blocking agents fall generally into 2 classes, *depolarizing* and *competitive/nondepolarizing*. At present, only a single depolarizing agent, succinylcholine (ANECTINE, QUELICIN), is in general clinical use; multiple competitive or nondepolarizing agents are available (*see* Table 11–2).

See the 12th edition of the parent text for the history, sources, and chemistry of curare, the prototypical South American arrow poison and neuromuscular blocking agent, the action of which was described by Claude Bernard in the 1850s. The 12th edition also shows the structures of the various classes of depolarizing and competitive neuromuscular blockers in Figure 11–3.

Pharmacological Effects

SKELETAL MUSCLE. *Competitive antagonists* bind the nicotinic ACh receptor of the motor endplate and thereby competitively block the binding of ACh. The *depolarizing agents*, such as succinylcholine, depolarize the membrane by opening channels in the same manner as ACh. However, they persist longer at the neuromuscular junction primarily because of their resistance to AChE. The depolarization is thus longer lasting, resulting in a brief period of repetitive excitation that may elicit transient and repetitive muscle excitation (fasciculations), followed by block of neuromuscular transmission and flaccid paralysis (called *phase I block*).

The block arises because, after an initial opening, peri-junctional Na^{+} channels close and will not reopen until the endplate is repolarized. At this point, neural release of ACh results in the binding of ACh to receptors on an already depolarized endplate. These closed perijunctional channels keep the depolarization signal from affecting downstream channels and effectively shield the rest of the muscle from activity at the motor endplate. The characteristics of depolarization and competitive blockade are contrasted in Table 11–3.

Under clinical conditions, with increasing concentrations of succinylcholine and over time, the block may convert slowly from a depolarizing phase I block to a nondepolarizing, *phase II block*. While the response to peripheral stimulation during phase II block resembles that of the competitive agents, reversal of phase II

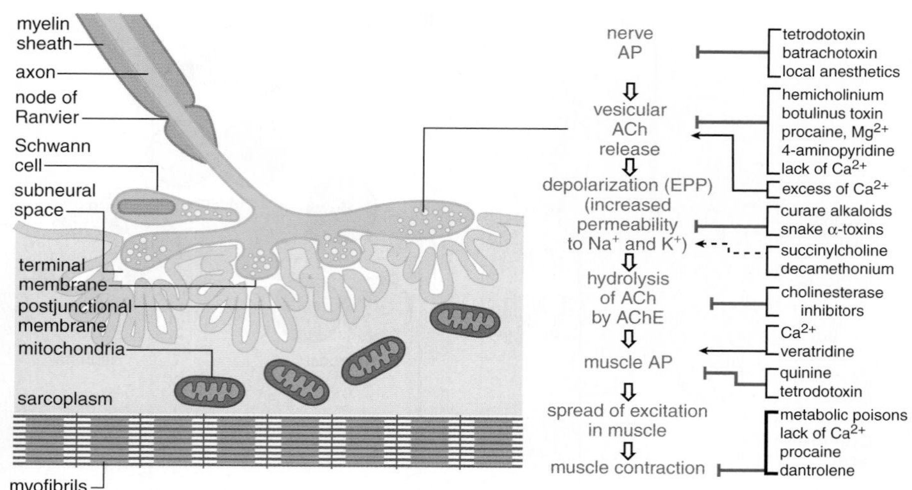

Figure 11–3 *A pharmacologist's view of the motor end plate.* The structures of the motor end plate (left side of figure) facilitate the series of physiological events leading from nerve action potential (AP) to skeletal muscle contraction (center column). Pharmacological agents can modify neurotransmission and excitation-contraction coupling at myriad sites (righthand column). ←——, enhancement; ⊢——, blockade; ←- - - -, depolarization and phase II block.

block by administration of anticholinesterase (anti-ChE) agents (e.g., with neostigmine) is difficult to predict and should be undertaken with much caution. The characteristics of phase I and phase II blocks are shown in Table 11–1.

Sequence and Characteristics of Paralysis. Following intravenous injection of an appropriate dose of a *competitive blocking agent*, motor weakness progresses to a total flaccid paralysis. Small, rapidly moving muscles such as those of the eyes, jaw, and larynx relax before those of the limbs and trunk. Ultimately, the intercostal muscles and finally the diaphragm are paralyzed, and respiration then ceases. Recovery of muscles usually occurs in the reverse order to that of their paralysis, and thus the diaphragm ordinarily is the first muscle to regain function.

After a single intravenous dose of 10-30 mg of *succinylcholine*, muscle fasciculations, particularly over the chest and abdomen, occur briefly; then relaxation occurs within 1 min, becomes maximal within 2 min, and generally disappears within 5 min. Transient apnea usually occurs at the time of maximal effect. Muscle

Table 11–1

Clinical Responses and Monitoring of Phase I and Phase II Neuromuscular Blockade by Succinylcholine Infusion

RESPONSE	PHASE I	PHASE II
End-plate membrane potential	Depolarized to −55 mV	Repolarization toward −80 mV
Onset	Immediate	Slow transition
Dose-dependence	Lower	Usually higher or follows prolonged infusion
Recovery	Rapid	More prolonged
Train of four and tetanic stimulation	No fade	Fade[a]
Acetylcholinesterase inhibition	Augments	Reverses or antagonizes
Muscle response	Fasciculations → flaccid paralysis	Flaccid paralysis

[a]*Post-tetanic potentiation follows fade.*

relaxation of longer duration is achieved by continuous intravenous infusion. After infusion is discontinued, the effects of the drug usually disappear rapidly because of its efficient hydrolysis by plasma and hepatic butyrylcholinesterase. Muscle soreness may follow the administration of succinylcholine.

During prolonged depolarization, muscle cells may lose significant quantities of K^+ and gain Na^+, Cl^-, and Ca^{2+}. In patients with extensive injury to soft tissues, the efflux of K^+ following continued administration of succinylcholine can be life threatening. There are many conditions for which succinylcholine administration is contraindicated or should be undertaken with great caution. The change in the nature of the blockade produced by succinylcholine (from phase I to phase II) presents an additional complication with long-term infusions.

CNS. Tubocurarine and other quaternary neuromuscular blocking agents are virtually devoid of central effects following ordinary clinical doses because of their inability to penetrate the blood-brain barrier.

AUTONOMIC GANGLIA AND MUSCARINIC SITES. Neuromuscular blocking agents show variable potencies in producing ganglionic blockade. Ganglionic blockade by tubocurarine and other stabilizing drugs is reversed or antagonized by anti-ChE agents.

Clinical doses of tubocurarine produce partial blockade both at autonomic ganglia and at the adrenal medulla, which results in a fall in blood pressure and tachycardia. Pancuronium shows less ganglionic blockade at common clinical doses. Atracurium, vecuronium, doxacurium, pipecuronium, mivacurium, and rocuronium are even more selective. The maintenance of cardiovascular reflex responses usually is desired during anesthesia. Pancuronium has a vagolytic action, presumably from blockade of muscarinic receptors, which leads to tachycardia.

Of the depolarizing agents, succinylcholine at doses producing neuromuscular relaxation rarely causes effects attributable to ganglionic blockade. However, cardiovascular effects are sometimes observed, probably owing to the successive stimulation of vagal ganglia (manifested by bradycardia) and sympathetic ganglia (resulting in hypertension and tachycardia).

MAST CELLS AND HISTAMINE RELEASE. Tubocurarine produces typical histamine-like wheals when injected intracutaneously or intraarterially in humans, and some clinical responses to neuromuscular blocking agents (e.g., bronchospasm, hypotension, excessive bronchial and salivary secretion) appear to be caused by the release of histamine. Succinylcholine, mivacurium, and atracurium also cause histamine release, but to a lesser extent unless administered rapidly. The ammonio steroids, pancuronium, vecuronium, pipecuronium, and rocuronium, have even less tendency to release histamine after intradermal or systemic injection. Histamine release typically is a direct action of the muscle relaxant on the mast cell rather than IgE-mediated anaphylaxis.

ABSORPTION, DISTRIBUTION, AND ELIMINATION

Quaternary ammonium neuromuscular blocking agents are very poorly absorbed from the GI tract. Absorption is quite adequate from intramuscular sites. Rapid onset is achieved with intravenous administration. The more potent agents must be given in lower concentrations, and diffusional requirements slow their rate of onset.

When long-acting competitive blocking agents such as D-tubocurarine and pancuronium are administered, blockade may diminish after 30 min owing to redistribution of the drug, yet residual blockade and plasma levels of the drug persist. Subsequent doses show diminished redistribution. Long-acting agents may accumulate with multiple doses.

The ammonio steroids contain ester groups that are hydrolyzed in the liver. Typically, the metabolites have about one-half the activity of the parent compound and contribute to the total relaxation profile. Ammonio steroids of intermediate duration of action, such as vecuronium and rocuronium (Table 11–2), are cleared more rapidly by the liver than is pancuronium. The more rapid decay of neuromuscular blockade with compounds of intermediate duration argues for sequential dosing of these agents rather than administering a single dose of a long-duration neuromuscular blocking agent.

Atracurium is converted to less active metabolites by plasma esterases and spontaneous Hofmann elimination. Cisatracurium is also subject to this spontaneous degradation. Because of these alternative routes of metabolism, atracurium and cisatracurium do not exhibit an increased $t_{1/2}$ in patients with impaired renal function and therefore are good choices in this setting.

The extremely brief duration of action of succinylcholine is due largely to its rapid hydrolysis by the butyrylcholinesterase synthesized by the liver and found in the plasma. Among the occasional patients who exhibit prolonged apnea following the administration of succinylcholine or mivacurium, most have an atypical plasma cholinesterase or a deficiency of the enzyme owing to allelic variations, hepatic or renal disease, or a nutritional disturbance; however, in some, the enzymatic activity in plasma is normal.

Gantacurium is degraded by 2 chemical mechanisms, a rapid cysteine adduction and a slower hydrolysis of the ester bond adjacent to the chlorine. Both processes are purely chemical and hence not dependent on enzymatic activities. The adduction process has a $t_{1/2}$ of 1-2 min and is likely the basis for the ultrashort duration of action of gantacurium. Administration of exogenous cysteine, which may have excitotoxic side effects, can accelerate the antagonism of gantacurium-induced neuromuscular blockade.

CLINICAL PHARMACOLOGY

CHOICE OF AGENT

Therapeutic selection of a neuromuscular blocking agent should be based on achieving a pharmacokinetic profile consistent with the duration of the interventional procedure and minimizing cardiovascular compromise or other side effects, with attention to drug-specific modes of elimination in patients with renal or hepatic failure (*see* Table 11–2).

Table 11–2

Classification of Neuromuscular Blocking Agents

AGENT	CHEMICAL CLASS	DURATION, TYPE	ONSET (min)[a]	DURATION (min)[a]	MODE OF ELIMINATION
Succinylcholine	DCE	Ultrashort; depolarizing	0.8-1.4	6-11	Hydrolysis by plasma cholinesterases
D-Tubocurarine[b]	CBI	Long; competitive	6	80	Renal and hepatic elimination
Metocurine[b]	BIQ	Long; competitive	4	110	Renal elimination
Atracurium	BIQ	Intermediate; competitive	3	45	Hofmann elimination; esterase hydrolysis
Cisatracurium	BIQ	Intermediate; competitive	2-8	45-90	Hofmann and renal elimination
Doxacurium[b]	BIQ	Long; competitive	4-8	120	Renal elimination
Mivacurium	BIQ	Short; competitive	2-3	15-21	Hydrolysis by plasma cholinesterases
Pancuronium	AS	Long; competitive	3-4	85-100	Renal and hepatic elimination
Pipecuronium[b]	AS	Long; competitive	3-6	30-90	Renal elimination; hepatic metabolism/ clearance
Rocuronium	AS	Intermediate; competitive	0.9-1.7	36-73	Hepatic elimination
Vecuronium	AS	Intermediate; competitive	2-3	40-45	Hepatic and renal elimination
Gantacurium[c]	MOCF	Ultrashort, competitive	1-2	5-10	cysteine adduction, ester hydrolysis

AS, ammonio steroid; BIQ, benzylisoquinoline; CBI (natural alkaloid), cyclic benzylisoquinoline; DCE, Dicholine ester; MOCF, assymetric mixed-onium chlorofumarate.

[a]Time of onset and clinical duration achieved from dose ranges in Table 11–3.

[b]D-Tubocurarine, doxacurium, metocurine, and pipecuronium are no longer available in the U.S.

[c]Gantacurium is investigational.

Table 11–3

Dosing Ranges for Neuromuscular Blocking Agents

AGENT	INITIATION DOSE (mg/kg)	MAINTENANCE DOSE: INTERMITTENT INJECTION (mg/kg)	MAINTENANCE DOSE: CONTINUOUS INFUSION (μg/kg/min)
Succinylcholine	0.5-1	0.04-0.07	N/A
D-Tubocurarine[a]	0.6	0.25-0.5	2-3
Metocurine[a]	0.4	0.5-1	N/A
Atracurium	0.5	0.08-0.1	5-10
Cisatracurium	0.1-0.4	0.03	1-3
Mivacurium	0.15-0.25	0.1	9-10
Doxacurium[a]	0.03-0.06	0.005-0.01	N/A
Pancuronium	0.08-0.1	0.01-0.015	1
Rocuronium	0.6-1.2	0.1-0.2	10-12
Vecuronium	0.1	0.01-0.015	0.8-1
Gantacurium[a]	0.2-0.5	N/A	N/A

[a]*Not commercially available in the U.S.*

Two characteristics are useful in distinguishing side effects and pharmacokinetic behavior of neuromuscular blocking agents:

- **Duration of drug action.** These agents are categorized as long-, intermediate-, or short-acting agents. Often, the long-acting agents are the more potent, requiring the use of low concentrations (Table 11–3). The necessity of administering potent agents in low concentrations delays their onset.
- **The chemical nature of the agents (Table 11–2).** Apart from a shorter duration of action, newer agents exhibit greatly diminished frequency of side effects, chief of which are ganglionic blockade, block of vagal responses, and histamine release.

The prototypical ammonio steroid, pancuronium, induces virtually no histamine release; however, it blocks muscarinic receptors, and this antagonism is manifested primarily in vagal blockade and tachycardia. Tachycardia is eliminated in the newer ammonio steroids, vecuronium and rocuronium. The benzylisoquinolines appear to be devoid of vagolytic and ganglionic blocking actions but show a slight propensity to cause histamine release. The unusual metabolism of the prototype compound atracurium and its congener mivacurium confers special indications for use of these compounds. For example, atracurium's disappearance from the body depends on hydrolysis of the ester moiety by plasma esterases and by a spontaneous or Hofmann degradation (cleavage of the *N*-alkyl portion in the benzylisoquinoline). Hence 2 routes for degradation are available, both of which remain functional in renal failure. Mivacurium is extremely sensitive to catalysis by cholinesterase or other plasma hydrolases, accounting for its short duration of action. Side effects are not yet fully characterized for gantacurium, but transient adverse cardiovascular effects suggestive of histamine release have been observed at doses over 3 times the ED_{95}.

Uses

Muscle Relaxation. The main clinical use of the neuromuscular blocking agents is as an adjuvant in surgical anesthesia to obtain relaxation of skeletal muscle, particularly of the abdominal wall, to facilitate operative manipulations. With muscle relaxation no longer dependent on the depth of general anesthesia, a much lighter level of anesthesia suffices. Thus, the risk of respiratory and cardiovascular depression is minimized, and post-anesthetic recovery is shortened. Neuromuscular blocking agents of short duration often are used to facilitate endotracheal intubation and have been used to facilitate laryngoscopy, bronchoscopy, and esophagoscopy in combination with a general anesthetic agent. Neuromuscular blocking agents are administered parenterally, nearly always intravenously.

Measurement of Neuromuscular Blockade in Humans. Assessment of neuromuscular block usually is performed by stimulation of the ulnar nerve. Responses are monitored from compound action potentials or muscle tension developed in the adductor pollicis (thumb) muscle. Responses to repetitive or tetanic stimuli are most useful for evaluation of blockade of transmission. Rates of onset of blockade and recovery are more rapid in the airway musculature (jaw, larynx, and diaphragm) than in the thumb. Hence, tracheal intubation can be performed before onset of complete block at the adductor pollicis, whereas partial recovery of function of this muscle allows sufficient recovery of respiration for extubation.

Preventing Trauma During Electroshock Therapy. Electroconvulsive therapy (ECT) of psychiatric disorders occasionally is complicated by trauma to the patient; the seizures induced may cause dislocations or fractures. Inasmuch as the muscular component of the convulsion is not essential for benefit from the procedure, neuromuscular blocking agents, usually succinylcholine, and a short-acting barbiturate, usually methohexital or thiopental, are employed.

Control of Muscle Spasms and Rigidity. Botulinum toxins and dantrolene act peripherally to reduce muscle contraction; a variety of other agents act centrally to reduce skeletal muscle tone and spasm. Onabotulinum toxin A (BOTOX), abobotulinum toxin A (DYSPORT), and rimabotulinum toxin B (MYOBLOC), by blocking ACh release, produce flaccid paralysis of skeletal muscle and diminished activity of parasympathetic and sympathetic cholinergic synapses. Inhibition lasts from several weeks to 3-4 months, and restoration of function requires nerve sprouting.

Originally approved for the treatment of the ocular conditions of strabismus and blepharospasm and for hemifacial spasms, botulinum toxin has been used to treat spasms and dystonias, and spasms associated with the lower esophageal sphincter and anal fissures. Botox treatments also have become a popular cosmetic procedure for those seeking a wrinkle-free face. Like the bloom of youth, the reduction of wrinkles is temporary; unlike the bloom of youth, the effect of Botox can be renewed by readministration. The FDA has issued a safety alert, warning of respiratory paralysis from unexpected spread of the toxin from the site of injection (uses are described in Chapter 65).

Dantrolene (DANTRIUM, others) inhibits Ca^{2+} release from the sarcoplasmic reticulum of skeletal muscle by limiting the capacity of Ca^{2+} and calmodulin to activate RYR1. Because of its efficacy in managing an acute attack of malignant hyperthermia (described under "Toxicology"), dantrolene has been used experimentally in the treatment of muscle rigidity and hyperthermia in neuroleptic malignant syndrome (NMS). Dantrolene is also used in treatment of spasticity and hyperreflexia. With its peripheral action, it causes a generalized weakness. Thus, its use should be reserved to nonambulatory patients with severe spasticity. Hepatotoxicity has been reported with continued use, requiring liver function tests.

Synergisms and Antagonisms. The comparison of interactions between competitive and depolarizing neuromuscular blocking agents is instructive (Table 11–4) and a good test of one's understanding of the drugs' actions. In addition, many other drugs affect transmission at the neuromuscular junction, and thus can affect the choice and dosage of neuromuscular blocking agent used.

Because the anti-ChE agents neostigmine, pyridostigmine, and edrophonium preserve endogenous ACh and also act directly on the neuromuscular junction, they have been used in the treatment of overdosage

Table 11–4

Comparison of Competitive (D-Tubocurarine) and Depolarizing (Decamethonium) Blocking Agents

	D-TUBOCURARINE	DECAMETHONIUM
Effect of D-tubocurarine administered previously	Additive	Antagonistic
Effect of decamethonium administered previously	No effect, or antagonistic	Some tachyphylaxis; but may be additive
Effect of anticholinesterase agents on block	Reversal of block	No reversal
Effect on motor end plate	Elevated threshold to acetylcholine; no depolarization	Partial, persisting depolarization
Initial excitatory effect on striated muscle	None	Transient fasciculations
Character of muscle response to indirect tetanic stimulation during *partial* block	Poorly sustained contraction	Well-sustained contraction

with competitive blocking agents. Similarly, on completion of the surgical procedure, many anesthesiologists employ neostigmine or edrophonium to reverse and decrease the duration of competitive neuromuscular blockade. A muscarinic antagonist (atropine or glycopyrrolate) is used concomitantly to prevent stimulation of muscarinic receptors and thereby to avoid slowing of the heart rate. Anti-ChE agents will not reverse depolarizing neuromuscular blockade and, in fact, can enhance it.

Many inhalational anesthetics exert a stabilizing effect on the postjunctional membrane and therefore potentiate the activity of competitive blocking agents. Consequently, when such blocking drugs are used for muscle relaxation as adjuncts to these anesthetics, their doses should be reduced. The rank of order of potentiation is desflurane > sevoflurane > isoflurane > halothane > nitrous oxide-barbiturate-opioid or propofol anesthesia.

Aminoglycoside antibiotics produce neuromuscular blockade by inhibiting ACh release from the preganglionic terminal (through competition with Ca^{2+}) and to a lesser extent by noncompetitively blocking the receptor. The blockade is antagonized by Ca^{2+} salts but only inconsistently by anti-ChE agents (*see* Chapter 54). The tetracyclines also can produce neuromuscular blockade, possibly by chelation of Ca^{2+}. Additional antibiotics that have neuromuscular blocking action, through both presynaptic and postsynaptic actions, include polymyxin B, colistin, clindamycin, and lincomycin. Ca^{2+} channel blockers enhance neuromuscular blockade produced by both competitive and depolarizing antagonists. When neuromuscular blocking agents are administered to patients receiving these agents, dose adjustments should be considered.

Miscellaneous drugs that may have significant interactions with either competitive or depolarizing neuromuscular blocking agents include trimethaphan, lithium, opioid analgesics, procaine, lidocaine, quinidine, phenelzine, carbamazepine, phenytoin, propranolol, dantrolene, azathioprine, tamoxifen, magnesium salts, corticosteroids, digitalis glycosides, chloroquine, catecholamines, and diuretics.

TOXICOLOGY

The important untoward responses of the neuromuscular blocking agents include prolonged apnea, cardiovascular collapse, those resulting from histamine release, and rarely, anaphylaxis. Related factors may include alterations in body temperature; electrolyte imbalance, particularly of K^+; low plasma butyrylcholinesterase levels, resulting in a reduction in the rate of destruction of succinylcholine; the presence of latent myasthenia gravis or of malignant disease such as small cell carcinoma of the lung with Eaton-Lambert myasthenic syndrome; reduced blood flow to skeletal muscles, causing delayed removal of the blocking drugs; and decreased elimination of the muscle relaxants secondary to hepatic dysfunction (cisatracurium, rocuronium, vecuronium) or reduced renal function (pancuronium). Great care should be taken when administering neuromuscular blockers to dehydrated or severely ill patients. Depolarizing agents can cause rapid release of K^+ from intracellular sites; this may be a factor in production of the prolonged apnea in patients who receive these drugs while in electrolyte imbalance. Succinylcholine-induced hyperkalemia is a life-threatening complication of that drug.

MALIGNANT HYPERTHERMIA. Malignant hyperthermia is a potentially life-threatening event triggered by the administration of certain anesthetics and neuromuscular blocking agents. The clinical features include contracture, rigidity, and heat production from skeletal muscle resulting in severe hyperthermia (increases of up to 1°C/5 min), accelerated muscle metabolism, metabolic acidosis, and tachycardia. Uncontrolled release of Ca^{2+} from the sarcoplasmic reticulum of skeletal muscle is the initiating event. Although the halogenated hydrocarbon anesthetics (e.g., halothane, isoflurane, and sevoflurane) and succinylcholine alone have been reported to precipitate the response, most of the incidents arise from the combination of depolarizing blocking agent and anesthetic. Susceptibility to malignant hyperthermia, an autosomal dominant trait, is associated with certain congenital myopathies such as *central core disease*. In the majority of cases, however, no clinical signs are visible in the absence of anesthetic intervention.

Treatment entails intravenous administration of dantrolene (DANTRIUM, others), which blocks Ca^{2+} release from the sarcoplasmic reticulum of skeletal muscle (*see* "Control of Muscle Spasms and Rigidity" earlier in the chapter). Rapid cooling, inhalation of 100% O_2, and control of acidosis should be considered adjunct therapy in malignant hyperthermia.

RESPIRATORY PARALYSIS. Treatment of respiratory paralysis arising from an adverse reaction or overdose of a neuromuscular blocking agent should be by positive-pressure artificial respiration with oxygen and maintenance of a patent airway until recovery of normal respiration is ensured. With the competitive blocking agents, this may be hastened by the administration of neostigmine methylsulfate (0.5-2 mg IV) or edrophonium (10 mg IV, repeated as required up to a total of 40 mg).

INTERVENTIONAL STRATEGIES FOR OTHER TOXIC EFFECTS. Neostigmine effectively antagonizes only the skeletal muscular blocking action of the competitive blocking agents and may aggravate such side effects as hypotension or induce bronchospasm. In such circumstances, sympathomimetic amines may be given to support the blood pressure. Atropine or glycopyrrolate is administered to counteract muscarinic stimulation. Antihistamines are definitely beneficial to counteract the responses that follow the release of histamine, particularly when administered before the neuromuscular blocking agent.

REVERSAL OF EFFECTS BY CHELATION THERAPY. Sugammadex (BRIDION), a modified γ-cyclodextrin, is a chelating agent specific for rocuronium and vecuronium. Sugammadex at doses >2 mg/kg is able to reverse neuromuscular blockade from rocuronium within 3 min. In patients with impaired renal function, sugammadex clearance is markedly reduced and this agent should be avoided. Sugammadex is approved for clinical use in Europe but not yet in the U.S. Side effects include dysgeusia and rare hypersensitivity.

GANGLIONIC NEUROTRANSMISSION

Neurotransmission in autonomic ganglia involves release of ACh and the rapid depolarization of postsynaptic membranes via the activation of neuronal nicotinic (N_n) receptors by ACh. Intracellular recordings from postganglionic neurons indicate that at least 4 different changes in postsynaptic membrane potential can be elicited by stimulation of the preganglionic nerve (Figure 11–4):

- An initial excitatory postsynaptic potential (EPSP, via nicotinic receptors) that may result in an action potential
- An inhibitory postsynaptic potential (IPSP) mediated by M_2 muscarinic receptors
- A secondary slow EPSP mediated by M_1 muscarinic receptors
- A late, slow EPSP mediated by myriad peptides

There are multiple nicotinic receptor subunits (e.g., α3, α5, α7, β2, and β4) in ganglia, with α3 and β2 being most abundant. The ganglionic nicotinic ACh receptors are sensitive to classical blocking agents such as hexamethonium and trimethaphan.

An action potential is generated in the postganglionic neuron when the initial EPSP attains a critical amplitude. Unlike the neuromuscular junction, discrete endplates with focal localization of receptors do not exist in ganglia; rather, the dendrites and nerve cell bodies contain the receptors. The characteristics of nicotinic-receptor channels of the ganglia and the neuromuscular junction are quite similar.

The events that follow the initial depolarization (IPSP; slow EPSP; late, slow EPSP) are insensitive to hexamethonium or other N_n antagonists. Electrophysiological and neurochemical evidence suggests that catecholamines participate in the generation of the IPSP. Dopamine and norepinephrine cause hyperpolarization of

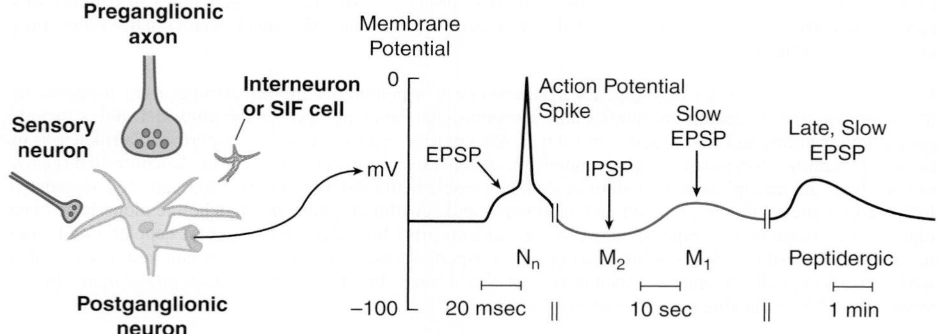

Figure 11–4 *Postsynaptic potentials recorded from an autonomic postganglionic nerve cell body after stimulation of the preganglionic nerve fiber.* The preganglionic nerve releases ACh onto postganglionic cells. The initial EPSP results from the inward Na^+ current (and perhaps Ca^{2+} current) through the nicotinic receptor channel. If the EPSP is of sufficient magnitude, it triggers an action potential spike, which is followed by a slow IPSP, a slow EPSP, and a late, slow EPSP. The slow IPSP and slow EPSP are not seen in all ganglia. The electrical events subsequent to the initial EPSP are thought to modulate the probability that a subsequent EPSP will reach the threshold for triggering a spike. Other interneurons, such as catecholamine-containing, small intensely fluorescent (SIF) cells, and axon terminals from sensory, afferent neurons also release transmitters and that may influence the slow potentials of the postganglionic neuron. There are cholinergic, peptidergic, adrenergic, and amino acid receptors on the dendrites and soma of the postganglionic neuron and the interneurons. The preganglionic fiber releases ACh and peptides; the interneurons store and release catecholamines, amino acids, and peptides; the sensory afferent nerve terminals release peptides. The initial EPSP is mediated through nicotinic (N_n) receptors, the slow IPSP and EPSP through M_2 and M_1 muscarinic receptors, and the late, slow EPSP through various peptidergic receptors.

ganglia; however, in some ganglia IPSPs are mediated by M_2 muscarinic receptors. The slow EPSP is generated by ACh activation of M_1 (G_q-coupled) muscarinic receptors and is blocked by atropine and M_1-selective antagonists (*see* Chapter 9).

Secondary synaptic events modulate the initial EPSP. A variety of peptides, including gonadotropin-releasing hormone, substance P, angiotensin, calcitonin gene–related peptide, vasoactive intestinal polypeptide, neuropeptide Y, and enkephalins, have been identified in ganglia by immunofluorescence. They appear localized to particular cell bodies, nerve fibers, or SIF cells, are released on nerve stimulation, and are presumed to mediate the late slow EPSP. Other neurotransmitter substances (e.g., 5HT and GABA) can modify ganglionic transmission.

GANGLIONIC-STIMULATING DRUGS

Drugs that stimulate cholinergic receptor sites on autonomic ganglia have been essential for analyzing the mechanism of ganglionic function; however, these ganglionic agonists have very limited therapeutic use. They can be grouped into 2 categories. The first group consists of drugs with nicotinic specificity, including nicotine, lobeline, tetramethylammonium (TEA), and dimethylphenylpiperazinium (DMPP). Nicotine's excitatory effects on ganglia are rapid in onset, are blocked by ganglionic nicotinic-receptor antagonists, and mimic the initial EPSP. The second group consists of muscarinic receptor agonists such as muscarine, McN-A-343, and methacholine (*see* Chapter 9); their excitatory effects on ganglia are delayed in onset, blocked by atropine-like drugs, and mimic the slow EPSP.

NICOTINE

Nicotine is of considerable medical significance because of its toxicity, presence in tobacco, and propensity for conferring a dependence on its users. The chronic effects of nicotine and the untoward effects of the chronic use of tobacco are considered in Chapter 24.

PHARMACOLOGICAL ACTIONS. In addition to the actions of nicotine on a variety of neuroeffector and chemosensitive sites, the alkaloid can both stimulate and desensitize receptors. The ultimate response of any 1 system represents the summation of stimulatory and inhibitory effects of nicotine. Nicotine can increase heart rate by excitation of sympathetic ganglia or by paralysis of parasympathetic cardiac ganglia, and it can slow heart rate by paralysis of sympathetic or stimulation of parasympathetic cardiac ganglia. The effects of the drug on the chemoreceptors of the carotid and aortic bodies and on regions of the CNS also can influence heart rate, as can the compensatory baroreceptor reflexes resulting from changes in blood pressure caused by nicotine. Finally, nicotine elicits a discharge of epinephrine from the adrenal medulla, which accelerates heart rate and raises blood pressure.

Peripheral Nervous System. The major action of nicotine consists initially of transient stimulation and subsequently of a more persistent depression of all autonomic ganglia. Small doses of nicotine stimulate the ganglion cells directly and may facilitate impulse transmission. Following larger doses, the initial stimulation is followed by a blockade of transmission. Whereas stimulation of the ganglion cells coincides with their depolarization, depression of transmission by adequate doses of nicotine occurs both during the depolarization and after it has subsided. Nicotine also possesses a biphasic action on the adrenal medulla: small doses evoke the discharge of catecholamines; larger doses prevent their release in response to splanchnic nerve stimulation.

The effects of high doses of nicotine on the neuromuscular junction are similar to those on ganglia. However, the stimulant phase is obscured largely by the rapidly developing paralysis. In the latter stage, nicotine also produces neuromuscular blockade by receptor desensitization.

Nicotine, like ACh, stimulates a number of sensory receptors. These include mechanoreceptors that respond to stretch or pressure of the skin, mesentery, tongue, lung, and stomach; chemoreceptors of the carotid body; thermal receptors of the skin and tongue; and pain receptors. Prior administration of hexamethonium prevents stimulation of the sensory receptors by nicotine but has little, if any, effect on the activation of sensory receptors by physiological stimuli.

CNS. Nicotine markedly stimulates the CNS. Low doses produce weak analgesia; with higher doses, tremors leading to convulsions at toxic doses are evident. The excitation of respiration is a prominent action of nicotine: large doses act directly on the medulla oblongata, whereas smaller doses augment respiration reflexly by excitation of the chemoreceptors of the carotid and aortic bodies. Stimulation of the CNS with large doses is followed by depression, and death results from failure of respiration owing to both central paralysis and peripheral blockade of the diaphragm and intercostal muscles that facilitate respiration.

Nicotine induces vomiting by both central and peripheral actions. The primary sites of action of nicotine in the CNS are prejunctional, causing the release of other transmitters. The stimulatory and pleasure–reward actions of nicotine appear to result from release of excitatory amino acids, dopamine, and other biogenic amines from various CNS centers. Release of excitatory amino acids may account for much of nicotine's stimulatory action. Chronic exposure to nicotine in several systems causes a marked increase in the density or number of nicotinic receptors, possibly contributing to tolerance and dependence.

Cardiovascular System. In general, the cardiovascular responses to nicotine are due to stimulation of sympathetic ganglia and the adrenal medulla, together with the discharge of catecholamines from sympathetic nerve endings. Contributing to the sympathomimetic response to nicotine is the activation of chemoreceptors of the aortic and carotid bodies, which reflexly results in vasoconstriction, tachycardia, and elevated blood pressure.

GI Tract. The combined activation of parasympathetic ganglia and cholinergic nerve endings by nicotine results in increased tone and motor activity of the bowel. Nausea, vomiting, and occasionally diarrhea are observed following systemic absorption of nicotine in an individual who has not been exposed to nicotine previously.

Exocrine Glands. Nicotine causes an initial stimulation of salivary and bronchial secretions that is followed by inhibition.

ABSORPTION, DISTRIBUTION, AND ELIMINATION. Nicotine is readily absorbed from the respiratory tract, buccal membranes, and skin. Severe poisoning has resulted from percutaneous absorption. As a relatively strong base, nicotine has limited absorption from the stomach. Intestinal absorption is far more efficient. Nicotine in chewing tobacco, because it is absorbed more slowly than inhaled nicotine, has a longer duration of effect. The average cigarette contains 6-11 mg nicotine and delivers ~1-3 mg nicotine systemically to the smoker; bioavailability can increase as much as 3-fold with the intensity of puffing and technique of the smoker.

Approximately 80-90% of nicotine is altered in the body, mainly in the liver but also in the kidney and lung. Cotinine is the major metabolite. The $t_{1/2}$ of nicotine following inhalation or parenteral administration is ~2 h. Nicotine and its metabolites are eliminated rapidly by the kidney. The rate of urinary excretion of nicotine diminishes when the urine is alkaline. Nicotine also is excreted in the milk of lactating women who smoke; the milk of heavy smokers may contain 0.5 mg/L.

ACUTE NICOTINE POISONING. Poisoning from nicotine may occur from accidental ingestion of nicotine-containing insecticide sprays or in children from ingestion of tobacco products. The acutely fatal dose of nicotine for an adult is probably ~60 mg. Smoking tobacco usually contains 1-2% nicotine. Apparently, the gastric absorption of nicotine from tobacco taken by mouth is delayed because of slowed gastric emptying, so vomiting caused by the central effect of the initially absorbed fraction may remove much of the tobacco remaining in the GI tract.

The onset of symptoms of acute, severe nicotine poisoning is rapid; they include nausea, salivation, abdominal pain, vomiting, diarrhea, cold sweat, headache, dizziness, disturbed hearing and vision, mental confusion, and marked weakness. Faintness and prostration ensue; the blood pressure falls; breathing is difficult; the pulse is weak, rapid, and irregular; and collapse may be followed by terminal convulsions. Death may result within a few minutes from respiratory failure.

Therapy. Vomiting may be induced, or gastric lavage should be performed. Alkaline solutions should be avoided. A slurry of activated charcoal is then passed through the tube and left in the stomach. Respiratory assistance and treatment of shock may be necessary.

SMOKING CESSATION. Two goals of the pharmacotherapy of smoking cessation are the reduction of the craving for nicotine and inhibition of the reinforcing effects of nicotine. Myriad approaches and drug regimens are used, including nicotine replacement, bupropion (*see* Chapter 15), and nicotinic ACh receptor agonists (*see* Chapters 15 and 24).

Varenicline (CHANTIX) has been recently introduced as an aid to smoking cessation. The drug interacts with nicotinic ACh receptors. In model systems, varenicline is a partial agonist at $\alpha_4\beta_2$ receptors and a full agonist at the α_7 subtype, with weak activity toward $\alpha_3\beta_2$- and α_6-containing receptors. The drug is effective clinically; however, it is not benign: the FDA has issued a warning about mood and behavioral changes associated with its use.

Nicotine itself is available in several dosage forms to help achieve abstinence from tobacco use. Nicotine is marketed for over-the-counter use as a gum or lozenge (NICOTINE POLACRILEX, NICORETTE, COMMIT, THRIVE, others), transdermal patch (NICODERM, HABITROL, others), a nasal spray (NICOTROL), or a vapor inhaler

(NICOTROL). The efficacy of these dosage forms in producing abstinence from smoking is enhanced when linked to counseling and motivational therapy.

GANGLIONIC BLOCKING DRUGS

There are 2 categories of agents that block ganglionic nicotinic receptors. The prototype of the first group, nicotine, initially stimulates the ganglia by an ACh-like action and then blocks them by causing a persistent depolarization. Compounds in the second category (e.g., *trimethaphan* and *hexamethonium*) impair transmission. Trimethaphan acts by competition with ACh, analogous to the mechanism of action of curare at the neuromuscular junction. Hexamethonium appears to block the channel after it opens; this action shortens the duration of current flow because the open channel either becomes occluded or closes. Thus the initial EPSP is blocked, and ganglionic transmission is inhibited. The diverse chemicals that block autonomic ganglia without first causing stimulation are:

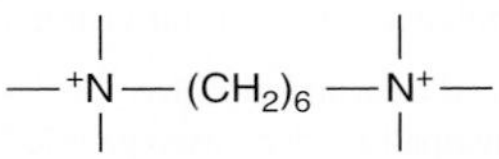

$-{}^{+}N-(CH_2)_6-N^{+}-$

HEXAMETHONIUM (C6)

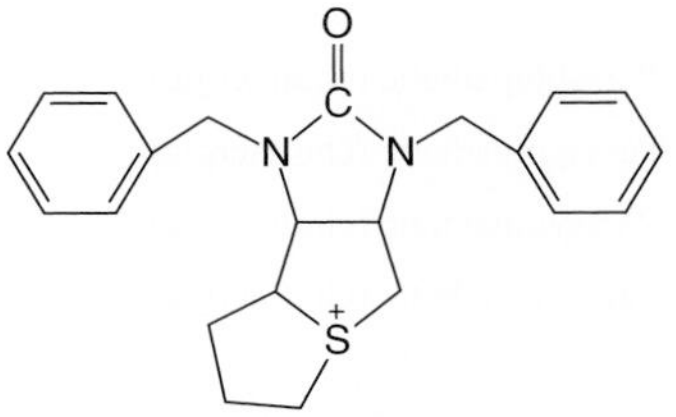

TRIMETHAPHAN

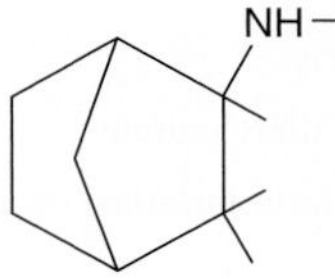

MECAMYLAMINE

Ganglionic blocking agents were the first effective therapy for the treatment of hypertension. However, due to the role of ganglionic transmission in both sympathetic and parasympathetic neurotransmission, the antihypertensive action of ganglionic blocking agents was accompanied by numerous undesirable side effects. Mecamylamine, a secondary amine, is currently licensed as an orphan drug for Tourette syndrome.

PHARMACOLOGICAL PROPERTIES. Nearly all the physiological alterations observed after the administration of ganglionic blocking agents can be anticipated with reasonable accuracy by a careful inspection of Figure 8–1 and Table 8–1, and by knowing which division of the autonomic nervous system exercises dominant control of various organs (Table 11–5). For example, blockade of sympathetic ganglia interrupts adrenergic control of arterioles and results in vasodilation, improved peripheral blood flow in some vascular beds, and a fall in blood pressure.

Generalized ganglionic blockade also may result in atony of the bladder and GI tract, cycloplegia, xerostomia, diminished perspiration, and by abolishing circulatory reflex pathways, postural hypotension. These changes represent the generally undesirable features of ganglionic blockade that severely limit the therapeutic efficacy of ganglionic blocking agents.

Cardiovascular System. Existing sympathetic tone is critical in determining the degree to which blood pressure is lowered by ganglionic blockade; thus, blood pressure may be decreased only minimally in recumbent normotensive subjects but may fall markedly in sitting or standing subjects. Postural hypotension limits the use of ganglionic blockers in ambulatory patients.

Changes in heart rate following ganglionic blockade depend largely on existing vagal tone. In humans, mild tachycardia usually accompanies the hypotension, a sign that indicates fairly complete ganglionic blockade. However, a decrease may occur if the heart rate is high initially.

Cardiac output often is reduced by ganglionic blocking drugs in patients with normal cardiac function, as a consequence of diminished venous return resulting from venous dilation and peripheral pooling of blood. In patients with cardiac failure, ganglionic blockade frequently results in increased cardiac output owing to a reduction in peripheral resistance. In hypertensive subjects, cardiac output, stroke volume, and left ventricular work are diminished. Although total systemic vascular resistance is decreased in patients who receive ganglionic blocking agents, changes in blood flow and vascular resistance of individual vascular beds are variable. Reduction of cerebral blood flow is small unless mean systemic blood pressure falls below 50-60 mm Hg. Skeletal muscle blood flow is unaltered, but splanchnic and renal blood flow decrease.

ABSORPTION, DISTRIBUTION, AND ELIMINATION. The absorption of quaternary ammonium and sulfonium compounds from the enteric tract is incomplete and unpredictable. This is due both to the limited ability of these ionized substances to penetrate cell membranes and to the depression of propulsive movements of the

Table 11–5

Usual Predominance of Sympathetic or Parasympathetic Tone at Various Effector Sites, and Consequences of Autonomic Ganglionic Blockade

SITE	PREDOMINANT TONE	EFFECT OF GANGLIONIC BLOCKADE
Arterioles	Sympathetic (adrenergic)	Vasodilation; increased peripheral blood flow; hypotension
Veins	Sympathetic (adrenergic)	Dilation: peripheral pooling of blood; decreased venous return; decreased cardiac output
Heart	Parasympathetic (cholinergic)	Tachycardia
Iris	Parasympathetic (cholinergic)	Mydriasis
Ciliary muscle	Parasympathetic (cholinergic)	Cycloplegia—focus to far vision
Gastrointestinal tract	Parasympathetic (cholinergic)	Reduced tone and motility; constipation; decreased gastric and pancreatic secretions
Urinary bladder	Parasympathetic (cholinergic)	Urinary retention
Salivary glands	Parasympathetic (cholinergic)	Xerostomia
Sweat glands	Sympathetic (cholinergic)	Anhidrosis
Genital tract	Sympathetic and parasympathetic	Decreased stimulation

small intestine and gastric emptying. Although the absorption of mecamylamine is less erratic, reduced bowel activity and paralytic ileus are a danger. After absorption, the quaternary ammonium- and sulfonium-blocking agents are confined primarily to the extracellular space and are excreted mostly unchanged by the kidney. Mecamylamine concentrates in the liver and kidney and is excreted slowly in an unchanged form.

UNTOWARD RESPONSES AND SEVERE REACTIONS. Among the milder untoward responses observed are visual disturbances, dry mouth, conjunctival suffusion, urinary hesitancy, decreased potency, subjective chilliness, moderate constipation, occasional diarrhea, abdominal discomfort, anorexia, heartburn, nausea, eructation, and bitter taste and the signs and symptoms of syncope caused by postural hypotension. More severe reactions include marked hypotension, constipation, syncope, paralytic ileus, urinary retention, and cycloplegia.

For a complete Bibliographical Listing see Goodman & Gilman's ***The Pharmacological Basis of Therapeutics***, 12th ed., or Goodman & Gilman Online at www.AccessMedicine.com.

Adrenergic Agonists and Antagonists

Catecholamines and Sympathomimetic Drugs

Catecholamines and sympathomimetic drugs are classified as *direct-acting, indirect-acting*, or *mixed-acting sympathomimetics* (Figure 12–1).

Direct-acting sympathomimetic drugs act directly on 1 or more of the adrenergic receptors. These agents may exhibit considerable selectivity for a specific receptor subtype (e.g., phenylephrine for α_1, terbutaline for β_2) or may have no or minimal selectivity and act on several receptor types (e.g., epinephrine for α_1, α_2, β_1, β_2, and β_3 receptors; norepinephrine for α_1, α_2, and β_1 receptors).

Indirect-acting drugs increase the availability of norepinephrine (NE) or epinephrine (EPI) to stimulate adrenergic receptors by several mechanisms:

- By releasing or displacing NE from sympathetic nerve varicosities
- By inhibiting the transport of NE into sympathetic neurons (e.g., cocaine), thereby increasing the dwell time of the transmitter at the receptor
- By blocking the metabolizing enzymes, *monoamine oxidase* (MAO) (e.g., pargyline) or *catechol-O-methyltransferase* (COMT) (e.g., entacapone), effectively increasing transmitter supply

Drugs that indirectly release NE and also directly activate receptors are referred to as *mixed-acting sympathomimetic drugs* [e.g., ephedrine, dopamine (DA)].

A feature of direct-acting sympathomimetic drugs is that their responses are not reduced by prior treatment with *reserpine* or *guanethidine*, which deplete NE from sympathetic neurons. After transmitter depletion, the actions of direct-acting sympathomimetic drugs actually may increase because the loss of the neurotransmitter induces compensatory changes that upregulate receptors or enhance the signaling pathway. In contrast,

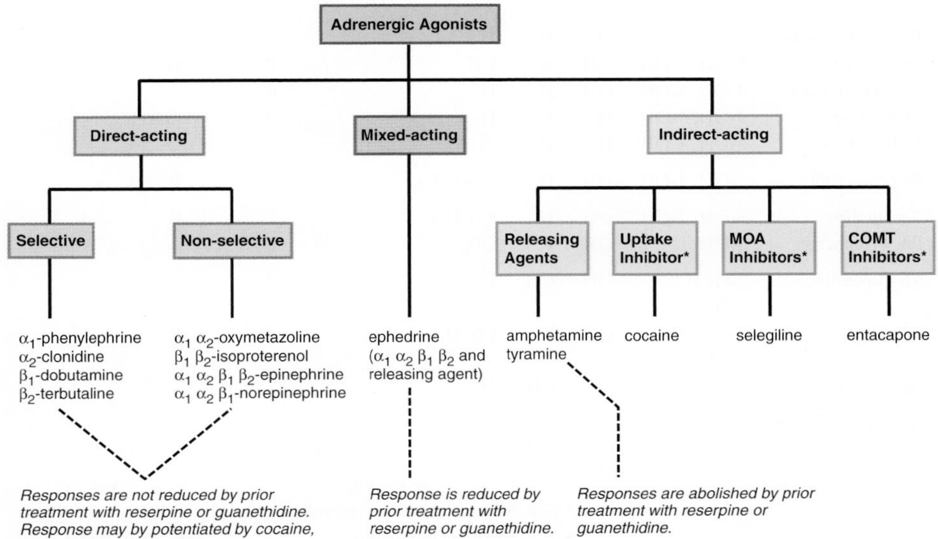

Figure 12–1 *Classification of adrenergic receptor agonists (sympathomimetic amines) and drugs that produce sympathomimetic-like effects. For each category, a prototypical drug is shown. (*Not actually sympathetic drugs but produce sympathomimetic-like effects.)*

the responses of indirect-acting sympathomimetic drugs (e.g., amphetamine, tyramine) are abolished by prior treatment with reserpine or guanethidine. The cardinal feature of mixed-acting sympathomimetic drugs is that their effects are blunted, but not abolished, by prior treatment with reserpine or guanethidine.

Because the actions of NE are more pronounced on α and β_1 receptors than on β_2 receptors, many non-catecholamines that release NE have predominantly α receptor–mediated and cardiac effects. However, certain non-catecholamines with both direct and indirect effects on adrenergic receptors show significant β_2 activity and are used clinically for these effects. Thus, ephedrine, although dependent on release of NE for some of its effects, relieves bronchospasm by its action on β_2 receptors in bronchial smooth muscle, an effect not seen with NE. Moreover, some non-catecholamines (e.g., phenylephrine) act primarily and directly on target cells. It therefore is impossible to predict precisely the effects of non-catecholamines solely on their ability to provoke NE release.

CHEMISTRY AND STRUCTURE-ACTIVITY RELATIONSHIP OF SYMPATHOMIMETIC AMINES. β-Phenylethylamine (Table 12–1) can be viewed as the parent compound of the sympathomimetic amines, consisting of a benzene ring and an ethylamine side chain. The structure permits substitutions to be made on the aromatic ring, the α- and β-carbon atoms, and the terminal amino group to yield a variety of compounds with sympathomimetic activity. *NE, EPI, DA, isoproterenol*, and a few other agents have hydroxyl groups substituted at positions 3 and 4 of the benzene ring. Since *o*-dihydroxybenzene is also known as *catechol*, sympathomimetic amines with these hydroxyl substitutions in the aromatic ring are termed *catecholamines*.

Many directly acting sympathomimetic drugs influence both α and β receptors, but the ratio of activities varies among drugs in a continuous spectrum from predominantly α activity (phenylephrine) to predominantly β activity (isoproterenol) (*see* Table 12–1).

Catecholamines have only a brief duration of action and are ineffective when administered orally, because they are rapidly inactivated in the intestinal mucosa and in the liver before reaching the systemic circulation (*see* Chapter 8). Compounds without 1 or both hydroxyl substituents are not acted on by COMT, and their oral effectiveness and duration of action are enhanced.

Table 12–1

Chemical Structures and Major Effects of Some Sympathomimetic Drugs

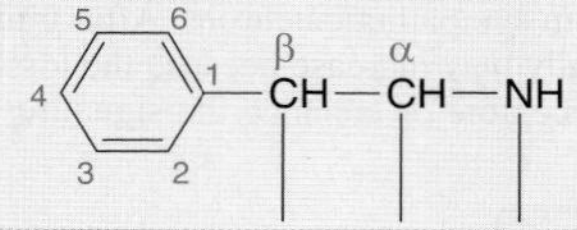

	(ring positions 1–6)	β CH—	α CH—	NH	MAIN CLINICAL USES							
					α RECEPTOR				β RECEPTOR			CNS
					A	N	P	V	B	C	U	
Phenylethylamine		H	H	H								
Epinephrine	3-OH, 4-OH	OH	H	CH_3	A		P	V	B	C		
Norepinephrine	3-OH, 4-OH	OH	H	H			P					
Dopamine	3-OH, 4-OH	H	H	H			P					
Dobutamine	3-OH, 4-OH	H	H	1						C		
Isoproterenol	3-OH, 4-OH	OH	H	$CH(CH_3)_2$					B	C		
Terbutaline	3-OH, 5-OH	OH	H	$C(CH_3)_3$					B		U	
Phenylephrine	3-OH	OH	H	CH_3		N	P					
Methoxamine	2-OCH_3, 5-OCH_3	OH	CH_3	H			P					
Albuterol	3-CH_2OH, 4-OH	OH	H	$C(CH_3)_3$					B		U	
Amphetamine		H	CH_3	H								+
Methamphetamine		H	CH_3	CH_3								+
Ephedrine		OH	CH_3	CH_3		N	P		B	C		

α Activity
A = Allergic reactions (includes action)
N = Nasal decongestion
P = Pressor (may include action)
V = Other local vasoconstriction

β Activity
B = Bronchodilator
C = Cardiac
U = Uterus

CNS = Central nervous system activity

PHYSIOLOGICAL BASIS OF ADRENERGIC RECEPTOR FUNCTION. An important factor in the response of any cell or organ to sympathomimetic amines is the density and proportion of α and β adrenergic receptors. For example, NE has relatively little capacity to increase bronchial airflow, since the receptors in bronchial smooth muscle are largely of the β_2 subtype. In contrast, isoproterenol and EPI are potent bronchodilators. Cutaneous blood vessels physiologically express almost exclusively α receptors; thus, NE and EPI cause constriction of such vessels, whereas isoproterenol has little effect. The smooth muscle of blood vessels that supply skeletal muscles has both β_2 and α receptors; activation of β_2 receptors causes vasodilation, and stimulation of α receptors constricts these vessels. In such vessels, the threshold concentration for activation of β_2 receptors by EPI is lower than that for α receptors, but when both types of receptors are activated at high concentrations of EPI, the response to α receptors predominates. Physiological concentrations of EPI primarily cause vasodilation.

The ultimate response of a target organ to sympathomimetic amines is dictated by the direct effects of the agents and the reflex homeostatic adjustments of the organism. Many sympathomimetic amines produce a rise in arterial blood pressure caused by stimulation of vascular α adrenergic receptors. This stimulation elicits compensatory reflexes that are mediated by the carotid–aortic baroreceptor system. As a result, sympathetic tone is diminished and vagal tone is enhanced; each of these responses leads to slowing of the heart rate. Conversely, when a drug (e.g., a β_2 agonist) lowers mean blood pressure at the mechanoreceptors of the carotid sinus and aortic arch, the baroreceptor reflex works to restore pressure by reducing parasympathetic (vagal) outflow from the CNS to the heart, and increasing sympathetic outflow to the heart and vessels.

FALSE-TRANSMITTER CONCEPT. This hypothesis is a possible explanation for some of the effects of MAO inhibitors. Phenylethylamines normally are synthesized in the GI tract as a result of the action of bacterial *tyrosine decarboxylase*. The *tyramine* formed in this fashion usually is oxidatively deaminated in the GI tract and the liver. However, when an MAO inhibitor is administered, tyramine may be absorbed systemically and transported into sympathetic nerve terminals, where its catabolism again is prevented because of the inhibition of MAO at this site; the tyramine then is β-hydroxylated to *octopamine*, which is stored in vesicles. As a consequence, NE gradually is displaced by octopamine, and stimulation of the nerve terminal results in the release of a relatively small amount of NE along with a fraction of octopamine. The latter amine has relatively little ability to activate either α or β receptors. Thus, a functional impairment of sympathetic transmission parallels long-term administration of MAO inhibitors.

Despite such functional impairment, patients who have received MAO inhibitors may experience severe hypertensive crises if they ingest cheese, beer, or red wine. These and related foods, which are produced by fermentation, contain a large quantity of tyramine, and to a lesser degree, other phenylethylamines. When GI and hepatic MAO are inhibited, the large quantity of tyramine that is ingested is absorbed rapidly and reaches the systemic circulation in high concentration. A massive and precipitous release of NE can result, with consequent hypertension that can be severe enough to cause myocardial infarction or a stroke (*see* Chapter 15).

ENDOGENOUS CATECHOLAMINES

EPINEPHRINE

EPI (adrenaline) is a potent stimulant of both α and β adrenergic receptors. Most of the responses listed in Table 8–1 are seen after injection of EPI, although the occurrence of sweating, piloerection, and mydriasis depends on the physiological state of the subject. Particularly prominent are the actions on the heart and on vascular and other smooth muscle.

BLOOD PRESSURE. EPI is one of the most potent vasopressor drugs known. If a pharmacological dose is given rapidly *by an intravenous route*, it evokes a characteristic effect on blood pressure, which rises rapidly to a peak that is proportional to the dose. The increase in systolic pressure is greater than the increase in diastolic pressure, so that the pulse pressure increases. As the response wanes, the mean pressure may fall below normal before returning to control levels.

The mechanism of the rise in blood pressure due to EPI is:

- A direct myocardial stimulation that increases the strength of ventricular contraction (*positive inotropic action*)
- An increased heart rate (*positive chronotropic action*)
- Vasoconstriction in many vascular beds—especially in the *precapillary resistance vessels* of skin, mucosa, and kidney—along with marked constriction of the veins

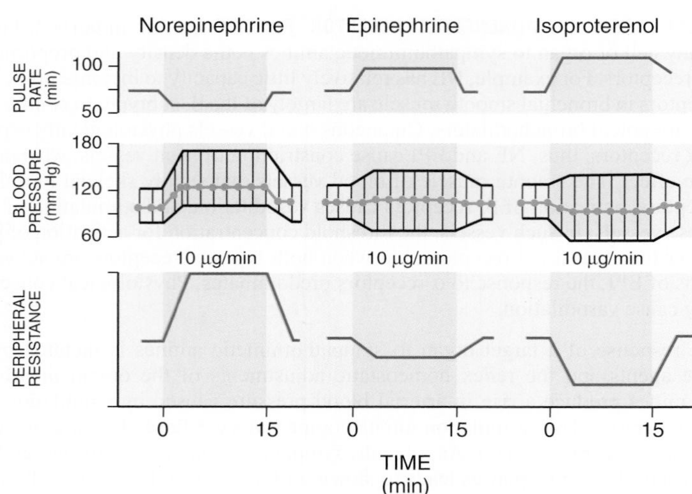

Figure 12–2 *Effects of intravenous infusion of norepinephrine, epinephrine, or isoproterenol in humans.* (Modified from Allwood MJ, Cobbold AF, Ginsberg J. Peripheral vascular effects of noradrenaline, isopropylnoradrenaline, and dopamine. *Br Med Bull,* 1963;19:132-136. With permission from Oxford University Press.)

The pulse rate, at first accelerated, may be slowed markedly at the height of the rise of blood pressure by compensatory vagal discharge (baroreceptor reflex). Small doses of EPI (0.1 μg/kg) may cause the blood pressure to fall. The depressor effect of small doses and the biphasic response to larger doses are due to greater sensitivity to EPI of vasodilator β_2 receptors than of constrictor α receptors.

Absorption of EPI after *subcutaneous injection* is slow due to local vasoconstrictor action; the effects of doses as large as 0.5-1.5 mg can be duplicated by intravenous infusion at a rate of 10-30 μg/min. There is a moderate increase in systolic pressure due to increased cardiac contractile force and a rise in cardiac output (Figure 12–2). Peripheral resistance decreases, owing to a dominant action on β_2 receptors of vessels in skeletal muscle, where blood flow is enhanced; as a consequence, diastolic pressure usually falls. Because the mean blood pressure is not, as a rule, greatly elevated, compensatory baroreceptor reflexes do not appreciably antagonize the direct cardiac actions. Heart rate, cardiac output, stroke volume, and left ventricular work per beat are increased as a result of direct cardiac stimulation and increased venous return to the heart, which is reflected by an increase in right atrial pressure. The details of the effects of intravenous infusion of EPI, NE, and isoproterenol in humans are compared in Table 12–2 and Figure 12–2.

VASCULAR EFFECTS. In the vasculature, EPI acts chiefly on the smaller arterioles and precapillary sphincters, although veins and large arteries also respond to the drug. Various vascular beds react differently, which results in a substantial redistribution of blood flow. Injected EPI markedly decreases cutaneous blood flow, constricting precapillary vessels and small venules. Cutaneous vasoconstriction accounts for a marked decrease in blood flow in the hands and feet. Blood flow to skeletal muscles is increased by therapeutic doses in humans. This is due in part to a powerful β_2-mediated vasodilator action that is only partially counterbalanced by a vasoconstrictor action on the α receptors that also are present in the vascular bed.

The effect of EPI on cerebral circulation is related to systemic blood pressure. In usual therapeutic doses, the drug has relatively little constrictor action on cerebral arterioles. Indeed, autoregulatory mechanisms tend to limit the increase in cerebral blood flow caused by increased blood pressure.

Doses of EPI that have little effect on mean arterial pressure consistently increase renal vascular resistance and reduce renal blood flow by as much as 40%. Since the glomerular filtration rate is only slightly and variably altered, the filtration fraction is consistently increased. Excretion of Na^+, K^+, and Cl^- is decreased; urine volume may be increased, decreased, or unchanged. Maximal tubular reabsorptive and excretory capacities are unchanged. The secretion of renin is increased as a consequence of a direct action of EPI on β_1 receptors in the juxtaglomerular apparatus. Arterial and venous pulmonary pressures are raised. Although direct pulmonary vasoconstriction occurs, redistribution of blood from the systemic to the pulmonary circulation, due to

Table 12–2

Comparative Effects of Infusion of Epinephrine and Norepinephrine in Humans[a]

EFFECT	EPI	NE
Cardiac		
Heart rate	+	–[b]
Stroke volume	++	++
Cardiac output	+++	0,–
Arrhythmias	++++	++++
Coronary blood flow	++	++
Blood Pressure		
Systolic arterial	+++	+++
Mean arterial	+	++
Diastolic arterial	+,0,–	++
Mean pulmonary	++	++
Peripheral Circulation		
Total peripheral resistance	–	++
Cerebral blood flow	+	0,–
Muscle blood flow	+++	0,–
Cutaneous blood flow	–	–
Renal blood flow	–	–
Splanchnic blood flow	+++	0,+
Metabolic Effects		
O_2 consumption	++	0,+
Blood glucose	+++	0,+
Blood lactic acid	+++	0,+
Eosinopenic response	+	0
CNS		
Respiration	+	+
Subjective sensations	+	+

EPI, epinephrine; NE, norepinephrine; +, increase; 0, no change; –, decrease; –[b], after atropine.
[a]0.1-0.4 μg/kg per minute.
Source: After Goldenberg M, Aranow H Jr, Smith AA, Faber M. Pheochromocytoma and essential hypertensive vascular disease. Arch Intern Med 1950;86;823-836.

constriction of the more powerful musculature in the systemic great veins, doubtless plays an important part in the increase in pulmonary pressure. Very high concentrations of EPI may cause pulmonary edema precipitated by elevated pulmonary capillary filtration pressure and possibly by "leaky" capillaries.

Coronary blood flow is enhanced by EPI or by cardiac sympathetic stimulation under physiological conditions. The increased flow, which occurs even with doses that do not increase the aortic blood pressure, is the result of 2 factors. The first is the increased relative duration of diastole at higher heart rates; this is partially offset by decreased blood flow during systole because of more forceful contraction of the surrounding myocardium and an increase in mechanical compression of the coronary vessels. The increased flow during diastole is further enhanced if aortic blood pressure is elevated by EPI; as a consequence, total coronary flow may be increased. The second factor is a metabolic dilator effect that results from the increased strength of contraction and myocardial O_2 consumption due to the direct effects of EPI on cardiac myocytes. This vasodilation is mediated in part by adenosine released from cardiac myocytes, which tends to override a direct vasoconstrictor effect of EPI that results from activation of α receptors in coronary vessels.

CARDIAC EFFECTS. EPI is a powerful cardiac stimulant. It acts directly on the predominant β_1 receptors of the myocardium and of the cells of the pacemaker and conducting tissues; β_2, β_3, and α receptors also are present in the heart. Direct responses to EPI include increases in contractile force, accelerated rate of rise of isometric tension, enhanced rate of relaxation, decreased time to peak tension, increased excitability, acceleration of the rate of spontaneous beating, and induction of automaticity in specialized regions of the heart. In accelerating the heart, EPI preferentially shortens systole so that the duration of diastole usually is not reduced.

EPI normally shortens the refractory period of the human atrioventricular (AV) node by direct effects on the heart, although doses of EPI that slow the heart through reflex vagal discharge may indirectly tend to prolong it. EPI also decreases the grade of AV block that occurs as a result of disease, drugs, or vagal stimulation. Depression of sinus rate and AV conduction by vagal discharge probably plays a part in EPI-induced ventricular arrhythmias, because various drugs that block the vagal effect confer some protection. The actions of EPI in enhancing cardiac automaticity are effectively antagonized by β receptor antagonists such as propranolol. However, α_1 receptors exist in most regions of the heart, and their activation prolongs the refractory period and strengthens myocardial contractions. Cardiac arrhythmias have been seen in patients after inadvertent intravenous administration of conventional subcutaneous doses of EPI. EPI as well as other catecholamines may cause myocardial cell death, particularly after intravenous infusions. Acute toxicity is associated with contraction band necrosis and other pathological changes; prolonged sympathetic stimulation of the heart, such as in congestive cardiomyopathy, may promote apoptosis of cardiomyocytes.

EFFECTS ON SMOOTH MUSCLES. The effects of EPI on the smooth muscles of different organs and systems depend on the type of adrenergic receptor in the muscle (*see* Table 8–1). In general, EPI relaxes GI smooth muscle due to activation of both α and β receptors. Intestinal tone and the frequency and amplitude of spontaneous contractions are reduced. The stomach usually is relaxed and the pyloric and ileocecal sphincters are contracted, but these effects depend on the preexisting tone of the muscle. If tone already is high, EPI causes relaxation; if low, contraction.

The responses of uterine muscle to EPI vary with species, phase of the sexual cycle, state of gestation, and dose given. During the last month of pregnancy and at parturition, EPI inhibits uterine tone and contractions (*see* Chapter 66). EPI relaxes the detrusor muscle of the bladder as a result of activation of β receptors and contracts the trigone and sphincter muscles owing to its α-agonist activity. This can result in hesitancy in urination and may contribute to retention of urine in the bladder. Activation of smooth muscle contraction in the prostate promotes urinary retention.

RESPIRATORY EFFECTS. EPI has a powerful bronchodilator action, most evident when bronchial muscle is contracted because of disease, as in bronchial asthma, or in response to drugs or various autacoids.

The beneficial effects of EPI in asthma also may arise from inhibition of antigen-induced release of inflammatory mediators from mast cells, and to a lesser extent from diminution of bronchial secretions and congestion within the mucosa. Inhibition of mast cell secretion is mediated by β_2 receptors, while the effects on the mucosa are mediated by α receptors. however, glucocorticoids have much more profound anti-inflammatory effects (*see* Chapters 33 and 34).

EFFECTS ON THE CNS. EPI, a polar compound, penetrates poorly into the CNS and hence is not a powerful CNS stimulant. While the drug may cause restlessness, apprehension, headache, and tremor in many persons, these effects in part may be secondary to the effects of EPI on the cardiovascular system, skeletal muscles, and intermediary metabolism; that is, they may be the result of somatic manifestations of anxiety.

METABOLIC EFFECTS. EPI elevates the concentrations of glucose and lactate in blood (*see* Chapter 8). Insulin secretion is inhibited through an interaction with α_2 receptors and is enhanced by activation of β_2 receptors; the predominant effect seen with EPI is inhibition. Glucagon secretion is enhanced by an action on the β receptors of the α cells of pancreatic islets. EPI also decreases the uptake of glucose by peripheral tissues. EPI stimulates glycogenolysis in most tissues through β receptors. EPI raises the concentration of free fatty acids in blood by stimulating β receptors in adipocytes. The calorigenic action of EPI (increase in metabolism) is reflected in humans by an increase of 20-30% in O_2 consumption after conventional doses.

MISCELLANEOUS EFFECTS. EPI reduces circulating plasma volume by loss of protein-free fluid to the extracellular space, thereby increasing hematocrit and plasma protein concentration. EPI rapidly increases the number of circulating polymorphonuclear leukocytes, likely due to β receptor–mediated demargination of these cells. EPI accelerates blood coagulation and promotes fibrinolysis. EPI stimulates lacrimation and a scanty mucus secretion from salivary glands. EPI also acts directly on white, fast-twitch muscle fibers to prolong the active state, thereby increasing peak tension.

EPI promotes a fall in plasma K^+, largely due to stimulation of K^+ uptake into cells, particularly skeletal muscle, due to activation of β_2 receptors. This is associated with decreased renal K^+ excretion.

ABSORPTION, FATE, AND EXCRETION. EPI is ineffective after oral administration. Absorption from subcutaneous tissues occurs relatively slowly. Absorption is more rapid after intramuscular injection. When concentrated solutions are nebulized and inhaled, the actions of the drug largely are restricted to the respiratory tract; however, systemic reactions such as arrhythmias may occur, particularly if larger amounts are used. EPI is rapidly inactivated in the liver by COMT and MAO (*see* Figure 8–7 and Table 8–4).

EPI is available in a variety of formulations geared for different routes of administration, including self-administration for anaphylactic reactions (EpiPen). EPI is unstable in alkaline solution; when exposed to air or light, it turns pink from oxidation to adrenochrome and then brown from formation of polymers. EPI injection is available in 1 mg/mL (1:1000), 0.1 mg/mL (1:10,000), and 0.5 mg/mL (1:2000) solutions. Subcutaneous dose ranges from 0.3-0.5 mg. The intravenous route is used cautiously if an immediate and reliable effect is mandatory. If the solution is given by vein, it must be adequately diluted and injected very slowly.

TOXICITY, ADVERSE EFFECTS, AND CONTRAINDICATIONS. EPI may cause restlessness, throbbing headache, tremor, and palpitations. The effects rapidly subside with rest, quiet, recumbency, and reassurance. More serious reactions include cerebral hemorrhage and cardiac arrhythmias. The use of large doses or the accidental, rapid intravenous injection of EPI may result in cerebral hemorrhage from the sharp rise in blood pressure. Angina may be induced by EPI in patients with coronary artery disease. The use of EPI generally is contraindicated in patients who are receiving nonselective β receptor antagonists, because its unopposed actions on vascular α_1 receptors may lead to severe hypertension and cerebral hemorrhage.

THERAPEUTIC USES. A major use of EPI is to provide rapid, emergency relief of hypersensitivity reactions, including anaphylaxis, to drugs and other allergens. EPI also is used to prolong the action of local anesthetics, presumably by decreasing local blood flow (*see* Chapter 20). Its cardiac effects may be of use in restoring cardiac rhythm in patients with cardiac arrest due to various causes. It also is used as a topical hemostatic agent on bleeding surfaces such as in the mouth or in bleeding peptic ulcers during endoscopy of the stomach and duodenum. Inhalation of EPI may be useful in the treatment of post-intubation and infectious croup.

NOREPINEPHRINE

Norepinephrine (levarterenol, *l*-noradrenaline, NE) is a major chemical mediator liberated by mammalian postganglionic sympathetic nerves (*see* Table 12–1).

NE constitutes 10-20% of the catecholamine content of human adrenal medulla and as much as 97% in some pheochromocytomas.

PHARMACOLOGICAL PROPERTIES. The pharmacological actions of NE and EPI are compared in Table 12–2. Both drugs are direct agonists on effector cells; their actions differ mainly in the ratio of their effectiveness in stimulating α and β_2 receptors. They are approximately equipotent in stimulating β_1 receptors. NE is a potent α agonist, has relatively little action on β_2 receptors, and is somewhat less potent than EPI on the α receptors of most organs.

ABSORPTION, FATE, AND EXCRETION. NE, like EPI, is ineffective when given orally and is absorbed poorly from sites of subcutaneous injection. It is rapidly inactivated in the body by uptake and the actions of COMT and MAO. Small amounts normally are found in the urine. The excretion rate may be greatly increased in patients with pheochromocytoma.

CARDIOVASCULAR EFFECTS. In response to infused NE (*see* Figure 12–2), systolic and diastolic pressures, and usually pulse pressure, are increased. Cardiac output is unchanged or decreased, and total peripheral resistance is raised. Compensatory vagal reflex activity slows the heart, overcoming a direct cardioaccelerator action, and stroke volume is increased. The peripheral vascular resistance increases in most vascular beds, and renal blood flow is reduced. NE constricts mesenteric vessels and reduces splanchnic and hepatic blood flow. Coronary flow usually is increased, probably owing both to indirectly induced coronary dilation, as with EPI, and to elevated blood pressure. Although generally a poor β_2 receptor agonist, NE may increase coronary blood flow directly by stimulating β_2 receptors on coronary vessels. Patients with Prinzmetal variant angina pectoris may be supersensitive to the α adrenergic vasoconstrictor effects of NE.

ADVERSE EFFECTS AND PRECAUTIONS. The untoward effects of NE are similar to those of EPI, although there typically is greater elevation of blood pressure with NE. Care must be taken that necrosis and sloughing do not occur at the site of intravenous injection owing to extravasation of the drug. Impaired circulation at injection sites may be relieved by infiltrating the area with phentolamine, an α receptor antagonist. Blood pressure must be determined frequently during the infusion and particularly during adjustment of the rate of the infusion. Reduced blood flow to organs such as kidney and intestines is a constant danger with the use of NE.

THERAPEUTIC USES AND STATUS. NE (LEVOPHED, others) is used as a vasoconstrictor to raise or support blood pressure under certain intensive care conditions (discussed below).

DOPAMINE

DA (*see* Table 12–1) is the immediate metabolic precursor of NE and EPI; it is a central neurotransmitter important in the regulation of movement (*see* Chapters 14, 16, and 22) and possesses important intrinsic pharmacological properties. In the periphery, it is synthesized in epithelial cells of the proximal tubule and is thought to exert local diuretic and natriuretic effects. DA is a substrate for both MAO and COMT and thus is ineffective when administered orally.

PHARMACOLOGICAL PROPERTIES.

Cardiovascular Effects. The cardiovascular effects of DA are mediated by several distinct types of receptors that vary in their affinity for DA (*see* Chapter 13). At low concentrations, the primary interaction of DA is with vascular D_1 receptors, especially in the renal, mesenteric, and coronary beds. By activating adenylyl cyclase and raising intracellular concentrations of cyclic AMP, D_1 receptor stimulation leads to vasodilation. Infusion of low doses of DA causes an increase in glomerular filtration rate, renal blood flow, and Na^+ excretion. Activation of D_1 receptors on renal tubular cells decreases Na^+ transport by cyclic AMP-dependent and cyclic AMP-independent mechanisms. The renal tubular actions of DA that cause natriuresis may be augmented by the increase in renal blood flow and the small increase in the glomerular filtration rate that follow its administration. The resulting increase in hydrostatic pressure in the peritubular capillaries and reduction in oncotic pressure may contribute to diminished reabsorption of Na^+ by the proximal tubular cells. As a consequence, DA has pharmacologically appropriate effects in the management of states of low cardiac output associated with compromised renal function, such as severe congestive heart failure.

At higher concentrations, DA exerts a positive inotropic effect on the myocardium, acting on β_1 adrenergic receptors. DA also causes the release of NE from nerve terminals, which contributes to its effects on the heart. Tachycardia is less prominent during infusion of DA than of isoproterenol. DA usually increases systolic blood pressure and pulse pressure and either has no effect on diastolic blood pressure or increases it slightly. Total peripheral resistance usually is unchanged when low or intermediate doses of DA are given. At high concentrations, DA activates vascular α_1 receptors, leading to more general vasoconstriction.

PRECAUTIONS, ADVERSE REACTIONS, AND CONTRAINDICATIONS. Before DA is administered to patients in shock, hypovolemia should be corrected by transfusion of whole blood, plasma, or other appropriate fluid. Untoward effects due to overdosage generally are attributable to excessive sympathomimetic activity (although this also may be the response to worsening shock). Nausea, vomiting, tachycardia, anginal pain, arrhythmias, headache, hypertension, and peripheral vasoconstriction may be encountered during DA infusion. Extravasation of large amounts of DA during infusion may cause ischemic necrosis and sloughing. Rarely, gangrene of the fingers or toes has followed prolonged infusion of the drug. DA should be avoided if the patient has received an MAO inhibitor. Careful adjustment of dosage also is necessary in patients who are taking tricyclic antidepressants.

THERAPEUTIC USES. DA is used in the treatment of severe congestive heart failure, particularly in patients with oliguria and low or normal peripheral vascular resistance. The drug may improve physiological parameters in the treatment of cardiogenic and septic shock. While DA may acutely improve cardiac and renal function in severely ill patients with chronic heart disease or renal failure, there is relatively little evidence supporting long-term benefit in clinical outcome.

Dopamine hydrochloride is used only intravenously, administered at a rate of 2-5 μg/kg/min; this rate may be increased gradually up to 20-50 μg/kg/min as necessary. During the infusion, patients require clinical assessment of myocardial function, perfusion of vital organs such as the brain, and the production of urine. Reduction in urine flow, tachycardia, or the development of arrhythmias may be indications to slow or terminate the infusion. The duration of action of DA is brief, and hence the rate of administration can be used to control the intensity of effect.

Related drugs include *fenoldopam* and *dopexamine*. Fenoldopam (CORLOPAM, others), a benzazepine derivative, is a rapidly acting vasodilator used for control of severe hypertension (e.g., malignant hypertension with end-organ damage) in hospitalized patients for ≤48 h. Fenoldopam is an agonist for peripheral D_1 receptors and binds with moderate affinity to α_2 adrenergic receptors; it has no significant affinity for D_2 receptors or α_1 or β adrenergic receptors. Fenoldopam is a racemic mixture; the R-isomer is the active component. It dilates a variety of blood vessels, including coronary arteries, afferent and efferent arterioles in the kidney, and mesenteric arteries. Less than 6% of an orally administered dose is absorbed because of extensive first-pass metabolism. The elimination $t_{1/2}$ of intravenously infused fenoldopam is ~10 min. Adverse effects are related to the vasodilation and include headache, flushing, dizziness, and tachycardia or bradycardia.

Dopexamine (DOPACARD) is a synthetic analog related to DA with intrinsic activity at dopamine D_1 and D_2 receptors as well as at β_2 receptors; it may have other effects such as inhibition of catecholamine uptake. It has favorable hemodynamic actions in patients with severe congestive heart failure, sepsis, and shock. In patients with low cardiac output, dopexamine infusion significantly increases stroke volume with a decrease in systemic vascular resistance. Tachycardia and hypotension can occur, but usually only at high infusion rates. Dopexamine is not currently available in the U.S.

β ADRENERGIC RECEPTOR AGONISTS

β agonists play a major role only in the treatment of bronchoconstriction in patients with asthma (reversible airway obstruction) or chronic obstructive pulmonary disease (COPD). Minor uses include management of preterm labor, treatment of complete heart block in shock, and short-term treatment of cardiac decompensation after surgery or in patients with congestive heart failure or myocardial infarction. β Receptor agonists may be used to stimulate the rate and force of cardiac contraction. The chronotropic effect is useful in the emergency treatment of arrhythmias such as torsade de pointes, bradycardia, or heart block (*see* Chapter 29).

ISOPROTERENOL

Isoproterenol (*see* Table 12–1) is a potent, nonselective β receptor agonist with very low affinity for α receptors. Consequently, isoproterenol has powerful effects on all β receptors and almost no action at α receptors.

PHARMACOLOGICAL ACTIONS. The major cardiovascular effects of isoproterenol (compared with EPI and NE) are illustrated in Figure 12–2. IV infusion of isoproterenol lowers peripheral vascular resistance, primarily in skeletal muscle but also in renal and mesenteric vascular beds. Diastolic blood pressure falls. Systolic blood pressure may remain unchanged or rise, although mean arterial pressure typically falls. Cardiac output is increased because of the positive inotropic and chronotropic effects of the drug in the face of diminished peripheral vascular resistance. The cardiac effects of isoproterenol may lead to palpitations, sinus tachycardia, and more serious arrhythmias.

Isoproterenol relaxes almost all varieties of smooth muscle when the tone is high, but this action is most pronounced on bronchial and GI smooth muscle. It prevents or relieves bronchoconstriction. Its effect in asthma may be due in part to an additional action to inhibit antigen-induced release of histamine and other mediators of inflammation; this action is shared by β_2-selective stimulants.

ABSORPTION, FATE, AND EXCRETION. Isoproterenol is readily absorbed when given parenterally or as an aerosol. It is metabolized primarily in the liver and other tissues by COMT. Isoproterenol is a relatively poor substrate for MAO and is not taken up by sympathetic neurons to the same extent as are EPI and NE. The duration of action of isoproterenol therefore may be longer than that of EPI, but it still is brief.

TOXICITY AND ADVERSE EFFECTS. Palpitations, tachycardia, headache, and flushing are common. Cardiac ischemia and arrhythmias may occur, particularly in patients with underlying coronary artery disease.

THERAPEUTIC USES. Isoproterenol (ISUPREL, others) may be used in emergencies to stimulate heart rate in patients with bradycardia or heart block, particularly in anticipation of inserting an artificial cardiac pacemaker or in patients with the ventricular arrhythmia torsade de pointes. In disorders such as asthma and shock, isoproterenol largely has been replaced by other sympathomimetic drugs (*see* below and Chapter 36).

DOBUTAMINE

The pharmacological effects of *dobutamine* (*see* Table 12–1) are due to direct interactions with α and β receptors and are complex.

Dobutamine possesses a center of asymmetry; both enantiomeric forms are present in the racemic mixture used clinically. The (–) isomer of dobutamine is a potent agonist at α_1 receptors and is capable of causing marked pressor responses; (+)-dobutamine is a potent α_1 receptor antagonist, which can block the effects of (–)-dobutamine. Both isomers are full agonists at β receptors, but the (+) isomer is a more potent β receptor agonist than the (–) isomer (~10-fold).

CARDIOVASCULAR EFFECTS. The cardiovascular effects of racemic dobutamine are a composite of the pharmacological properties of the (−) and (+) stereoisomers. Dobutamine has relatively more prominent inotropic than chronotropic effects on the heart compared to isoproterenol. Although not completely understood, this useful selectivity may arise because peripheral resistance is relatively unchanged. Alternatively, cardiac α_1 receptors may contribute to the inotropic effect. At equivalent inotropic doses, dobutamine enhances automaticity of the sinus node to a lesser extent than does isoproterenol; however, enhancement of atrioventricular and intraventricular conduction is similar for both drugs.

ADVERSE EFFECTS. Blood pressure and heart rate may increase significantly during dobutamine administration requiring reduction of infusion rate. Patients with a history of hypertension may exhibit an exaggerated pressor response more frequently. Because dobutamine facilitates AV conduction, patients with atrial fibrillation are at risk of marked increases in ventricular response rates; digoxin or other measures may be required to prevent this from occurring. Some patients may develop ventricular ectopic activity. As with any inotropic agent, dobutamine may increase the size of a myocardial infarct by increasing myocardial O_2 demand. The efficacy of dobutamine over a period of more than a few days is uncertain; there is evidence for the development of tolerance.

THERAPEUTIC USES. Dobutamine (DOBUTREX) is indicated for the short-term treatment of cardiac decompensation that may occur after cardiac surgery or in patients with congestive heart failure or acute myocardial infarction. Dobutamine increases cardiac output and stroke volume in such patients, usually without a marked increase in heart rate. Alterations in blood pressure or peripheral resistance usually are minor. An infusion of dobutamine in combination with echocardiography is useful in the noninvasive assessment of patients with coronary artery disease.

Dobutamine has a $t_{1/2}$ ~2 min; the onset of effect is rapid, steady-state concentrations are achieved within 10 min, and major metabolites are conjugates of dobutamine and 3-*O*-methyldobutamine. The rate of infusion required to increase cardiac output is 2.5-10 μg/kg/min; higher infusion rates occasionally are required. The rate and duration of the infusion are determined by the clinical and hemodynamic responses of the patient.

β_2-SELECTIVE ADRENERGIC RECEPTOR AGONISTS

In the treatment of asthma or COPD, drugs with preferential affinity for β_2 receptors compared with β_1 receptors have been developed. The selectivity, however, is not absolute, and is lost at high concentrations of these drugs. Moreover up to 40% of the β receptors in the human heart are β_2 receptors, activation of which can cause cardiac stimulation. A useful strategy to enhance preferential activation of pulmonary β_2 receptors is the administration by inhalation of small doses of the drug in aerosol form. This approach typically leads to effective activation of β_2 receptors in the bronchi but very low systemic drug concentrations. Consequently, there is less potential to activate cardiac β_1 or β_2 receptors or to stimulate β_2 receptors in skeletal muscle, which can cause tremor and thereby limit oral therapy.

Administration of β agonists by aerosol (*see* Chapter 36) typically leads to a very rapid therapeutic response, generally within minutes, although some agonists such as salmeterol have a delayed onset of action. Only ~10% of an inhaled dose actually enters the lungs; much of the remainder is swallowed and ultimately may be absorbed.

In the treatment of asthma and COPD, β receptor agonists are used to activate pulmonary receptors that relax bronchial smooth muscle and decrease airway resistance. β receptor agonists also may suppress the release of leukotrienes and histamine from mast cells in lung tissue, enhance mucociliary function, and decrease microvascular permeability.

SHORT-ACTING β_2 ADRENERGIC AGONISTS

METAPROTERENOL. *Metaproterenol* (called *orciprenaline* in Europe), along with *terbutaline* and *fenoterol*, belongs to the structural class of resorcinol bronchodilators that have hydroxyl groups at positions 3 and 5 of the phenyl ring (rather than at positions 3 and 4 as in catechols) (*see* Table 12–1). Consequently, metaproterenol is resistant to methylation by COMT. It is excreted primarily as glucuronic acid conjugates. Metaproterenol is considered to be β_2-selective, although it probably is less selective than albuterol or terbutaline and hence is more prone to cause cardiac stimulation.

Effects occur within minutes of inhalation and persist for several hours. After oral administration, onset of action is slower, but effects last 3-4 h. Metaproterenol is used for the long-term treatment of obstructive airway diseases, asthma, and for treatment of acute bronchospasm. Side effects are similar to the short- and intermediate-acting sympathomimetic bronchodilators.

ALBUTEROL. Albuterol (VENTOLIN-HFA, PROVENTIL-HFA, others; *see* Table 12–1) is a selective β_2 receptor agonist with pharmacological properties and therapeutic indications similar to those of terbutaline. It is administered either by inhalation or orally for the symptomatic relief of bronchospasm.

When administered by inhalation, it produces significant bronchodilation within 15 min, and effects persist for 3-4 h. The cardiovascular effects of albuterol are considerably weaker than those of isoproterenol when doses that produce comparable bronchodilation are administered by inhalation. Oral albuterol has the potential to delay preterm labor. Although rare, CNS and respiratory side effects are sometimes observed.

LEVALBUTEROL. Levalbuterol (XOPENEX) is the R-enantiomer of albuterol that is a used to treat asthma and COPD. Levalbuterol is β_2-selective and acts like other β_2 adrenergic agonists and has similar pharmacokinetic and pharmacodynamics properties to albuterol.

PIRBUTEROL. Pirbuterol is a relatively selective β_2 agonist. Pirbuterol acetate (MAXAIR) is available for inhalation therapy; dosing is typically every 4-6 h.

TERBUTALINE. Terbutaline is a β_2-selective bronchodilator. It contains a resorcinol ring and thus is not a substrate for COMT methylation. It is effective when taken orally, subcutaneously, or by inhalation (not marketed for inhalation in the U.S.).

Effects are observed rapidly after inhalation or parenteral administration; after inhalation its action may persist 3-6 h. With oral administration, the onset of effect may be delayed 1-2 h. Terbutaline (BRETHINE, others) is used for the long-term treatment of obstructive airway diseases and for treatment of acute bronchospasm, and also is available for parenteral use for the emergency treatment of status asthmaticus (*see* Chapter 36).

ISOETHARINE. Isoetharine selectivity for β_2 receptors may not approach that of some of the other agents. Although resistant to metabolism by MAO, it is a catecholamine and thus is a good substrate for COMT. It is used only by inhalation for the treatment of acute episodes of bronchoconstriction. Isoetharine is not marketed in the U.S.

BITOLTEROL. Bitolterol (TORNALATE) is a β_2 agonist in which the hydroxyl groups in the catechol moiety are protected by esterification. Esterases in the lung and other tissues hydrolyze this prodrug to the active form, colterol, or terbutylnorepinephrine. The duration of effect of bitolterol after inhalation ranges from 3-6 h. Bitolterol has been discontinued in the U.S.

FENOTEROL. Fenoterol (BEROTEC) is a β_2-selective receptor agonist. After inhalation, it has a prompt onset of action, and its effect typically is sustained for 4-6 h. The possible association of fenoterol use with increased deaths from asthma, although controversial, has led to its withdrawal from the market.

PROCATEROL. Procaterol (MASCACIN, others) is a β_2-selective receptor agonist. After inhalation, it has a prompt onset of action that is sustained for ~5 h. Procaterol is not available in the U.S.

LONG-ACTING β_2 ADRENERGIC AGONISTS (LABA)

SALMETEROL. Salmeterol (SEREVENT) is a β_2-selective agonist with a prolonged duration of action (>12 h); it has at least 50-fold greater selectivity for β_2 receptors than albuterol. It provides symptomatic relief and improves lung function and quality of life in patients with COPD. It has additive effects when used in combination with inhaled ipratropium or oral theophylline. It is highly lipophilic and has a sustained duration of action. It also may have anti-inflammatory activity.

Salmeterol is metabolized by CYP3A4 to α-hydroxy-salmeterol, which is eliminated primarily in the feces. The onset of action of inhaled salmeterol is relatively slow, so it is not suitable monotherapy for acute breakthrough attacks of bronchospasm. Salmeterol generally is well tolerated. Salmeterol should not be used more than twice daily (morning and evening) and should not be used to treat acute asthma symptoms, which should be treated with a short-acting β_2 agonist (e.g., albuterol) when breakthrough symptoms occur despite twice-daily use of salmeterol. The use of LABA is recommended only for patients in whom inhaled corticosteroids alone either have failed to achieve good asthma control or for initial therapy.

FORMOTEROL. Formoterol (FORADIL, others) is a long-acting β_2-selective receptor agonist. Significant bronchodilation occurs within minutes of inhalation of a therapeutic dose, which may persist for up to 12 h. It is highly lipophilic and has high affinity for β_2 receptors. Its major advantage over many other β_2-selective agonists is this prolonged duration of action. Formoterol is FDA-approved for treatment of asthma, bronchospasm, prophylaxis of exercise-induced bronchospasm, and COPD. It can be used concomitantly with short-acting β_2 agonists, glucocorticoids (inhaled or systemic), and theophylline.

ARFORMOTEROL. Arformoterol (BROVANA), the (R,R) enantiomer of formoterol, is a selective long-acting β_2 agonist that has twice the potency of racemic formoterol. It is used for the long-term treatment of bronchoconstriction in patients with COPD, including chronic bronchitis and emphysema. Systemic exposure to arformoterol is due to pulmonary absorption with plasma levels reaching peak levels in 0.25-1 h. Plasma protein binding is 52-65%. It is primarily metabolized by CYP2D6 and CYP2C19. It does not inhibit any of the common CYPs.

INDACATEROL. Indacaterol is a once-daily long-acting β adrenergic agonist, classified as an *ultra-LABA*, was recently approved for treatment of COPD.

It has a fast onset of action, long duration, and appears well tolerated. Indacaterol behaves as a potent β_2 agonist with high intrinsic efficacy, which, in contrast to salmeterol, does not antagonize the bronchorelaxant effect of short-acting β_2 adrenergic agonists. Evidence indicates that indacaterol has a longer duration of action than salmeterol and formoterol. Indacaterol is not indicated for the treatment of asthma.

Carmoterol is also an ultra-LABA that is currently in phase III clinical trials in the U.S.

RITODRINE. Ritodrine is a β_2-selective agonist that was developed specifically for use as a uterine relaxant. Nevertheless, its pharmacological properties closely resemble those of the other agents in this group.

The pharmacokinetic properties of ritodrine are complex and incompletely defined, especially in pregnant women. Ritodrine may be administered intravenously to selected patients to arrest premature labor. However, β_2-selective agonists may not have clinically significant benefits on perinatal mortality and may actually increase maternal morbidity. Ritodrine is not available in the U.S. *See* Chapter 66 for the pharmacology of tocolytic agents.

ADVERSE EFFECTS OF β_2-SELECTIVE AGONISTS. The major adverse effects of β receptor agonists occur as a result of excessive activation of β receptors. Patients with underlying cardiovascular disease are particularly at risk for significant reactions. However, the likelihood of adverse effects can be greatly decreased in patients with lung disease by administering the drug by inhalation.

Tremor is a relatively common adverse effect of the β_2-selective receptor agonists. Tolerance generally develops to this effect. This adverse effect can be minimized by starting oral therapy with a low dose of drug and progressively increasing the dose as tolerance to the tremor develops. Feelings of restlessness, apprehension, and anxiety may limit therapy with these drugs, particularly oral or parenteral administration.

Tachycardia is a common adverse effect of systemically administered β receptor agonists. Stimulation of heart rate occurs primarily by means of β_1 receptors. During a severe asthma attack, heart rate actually may decrease during therapy with a β agonist, presumably because of improvement in pulmonary function with consequent reduction in endogenous cardiac sympathetic stimulation. In patients without cardiac disease, β agonists rarely cause significant arrhythmias or myocardial ischemia; however, patients with underlying coronary artery disease or preexisting arrhythmias are at greater risk. The risk of adverse cardiovascular effects also is increased in patients who are receiving MAO inhibitors. In general, at least 2 weeks should elapse between the use of MAO inhibitors and administration of β_2 agonists or other sympathomimetics.

When given parenterally, these drugs may increase the concentrations of plasma glucose, lactate, and free fatty acids and decrease the concentration of K^+. The decrease in K^+ concentration is especially important in patients with cardiac disease taking digoxin and diuretics. In some diabetic patients, hyperglycemia may be worsened and higher doses of insulin may be required. These adverse effects are far less likely with inhalation therapy.

β_3-SELECTIVE ADRENERGIC RECEPTOR AGONISTS

MIRABEGRON. (MYRBETRIQ), a selective β_3 adrenergic agonist, is approved for the treatment of overactive bladder (urinary urgency, frequency, urge incontinence). The drug activates β_3 adrenergic receptors on the detrusor muscle of the bladder to facilitate filling of the bladder and storage of urine. The drug is administered orally with a starting dose of 25 mg once daily. Side effects may include hypertension, nasopharyngitis, urinary tract infection, and headache. Mirabegron is an inhibitor of CYPs 2D6 and 3A.

α_1-SELECTIVE ADRENERGIC RECEPTOR AGONISTS

Activation of α adrenergic receptors in vascular smooth muscle results in contraction, causing increases in peripheral vascular resistance and increases in blood pressure. Although the clinical utility of these drugs is limited, they may be useful in the treatment of some patients with hypotension, including orthostatic hypotension, or shock. *Phenylephrine* and *methoxamine* (discontinued in the U.S.) are direct-acting vasoconstrictors and are selective activators of α_1 receptors. *Mephentermine* and *metaraminol* act both directly and indirectly. *Midodrine* is a prodrug that is converted, after oral administration, to *desglymidodrine*, a direct-acting α_1 agonist.

PHENYLEPHRINE. Phenylephrine (NEO-SYNEPHRINE, others) is a α_1-selective agonist; it activates β receptors only at much higher concentrations. The drug causes marked arterial vasoconstriction during intravenous infusion. Phenylephrine (NEO-SYNEPHRINE, others) also is used as a nasal decongestant and as a mydriatic in various nasal and ophthalmic formulations (*see* Chapter 64).

MEPHENTERMINE. Mephentermine acts both directly and indirectly. After an intramuscular injection, the onset of action is prompt (within 5-15 min), and effects may last for several hours. Because the drug releases NE, cardiac contraction is enhanced, and cardiac output and systolic and diastolic pressures usually are increased. The change in heart rate is variable, depending on the degree of vagal tone. Adverse effects are related to CNS stimulation, excessive rises in blood pressure, and arrhythmias. Mephentermine is used to prevent hypotension, which frequently accompanies spinal anesthesia. The drug has been discontinued in the U.S.

METARAMINOL. Metaraminol exerts direct effects on vascular α adrenergic receptors. Metaraminol also is an indirectly acting agent that stimulates the release of NE. The drug has been used in the treatment of hypotensive states or off-label to relieve attacks of paroxysmal atrial tachycardia, particularly those associated with hypotension (*see* Chapter 29).

MIDODRINE. Midodrine (PROAMATINE, others) is an orally effective α_1 receptor agonist. It is a prodrug, converted to an active metabolite, desglymidodrine. Midodrine-induced rises in blood pressure are associated with both arterial and venous smooth muscle contraction. A frequent complication in these patients is supine hypertension. This can be minimized by administering the drug during periods when the patient will remain upright, and elevating the head of the bed. Typical dosing, achieved by careful titration of blood pressure responses, varies between 2.5 and 10 mg thrice daily.

α_2-SELECTIVE ADRENERGIC RECEPTOR AGONISTS

α_2-Selective adrenergic agonists are used primarily for the treatment of systemic hypertension. Their efficacy as antihypertensive agents is somewhat surprising, as many blood vessels contain postsynaptic α_2 adrenergic receptors that promote vasoconstriction (*see* Chapter 8). Clonidine, the prototypic α_2 agonist, lowers blood pressure by activation of α_2 receptors in the CNS. Some α_2 agonists are used to reduce intraocular pressure.

CLONIDINE

Intravenous infusion of clonidine causes an acute rise in blood pressure, because of activation of postsynaptic α_2 receptors in vascular smooth muscle. This transient vasoconstriction (not usually seen with oral administration) is followed by a more prolonged hypotensive response that results from decreased sympathetic outflow from the CNS. The effect appears to result, at least in part, from activation of α_2 receptors in the lower brainstem region. Clonidine also stimulates parasympathetic outflow, which may contribute to the slowing of heart rate. In addition, some of the antihypertensive effects of clonidine may be mediated by activation of presynaptic α_2 receptors that suppress the release of NE, ATP, and NPY from postganglionic sympathetic nerves. Clonidine decreases the plasma concentration of NE and reduces its excretion in the urine.

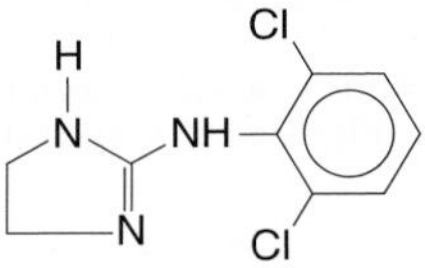

H N NH Cl N Cl

CLONIDINE

ABSORPTION, FATE, AND EXCRETION. Clonidine is well absorbed after oral administration, with bioavailability ~100%. Peak concentration in plasma and the maximal hypotensive effect are observed 1-3 h after an oral dose. The elimination $t_{1/2}$ is 6-24 h (mean of ~12 h). About half of an administered dose can be recovered unchanged in the urine; the $t_{1/2}$ of the drug may increase with renal failure. A transdermal delivery patch permits continuous administration of clonidine as an alternative to oral therapy. The drug is released at an approximately constant rate for a week; 3-4 days are required to reach steady-state concentrations in plasma. When the patch is removed, plasma concentrations remain stable for ~8 h and then decline gradually over a period of several days; this decrease is associated with a rise in blood pressure.

ADVERSE EFFECTS. The major adverse effects of clonidine are dry mouth and sedation, which may diminish in intensity after several weeks of therapy. Sexual dysfunction also may occur. Marked bradycardia is observed in some patients. These effects of clonidine frequently are related to dose, and their incidence may be lower with transdermal administration of clonidine. About 15-20% of patients develop contact dermatitis when using the transdermal system. Withdrawal reactions follow abrupt discontinuation of long-term therapy with clonidine in some hypertensive patients (*see* Chapter 27).

THERAPEUTIC USES. The major therapeutic use of clonidine (CATAPRES, others) is in the treatment of hypertension (*see* Chapter 27). Clonidine also has apparent efficacy in the off-label treatment of a range of other disorders: in reducing diarrhea in some diabetic patients with autonomic neuropathy, in treating and preparing addicted subjects for withdrawal from narcotics, alcohol, and tobacco (*see* Chapter 24) by ameliorating some of the adverse sympathetic nervous activity associated with withdrawal and decreasing craving for the drug, in reducing the incidence of menopausal hot flashes (transdermal application of CATAPRES). Acute administration of clonidine has been used in the differential diagnosis of patients with hypertension and suspected pheochromocytoma. Among the other off-label uses of clonidine are atrial fibrillation, attention deficit hyperactivity disorder (ADHD), constitutional growth delay in children, cyclosporine-associated nephrotoxicity, Tourette syndrome, hyperhidrosis, mania, posthepatic neuralgia, psychosis, restless leg syndrome, ulcerative colitis, and allergy-induced inflammatory reactions in patients with extrinsic asthma.

APRACLONIDINE. *Apraclonidine* (IOPIDINE) is a relatively selective α_2 receptor agonist that is used topically to reduce intraocular pressure with minimal systemic effects.

Apraclonidine does not cross the blood-brain barrier and is more useful than clonidine for ophthalmic therapy. Apraclonidine is useful as short-term adjunctive therapy in glaucoma patients whose intraocular pressure is not well controlled by other pharmacological agents. The drug also is used to control or prevent elevations in intraocular pressure that occur in patients after laser trabeculoplasty or iridotomy (*see* Chapter 64).

BRIMONIDINE. *Brimonidine* (ALPHAGAN, others) is a clonidine derivative and α_2-selective agonist that is administered ocularly to lower intraocular pressure in patients with ocular hypertension or open-angle glaucoma. Unlike apraclonidine, brimonidine can cross the blood-brain barrier and can produce hypotension and sedation, although these CNS effects are slight compared to those of clonidine.

GUANFACINE. *Guanfacine* (TENEX, others) is an α_2 receptor agonist that is more selective for α_2 receptors than is clonidine. Guanfacine lowers blood pressure by activation of brainstem receptors with resultant suppression of sympathetic activity. A sustained-release form (INTUNIV) is FDA-approved for treatment of ADHD in children ages 6-17 years. Guanfacine and clonidine appear to have similar efficacy for the treatment of hypertension and similar pattern of adverse effects. A withdrawal syndrome may occur after the abrupt discontinuation, but it is less frequent and milder than the syndrome that follows clonidine withdrawal; this difference may relate to the longer $t_{1/2}$ of guanfacine.

GUANABENZ. Guanabenz (WYTENSIN, others) is a centrally acting α_2 agonist that decreases blood pressure by a mechanism similar to those of clonidine and guanfacine. Guanabenz has a $t_{1/2}$ of 4-6 h and is extensively metabolized by the liver; dosage adjustment may be necessary in patients with hepatic cirrhosis. The adverse effects caused by guanabenz are similar to those seen with clonidine.

METHYLDOPA. Methyldopa (α-methyl-3,4-dihydroxyphenylalanine) is a centrally acting antihypertensive agent. It is metabolized to α-methylnorepinephrine in the brain, and this compound is thought to activate central α_2 receptors and lower blood pressure in a manner similar to that of clonidine (*see* Chapter 27).

TIZANIDINE. Tizanidine (ZANAFLEX, others) is a muscle relaxant used for the treatment of spasticity associated with cerebral and spinal disorders. It is also an α_2 agonist with some properties similar to those of clonidine.

MISCELLANEOUS SYMPATHOMIMETIC AGONISTS

AMPHETAMINE

Amphetamine, racemic β-phenylisopropylamine (*see* Table 12–1), has powerful CNS stimulant actions and α and β receptor stimulation in the periphery. Unlike EPI, it is effective after oral administration and its effects last for several hours.

CARDIOVASCULAR SYSTEM. Amphetamine given orally raises both systolic and diastolic blood pressure. Heart rate often is reflexly slowed; with large doses, cardiac arrhythmias may occur.

OTHER SMOOTH MUSCLES. In general, smooth muscles respond to amphetamine as they do to other sympathomimetic amines. The contractile effect on the sphincter of the urinary bladder is particularly marked, and for this reason amphetamine has been used in treating enuresis and incontinence. Pain and difficulty in micturition occasionally occur. The GI effects of amphetamine are unpredictable. If enteric activity is pronounced, amphetamine may cause relaxation and delay the movement of intestinal contents; if the gut already is relaxed, the opposite effect may occur. The response of the human uterus varies, but there usually is an increase in tone.

CNS. Amphetamine is one of the most potent sympathomimetic amines in stimulating the CNS. It stimulates the medullary respiratory center, lessens the degree of central depression caused by various drugs, and produces other signs of CNS stimulation. In eliciting of CNS excitatory effects, the *d*-isomer (dextroamphetamine) is 3-4 times more potent than the *l*-isomer. The psychic effects depend on the dose and the mental state and personality of the individual. The main results of an oral dose of 10-30 mg include wakefulness, alertness, and a decreased sense of fatigue; elevation of mood, with increased initiative, self-confidence, and ability to concentrate; often, elation and euphoria; and increase in motor and speech activities. Performance of simple mental tasks is improved, but, although more work may be accomplished, the number of errors may increase. Physical performance (e.g., in athletes) is improved, and the drug often is abused for this purpose. These effects are variable and may be reversed by overdosage or repeated usage. Prolonged use or large doses are nearly always followed by depression and fatigue. Many individuals given amphetamine experience headache, palpitation, dizziness, vasomotor disturbances, agitation, confusion, dysphoria, apprehension, delirium, or fatigue (*see* Chapter 24).

FATIGUE AND SLEEP. In general, amphetamine prolongs the duration of adequate performance before fatigue appears, and the effects of fatigue are at least partly reversed. Amphetamine reduces the frequency of attention lapses that impair performance after prolonged sleep deprivation and thus improves execution of tasks requiring sustained attention. The need for sleep may be postponed, but it cannot be avoided indefinitely. When the drug is discontinued after long use, the pattern of sleep may take as long as 2 months to return to normal.

ANALGESIA. Amphetamine and some other sympathomimetic amines have a small analgesic effect, but it is not sufficiently pronounced to be therapeutically useful. However, amphetamine can enhance the analgesia produced by opiates.

Respiration. Amphetamine stimulates the respiratory center, increasing the rate and depth of respiration. In normal individuals, usual doses of the drug do not appreciably increase respiratory rate or minute volume. Nevertheless, when respiration is depressed by centrally acting drugs, amphetamine may stimulate respiration.

Depression of Appetite. Amphetamine and similar drugs have been used for the treatment of obesity. Weight loss is almost entirely due to reduced food intake and only in small measure to increased metabolism. In humans, tolerance to the appetite suppression develops rapidly.

Mechanisms of Action in the CNS. Amphetamine exerts its effects in the CNS by releasing biogenic amines from their storage sites in nerve terminals. The neuronal dopamine transporter (DAT) and the vesicular monoamine transporter 2 (VMAT2) appear to be 2 of the principal targets of amphetamine's action. The alerting effect of amphetamine, its anorectic effect, and at least a component of its locomotor-stimulating action presumably are mediated by release of NE from central noradrenergic neurons. Some aspects of locomotor activity and the stereotyped behavior induced by amphetamine probably are a consequence of the release of DA from dopaminergic nerve terminals, particularly in the neostriatum. Higher doses are required to produce the behavioral effects. With still higher doses of amphetamine, disturbances of perception and overt psychotic behavior occur, possibly due to release of 5HT from serotonergic neurons and of DA in the mesolimbic system.

TOXICITY AND ADVERSE EFFECTS. The acute toxic effects of amphetamine usually are extensions of its therapeutic actions, and as a rule result from overdosage. CNS effects commonly include restlessness, dizziness, tremor, hyperactive reflexes, talkativeness, tenseness, irritability, weakness, insomnia, fever, and sometimes euphoria. Confusion, aggressiveness, changes in libido, anxiety, delirium, paranoid hallucinations, panic states, and suicidal or homicidal tendencies occur, especially in mentally ill patients. However, these psychotic effects can be elicited in any individual if sufficient quantities of amphetamine are ingested for a prolonged period. Fatigue and depression usually follow central stimulation. Cardiovascular effects are common and include headache, chilliness, pallor or flushing, palpitation, cardiac arrhythmias, anginal pain, hypertension or hypotension, and circulatory collapse. Excessive sweating occurs. GI symptoms include dry mouth, metallic taste, anorexia, nausea, vomiting, diarrhea, and abdominal cramps. Fatal poisoning usually terminates in convulsions and coma, and cerebral hemorrhages are the main pathological findings.

The toxic dose of amphetamine varies widely; occasionally occurring after as little as 2 mg, but rare with <15 mg. Severe reactions have occurred with 30 mg, yet doses of 400-500 mg are not uniformly fatal. Larger doses can be tolerated after chronic use of the drug. Treatment of acute amphetamine intoxication may include acidification of the urine by administration of ammonium chloride to enhance the rate of elimination. Sedatives may be required for the CNS symptoms. Severe hypertension may require administration of sodium nitroprusside or an α adrenergic receptor antagonist. Chronic intoxication with amphetamine causes symptoms similar to those of acute overdosage. Weight loss may be marked. A psychotic reaction with vivid hallucinations and paranoid delusions, often mistaken for schizophrenia, is the most common serious effect. Recovery is rapid after withdrawal of the drug, but occasionally the condition becomes chronic, with amphetamine hastening the onset of incipient schizophrenia. Amphetamines are schedule II drugs and should be used only under medical supervision. Amphetamine use is inadvisable in patients with anorexia, insomnia, asthenia, psychopathic personality, or a history of homicidal or suicidal tendencies.

DEPENDENCE AND TOLERANCE. Psychological dependence often occurs when amphetamine or dextroamphetamine is used chronically, as discussed in Chapter 24. Tolerance almost invariably develops to the anorexigenic effect of amphetamines, and often is seen also in the need for increasing doses to maintain improvement of mood in psychiatric patients. Development of tolerance is not invariable, and cases of narcolepsy have been treated for years without requiring an increase in the initially effective dose.

THERAPEUTIC USES. Amphetamine is used chiefly for its CNS effects. Dextroamphetamine is FDA-approved for the treatment of narcolepsy and ADHD (*see* below).

METHAMPHETAMINE

Methamphetamine (DESOXYN; *see* Table 12–1) acts centrally to release DA and other biogenic amines, and to inhibit neuronal and vesicular monoamine transporters as well as MAO. Small doses have prominent central stimulant effects without significant peripheral actions; somewhat larger doses produce a sustained rise in systolic and diastolic blood pressures, due mainly to cardiac stimulation. Methamphetamine is a schedule II drug and has high potential for abuse (*see* Chapter 24).

METHYLPHENIDATE

Methylphenidate is structurally related to amphetamine.

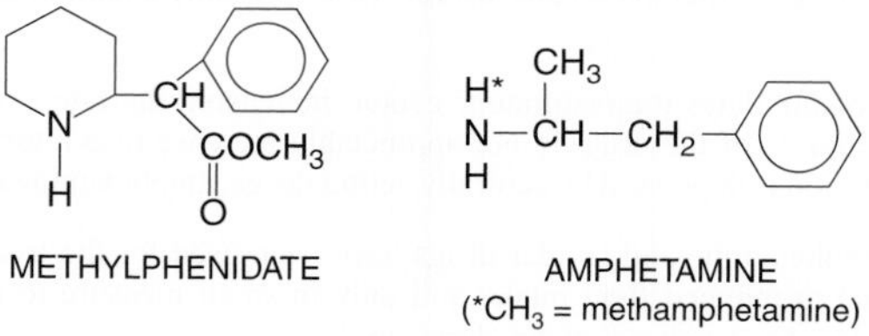

CH, N, H, $COCH_3$, O

METHYLPHENIDATE

CH_3, H*, N—CH—CH_2—, H

AMPHETAMINE
(*CH_3 = methamphetamine)

Methylphenidate (RITALIN, others) is a mild CNS stimulant with more prominent effects on mental than on motor activities. However, large doses produce signs of generalized CNS stimulation that may lead to convulsions. In pharmacological properties, it resembles amphetamines. Methylphenidate also shares the abuse potential of the amphetamines and is listed as a schedule II controlled substance in the U.S. Methylphenidate is effective in the treatment of narcolepsy and ADHD. The use of methylphenidate is contraindicated in patients with glaucoma.

DEXMETHYLPHENIDATE. Dexmethylphenidate (FOCALIN) is the *d*-threo enantiomer of racemic methylphenidate. It is FDA-approved as a schedule II drug for the treatment of ADHD.

PEMOLINE. Pemoline (CYLERT, others) is structurally dissimilar to methylphenidate but elicits similar changes in CNS function with minimal effects on the cardiovascular system. It is employed in treating ADHD. It can be given once daily because of its long $t_{1/2}$. Clinical improvement may require treatment for 3-4 weeks. Use of pemoline has been associated with severe hepatic failure and was discontinued in the U.S. in 2006.

EPHEDRINE

Ephedrine is an agonist at both α and β receptors; in addition, it enhances release of NE from sympathetic neurons and thus is a mixed-acting sympathomimetic (*see* Table 12–1 and Figure 12–1).

Only *l*-ephedrine and racemic ephedrine are used clinically. Ephedrine is effective after oral administration. The drug stimulates heart rate and cardiac output and variably increases peripheral resistance; as a result, ephedrine usually increases blood pressure. Activation of β receptors in the lungs promotes bronchodilation. Ephedrine is a potent CNS stimulant. After oral administration, the effects of the drug persist for several hours.

THERAPEUTIC USES AND TOXICITY. The use of ephedrine as a bronchodilator in patients with asthma has become less extensive with the development of β_2-selective agonists. Ephedrine has been used to promote urinary continence. Ephedrine also has been used to treat the hypotension that may occur with spinal anesthesia.

Untoward effects of ephedrine include hypertension and insomnia. Concerns have been raised about the safety of ephedrine. Large amounts of herbal preparations containing ephedrine (ma huang, ephedra) are used around the world. The considerable variability in the content of ephedrine in these preparations is a cause for concern and can lead to inadvertent consumption of dangerous doses of ephedrine and its isomers. The Combat Methamphetamine Epidemic Act of 2005 regulates the sale of ephedrine, phenylpropanolamine, and pseudoephedrine, which can be used as precursors in the illicit manufacture of amphetamine and methamphetamine.

OTHER SYMPATHOMIMETIC AGENTS

Several sympathomimetic drugs are used primarily as vasoconstrictors for local application to the nasal mucous membrane or the eye: propylhexedrine (BENZEDREX, others), naphazoline (PRIVINE, NAPHCON, others), oxymetazoline (AFRIN, OCUCLEAR, others), and xylometazoline (OTRIVIN, others). Phenylephrine, pseudoephedrine (SUDAFED, others) (a stereoisomer of ephedrine), and phenylpropanolamine have been used most commonly in oral preparations for the relief of nasal congestion. Phenylpropanolamine shares the pharmacological properties of ephedrine and is approximately equal in potency except that it causes less CNS stimulation. Because phenylpropanolamine may increase the risk of hemorrhagic stroke, the drug is no longer licensed for marketing in the U.S.

THERAPEUTIC USES OF SYMPATHOMIMETIC DRUGS

SHOCK. Shock is an immediately life-threatening impairment of delivery of oxygen and nutrients to the organs of the body. Causes of shock include hypovolemia (due to dehydration or blood loss), cardiac failure (extensive myocardial infarction, severe arrhythmia), obstruction to cardiac output, and peripheral circulatory dysfunction (sepsis or anaphylaxis). The treatment of shock consists of reversing the underlying pathogenesis as well as nonspecific measures aimed at correcting hemodynamic abnormalities. The accompanying fall in blood pressure generally leads to marked activation of the sympathetic nervous system. This, in turn, causes peripheral vasoconstriction and an increase in the rate and force of cardiac contraction. In the initial stages of shock these mechanisms may maintain blood pressure and cerebral blood flow, although blood flow to the kidneys, skin, and other organs may be decreased, leading to impaired production of urine and metabolic acidosis.

The initial therapy of shock involves basic life-support measures. It is essential to maintain blood volume, which often requires monitoring of hemodynamic parameters. Specific therapy (e.g., antibiotics for patients in septic shock) should be initiated immediately. If these measures do not lead to an adequate therapeutic response, it may be necessary to use vasoactive drugs. Many of these pharmacological approaches, while apparently clinically reasonable, are of uncertain efficacy. Adrenergic receptor agonists may be used in an attempt to increase myocardial contractility or to modify peripheral vascular resistance. In general terms, β receptor agonists increase heart rate and force of contraction, α receptor agonists increase peripheral vascular resistance, and DA promotes dilation of renal and splanchnic vascular beds, in addition to activating β and α receptors.

Cardiogenic shock due to myocardial infarction has a poor prognosis; therapy is aimed at improving peripheral blood flow. Medical intervention is designed to optimize cardiac filling pressure (preload), myocardial contractility, and peripheral resistance (afterload). Preload may be increased by administration of intravenous fluids or reduced with drugs such as diuretics and nitrates. A number of sympathomimetic amines have been used to increase the force of contraction of the heart. Some of these drugs have disadvantages: isoproterenol is a powerful chronotropic agent and can greatly increase myocardial O_2 demand; NE intensifies peripheral vasoconstriction; and EPI increases heart rate and may predispose the heart to dangerous arrhythmias. DA is an effective inotropic agent that causes less increase in heart rate than does isoproterenol. DA also promotes renal arterial dilation; this may be useful in preserving renal function. When given in high doses (>10-20 μg/kg/min), DA activates α receptors, causing peripheral and renal vasoconstriction. Dobutamine has complex pharmacological actions that are mediated by its stereoisomers; the clinical effects of the drug are to increase myocardial contractility with little increase in heart rate or peripheral resistance.

In some patients, hypotension is so severe that vasoconstricting drugs are required to maintain a blood pressure that is adequate for CNS perfusion. α Agonists have been used for this purpose. This approach may be advantageous in patients with hypotension due to failure of the sympathetic nervous system (e.g., after spinal anesthesia or injury). However, in patients with other forms of shock, such as cardiogenic shock, reflex vasoconstriction generally is intense, and α receptor agonists may further compromise blood flow to organs such as the kidneys and gut and adversely increase the work of the heart. Vasodilating drugs such as nitroprusside are more likely to improve blood flow and decrease cardiac work in such patients by decreasing afterload if a minimally adequate blood pressure can be maintained.

The hemodynamic abnormalities in septic shock are complex and poorly understood. Most patients with septic shock initially have low or barely normal peripheral vascular resistance, possibly owing to excessive effects of endogenously produced NO as well as normal or increased cardiac output. If the syndrome progresses, myocardial depression, increased peripheral resistance, and impaired tissue oxygenation occur. The primary treatment of septic shock is antibiotics. Therapy with drugs such as DA or dobutamine is guided by hemodynamic monitoring.

HYPOTENSION. Drugs with predominantly α agonist activity can be used to raise blood pressure in patients with decreased peripheral resistance in conditions such as spinal anesthesia or intoxication with antihypertensive medications. However, hypotension per se is not an indication for treatment with these agents unless there is inadequate perfusion of organs such as the brain, heart, or kidneys. Furthermore, adequate replacement of fluid or blood may be more appropriate than drug therapy for many patients with hypotension.

Patients with orthostatic hypotension often represent a pharmacological challenge. Therapeutic approaches include physical maneuvers and a variety of drugs (fludrocortisone, prostaglandin synthesis inhibitors, somatostatin analogs, caffeine, vasopressin analogs, DA antagonists, and some sympathomimetic drugs). The ideal agent would enhance venous constriction prominently and produce relatively little arterial constriction so as to avoid supine hypertension. No such agent currently is available. Drugs used include α_1 agonists and indirect-acting agents. Midodrine shows promise in treating this disorder.

HYPERTENSION. Centrally acting α_2 agonists such as clonidine are useful in the treatment of hypertension. Drug therapy of hypertension is discussed in Chapter 27.

ALLERGIC REACTIONS. EPI is the drug of choice to reverse the manifestations of serious acute hypersensitivity reactions (e.g., from food, bee sting, or drug allergy).

A subcutaneous injection of EPI rapidly relieves itching, hives, and swelling of lips, eyelids, and tongue. In some patients, careful intravenous infusion of EPI may be required to ensure prompt pharmacological effects. In addition to its cardiovascular effects, EPI is thought to activate β receptors that suppress the release from mast cells of mediators such as histamine and leukotrienes. EPI auto-injectors (EPIPEN, others) are employed widely for the emergency self-treatment of anaphylaxis.

CARDIAC ARRHYTHMIAS. Cardiopulmonary resuscitation in patients with cardiac arrest due to ventricular fibrillation, electromechanical dissociation, or asystole may be facilitated by drug treatment. EPI is an important therapeutic agent in patients with cardiac arrest. α Agonists also help to preserve cerebral blood flow during resuscitation. Consequently, during external cardiac massage, EPI facilitates distribution of the limited cardiac output to the cerebral and coronary circulations. The optimal dose of EPI in patients with cardiac arrest is unclear. Once a cardiac rhythm has been restored, it may be necessary to treat arrhythmias, hypotension, or shock.

LOCAL VASCULAR EFFECTS. EPI is used in many surgical procedures in the nose, throat, and larynx to shrink the mucosa and improve visualization by limiting hemorrhage. Simultaneous injection of EPI with local anesthetics retards the absorption and increases the duration of anesthesia (*see* Chapter 20). Injection of α agonists into the penis may be useful in reversing priapism, a complication of the use of α receptor antagonists or PDE5 inhibitors (e.g., sildenafil) in the treatment of erectile dysfunction. Both phenylephrine and oxymetazoline are efficacious vasoconstrictors when applied locally during sinus surgery.

NASAL DECONGESTION. α Receptor agonists are used extensively as nasal decongestants. α Agonists may be administered either orally or topically. Sympathomimetic decongestants should be used with great caution in patients with hypertension and in men with prostatic enlargement, and they are contraindicated in patients who are taking MAO inhibitors. Oral decongestants are much less likely to cause rebound congestion but carry a greater risk of inducing adverse systemic effects. Patients with uncontrolled hypertension or ischemic heart disease generally should avoid the oral consumption of OTC products or herbal preparations containing sympathomimetic drugs.

ASTHMA. Use of β adrenergic agonists in the treatment of asthma and COPD is discussed in Chapter 36.

OPHTHALMIC USES. Ophthalmic use is discussed in Chapter 64.

NARCOLEPSY AND RELATED SYNDROMES. Narcolepsy is characterized by hypersomnia. Some patients respond to treatment with tricyclic antidepressants or MAO inhibitors. Alternatively, CNS stimulants such as amphetamine, dextroamphetamine, or methamphetamine may be useful. Therapy with amphetamines is complicated by the risk of abuse and the likelihood of the development of tolerance and behavioral changes. Modafinil (PROVIGIL), a CNS stimulant, may have benefit in narcolepsy. In the U.S., it is a schedule IV controlled substance. Its mechanism of action in narcolepsy is unclear. Armodafinil (NUVIGIL), the R-enantiomer of modafinil (a mixture of R- and S-enantiomers) is also indicated for narcolepsy.

WEIGHT REDUCTION. Amphetamine promotes weight loss by suppressing appetite rather than by increasing energy expenditure. Other anorexic drugs include methamphetamine, dextroamphetamine, phentermine, benzphetamine, phendimetrazine, phenmetrazine, diethylpropion, mazindol, phenylpropanolamine, and sibutramine (a mixed adrenergic/serotonergic drug). Phenmetrazine, mazindol, and phenylpropanolamine have been discontinued in the U.S. Available evidence does not support the isolated use of these drugs in the absence of a more comprehensive program that stresses exercise and modification of diet.

ATTENTION DEFICIT HYPERACTIVITY DISORDER. This syndrome, usually first evident in childhood, is characterized by excessive motor activity, difficulty in sustaining attention, and impulsiveness. A variety of stimulant drugs have been used in the treatment of ADHD, and they are particularly indicated in moderate-to-severe cases. *Methylphenidate* is effective in children with ADHD and is the most common intervention. Treatment may start with a dose of 5 mg of methylphenidate in the morning and at lunch; the dose is increased gradually over a period of weeks depending on the response as judged by parents, teachers, and the clinician. The total daily dose generally should not exceed 60 mg; because of its short duration of action, most children require 2 or 3 doses of methylphenidate each day. Sustained-release preparations of *dextroamphetamine*, *methylphenidate* (RITALIN SR, CONCERTA, METADATE), *methylphenidate hydrochloride* (QUILLIVANT XR) *dexmethylphenidate* (FOCALIN XR), and *amphetamine* (ADDERALL XR) may be used once daily in children and adults. *Lisdexamfetamine* (VYVANSE) can be administered once daily and a transdermal formulation of methylphenidate (DAYTRANA) is marketed for daytime use. Potential adverse effects of these medications include insomnia, abdominal pain, anorexia, and weight loss that may be associated with suppression of growth in children. A sustained release formulation of *guanfacine* (INTUNIV), an α_{2A} receptor agonist, has been approved for use in children (ages 6-17 years) in treating ADHD.

Adrenergic Receptor Antagonists

Adrenergic receptor *antagonists* inhibit the interaction of NE, EPI, and other sympathomimetic drugs with α and β receptors (Figure 12–3). Additional background material is presented in Chapter 8. Agents that block DA receptors are considered in Chapter 13.

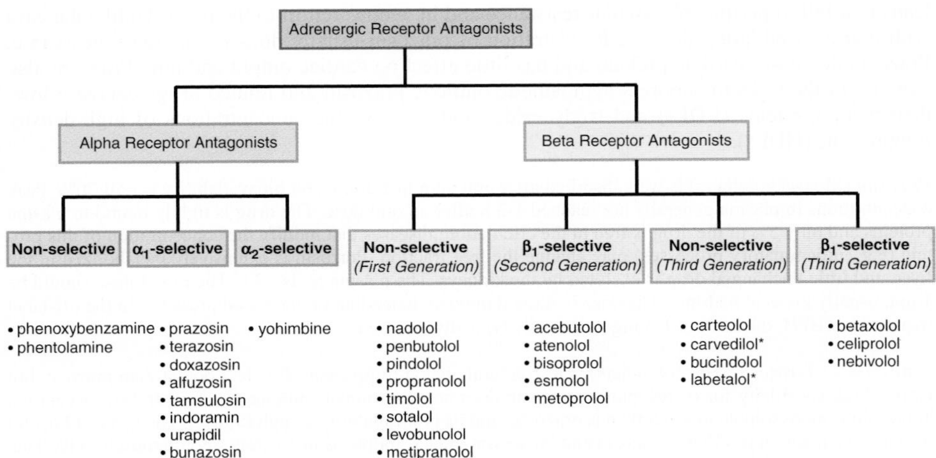

Figure 12–3 *Classification of adrenergic receptor antagonists.* Drugs marked by an asterisk (*) also block α_1 receptors.

The α_1 receptors mediate contraction of arterial, venous, and visceral smooth muscle, while the α_2 receptors are involved in suppressing sympathetic output, increasing vagal tone, facilitating platelet aggregation, inhibiting NE and ACh release from nerve endings, and regulating metabolic effects (e.g., suppression of insulin secretion and inhibition of lipolysis). The α_2 receptors also mediate contraction of some arteries and veins.

Some of the most important effects of α receptor antagonists observed clinically are on the cardiovascular system. α Receptor antagonists have a wide spectrum of pharmacological specificities and are chemically heterogeneous. Some of these drugs have markedly different affinities for α_1 and α_2 receptors. More recently, agents that discriminate among the various subtypes of a particular receptor have become available; e.g., tamsulosin has higher potency at α_{1A} than at α_{1B} receptors.

α_1 RECEPTOR ANTAGONISTS

GENERAL PHARMACOLOGICAL PROPERTIES. Blockade of α_1 receptors inhibits vasoconstriction induced by endogenous catecholamines; vasodilation may occur in both arteriolar resistance vessels and veins. The result is a fall in blood pressure due to decreased peripheral resistance. The magnitude of such effects depends on the activity of the sympathetic nervous system at the time the antagonist is administered, and thus is less in supine than in upright subjects. For most α receptor antagonists, the fall in blood pressure is opposed by baroreceptor reflexes that cause increases in heart rate and cardiac output, as well as fluid retention (effects largely inhibited by β antagonists). These reflexes are exaggerated if the antagonist also blocks α_2 receptors on peripheral sympathetic nerve endings, leading to enhanced release of NE and increased stimulation of postsynaptic β_1 receptors in the heart and on juxtaglomerular cells (*see* Chapter 8). Blockade of α_1 receptors can alleviate some of the symptoms of benign prostatic hyperplasia (BPH). The prostate and lower urinary tract tissues exhibit a high proportion of α_{1A} receptors.

AVAILABLE AGENTS

PRAZOSIN AND RELATED DRUGS. Due in part to its greater α_1 receptor selectivity, this class of α receptor antagonists exhibits greater clinical utility and has largely replaced the nonselective haloalkylamine (e.g., phenoxybenzamine) and imidazoline (e.g., phentolamine) α receptor antagonists. Prazosin is the prototypical α_1-selective antagonist.

The affinity of prazosin for α_1 adrenergic receptors is ~1000-fold greater than that for α_2 adrenergic receptors. Prazosin has similar potencies at α_{1A}, α_{1B}, and α_{1D} subtypes. Prazosin, doxazosin, and tamsulosin, frequently are used for the treatment of hypertension (*see* Chapter 27).

PHARMACOLOGICAL PROPERTIES

The major effects of prazosin result from its blockade of α_1 receptors in arterioles and veins. This leads to a fall in peripheral vascular resistance and in venous return to the heart. Unlike the case with many vasodilating drugs, administration of prazosin usually does not increase heart rate. Prazosin decreases cardiac preload and has little effect on cardiac output and rate. Prazosin also may act in the CNS to suppress sympathetic outflow. Prazosin and related drugs decrease low-density lipoproteins (LDLs) and triglycerides and increase the concentrations of high-density lipoproteins (HDLs).

Prazosin (MINIPRESS, others) is well absorbed after oral administration, and bioavailability is ~50-70%. Peak concentrations in plasma generally are reached 1-3 h after an oral dose. The drug is tightly bound to plasma proteins and only 5% of the drug is free in the circulation; diseases that modify the concentration of this protein (e.g., inflammatory processes) may change the free fraction. Prazosin is extensively metabolized in the liver, and little unchanged drug is excreted by the kidneys. The plasma $t_{1/2}$ is ~3 h. The initial dose should be 1 mg, usually given at bedtime. The dose is titrated upward depending on the blood pressure. In the off-label treatment of BPH, doses from 1-5 mg twice daily typically are used.

TERAZOSIN. *Terazosin* (HYTRIN, others) is a structural analog of prazosin. It is less potent than prazosin but retains high specificity for α_1 receptors; terazosin does not discriminate among α_{1A}, α_{1B}, and α_{1D} receptors. Terazosin is more soluble in water than is prazosin, and its bioavailability is high (>90%). The $t_{1/2}$ is ~12 h, and its duration of action is >18 h. Terazosin and doxazosin induce apoptosis in prostate smooth muscle cells. This apoptosis may lessen the symptoms associated with chronic BPH. The apoptotic effect of terazosin and doxazosin appears to be related to the quinazoline moiety rather than α_1 receptor antagonism. An initial first dose of 1 mg is recommended, that is titrated upward depending on the therapeutic response. Doses of 10 mg/day may be required for maximal effect in BPH.

DOXAZOSIN. *Doxazosin* (CARDURA, others) is a structural analog of prazosin and a highly selective antagonist at α_1 receptors. It is nonselective among α_1 receptor subtypes. The $t_{1/2}$ of doxazosin is ~20 h, and its duration of action may extend to 36 h. Bioavailability and extent of metabolism of doxazosin and prazosin are similar. Doxazosin is given initially as a 1-mg dose in the treatment of hypertension or BPH. Doxazosin also may have beneficial actions in the long-term management of BPH related to apoptosis.

ALFUZOSIN. *Alfuzosin* (UROXATRAL) is α_1 receptor antagonist with similar affinity at all of the α_1 receptor subtypes. It is used in treating BPH but not for treatment of hypertension. Its bioavailability is ~64%; it has a $t_{1/2}$ of 3-5 h. Alfuzosin is a substrate of CYP3A4. The recommended dosage is one 10-mg extended-release tablet daily to be taken after the same meal each day.

TAMSULOSIN. *Tamsulosin* (FLOMAX), is an α_1 receptor antagonist with some selectivity for α_{1A} (and α_{1D}) subtypes compared to the α_{1B} subtype. This selectivity may favor blockade of α_{1A} receptors in prostate. Tamsulosin is efficacious in the treatment of BPH with little effect on blood pressure. Tamsulosin is well absorbed, is extensively metabolized by CYPs, and has a $t_{1/2}$ of 5-10 h. Tamsulosin may be administered at a 0.4-mg starting dose. Abnormal ejaculation is an adverse effect of tamsulosin.

SILODOSIN. *Silodosin* (RAPAFLO) exhibits selectivity for the α_{1A} over the α_{1B} receptor. The drug is metabolized by UGT2B7; coadministration with inhibitors of this enzyme (e.g., probenecid, valproic acid, fluconazole) increases systemic exposure to silodosin. The drug is approved for the treatment of BPH. The chief side effect of silodosin is retrograde ejaculation (in 28% of those treated). Silodosin is available as 4-mg and 8-mg capsules.

ADVERSE EFFECTS

An adverse effect of prazosin and its congeners is the first-dose effect; marked postural hypotension and syncope sometimes are seen 30-90 min after the initial dose of prazosin. The risk of the first-dose phenomenon is minimized by limiting the initial dose (e.g., 1 mg at bedtime), by increasing the dosage slowly, and by introducing additional antihypertensive drugs cautiously. Nonspecific adverse effects such as headache, dizziness, and asthenia rarely limit treatment with prazosin.

THERAPEUTIC USES

Hypertension. Prazosin and its congeners have been used successfully in the treatment of essential hypertension (*see* Chapter 27).

Congestive Heart Failure. α Receptor antagonists have been used in the treatment of congestive heart failure, but are not the drugs of choice.

Benign Prostatic Hyperplasia. BPH produces symptomatic urethral obstruction that leads to weak stream, urinary frequency, and nocturia. α_1 Receptors in the trigone muscle of the bladder and urethra contribute to the resistance to outflow of urine; prazosin reduces this. *Finasteride* (PROPECIA, PROSCAR, others) and *dutasteride* (AVODART), 2 drugs that inhibit conversion of testosterone to dihydrotestosterone (*see* Chapter 41) and can reduce prostate volume in some patients, are approved as monotherapy and in combination with α receptor antagonists. α_1-Selective antagonists have efficacy in BPH owing to relaxation of smooth muscle in the bladder neck, prostate capsule, and prostatic urethra. Combination therapy with doxazosin and finasteride reduces the risk of overall clinical progression of BPH significantly more than treatment with either drug alone. Tamsulosin at the recommended dose of 0.4 mg daily and silodosin at 0.8 mg are less likely to cause orthostatic hypotension than are the other drugs. The predominant α_1 subtype expressed in the human prostate is the α_{1A} receptor.

Other Disorders. Some studies indicate that prazosin can decrease the incidence of digital vasospasm in patients with Raynaud's disease; however, its relative efficacy as compared with Ca^{2+} channel blockers is not known. Prazosin may have some benefit in patients with other vasospastic disorders. Prazosin may be useful for the treatment of patients with mitral or aortic valvular insufficiency, presumably by reducing afterload.

α_2 ADRENERGIC RECEPTOR ANTAGONISTS

Activation of presynaptic α_2 receptors inhibits the release of NE and other cotransmitters from peripheral sympathetic nerve endings. Activation of α_2 receptors in the CNS inhibits sympathetic nervous system activity and leads to a fall in blood pressure. Blockade of α_2 receptors with selective antagonists such as *yohimbine* thus can increase sympathetic outflow and potentiate the release of NE from nerve endings. Antagonists that also block α_1 receptors give rise to similar effects on sympathetic outflow and release of NE, but the net increase in blood pressure is prevented by inhibition of vasoconstriction.

Although certain vascular beds contain α_2 receptors that promote contraction of smooth muscle, these receptors are preferentially stimulated by circulating catecholamines, whereas α_1 receptors are activated by NE released from sympathetic nerve fibers. The physiological role of vascular α_2 receptors in the regulation of blood flow within various vascular beds is uncertain. The α_2 receptors contribute to smooth muscle contraction in the human saphenous vein, whereas α_1 receptors are more prominent in dorsal hand veins. The effects of α_2 receptor antagonists on the cardiovascular system are dominated by actions in the CNS and on sympathetic nerve endings.

YOHIMBINE. Yohimbine (YOCON, APHRODYNE) is a competitive antagonist that is selective for α_2 receptors. Yohimbine enters the CNS, where it acts to increase blood pressure and heart rate; it also enhances motor activity and produces tremors. Yohimbine also antagonizes effects of 5HT.

In the past, it was used to treat male sexual dysfunction. Some studies suggest that yohimbine also may be useful for diabetic neuropathy and postural hypotension. In the U.S., yohimbine may be sold as a dietary supplement; however, labeling claims that it will increase sexual desire or performance are prohibited.

NONSELECTIVE α ADRENERGIC ANTAGONISTS: PHENOXYBENZAMINE AND PHENTOLAMINE

Phenoxybenzamine and *phentolamine* are nonselective α receptors antagonists. Phenoxybenzamine produces an irreversible antagonism; phentolamine produces a competitive antagonism.

Phenoxybenzamine and phentolamine cause a progressive decrease in peripheral resistance, an increase in cardiac output (due in part to reflex sympathetic nerve stimulation), and enhanced release of NE from cardiac sympathetic nerve due to antagonism of presynaptic α_2 receptors. Postural hypotension, a prominent feature accompanied by reflex tachycardia that can precipitate cardiac arrhythmias, severely limits the use of these drugs to treat essential hypertension. The α_1-selective antagonists have replaced the classical α-blockers in the management of essential hypertension. Phenoxybenzamine and phentolamine are still marketed for several specialized uses.

Therapeutic Uses. A use of phenoxybenzamine (DIBENZYLINE) is in the treatment of pheochromocytoma, which are tumors of the adrenal medulla and sympathetic neurons that secrete enormous quantities of catecholamines. Phenoxybenzamine is often used in preparing the patient for surgical removal of the tumor. A conservative approach is to initiate treatment with phenoxybenzamine (at a dosage of 10 mg twice daily) 1-3 weeks before the operation. The dose is increased every other day until the desired effect on blood pressure is achieved. Prolonged treatment with phenoxybenzamine may be necessary in patients with inoperable or malignant pheochromocytoma. In some patients, particularly those with malignant disease, administration of metyrosine, a competitive inhibitor of tyrosine hydroxylase, may be a useful adjuvant (*see* Chapter 8). β Receptor antagonists also are used but only after the administration of an α receptor antagonist.

Phentolamine can also be used in short-term control of hypertension in patients with pheochromocytoma. Phentolamine has been used locally to prevent dermal necrosis after the inadvertent extravasation of an α receptor agonist.

Toxicity and Adverse Effects. Hypotension is the major adverse effect of phenoxybenzamine and phentolamine. In addition, reflex cardiac stimulation may cause alarming tachycardia, cardiac arrhythmias, and ischemic cardiac events, including myocardial infarction. Reversible inhibition of ejaculation may occur due to impaired smooth muscle contraction in the vas deferens and ejaculatory ducts. Phenoxybenzamine is mutagenic in the Ames test.

ADDITIONAL α ADRENERGIC RECEPTOR ANTAGONISTS

Ergot Alkaloids. The ergot alkaloids were the first adrenergic receptor antagonists to be discovered. Information about the ergot alkaloids can be found in Chapter 13.

INDORAMIN. *Indoramin* is a selective, competitive α_1 receptor antagonist that also antagonizes H_1- and 5HT receptors. As an α_1-selective antagonist, indoramin lowers blood pressure with minimal tachycardia. The drug also decreases the incidence of attacks of Raynaud phenomenon. Some of the adverse effects of indoramin include sedation, dry mouth, and failure of ejaculation. Indoramin is not available in the U.S.

KETANSERIN. *Ketanserin*, a 5HT/α_1 receptor antagonist not available in the U.S., is discussed in Chapter 13.

URAPIDIL. *Urapidil* is a selective α_1 receptor antagonist that is not commercially available in the U.S. Blockade of peripheral α_1 receptors appears to be primarily responsible for the hypotension produced by urapidil, although it has actions in the CNS as well.

BUNAZOSIN. *Bunazosin* is an α_1-selective antagonist of the quinazoline class that can lower blood pressure in patients with hypertension; this agent is not available in the U.S.

NEUROLEPTIC AGENTS. Chlorpromazine, haloperidol, and other neuroleptic drugs of the phenothiazine and butyrophenone types produce significant blockade of both α and D_2 receptors.

β ADRENERGIC RECEPTOR ANTAGONISTS

β Antagonists can be distinguished by the following properties:

- Relative affinity for β_1 and β_2 receptors
- Intrinsic sympathomimetic activity
- Blockade of α receptors
- Differences in lipid solubility
- Capacity to induce vasodilation
- Pharmacokinetic parameters

β Adrenergic receptor antagonists are classified as non–subtype-selective (first generation), β_1-selective (second generation), and non–subtype or subtype-selective *with additional cardiovascular actions* (third generation). These latter drugs have additional cardiovascular properties (especially vasodilation) that seem unrelated to β blockade. Table 12–3 summarizes important pharmacological and pharmacokinetic properties of β receptor antagonists.

Several β receptor antagonists also have local anesthetic or membrane-stabilizing activity that is independent of β-blockade. Such drugs include propranolol, acebutolol, and carvedilol. Pindolol, metoprolol, betaxolol, and labetalol have slight membrane-stabilizing effects.

Table 12–3

Pharmacological/Pharmacokinetic Properties of β Adrenergic Receptor Blocking Agents

DRUG	MEMBRANE STABILITY	IAA	LIPID SOLUBILITY	% ABSORPTION	% ORAL AVAILABILITY	PLASMA $t_{1/2}$ (h)
Classical non-selective β blockers: First generation						
Nadolol	0	0	Low	30	30-50	20-24
Penbutolol	0	+	High	~100	~100	~5
Pindolol	+	+++	Low	>95	~100	3-4
Propranolol	++	0	High	<90	30	3-5
Timolol	0	0	Low/moderate	90	75	4
β_1-Selective β blockers: Second generation						
Acebutolol	+	+	Low	90	20-60	3-4
Atenolol	0	0	Low	90	50-60	6-7
Bisoprolol	0	0	Low	≤90	80	9-12
Esmolol	0	0	Low	NA	NA	0.15
Metoprolol	+[a]	0	Moderate	~100	40-50	3-7
Non-selective β blockers with additional actions: Third generation						
Carteolol	0	++	Low	85	85	6
Carvedilol	++	0	Moderate	>90	~30	7-10
Labetalol	+	+	Low	>90	~33	3-4
β_1-selective β blockers with additional actions: Third generation						
Betaxolol	+	0	Moderate	>90	~80	15
Celiprolol	0	+	Low	~74	30-70	5
Nebivolol	0	0	Low	NA	NA	11-30

IAA, intrinsic agonist activity.
[a]*Detectable only at doses much greater than required for β blockade.*

CARDIOVASCULAR SYSTEM. The major therapeutic effects of β receptor antagonists are on the cardiovascular system. It is important to distinguish the effects in normal subjects from those in subjects with cardiovascular disease such as hypertension or myocardial ischemia.

Because catecholamines have positive chronotropic and inotropic actions, β receptor antagonists slow the heart rate and decrease myocardial contractility. When tonic stimulation of β receptors is low, this effect is correspondingly modest. However, when the sympathetic nervous system is activated, as during exercise or stress, β receptor antagonists attenuate the expected rise in heart rate. Short-term administration of β receptor antagonists such as propranolol decreases cardiac output; peripheral resistance increases in proportion to maintain blood pressure as a result of blockade of vascular β_2 receptors and compensatory reflexes, such as increased sympathetic nervous system activity, leading to activation of vascular α receptors. With long-term use of β antagonists, total peripheral resistance returns to initial values or decreases in patients with hypertension. With β antagonists that also are α_1 receptor antagonists (e.g., labetalol, carvedilol, and bucindolol), cardiac output is maintained with a greater fall in peripheral resistance.

β Receptor antagonists have significant effects on cardiac rhythm and automaticity, which involves blockade of both β_1 receptors and β_2 receptors. β Receptor antagonists reduce sinus rate, decrease the spontaneous rate of depolarization of ectopic pacemakers, slow conduction in the atria and in the AV node, and increase the functional refractory period of the AV node.

ACTIVITY AS ANTIHYPERTENSIVE AGENTS. β Receptor antagonists generally do not reduce blood pressure in patients with normal blood pressure. However, these drugs lower blood pressure in patients with hypertension. Reduction of β_1-stimulated renin release from the juxtaglomerular cells is a putative contributing mechanism (*see* Chapter 26). Because presynaptic β receptors enhance the release of NE from sympathetic neurons, diminished release of NE from β blockade is a possible response. Long-term administration of β-blockers to hypertensive patients ultimately leads to a fall in peripheral vascular resistance.

Some β antagonists have additional effects that may contribute to their capacity to lower blood pressure. These drugs all produce peripheral vasodilation; properties that have been proposed to contribute to this effect include production of NO, activation of β_2 receptors, blockade of α_1 receptors, blockade of Ca^{2+} entry, opening of K^+ channels, and antioxidant activity (Table 12–4 and Figure 12–4). These mechanisms appear to contribute to the antihypertensive effects by enhancing hypotension, increasing peripheral blood flow, and decreasing afterload. Celiprolol and nebivolol also have been observed to produce vasodilation and thereby reduce preload.

Propranolol and other nonselective β receptor antagonists inhibit the vasodilation caused by isoproterenol and augment the pressor response to EPI. This is particularly significant in patients with pheochromocytoma, in whom β receptor antagonists should be used only after adequate α receptor blockade has been established.

PULMONARY SYSTEM. Nonselective β receptor antagonists such as propranolol block β_2 receptors in bronchial smooth muscle. This usually has little effect on pulmonary function in normal individuals. However, in

Table 12–4

Third-Generation β Receptor Antagonists with Putative Additional Mechanisms of Vasodilation

NITRIC OXIDE PRODUCTION	β_2 RECEPTOR AGONISM	α_1 RECEPTOR ANTAGONISM	Ca^{2+} ENTRY BLOCKADE	K^+ CHANNEL OPENING	ANTIOXIDANT ACTIVITY
Celiprolol[a]	Celiprolol[a]	Carvedilol	Carvedilol	Tilisolol[a]	Carvedilol
Nebivolol	Carteolol	Bucindolol[a]	Betaxolol		
Carteolol	Bopindolol[a]	Bevantolol[a]	Bevantolol[a]		
Bopindolol[a]		Nipradilol[a]			
Nipradilol[a]		Labetalol			

[a] *Not currently available in the U.S., where most are under investigation for use.*

SECTION II NEUROPHARMACOLOGY

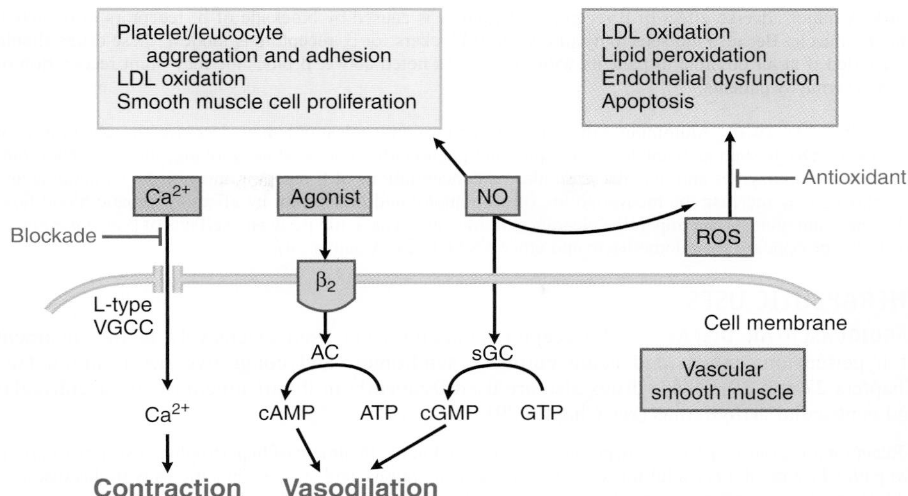

Figure 12–4 *Mechanisms underlying actions of vasodilating β blockers in blood vessels.* (ROS, reactive oxygen species; sGC, soluble guanylyl cyclase; AC adenylyl cyclase; L-type VGCC, L-type voltage-gated Ca^{2+} channel.) (Modified with permission from Toda N. Vasodilating β-adrenoreceptor blockers as cardiovascular therapeutics. *Pharmacol Ther*, 2003;100:215-234. Copyright © Elsevier.)

patients with COPD, such blockade can lead to life-threatening bronchoconstriction. Although β_1-selective antagonists or antagonists with intrinsic sympathomimetic activity are less likely than propranolol to increase airway resistance in patients with asthma, these drugs should be used only with great caution, if at all, in patients with bronchospastic diseases.

METABOLIC EFFECTS. Catecholamines promote glycogenolysis and mobilize glucose in response to hypoglycemia. Nonselective β blockers may delay recovery from hypoglycemia in type 1 (insulin-dependent) diabetes mellitus, but infrequently in type 2 diabetes mellitus. β Receptor antagonists can interfere with the counter-regulatory effects of catecholamines secreted during hypoglycemia by blunting the perception of symptoms such as tremor, tachycardia, and nervousness. Use β adrenergic receptor antagonists with great caution in patients with labile diabetes and frequent hypoglycemic reactions; if such a drug is indicated, use a β_1-selective antagonist.

β Receptor antagonists can attenuate the release of free fatty acids from adipose tissue. Nonselective β receptor antagonists consistently reduce HDL cholesterol, increase LDL cholesterol, and increase triglycerides. In contrast, β_1-selective antagonists, including celiprolol, carteolol, nebivolol, carvedilol, and bevantolol, reportedly improve the serum lipid profile of dyslipidemic patients. Propranolol and atenolol increase triglycerides, whereas chronic celiprolol, carvedilol, and carteolol reduce plasma triglycerides. In contrast to classical β-blockers, which decrease insulin sensitivity, the vasodilating β receptor antagonists (e.g., celiprolol, nipradilol, carteolol, carvedilol, and dilevalol) increase insulin sensitivity in patients with insulin resistance.

Other Effects. β Receptor antagonists block catecholamine-induced tremor. They also block inhibition of mast-cell degranulation by catecholamines.

ADVERSE EFFECTS AND PRECAUTIONS

The most common adverse effects of β receptor antagonists arise as pharmacological consequences of blockade of β receptors. β Receptor blockade may cause or exacerbate heart failure in patients with compensated heart failure, acute myocardial infarction, or cardiomegaly. Nonetheless, there is convincing evidence that chronic administration of β receptor antagonists is efficacious in prolonging life in the therapy of heart failure in selected patients (*see* Chapter 28). The use of β adrenergic receptor antagonists is contraindicated in patients with asthma, COPD, sinus bradycardia, and cardiogenic shock.

Bradycardia is a normal response to β receptor blockade; however, in patients with partial or complete AV conduction defects, β antagonists may cause life-threatening bradyarrhythmias. *Abrupt discontinuation of β receptor antagonists after long-term treatment can exacerbate angina and may increase the risk of sudden death*. A major adverse effect of β receptor antagonists is caused by blockade of β_2 receptors in bronchial smooth muscle. Because the selectivity of current β blockers for β_1 receptors is modest, these drugs should be avoided if at all possible in patients with asthma. As noted above, β blockade may blunt recognition of hypoglycemia by patients.

DRUG INTERACTIONS. Aluminum salts, cholestyramine, and colestipol may decrease the absorption of β-blockers. Drugs such as phenytoin, rifampin, and phenobarbital, as well as smoking, induce hepatic biotransformation enzymes and may decrease plasma concentrations of β receptor antagonists. Cimetidine and hydralazine may increase the bioavailability of propranolol and metoprolol by affecting hepatic blood flow. β Receptor antagonists can impair the clearance of lidocaine. The antihypertensive effects of β receptor antagonists can be opposed by indomethacin and other NSAIDs (*see* Chapter 34).

THERAPEUTIC USES

CARDIOVASCULAR DISEASES. β Receptor antagonists are used extensively in the treatment of hypertension, angina and acute coronary syndromes, and congestive heart failure (*see* Chapters 27 and 28). These drugs also are used frequently in the treatment of supraventricular and ventricular arrhythmias (*see* Chapter 29).

β Receptor antagonists, particularly propranolol, are used in the treatment of hypertrophic obstructive cardiomyopathy. Propranolol is useful for relieving angina, palpitations, and syncope in patients with this disorder. β-blockers also may attenuate catecholamine-induced cardiomyopathy in pheochromocytoma.

GLAUCOMA. β Receptor antagonists are very useful in the treatment of chronic open-angle glaucoma.

Six drugs are currently available: carteolol (OCUPRESS, others), betaxolol (BETOPTIC, others), levobunolol (BETAGAN, others), metipranolol (OPTIPRANOLOL, others), timolol (TIMOPTIC, others), and levobetaxolol (BETAXON). These agents decrease the production of aqueous humor. Glaucoma and therapies are presented in Chapter 64.

OTHER USES. β Receptor antagonists control many of the cardiovascular signs and symptoms of hyperthyroidism and are useful adjuvants to more definitive therapy. In addition, propranolol inhibits the peripheral conversion of thyroxine to triiodothyronine, an effect that may be independent of β receptor blockade (*see* Chapter 39). Propranolol, timolol, and metoprolol are effective for the prophylaxis of migraine. Tachycardia, muscle tremors, and other evidence of increased sympathetic activity are reduced by β-blockers.

NONSELECTIVE β ADRENERGIC RECEPTOR ANTAGONISTS

PROPRANOLOL

Propranolol interacts with β_1 and β_2 receptors with equal affinity, lacks intrinsic sympathomimetic activity, and does not block α receptors.

Propranolol is used for the treatment of hypertension and angina. The initial oral dose is 40-80 mg/day, titrated upward until the optimal response is obtained (typically <320 mg/day). Propranolol also is used for supraventricular arrhythmias/tachycardias, ventricular arrhythmias/tachycardias, premature ventricular contractions, digitalis-induced tachyarrhythmias, myocardial infarction, pheochromocytoma, essential tremor, and the prophylaxis of migraine. It also is used for several off-label indications including parkinsonian tremors (sustained-release only), akathisia induced by antipsychotic drugs, variceal bleeding in portal hypertension, and anxiety disorder.

Propranolol is highly lipophilic and is almost completely absorbed after oral administration. The drug is highly metabolized by the liver during its first passage through the portal circulation; on average, only ~25% reaches the systemic circulation. Individual variation in hepatic clearance of propranolol contributes to enormous variability in plasma concentrations (~20-fold) after oral administration. The degree of hepatic extraction of propranolol declines as the dose is increased. The bioavailability of propranolol may be increased by the concomitant ingestion of food. Propranolol readily enters the CNS. Sustained-release formulations of propranolol (INDERAL LA, others) have been developed to maintain therapeutic concentrations of propranolol in plasma throughout a 24-h period.

NADOLOL

Nadolol (CORGARD, others) is a long-acting antagonist with equal affinity for β_1 and β_2 receptors.

A distinguishing characteristic of nadolol is its relatively long $t_{1/2}$. It can be used to treat hypertension and angina pectoris. Unlabeled uses have included migraine prophylaxis, parkinsonian tremors, and variceal bleeding in portal hypertension. The $t_{1/2}$ of the drug in plasma is ~20 h. Nadolol is largely excreted intact in the urine and may accumulate in patients with renal failure.

TIMOLOL

Timolol (BLOCADREN, others) is a potent, nonselective β receptor antagonist used for hypertension, congestive heart failure, acute myocardial infarction, and migraine prophylaxis.

The ocular formulation of timolol (TIMOPTIC, others), used for the treatment of glaucoma, may be extensively absorbed systemically (*see* Chapter 64); adverse effects can occur in susceptible patients, such as those with asthma or congestive heart failure.

PINDOLOL

Pindolol (VISKEN, others) is a nonselective β receptor antagonist with intrinsic sympathomimetic activity.

Pindolol has low membrane-stabilizing activity and low lipid solubility. It is a weak partial β agonist; such drugs may be preferred as antihypertensive agents in individuals with diminished cardiac reserve or a propensity for bradycardia. It is used to treat angina pectoris and hypertension.

β_1-SELECTIVE ADRENERGIC RECEPTOR ANTAGONISTS

METOPROLOL

Metoprolol (LOPRESSOR, others) is a β_1-selective receptor antagonist.

It is highly absorbed after oral administration, but bioavailability is relatively low (~40%) because of first-pass metabolism. Plasma concentrations of the drug vary widely (up to 17-fold) possibly due to genetically determined differences in the rate of metabolism in the liver by CYP2D6. The $t_{1/2}$ of metoprolol is 3-4 h, but can double in CYP2D6 poor metabolizers who have a 5X higher risk for developing adverse effects. An extended-release formulation (TOPROL XL) is available for once-daily administration.

For the treatment of hypertension, the usual initial dose is 100 mg/day. The drug sometimes is effective when given once daily, although it frequently is used in 2 divided doses. Dosage may be increased at weekly intervals until optimal reduction of blood pressure is achieved. Metoprolol generally is used in 2 divided doses for the treatment of stable angina. For the initial treatment of patients with acute myocardial infarction, an intravenous formulation of metoprolol tartrate is available. Metoprolol generally is contraindicated for the treatment of acute myocardial infarction in patients with heart rates of <45 beats/min, heart block greater than first-degree (PR interval ≥0.24 second), systolic blood pressure <100 mm Hg, or moderate to severe heart failure. Metoprolol also has been proven to be effective in chronic heart failure.

ATENOLOL

Atenolol (TENORMIN, others) is a β_1-selective antagonist.

Atenolol is incompletely absorbed (~50%) and is excreted largely unchanged in the urine with elimination $t_{1/2}$ ~5-8 h. The drug accumulates in patients with renal failure, and dosage should be adjusted for patients whose creatinine clearance is <35 mL/min. The initial dose of atenolol for the treatment of hypertension usually is 50 mg/day, given once daily, and may be increased to 100 mg. Atenolol has been shown to be efficacious, in combination with a diuretic, in elderly patients with isolated systolic hypertension.

ESMOLOL

Esmolol (BREVIBLOC, others) is a β_1-selective antagonist with a rapid onset and a very short duration of action.

Esmolol is used when β-blockade of short duration is desired or in critically ill patients in whom adverse effects of bradycardia, heart failure, or hypotension may necessitate rapid withdrawal of the drug. Esmolol is given by slow IV injection. The drug is hydrolyzed rapidly by esterases in erythrocytes and has a $t_{1/2}$ of ~8 min. Peak hemodynamic effects occur within 6-10 min of administration of a loading dose, and there is substantial attenuation of β blockade within 20 min of stopping an infusion. Because esmolol is used in urgent settings where immediate onset of β blockade is warranted, a partial loading dose typically is administered, followed by a continuous infusion of the drug. If an adequate therapeutic effect is not observed within 5 min, the same loading dose is repeated, followed by a maintenance infusion at a higher rate. This process may need to be repeated to approach desired end point (e.g., lowered heart rate or blood pressure).

ACEBUTOLOL. Acebutolol (SECTRAL, others) is a β_1-selective antagonist with some intrinsic sympathomimetic and membrane-stabilizing activity. Acebutolol is well absorbed, and undergoes significant first-pass metabolism to an active metabolite, *diacetolol*, which accounts for most of the drug's activity. Acebutolol has been used to treat hypertension, cardiac arrhythmias, and acute myocardial infarction. The initial dose in hypertension is 400 mg/day; given as a single or 2 divided doses. Optimal responses usually occur with doses of 400-800 mg per day (range, 200-1200 mg).

BISOPROLOL. Bisoprolol (ZEBETA) is a highly selective β_1 receptor antagonist that is approved for the treatment of hypertension. Bisoprolol can be considered a standard treatment option when selecting a β-blocker for use in combination with ACE inhibitors and diuretics in patients with chronic heart failure and in treating hypertension. Bisoprolol generally is well tolerated; side effects include dizziness, bradycardia, hypotension, and fatigue. It is eliminated by renal excretion (50%) and liver metabolism (50%).

BETAXOLOL. Betaxolol (BETOPTIC, LOKERN, KERLONE, others) is a selective β_1 receptor antagonist with slight membrane-stabilizing properties. Betaxolol is used to treat hypertension, angina pectoris, and glaucoma. It is usually well tolerated and side effects are mild and transient. In glaucoma it reduces intraocular pressure.

β RECEPTOR ANTAGONISTS WITH ADDITIONAL CARDIOVASCULAR EFFECTS (THIRD-GENERATION β-BLOCKERS)

Third-generation β-blockers possess vasodilating actions produced through a variety of mechanisms (*see* Table 12–4 and Figure 12–4).

LABETALOL

Labetalol (NORMODYNE, TRANDATE, others) is representative of a class of drugs that act as competitive antagonists at both α_1 and β receptors. The pharmacological properties of the drug are complex, because each isomer displays different relative activities.

The properties of the mixture include selective blockade of α_1 receptors (as compared with the α_2 subtype), blockade of β_1 and β_2 receptors, partial agonist activity at β_2 receptors, and inhibition of neuronal uptake of NE (cocaine-like effect) (*see* Chapter 8). The potency of the mixture for β blockade is 5-10 fold that for α_1 blockade. The actions of labetalol on both α_1 and β receptors contribute to the fall in blood pressure observed in patients with hypertension. α_1 Receptor blockade leads to relaxation of arterial smooth muscle and vasodilation. β_1 Blockade contributes to a fall in blood pressure, in part by blocking reflex sympathetic stimulation of the heart. The intrinsic sympathomimetic activity of labetalol at β_2 receptors may contribute to vasodilation.

Labetalol is available in oral form for therapy of chronic hypertension and as an intravenous formulation for use in hypertensive emergencies. Labetalol has been associated with hepatic injury in a limited number of patients.

CARVEDILOL

Carvedilol (COREG) blocks β_1, β_2, and α_1 receptors, and also has antioxidant and anti-inflammatory effects. Carvedilol produces vasodilation.

Carvedilol is extremely liphophic and is able to protect cell membranes from lipid peroxidation. At high doses, carvedilol exerts Ca^{2+} channel-blocking activity. Carvedilol does not increase β receptor density. Carvedilol improves ventricular function and reduces mortality and morbidity in patients with mild to severe congestive heart failure. Carvedilol is rapidly absorbed following oral administration, with peak plasma concentrations occurring in 1-2 h. No significant changes in the pharmacokinetics of carvedilol are seen in elderly patients with hypertension, and no change in dosage is needed in patients with moderate to severe renal insufficiency. Due to its extensive oxidative metabolism by the liver, carvedilol's pharmacokinetics can be profoundly affected by drugs that induce or inhibit oxidation. These include the inducer, rifampin, and inhibitors such as cimetidine, quinidine, fluoxetine, and paroxetine.

BUCINDOLOL. Bucindolol (SANDONORM) is a third-generation nonselective β adrenergic antagonist with weak α_1 adrenergic blocking properties. Bucindolol reduces afterload and increases plasma HDL cholesterol, but does not affect plasma triglycerides. Bucindolol is extensively metabolized by the liver and has a $t_{1/2}$ of ~8 h. A new drug application is under review with the FDA.

CELIPROLOL. Celiprolol (SELECTOL) is a cardioselective β receptor antagonist with weak vasodilating and bronchodilating effects attributed to partial selective β_2 agonist activity. It may antagonize peripheral α_2 adrenergic receptor activity, promote NO production, and inhibit oxidative stress. It is largely unmetabolized and is excreted unchanged in the urine and feces. Celiprolol is used for treatment of hypertension and angina.

NEBIVOLOL. Nebivolol (BYSTOLIC) is a selective β_1 receptor antagonist, has endothelial NO-mediated vasodilator activity, and is approved for treatment of hypertension. The *d*-isomer is the active β-blocking component; the *l*-isomer is responsible for enhancing production of NO. It is lipophilic, and concomitant administration of chlorthalidone, hydrochlorothiazide, theophylline, or digoxin with nebivolol may reduce its extent of absorption. The NO-dependent vasodilating action of nebivolol and its high β_1 adrenergic receptor selectivity likely contribute to the drug's efficacy and improved tolerability (e.g., less fatigue and sexual dysfunction) as an antihypertensive agent. Metabolism occurs via CYP2D6.

OTHER β ADRENERGIC RECEPTOR ANTAGONISTS. There are numerous β adrenergic receptor antagonists on the market as ophthalmologic preparations for the treatment of glaucoma (*see* Chapter 64).

For a complete Bibliographical Listing see Goodman & Gilman's ***The Pharmacological Basis of Therapeutics***, 12th ed., or Goodman & Gilman Online at www.AccessMedicine.com.

chapter 13 5-Hydroxytryptamine (Serotonin) and Dopamine

5-Hydroxytryptamine (5HT, serotonin) and dopamine (DA) have prominent actions in the CNS and the periphery. Fourteen 5HT receptor subtypes and five DA receptor subtypes have been delineated by pharmacological analyses and cDNA cloning. The availability of cloned receptors has allowed the development of subtype-selective drugs and the elucidation of actions of these neurotransmitters at a molecular level.

5-HYDROXYTRYPTAMINE

5HT is found in high concentrations in enterochromaffin cells throughout the GI tract, in storage granules in platelets, and broadly throughout the CNS. 5HT regulates smooth muscle in the cardiovascular system and the GI tract and enhances platelet aggregation.

SYNTHESIS AND METABOLISM OF 5HT. 5HT is synthesized by a 2-step pathway from the *tryptophan* (Figure 13–1).

Tryptophan is actively transported into the brain by a carrier protein. Levels of tryptophan in the brain reflect its plasma concentration and the plasma concentrations of amino acids that compete for the same transporter. *Tryptophan hydroxylase*, the rate-limiting enzyme in the synthetic pathway, converts tryptophan to L-5-hydroxytryptophan; the enzyme is not regulated by end-product inhibition. Brain tryptophan hydroxylase is not generally saturated with substrate; consequently, the concentration of tryptophan in the brain influences the synthesis of 5HT.

Aromatic L-amino acid decarboxylase (AADC) converts L-5-hydroxytryptophan to 5HT; it is widely distributed and has broad substrate specificity. The synthesized product, 5HT, is accumulated in secretory granules by a *vesicular monoamine transporter* (VMAT2); vesicular 5HT is released by *exocytosis* from *serotonergic neurons*. In the nervous system, the action of released 5HT is terminated via neuronal uptake by a specific 5HT transporter (SERT), localized in the membrane of serotonergic axon terminals and in the membrane of platelets. This uptake system is the means by which platelets acquire 5HT, since they lack the enzymes required for 5HT synthesis. The amine transporters are distinct from VMAT2, which concentrates amines in intracellular storage vesicles and is a nonspecific amine carrier, whereas the 5HT transporter is specific.

The principal route of metabolism of 5HT involves oxidative deamination by *monoamine oxidase* (MAO); the aldehyde intermediate thus formed is converted to 5-hydroxyindole acetic acid (5-HIAA) by *aldehyde dehydrogenase* (*see* Figure 13–1). 5-HIAA is actively transported out of the brain by a process that is sensitive to the nonspecific transport inhibitor, *probenecid*. 5-HIAA from brain and peripheral sites of 5HT storage and metabolism is excreted in the urine along with small amounts of 5-hydroxytryptophol sulfate or glucuronide conjugates. The usual range of urinary excretion of 5-HIAA by a normal adult is 2-10 mg daily. Ingestion of ethanol results in elevated amounts of $NADH_2$ (*see* Chapter 23), which diverts 5-hydroxyindole acetaldehyde from the oxidative route to the reductive pathway and tends to increase the excretion of 5-hydroxytryptophol and correspondingly reduce the excretion of 5-HIAA.

Of the 2 isoforms of monoamine oxidase (MAO; *see* Chapter 8), MAO-A preferentially metabolizes 5HT and NE. Dopamine and tryptamine are metabolized equally well by both isoforms. Neurons contain both isoforms of MAO, localized primarily in the outer membrane of mitochondria. MAO-B is the principal isoform in platelets, which contain large amounts of 5HT.

PHYSIOLOGICAL FUNCTIONS OF SEROTONIN

MULTIPLE 5HT RECEPTORS

The multiple 5HT receptor subtypes cloned comprise the largest known neurotransmitter-receptor family. The 5HT receptor subtypes are expressed in distinct but often overlapping patterns and are coupled to different transmembrane-signaling mechanisms (Table 13–1).

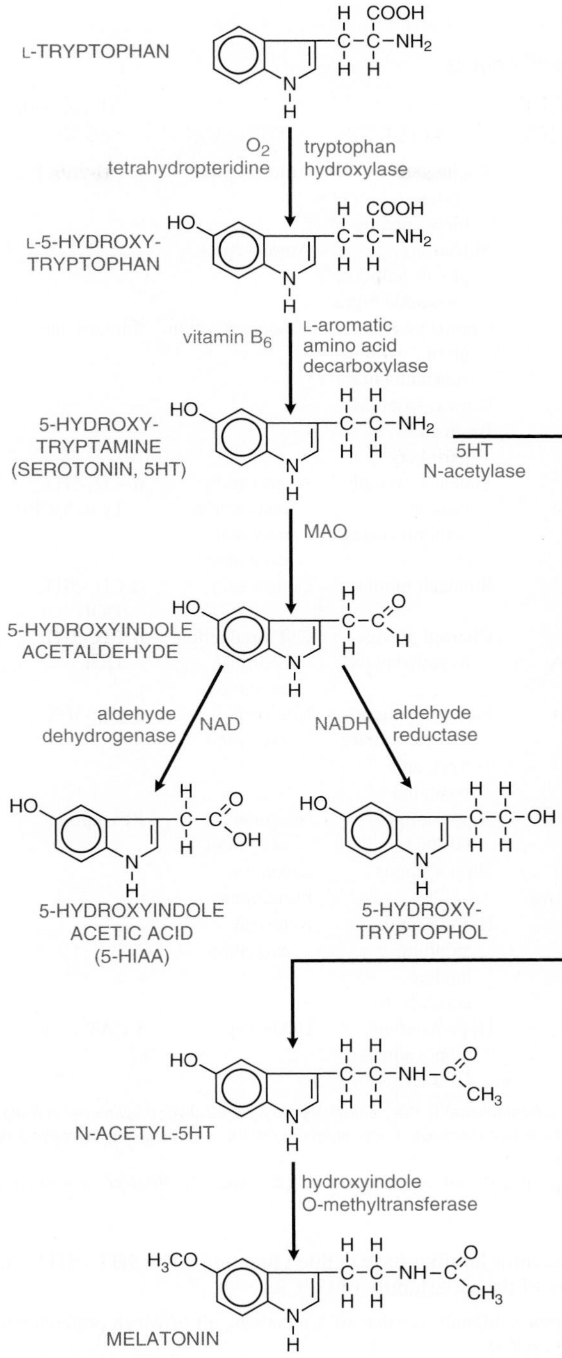

L-TRYPTOPHAN

O_2
tetrahydropteridine
tryptophan
hydroxylase

L-5-HYDROXY-
TRYPTOPHAN

vitamin B_6
L-aromatic
amino acid
decarboxylase

5-HYDROXY-
TRYPTAMINE
(SEROTONIN, 5HT)

5HT
N-acetylase

MAO

5-HYDROXYINDOLE
ACETALDEHYDE

aldehyde
dehydrogenase
NAD

NADH
aldehyde
reductase

5-HYDROXYINDOLE
ACETIC ACID
(5-HIAA)

5-HYDROXY-
TRYPTOPHOL

N-ACETYL-5HT

hydroxyindole
O-methyltransferase

MELATONIN

Figure 13–1 *Synthesis and inactivation of serotonin.* Enzymes are identified in *red* lettering, and cofactors are shown in *blue*.

Table 13–1

Serotonin Receptor Subtypes

SUBTYPE	SIGNALING EFFECTOR	LOCALIZATION	FUNCTION	SELECTIVE AGONIST	SELECTIVE ANTAGONIST
$5HT_{1A}$	↓ AC	Raphe nuclei, cortex, hippocampus	Autoreceptor	8-OH-DPAT	WAY 100135
$5HT_{1B}$[a]	↓ AC	Subiculum, globus pallidus, substantia nigra	Autoreceptor	—	—
$5HT_{1D}$	↓ AC	Cranial vessels, globus pallidus, substantia nigra	Vasoconstriction	Sumatriptan	—
$5HT_{1E}$	↓ AC	Cortex, striatum	—	—	—
$5HV_{1F}$[b]	↓ AC	Brain and periphery	—	—	—
$5HT_{2A}$[c]	↑ PLC, PLA_2	Platelets, smooth muscle, cerebral cortex	Aggregation, contraction, neuronal excitation	α-CH_3-5HT, DOI, MCPP	Ketanserin, LY53857
$5HT_{2B}$	↑ PLC	Stomach fundus	Contraction	α-CH_3-5HT, DOI	LY53857
$5HT_{2C}$	↑ PLC, PLA_2	Choroid plexus, hypothalamus	CSF production, neuronal excitation	α-CH_3-5HT, DOI	LY53857, Mesulergine
$5HT_3$[d]	cations	Parasympathetic nerves, solitary tract, area postrema	Neuronal excitation	2-CH_3-5HT	Ondansetron, tropisetron
$5HT_4$	↑ AC	Hippocampus, GI tract	Neuronal excitation	Renzapride	GR 113808
$5HT_{5A}$	↓ AC	Hippocampus	Unknown	—	—
$5HT_{5B}$	Unknown	—	Pseudogene	—	—
$5HT_6$	↑ AC	Hippocampus, striatum, nucleus accumbens	Neuronal excitation	—	SB 271046
$5HT_7$	↑ AC	Hypothalamus, hippocampus, GI tract	Unknown	5-CAT	

AC, adenylyl cyclase; PLC, phospholipase C; PLA_2; phospholipase A_2; 8-OH-DPAT, 8-hydroxy-(2-N,N-dipropylamino)-tetraline; DOI, 1-(2,5-dimethoxy-4-iodophenyl) isopropylamine; MCPP, metachlorphenylpiperazine; MK212; 5-CAT, 5-carboxamino-tryptamine.

[a]Also referred to as $5HT_{1D\beta}$. [b]Also referred to as $5HT_{1E\beta}$. [c]Aka the D receptor. [d]a 5HT-gated ion channel, aka the M receptor.

Four of seven 5HT receptor families have defined functions. The $5HT_1$, $5HT_2$, and $5HT_{4–7}$ receptor families are members of the superfamily of GPCRs.

- The $5HT_1$-receptor subfamily consists of 5 members, all of which preferentially couple to $G_{i/o}$ and inhibit adenylyl cyclase.
- The 3 subtypes of $5HT_2$ receptors couple to G_q/G_{11} proteins and activate the PLC-DAG/IP_3-Ca^{2+}-PKC pathway. $5HT_{2A}$ and $5HT_{2C}$ receptors also activate phospholipase A_2, promoting the release of arachidonic acid.
- The $5HT_3$ receptor is the only monoamine neurotransmitter receptor that functions as a ligand-operated ion channel. Activation of $5HT_3$ receptors elicits a rapidly desensitizing depolarization, mediated by the gating of cations.
- $5HT_4$ receptors couple to G_s to activate adenylyl cyclase and increase intracellular cyclic AMP.

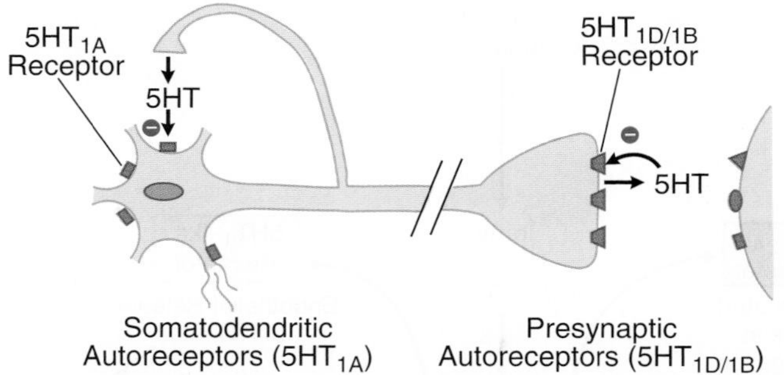

Figure 13–2 *Two classes of 5HT autoreceptors with differential localizations.* Somatodendritic $5HT_{1A}$ autoreceptors decrease raphe cell firing when activated by 5HT released from axon collaterals of the same or adjacent neurons. The receptor subtype of the presynaptic autoreceptor on axon terminals in the forebrain has different pharmacological properties and has been classified as $5HT_{1D}$ (in humans) or $5HT_{1B}$ (in rodents). This receptor modulates the release of 5HT. Postsynaptic $5HT_1$ receptors are also indicated.

The $5HT_{1A}$, $5HT_{1B}$, and $5HT_{1D}$ receptor subtypes also activate a receptor-operated K^+ channel and inhibit a voltage-gated Ca^{2+} channel. The $5HT_{1A}$ receptor is found in the raphe nuclei of the brainstem, where it functions as an inhibitory somatodendritic autoreceptor on cell bodies of serotonergic neurons (Figure 13–2). The $5HT_{1D/1B}$ receptor functions as an autoreceptor on axon terminals, inhibiting 5HT release. $5HT_{1D}$ receptors, abundantly expressed in the substantia nigra and basal ganglia, regulate the firing rate of DA-containing cells and the release of DA at axonal terminals.

$5HT_{2A}$ receptors are broadly distributed in the CNS (primarily in serotonergic terminal areas, with high densities in prefrontal and parietal areas, and somatosensory cortex), as well as in blood platelets (Figure 13–3) and smooth muscle cells. The $5HT_{2C}$ receptor has been implicated in the control of cerebrospinal fluid production and in feeding behavior and mood.

$5HT_3$ receptors are located on parasympathetic terminals in the GI tract, including vagal and splanchnic afferents. In the CNS, a high density of $5HT_3$ receptors occurs in the solitary tract nucleus and the area postrema. $5HT_3$ receptors in both the GI tract and the CNS participate in the emetic response, providing a basis for the antiemetic property of $5HT_3$ receptor antagonists.

In the CNS, $5HT_4$ receptors are found on neurons of the superior and inferior colliculi and in the hippocampus. In the GI tract, $5HT_4$ receptors are located on neurons of the myenteric plexus and on smooth muscle and secretory cells. In the GI tract, stimulation of the $5HT_4$ receptor is thought to evoke secretion and to facilitate the peristaltic reflex. The latter effect may explain the utility of prokinetic benzamides in GI disorders (*see* Chapter 46).

Two subtypes of the $5HT_5$ receptor have been cloned; although the $5HT_{5A}$ receptor has been shown to inhibit adenylyl cyclase, functional coupling of the cloned $5HT_{5B}$ receptor has not yet been described. Two other cloned receptors, $5HT_6$ and $5HT_7$, are linked to activation of adenylyl cyclase. $5HT_7$ receptors may play a role in the relaxation of smooth muscle in the GI tract and the vasculature. The atypical antipsychotic drug clozapine has a high affinity for $5HT_6$ and $5HT_7$ receptors; whether this property is related to the broader effectiveness of clozapine compared to conventional antipsychotic drugs is not known (*see* Chapter 16).

ACTIONS OF 5HT IN PHYSIOLOGICAL SYSTEMS

PLATELETS. Platelets differ from other formed elements of blood in expressing mechanisms for uptake, storage, and endocytotic release of 5HT. 5HT is not synthesized in platelets, but is taken up from the circulation and stored in secretory granules by active transport, similar to the uptake and storage of serotonin by serotonergic nerve terminals.

Thus, Na^+-dependent transport across the platelet plasma membrane via the 5HT transporter is followed by VMAT2-mediated uptake into storage granules creating a gradient of 5HT as high as 1000:1 with an internal concentration of 0.6 M in the storage vesicles.

When platelets make contact with injured endothelium (*see* Chapter 30), they release substances that promote platelet aggregation, and secondarily, they release 5HT (*see* Figure 13–3). 5HT binds to platelet $5HT_{2A}$ receptors and elicits a weak aggregation response that is markedly augmented by the presence of collagen. If the damaged blood vessel is injured to a depth where vascular

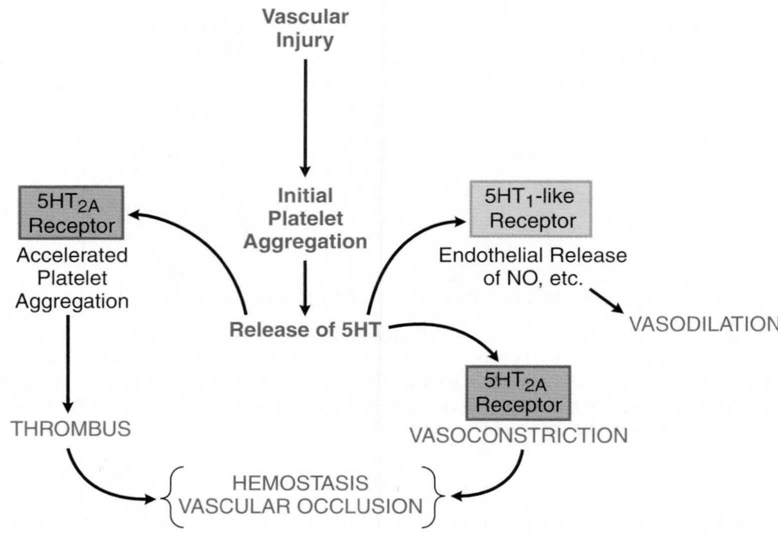

Figure 13–3 *The local influences of platelet 5HT.* The release of 5HT stored in platelets is triggered by aggregation. The local actions of 5HT include feedback actions on platelets (shape change and accelerated aggregation) mediated by interaction with platelet $5HT_{2A}$ receptors, stimulation of NO production mediated by $5HT_1$-like receptors on vascular endothelium, and contraction of vascular smooth muscle mediated by $5HT_{2A}$ receptors. These influences act in concert with many other mediators that are not shown to promote thrombus formation and hemostasis. *See* Chapter 30 for details of adhesion and aggregation of platelets and factors contributing to thrombus formation and blood clotting.

smooth muscle is exposed, 5HT exerts a direct vasoconstrictor effect, thereby contributing to hemostasis, which is enhanced by locally released autocoids (thromboxane A_2, kinins, and vasoactive peptides). Conversely, 5HT may interact with endothelial cells to stimulate production of NO and antagonize its own vasoconstrictor action, as well as the vasoconstriction produced by other locally released agents.

CARDIOVASCULAR SYSTEM. The classical response of blood vessels to 5HT is contraction, particularly in the splanchnic, renal, pulmonary, and cerebral vasculatures. 5HT also induces a variety of responses by the heart that are the result of activation of multiple 5HT receptor subtypes, stimulation or inhibition of autonomic nerve activity, or dominance of reflex responses to 5HT.

Thus, 5HT has positive inotropic and chronotropic actions on the heart that may be blunted by simultaneous stimulation of afferent nerves from baroreceptors and chemoreceptors. Activation of $5HT_3$ receptors on vagus nerve endings elicits the Bezold-Jarisch reflex, causing extreme bradycardia and hypotension. The local response of arterial blood vessels to 5HT also may be inhibitory, the result of the stimulation of endothelial NO production and prostaglandin synthesis and blockade of NE release from sympathetic nerves. Conversely, 5HT amplifies the local constrictor actions of NE, ANGII, and histamine, which reinforce the hemostatic response to 5HT.

GI TRACT. Enterochromaffin cells in the gastric mucosa are the site of the synthesis and most of the storage of 5HT in the body and are the source of circulating 5HT. Motility of gastric and intestinal smooth muscle may be either enhanced or inhibited by at least 6 subtypes of 5HT receptors (Table 13–2).

Basal release of enteric 5HT is augmented by mechanical stretching, such as that caused by food, and by efferent vagal stimulation. Released 5HT enters the portal vein and is subsequently metabolized by MAO-A in the liver. 5HT that survives hepatic oxidation may be captured by platelets or rapidly removed by the endothelium of lung capillaries and inactivated. 5HT released from enterochromaffin cells also acts locally to regulate GI function. Abundant $5HT_3$ receptors on vagal and other afferent neurons and on enterochromaffin cells play a pivotal role in emesis (*see* Chapter 46). Enteric 5HT triggers peristaltic contraction when released in response to acetylcholine, sympathetic nerve stimulation, increases in intraluminal pressure, and lowered pH.

Table 13–2

Some Actions of 5HT in the Gastrointestinal Tract

SITE	RESPONSE	RECEPTOR
Enterochromaffin cells	Release of 5HT	$5HT_3$
	Inhibition of 5HT release	$5HT_4$
Enteric ganglion cells (presynaptic)	Release of ACh	$5HT_4$
	Inhibition of ACh release	$5HT_{1P}$, $5HT_{1A}$
Enteric ganglion cells (postsynaptic)	Fast depolarization	$5HT_3$
	Slow depolarization	$5HT_{1P}$
Smooth muscle, intestinal	Contraction	$5HT_{2A}$
Smooth muscle, stomach fundus	Contraction	$5HT_{2B}$
Smooth muscle, esophagus	Contraction	$5HT_4$

ACh, acetylcholine.

CNS. All of the cloned 5HT receptors are expressed in the brain; 5HT influences a multitude of brain functions, including sleep, cognition, sensory perception, motor activity, temperature regulation, nociception, mood, appetite, sexual behavior, and hormone secretion. The roles of specific 5HT receptors in these functions have been defined in receptor knockout mice (Table 13–3).

The principal cell bodies of 5HT neurons are located in raphe nuclei of the brainstem and project throughout the brain and spinal cord (*see* Chapter 14). In addition to being released at discrete synapses, release of serotonin also seems to occur at sites of axonal *varicosities* that do not form distinct synaptic contacts. 5HT released at nonsynaptic varicosities is thought to diffuse to outlying targets, rather than acting on discrete synaptic targets, perhaps acting as a neuromodulator as well as a neurotransmitter (*see* Chapter 14). Serotonergic nerve terminals contain the proteins needed to synthesize 5HT from L-tryptophan. Newly formed 5HT is rapidly accumulated in synaptic vesicles (through VMAT2), where it is protected from MAO. 5HT released by nerve-impulse flow is reaccumulated into the presynaptic terminal by the 5HT transporter, SERT (SLC6A4; *see* Chapter 5). Presynaptic reuptake is a highly efficient mechanism for terminating the action of 5HT released by nerve-impulse flow. MAO localized in postsynaptic elements and surrounding cells rapidly inactivates 5HT that escapes neuronal reuptake and storage.

ELECTROPHYSIOLOGY. The physiological consequences of 5HT release vary with the brain area and the neuronal element involved, as well as with the 5HT receptor subtype(s) expressed (Table 13–4).

Table 13–3

Physiological Roles of 5HT Receptors Defined by Phenotypes in Knockout Mice

	$5HT_{1A}$	$5HT_{1B}$	$5HT_{2A}$	$5HT_{2B}$	$5HT_{2C}$	$5HT_3$	$5HT_4$	$5HT_{5A}$	$5HT_6$	$5HT_7$
Anxiety	↑		↓							
Aggression		↑								
Heart defects				Lethal						
Food intake					↑					
Seizure susceptibility					↑		↑			
Nociception						↓				
Exploratory activity								↑		
Ethanol sensitivity									↓	
Thermo-regulation										↓

Arrow indicates direction of alteration of the trait.
See Table 13–2 of parent text, 12th edition, for references.

Table 13–4

Electrophysiological Effects of 5HT Receptors

SUBTYPE	RESPONSE
$5HT_{1A,B}$	Increase K^+ conductance Hyperpolarization
$5HT_{2A}/5HT_{2C}$	Decrease K^+ conductance Slow depolarization
$5HT_3$	Gating of Na^+, K^+ Fast depolarization
$5HT_4$	Decrease K^+ conductance Slow depolarization

BEHAVIOR

SLEEP-WAKE CYCLE. 5HT plays a role in sleep-wake cycle.

Depletion of 5HT with *p-Chlorophenylalanine*, a tryptophan hydroxylase inhibitor, elicits insomnia that is reversed by the 5HT precursor, 5-hydroxytryptophan. Conversely, treatment with L-tryptophan or with nonselective 5HT agonists accelerates sleep onset and prolongs total sleep time. 5HT antagonists reportedly can increase and decrease slow-wave sleep, probably reflecting interacting or opposing roles for subtypes of 5HT receptors. One relatively consistent finding in humans and in laboratory animals is an increase in slow-wave sleep following administration of a selective $5HT_{2A/2C}$-receptor antagonist such as ritanserin.

AGGRESSION AND IMPULSIVITY. 5HT serves a critical role in aggression and impulsivity.

Human studies reveal a correlation between low cerebrospinal fluid 5-HIAA and violent impulsivity and aggression. Knockout mice lacking the $5HT_{1B}$ receptor exhibit extreme aggression, suggesting either a role for $5HT_{1B}$ receptors in the development of neuronal pathways important in aggression or a direct role in the mediation of aggressive behavior. A human genetic study identified a point mutation in the gene encoding MAO-A, which was associated with extreme aggressiveness and mental retardation; this has been confirmed in knockout mice lacking MAO-A.

ANXIETY AND DEPRESSION. The effects of 5HT–active drugs in anxiety and depressive disorders, like the effects of selective serotonin reuptake inhibitors (SSRIs), strongly suggest a role for 5HT in the neurochemical mediation of these disorders.

Inhibition of neuronal reuptake of 5HT via the transporter SERT (SLC6A4) prolongs the dwell-time of 5HT in the synapse. SSRIs, such as fluoxetine (PROZAC, others), potentiate and prolong the action of 5HT released by neuronal activity. When coadministered with L-5-hydroxytryptophan, SSRIs elicit a profound activation of serotonergic responses. SSRIs (citalopram [CELEXA], escitalopram [LEXAPRO], fluoxetine, fluvoxamine, paroxetine [PAXIL], and sertraline [ZOLOFT]) are the most widely used treatment for endogenous depression (*see* Chapter 15).

APPETITE. *Sibutramine* (MERIDIA), an inhibitor of the reuptake of 5HT, NE, and DA, is used as an appetite suppressant in the management of obesity.

Sibutramine is classified as a selective serotonin-norepinephrine reuptake inhibitor (SNRI). Other SNRIs include duloxetine (CYMBALTA; approved for depression, anxiety, peripheral neuropathy, and fibromyalgia), venlafaxine (EFFEXOR; approved for the treatment of depression, anxiety, and panic disorders), desvenlafaxine (PRISTIQ; approved for depression), and milnacipran (SAVELLA; approved for fibromyalgia).

5HT RECEPTOR AGONISTS AND ANTAGONISTS

5HT RECEPTOR AGONISTS

Direct-acting 5HT receptor agonists have widely different chemical structures, as well as diverse pharmacological properties and are used in the pharmacotherapy of migraine, anxiety, depression, chemotherapy-induced emesis, and disorders of GI motility (Table 13–5).

Table 13–5

Serotonergic Drugs: Primary Actions and Clinical Indications

RECEPTOR	ACTION	DRUG EXAMPLES	CLINICAL DISORDER
$5HT_{1A}$	Partial agonist	Buspirone, ipsaperone	Anxiety, depression
$5HT_{1D}$	Agonist	Sumatriptan	Migraine
$5HT_{2A/2C}$	Antagonist	Methysergide, risperidone, ketanserin	Migraine, depression, schizophrenia
$5HT_3$	Antagonist	Ondansetron	Chemotherapy-induced emesis
$5HT_4$	Agonist	Cisapride	GI disorders
SERT (5HT transporter)	Inhibitor	Fluoxetine, sertraline	Depression, obsessive-compulsive disorder, panic disorder, social phobia, posttraumatic stress disorder

5HT RECEPTOR AGONISTS AND MIGRAINE. 5HT seems to be a key mediator in the pathogenesis of migraine. Consistent with the 5HT hypothesis of migraine, 5HT receptor agonists are a mainstay for *acute* treatment of migraine headaches. The efficacy of antimigraine drugs varies with the absence or presence of aura, duration of the headache, its severity and intensity, and as yet undefined environmental and genetic factors.

$5HT_{1B/1D}$ RECEPTOR AGONISTS: THE TRIPTANS. The triptans are indole derivatives that are effective, acute antimigraine agents. Their capacity to decrease the nausea and vomiting of migraine is an important advance in the treatment of the condition. Available compounds include almotriptan (AXERT), eletriptan (RELPAX), frovatriptan (FROVA), naratriptan (AMERGE), rizatriptan (MAXALT, others), sumatriptan (IMITREX, others), and zolmitriptan (ZOMIG). Sumatriptan for migraine headaches is also marketed in a fixed-dose combination with naproxen (TREXIMET).

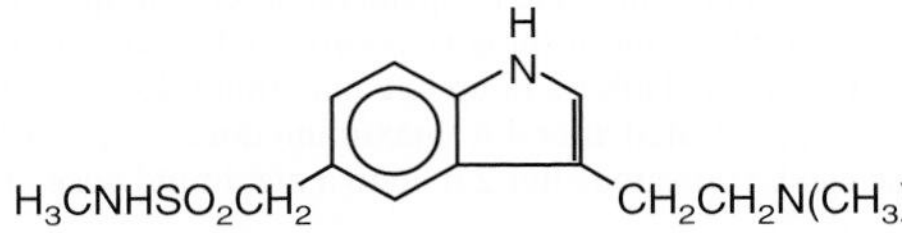

H

N

$H_3CNHSO_2CH_2$ $CH_2CH_2N(CH_3)_2$

SUMATRIPTAN

Pharmacological Properties. The pharmacological effects of the triptans appear to be limited to the $5HT_1$ family of receptors, providing evidence that this receptor subclass plays an important role in the acute relief of a migraine attack. The triptans interact potently with $5HT_{1B}$ and $5HT_{1D}$ receptors and have a low or no affinity for other subtypes of 5HT receptors, as well as α_1 and α_2 adrenergic, β adrenergic, dopaminergic, muscarinic cholinergic, and benzodiazepine receptors. Clinically effective doses of the triptans correlate well with their affinities for both $5HT_{1B}$ and $5HT_{1D}$ receptors, supporting the hypothesis that $5HT_{1B}$ and/or $5HT_{1D}$ receptors are the most likely receptors involved in the mechanism of action of acute antimigraine drugs.

Mechanism of Action. The mechanism of the efficacy of $5HT_{1B/1D}$ agonists in migraine is not resolved. One hypothesis of migraine suggests that unknown events lead to the abnormal dilation of carotid arteriovenous anastomoses in the head and shunting of carotid arterial blood flow, producing cerebral ischemia and hypoxia perceived as migraine pain; activation of $5HT_{1B/1D}$ receptors may cause constriction of intracranial blood vessels including arteriovenous anastomoses, closing the shunts and restoring blood flow to the brain. An alternative hypothesis proposes that both $5HT_{1B}$ and $5HT_{1D}$ receptors serve as presynaptic autoreceptors that may block the release of pro-inflammatory neuropeptides from the nerve terminal in the perivascular space, which could account for their efficacy in the acute treatment of migraine.

Absorption, Fate, and Excretion. When given subcutaneously, sumatriptan reaches its peak plasma concentration in ~12 min. Following oral administration, peak plasma concentrations occur within 1-2 h. Bioavailability following the subcutaneous route of administration is ~97%; after oral administration or nasal spray, bioavailability is only 14-17%. The elimination $t_{1/2}$ is ~1-2 h. Sumatriptan is metabolized predominantly by MAO-A, and its metabolites are excreted in the urine.

Zolmitriptan reaches its peak plasma concentration 1.5-2 h after oral administration. Zolmitriptan is converted to an active *N*-desmethyl metabolite, which has severalfold higher affinity for $5HT_{1B}$ and $5HT_{1D}$ receptors than does the parent drug. Both the metabolite and the parent drug have half-lives of 2-3 h.

Naratriptan, administered orally, reaches its peak plasma concentration in 2-3 h. It is the second longest acting of the triptans, with a $t_{1/2}$ of ~6 h. Fifty percent of an administered dose of naratriptan is excreted unchanged in the urine, and ~30% is excreted as products of oxidation by CYPs.

Rizatriptan reaches peak plasma levels within 1-1.5 h after oral ingestion of the drug. An orally disintegrating dosage form has a somewhat slower rate of absorption. The principal route of metabolism of rizatriptan is by oxidative deamination by MAO-A.

Adverse Effects and Contraindications. Rare but serious cardiac events have been associated with the administration of $5HT_1$ agonists, including coronary artery vasospasm, transient myocardial ischemia, atrial and ventricular arrhythmias, and myocardial infarction, predominantly in patients with risk factors for coronary artery disease. In general, however, only minor side effects are seen with the triptans in the acute treatment of migraine. After subcutaneous injection of sumatriptan, patients often experience irritation at the site of injection (transient mild pain, stinging, or burning sensations). The most common side effect of sumatriptan nasal spray is a bitter taste. Orally administered triptans can cause paresthesias; asthenia and fatigue; flushing; feelings of pressure, tightness, or pain in the chest, neck, and jaw; drowsiness; dizziness; nausea; and sweating.

Because triptans may cause an acute, usually small, increase in blood pressure, they also are contraindicated in patients with uncontrolled hypertension. Naratriptan is contraindicated in patients with severe renal or hepatic impairment. Rizatriptan should be used with caution in patients with renal or hepatic disease but is not contraindicated in such patients. Eletriptan is contraindicated in hepatic disease. Almotriptan, rizatriptan, sumatriptan, and zolmitriptan are contraindicated in patients who have taken an MAO inhibitor within the preceding 2 weeks, and all triptans are contraindicated in patients with near-term prior exposure to ergot alkaloids or other 5HT agonists.

TRIPTANS IN TREATMENT OF MIGRAINE. The triptans are effective in the acute treatment of migraine (with or without aura).

Approximately 70% of individuals report significant headache relief from a 6-mg subcutaneous dose of sumatriptan. This dose may be repeated once within a 24-h period. The oral dose of sumatriptan is 25-100 mg, which may be repeated after 2 h up to a total dose of 200 mg over a 24-h period. When administered by nasal spray, from 5-20 mg of sumatriptan is recommended, repeatable after 2 h up to a maximum dose of 40 mg over a 24-h period. The onset of action with nasal spray is as early as 15 min. Zolmitriptan is given orally in a dose of 1.25-2.5 mg, which can be repeated after 2 h, up to a maximum dose of 10 mg over 24 h. Naratriptan is given orally in a dose of 1-2.5 mg, repeated after 4 h (maximum dose 5 mg/ 24-h period). The oral dose of rizatriptan is 5-10 mg. The dose can be repeated after 2 h up to a maximum dose of 30 mg over a 24-h period.

ERGOT ALKALOIDS. Ergot is the product of a fungus (*Claviceps purpurea*) that grows on rye and other grains. The pharmacological effects of the ergot alkaloids are varied and complex; in general, the effects result from their actions as partial agonists or antagonists at serotonergic, dopaminergic, and adrenergic receptors. The history, chemistry, and pharmacological properties of the ergot alkaloids are covered in detail in Chapter 13 of the 12th edition of the parent text. The main uses of the ergot alkaloids are:

- In treatment of migraine (ergotamine tartrate and dihydroergotamine mesylate, in many dosage formulations; methysergide for prophylaxis)
- To control the secretion of prolactin (*bromocriptine*, taking advantage of its DA agonist effect)
- To increase uterine tone (all natural ergot alkaloids have this effect but ergonovine and its semisynthetic derivative methylergonovine have replaced other ergot preparations as uterine-stimulating agents in obstetrics)

ERGOT IN THE TREATMENT OF MIGRAINE. The multiple pharmacological effects of ergot alkaloids have complicated the determination of their precise mechanism of action in the acute treatment of migraine. The actions of ergot alkaloids at $5HT_{1B/1D}$ receptors likely mediate their *acute* antimigraine effects. The use of ergot alkaloids for migraine should be restricted to patients having frequent, moderate migraine or infrequent, severe migraine attacks. Ergot preparations should be administered as soon as possible after the onset of a headache. GI absorption of ergot alkaloids is erratic, perhaps contributing to the large variation in patient response to these drugs.

USE OF ERGOT ALKALOIDS IN POSTPARTUM HEMORRHAGE. All of the natural ergot alkaloids markedly increase the motor activity of the uterus. As the dose is increased, contractions become more forceful and prolonged, resting tone is dramatically increased, and sustained contracture can result. This characteristic is quite compatible with their use postpartum or after abortion to control bleeding and maintain uterine contraction. In current obstetric practice, ergot alkaloids are used primarily to prevent postpartum hemorrhage.

ADVERSE EFFECTS AND CONTRAINDICATIONS OF ERGOT ALKALOIDS. Ergot alkaloids are contraindicated in women who are, or may become, pregnant because the drugs may cause fetal distress and miscarriage. Ergot alkaloids also are contraindicated in patients with peripheral vascular disease, coronary artery disease, hypertension, impaired hepatic or renal function, and sepsis. Ergot alkaloids should not be taken within 24 h of the use of the triptans or used with other drugs that can cause vasoconstriction.

METHYSERGIDE. Methysergide (SANSERT; 1-methyl-*d*-lysergic acid butanolamide) interacts with $5HT_1$ receptors, but its therapeutic effects appear primarily to reflect blockade of $5HT_{2A}$ and $5HT_{2C}$ receptors.

Although methysergide is an ergot derivative, it has only weak vasoconstrictor and oxytocic activity. Methysergide is used for the prophylactic treatment of migraine and other vascular headaches. A potentially serious complication of prolonged treatment is inflammatory fibrosis, giving rise to various syndromes that include pleuropulmonary fibrosis, and coronary and endocardial fibrosis. Usually the fibrosis regresses after drug withdrawal, although persistent cardiac valvular damage has been reported. If methysergide is used chronically, treatment should be interrupted for 3 weeks or more every 6 months. Methysergide is not available in the U.S.

D-LYSERGIC ACID DIETHYLAMIDE (LSD). LSD is a nonselective 5HT agonist. This ergot derivative profoundly alters human behavior, eliciting sensory distortion (especially visual) and hallucinations at doses as low as 1 μg/kg. The potent, mind-altering effects of LSD explain its abuse by humans.

LSD interacts with brain 5HT receptors as an agonist/partial agonist. LSD mimics 5HT at $5HT_{1A}$ autoreceptors on raphe cell bodies, producing a marked slowing of the firing rate of serotonergic neurons. In the raphe, LSD and 5HT are equi-effective; however, in areas of serotonergic axonal projections (such as visual relay centers), LSD is far less effective than is 5HT. In an animal behavioral model, the discriminative stimulus effects of LSD and other hallucinogenic drugs appear to be mediated by activation of $5HT_{2A}$ receptors. LSD also interacts potently with many other 5HT receptors, including cloned receptors whose functions have not yet been determined. The hallucinogenic phenethylamine derivatives are selective $5HT_{2A/2C}$ receptor agonists. Current theories of the mechanism of action of LSD and other hallucinogens focus on $5HT_{2A}$ receptor-mediated disruption of thalamic gating with sensory overload of the cortex. Positron emission tomography imaging studies revealed that administration of the hallucinogen psilocybin (the active component of "shrooms") mimics the pattern of brain activation found in schizophrenic patients experiencing hallucinations. This action of psilocybin is blocked by pretreatment with a $5HT_{2A/2C}$ antagonist.

BUSPIRONE (BUSPAR, others). Buspirone, gepirone, and ipsapirone are selective partial agonists at $5HT_{1A}$ receptors. Buspirone has been effective in the treatment of anxiety (*see* Chapter 15). Buspirone mimics the antianxiety properties of benzodiazepines but does not interact with $GABA_A$ receptors and or display the sedative and anticonvulsant properties of benzodiazepines.

VILAZODONE (VIIBRYD). Vilazadone is an SSRI and a partial agonist at the $5HT_{1A}$ receptor. It is FDA-approved in adults for treatment of major depressive disorder.

m-CHLOROPHENYLPIPERAZINE (mCPP). The actions of mCPP in vivo primarily reflect activation of $5HT_{1B}$ and/or $5HT_{2A/2C}$ receptors; mCPP is an active metabolite of the antidepressant drug trazodone.

Animal studies suggest a greater involvement of the $5HT_{2C}$ receptor in the anxiogenic actions of mCPP. mCPP elevates cortisol and prolactin secretion, probably through a combination of $5HT_1$ and $5HT_{2A/2C}$ receptor activation. It also increases growth hormone secretion, apparently by a 5HT independent mechanism.

LORCASERIN (BELVIQ). Lorcaserin is a $5HT_{2C}$ receptor agonist approved for weight loss.

The drug is thought to decrease food consumption and promote satiety by selectively activating $5HT_{2C}$ receptors on anorexigenic proopiomelanocortin (POMC) neurons in the arcuate nucleus of the hypothalamus.

5HT RECEPTOR ANTAGONISTS

The properties of 5HT receptor antagonists vary widely. Ergot alkaloids and related compounds tend to be nonspecific 5HT receptor antagonists; however, a few ergot derivatives, such as metergoline, bind preferentially to members of the $5HT_2$ receptor family. A number of selective antagonists for $5HT_{2A/2C}$ and $5HT_3$ receptors are currently available. Ketanserin is the prototypic $5HT_{2A}$ receptor antagonist. A large series of $5HT_3$ receptor antagonists are being explored for treatment of various GI disturbances (e.g., ondansetron [ZOFRAN, others], dolasetron [ANZEMET], granisetron

[Kytril, others], and palonosetron [Aloxi]). All $5HT_3$ receptor antagonists have proven to be highly efficacious in the treatment of chemotherapy-induced nausea, and alosetron (Lotronex) is licensed for irritable bowel syndrome (*see* Chapter 46).

KETANSERIN. Ketanserin (Sufrexal, others) potently blocks $5HT_{2A}$ receptors, less potently blocks $5HT_{2C}$ receptors, and has no significant effect on $5HT_3$ or $5HT_4$ receptors or any members of the $5HT_1$-receptor family. Ketanserin also blocks α adrenergic receptors and histamine H_1 receptors.

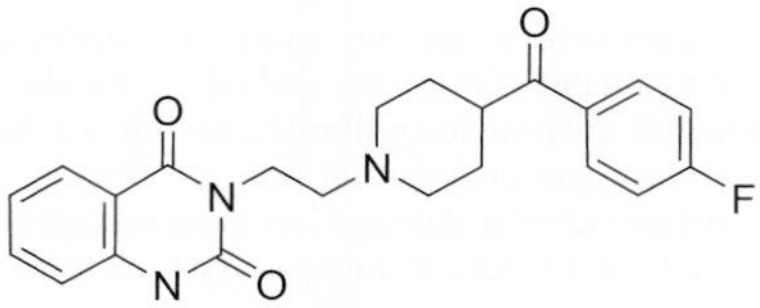

KETANSERIN

Ketanserin lowers blood pressure in patients with hypertension, causing a reduction comparable to that seen with β adrenergic receptor antagonists or diuretics. This effect likely relates to its blockade of α_1 adrenergic receptors. Ketanserin inhibits 5HT-induced platelet aggregation. Its oral bioavailability is ~50%, and its plasma $t_{1/2}$ is 12-25 h. The primary mechanism of inactivation is hepatic metabolism. Ketanserin is not marketed in the U.S. Chemical relatives of *ketanserin* such as *ritanserin* are more selective $5HT_{2A}$ receptor antagonists with low affinity for α_1 adrenergic receptors. Ritanserin, as well as most other $5HT_{2A}$ receptor antagonists, also potently antagonize $5HT_{2C}$ receptors.

ATYPICAL ANTIPSYCHOTIC DRUGS. Clozapine (Clozaril, others), a $5HT_{2A/2C}$ receptor antagonist, represents a class of atypical antipsychotic drugs with reduced incidence of extrapyramidal side effects compared to the classical neuroleptics (*see* Chapter 16). Clozapine also has a high affinity for subtypes of DA receptors.

A common strategy for the design of atypical antipsychotic drugs is to combine $5HT_{2A/2C}$ and dopamine D_2 receptor–blocking actions in the same molecule. Risperidone (Risperdal, others) is a potent $5HT_{2A}$ and D_2 receptor antagonist. Low doses of risperidone have been reported to attenuate negative symptoms of schizophrenia with a low incidence of extrapyramidal side effects.

CYPROHEPTADINE. *Cyproheptadine* is an effective H_1-receptor antagonist. Cyproheptadine blocks 5HT activity on smooth muscle by binding to $5HT_{2A}$ receptors. In addition, it has weak anticholinergic activity and possesses mild CNS depressant properties.

Cyproheptadine shares the properties and uses of other H_1-receptor antagonists (*see* Chapter 32). The 5HT blocking actions of cyproheptadine explain its value in the off-label uses for postgastrectomy dumping syndrome, intestinal hypermotility of carcinoid, and migraine prophylaxis. Cyproheptadine is not a preferred treatment for these conditions.

METHYSERGIDE. Methysergide has both agonist and antagonist activities at multiple 5HT receptors. *See* its section, above.

CLINICAL MANIPULATION OF 5HT LEVELS: SEROTONIN SYNDROME

Excessive elevation of 5HT levels in the body can cause *serotonin syndrome*, a constellation of symptoms sometimes observed in patients starting new or increased antidepressant therapy or combining an SSRI with an NE reuptake inhibitor or a triptan (for migraine). Symptoms may include restlessness, confusion, shivering, tachycardia, diarrhea, muscle twitches/rigidity, fever, seizures, loss of consciousness, and death.

DOPAMINE

The highest concentrations of DA are found in the brain; DA stores are also present peripherally in the adrenal medulla and the transmitter is detectable in the plexuses of the GI tract and in enteric nervous system. DA modulates peripheral vascular tone, renal perfusion, and heart rate.

DA consists of a catechol moiety linked to an ethyl amine, leading to its classification as a catecholamine. DA is closely related to melanin, a pigment that is formed by oxidation of DA, tyrosine, or L-dopa. Melanin exists in the skin and cuticle and gives the substantia nigra its namesake dark color. Both DA and L-dopa are readily oxidized by nonenzymatic pathways to form cytotoxic reactive oxygen species (ROS) and quinones. DA- and DOPA-quinones form adducts with α-synuclein, a major constituent of Lewy bodies in Parkinson disease (*see* Chapter 22). DA is a polar molecule that does not readily cross the blood-brain barrier.

SYNTHESIS AND METABOLISM OF DA. The biosynthesis and metabolism of DA are summarized by Figure 13–4.

Phenylalanine and tyrosine are the precursors of DA. For the most part, mammals convert dietary phenylalanine to tyrosine by *phenylalanine hydroxylase*. Tyrosine crosses readily into the brain through uptake; normal brain levels of tyrosine are typically saturating. Conversion of tyrosine to L-dopa (3,4-dihydroxyphenylalanine) by the enzyme *tyrosine hydroxylase* is the rate-limiting step in the synthesis of DA (as in NE synthesis; *see* Chapter 8). Once generated, L-dopa is rapidly converted to DA by AADC, the same enzyme that generates 5HT from L-5-hydroxytryptophan. Unlike DA, L-dopa readily crosses the blood-brain barrier and is converted to DA in the brain, which explains its utility in therapy for Parkinson disease (*see* Chapter 22). Diminished levels of phenylalanine hydroxylase lead to high levels of phenylalanine, producing a condition known as *phenylketonuria*, which must be controlled by dietary restrictions in order to avoid intellectual impairment.

THE DOPAMINERGIC SYNAPSE. The neurochemical events that underlie DA neurotransmission are summarized in Figure 13–5.

In dopaminergic neurons, synthesized DA is packaged into secretory vesicles (or into granules within adrenal chromaffin cells) by the vesicular monoamine transporter, VMAT2. By contrast, in adrenergic or noradrenergic cells, the DA is not packaged; instead, it is converted to NE by DA β-hydroxylase and, in adrenergic cells, further altered to epinephrine in cells expressing phenylethanolamine *N*-methyltransferase (*see* Chapter 8). Synaptically released DA is subject to transporter clearance and metabolism. The DA transporter (DAT) is not selective for DA; moreover, DA can also be cleared from the synapse by the NE transporter, NET. Reuptake of DA by DAT is the primary mechanism for termination of DA action, and allows for either vesicular repackaging of transmitter or metabolism. The DA transporter is regulated by phosphorylation, offering the potential for DA to regulate its own uptake.

The DA transporter is predominantly localized perisynaptically so that DA is cleared at a distance from its release site. The DA transporter is a site of action for cocaine and methamphetamine. The DA transporter is also the molecular target for some neurotoxins, including 6-hydroxydopamine and 1-methyl-4-phenylpyridinium (MPP+), the neurotoxic metabolite of 1-methyl-4-phenyl-1,2,3,6-tetrahydropyridine (MPTP). Following uptake into dopaminergic neurons, MPP+ and 6-hydroxydopamine elicit intra- and extracellular DA release, ultimately resulting in neuronal death. This selective dopaminergic degeneration mimics Parkinson disease, and serves as an animal model for this disorder.

Metabolism of DA occurs primarily by MAO localized in both pre- and postsynaptic elements. MAO acts on DA to generate an inactive aldehyde derivative by oxidative deamination (*see* Figures 13–4 and 13–5), which is subsequently metabolized by aldehyde dehydrogenase to form 3,4-dihydroxyphenylacetic acid (DOPAC). DOPAC can be further metabolized by COMT to form homovanillic acid (HVA). COMT can convert DA to 3-methoxytyramine, which is subsequently converted to HVA by MAO. DOPAC, and HVA, as well as DA, are excreted in the urine.

COMT in the periphery also metabolizes L-dopa to 3-O-methyldopa, which then competes with L-dopa for uptake into the CNS. Consequently, L-dopa given in the treatment of Parkinson disease must be coadministered with peripheral COMT inhibitors to preserve L-dopa and allow sufficient entry into the CNS (*see* Chapter 22).

PHYSIOLOGICAL FUNCTIONS OF DOPAMINE

MULTIPLE DA RECEPTORS

Five distinct GPCRs have been cloned and determined to mediate the actions of DA. The family of DA receptors is divided into the D1 and D2 subfamilies based on their effector-coupling profiles (Figure 13–6).

The D1 subfamily consists of the D_1 and D_5 receptor subtypes; both are GPCRs that couple to G_s to stimulate cellular cyclic AMP production couple, but they differ in their pharmacological profiles.

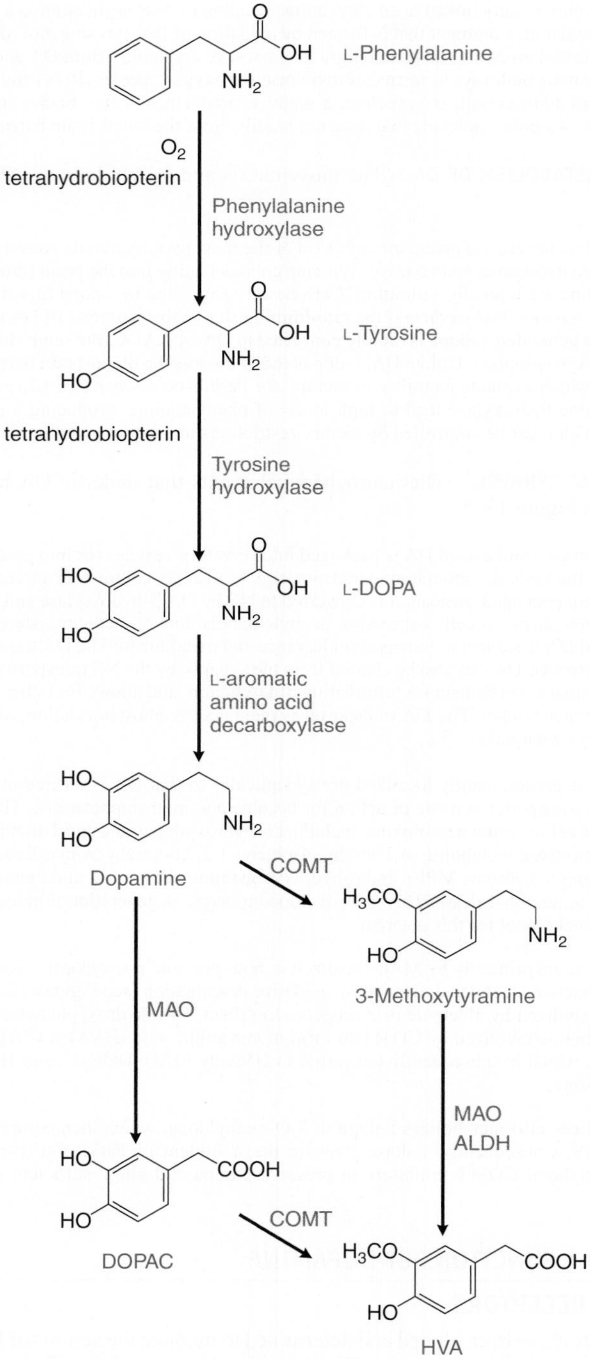

L-Phenylalanine

O_2
tetrahydrobiopterin
Phenylalanine hydroxylase

L-Tyrosine

tetrahydrobiopterin
Tyrosine hydroxylase

L-DOPA

L-aromatic amino acid decarboxylase

Dopamine

COMT

3-Methoxytyramine

MAO

MAO
ALDH

DOPAC

COMT

HVA

Figure 13–4 *Synthesis and inactivation of dopamine.* Enzymes are identified in *blue* lettering, and cofactors are shown in *black* letters. *See* legend to Figure 13–5 for key to abbreviations.

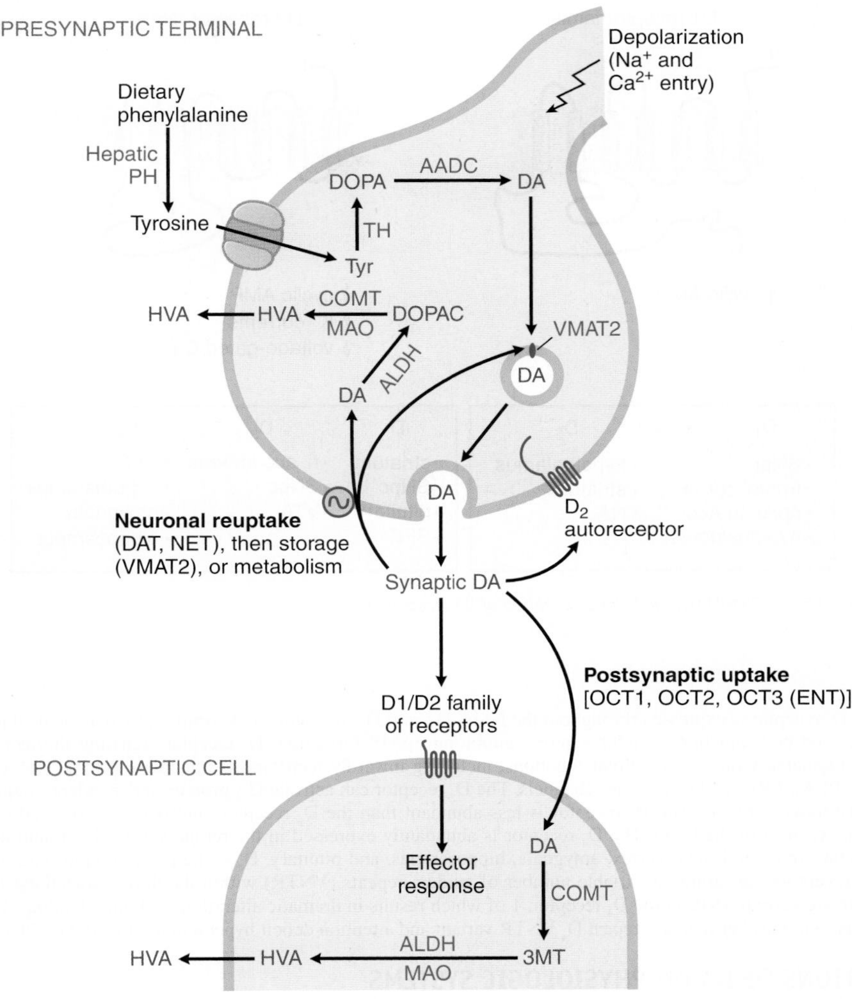

Figure 13–5 *Dopaminergic nerve terminal.* Dopamine (DA) is synthesized from tyrosine in the nerve terminal by the sequential actions of tyrosine hydrolase (TH) and aromatic amino acid decarboxylase (AADC). DA is sequestered by vesicular monoamine transporter (VMAT2) in storage granules and released by exocytosis. Synaptic DA activates presynaptic autoreceptors and postsynaptic D_1 and D_2 receptors. Synaptic DA may be taken up into the neuron via the DA and NE transporters (DAT, NET), or removed by postsynaptic uptake via OCT3 transporters. Cytosolic DA is subject to degradation by monoamine oxidase (MAO) and aldehyde dehydrogenase (ALDH) in the neuron, and by catechol-*O*-methyltransferase (COMT) and MAO/ALDH in nonneuronal cells; the final metabolic product is homovanillic acid (HVA). PH, phenylalanine hydroxylase. *See* structures in Figure 13–4.

The D_1 receptor is the most highly conserved and the most highly expressed of the DA receptors. The highest levels of D_1 receptor protein are found within the CNS. The neostriatum expresses the highest levels of D_1 receptor but does not express any detectable $G\alpha_s$. In this region, the D_1 receptor appears to couple to G_{olf} to increase levels of cAMP and its downstream effectors. The D_1 receptor is also located in the kidney, retina, and cardiovascular system. The D_5 gene is polymorphic; several functional single nucleotide polymorphisms (SNPs) within the transmembrane domains alter binding properties of numerous ligands, including DA. The D_5 receptor is most highly expressed in the substantia nigra, hypothalamus, striatum, cerebral cortex, nucleus accumbens, and olfactory tubercle.

The D2 subfamily contains the D_2, D_3, and D_4 receptors. All reduce intracellular cyclic AMP production by coupling to $G_{i/o}$ proteins, but they diverge in amino acid sequence and pharmacology.

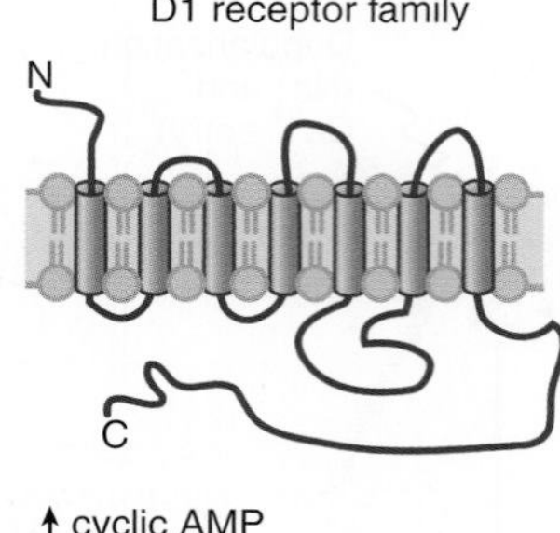

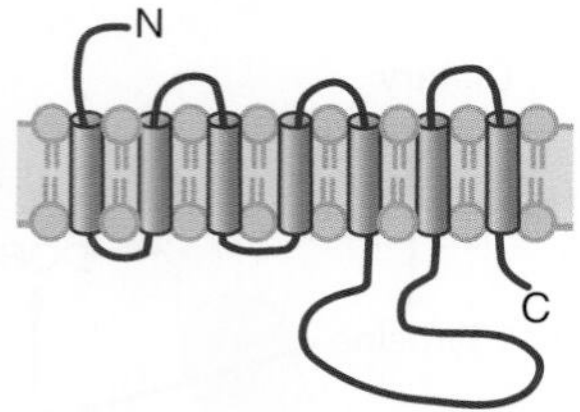

D_1	D_5	D_2	D_3	D_4
• SNpr	• hypothalamus	• striatum	• n. accumbens	• PFC
• frontal cortex	• striatum	• SNpc	• SNpc	• hypothalamus
• nucleus Acc	• NAc	• pituitary	• VTA	• amygdala
• hypothalamus		• PFC		• hippocampus

Figure 13–6 *Distribution and characterization of DA receptors in the CNS.*

The D_2 receptor is expressed throughout the brain. D_{2S} and D_{2L} receptors have similar pharmacological properties and both function as autoreceptors, inhibiting cAMP formation. D_2 receptor signaling through Gβγ also regulates a variety of cellular functions, including inwardly rectifying K^+ channels, N-type Ca^{2+} channels, PLA_2, ERK, and L-type Ca^{2+} channels. The D_2 receptor can activate $G_{i/o}$ proteins independent of agonist (constitutive activity). The D_3 receptor is less abundant than the D_2 receptor, and is only expressed in the limbic regions of the brain. The D_4 receptor is abundantly expressed in the retina, and is also found in the hypothalamus, prefrontal cortex, amygdala, hippocampus, and pituitary. D_4 is the most polymorphic of the DA receptors, containing a variable number of tandem repeats (VNTR) within the third intracellular loop. There are several SNPs in the D_4 receptor, 1 of which results in dramatic alterations in ligand binding. There are associations between a 7-repeat D_4 VNTR variant and attention deficit hyperactivity disorder (ADHD).

ACTIONS OF DA ON PHYSIOLOGIC SYSTEMS

HEART AND VASCULATURE. At low concentrations, circulating DA primarily stimulates vascular D_1 receptors, causing vasodilation and reducing cardiac afterload. The net result is a decrease in blood pressure and an increase in cardiac contractility. As circulating DA concentrations rise, DA is able to activate β adrenergic receptors to further increase cardiac contractility.

At very high concentrations, circulating DA activates α adrenergic receptors in the vasculature, thereby causing vasoconstriction; thus, high concentrations of DA increase blood pressure. Clinically, DA administration is used to treat severe congestive heart failure, sepsis, or cardiogenic shock. It is only administered intravenously and is not considered a long-term treatment.

KIDNEY. DA is a paracrine/autocrine transmitter in the kidney and binds to both receptors of both the D1 and D2 subfamily. Renal DA primarily serves to increase natriuresis, though it can also increase renal blood flow and glomerular filtration. Under basal sodium conditions, DA regulates Na^+ excretion by inhibiting the activity of various Na^+ transporters, including the apical Na^+-H^+ exchanger and the basolateral Na^+,K^+-ATPase. Activation of D_1 receptors increases renin secretion, whereas DA, acting on D_3 receptors, reduces renin secretion. Abnormalities in the DA system and its receptors have been implicated in human hypertension.

PITUITARY GLAND. DA is the primary regulator of prolactin secretion from the pituitary gland. DA released from the hypothalamus into the hypophyseal portal blood supply acts on lactotroph D_{2S} and D_{2L} receptors to decrease prolactin secretion (*see* Chapter 38).

CATECHOLAMINE RELEASE. Both D_1 and D_2 receptors modulate the release of NE and EPI. The D_2 receptor provides tonic inhibition of EPI release from chromaffin cells of the adrenal medulla, and of NE release from sympathetic nerve terminals. In contrast, the D_1 receptor promotes the release of catecholamines from the adrenal medulla.

CNS. There are 3 major groups of DA projections in the brain (Figure 13–7): mesocortico/mesolimbic (originating in the ventral tegmental area), nigrostriatal (originating in the substantia nigra pars compacta) and tuberoinfundibular (originating in the hypothalamus). The physiological processes under dopaminergic control include reward, emotion, cognition, memory, and motor activity. Dysregulation of the dopaminergic system is critical in a number of disease states, including Parkinson disease, Tourette syndrome, bipolar depression, schizophrenia, ADHD, and addiction/substance abuse.

The mesolimbic pathway is associated with reward and, less so, with learned behaviors. Dysfunction in this pathway is associated with addiction, schizophrenia, and psychoses (including bipolar depression), and learning deficits. The mesocortical projections are important for "higher-order" cognitive functions including motivation, reward, emotion, and impulse control; they are also implicated in psychoses, including schizophrenia, and in ADHD. The nigrostriatal pathway is a key regulator of movement (*see* Chapter 22). Impairments in this pathway are evident in Parkinson disease and underlie detrimental movement side effects associated with dopaminergic therapy, including tardive dyskinesia. DA released in the tuberoinfundibular pathway is carried by the hypophyseal blood supply to the pituitary, where it regulates prolactin secretion.

ELECTROPHYSIOLOGY. DA is not a classical excitatory or inhibitory neurotransmitter; rather, DA acts as a modulator of neurotransmission. D_1-like receptor activation modulates Na^+, as well as N-, P- and L-type Ca^{2+} currents, via a PKA-dependent pathway. D_2 receptors regulate K^+ currents. DA also modulates the activity of ligand-gated ion channels, including NMDA and AMPA receptors.

Dopaminergic neurons are strongly influenced by *excitatory glutamate and inhibitory GABA input*. In general, glutamate inputs enable burstlike firing of dopaminergic neurons, resulting in high concentrations of synaptic DA. GABA inhibition of DA neurons causes a tonic, basal level of DA release into the synapse. DA release also modulates GABA and glutamate neurons, thus providing an additional level of interaction between DA and other neurotransmitters. Strong phasic or slow tonic release of DA, and the subsequent activation of DA receptors, has differential effects on the induction of long-term potentiation (LTP) and long-term depression (LTD). In the striatum, phasic activation of DA neurons and stimulation of D_1 receptors favors LTP induction, while tonic DA release with concomitant activation of both D_1- and D_2-like receptors favors LTD.

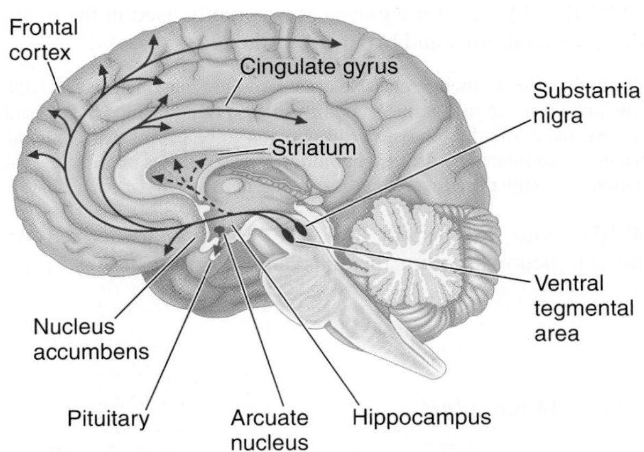

Figure 13–7 *Major dopaminergic projections in the CNS.*

- The nigrostriatal (or mesostriatal) pathway. Neurons in the substantia nigra pars compacta (SNc) project to the dorsal striatum (*upward dashed blue arrows*); this is the pathway that degenerates in Parkinson disease.
- The mesocortico/mesolimbic pathway. Neurons in the ventral tegmental area project to the ventral striatum (nucleus accumbens), olfactory bulb, amygdala, hippocampus, orbital and medial prefrontal cortex, and cingulate gyrus (*solid blue arrows*).
- The tuberoinfundibular pathway. Neurons in the arcuate nucleus of the hypothalamus project by the tuberoinfundibular pathway in the hypothalamus, from which DA is delivered to the anterior pituitary (*red arrows*).

ROLES OF DA IN BEHAVIOR

LOCOMOTION: MODELS OF PARKINSON DISEASE (PD). In the early 1980s, several young people in California developed rapid-onset parkinsonism. All of the affected individuals had injected a synthetic analog of meperidine that was contaminated with MPTP. MPTP is metabolized by MAO-B to the neurotoxic MPP^+. Because of the high specificity of MPP^+ for the DA transporter, neuronal death is largely restricted to the substantia nigra and ventral tegmental area, resulting in a phenotype remarkably similar to Parkinson disease.

6-Hydroxydopamine (6-OHDA) is similar to MPTP in both mechanism of action and utility in animal models. Lesioning animals with MPTP or 6-OHDA results in tremor, grossly diminished locomotor activity, and rigidity. As with Parkinson disease, these motor deficits are alleviated with L-dopa therapy or dopaminergic agonists.

Other pharmacological agents are also known to alter locomotor activity via dopaminergic actions, including cocaine and amphetamine. These drugs bind to DAT and inhibit reuptake of synaptic DA.

Studies with D_1 receptor knockout mice indicate that the D_1 receptor, but not the D_5 receptor, is primarily responsible for the increase in locomotor activity that occurs following administration of D1-family agonists. D_2 receptor knockout mice display marked reductions in locomotor activity, initiation of movement, and rearing behaviors. This reduction in motor activity is also present in mice that are specifically lacking only the D_{2L} receptor. The D_3 and D_4 receptor knockout animals display unique locomotor alterations in response to novel environments.

REWARD: IMPLICATIONS IN ADDICTION. In general, drugs of abuse cause increased DA levels in the nucleus accumbens, an area critical for rewarded behaviors. This role for mesolimbic DA in addiction has led to numerous studies on abused drugs in DA receptor knockout mice that suggest complex roles of D_1, D_2, and D_3 receptors in addiction that are reviewed in the parent text.

COGNITION, LEARNING, AND MEMORY. Mice lacking the D_1 receptor display deficits in multiple forms of memory. Other findings in animal models imply an important role for the D_2 receptor in disorders with defects in sensorimotor gating, most notably schizophrenia. Indeed, many of the antipsychotic drugs used in the treatment of schizophrenia are high affinity antagonists for the D_2 receptor.

DA RECEPTOR AGONISTS AND ANTAGONISTS

DA RECEPTOR AGONISTS. DA receptor agonists are currently used in the treatment of Parkinson disease (PD), restless leg syndrome, and hyperprolactinemia.

One of the primary limitations to the therapeutic use of dopaminergic agonists is the lack of receptor subtype selectivity. Recent advances in receptor-ligand structure-function relationships have enabled the development of subtype-specific drugs, many of which have already proven to be useful experimental tools (Table 13–6). DA receptor activity can be modulated by drugs that bind to allosteric sites on the receptor, thereby enhancing or decreasing endogenous DA signaling in a receptor-specific manner.

DA RECEPTOR AGONISTS AND PARKINSON DISEASE. PD is characterized by extensive degeneration of dopaminergic neurons within the substantia nigra, resulting in tremor, rigidity, and

Table 13–6

Experimental Tools at DA Receptors

	AGONIST	ANTAGONIST
D1-like	Dihydrexidine	SCH23390
	SKF38393	SKF83566
D2-like	7-OH-DPAT	Sulpiride
D_3	7-OH-PIPAT	U99194
		BP-897
D_4	PD168077	L-745,870
D_5	ADTN	—

bradykinesia. The principal pharmacotherapy for PD is L-dopa, but limitations to its therapeutic effects (*see* Chapter 22) have generated intense interest in developing alternative therapies for PD, with the intent of either delaying the usage of L-dopa or alleviating its side effects. DA agonists can be used in conjunction with lower doses of L-dopa in a combined therapy approach. Two general classes of dopaminergic agonists are used in the treatment of PD: ergots and non-ergots. The use of these drugs in the management of PD is described in Chapter 22.

D_1/D_2 RECEPTOR AGONISTS: ERGOT ALKALOIDS. Ergot derivatives act on several different neurotransmitter systems, including DA, 5HT, and adrenergic receptors. *Bromocriptine* (PARLODEL) and pergolide (PERMAX) have been used for the treatment of PD; however, their use is associated with risk for serious cardiac complications.

Bromocriptine is a potent D_2 receptor agonist and a weak D_1 antagonist. Pergolide is a partial agonist of D_1 receptors and a strong D2-family agonist with high affinity for both D_2 and D_3 receptor subtypes. Ergot derivatives are commonly reported to cause unpleasant side effects, including nausea, dizziness, and hallucinations. Pergolide was removed from the U.S. market as therapy for PD after as it was associated with an increased risk for valvular heart disease.

ERGOT ALKALOIDS IN THE TREATMENT OF HYPERPROLACTINEMIA. The ergot-based DA agonists bromocriptine and *cabergoline* (DOSTINEX) are used in the treatment of hyperprolactinemia. Both are strong agonists at D_2 receptors, with lower affinity for D_1, 5HT, and α adrenergic receptors; both activate D_2 receptors in the pituitary to reduce prolactin secretion. The risk of valvular heart disease in ergot therapy is not associated with the lower doses used in treating hyperprolactinemia. The use of bromocriptine and cabergoline in the management of hyperprolactinemia is described in Chapter 38.

D_1/D_2 RECEPTOR AGONISTS (NON-ERGOT ALKALOIDS). *Apomorphine* (APOKYN) is approved for the treatment of PD. Apomorphine binds with the order of potency $D_4 > D_2 > D_3 > D_5$, and with lower affinity to D_1, α adrenergic, $5HT_{1A}$, and $5HT_2$ receptors. Apomorphine is most commonly used in combination with L-dopa to surmount the sudden "off" periods that can occur after long-term L-dopa treatment.

Rotigotine is offered in a transdermal patch (NEUPRO) that is approved for the treatment of PD and restless leg syndrome (RLS). Rotigotine preferentially binds to D_2 and D_3 receptors and has much lower affinity for D_1 receptors. In addition, rotigotine is an agonist at $5HT_{1A}$ and $5HT_2$ receptors, and an antagonist at α_2 adrenergic receptors.

D_2 FAMILY RECEPTOR AGONISTS (NON-ERGOT ALKALOIDS). Pramipexole (MIRAPEX) and ropinirole (REQUIP) are agonists at all D_2 family receptors and also bind with highest affinity to the D_3 receptor subtype. In addition to its utility in the treatment of PD, ropinirole has also been FDA-approved as pharmacotherapy for RLS. Mild dopaminergic hypofunction has been noted in patients with RLS.

D_4 RECEPTOR AGONISTS AND ADHD. The D_4 receptor is significant in ADHD; there is an association between the 7-repeat D_4 VNTR variant and patients with ADHD. D_4-selective agonists show significant promise for the next generation of ADHD therapy.

DA RECEPTOR ANTAGONISTS

As with the DA receptor agonists, a lack of subtype-specific antagonists has limited the therapeutic utility of this group of ligands. Selective antagonists are now available as experimental tools (*see* Table 13–6). Many subtype-selective antagonists are in early stages of preclinical testing for therapeutic utility.

DA RECEPTOR ANTAGONISTS AND SCHIZOPHRENIA. DA receptor antagonists are a mainstay in the pharmacotherapy of schizophrenia. While many neurotransmitter systems likely contribute to the complex pathology of schizophrenia (*see* Chapter 16), DA dysfunction is considered the basis of this disorder. The DA hypothesis of schizophrenia has its origins in the characteristics of the drugs used to treat this disorder: All antipsychotic compounds used clinically have high affinity for DA receptors. The drugs used to treat schizophrenia are classified as either typical (first generation) antipsychotics or atypical antipsychotics (characterized by lack of extrapyramidal side effects). Most atypical antipsychotics are low affinity antagonists at the D_2 receptor and high affinity antagonists or inverse agonists at the $5HT_{2A}$ receptor. Some of the newer drugs in development do not fit into this classification scheme, including the D_1-selective agonist, dihydrexidine.

Typical Antipsychotics. The first antipsychotic drug used to treat schizophrenia was *chlorpromazine* (THORAZINE). Its antipsychotic properties were attributed to its antagonism of DA receptors, especially the D_2 receptor. More D_2-selective ligands were developed to improve the antipsychotic properties, including haloperidol (HALDOL) and similar D_2-selective drugs (*see* Chapter 16).

Atypical Antipsychotics. This class of antipsychotic drugs originated with *clozapine* (FAZACLO). The lack of extrapyramidal side effects has been attributed to a much lower affinity for the D_2 receptor compared to the typical antipsychotics. Atypical agents are also less likely to stimulate prolactin production. Clozapine has higher affinity for the D_4 receptor. Most atypical antipsychotics are low affinity antagonists at the D_2 receptor and high affinity antagonists or inverse agonists at the $5HT_{2A}$ receptor.

Aripiprazole (ABILIFY) has fewer side effects than earlier atypical antipsychotics. Aripiprazole diverges from the traditional atypical profile in 2 ways: first, it has higher affinity for D_2 receptors than for $5HT_{2A}$ receptors; second, it is a partial agonist at D_2 receptors. As a partial agonist, aripiprazole may diminish the subcortical DA hyperfunction by competing with DA for receptor binding, while simultaneously enhancing dopaminergic neurotransmission in the prefrontal cortex by acting as an agonist. The dual mechanism afforded by a partial agonist may thus treat both the positive and negative symptoms associated with schizophrenia.

D_3 RECEPTOR ANTAGONISTS AND DRUG ADDICTION. D_3-selective antagonists show promise in the treatment of addiction.

For a complete Bibliographical Listing see Goodman & Gilman's ***The Pharmacological Basis of Therapeutics***, 12th ed., or Goodman & Gilman Online at www.AccessMedicine.com.

Neurotransmission and the Central Nervous System

ORGANIZATIONAL PRINCIPLES OF THE CNS

The brain is a complex assembly of interacting neurons and nuclei that regulate their own and each other's activities in a dynamic fashion, generally through chemical neurotransmission. It is useful to examine the major anatomical regions of the CNS and their associations with specific neurotransmitter systems and the effect of pharmacological agents thereon.

CELLULAR ORGANIZATION OF THE BRAIN

Neurons. Neurons are classified according to function (sensory, motor, or interneuron), location, the identity of the transmitter they synthesize and release or the class or classes of receptor expressed on the cell surface. Neurons exhibit the cytological characteristics of highly active secretory cells with large nuclei: large amounts of smooth and rough endoplasmic reticulum; and frequent clusters of specialized smooth endoplasmic reticulum (Golgi complex), in which secretory products of the cell are packaged into membrane-bound organelles for transport from the perikaryon to the axon or dendrites. The sites of interneuronal communication in the CNS are termed *synapses*. Like peripheral "junctions," central synapses are denoted by accumulations of tiny (50-150 nm) *synaptic vesicles*. The proteins of these vesicles have specific roles in transmitter storage, vesicle docking, and secretion and re-storage of transmitter.

Support Cells. Neurons in the CNS are outnumbered by support cells, including macroglia, microglia, vascular elements, the cerebrospinal fluid (CSF)-forming cells of the choroid plexus found within the intracerebral ventricular system, and the meninges, which cover the surface of the brain and comprise the CSF-containing envelope. Macroglia are the most abundant support cells; some are categorized as *astrocytes* (cells interposed between the vasculature and the neurons, often surrounding individual compartments of synaptic complexes). Astrocytes play a variety of metabolic support roles including furnishing energy intermediates and supplementary removal of neurotransmitters following release. The *oligodendroglia*, a second prominent category of macroglia, are myelin-producing cells. Myelin, made up of multiple layers of compacted membranes, insulate segments of axons bioelectrically and permit nondecremental propagation of action potentials. Microglia are derived from mesoderm and are related to the macrophage/monocyte lineage. Some microglia reside within the brain, while additional cells of this class may be recruited to the brain during periods of inflammation following either microbial infection or brain injury.

BLOOD-BRAIN BARRIER. The *blood-brain barrier* (BBB) is an important boundary between the periphery and the CNS that forms a permeability barrier to the passive diffusion of substances from the bloodstream into the CNS. The BBB diminishes the rate of access of many chemicals from plasma to the brain and is the localization of several drug export systems in the cells that constitute the BBB (*see* Chapter 5). An exception exists for lipophilic molecules, which diffuse fairly freely across the BBB and accumulate in the brain.

This barrier, nonexistent in the peripheral nervous system, is much less prominent in the hypothalamus and in several small, specialized organs (the circumventricular organs) lining the third and fourth ventricles of the brain: the median eminence, area postrema, pineal gland, subfornical organ, and subcommissural organ.

Selective barriers to permeation into and out of the brain also exist for small, charged molecules such as neurotransmitters, their precursors and metabolites, and some drugs. These diffusional barriers are viewed as a combination of the partition of solute across the vasculature (which governs passage by definable properties such as molecular weight, charge, and lipophilicity) and the presence or absence of energy-dependent transport systems (*see* Chapter 5). Important exceptions are the specific uptake transporters for amino acids, one of which contributes to the therapeutic utility of L-dopa in the treatment of Parkinson disease.

The brain clears metabolites of transmitters into the fluid-containing lateral ventricles by excretion via the acid transport system of the choroid plexus. Substances that rarely gain access to the brain from the bloodstream often can reach the brain when injected directly into the cerebrospinal fluid. Under certain conditions, it may be possible to open the BBB, at least transiently, to permit the entry of chemotherapeutic agents. Cerebral ischemia and inflammation also modify the BBB, increasing access to substances that ordinarily would not affect the brain.

A central concept of neuropsychopharmacology is that drugs that influence behavior and improve the functional status of patients with neurological or psychiatric diseases act by enhancing or blunting the effectiveness of specific transmitters and channels.

Identified targets for centrally acting drugs include *ion channels* that mediate change in excitability induced by neurotransmitters, *neurotransmitter receptors*, and *transport proteins* that reaccumulate released transmitter. The *transport* proteins include those selective for NE, dopamine, and serotonin (NET, DAT, and SERT) that accumulate released transmitter and those that package it for reuse (e.g., VMAT2). Inhibition of *reuptake* increases the concentration and dwell time of transmitter in the synaptic space (e.g., as do serotonin selective reuptake inhibitors and cocaine). Inhibition of *vesicular storage* leads to depletion of releasable neurotransmitter (e.g., inhibition of VMAT2 and NE storage by reserpine).

An understanding at the systems level is required to assemble the structural and functional properties of specific central transmitter systems, linking the neurons that make and release a given neurotransmitter to its behavioral effects. The entire concept of animal models of human psychiatric diseases rests on the assumption that scientists can appropriately infer from observations of behavior and physiology (heart rate, respiration, locomotion, etc.) that the states experienced by animals are equivalent to the emotional states experienced by human beings expressing similar physiological changes.

IDENTIFICATION OF CENTRAL TRANSMITTERS. The criteria for identification of central transmitters require the same data set used to establish the transmitters of the autonomic nervous system (*see* Chapter 8):

- *The transmitter must be shown to be present in the presynaptic terminals of the synapse and in the neurons from which those presynaptic terminals arise.*
- *The transmitter must be released from the presynaptic nerve concomitantly with presynaptic nerve activity.*
- *When applied experimentally to target cells, the effects of the putative transmitter must be identical to the effects of stimulating the presynaptic pathway.*
- *Specific pharmacological agonists and antagonists should mimic and antagonize, respectively, the measured functions of the putative transmitter with appropriate affinities and order of potency.*

Many brain and spinal cord terminals contain more than 1 transmitter substance. Coexisting substances (presumed to be released together) may either act jointly on the postsynaptic membrane, or may act presynaptically to affect release of transmitter from the presynaptic terminal. Clearly, if more than 1 substance transmits information, no single agonist or antagonist would be expected to faithfully mimic or fully antagonize activation of a given presynaptic element. Co-storage and co-release of ATP and NE are an example. In addition to being released as a cotransmitter with other biogenic amines, ATP and adenosine have been shown to mediate diverse effects through interactions with *purinergic* receptors.

MANY NEUROTRANSMITTERS AND DRUGS ACT ON IDENTIFIED NEURONAL MACROMOLECULES

A number of molecular mechanisms link receptor occupancy to biological responses (*see* Chapter 3). The most commonly seen post-receptor events are changes in *ion flux through channels* formed by a multi-subunit receptor complex and the alteration of intracellular signaling via transmembrane receptor systems.

ION CHANNELS. The electrical excitability of neurons is achieved through modification of ion channels in neuronal plasma membranes. Na^+, K^+, and Ca^{2+}, as well as Cl^- anions, are regulated in their flow through highly discriminative ion channels. These channels are grouped structurally and termed voltage-dependent channels (Figure 14–1), and Cl^- channels (Figure 14–2). Ligand-gated ion channels, regulated by the binding of neurotransmitters, form another distinct group of ion channels; a prominent example is the nicotinic acetylcholine receptor, a Na^+ channel when activated (*see* Figures 11–1 and 11–2).

Two other families of channels regulate ion fluxes: *cyclic nucleotide–gated* (CNG) *channels*, and *transient receptor potential (TRP) channels*. CNG channels consist of 2 groups:

- The CNG channels, which play important roles in sensory transduction for olfactory and photoreceptors
- The hyperpolarization-activated, cyclic nucleotide–gated (HCN) channels

HCN channels are cation channels that open with hyperpolarization and close with depolarization; upon direct binding of cyclic AMP or cyclic GMP, the activation curves for the channels are shifted to more hyperpolarized potentials. These channels play essential roles in cardiac pacemaker cells and presumably in rhythmically discharging neurons.

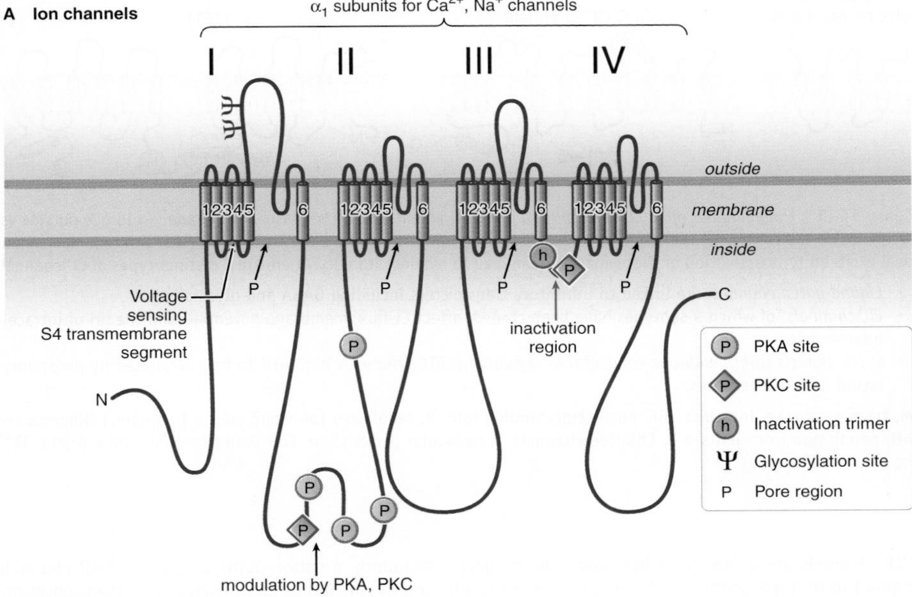

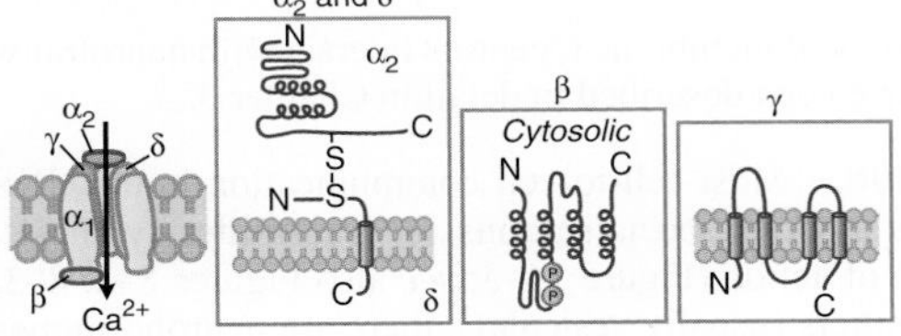

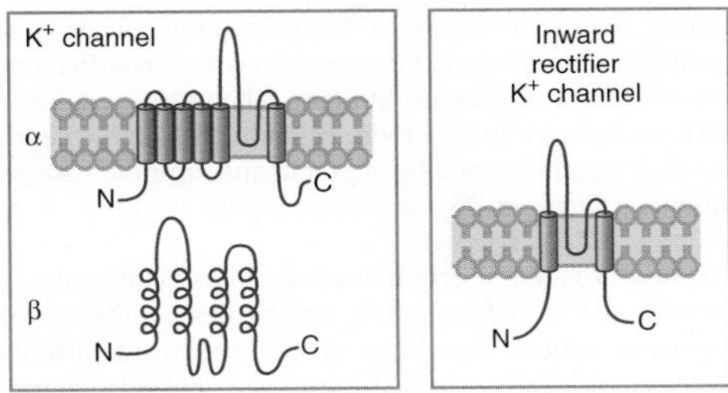

Figure 14–1 *Structural similarities of voltage-dependent Na^+, Ca^{2+}, and K^+ channels.* **A.** The α subunit in both Ca^{2+} and Na^+ channels contains 4 subunits, each with 6 transmembrane hydrophobic domains. The hydrophobic regions that connect segments 5 and 6 in each domain form the pore of the channel. Segment 4 in each domain includes the voltage-sensor. (Adapted with permission from Catterall W. *Neuron*, 2000;26:13–25. © Elsevier.) **B.** The Ca^{2+} channel also requires several auxiliary small proteins (α_2, β, γ, and δ); α_2 and δ subunits are linked by a disulfide bond. Regulatory subunits also exist for Na^+ channels. **C.** Voltage-sensitive K^+ channels (K_v) and the rapidly activating K^+ channel (K_A) share a similar putative hexaspanning structure resembling in overall configuration 1 repeat unit within the Na^+ and Ca^{2+} channel structure; the inwardly rectifying K^+ channel protein (K_{ir}) retains the general configuration of just loops 5 and 6. Regulatory β subunits (cytosolic) can alter K_v channel functions. Voltage-dependent channels provide for rapid changes in ion permeability along axons and within dendrites and for excitation-secretion coupling that releases neurotransmitters from presynaptic sites. The transmembrane Na^+ gradient (~140 mM outside vs. ~14 mM inside the cell) means that increases in permeability to Na^+ causes *depolarization*. In contrast, the K^+ gradient (~4 mM outside the cell vs. ~120 mM inside) is such that increased permeability to K^+ results in *hyperpolarization*. Changes in the concentration of intracellular Ca^{2+} (extracellular free Ca^{2+}: 1.25 mM; intracellular Ca^{2+}: resting ~100 nM, rising to ~1 μM when Ca^{2+} entry is stimulated) affects multiple processes in the cell and are critical in the release of neurotransmitters.

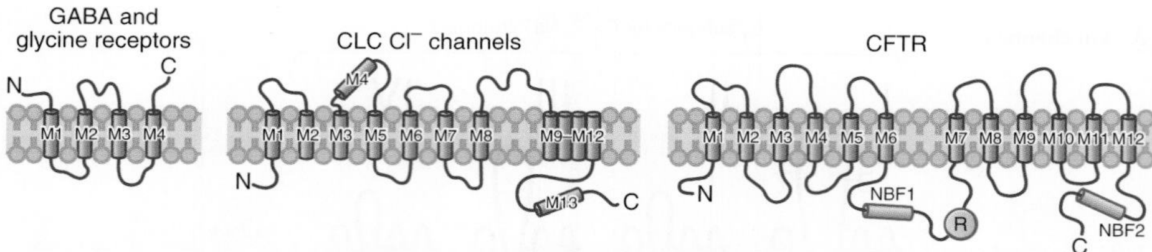

Figure 14–2 *Three families of Cl⁻ channel.* Due to the Cl⁻ gradient across the plasma membrane (~116 mM outside vs. 20 mM inside the cell), activation of Cl⁻ channels causes an inhibitory postsynaptic potential (IPSP) that dampens neuronal excitability; inactivation of these channels can lead to hyperexcitability. There are 3 distinct types of Cl⁻ channel:

- *Ligand-gated channels* are linked to inhibitory transmitters including GABA and glycine.
- *ClC channels*, of which 9 subtypes have been cloned, affect Cl-flux, membrane potential, and the pH of intracellular vesicles.
- *Cystic fibrosis transmembrane conductance regulated (CFTR) channels* bind ATP and are regulated by phosphorylation of serine residues.

(M, transmembrane domains; NBF, nucleotide-binding fold; R, regulatory [phosphorylation] domain.) (Reproduced with permission from Jentsch J. Chloride channels: A molecular perspective. *Curr Opin Neurobiol,* 1996;6:303–310. Copyright © Elsevier.)

TRP channels are a family of hexaspanning receptors containing a cation-permeable pore. TRP channels respond to multiple stimuli and function in sensory physiology, including thermosensation, osmosensation, and taste. Members of the IRPV subfamily (vanilloid receptors) interact with ligands such as the endogenous cannabinoid anandamide and capsaicin, a "hot" or "irritant" component of chili peppers.

TRANSMEMBRANE RECEPTOR SYSTEMS. A variety of membrane receptors interact with neurotransmitters and neurohormones. These systems have been described in detail in Chapter 3.

CELL SIGNALING AND SYNAPTIC TRANSMISSION. Most cell-to-cell communication in the CNS involves chemical transmission that requires a series specializations for transmitter synthesis, storage, release, recognition, and termination of action (Figure 14–3; *see* also Figures 8–2, 8–3, and 8–5). In addition to primary neurotransmitters (usually vesicular), there are neurohormones neuromodulators, and neurotrophic factors that influence CNS function:

NEUROHORMONES. The anterior and posterior pituitary secrete a variety of hormones and releasing factors. Hypothalamic neurons affecting the anterior pituitary release their hormones into the hypothalamic–adenohypophyseal portal blood system, which delivers them to the anterior pituitary, where they regulate the release of trophic hormones (i.e., ACTH, FSH, GH, LH, prolactin) into the blood. Other hypothalamic neurons project onto the posterior pituitary, where they release their peptide contents, oxytocin and arginine vasopressin (antidiuretic hormone) into the systemic circulation (*see* Chapters 25 and 38 and Figure 38–1).

NEUROMODULATORS. The distinctive feature of a modulator is that it originates from nonsynaptic sites, yet influences the excitability of nerve cells. Substances such as CO and ammonia, arising from active neurons or glia, are potential modulators acting through non-synaptic actions. Similarly, circulating steroid hormones, steroids produced in the nervous system (i.e., neurosteroids), locally released adenosine, and other purines, eicosanoids, and nitric oxide (NO) are regarded as modulators and/or neurotransmitters.

NEUROTROPHIC FACTORS. Neurotrophic factors are substances produced within the CNS by neurons, astrocytes, microglia, or inflammatory or immune cells that assist neurons in their attempts to repair damage. Seven categories of neurotrophic peptides are recognized:

- *Classic neurotrophins* (nerve growth factor, brain-derived neurotrophic factor, and the related neurotrophins)
- *Neuropoietic factors*, (e.g., cholinergic differentiation factor [also called leukemia inhibitory factor], ciliary neurotrophic factor, and some interleukins)
- Growth factor peptides, such as epidermal growth factor, transforming growth factors α and β, glial cell–derived neurotrophic factor, and activin A
- Fibroblast growth factors
- Insulin-like growth factors
- Platelet-derived growth factors
- Axon guidance molecules, some of which also affect cells of the immune system

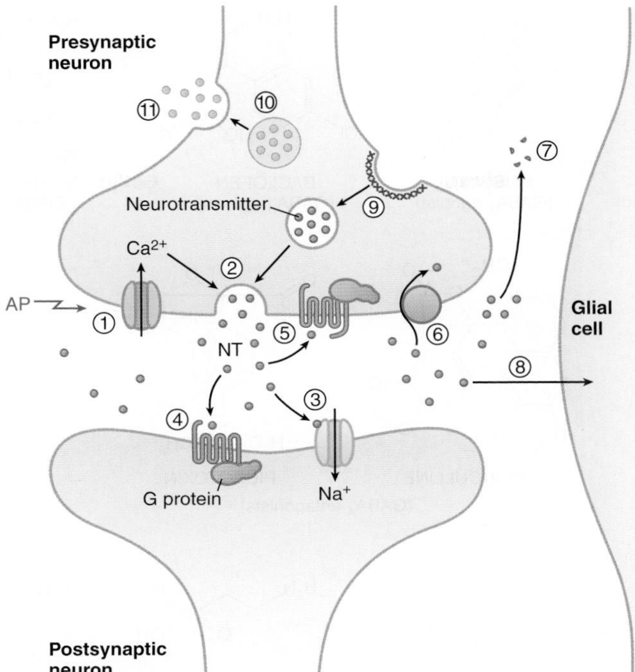

Figure 14–3 *Transmitter release, action, and inactivation.* Depolarization opens voltage-dependent Ca^{2+} channels in the presynaptic nerve terminal. (1) The influx of Ca^{2+} during an action potential (AP) triggers (2) the exocytosis of small synaptic vesicles that store neurotransmitter (NT) involved in fast neurotransmission. Released neurotransmitter interacts with receptors in the postsynaptic membranes that either couple directly with ion channels (3) or act through second messengers, such as (4) GPCRs. Neurotransmitter receptors in the presynaptic nerve terminal membrane (5) can inhibit or enhance subsequent exocytosis. Released neurotransmitter is inactivated by reuptake into the nerve terminal by (6) a transport protein coupled to the Na^+ gradient (e.g., for DA, NE, and GABA), or by (7) degradation (ACh, peptides), or by (8) uptake and metabolism by glial cells (Glu). The synaptic vesicle membrane is recycled by (9) clathrin-mediated endocytosis. Neuropeptides and proteins are stored in (10) larger, dense core granules within the nerve terminal. These dense core granules are released from (11) sites distinct from active zones after repetitive stimulation.

CENTRAL NEUROTRANSMITTERS

Neurotransmitters can be discussed by chemical categories: amino acids, amines, and neuropeptides. Other substances that may participate in central synaptic transmission include purines (such as adenosine and ATP), NO, and arachidonic acid derivatives.

AMINO ACIDS. The CNS contains uniquely high concentrations of certain amino acids, notably glutamate and γ-aminobutyric acid (GABA) that potently alter neuronal firing. They are ubiquitously distributed within the brain and they produce prompt, powerful, and readily reversible but redundant effects on neurons. The dicarboxylic amino acids (e.g., glutamate and aspartate) produce excitation, while the monocarboxylic amino acids (e.g., GABA, glycine, β-alanine, and taurine) cause inhibition. Following the emergence of selective antagonists, identification of selective receptors and receptor subtypes became possible. Figure 14–4 shows these amino acid transmitters and their drug congeners.

GABA. GABA receptors have been divided into 3 main types:

- The *$GABA_A$ receptor* (the most prominent GABA receptor subtype), a ligand-gated Cl-ion channel, or *ionotropic receptor*
- The *$GABA_B$ receptor*, a GPCR, or metabotropic receptor
- The *$GABA_C$ receptor*, a transmitter-gated Cl-channel

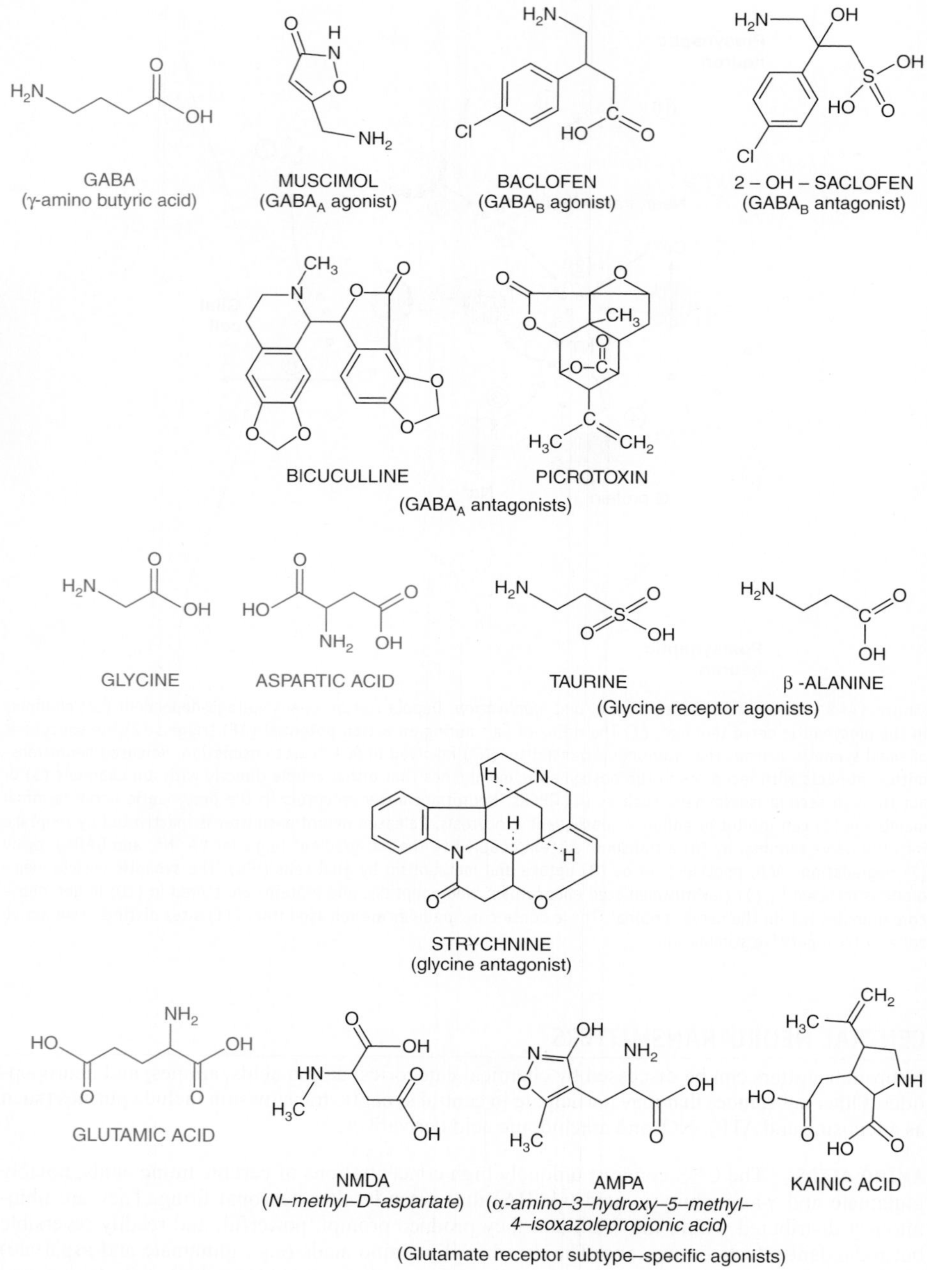

GABA
(γ-amino butyric acid)

MUSCIMOL
($GABA_A$ agonist)

BACLOFEN
($GABA_B$ agonist)

2 – OH – SACLOFEN
($GABA_B$ antagonist)

BICUCULLINE

PICROTOXIN

($GABA_A$ antagonists)

GLYCINE

ASPARTIC ACID

TAURINE

β -ALANINE

(Glycine receptor agonists)

STRYCHNINE
(glycine antagonist)

GLUTAMIC ACID

NMDA
(*N–methyl–D–aspartate*)

AMPA
(α*-amino–3–hydroxy–5–methyl–4–isoxazolepropionic acid*)

KAINIC ACID

(Glutamate receptor subtype–specific agonists)

Figure 14–4 *Amino acid transmitters and congeners.*

$GABA_A$ receptor has been extensively characterized as the site of action of many neuroactive drugs, notably benzodiazepines, barbiturates, ethanol, anesthetic steroids, and volatile anesthetics (Figure 14–5). The $GABA_A$ receptor is probably pentameric or tetrameric in structure, with subunits that assemble around a central pore. The major form of the $GABA_A$ receptor contains at least 3 different subunits α, β, and γ, with likely stoichiometry of 2α, 2β, 1γ. All 3 subunits are required to interact with benzodiazepines with the profile expected of a native $GABA_A$ receptor.

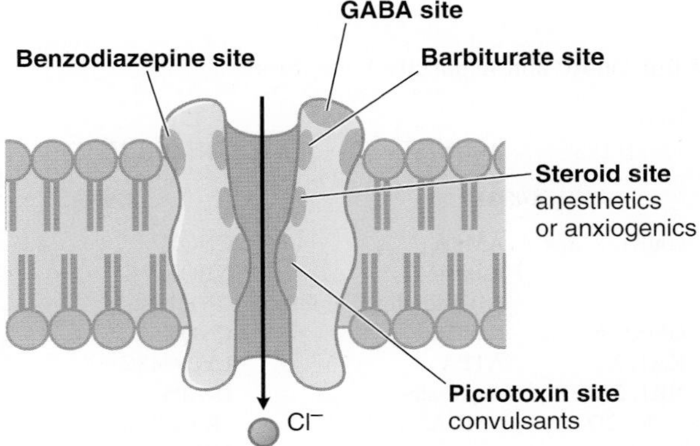

Figure 14–5 *Pharmacologic binding sites on the $GABA_A$ receptor.* (Reproduced with permission from Nestler EJ, Hyman SE, Malenka RC, eds. *Molecular Neuropharmacology*. New York: McGraw-Hill, 2009, p 135. © 2009 by The McGraw-Hill Companies, Inc.)

The $GABA_B$ or metabotropic GABA receptors interact with G_i to inhibit adenylyl cyclase, activate K^+ channels, and reduce Ca^{2+} conductance and with G_q to enhance PLC activity. Presynaptic $GABA_B$ receptors function as autoreceptors, inhibiting GABA release, and may play the same role on neurons releasing other transmitters. The $GABA_C$ receptor is less widely distributed than the A and B subtypes. GABA is more potent by an order of magnitude at $GABA_C$ than at $GABA_A$ receptors, and a number of $GABA_B$ agonists (e.g., baclofen) and modulators (e.g., benzodiazepines and barbiturates) do not interact with $GABA_C$ receptors. $GABA_C$ receptors are found in the retina, spinal cord, superior colliculus, and pituitary.

GABA mediates the inhibitory actions of local interneurons in the brain and may also mediate presynaptic inhibition within the spinal cord. GABA-containing neurons frequently coexpress 1 or more neuropeptides.

The most useful compounds for confirmation of GABA-mediated effects have been *bicuculline* and *picrotoxin*; however, many convulsants whose actions previously were unexplained (including *penicillin* and pentylenetetrazol) are relatively selective antagonists of the action of GABA. Useful therapeutic effects have not yet been obtained through the use of agents that mimic GABA (such as *muscimol*), inhibit its active reuptake (such as *2,4-diaminobutyrate*, *nipecotic acid*, and *guvacine*), or alter its turnover (such as *aminooxyacetic acid*).

GLYCINE. Many of the features described for the $GABA_A$ receptor family also apply to the inhibitory glycine receptor, which is prominent in the brainstem and spinal cord. Multiple subunits assemble into a variety of glycine receptor subtypes, the complete functional significance of which is not known.

GLUTAMATE AND ASPARTATE. Glutamate and aspartate have powerful excitatory effects on neurons in virtually every region of the CNS. Glutamate receptors are classed functionally either as *ligand-gated ion channel (ionotropic) receptors* or as *metabotropic GPCRs* (Table 14–1). The ligand-gated ion channels are further classified into *N*-methyl-D-aspartate (NMDA) receptors and non-NMDA receptors. The non-NMDA receptors include the *α-amino-3-hydroxy-5-methyl-4-isoxazole propionic acid (AMPA)*, and *kainic acid (KA) receptors*.

NMDA receptor agonists include open-channel blockers such as phencyclidine (PCP or "angel dust"); antagonists include 5,7-dichlorokynurenic acid, which acts at an allosteric glycine-binding site, and ifenprodil, which may act as a closed-channel blocker. The activity of NMDA receptors is sensitive to pH and to modulation by a variety of endogenous agents including Zn^{2+}, some neurosteroids, arachidonic acid, redox reagents, and polyamines such as spermine. NMDA receptors are involved in normal synaptic transmission; activation of NMDA receptors is associated more closely with the induction of various forms of synaptic plasticity rather than with fast point-to-point signaling in the brain.

AMPA and kainate receptors mediate fast depolarization at glutamatergic synapses in the brain and spinal cord. AMPA or kainate receptors and NMDA receptors may be colocalized at many glutamatergic synapses.

Table 14–1

Classification of Glutamate and Aspartate Receptors[a]

FUNCTIONAL CLASSES	GENE FAMILIES	AGONISTS	ANTAGONISTS	
Ionotropic				
AMPA	GluR1, 2, 3, 4	AMPA Kainate (s) -5-fluorowillardine	CNQX NBQX GYK153655	
Kainate	GluR5, 6, 7 KA1, 2	Kainate ATPA	CNQX LY294486	
NMDA	NR1, 2A, 2B, 2C, 2D	Aspartate NMDA	D-AP5 2R-CPPene MK-801 Ketamine Phencyclidine D-aspartate	
Metabotropic				INTRACELLULAR SIGNALING
Group 1	mGluR1 mGluR5	3,5-DHPG, quisqalate	AIDA CBPG	↑ G_q-PLC-IP_3-Ca^{2+}
Group 2	mGluR2 mGluR3	APDC, MGS0028 DCG-IV, LY354740	EGLU PCCG-4	↑ G_i-AC (↓ cAMP)
Group 3	mGluR4 mGluR6 mGluR7 mGluR8	L-AP-4 L-AP4 L-AP4 L-AP4, (S)-3,4-DCPG	MAP4 MPPG LY341495	↑ G_i-AC (↓ cAMP)

[a]*Glutamate is the principal agonist at both ionotropic and metabotropic receptors for glutamate and aspartate. CNQX, 6-Cyano-7-nitroquinoxaline-2,3-dione; NBQX, 1,2,3,4-Tetrahydro-6-nitro-2,3-dioxo-benzo[f]quinoxaline-7-sulfonamide; D-AP5, D-2-amino-5-phosphonovaleric acid; AIDA, 1-aminoindan-1,5-dicarboxylic acid; CBPG, (S)-(+)-2-(3′-carboxybicyclo(1.1.1)pentyl)-glycine; EGLU, (2S)-α-ethylglutamic acid; PCCG-4, phenylcarboxycyclopropyl-glycine; MAP4, (S)-amino-2-methyl-4-phosphonobutanoic acid; MPPG, (RS)-a-methyl-4-phosphonophenylglycine; AMPA, α-amino-3-hydroxy-5-methyl-4-isoxazolepropionic acid; ATPA, 2-amino-3(3-hydroxy-5-tert-butylisoxa-zol-4-yl)propanoic acid; NMDA, N-methyl-D-aspartate; 3,5-DHPG, 3,5-dihydroxyphenylglycine; DCG-IV, dicarboxycyclopropyl)glycine; L-AP-4, L-2-amino-4-phosphonobutiric acid; (S)-3,4-DCPG, (S)-3,4-dicarboxyphenylglycine.*

A well-characterized phenomenon involving NMDA receptors is the induction of long-term potentiation (LTP) and its converse, long-term depression (LTD) (Figure 14–6).

GLUTAMATE EXCITOTOXICITY. High concentrations of glutamate lead to neuronal cell death (Figure 14–7). The cascade of events leading to neuronal death is thought to be triggered by excessive activation of NMDA or AMPA/kainate receptors, allowing significant influx of Ca^{2+} into neurons. Glutamate-mediated excitotoxicity may underlie the damage that occurs after ischemia or hypoglycemia in the brain, during which a massive release and impaired reuptake of glutamate in the synapse leads to excess stimulation of glutamate receptors and subsequent cell death. NMDA receptor antagonists can attenuate neuronal cell death induced by activation of these receptors.

ACETYLCHOLINE. The effects of ACh result from interaction with a mixture of nicotinic and muscarinic receptors. Nicotinic ACh receptors (*see* Figures 11–1 and 11–2) are found in autonomic ganglia, the adrenal gland, and in the CNS. Their activation by ACh results in a rapid increase in the influx of Na^+, depolarization, and the activation of voltage-sensitive Ca^{2+} influx. There are 5 subtypes of muscarinic receptors, all of which are expressed in the brain. M_1, M_3, and M_5 couple to G_q while the M_2 and M_4 receptors couple to G_i (Table 14–2).

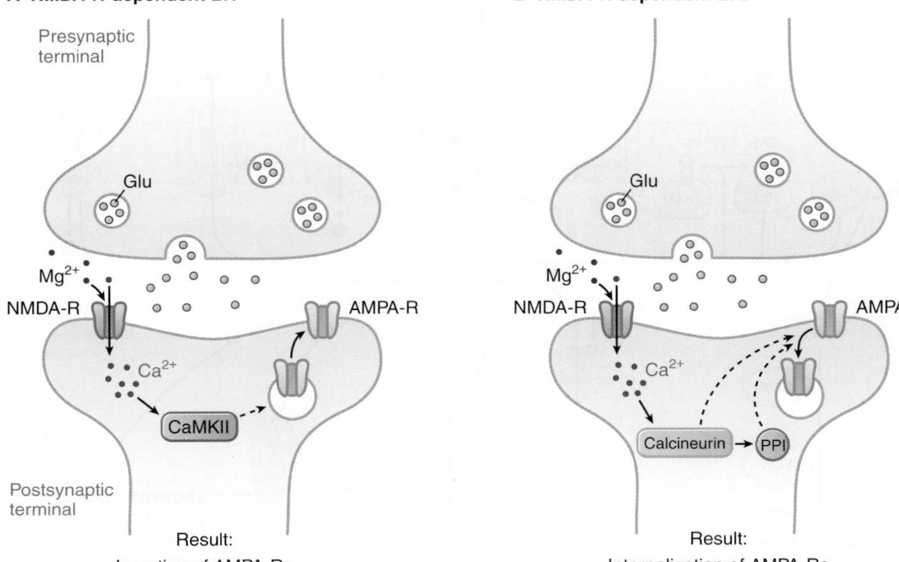

Figure 14–6 *NMDA receptor-dependent LTP and LTD.* LTP refers to a prolonged (hours to days) increase in the size of a postsynaptic response to a presynaptic stimulus of given strength. Activation of NMDA receptors is obligatory for the induction of LTP that occurs in the hippocampus. NMDA receptors normally are blocked by Mg^{2+} at resting membrane potentials. Thus, activation of NMDA receptors requires glutamate binding and the simultaneous depolarization of the postsynaptic membrane. This is achieved by activation of AMPA/kainate receptors at nearby synapses involving inputs from different neurons. AMPA receptors also are dynamically regulated to affect their sensitivity to the synergism with NMDA. Thus, NMDA receptors may function as coincidence detectors, being activated only when there is simultaneous firing of 2 or more neurons. LTD is the converse of LTP. **A.** NMDA receptor-dependent LTP requires post synaptic NMDA receptor activation leading to a rise in Ca^{2+} and activation of CaM kinase II (CaMKII). AMPA receptor insertion into the postsynaptic membrane is a major mechanism underlying LTP expression. **B.** NMDA receptor-dependent LTD is triggered by Ca^{2+} entry through postsynaptic NMDA receptor channels, leading to increases in the activity of the protein phosphatases calcineurin and PP1. LTD occurs when postsynaptic AMPA receptors are internalized. (Redrawn with permission from Nestler EJ, Hyman SE, Malenka RC, eds. *Molecular Neuropharmacology*. New York: McGraw-Hill, 2009, p 132. © 2009 by The McGraw-Hill Companies, Inc.)

CATECHOLAMINES. The brain contains separate neuronal systems that use 3 different catecholamines—dopamine (DA), NE, and epinephrine (EPI). Each system is anatomically distinct and serves separate, functional roles within its field of innervation.

DOPAMINE. More than half the CNS content of catecholamine is DA. The 5 receptors for DA are GPCRs that regulate adenylyl cyclase activity via coupling to G_s (D_1 and D_5) and G_i (D_{2-4}) (Table 14–3). DA-containing pathways and receptors have been implicated in the pathophysiology of schizophrenia and Parkinson disease and in the side effects seen following pharmacotherapy of these disorders (*see* Chapters 16 and 22).

Large amounts of DA are found in the basal ganglia. There are 3 major DA-containing pathways in the CNS: the nigrostriatal, the mesocortical/mesolimbic, and the tuberoinfundibular, as described in Chapter 13 and depicted in Figure 13–7.

NOREPINEPHRINE. Both α and β adrenergic receptors subtypes are present in the CNS; all are GPCRs (Table 14–4; *see* also Chapter 8).

β receptors couple to G_s and thence to adenylyl cyclase. α_1 Adrenergic receptors are coupled to G_q, resulting in stimulation of the PLC-IP_3/DAG-Ca^{2+}-PKC pathway, and are associated predominantly with neurons. α_1 Receptors on noradrenergic target neurons respond to NE with *depolarizing responses* because of decreases in K^+ conductance. α_2 Adrenergic receptors are found on glial and vascular elements, as well as on neurons. They are prominent on noradrenergic neurons, where they presumably couple to G_i, inhibit

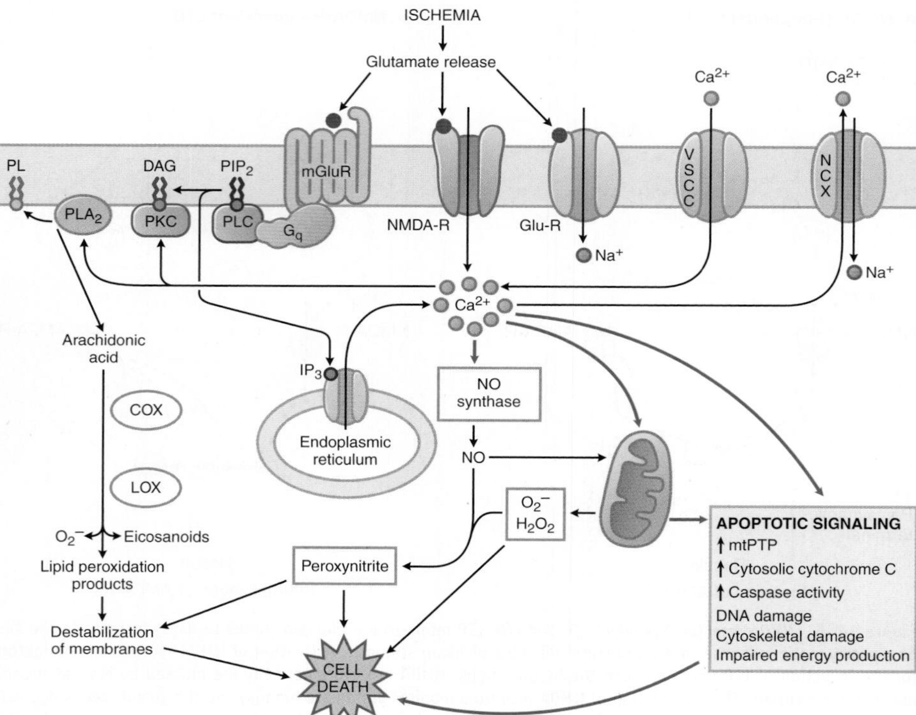

Figure 14–7 *Mechanisms contributing to neuronal injury during ischemia-reperfusion-induced glutamate release.* Several pathways contribute to excitotoxic neuronal injury in ischemia, with excess cytosolic Ca^{2+} playing a precipitating role. *DAG,* diacylglycerol; *GluR,* AMPA/kainate type of glutamate receptors; IP_3, inositol trisphosphate; *mGluR,* metabotropic glutamate receptor; *NMDA- R, N*—methyl-D-aspartate receptor; O_2^-, superoxide radical; PIP_2, phosphatidylinositol 4,5-bisphosphate; PKC, protein kinase C; PL, phospholipids, PLA_2/C phospholipases, VSCC, voltage-sensitive Ca^{2+} channel. COX, cyclooxygenase; LOX, lipoxygenase; NCX, Na^+/Ca^{2+} exchanger; mtPTP, mitochondrial permeability transition pore. (Reproduced with permission from Dugan LL, Kim-Han JS: Hypoxic-ischemic brain injury and oxidative stress, in Siegel GS, Albers RW, Brady S, Price D, eds. *Basic Neurochemistry: Molecular, Cellular, and Medical Aspects,* 7th ed. Burlington, MA: Elsevier Academic Press, 2006, p 564. © 2006, American Society for Neurochemistry.)

adenylyl cyclase, and mediate a *hyperpolarizing response* due to enhancement of an inwardly rectifying K^+ channel (via βγ heterodimer). α_2 Receptors are located presynaptically where they function as inhibitory autoreceptors. The antihypertensive effects of clonidine may result from stimulation of such autoreceptors.

There are relatively large amounts of NE within the hypothalamus and in certain parts of the limbic system, such as the central nucleus of the amygdala and the dentate gyrus of the hippocampus. NE also is present in

Table 14–2

Subtypes of Muscarinic Receptors in the CNS

SUBTYPE	SELECTIVE ANTAGONISTS	G-PROTEIN FAMILY	LOCALIZATION IN THE CNS
M_1	pirenzepine, telenzepine, 4-DAMP	G_q	cortex, hippocampus, striatum
M_2	AF-Dx-384, methoctramine	G_i	basal forebrain, thalamus
M_3	darifenacin, 4-DAMP	G_q	cortex, hippocampus, thalamus
M_4	AF-Dx384, 4-DAMP	G_i	cortex, hippocampus, striatum
M_5	4-DAMP	G_q	substantia nigra

Non-selective agonists include carbachol, pilocarpine, and oxotremorine. Non-selective antagonists include atropine and scopolamine. McN-A-3436 is a selective agonist at the M_1 receptor. 4-DAMP, 4-diphenylacetoxy-N-methylpiperidine.

Table 14–3

Dopamine Receptors in the CNS

RECEPTOR	AGONISTS	ANTAGONISTS	G-PROTEIN FAMILY	AREAS OF LOCALIZATION
D_1	SKF82958 SKF81297	SCH23390 SKF83566; haloperidol	G_s	neostriatum; cerebral cortex; olfactory tubercle; nucleus accumbens
D_2	Bromocriptine, apomorphine	Raclopride, sulpiride, haloperidol	G_i	neostriatum; olfactory tubercle; nucleus accumbens
D_3	Quinpirole 7-OH-DPAT	Raclopride	G_i	nucleus accumbens; islands of Calleja
D_4		Clozapine, L-745,870, sonepiprazole	G_i	midbrain; amygdala; hippocampus; hypothalamus
D_5	SKF38393	SCH23390	G_s	

7-OH-DPAT, 7-hydroxy-N,N-di-n-propyl-2-aminotetralin.

significant amounts in most brain regions. Mapping studies indicate that noradrenergic neurons of the locus ceruleus innervate specific target cells in a large number of cortical, subcortical, and spinomedullary fields.

EPINEPHRINE. EPI-containing neurons are found in the medullary reticular formation. Their physiological properties have not been identified.

5-HYDROXYTRYPTAMINE (SEROTONIN; 5HT). There are 5 types of 5HT receptors, with 14 distinct subtypes (Table 14–5). These subtypes exhibit characteristic ligand-binding profiles,

Table 14–4

Adrenergic Receptors in the CNS

RECEPTOR	AGONIST	ANTAGONIST	G-PROTEIN FAMILY	AREAS OF LOCALIZATION IN THE BRAIN
α_{1A}	A61603 phenylephrine oxymetazoline	nigulpidine prazosin 5-methylurapidil	G_q	cortex, hippocampus
α_{1B}	phenylephrine oxymetazoline	spiperone prazosin, (+)-cyclazosin	G_q	cortex brainstem
α_{1D}	phenylephrine oxymetazoline	A-119637 tamsulosin	G_q	cortex
α_{2A}	oxymetazoline clonidine	yohimbine, rauwolscine, bromocriptine	G_i	locus ceruleus and hippocampus
α_{2B}	clonidine dexmedetomidine	yohimbine, rauwolscine, lisuride	G_i	diencephalon
α_{2C}	clonidine	yohimbine, rauwolscine, lisuride	G_i	widely distributed
β_1	CGP 12177 prenalterol	alprenolol betaxolol, metoprolol	G_s	cortex and hypothalamus
β_2	fenoterol salmeterol	propranolol ICI118551	G_s	cerebellum, hippocampus, cortex
β_3	carazolol	carvedilol, tertalolol	? G_s	unknown

Table 14–5

5HT Receptors in the CNS

RECEPTOR	AGONISTS	ANTAGONISTS	TRANSDUCER	LOCALIZATION
$5HT_{1A}$	8-OH-DPAT, buspirone, lisuride	WAY 100135, NAD 299	G_i	hippocampus, septum, amygdala, dorsal raphe, cortex
$5HT_{1B}$	sumatriptan, dihydroergota-mine, oxymetazoline	GR-127935, ketanserin	G_i	substantia nigra, basal ganglia
$5HT_{1D}$	sumatriptan, dihydroergotamine, oxymetazoline	GR127935, methysergide, L-772405	G_i	substantia nigra, striatum, nucleus accumbens, hippocampus
$5HT_{1E}$	eletriptan, ORG-5222		G_i	
$5HT_{1F}$	LY334370, naratriptan	methysergide	G_i	dorsal raphe, hippocampus, cortex
$5HT_{2A}$	DMT, DOB, DOI, ergotamine, LSD	amoxapine, chlorpro-mazine, ketanserin	G_q	cortex, olfactory tubercle, claustrum
$5HT_{2B}$	cabergoline, 5-MeOT	clozapine, lisuride, LY53857	G_q	not located in the brain
$5HT_{2C}$	ergotamine, DOI, lisuride	amoxepine, fluoxetine, mesulergine	G_q	basal ganglia, choroid plexus, substantia nigra
$5HT_3$		ondansetron, granisetron	Ligand-gated ion channel	spinal cord, cortex, hippocampus, brainstem nuclei
$5HT_4$	cisapride, metoclopramide	GR113808, SB204070	G_s	hippocampus, nucleus accumbens striatum, substantia nigra
$5HT_{5A}$		methiothepin	G_s	cortex, hippocampus, cerebellum
$5HT_{5B}$		ergotamine, methiothepin	$?G_i$	habenula, hippocampal CA1
$5HT_6$	bromocriptine	methiothepin, clozapine, amiltriptyline	G_s	striatum, olfactory tubercle, cortex, hippocampus
$5HT_7$	pergolide, 5-MeOT	methiothepin, clozapine, metergoline	G_s	hypothalamus, thalamus, cortex, suprachiasmatic nucleus

8-OH-DPAT, 8-hydroxy-N,N-dipropyl-2-aminotetralin; DOB, 2,5-Dimethoxy-4-bromoamphetamine; DOI, (±)-2,5-dimethoxy-4-iodoamphetamine; DMT, N,N-dimethyltryptamine; 5-MeOT, 2-(5-methoxy-1H-indol-3-yl) ethanamine; LSD, Lysergic acid diethylamide.

couple to different intracellular signaling systems, exhibit subtype-specific distributions within the CNS, and mediate distinct behavioral effects of 5HT. All 5HT receptors are GPCRs coupling to a variety of G-protein α subunits *except* the $5HT_3$ receptor, which is a ligand-gated ion channel. The localizations and properties of 5HT receptors are summarized in Table 13–1, their physiological roles in various CNS activities in Table 13–2, the electrophysiological events

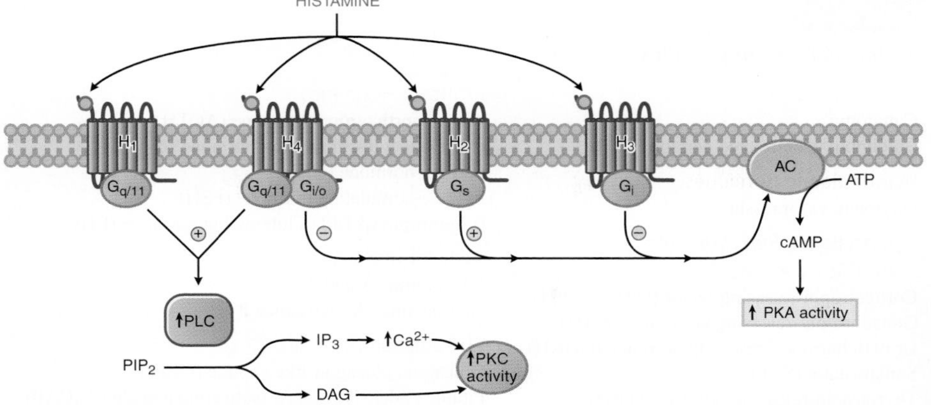

Figure 14–8 *Main signaling pathways for histamine receptors.* Histamine can couple to a variety of G protein-linked signal transduction pathways via 4 different receptors. The H_1 receptor and some H_4 receptors activate phosphatidylinositol turnover via $G_{q/11}$. The other receptors couple either positively (H_2 receptor) or negatively (H_3 and H_4 receptor) to adenylyl cyclase activity via G_s and $G_{i/o}$.

associated with receptor activation in Table 13–4, and aspects of their clinical pharmacology in Table 13–5.

In mammalian CNS, neurons containing 5HT are found in 9 nuclei lying in or adjacent to the midline (raphe) regions of the pons and upper brainstem. Cells receiving cytochemically demonstrable 5HT input, such as the suprachiasmatic nucleus, ventrolateral geniculate body, amygdala, and hippocampus, exhibit a uniform and dense investment of serotonergic terminals.

HISTAMINE. Four subtypes of histamine receptors have been described; all are GPCRs coupling to regulate adenylyl cyclase and PLC as described in Figure 14–8. *H_1 receptors*, the most prominent, are located on glia and vessels as well as on neurons. *H_3 receptors*, which have the greatest sensitivity to histamine, are localized primarily in basal ganglia and olfactory regions in rat brain. *H_4 receptors* are expressed on cells of hematopoietic origin: eosinophils, T cells, mast cells, basophils, and dendritic cells. H_4 receptors are postulated to play a role in inflammation and chemotaxis. For details, consult Chapter 32.

Histaminergic neurons are located in the ventral posterior hypothalamus; they give rise to long ascending and descending tracts that are typical of the patterns characteristic of other aminergic systems. The histaminergic system is thought to affect arousal, body temperature, and vascular dynamics.

PEPTIDES. A remarkable array of neurotransmitters and neuromodulators have been described (Table 14–6). While some CNS peptides (*see* Table 14–6) may function on their own, most are now thought to act primarily in concert with coexisting transmitters (biogenic amines and amino acids), but their release can be independently regulated (*see* Figure 14–3). Many neuropeptides act via GPCRs (Table 14–7).

Peptide synthesis takes place primarily in perikarya and the resulting peptide is then transported to nerve terminals. Single genes can, through posttranslational modifications, give rise to multiple neuropeptides. For example, proteolytic processing of proopiomelanocortin (POMC) gives rise to ACTH, α- , γ- , and β-MSH, and β-endorphin (Figure 14–9). In addition, alternative splicing of RNA transcripts may result in distinct mRNA species (e.g., calcitonin and calcitonin gene-related peptide [CGRP]).

CANNABINOIDS. Delta-9-tetrahydrocannabinol (THC) is 1 of several active substances in marijuana (Figure 14–10). The primary pharmacologic effects of THC follow its interaction with *CB_1 receptors* in the CNS and *CB_2 receptors* in the periphery. Both CB_1 and CB_2 receptors are linked to G_i and thence to inhibition of adenylyl cyclase activity. The natural endogenous ligands for these receptors are arachidonic acid derivatives including *anandamide* and *2-arachidonyl glycerol* (*see* Figure 14–10).

Table 14–6

Examples of Neuropeptides

Calcitonin Family	**Pituitary Hormones**
Calcitonin	Adrenocorticotropic hormone (ACTH)
Calcitonin gene-related peptide (CGRP)	α-Melanocyte-stimulating hormone (α-MSH)
Hypothalamic Hormones	Growth hormone (GH)
Oxytocin, vasopressin	Follicle-stimulating hormone (FSH)
Hypothalamic Releasing and Inhibitory Hormones	β-lipotropin (β-LPH), luteinizing hormone (LH)
Corticotropin-releasing factor (CRF or CRH)	**Tachykinins**
Gonadotropin-releasing hormone (GnRH)	Neurokinins A and B
Growth hormone-releasing hormone (GHRH)	Neuropeptide K, substance P
Somatostatin (SST)	**VIP-Glucagon Family**
Thyrotropin-releasing hormone (TRH)	Glucagon, glucagon-like peptide (GLP-1)
Neuropeptide Y Family	Pituitary adenylyl cyclase–activating peptide (PACAP)
Neuropeptide Y (NPY)	Vasoactive intestinal polypeptide (VIP)
Neuropeptide YY (PYY)	**Other Peptides**
Pancreatic polypeptide (PP)	Agouti-related peptide (ARP)
Opioid Peptides	Bombesin, bradykinin (BK)
β-endorphin (also pituitary hormone)	Cholecystokinin (CCK)
Dynorphin peptides	Cocaine/amphetamine-regulated transcript (CART)
Leu-enkephalin, *met*-enkephalin	Galanin, ghrelin
	Melanin-concentrating hormone (MCH)
	Neurotensin, nerve growth factor (NGF)
	Orexins, orphanin FQ (nociceptin)

Source: Modified with permission from Nestler EJ, Hyman SE, Malenka RC, eds. Molecular Neuropharmacology. New York: McGraw-Hill, 2009, p 184, Table 7–1. © 2009 by The McGraw-Hill Companies, Inc.

THC has dramatic short-term effects, including causing feelings of euphoria and altered sensory perception. CB_1 receptors are found primarily in the basal ganglia, hippocampus, cerebellum, and cerebral cortex; activation of CB_1 receptors results in inhibition of glutamate release. Some nonneuronal cells and tissues also express CB_1 receptors, including leukocytes and testis. CB_2 receptors are expressed in the spleen, tonsils, bone marrow, and on peripheral blood leukocytes.

Efforts to develop CB_1 antagonists like rimonabant (*see* Figure 14–10) have focused on possible treatments for drug addiction and obesity. Efforts are also underway to develop agonists that interact with CB_1 and CB_2 receptors for the relief of pain. THC (dronabinol [MARINOL]) is sometimes used in the control of nausea and moderate pain (*see* Chapter 46).

PURINES. Adenosine, ATP, UDP, and UTP have roles as extracellular signaling molecules. ATP is a component of the adrenergic storage vesicles and is released along with catecholamines. Intracellular nucleotides may also reach the cell surface by other means, and extracellular adenosine can result from cellular release and metabolism of ATP.

Extracellular nucleotides and adenosine act on a family of purinergic receptors that is divided into 2 classes, P1 and P2 (Table 14–8). P1 receptors are GPCRs that interact with adenosine; 2 of these receptors (A_1 and A_3) couple to G_i and 2 (A_{2a} and A_{2b}) couple to G_s; methylxanthines antagonize A_1 and A_3 receptors. Activation of A_1 receptors is associated with inhibition of adenylyl cyclase, activation of K^+ currents, and in some instances, with activation of PLC; stimulation of A_2 receptors activates adenylyl cyclase. The P2 class includes a large number of P2X receptors that are ligand-gated ion channels and the P2Y receptors, a large subclass of GPCRs that couple to G_q or G_i. The $P2Y_{14}$ receptor is expressed in the CNS; it interacts with UDP-glucose and may couple to G_q. The $P2Y_{12}$ receptor is important clinically: inhibition of this receptor in platelets inhibits platelet aggregation.

Although many of these receptors have been detected in brain, most of the current interest stems from pharmacological rather than physiological observations. Adenosine can act presynaptically throughout the cortex and hippocampal formation to inhibit the release of amine and amino acid transmitters. ATP-regulated responses have been linked pharmacologically to a variety of pathophysiological functions, including anxiety, stroke,

Table 14–7

Peptide Transmitters and Receptors

PEPTIDE	RECEPTOR	AGONISTS	EFFECTOR MECHANISM	ANTAGONISTS
Opioid	δ	DADLE, diprenorphine	↑ G_i-AC (↓ cAMP)	naltriben, naltrindole
	κ	bremazocine, etorphine		nalmefene, naltrexone
	μ	DAMGO, etorphine		diprenorphine, naltrexone
Somatostatin	SST_1	CST-17	↑ G_i-AC (↓ cAMP)	SRA880
	SST_2	BIM 23059		D-Tyr8-CYN 154806
	SST_3	BIM 23066		sst3-ODN-8
	SST_4	CGP 23996		
	SST_5	BIM 23313		L-Tyr8-CYN 154806
Neurotensin	NTS1	EISAI-1, JMV431	↑ G_q -PLC	SR142948A
	NTS2	levocabastine		
Oxenin	OX_1		↑ G_q -PLC	SB-410220
	OX_2			
Tachykinin	NK_1	Substance P methyl ester	↑ G_q -PLC	
	NK_2	β-{ala²}$NKA_{4\text{-}10}$		
	NK_3	GR138676		
CCK	CCK_1	ARL-15849, SR14613	↑ G_q-PLC	FK-480, lintitript
	CCK_2	BC-264, PBC-264		Triglumide, PD-149164
NPY	Y_1		↑ G_i-AC (↓ cAMP)	GR231118
	Y_2		↓ cAMP	BIIE0246
	Y_4		↑ G_q-PLC	
	Y_5		↑ G_i-AC (↓ cAMP)	CGP 71683A

DADLE, 2-Alanyl-Leucine enkephalin; DAMGO, 2-Ala-4-MePhe-5-Gly-enkephalin

and epilepsy. A_2 receptors and dopamine D_2 receptors appear to be functionally antagonistic, leading to investigation of A_{2a} antagonists as adjunctive therapy for Parkinson disease.

LIPID MEDIATORS. *Arachidonic acid*, normally stored within the cell membrane as a glycerol ester, can be liberated during phospholipid hydrolysis (by pathways involving phospholipases A_2, C, and D). Arachidonic acid can be converted to highly reactive regulators by 3 major enzymatic pathways (*see* Chapter 33): *cyclooxygenases* (leading to prostaglandins and thromboxane), *lipoxygenases* (leading to the leukotrienes and other transient catabolites of eicosatetraenoic acid), and *CYPs* (which are inducible and also expressed at low levels in brain). Arachidonic acid metabolites have been implicated as diffusible modulators in the CNS, possibly involved with the formation of LTP and other forms of neuronal plasticity.

NITRIC OXIDE (NO) AND CARBON MONOXIDE (CO). Both constitutive and inducible forms of NOS are expressed in the brain. The application of inhibitors of NOS (e.g., methylarginine) and of NO donors (such as nitroprusside) suggests the involvement of NO in a host of CNS phenomena, including LTP, activation of soluble guanylyl cyclase, neurotransmitter release, and enhancement of glutamate (NMDA)-mediated neurotoxicity. CO, generated in neurons, is another diffusable gas that may act as intracellular messenger stimulating soluble guanylyl cyclase.

CYTOKINES. Cytokines are a family of polypeptide regulators. The effects of cytokines are regulated by the conditions imposed by other cytokines, interacting as a network with variable effects leading to synergistic, additive, or opposing actions. Tissue-produced peptides, termed *chemokines*, serve to attract immune and inflammatory cells into interstitial spaces. These special cytokines have received attention as potential regulators of nervous system inflammation (as in early stages of dementia, following infection with human immunodeficiency virus, and during recovery from traumatic injury). Neurons and astrocytes may be induced under some pathophysiological conditions to express cytokines or other growth factors.

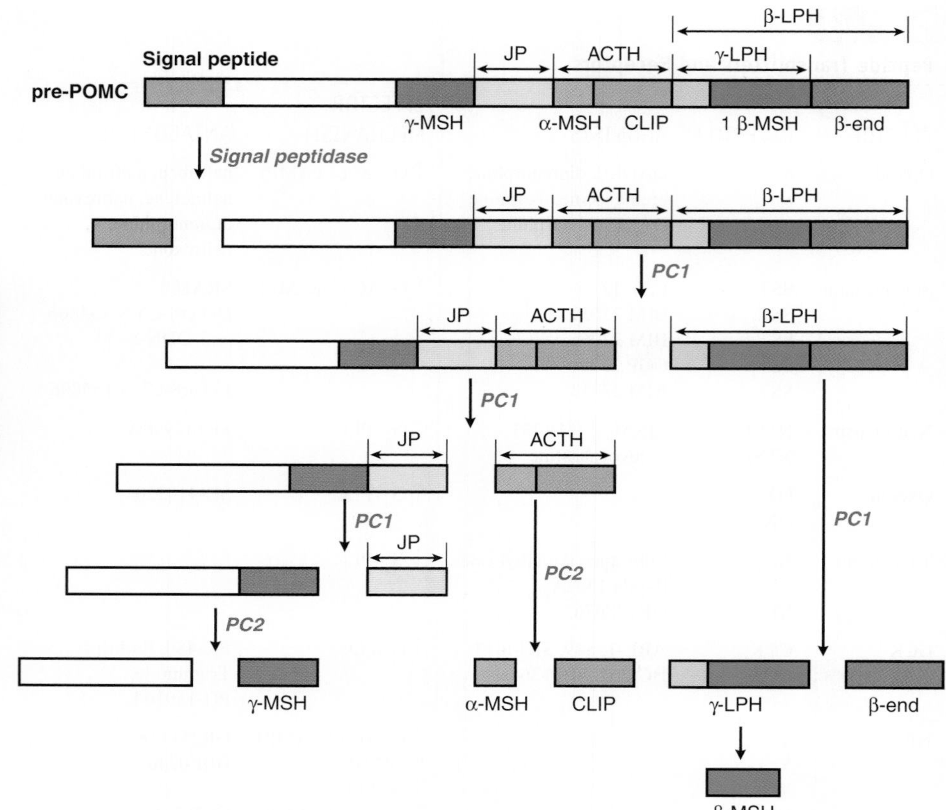

Figure 14–9 *Proteolytic processing of proopiomelanocortin (POMC).* After removal of the signal peptide from pre-POMC, the remaining propeptide undergoes endoproteolysis by prohormone convertases 1 and 2 (PC1 and PC2) at dibasic residues. PC1 liberates the bioactive peptides adrenocorticotropic hormone (ACTH), β-endorphin (β end), and γ-lipotrophic hormone (γ-LPH). PC2 cleaves ACTH into corticotrophin-like intermediate lobe peptide (CLIP) and α-melanocyte stimulating hormone (α-MSH) and also releases γ-MSH from the N-terminal portion of the propeptide. The joining peptide (JP) is the region between ACTH and γ-MSH. β-MSH is formed by cleavage of γ-LPH. Some of the resulting peptides are amidated or acetylated before they become fully active.

ACTIONS OF DRUGS IN THE CNS

SPECIFICITY AND NONSPECIFICITY OF CNS DRUG ACTIONS. The effect of a drug in the CNS is termed specific when it affects an identifiable molecular mechanism unique to target cells that bear receptors for that drug. Even a drug that is highly specific when tested at low concentrations may exhibit nonspecific actions at higher doses. In general, the more potent a drug at its desired target, the lower the probability that it will have off-target effects. Conversely, even drugs that have a broad spectrum of activity may not act identically at all levels of the CNS. For example, sedatives, hypnotics, and general anesthetics would have very limited utility if central neurons that control the respiratory and cardiovascular systems were especially sensitive to their actions. *The specificity of a drug's action is frequently overestimated. This is partly due to the fact that drugs are often identified with the effect that is implied by the class name.*

GENERAL (NONSPECIFIC) CNS DEPRESSANTS. This category includes the anesthetic gases and vapors, the aliphatic alcohols, and some hypnotic-sedative drugs. These agents share the capacity to depress excitable tissue at all levels of the CNS, leading to a decrease in the amount of transmitter released by the nerve impulse, as well as to general depression of postsynaptic responsiveness and ion flux. At sub-anesthetic concentrations, these agents (e.g., ethanol) can exert relatively specific effects on certain groups of neurons, which may account for differences in their behavioral effects, especially the propensity to produce dependence.

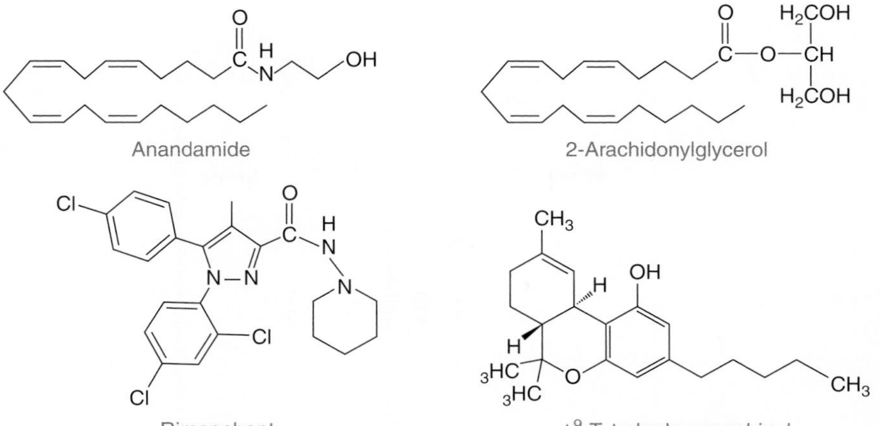

Figure 14–10 *Cannabinoid receptor ligands.* Anandamide and 2-arachidonylglycerol are endogenous agonists. Rimonabant is a synthetic CB receptor antagonist. Δ^9-tetrahydrocannabinol is a CB agonist derived from marijuana.

GENERAL (NONSPECIFIC) CNS STIMULANTS. This category includes *pentylenetetrazol* and related agents that are capable of powerful excitation of the CNS, and the methylxanthines, which have a much weaker stimulant action. Stimulation may be accomplished by 1 of 2 general mechanisms: (1) blockade of inhibition or (2) direct neuronal excitation that may involve increased transmitter release or more prolonged transmitter action, as occurs when the reuptake of a released transmitter is inhibited.

DRUGS THAT SELECTIVELY MODIFY CNS FUNCTION. The agents in this group may cause either depression or excitation. In some instances, a drug may produce both effects simultaneously on different systems. The principal classes of these CNS drugs are anticonvulsants, drugs used in treating Parkinson disease, opioid and nonopioid analgesics, appetite suppressants, antiemetics, analgesic-antipyretics, certain stimulants, antidepressants, antimanic and antipsychotic agents, tranquilizers, sedatives and hypnotics, and medications employed in the treatment of Alzheimer disease (cholinesterase inhibitors and anti-glutamate neuroprotectants). Even if selectivity of action is remarkable, a drug usually affects several CNS functions to varying degrees.

GENERAL CHARACTERISTICS OF CNS DRUGS. Combinations of centrally acting drugs frequently are administered to therapeutic advantage (e.g., an anticholinergic drug and levodopa for Parkinson disease). However, other combinations of drugs may be detrimental because of potentially dangerous additive or mutually antagonistic effects. The effects of a CNS drug may be additive with the physiological state and the effects of other depressant and stimulant drugs. For example, anesthetics are less effective in a hyperexcitable subject than in a normal patient; the converse is true for stimulants. In general, the depressant effects of drugs from different categories are additive (e.g., the potentially fatal combination of barbiturates or benzodiazepines with ethanol), as are the effects of stimulants. Therefore, respiration depressed by morphine is further impaired by depressant drugs, while stimulant drugs can augment the excitatory effects of morphine to produce vomiting and convulsions.

Antagonism between depressants and stimulants is variable. Some instances of true pharmacological antagonism among CNS drugs are known; for example, opioid antagonists can selectively antagonize the effects of opioid analgesics. However, the antagonism exhibited between 2 CNS drugs is most often physiological in nature. For example, an individual whose CNS is depressed by an opiate cannot be returned entirely to normal by stimulation with caffeine.

The selective effects of drugs on specific neurotransmitter systems may be additive or competitive. The potential for drug interactions must be considered whenever such drugs are concurrently administered. To minimize such interactions, a drug-free period may be required when modifying therapy; in fact, development of desensitized and supersensitive states with prolonged therapy may limit the speed with which 1 drug may be halted and another started. An excitatory effect is commonly observed with low concentrations of certain depressant drugs due either to depression of inhibitory systems or to a transient increase in the release of excitatory transmitters. Examples include the stage of excitement seen during induction of general anesthesia. The excitatory phase typically occurs with low concentrations of the depressant; uniform depression ensues with increasing

Table 14–8

Characteristics of Purinergic Receptors

CLASS	RECEPTOR SUBTYPE							
P1 (adenosine)	A_1	A_{2A}	A_{2B}	A_3				
Transducer	G_i	G_s	G_s	G_i				
Agonists	CPA	CGS21680		1B-MECA				
Antagonists	CPX	SCH58261	MRS-1754					
P2X (ionotropic)	$P2X_1$	$P2X_2$	$P2X_3$	$P2X_4$	$P2X_5$	$P2X_6$	$P2X_7$	
Substrate Specificity	ATP>ADP	ATP	ATP	ATP>CTP	ATP	unknown	ATP	
Antagonist	NF449	NF279	TNP-ATP	protons	PPADS	none known	Brilliant Blue G	
P2Y (metabotropic)	$P2Y_1$	$P2Y_2$	$P2Y_4$	$P2Y_6$	$P2Y_{11}$	$P2Y_{12}$	$P2Y_{13}$	$P2Y_{14}$
Transducer	G_q	G_q, G_i	G_q, G_i	G_q	G_q	G_i	G_i	G_i
Substrate specificity	ADP, ATP, ApoA	ATP=UTP	UTP>ATP	UDP	ATP>ADP	ADP	ADP	UDP-glucose[a]

[a]$P2Y_{14}$ binds UDP-glucose, UDP-galactose, and/or UDP-acetylglucosamine.

NECA is a non-selective agonist of P1 receptors.

CPA, N6-cyclopentyladenosine; CPX, 8-cyclopentyl-l,3-dipropylxanthine; 1B-MECA, N6-(3-iodobenzyl)-adenosine-5α-N-methylcarboxamide; NECA, l-(6-amino-9H-purin-9-yl)-l-deoxy-N-ethyl-β-D-ribofuronamide; PPADS, Pyridoxalphosphate-6-azophenyl-2′,4′-disulfonic acid; TNP-ATP, 2′,3′-0-(2,4,6-trinitrophenyl)adenosine-5′-triphosphate.

drug concentration. The excitatory effects can be minimized, when appropriate, by pretreatment with a depressant drug that is devoid of such effects (e.g., benzodiazepines in preanesthetic medication). Acute, excessive stimulation of the cerebrospinal axis normally is followed by depression, which is in part a consequence of neuronal fatigue and exhaustion of stores of transmitters. Postictal depression is additive with the effects of depressant drugs. Acute, drug-induced depression generally is not followed by stimulation. However, chronic drug-induced sedation or depression may be followed by prolonged hyperexcitability on abrupt withdrawal of the medication (barbiturates or alcohol). This type of hyperexcitability can be controlled effectively by the same or another depressant drug (*see* Chapters 17, 23, and 24).

For a complete Bibliographical Listing *see* Goodman & Gilman's ***The Pharmacological Basis of Therapeutics***, 12th ed., or Goodman & Gilman Online at www.AccessMedicine.com.

Drug Therapy of Depression and Anxiety Disorders

Depression and anxiety disorders are the most common mental illnesses, each affecting in excess of 10-15% of the population at some time in their lives. With the advent of more selective and safer drugs, the use of antidepressants and anxiolytics has moved from the domain of psychiatry to other medical specialties, including primary care. *The relative safety of the majority of commonly used antidepressants and anxiolytics notwithstanding, their optimal use requires a clear understanding of their mechanisms of action, pharmacokinetics, potential drug interactions, and the differential diagnosis of psychiatric illnesses.*

A confluence of symptoms of depression and anxiety may affect an individual patient; some of the drugs discussed here are effective in treating both disorders, suggesting common underlying mechanisms of pathophysiology and response to pharmacotherapy. In large measure, our current understanding of pathophysiological mechanisms underlying depression and anxiety has been inferred from the mechanisms of action of psychopharmacological compounds (*see* Chapter 14). While depression and anxiety disorders comprise a wide range of symptoms, including changes in mood, behavior, somatic function, and cognition, some progress has been made in developing animal models that respond with some sensitivity and selectivity to antidepressant or anxiolytic drugs. The last half century has seen notable advances in the discovery and development of drugs for treating depression and anxiety.

CHARACTERIZATION OF DEPRESSIVE AND ANXIETY DISORDER

SYMPTOMS OF DEPRESSION

Depression is classified as major depression (i.e., unipolar depression) or bipolar depression (i.e., manic depressive illness); bipolar depression and its treatment are discussed in Chapter 16. Lifetime risk of unipolar depression is ~15%. Females are affected twice as frequently as males. Depressive episodes are characterized by sad mood, pessimistic worry, diminished interest in normal activities, mental slowing and poor concentration, insomnia or increased sleep, significant weight loss or gain due to altered eating and activity patterns, psychomotor agitation or retardation, feelings of guilt and worthlessness, decreased energy and libido, and suicidal ideation, occurring most days for a period of at least 2 weeks. In some cases, the primary complaint of patients involves somatic pain or other physical symptoms and can present a diagnostic challenge for primary care physicians. Depressive symptoms also can occur secondary to other illnesses such as hypothyroidism, Parkinson disease, and inflammatory conditions. Further, depression often complicates the management of other medical conditions (e.g., severe trauma, cancer, diabetes, and cardiovascular disease, especially myocardial infarction).

Depression is underdiagnosed and undertreated. Approximately 10-15% of those with severe depression attempt suicide at some time. Thus, it is important that symptoms of depression be recognized and treated in a timely manner. Furthermore, the response to treatment must be assessed and decisions made regarding continued treatment with the initial drug, dose adjustment, adjunctive therapy, or alternative medication.

SYMPTOMS OF ANXIETY. Anxiety disorder symptoms include generalized anxiety disorder, obsessive-compulsive disorder, panic disorder, posttraumatic stress disorder (PTSD), separation anxiety disorder, social phobia, specific phobias, and acute stress. In general, symptoms of anxiety that lead to pharmacological treatment are those that interfere significantly with normal function. Symptoms of anxiety also are often associated with depression and other medical conditions.

Anxiety is a normal human emotion that serves an adaptive function from a psychobiological perspective. However, in the psychiatric setting, feelings of fear or dread that are unfocused (e.g., generalized anxiety disorder) or out of scale with the perceived threat (e.g., specific phobias) often require treatment. Drug treatment includes acute drug administration to manage episodes of anxiety, and chronic or repeated treatment to manage unrelieved and continuing anxiety disorders.

ANTIDEPRESSANT DRUGS

In general, antidepressants enhance serotonergic or noradrenergic transmission. Sites of interaction of antidepressant drugs with noradrenergic and serotonergic neurons are depicted in Figure 15–1. Table 15–1 summarizes the actions of the most widely used antidepressants. The most commonly used medications, often referred to as second-generation antidepressants, are the selective serotonin reuptake inhibitors (SSRIs) and the serotonin-norepinephrine reuptake inhibitors (SNRIs), which have greater efficacy and safety compared to the first-generation

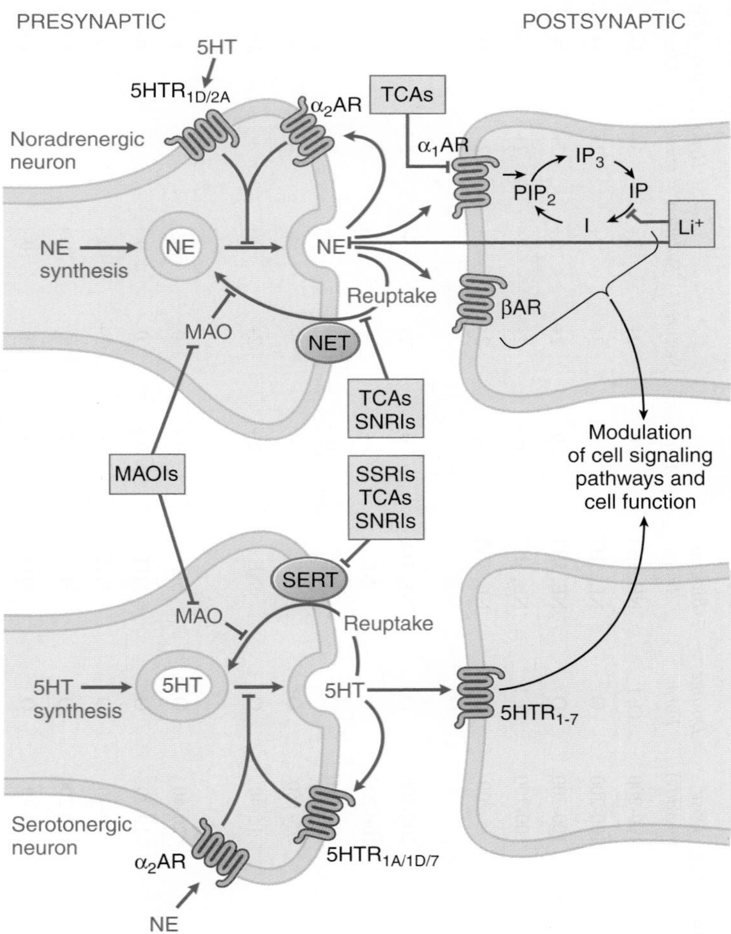

Figure 15–1 *Sites of action of antidepressants at noradrenergic (top) and serotonergic (bottom) nerve terminals.* SSRIs, SNRIs, and TCAs increase noradrenergic or serotonergic neurotransmission by blocking the NE or 5HT transporter at presynaptic terminals (NET, SERT). MAOIs inhibit the catabolism of NE and 5HT. Trazodone and related drugs have direct effects on 5HT receptors that contribute to their clinical effects. Chronic treatment with a number of antidepressants desensitizes presynaptic autoreceptors and heteroreceptors, producing long-lasting changes in monoaminergic neurotransmission. Post-receptor effects of antidepressant treatment, including modulation of GPCR signaling and activation of protein kinases and ion channels, are involved in the mediation of the long-term effects of antidepressant drugs. Note that NE and 5HT also affect each other's neurons.

Table 15–1

Antidepressants: Dose and Dosage Forms, and Side Effects

CLASS/Agent	ADMINISTRATION		MEDIATOR	SIDE EFFECTS								
NE Reuptake Inhibitors: *3° Amine Tricyclics*	*Dose*[a] *(mg/day)*	*Dosage Form*	*Biogenic Amine*	*Agitation*	*Seizures*	*Sedation*	*Hypo-tension*	*Anti-ACh Effects*	*GI Effects*	*Weight Gain*	*Sexual Effects*	*Cardiac Effects*
Amitriptyline	100-200	O, I	NE, 5HT	0	2+	3+	3+	3+	0/+	2+	2+	3+
Clomipramine	100-200	O	NE, 5HT	0	3+	2+	2+	3+	+	2+	3+	3+
Doxepin	100-200	O	NE, 5HT	0	2+	3+	2+	2+	0-+	2+	2+	3+
Imipramine	100-200	O, I	NE, 5HT	0/+	2+	2+	2+	2+	0/+	2+	2+	3+
(+)-Trimipramine	75-200	O	NE, 5HT	0	2+	3+	2+	3+	0/+	2+	2+	3+
2° Amine Tricyclics												
Amoxapine	200-300	O	NE, DA	0	2+	+	2+	+	0/+	+	2+	2+
Desipramine	100-200	O	NE	+	+	0/+	+	+	0/+	+	2+	2+
Maprotiline	100-150	O	NE	0/+	3+	2+	2+	2+	0/+	+	2+	2+
Nortriptyline	75-150	O	NE	0	+	+	+	+	0/+	+	2+	2+
Protriptyline	15-40	O	NE	2+	2+	0/+	+	2+	0/+	+	2+	3+
SSRIs												
(±)-Citalopram	20-40	O	5HT	0/+	0	0/+	0	0	3+	0	3+	0
(+)-Escitalopram	10-20	O	5HT	0/+	0	0/+	0	0	3+	0	3+	0
(±)-Fluoxetine	20-40	O	5HT	+	0/+	0/+	0	0	3+	0/+	3+	0/+
Fluvoxamine	100-200	O	5HT	0	0	0/+	0	0	3+	0	3+	0
(−)-Paroxetine	20-40	O	5HT	+	0	0/+	0	0/+	3+	0	3+	0
(+)-Sertraline	100-150	O	5HT	+	0	0/+	0	0	3+	0	3+	0
(±)-Venlafaxine	75-225	O	5HT, NE	0/+	0	0	0	0	3+	0	3+	0/+

Atypical Antidepressants	*Dose*[a] *(mg/day)*	*Dosage Form*	*Biogenic Amine*	*Agitation*	*Seizures*	*Sedation*	*Hypo-tension*	*Anti-ACh Effects*	*GI Effects*	*Weight Gain*	*Sexual Effects*	*Cardiac Effects*
(−)-Atomoxetine	40-80	O	NE	0	0	0	0	0	0/+	0	0	0
Bupropion	200-300	O	DA, ?NE	3+	4+	0	0	0	2+	0	0	0
(+)-Duloxetine	80-100	O	NE, 5HT	+	0	0/+	0/+	0	0/+	0/+	0/+	0/+
(±)-Mirtazapine	15-45	O	5HT, NE	0	0	4+	0/+	0	0/+	0/+	0	0
Nefazodone	200-400	O	5HT	0	0	3+	0	0	2+	0/+	0/+	0/+
Trazodone	150-200	O	5HT	0	0	3+	0	0	2+	+	+	0/+
MAO Inhibitors												
Phenelzine	30-60	O	NE, 5HT, DA	0/+	0	+	+	0	0/+	+	3+	0
Tranylcypromine	20-30	O	NE, 5HT, DA	2+	0	0	+	0	0/+	+	2+	0
(−)-Selegiline	10	O	DA, ?NE, ?5HT	0	0	0	0	0	0	0	+	0

Note: Selegiline is approved for early Parkinson disease, but may have antidepressant effects, especially at daily doses 20 mg, and is under investigation for administration by transdermal patch.

[a]Both higher and lower doses are sometimes used, depending on an individual patient's needs and response to the drug; see the literature and FDA-approved dosage recommendations.

[b]Children, 0.5–1 mg/kg, up to 70 kg; see black box warning.

O, oral tablet or capsule; I, injectable; NE, norepinephrine; 5HT, serotonin; DA, dopamine; 0, negligible; 0/+, minimal; +, mild; 2+, moderate; 3+, moderately severe; 4+, severe.

Other significant side effects for individual drugs are described in the text.

drugs, which include monoamine oxidase inhibitors (MAOIs) and tricyclic antidepressants (TCAs).

In monoamine systems, inhibition of reuptake can enhance neurotransmission, presumably by slowing clearance of the transmitter from the synapse and prolonging the dwell-time of the transmitter in the synapse. Reuptake inhibitors inhibit either SERT, the neuronal serotonin (5-hydroxytryptamine [5HT]) transporter; NET, the neuronal norepinephrine (NE) transporter; or both. Similarly, MAOIs and TCAs enhance monoaminergic neurotransmission: the MAOIs by inhibiting monoamine metabolism and thereby enhancing neurotransmitter storage in secretory granules, the TCAs by inhibiting 5HT and NE reuptake

Long-term effects of antidepressant drugs evoke regulatory mechanisms that enhance the effectiveness of therapy. These responses include increased adrenergic or serotonergic receptor density or sensitivity, increased receptor-G protein coupling and cyclic nucleotide signaling, induction of neurotrophic factors, and increased neurogenesis in the hippocampus. Persistent antidepressant effects depend on the continued inhibition of 5HT or NE transporters, or enhanced serotonergic or noradrenergic neurotransmission achieved by an alternative pharmacological mechanism. Compelling evidence suggests that sustained signaling via NE or 5HT increases the expression of specific downstream gene products, particularly brain-derived neurotrophic factor (BDNF), which appears to be related to the ultimate mechanism of action of these drugs.

CLINICAL CONSIDERATIONS WITH ANTIDEPRESSANT DRUGS

Antidepressant drug treatment has generally a "therapeutic lag" lasting 3-4 weeks before a measurable therapeutic response becomes evident. After the successful initial treatment phase, a 6-12–month maintenance treatment phase is typical, after which the drug is gradually withdrawn. If a patient is chronically depressed (i.e., >2 years), lifelong treatment with an antidepressant is advisable.

A controversial issue regarding the use of all antidepressants is their relationship to suicide. Data establishing a clear link between antidepressant treatment and suicide are lacking. However, the FDA has issued a "black box" warning regarding the use of SSRIs and a number of other antidepressants in children and adolescents due to the possibility of an association between antidepressant treatment and suicide. For seriously depressed patients, the risk of not being on an effective antidepressant drug outweighs the risk of being treated with one.

SELECTIVE SEROTONIN REUPTAKE INHIBITORS

The SSRIs are effective in treating major depression. SSRIs also are anxiolytics with demonstrated efficacy in the treatment of generalized anxiety, panic, social anxiety, and obsessive-compulsive disorders. *Sertraline* and *paroxetine* are approved for the treatment of PTSD. SSRIs also are used for treatment of premenstrual dysphoric syndrome and for preventing vasovagal symptoms in postmenopausal women.

SERT mediates the reuptake of serotonin into the presynaptic terminal; neuronal uptake is the primary process by which neurotransmission via 5HT is terminated (*see* Figure 15–1). SSRIs block reuptake and prolong serotonergic neurotransmission. SSRIs used clinically are relatively selective for inhibition of SERT relative to NET (Table 15–2; not shown is vilazodone [VIIBRYD], an SSRI and partial $5HT_{1A}$ agonist, recently approved by the FDA for treatment of major depression).

SSRI treatment causes stimulation of $5HT_{1A}$ and $5HT_7$ autoreceptors on cell bodies in the raphe nucleus and of $5HT_{1D}$ autoreceptors on serotonergic terminals, and this reduces serotonin synthesis and release toward predrug levels. With repeated treatment with SSRIs, there is a gradual downregulation and desensitization of these autoreceptor mechanisms. In addition, downregulation of postsynaptic $5HT_{2A}$ receptors may contribute to antidepressant efficacy directly or by influencing the function of noradrenergic and other neurons via serotonergic heteroreceptors. Other postsynaptic 5HT receptors likely remain responsive to increased synaptic concentrations of 5HT and contribute to the therapeutic effects of the SSRIs.

Later-developing effects of SSRI treatment also may be important in mediating ultimate therapeutic responses. These include sustained increases in cyclic AMP signaling and phosphorylation of the nuclear transcription factor CREB, as well as increases in the expression of trophic factors such as BDNF, and increases of neurogenesis from progenitor cells in the hippocampus and subventricular zone. Repeated treatment with SSRIs reduces the expression of SERT, resulting in reduced clearance of released 5HT and increased serotonergic neurotransmission.

Table 15–2

Selectivity of Antidepressants at the Human Biogenic Amine Transporters

DRUG	SELECTIVITY	DRUG	SELECTIVITY
NE Selective	NET *vs* SERT	5HT Selective	SERT *vs* NET
Oxaprotiline	800	*S*-Citalopram	7127
Maprotiline	532	*R,S*-Citalopram	3643
Viloxazine	109	Sertraline	1390
Nomifensine	64	Fluvoxamine	591
Desipramine	22	Paroxetine	400
Protriptyline	14	Fluoxetine	305
Atomoxetine	12	Clomipramine	123
Reboxetine	8.3	Venlafaxine	116
Nortriptyline	4.2	Zimelidine	60
Amoxapine	3.6	Trazodone	52
Doxepin	2.3	Imipramine	26
DA Selective	DAT *vs* NET	Amitriptyline	8.0
Bupropion	1000	Duloxetine	7.0
		Dothiepin	5.5
		Milnacipran	1.6

Selectivity is defined as ratio of the relevant K_i values (SERT/NET, NET/SERT, NET/DAT). Bupropion is selective for the DAT relative to the NET and SERT.
See 12th edition of parent text, Table 15–2, for references.

SEROTONIN-NOREPINEPHRINE REUPTAKE INHIBITORS

Four medications with a nontricyclic structure that inhibit the reuptake of both 5HT and NE have been approved for use in the U.S. for treatment of depression, anxiety disorders, and pain: venlafaxine and its demethylated metabolite, desvenlafaxine; duloxetine; and milnacipran.

SNRIs inhibit both SERT and NET (*see* Table 15–2) and cause enhanced serotonergic and/or noradrenergic neurotransmission. Similar to the action of SSRIs, the initial inhibition of SERT induces activation of $5HT_{1A}$ and $5HT_{1D}$ autoreceptors. This action decreases serotonergic neurotransmission by a negative feedback mechanism until these serotonergic autoreceptors are desensitized. Then, the enhanced serotonin concentration in the synapse can interact with postsynaptic 5HT receptors. SNRIs were developed with the rationale that they might improve overall treatment response compared to SSRIs. Specifically, the remission rate for venlafaxine appears slightly better than for SSRIs in head-to-head trials. Duloxetine, in addition to being approved for use in the treatment of depression and anxiety, also is used for treatment of fibromyalgia and neuropathic pain associated with peripheral neuropathy. Off-label uses include stress urinary incontinence (duloxetine), autism, binge eating disorders, hot flashes, pain syndromes, premenstrual dysphoric disorders, and PTSDs (venlafaxine).

SEROTONIN RECEPTOR ANTAGONISTS

Several antagonists of the $5HT_2$ family of receptors are effective antidepressants. These includes 2 close structural analogues, trazodone and nefazodone, as well as mirtazapine (REMERON, others) and mianserin (not marketed in the U.S.).

The efficacy of trazodone may be somewhat more limited than the SSRIs; however, low doses of trazodone (50-100 mg) have been used widely both alone and concurrently with SSRIs or SNRIs to treat insomnia. Both mianserin and mirtazapine are quite sedating and are treatments of choice for some depressed patients with insomnia. Trazodone blocks the $5HT_2$ and α_1-adrenergic receptors. Trazodone also inhibits the serotonin transporter, but is markedly less potent for this action relative to its blockade of $5HT_{2A}$ receptors. Similarly, the most potent pharmacological action of nefazodone also is the blockade of the $5HT_2$ receptors. Both mirtazapine and mianserin potently block histamine H_1 receptors. They also have some affinity for α_2-adrenergic receptors. Their affinities for $5HT_{2A}$, $5HT_{2C}$, and $5HT_3$ receptors are high, though less so than for histamine H_1 receptors. Both of these drugs have been shown to increase the antidepressant response when combined with SSRIs compared to the action of the SSRIs alone.

BUPROPION

Bupropion (WELLBUTRIN, others) is discussed separately because it appears to act via multiple mechanisms. It enhances both noradrenergic and dopaminergic neurotransmission via inhibition of reuptake (by NET and also by DAT, although effects on this transporter are not potent in animal studies) (*see* Table 15–2). Its mechanism of action may also involve the presynaptic release of NE and DA and effects on VMAT2, the vesicular monoamine transporter (*see* Figure 8–6). The hydroxybupropion metabolite may contribute to the therapeutic effects of bupropion: This metabolite appears to have a similar pharmacology and is present in substantial levels. Bupropion is indicated for the treatment of depression, prevention of seasonal depressive disorder, and as a smoking cessation treatment (under the ZYBAN brand). Bupropion has effects on sleep EEG that are opposite those of most antidepressant drugs. Bupropion may improve symptoms of attention deficit hyperactivity disorder (ADHD) and has been used off-label for neuropathic pain and weight loss. Clinically, bupropion is widely used in combination with SSRIs to obtain a greater antidepressant response; however, there are very limited clinical data providing strong support for this practice.

ATYPICAL ANTIPSYCHOTICS

In addition to their use in schizophrenia, bipolar depression, and major depression with psychotic disorders, atypical antipsychotics have gained further, off-label use for major depression without psychotic features. The combination of aripiprazole (ABILIFY) with SSRIs and SNRIs and a combination of olanzapine and the SSRI fluoxetine (SYMBYAX) have been approved by the FDA for treatment-resistant major depression (i.e., following an inadequate response to at least 2 different antidepressants).

The initial recommended dose of aripiprazole is 2-5 mg/day with a recommended maximal dose of 15 mg/day following increments of no more than 5 mg/day every week. The olanzapine-fluoxetine combination is available in fixed-dose combinations of either 6 or 12 mg of olanzapine and 25 or 50 mg of fluoxetine. Quetiapine (SEROQUEL) may have either primary antidepressant actions on its own or adjunctive benefit for treatment-resistant depression; it is used off-label for insomnia. The mechanism of action and adverse effects of the atypical antipsychotics are described in detail in Chapter 16. The major risks of these agents are weight gain and metabolic syndrome, a greater problem for quetiapine and olanzapine than for aripiprazole.

TRICYCLIC ANTIDEPRESSANTS

TCAs may cause serious side effects and generally are not used as first-line drugs for the treatment of depression. TCAs and first-generation antipsychotics are synergistic for the treatment of psychotic depression. Tertiary amine TCAs (e.g., doxepin, amitriptyline) have been used for many years in relatively low doses for treating insomnia. In addition, because of the role of norepinephrine and serotonin in pain transmission, these drugs are commonly used to treat a variety of pain conditions.

The pharmacological action of TCAs is antagonism of serotonin and norepinephrine transporters (*see* Table 15–2). In addition to inhibiting NET somewhat selectively (desipramine, nortriptyline, protriptyline, amoxapine) or both SERT and NET (imipramine, amitriptyline), these drugs also block other receptors (H_1, $5HT_2$, α_1, and muscarinic). Given the superior activity of clomipramine over SSRIs, some combination of these additional pharmacological actions may contribute to the therapeutic effects of TCAs. One TCA, amoxapine, also is a dopamine-receptor antagonist; its use, unlike that of other TCAs, poses some risk for the development of extrapyramidal side effects such as tardive dyskinesia.

MONOAMINE OXIDASE INHIBITORS

MAOIs have efficacy equivalent to that of the TCAs but are rarely used because of their toxicity and major drug and food interactions. The MAOIs approved for treatment of depression include tranylcypromine (PARNATE, others), phenelzine (NARDIL), and isocarboxazid (MARPLAN). Selegiline (EMSAM) is available as a transdermal patch; transdermal delivery may reduce the risk for diet-associated hypertensive reactions.

The MAOIs nonselectively and irreversibly inhibit both MAO-A and MAO-B, which are located in the mitochondria and metabolize monoamines, including 5HT and NE (*see* Chapter 8). Selegiline inhibits MAO-B at lower doses, with effects on MAO-A at higher doses. Selegiline also is a reversible inhibitor of MAO, which may reduce the potential for serious adverse drug and food interactions. While both MAO-A and MAO-B are involved in metabolizing 5HT, only MAO-B is found in serotonergic neurons (*see* Chapter 13).

PHARMACOKINETICS

The metabolism of most antidepressants is mediated by hepatic CYPs (Table 15–3). Some antidepressants inhibit the clearance of other drugs by the CYP system, and this possibility of drug interactions should be a significant factor in considering the choice of agents.

SELECTIVE SEROTONIN REUPTAKE INHIBITORS. All of the SSRIs are orally active and possess elimination half-lives consistent with once-daily dosing. In the case of fluoxetine, the combined action of the parent and the desmethyl metabolite norfluoxetine allows for a once-weekly formulation (PROZAC WEEKLY). CYP2D6 is involved in the metabolism of most SSRIs and the SSRIs are at least moderately potent inhibitors of this isoenzyme. This creates a significant potential for drug interaction for postmenopausal women taking the breast cancer drug and estrogen antagonist, tamoxifen (*see* Chapter 63). Because venlafaxine and desvenlafaxine are weak inhibitors of CYP2D6, these antidepressants are not contraindicated in this clinical situation. However, care should be used in combining SSRIs with drugs that are metabolized by CYPs.

SEROTONIN-NOREPINEPHRINE REUPTAKE INHIBITORS. Both immediate-release and extended-release (tablet or capsule) preparations of venlafaxine (EFFEXOR XR, others) produces steady state-levels of drug in plasma within 3 days. The elimination half-lives for the parent venlafaxine and its active and major metabolite desmethyl venlafaxine are 5 and 11 h, respectively. Desmethyl venlafaxine is eliminated by hepatic metabolism and by renal excretion. Venlafaxine dose reductions are suggested for patients with renal or hepatic impairment. Duloxetine has a $t_{1/2}$ of 12 h. Duloxetine is not recommended for those with end-stage renal disease or hepatic insufficiency.

SEROTONIN RECEPTOR ANTAGONISTS. Mirtazapine has an elimination $t_{1/2}$ of 16-30 h. Thus, dose changes are suggested no more often than 1-2 weeks. The recommended initial dosing of mirtazapine is 15 mg/day with a maximal recommended dose of 45 mg/day. Clearance of mirtazapine is decreased in the elderly and in patients with moderate to severe renal or hepatic impairment. Pharmacokinetics and adverse effects of mirtazapine may have an enantiomer-selective component. Steady-state trazodone is observed within 3 days following dosing regimen. Trazodone typically is started at 150 mg/day in divided doses with 50 mg increments every 3-4 days. The maximally recommended dose is 400 mg/day for outpatients and 600 mg/day for inpatients. Nefazodone has a $t_{1/2}$ of only 2-4 h; its major metabolite hydroxynefazodone has a $t_{1/2}$ of 1.5-4 h.

BUPROPION. Bupropion elimination has a $t_{1/2}$ of 21 h and involves both hepatic and renal routes. Patients with severe hepatic cirrhosis should receive a maximum dose of 150 mg every other day while consideration for a decreased dose should also be made in cases of renal impairment.

TRICYCLIC ANTIDEPRESSANTS. The TCAs, or their active metabolites, have plasma half-lives of 8-80 h; this makes once-daily dosing possible for most of the compounds. Steady-state concentrations occur within several days to several weeks of beginning treatment. TCAs are largely eliminated by hepatic CYPs (*see* Table 15–3). Dosage adjustments of TCAs are typically made according to patient's clinical response, not based on plasma levels. Nonetheless, monitoring the plasma exposure has an important relationship to treatment response: there is a relatively narrow therapeutic window. About 7% of patients metabolize TCAs slowly due to a variant CYP2D6 isoenzyme, causing a 30-fold difference in plasma concentrations among different patients given the same TCA dose. To avoid toxicity in "slow metabolizers," plasma levels should be monitored and doses adjusted downward.

MONOAMINE OXIDASE INHIBITORS. MAOIs are metabolized by acetylation. A significant portion of the population (50% of the Caucasian population and an even higher percentage among Asians) are "slow acetylators" and will exhibit elevated plasma levels. The nonselective MAOIs used in the treatment of depression are irreversible inhibitors; thus, it takes up to 2 weeks for MAO activity to recover, even though the parent drug is excreted within 24 h. Recovery of normal enzyme function is dependent on synthesis and transport of new MAO to monoaminergic nerve terminals. Despite this irreversible enzyme inhibition, MAOIs require daily dosing.

ADVERSE EFFECTS

SELECTIVE SEROTONIN REUPTAKE INHIBITORS. The SSRIs have no major cardiovascular side effects. The SSRIs are generally free of antimuscarinic side effects (dry mouth, urinary retention, confusion), do not block histamine or α-adrenergic receptors, and are not sedating (Table 15–4).

Table 15–3

Disposition of Antidepressants

DRUG	ELIMINATION $t_{1/2}$ (h) OF PARENT DRUG *(of active metabolite)*	TYPICAL C_P (ng/mL)	PREDOMINANT CYP INVOLVED IN METABOLISM
Tricyclic Antidepressants			
Amitriptyline	16 *(30)*	100-250	2D6, 2C19, 3A3/4 1A2
Amoxapine	8 *(30)*	200-500	
Clomipramine	32 *(70)*	150-500	
Desipramine	30	125-300	
Doxepin	18 *(30)*	150-250	
Imipramine	12 *(30)*	175-300	
Maprotiline	48	200-400	
Nortriptyline	31	60-150	
Protriptyline	80	100-250	
Trimipramine	16 *(30)*	100-300	
Selective Serotonin Reuptake Inhibitors			
R,S-Citalopram	36	75-150	3A4, 2C19
S-Citalopram	30	40-80	3A4, 2C19
Fluoxetine	53 *(240)*	100-500	2D6, 2C9
Fluvoxamine	18	100-200	2D6, 1A2, 3A4, 2C9
Paroxetine	17	30-100	2D6
Sertraline	23 *(66)*	25-50	2D6
Serotonin-Norepinephrine Reuptake Inhibitors			
Duloxetine	11	—	2D6
Venlafaxine	5 *(11)*	—	2D6, 3A4
Other Antidepressants			
Atomoxetine	5-20; child, 3	—	2D6, 3A3/4
Bupropion	11	75-100	2B6
Mirtazapine	16	—	2D6
Nefazodone	2-4	—	3A3/4
Reboxetine	12	—	—
Trazodone	6	800-1600	2D6

Values shown are elimination $t_{1/2}$ values for a number of clinically used antidepressant drugs; numbers in parentheses are $t_{1/2}$ values of active metabolites. Fluoxetine (2D6), fluvoxamine (1A2, 2C8, 3A3/4), paroxetine (2D6), and nefazodone (3A3/4) are potent inhibitors of CYPs; sertraline (2D6), citalopram (2C19), and venlafaxine are less potent inhibitors. Plasma concentrations are those observed at typical clinical doses. Information was obtained from manufacturers' summaries and Appendix II of the parent text, which the reader should consult for important details.

Adverse side effects of SSRIs from excessive stimulation of brain $5HT_2$ receptors may result in insomnia, increased anxiety, irritability, and decreased libido, effectively worsening prominent depressive symptoms. Excess activity at spinal $5HT_2$ receptors causes sexual side effects including erectile dysfunction, anorgasmia, and ejaculatory delay; these effects may be more prominent with paroxetine. Stimulation of $5HT_3$ receptors in the CNS and periphery contributes to GI effects, which are usually limited to nausea but may include diarrhea and emesis. Some patients experience an increase in anxiety, especially with the initial dosing of SSRIs. With

Table 15–4

Potencies of Selected Antidepressants at Muscarinic, Histamine H_1, and Alpha$_1$ Adrenergic Receptors

	RECEPTOR TYPE		
DRUG	MUSCARINIC CHOLINERGIC	HISTAMINE H_1	α_1 ADRENERGIC
Amytriptyline	18	1.1	27
Amoxapine	1000	25	50
Atomoxetine	≥1000	≥1000	≥1000
Bupropion	40,000	6700	4550
R,S-Citalopram	1800	380	1550
S-Citalopram	1240	1970	3870
Clomipramine	37	31.2	39
Desipramine	196	110	130
Doxepin	83.3	0.24	24
Duloxetine	3000	2300	8300
Fluoxetine	2000	6250	5900
Fluvoxamine	24,000	>100,000	7700
Imipramine	91	11.0	91
Maprotiline	560	2.0	91
Mirtazapine	670	0.1	500
Nefazodone	11,000	21	25.6
Nortriptyline	149	10	58.8
Paroxetine	108	22,000	>100,000
Protriptyline	25	25	130
Reboxetine	6700	312	11,900
Sertraline	625	24,000	370
Trazodone	>100,000	345	35.7
Trimipramine	59	0.3	23.8
Venlafaxine	>100,000	>100,000	>100,000

Values are experimentally determined potencies (K_i values, nM) for binding to receptors that contribute to common side effects of clinically used antidepressant drugs: muscarinic cholinergic receptors (e.g., dry mouth, urinary retention, confusion), histamine H_1 receptors (sedation), and α_1-adrenergic receptors (orthostatic hypotension, sedation). Source: Data adapted from Leonard BE, Richelson E. Synaptic effects of anitdepressants. In, Schizophrenia and Mood Disorders: The New Drug Therapies in Clinical Practice. (Buckley PF, Waddington JL, eds.) Butterworth- Heinemann, Boston, 2000, pp. 67–84.

continued treatment, some patients also report a dullness of intellectual abilities and concentration. In general, there is not a strong relationship between SSRI serum concentrations and therapeutic efficacy. Thus, dosage adjustments are based more on evaluation of clinical response and management of side effects.

Sudden withdrawal of antidepressants can precipitate a withdrawal syndrome. For SSRIs or SNRIs, the symptoms of withdrawal may include dizziness, headache, nervousness, nausea, and insomnia. This withdrawal syndrome appears most intense for paroxetine and venlafaxine compared to other antidepressants due to their relatively short half-lives and, in the case of paroxetine, lack of active metabolites. Conversely, the active metabolite of fluoxetine, norfluoxetine, has such a long $t_{1/2}$ (1-2 weeks) that few patients experience any withdrawal symptoms when discontinuing fluoxetine.

Unlike the other SSRIs, paroxetine is associated with an increased risk of congenital cardiac malformations when administered in the first trimester of pregnancy. Venlafaxine also is associated with an increased risk of perinatal complications.

SEROTONIN-NOREPINEPHRINE REUPTAKE INHIBITORS. SNRIs have a side effect profile similar to that of the SSRIs, including nausea, constipation, insomnia, headaches, and sexual dysfunction. The immediate release formulation of venlafaxine can induce sustained diastolic hypertension (diastolic blood pressure >90 mm Hg at consecutive weekly visits) in 10-15% of patients at higher doses; this risk is reduced with the extended-release form. This effect of venlafaxine may not be associated simply with inhibition of NET, since duloxetine does not share this side effect.

SEROTONIN RECEPTOR ANTAGONISTS. The main side effects of mirtazapine, seen in >10% of the patients, are somnolence, increased appetite, and weight gain. A rare side effect of mirtazapine is agranulocytosis. Trazodone use is associated with priapism in rare instances. Nefazodone was voluntarily withdrawn from the market after rare cases of liver failure were associated with its use. Generic nefazodone is still available in the U.S.

BUPROPION. At doses higher than that recommended for depression (450 mg/day), the risk of seizures increases significantly. The use of extended-release formulations often blunts the maximum concentration observed after dosing and minimizes the chance of reaching drug levels associated with an increased risk of seizures.

TRICYCLIC ANTIDEPRESSANTS. TCAs are potent antagonists at histamine H_1 receptors; H_1-receptor antagonism contributes to the sedative effects of TCAs (*see* Table 15–4). Antagonism of muscarinic acetylcholine receptors contributes to cognitive dulling as well as a range of adverse effects mediated by the parasympathetic nervous system (blurred vision, dry mouth, tachycardia, constipation, difficulty urinating). Some tolerance does occur for these anticholinergic effects. Antagonism of α_1 adrenergic receptors contributes to orthostatic hypotension and sedation. Weight gain is another side effect of this class of antidepressants.

TCAs also have quinidine-like effects on cardiac conduction that can be life threatening with overdose and limit the use of TCAs in patients with coronary heart disease. This is the primary reason that only a very limited supply should be available to the patient at any given time. Like other antidepressant drugs, TCAs also lower the seizure threshold.

MONOAMINE OXIDASE INHIBITORS. Hypertensive crisis resulting from food or drug interactions is one of the life-threatening toxicities associated with use of the MAOIs. Foods containing tyramine are a contributing factor. MAO-A within the intestinal wall and MAO-A and MAO-B in the liver normally degrade dietary tyramine. When MAO-A is inhibited, the ingestion of tyramine-containing foods leads to accumulation of tyramine in adrenergic nerve endings and neurotransmitter vesicles and induces norepinephrine and epinephrine release. The released catecholamines stimulate postsynaptic receptors in the periphery, increasing blood pressure to dangerous levels. The use of prescription or over-the-counter medications that contain sympathomimetic compounds also result in a potentially life-threatening elevation of blood pressure. In comparison to tranylcypromine and isocarboxazid, the selegiline transdermal patch is better tolerated and safer. Another serious, life-threatening issue with chronic administration of MAOIs is hepatotoxicity.

MAO-A inhibitors are efficacious in treating depression. However, MAO-B inhibitors such as selegiline (with oral formulations) are effective in treating depression only when given at doses that block both MAO-A and MAO-B. While not available in the U.S., reversible inhibitors of MAO-A (RIMAs, such as moclobemide) have been developed. Because these drugs are selective for MAO-A, significant MAO-B activity remains. Further, since the inhibition of MAO-A by RIMAs is reversible and competitive, as concentrations of tyramine rise, enzyme inhibition is surmounted. Thus, RIMAs produce antidepressant effects with reduced risk of tyramine-induced hypertensive crisis.

DRUG INTERACTIONS

Many of these drugs are metabolized by hepatic CYPs, especially CYP2D6. Thus, other agents that are substrates or inhibitors of CYP2D6 can increase plasma concentrations of the primary drug. The combination of other classes of antidepressant agents with MAOIs is inadvisable and can lead to serotonin syndrome.

SELECTIVE SEROTONIN REUPTAKE INHIBITORS. Paroxetine and, to a lesser degree, fluoxetine are potent inhibitors of CYP2D6. The other SSRIs, outside of fluvoxamine, are at least moderate inhibitors of CYP2D6. This inhibition can result in disproportionate increases in plasma concentrations of drugs metabolized by CYP2D6 when doses of these drugs are increased. Fluvoxamine directly inhibits CYP1A2 and CYP2C19; fluoxetine and fluvoxamine also inhibit CYP3A4. A prominent interaction is the increase in TCA exposure that may be observed during coadministration of TCAs and SSRIs.

MAOIs enhance the effects of SSRIs due to inhibition of serotonin metabolism. Administration of these drugs together can produce synergistic increases in extracellular brain serotonin, leading to the serotonin syndrome. Symptoms of the serotonin syndrome include hyperthermia, muscle rigidity, myoclonus, tremors, autonomic instability, confusion, irritability, and agitation; this can progress toward coma and death. Other drugs that may induce the serotonin syndrome include substituted amphetamines such as methylenedioxymethamphetamine (Ecstasy), which directly releases serotonin from nerve terminals.

SSRIs should not be started until at least 14 days following discontinuation of treatment with an MAOI; this allows for synthesis of new MAO. For all SSRIs but fluoxetine, at least 14 days should pass prior to beginning treatment with an MAOI following the end of treatment with an SSRI. Because the active metabolite norfluoxetine has a $t_{1/2}$ of 1-2 weeks, at least 5 weeks should pass between stopping fluoxetine and beginning an MAOI.

SEROTONIN-NOREPINEPHRINE REUPTAKE INHIBITORS. While 14 days are suggested to elapse from ending MAOI therapy and starting venlafaxine treatment, an interval of only 7 days is considered safe. Duloxetine has a similar interval to initiation following MAOI therapy, but requires only a 5-day waiting period to begin MAOI treatment after ending duloxetine. Failure to observe these required waiting periods can result in the serotonin syndrome.

SEROTONIN RECEPTOR ANTAGONISTS. Trazodone dosing may need to be lowered when given together with drugs that inhibit CYP3A4. Mirtazapine is metabolized by CYPs 2D6, 1A2, and 3A4. Trazodone and nefazodone are weak inhibitors of serotonin uptake and should not be administered with MAOIs due to concerns about the serotonin syndrome.

BUPROPION. The major route of metabolism for bupropion is CYP2B6. While there does not appear to be any evidence for metabolism by CYP2D6 and this drug is frequently administered with SSRIs, the potential for interactions with drugs metabolized by CYP2D6 should be kept in mind until the safety of the combination is firmly established.

TRICYCLIC ANTIDEPRESSANTS. Drugs that inhibit CYP2D6, such as SSRIs, may increase plasma exposures of TCAs. Other drugs that may act similarly are phenothiazine antipsychotic agents, type 1C anti-arrhythmic drugs, and other drugs with antimuscarinic, antihistaminic, and α-adrenergic antagonistic effects. TCAs can potentiate the actions of sympathomimetic amines and should not be used concurrently with MAOIs or within 14 days of stopping MAOIs.

MONOAMINE OXIDASE INHIBITORS. CNS depressants including meperidine and other narcotics, alcohol, and anesthetic agents should not be used with MAOIs. Meperidine and other opioid agonists in combination with MAOIs also induce the serotonin syndrome. SSRIs and SNRIs are contraindicated in patients on MAOIs to avoid the serotonin syndrome. In general, other antidepressants such as TCAs and bupropion also should be avoided in patients taking an MAOI.

ANXIOLYTIC DRUGS

Primary treatments for anxiety-related disorders include the SSRIs, SNRIs, benzodiazepines, buspirone, and β adrenergic antagonists. The SSRIs and the SNRI venlafaxine have anxiolytic activity with chronic treatment. The benzodiazepines are effective anxiolytics as both acute and chronic treatment. Buspirone, like the SSRIs, is effective following chronic treatment. It acts, at least in part, via the serotonergic system, where it is a partial agonist at $5HT_{1A}$ receptors. Buspirone also has antagonistic effects at dopamine D_2 receptors, but the relationship between this effect and its clinical actions is uncertain. β adrenergic antagonists (e.g., propranolol and nadolol) are occasionally used for performance anxiety such as fear of public speaking; their use is limited due to significant side effects such as hypotension.

The antihistamine hydroxyzine and various sedative-hypnotic agents have been used as anxiolytics, but are generally not recommended because of their side effect profiles. Hydroxyzine, which produces short-term sedation, is used in patients who cannot use other types of anxiolytics (e.g., those with a history of drug or alcohol abuse where benzodiazepines would be avoided). Chloral hydrate has been used for situational anxiety, but there is a narrow dose range where anxiolytic effects are observed in the absence of significant sedation, and, therefore, the use of chloral hydrate is not recommended.

CLINICAL CONSIDERATIONS WITH ANXIOLYTIC DRUGS. The choice of pharmacological treatment for anxiety is dictated by the specific anxiety-related disorders and the clinical need for acute anxiolytic effects. The benzodiazepines and β adrenergic antagonists are effective acutely. Chronic treatment with SSRIs, SNRIs, and buspirone is required to produce and sustain anxiolytic effects.

Benzodiazepines, such as alprazolam, chlordiazepoxide, clonazepam, clorazepate, diazepam, lorazepam, and oxazepam, are effective in the treatment of generalized anxiety disorder, panic disorder, and situational anxiety. In addition to their anxiolytic effects, benzodiazepines produce sedative, hypnotic, anesthetic, anticonvulsant, and muscle relaxant effects. The benzodiazepines also impair cognitive performance and memory, adversely affect motor control, and potentiate the effects of other sedatives including alcohol. The anxiolytic effects of this class of drugs are mediated by allosteric interactions with the pentameric benzodiazepine-$GABA_A$ receptor complex, in particular those $GABA_A$ receptors comprised of α2, α3, and α5 subunits (*see* Chapters 14 and 17). The primary effect of the anxiolytic benzodiazepines is to enhance the inhibitory effects of the neurotransmitter GABA. The use of benzodiazepines in the treatment of anxiety has the potential for habituation, dependence, and abuse. Withdrawal of benzodiazepines after chronic treatment, particularly those with short durations of action, can include increased anxiety and seizures. For this reason, it is important that discontinuation be carried out in a gradual manner.

Benzodiazepines cause many adverse effects, including sedation, mild memory impairments, decreased alertness, and slowed reaction time. Occasionally, paradoxical reactions can occur with benzodiazepines such as increases in anxiety, sometimes reaching panic attack proportions. Other pathological reactions can include irritability, aggression, or behavioral disinhibition. Amnesic reactions (i.e., loss of memory for particular periods) can also occur. Benzodiazepines should not be used in pregnant women; there have been rare reports of craniofacial defects. In addition, benzodiazepines taken prior to delivery may result in sedated, underresponsive newborns and prolonged withdrawal reactions. In the elderly, benzodiazepines increase the risk for falls and must be used cautiously. These drugs are safer than classical sedative-hypnotics in overdosage and typically are fatal only if combined with other CNS depressants.

Benzodiazepines have some abuse potential. When these agents are abused, it is generally in a multidrug abuse pattern. In fact, the primary reason for misuse of these agents often is failed attempts to control anxiety. Tolerance to the anxiolytic effects develops with chronic administration, with the result that some patients escalate the dose of benzodiazepines over time. Ideally, benzodiazepines should be used for short periods of time and in conjunction with other medications (e.g., SSRIs) or evidence-based psychotherapies (e.g., cognitive behavioral therapy for anxiety disorders).

SSRIs and the SNRI venlafaxine are first-line treatments for most types of anxiety disorders, except when an acute drug effect is desired; fluvoxamine is approved only for obsessive-compulsive disorder. As for their antidepressant actions, the anxiolytic effects of these drugs become manifest following chronic treatment. Other drugs with actions on serotonergic neurotransmission, including trazodone, nefazodone, and mirtazapine, also are used in the treatment of anxiety disorders. Details regarding the pharmacology of these classes of were presented earlier. Both SSRIs and SNRIs are beneficial in specific anxiety conditions such as generalized anxiety disorder, social phobias, obsessive-compulsive disorder, and panic disorder. These effects appear to be related to the capacity of serotonin to regulate the activity of brain structures such as amygdala and locus coeruleus that are thought to be involved in the genesis of anxiety. Anxious patients appear to be particularly prone to severe discontinuation reactions with certain medications such as venlafaxine and paroxetine; therefore, slow off-tapering is required.

Buspirone requires chronic treatment for effectiveness. Buspirone is primarily effective in the treatment of generalized anxiety disorder, but not for other anxiety disorders.

For a complete Bibliographical Listing see Goodman & Gilman's ***The Pharmacological Basis of Therapeutics***, 12th ed., or Goodman & Gilman Online at www.AccessMedicine.com.

Pharmacotherapy of Psychosis and Mania

Psychosis is a symptom of mental illnesses characterized by a distorted or nonexistent sense of reality. Common psychotic disorders include mood disorders (major depression or mania) with psychotic features, substance-induced psychosis, dementia with psychotic features, delirium with psychotic features, brief psychotic disorder, delusional disorder, schizoaffective disorder, and schizophrenia. Schizophrenia has a worldwide prevalence of 1%, but patients with schizophrenia exhibit features that extend beyond those seen in other psychotic illnesses. The *positive symptoms* of psychotic disorders include: hallucinations, delusions, disorganized speech, and disorganized or agitated behavior. Schizophrenia patients also suffer from *negative symptoms* (apathy, avolition, alogia), and *cognitive deficits*, particularly deficits in working memory, processing speed, and social cognition.

The dopamine (DA) hypothesis of psychosis was derived from the discovery that chlorpromazine and reserpine exhibited therapeutic antipsychotic properties in schizophrenia by decreasing dopaminergic neurotransmission. The DA overactivity hypothesis led to the development of the first therapeutic class of antipsychotic agents, now referred to as *typical or first-generation antipsychotic drugs. The term "neuroleptic" refers to typical antipsychotic drugs that act through D_2 receptor blockade but are associated with extrapyramidal side effects.*

The DA hypothesis has its limitations: it does not account for the cognitive deficits associated with schizophrenia and does not explain the psychotomimetic effects of LSD (e.g., *d*-lysergic acid, a potent serotonin $5HT_2$ receptor agonist) or the effects of phencyclidine and ketamine, antagonists of the *N*-methyl-D-aspartate (NMDA) glutamate receptor. Advances in treatment have emerged from exploration of alternative (non-dopaminergic) mechanisms for psychosis and from experience with atypical antipsychotic agents such as clozapine. *The newer atypical antipsychotics potently antagonize the $5HT_2$ receptor, while blocking D_2 receptors less potently than older typical antipsychotic agents, resulting in antipsychotic efficacy with limited extrapyramidal side effects.* Promising medications target glutamate and $5HT_7$ receptor subtypes, receptors for γ-aminobutyric acid (GABA) and acetylcholine (both muscarinic and nicotinic), and peptide hormone receptors (e.g., oxytocin).

PHARMACOTHERAPY

The 12th edition of the parent text reviews the relevant pathophysiology and the general goals of pharmacotherapy of psychosis and mania. Regardless of the underlying pathology, the immediate goal of antipsychotic treatment is a decrease in the acute symptoms that induce patient distress, particularly behavioral symptoms (e.g., hostility, agitation) that may present a danger to the patient or others. The dosing, route of administration, and choice of antipsychotic depend on the underlying disease state, clinical acuity, drug-drug interactions with concomitant medications, and patient sensitivity to short- or long-term adverse effects. With the exception of clozapine's superior efficacy in treatment-refractory schizophrenia, neither the clinical presentation nor biomarkers predict the likelihood of response to a specific antipsychotic class or agent. As a result, avoidance of adverse effects based upon patient and drug characteristics and exploitation of certain medication properties (e.g., sedation related to histamine H_1 or muscarinic antagonism) are the principal determinants for choosing initial antipsychotic therapy.

All commercially available antipsychotic drugs reduce dopaminergic neurotransmission (Figure 16–1). Chlorpromazine and other early low-potency typical antipsychotic agents are also profoundly sedating, a feature that used to be considered relevant to their therapeutic pharmacology. The development of the high-potency typical antipsychotic agent haloperidol, a drug with limited H_1 and M_1 affinity and significantly less sedative effect, demonstrate that sedation is not necessary for antipsychotic activity, although at times desirable.

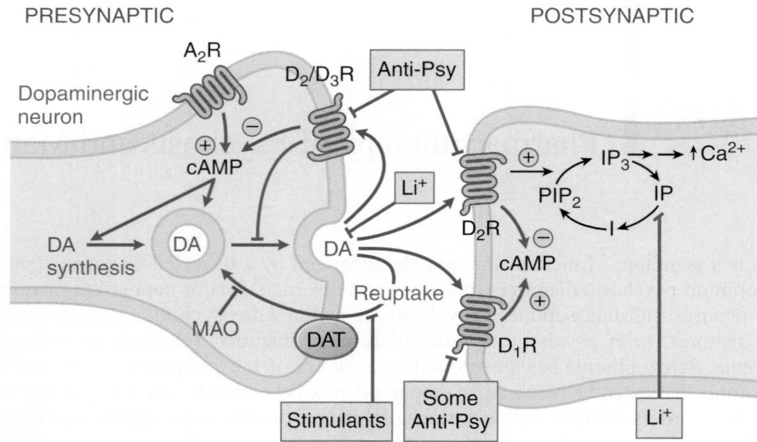

Figure 16–1 *Sites of action of antipsychotic agents and Li^+*. Following exocytotic release, DA interacts with both postsynaptic receptors and presynaptic autoreceptors. Termination of DA action occurs primarily by reuptake into presynaptic terminals via the DA transporter DAT, with secondary deamination by mitochondrial monoamine oxidase (MAO). Stimulation of postsynaptic D_1 receptors activates the G_s-adenylyl cyclase-cAMP pathway. D_2 receptors couple through G_i to inhibit adenylyl cyclase and through G_q to activate the PLC-IP_3-Ca^{2+} pathway. Activation of the G_i pathway can also activate K^+ channels, leading to hyperpolarization. Li^+ inhibits the phosphatase that liberates inositol (I) from inositol phosphate (IP). Li^+ can also inhibit depolarization-evoked release of DA and NE, but not 5HT. D_2-like autoreceptors suppress synthesis of DA by diminishing phosphorylation of rate-limiting tyrosine hydroxylase (TH), and by limiting DA release. In contrast, presynaptic A_2 adenosine receptors (A_2R) activate the AC-cAMP-PKA pathway, thereby enhancing TH activity. All antipsychotic agents act at D_2 receptors and autoreceptors; some also block D_1 receptors (*see* Table 16–2). Stimulant agents inhibit DA reuptake by DAT, thereby prolonging the dwell time of synaptic DA. Initially in antipsychotic treatment, DA neurons release more DA, but following repeated treatment, they enter a state of physiological depolarization inactivation, with diminished production and release of DA, in addition to continued receptor blockade. ——┤, inhibition or blockade; +, elevation of activity; –, reduction of activity.

SHORT-TERM TREATMENT

DELIRIUM AND DEMENTIA. Disease variables have considerable influence on selection of antipsychotic agents. Psychotic symptoms of delirium or dementia are generally treated with low medication doses, although doses may have to be repeated at frequent intervals initially to achieve adequate behavioral control. Despite widespread clinical use, not a single antipsychotic drug has received approval for dementia-related psychosis. Moreover, all antipsychotic drugs carry warnings that they may increase mortality in this setting. Because anticholinergic drug effects may worsen delirium and dementia, high-potency typical antipsychotic drugs (e.g., haloperidol) or atypical antipsychotic agents with limited antimuscarinic properties (e.g., risperidone) are often the drugs of choice.

The best tolerated doses in dementia patients are one-fourth of adult schizophrenia doses. Extrapyramidal neurological symptoms (EPSs), orthostasis, and sedation are particularly problematic in this patient population (*see* Chapter 22). Significant antipsychotic benefits are usually seen in acute psychosis within 60-120 min after drug administration. Oral dissolving tablet (ODT) preparations for risperidone, aripiprazole, and olanzapine, or liquid concentrate forms of risperidone or aripiprazole, are options for some patients. The dissolving tablets adhere to any moist tongue or oral surface, cannot be spit out, and are then swallowed along with oral secretions. Intramuscular (IM) administration of ziprasidone, aripiprazole, or olanzapine represents an option for treating agitated and minimally cooperative patients, and presents less risk for drug-induced parkinsonism than haloperidol. QT_c prolongation associated with intramuscular droperidol and intravenous administration of haloperidol have curtailed use of those particular formulations.

MANIA. All atypical antipsychotic agents with the exception of clozapine and iloperidone have indications for acute mania, and doses are titrated rapidly to the maximum recommended dose over the first 24-72 h of treatment. Acute mania patients with psychosis require very high daily

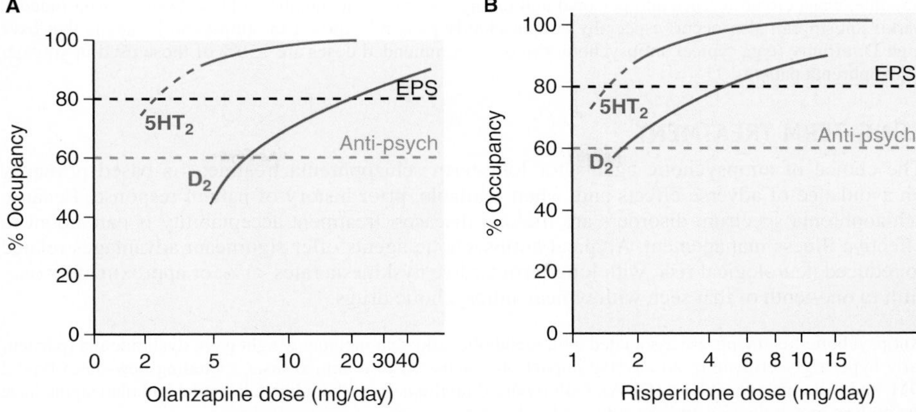

Figure 16–2 *Receptor occupancy and clinical response for antipsychotic agents.* Typically, D_2 receptor occupancy by the drug >60% provides antipsychotic effects; receptor occupancy >80% causes extrapyramidal symptoms (EPS). Atypical agents combine weak D_2 receptor blockade with more potent $5HT_{2A}$ antagonism/inverse agonism. Inverse agonism at $5HT_2$ receptor subtypes may contribute to the reduced EPS risk of olanzapine (Panel A) and risperidone (Panel B) and efficacy at lower D_2 receptor occupancy (olanzapine, Panel A). Aripiprazole is a partial D_2 agonist that can achieve only 75% functional blockade.

doses. Clinical response (decreased psychomotor agitation and irritability, increased sleep, and reduced or absent delusions and hallucinations) usually occurs within 7 days. Patients with mania may need to continue on antipsychotic treatment for many months after the resolution of psychotic and manic symptoms, typically in combination with a mood stabilizer such as lithium or valproic acid preparations. Combining an antipsychotic agent with a mood stabilizer often improves control of manic symptoms, and further reduces the risk of relapse. Weight gain from the additive effects of antipsychotic agents and mood stabilizers (lithium, valproic acid) presents a significant clinical problem.

MAJOR DEPRESSION. Patients with major depressive disorder with psychotic features require lower than average doses of antipsychotic drugs, given in combination with an antidepressant. Most antipsychotic drugs show limited antidepressant benefit as monotherapy agents. However, atypical antipsychotic agents are efficacious as adjunct therapy in treatment-resistant depression. Their clinical efficacy may be related to the fact that almost all atypical antipsychotic medications are potent $5HT_{2A}$ antagonists (Figure 16–2).

$5HT_{2A}$ and $5HT_{2C}$ antagonism facilitates DA release and increases noradrenergic outflow from the locus coeruleus. Administration of $5HT_{2A}$ and $5HT_{2C}$ antagonists in the form of low doses of atypical antipsychotic agents, along with selective serotonin reuptake inhibitors (SSRIs), increases responses rates in SSRI nonresponders. A combination preparation of low-dose olanzapine and fluoxetine is approved for bipolar depression, and low-dose risperidone (i.e., 1 mg) increases clinical response rates when added to existing SSRI treatment in SSRI nonresponders. Aripiprazole is FDA-approved for adjunctive use in antidepressant nonresponders, again at low doses (2-15 mg). Aripiprazole and most other antipsychotic drugs are ineffective as monotherapy for bipolar depression, with quetiapine being the sole exception.

SCHIZOPHRENIA. Newer, atypical antipsychotic agents offer a better neurological side-effect profile than typical antipsychotic drugs. Atypical agents show markedly reduced EPS risk compared to typical antipsychotic agents. Excessive D_2 blockade increases risk for motor neurological effects (e.g., muscular rigidity, bradykinesia, tremor, akathisia), slows mentation (bradyphrenia), and interferes with central reward pathways, resulting in patient complaints of anhedonia. In acute psychosis, sedation may be desirable, but the use of a sedating antipsychotic drug may interfere with a patient's cognitive function and social reintegration.

Schizophrenia patients have a 2-fold higher prevalence of metabolic syndrome and type 2 diabetes mellitus (DM) and twice the rate of cardiovascular (CV) related mortality than the general population. Consensus guidelines recommend baseline determination of serum glucose, lipids, weight, blood pressure, and when possible, waist circumference and personal and family histories of metabolic and CV disease. Drug-induced parkinsonism can also occur, especially among elderly patients exposed to antipsychotic agents that have high D_2 affinity (e.g., typical antipsychotic drugs); recommended doses are ~50% of those used in younger schizophrenia patients.

LONG-TERM TREATMENT

The choice of antipsychotic agents for long-term schizophrenia treatment is based primarily on avoidance of adverse effects and, when available, prior history of patient response. Because schizophrenia spectrum disorders are lifelong diseases, treatment acceptability is paramount to effective illness management. Atypical antipsychotic agents offer significant advantages related to reduced neurological risk, with long-term tardive dyskinesia rates <1%, or approximately one-fifth to one-tenth of that seen with typical antipsychotic drugs.

Antipsychotic treatments are associated with metabolic risks that include: weight gain, dyslipidemia (particularly hypertriglyceridemia), an adverse impact on glucose-insulin homeostasis, including new-onset type 2 DM, and diabetic ketoacidosis (DKA), with reported fatalities from the latter. Clozapine and olanzapine have the highest metabolic risk and are only used as last resort.

Acutely psychotic patients usually respond within hours after drug administration, but weeks may be required to achieve maximal drug response, especially for negative symptoms. Usual dosages for acute and maintenance treatment are noted in Table 16–1. Treatment-limiting adverse effects may include weight gain, sedation, orthostasis, and EPS, which to some degree can be predicted based on the potencies of the selected agent to inhibit neurotransmitter receptors (Table 16–2). The detection of dyslipidemia or hyperglycemia is based on laboratory monitoring (*see* Table 16–1). Certain adverse effects such as hyperprolactinemia, EPS, orthostasis, and sedation may respond to dose reduction, but metabolic abnormalities improve only with discontinuation of the drug and switching to a more metabolically benign medication. Patients with refractory schizophrenia on clozapine are not good candidates for switching because they are resistant to other medications (*see* the definition of refractory schizophrenia below).

The common problem of medication nonadherence among schizophrenia patients has led to the development of long-acting injectable (LAI) antipsychotic medications, often referred to as *depot antipsychotics*. There are currently 4 available LAI forms in the U.S.: decanoate esters of fluphenazine and haloperidol, risperidone-impregnated microspheres, and paliperidone palmitate. Patients receiving LAI antipsychotic medications show consistently lower relapse rates compared to patients receiving comparable oral forms and may suffer fewer adverse effects.

Lack of response to adequate antipsychotic drug doses for adequate periods of time may indicate treatment-refractory illness. Refractory schizophrenia is defined using the Kane criteria: failed 6-week trials of 2 separate agents and a third trial of a high-dose typical antipsychotic agent (e.g., haloperidol or fluphenazine 20 mg/day). In this patient population, response rates to typical antipsychotic agents, defined as 20% symptom reduction using standard rating scales (e.g., Positive and Negative Syndrome Scale [PANSS]), are 0%, and for any atypical antipsychotic except clozapine, are <10%. The therapeutic clozapine dose for a specific patient is not predictable, but various studies have found correlations between trough serum clozapine levels >327-504 ng/mL and likelihood of clinical response. When therapeutic serum concentrations are reached, response to clozapine occurs within 8 weeks.

Clozapine has numerous other adverse effects. These include agranulocytosis risk that mandates routine ongoing hematological monitoring, high metabolic risk, dose-dependent lowering of the seizure threshold, orthostasis, sedation, anticholinergic effects (especially constipation), and sialorrhea related to muscarinic agonism at M_4 receptors. As a result, clozapine use is limited to refractory schizophrenia patients. Electroconvulsive therapy is considered a treatment of last resort in refractory schizophrenia and is rarely employed.

PHARMACOLOGY OF ANTIPSYCHOTIC AGENTS

Tables 16–1 and 16–2 summarize the drug classes, dose ranges, severity metabolic side effects, and potencies at important CNS receptors for a variety of antipsychotic agents.

The introduction of clozapine stimulated research into agents with antipsychotic activity and low EPS risk. This search led to a series of atypical antipsychotic agents with certain pharmacological similarities to clozapine: namely lower affinity for D_2 receptors than typical antipsychotic drugs and high $5HT_2$ antagonist effects. Currently available atypical antipsychotic medications include the structurally related olanzapine, quetiapine, and clozapine; risperidone, its active metabolite paliperidone, and iloperidone; ziprasidone; lurasidone; asenapine, and aripiprazole (*see* Table 16–1).

Table 16–1

Drugs for Psychosis and Schizophrenia: Dosing and Metabolic Risk Profile[a]

GENERIC NAME **Dosage Forms**	ORAL DOSAGE (mg/day) ACUTE PSYCHOSIS 1ST Episode	Chronic	MAINTENANCE 1ST Episode	Chronic	METABOLIC SIDE EFFECTS ↑Weight	Lipids	Glucose
Phenothiazines							
Chlorpromazine ***O, S, IM***	200-600	400-800	150-600	250-750	+++	+++	++
Perphenazine ***O, S, IM***	12-50	24-48	12-48	24-60	+/–	–	–
Trifluoperazine ***O, S, IM***	5-30	10-40	2.5-20	10-30	+/–	–	–
Fluphenazine ***O, S, IM***	2.5-15	5-20	2.5-10	5-15	+/–	–	–
decanoate ***Depot IM***	Not for acute use		5-75 mg/2 wks		+/–	–	–
Other Typical Agents							
Molindone ***O, S***	15-50	30-60	15-50	30-60	–	–	–
Loxapine ***O, S, IM***	15-50	30-60	15-50	30-60	+	–	–
Haloperidol ***O, S, IM***	2.5-10	5-20	2.5-10	5-15	+/–	–	–
decanoate ***Depot IM***	Not for acute use		100-300 mg/month		+/–	–	–
Atypical Antipsychotic Agents							
Aripiprazole ***O, S, ODT, IM***	10-20	15-30	10-20	15-30	+/–	–	–
Asenapine ***ODT***	10	10-20	10	10-20	+/–	–	–
Clozapine ***O, ODT***	200-600	400-900	200-600	300-900	++++	+++	+++
Iloperidone ***O***		12-24[b]		8-16	+	+/–	+/–
Olanzapine ***O, ODT, IM***	7.5-20	10-30	7.5-15	15-30	++++	+++	+++
Paliperidone ***O***	6-9	6-12	3-9	6-15	+	+/–	+/–
palmitate ***Depot IM***[c]	See note[c] on dosing				+	+/–	+/–
Quetiapine ***O***	200-600	400-900	200-600	300-900	+	+	+/–
Risperidone ***O, S, ODT***	2-4	3-6	2-6	3-8	+	+/–	+/–
RISPERDAL CONSTA ***Depot IM***	Not for acute use		25-50 mg/2 wks				
Sertindole ***O***[d]	4-16	12-20	12-20	12-32	+/–	–	–
Ziprasidone ***O, IM***[e]	120-160	120-200	80-160	120-200	+/–	–	–

Dosage Forms: *O, tablet; S, solution; IM, acute intramuscular; ODT, orally dissolving tablet.*

[a]*For further information, see optimizing pharmacologic treatment of psychotic disorders.* J Clin Psychiatry, ***2003***, 64(Suppl 12):*2–97.*

Doses in first-episode, younger, or antipsychotic-naïve patients are lower than for chronic schizophrenia patients. Dose in elderly patients is ~50% of that used in younger adults; dosing for dementia-related psychosis is ~25%.

[b]*Due to orthostasis risk, dose titration of iloperidone is 1 mg 2× daily on day 1, increasing to 2, 4, 6, 8, 10, and 12 mg 2× daily on days 2–7 (as needed).*

[c]*In acute schizophrenia, deltoid IM loading doses of 234 mg at day 1 and 156 mg at day 8 provide paliperidone levels equivalent to 6 mg oral paliperidone during the first week, and peaking on day 15 at a level comparable to 12 mg oral paliperidone. No oral antipsychotic needed in first week. Maintenance IM doses can be given every 4 weeks after day 8. Maintenance dose options: 39 to 234 mg every 4 weeks. Failure to give initiation doses (except for those switching from depot) will result in subtherapeutic levels for months.*

[d]*Not available in the U.S.*

[e]*Oral dose must be given with food to facilitate absorption.*

MECHANISM OF ACTION. All clinically available antipsychotics are antagonists at dopamine D_2 receptors. This reduction in dopaminergic neurotransmission is achieved through D_2 antagonism or partial D_2 agonism (e.g., aripiprazole).

Aripiprazole has an affinity for D_2 receptors only slightly less than DA itself, but its intrinsic activity is ~25% that of DA. That is, when DA is incubated with increasing concentrations of aripiprazole, maximal inhibition

Table 16–2

Potencies of Antipsychotic Agents at Neurotransmitter Receptors[a]

	DOPAMINE	SEROTONIN			$5HT_{2A}/D_2$	DOPAMINE		MUSCARINIC	ADRENERGIC		HISTAMINE
	D_2	$5HT_{1A}$	$5HT_{2A}$	$5HT_{2C}$	RATIO	D_1	D_4	M_1	α_{1A}	α_{2A}	H_1
Typical Agents											
Haloperidol	1.2	2100	57	4500	47	120	5.5	>10,000	12	1130	1700
Fluphenazine	0.8	1000	3.2	990	3.9	17	29	1100	6.5	310	14
Thiothixene	0.7	410	50	1360	72	51	410	>10,000	12	80	8
Perphenazine	0.8	420	5.6	130	7.4	37	40	1500	10	810	8.0
Loxapine	11	2550	4.4	13	0.4	54	8.1	120	42	150	4.9
Molindone	20	3800	>5000	10,000	>250	>10,000	>2000	>10,000	2600	1100	2130
Thioridazine	8.0	140	28	53	3.5	94	6.4	13	3.2	130	16
Chlorpromazine	3.6	2120	3.6	16	1	76	12	32	0.3	250	3.1
Atypical Agents											
Asenapine[b]	1.4	2.7	0.1	0.03	0.05	1.4	1.1	>10,000	1.2	1.2	1.0
Ziprasidone	6.8	12	0.6	13	0.1	30	39	>10,000	18	160	63
Sertindole[b]	2.7	280	0.4	0.90	0.2	12	13	>5000	1.8	640	130
Zotepine[b]	8.0	470	2.7	3.2	0.3	71	39	330	6.0	210	3.2
Risperidone	3.2	420	0.2	50	0.05	240	7.3	>10,000	5.0	16	20
Paliperidone	4.2	20	0.7	48	0.2	41	54	>10,000	2.5	4.7	19
Iloperidone	6.3	90	5.6	43	0.9	130	25	4900	0.3	160	12
Aripiprazole	1.6	6.0	8.7	22	5.0	1200	510	6800	26	74	28
Sulpiride[b]	6.4	>10,000	>10,000	>10,000	>1000	>10,000	54	>10,000	>10000	>5000	>10,000
Olanzapine	31	2300	3.7	10	0.1	70	18	2.5	110	310	2.2
Quetiapine	380	390	640	1840	2.0	990	2020	37	22	2900	6.9
Clozapine	160	120	5.4	9.4	0.03	270	24	6.2	1.6	90	1.1

[a]Data are averaged K_i values (nM) from published sources determined by competition with radioligands for binding to the indicated cloned human receptors. Data derived from receptor binding to human or rat brain tissue is used when cloned human receptor data is lacking.

[b]Not available in the U.S.

Source: NIMH Psychoactive Drug Screening Program (PDSP) K_i Database: http://pdsp.med.unc.edu/pdsp.php (Accessed June 30, 2009).

of D_2 activity do not exceed 25% of the DA response, the level of agonism provided by aripiprazole. Aripiprazole's capacity to stimulate D_2 receptors in brain areas where synaptic DA levels are limited (e.g., PFC neurons) or decrease dopaminergic activity when DA concentrations are high (e.g., mesolimbic cortex) is thought to be the basis for its clinical effects in schizophrenia. Even with 100% receptor occupancy, aripiprazole's intrinsic dopaminergic agonism can generate a 25% postsynaptic signal, implying a maximal 75% reduction in DA neurotransmission, below the 78% threshold that triggers EPS in most individuals.

The pharmacological basis for the clinical efficacy atypical antipsychotics without EPS induction results from a significantly weaker D_2 antagonism, combined with potent $5HT_2$ antagonism. Clozapine possesses activity at other receptors including antagonism and agonism at various muscarinic receptor subtypes and antagonism at dopamine D_4 receptors. However D_4 antagonists that do not have D_2 antagonism lack antipsychotic activity. Clozapine's active metabolite, *N*-desmethylclozapine, is a potent muscarinic M_1 agonist.

The glutamate hypofunction hypothesis of schizophrenia has led to novel animal models that examine the influence of antipsychotic agents with agonist properties at metabotropic glutamate receptors $mGlu_2$ and $mGlu_3$ and other subtypes. Atypical antipsychotic drugs are better than typical antipsychotic medications at reversing the negative symptoms, cognitive deficits and social withdrawal induced by glutamate antagonists.

DOPAMINE RECEPTOR OCCUPANCY AND BEHAVIORAL EFFECTS. Excessive dopaminergic functions in the limbic system are central to the positive symptoms of psychosis. The behavioral effects and the time course of antipsychotic response parallel the rise in D_2 occupancy and include calming of psychomotor agitation, decreased hostility, decreased social isolation, and less interference from disorganized or delusional thought processes and hallucinations. Occupation of >78% of D_2 receptors in the basal ganglia is associated with a risk of EPS across all DA antagonist antipsychotic agents, while occupancies in the range of 60-75% are associated with antipsychotic efficacy (*see* Figure 16–2). With the exception of aripiprazole, all atypical antipsychotic drugs at low doses have much greater occupancy of $5HT_{2A}$ receptors (e.g., 75-99%) than typical agents (*see* Table 16–2).

D_3 and D_4 Receptors in the Basal Ganglia and Limbic System. D_3 and D_4 receptors are preferentially expressed in limbic areas. The D_4 receptors, which are preferentially localized in cortical and limbic brain regions in low abundance, are upregulated after repeated administration of most typical and atypical antipsychotic drugs. These receptors may contribute to clinical antipsychotic actions, but agents that are D_4 selective (e.g., sonepiprazole) or mixed $D_4/5HT_{2A}$ antagonists (e.g., fananserin) lack antipsychotic efficacy in clinical studies.

D_3 receptors are unlikely to play a pivotal role in antipsychotic drug actions. The subtle and atypical functional activities of cerebral D_3 receptors suggest that D_3 agonists rather than antagonists may have useful psychotropic effects, particularly in antagonizing stimulant-reward and dependence behaviors.

The Role of Non-Dopamine Receptors for Atypical Antipsychotic Agents. The concept of atypicality was initially based on clozapine's absence of EPS within the therapeutic range, combined with a prominent role of $5HT_2$ receptor antagonism. As subsequent agents were synthesized using clozapine's $5HT_2/D_2$ ratio as a model, most of which possessed greater D_2 affinity and EPS risk than clozapine, there has been considerable debate on the definition of an atypical antipsychotic agent and its necessary properties. Nonetheless, the term "atypical" persists in common usage and designates lesser (but not absent) EPS risk and other decreased effects of excessive D_2 antagonism.

Antipsychotic agents with appreciable $5HT_2$ affinity have significant effects at both $5HT_{2A}$ and $5HT_{2C}$ receptors with individual medications varying in their relative potencies at each subtype. As discussed previously, atypical antipsychotic agents exhibit potent functional antagonism at both subtypes of $5HT_2$ receptors, but in vitro assays suggest that these effects result from inverse agonism at these G-coupled receptors.

TOLERANCE AND PHYSICAL DEPENDENCE. As defined in Chapter 24, antipsychotic drugs are not addicting; however, tolerance to the antihistaminic and anticholinergic effects of antipsychotic agents usually develops over days or weeks.

ABSORPTION, DISTRIBUTION, AND ELIMINATION. Most antipsychotic drugs are highly lipophilic, highly membrane- or protein-bound, and accumulate in the brain, lung, and other tissues with a rich blood supply. They also enter the fetal circulation and breast milk. Despite half-lives that may be short, the biological effects of single doses of most antipsychotic medications usually persist for at least 24 h, permitting once-daily dosing for many agents once the patient has adjusted to initial side effects.

Absorption for most agents is quite high, and concurrent administration of anticholinergic anti-parkinsonian agents does not appreciably diminish intestinal absorption. Most ODTs and liquid preparations provide similar pharmacokinetics. Asenapine remains the only exception; it is available only as an ODT preparation administered sublingually, and all absorption occurs via oral mucosa, with bioavailability of 35% by this route. If asenapine is swallowed, the first pass effect is >98%, indicating that drug swallowed with oral secretions is not bioavailable. IM administration avoids much of the first-pass enteric metabolism and provides measurable concentrations in plasma within 15-30 min. Most agents are highly protein bound, but this protein binding may include glycoprotein sites. Antipsychotic medications are predominantly highly lipophilic with apparent volumes of distribution as high as 20 L/kg.

Elimination from the plasma may be more rapid than from sites of high lipid content and binding, notably the CNS. Slow removal of drug may contribute to the typical delay of exacerbation of psychosis after stopping drug treatment. Depot decanoate esters of fluphenazine and haloperidol, paliperidone palmitate, as well as risperidone-impregnated microspheres, are absorbed and eliminated much more slowly than are oral preparations. For example, the $t_{1/2}$ of oral fluphenazine is ~20 h, while the IM decanoate ester has a $t_{1/2}$ of 14.3 days; oral haloperidol has a $t_{1/2}$ of 24-48 h in CYP2D6-extensive metabolizers, while haloperidol decanoate has a $t_{1/2}$ of 21 days; paliperidone palmitate has a $t_{1/2}$ of 25-49 days compared to an oral paliperidone $t_{1/2}$ of 23 h. Clearance of fluphenazine and haloperidol decanoate following repeated dosing can require 6-8 months. Effects of LAI *risperidone* (RISPERDAL CONSTA) are delayed for 4 weeks because of slow biodegradation of the microspheres and persist for at least 4-6 weeks after the injections are discontinued. The dosing regimen recommended for starting patients on LAI paliperidone generates therapeutic levels in the first week, obviating the need for routine oral antipsychotic supplementation.

With the exception of asenapine, paliperidone, and ziprasidone, all antipsychotic drugs undergo extensive phase I metabolism by CYPs and subsequent phase II glucuronidation, sulfation, and other conjugations. Hydrophilic metabolites of these drugs are excreted in the urine and to some extent in the bile. Most oxidized metabolites of antipsychotic drugs are biologically inactive; a few (e.g., P88 metabolite of iloperidone, hydroxy metabolite of haloperidol, 9-OH risperidone, *N*-desmethylclozapine, and dehydroaripiprazole) are active. These active metabolites may contribute to biological activity of the parent compound and complicate correlating serum drug levels with clinical effects. Table 16–3 in the 12th edition of the parent text outlines the metabolic pathways of selected agents in common use.

THERAPEUTIC USES

Antipsychotic agents are also used in several nonpsychotic neurological disorders and as antiemetics.

ANXIETY DISORDERS. Adjunctive treatments with antipsychotic drugs are beneficial in obsessive-compulsive disorder (OCD) and posttraumatic stress disorder (PTSD). Adjunctive low-dose quetiapine, olanzapine, and particularly risperidone significantly reduce the overall level of symptoms in SSRI-resistant PTSD, and OCD patients with limited response to the standard 12-week regimen of high-dose SSRI also benefit from adjunctive risperidone (mean dose 2.2 mg), even in the presence of comorbid tic disorders. For generalized anxiety disorder, double-blind placebo-controlled clinical trials demonstrate efficacy for quetiapine as monotherapy, and for adjunctive low-dose risperidone.

TOURETTE DISORDER. The ability of antipsychotic drugs to suppress tics in patients with Tourette disorder relates to reduced D_2 neurotransmission in basal ganglia sites. While lacking FDA approval for tic disorders, risperidone and aripiprazole have indications for child and adolescent schizophrenia and bipolar disorder (acute mania) treatment, and these agents (as well as ziprasidone) have published data supporting their use for tic suppression.

HUNTINGTON DISEASE. Huntington disease is associated with basal ganglia pathology. DA blockade can suppress the severity of choreoathetotic movements, but is not strongly endorsed due to the risks associated of excessive DA antagonism that outweigh the marginal benefit. Inhibition of the vesicular monoamine transporter type 2 (VMAT2) with tetrabenazine has replaced DA receptor blockade in the management of chorea (*see* Chapter 22).

AUTISM. Risperidone has FDA approval for irritability associated with autism in child and adolescent patients ages 5-16, with common use for disruptive behavior problems in autism and other forms of mental retardation. Initial risperidone daily doses are 0.25 mg for patients weighing <20 kg, and 0.5 mg for others, with a target dose of 0.5 mg/day in those <20 kg weight, and 1.0 mg/day for other patients, with a range 0.5-3.0 mg/day.

Table 16–3

Neurological Side Effects of Antipsychotic Drugs

REACTION	FEATURES	TIME OF ONSET AND RISK INFO	PROPOSED MECHANISM	TREATMENT
Acute dystonia	Spasm of muscles of tongue, face, neck, back	Time: 1-5 days. Young, antipsychotic naïve patients at highest risk	Acute DA antagonism	Anti-parkinsonian agents are diagnostic and curative[a]
Akathisia	Subjective and objective restlessness; *not* anxiety or "agitation"	Time: 5-60 days	Unknown	Reduce dose or change drug; clonazepam, propranolol more effective than anti-parkinsonian agents[b]
Parkinsonism	Bradykinesia, rigidity, variable tremor, mask facies, shuffling gait	Time: 5-30 days. Elderly at greatest risk	DA antagonism	Dose reduction; change medication; anti-parkinsonian agents[c]
Neuroleptic malignant syndrome	Extreme rigidity, fever, unstable BP, myoglobinemia; can be fatal	Time: weeks–months. Can persist for days after stopping antipsychotic	DA antagonism	Stop antipsychotic immediately; supportive care; dantrolene and bromocriptine[d]
Perioral tremor ("rabbit syndrome")	Perioral tremor (may be a late variant of parkinsonism)	Time: months or years of treatment	Unknown	Anti-parkinsonian agents often help[c]
Tardive dyskinesia	Orofacial dyskinesia; rarely widespread choreoathetosis or dystonia	Time: months, years of treatment. Elderly at 5-fold greater risk. Risk ∝ potency of D_2 blockade	Postsynaptic DA receptor supersensitivity, upregulation	Prevention crucial; treatment unsatisfactory. May be reversible with early recognition and drug discontinuation

[a]Treatment: diphenhydramine 25-50 mg IM, or benztropine 1-2 mg IM. Due to long antipsychotic $t_{1/2}$, may need to repeat, or follow with oral medication.
[b]Propranolol often effective in relatively low doses (20-80 mg/day in divided doses). β_1 Selective adrenergic receptor antagonists are less effective. Non-lipophilic β adrenergic antagonists have limited CNS penetration and are of no benefit (e.g., atenolol).
[c]Use of amantadine avoids anticholinergic effects of benztropine or diphenhydramine.
[d]Despite the response to dantrolene, there is no evidence of abnormal Ca^{2+} transport in skeletal muscle; with persistent antipsychotic effects (e.g., long-acting injectable agents), bromocriptine may be tolerated in large doses (10-40 mg/day). Anti-parkinsonian agents are not effective.

ANTIEMETIC USE. Most antipsychotic drugs protect against the nausea- and emesis-inducing effects of DA agonists. Drugs or other stimuli that cause emesis by an action on the nodose ganglion, or locally on the GI tract, are not antagonized by antipsychotic drugs, but potent piperazines and butyrophenones are sometimes effective against nausea caused by vestibular stimulation. The commonly used antiemetic phenothiazines are weak DA antagonists (e.g., prochlorperazine) without antipsychotic activity, but can be associated with EPS or akathisia.

ADVERSE EFFECTS PREDICTED BY MONOAMINE RECEPTOR AFFINITIES (*SEE* TABLE 16–2)

Dopamine D_2 Receptor. With the exception of the D_2 partial agonist aripiprazole, all other antipsychotic agents possess D_2 antagonist properties, the strength of which determines the likelihood for EPS, akathisia, long-term tardive dyskinesia risk, and hyperprolactinemia. The manifestations of EPS are described in Table 16–3, along with the usual treatment approach. Acute dystonic reactions occur in the early hours and days of treatment with highest risk among younger patients (peak incidence ages 10-19), especially antipsychotic drug-naïve individuals, in response to abrupt decreases in nigrostriatal D_2 neurotransmission. The dystonia typically involves head and neck muscles, the tongue, and in its severest form, the oculogyric crisis, extraocular muscles, and is very frightening to the patient.

Parkinsonism resembling its idiopathic form occurs when striatal D_2 occupancy exceeds 78%. Clinically, there is a generalized slowing and impoverishment of volitional movement (bradykinesia) with masked facies and reduced arm movements during walking. The syndrome characteristically evolves gradually over days to weeks as the risk of acute dystonia diminishes. The treatment of acute dystonia and antipsychotic-induced parkinsonism involves the use of antiparkinsonian agents, although dose reduction should be considered as the initial strategy for parkinsonism. Muscarinic cholinergic receptors modulate nigrostriatal DA release, with blockade increasing synaptic DA availability. Important issues in the use of anticholinergics include the negative impact on cognition and memory, peripheral antimuscarinic adverse effects (e.g., urinary retention, dry mouth, cycloplegia, etc.), and the relative risk of exacerbating tardive dyskinesia.

Amantadine (SYMMETREL), originally marketed as an antiviral agent toward influenza A, represents the most commonly used nonanticholinergic medication for antipsychotic-induced parkinsonism. Its mechanism of action is unclear but appears to involve presynaptic DA reuptake blockade, facilitation of DA release, postsynaptic DA agonism, and receptor modulation.

Tardive dyskinesia is a situation of increased nigrostriatal dopaminergic activity as the result of postsynaptic receptor supersensitivity and upregulation from chronically high levels of postsynaptic D_2 blockade (and possible direct toxic effects of high-potency DA antagonists). Tardive dyskinesia is characterized by stereotyped, repetitive, painless, involuntary, quick choreiform (tic-like) movements of the face, eyelids (blinks or spasm), mouth (grimaces), tongue, extremities, or trunk. The dyskinetic movements can be suppressed partially by use of a potent DA antagonist, but such interventions over time may worsen the severity. Switching patients from potent D_2 antagonists to weaker agents, especially clozapine has at times proven effective. When possible, drug discontinuation may be beneficial, but usually cannot be offered to schizophrenia patients.

Akathisia is seen quite commonly during treatment with high doses of high potency typical antipsychotic drugs, but also can be seen with atypical agents, including those with weak D_2 affinities (e.g., quetiapine), and aripiprazole. Despite the association with D_2 blockade, akathisia does not have a robust response to antiparkinsonian drugs, so other treatment strategies must be employed, including the use of high-potency benzodiazepines (e.g., clonazepam), nonselective β-blockers with good CNS penetration (e.g., propranolol), and also dose reduction, or switching to another antipsychotic agent. That clonazepam and propranolol have significant cortical activity and are ineffective for other forms of EPS, points to an extrastriatal origin for akathisia symptoms.

The rare neuroleptic malignant syndrome (NMS) resembles a very severe form of parkinsonism, with signs of autonomic instability (hyperthermia and labile pulse, blood pressure, and respiration rate), stupor, elevation of creatine kinase in serum, and sometimes myoglobinemia with potential nephrotoxicity. The prevalence of this reaction is greater when relatively high doses of potent agents are used, especially when they are administered parenterally.

Hyperprolactinemia results from blockade of the pituitary actions of the tuberoinfundibular dopaminergic neurons that deliver DA to the anterior pituitary. D_2 receptors on lactotropes in the anterior pituitary mediate the tonic prolactin-inhibiting action of DA. Correlations between the D_2 potency of antipsychotic drugs and prolactin elevations are excellent. With the exception of risperidone and paliperidone, atypical antipsychotic agents show limited (asenapine, iloperidone, olanzapine, quetiapine, ziprasidone) to almost no effects (clozapine, aripiprazole) on prolactin secretion.

H_1 Receptors. Central antagonism of H_1 receptors is associated with 2 major adverse effects: sedation and weight gain via appetite stimulation. Examples of sedating antipsychotic drugs include low-potency typical agents such as chlorpromazine and thioridazine, and the atypical agents clozapine and quetiapine. The sedating effect is easily predicted by their high H_1 receptor affinities (*see* Table 16–2). Some tolerance to the sedative properties will develop.

M_1 Receptors. Muscarinic antagonism is responsible for the central and peripheral anticholinergic effects of medications. Most of the atypical antipsychotic drugs have no muscarinic affinity and no appreciable anticholinergic effects, while clozapine and low-potency phenothiazines have significant anticholinergic adverse effects (*see* Table 16–2). Quetiapine has modest muscarinic affinity, but its active metabolite norquetiapine is likely responsible for anticholinergic complaints. Clozapine is particularly associated with significant constipation. Routine use of stool softeners, and repeated inquiry into bowel habits are necessary to prevent serious intestinal obstruction from undetected constipation. Medications with significant anticholinergic properties should be particularly avoided in elderly patients, especially those with dementia or delirium.

***α_1* Receptors.** α_1 Adrenergic antagonism is associated with risk of orthostatic hypotension and can be particularly problematic for elderly patients who have poor vasomotor tone. Compared to high-potency typical agents, low-potency typical agents have significantly greater affinities for α_1 receptors and greater risk for orthostasis. While risperidone has a K_i that indicates greater α_1 adrenergic affinity than chlorpromazine, thioridazine, clozapine, and quetiapine, in clinical practice risperidone is used at 0.01-0.005 times the dosages of these medications, and thus causes a relatively lower incidence of orthostasis in nonelderly patients. Since clozapine-treated patients have few other antipsychotic options, the potent mineralocorticoid fludrocortisone is sometimes tried at the dose of 0.1 mg/day as a volume expander.

ADVERSE EFFECTS NOT PREDICTED BY MONOAMINE RECEPTOR AFFINITIES

ADVERSE METABOLIC EFFECTS. Such effects have become the area of greatest concern during long-term antipsychotic treatment, paralleling the overall concern for high prevalence of prediabetic conditions and type 2 DM, and 2-fold greater CV mortality among patients with schizophrenia. Aside from weight gain, the 2 predominant metabolic adverse effects seen with antipsychotic drugs are dyslipidemia, primarily elevated serum triglycerides, and impairments in glycemic control.

Low-potency phenothiazines were known to elevate serum triglyceride values, but this effect was not seen with high-potency agents. As atypical antipsychotic drugs became more widely used, significant increases in fasting triglyceride levels were noted during clozapine and olanzapine exposure, and to a lesser extent, with quetiapine. Mean increases during chronic treatment of 50-100 mg/dL are common, with serum triglyceride levels exceeding 7000 mg/dL in some patients. Effects on total cholesterol and cholesterol fractions are significantly less, but show expected associations related to agents of highest risk: clozapine, olanzapine, and quetiapine. Risperidone and paliperidone have fewer effects on serum lipids, while asenapine, iloperidone, aripiprazole, and ziprasidone appear to have none. Weight gain in general may induce deleterious lipid changes, but there is compelling evidence to indicate that antipsychotic-induced hypertriglyceridemia is a weight-independent adverse event that temporally occurs within weeks of starting an offending medication, and which similarly resolves within 6 weeks after medication discontinuation.

In individuals not exposed to antipsychotic drugs, elevated fasting triglycerides are a direct consequence of insulin resistance since insulin-dependent lipases in fat cells are normally inhibited by insulin. Elevated fasting triglyceride levels thus become a sensitive marker of insulin resistance, leading to the hypothesis that the triglyceride increases seen during antipsychotic treatment are the result of derangements in glucose-insulin homeostasis. Analysis of the FDA MedWatch database found that reversibility was high upon drug discontinuation (~78%) for olanzapine- and clozapine-associated diabetes and ketoacidosis, supporting the contention of a drug effect. Comparable rates for risperidone and quetiapine were significantly lower. The mechanism by which antipsychotic drugs disrupt glucose-insulin homeostasis is not known.

Antipsychotics increase risk for metabolic disorders among patients with schizophrenia, and the medication itself seems to be the primary modifiable risk factor. As a result, all atypical antipsychotic drugs have a hyperglycemia warning in the drug label in the U.S., although there is essentially no evidence that asenapine, iloperidone, aripiprazole, and ziprasidone cause hyperglycemia. Clinicians should obtain baseline metabolic data, including fasting glucose, lipid panel, and also waist circumference, given the known association between central obesity and future type 2 diabetes risk. Ongoing follow-up of metabolic parameters is commonly built into psychiatric charts and community mental health clinic procedures to insure that all patients receive some level of metabolic monitoring.

ADVERSE CARDIAC EFFECTS. Ventricular arrhythmias and sudden cardiac death (SCD) are a concern with the use of antipsychotic agents.

Most of the older antipsychotic agents (e.g., thioridazine) inhibit cardiac K^+ channels, and all antipsychotic medications marketed in the U.S. carry a class label warning regarding QTc prolongation. A black box warning exists for thioridazine, mesoridazine, pimozide, IM droperidol, and IV (but not oral or IM) haloperidol due to reported cases of torsade de pointes and subsequent fatal ventricular arrhythmias. Although the newer atypical agents are thought to have less effects on heart electrophysiology compared to the typical agents, a recent retrospective study found a dose-dependent increased risk for SCD among antipsychotic users of newer and older agents alike compared to antipsychotic nonusers, with a relative risk of 2.

Other Adverse Effects. Seizure risk is an unusual adverse effect of antipsychotic drugs. In the U.S., there is a class label warning for seizure risk on all antipsychotic agents, with reported incidences well below 1%. Among commonly used newer antipsychotic drugs, only clozapine has a dose-dependent seizure risk, with an incidence of 3-5% per year. Seizure disorder patients who commence antipsychotic treatment must receive adequate prophylaxis, with consideration given to avoiding carbamazepine and phenytoin due to their capacity to induce CYPs and P-glycoprotein. Carbamazepine is also contraindicated during clozapine treatment due to its bone marrow effects, particularly leukopenia. Redistribution and increased spacing of doses to minimize high peak serum clozapine levels can help, but patients may eventually require antiseizure medication. Valproic acid derivatives (e.g., divalproex sodium) are often used, but will compound clozapine-associated weight gain.

Clozapine possesses a host of unusual adverse effects aside from seizure induction, the most concerning of which is agranulocytosis. Clozapine's introduction in the U.S. was based on its efficacy in refractory schizophrenia, but came with FDA-mandated CBC monitoring that is overseen by industry-created registries. Now that several generic forms of clozapine are available in addition to proprietary CLOZARIL, clinicians must verify with each manufacturer the history of prior exposure. Increased risk is associated with certain HLA types and advanced age.

While rarely used due to its risk of QTc prolongation, thioridazine is also associated with pigmentary retinopathy at daily doses ≥800 mg/day. Low-potency phenothiazines are associated with the development of photosensitivity, which necessitated warnings regarding sun exposure. Phenothiazines are also associated with development of a cholestatic picture on laboratory assessments (e.g., elevated alkaline phosphatase), and rarely elevations in hepatic transaminases.

Increased Mortality in Dementia Patients. All antipsychotic agents carry a mortality warning in the drug label regarding their use in dementia patients. Mortality is due to heart failure, sudden death, or pneumonia. Overdose with typical antipsychotic agents is of particular concern with *low*-potency agents (e.g., chlorpromazine) due to the risk of torsade de pointes, sedation, anticholinergic effects, and orthostasis. Patients who overdose on *high*-potency typical antipsychotic drugs (e.g., haloperidol) and the substituted benzamides are at greater risk for EPS due to the high D_2 affinity, but also must be observed for ECG changes.

DRUG-DRUG INTERACTIONS. Antipsychotic agents are not significant inhibitors of CYP enzymes with a few notable exceptions (chlorpromazine, perphenazine, and thioridazine inhibit CYP 2D6). The plasma half-lives of a number of these agents are altered by induction or inhibition of hepatic CYPs and by genetic polymorphisms that alter specific CYP activities (Table 7–3; *see also* Table 16–3 in the parent text, 12th edition). Smoking causes upregulation in CYP1A2 activity, and changes in smoking status can be especially problematic for clozapine-treated patients and will alter serum levels by 50% or more.

USE IN PEDIATRIC POPULATIONS. Both risperidone and aripiprazole have indications for child and adolescent bipolar disorder (acute mania) for ages 10-17, and for adolescent schizophrenia (ages 13-17). Risperidone and aripiprazole are FDA-approved for irritability associated with autism in child and adolescent patients ages 5-16. Antipsychotic drug-naïve patients and younger patients are more susceptible to EPS and to weight gain. Use of the minimum effective dose can minimize EPS risk.

USE IN GERIATRIC POPULATIONS. The increased sensitivity to EPS, orthostasis, sedation, and anticholinergic effects are important issues for the geriatric population, and often dictate the choice of antipsychotic medication. Avoidance of drug-drug interactions is also important, as older patients on numerous concomitant medications have multiple opportunities for interactions. Elderly patients have an increased risk for tardive dyskinesia and parkinsonism. Increased risk for cerebrovascular events and all-cause mortality is also seen in elderly patients with dementia. Compared to younger patients, antipsychotic-induced weight gain is lower in elderly patients.

USE DURING PREGNANCY AND LACTATION. Antipsychotic agents carry pregnancy class B or C warnings. Human data indicate no patterns of toxicity and no consistent increased rates of malformations. Haloperidol is often cited as the agent with the best safety record based on decades of accumulated human exposure reports. Antipsychotic drugs are designed to cross the blood-brain barrier, and all have high rates of placental passage. *Use in lactation presents a separate set of concerns due to the low level of infant hepatic catabolic activity in the first 2 postpartum months. The inability of the newborn to adequately metabolize xenobiotics presents a significant risk for antipsychotic drug toxicity.*

TREATMENT OF MANIA

Mania is a period of elevated, expansive, or irritable mood with coexisting symptoms of increased energy and goal-directed activity, and decreased need for sleep. Mania represents 1 pole of what had been termed manic-depressive illness, but is now referred to as bipolar disorder. Mania may be induced by medications (e.g., DA agonists, antidepressants, stimulants) or substances of abuse, primarily cocaine and amphetamines, although periods of substance-induced mania should not be relied on solely to make a diagnosis of bipolar disorder.

Mania is distinguished from its less severe form, hypomania, by the fact that hypomania, by definition, does not result in functional impairment or hospitalization, and is not associated with psychotic symptoms. Patients who experience periods of hypomania and major depression have bipolar II disorder, those with mania at any time, bipolar I, and those with hypomania, but less severe forms of depression, cyclothymia. The prevalence of bipolar I disorder is roughly 1% of the population, and the prevalence of all forms of bipolar disorder 3-5%. Genetics studies of bipolar disorder have yielded several loci of interest associated with disease risk and predictors of treatment response, but the data are not yet at the phase of clinical application.

There is no medication designed to treat the full spectrum of bipolar disorder. While many classes of agents demonstrate efficacy in acute mania, including lithium, antipsychotic drugs, and certain anticonvulsants, no medication has surpassed lithium's efficacy for prophylaxis of future manic and depressive phases of bipolar disorder, and no other medication has demonstrated lithium's reduction in suicidality among bipolar patients.

PHARMACOLOGICAL PROPERTIES OF AGENTS FOR MANIA

ANTIPSYCHOTIC AGENTS. The chemistry and pharmacology of antipsychotic medications are addressed earlier in this chapter.

ANTICONVULSANTS. The pharmacology and chemistry of the anticonvulsants with significant data for acute mania (valproic acid compounds, carbamazepine) and for bipolar maintenance (lamotrigine) are covered in Chapter 21. These compounds are of diverse chemical classes, but share the common property of functional blockade of voltage-gated Na^+ channels, albeit with differing binding sites. These anticonvulsants have varying affinities for voltage-dependent Ca^{2+} channels, and differ in their ability to facilitate GABA-ergic (valproate) or inhibit glutamatergic neurotransmission (lamotrigine).

LITHIUM. Salts of the monovalent cation lithium (Li^+) share some characteristics with those of Na^+ and K^+. Traces of the ion occur normally in animal tissues, but it has no known physiological role. Lithium carbonate and lithium citrate are used therapeutically in the U.S.

Hypotheses for the Mechanism of Action of Lithium, and Relationship to Anticonvulsants. In animal brain tissue, Li^+ at concentrations of 1-10 mEq/L inhibits the depolarization-provoked and Ca^{++}-dependent release of NE and DA, but not 5HT, from nerve terminals. Li^+ may even transiently enhance release of 5HT. Li^+ modifies some hormonal responses mediated by adenylyl cyclase or PLC in other tissues, including the actions of vasopressin and thyroid-stimulating hormone on their peripheral target tissues. Li^+ can inhibit the effects of receptor-blocking agents that cause supersensitivity in such systems. In part, the actions of Li^+ may reflect its ability to interfere with the activity of both stimulatory and inhibitory G proteins (G_s and G_i) by keeping them in their inactive $\alpha\beta\gamma$ trimeric states.

Lithium's therapeutic efficacy may involve inhibition of inositol monophosphatase of the phosphatidylinositol pathway (*see* Figure 16–1), leading to decreased cerebral inositol concentrations (*see* Chapter 3). Further support for the role of inositol signaling in mania rests on the finding that valproate, and valproate derivatives, decrease intracellular inositol concentrations. Li^+ treatment also leads to consistent decreases in the functioning of protein kinases in brain tissue, including PKC, particularly isoforms α and β. This effect is also shared with valproic acid (particularly for PKC) but not with carbamazepine. The impact of Li^+ or valproate on PKC activity may secondarily alter the release of amine neurotransmitters and hormones as well as the activity of tyrosine hydroxylase. The proposed mechanism of PKC inhibition has been the basis for therapeutic trials of tamoxifen, a selective estrogen receptor modulator that is also a potent centrally active PKC inhibitor. In acutely manic bipolar I patients, tamoxifen has shown evidence of efficacy as adjunctive treatment.

Both Li^+ and valproate treatment inhibit the activity of glycogen synthase kinase-3β (GSK-3β). GSK-3β inhibition increases hippocampal levels of β-catenin, a function implicated in mood stabilization. GSK-3β regulates mood stabilizer-induced axonal growth and synaptic remodeling and modulates brain-derived neurotrophic factor response. Li^+ and valproate reduce arachidonic acid turnover in brain membrane phospholipids, and Li^+ also decreases gene expression of PLA_2 and decreases levels of COX-2.

ABSORPTION, DISTRIBUTION, AND ELIMINATION. Li^+ is absorbed readily and almost completely from the GI tract. Peak plasma concentrations achieved 2-4 h after an oral dose. Slow-release preparations of lithium carbonate minimize early peaks in plasma concentrations, and may decrease local GI adverse effects, but the increased trough levels may increase the risk for nephrogenic diabetes insipidus. Li^+ initially is distributed in the extracellular fluid, and gradually accumulates in various tissues. The concentration gradient across plasma membranes is much smaller than those for Na^+ and K^+. The final volume of distribution (0.7-0.9 L/kg) approaches that of total body water. Passage through the blood-brain barrier is slow, and at steady state, the concentration of Li^+ in the cerebrospinal fluid and in brain tissue is ~40-50% of the concentration in plasma.

Approximately 95% of a single dose of Li^+ is eliminated in the urine. From 33-66% of an acute dose is excreted during the first 6-12 h, followed by slow excretion over the next 10-14 days. The elimination $t_{1/2}$ averages 20-24 h. Steady state is achieved after ~5 half-lives. Loading with Na^+ produces a small enhancement of Li^+ excretion, but Na^+ depletion promotes a clinically important degree of Li^+ retention. Li^+ is completely filtered, and 80% is reabsorbed in the proximal tubules. Heavy sweating leads to a preferential secretion of Li^+ over Na^+; however, the repletion of excessive sweating using free water without electrolytes can cause hyponatremia, and promote Li^+ retention. Thiazide diuretics deplete Na^+ and reduce Li^+ clearance that may result in toxic levels. The K^+-sparing diuretics triamterene, spironolactone, and amiloride have modest effects on the excretion of Li^+. Less than 1% of ingested Li^+ leaves the human body in the feces; 4-5% is secreted in sweat. Li^+ is secreted in saliva in concentrations about twice those in plasma, while its concentration in tears is about equal to that in plasma. Li^+ is secreted in human milk, but serum levels in breast-fed infants are ~20% that of maternal levels, and are not associated with notable behavioral effects.

SERUM LEVEL MONITORING AND DOSE. Because of the low therapeutic index for Li^+, periodic determination of serum concentrations is crucial.

Concentrations considered to be effective and acceptably safe are between 0.6 and 1.5 mEq/L. The range of 1.0-1.5 mEq/L is favored for treatment of acutely manic or hypomanic patients. Somewhat lower values (0.6-1.0 mEq/L) are considered adequate and are safer for long-term prophylaxis. Serum concentrations of Li^+ have been found to follow a clear dose-effect relationship between 0.4 and 1.0 mEq/L, but with a corresponding dose-dependent rise in polyuria and tremor as indices of adverse effects. Nonetheless, patients who maintain trough levels of 0.8-1.0 mEq/L experience decreased relapse risk compared to those maintained at lower serum concentrations.

THERAPEUTIC USES

DRUG TREATMENT OF BIPOLAR DISORDER. Treatment with Li^+ ideally is conducted in patients with normal cardiac and renal function. Li^+ is the only mood stabilizer with data on suicide reduction in bipolar patients, and Li^+ also has abundant efficacy data for augmentation in unipolar depressive patients who are inadequate responders to antidepressant therapy.

DRUG TREATMENT OF MANIA. While Li^+, valproate, and carbamazepine have efficacy in acute mania, in clinical practice these are usually combined with atypical antipsychotic drugs, due to their delayed onset of action. Li^+, carbamazepine, and valproic acid preparations are only effective with daily dosing that maintains adequate serum levels, and require serum level monitoring. Acute IM forms of olanzapine, ziprasidone, and aripiprazole can be used to achieve rapid control of psychosis and agitation. Benzodiazepines are often used adjunctively for agitation and sleep induction.

A 600-mg loading dose of Li^+ can be given to hasten the time to steady state. Acutely manic patients may require higher dosages to achieve therapeutic serum levels, and downward adjustment may be necessary once the patient is euthymic.

The anticonvulsant sodium valproate provides more rapid antimanic effects than Li^+, with therapeutic benefit seen within 3-5 days. The most common form of valproate in use is divalproex sodium, preferred over valproic acid due to lower incidence of GI and other adverse effects. Divalproex is initiated at 25 mg/kg once daily and titrated to effect or the desired serum concentration. Serum concentrations of 90-120 μg/mL show the best response in clinical studies. With immediate release forms of valproic acid and divalproex sodium, 12-h troughs are used to guide treatment. With the extended-release divalproex preparation, patients respond best when the 24-h trough levels are in the high therapeutic range.

Carbamazepine is effective for acute mania. Immediate release forms of carbamazepine cannot be loaded or rapidly titrated over 24 h due to the development of neurological adverse effects such as dizziness or ataxia. The extended-release form is better tolerated and effective as monotherapy with once-daily dosing. Carbamazepine response rates are lower than those for valproate compounds or Li^+; nevertheless, certain individuals respond to carbamazepine after failing Li^+ and valproate. Initial doses are 400 mg/day, with the larger dose given at bedtime due to the sedating properties of carbamazepine. Titration proceeds by

200-mg increments every 24-48 h based on clinical response and serum trough levels. Due to increased risk of Stevens-Johnson syndrome in Asian individuals, HLA testing must be performed prior to treatment in populations at risk.

PROPHYLACTIC TREATMENT OF BIPOLAR DISORDER. Both aripiprazole and olanzapine are effective as monotherapy for mania prophylaxis, but olanzapine use is eschewed out of concern for metabolic effects, and aripiprazole shows no benefit for prevention of depressive relapse. LAI risperidone is also approved for bipolar maintenance treatment to be used adjunctively with Li^+ or valproate, or as monotherapy. Clozapine can be beneficial in refractory mania patients as adjunctive therapy and as monotherapy.

Bipolar disorder is a lifetime illness with high recurrence rates. Stopping mood stabilizer therapy can be considered in patients who have experienced only 1 lifetime manic episode, and who have been euthymic for extended periods. Discontinuation of maintenance Li^+ treatment in bipolar I patients carries a high risk of early recurrence and of suicidal behavior over a period of several months. This risk may be moderated by slow, gradual removal of Li^+, while rapid discontinuation should be avoided unless dictated by medical emergencies.

OTHER USES OF LITHIUM. Li^+ has been shown to be effective as adjunct therapy in treatment-resistant major depression. Clinical data also support Li^+ use as monotherapy for unipolar depression. Meta-analyses indicate that lithium's benefit on suicide reduction extends to unipolar mood disorder patients. While maintenance Li^+ levels of 0.6-1.0 mEq/L are used for bipolar prophylaxis, a lower range (0.4-0.8 mEq/L) is recommended for antidepressant augmentation.

INTERACTIONS WITH OTHER DRUGS. Interactions between Li^+ and diuretics (especially thiazides spironolactone and amiloride), angiotensin-converting enzyme inhibitors, and nonsteroidal anti-inflammatory agents have been discussed earlier. Amiloride has been used safely to reverse the syndrome of nephrogenic diabetes insipidus associated with Li^+ therapy, but requires careful monitoring and Li^+ dosage reduction to prevent lithium toxicity.

ADVERSE EFFECTS

CNS Effects. The most common CNS effect of Li^+ in the therapeutic dose range is fine postural hand tremor. Severity and risk for tremor are dose-dependent, with incidence ranging from 15-70%. In addition to the avoidance of caffeine and other agents that increase tremor amplitude, therapeutic options include dose reduction (bearing in mind the increased relapse risk with lower serum Li^+ levels), or β adrenergic blockade. Valproate treatment has a similar problem, and the approach to valproate-induced tremor is identical. At peak serum (and CNS) levels, some individuals may complain of incoordination, ataxia, or slurred speech, which can be avoided by dosing Li^+ at bedtime. Li^+ routinely causes EEG changes characterized by diffuse slowing, widened frequency spectrum, and potentiation with disorganization of background rhythm. Seizures have been reported in nonepileptic patients with therapeutic plasma concentrations of Li^+. Li^+ treatment has also been associated with increased risk of post-ECT confusion, and is generally tapered off prior to a course of ECT.

Li^+ (and valproate) treatment results in significant weight gain, a problem that is magnified by concurrent use of antipsychotic drugs.

Renal Effects. The kidneys' ability to concentrate urine decreases during Li^+ therapy, and ~60% of individuals exposed to Li^+ experience some form of polyuria and compensatory polydipsia. The mechanism of polyuria is unclear, but the result is decreased vasopressin stimulation of renal reabsorption of water, and the clinical picture of nephrogenic diabetes insipidus. Mean 24-h urinary volumes of 3 L/day are common among long-term Li^+ users, but Li^+ discontinuation or a switch to single daily dosing may reverse the effect on renal concentrating ability in patients with <5 years of Li^+ exposure. Renal function should be monitored with biannual serum blood urea nitrogen and creatinine levels, calculation of estimated GFR using standard formulas, and annual measurement of 24-h urinary volume.

Thyroid and Endocrine Effects. A small number of patients on Li^+ develop a benign, diffuse, nontender thyroid enlargement suggestive of compromised thyroid function, although many of these patients will have normal thyroid function. Measurable effects of Li^+ on thyroid indices are seen in a fraction of patients: 7-10% develop overt hypothyroidism, and 23% have subclinical disease, with women at 3-9 times greater risk. Ongoing monitoring of TSH and free T_4 is recommended throughout the course of Li^+ treatment.

ECG Effects. The prolonged use of Li^+ causes a benign and reversible T-wave flattening in ~20% of patients and the appearance of U waves, effects unrelated to depletion of Na^+ or K^+. Li^+-induced effects on cardiac conduction and pacemaker automaticity become pronounced during overdose and lead to sinus bradycardia, atrioventricular blocks, and possible CV compromise. Routine ECG monitoring may be considered in older patients, particularly those with a history of arrhythmia or coronary heart disease.

Skin Effects. Allergic reactions such as dermatitis, folliculitis, and vasculitis can occur with Li^+ administration. Worsening of acne vulgaris, psoriasis, and other dermatological conditions are usually treatable by topical measures, but in some may improve only upon discontinuation of Li^+. Some patients on Li^+ (and valproate) may experience alopecia.

PREGNANCY AND LACTATION. Li^+ is classified as risk category D. The use of Li^+ in early pregnancy may be associated with an increase in the incidence of CV anomalies of the newborn, especially Ebstein malformation. Although the anticonvulsants valproic acid and carbamazepine are also pregnancy risk category D, these agents are associated with irreversible neural tube defects. Potentially safer treatments for acute mania include antipsychotic drugs or ECT.

In pregnancy, maternal polyuria may be exacerbated by Li^+. Concomitant use of Li^+ with medications that waste Na^+ or a low-Na^+ diet during pregnancy can contribute to maternal and neonatal Li^+ intoxication. Li^+ freely crosses the placenta, and fetal or neonatal Li^+ toxicity may develop when maternal blood levels are within the therapeutic range. Fetal Li^+ exposure is associated with neonatal goiter, CNS depression, hypotonia ("floppy baby" syndrome), and cardiac murmur. Most recommend withholding lithium therapy for 24-48 h before delivery.

Other Effects. A benign, sustained increase in circulating polymorphonuclear leukocytes (12,000-15,000 cells/mm^3) occurs during the chronic use of Li^+ and is reversed within a week after termination of treatment. Some patients complain of a metallic taste, making food less palatable. Myasthenia gravis may worsen during treatment with Li^+.

ACUTE TOXICITY AND OVERDOSE. Acute intoxication is characterized by vomiting, profuse diarrhea, coarse tremor, ataxia, coma, and convulsions. Symptoms of milder toxicity include nausea, vomiting, abdominal pain, diarrhea, sedation, and fine tremor. The more serious effects involve the nervous system and include mental confusion, hyperreflexia, gross tremor, dysarthria, seizures, and cranial nerve and focal neurological signs, progressing to coma and death. Sometimes both cognitive and motor neurological damage may be irreversible, with persistent cerebellar tremor being the most common. Other toxic effects are cardiac arrhythmias, hypotension, and albuminuria.

USE IN PEDIATRIC AND GERIATRIC POPULATIONS

Pediatric Use. Only Li^+ has FDA approval for child/adolescent bipolar disorder for ages ≥12 years. Recently, aripiprazole and risperidone were FDA-approved for acute mania in children and adolescents ages 10-17. Children and adolescents have higher volumes of body water and higher GFR than adults. The resulting shorter $t_{1/2}$ of Li^+ demands dosing increases on a mg/kg basis, and multiple daily dosing is often required. As with adults, ongoing monitoring of renal and thyroid function is important. A number of studies suggest that valproate has efficacy comparable to that of Li^+ for mania in children or adolescents. As with Li^+, weight gain and tremor can be problematic. Ongoing monitoring of platelets and liver function tests, in addition to serum drug levels, is recommended.

Geriatric Use. The majority of older patients on Li^+ therapy are maintained for years on the medication. Age-related reductions in total body water and creatinine clearance reduce the safety margin for Li^+ treatment in older patients. Li^+ toxicity occurs more frequently in elderly patients, in part as the result of concurrent use of loop diuretics and angiotensin-converting enzyme inhibitors. Anticonvulsants, especially extended-release divalproex, are a reasonable alternative to Li^+. Elderly patients who are drug-naïve may be more sensitive to CNS adverse effects.

MAJOR DRUGS AVAILABLE IN THE CLASS

FORMULATIONS. Most Li^+ preparations currently used in the U.S. are tablets or capsules of lithium carbonate in strengths of 150, 300, and 600 mg. Slow-release preparations of lithium carbonate also are available in strengths of 300 and 450 mg, as is lithium citrate syrup (with 8 mEq of Li^+/5 mL citrate liquid, equivalent to 300 mg of lithium carbonate). Because slow-release forms carry an increased risk for polyuria, their use should be limited to patients who experience GI side effects related to rapid absorption.

For a complete Bibliographical Listing see Goodman & Gilman's ***The Pharmacological Basis of Therapeutics***, 12th ed., or Goodman & Gilman Online at www.AccessMedicine.com.

chapter 17 Hypnotics and Sedatives

The CNS depressants discussed in this chapter include benzodiazepines, other benzodiazepine receptor agonists (the "Z compounds"), barbiturates, and sedative-hypnotic agents of diverse chemical structure. Older sedative-hypnotic drugs depress the CNS in a dose-dependent fashion, progressively producing a spectrum of responses from mild sedation to coma and death. A *sedative* drug decreases activity, moderates excitement, and calms the recipient, whereas a *hypnotic* drug produces drowsiness and facilitates the onset and maintenance of a state of sleep that resembles natural sleep in its electroencephalographic characteristics and from which the recipient can be aroused easily.

Sedation is a side effect of many drugs that are not general CNS depressants (e.g., antihistamines and antipsychotic agents). Although such agents can intensify the effects of CNS depressants, they usually produce more specific therapeutic effects at concentrations far lower than those causing substantial CNS depression. The benzodiazepine sedative-hypnotics resemble such agents; although coma may occur at very high doses, neither surgical anesthesia nor fatal intoxication is produced by benzodiazepines in the absence of other drugs with CNS-depressant actions; an important exception is midazolam, which has been associated with decreased tidal volume and respiratory rate. Moreover, specific antagonists of benzodiazepines exist. This constellation of properties sets the benzodiazepine receptor agonists apart from other sedative-hypnotic drugs and imparts a measure of safety such that benzodiazepines and the newer Z compounds have largely displaced older agents for the treatment of insomnia and anxiety.

The sedative-hypnotic drugs that do not specifically target the benzodiazepine receptor belong to a group of agents that depress the CNS in a dose-dependent fashion, progressively producing calming or drowsiness (sedation), sleep (pharmacological hypnosis), unconsciousness, coma, surgical anesthesia, and fatal depression of respiration and cardiovascular regulation. They share these properties with a large number of chemicals, including general anesthetics (*see* Chapter 19) and alcohols, most notably ethanol (*see* Chapter 23).

BENZODIAZEPINES

All benzodiazepines in clinical use promote the binding of the major inhibitory neurotransmitter γ-aminobutyric acid (GABA) to the $GABA_A$ receptor, a multi-subunit, ligand-gated chloride channel. GABA binding induces the Cl^- current through these channels (*see* Figure 14–6).

Pharmacological data suggest heterogeneity among sites of binding and action of benzodiazepines; different subunit combinations comprise the GABA-gated chloride channels expressed in different neurons. Receptor subunit composition appears to govern the interaction of various allosteric modulators with these channels, giving hope to efforts to find agents displaying different combinations of benzodiazepine-like properties that reflect selective actions on 1 or more subtypes of $GABA_A$ receptors. A number of distinct mechanisms of action are thought to contribute to the sedative-hypnotic, muscle-relaxant, anxiolytic, and anticonvulsant effects of the benzodiazepines, and specific subunits of the $GABA_A$ receptor are responsible for specific pharmacological properties of benzodiazepines. While only the benzodiazepines used primarily for hypnosis are discussed in detail, this chapter describes the general properties of the group and important differences among individual agents (*see* also Chapters 15 and 21).

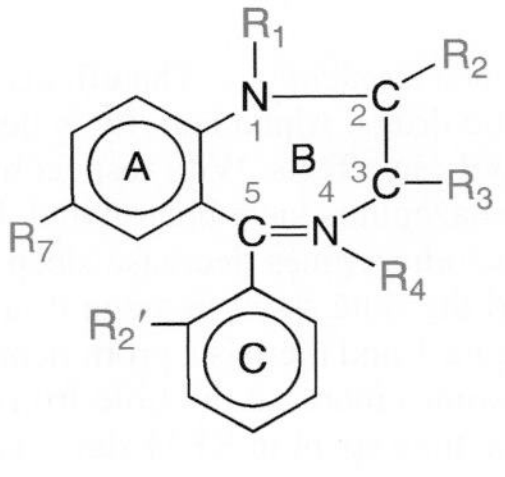

R1
N
1
2
C
R2
A
B
5
4
3
C—R3
R7
C=N
R4
R2′
C

Benzodiazepine refers to the portion of the this structure composed of a benzene ring (A) fused to a 7-membered diazepine ring (B). Because all the important benzodiazepines contain a 5-aryl substituent (ring C) and a 1,4-diazepine ring, the term has come to mean the 5-aryl-1,4-benzodiazepines. Numerous modifications in the structure of the ring systems and substituents have yielded compounds with similar activities, including flumazenil (ROMAZICON, in which ring C is replaced with a keto function at position 5 and a methyl substituent is added at position 4), a benzodiazepine receptor antagonist. A large number of nonbenzodiazepine compounds compete with classic benzodiazepines and flumazenil for binding at specific sites in the CNS (e.g., β-carbolines, zolpidem, eszopiclone).

PHARMACOLOGICAL PROPERTIES

Virtually all effects of the benzodiazepines result from their actions on the CNS. The most prominent of these effects are sedation, hypnosis, decreased anxiety, muscle relaxation, anterograde amnesia, and anticonvulsant activity. Only 2 effects of these drugs result from peripheral actions: coronary vasodilation, seen after intravenous administration of therapeutic doses of certain benzodiazepines, and neuromuscular blockade, seen only with very high doses.

CNS. While benzodiazepines depress activity at all levels of the neuraxis, some structures are affected preferentially. The benzodiazepines do not produce the same degrees of neuronal depression produced by barbiturates and volatile anesthetics. All the benzodiazepines have similar pharmacological profiles. Nevertheless, the drugs differ in selectivity, and the clinical usefulness of individual benzodiazepines thus varies considerably.

As the dose of a benzodiazepine is increased, sedation progresses to hypnosis and then to stupor. The clinical literature often refers to the "anesthetic" effects and uses of certain benzodiazepines, but the drugs do not cause a true general anesthesia because awareness usually persists, and immobility sufficient to allow surgery cannot be achieved. Nonetheless, at "preanesthetic" doses, there is amnesia for events subsequent to administration of the drug. Despite to separate the anxiolytic actions of benzodiazepines from their sedative-hypnotic effects, distinguishing between these behaviors is problematic. Measurements of anxiety and sedation are difficult in humans, and the validity of animal models for anxiety and sedation is uncertain. The existence of multiple benzodiazepine receptors may explain in part the diversity of pharmacological responses in different species.

Tolerance to Benzodiazepines. Studies on tolerance in laboratory animals often are cited to support the belief that disinhibitory effects of benzodiazepines are distinct from their sedative-ataxic effects. Although most patients who ingest benzodiazepines chronically report that drowsiness wanes over a few days, tolerance to the impairment of some measures of psychomotor performance (e.g., visual tracking) usually is not observed. Whether tolerance develops to the anxiolytic effects of benzodiazepines remains a subject of debate. Many patients can maintain themselves on a fairly constant dose; increases or decreases in dosage appear to correspond with changes in problems or stresses. Conversely, some patients either do not reduce their dosage when stress is relieved or steadily escalate dosage. Such behavior may be associated with the development of drug dependence (*see* Chapter 24).

Some benzodiazepines induce muscle hypotonia without interfering with normal locomotion and can decrease rigidity in patients with cerebral palsy. Clonazepam in nonsedative doses does cause muscle relaxation, but diazepam and most other benzodiazepines do not. Tolerance occurs to the muscle relaxant and ataxic effects of these drugs.

Clonazepam, nitrazepam, and nordazepam have more selective anticonvulsant activity than most other benzodiazepines. Benzodiazepines also suppress photic seizures in baboons and ethanol-withdrawal seizures in humans. However, the development of tolerance to the anticonvulsant effects has limited the usefulness of benzodiazepines in the treatment of recurrent seizure disorders in humans (*see* Chapter 21).

Although analgesic effects of benzodiazepines have been observed in experimental animals, only transient analgesia is apparent in humans after intravenous administration. Such effects actually may involve the production of amnesia. Unlike barbiturates, benzodiazepines do not cause hyperalgesia.

Effects on the Electroencephalogram (EEG) and Sleep Stages. The effects of benzodiazepines on the waking EEG resemble those of other sedative-hypnotic drugs. Alpha activity is decreased, but there is an increase in low-voltage fast activity. Tolerance occurs to these effects. With respect to sleep, some differences in the patterns of effects exerted by the various benzodiazepines have been noted, but benzodiazepine use usually imparts a sense of deep or refreshing sleep. Benzodiazepines decrease sleep latency, especially when first used, and diminish the number of awakenings and the time spent in stage 0 (a stage of wakefulness). Time in stage 1 (descending drowsiness) usually is decreased, and there is a prominent decrease in the time spent in slow-wave sleep (stages 3 and 4). Most benzodiazepines increase the time from onset of spindle sleep to the first burst of rapid-eye-movement (REM) sleep; the time spent in REM sleep usually is shortened, however, the number of cycles of REM sleep usually is increased, mostly late in the sleep time. Zolpidem and zaleplon suppress REM sleep to a lesser extent than do benzodiazepines and thus may be superior to benzodiazepines for use as hypnotics.

Despite the shortening of stage 4 and REM sleep, benzodiazepine administration typically increases total sleep time, largely by increasing the time spent in stage 2 (which is the major fraction of non-REM sleep). The effect is greatest in subjects with the shortest baseline total sleep time. In addition, despite the increased number of REM cycles, the number of shifts to lighter sleep stages (1 and 0) and the amount of body movement are diminished. Nocturnal peaks in the secretion of growth hormone, prolactin, and luteinizing hormone are not affected. During chronic nocturnal use of benzodiazepines, the effects on the various stages of sleep usually decline within a few nights. When such use is discontinued, the pattern of drug-induced changes in sleep parameters may "rebound," and an increase in the amount and density of REM sleep may be especially prominent. If the dosage has not been excessive, patients usually will note only a shortening of sleep time rather than an exacerbation of insomnia.

MOLECULAR TARGETS FOR BENZODIAZEPINE ACTIONS IN THE CNS. Benzodiazepines act at $GABA_A$ receptors by binding directly to a specific site that is distinct from that of GABA binding (*see* Figure 14–6). Unlike barbiturates, benzodiazepines do not activate $GABA_A$ receptors directly; rather, benzodiazepines act allosterically by modulating the effects of GABA. Benzodiazepines and GABA analogs bind to their respective sites on brain membranes with nanomolar affinity. Benzodiazepines modulate GABA binding, and GABA alters benzodiazepine binding in an allosteric fashion.

Benzodiazepines and related compounds can act as agonists, antagonists, or inverse agonists at the benzodiazepine-binding site on $GABA_A$ receptors. Agonists at the binding site increase, and inverse agonists decrease, the amount of chloride current generated by $GABA_A$-receptor activation. Agonists at the benzodiazepine binding site shift the GABA concentration-response curve to the left, whereas inverse agonists shift the curve to the right. Both these effects are blocked by antagonists at the benzodiazepine binding site. In the absence of an agonist or inverse agonist for the benzodiazepine binding site, an antagonist for this binding site does not affect $GABA_A$ receptor function. One such antagonist, flumazenil, is used clinically to reverse the effects of high doses of benzodiazepines. The behavioral and electrophysiological effects of benzodiazepines also can be reduced or prevented by prior treatment with antagonists at the GABA binding site (e.g., bicuculline).

Each $GABA_A$ receptor is believed to consist of a pentamer of homologous subunits. Thus far 16 different subunits have been identified and classified into 7 subunit families. The exact subunit structures of native GABA receptors still are unknown; most GABA receptors are likely of α, β, and γ subunits that co-assemble with some uncertain stoichiometry. The multiplicity of subunits generates heterogeneity in $GABA_A$ receptors and is responsible, at least in part, for the pharmacological diversity in benzodiazepine effects in behavioral, biochemical, and functional studies. An understanding of which $GABA_A$ receptor subunits are responsible for particular effects of benzodiazepines in vivo is emerging from KO animal studies. The attribution of specific behavioral effects of benzodiazepines to individual receptor subunits will, hopefully, aid in the development of new compounds exhibiting fewer undesired side effects.

$GABA_A$ Receptor-Mediated Electrical Events. Benzodiazepines exert their major actions by increasing the gain of inhibitory neurotransmission mediated by $GABA_A$ receptors. Enhancement of GABA-induced chloride currents by benzodiazepines results primarily from an increase in the frequency of bursts of Cl^- channel opening produced by submaximal amounts of GABA. At therapeutically relevant concentrations, benzodiazepines potentiate inhibitory synaptic transmission measured after stimulation of afferent fibers.

The remarkable safety of the benzodiazepines likely relates to the fact that their effects in vivo depend on the presynaptic release of GABA; in the absence of GABA, benzodiazepines have no effects on $GABA_A$ receptor function. This is in distinction to barbiturates, which also enhance the effects of GABA at low concentrations, *but, in addition,* directly activate GABA receptors at higher concentrations, which can lead to profound CNS depression.

The behavioral and sedative effects of benzodiazepines can be ascribed in part to potentiation of GABA-ergic pathways that serve to regulate the firing of monoamine-containing neurons known to promote behavioral arousal and to be important mediators of the inhibitory effects of fear and punishment on behavior. Finally, inhibitory effects on muscular hypertonia or the spread of seizure activity can be rationalized by potentiation of inhibitory GABA-ergic circuits at various levels of the neuraxis. The magnitude of the effects produced by benzodiazepines varies widely depending on such factors as the types of inhibitory circuits that are operating, the sources and intensity of excitatory input, and the manner in which experimental manipulations are performed and assessed. Accordingly, benzodiazepines markedly prolong the period after brief activation of recurrent GABA-ergic pathways during which neither spontaneous nor applied excitatory stimuli can evoke neuronal discharge; this effect is reversed by the $GABA_A$ receptor antagonist bicuculline (*see* Figure 14–5).

Respiration. Hypnotic doses of benzodiazepines are without effect on respiration in normal subjects, but special care must be taken in the treatment of children and individuals with impaired hepatic function. At higher doses, such as those used for preanesthetic medication or for endoscopy, benzodiazepines slightly depress alveolar ventilation and cause respiratory acidosis as the result of a decrease in hypoxic rather than hypercapnic drive; these effects are exaggerated in patients with chronic obstructive pulmonary disease (COPD), and alveolar hypoxia and CO_2 narcosis may result. These drugs can cause apnea during anesthesia or when given with opioids. Patients severely intoxicated with benzodiazepines only require respiratory assistance when they also have ingested another CNS-depressant drug, most commonly ethanol.

In contrast, hypnotic doses of benzodiazepines may worsen sleep-related breathing disorders by adversely affecting control of the upper airway muscles or by decreasing the ventilatory response to CO_2. The latter effect may cause hypoventilation and hypoxemia in some patients with severe COPD. In patients with obstructive sleep apnea (OSA), hypnotic doses of benzodiazepines may decrease muscle tone in the upper airway and exaggerate the impact of apneic episodes on alveolar hypoxia, pulmonary hypertension, and cardiac ventricular load. Benzodiazepines may promote the appearance of episodes of apnea during REM sleep (associated with decreases in oxygen saturation) in patients recovering from a myocardial infarction; however, no impact of these drugs on survival of patients with cardiac disease has been reported.

Cardiovascular System. The cardiovascular effects of benzodiazepines are minor in normal subjects except in severe intoxication. In preanesthetic doses, all benzodiazepines decrease blood pressure and increase heart rate. With midazolam, effects appear to be secondary to a decrease in peripheral resistance; with diazepam, effects are secondary to a decrease in left ventricular work and cardiac output. Diazepam increases coronary flow, possibly by an action to increase interstitial concentrations of adenosine, and the accumulation of this cardiodepressant metabolite also may explain the negative inotropic effects of the drug. In large doses, midazolam decreases cerebral blood flow and oxygen assimilation considerably.

GI Tract. Benzodiazepines are thought by some gastroenterologists to improve a variety of "anxiety-related" GI disorders. Diazepam markedly decreases nocturnal gastric secretion in humans. Other drug classes are considerably more effective in acid-peptic disorders (*see* Chapter 45).

ABSORPTION, FATE, AND EXCRETION. All the benzodiazepines are absorbed completely (clorazepate is decarboxylated rapidly in gastric juice to *N*-desmethyldiazepam [nordazepam], which subsequently is absorbed completely). Drugs active at the benzodiazepine receptor may be divided into 4 categories based on their elimination $t_{1/2}$:

- Ultra-short-acting benzodiazepines
- Short-acting agents ($t_{1/2}$ <6 h), including triazolam, the non-benzodiazepine zolpidem ($t_{1/2}$ ~2 h), and eszopiclone ($t_{1/2}$ 5-6 h)
- Intermediate-acting agents ($t_{1/2}$ 6-24 h), including estazolam and temazepam
- Long-acting agents ($t_{1/2}$ >24 h), including flurazepam, diazepam, and quazepam

Flurazepam itself has a short $t_{1/2}$ (~2.3 h), but a major active metabolite, *N*-des-alkyl-flurazepam, is long-lived ($t_{1/2}$ 47-100 h); such features complicate the classification of individual benzodiazepines.

The benzodiazepines and their active metabolites bind to plasma proteins. The extent of binding correlates strongly with lipid solubility and ranges from ~70% for alprazolam to nearly 99% for diazepam. The concentration in the cerebrospinal fluid is approximately equal to the concentration of free drug in plasma. The plasma concentrations of most benzodiazepines exhibit patterns that are consistent with 2-compartment models, but 3-compartment models appear to be more appropriate for the compounds with the highest lipid solubility. Accordingly, there is rapid uptake of benzodiazepines into the brain and other highly perfused organs after intravenous administration (or oral administration of a rapidly absorbed compound); rapid uptake is followed by a phase of redistribution into tissues that are less well perfused, especially muscle and fat. Redistribution is most rapid for drugs with the highest lipid solubility. The kinetics of redistribution of diazepam and other lipophilic benzodiazepines are complicated by enterohepatic circulation. The volumes of distribution of the benzodiazepines are large and in many cases are increased in elderly patients. These drugs cross the placental barrier and are secreted into breast milk.

Benzodiazepines are metabolized extensively by hepatic CYPs, particularly CYPs 3A4 and 2C19. Some benzodiazepines, such as oxazepam, are conjugated directly and are not metabolized by these enzymes. Erythromycin, clarithromycin, ritonavir, itraconazole, ketoconazole, nefazodone, and grapefruit juice are inhibitors of CYP3A4 (*see* Chapter 6) and can affect the metabolism of benzodiazepines. Because active metabolites of some benzodiazepines are biotransformed more slowly than are the parent compounds, the duration of action of many benzodiazepines bears little relationship to the $t_{1/2}$ of elimination of the parent drug that was administered, as noted above for flurazepam. Conversely, the rate of biotransformation of agents that are inactivated by the initial reaction is an important determinant of their duration of action; these agents include oxazepam, lorazepam, temazepam, triazolam, and midazolam.

Because the benzodiazepines apparently do not significantly induce the synthesis of hepatic CYPs, their chronic administration usually does not result in the accelerated metabolism of other substances or of the benzodiazepines. Cimetidine and oral contraceptives inhibit *N*-dealkylation and 3-hydroxylation of benzodiazepines. Ethanol, isoniazid, and phenytoin are less effective in this regard. These reactions usually are reduced to a greater extent in elderly patients and in patients with chronic liver disease than are those involving conjugation.

PHARMACOKINETICS AND THE IDEAL HYPNOTIC. An ideal hypnotic agent would have a rapid onset of action when taken at bedtime, a sufficiently sustained action to facilitate sleep throughout the night, and no residual action by the following morning. Among the benzodiazepines that are used commonly as hypnotic agents, triazolam theoretically fits this description most closely. Because of the slow rate of elimination of desalkylflurazepam, flurazepam (or quazepam) might seem to be unsuitable for this purpose. In practice, there appear to be some disadvantages to the use of agents that have a relatively rapid rate of disappearance, including the early-morning insomnia that is experienced by some patients and a greater likelihood of rebound insomnia on drug discontinuation. With careful selection of dosage, flurazepam and other benzodiazepines with slower rates of elimination than triazolam can be used effectively.

THERAPEUTIC USES

The therapeutic uses and routes of administration of individual benzodiazepines that are marketed in the U.S. are summarized in Table 17–1. Most benzodiazepines can be used interchangeably. For example, diazepam can be used for alcohol withdrawal, and most benzodiazepines work as hypnotics. Benzodiazepines that are useful as anticonvulsants have a long $t_{1/2}$, and rapid entry into the brain is required for efficacy in treatment of status epilepticus. A short elimination $t_{1/2}$ is desirable for hypnotics. Antianxiety agents, in contrast, should have a long $t_{1/2}$ despite the drawback of the risk of neuropsychological deficits caused by drug accumulation.

UNTOWARD EFFECTS. At peak concentration in plasma, hypnotic doses of benzodiazepines cause varying degrees of light-headedness, lassitude, increased reaction time, motor incoordination, impairment of mental and motor functions, confusion, and anterograde amnesia. Cognition appears to be affected less than motor performance. *All of these effects can greatly impair driving and other psychomotor skills, especially if combined with ethanol.* When the drug is given at the intended time of sleep, the persistence of these effects during the waking hours is adverse. The intensity and incidence of CNS toxicity generally increase with age. Other common side effects of benzodiazepines are weakness, headache, blurred vision, vertigo, nausea and vomiting, epigastric distress, and diarrhea; joint pains, chest pains, and incontinence are much rarer. Anticonvulsant benzodiazepines sometimes increase the frequency of seizures in patients with epilepsy.

ADVERSE PSYCHOLOGICAL EFFECTS. Benzodiazepines may cause paradoxical effects. Flurazepam occasionally increases the incidence of nightmares—especially during the first week of use—and sometimes causes garrulousness, anxiety, irritability, tachycardia, and sweating. Amnesia, euphoria, restlessness, hallucinations, sleep-walking, sleep-talking, other complex behaviors, and hypomanic behavior have been reported to occur during use of various benzodiazepines. Bizarre uninhibited behavior has been noted in some users, whereas hostility and rage may occur in others; collectively, these are sometimes referred to as *disinhibition* or *dyscontrol reactions*. Paranoia, depression, and suicidal ideation also occasionally may accompany the use of these agents. Such paradoxical or disinhibition reactions are rare and appear to be dose related. Because of reports of an increased incidence of confusion and abnormal behaviors, triazolam has been banned in the U.K., although the FDA declared triazolam to be safe and effective in low doses of 0.125-0.25 mg.

Chronic benzodiazepine use poses a risk for development of dependence and abuse. Abuse of benzodiazepines includes the use of flunitrazepam (Rohypnol; not licensed for use in the U.S.) as a "date-rape drug." Withdrawal symptoms may include temporary intensification of the problems that originally prompted their use (e.g., insomnia or anxiety). Dysphoria, irritability, sweating, unpleasant dreams, tremors, anorexia, and faintness or dizziness also may occur, especially when withdrawal of the benzodiazepine occurs abruptly. Despite their adverse effects, benzodiazepines are relatively safe drugs. Ethanol is a common contributor to deaths involving benzodiazepines, and true coma is uncommon in the absence of another CNS depressant. Benzodiazepines can further compromise respiration in patients with COPD or obstructive sleep apnea (OSA).

A wide variety of serious allergic, hepatotoxic, and hematologic reactions to the benzodiazepines may occur, but the incidence is quite low; these reactions have been associated with the use of flurazepam, triazolam, and temazepam. Large doses taken just before or during labor may cause hypothermia, hypotonia, and mild respiratory depression in the neonate. Abuse by the pregnant mother can result in a withdrawal syndrome in the newborn.

Except for additive effects with other sedative or hypnotic drugs, reports of clinically important pharmacodynamic interactions between benzodiazepines and other drugs have been infrequent. Ethanol increases both the

Table 17–1

Therapeutic Uses of Benzodiazepines

COMPOUND	ROUTES OF ADMINISTRATION[a]	EXAMPLES OF THERAPEUTIC USES[b]	COMMENTS	$t_{1/2}$ (h)[c]	USUAL SEDATIVE-HYPNOTIC DOSE, mg[d]
Alprazolam	Oral	Anxiety disorders, agoraphobia	Withdrawal symptoms may be especially severe	12±2	—
Chlordiazepoxide	Oral, IM, IV	Anxiety disorders, management of alcohol withdrawal, anesthetic premedication	Long-acting and self-tapering because of active metabolites	10±3.4	50-100, 1-4 × daily[e]
Clonazepam	Oral	Seizure disorders, adjunctive treatment in acute mania and certain movement disorders	Tolerance develops to anticonvulsant effects	23±5	—
Clorazepate	Oral	Anxiety disorders, seizure disorders	Prodrug; activity due to formation of nordazepam during absorption	2.0±0.9	3.75-20, 2-4 × daily[e]
Diazepam	Oral, IM, IV, rectal	Anxiety disorders, status epilepticus, skeletal muscle relaxation, anesthetic premedication	Prototypical benzodiazepine	43±13	5-10, 3-4 × daily[e]
Estazolam	Oral	Insomnia	Contains triazolo ring; adverse effects may be similar to those of triazolam	10–24	1-2
Flurazepam	Oral	Insomnia	Active metabolites accumulate with chronic use	74±24	15-30
Lorazepam	Oral, IM, IV	Anxiety disorders, preanesthetic medication	Metabolized solely by conjugation	14±5	2-4
Midazolam	IV, IM	Preanesthetic and intraoperative medication	Rapidly inactivated	1.9±0.6	—[f]
Oxazepam	Oral	Anxiety disorders	Metabolized solely by conjugation	8.0±2.4	15-30, 3-4 × daily[e]
Quazepam	Oral	Insomnia	Active metabolites accumulate with chronic use	39	7.5-15
Temazepam	Oral	Insomnia	Metabolized mainly by conjugation	11±6	7.5-30
Triazolam	Oral	Insomnia	Rapidly inactivated; may cause disturbing daytime side effects	2.9±1.0	0.125-0.25

[a] *IM, intramuscular injection; IV, intravenous administration; qd, once a day; bid, twice a day; tid, three times a day; qid, four times a day.*

[b] *The therapeutic uses are identified as examples to emphasize that most benzodiazepines can be used interchangeably. In general, the therapeutic uses of a given benzodiazepine are related to its $t_{1/2}$ and may not match the marketed indications. The issue is addressed more extensively in the text.*

[c] *Half-life of active metabolite may differ. See Appendix II for additional information.*

[d] *For additional dosage information, see Chapter 13 (anesthesia), Chapter 17 (anxiety), and Chapter 19 (seizure disorders).*

[e] *Approved as a sedative-hypnotic only for management of alcohol withdrawal; doses in a nontolerant individual would be smaller.*

[f] *Recommended doses vary considerably depending on specific use, condition of patient, and concomitant administration of other drugs.*

rate of absorption of benzodiazepines and the associated CNS depression. Valproate and benzodiazepines in combination may cause psychotic episodes. Pharmacokinetic interactions were discussed earlier.

NOVEL BENZODIAZEPINE RECEPTOR AGONISTS

Hypnotics in this class are commonly referred to as "Z compounds." They include zolpidem (AMBIEN), zaleplon (SONATA), zopiclone (not marketed in the U.S.), and eszopiclone (LUNESTA), which is the S(+) enantiomer of zopiclone. Although the Z compounds are structurally unrelated to each other and to benzodiazepines, their therapeutic efficacy as hypnotics is due to agonist effects on the benzodiazepine site of the $GABA_A$ receptor. Compared to benzodiazepines, Z compounds are less effective as anticonvulsants or muscle relaxants, which may be related to their relative selectivity for $GABA_A$ receptors containing the α_1 subunit. Over the last decade, Z compounds have largely replaced benzodiazepines in the treatment of insomnia. Z compounds were initially promoted as having less potential for dependence and abuse than traditional benzodiazepines. However, based on postmarketing clinical experience with zopiclone and zolpidem, tolerance and physical dependence can be expected during long-term use of Z compounds, especially with higher doses. Zopiclone and its isomers are classified as schedule IV drugs in the U.S. The clinical presentation of overdose with Z compounds is similar to that of benzodiazepine overdose and can be treated with the benzodiazepine antagonist flumazenil.

Zaleplon and zolpidem are effective in relieving sleep-onset insomnia. Both drugs are FDA-approved for use as long as to 7-10 days at a time. Zaleplon and zolpidem have sustained hypnotic efficacy without occurrence of rebound insomnia on abrupt discontinuation. Zaleplon and zolpidem have similar degrees of efficacy. Zolpidem has a $t_{1/2}$ of ~2 h, which is sufficient to cover most of a typical 8-h sleep period, and is presently approved for bedtime use only. Zaleplon has a shorter $t_{1/2}$ ~1 h, which offers the possibility for safe dosing later in the night, within 4 h of the anticipated rising time. Zaleplon and zolpidem differ in residual side effects; late-night administration of zolpidem has been associated with morning sedation, delayed reaction time, and anterograde amnesia, whereas zaleplon does not differ from placebo.

ZALEPLON. Zaleplon (SONATA, generic) is a nonbenzodiazepine and is a member of the pyrazolopyrimidine class. Zaleplon preferentially binds to the benzodiazepine-binding site on $GABA_A$ receptors containing the α_1 receptor subunit. Zaleplon is absorbed rapidly and reaches peak plasma concentrations in ~1 h. Its bioavailability is ~30% because of presystemic metabolism. Zaleplon is metabolized largely by aldehyde oxidase and to a lesser extent by CYP3A4. Its oxidative metabolites are converted to glucuronides and eliminated in urine. Less than 1% of zaleplon is excreted unchanged in urine. None of zaleplon's metabolites are pharmacologically active. Zaleplon is usually administered in 5-, 10-, or 20-mg doses.

ZOLPIDEM. Zolpidem (AMBIEN, others) is a non-benzodiazepine sedative-hypnotic drug. The actions of zolpidem are due to agonist effects on $GABA_A$ receptors and generally resemble those of benzodiazepines. Zolpidem has little effect on the stages of sleep in normal human subjects. The drug is effective in shortening sleep latency and prolonging total sleep time in patients with insomnia. After discontinuation of zolpidem, the beneficial effects on sleep reportedly persist for up to 1 week, but mild rebound insomnia on the first night also has occurred. Tolerance and physical dependence are rare. Nevertheless, zolpidem is approved only for the short-term treatment of insomnia. At therapeutic doses (5-10 mg), zolpidem infrequently produces residual daytime sedation or amnesia, and the incidence of other adverse effects also is low. As with the benzodiazepines, large overdoses of zolpidem do not produce severe respiratory depression unless other agents (e.g., ethanol) also are ingested. Hypnotic doses increase the hypoxia and hypercarbia of patients with OSA.

Zolpidem is absorbed readily from the GI tract; first-pass hepatic metabolism results in an oral bioavailability of ~70%, but this value is lower when the drug is ingested with food. Zolpidem is eliminated almost entirely by conversion to inactive products in the liver, largely through oxidation of the methyl groups on the phenyl and imidazopyridine rings to the corresponding carboxylic acids. Its plasma $t_{1/2}$ is ~2 h in individuals with normal hepatic blood flow or function. This value may be increased 2-fold or more in those with cirrhosis and also tends to be greater in older patients; adjustment of dosage often is necessary in both categories of patients. Although little or no unchanged zolpidem is found in the urine, elimination of the drug is slower in patients with chronic renal insufficiency largely owing to an increase in its apparent volume of distribution.

ESZOPICLONE. Eszopiclone (LUNESTA) is the active S(+) enantiomer of zopiclone. Eszopiclone has no structural similarity to benzodiazepines, zolpidem, or zaleplon. Eszopiclone is believed to exert its sleep-promoting effects through its enhancement of $GABA_A$ receptor function at the benzodiazepine binding site. Eszopiclone is used for the long-term treatment of insomnia and for sleep maintenance. It is available in 1-, 2-, or 3-mg tablets. Eszopiclone decreases the latency to onset of sleep. In clinical studies, no tolerance was observed; no signs of serious withdrawal, such as seizures or rebound insomnia, were seen on discontinuation of the drug (however, there are such reports for zopiclone, the racemate used outside the U.S.). Mild withdrawal consisting of abnormal dreams, anxiety, nausea, and upset stomach can occur (rate ≤2%). A minor reported adverse effect of eszopiclone was a bitter taste. Eszopiclone is a schedule IV controlled substance in the U.S.

Eszopiclone is absorbed rapidly after oral administration, with a bioavailability of ~80%; it is metabolized by CYPs 3A4 and 2E1 and has a $t_{1/2}$ of ~6 h.

FLUMAZENIL: A BENZODIAZEPINE RECEPTOR ANTAGONIST

Flumazenil (ROMAZICON, generic), the only member of this class, is an imidazobenzodiazepine that binds with high affinity to specific sites on the $GABA_A$ receptor, where it competitively antagonizes the binding and allosteric effects of benzodiazepines and other ligands. Flumazenil antagonizes both the electrophysiological and behavioral effects of agonist and inverse-agonist benzodiazepines and β-carbolines.

Flumazenil is available only for intravenous administration. Flumazenil is eliminated almost entirely by hepatic metabolism to inactive products with a $t_{1/2}$ of ~1 h; the duration of clinical effects usually is only 30-60 min. Although absorbed rapidly after oral administration, <25% of the drug reaches the systemic circulation owing to extensive first-pass hepatic metabolism; effective oral doses are apt to cause headache and dizziness. The administration of a series of small injections is preferred to a single bolus injection. A total of 1 mg flumazenil given over 1-3 min usually is sufficient to abolish the effects of therapeutic doses of benzodiazepines. Additional courses of treatment with flumazenil may be needed within 20-30 min should sedation reappear.

The primary indications for the use of flumazenil are the management of suspected benzodiazepine overdose and the reversal of sedative effects produced by benzodiazepines administered during either general anesthesia or diagnostic and/or therapeutic procedures. Flumazenil is not effective in single-drug overdoses with either barbiturates or tricyclic antidepressants or in patients who had been taking benzodiazepines for protracted periods and in whom tolerance and/or dependence may have developed. The administration of flumazenil in these settings may be associated with the onset of seizures, especially in patients poisoned with tricyclic antidepressants.

MELATONIN CONGENERS

RAMELTEON. Ramelteon (ROZEREM) is a synthetic tricyclic analog of melatonin, approved in the U.S. for the treatment of insomnia, specifically difficulties of sleep onset.

Mechanism of Action. Melatonin levels in the suprachiasmatic nucleus rise and fall in a circadian fashion, with concentrations increasing in the evening as an individual prepares for sleep, and then reaching a plateau and ultimately decreasing as the night progresses. Two GPCRs for melatonin, MT_1 and MT_2, occur in the suprachiasmatic nucleus, each playing a different role in sleep. Binding of agonists such as melatonin to MT_1 receptors promotes the onset of sleep; melatonin binding to MT_2 receptors shifts the timing of the circadian system. Ramelteon binds to both MT_1 and MT_2 receptors with high affinity but, unlike melatonin, it does not bind appreciably to quinone reductase 2, the structurally unrelated MT_3 receptor. Ramelteon is not known to bind to any other classes of receptors.

Clinical Pharmacology. Prescribing guidelines suggest that an 8-mg tablet be taken ~30 min before bedtime. Ramelteon is rapidly absorbed from the GI tract. Because of the significant first-pass metabolism that occurs after oral administration, ramelteon bioavailability is <2%. The drug is largely metabolized by hepatic CYPs 1A2, 2C, and 3A4, with $t_{1/2}$ of ~2 h in humans. Of the 4 metabolites, one, M-II, acts as an agonist at MT_1 and MT_2 receptors and may contribute to the sleep-promoting effects of ramelteon. Ramelteon is efficacious in combating both transient and chronic insomnia. Studies indicate that the drug is generally well tolerated by patients and does not impair next-day cognitive function. Sleep latency was consistently found to be shorter in patients given ramelteon compared to placebo controls. No evidence of rebound insomnia or withdrawal effects were noted upon ramelteon withdrawal. Unlike most agents mentioned in this chapter, ramelteon is not a controlled substance.

BARBITURATES

The barbiturates were once used extensively as sedative-hypnotic drugs. Except for a few specialized uses, they have been largely replaced by the much safer benzodiazepines. Table 17–2 lists the common barbiturates and their pharmacological properties.

Table 17–2

Major Pharmacological Properties of Selected Barbiturates

COMPOUND	DOSAGE FORMS	$t_{1/2}$ (h)	THERAPEUTIC USES	COMMENTS
Amobarbital	IM, IV	10-40	Insomnia, pre-op sedation, emergency management of seizures	Only Na^+ salt administered parenterally
Butabarbital	Oral	35-50	Insomnia, pre-op sedation	Redistribution shortens duration of action of single dose to 8 hours
Mephobarbital	Oral	10-70	Seizure disorders, daytime sedation	Second-line anticonvulsant
Methohexital	IV	3-5[a]	Induction and maintenance of anesthesia	Only Na^+ salt available; single dose provides 5-7 min of anesthesia[a]
Pentobarbital	Oral, IM, IV, rectal	15-50	Insomnia, pre-op sedation, emergency management of seizures	Only Na^+ salt administered parenterally
Phenobarbital	Oral, IM, IV	80-120	Seizure disorders, status epilepticus, daytime sedation	First-line anticonvulsant; only Na^+ salt administered parenterally
Secobarbital	Oral	15-40	Insomnia, preoperative sedation	Only Na^+ salt available
Thiopental	IV	8-10[a]	Induction/maintenance of anesthesia, pre-op sedation, emergency management of seizures	Only Na^+ salt available; single dose provides brief of anesthesia[a]

[a]*Terminal $t_{1/2}$ due to hepatic metabolism; redistribution following parenteral administration produces effects lasting only a few minutes.*

Barbiturates are derivatives of this parent structure:

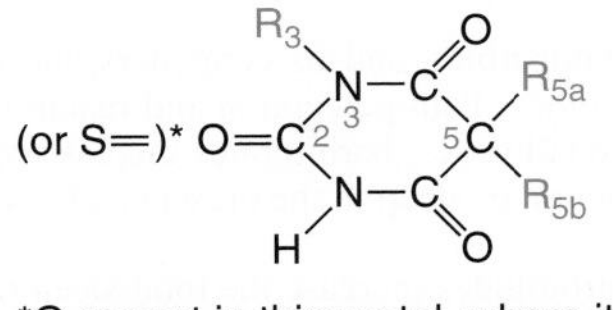

*O except in thiopental, where it is replaced by S.

The presence of alkyl or aryl groups at position 5 confers sedative-hypnotic and sometimes other activities. Barbiturates in which the oxygen at C2 is replaced by sulfur sometimes are called *thiobarbiturates.* These compounds are more lipid-soluble than the corresponding *oxybarbiturates.* In general, structural changes that increase lipid solubility decrease duration of action, decrease latency to onset of activity, accelerate metabolic degradation, and increase hypnotic potency.

PHARMACOLOGICAL PROPERTIES

The barbiturates reversibly depress the activity of all excitable tissues. The CNS is exquisitely sensitive, and even when barbiturates are given in anesthetic concentrations, direct effects on peripheral excitable tissues are weak. However, serious deficits in cardiovascular and other peripheral functions occur in acute barbiturate intoxication.

ABSORPTION, FATE, AND EXCRETION. For sedative-hypnotic use, the barbiturates usually are administered orally (*see* Table 17–2). Na^+ salts are absorbed more rapidly than the corresponding free acids, especially from liquid formulations. The onset of action varies from 10-60 min, and is delayed by the presence of food. Intramuscular injections of solutions of the Na^+ salts should be placed deeply into large muscles to avoid the pain and possible necrosis that can result at more superficial sites. The intravenous route usually is reserved for the management of status epilepticus (phenobarbital sodium) or for the induction and/or maintenance of general anesthesia (e.g., thiopental or methohexital). Barbiturates are distributed widely and readily cross the placenta. Uptake into less vascular tissues, especially muscle and fat, leads to a decline in the concentration of barbiturate in the plasma and brain. With thiopental and methohexital, this results in the awakening of patients within 5-15 min of the injection of the usual anesthetic doses (*see* Chapter 19).

Except for the less lipid-soluble aprobarbital and phenobarbital, nearly complete metabolism and/or conjugation of barbiturates in the liver precedes their renal excretion. The oxidation of radicals at C5 is the most important biotransformation that terminates biological activity. In some instances (e.g., phenobarbital), *N*-glycosylation is an important metabolic pathway. Other biotransformations include *N*-hydroxylation, desulfuration of thiobarbiturates to oxybarbiturates, opening of the barbituric acid ring, and *N*-dealkylation of *N*-alkyl barbiturates to active metabolites (e.g., mephobarbital to phenobarbital). About 25% of phenobarbital and nearly all of aprobarbital are excreted unchanged in the urine.

The metabolic elimination of barbiturates is more rapid in young people than in the elderly and infants, and $t_{1/2}$ are increased during pregnancy partly because of the expanded volume of distribution. Chronic liver disease often increases the $t_{1/2}$ of the biotransformable barbiturates. Repeated administration, especially of phenobarbital, shortens the $t_{1/2}$ of barbiturates that are metabolized as a result of the induction of microsomal enzymes.

The barbiturates commonly used as hypnotics in the U.S. have $t_{1/2}$ *values such that the drugs are not fully eliminated in 24 h (see Table 17–2). Thus, these barbiturates will accumulate during repetitive administration unless appropriate adjustments in dosage are made. Furthermore, the persistence of the drug in plasma during the day favors the development of tolerance and abuse.*

CENTRAL NERVOUS SYSTEM

Sites and Mechanisms of Action on the CNS. Barbiturates act throughout the CNS; nonanesthetic doses preferentially suppress polysynaptic responses. Facilitation is diminished, and inhibition usually is enhanced. The site of inhibition is either postsynaptic, as at cortical and cerebellar pyramidal cells and in the cuneate nucleus, substantia nigra, and thalamic relay neurons, or presynaptic, as in the spinal cord. Enhancement of inhibition occurs primarily at synapses where neurotransmission is mediated by GABA acting at $GABA_A$ receptors. Mechanisms underlying the actions of barbiturates on $GABA_A$ receptors appear to be distinct from those of either GABA or the benzodiazepines. Barbiturates activate inhibitory $GABA_A$ receptors and inhibit excitatory AMPA/kainate receptors, These actions can explain their CNS-depressant effects. For details, see the 12th edition of the parent text.

Barbiturates can produce all degrees of depression of the CNS, ranging from mild sedation to general anesthesia (*see* Chapter 19). Certain barbiturates, particularly those containing a 5-phenyl substituent (e.g., phenobarbital and mephobarbital), have selective anticonvulsant activity (*see* Chapter 21). The anti-anxiety properties of the barbiturates are inferior to those exerted by the benzodiazepines.

Except for the anticonvulsant activities of phenobarbital and its congeners, the barbiturates possess a low degree of selectivity and a narrow therapeutic index. Pain perception and reaction are relatively unimpaired until the moment of unconsciousness, and in small doses, barbiturates increase reactions to painful stimuli. Hence, they cannot be relied on to produce sedation or sleep in the presence of even moderate pain.

Effects on Stages of Sleep. Hypnotic doses of barbiturates increase the total sleep time and alter the stages of sleep in a dose-dependent manner. Like the benzodiazepines, these drugs decrease sleep latency, the number of awakenings, and the durations of REM and slow-wave sleep. During repetitive nightly administration, some tolerance to the effects on sleep occurs within a few days, and the effect on total sleep time may be reduced by as much as 50% after 2 weeks of use. Discontinuation leads to rebound increases in all the parameters reported to be decreased by barbiturates.

Tolerance. With chronic administration of gradually increasing doses, pharmacodynamic tolerance continues to develop over a period of weeks to months, depending on the dosage schedule, whereas pharmacokinetic tolerance reaches its peak in a few days to a week. Tolerance to the effects on mood, sedation, and hypnosis occurs more readily and is greater than that to the anticonvulsant and lethal effects; thus, as tolerance increases, the therapeutic index decreases. Pharmacodynamic tolerance to barbiturates confers cross-tolerance to all general CNS-depressant drugs, including ethanol.

Abuse and Dependence. Like other CNS depressant drugs, barbiturates are abused, and some individuals develop a dependence on them (*see* Chapter 24). Moreover, the barbiturates may have euphoriant effects.

Peripheral Nervous Structures. Barbiturates selectively depress transmission in autonomic ganglia and reduce nicotinic excitation by choline esters. This effect may account, at least in part, for the fall in blood pressure produced by intravenous oxybarbiturates and by severe barbiturate intoxication. At skeletal neuromuscular junctions, the blocking effects of both tubocurarine and decamethonium are enhanced during barbiturate anesthesia. These actions probably result from the capacity of barbiturates at hypnotic or anesthetic concentrations to inhibit the passage of current through nicotinic cholinergic receptors. Several distinct mechanisms appear to be involved, and little stereoselectivity is evident.

RESPIRATION. Barbiturates depress both the respiratory drive and the mechanisms responsible for the rhythmic character of respiration. The neurogenic drive is essentially eliminated by a dose 3 times greater than that used normally to induce sleep. Such doses also suppress the hypoxic drive and, to a lesser extent, the chemoreceptor drive. However, the margin between the lighter planes of surgical anesthesia and dangerous respiratory depression is sufficient to permit the ultra-short-acting barbiturates to be used, with suitable precautions, as anesthetic agents. The barbiturates only slightly depress protective reflexes until the degree of intoxication is sufficient to produce severe respiratory depression. Coughing, sneezing, hiccoughing, and laryngospasm may occur when barbiturates are employed as intravenous anesthetic agents.

CARDIOVASCULAR SYSTEM. When given orally in sedative or hypnotic doses, barbiturates do not produce significant overt cardiovascular effects. In general, the effects of thiopental anesthesia on the cardiovascular system are benign in comparison with those of the volatile anesthetic agents; there usually is either no change or a fall in mean arterial pressure (*see* Chapter 19).

Other cardiovascular changes often noted when thiopental and other intravenous thiobarbiturates are administered after conventional preanesthetic medication include decreased renal and cerebral blood flow with a marked fall in CSF pressure. Although cardiac arrhythmias are observed only infrequently, intravenous anesthesia with barbiturates can increase the incidence of ventricular arrhythmias, especially when epinephrine and halothane also are present. Anesthetic concentrations of barbiturates have direct electrophysiological effects on the heart; in addition to depressing Na^+ channels, they reduce the function of at least 2 types of K^+ channels. However, direct depression of cardiac contractility occurs only when doses several times those required to cause anesthesia are administered.

GI TRACT. The oxybarbiturates tend to decrease the tone of the GI musculature and the amplitude of rhythmic contractions. A hypnotic dose does not significantly delay gastric emptying in humans. The relief of various GI symptoms by sedative doses is probably largely due to the central-depressant action.

LIVER. The effects vary with the duration of exposure to the barbiturate. *Acutely,* the barbiturates combine with several CYPs and inhibit the biotransformation of a number of other drugs and endogenous substrates, such as steroids; other substrates may reciprocally inhibit barbiturate biotransformations.

Chronic administration of barbiturates markedly increases the protein and lipid content of the hepatic smooth endoplasmic reticulum, as well as the activities of glucuronyl transferase and CYPs 1A2, 2C9, 2C19, and 3A4. The induction of these enzymes increases the metabolism of a number of drugs and endogenous substances, including steroid hormones, cholesterol, bile salts, and vitamins K and D. This also results in an increased rate of barbiturate metabolism, which partly accounts for tolerance to barbiturates. The inducing effect is not limited to the microsomal enzymes; e.g., there are increases in δ-aminolevulinic acid (ALA) synthetase, a mitochondrial enzyme, and aldehyde dehydrogenase, a cytosolic enzyme. The effect of barbiturates on ALA synthetase can cause dangerous disease exacerbations in persons with intermittent porphyria.

KIDNEY. Severe oliguria or anuria may occur in acute barbiturate poisoning largely as a result of the marked hypotension.

THERAPEUTIC USES

The major uses of individual barbiturates are listed in Table 17–2. As with the benzodiazepines, the selection of a particular barbiturate for a given therapeutic indication is based primarily on pharmacokinetic considerations. Benzodiazepines and other compounds for sedation have largely replaced barbiturates.

UNTOWARD EFFECTS

After-Effects. Drowsiness may last for only a few hours after a hypnotic dose of barbiturate, but residual CNS depression sometimes is evident the following day, and subtle distortions of mood and impairment of judgment and fine motor skills may be demonstrable. Residual effects also may take the form of vertigo, nausea, vomiting, or diarrhea, or sometimes may be manifested as overt excitement.

Paradoxical Excitement. In some persons, barbiturates produce excitement rather than depression, and the patient may appear to be inebriated. This type of idiosyncrasy is relatively common among geriatric and debilitated patients and occurs most frequently with phenobarbital and *N*-methylbarbiturates. Barbiturates may cause restlessness, excitement, and even delirium when given in the presence of pain and may worsen a patient's perception of pain.

Hypersensitivity. Allergic reactions occur, especially in persons with asthma, urticaria, angioedema, or similar conditions. Hypersensitivity reactions include localized swellings, particularly of the eyelids, cheeks, or lips, and erythematous dermatitis. Rarely, exfoliative dermatitis may be caused by phenobarbital and can prove fatal; the skin eruption may be associated with fever, delirium, and marked degenerative changes in the liver and other parenchymatous organs.

DRUG INTERACTIONS. Barbiturates combine with other CNS depressants to cause severe depression; ethanol is the most frequent offender, and interactions with first-generation antihistamines also are common. Isoniazid, methylphenidate, and monoamine oxidase inhibitors also increase the CNS-depressant effects.

Barbiturates competitively inhibit the metabolism of certain other drugs; however, the greatest number of drug interactions results from induction of hepatic CYPs (as described above) and the accelerated disappearance of many drugs and endogenous substances. Hepatic enzyme induction enhances metabolism of endogenous steroid hormones, which may cause endocrine disturbances, as well as of oral contraceptives, which may result in unwanted pregnancy. Barbiturates also induce the hepatic generation of toxic metabolites of chlorocarbons (chloroform, trichloroethylene, carbon tetrachloride) and consequently promote lipid peroxidation, which facilitates periportal necrosis of the liver caused by these agents.

Other Untoward Effects. Because barbiturates enhance porphyrin synthesis, they are absolutely contraindicated in patients with acute intermittent porphyria or porphyria variegata. Hypnotic doses, in the presence of pulmonary insufficiency are contraindicated. Rapid intravenous injection of a barbiturate may cause cardiovascular collapse before anesthesia ensues. Blood pressure can fall to shock levels; even slow intravenous injection of barbiturates often produces apnea and occasionally laryngospasm, coughing, and other respiratory difficulties.

BARBITURATE POISONING. Most of the cases are the result of attempts at suicide, but some are from accidental poisonings in children or in drug abusers. The lethal dose of barbiturate varies, but severe poisoning is likely to occur when >10 times the full hypnotic dose has been ingested at once. The lethal dose becomes lower if alcohol or other depressant drugs also are present. The treatment of acute barbiturate intoxication is based on general supportive measures, which are applicable in most respects to poisoning by any CNS depressant. If renal and cardiac functions are satisfactory, and the patient is hydrated, forced diuresis and alkalinization of the urine will hasten the excretion of phenobarbital. *See* Chapter 4, *Drug Toxicity and Poisoning*.

MISCELLANEOUS SEDATIVE-HYPNOTIC DRUGS

Many drugs with diverse structures have been used for their sedative-hypnotic properties, including ramelteon, chloral hydrate, meprobamate, and paraldehyde. With the exception of ramelteon and meprobamate, the pharmacological actions of these drugs generally resemble those of the barbiturates: they all are general CNS depressants that can produce profound hypnosis with little or no analgesia; their effects on the stages of sleep are similar to those of the barbiturates; their therapeutic index is limited, and acute intoxication, which produces respiratory depression and hypotension, is managed similarly to barbiturate poisoning; their chronic use can result in tolerance and physical dependence; and the syndrome after chronic use can be severe and life-threatening.

CHLORAL HYDRATE. Chloral hydrate may be used to treat patients with paradoxical reactions to benzodiazepines. Chloral hydrate is reduced rapidly to the active compound, trichloroethanol (CCl_3CH_2OH), largely by hepatic alcohol dehydrogenase. Its pharmacological effects probably are caused by trichloroethanol, which can exert barbiturate-like effects on $GABA_A$ receptor channels in vitro.

Chloral hydrate is best known in the U.S. as a literary poison, the "knock-out drops" added to a strong alcoholic beverage to produce a "Mickey Finn" or "Mickey," a cocktail given to an unwitting imbiber to render him malleable or unconscious, most famously Sam Spade in Dashiell Hammett's 1930 novel, *The Maltese Falcon*. Now that detectives drink white wine rather than whiskey, this off-label use of chloral hydrate has waned.

MEPROBAMATE. Meprobamate a *bis*-carbamate ester, was introduced as an antianxiety agent and this remains its only approved use in the U.S. However, it also became popular as a sedative-hypnotic agent. The pharmacological properties of meprobamate resemble those of the benzodiazepines in a number of ways. Meprobamate can release suppressed behaviors in experimental animals at doses that cause little impairment of locomotor activity, and although it can cause depression of the CNS, it cannot produce anesthesia. Large doses of meprobamate cause severe respiratory depression, hypotension, shock, and heart failure. Meprobamate appears to have a mild analgesic effect in patients with musculoskeletal pain, and it enhances the analgesic effects of other drugs.

Meprobamate is well absorbed when administered orally. Nevertheless, an important aspect of intoxication with meprobamate is the formation of gastric bezoars consisting of undissolved meprobamate tablets; hence treatment may require endoscopy, with mechanical removal of the bezoar. Most of the drug is metabolized in the liver, mainly to a side-chain hydroxy derivative and a glucuronide; the kinetics of elimination may depend on the dose. The $t_{1/2}$ of meprobamate may be prolonged during its chronic administration, even though the drug can induce some hepatic CYPs.

The major unwanted effects of the usual sedative doses of meprobamate are drowsiness and ataxia; larger doses impair learning and motor coordination and prolongation of reaction time. Meprobamate enhances the CNS depression produced by other drugs. The abuse of meprobamate has continued despite a substantial decrease in the clinical use of the drug. Carisoprodol (SOMA), a skeletal muscle relaxant whose active metabolite is meprobamate, also has abuse potential and has become a popular "street drug."

PARALDEHYDE. Paraldehyde is a polymer of acetaldehyde, basically a cyclic polyether. It has a strong odor and a disagreeable taste. Orally, it is irritating to the throat and stomach, and it is not administered parenterally because of its injurious effects on tissues. Use of paraldehyde has been discontinued in the U.S.

OTHER AGENTS. *Etomidate* (AMIDATE, generic) is used in the U.S. and other countries as an intravenous anesthetic, often in combination with fentanyl. It is advantageous because it lacks pulmonary and vascular depressant activity, although it has a negative inotropic effect on the heart. Its pharmacology and anesthetic uses are described in Chapter 19. *Clomethiazole* has sedative, muscle relaxant, and anticonvulsant properties. Given alone, its effects on respiration are slight, and the therapeutic index is high. However, deaths from adverse interactions with ethanol are relatively frequent. *Propofol* (DIPRIVAN) is a rapidly acting and highly lipophilic diisopropylphenol used in the induction and maintenance of general anesthesia (*see* Chapter 19), as well as in the maintenance of long-term sedation.

NONPRESCRIPTION HYPNOTIC DRUGS. The antihistamines diphenhydramine and doxylamine are FDA-approved as ingredients in over-the-counter (OTC) nonprescription sleep aids. With elimination $t_{1/2}$ of ~9-10 h, these antihistamines can be associated with prominent residual daytime sleepiness when taken the prior evening as a sleep aid.

MANAGEMENT OF INSOMNIA

The "perfect" hypnotic would allow sleep to occur with normal sleep architecture rather than produce a pharmacologically altered sleep pattern. It would not cause next-day effects, either of rebound anxiety or of continued sedation. It would not interact with other medications. It could be used chronically without causing dependence or rebound insomnia on discontinuation. Controversy in the management of insomnia revolves around 2 issues:

- Pharmacological versus nonpharmacological treatment
- Use of short-acting versus long-acting hypnotics

CATEGORIES OF INSOMNIA

- *Transient insomnia* lasts <3 days and usually is caused by a brief environmental or situational stressor.
- *Short-term insomnia* lasts from 3 days to 3 weeks and usually is caused by a personal stressor such as illness, grief, or job problems. Hypnotics are best used intermittently during this time, with the patient skipping a dose after 1-2 nights of good sleep.
- *Long-term insomnia* is insomnia that has lasted for >3 weeks; no specific stressor may be identifiable.

Insomnia Accompanying Major Psychiatric Illnesses. The insomnia caused by major psychiatric illnesses often responds to specific pharmacological treatment for that illness. In major depressive episodes with insomnia, e.g., the selective serotonin reuptake inhibitors, which may cause insomnia as a side effect, usually will result in improved sleep because they treat the depressive syndrome. In patients whose depression is responding to the serotonin reuptake inhibitor but who have persistent insomnia as a side effect of the medication, judicious use of evening trazodone may improve sleep, as well as augment the antidepressant effect of the reuptake inhibitor. However, the patient should be monitored for priapism, orthostatic hypotension, and arrhythmias.

Adequate control of anxiety in patients with anxiety disorders often produces adequate resolution of the accompanying insomnia. The profound insomnia of patients with acute psychosis owing to schizophrenia or mania usually responds to dopamine-receptor antagonists (*see* Chapters 13 and 16). Benzodiazepines often are used adjunctively in this situation to reduce agitation and improved sleep.

Insomnia Accompanying Other Medical Illnesses. For long-term insomnia owing to other medical illnesses, adequate treatment of the underlying disorder, such as congestive heart failure, asthma, or COPD, may resolve the insomnia. Adequate pain management in conditions of chronic pain will treat both the pain and the insomnia and may make hypnotics unnecessary. *Adequate attention to sleep hygiene, including reduced caffeine intake, avoidance of alcohol, adequate exercise, and regular sleep and wake times, often will reduce the insomnia.*

Long-Term Insomnia. Nonpharmacological treatments are important for all patients with long-term insomnia. These include education about sleep hygiene, relaxation training, and behavioral-modification approaches, such as sleep-restriction and stimulus-control therapies.

Long-term hypnotic use leads to a decrease in effectiveness and may produce rebound insomnia on discontinuance. Almost all hypnotics change sleep architecture. The barbiturates reduce REM sleep; the benzodiazepines reduce slow-wave non-REM sleep and, to a lesser extent, REM sleep. While the significance of these findings is not clear, there is an emerging consensus that slow-wave sleep is particularly important for physical restorative processes. REM sleep may aid in the consolidation of learning. The blockade of slow-wave sleep by benzodiazepines may partly account for their diminishing effectiveness over the long term, and it also may explain their effectiveness in blocking sleep terrors, a disorder of arousal from slow-wave sleep.

Long-acting benzodiazepines can cause next-day confusion, whereas shorter-acting agents can produce rebound next-day anxiety. Paradoxically, the acute amnestic effects of benzodiazepines may be responsible for the patient's subsequent report of restful sleep. Anterograde amnesia may be more common with triazolam. Hypnotics should not be given to patients with sleep apnea, especially of the obstructive type, because these agents decrease upper airway muscle tone while also decreasing the arousal response to hypoxia.

Insomnia in Older Patients. The elderly, like the very young, tend to sleep in a *polyphasic* (multiple sleep episodes per day) pattern rather than the *monophasic* pattern characteristic of younger adults. This pattern makes assessment of adequate sleep time difficult. Changes in the pharmacokinetic profiles of hypnotic agents occur in the elderly because of reduced body water, reduced renal function, and increased body fat, leading to a longer $t_{1/2}$ for benzodiazepines. A dose that produces pleasant sleep and adequate daytime wakefulness during week 1 may produce daytime confusion and amnesia by week 3 as the level continues to rise, particularly with long-acting hypnotics.

MANAGEMENT OF PATIENTS AFTER LONG-TERM TREATMENT WITH HYPNOTIC AGENTS. If a benzodiazepine has been used regularly for >2 weeks, it should be tapered rather than discontinued abruptly. In some patients on hypnotics with a short $t_{1/2}$, it is easier to switch first to a hypnotic with a long $t_{1/2}$ and then to taper.

PRESCRIBING GUIDELINES FOR THE MANAGEMENT OF INSOMNIA. Hypnotics that act at $GABA_A$ receptors, including the benzodiazepine hypnotics and the newer agents zolpidem, zopiclone, and zaleplon, are preferred to barbiturates because they have a greater therapeutic index, have smaller effects on sleep architecture, and have less abuse potential. Compounds with a shorter $t_{1/2}$ are favored in patients with sleep-onset insomnia but without significant daytime anxiety who need to function at full effectiveness during the day. These compounds also are appropriate for the elderly because of a decreased risk of falls and respiratory depression. Benzodiazepines with longer $t_{1/2}$ are favored for patients who have significant daytime anxiety. However, longer-acting benzodiazepines can be associated with next-day cognitive impairment or delayed daytime cognitive impairment (after 2-4 weeks of treatment) as a result of drug accumulation with repeated administration.

Older agents such as barbiturates, chloral hydrate, and meprobamate should be avoided for the management of insomnia. They have high abuse potential and are dangerous in overdose.

For a complete Bibliographical Listing see Goodman & Gilman's ***The Pharmacological Basis of Therapeutics***, 12th ed., or Goodman & Gilman Online at www.AccessMedicine.com.

Opioids, Analgesia, and Pain Management

Pain is a component of virtually all clinical pathologies, and management of pain is a primary clinical imperative. Opioids are a mainstay of pain treatment, but depending upon the pain state, therapy may involve NSAIDs, anticonvulsants, or antidepressants.

The term *opiate* refers to compounds structurally related to products found in opium derived from the resin of the opium poppy, *Papaver somniferum*. Opiates include the natural plant alkaloids, such as morphine, codeine, thebaine, and many semisynthetic derivatives. An *opioid* is any agent that has the functional and pharmacological properties of an opiate. Endogenous opioids are naturally occurring ligands for opioid receptors found in animals. The term *endorphin* is used synonymously with *endogenous opioid peptides* but also refers to a specific endogenous opioid, β-*endorphin*. Although the term *narcotic* originally referred to any drug that induced narcosis or sleep, the word has become associated with opioids and is often used in a legal context to refer to substances with abuse or addictive potential.

ENDOGENOUS OPIOID PEPTIDES

Several distinct families of endogenous opioids peptides have been identified: principally the *enkephalins, endorphins,* and *dynorphins* (Table 18–1). These families have several common properties:

- Each derives from a distinct precursor protein, pre-pro-opiomelanocortin (pre-POMC), preproenkephalin, and preprodynorphin, respectively, encoded by a corresponding gene.
- Each precursor is subject to complex cleavages by distinct trypsin-like enzymes, and to a variety of posttranslational modifications resulting in the synthesis of multiple peptides, some of which are active.
- Most opioid peptides with activity at a receptor share the common amino-terminal sequence of Tyr-Gly-Gly-Phe-(Met or Leu) followed by various C-terminal extensions yielding peptides of 5-31 residues; the endomorphins, with different terminal sequences, are exceptions.

The opioid peptide precursors are a protean family (Figure 18–1). The major opioid peptide derived from *POMC* is *the potent opioid agonist,* β-*endorphin*. The *POMC* sequence also is processed into a variety of nonopioid peptides including adrenocorticotropic hormone (ACTH), melanocyte-stimulating hormone (α-MSH), and β-lipotropin (β-LPH). Although β-endorphin contains the sequence for met-enkephalin at its amino terminus, it is not converted to this peptide. *Proenkephalin* contains multiple copies of *met-enkephalin*, as well as a single copy of *leu-enkephalin*. *Prodynorphin* contains 3 peptides of differing lengths that all begin with the leu-enkephalin sequence: *dynorphin A, dynorphin B, and neoendorphin*. *Nociceptin peptide* or *orphanin FQ* (now termed N/OFQ) shares structural similarity with dynorphin A.

Endomorphins belong to a novel family of peptides that include*: endomorphin-1* (Tyr-Pro-Trp-Phe-NH_2) and *endomorphin-2* (Tyr-Pro-Phe-Phe-NH_2). Endomorphins have an atypical structure and display selectivity towards the μ opioid receptor. *Several points should be stressed*:

- Not all cells that make a given opioid prohormone precursor store and release the same mixture of opioid peptides; this results from differential processing secondary to variations in the cellular complement of peptidases that produce and degrade the active opioid fragments.
- Processing of these peptides is altered by physiological demands, leading to the release of a different mix of posttranslationally derived peptides by a given cell under different conditions.
- Opioid peptides are found in plasma and reflect release from secretory systems such as the pituitary and the adrenals that do not reflect neuraxial release. Conversely, levels of these peptides in brain/spinal cord and in cerebrospinal fluid (CSF) arise from neuraxial systems and not from peripheral systems.

OPIOID RECEPTORS

The 3 opioid receptors—μ, δ, and κ (MOR, DOR, and KOR)—belong to the rhodopsin family of GPCRs (*see* Chapter 3) and share extensive sequence homologies (55-58%). Highly selective agonists have been developed that show specific affinity for the respective binding site (e.g., DAMGO

Table 18–1

Endogenous Opioid Peptides

OPIOID LIGANDS	RECEPTOR TYPES μ	δ	κ
Met-enkephalin (**Tyr-Gly-Gly-Phe-Met**)	++	+++	
Leu-enkephalin (**Tyr-Gly-Gly-Phe-Leu**)	++	+++	
β-Endorphin (**Tyr-Gly-Gly-Phe-Met**-Thr-Ser-Glu-Lys-Ser-Gln-Thr-Pro-Leu-Val-Thr-Leu-Phe-Lys-Asn-Ala-Ile-Ile-Lys-Asn-Ala-Tyr-Lys-Lys-Gly-Glu)	+++	+++	
Dynorphin A (**Tyr-Gly-Gly-Phe-Leu**-Arg-Arg-Ile-Arg-Pro-Lys-Leu-Lys-Trp-Asp-Asn-Gln)	++		+++
Dynorphin B (**Tyr-Gly-Gly-Phe-Leu**-Arg-Arg-Gln-Phe-Lys-Val-Val-Thr)	+	+	+++
α-Neoendorphin (**Tyr-Gly-Gly-Phe-Leu**-Arg-Lys-Tyr-Pro-Lys)	+	+	+++
Endomorphin-1 (Tyr-Pro-Trp-Phe-NH_2)	+++		
Nociceptin (orphanin FQ) (Phe-Gly-Gly-Phe-Thr-Gly-Ala-Arg-Lys-Ser-Ala-Arg-Lys-Leu-Ala-Asn-Gln)	–	–	–

+, agonist; –, antagonist. + < ++ < +++ in potency.

Source: Reproduced with permission from Raynor K et al. Pharmacological characterization of the cloned kappa-, delta-, and mu-opioid receptors. Mol Pharmacol, 1994;45:330–334.

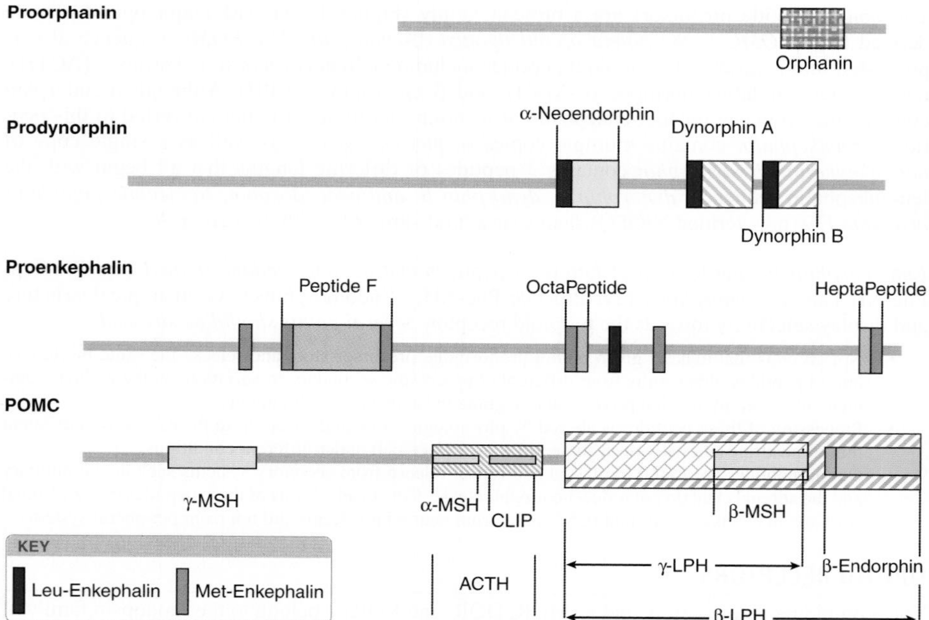

Figure 18–1 *Peptide precursors.* (Reproduced with permission from Akil H, Owens C, Gustein H, et al. Endogenous opioids: Overview and current issues. *Drug Alcohol Depend*, 1998;51:127-140. Copyright © Elsevier.)

Table 18–2
Opioid Agonists

OPIOID LIGANDS	RECEPTOR TYPES μ	δ	κ
Etorphine	+++	+++	+++
Fentanyl	+++		
Hydromorphone	+++		+
Levorphanol	+++		
Methadone	+++		
Morphine[a]	+++		+
Sufentanil	+++	+	+
DAMGO[a] ([D-Ala^2,MePhe^4,Gly(ol)^5] enkephalin)	+++		
DPDPE[b] ([D-Pen^2,D-Pen^5]enkephalin)		++	
[D-Ala^2,Glu^4]deltorphin		++	
DSLET ([D-Ser^2,Leu^5]enkephalin-Thr^6)	+	++	
SNC80		++	
Bremazocine	+++	++	+++
Buprenorphine	P		– –
Butorphanol	P		+++
Ethylketocyclazocine	P	+	+++
Nalbuphine	– –		++
Spiradoline[c]	+		+++
U50,488[c]			+++
U69,593[c]			+++

+, agonist; –, antagonist; P, partial agonist. + < ++ < +++ in potency.
[a]Protoypical μ-preferring. [b]Prototypical δ-preferring. [c]Prototypical κ-preferring.
Source: Reproduced with permission from Raynor K et al. Pharmacological characterization of the cloned kappa-, delta-, and mu-opioid receptors. Mol Pharmacol, 1994;45:330–334.

for μ, DPDPE for δ, and U-50,488, and U-69,593 for κ) (Table 18–2). Commonly used antagonists (Table 18–3) include cyclic analogs of somatostatin such as CTOP as a μ receptor antagonist, a derivative of naloxone called naltrindole as a δ receptor antagonist, and a bivalent derivative of naltrexone called nor-binaltorphimine (nor-BNI) as a κ-receptor antagonist.

In the membrane, opiate receptors can form both homo- and heterodimers. Dimerization can alter the pharmacological properties of the respective receptors. Splice variants exist within each of the 3 opioid receptor families, and this alternative splicing of receptor transcripts may be crucial for the diversity of opioid receptors. Given the functional importance of the intracellular components of the GPCRs, it is not surprising that significant differences exist for the receptor isoforms in terms of agonist-induced G protein activation and receptor internalization.

An opiate receptor-like protein (ORL1 or NOP) was cloned based on its structural homology (48-49% identity) to other members of the opioid receptor family; it is G-protein coupled, has an endogenous ligand (nociception/orphanin, FQ: N/OFQ), but does not display an opioid pharmacology.

Table 18–3

Opioid Antagonists

OPIOID LIGANDS	RECEPTOR TYPES μ	δ	κ
Naloxone[a]	− − −	−	− −
Naltrexone[a]	− − −	−	− − −
CTOP[b]	− − −		
Diprenorphine	− − −	− −	− − −
β-Funaltrexamine[b,c]	− − −	−	++
Naloxonazine	− − −	−	−
nor-Binaltorphimine	−	−	− − −
Naltrindole[d]	−	− − −	−
Naloxone benzoylhydrazone	− − −	−	−

+, agonist; −, antagonist. − < − − < − − − in potency.
[a]Universal ligand. [b]Prototypical μ-preferring. [c]Irreversible ligand. [d]Prototypical δ-preferring.
Source: Reproduced with permission from Raynor K et al. Pharmacological characterization of the cloned kappa-, delta-, and mu-opioid receptors. Mol Pharmacol, 1994;45:330–334.

OPIATE RECEPTOR SIGNALING

The μ, δ, and κ receptors couple through pertussis toxin-sensitive, G_i/G_o proteins (but occasionally to G_s or G_z). Upon receptor activation, the G_i/G_o coupling results in a large number of intracellular events, including:

- Inhibition of adenylyl cyclase activity
- Reduced opening of voltage-gated Ca^{2+} channels (reduces neurotransmitter release from presynaptic terminals)
- Stimulation of K^+ current through several channels including G protein-activated inwardly rectifying K^+ channels (GIRKs) (hyperpolarizes and inhibits postsynaptic neurons)
- Activation of PKC and PLC_β

FUNCTIONAL CONSEQUENCES OF ACUTE AND CHRONIC OPIATE RECEPTOR ACTIVATION

The loss of effect with exposure to opiates occurs over short- and long-term intervals.

INTERNALIZATION. μ and δ receptors can undergo rapid agonist-mediated internalization via a classic endocytic, β-arrestin-mediated pathway, whereas κ receptors do not internalize after prolonged agonist exposure. Internalization of the μ and δ receptors may be induced differentially as a function of the structure of the ligand.

DESENSITIZATION. In the face of a transient activation (minutes to hours), acute tolerance or desensitization occurs that is specific for that receptor and disappears with a time course parallel to the clearance of the agonist. Short-term desensitization probably involves phosphorylation of the receptors resulting in an uncoupling of the receptor from its G-protein and/or internalization of the receptor.

TOLERANCE. Here tolerance refers to a decrease in the apparent effectiveness of a drug with continuous or repeated agonist administration (days to weeks), that, following removal of the agonist, disappears over several weeks. This tolerance is reflected by a reduction in the maximum achievable effect or a right shift in the dose-effect curve. This loss of effect with persistent exposure to an opiate agonist has several key properties:

- Different physiological responses develop tolerance at different rates. Thus, at the organ system level, some end points show little or no tolerance development (pupillary miosis), some show moderate tolerance (constipation, emesis, analgesia, sedation), and some show rapid tolerance (euphorigenic).
- In general, opiate agonists of a given class will typically show a reduced response in a system rendered tolerant to another agent of that class (e.g., cross-tolerance between the μ agonists, such as morphine and fentanyl). This cross-tolerance is not consistent or complete, thereby forming the basis for the switching between opioid drugs in clinical therapy.

DEPENDENCE. Dependence represents a state of adaptation manifested by receptor/drug class-specific withdrawal syndrome produced by cessation of drug exposure (e.g., by drug abstinence) or administration of an antagonist (e.g., naloxone). At the organ system level, withdrawal is manifested by significant somatomotor and autonomic outflow (reflected by agitation, hyperalgesia, hyperthermia, hypertension, diarrhea, pupillary dilation, and release of virtually all pituitary and adrenomedullary hormones) and by affective symptoms (dysphoria, anxiety, and depression).

ADDICTION. Addiction is a behavioral pattern characterized by compulsive use of a drug. The positive, rewarding effects of opiates are considered to be the driving component for initiating the recreational use of opiates. This positive reward property is subject to the development of tolerance. Given the aversive nature of withdrawal symptoms, avoidance and alleviation of withdrawal symptoms may become a primary motivation for compulsive drug taking. Drug dependence is *not* synonymous with drug addiction. Tolerance and dependence are physiological responses seen in all patients but are not predictors of addiction (*see* Chapter 24). For example, cancer pain often requires prolonged treatment with high doses of opioids, leading to tolerance and dependence. Yet abuse in this setting is considered to be unusual.

MECHANISMS OF TOLERANCE/DEPENDENCE-WITHDRAWAL. The mechanisms underlying chronic tolerance and dependence/withdrawal are controversial. Several types of events may to contribute.

Receptor Disposition. Acute desensitization or receptor internalization may play a role in the initiation of chronic tolerance but is not sufficient to explain persistent changes observed with chronic exposure. Thus, morphine, unlike other μ agonists, does not promote μ receptor internalization or receptor phosphorylation and desensitization. Receptor desensitization and downregulation are agonist specific. Endocytosis and sequestration of receptors do not invariably lead to receptor degradation but can also result in receptor dephosphorylation and recycling to the surface of the cell. Accordingly, opioid tolerance may not be related to receptor desensitization but rather to a lack of desensitization. Agonists that rapidly internalize opioid receptors also would rapidly desensitize signaling, but this desensitization would be at least partially reset by recycling of "reactivated" opioid receptors.

Adaptation of Intracellular Signaling Mechanisms in the Opioid Receptor-Bearing Neurons. Coupling of MOR to cellular effectors, such as inhibition of adenylyl cyclase, activation of inwardly rectifying K^+ channels, inhibition of Ca^{2+} currents, and inhibition of terminal release of transmitters demonstrates functional uncoupling of receptor occupancy from effector function. Importantly, the chronic opioid effect initiates adaptive counter-regulatory change. The best example of such cellular counter-regulatory processes is the rebound increase in cellular cyclic AMP levels produced by "superactivation" of adenylyl cyclase and upregulation of the amount of enzyme.

System Level Counter-Adaptation. With chronic opiate exposure, there is a loss of drug effect; this may reflect an enhanced excitability of the regulated link. Thus, tolerance to the analgesic action of chronically administered μ opiates may result in an activation of bulbospinal pathways that increases the excitability of spinal dorsal horn pain transmission linkages. With chronic opiate exposure, opiate receptor occupancy will lead to the activation of PKC, which can phosphorylate and, accordingly, enhance the activation of local NMDA glutamate receptors (*see* Chapter 14). These receptors mediate a facilitated state leading to enhanced spinal pain processing. Blocking of these receptors can at least partially attenuate the loss of analgesic efficacy with continued opiate exposure. These system level counter-adaptation hypotheses represent mechanisms that may apply to specific systems (e.g., pain modulation) but not necessarily to others (e.g., sedation or miosis).

EFFECTS OF CLINICALLY USED OPIOIDS

Opiates, depending on their receptor specificities, produce a variety of effects consistent with the role played by the organ systems with which the receptors are associated. Although the primary clinical use of opioids is for their pain-relieving properties, opioids produce a host of other effects. This is not surprising in view of the wide distribution of opioid receptors in the brain and the periphery.

ANALGESIA. Morphine-like drugs produce *analgesia*, *drowsiness*, and *euphoria* (changes in mood, and mental clouding). When therapeutic doses of morphine are given to patients with pain, they report the pain to be less intense or entirely gone. In addition to relief of distress, some patients may experience euphoria. Analgesia often occurs without loss of consciousness, though drowsiness commonly occurs. Morphine at these doses does not have anticonvulsant activity and usually does not cause slurred speech, emotional lability, or significant motor uncoordination. When morphine in an analgesic dose is given to normal, pain-free individuals, the patients may report the drug experience to be frankly unpleasant. There may be drowsiness, difficulty in mentation, apathy, and lessened physical activity. As the dose is increased, the subjective, analgesic, and toxic effects, including respiratory depression, become more pronounced. The relief of pain by morphine-like opioids is selective in that other sensory modalities, such as light touch, proprioception, and the sense of moderate temperatures, are unaffected. Low doses of morphine produce reductions in the affective but not the perceived intensity of pain. Continuous dull pain (as generated by tissue injury and inflammation) is relieved more effectively than sharp intermittent (incident) pain, such as that associated with the movement of an inflamed joint, but with sufficient amounts of opioid it is possible to relieve even the severe piercing pain associated with acute renal or biliary colic.

PAIN STATES AND MECHANISMS UNDERLYING DIFFERENT PAIN STATES

Acute Nociception. Acute activation of small high-threshold sensory afferents (Aδ and C fibers) generates transient input into the spinal cord, which in turn leads to activation of neurons that project contralaterally to the thalamus and thence to the somatosensory cortex. A parallel spinofugal projection is to the medial thalamus and from there to the anterior cingulate cortex, part of the limbic system. The output produced by acutely activating this ascending system is sufficient to evoke pain reports. Examples of such stimuli include a hot coffee cup, a needle stick, or an incision.

Tissue Injury. Following tissue injury or local inflammation (e.g., local skin burn, toothache, rheumatoid joint), an ongoing pain state arises that is characterized by burning, throbbing, or aching and an abnormal pain response (hyperalgesia) and can be evoked by otherwise innocuous or mildly aversive stimuli (tepid bathwater on a sunburn; moderate extension of an injured joint). This pain typically reflects the effects of active factors (such as prostaglandins, bradykinin, cytokines, and H^+ ions, among many mediators) released into the injury site, which have the ability to activate the terminal of small high-threshold afferents (Aδ and C fibers) and to reduce the stimulus intensity required to activate these sensory afferents (peripheral sensitization). In addition, the ongoing afferent traffic initiated by the injury leads to the activation of spinal facilitatory cascades, yielding a greater output to the brain for any given input. This facilitation is thought to underlie the hyperalgesic states. Such tissue injury-evoked pain is often referred to as "nociceptive" pain (Figure 18–2).

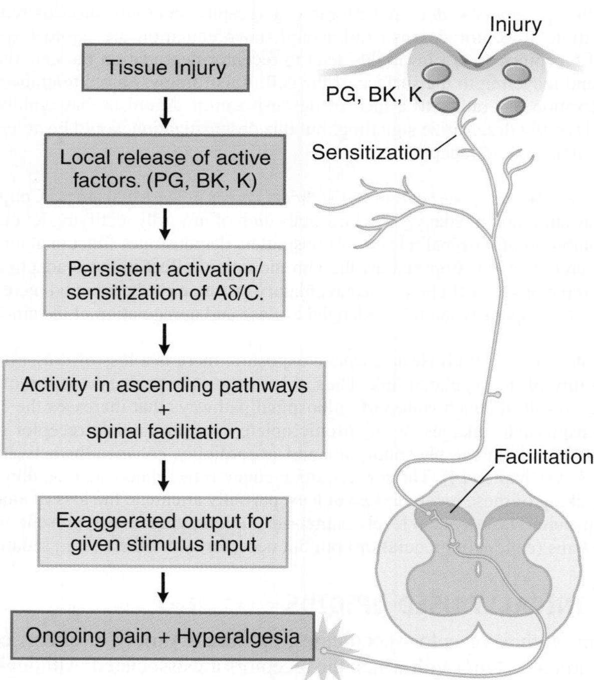

Figure 18–2 *Mechanisms of tissue injury-evoked nociception.*

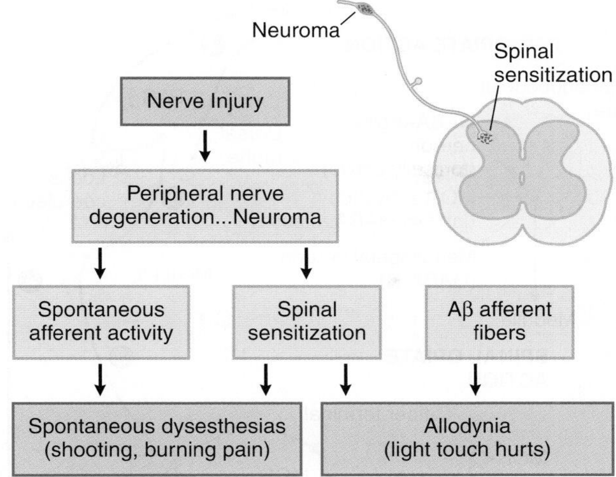

Figure 18–3 *Mechanisms of nerve injury-evoked nociception.*

Examples of such states would be burn, post-incision, abrasion of the skin, inflammation of the joint, and musculoskeletal injury.

Nerve Injury. Injury to the peripheral nerve yields complex anatomical and biochemical changes in the nerve and spinal cord that induce spontaneous dysesthesias (shooting, burning pain) and allodynia (light touch hurts). This nerve injury pain state may not depend on the activation of small afferents, but may be initiated by low-threshold sensory afferents (e.g., Aβ fibers). Such nerve injuries result in the development of ectopic activity arising from neuromas formed by nerve injury and the dorsal root ganglia of the injured axons as well as a dorsal horn reorganization, such that low-threshold afferent input carried by Aβ fibers evokes a pain state. Examples of such nerve injury-inducing events include nerve trauma or compression (carpal tunnel syndrome), chemotherapy (as for cancer), diabetes, and in the post-herpetic state (shingles). These pain states are said to be neuropathic (Figure 18–3). Many clinical pain syndromes, such as found in cancer, typically represent a combination of these inflammatory and neuropathic mechanisms. Although nociceptive pain usually is responsive to opioid analgesics, neuropathic pain is typically considered to respond less well to opioid analgesics.

Sensory Versus Affective Dimensions. When pain does not evoke its usual responses (anxiety, fear, panic, and suffering), a patient's ability to tolerate the pain may be markedly increased, even when the capacity to perceive the sensation is relatively unaltered. It is clear, however, that alteration of the emotional reaction to painful stimuli is not the sole mechanism of analgesia. Thus, intrathecal administration of opioids can produce profound segmental analgesia without causing significant alteration of motor or sensory function or subjective effects.

MECHANISMS OF OPIOID-INDUCED ANALGESIA. The analgesic actions of opiates after systemic delivery represent actions in the brain, spinal cord, and in some instances in the periphery.

Supraspinal Actions. Microinjections of morphine into the mesencephalic periaqueductal gray (PAG) matter region will block nociceptive responses; naloxone will reverse these effects. Several mechanisms exist whereby opiates with an action limited to the PAG may act to alter nociceptive transmission. These are summarized in Figure 18–4. MOR agonists block release of the inhibitory transmitter GABA from tonically active PAG systems that regulate activity in projections to the medulla. PAG projections to the medulla activate medullospinal release of NE and 5HT at the level of the spinal dorsal horn. This release can attenuate dorsal horn excitability. Interestingly, this PAG organization can also serve to increase excitability of dorsal raphe and locus coeruleus from which ascending serotonergic and noradrenergic projections to the limbic forebrain originate.

Spinal Opiate Action. A local action of opiates in the spinal cord will selectively depress the discharge of spinal dorsal horn neurons evoked by small (high-threshold) but not large (low-threshold) afferent nerve fibers. Intrathecal administration of opioids in animals ranging from mouse to human will reliably attenuate the response of the organism to a variety of somatic and visceral stimuli that otherwise evoke pain states. Specific opiate binding and receptor protein are limited for the most part to the substantia gelatinosa of the superficial dorsal horn, the region in which small, high-threshold sensory afferents show their principal termination. A significant proportion of these opiate receptors are associated with small peptidergic primary afferent C fibers; the remainder are on local dorsal horn neurons.

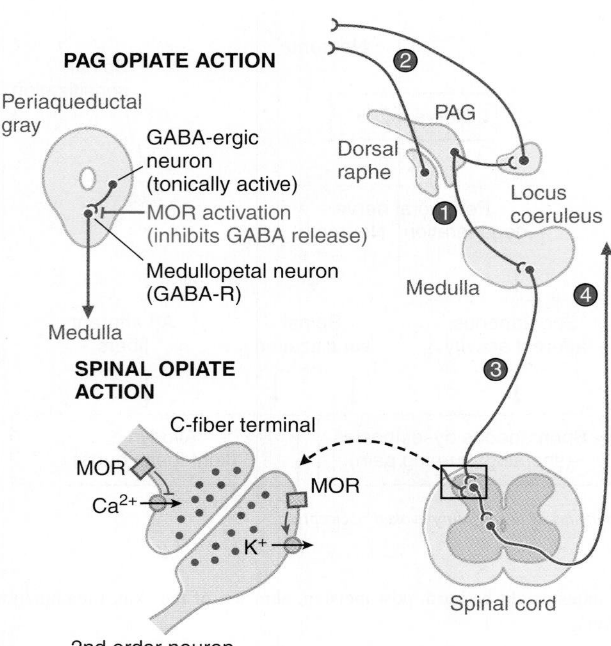

Figure 18–4 *Mechanisms of opiate action in producing analgesia. Top left*: Schematic of organization of opiate action in the periaqueductal gray. *Top right*: Opiate-sensitive pathways in PAG μ-opiate actions block the release of GABA from tonically active systems that otherwise regulate the projections to the medulla (1) leading to an activation of PAG outflow resulting in activation of forebrain (2) and spinal (3) monoamine receptors that regulate spinal cord projections (4), which provide sensory input to higher centers and mood. *Bottom left*: Schematic of primary afferent synapse with second-order dorsal horn spinal neuron, showing pre- and postsynaptic opiate receptors coupled to Ca^{2+} and K^+ channels, respectively. Opiate-receptor binding is highly expressed in the superficial spinal dorsal horn (substantia gelatinosa). These receptors are located presynaptically on the terminals of small primary afferents (C fibers) and postsynaptically on second-order neurons. Presynaptically, activation of MOR blocks the opening of the voltage-sensitive Ca^{2+} channel, which otherwise initiates transmitter release. Postsynaptically, MOR activation enhances opening of K^+ channels, leading to hyperpolarization. Thus, an opiate agonist acting at these sites jointly serves to attenuate the afferent-evoked excitation of the second-order neuron.

Spinal opiates reduce the release of primary afferent peptide transmitters such as substance P contained in small afferents. The presynaptic action corresponds to the ability of opiates to prevent the opening of voltage-sensitive Ca^{2+} channels, thereby preventing transmitter release. A postsynaptic action is demonstrated by the ability of opiates to block excitation of dorsal horn neurons directly evoked by glutamate, reflecting a direct activation of dorsal horn projection neurons. The activation of K^+ channels in these postsynaptic neurons, leading to hyperpolarization, is consistent with a direct postsynaptic inhibition. The joint capacity of spinal opiates to reduce the release of excitatory neurotransmitters from C fibers and to decrease the excitability of dorsal horn neurons is believed to account for the powerful and selective effect of opiates on spinal nociceptive processing. A variety of opiates delivered spinally (intrathecally or epidurally) can induce a powerful analgesia that is reversed by low doses of systemic naloxone.

Peripheral Action. Direct application of opiates to a peripheral nerve can, in fact, produce a local anesthetic-like action at high concentrations, but this is not naloxone reversible and is believed to reflect a "nonspecific" action. Conversely, direct injection of these agents into peripheral sites have demonstrated that under conditions of inflammation, where there is an increased terminal sensitivity leading to an exaggerated pain response (e.g., hyperalgesia), the local action of opiates can exert a normalizing effect on the exaggerated thresholds. Whether the effects are uniquely on the afferent terminal, whether the opiate acts on inflammatory cells that release products that sensitize the nerve terminal, or both, is not known.

MOOD ALTERATIONS AND REWARDING PROPERTIES. The mechanisms by which opioids produce euphoria, tranquility, and other alterations of mood (including rewarding properties) are complex and not entirely clear. Neural systems that mediate opioid reinforcement overlap with, but are distinct from, those involved

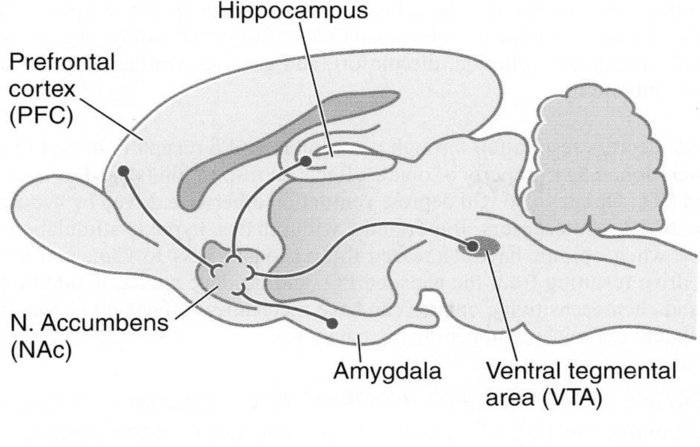

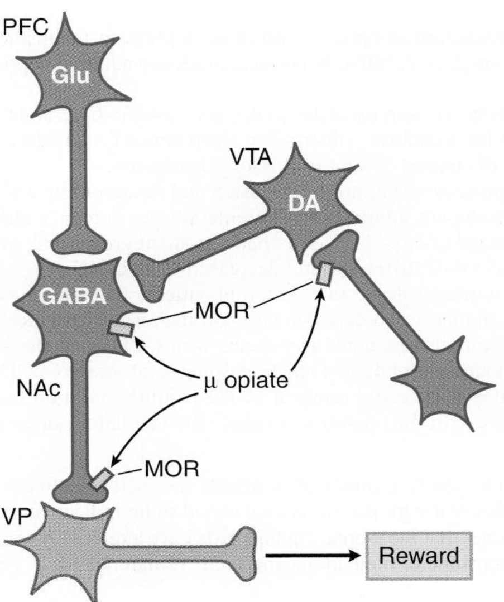

Figure 18–5 *Schematic pathways underlying rewarding properties of opiates. Upper panel*: This sagittal section of rat brain shows DA and GABA inputs from the ventral tegmental area (VTA) and prefrontal cortex (PFC), respectively, into the nucleus accumbens (NAc). *Lower panel*: Neurons are labeled with their primary neurotransmitters. At a cellular level, MOR agonists reduce excitability and transmitter release at the sites indicated by inhibiting Ca^{2+} influx and enhancing K^+ current (*see* Figure 18–4). Thus, opiate-induced inhibition in the VTA on GABA-ergic interneurons or in the NAc reduce GABA-mediated inhibition and increase outflow from the ventral pallidum (VP), which appears to correlate with a positive reinforcing state (enhanced reward).

in physical dependence and analgesia. Behavioral and pharmacological data point to a pivotal role of the mesocorticolimbic dopamine system that projects to the nucleus accumbens (NAc) in drug-induced reward and motivation (Figure 18–5).

RESPIRATION. Although effects on respiration are readily demonstrated, clinically significant respiratory depression rarely occurs with standard analgesic doses in the absence of other contributing variables (discussed in the next sections). It should be stressed, however, that *respiratory depression represents the primary cause of morbidity secondary to opiate therapy*. In humans, death from opiate poisoning is nearly always due to respiratory arrest or obstruction. Opiates depress all phases of respiratory activity (rate, minute volume, and tidal exchange) and produce irregular and aperiodic breathing. The diminished respiratory volume is due primarily to a slower rate of breathing; with toxic amounts of opioids, the rate may fall to 3-4 breaths/min. Thus, opioids must be used with caution in patients with asthma, chronic obstructive pulmonary disease (COPD), cor pulmonale, decreased respiratory reserve, preexisting respiratory depression, hypoxia, or hypercapnia to avoid apnea due to a decrease in respiratory drive coinciding with an increased airway resistance. Although respiratory depression is not considered to be a favorable therapeutic effect of opiates, their ability to suppress respiratory drive is used to therapeutic advantage to treat dyspnea resulting, e.g., in patients with COPD, where air hunger leads to extreme agitation, discomfort, and gasping; similarly, opiates find use in patients who require artificial ventilation.

Morphine-like opioids depress respiration through μ receptors and δ receptors in part by a direct depressant effect on rhythm generation. A key property of opiate effects on respiration is the depression of the ventilatory response to increased CO_2. Opiates also will depress ventilation otherwise driven by hypoxia through an effect on carotid and aortic body chemosensors. Importantly, with opiates, hypoxic stimulation of chemoreceptors still may be effective when opioids have decreased the responsiveness to CO_2, and inhalation of O_2 may remove the residual drive resulting from the elevated PO_2 and produce apnea. In addition to the effect upon respiratory rhythm and chemosensitivity, opiates can have mechanical effects on airway function by increasing chest wall rigidity and diminishing upper airway patency.

FACTORS EXACERBATING OPIATE-INDUCED RESPIRATORY DEPRESSION. A number of factors are recognized as increasing the risk of opiate-related respiratory depression even at therapeutic doses:

- ***Other medications.*** The combination of opiates with other depressant medications, such as general anesthetics, tranquilizers, alcohol, or sedative-hypnotics, produces additive depression of respiratory activity.
- ***Sleep.*** Natural sleep decreases the sensitivity of the medullary center to CO_2, and the depressant effects of morphine and sleep are at least additive. Obstructive sleep apnea is considered to be an important risk factor for increasing the likelihood of fatal respiratory depression.
- ***Age.*** Newborns can show significant respiratory depression and desaturation; and this may be evident in lower Apgar scores if opioids are administered parenterally to women within 2-4 h of delivery because of transplacental passage of opioids. Elderly patients are at greater risk of depression because of reduced lung elasticity, chest wall stiffening, and decreased vital capacity.
- ***Disease.*** Opiates may cause a greater depressant action in patients with chronic cardiopulmonary or renal diseases because they can manifest a desensitization of the response to increased CO_2.
- ***COPD.*** Enhanced depression can also be noted in patients with COPD and sleep apnea secondary to diminished hypoxic drive (although morphine can relieve gasping in late-stage COPD by this mechanism).
- ***Relief of Pain.*** Pain stimulates respiration; removal of the painful condition (as with the analgesia resulting from the therapeutic use of the opiate) will reduce the ventilatory drive and lead to apparent respiratory depression.

Respiratory depression produced by any opiate agonist can be readily reversed by delivery of an opiate antagonist. Opiate antagonist reversal in the somnolent patient is considered to be indicative of an opiate-mediated somnolence. It is important to remember that most opiate antagonists have a relatively short duration of action as compared to an agonist such as morphine or methadone and fatal "re-narcotization" can occur if vigilance is not exercised.

NEUROENDOCRINE EFFECTS. The regulation of the release of hormones and factors from the pituitary is under complex regulation by opiate receptors in the hypothalamic-pituitary-adrenal (HPA) axis. Broadly considered, morphine-like opioids block the release of a large number of HPA hormones.

Sex Hormones. In males, acute opiate therapy reduces plasma cortisol, testosterone, and gonadotrophins. Inhibition of adrenal function is reflected by reduced cortisol production and reduced adrenal androgens (dehydroepiandrosterone, DHEA). In females, morphine will additionally result in lower LH and FSH release. In both males and females, chronic therapy can result in endocrinopathies, including hypogonadotrophic hypogonadism. In men, this may result in decreased libido and, with extended exposure, reduced secondary sex characteristics. In women these exposures are associated with menstrual cycle irregularities. These changes are reversible with removal of the opiate.

Prolactin. Prolactin release from the anterior pituitary is under inhibitory control by DA released from neurons of the arcuate nucleus. MOR agonists act presynaptically on these DA-releasing terminals to inhibit DA release and thereby increase plasma prolactin.

Antidiuretic Hormone and Oxytocin. KOR agonists inhibit the release of oxytocin and antidiuretic hormone (and cause prominent diuresis). It should be noted that agents such as morphine may yield a hypotension secondary to histamine release and this would, by itself, promote ADH release.

MIOSIS. MOR agonists induce pupillary constriction (miosis) in the awake state and block pupillary reflex dilation during anesthesia. The parasympathetic outflow is locally regulated by GABA-ergic interneurons. Opiates are believed to block the GABA-ergic interneuron-mediated inhibition.

SEIZURES AND CONVULSIONS. In older children and adults, moderately higher doses of opiates produce EEG slowing. In the newborn, morphine has been shown to produce epileptiform activity and occasionally seizure activity. Several mechanisms are most certainly involved in these excitatory actions:

- *Inhibition of inhibitory interneurons*. Morphine-like drugs excite certain groups of neurons, especially hippocampal pyramidal cells, probably from inhibition of the release of GABA by interneurons.
- *Direct stimulatory effects*.
- *Actions mediated by non-opioid receptors*. The metabolites of several opiates (morphine-3-glucuronide, normeperidine) have been implicated in seizure activity.

COUGH. Morphine and related opioids depress the cough reflex at least in part by a direct effect on a cough center in the medulla and this can be achieved without altering the protective glottal function. Cough is a protective reflex evoked by airway stimulation. It involves rapid expression of air against a transiently closed glottis.

NAUSEANT AND EMETIC EFFECTS. Nausea and vomiting produced by morphine-like drugs are side effects caused by direct stimulation of the chemoreceptor trigger zone for emesis in the area postrema of the medulla.

CARDIOVASCULAR SYSTEM. In the supine patient, therapeutic doses of morphine-like opioids have no major effect on blood pressure or cardiac rate and rhythm. Such doses can, however, produce peripheral vasodilation, reduced peripheral resistance, and an inhibition of baroreceptor reflexes. Thus, when supine patients assume the head-up position, orthostatic hypotension and fainting may occur. The peripheral arteriolar and venous dilation produced by morphine involves several mechanisms:

- Morphine induces release of histamine from mast cells, leading to vasodilation; this effect is reversed by naloxone but only partially blocked by H_1 antagonists
- Morphine blunts reflex vasoconstriction caused by increased P_{CO_2}

Morphine may exert its therapeutic effect in the treatment of angina pectoris and acute myocardial infarction by decreasing preload, inotropy, and chronotropy, thus favorably altering determinants of myocardial O_2 consumption. Morphine has been shown to produce cardioprotective effects. Morphine can mimic the phenomenon of ischemic preconditioning, where a short ischemic episode paradoxically protects the heart against further ischemia. This effect appears to be mediated through receptors signaling through a mitochondrial ATP-sensitive K^+ channel in cardiac myocytes; the effect also is produced by other GPCRs signaling through G_i. Morphine-like opioids should be used with caution in patients who have decreased blood volume because these agents can aggravate hypovolemic shock. Morphine should be used with great care in patients with cor pulmonale; deaths after ordinary therapeutic doses have been reported. Concurrent use of certain phenothiazines may increase the risk of morphine-induced hypotension.

MOTOR TONE. High doses of opioids, as used for anesthetic induction, produce muscular rigidity. Myoclonus, ranging from mild twitching to generalized spasm, is an occasional side effect, which has been reported with all clinical opiate agonists; it is particularly prevalent in patients receiving high doses. Increase motor tone and rigidity are reversed by opiate antagonists.

GI TRACT. Between 40% and 95% of patients treated with opioids develop constipation and changes in bowel function. Opioid receptors are densely distributed in enteric neurons between the myenteric and submucosal plexi and on a variety of secretory cells.

Esophagus. Morphine inhibits lower esophageal sphincter relaxation induced by swallowing and by esophageal distension; the effect is believed to be centrally mediated.

Stomach. Morphine increases in tonic contracture of the antral musculature and upper duodenum and reduces resting tone in the musculature of the gastric reservoir, thereby prolonging gastric emptying time and increasing the likelihood of esophageal reflux. Passage of the gastric contents through the duodenum may be delayed by as much as 12 h, and the absorption of orally administered drugs is retarded. Morphine and other agonists usually decrease secretion of hydrochloric acid.

Intestine. Morphine reduces propulsatile activity in the small and large intestine and diminishes intestinal secretions. Opiate agonists suppress rhythmic inhibition of muscle tone leading to concurrent increases in basal tone in the circular muscle of the small and large intestine. This results in enhanced high-amplitude phasic contractions, which are nonpropulsive. The upper part of the small intestine, particularly the duodenum, is affected more than the ileum. A period of relative atony may follow the hypertonicity. The reduced rate of passage of the intestinal contents, along with reduced intestinal secretion, leads to increased water absorption, increasing viscosity of the bowel contents, and constipation. The tone of the anal sphincter is augmented greatly, and reflex relaxation in response to rectal distension is reduced. Patients who take opioids chronically remain constipated. Intestinal secretion arises from activation of enterocytes by local cholinergic submucosal plexus secretomotor neurons. Opioids act though μ/δ receptors on these secretomotor neurons to inhibit their excitatory output to the enterocytes and thereby reduce intestinal secretion.

Biliary Tract. Morphine constricts the sphincter of Oddi, and the pressure in the common bile duct may rise >10-fold within 15 min. Fluid pressure also may increase in the gallbladder and produce symptoms that may vary from epigastric distress to typical biliary colic. All opioids can cause biliary spasm. Some patients with biliary colic experience exacerbation rather than relief of pain when given opioids. Spasm of the sphincter of Oddi probably is responsible for elevations of plasma amylase and lipase that occur sometimes after morphine administration.

OTHER SMOOTH MUSCLE

Ureter and Urinary Bladder. Morphine inhibits the urinary voiding reflex and increases the tone of the external sphincter with a resultant increase in the volume of the bladder. Tolerance develops to these effects of opioids on the bladder. Clinically, opiate-mediated inhibition of micturition can be of such clinical severity that catheterization sometimes is required after therapeutic doses of morphine, particularly with spinal drug administration. Importantly, the inhibition of systemic opiate effects on micturition is reversed by peripherally restricted antagonists.

Uterus. Morphine may prolong labor. If the uterus has been made hyperactive by oxytocics, morphine tends to restore the contractions to normal.

SKIN. Therapeutic doses of morphine cause dilation of cutaneous blood vessels. The skin of the face, neck, and upper thorax frequently becomes flushed. These changes may be due in part to the release of histamine and may be responsible for the sweating and some of the pruritus that commonly follow the systemic administration of morphine (described later). Histamine release probably accounts for the urticaria commonly seen at the site of injection. Itching is readily seen with morphine and meperidine but to a much lesser extent with oxymorphone, methadone, fentanyl, or sufentanil. This pruritus can be caused by systemic as well as intraspinal injections of opioids, but it is more intense after epidural or intrathecal administration.

IMMUNE SYSTEM. Opioids modulate immune function by direct effects on cells of the immune system and indirectly through centrally mediated neuronal mechanisms. The acute central immunomodulatory effects of opioids may be mediated by activation of the sympathetic nervous system; the chronic effects of opioids may involve modulation of the HPA axis. Direct effects on immune cells may involve unique variants of the classical neuronal opioid receptors, with μ receptor variants being most prominent. A proposed mechanism for the immune suppressive effects of morphine on neutrophils is through NO–dependent inhibition of NF-kB activation. Activation of MAP kinase also may play a role.

TEMPERATURE REGULATION. Opioids alter the equilibrium point of the hypothalamic heat-regulatory mechanisms such that body temperature usually falls slightly. Agonists at the μ receptor (e.g., alfentanil and meperidine), acting in the CNS, result in slightly increased thresholds for sweating and significantly lower the threshold temperatures for evoking vasoconstriction and shivering.

FUNCTIONAL OPIOID DRUG TYPES

Most of the clinically used opioid agonists presented in Table 18–4 are relatively selective for MOR. They produce analgesia, affect mood and rewarding behavior, and alter respiratory, cardiovascular, GI, and neuroendocrine function. KOR agonists, with few exceptions (e.g., butorphanol), are not typically employed for long-term therapy as they may produce dysphoric and psychotomimetic effects. DOR agonists have not found clinical utility, and NOP agonists lack analgesic effects. Opiates that are relatively receptor selective at lower doses will interact with additional receptor types when given at high doses, especially as doses are escalated to overcome tolerance.

The mixed agonist–antagonist agents frequently interact with more than 1 receptor class at usual clinical doses. A "ceiling effect" limiting the amount of analgesia attainable often is seen with these drugs, such as buprenorphine, which is approved for the treatment of opioid dependence. Some mixed agonist–antagonist drugs, such as pentazocine and nalorphine (not available in the U.S.), can precipitate withdrawal in opioid-tolerant patients. For these reasons, except for the sanctioned use of buprenorphine to manage opioid addiction, the clinical use of mixed agonist–antagonist drugs is generally limited.

The dosing guidelines and duration of action for the numerous drugs that are part of opioid therapy are summarized in Table 18–4.

MORPHINE. Morphine remains the standard against which new analgesics are measured.

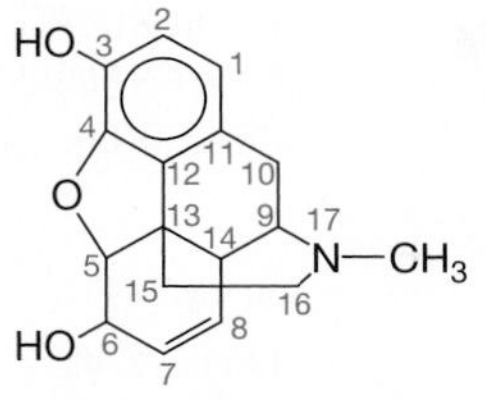

HO 3 2 1 4 12 11 10 O 13 9 17 14 N—CH_3 5 15 16 HO 6 8 7

Morphine

Morphine is obtained from opium or extracted from poppy straw. Powdered opium contains a number of alkaloids; only a few—morphine, codeine, and papaverine—have clinical utility. These alkaloids are divided into 2 distinct chemical classes, phenanthrenes and benzylisoquinolines. The principal phenanthrenes are morphine (10% of opium), codeine (0.5%), and thebaine (0.2%). The principal benzylisoquinolines are papaverine (1%) (a smooth muscle relaxant) and noscapine (6%). Many semisynthetic derivatives are made by relatively simple modifications of morphine or thebaine.

Absorption. Opioids are absorbed from the GI tract; absorption through the rectal mucosa is adequate and a few agents (e.g., morphine, hydromorphone) are available in suppositories. The more lipophilic opioids are absorbed readily through the nasal or buccal mucosa. Those with the greatest lipid solubility also can be absorbed transdermally. Opioids, particularly morphine, have been widely used for spinal delivery to produce analgesia through a spinal action. These agents display useful transdural movement adequate to permit their use epidurally.

With most opioids, including morphine, the effect of a given dose is less after oral than after parenteral administration because of variable but significant first-pass metabolism in the liver. For example, the bioavailability of oral preparations of morphine is only ~25%. The shape of the time-effect curve also varies with the route of administration, so the duration of action often is somewhat longer with the oral route. If adjustment is made for variability of first-pass metabolism and clearance, adequate relief of pain can be achieved with oral administration of morphine. Satisfactory analgesia in cancer patients is associated with a very broad range of steady-state concentrations of morphine in plasma (16-364 ng/mL). When morphine and most opioids are given intravenously, they act promptly. Compared with more lipid-soluble opioids such as codeine, heroin, and methadone, morphine crosses the blood-brain barrier at a considerably lower rate.

Distribution and Metabolism. About one-third of morphine in the plasma is protein-bound after a therapeutic dose. Morphine itself does not persist in tissues, and 24 h after the last dose, tissue concentrations are low. The major pathway for the metabolism of morphine is conjugation with glucuronic acid. The 2 major metabolites formed are morphine-6-glucuronide and morphine-3-glucuronide. Morphine-6-glucuronide has pharmacological actions indistinguishable from those of morphine. With chronic administration, the 6-glucuronide accounts for a significant portion of morphine's analgesic actions. Morphine-6-glucuronide is excreted by the kidney. In renal failure, the levels of morphine-6-glucuronide can accumulate, perhaps explaining morphine's potency and long duration in patients with compromised renal function. In adults, the $t_{1/2}$ of morphine is ~2 h; the $t_{1/2}$ of morphine-6-glucuronide is somewhat longer. Children achieve adult renal function values by 6 months of age. In elderly patients, lower doses of morphine are recommended based on a smaller volume of distribution and the general decline in renal function. Morphine-3-glucuronide has little affinity for opioid receptors but may contribute to excitatory effects of morphine. N-Dealkylation also is important in the metabolism of some congeners of morphine.

Excretion. Morphine is eliminated by glomerular filtration, primarily as morphine-3-glucuronide; 90% of the total excretion takes place during the first day. Very little morphine is excreted unchanged.

CODEINE. In contrast to morphine, codeine is ~60% as effective orally as parenterally as an analgesic and as a respiratory depressant. Codeine analogs such as levorphanol, oxycodone, and methadone have a high ratio of oral-to-parenteral potency. The greater oral efficacy of these drugs reflects lower first-pass metabolism in the liver. Once absorbed, codeine is metabolized by the liver, and its metabolites are excreted chiefly as inactive forms in the urine. A small fraction (~10%) of administered codeine is O-demethylated to morphine, and free and conjugated morphine can be found in the urine after therapeutic doses of codeine. Codeine has an exceptionally low affinity for opioid receptors, and the analgesic effect of codeine is due to its conversion to

Table 18–4

Dosing Data for Clinically Employed Opioid Analgesics *(Continued on next page)*

DRUG	APPROXIMATE EQUIANALGESIC ORAL DOSE	APPROXIMATE EQUIANALGESIC PARENTERAL DOSE
Opioid Agonists		
Morphine	30 mg/3–4h	10 mg/3–4h
Codeine	130 mg/3–4h	75 mg/3–4h
Hydromophone	6 mg/3–4h	1.5 mg/3–4h
Hydrocodone (typically with acetominophen)	30 mg/3–4h	Not available
Levorphanol	4 mg/6–8h	2 mg/6–8h
Meperidine	300 mg/2–3h	100 mg/3h
Methadone	10 mg/6–8h	10 mg/6–8h
Oxycodone	20 mg/3–4h	Not available
Oxymorphone	10 mg/3–4h	1 mg/3–4h
Propoxyphene	130 mg	Not available
Tramadol	100 mg	100 mg
Fentanyl Transdermal 72-hour patch (25 μg/h) = morphine 50 mg/24h		
Opioid Agonist-Antagonists or Partial Agonists		
Buprenorphine	Not available	0.3–0.4 mg/6–8h
Butorphanol	Not available	2 mg/3–4h
Nalbuphine	Not available	10 mg/3–4h

These data are merely guidelines. Clinical response must be the guide for each patient, with consideration to hepatic and renal function, disease, age, concurrent medications (their effects and dose limitations [acetaminophen, 3 g/day for adults]), and other factors that could modify pharmacokinetics and drug response. Recommended start doses are approximately but not precisely equianalgesic and are driven by doses available from manufacturers. Transdermal fentanyl is contraindicated for acute pain and in patients receiving <60 mg oral morphine equivalent per day. Use Table 18–8 for converting morphine to methadone dosing.

For morphine, hydromorphone, and oxymorphone, rectal administration is an alternate route for patients unable to take oral medications, but equianalgesic doses may differ from oral and parenteral doses because of pharmacokinetic differences.

morphine. However, codeine's antitussive actions may involve distinct receptors that bind codeine itself, and codeine is commonly employed for the management of cough. The $t_{1/2}$ of codeine in plasma is 2-4 h.

CYP2D6 catalyzes the conversion of codeine to morphine. Genetic polymorphisms in CYP2D6 lead to the inability to convert codeine to morphine, thus making codeine ineffective as an analgesic for ~10% of the Caucasian population. Other polymorphisms (e.g., the CYP2D6*2×2 genotype) can lead to ultrarapid metabolism and thus increased sensitivity to codeine's effects due to higher than expected serum morphine levels. Thus, it is important to consider the possibility of metabolic enzyme polymorphism in any patient who experiences toxicity or does not receive adequate analgesia from codeine or other opioid prodrugs (e.g., hydrocodone and oxycodone).

HEROIN. Heroin (diacetylmorphine) is rapidly hydrolyzed to 6-monoacetylmorphine (6-MAM), which in turn is hydrolyzed to morphine. Heroin and 6-MAM are more lipid soluble than morphine and enter the brain more readily. Evidence suggests that morphine and 6-MAM are responsible for the pharmacological actions of heroin. Heroin is excreted mainly in the urine largely as free and conjugated morphine.

Table 18–4

Dosing Data for Clinically Employed Opioid Analgesics (*Continued*)

RECOMMENDED STARTING DOSE (adults >50 kg)		RECOMMENDED STARTING DOSE (children and adults <50 kg)	
ORAL	PARENTERAL	ORAL	PARENTERAL
15 mg/3–4h	5 mg/3–4h	0.3 mg/kg/3–4h	0.1 mg/kg/3–4h
30 mg/3–4h	30 mg/2h (IM/SC)	0.5 mg/kg/3–4h	Not recommended
2 mg/3–4h	0.5 mg/3–4h	0.03 mg/kg/3–4h	0.005 mg/kg/3–4h
5 mg/3–4h	Not available	0.1 mg/kg/3–4h	Not available
4 mg/6–8h	2 mg/6–8h	0.04 mg/kg/6–8h	0.02 mg/kg/6–8h
Not recommended	50 mg/3h	Not recommended	0.75 mg/kg/2–3h
5 mg/12h	Not recommended	0.1 mg/kg/12h	Not recommended
5 mg/3–4h	Not available	0.1 mg/kg/3–4h	Not available
5 mg/3–4h	1 mg/3–4h	0.1 mg/kg/3–4h	Not recommended
65 mg/4–6h	Not available	Not recommended	Not recommended
50–100 mg/6h	50–100 mg/6h	Not recommended	Not recommended
Not available	0.4 mg/6–8h	Not available	0.004 mg/kg/6–8h
Not available	2 mg/3–4h	Not available	Not recommended
Not available	10 mg/3–4h	Not available	0.1 mg/kg/3–4h

Doses listed for patients with body weight less than 50 kg cannot be used as initial starting doses in babies less than 6 months of age; consult the Department of Health and Human Services Clinical Practice Guideline #1, Acute Pain Management: Operative or Medical Procedures and Trauma, *section on neonates, for recommendations.*
See legend to Table 18–2 in 12th edition of parent text for additional precautions and comparative information.
Source: Modified from Agency for Healthcare Policy and Research, 1992.

UNTOWARD EFFECTS AND PRECAUTIONS

Morphine and related opioids produce a wide spectrum of unwanted effects, including respiratory depression, nausea, vomiting, dizziness, mental clouding, dysphoria, pruritus, constipation, increased pressure in the biliary tract, urinary retention, and hypotension. Rarely, a patient may develop delirium. Increased sensitivity to pain after analgesia has worn off and between-dose withdrawal also may occur.

A number of factors may alter a patient's sensitivity to opioid analgesics, including the integrity of the blood-brain barrier. Morphine is hydrophilic, so proportionately less morphine normally crosses into the CNS than with more lipophilic opioids. In neonates or when the blood-brain barrier is compromised, lipophilic opioids may give more predictable clinical results than morphine. In adults, the duration of the analgesia produced by morphine increases progressively with age; however, the degree of analgesia that is obtained with a given dose changes little. The patient with severe pain may tolerate larger doses of morphine. However, as the pain subsides, the patient may exhibit sedation and even respiratory depression as the stimulatory effects of pain are diminished.

All opioid analgesics are metabolized by the liver and should be used with caution in patients with hepatic disease. Renal disease also significantly alters the pharmacokinetics of morphine, codeine, dihydrocodeine, meperidine, and propoxyphene. Although single doses of morphine are well tolerated, the active metabolite, morphine-6-glucuronide, may accumulate with continued dosing, and symptoms of opioid overdose may result. This metabolite also may accumulate during repeated administration of codeine to patients with impaired renal function.

Morphine and related opioids must be used cautiously in patients with compromised respiratory function (e.g., emphysema, kyphoscoliosis, severe obesity). The respiratory-depressant effects of opioids and the related capacity to elevate intracranial pressure must be considered in the presence of head injury or an already elevated intracranial pressure. Patients with reduced blood volume are more susceptible to the vasodilating effects of morphine and related drugs, and these agents must be used cautiously in patients with hypotension from any cause.

Morphine causes histamine release, which can cause bronchoconstriction and vasodilation. Morphine has the potential to precipitate or exacerbate asthmatic attacks and should be avoided in patients with a history of asthma. Other receptor agonists associated with a lower incidence of histamine release, such as the fentanyl derivatives, may be better choices for such patients. Opioid analgesics may evoke allergic phenomena, the effects usually are manifested as urticaria and other types of skin rashes.

LEVORPHANOL

Levorphanol (LEVO-DROMORAN) is the principal available opioid agonist of the morphinan series.

The D-isomer (dextrorphan) is devoid of analgesic action but has inhibitory effects at NMDA receptors. It has affinity at the MOR, KOR, and DORs and is available for intravenous (IV), intramuscular (IM), and oral administration. The pharmacological effects of levorphanol closely parallel those of morphine. However, clinical reports suggest that it may produce less nausea and vomiting. Levorphanol is metabolized less rapidly than morphine and has a $t_{1/2}$ of 12-16 h; repeated administration at short intervals may thus lead to accumulation of the drug in plasma.

MEPERIDINE, DIPHENOXYLATE, LOPERAMIDE

These agents are MOR agonists with principal pharmacological effects on the CNS and neural elements in the bowel.

MEPERIDINE

Meperidine is predominantly an MOR agonist that produces a pattern of effects similar but not identical to those already described for morphine.

CNS Actions. Meperidine is a potent MOR agonist yielding strong analgesic actions. Meperidine causes pupillary constriction, increases the sensitivity of the labyrinthine apparatus, and has effects on the secretion of pituitary hormones similar to those of morphine. Meperidine sometimes causes CNS excitation, characterized by tremors, muscle twitches, and seizures; these effects are due largely to accumulation of a metabolite, normeperidine. Meperidine has well-known local anesthetic properties, particularly noted after epidural administration. As with morphine, respiratory depression is responsible for an accumulation of CO_2, which in turn leads to cerebrovascular dilation, increased cerebral blood flow, and elevation of cerebrospinal fluid pressure.

Cardiovascular System. The effects of meperidine on the cardiovascular system generally resemble those of morphine, including the ability to release histamine following parenteral administration. Intramuscular administration of meperidine does not affect heart rate significantly, but IV administration frequently produces a marked increase in heart rate.

Smooth Muscle, GI Tract. Meperidine does not cause as much constipation as does morphine, even when given over prolonged periods of time; this may be related to its greater ability to enter the CNS, thereby producing analgesia at lower systemic concentrations. As with other opioids, clinical doses of meperidine slow gastric emptying sufficiently to delay absorption of other drugs significantly. The uterus of a nonpregnant woman usually is mildly stimulated by meperidine. Administered before an oxytocic, meperidine does not exert any antagonistic effect.

ADME. Meperidine is absorbed by all routes of administration. The peak plasma concentration usually occurs at ~45 min, but the range is wide. After oral administration, only ~50% of the drug escapes first-pass metabolism to enter the circulation, and peak concentrations in plasma usually are observed in 1-2 h. Meperidine is metabolized chiefly in the liver, with a $t_{1/2}$ ~3 h. In patients with cirrhosis, the bioavailability of meperidine (the N-demethyl metabolite) is increased to as much as 80%, and the $t_{1/2}$ of both meperidine and normeperidine are prolonged. Only a small amount of meperidine is excreted unchanged.

UNTOWARD EFFECTS, PRECAUTIONS, AND CONTRAINDICATIONS. The overall incidence of untoward effects are similar to those observed after equianalgesic doses of morphine, except that constipation and urinary retention may be less common. Patients who experience nausea and vomiting with morphine may not do so with meperidine; the converse also may be true. In patients or addicts who are tolerant to the depressant effects of meperidine, large doses repeated at short intervals may produce an excitatory syndrome including hallucinations, tremors, muscle twitches, dilated pupils, hyperactive reflexes, and convulsions. These excitatory symptoms are due to the accumulation of normeperidine, which has a $t_{1/2}$ of 15-20 h, compared to 3 h for meperidine. Decreased renal or hepatic function increases the likelihood of toxicity. As a result of these properties, meperidine is not recommended for the treatment of chronic pain because of concerns over metabolite toxicity. It should not be used for longer than 48 h or in doses >600 mg/day.

INTERACTIONS WITH OTHER DRUGS. Severe reactions may follow the administration of meperidine to patients being treated with MAO inhibitors. Two basic types of interactions can be observed. The more prominent is an excitatory reaction ("serotonin syndrome") with delirium, hyperthermia, headache, hyper- or hypotension, rigidity, convulsions, coma, and death. This reaction may be due to the ability of meperidine to block neuronal reuptake of 5HT, resulting in serotonergic overactivity. Conversely, the MAO inhibitor interaction with meperidine may resemble acute narcotic overdose owing to the inhibition of hepatic CYPs. Therefore, meperidine and its congeners are contraindicated in patients taking MAO inhibitors or within 14 days after discontinuation of an MAO inhibitor. Dextromethorphan (an analog of levorphanol used as a nonnarcotic cough suppressant) also inhibits neuronal 5HT uptake and must be avoided in these patients.

Chlorpromazine increases the respiratory-depressant effects of meperidine, as do tricyclic antidepressants (but not diazepam). Concurrent administration of drugs such as promethazine or chlorpromazine also may greatly enhance meperidine-induced sedation without slowing clearance of the drug. Treatment with phenobarbital or phenytoin increases systemic clearance and decreases oral bioavailability of meperidine. As with morphine, concomitant administration of amphetamine has been reported to enhance the analgesic effects of meperidine and its congeners while counteracting sedation.

THERAPEUTIC USES. The major use of meperidine is for analgesia. The analgesic effects of meperidine are detectable ~15 min after oral administration, peak in 1-2 h, and subside gradually. The onset of analgesic effect is faster (within 10 min) after subcutaneous or IM administration, and the effect reaches a peak in ~1 h, corresponding closely to peak concentrations in plasma. In clinical use, the duration of effective analgesia is ~1.5-3 h. In general, 75-100 mg meperidine hydrochloride (pethidine, DEMEROL, others) given parenterally is approximately equivalent to 10 mg morphine. In terms of total analgesic effect, meperidine is about one-third as effective when given orally as when administered parenterally.

Single doses of meperidine can be effective in the treatment of postanesthetic shivering. Meperidine, 25-50 mg, is used frequently with antihistamines, corticosteroids, acetaminophen, or NSAIDs to prevent or ameliorate infusion-related rigors and shaking chills that accompany the IV administration of agents such as amphotericin B, aldesleukin (interleukin-2), trastuzumab, and alemtuzumab. Meperidine crosses the placental barrier and even in reasonable analgesic doses causes a significant increase in the percentage of babies who show delayed respiration, decreased respiratory minute volume, or decreased O_2 saturation or who require resuscitation. Fetal and maternal respiratory depression induced by meperidine can be treated with naloxone.

DIPHENOXYLATE

Diphenoxylate is a meperidine congener that has a definite constipating effect in humans. Its only approved use is in the treatment of diarrhea (*see* Chapter 46). Diphenoxylate is unusual in that even its salts are virtually insoluble in aqueous solution, thus reducing the probability of abuse by the parenteral route. Diphenoxylate hydrochloride is available only in combination with atropine sulfate (LOMOTIL, others). The recommended daily dosage of diphenoxylate for the treatment of diarrhea in adults is 20 mg in divided doses. Difenoxin a metabolite of diphenoxylate, is marketed in a fixed dose with atropine (MOTOFEN) for the management of diarrhea.

LOPERAMIDE

Loperamide (IMODIUM, others), like diphenoxylate, is a piperidine derivative. It slows GI motility by effects on the circular and longitudinal muscles of the intestine. Part of its antidiarrheal effect may be due to a reduction of GI secretion. In controlling chronic diarrhea, loperamide is as effective as diphenoxylate and little tolerance develops to its constipating effect. Concentrations of drug in plasma peak ~4 h after ingestion. The apparent elimination $t_{1/2}$ is 7-14 h. Loperamide is poorly absorbed after oral administration and, in addition, apparently does not penetrate well into the brain due to the exporting activity of P-glycoprotein, which is widely expressed in the brain endothelium. The usual dosage is 4-8 mg/day; the daily dose should not exceed 16 mg.

FENTANYL

Fentanyl is a synthetic opioid related to the phenylpiperidines. The actions of fentanyl and its congeners, sufentanil, remifentanil, and alfentanil, are similar to those of other MOR agonists. Fentanyl and sufentanil are very important drugs in anesthetic practice because of their relatively short time to peak analgesic effect, rapid termination of effect after small bolus doses, and cardiovascular safety and their capacity to significantly reduce the dosing requirement for the volatile agents (*see* Chapter 19). In addition to a role in anesthesia, fentanyl also is used in the management of severe pain states.

PHARMACOLOGICAL PROPERTIES

CNS. Fentanyl and its congeners are all extremely potent analgesics and typically exhibit a very short duration of action when given parenterally. As with other opioids, nausea, vomiting, and itching can be observed. Muscle rigidity, while possible after all narcotics, appears to be more common after the high doses used in anesthetic induction. Rigidity can be treated with depolarizing or nondepolarizing neuromuscular blocking agents while controlling the patient's ventilation. Care must be taken to make sure that the patient is not simply immobilized but aware. Respiratory depression is similar to that observed with other MOR agonists, but onset is more rapid. As with analgesia, respiratory depression after small doses is of shorter duration than with morphine but of similar duration after large doses or long infusions. Delayed respiratory depression also can be seen after the use of fentanyl or sufentanil, possibly owing to enterohepatic circulation.

Cardiovascular System. Fentanyl and its derivatives decrease heart rate and mildly decrease blood pressure. However, these drugs do not release histamine and direct depressant effects on the myocardium are minimal.

ADME. These agents are highly lipid soluble and rapidly cross the blood-brain barrier. This is reflected in the $t_{1/2}$ for equilibration between the plasma and CSF of ~5 min for fentanyl and sufentanil. The levels in plasma and CSF decline rapidly owing to redistribution of fentanyl from highly perfused tissue groups to other tissues, such as muscle and fat. As saturation of less well-perfused tissue occurs, the duration of effect of fentanyl and sufentanil approaches the length of their elimination $t_{1/2}$, 3-4 h. Fentanyl and sufentanil undergo hepatic metabolism and renal excretion. With the use of higher doses or prolonged infusions, the drugs accumulate, these clearance mechanisms become progressively saturated, and fentanyl and sufentanil become longer acting.

THERAPEUTIC USES. Fentanyl citrate (SUBLIMAZE, others) and sufentanil citrate (SUFENTA, others) have widespread popularity as anesthetic adjuvants (*see* Chapter 19), administered intravenously, epidurally, or intrathecally. Fentanyl is ~100 times more potent than morphine; sufentanil is ~1000 times more potent than morphine. The time to peak analgesic effect after IV administration of fentanyl and sufentanil (~5 min) is notably less than that for morphine and meperidine (~15 min). Recovery from analgesic effects also occurs more quickly. However, with larger doses or prolonged infusions, the effects of these drugs become more lasting, with durations of action becoming similar to those of longer-acting opioids.

The use of fentanyl and sufentanil in chronic pain treatment has become more widespread. Transdermal patches (DURAGESIC, others) that provide sustained release of fentanyl for 48-72 h are available. However, factors promoting increased absorption (e.g., fever) can lead to relative overdosage and increased side effects. Transbuccal absorption by the use of buccal tablets, and lollipop-like lozenges permits rapid absorption and has found use in the management of acute incident pain (FENTORA, ACTIQ, ONSOLIS, others) and for the relief of breakthrough cancer pain. As fentanyl is poorly absorbed in the GI tract, the optimal absorption is through buccal absorption. Epidural use of fentanyl and sufentanil for postoperative or labor analgesia is popular. A combination of epidural opioids with local anesthetics permits reduction in the dosage of both components.

REMIFENTANIL

The pharmacological properties of remifentanil are similar to those of fentanyl and sufentanil. Remifentanil produces similar incidences of nausea, vomiting, and dose-dependent muscle rigidity.

ADME. Remifentanil has a more rapid onset of analgesic action than fentanyl or sufentanil. Analgesic effects occur within 1-1.5 min following IV administration. Peak respiratory depression after bolus doses of remifentanil occurs after 5 min. Remifentanil is metabolized by plasma esterases, with a $t_{1/2}$ of 8-20 min; thus, elimination is independent of hepatic metabolism or renal excretion. Age and weight can affect clearance of remifentanil. After 3- to 5-h infusions of remifentanil, recovery of respiratory function can be seen within 3-5 min; full recovery from all effects of remifentanil is observed within 15 min. The primary metabolite, remifentanil acid, has 0.05-0.025% of the potency of the parent compound, and is excreted renally.

THERAPEUTIC USES. Remifentanil hydrochloride (ULTIVA) is useful for short, painful procedures that require intense analgesia and blunting of stress responses; the drug is routinely given by continuous IV infusion because its short duration of action. When postprocedural analgesia is required, remifentanil alone is a poor choice. In this situation, either a longer-acting opioid or another analgesic modality should be combined with remifentanil for prolonged analgesia, or another opioid should be used. Remifentanil is not used intraspinally because of its formulation with glycine, an inhibitory transmitter in the spinal dorsal horn.

METHADONE AND PROPOXYPHENE

METHADONE

Methadone is a long-acting MOR agonist with pharmacological properties qualitatively similar to those of morphine. The analgesic activity of methadone, a racemate, is almost entirely the result of its content of L-methadone, which is 8-50 times more potent than the D-isomer. D-methadone also lacks significant respiratory depressant action and addiction liability but possesses antitussive activity.

MAJOR EFFECTS; SIDE EFFECTS. The outstanding properties of methadone are its analgesic activity, its efficacy by the oral route, its extended duration of action in suppressing withdrawal symptoms in physically dependent individuals, and its tendency to show persistent effects with repeated administration. Miotic and respiratory-depressant effects can be detected for >24 h after a single dose; on repeated administration, marked sedation is seen in some patients. Effects on cough, bowel motility, biliary tone, and the secretion of pituitary hormones are qualitatively similar to those of morphine. Side effects are similar to those described for morphine. Rifampin and phenytoin accelerate the metabolism of methadone and can precipitate withdrawal symptoms. Unlike other opioids, methadone is associated with the prolonged QT syndrome and is additive with agents known to prolong the QT interval.

ADME. Methadone is absorbed well from the GI tract and can be detected in plasma within 30 min of oral ingestion; it reaches peak concentrations at ~4 h. Peak concentrations occur in brain within 1-2 h of subcutaneous or IM administration, and this correlates well with the intensity and duration of analgesia. Methadone also can be absorbed from the buccal mucosa. Methadone undergoes extensive biotransformation in the liver. The major metabolites, pyrrolidine and pyrroline, are excreted in the urine and the bile along with small amounts of unchanged drug. The amount of methadone excreted in the urine is increased when the urine is acidified. The $t_{1/2}$ of methadone is long, 15-40 h. Methadone appears to be firmly bound to protein in various tissues, including brain. After repeated administration, there is gradual accumulation in tissues. When administration is discontinued, low concentrations are maintained in plasma by slow release from extravascular binding sites; this process probably accounts for the relatively mild but protracted withdrawal syndrome.

THERAPEUTIC USES. The primary uses of methadone hydrochloride (DOLOPHINE, others) are relief of chronic pain, treatment of opioid abstinence syndromes, and treatment of heroin users. The onset of analgesia occurs 10-20 min after parenteral administration and 30-60 min after oral medication. The typical oral dose is 2.5-10 mg repeated every 8-12 h as needed depending on the severity of the pain and the response of the patient. Care must be taken when increasing the dosage because of the prolonged $t_{1/2}$ of the drug and its tendency to accumulate over a period of several days with repeated dosing. The peak respiratory depressant effects of methadone typically occur later and persist longer than peak analgesia, so it is necessary to exercise vigilance and strongly caution patients against self-medicating with CNS depressants, particularly during treatment initiation and dose titration. Methadone should not be used in labor. Despite its longer plasma $t_{1/2}$, the duration of the analgesic action of single doses is essentially the same as that of morphine. With repeated use, cumulative effects are seen, so either lower dosages or longer intervals between doses become possible.

Because of its oral bioavailability and long $t_{1/2}$, methadone has been widely implemented as a replacement modality to treat heroin dependence. Methadone, like other opiates, will produce tolerance and dependence. Thus, addicts who receive daily subcutaneous or oral therapy develop partial tolerance to the nauseant, anorectic, miotic, sedative, respiratory-depressant, and cardiovascular effects of methadone. Many former heroin users treated with oral methadone show virtually no overt behavioral effects. Development of physical dependence during the long-term administration of methadone can be demonstrated following abrupt drug withdrawal or by administration of an opioid antagonist. Likewise, subcutaneous administration of methadone to former opioid addicts produces euphoria equal in duration to that caused by morphine, and its overall abuse potential is comparable with that of morphine.

PROPOXYPHENE

Propoxyphene is structurally related to methadone. Its analgesic effect resides in the D-isomer. However, L-propoxyphene seems to have some antitussive activity.

PHARMACOLOGICAL ACTIONS. Although slightly less selective than morphine, propoxyphene binds primarily to MOR and produces analgesia and other CNS effects that are similar to those seen with morphine-like opioids. At equianalgesic doses, the incidence of side effects such as nausea, anorexia, constipation, abdominal pain, and drowsiness are similar to those of codeine. As an analgesic, propoxyphene is about one-half to two-thirds as potent as codeine given orally. A dose of 90-120 mg of propoxyphene hydrochloride administered orally provides the analgesic effects of 60 mg of codeine, a dose that usually produces about as much analgesia as 600 mg aspirin. Combinations of propoxyphene and aspirin, like combinations of codeine and aspirin, afford a higher level of analgesia than does either agent given alone. Given orally, propoxyphene is approximately one-third as potent as orally administered codeine in depressing respiration. Larage toxic doses may produce convulsions in addition to respiratory depression. Naloxone antagonizes the respiratory-depressant, convulsant, and some of the cardiotoxic effects of propoxyphene.

ADME. After oral administration, peak plasma concentrations occur at 1-2 h. There is great variability between subjects in the rate of clearance. The average $t_{1/2}$ of propoxyphene in plasma after a single dose is 6-12 h, which is longer than that of codeine. In humans, the major route of metabolism is N-demethylation to yield norpropoxyphene. The $t_{1/2}$ of norpropoxyphene is ~30 h; it may accumulate with repeated doses and cause some toxicity.

Higher than expected serum levels of propoxyphene will occur from the concomitant administration of strong CYP3A4 inhibitors (e.g., ritonavir, ketoconazole, itraconazole, clarithromycin, nelfinavir, nefazodone, amiodarone, amprenavir, aprepitant, diltiazem, erythromycin, fluconazole, fosamprenavir, grapefruit juice, and verapamil). Propoxyphene alternatives should be considered for patients receiving a strong CYP3A4 inhibitor and others at risk for overdose, particularly those with preexisting heart disease.

TOLERANCE AND DEPENDENCE. Very large doses (800 mg propoxyphene hydrochloride [DARVON, others] or 1200 mg of the napsylate [DARVON-N] per day) reduce the intensity of the morphine withdrawal syndrome somewhat less effectively than do 1500 mg doses of codeine. Maximal tolerated doses are equivalent to daily doses of 20-25 mg morphine given subcutaneously. The use of higher doses of propoxyphene is accompanied by untoward effects including toxic psychoses. Very large doses produce some respiratory depression in morphine-tolerant addicts, suggesting that cross-tolerance between propoxyphene and morphine is incomplete. Abrupt discontinuation of chronically administered propoxyphene hydrochloride (up to 800 mg/day given for almost 2 months) results in mild abstinence phenomena, and large oral doses (300-600 mg) produce subjective effects that are considered pleasurable by post-addicts. The drug is quite irritating when administered either intravenously or subcutaneously, so abuse by these routes results in severe damage to veins and soft tissues.

THERAPEUTIC USES. The European Medicines Agency has concluded that the benefits of dextropropoxyphene do not outweigh the risks, that dextropropoxyphene-containing medicines are weak painkillers with a narrow therapeutic index and limited effectiveness in the treatment of pain, and that acetaminophen-containing combinations with dextropropoxyphene are no more effective than acetaminophen alone. Consequently, the Agency has recommended a gradual withdrawal of marketing authorization throughout the E.U. In the U.S., the FDA has asked companies to voluntarily remove propoxyphene-containing products from the market due to concerns related to cardiotoxic effects of the drug at therapeutic doses.

OTHER OPIOID AGONISTS

TRAMADOL. Tramadol (ULTRAM) is a synthetic codeine analog that is a weak MOR agonist. Part of its analgesic effect is produced by inhibition of uptake of NE and 5HT. In the treatment of mild to moderate pain, tramadol is as effective as morphine or meperidine. However, for the treatment of severe or chronic pain, tramadol is less effective. Tramadol is as effective as meperidine in the treatment of labor pain and may cause less neonatal respiratory depression.

ADME. Tramadol is 68% bioavailable after a single oral dose and 100% available when administered intramuscularly. Its affinity for the μ-opioid receptor is only 1/6000 that of morphine. The primary O-demethylated metabolite of tramadol is 2-4 times more potent than the parent drug and may account for part of the analgesic effect. Tramadol is supplied as a racemate that is more effective than either enantiomer alone. The (+)-enantiomer binds to the receptor and inhibits 5HT uptake. The (−)-enantiomer inhibits NE uptake and stimulates α_2 adrenergic receptors. Tramadol undergoes extensive hepatic metabolism by a number of pathways, including CYP2D6 and CYP3A4, as well as by conjugation with subsequent renal excretion. The elimination $t_{1/2}$ is 6 h for tramadol and 7.5 h for its active metabolite. Analgesia begins within an hour of oral dosing and peaks within 2-3 h. The duration of analgesia is ~6 h. The maximum recommended daily dose is 400 mg.

Side Effects; Adverse Effects. Side effects of tramadol include nausea, vomiting, dizziness, dry mouth, sedation, and headache. Respiratory depression appears to be less than with equianalgesic doses of morphine, and the degree of constipation is less than that seen after equivalent doses of codeine. Tramadol can cause seizures and possibly exacerbate seizures in patients with predisposing factors. Tramadol-induced respiratory depression is reversed by naloxone. Precipitation of withdrawal necessitates that tramadol be tapered prior to discontinuation. Tramadol should not be used in patients taking MAO inhibitors, SSRIs, or other drugs that lower the seizure threshold.

TAPENTADOL. Tapentadol (NUCYNTA) is structurally and mechanistically similar to tramadol. It displays a mild opioid activity and possesses monoamine reuptake inhibitor activity. It is considered similar to tramadol in activity, efficacy, and side-effect profile.

OPIOID AGONISTS/ANTAGONISTS AND PARTIAL AGONISTS

Drugs such as *nalbuphine* and *butorphanol* are competitive MOR antagonists but exert their analgesic actions by acting as agonists at KOR receptors. *Pentazocine* qualitatively resembles these drugs, but it may be a weaker MOR receptor antagonist or partial agonist while retaining its KOR agonist activity. *Buprenorphine*, however, is a partial agonist at MOR. The stimulus for the development of mixed agonist–antagonist drugs was a desire for analgesics with less respiratory depression and addictive potential. However, the clinical use of these compounds is limited by undesirable side effects and limited analgesic effects.

PENTAZOCINE

Pentazocine was synthesized as part of a deliberate effort to develop an effective analgesic with little or no abuse potential. It has agonistic actions and weak opioid antagonistic activity.

PHARMACOLOGICAL ACTIONS AND SIDE EFFECTS. The pattern of CNS effects produced by pentazocine generally is similar to that of the morphine-like opioids, including analgesia, sedation, and respiratory depression. The analgesic effects of pentazocine are due to agonistic actions at KOR. Higher doses of pentazocine (60-90 mg) elicit dysphoric and psychotomimetic effects; these effects may be reversible by naloxone. The cardiovascular responses to pentazocine differ from those seen with typical receptor agonists, in that high doses cause an increase in blood pressure and heart rate. Pentazocine acts as a weak antagonist or partial agonist at MOR. Pentazocine does not antagonize the respiratory depression produced by morphine. However, when given to patients dependent on morphine or other MOR agonists, pentazocine may precipitate withdrawal. Ceiling effects for analgesia and respiratory depression are observed at doses above 50-100 mg of pentazocine.

THERAPEUTIC USES. Pentazocine lactate (TALWIN) injection is indicated for the relief of moderate to severe pain and is also used as a preoperative medication and as a supplement to anesthesia. Pentazocine tablets for oral use are only available in fixed-dose combinations with acetaminophen (TALACEN, others) or naloxone (TALWIN NX). Combination of pentazocine with naloxone reduces the potential misuse of tablets as a source of injectable pentazocine by producing undesirable effects in subjects dependent on opioids. An oral dose of ~50 mg pentazocine results in analgesia equivalent to that produced by 60 mg of codeine orally.

NALBUPHINE

Nalbuphine is a KOR agonist-MOR antagonist opioid with effects that qualitatively resemble those of pentazocine; however, nalbuphine produces fewer dysphoric side effects than pentazocine.

PHARMACOLOGICAL ACTIONS AND SIDE EFFECTS. An IM dose of 10 mg nalbuphine is equianalgesic to 10 mg morphine, with similar onset and duration of analgesic and subjective effects. Nalbuphine depresses respiration as much as do equianalgesic doses of morphine; however, nalbuphine exhibits a ceiling effect such that increases in dosage beyond 30 mg produce no further respiratory depression or analgesia. In contrast to pentazocine and butorphanol, 10 mg nalbuphine given to patients with stable coronary artery disease does not produce an increase in cardiac index, pulmonary arterial pressure, or cardiac work, and systemic blood pressure is not significantly altered; these indices also are relatively stable when nalbuphine is given to patients with acute myocardial infarction. Nalbuphine produces few side effects at doses of 10 mg or less; sedation, sweating, and headache are the most common. At much higher doses (70 mg), psychotomimetic side effects (e.g., dysphoria, racing thoughts, and distortions of body image) can occur. Nalbuphine is metabolized in the liver and has a plasma $t_{1/2}$ of 2-3 h. Nalbuphine is 20-25% as potent when administered orally as when given intramuscularly. Prolonged administration of nalbuphine can produce physical dependence. The withdrawal syndrome is similar in intensity to that seen with pentazocine.

THERAPEUTIC USE. Nalbuphine hydrochloride (NUBAIN, others) is used to produce analgesia. Because it is an agonist–antagonist, administration to patients who have been receiving morphine-like opioids may create difficulties unless a brief drug-free interval is interposed. The usual adult dose is 10 mg parenterally every 3-6 h; this may be increased to 20 mg in nontolerant individuals. A caveat: Agents that act through the KOR have been reported to be relatively more effective in women than in men.

BUTORPHANOL

Butorphanol is a morphinan congener with a profile of actions similar to those of pentazocine and nalbuphine: KOR agonist and MOR antagonist.

PHARMACOLOGICAL ACTIONS AND SIDE EFFECTS. In postoperative patients, a parenteral dose of 2-3 mg butorphanol produces analgesia and respiratory depression approximately equal to that produced by 10 mg morphine or 80-100 mg meperidine. The plasma $t_{1/2}$ of butorphanol is ~3 h. Like pentazocine, analgesic doses of butorphanol produce an increase in pulmonary arterial pressure and in the work of the heart; systemic arterial pressure is slightly decreased. The major side effects of butorphanol are drowsiness, weakness, sweating, feelings of floating, and nausea. While the incidence of psychotomimetic side effects is lower than that with equianalgesic doses of pentazocine, they are qualitatively similar. Nasal administration is associated with drowsiness and dizziness. Physical dependence can occur.

THERAPEUTIC USE. Butorphanol tartrate (STADOL, others) is used for the relief of acute pain (e.g., postoperative), and because of its potential for antagonizing MOR agonists should not be used in combination. Because of its side effects on the heart, it is less useful than morphine or meperidine in patients with congestive heart failure or myocardial infarction. The usual dose is 1-4 mg of the tartrate given intramuscularly, or 0.5-2 mg given intravenously, every 3-4 h. A nasal formulation is available and has proven to be effective in pain relief, including migraine pain.

BUPRENORPHINE

Buprenorphine is a highly lipophilic MOR agonist, 25-50 times more potent than morphine. It is a partial MOR agonist (e.g., has limited intrinsic activity) and accordingly can display antagonism when used in conjunction with a full agonist.

PHARMACOLOGICAL ACTIONS. Buprenorphine produces analgesia and other CNS effects that are qualitatively similar to those of morphine. About 0.4 mg buprenorphine is equianalgesic with 10 mg morphine given intramuscularly. Some of the subjective and respiratory-depressant effects are unequivocally slower in onset and last longer than those of morphine. Buprenorphine is a partial MOR agonist; thus, it may cause symptoms of abstinence in patients who have been receiving μ receptor agonists for several weeks. It antagonizes the respiratory depression produced by anesthetic doses of fentanyl about as well as naloxone without completely reversing opioid pain relief. The respiratory depression and other effects of buprenorphine can be prevented by prior administration of naloxone, but they are not readily reversed by high doses of naloxone once the effects have been produced, probably due to slow dissociation of buprenorphine from opioid receptors. The $t_{1/2}$ for dissociation from the receptor is 166 min for buprenorphine, as opposed to 7 min for fentanyl. Therefore, plasma levels of buprenorphine may not parallel clinical effects. Cardiovascular and other side effects (e.g., sedation, nausea, vomiting, dizziness, sweating, and headache) appear to be similar to those of morphine-like opioids.

Administered sublingually, buprenorphine (0.4-0.8 mg) produces satisfactory analgesia in postoperative patients. Concentrations in blood peak within 5 min of IM injection and within 1-2 h of oral or sublingual administration. While the plasma $t_{1/2}$ in plasma is ~3 h, this value bears little relationship to the rate of disappearance of effects. Both N-dealkylated and conjugated metabolites are detected in the urine, but most of the drug is excreted unchanged in the feces. When buprenorphine is discontinued, a withdrawal syndrome develops that is delayed in onset for 2-14 days and persists for 1-2 weeks.

THERAPEUTIC USES. Buprenorphine (BUPRENEX) injection is indicated for use as an analgesic. Oral formulations of buprenorphine (SUBUTEX) and buprenorphine in fixed-dose combination with naloxone (SUBOXONE) are used for treatment of opioid dependence. The usual IM or IV dose for analgesia is 0.3 mg given every 6 h. Buprenorphine is metabolized to norbuprenorphine by CYP3A4 and should not be taken with known inhibitors of CYP3A4 (e.g., azole antifungals, macrolide antibiotics, and HIV protease inhibitors), or drugs that induce CYP3A4 activity (e.g., certain anticonvulsants and rifampin).

OPIOID ANTAGONISTS

A variety of agents bind competitively to 1 or more of the opioid receptors, display little or no intrinsic activity, and robustly antagonize the effects of receptor agonists.

Relatively minor changes in the structure of an opioid can convert a drug that is primarily an agonist into 1 with antagonistic actions at 1 or more types of opioid receptors. Simple substitutions transform morphine to nalorphine, levorphanol to levallorphan, and oxymorphone to naloxone (NARCAN, others) or naltrexone (REVIA, VIVITROL, others). In some cases, congeners are produced that are competitive antagonists at MOR but that also have agonistic actions at KORs; nalorphine and levallorphan have such properties. Other congeners, especially naloxone and naltrexone, appear to be devoid of agonistic actions and interact with all types of opioid receptors, albeit with somewhat different affinities. Nalmefene (not marketed in the U.S.) is a relatively pure MOR antagonist that is more potent than naloxone. The majority of these agents are relatively lipid soluble and have excellent CNS bioavailability after systemic delivery. A recognition that there was a need for antagonism limited to peripheral sites led to the development of agents that have poor CNS bioavailability such as methylnaltrexone (RELISTOR).

PHARMACOLOGICAL PROPERTIES

Opioid antagonists have obvious therapeutic utility in the treatment of opioid overdose. Under ordinary circumstances, these opioid antagonists produce few effects in the absence of an exogenous agonist. However, under certain conditions (e.g., shock), when the endogenous opioid systems are activated, the administration of an opioid antagonist alone may have visible consequences.

EFFECTS IN THE ABSENCE OF OPIOID AGONISTS. Subcutaneous doses of naloxone up to 12 mg produce no discernible effects in humans, and 24 mg causes only slight drowsiness. Naltrexone also is a relatively pure antagonist but with higher oral efficacy and a longer duration of action. The effects of opiate receptor antagonists are usually both subtle and limited. Most likely this reflects the low levels of tonic activity and organizational complexity of the opioid systems in various physiologic systems. Opiate antagonism in humans is associated with variable effects ranging from no effect to a mild hyperalgesia. A number of studies have, however, suggested that agents such as naloxone appear to attenuate the analgesic effects of placebo medications and acupuncture.

Endogenous opioid peptides participate in the regulation of pituitary secretion apparently by exerting tonic inhibitory effects on the release of certain hypothalamic hormones (*see* Chapter 38). Thus, the administration of naloxone or naltrexone increases the secretion of gonadotropin-releasing hormone and corticotropin-releasing hormone and elevates the plasma concentrations of LH, FSH, and ACTH, as well as the steroid hormones produced by their target organs. Naloxone stimulates the release of prolactin in women. Endogenous opioid peptides probably have some role in the regulation of feeding or energy metabolism; however, naltrexone does not accelerate weight loss in very obese subjects, even though short-term administration of opioid antagonists reduces food intake in lean and obese individuals. Long-term administration of antagonists increases the density of opioid receptors in the brain and causes a temporary exaggeration of responses to the subsequent administration of opioid agonists.

EFFECTS IN THE PRESENCE OF OPIOID AGONISTS

Antagonistic Effects. Small doses (0.4-0.8 mg) of naloxone given intramuscularly or intravenously prevent or *promptly* reverse the effects of receptor agonists. In patients with respiratory depression, an increase in respiratory rate is seen within 1-2 min. Sedative effects are reversed, and blood pressure, if depressed, returns to normal. Higher doses of naloxone are required to antagonize the respiratory-depressant effects of buprenorphine; 1 mg naloxone intravenously completely blocks the effects of 25 mg heroin. Naloxone reverses the psychotomimetic and dysphoric effects of agonist–antagonist agents such as pentazocine, but much higher doses (10-15 mg) are required. The duration of antagonistic effects depends on the dose but usually is 1-4 h. Antagonism of opioid effects by naloxone often is accompanied by an "overshoot" phenomenon. For example, respiratory rate depressed by opioids transiently becomes higher than that before the period of depression. Rebound release of catecholamines may cause hypertension, tachycardia, and ventricular arrhythmias. Pulmonary edema also has been reported.

Effects in Opioid-Dependent Patients. In subjects who are dependent on morphine-like opioids, small subcutaneous doses of naloxone (0.5 mg) precipitate a moderate to severe withdrawal syndrome that is very similar to that seen after abrupt withdrawal of opioids, except that the syndrome appears within minutes of administration and subsides in ~2 h. The severity and duration of the syndrome are related to the dose of the antagonist and to the degree and type of dependence. Naloxone produces overshoot phenomena suggestive of early acute physical dependence 6-24 h after a single dose of a μ agonist.

ADME

Although absorbed readily from the GI tract, naloxone is almost completely metabolized by the liver before reaching the systemic circulation and thus must be administered parenterally. The $t_{1/2}$ of naloxone is ~1 h, but its clinically effective duration of action can be even less. Compared with naloxone, naltrexone has more efficacy by the oral route, and its duration of action approaches 24 h after moderate oral doses. Peak concentrations in plasma are reached within 1-2 h and then decline with an apparent $t_{1/2}$ of ~3 h. Naltrexone is metabolized to 6-naltrexol, which is a weaker antagonist with longer $t_{1/2}$, ~13 h. Naltrexone is much more potent than naloxone, and 100-mg oral doses given to patients addicted to opioids produce concentrations in tissues sufficient to block the euphorigenic effects of 25-mg IV doses of heroin for 48 h. Methylnaltrexone is similar to naltrexone; it is converted to methyl-6-naltrexol isomers and eliminated primarily as the unchanged drug with active renal secretion. The $t_{1/2}$ of methylnaltrexone is ~8 h.

THERAPEUTIC USES

TREATMENT OF OPIOID OVERDOSAGE. Opioid antagonists, particularly naloxone, have an established use in the treatment of opioid-induced toxicity, especially respiratory depression. Its specificity is such that reversal by naloxone is virtually diagnostic for the contribution of an opiate to the depression. Naloxone acts rapidly to reverse the respiratory depression associated with high doses of opioids. It should be titrated cautiously because it also can precipitate withdrawal in dependent subjects and cause undesirable cardiovascular side effects. The duration of action of naloxone is relatively short, and it often must be given repeatedly or by continuous infusion. Opioid antagonists also have been employed effectively to decrease neonatal respiratory depression secondary to the IV or IM administration of opioids to the mother. In the neonate, the initial dose is 10 μg/kg given intravenously, intramuscularly, or subcutaneously.

MANAGEMENT OF CONSTIPATION. The peripherally limited antagonists such as methylnaltrexone have a very important role in the management of the constipation and the reduced GI motility present in the patient undergoing chronic opioid therapy (as for chronic pain or methadone maintenance). Other strategies for the management of opioid-induced constipation are described in Chapter 46.

MANAGEMENT OF ABUSE SYNDROMES. There is interest in the use of opiate antagonists such as naltrexone as an adjuvant in treating a variety of nonopioid dependency syndromes such as alcoholism (*see* Chapters 23 and 24), where an opiate antagonist decreases the chance of relapse. Interestingly, patients with a single nucleotide polymorphism (SNP) in the MOR gene have significantly lower relapse rates to alcoholism when treated with naltrexone. Naltrexone is FDA-approved for treatment of alcoholism.

CENTRALLY ACTIVE ANTITUSSIVES

Cough is a useful physiological mechanism that serves to clear the respiratory passages of foreign material and excess secretions. It should not be suppressed indiscriminately. There are, however, situations in which cough does not serve any useful purpose but may, instead, annoy the patient, prevent rest and sleep, or hinder adherence to otherwise beneficial medication regimens (e.g., angiotensin-converting enzyme [ACE] inhibitor-induced cough). In such situations, the physician should try to substitute a drug with a different side-effect profile (e.g., an AT1 antagonist in place of an ACE inhibitor) or add an antitussive agent that will reduce the frequency or intensity of the coughing. A number of drugs reduce cough as a result of their central actions, including opioid analgesics (codeine, hydrocodone, and dihydrocodeine are most commonly used). Cough suppression often occurs with lower doses of opioids than those needed for analgesia. A 10- or 20-mg oral dose of codeine, although ineffective for analgesia, produces a demonstrable antitussive effect, and higher doses produce even more suppression of chronic cough. A few other antitussive agents are noted below.

DEXTROMETHORPHAN

Dextromethorphan (D-3-methoxy-N-methylmorphinan) is the D-isomer of the codeine analog methorphan; however, unlike the L-isomer, it has no analgesic or addictive properties and does not act through opioid receptors. The drug acts centrally to elevate the threshold for coughing. Its effectiveness in patients with pathological cough has been demonstrated in controlled studies; its potency is nearly equal to that of codeine, but dextromethorphan produces fewer subjective and GI side effects. In therapeutic dosages, the drug does not inhibit ciliary activity, and its antitussive effects persist for 5-6 h. Its toxicity is low, but extremely high doses may produce CNS depression. The average adult dosage of dextromethorphan hydrobromide is 10-30 mg 3-6 times daily, not to exceed 120 mg daily. The drug is marketed for over-the-counter sale in liquids, syrups, capsules, soluble strips, lozenges, and freezer pops or in combinations with antihistamines, bronchodilators, expectorants, and decongestants. An extended-release dextromethorphan suspension (DELSYM) is approved for twice-daily administration.

Although dextromethorphan is known to function as an NMDA receptor antagonist, the dextromethorphan binding sites are not limited to the known distribution of NMDA receptors. Thus, the mechanism by which dextromethorphan exerts its antitussive effect still is not clear.

OTHER ANTITUSSIVES. Pholcodine [3-O-(2-morpholinoethyl) morphine] is used clinically in many countries outside the U.S. Although structurally related to the opioids, pholcodine has no opioid-like actions. Pholcodine is at least as effective as codeine as an antitussive; it has a long $t_{1/2}$ and can be given once or twice daily.

Benzonatate (TESSALON, others) is a long-chain polyglycol derivative chemically related to procaine and believed to exert its antitussive action on stretch or cough receptors in the lung, as well as by a central mechanism. It is available in oral capsules and the dosage is 100 mg 3 times daily; doses as high as 600 mg daily have been used safely.

ROUTES OF ANALGESIC DRUG ADMINISTRATION

In addition to the traditional oral and parenteral formulations for opioids, many other methods of administration have been developed in an effort to improve therapeutic efficacy while minimizing side effects.

PATIENT-CONTROLLED ANALGESIA (PCA). With this modality, the patient has limited control of the dosing of opioid from an infusion pump programmed within tightly mandated parameters. PCA can be used for IV, epidural, or intrathecal administration of opioids. This technique avoids delays inherent in administration by a caregiver and generally permits better alignment between pain control and individual differences in pain perception and responsiveness to opioids.

SPINAL DELIVERY. Administration of opioids into the epidural or intrathecal space provides more direct access to the first pain-processing synapse in the dorsal horn of the spinal cord. This permits the use of doses substantially lower than those required for oral or parenteral administration (Table 18–5).

Epidural and intrathecal opioids have their own dose-dependent side effects, such as pruritus, nausea, vomiting, respiratory depression, and urinary retention. Hydrophilic opioids such as morphine (DURAMORPH, others) have a longer residence times in the cerebrospinal fluid; as a consequence, after intrathecal or epidural morphine, delayed respiratory depression can be observed for as long as 24 h after a bolus dose. The risk of delayed respiratory depression is reduced with more lipophilic opioids. Use of intraspinal opioids in the opioid-naïve patient is reserved for postoperative pain control in an inpatient monitored setting. Epidural administration of opioids has become popular in the management of postoperative pain and for providing analgesia during labor and delivery. Lower systemic opioid levels are achieved with epidural opioids, leading to less placental transfer and less potential for respiratory depression of the newborn. Agents approved for spinal delivery are certain preservative-free formulations of morphine sulfate (DURAMORPH, DEPODUR, others) and sufentanil (SUFENTA). The spinal route of delivery

Table 18–5

Epidural or Intrathecal Opioids for the Treatment of Acute (Bolus) or Chronic (Infusion) Pain

DRUG	SINGLE DOSE (mg)[a]	INFUSION RATE (mg/h)[b]	ONSET (min)	DURATION OF EFFECT OF SINGLE DOSE (h)[c]
Epidural				
Morphine	1-6	0.1-1.0	30	6-24
Meperidine	20-150	5-20	5	4-8
Methadone	1-10	0.3-0.5	10	6-10
Hydromorphone	1-2	0.1-0.2	15	10-16
Fentanyl	0.025-0.1	0.025-0.10	5	2-4
Sufentanil	0.01-0.06	0.01-0.05	5	2-4
Alfentanil	0.5-1	0.2	15	1-3
Subarachnoid (Intrathecal)				
Morphine	0.1-0.3		15	8-24+
Fentanyl	0.005-0.025		5	3-6

[a]*Low doses may be effective when administered to the elderly or when injected in the thoracic region.*
[b]*If combining with a local anesthetic, consider using 0.0625% bupivacaine.*
[c]*Duration of analgesia varies widely; higher doses produce longer duration. With the exception of epidural/intrathecal morphine or epidural sufentanil, all other spinal opioid use is considered to be off label.*
Source: Adapted from International Association for the Study of Pain, 1992.

represents a novel environment wherein the neuraxis may be exposed to exceedingly high concentrations of an agent for an extended period of time; safety by another route (e.g., PO, IV) may not translate to safety after spinal delivery.

Intraspinal narcotics often are combined with other agents that include local anesthetics, N-type Ca^{2+} channel blockers (e.g., ziconotide), α_2 adrenergic agonists, and $GABA_B$ agonists. The synergy between drugs with different mechanisms allows the use of lower concentrations of both agents, minimizing side effects and opioid-induced complications.

RECTAL ADMINISTRATION. This route is an alternative for patients with difficulty swallowing or other oral pathology and who prefer a less invasive route than parenteral administration. This route is not well tolerated by most children. Onset of action is within 10 min. In the U.S., only morphine and hydromorphone are available in rectal suppository formulations.

ORAL TRANSMUCOSAL ADMINISTRATION. Opioids can be absorbed through the oral mucosa more rapidly than through the stomach. Bioavailability is greater owing to avoidance of first-pass metabolism, and lipophilic opioids are absorbed better by this route than are hydrophilic compounds such as morphine. A transmucosal delivery system that suspends fentanyl in a dissolvable sugar-based lollipop (ACTIQ, others) or rapidly dissolving buccal tablet (FENTORA) and a buccal fentanyl "film" are FDA-approved for the treatment of cancer pain (ONSOLIS).

TRANSNASAL ADMINISTRATION. Butorphanol, a KOR agonist/MOR antagonist, has been employed intranasally. A transnasal pectin-based fentanyl spray is currently in clinical trials for the treatment of cancer-related pain. Administration is well tolerated and pain relief occurs within 10 min of delivery.

TRANSDERMAL ADMINISTRATION. Transdermal fentanyl patches are approved for use in sustained pain. The opioid permeates the skin, and a "depot" is established in the stratum corneum layer. However, fever and external heat sources (heating pads, hot baths) can increase absorption of fentanyl and potentially lead to an overdose. This modality is well suited for cancer pain treatment because of its ease of use, prolonged duration of action, and stable blood levels. There may be great variability in plasma levels after a given dose. The plasma $t_{1/2}$ after patch removal is ~17 h. Thus, if excessive sedation or respiratory depression is experienced, antagonist infusions may need to be maintained for an extended period. Dermatological side effects from the patches, such as rash and itching, usually are mild. Opiate-addicted patients have been known to chew the patches and receive an overdose.

THERAPEUTIC CONSIDERATIONS

Management of pain is an important element in any therapeutic intervention. Failure to adequately manage pain can have important negative consequences on physiological function such as autonomic hyperreactivity (increased blood pressure, heart rate, suppression of gastrointestinal motility, reduced secretions), reduced mobility leading to deconditioning, muscle wasting, joint stiffening, and decalcification, and can contribute to deleterious changes in the psychological state (depression, helplessness syndromes, anxiety). By many hospital accrediting organizations, and by law in many states, appropriate pain assessment and adequate pain management are considered to be standard of care, with pain being considered the "fifth vital sign."

GUIDELINES FOR OPIATE DOSING

The World Health Organization provides a 3-step ladder as a guide to treat both cancer pain and chronic noncancer pain (Table 18–6). The 3-step ladder encourages the use of more conservative therapies before initiating opioid therapy. Weaker opioids can be supplanted by stronger opioids in cases of moderate and severe pain. Antidepressants such as duloxetine and amitriptyline that are used in the treatment of chronic neuropathic pain have limited intrinsic analgesic actions in acute pain; however, antidepressants may enhance morphine-induced analgesia. In the presence of severe pain, the opioids should be considered sooner rather than later.

Numerous societies and agencies have published guidelines for the use of strong opioids in treating pain. While slightly different in particulars, all guidelines to date share the criteria of Table 18–7. Methadone dosing is considered separately in Table 18–8.

Suggestions for the oral and parenteral dosing of commonly used opioids (*see* Table 18–2) are only guidelines. They are typically constructed with the use of these agents in the management of acute (e.g., postoperative) pain in opioid-naïve patients. A number of factors will contribute to the dosing requirement (described in subsequent sections).

Table 18–6

World Health Organization Analgesic Ladder[a]

Step 1 Mild to Moderate Pain

Non-opioid ± adjuvant agent

- Acetaminophen or an NSAID should be used, unless contraindicated. Adjuvant agents are those that enhance analgesic efficacy, treat concurrent symptoms that exacerbate pain, and/or provide independent analgesic activity for specific types of pain.

Step 2 Mild to Moderate Pain or Pain Uncontrolled after Step 1

Short-acting opioid as required ± non-opioid around the clock (ATC) ± adjuvant agent

- Morphine, oxycodone, or hydromorphone should be added to acetaminophen or an NSAID for maximum flexibility of opioid dose.

Step 3 Moderate to Severe Pain or Pain Uncontrolled after Step 2

Sustained release/long-acting opioid ATC or continuous infusion + short-acting opioid as required ± non-opioid ± adjuvant agent

- Sustained release oxycodone, morphine, oxymorphone, or transdermal fentanyl is indicated.

[a]*http://www.who.int/cancer/palliative/painladder/en/*

VARIABLES MODIFYING THE THERAPEUTIC RESPONSE TO OPIATES

There is substantial individual variability in responses to opioids. A standard IM dose of 10 mg morphine sulfate will relieve severe pain adequately in only 2 of 3 patients. The minimal effective analgesic concentration for opioids, such as morphine, meperidine (pethidine), alfentanil, and sufentanil, varies among patients by factors of 5-10.

The 12th edition of the parent text covers a variety of issues that can affect patient response to opiates, including physical condition of the patient, disease, intensity of pain, type of pain, acuity and chronicity of pain, opioid tolerance, pharmacokinetic variables, and genetic factors. These factors will affect the choice of agent and mode of delivery. Other considerations include opioid rotation (changing to a different opioid when the patient fails to achieve benefit or side effects become limiting before analgesia is sufficient), and combination therapy.

Certain opiate combinations are useful. For example, in a chronic pain state with periodic incident or breakthrough pain, the patient might receive a slow-release formulation of morphine for baseline pain relief and

Table 18–7

Guidelines for the Use of Opioids to Treat Chronic Pain

- *Evaluation of the patient*: A complete medical history and physical must be conducted and documented in the medical record.
- *Treatment plan*: The treatment plan should state objectives that are used to determine treatment success.
- *Informed consent and agreement*: The physician should discuss the risks, benefits, and alternatives to chronic opioid therapy with the patient. Many practitioners have developed an "opioid contract" that outlines the responsibilities of the physician and the patient for continued prescription of controlled substances.
- *Periodic review*: At reasonable intervals, the patient should be seen by the physician to review the course of treatment and document results of consultation, diagnostic, testing, laboratory results, and the success of treatment.
- *Consultation*: The physician should refer the patient for consultation when appropriate.
- *Documentation/medical records*: The physician should keep actual and complete medical records that include: (a) medical history and physical examination; (b) diagnostic, therapeutic, and laboratory results; (c) evaluations and consultations; (d) treatment objectives; (e) discussion of risks and benefits; (f) treatment; (g) medications including date, type, dosage, and quantity prescribed; (h) instructions and agreements; and (i) periodic reviews.
- *Compliance with controlled substances law and regulations*: To prescribe, dispense, or administer controlled substances, the physician must be licensed in the state and comply with applicable state and federal regulations.

Table 18–8

Oral Morphine to Methadone Conversion Guidelines

DAILY MORPHINE DOSE (mg/24 h, oral)	CONVERSION RATIOS MORPHINE : METHADONE (oral) (oral)
<100	6 : 1
101-300	8 : 1
301-600	10 : 1
601-800	12 : 1
801-1000	15 : 1
>1001	20 : 1

Note: When converting from methadone to morphine, use 3:1 conversion.

the acute incident pain may be managed with a rapid-onset/short-lasting formulation such as buccal fentanyl. For inflammatory or nociceptive pain, opioids may be usefully combined with other analgesic agents, such as NSAIDs or acetaminophen (Table 18–9). In some situations, NSAIDs can provide analgesia equal to that produced by 60 mg codeine. In the case of neuropathic pain, other drug classes may be useful in combination with the opiate. For example, antidepressants that block amine reuptake, such as amitriptyline or duloxetine, and anticonvulsants such as gabapentin, may enhance the analgesic effect and may be synergistic in some pain states.

NONANALGESIC THERAPEUTIC USES OF OPIOIDS

DYSPNEA. Morphine is used to alleviate the dyspnea of acute left ventricular failure and pulmonary edema, and the response to IV morphine may be dramatic. The mechanism underlying this relief is not clear. It may involve an alteration of the patient's reaction to impaired respiratory function and an indirect reduction of the work of the heart owing to reduced fear and apprehension. However, it is more probable that the major benefit is due to cardiovascular effects, such as decreased peripheral resistance and an increased capacity of the peripheral and splanchnic vascular compartments. Nitroglycerin, which also causes vasodilation, may be superior to morphine in this condition. In patients with normal blood gases but severe breathlessness owing to chronic obstruction of airflow ("pink puffers"), dihydrocodeine, 15 mg orally before exercise, reduces the feeling of breathlessness and increases exercise tolerance. Nonetheless, opioids generally are contraindicated in pulmonary edema unless severe pain also is present.

ANESTHETIC ADJUVANTS. High doses of opioids, notably fentanyl and sufentanil, are widely used as the primary anesthetic agents in many surgical procedures. They have powerful "MAC-sparing" effects, e.g., they reduce the concentrations of volatile anesthetic otherwise required to produce an adequate anesthetic depth. Although respiration is so depressed that physical assistance is required, patients can retain consciousness. Therefore, when using an opioid as the primary anesthetic agent, use it in conjunction with an agent that results in unconsciousness and produces amnesia such as the benzodiazepines or low concentrations of volatile anesthetics. High doses of opiate also result in prominent rigidity of the chest wall and masseters requiring concurrent treatment with muscle relaxants to permit intubations and ventilation.

TREATMENT OF ACUTE OPIOID TOXICITY

Acute opioid toxicity may result from clinical overdosage, accidental overdosage, or attempts at suicide. Occasionally, a delayed type of toxicity may occur from the injection of an opioid into chilled skin areas or in patients with low blood pressure and shock. The drug is not fully absorbed, and therefore, a subsequent dose may be given. When normal circulation is restored, an excessive amount may be absorbed suddenly. In nontolerant individuals, serious toxicity with methadone may follow the oral ingestion of 40-60 mg. In the case of morphine, a normal, pain-free adult is not likely to die after oral doses <120 mg or to have serious toxicity with <30 mg parenterally.

SYMPTOMS AND DIAGNOSIS. The patient who has taken an overdose of an opioid usually is stuporous or, if a large overdose has been taken, may be in a profound coma. The respiratory rate will be very low, or the patient may be apneic, and cyanosis may be present. If adequate oxygenation is restored early, the blood

Table 18–9

Summary of Drug Target and Site of Action of Common Drug Classes and Relative Efficacy by Pain State

DRUG CLASS (examples)	DRUG ACTION	SITE OF ACTION[a]	RELATIVE EFFICACY IN PAIN STATES[a]
NSAIDs (ibuprofen, aspirin, acetominophen)	Nonspecific COX inhibitors	Peripheral and spinal	Tissue injury >> acute stimuli = nerve injury = 0
COX 2 inhibitor (celecoxib)	COX2-selective inhibitor	Peripheral and spinal	Tissue injury >> acute stimuli = nerve injury = 0
Opioids (morphine)	μ receptor agonist	Supraspinal and spinal	Tissue injury = acute stimuli ≥ nerve injury > 0 (*see* this chapter)
Anticonvulsants (gabapentin)	Na^+ channel block, $\alpha_2\delta$ subunit of Ca^{2+} channel	Supraspinal and spinal	Nerve injury > tissue injury = acute stimuli = 0
Tricyclic antidepressants (amitryptiline)	Inhibit uptake of 5HT/NE	Supraspinal and spinal	Nerve injury ≥ tissue injury >> acute stimuli = 0

[a]*As defined by studies in preclinical models. See 12th edition of parent text, Table 18–8.*

pressure will improve; if hypoxia persists untreated, there may be capillary damage, and measures to combat shock may be required. The pupils will be symmetrical and pinpoint in size; however, if hypoxia is severe, they may be dilated. Urine formation is depressed. Body temperature falls, and the skin becomes cold and clammy. The skeletal muscles are flaccid, the jaw is relaxed, and the tongue may fall back and block the airway. Frank convulsions occasionally may be noted in infants and children. When death occurs, it is nearly always from respiratory failure. Even if respiration is restored, death still may occur as a result of complications that develop during the period of coma, such as pneumonia or shock.

TREATMENT. The first step is to establish a patent airway and ventilate the patient. Opioid antagonists can produce dramatic reversal of the severe respiratory depression, and the antagonist naloxone is the treatment of choice. However, care should be taken to avoid precipitating withdrawal in dependent patients, who may be extremely sensitive to antagonists. The safest approach is to dilute the standard naloxone dose (0.4 mg) and slowly administer it intravenously, monitoring arousal and respiratory function. With care, it usually is possible to reverse the respiratory depression without precipitating a major withdrawal syndrome. If no response is seen with the first dose, additional doses can be given. Patients should be observed for rebound increases in sympathetic nervous system activity, which may result in cardiac arrhythmias and pulmonary edema. For reversing opioid poisoning in children, the initial dose of naloxone is 0.01 mg/kg. If no effect is seen after a total dose of 10 mg, one can reasonably question the accuracy of the diagnosis. Pulmonary edema sometimes associated with opioid overdosage may be countered by positive-pressure respiration. Tonic-clonic seizures, occasionally seen as part of the toxic syndrome with meperidine, propoxyphene, and tramadol, are ameliorated by treatment with naloxone.

The presence of general CNS depressants does not prevent the salutary effect of naloxone, and in cases of mixed intoxications, the situation will be improved largely owing to antagonism of the respiratory-depressant effects of the opioid (however, some evidence indicates that naloxone and naltrexone also may antagonize some of the depressant actions of sedative-hypnotics). One need not attempt to restore the patient to full consciousness. The duration of action of the available antagonists is shorter than that of many opioids; hence patients can slip back into coma. This is particularly important when the overdosage is due to methadone. The depressant effects of these drugs may persist for 24-72 h, and fatalities have occurred as a result of premature discontinuation of naloxone. In cases of overdoses of these drugs, a continuous infusion of naloxone should be considered. Toxicity owing to overdose of pentazocine and other opioids with mixed actions may require higher doses of naloxone.

For a complete Bibliographical Listing see Goodman & Gilman's ***The Pharmacological Basis of Therapeutics***, 12th ed., or Goodman & Gilman Online at www.AccessMedicine.com.

General Anesthetics and Therapeutic Gases

General Anesthetics

General anesthetics depress the central nervous system to a sufficient degree to permit the performance of surgery and unpleasant procedures. General anesthetics have low therapeutic indices and thus require great care in administration. The selection of specific drugs and routes of administration to produce general anesthesia is based on their pharmacokinetic properties and on the secondary effects of the various drugs, in the context of the proposed diagnostic or surgical procedure and with the consideration of the individual patient's age, and associated medical condition.

GENERAL PRINCIPLES OF SURGICAL ANESTHESIA

The administration of general anesthesia is driven by 3 general objectives:

1. *Minimizing the potentially deleterious direct and indirect effects of anesthetic agents and techniques*
2. *Sustaining physiologic homeostasis during surgical procedures* that may involve major blood loss, tissue ischemia, reperfusion of ischemic tissue, fluid shifts, exposure to a cold environment, and impaired coagulation
3. *Improving postoperative outcomes* by choosing techniques that block or treat components of the surgical stress response, which may lead to short- or long-term sequelae

HEMODYNAMIC EFFECTS OF GENERAL ANESTHESIA. The most prominent physiological effect of anesthesia induction is a decrease in systemic arterial blood pressure. The causes include direct vasodilation, myocardial depression, or both; a blunting of baroreceptor control; and a generalized decrease in central sympathetic tone. Agents vary in the magnitude of their specific effects, but in all cases the hypotensive response is enhanced by underlying volume depletion or preexisting myocardial dysfunction.

RESPIRATORY EFFECTS OF GENERAL ANESTHESIA. Nearly all general anesthetics reduce or eliminate both ventilatory drive and the reflexes that maintain airway patency. Therefore, ventilation generally must be assisted or controlled for at least some period during surgery. The gag reflex is lost, and the stimulus to cough is blunted. Lower esophageal sphincter tone also is reduced, so both passive and active regurgitation may occur. Endotracheal intubation has been a major reason for a decline in the number of aspiration deaths during general anesthesia. Muscle relaxation is valuable during the induction of general anesthesia where it facilitates management of the airway, including endotracheal intubation. Neuromuscular blocking agents commonly are used to effect such relaxation (*see* Chapter 11). Alternatives to an endotracheal tube include a face mask and a laryngeal mask, an inflatable mask placed in the oropharynx forming a seal around the glottis.

HYPOTHERMIA. Patients commonly develop hypothermia (body temperature <36°C) during surgery. The reasons include low ambient temperature, exposed body cavities, cold intravenous (IV) fluids, altered thermoregulatory control, and reduced metabolic rate. Metabolic rate and total body oxygen consumption decrease with general anesthesia by ~30%, reducing heat generation. Hypothermia may lead to an increase in perioperative morbidity. Prevention of hypothermia is a major goal of anesthetic care.

NAUSEA AND VOMITING. Nausea and vomiting continue to be significant problems following general anesthesia and are caused by an action of anesthetics on the chemoreceptor trigger zone and the brainstem vomiting center, which are modulated by serotonin (5HT), histamine, ACh, and dopamine (DA). The $5HT_3$ receptor antagonists, ondansetron and dolasetron (*see* Chapters 13 and 46), are very effective in suppressing nausea and vomiting. Common treatments also include droperidol, metoclopramide, dexamethasone, and avoidance of N_2O. The use of propofol as an induction agent and the nonsteroidal anti-inflammatory drug ketorolac as a substitute for opioids may decrease the incidence and severity of postoperative nausea and vomiting.

OTHER EMERGENCE AND POSTOPERATIVE PHENOMENA. Hypertension and tachycardia are common as the sympathetic nervous system regains its tone and is enhanced by pain. Myocardial ischemia can appear or worsen during emergence in patients with coronary artery disease. Emergence excitement occurs in 5-30% of patients and is characterized by tachycardia, restlessness, crying, moaning, and thrashing. Neurologic signs, including delirium, spasticity, hyperreflexia, and Babinski sign, are often manifest in the patient emerging from anesthesia. Postanesthesia shivering occurs frequently because of core hypothermia. A small dose of meperidine (12.5 mg) lowers the shivering trigger temperature and effectively stops the activity. The incidence of all of these emergence phenomena is greatly reduced with opioids and α_2 agonists (dexmedetomidine).

Airway obstruction may occur during the postoperative period because residual anesthetic effects. Pulmonary function is reduced following all types of anesthesia and surgery, and hypoxemia may occur. Pain control can be complicated in the immediate postoperative period and respiratory suppression associated with opioids can be problematic. Regional anesthetic techniques are an important part of a perioperative approach that employs local anesthetic wound infiltration; epidural, spinal, and plexus blocks; and nonsteroidal anti-inflammatory drugs, opioids, α_2 adrenergic receptor agonists, and NMDA receptor antagonists.

ACTIONS AND MECHANISMS OF GENERAL ANESTHETICS

THE ANESTHETIC STATE

The components of the anesthetic state include:

- *Amnesia*
- *Immobility* in response to noxious stimulation
- *Attenuation of autonomic responses* to noxious stimulation
- *Analgesia*
- *Unconsciousness*

The potency of general anesthetic agents is measured by determining the concentration of general anesthetic that prevents movement in response to surgical stimulation. For inhalational anesthetics, anesthetic potency is measured in *MAC units*, with 1 MAC defined as the minimum alveolar concentration that prevents movement in response to surgical stimulation in 50% of subjects. The strengths of MAC as a measurement are that:

- Alveolar concentrations can be monitored continuously by measuring end-tidal anesthetic concentration using infrared spectroscopy or mass spectrometry.
- It provides a direct correlate of the free concentration of the anesthetic at its site(s) of action in the CNS.
- It is a simple-to-measure end point that reflects an important clinical goal.

End points other than immobilization also can be used to measure anesthetic potency. For example, the ability to respond to verbal commands (MAC_{awake}) and the ability to form memories also have been correlated with alveolar anesthetic concentration. Verbal response and memory formation are suppressed at a fraction of MAC. The ratio of the anesthetic concentrations required to produce amnesia and immobility vary significantly among different inhalational anesthetic agents (nitrous oxide versus isoflurane).

Generally, the potency of IV agents is defined as the free plasma concentration (at equilibrium) that produces loss of response to surgical incision (or other end points) in 50% of subjects.

MECHANISMS OF ANESTHESIA

CELLULAR MECHANISMS OF ANESTHESIA. General anesthetics produce 2 important physiologic effects at the cellular level:

- The inhalational anesthetics can hyperpolarize neurons. This may be an important effect on neurons serving a pacemaker role and on pattern-generating circuits.
- Both inhalational and IV anesthetics have substantial effects on synaptic transmission and much smaller effects on action-potential generation or propagation.

Inhalational anesthetics inhibit excitatory synapses and enhance inhibitory synapses in various preparations. The inhalational anesthetic isoflurane clearly can inhibit neurotransmitter release, while the small reduction in presynaptic action potential amplitude produced by isoflurane (3% reduction at MAC concentration) substantially inhibits neurotransmitter release. Inhalational anesthetics also can act postsynaptically, altering the response to released neurotransmitter. These actions are thought to be due to specific interactions of anesthetic agents with neurotransmitter receptors.

Intravenous anesthetics produce a narrower range of physiological effects. Their predominant actions are at the synapse, where they have profound and relatively specific effects on the postsynaptic response to released neurotransmitter. Most of the IV agents act predominantly by enhancing inhibitory neurotransmission, whereas ketamine predominantly inhibits excitatory neurotransmission at glutamatergic synapses.

MOLECULAR ACTIONS OF GENERAL ANESTHETICS. Most IV general anesthetics act predominantly through $GABA_A$ receptors and perhaps through some interactions with other ligand-gated ion channels such as NMDA receptors and 2-pore K^+ channels.

Chloride channels gated by the inhibitory $GABA_A$ receptors (*see* Figures 14–3 and 14–6) are sensitive to a wide variety of anesthetics, including the halogenated inhalational agents and many IV agents (propofol, barbiturates, etomidate, and neurosteroids). At clinical concentrations, general anesthetics increase the sensitivity of the $GABA_A$ receptor to GABA, thus enhancing inhibitory neurotransmission and depressing nervous system activity. The action of anesthetics on the $GABA_A$ receptor probably is mediated by binding of the anesthetics to specific sites on the $GABA_A$-receptor protein (but they do not compete with GABA for its binding site on the receptor). The capacity of propofol and etomidate to inhibit the response to noxious stimuli is mediated by a specific site on the β_3 subunit of the $GABA_A$ receptor, whereas the sedative effects of these anesthetics are mediated by on the β_2 subunit.

Structurally related to the $GABA_A$ receptors are other ligand-gated ion channels including *glycine receptors* and neuronal *nicotinic ACh receptors*. Glycine receptors may play a role in mediating inhibition by anesthetics of responses to noxious stimuli. Inhalational anesthetics enhance the capacity of glycine to activate *glycine-gated chloride channels* (glycine receptors), which play an important role in inhibitory neurotransmission in the spinal cord and brainstem. Propofol, neurosteroids, and barbiturates also potentiate glycine-activated currents, whereas etomidate and ketamine do not. Subanesthetic concentrations of the inhalational anesthetics inhibit some classes of neuronal nicotinic ACh receptors, which seem to mediate other components of anesthesia such as analgesia or amnesia.

Ketamine, nitrous oxide, cyclopropane, and xenon are the only general anesthetics that do not have significant effects on $GABA_A$ or glycine receptors. These agents inhibit a different type of ligand-gated ion channel, the NMDA receptor (*see* Figure 14–7 and Table 14–1). NMDA receptors are glutamate-gated cation channels that are somewhat selective for Ca^{++} and are involved in long-term modulation of synaptic responses (long-term potentiation) and glutamate-mediated neurotoxicity.

Halogenated inhalational anesthetics activate some members of a class of K^+ channels known as *2-pore domain channels*; other 2-pore domain channel family members are activated by xenon, nitrous oxide, and cyclopropane. These channels are located in both presynaptic and postsynaptic sites. The postsynaptic channels may be the molecular locus through which these agents hyperpolarize neurons.

Anatomic Sites of Anesthetic Action. In principle, general anesthetics could interrupt nervous system function at myriad levels, including peripheral sensory neurons, the spinal cord, the brainstem, and the cerebral cortex. Most anesthetics cause, with some exceptions, a global reduction in cerebral metabolic rate (CMR) and in cerebral blood flow (CBF). A consistent feature of general anesthesia is a suppression of metabolism in the thalamus, which serves as a major relay by which sensory input from the periphery ascends to the cortex. Suppression of thalamic activity may serve as a switch between the awake and anesthetized states. General anesthesia also results in the suppression of activity in specific regions of the cortex, including the mesial parietal cortex, posterior cingulate cortex, precuneus, and inferior parietal cortex.

Similarities between natural sleep and the anesthetized state suggest that anesthetics might also modulate endogenous sleep regulating pathways, which include ventrolateral preoptic (VLPO) and tuberomammillary nuclei. VLPO projects inhibitory GABA-ergic fibers to ascending arousal nuclei, which in turn project to the cortex, forebrain, and subcortical areas; release of histamine, 5HT, orexin, NE, and ACh mediate wakefulness. Intravenous and inhalational agents with activity at $GABA_A$ receptors can increase the inhibitory effects of VLPO, thereby suppressing consciousness. Dexmedetomidine, an α_2 agonist, also increases VLPO-mediated inhibition by suppressing the inhibitory effect of locus ceruleus neurons on VLPO. Finally, both IV and inhalational anesthetics depress hippocampal neurotransmission, a probable locus for their amnestic effects.

PARENTERAL ANESTHETICS

Parenteral anesthetics are the most common drugs used for anesthetic induction of adults. Their lipophilicity, coupled with the relatively high perfusion of the brain and spinal cord, results in rapid onset and short duration after a single bolus dose. These drugs ultimately accumulate in fatty tissue. Each anesthetic has its own unique set of properties and side effects (Tables 19–1 and 19–2). Propofol and thiopental are the 2 most commonly used parenteral agents. Propofol is advantageous for procedures where rapid return to a preoperative mental status is desirable. Thiopental has a long-established track record of safety. Etomidate usually is reserved for patients at risk for hypotension and/or myocardial ischemia. Ketamine is best suited for patients with asthma or for children undergoing short, painful procedures.

PHARMACOKINETIC PRINCIPLES

Parenteral anesthetics are small, hydrophobic, substituted aromatic or heterocyclic compounds (Figure 19–1). Hydrophobicity is the key factor governing their pharmacokinetics. After a single IV bolus, these drugs preferentially partition into the highly perfused and lipophilic tissues of

Table 19–1

Pharmacological Properties of Parenteral Anesthetics

DRUG	IV Induction Dose (mg/kg)	Minimal Hypnotic Level (μg/mL)	Induction Dose Duration (min)	$t_{1/2}\beta$ (h)	*CL* (mL/min/kg)	Protein Binding (%)	V_{SS} (L/kg)
Thiopental	3-5	15.6	5-8	12.1	3.4	85	2.3
Methohexital	1-2	10	4-7	3.9	10.9	85	2.2
Propofol	1.5-2.5	1.1	4-8	1.8	30	98	2.3
Etomidate	0.2-0.4	0.3	4-8	2.9	17.9	76	2.5
Ketamine	0.5-1.5	1	10-15	3.0	19.1	27	3.1

$t_{1/2}\beta$, β phase half-life; CL, clearance; V_{ss}, volume of distribution at steady state; EDTA, ethylenediaminetetraacetic acid; Na-MBS, Na-metabisulfite; PG, propylene glycol; PL, phospholipid.

the brain and spinal cord where they produce anesthesia within a single circulation time. Subsequently blood levels fall rapidly, resulting in drug redistribution out of the CNS back into the blood. The anesthetic then diffuses into less perfused tissues such as muscle and viscera, and at a slower rate into the poorly perfused but very hydrophobic adipose tissue. Termination of anesthesia after single boluses of parenteral anesthetics primarily reflects redistribution out of the CNS rather than metabolism (Figure 19–2).

After redistribution, anesthetic blood levels fall according to a complex interaction between the metabolic rate and the amount and lipophilicity of the drug stored in the peripheral compartments. Thus, parenteral anesthetic half-life are "context-sensitive," and the degree to which a $t_{1/2}$ is contextual varies greatly from drug to drug, as might be predicted based on their differing hydrophobicities and metabolic clearances (Figure 19–3; *see* Table 19–1). For example, after a single bolus of thiopental, patients usually emerge from anesthesia within 10 min; however, a patient may require more than a day to awaken from a prolonged thiopental infusion. Most individual variability in sensitivity to parenteral anesthetics can be accounted for by pharmacokinetic factors. For example, in patients with lower cardiac output, the relative perfusion of the brain and the fraction of anesthetic dose delivered to the brain are higher; thus, patients in septic shock or with cardiomyopathy usually require lower doses of anesthetic. The elderly also typically require a smaller anesthetic dose, primarily because of a smaller initial volume of distribution.

SPECIFIC PARENTERAL AGENTS

PROPOFOL, FOSPROPOFOL

Propofol is the most commonly used parenteral anesthetic in the U.S. Fospropofol is a prodrug form that is converted to propofol in vivo. The clinical pharmacological properties of propofol are summarized in Table 19–1.

Table 19–2

Some Pharmacological Effects of Parenteral Anesthetics[a]

DRUG	CBF	$CMRo_2$	ICP	MAP	HR	CO	RR	$\dot{V}_E$
Thiopental	---	---	---	-	+	-	-	--
Etomidate	---	---	---	0	0	0	-	-
Ketamine	++	0	++	+	++	+	0	0
Propofol	---	---	---	--	+	-	--	---

CBF, cerebral blood flow; $CMRo_2$, cerebral oxygen consumption; ICP, intracranial pressure; MAP, mean arterial pressure; HR, heart rate; CO, cardiac output; RR, respiratory rate; $\dot{V}_E$, minute ventilation.

[a]Typical effects of a single induction dose in humans; see text for references. Qualitative scale from --- to +++ signifies slight, moderate, or large decrease or increase, respectively; 0 indicates no significant change.

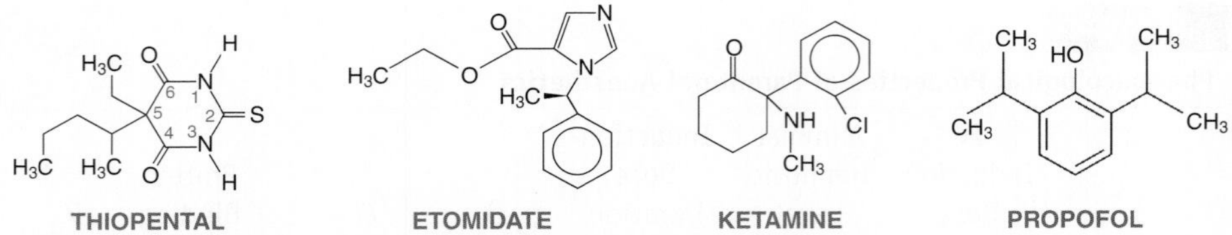

THIOPENTAL ETOMIDATE KETAMINE PROPOFOL

Figure 19–1 *Structures of some parenteral anesthetics.*

CHEMISTRY AND FORMULATIONS. The active ingredient in propofol, 2,6-diisopropylphenol, is an oil at room temperature and insoluble in aqueous solutions. Propofol is formulated for IV administration as a 1% (10 mg/mL) emulsion in 10% soybean oil, 2.25% glycerol, and 1.2% purified egg phosphatide. In the U.S., disodium EDTA (0.05 mg/mL) or sodium metabisulfite (0.25 mg/mL) is added to inhibit bacterial growth. Propofol should be administered within 4 h of its removal from sterile packaging; unused drug should be discarded. The lipid emulsion formulation of propofol is associated with significant pain on injection and hyperlipidemia. A new aqueous formulation of propofol, fospropofol, which is not associated with these adverse effects, has recently been approved for use for sedation in patients undergoing diagnostic procedures. Fospropofol, which itself is inactive, is a phosphate ester prodrug of propofol that is hydrolyzed by endothelial alkaline phosphatases to yield propofol, phosphate, and formaldehyde. The formaldehyde is rapidly converted to formic acid, which then is metabolized by tetrahydrofolate dehydrogenase to CO_2 and water.

DOSAGE AND CLINICAL USE. The induction dose of propofol (DIPRIVAN, others) in a healthy adult is 2-2.5 mg/kg. Dosages should be reduced in the elderly and in the presence of other sedatives and increased in young children. Because of its reasonably short elimination $t_{1/2}$, propofol often is used for maintenance of anesthesia as well as for induction. For short procedures, small boluses (10-50% of the induction dose) every 5 min or as needed are effective. An infusion of propofol produces a more stable drug level (100-300 μg/kg/min)

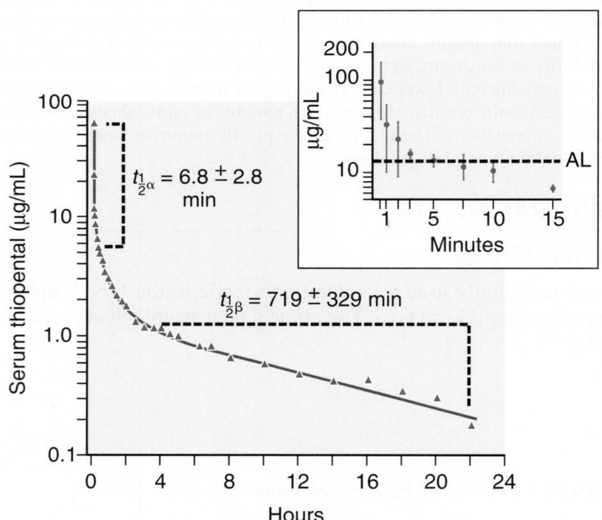

Figure 19–2 *Thiopental serum levels after a single intravenous induction dose.* Thiopental serum levels after a bolus can be described by two time constants, $t_{1/2}\alpha$ and $t_{1/2}\beta$. The initial fall is rapid ($t_{1/2\alpha}$<10 min) and is due to redistribution of drug from the plasma and the highly perfused brain and spinal cord into less well-perfused tissues such as muscle and fat. During this redistribution phase, serum thiopental concentration falls to levels at which patients awaken (AL, awakening level; see inset—the average thiopental serum concentration in 12 patients after a 6-mg/kg intravenous bolus of thiopental). Subsequent metabolism and elimination is much slower and is characterized by a half-life ($t_{1/2}$ β) of more than 10 hours. (Adapted with permission from Burch PG, and Stanski DR, The role of metabolism and protein binding in thiopental anesthesia. *Anesthesiology*, **1983**, 58:146–152. Copyright Lippincott Williams & Wilkins. http://lww.com.)

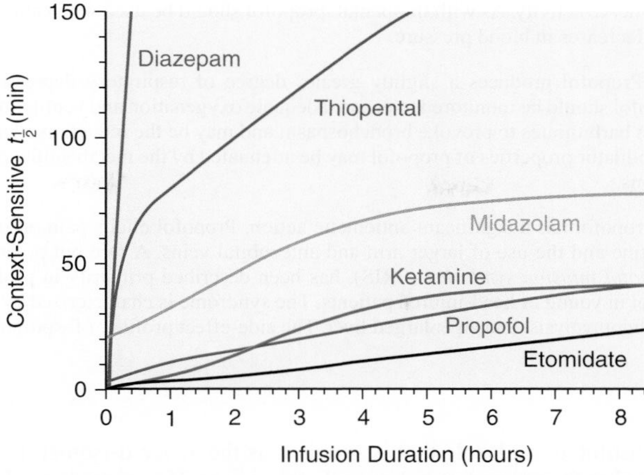

Figure 19–3 *Context-sensitive half-time of general anesthetics.* The duration of action of single intravenous doses of anesthetic/hypnotic drugs is similarly short for all and is determined by redistribution of the drugs away from their active sites (*see* Figure 19–2). However, after prolonged infusions, drug half-lives and durations of action are dependent on a complex interaction between the rate of redistribution of the drug, the amount of drug accumulated in fat, and the drug's metabolic rate. This phenomenon has been termed the *context-sensitive half-time*; that is, the $t_{1/2}$ of a drug can be estimated only if one knows the context—the total dose and over what time period it has been given. Note that the half-times of some drugs such as etomidate, propofol, and ketamine increase only modestly with prolonged infusions; others (e.g., diazepam and thiopental) increase dramatically. (Reproduced with permission from Reves JG, Glass PSA, Lubarsky DA, et al: Intravenous anesthetics, in Miller RD, et al, (eds): *Miller's Anesthesia*, 7th ed. Philadelphia: Churchill Livingstone, 2010, p 718. Copyright © Elsevier.)

and is better suited for longer-term anesthetic maintenance. Sedating doses of propofol are 20-50% of those required for general anesthesia. Fospropofol produces dose-dependent sedation and can be administered in otherwise healthy individuals at 2-8 mg/kg intravenously (delivered either as a bolus or by a short infusion over 5-10 min). The optimum dose for sedation is ~6.5 mg/kg. This results in a loss of consciousness in ~10 min. The duration of the sedative effect is ~45 min.

PHARMACOKINETICS AND METABOLISM. Onset and duration of anesthesia after a single bolus are similar to thiopental. Propofol has a context-sensitive $t_{1/2}$ of ~10 min with an infusion lasting 3 h and ~40 min for infusions lasting up to 8 h (*see* Figure 19–3). Propofol's shorter duration of action after infusion can be explained by its very high clearance, coupled with the slow diffusion of drug from the peripheral to the central compartment.

Propofol is metabolized in the liver by conjugation to sulfate and glucuronide to less active metabolites that are renally excreted. Propofol is highly protein bound, and its pharmacokinetics, like those of the barbiturates, may be affected by conditions that alter serum protein levels. Clearance of propofol is reduced in the elderly. In neonates, propofol clearance is also reduced. By contrast, in young children, a more rapid clearance in combination with a larger central volume may necessitate larger doses of propofol for induction and maintenance of anesthesia.

The $t_{1/2}$ for hydrolysis of fospropofol is 8 min; the drug has a small volume of distribution and a terminal $t_{1/2}$ ~46 min.

SIDE EFFECTS

Nervous System. The sedation and hypnotic actions of propofol are mediated by its action on $GABA_A$ receptors; agonism at these receptors results in an increased chloride conduction and hyperpolarization of neurons. Propofol suppresses the EEG, and in sufficient doses, can produce burst suppression of the EEG. Propofol decreases cerebral metabolic rate of O_2 consumption ($CMRO_2$), CBF, and intracranial and intraocular pressures by about the same amount as thiopental. Like thiopental, propofol has been used in patients at risk for cerebral ischemia; however, no human outcome studies have been performed to determine its efficacy as a neuroprotectant.

Cardiovascular System. Propofol produces a dose-dependent decrease in blood pressure that is significantly greater than that produced by thiopental. The fall in blood pressure can be explained by both vasodilation and possibly mild depression of myocardial contractility. Propofol appears to blunt the baroreceptor reflex and reduce sympathetic nerve activity. As with thiopental, propofol should be used with caution in patients at risk for or intolerant of decreases in blood pressure.

Respiratory System. Propofol produces a slightly greater degree of respiratory depression than thiopental. Patients given propofol should be monitored to ensure adequate oxygenation and ventilation. Propofol appears to be less likely than barbiturates to provoke bronchospasm and may be the induction agent of choice in asthmatics. The bronchodilator properties of propofol may be attenuated by the metabisulfite preservative in some propofol formulations.

Other Side Effects. Propofol has a significant antiemetic action. Propofol elicits pain on injection that can be reduced with lidocaine and the use of larger arm and antecubital veins. A rare but potentially fatal complication, termed *propofol infusion syndrome* (PRIS), has been described primarily in prolonged, higher-dose infusions of propofol in young or head-injured patients. The syndrome is characterized by metabolic acidosis, hyperlipidemia, rhabdomyolysis, and an enlarged liver. The side-effect profile of fospropofol is similar to that of propofol.

ETOMIDATE

Etomidate is a substituted imidazole that is supplied as the active d-isomer. Etomidate is poorly soluble in water and is formulated as a 2 mg/mL solution in 35% propylene glycol. Unlike thiopental, etomidate does not induce precipitation of neuromuscular blockers or other drugs frequently given during anesthetic induction.

DOSAGE AND CLINICAL USE. Etomidate (AMIDATE, others) is primarily used for anesthetic induction of patients at risk for hypotension. Induction doses of etomidate (*see* Table 19–1) are accompanied by a high incidence of pain on injection and myoclonic movements. Lidocaine effectively reduces the pain of injection, while myoclonic movements can be reduced by premedication with either benzodiazepines or opiates. Etomidate is pharmacokinetically suitable for off-label infusion for anesthetic maintenance (10 μg/kg/min) or sedation (5 μg/kg/min); however, long-term infusions are not recommended.

PHARMACOKINETICS AND METABOLISM. An induction dose of etomidate has a rapid onset; redistribution limits the duration of action. Metabolism occurs in the liver, primarily to inactive compounds. Elimination is both renal (78%) and biliary (22%). Compared to thiopental, the duration of action of etomidate increases less with repeated doses (*see* Figure 19–3).

SIDE EFFECTS

Nervous System. Etomidate produces hypnosis and has no analgesic effects. The effects of etomidate on CBF, metabolism, and intracranial and intraocular pressures are similar to those of thiopental (without dropping mean arterial blood pressure). Etomidate produces increased EEG activity in epileptogenic foci and has been associated with seizures.

Cardiovascular System. Cardiovascular stability after induction is a major advantage of etomidate over either barbiturates or propofol. Induction doses of etomidate typically produce a small increase in heart rate and little or no decrease in blood pressure or cardiac output etomidate has little effect on coronary perfusion pressure while reducing myocardial O_2 consumption.

Respiratory and Other Side Effects. The degree of respiratory depression due to etomidate appears to be less than that due to thiopental. Like methohexital, etomidate may induce hiccups but does not significantly stimulate histamine release. Etomidate has been associated with nausea and vomiting. The drug also inhibits adrenal biosynthetic enzymes required for the production of cortisol and some other steroids. Thus, while etomidate is not recommended for long-term infusion, it appears safe for anesthetic induction and has some unique advantages in patients prone to hemodynamic instability.

KETAMINE

Ketamine is an arylcyclohexylamine, a congener of phencyclidine. Ketamine is supplied as a mixture of the R+ and S-isomers even though the S-isomer is more potent with fewer side effects. Although more lipophilic than thiopental, ketamine is water-soluble.

DOSAGE AND CLINICAL USE. Ketamine (KETALAR, others) it useful for anesthetizing patients at risk for hypotension and bronchospasm and for certain pediatric procedures. However, significant side effects limit its routine use. Ketamine rapidly produces a hypnotic state quite distinct from that of other anesthetics. Patients have profound analgesia, unresponsiveness to commands, and amnesia, but may have their eyes open, move their limbs involuntarily, and breathe spontaneously. This cataleptic state has been termed *dissociative anesthesia.* The administration of ketamine has been shown to reduce the development of tolerance to long-term opioid use. Ketamine typically is administered intravenously but also is effective by intramuscular, oral, and rectal routes. Ketamine does not elicit pain on injection or true excitatory behavior as described for methohexital, although involuntary movements produced by ketamine can be mistaken for anesthetic excitement.

PHARMACOKINETICS AND METABOLISM. The onset and duration of an induction dose of ketamine are determined by the same distribution/redistribution mechanisms operant for all the other parenteral anesthetics. Ketamine is hepatically metabolized to norketamine, which has reduced CNS activity; norketamine is further metabolized and excreted in urine and bile. Ketamine has a large volume of distribution and rapid clearance that make it suitable for continuous infusion without the lengthening in duration of action seen with thiopental (*see* Table 19–1 and Figure 19–3). Protein binding is much lower with ketamine than with the other parenteral anesthetics.

SIDE EFFECTS

Nervous System. Ketamine has indirect sympathomimetic activity and produces distinct behavioral effects. The ketamine-induced cataleptic state is accompanied by nystagmus with pupillary dilation, salivation, lacrimation, and spontaneous limb movements with increased overall muscle tone. Patients are amnestic and unresponsive to painful stimuli. Ketamine produces profound analgesia, a distinct advantage over other parenteral anesthetics. Unlike other parenteral anesthetics, ketamine increases CBF and intracranial pressure (ICP) with minimal alteration of cerebral metabolism. The effects of ketamine on CBF can be readily attenuated by the simultaneous administration of sedative-hypnotic agents.

Emergence delirium, characterized by hallucinations, vivid dreams, and delusions, is a frequent complication of ketamine that can result in serious patient dissatisfaction and can complicate postoperative management. Benzodiazepines reduce the incidence of emergence delirium.

Cardiovascular System. Unlike other anesthetics, induction doses of ketamine typically increase blood pressure, heart rate, and cardiac output. The cardiovascular effects are indirect and are most likely mediated by inhibition of both central and peripheral catecholamine reuptake. Ketamine has direct negative inotropic and vasodilating activity, but these effects usually are overwhelmed by the indirect sympathomimetic action. Thus, ketamine is a useful drug, along with etomidate, for patients at risk for hypotension during anesthesia. While not arrhythmogenic, ketamine increases myocardial O_2 consumption and is not an ideal drug for patients at risk for myocardial ischemia.

Respiratory System. The respiratory effects of ketamine are perhaps the best indication for its use. Induction doses of ketamine produce small and transient decreases in minute ventilation, but respiratory depression is less severe than with other general anesthetics. Ketamine is a potent bronchodilator and is particularly well suited for anesthetizing patients at high risk for bronchospasm.

BARBITURATES

CHEMISTRY AND FORMULATIONS. Barbiturates are derivatives of barbituric acid with either an oxygen or a sulfur at the 2-position (*see* Figure 19–1 and Chapter 17). The 3 barbiturates most commonly used in clinical anesthesia are sodium *thiopental*, *thiamylal*, and *methohexital*. Sodium thiopental (PENTOTHAL, others) has been used most frequently for inducing anesthesia. Thiamylal (SURITAL) is licensed in the U.S. only for veterinary use. Barbiturates are supplied as racemic mixtures despite enantioselectivity in their anesthetic potency. Barbiturates are formulated as the sodium salts with 6% sodium carbonate and reconstituted in water or isotonic saline to produce 2.5% (thiopental), 2% (thiamylal), or 1% (methohexital) alkaline solutions ($10 \leq pH \leq 11$). *Mixing barbiturates with drugs in acidic solutions during anesthetic induction can result in precipitation of the barbiturate as the free acid; thus, standard practice is to delay the administration of other drugs until the barbiturate has cleared the IV tubing.*

PHARMACOLOGICAL PROPERTIES. The pharmacological properties and other therapeutic uses of the barbiturates are presented in Chapter 17. Table 17–2 lists the common barbiturates with their clinical pharmacological properties.

DOSAGES AND CLINICAL USE. Recommended IV dosing for parenteral barbiturates in a healthy young adult is given in Table 19–1.

PHARMACOKINETICS AND METABOLISM. The principal mechanism limiting anesthetic duration after single doses is redistribution of these hydrophobic drugs from the brain to other tissues. However, after multiple doses or infusions, the duration of action of the barbiturates varies considerably depending on their clearances. *See* Table 19–1 for pharmacokinetic parameters.

Methohexital differs from the other two IV barbiturates in its much more rapid clearance; thus, it accumulates less during prolonged infusions. Because of their slow elimination and large volumes of distribution, prolonged infusions or very large doses of thiopental and thiamylal can produce unconsciousness lasting several days. All 3 barbiturates are primarily eliminated by hepatic metabolism and renal excretion of inactive metabolites; a small fraction of thiopental undergoes desulfuration to the longer-acting hypnotic pentobarbital. These drugs are highly protein bound. Hepatic disease or other conditions that reduce serum protein concentration will increase the initial free concentration and hypnotic effect of an induction dose.

SIDE EFFECTS

Nervous System. Barbiturates suppress the EEG and can produce burst suppression of the EEG. They reduce the CMR, as measured by $CMRO_2$, in a dose-dependent manner. As a consequence of the decrease in $CMRO_2$, CBF and ICP are similarly reduced. Presumably in part due to their CNS depressant activity, barbiturates are effective anticonvulsants. Thiopental in particular is a proven medication in the treatment of status epilepticus. Methohexital can increase ictal activity, and seizures have been described in patients who received doses sufficient to produce burst suppression of the EEG. This property makes methohexital a good choice for anesthesia in patients who undergo electroconvulsive therapy.

Cardiovascular System. The anesthetic barbiturates produce dose-dependent decreases in blood pressure. The effect is due primarily to vasodilation, particularly venodilation, and to a lesser degree to a direct decrease in cardiac contractility. Typically, heart rate increases as a compensatory response to a lower blood pressure, although barbiturates also blunt the baroreceptor reflex. Thiopental maintains the ratio of myocardial O_2 supply to demand in patients with coronary artery disease within a normal blood pressure range. Hypotension can be severe in patients with an impaired ability to compensate for venodilation such as those with hypovolemia, cardiomyopathy, valvular heart disease, coronary artery disease, cardiac tamponade, or β adrenergic blockade. None of the barbiturates has been shown to be arrhythmogenic.

Respiratory System. Barbiturates are respiratory depressants. Induction doses of thiopental decrease minute ventilation and tidal volume, with a smaller and inconsistent decrease in respiratory rate. Reflex responses to hypercarbia and hypoxia are diminished by anesthetic barbiturates; at higher doses or in the presence of other respiratory depressants such as opiates, apnea can result. Compared to propofol, barbiturates produce a higher incidence of wheezing in asthmatics, attributed to histamine release from mast cells, during induction of anesthesia.

Other Side Effects. Short-term administration of barbiturates has no clinically significant effect on the hepatic, renal, or endocrine systems. True allergies to barbiturates are rare; however, direct drug-induced histamine release is occasionally seen. Barbiturates can induce fatal attacks of porphyria in patients with acute intermittent or variegate porphyria and are contraindicated in such patients. Methohexital can produce pain on injection to a greater degree than thiopental. Inadvertent intraarterial injection of thiobarbiturates can induce a severe inflammatory and potentially necrotic reaction that can threaten limb survival. Methohexital and to a lesser degree other barbiturates can produce excitatory symptoms on induction such as cough, hiccup, muscle tremors, twitching, and hypertonus.

INHALATIONAL ANESTHETICS

A wide variety of gases and volatile liquids can produce anesthesia. The structures of the currently used inhalational anesthetics are shown in Figure 19–4. The inhalational anesthetics have therapeutic indices (LD_{50}/ED_{50}) that range from 2-4, making these among the most dangerous drugs in clinical use. The toxicity of these drugs is largely a function of their side effects, and each of the

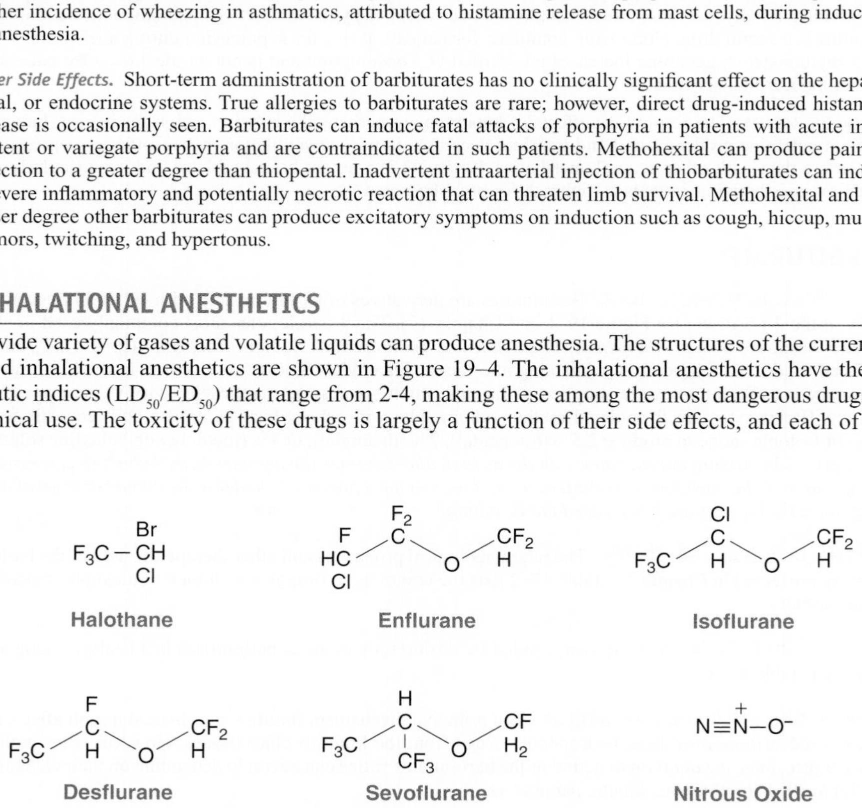

Halothane

Enflurane

Isoflurane

Desflurane

Sevoflurane

Nitrous Oxide

Figure 19–4 *Structures of inhalational general anesthetics.* Note that all inhalational general anesthetic agents except nitrous oxide and halothane are ethers, and that fluorine progressively replaces other halogens in the development of the halogenated agents. All structural differences are associated with important differences in pharmacological properties.

Table 19–3

Properties of Inhalational Anesthetic Agents

AGENT	MAC[a] (vol %)	MAC_{AWAKE}[b] (vol %)	VAPOR PRESSURE (mm Hg, 20°C)	PARTITION COEFFICIENT AT 37°C Blood Gas	Brain Blood	Fat Blood	% RECOVERED AS METABOLITES
Halothane	0.75	0.41	243	2.3	2.9	51	20
Isoflurane[c]	1.2	0.4	250	1.4	2.6	45	0.2
Enflurane	1.6	0.4	175	1.8	1.4	36	2.4
Sevoflurane	2	0.6	160	0.65	1.7	48	3
Desflurane	6	2.4	664	0.45	1.3	27	0.02
N_2O[c]	105	60.0	Gas	0.47	1.1	2.3	0.004
Xe	71	32.6	Gas	0.12	—	—	0

[a]*MAC (minimum alveolar concentration) values are expressed as vol %, the percentage of the atmosphere that is anesthetic. A value of MAC > 100% means that hyperbaric conditions would be required.*

[b]*MAC_{AWAKE} is the concentration at which appropriate responses to commands are lost.*

[c]*EC_{50} for memory suppression (vol %): isoflurane, 0.24; N_2O, 52.5; values not available for other agents.*

inhalational anesthetics has a unique side-effect profile. Hence, the selection of an inhalational anesthetic often is based on matching a patient's pathophysiology with drug side-effect profiles.

Table 19–3 lists the widely varying physical properties of the inhalational agents in clinical use. Ideally, an inhalational agent would produce a rapid induction of anesthesia and a rapid recovery following discontinuation.

PHARMACOKINETIC PRINCIPLES

Inhalational agents behave as gases rather than as liquids and thus require different pharmacokinetic constructs to be used in analyzing their uptake and distribution. Inhalational anesthetics distribute between tissues (or between blood and gas) such that equilibrium is achieved when the partial pressure of anesthetic gas is equal in the 2 tissues. When a person has breathed an inhalational anesthetic for a sufficiently long time that all tissues are equilibrated with the anesthetic, the partial pressure of the anesthetic in all tissues will be equal to the partial pressure of the anesthetic in inspired gas. While the partial pressure of the anesthetic may be equal in all tissues, the concentration of anesthetic in each tissue will be different. Indeed, anesthetic partition coefficients are defined as the ratio of anesthetic concentration in 2 tissues when the partial pressures of anesthetic are equal in the 2 tissues. Blood:gas, brain:blood, and fat:blood partition coefficients for the various inhalational agents are listed in Table 19–3. These partition coefficients show that inhalational anesthetics are more soluble in some tissues (e.g., fat) than they are in others (e.g., blood).

In clinical practice, equilibrium is achieved when the partial pressure in inspired gas is equal to the partial pressure in end-tidal (alveolar) gas. For inhalational agents that are not very soluble in blood or any other tissue, equilibrium is achieved quickly, as illustrated for nitrous oxide in Figure 19–5. If an agent is more soluble in a tissue such as fat, equilibrium may take many hours to reach. This occurs because fat represents a huge anesthetic reservoir that will be filled slowly because of the modest blood flow to fat. Anesthesia is produced when anesthetic partial pressure in brain is equal to or greater than MAC. Because the brain is well perfused, anesthetic partial pressure in brain becomes equal to the partial pressure in alveolar gas (and in blood) over the course of several minutes. Therefore, anesthesia is achieved shortly after alveolar partial pressure reaches MAC.

Elimination of inhalational anesthetics is largely the reverse process of uptake. For inhalational agents with high blood and tissue solubility, recovery will be a function of the duration of anesthetic administration. This occurs because the accumulated amounts of anesthetic in the fat reservoir will prevent blood (and therefore alveolar) partial pressures from falling rapidly. Patients will be arousable when alveolar partial pressure reaches MAC_{awake}, a partial pressure somewhat lower than MAC (*see* Table 19–3).

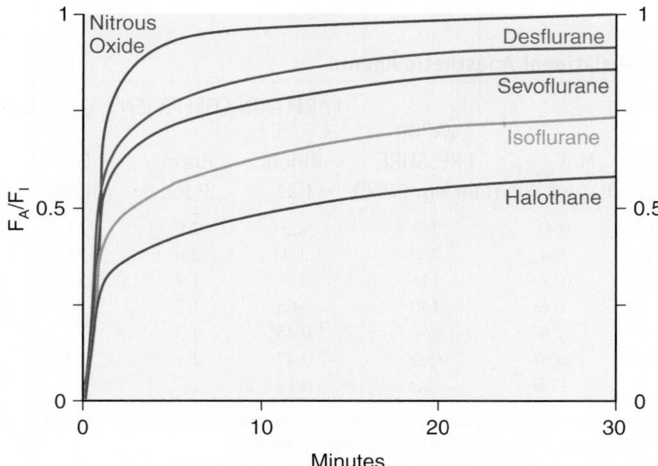

Figure 19–5 *Uptake of inhalational general anesthetics*. The rise in end-tidal alveolar (F_A) anesthetic concentration toward the inspired (F_I) concentration is most rapid with the least soluble anesthetics, nitrous oxide and desflurane, and slowest with the most soluble anesthetic, halothane. All data are from human studies. (Reproduced with permission from Eger EI, II. Inhaled anesthetics: Uptake and distribution, in Miller RD et al, eds. *Miller's Anesthesia*, 7th ed. Philadelphia: Churchill Livingstone, 2010, p 540. Copyright © Elsevier.)

HALOTHANE

Halothane is a volatile liquid at room temperature and must be stored in a sealed container. Because halothane is a light-sensitive compound, it is marketed in amber bottles with thymol added as a preservative. Mixtures of halothane with O_2 or air are neither flammable nor explosive.

PHARMACOKINETICS. Halothane has a relatively high blood:gas partition coefficient and high fat:blood partition coefficient. Induction with halothane is relatively slow, and the alveolar halothane concentration remains substantially lower than the inspired halothane concentration for many hours of administration. Because halothane is soluble in fat and other body tissues, it will accumulate during prolonged administration.

Approximately 60-80% of halothane taken up by the body is eliminated unchanged by the lungs in the first 24 h after its administration. A substantial amount of the halothane not eliminated in exhaled gas is biotransformed by hepatic CYPs. The major metabolite of halothane is trifluoroacetic acid, which is formed by removal of bromine and chlorine ions. Trifluoroacetic acid, bromine, and chlorine all can be detected in the urine. Trifluoroacetylchloride, an intermediate in oxidative metabolism of halothane, can trifluoroacetylate several proteins in the liver. An immune reaction to these altered proteins may be responsible for the rare cases of fulminant halothane-induced hepatic necrosis.

CLINICAL USE. Halothane is used for maintenance of anesthesia. It is well tolerated for inhalation induction of anesthesia, most commonly in children. The use of halothane in the U.S. has diminished because of the introduction of newer inhalational agents with better pharmacokinetic and side-effect profiles. Halothane continues to be extensively used in children because it is well tolerated and its side effects appear to be diminished in children. Halothane has a low cost and is still widely used in developing countries.

SIDE EFFECTS

Cardiovascular System. Halothane induces a dose-dependent reduction in arterial blood pressure. Mean arterial pressure typically decreases ~20-25% at MAC concentrations of halothane, primarily as a result of direct myocardial depression leading to reduced cardiac output and attenuation of baroreceptor reflex function. Halothane-induced reductions in blood pressure and heart rate generally disappear after several hours of constant halothane administration, presumably because of progressive sympathetic stimulation. Halothane does not cause a significant change in systemic vascular resistance but does dilates the vascular beds of the skin and brain. Halothane inhibits autoregulation of renal, splanchnic, and CBF, leading to reduced perfusion of these organs in the face of reduced blood pressure. Coronary autoregulation is largely preserved during halothane anesthesia. Halothane inhibits hypoxic pulmonary vasoconstriction, leading to increased perfusion to poorly ventilated regions of the lung and an increased alveolar:arterial O_2 gradient. Sinus bradycardia and atrioventricular rhythms occur frequently during halothane anesthesia but usually are benign. These rhythms result mainly from a direct depressive effect of halothane on sinoatrial node discharge. Halothane also can sensitize the myocardium to the arrhythmogenic effects of epinephrine.

Respiratory System. Spontaneous respiration is rapid and shallow during halothane anesthesia. The decreased alveolar ventilation results in an elevation in arterial CO_2 tension from 40 mm Hg to >50 mm Hg at 1 MAC. The elevated CO_2 does not provoke a compensatory increase in ventilation, because halothane causes a concentration-dependent inhibition of the ventilatory response to CO_2. This action of halothane is thought to be mediated by depression of central chemoceptor mechanisms. Halothane also inhibits peripheral chemoceptor responses to arterial hypoxemia. Thus, neither hemodynamic (tachycardia and hypertension) nor ventilatory responses to hypoxemia are observed during halothane anesthesia, making it prudent to monitor arterial O_2 directly.

Nervous System. Halothane dilates the cerebral vasculature, increasing CBF and cerebral blood volume. This can result in an increase in ICP, especially in patients with space-occupying intracranial masses, brain edema, or preexisting intracranial hypertension. Halothane attenuates autoregulation of CBF in a dose-dependent manner.

Muscle. Halothane causes some relaxation of skeletal muscle by its central depressant effects. Halothane also potentiates the actions of nondepolarizing muscle relaxants (curariform drugs; *see* Chapter 11), increasing both their duration of action and the magnitude of their effect. Halothane and the other halogenated inhalational anesthetics can trigger malignant hyperthermia. This syndrome frequently is fatal and is treated by immediate discontinuation of the anesthetic and administration of dantrolene. Halothane relaxes uterine smooth muscle, a useful property for manipulation of the fetus (version) in the prenatal period and for delivery of retained placenta.

Kidney. Patients anesthetized with halothane usually produce a small volume of concentrated urine. This is the consequence of halothane-induced reduction of renal blood flow and glomerular filtration rate, which may be reduced by 40-50% at 1 MAC. Halothane-induced changes in renal function are fully reversible and are not associated with long-term nephrotoxicity.

Liver and GI Tract. Halothane reduces splanchnic and hepatic blood flow. Halothane can produce fulminant hepatic necrosis (*halothane hepatitis*) in ~1 in 10,000 patients receiving halothane and is referred to as halothane *hepatitis*. This syndrome (with a 50% fatality rate) is characterized by fever, anorexia, nausea, and vomiting, developing several days after anesthesia and can be accompanied by a rash and peripheral eosinophilia. Halothane hepatitis may be the result of an immune response to hepatic proteins that become trifluoroacetylated as a consequence of halothane metabolism.

ISOFLURANE

Isoflurane (FORANE, others) is a volatile liquid at room temperature and is neither flammable nor explosive in mixtures of air or oxygen.

PHARMACOKINETICS. Isoflurane has a blood:gas partition coefficient substantially lower than that of halothane or enflurane. Consequently, induction with isoflurane and recovery from isoflurane are relatively faster. More than 99% of inhaled isoflurane is excreted unchanged by the lungs. Isoflurane does not appear to be a mutagen, teratogen, or carcinogen.

CLINICAL USE. Isoflurane is a commonly used inhalational anesthetic worldwide. It is typically used for maintenance of anesthesia *after induction* with other agents because of its pungent odor, but induction of anesthesia can be achieved in <10 min with an inhaled concentration of 3% isoflurane in O_2; this concentration is reduced to 1-2% (~1-2 MAC) for maintenance of anesthesia. The use of adjunct agents such as opioids or nitrous oxide reduces the concentration of isoflurane required for surgical anesthesia.

SIDE EFFECTS

Cardiovascular System. Isoflurane produces a concentration-dependent decrease in arterial blood pressure; cardiac output is well maintained; hypotension is the result of decreased systemic vascular resistance. Isoflurane produces vasodilation in most vascular beds, with particularly pronounced effects in skin and muscle. Isoflurane is a potent coronary vasodilator, simultaneously producing increased coronary blood flow and decreased myocardial O_2 consumption. Isoflurane significantly attenuates baroreceptor function. Patients anesthetized with isoflurane generally have mildly elevated heart rates as a compensatory response to reduced blood pressure; however, rapid changes in isoflurane concentration can produce both transient tachycardia and hypertension due to isoflurane-induced sympathetic stimulation.

Respiratory System. Isoflurane produces concentration-dependent depression of ventilation. Isoflurane is particularly effective at depressing the ventilatory response to hypercapnia and hypoxia. Although isoflurane is an effective bronchodilator, it also is an airway irritant and can stimulate airway reflexes during induction of anesthesia, producing coughing and laryngospasm.

Nervous System. Isoflurane dilates the cerebral vasculature, producing increased CBF; this vasodilating activity is less than that of either halothane or enflurane. There is a modest risk of an increase in ICP in patients with preexisting intracranial hypertension. Isoflurane reduces $CMRO_2$ in a dose-dependent manner.

Muscle. Isoflurane produces some relaxation of skeletal muscle by its central effects. It also enhances the effects of both depolarizing and nondepolarizing muscle relaxants. Like other halogenated inhalational anesthetics, isoflurane relaxes uterine smooth muscle and is not recommended for analgesia or anesthesia for labor and vaginal delivery.

Kidney. Isoflurane reduces renal blood flow and glomerular filtration rate, resulting in a small volume of concentrated urine.

Liver and GI Tract. Splanchnic and hepatic blood flows are reduced with increasing doses of isoflurane as systemic arterial pressure decreases. There are no reported incidences of hepatic toxicity.

ENFLURANE

Enflurane (ETHRANE, others) is a clear, colorless liquid at room temperature with a mild, sweet odor. Like other inhalational anesthetics, it is volatile and must be stored in a sealed bottle. It is nonflammable and nonexplosive in mixtures of air or oxygen.

PHARMACOKINETICS. Because of its relatively high blood:gas partition coefficient, induction of anesthesia and recovery from enflurane are relatively slow. Enflurane is metabolized to a modest extent, with 2-8% of absorbed enflurane undergoing oxidative metabolism in the liver by CYP2E1. Fluoride ions are a by-product of enflurane metabolism, but plasma fluoride levels are low and nontoxic. Patients taking isoniazid exhibit enhanced metabolism of enflurane with consequent elevation of serum fluoride.

CLINICAL USE. Isoflurane is primarily utilized for maintenance rather than induction of anesthesia. Surgical anesthesia can be induced with enflurane in <10 min with an inhaled concentration of 4% in oxygen, and maintained with concentrations from 1.5-3%. Enflurane concentrations required to produce anesthesia are reduced when it is coadministered with nitrous oxide or opioids.

SIDE EFFECTS

Cardiovascular System. Enflurane causes a concentration-dependent decrease in arterial blood pressure, due in part, to depression of myocardial contractility, with some contribution from peripheral vasodilation. Enflurane has minimal effects on heart rate.

Respiratory System. The respiratory effects of enflurane are similar to those of halothane. Enflurane produces a greater depression of the ventilatory responses to hypoxia and hypercarbia than do either halothane or isoflurane. Enflurane, like other inhalational anesthetics, is an effective bronchodilator.

Nervous System. Enflurane is a cerebral vasodilator and can increase ICP in some patients; it also reduces $CMRO_2$. High concentrations of enflurane or profound hypocarbia during enflurane anesthesia can result in electrical seizure activity that may be accompanied by peripheral motor manifestations. The seizures are self-limited and are not thought to produce permanent damage. Epileptic patients are not particularly susceptible to enflurane-induced seizures; nonetheless, enflurane generally is not used in patients with seizure disorders.

Muscle. Enflurane produces significant skeletal muscle relaxation in the absence of muscle relaxants. It also significantly enhances the effects of nondepolarizing muscle relaxants. As with other inhalational agents, enflurane relaxes uterine smooth muscle.

Kidney. Enflurane reduces renal blood flow, glomerular filtration rate, and urinary output. These effects are rapidly reversed upon drug discontinuation. There is scant evidence of long-term nephrotoxicity following enflurane use, and it is safe to use in patients with renal impairment, provided that the depth of enflurane anesthesia and the duration of administration are not excessive.

Liver and GI Tract. Enflurane reduces splanchnic and hepatic blood flow in proportion to reduced arterial blood pressure. Enflurane does not appear to alter liver function or to be hepatotoxic.

DESFLURANE

Desflurane (SUPRANE) is a highly volatile liquid at room temperature (vapor pressure = 681 mm Hg) and must be stored in tightly sealed bottles. Delivery of a precise concentration of desflurane requires the use of a specially heated vaporizer that delivers pure vapor that then is diluted appropriately with other gases (O_2, air, or N_2O). Desflurane is nonflammable and nonexplosive in mixtures of air or O_2.

PHARMACOKINETICS. Desflurane has a very low blood:gas partition coefficient (0.42) and also is not very soluble in fat or other peripheral tissues. Thus, the alveolar and blood concentrations rapidly rise to the level of inspired concentration, providing rapid induction of anesthesia and rapid changes in depth of anesthesia following changes in the inspired concentration. Emergence from desflurane anesthesia also is very rapid. Desflurane is minimally metabolized; >99% of absorbed desflurane is eliminated unchanged through the lungs.

CLINICAL USE. Desflurane is a widely used anesthetic for outpatient surgery because of its rapid onset of action and rapid recovery. The drug irritates the tracheobronchial tree and can provoke coughing, salivation, and bronchospasm. Anesthesia therefore usually is induced with an IV agent, with desflurane subsequently administered for maintenance of anesthesia. Maintenance of anesthesia usually requires inhaled concentrations of 6-8% (~1 MAC). Lower concentrations of desflurane are required if it is coadministered with nitrous oxide or opioids.

SIDE EFFECTS

Cardiovascular System. Desflurane produces hypotension primarily by decreasing systemic vascular resistance. Cardiac output is well preserved, as is blood flow to the major organ beds (splanchnic, renal, cerebral, and coronary). Transient tachycardia is often noted with abrupt increases in desflurane's delivered concentration, a result of this desflurane-induced stimulation of the sympathetic nervous system. The hypotensive effects of desflurane do not wane with increasing duration of administration.

Respiratory System. Desflurane causes a concentration-dependent increase in respiratory rate and a decrease in tidal volume. At low concentrations (<1 MAC) the net effect is to preserve minute ventilation. Desflurane concentrations >1 MAC depress minute ventilation, resulting in elevated arterial CO_2 tension (Pa_{CO2}). Desflurane is a bronchodilator. However, it also is a strong airway irritant, and can cause coughing, breath-holding, laryngospasm, and excessive respiratory secretions. *Because of its irritant properties, desflurane is not used for induction of anesthesia.*

Nervous System. Desflurane decreases cerebral vascular resistance and $CMRO_2$. Burst suppression of the EEG is achieved with ~2 MAC desflurane; at this level, $CMRO_2$ is reduced by ~50%. Under conditions of normocapnia and normotension, desflurane produces an increase in CBF and can increase ICP in patients with poor intracranial compliance. The vasoconstrictive response to hypocapnia is preserved during desflurane anesthesia, and increases in ICP thus can be prevented by hyperventilation.

Muscle, Kidney, Liver and GI Tract. Desflurane produces direct skeletal muscle relaxation as well as enhancing the effects of nondepolarizing and depolarizing neuromuscular blocking agents. Consistent with its minimal metabolic degradation, desflurane has no reported nephrotoxicity or hepatotoxicity.

Desflurane and Carbon Monoxide. Inhaled anesthetics are administered via a system that permits unidirectional flow of gas and rebreathing of exhaled gases. To prevent rebreathing of CO_2 (which can lead to hypercarbia), CO_2 absorbers are incorporated into the anesthesia delivery circuits. With almost complete desiccation of the CO_2 absorbents, substantial quantities of CO can be produced. This effect is greatest with desflurane and can be prevented by the use of well-hydrated, fresh CO_2 absorbent.

SEVOFLURANE

Sevoflurane (ULTANE, others) is a clear, colorless, volatile liquid at room temperature and must be stored in a sealed bottle. It is nonflammable and nonexplosive in mixtures of air or oxygen. However, sevoflurane can undergo an exothermic reaction with desiccated CO_2 absorbent (BARALYME) to produce airway burns or spontaneous ignition, explosion, and fire.

Sevoflurane must not be not used with an anesthesia machine in which the CO_2 absorbent has been dried by prolonged gas flow through the absorbent. The reaction of sevoflurane with desiccated CO_2 absorbent also can produce CO, which can result in serious patient injury.

PHARMACOKINETICS. The low solubility of sevoflurane in blood and other tissues provides for rapid induction of anesthesia and rapid changes in anesthetic depth following changes in delivered concentration. Approximately 3% of absorbed sevoflurane is metabolized in the liver by CYP2E1, with the predominant product being hexafluoroisopropanol. Hepatic metabolism of sevoflurane also produces inorganic fluoride. Interaction of sevoflurane with soda lime also produces decomposition products that may be toxic such as compound A, pentafluoroisopropenyl fluoromethyl ether (*see* "Kidney" under "Side Effects").

CLINICAL USE. Sevoflurane is widely used, particularly for outpatient anesthesia, because of its rapid recovery profile, and because it is not irritating to the airway. Induction of anesthesia is rapidly achieved using inhaled concentrations of 2-4% sevoflurane.

SIDE EFFECTS

Cardiovascular System. Sevoflurane produces concentration-dependent decreases in arterial blood pressure (due to systemic vasodilation) and cardiac output. Sevoflurane does not produce tachycardia and thus may be a preferable agent in patients prone to myocardial ischemia.

Respiratory System. Sevoflurane produces a concentration-dependent reduction in tidal volume and increase in respiratory rate in spontaneously breathing patients. The increased respiratory frequency does not compensate for reduced tidal volume, with the net effect being a reduction in minute ventilation and an increase in Pa_{CO2}. Sevoflurane is not irritating to the airway and is a potent bronchodilator. As a result, sevoflurane is the most effective clinical bronchodilator of the inhalational anesthetics.

Nervous System. Sevoflurane produces effects on cerebral vascular resistance, $CMRO_2$, and CBF that are very similar to those produced by isoflurane and desflurane. Sevoflurane can increase ICP in patients with poor intracranial compliance, the response to hypocapnia is preserved during sevoflurane anesthesia, and increases in ICP can be prevented by hyperventilation. In children, sevoflurane is associated with delirium upon emergence from anesthesia. This delirium is short lived and without any reported adverse long-term sequelae.

Muscle. Sevoflurane produces skeletal muscle relaxation and enhances the effects of nondepolarizing and depolarizing neuromuscular blocking agents.

Kidney. Controversy has surrounded the potential nephrotoxicity of compound A, which is produced by interaction of sevoflurane with the CO_2-absorbent soda lime. Biochemical evidence of transient renal injury has been reported in human volunteers. Large clinical studies have shown no evidence of increased serum creatinine, blood urea nitrogen, or any other evidence of renal impairment following sevoflurane administration. *The FDA recommends that sevoflurane be administered with fresh gas flows of at least 2 L/min to minimize accumulation of compound A.*

Liver and GI Tract. Sevoflurane is not known to cause hepatotoxicity or alterations of hepatic function tests.

NITROUS OXIDE

Nitrous oxide (N_2O) is a colorless, odorless gas at room temperature. N_2O is sold in steel cylinders and must be delivered through calibrated flow meters provided on all anesthesia machines. N_2O is neither flammable nor explosive, but it does support combustion as actively as oxygen does when it is present in proper concentration with a flammable anesthetic or material.

PHARMACOKINETICS. N_2O is very insoluble in blood and other tissues. This results in rapid equilibration between delivered and alveolar anesthetic concentrations and provides for rapid induction of anesthesia and rapid emergence following discontinuation of administration. The rapid uptake of N_2O from alveolar gas serves to concentrate coadministered halogenated anesthetics; this effect (the "second gas effect") speeds induction of anesthesia. On discontinuation of N_2O administration, N_2O gas can diffuse from blood to the alveoli, diluting O_2 in the lung. This can produce an effect called *diffusional hypoxia. To avoid hypoxia, 100% O_2 rather than air should be administered when N_2O is discontinued.*

Almost all (99.9%) of the absorbed N_2O is eliminated unchanged by the lungs. N_2O can interact with the cobalt of vitamin B_{12}, thereby preventing vitamin B_{12} from acting as a cofactor for methionine synthase. Inactivation of methionine synthase can produce signs of vitamin B_{12} deficiency, including megaloblastic anemia and peripheral neuropathy, a particular concern in patients with malnutrition, vitamin B_{12} deficiency, or alcoholism. For this reason, N_2O is not used as a chronic analgesic or as a sedative in critical care settings.

CLINICAL USE. N_2O is a weak anesthetic agent that has significant analgesic effects. Surgical anesthetic depth is only achieved under hyperbaric conditions. By contrast, analgesia is produced at concentrations as low as 20%. The analgesic property of N_2O is a function of the activation of opioidergic neurons in the periaqueductal gray matter and the adrenergic neurons in the locus ceruleus. N_2O is frequently used in concentrations of ~50% to provide analgesia and mild sedation in outpatient dentistry. N_2O cannot be used at concentrations >80% because this limits the delivery of adequate O_2. Because of this limitation, N_2O is used primarily as an adjunct to other inhalational or IV anesthetics.

A major problem with N_2O is that it will exchange with N_2 in any air-containing cavity in the body. Moreover, because of their differential blood:gas partition coefficients, N_2O will enter the cavity faster than N_2 escapes, thereby increasing the volume and/or pressure in this cavity. Examples of air collections that can be expanded by N_2O include a pneumothorax, an obstructed middle ear, an air embolus, an obstructed loop of bowel, an intraocular air bubble, a pulmonary bulla, and intracranial air. N_2O should be avoided in these clinical settings.

SIDE EFFECTS

Cardiovascular System. Although N_2O produces a negative inotropic effect on heart muscle in vitro, depressant effects on cardiac function generally are not observed in patients because of the stimulatory effects of N_2O on the sympathetic nervous system. The cardiovascular effects of N_2O also are heavily influenced by the concomitant administration of other anesthetic agents. When N_2O is coadministered with halogenated inhalational anesthetics, it produces an increase in heart rate, arterial blood pressure, and cardiac output. In contrast, when N_2O is coadministered with an opioid, it generally decreases arterial blood pressure and cardiac output. N_2O also increases venous tone in both the peripheral and pulmonary vasculature. The effects of N_2O on pulmonary vascular resistance can be exaggerated in patients with preexisting pulmonary hypertension; thus, the drug generally is not used in these patients.

Respiratory System. N_2O causes modest increases in respiratory rate and decreases in tidal volume in spontaneously breathing patients. Even modest concentrations of N_2O markedly depress the ventilatory response to hypoxia. Thus, it is prudent to monitor arterial O_2 saturation directly in patients receiving or recovering from N_2O.

Nervous System. N_2O can significantly increase CBF and ICP. This cerebral vasodilatory capacity of N_2O is significantly attenuated by the simultaneous administration of IV agents such as opiates and propofol. By contrast, the combination of N_2O and inhaled agents results in greater vasodilation than the administration of the inhaled agent alone at equivalent anesthetic depth.

Muscle. N_2O does not relax skeletal muscle and does not enhance the effects of neuromuscular blocking drugs.

Kidney, Liver, and GI Tract. N_2O is not known have nephrotoxic or hepatotoxic effects.

XENON

Xenon (Xe), an inert gaseous element, is not approved for use in the U.S. and is unlikely to enjoy widespread use because it is a rare gas that cannot be manufactured and must be extracted from air; thus, xenon is expensive and available in limited quantities. Xenon, unlike other anesthetic agents, has minimal cardiorespiratory and other side effects.

Xenon is extremely insoluble in blood and other tissues, providing for rapid induction and emergence from anesthesia. It is sufficiently potent to produce surgical anesthesia when administered with 30% oxygen. However, supplementation with an IV agent such as propofol appears to be required for clinical anesthesia. Xenon is well tolerated in patients of advanced age. No long-term side effects from xenon anesthesia have been reported.

ANESTHETIC ADJUNCTS

A general anesthetic is usually given with adjuncts to augment specific components of anesthesia, permitting lower doses of general anesthetics with fewer side effects.

BENZODIAZEPINES

Benzodiazepines (*see* Chapter 17) can produce anesthesia similar to that of barbiturates, they are more commonly used for sedation rather than general anesthesia because prolonged amnesia and sedation may result from anesthetizing doses. As adjuncts, benzodiazepines are used for anxiolysis, amnesia, and sedation prior to induction of anesthesia or for sedation during procedures not requiring general anesthesia. The benzodiazepine most frequently used in the perioperative period is midazolam followed distantly by diazepam (VALIUM, others), and lorazepam (ATIVAN, others).

Midazolam is water soluble and typically is administered intravenously but also can be given orally, intramuscularly, or rectally; oral midazolam is particularly useful for sedation of young children. Midazolam produces minimal venous irritation (as opposed to diazepam and lorazepam, which are formulated in propylene glycol and are painful on injection, sometimes producing thrombophlebitis). Midazolam has the pharmacokinetic advantage, particularly over lorazepam, of being more rapid in onset and shorter in duration of effect. Sedative doses of midazolam (0.01-0.05 mg/kg intravenously) reach peak effect in ~2 min and provide sedation for ~30 min. Elderly patients tend to be more sensitive to and have a slower recovery from benzodiazepines. Midazolam is hepatically metabolized. Either for prolonged sedation or for general anesthetic maintenance, midazolam is more suitable for infusion than are other benzodiazepines, although its duration of action does significantly increase with prolonged infusions (*see* Figure 19–3). Benzodiazepines reduce CBF and metabolism but at equianesthetic doses are less potent in this respect than are barbiturates. Benzodiazepines modestly decrease blood pressure and respiratory drive, occasionally resulting in apnea.

α_2 ADRENERGIC AGONISTS. Dexmedetomidine (PRECEDEX) is a highly selective α_2 adrenergic receptor agonist used for short-term (<24 h) sedation of critically ill adults and for sedation prior to and during surgical or other medical procedures in nonintubated patients. Activation of the α_{2A} adrenergic receptor by dexmedetomidine produces both sedation and analgesia.

The recommended loading dose is 1 μg/kg given over 10 min, followed by infusion at a rate of 0.2-0.7 μg/kg/h. Reduced doses should be considered in patients with risk factors for severe hypotension. Dexmedetomidine is highly protein bound and is metabolized primarily in the liver; the glucuronide and methyl conjugates are excreted in the urine. Common side effects of dexmedetomidine include hypotension and bradycardia, attributed to decreased catecholamine release by activation peripherally and in the CNS of the α_{2A} receptor. Nausea and dry mouth also are common untoward reactions. At higher drug concentrations, the α_{2B} subtype is activated, resulting in hypertension and a further decrease in heart rate and cardiac output. Dexmedetomidine provides sedation and analgesia with minimal respiratory depression. However, dexmedetomidine does not appear to provide reliable amnesia and additional agents may be needed.

ANALGESICS

With the exception of ketamine, neither parenteral nor currently available inhalational anesthetics are effective analgesics. Analgesics typically are administered with general anesthetics to reduce anesthetic requirement and minimize hemodynamic changes produced by painful stimuli. Nonsteroidal anti-inflammatory drugs, COX-2 inhibitors, and acetaminophen (*see* Chapter 34) sometimes provide adequate analgesia for minor surgical procedures. However, opioids are the primary analgesics used during the perioperative period because of the rapid and profound analgesia they produce. Fentanyl (SUBLIMAZE, others), sufentanil (SUFENTA, others), alfentanil (ALFENTA, others), remifentanil (ULTIVA), meperidine (DEMEROL, others), and morphine are the major parenteral opioids used in the perioperative period. The primary analgesic activity of each of these drugs is produced by agonist activity at μ-opioid receptors (*see* Chapter 18).

The choice of a perioperative opioid is based primarily on duration of action, since, at appropriate doses, all produce similar analgesia and side effects. Remifentanil has an ultrashort duration of action (~10 min), accumulates minimally with repeated doses, and is particularly well suited for procedures that are briefly painful. Single doses of fentanyl, alfentanil, and sufentanil all have similar intermediate durations of action (30, 20, and 15 min, respectively), but recovery after prolonged administration varies considerably. Fentanyl's duration of action lengthens the most with infusion, sufentanil's much less so, and alfentanil's the least.

The frequency and severity of nausea, vomiting, and pruritus after emergence from anesthesia are increased by all opioids to about the same degree. A useful side effect of meperidine is its capacity to reduce shivering, a common problem during emergence from anesthesia; other opioids are not as efficacious against shivering, perhaps due to less κ-receptor agonism. Finally, opioids often are administered intrathecally and epidurally for management of acute and chronic pain (*see* Chapter 18). Neuraxial opioids with or without local anesthetics can provide profound analgesia for many surgical procedures; however, respiratory depression and pruritus usually limit their use to major operations.

NEUROMUSCULAR-BLOCKING AGENTS

The practical aspects of the use of neuromuscular blockers as anesthetic adjuncts are briefly described here. The detailed pharmacology of this drug class is presented in Chapter 11.

Depolarizing (e.g., succinylcholine) and nondepolarizing muscle relaxants (e.g., vecuronium) often are administered during the induction of anesthesia to relax muscles of the jaw, neck, and airway and thereby facilitate laryngoscopy and endotracheal intubation. Barbiturates will precipitate when mixed with muscle relaxants and should be allowed to clear from the IV line prior to injection of a muscle relaxant. The action of nondepolarizing muscle relaxants usually is antagonized, once muscle paralysis is no longer desired, with an acetylcholinesterase inhibitor such as neostigmine or edrophonium (*see* Chapter 10), in combination with a muscarinic receptor antagonist (e.g., glycopyrrolate or atropine; *see* Chapter 9) to offset the muscarinic activation resulting from esterase inhibition. Other than histamine release by some agents, nondepolarizing muscle relaxants used in this manner have few side effects. However, succinylcholine has multiple serious side effects (bradycardia, hyperkalemia, and severe myalgia) including induction of malignant hyperthermia in susceptible individuals.

Therapeutic Gases

OXYGEN

Oxygen (O_2) is essential to life. Hypoxia is a life-threatening condition in which O_2 delivery is inadequate to meet the metabolic demands of the tissues. Hypoxia may result from alterations in tissue perfusion, decreased O_2 tension in the blood, or decreased O_2 carrying capacity. In addition, hypoxia may result from restricted O_2 transport from the microvasculature to cells or impaired utilization within the cell. An inadequate supply of O_2 ultimately results in the cessation of aerobic metabolism and oxidative phosphorylation, depletion of high-energy compounds, cellular dysfunction, and death.

NORMAL OXYGENATION

O_2 makes up 21% of air, which at sea level represents a partial pressure of 21 kPa (158 mm Hg). While the fraction (percentage) of O_2 remains constant regardless of atmospheric pressure, the partial pressure of O_2 (Po_2) decreases with lower atmospheric pressure. Ascent to elevated altitude reduces the uptake and delivery of O_2 to the tissues, whereas, increases in atmospheric pressure (e.g., hyperbaric therapy or breathing at depth) raise the Po_2 in inspired air and increase gas uptake. As the air is delivered to the distal airways and alveoli, the Po_2 decreases by dilution with CO_2 and water vapor and by uptake into the blood.

Under ideal conditions, when ventilation and perfusion are well matched, the alveolar Po_2 will be ~14.6 kPa (110 mm Hg). The corresponding alveolar partial pressures of water and CO_2 are 6.2 kPa (47 mm Hg) and 5.3 kPa (40 mm Hg), respectively. Under normal conditions, there is complete equilibration of alveolar gas and capillary blood, and the Po_2 in end-capillary blood is typically within a fraction of a kPa of that in the alveoli. The Po_2 in arterial blood, however, is further reduced by venous admixture (shunt), the addition of mixed venous blood from the pulmonary artery, which has a Po_2 of ~5.3 kPa (40 mm Hg). Together, the diffusional barrier, ventilation–perfusion mismatches, and the shunt fraction are the major causes of the alveolar-to-arterial O_2 gradient, which is normally 1.3-1.6 kPa (10-12 mm Hg) when air is breathed and 4.0-6.6 kPa (30-50 mm Hg) when 100% O_2 is breathed. O_2 is delivered to the tissue capillary beds by the circulation and again follows a gradient out of the blood and into cells. Tissue extraction of O_2 typically reduces the Po_2 of venous blood by an additional 7.3 kPa (55 mm Hg). Although the Po_2 at the site of cellular O_2 utilization—the mitochondria—is not known, oxidative phosphorylation can continue at a Po_2 of only a few mm Hg.

In the blood, O_2 is carried primarily in chemical combination with hemoglobin and is to a small extent dissolved in solution. The quantity of O_2 combined with hemoglobin depends on the Po_2, as illustrated by the sigmoidal oxyhemoglobin dissociation curve (Figure 19–6). Hemoglobin is ~98% saturated with O_2 when air is breathed under normal circumstances, and it binds 1.3 mL of O_2 per gram when fully saturated. The steep slope of this curve with falling Po_2 facilitates unloading of O_2 from hemoglobin at the tissue level and reloading when desaturated mixed venous blood arrives at the lung. Shifting of the curve to the right with increasing temperature, increasing Pco_2, and decreasing pH, as is found in metabolically active tissues, lowers the O_2 saturation for the same Po_2 and thus delivers additional O_2 where and when it is most needed. However, the flattening of the curve with higher Po_2 indicates that increasing blood Po_2 by inspiring O_2-enriched mixtures

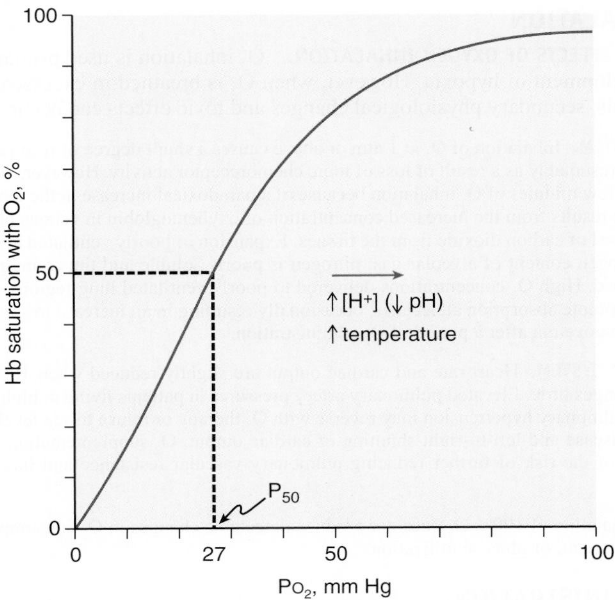

Figure 19–6 *Oxyhemoglobin dissociation curve for whole blood.* The relationship between Po_2 and hemoglobin (Hb) saturation is shown. The P_{50}, or the Po_2 resulting in 50% saturation, is indicated. An increase in temperature or a decrease in pH (as in working muscle) shifts this relationship to the right, reducing the hemoglobin saturation at the same Po_2 and thus aiding in the delivery of O_2 to the tissues.

can increase the amount of O_2 carried by hemoglobin only minimally. Because of the low solubility of O_2 (0.226 mL/L per kPa or 0.03 mL/L per mm Hg at 37°C), breathing 100% O_2 can increase the amount of O_2 dissolved in blood by only 15 mL/L, less than one-third of normal metabolic demands. However, if the inspired Po_2 is increased to 3 atm (304 kPa) in a hyperbaric chamber, the amount of dissolved O_2 is sufficient to meet normal metabolic demands even in the absence of hemoglobin (Table 19–4).

OXYGEN DEPRIVATION. *Hypoxemia* generally implies a failure of the respiratory system to oxygenate arterial blood. Classically, there are 5 causes of hypoxemia:

- Low inspired O_2 fraction (F_{IO_2})
- Increased diffusion barrier
- Hypoventilation
- Ventilation–perfusion mismatch
- Shunt or venous admixture

The term *hypoxia* denotes insufficient oxygenation of the tissues. In addition to failure of the respiratory system to oxygenate the blood adequately, a number of other factors can contribute to hypoxia at the tissue level. These may be divided into categories of O_2 delivery and O_2 utilization. O_2 delivery decreases globally when cardiac output falls or locally when regional blood flow is compromised, such as from a vascular occlusion (e.g., stenosis, thrombosis, or microvascular occlusion) or increased downstream pressure (e.g., compartment syndrome, venous stasis, or venous hypertension). Decreased O_2 carrying capacity of the blood likewise will reduce O_2 delivery, such as occurs with anemia, CO poisoning, or hemoglobinopathy. Finally, hypoxia may occur when transport of O_2 from the capillaries to the tissues is decreased (edema) or utilization of the O_2 by the cells is impaired (CN^- toxicity). Hypoxia produces a marked alteration in gene expression, mediated in part by hypoxia inducible factor-1α. The cellular consequences are discussed in Chapter 19 of the 12th edition of the parent text.

ADAPTATION TO HYPOXIA. Long-term hypoxia results in adaptive physiological changes; these have been studied most thoroughly in persons exposed to high altitude. Adaptations include increased numbers of pulmonary alveoli, increased concentrations of hemoglobin in blood and myoglobin in muscle, and a decreased ventilatory response to hypoxia. Short-term exposure to high altitude produces similar adaptive changes. In susceptible individuals, however, acute exposure to high altitude may produce *acute mountain sickness*, a syndrome characterized by headache, nausea, dyspnea, sleep disturbances, and impaired judgment progressing to pulmonary and cerebral edema. Mountain sickness is treated with rest and analgesics when mild or supplemental O_2, descent to lower altitude, or an increase in ambient pressure when more severe. Acetazolamide (a carbonic anhydrase inhibitor) and dexamethasone also may be helpful.

OXYGEN INHALATION

PHYSIOLOGICAL EFFECTS OF OXYGEN INHALATION. O_2 inhalation is used primarily to reverse or prevent the development of hypoxia. However, when O_2 is breathed in excessive amounts or for prolonged periods, secondary physiological changes and toxic effects can occur.

RESPIRATORY SYSTEM. Inhalation of O_2 at 1 atm or above causes a small degree of respiratory depression in normal subjects, presumably as a result of loss of tonic chemoreceptor activity. However, ventilation typically increases within a few minutes of O_2 inhalation because of a paradoxical increase in the tension of CO_2 in tissues. This increase results from the increased concentration of oxyhemoglobin in venous blood, which causes less efficient removal of carbon dioxide from the tissues. Expansion of poorly ventilated alveoli is maintained in part by the nitrogen content of alveolar gas; nitrogen is poorly soluble and thus remains in the airspaces while O_2 is absorbed. High O_2 concentrations delivered to poorly ventilated lung regions dilute the nitrogen content and can promote absorption atelectasis, occasionally resulting in an increase in shunt and a paradoxical worsening of hypoxemia after a period of O_2 administration.

CARDIOVASCULAR SYSTEM. Heart rate and cardiac output are slightly reduced when 100% O_2 is breathed; blood pressure changes little. Elevated pulmonary artery pressures in patients living at high altitude who have chronic hypoxic pulmonary hypertension may reverse with O_2 therapy or return to sea level. In neonates with congenital heart disease and left-to-right shunting of cardiac output, O_2 supplementation must be regulated carefully because of the risk of further reducing pulmonary vascular resistance and increasing pulmonary blood flow.

METABOLISM. Inhalation of 100% O_2 does not produce detectable changes in O_2 consumption, CO_2 production, respiratory quotient, or glucose utilization.

OXYGEN ADMINISTRATION

O_2 is supplied as a compressed gas in steel cylinders; purity of 99% is *medical grade*. For safety, O_2 cylinders and piping are color-coded (green in the U.S.), and some form of mechanical indexing of valve connections is used to prevent the connection of other gases to O_2 systems.

Table 19–4

The Carriage of Oxygen in Blood[a]

ARTERIAL P_{O_2} kPa (mm Hg)	ARTERIAL O_2 CONTENT (mL O_2/L)			MIXED VENOUS P_{O_2} kPa (mm Hg)	MIXED VENOUS O_2 CONTENT (mL O_2/L)			EXAMPLES
	DISSOLVED	BOUND TO HEMOGLOBIN	TOTAL		DISSOLVED	BOUND TO HEMOGLOBIN	TOTAL	
4.0 (30)	0.9	109	109.9	2.7 (20)	0.6	59	59.6	High altitude; respiratory failure breathing air
12.0 (90)	2.7	192	194.7	5.5 (41)	1.2	144	145.2	Normal person breathing air
39.9 (300)	9.0	195	204	5.9 (44)	1.3	153	154.3	Normal person breathing 50% O_2
79.7 (600)	18	196	214	6.5 (49)	1.5	163	164.5	Normal person breathing 100% O_2
239 (1800)	54	196	250	20.0 (150)	4.5	196	200.5	Normal person breathing hyperbaric O_2

[a]This table illustrates the carriage of oxygen in the blood under a variety of circumstances. As arterial O_2 tension increases, the amount of dissolved O_2 increases in direct proportion to the P_{O_2}, but the amount of oxygen bound to hemoglobin reaches a maximum of 196 mL O_2/liter (100% saturation of hemoglobin at 15 g/dL). Further increases in O_2 content require increases in dissolved oxygen. At 100% inspired O_2, dissolved O_2 still provides only a small fraction of total demand. Hyperbaric oxygen therapy is required to increase the amount of dissolved oxygen to supply all or a large part of metabolic requirements. Note that, during hyperbaric oxygen therapy, the hemoglobin in the mixed venous blood remains fully saturated with O_2. The figures in this table are approximate and are based on the assumptions of 15 g/dL hemoglobin, 50 mL O_2/liter whole-body oxygen extraction, and constant cardiac output. When severe anemia is present, arterial P_{O_2} remains the same, but arterial content is lower; oxygen extraction continues, resulting in lower O_2 content and tension in mixed venous blood. Similarly, as cardiac output falls significantly, the same oxygen extraction occurs from a smaller volume of blood and results in lower mixed venous oxygen content and tension.

O_2 is delivered by inhalation except during extracorporeal circulation, when it is dissolved directly into the circulating blood. Only a closed delivery system with an airtight seal to the patient's airway and complete separation of inspired from expired gases can precisely control F_{IO_2}. In all other systems, the actual delivered F_{IO_2} will depend on the ventilatory pattern (i.e., rate, tidal volume, inspiratory–expiratory time ratio, and inspiratory flow) and delivery system characteristics.

LOW-FLOW SYSTEMS. Low-flow systems, in which the O_2 flow is lower than the inspiratory flow rate, have a limited ability to raise the F_{IO_2} because they depend on entrained room air to make up the balance of the inspired gas. These devices typically deliver 24-28% F_{IO_2} at 2-3 L/min. Up to 40% F_{IO_2} is possible at higher flow rates, although this is poorly tolerated for more than brief periods because of mucosal drying.

HIGH-FLOW SYSTEMS. The most commonly used high-flow O_2 delivery device is the Venturi-style mask, which uses a specially designed mask insert to entrain room air reliably in a fixed ratio and thus provides a relatively constant F_{IO_2} at relatively high flow rates. Typically, each insert is designed to operate at a specific O_2 flow rate, and different inserts are required to change the F_{IO_2}. Lower delivered F_{IO_2} values use greater entrainment ratios, resulting in higher total (O_2 plus entrained air) flows to the patient, ranging from 80 L/min for 24% F_{IO_2} to 40 L/min at 50% F_{IO_2}. O_2 nebulizers, another type of Venturi-style device, provide patients with humidified O_2 at 35-100% F_{IO_2} at high flow rates. Finally, O_2 blenders provide high inspired O_2 concentrations at very high flow rates. These devices mix high-pressure compressed air and O_2 to achieve any concentration of O_2 from 21-100% at flow rates of up to 100 L/min. Despite the high flows, the delivery of high F_{IO_2} to an individual patient also depends on maintaining a tight-fitting seal to the airway and/or the use of reservoirs to minimize entrainment of diluting room air.

MONITORING OF OXYGENATION. Monitoring and titration are required to meet the therapeutic goal of O_2 therapy and to avoid complications and side effects. Although cyanosis is a physical finding of substantial clinical importance, it is not an early, sensitive, or reliable index of oxygenation. Noninvasive monitoring of arterial O_2 saturation can be achieved using transcutaneous pulse oximetry, in which O_2 saturation is measured from the differential absorption of light by oxyhemoglobin and deoxyhemoglobin and the arterial saturation determined from the pulsatile component of this signal. Pulse oximetry measures hemoglobin saturation and not P_{O_2}. It is not sensitive to increases in P_{O_2} that exceed levels required to saturate the blood fully. Pulse oximetry is very useful for monitoring the adequacy of oxygenation during procedures requiring sedation or anesthesia, rapid evaluation and monitoring of potentially compromised patients, and titrating O_2 therapy in situations where toxicity from O_2 or side effects of excess O_2 are of concern.

COMPLICATIONS OF OXYGEN THERAPY. In addition to the potential to promote absorption atelectasis and depress ventilation, high flows of dry O_2 can dry out and irritate mucosal surfaces of the airway and the eyes, as well as decrease mucociliary transport and clearance of secretions. Humidified O_2 thus should be used when prolonged therapy (>1 h) is required. Finally, any O_2-enriched atmosphere constitutes a fire hazard, and appropriate precautions must be taken. Hypoxemia can occur despite the administration of supplemental O_2. Therefore, it is essential that both O_2 saturation and adequacy of ventilation be assessed frequently.

THERAPEUTIC USES OF OXYGEN

CORRECTION OF HYPOXIA. The primary therapeutic use of O_2 is to correct hypoxia. Hypoxia is most commonly a manifestation of an underlying disease, and administration of O_2 thus should be viewed as temporizing therapy. Efforts must be directed at correcting the cause of the hypoxia. Hypoxia resulting from most pulmonary diseases can be alleviated at least partially by administration of O_2, allowing time for definitive therapy to reverse the primary process.

Reduction of Partial Pressure of an Inert Gas. Because nitrogen constitutes some 79% of ambient air, it also is the predominant gas in most gas-filled spaces in the body. In situations such as bowel distension from obstruction or ileus, intravascular air embolism, or pneumothorax, it is desirable to reduce the volume of air-filled spaces. Because nitrogen is relatively insoluble, inhalation of high concentrations of O_2 (and thus low concentrations of nitrogen) rapidly lowers the total-body partial pressure of nitrogen and provides a substantial gradient for the removal of nitrogen from gas spaces. Administration of O_2 for air embolism is additionally beneficial because it helps to relieve localized hypoxia distal to the vascular obstruction. In the case of *decompression sickness*, or *bends*, lowering the inert gas tension in blood and tissues by O_2 inhalation prior to or during a barometric decompression reduces the supersaturation that occurs after decompression so that bubbles do not form.

Hyperbaric Oxygen Therapy. O_2 can be administered at greater than atmospheric pressure in hyperbaric chambers. Clinical uses of hyperbaric O_2 therapy include the treatment of trauma, burns, radiation damage, infections, nonhealing ulcers, skin grafts, spasticity, and other neurological conditions. Hyperbaric O_2 may be useful in generalized hypoxia. In CO poisoning, hemoglobin (Hb) and myoglobin become unavailable for O_2 binding because of the high affinity of these proteins for CO. High P_{O_2} facilitates competition of O_2 for

Hb binding sites as CO is exchanged in the alveoli. In addition, hyperbaric O_2 increases the availability of dissolved O_2 in the blood (*see* Table 19–4). Adverse effects of hyperbaric O_2 therapy include middle ear barotrauma, CNS toxicity, seizures, lung toxicity, and aspiration pneumonia.

Hyperbaric O_2 therapy has 2 components: increased hydrostatic pressure and increased O_2 pressure. Both factors are necessary for the treatment of decompression sickness and air embolism. The hydrostatic pressure reduces bubble volume, and the absence of inspired nitrogen increases the gradient for elimination of nitrogen and reduces hypoxia in downstream tissues. Increased O_2 pressure at the tissue is the primary therapeutic goal for other indications for hyperbaric O_2. A small increase in Po_2 in ischemic areas enhances the bactericidal activity of leukocytes and increases angiogenesis. Repetitive brief exposures to hyperbaric O_2 may enhance therapy for chronic refractory osteomyelitis, osteoradionecrosis, crush injury, or the recovery of compromised skin and tissue grafts. Increased O_2 tension can be bacteriostatic and useful in the treatment for the spread of infection with *Clostridium perfringens* and clostridial myonecrosis (gas gangrene).

OXYGEN TOXICITY

O_2 can have deleterious actions at the cellular level. O_2 toxicity may result from increased production of hydrogen peroxide and reactive intermediates such as superoxide anion, singlet oxygen, and hydroxyl radicals that attack and damage lipids, proteins, and other macromolecules, especially those in biological membranes. A number of factors limit the toxicity of oxygen-derived reactive agents, including enzymes such as superoxide dismutase, glutathione peroxidase, and catalase, which scavenge toxic oxygen by-products, and reducing agents such as iron, glutathione, and ascorbate. These factors, however, are insufficient to limit the destructive actions of oxygen when patients are exposed to high concentrations over an extended time period. Tissues show differential sensitivity to oxygen toxicity, which is likely the result of differences in both their production of reactive compounds and their protective mechanisms.

RESPIRATORY TRACT. The pulmonary system is usually the first to exhibit toxicity, a function of its continuous exposure to the highest O_2 tensions in the body. Subtle changes in pulmonary function can occur within 8-12 h of exposure to 100% O_2. Increases in capillary permeability, which will increase the alveolar/arterial O_2 gradient and ultimately lead to further hypoxemia, and decreased pulmonary function can be seen after only 18 h of exposure. Serious injury and death, however, require much longer exposures. Pulmonary damage is directly related to the inspired O_2 tension, and concentrations of <0.5 atm appear to be safe over long time periods. The capillary endothelium is the most sensitive tissue of the lung. Endothelial injury results in loss of surface area from interstitial edema and leaks into the alveoli.

NERVOUS SYSTEM. Retinopathy of prematurity (ROP) is an eye disease in premature infants involving abnormal vascularization of the developing retina that can result from O_2 toxicity or relative hypoxia. CNS problems are rare, and toxicity occurs only under hyperbaric conditions where exposure exceeds 200 kPa (2 atm). Symptoms include seizures and visual changes, which resolve when O_2 tension is returned to normal. In premature neonates and those who have sustained in utero asphyxia, hyperoxia and hypocapnia are associated with worse neurologic outcomes.

CARBON DIOXIDE

CO_2 is produced by metabolism at approximately the same rate as O_2 is consumed. At rest, this value is ~3 mL/kg/min, but it may increase dramatically with exercise. CO_2 diffuses readily from the cells into the blood, where it is carried partly as bicarbonate ion (HCO_3^-), partly in chemical combination with hemoglobin and plasma proteins, and partly in solution at a partial pressure of ~6 kPa (46 mm Hg) in mixed venous blood. CO_2 is transported to the lung, where it is normally exhaled at the rate it is produced, leaving a partial pressure of ~5.2 kPa (40 mm Hg) in the alveoli and in arterial blood. An increase in Pco_2 results in a respiratory acidosis and may be due to decreased ventilation or the inhalation of CO_2, whereas an increase in ventilation results in decreased Pco_2 and a respiratory alkalosis. Since CO_2 is freely diffusible, the changes in blood Pco_2 and pH soon are reflected by intracellular changes in Pco_2 and pH and by widespread effects in the body, especially on respiration, circulation, and the CNS.

RESPIRATION. CO_2 is a rapid, potent stimulus to ventilation in direct proportion to the inspired CO_2. CO_2 stimulates breathing by acidifying central chemoreceptors and the peripheral carotid bodies. Elevated Pco_2 causes bronchodilation, whereas hypocarbia causes constriction of airway smooth muscle; these responses may play a role in matching pulmonary ventilation and perfusion.

CIRCULATION. The circulatory effects of CO_2 result from the combination of its direct local effects and its centrally mediated effects on the autonomic nervous system. The direct effect of CO_2 on the heart, diminished contractility, results from pH changes and a decreased myofilament Ca^{2+} responsiveness. The direct effect on systemic blood vessels results in vasodilation. CO_2 causes widespread activation of the sympathetic nervous system. The results of sympathetic nervous system activation generally are opposite to the local effects of carbon dioxide. The sympathetic effects consist of increases in cardiac contractility, heart rate, and vasoconstriction (*see* Chapter 12). The balance of opposing local and sympathetic effects, therefore, determines the total circulatory response to CO_2. The net effect of CO_2 inhalation is an increase in cardiac output, heart rate, and blood pressure. In blood vessels, however, the direct vasodilating actions of CO_2 appear more important, and total peripheral resistance decreases when the P_{CO_2} is increased. CO_2 also is a potent coronary vasodilator. Cardiac arrhythmias associated with increased P_{CO_2} are due to the release of catecholamines.

Hypocarbia results in opposite effects: decreased blood pressure and vasoconstriction in skin, intestine, brain, kidney, and heart. These actions are exploited clinically in the use of hyperventilation to diminish intracranial hypertension.

CNS. Hypercarbia depresses the excitability of the cerebral cortex and increases the cutaneous pain threshold through a central action. This central depression has therapeutic importance. For example, in patients who are hypoventilating from narcotics or anesthetics, increasing P_{CO_2} may result in further CNS depression, which in turn may worsen the respiratory depression. This positive-feedback cycle can have lethal consequences.

METHODS OF ADMINISTRATION. CO_2 is marketed in gray metal cylinders as the pure gas or as CO_2 mixed with O_2. It usually is administered at a concentration of 5-10% in combination with O_2 by means of a face mask. Another method for the temporary administration of CO_2 is by rebreathing, such as from an anesthesia breathing circuit or from something as simple as a paper bag.

THERAPEUTIC USES. CO_2 is used for insufflation during endoscopic procedures (e.g., laparoscopic surgery) because it is highly soluble and does not support combustion. CO_2 can be used to flood the surgical field during cardiac surgery. Because of its density, CO_2 displaces the air surrounding the open heart so that any gas bubbles trapped in the heart are CO_2 rather than insoluble N_2. It is used to adjust pH during cardiopulmonary bypass procedures when a patient is cooled.

Hypocarbia still has some uses in anesthesia; it constricts cerebral vessels, decreasing brain size slightly, and thus may facilitate the performance of neurosurgical operations. While short-term hypocarbia is effective for this purpose, sustained hypocarbia has been associated with worse outcomes in patients with head injury. Hypocarbia should be instituted with a clearly defined indication and normocarbia should be reestablished as soon the indication for hypocarbia no longer applies.

NITRIC OXIDE

Nitric oxide (NO) is a free-radical gas now known as a critical endogenous cell-signaling molecule with an increasing number of potential therapeutic applications.

Endogenous NO is produced from L-arginine by NO synthases (neural, inducible and endothelial) (*see* Chapter 3). In the vasculature, basal production of NO by endothelial cells is a primary determinant of resting vascular tone. NO causes vasodilation of smooth muscle cells and inhibition of platelet aggregation and adhesion. Impaired NO production is implicated in atherosclerosis, hypertension, cerebral and coronary vasospasm, ischemia–reperfusion injury, inflammation, and in mediating central nociceptive pathways. NO is rapidly inactivated in the circulation by oxyhemoglobin and by the reaction of NO with the heme iron, leading to the formation of nitrosyl-hemoglobin. Small quantities of methemoglobin are also produced and these are converted to the ferrous form of heme iron by cytochrome b5 reductase. The majority of inhaled NO is excreted in the urine in the form of nitrate.

THERAPEUTIC USES. Inhaled NO (iNO) selectively dilates the pulmonary vasculature and has potential as a therapy for numerous diseases associated with increased pulmonary vascular resistance. Inhaled NO is FDA-approved for only 1 indication, persistent pulmonary hypertension of the newborn.

DIAGNOSTIC USES. Inhaled NO can be used during cardiac catheterization to evaluate the pulmonary vasodilating capacity of patients with heart failure and infants with congenital heart disease. Inhaled NO also is used to determine the diffusion capacity (DL) across the alveolar–capillary unit. NO is more effective than CO_2 in this regard because of its greater affinity for hemoglobin and its higher water solubility at body temperature. NO is produced from the nasal passages and from the lungs of normal human subjects and can be detected in exhaled gas. The measurement of fractional exhaled NO (FeNO) is a noninvasive marker for airway inflammation with utility in the assessment of respiratory tract diseases including asthma, respiratory tract infection, and chronic lung disease.

TOXICITY. Administered at low concentrations (0.1-50 ppm), iNO appears to be safe and without significant side effects. Pulmonary toxicity can occur with levels higher than 50-100 ppm. NO is an atmospheric pollutant; the Occupational Safety and Health Administration places the 7-h exposure limit at 50 ppm. Part of the toxicity of NO may be related to its further oxidation to nitrogen dioxide (NO_2) in the presence of high concentrations of O_2.

The development of methemoglobinemia is a significant complication of inhaled NO at higher concentrations, and rare deaths have been reported with overdoses of NO. Methemoglobin concentrations should be monitored intermittently during NO inhalation. Inhaled NO can inhibit platelet function and has been shown to increase bleeding time in some clinical studies, although bleeding complications have not been reported. In patients with impaired function of the left ventricle, NO has a potential to further impair left ventricular performance by dilating the pulmonary circulation and increasing the blood flow to the left ventricle, thereby increasing left atrial pressure and promoting pulmonary edema formation.

The most important requirements for safe NO inhalation therapy include:

- Continuous measurement of NO and NO_2 concentrations using either chemiluminescence or electrochemical analyzers
- Frequent calibration of monitoring equipment
- Intermittent analysis of blood methemoglobin levels
- The use of certified tanks of NO
- Administration of the lowest NO concentration required for therapeutic effect

METHODS OF ADMINISTRATION. Courses of treatment of patients with inhaled NO are highly varied, extending from 0.1-40 ppm in dose and for periods of a few hours to several weeks in duration. The determination of dose response relationship on a frequent basis should assist in the titration of the optimum dose of NO. Commercial NO systems are available that will accurately deliver inspired NO concentrations between 0.1 and 80 ppm and simultaneously measure NO and NO_2 concentrations.

HELIUM

Helium (He) is an inert gas whose low density, low solubility, and high thermal conductivity provide the basis for its medical and diagnostic uses. Helium can be mixed with O_2 and administered by mask or endotracheal tube. Under hyperbaric conditions, it can be substituted for the bulk of other gases, resulting in a mixture of much lower density that is easier to breathe.

The primary uses of helium are in pulmonary function testing, the treatment of respiratory obstruction, laser airway surgery, as a label in imaging studies, and for diving at depth. Helium is also suited for determinations of residual lung volume, functional residual capacity, and related lung volumes. These measurements require a highly diffusible nontoxic gas that is insoluble and does not leave the lung by the bloodstream so that, by dilution, the lung volume can be measured. Helium can be added to O_2 to reduce turbulence due to airway obstruction since the density of helium is less than that of air and the viscosity of helium is greater than that of air. Mixtures of helium and O_2 reduce the work of breathing. Helium has high thermal conductivity, making it useful during laser surgery on the airway. Laser-polarized helium is used as an inhalational contrast agent for pulmonary magnetic resonance imaging. Optical pumping of hyperpolarized helium increases the signal from the gas in the lung to permit detailed imaging of the airways and inspired airflow patterns.

HYDROGEN SULFIDE

Hydrogen sulfide (H_2S), which has a characteristic rotten egg smell, is a colorless, flammable, water-soluble gas that is primarily considered a toxic agent due to its ability to inhibit mitochondrial respiration through blockade of cytochrome c oxidase. Inhibition of respiration is potentially toxic; however, if depression of respiration occurs in a controlled manner, it may allow nonhibernating species exposed to inhaled H_2S to enter a state akin to suspended animation (i.e., a slowing of cellular activity to a point where metabolic processes are inhibited but not terminal) and thereby increase tolerance to stress. H_2S also may cause activation of ATP-dependent K^+ channels, cause vasodilation properties, and serve as a free radical scavenger. H_2S has been shown to protect against whole-body hypoxia, lethal hemorrhage, and ischemia-reperfusion injury in various organs including the kidney, lung, liver, and heart. Currently, effort is underway for development of gas-releasing molecules that could deliver H_2S and other therapeutic gases to diseased tissue. H_2S in low quantities may have the potential to limit cell death.

For a complete Bibliographical Listing see Goodman & Gilman's ***The Pharmacological Basis of Therapeutics***, 12th ed., or Goodman & Gilman Online at www.AccessMedicine.com.

Local Anesthetics

Local anesthetics bind reversibly to a specific receptor site within the pore of the Na^+ channels in nerves and block ion movement through this pore. When applied locally to nerve tissue in appropriate concentrations, local anesthetics can act on any part of the nervous system and on every type of nerve fiber, reversibly blocking the action potentials responsible for nerve conduction.

CHEMISTRY AND STRUCTURE-ACTIVITY RELATIONSHIP. The most widely used agents today are procaine, lidocaine, bupivacaine, and tetracaine (Figure 20–1). These agents were synthesized as substitutes for cocaine, preserving the local anesthetic effect of cocaine but avoiding its toxicity and addictive properties. The typical local anesthetics contain hydrophilic and hydrophobic moieties that are separated by an intermediate ester or amide linkage. The hydrophilic group usually is a tertiary amine but also may be a secondary amine; the hydrophobic moiety must be aromatic. The nature of the linking group determines some of the pharmacological properties of these agents. For example, local anesthetics with an ester link are hydrolyzed readily by plasma esterases. Hydrophobicity increases both the potency and the duration of action of the local anesthetics; association of the drug at hydrophobic sites enhances the partitioning of the drug to its sites of action and decreases the rate of metabolism by plasma esterases and hepatic enzymes. In addition, the receptor site for these drugs on Na^+ channels is thought to be hydrophobic, so that receptor affinity for anesthetic agents is greater for more hydrophobic drugs. Hydrophobicity also increases toxicity, so that the therapeutic index is decreased for more hydrophobic drugs.

COCAINE

PROCAINE

TETRACAINE

LIDOCAINE

BUPIVACAINE

Figure 20–1 *Structural formulas of selected local anesthetics.* Most local anesthetics consist of a hydrophobic (aromatic) moiety (*black*), a linker region (*orange*), and a substituted amine (hydrophilic region, in *red*). Procaine is a prototypic ester-type local anesthetic; esters generally are well hydrolyzed by plasma esterases, contributing to the relatively short duration of action of drugs in this group. Lidocaine is a prototypic amide-type local anesthetic; these structures generally are more resistant to clearance and have longer durations of action. Figure 20–1 in 12th edition of the parent text shows additional variations on the basic structure.

Molecular size influences the rate of dissociation of local anesthetics from their receptor sites. Smaller drug molecules can escape from the receptor site more rapidly. This characteristic is important in rapidly firing cells, in which local anesthetics bind during action potentials and dissociate during the period of membrane repolarization. Rapid binding of local anesthetics during action potentials causes the frequency- and voltage-dependence of their action.

MECHANISM OF ACTION. Local anesthetics act at the cell membrane to prevent the generation and the conduction of nerve impulses. The major mechanism of action of local anesthetics involves their interaction with 1 or more specific binding sites within the Na^+ channel (*see* Figure 14–1A).

Local anesthetics block conduction by decreasing or preventing the large transient increase in the permeability of excitable membranes to Na^+ that normally is produced by membrane depolarization. This action of local anesthetics is due to their direct interaction with voltage-gated Na^+ channels. As the anesthetic action progressively develops in a nerve, the threshold for electrical excitability gradually increases, the rate of rise of the action potential declines, impulse conduction slows, and nerve conduction fails. Local anesthetics can block K^+ channels but this interaction requires higher concentrations of drug; thus, blockade of conduction is not accompanied by any large change in resting membrane potential.

FREQUENCY- AND VOLTAGE-DEPENDENCE OF LOCAL ANESTHETIC ACTION. A higher frequency of stimulation and more positive membrane potential cause a greater degree of anesthetic block. These frequency- and voltage-dependent effects of local anesthetics occur because the local anesthetic molecule in its charged form, gains access to its binding site within the pore only when the Na^+ channel is in an open state, and because the local anesthetic binds more tightly to and stabilizes the inactivated state of the Na^+ channel. The frequency dependence of local anesthetic action depends critically on the rate of dissociation from the receptor site in the pore of the Na^+ channel. A high frequency of stimulation is required for rapidly dissociating drugs so that drug binding during the action potential exceeds drug dissociation between action potentials.

DIFFERENTIAL SENSITIVITY OF NERVE FIBERS TO LOCAL ANESTHETICS. For most patients treatment with local anesthetics causes the sensation of pain to disappear first, followed by loss of the sensations of temperature, touch, deep pressure, and finally motor function (Table 20–1).

In general, autonomic fibers, small unmyelinated C fibers (mediating pain sensations), and small myelinated $A\delta$ fibers (mediating pain and temperature sensations) are blocked before the larger myelinated $A\gamma$, $A\beta$, and $A\alpha$ fibers (mediating postural, touch, pressure, and motor information) The precise mechanisms responsible for this apparent specificity of local anesthetic action on pain fibers are not known. *The differential rate of block exhibited by fibers mediating different sensations is of considerable practical importance in the use of local anesthetics.*

EFFECT OF pH. Local anesthetics tend to be only slightly soluble as unprotonated amines. Therefore, they generally are marketed as water-soluble salts, usually hydrochlorides. Inasmuch as the local anesthetics are weak bases (typical pK_a values range from 8-9), their hydrochloride salts are mildly acidic. This property increases the stability of the local anesthetic esters and the catecholamines added as vasoconstrictors. Under usual conditions of administration, the pH of the local anesthetic solution rapidly equilibrates to that of the extracellular fluids.

PROLONGATION OF ACTION BY VASOCONSTRICTORS. The duration of action of a local anesthetic is proportional to the time of contact with nerve. Consequently, maneuvers that keep the drug at the nerve prolong the period of anesthesia. In clinical practice, a vasoconstrictor, usually epinephrine, is often added to local anesthetics. The vasoconstrictor, by decreasing the rate of absorption, localizes the anesthetic at the desired site, and reduces systemic toxicity by allowing metabolism to keep pace with the rate at which it is absorbed into the circulation. It should be noted, however, that epinephrine also dilates skeletal muscle vascular beds through actions at β_2 adrenergic receptors, and therefore has the potential to increase systemic toxicity of anesthetic deposited in muscle tissue.

UNDESIRED EFFECTS OF LOCAL ANESTHETICS. Local anesthetics interfere with the function of all organs in which conduction or transmission of impulses occurs. Thus, they have important effects on the CNS, the autonomic ganglia, the neuromuscular junction, and all forms of muscle.

The danger of such adverse reactions is proportional to the concentration of local anesthetic achieved in the circulation. In general, in local anesthetics with chiral centers, the *S*-enantiomer is less toxic than the *R*-enantiomer.

CNS. Following absorption, local anesthetics may cause CNS stimulation, producing restlessness and tremor that may progress to clonic convulsions. Central stimulation is followed by depression; death usually is caused by respiratory failure. Benzodiazepines or rapidly acting barbiturates administered intravenously are the

Table 20–1

Susceptibility of Nerve Fibers to Local Anesthetics

TYPE	ANATOMIC LOCATION	DIAMETER (μm)	CONDUCTION VELOCITY (m/sec)	FUNCTION	CLINICAL SENSITIVITY TO BLOCK
Myelinated					
A fibers A α A β	Afferent to and efferent from muscles and joints	6–22	10–85	Motor and proprioception	+ ++
A γ	Efferent to muscle spindles	3–6	15–35	Muscle tone	++
A δ	Sensory roots and afferent peripheral nerves	1–4	5–25	Pain, temperature, touch	+++
B fibers	Preganglionic sympathetic	<3	3–15	Vaso-, viscero-, sudo-, pilo-motor	++++
Non-myelinated					
C fibers Sympathetic	Postganglionic sympathetic	0.3–1.3	0.7–1.3	Vaso-, viscero-, sudo-, pilo-motor	++++
Dorsal root	Sensory roots and afferent peripheral nerves	0.4–1.2	0.1–2	Pain, temperature, touch	++++

Source: Adapted with permission from Barash PG et al, eds. Clinical Anesthesia, 6th ed. Philadelphia: Lippincott Williams & Wilkins, 2009, p 533.

drugs of choice for both the prevention and arrest of convulsions (*see* Chapter 17). Lidocaine may produce dysphoria or euphoria and muscle twitching. Moreover, both lidocaine and procaine may produce a loss of consciousness that is preceded only by symptoms of sedation.

Cardiovascular System. Following systemic absorption, local anesthetics act on the cardiovascular system, primarily on the myocardium, where decreases in electrical excitability, conduction rate, and force of contraction occur. In addition, most local anesthetics cause arteriolar dilation. Untoward cardiovascular effects usually are seen only after high systemic concentrations are attained and effects on the CNS are produced; on rare occasions, lower doses of some local anesthetics will cause cardiovascular collapse and death. Ventricular tachycardia and fibrillation are relatively uncommon consequences of local anesthetics other than bupivacaine. Untoward cardiovascular effects of local anesthetic agents may result from their inadvertent intravascular administration, especially if epinephrine also is present.

Smooth Muscle. Local anesthetics depress contractions in the bowel. They also relax vascular and bronchial smooth muscle, although low concentrations initially may produce contraction. Spinal and epidural anesthesia and instillation of local anesthetics into the peritoneal cavity cause sympathetic nervous system paralysis, which can result in increased tone of GI musculature. Local anesthetics seldom depress uterine contractions during intrapartum regional anesthesia.

Neuromuscular Junction and Ganglionic Synapse. Local anesthetics also affect transmission at the neuromuscular junction. Procaine, e.g., can block the response of skeletal muscle to ACh at concentrations at which the muscle responds normally to direct electrical stimulation. Similar effects occur at autonomic ganglia. These effects are due to block of nicotinic ACh receptors by high concentrations of the local anesthetic.

HYPERSENSITIVITY TO LOCAL ANESTHETICS. Rare individuals are hypersensitive to local anesthetics. The reaction may manifest itself as an allergic dermatitis or a typical asthmatic attack. Hypersensitivity seems to occur more frequently with local anesthetics of the ester type and frequently extends to chemically related compounds. Local anesthetic preparations containing a vasoconstrictor also may elicit allergic responses due to the sulfite added as an antioxidant for the catecholamine/vasoconstrictor.

METABOLISM OF LOCAL ANESTHETICS. The metabolic fate of local anesthetics is of great practical importance, because their toxicity depends largely on the balance between their rates of absorption and elimination. The rate of absorption of many anesthetics can be reduced considerably by the incorporation of a vasoconstrictor agent in the anesthetic solution. However, the rate of degradation of local anesthetics varies greatly, and this is a major factor in determining the safety of a particular agent. Because toxicity is related to the concentration of free drug, binding of the anesthetic to proteins in the serum and to tissues reduces the concentration of free drug in the systemic circulation, and consequently reduces toxicity.

Some of the common local anesthetics (e.g., tetracaine) are esters; they are inactivated primarily by a plasma esterase. The liver also participates in hydrolysis of local anesthetics. Because spinal fluid contains little or no esterase, anesthesia produced by the intrathecal injection of an anesthetic agent will persist until the local anesthetic agent has been absorbed into the circulation. The amide-linked local anesthetics are, in general, degraded by the hepatic CYPs the initial reactions involving *N*-dealkylation and subsequent hydrolysis. With prilocaine, the initial step is hydrolytic, forming *o*-toluidine metabolites that can cause methemoglobinemia. The extensive use of amide-linked local anesthetics in patients with severe hepatic disease requires caution. The amide-linked local anesthetics are extensively (55-95%) bound to plasma proteins, particularly α_1-acid glycoprotein. Many factors increase (e.g., cancer, surgery, trauma, myocardial infarction, smoking, and uremia) or decrease (e.g., oral contraceptives) the level of this glycoprotein, thereby changing the amount of anesthetic delivered to the liver for metabolism and thus influencing systemic toxicity. Age-related changes in protein binding of local anesthetics also occur. The neonate is relatively deficient in plasma proteins that bind local anesthetics and thereby is more susceptible to toxicity. Uptake by the lung also may play an important role in the distribution of amide-linked local anesthetics in the body. Reduced cardiac output slows delivery of the amide compounds to the liver, reducing their metabolism and prolonging their plasma half-lives.

COCAINE

Cocaine, an ester of benzoic acid and methylecgonine, occurs in abundance in the leaves of the coca shrub.

PHARMACOLOGICAL ACTIONS AND PREPARATIONS. The clinically desired actions of cocaine are the blockade of nerve impulses, as a consequence of its local anesthetic properties, and local vasoconstriction, secondary to inhibition of local NE reuptake. Cocaine's high toxicity is due to reduced catecholamine uptake in both the central and peripheral nervous systems. Its euphoric properties are due primarily to inhibition of catecholamine uptake, particularly DA, in the CNS. Cocaine is used primarily for topical anesthesia of the upper respiratory tract, where its combination of both vasoconstrictor and local anesthetic properties provide anesthesia and shrinking of the mucosa. Cocaine hydrochloride is provided as a 1%, 4%, or 10% solution for topical application. Because of its abuse potential, cocaine is listed as a schedule II controlled substance by the U.S. Drug Enforcement Agency.

LIDOCAINE

Lidocaine (XYLOCAINE, others), an aminoethylamide, is the prototypical amide local anesthetic.

PHARMACOLOGICAL ACTIONS; PREPARATIONS. Lidocaine produces faster, more intense, longer-lasting, and more extensive anesthesia than does an equal concentration of procaine. Lidocaine is an alternative choice for individuals sensitive to ester-type local anesthetics. Lidocaine is absorbed rapidly after parenteral administration and from the GI and respiratory tracts. Although it is effective when used without any vasoconstrictor, epinephrine decreases the rate of absorption, such that the toxicity is decreased and the duration of action usually is prolonged. In addition to preparations for injection, lidocaine is formulated for topical, ophthalmic, mucosal, and transdermal use.

A lidocaine transdermal patch (LIDODERM) is used for relief of pain associated with postherpetic neuralgia. An oral patch (DENTIPATCH) is available for application to accessible mucous membranes of the mouth prior to superficial dental procedures. The combination of lidocaine (2.5%) and prilocaine (2.5%) in an occlusive dressing (EMLA, others) is used as an anesthetic prior to venipuncture, skin graft harvesting, and infiltration of anesthetics into genitalia. Lidocaine in combination with tetracaine (PLIAGLIS) in a formulation that generates a "peel" is approved for topical local analgesia prior to superficial dermatological procedures such as filler injections and laser-based treatments. Lidocaine in combination with tetracaine is marketed in a formulation that generates heat upon exposure to air (SYNERA), which is used prior to venous access and superficial dermatological procedures such as excision, electrodessication, and shave biopsy of skin lesions. The mild warming is intended to increase skin temperature by up to 5°C for the purpose of enhancing delivery of local anesthetic into the skin. Lidocaine is dealkylated in the liver by CYPs and metabolized to monoethylglycine and xylidide. Both metabolites retain local anesthetic activity.

TOXICITY. The side effects of lidocaine seen with increasing dose include drowsiness, tinnitus, dysgeusia, dizziness, and twitching. As the dose increases, seizures, coma, and respiratory depression and arrest will occur. Clinically significant cardiovascular depression usually occurs at serum lidocaine levels that produce marked CNS effects. The metabolites monoethylglycine xylidide and glycine xylidide may contribute to some of these side effects.

CLINICAL USES. Lidocaine has utility in almost any application where a local anesthetic of intermediate duration is needed. Lidocaine also is used as an anti-arrhythmic agent (*see* Chapter 29).

BUPIVACAINE

PHARMACOLOGICAL ACTIONS; PREPARATIONS. Bupivacaine (MARCAINE, SENSORCAINE, others), is a widely used amide local anesthetic. Bupivacaine is a potent agent capable of producing prolonged anesthesia. Its long duration of action plus its tendency to provide more sensory than motor block make it popular for providing prolonged analgesia during labor or the postoperative period. With indwelling catheters and continuous infusions, bupivacaine can be used to provide several days of effective analgesia.

TOXICITY. Bupivacaine is more cardiotoxic than equi-effective doses of lidocaine. Clinically, this is manifested by severe ventricular arrhythmias and myocardial depression after inadvertent intravascular administration. Although lidocaine and bupivacaine both rapidly block cardiac Na^+ channels during systole, bupivacaine dissociates much more slowly than does lidocaine during diastole, so a significant fraction of Na^+ channels at physiological heart rates remains blocked with bupivacaine at the end of diastole. Bupivacaine-induced cardiac toxicity can be very difficult to treat, and its severity is enhanced by coexisting acidosis, hypercarbia, and hypoxemia.

OTHER SYNTHETIC LOCAL ANESTHETICS

LOCAL ANESTHETICS SUITABLE FOR INJECTION

ARTICAINE. Articaine (SEPTOCAINE) is an amide local anesthetic approved in the U.S. for dental and periodontal procedures. Articaine exhibits a rapid onset (1-6 min) and duration of action of ~1 h.

CHLOROPROCAINE. Chloroprocaine (NESACAINE, others) is a chlorinated derivative of procaine. It has rapid onset and short duration of action and reduced acute toxicity due to its rapid metabolism (plasma $t_{1/2}$ ~25 seconds). A higher than expected incidence of muscular back pain following epidural anesthesia with 2-chloroprocaine has also been reported. This back pain is thought to be due to tetany in the paraspinous muscles, which may be a consequence of Ca^{2+} binding by the EDTA included as a preservative; the incidence of back pain appears to be related to the volume of drug injected and its use for skin infiltration.

MEPIVACAINE. Mepivacaine (CARBOCAINE, POLOCAINE, others) is an intermediate-acting amino amide. Its pharmacological properties are similar to those of lidocaine. Mepivacaine is more toxic to the neonate and thus is not used in obstetrical anesthesia. Mepivacaine is not effective as a topical anesthetic.

PRILOCAINE. Prilocaine (CITANEST) is an intermediate-acting amino amide. It has a pharmacological profile similar to that of lidocaine. It causes little vasodilation and thus can be used without a vasoconstrictor, and its increased volume of distribution reduces its CNS toxicity, making it suitable for intravenous regional blocks. The use of prilocaine is largely limited to dentistry because the drug can cause methemoglobinemia. This effect is a consequence of the metabolism of the aromatic ring to *o*-toluidine. Development of methemoglobinemia is dependent on the total dose administered, usually appearing after a dose of 8 mg/kg.

ROPIVACAINE. Ropivacaine (NAROPIN, others), an amino ethylamide, is slightly less potent than bupivacaine in producing anesthesia. In clinical studies, ropivacaine appears to be suitable for both epidural and regional anesthesia, with a duration of action similar to that of bupivacaine.

PROCAINE. Procaine (NOVOCAIN, others) is an amino ester. It is use now is confined to infiltration anesthesia and occasionally for diagnostic nerve blocks. This is because of its low potency, slow onset, and short duration of action. It is hydrolyzed in vivo to produce para-aminobenzoic acid, which inhibits the action of sulfonamides. Thus, large doses should not be administered to patients taking sulfonamide drugs.

TETRACAINE. Tetracaine (PONTOCAINE) is a long-acting amino ester. It is significantly more potent and has a longer duration of action than procaine. Tetracaine may exhibit increased systemic toxicity because it is more slowly metabolized than the other commonly used ester local anesthetics. It is widely used in spinal anesthesia when a drug of long duration is needed. Tetracaine also is incorporated into several topical anesthetic preparations. Tetracaine is rarely used in peripheral nerve blocks because of the large doses often necessary, its slow onset, and its potential for toxicity.

LOCAL ANESTHETICS USED PRIMARILY TO ANESTHETIZE MUCOUS MEMBRANES AND SKIN

Some anesthetics are either too irritating or too ineffective to be applied to the eye. However, they are useful as topical anesthetic agents on the skin and/or mucous membranes. These preparations are effective in the symptomatic relief of anal and genital pruritus, poison ivy rashes, and numerous other acute and chronic dermatoses. They sometimes are combined with a glucocorticoid or antihistamine and are available in a number of proprietary formulations.

DIBUCAINE. Dibucaine (NUPERCAINAL, others) is a quinoline derivative. Its toxicity resulted in its removal from the U.S. market as an injectable preparation; it retains wide popularity outside the U.S. as a spinal anesthetic. It currently is available as an over-the-counter ointment for use on the skin.

DYCLONINE. Dyclonine hydrochloride has a rapid onset of action and duration of effect comparable to that of procaine. It is absorbed through the skin and mucous membranes. Dyclonine is an active ingredient in a number of over-the-counter medications including sore throat lozenges (SUCRETS, others), a patch for cold sores (ORAJEL OVERNIGHT COLD SORE PATCH), and a 0.75% solution (SKIN SHIELD LIQUID BANDAGE).

PRAMOXINE. Pramoxine hydrochloride (TRONOTHANE, others) is a surface anesthetic agent that is not a benzoate ester. Its distinct chemical structure may help minimize the danger of cross-sensitivity reactions in patients allergic to other local anesthetics. Pramoxine produces satisfactory surface anesthesia and is reasonably well tolerated on the skin and mucous membranes.

ANESTHETICS OF LOW SOLUBILITY

Some local anesthetics are poorly soluble in water, and consequently are too slowly absorbed to be toxic. They can be applied directly to wounds and ulcerated surfaces, where they remain localized for long periods of time, producing a sustained anesthetic action. The most important member of the series is **benzocaine** (ethyl aminobenzoate; HURRICAINE, others). Benzocaine is incorporated into a large number of topical preparations. Benzocaine can cause methemoglobinemia; consequently, dosing recommendations must be followed carefully.

LOCAL ANESTHETICS LARGELY RESTRICTED TO OPHTHALMOLOGICAL USE

Most of the local anesthetics that have been described are too irritating for ophthalmological use. The 2 compounds used most frequently today are **proparacaine** (ALCAINE, OPHTHAINE, others) and **tetracaine** (*see* Figure 20–1). In addition to being less irritating during administration, proparacaine has the added advantage of bearing little antigenic similarity to the other benzoate local anesthetics. Thus, it sometimes can be used in individuals sensitive to the amino ester local anesthetics. For use in ophthalmology, these local anesthetics are instilled a single drop at a time. If anesthesia is incomplete, successive drops are applied until satisfactory conditions are obtained. The duration of anesthesia is determined chiefly by the vascularity of the tissue; thus, it is longest in normal cornea and shortest in inflamed conjunctiva. Long-term administration of topical anesthesia to the eye has been associated with retarded healing, pitting, and sloughing of the corneal epithelium, and predisposition of the eye to inadvertent injury; *see* Chapter 64.

CLINICAL USES OF LOCAL ANESTHETICS

Local anesthesia is the loss of sensation in a body part without the loss of consciousness or the impairment of central control of vital functions. It offers 2 major advantages. First, physiological perturbations associated with general anesthesia are avoided; second, neurophysiological responses to pain and stress can be modified beneficially. There is a poor relationship between the amount of local anesthetic injected and peak plasma levels in adults. Peak plasma levels vary widely depending on the area of injection. Thus, recommended maximum doses serve only as general guidelines.

TOPICAL ANESTHESIA

Anesthesia of mucous membranes of the nose, mouth, throat, tracheobronchial tree, esophagus, and genitourinary tract can be produced by direct application of aqueous solutions of salts of many local anesthetics or by suspension of the poorly soluble local anesthetics. Tetracaine (2%), lidocaine (2-10%), and cocaine (1-4%) typically are used. Cocaine is used only in the nose, nasopharynx, mouth, throat, and ear, where it uniquely produces vasoconstriction as well as anesthesia.

The shrinking of mucous membranes decreases operative bleeding while improving surgical visualization. Comparable vasoconstriction can be achieved with other local anesthetics by the addition of a low concentration of a vasoconstrictor such as phenylephrine (0.005%). *Maximal* safe total dosages for topical anesthesia in a healthy 70-kg adult are 300 mg for lidocaine, 150 mg for cocaine, and 50 mg for tetracaine. Peak anesthetic effect following topical application of cocaine or lidocaine occurs within 2-5 min (3-8 min with tetracaine), and anesthesia lasts for 30-45 min (30-60 min with tetracaine).

Local anesthetics are absorbed rapidly into the circulation following topical application to mucous membranes or denuded skin. Thus, topical anesthesia always carries the risk of systemic toxic reactions.

Use of eutectic mixtures of local anesthetics lidocaine (2.5%)/prilocaine (2.5%) (EMLA) and lidocaine (7%)/tetracaine (7%) (PLIAGLIS) bridges the gap between topical and infiltration anesthesia. The efficacy of each of these combinations lies in the fact that the mixture has a melting point less than that of either compound alone, existing at room temperature as an oil that can penetrate intact skin. These creams produce anesthesia to a maximum depth of 5 mm and are applied as a cream on intact skin under an occlusive dressing in advance (~30-60 min) of any procedure. These mixtures are effective for procedures involving skin and superficial subcutaneous structures (e.g., venipuncture and skin graft harvesting). These mixtures must not be used on mucous membranes or abraded skin, as rapid absorption across these surfaces may result in systemic toxicity.

INFILTRATION ANESTHESIA

Infiltration anesthesia is the injection of local anesthetic directly into tissue without taking into consideration the course of cutaneous nerves. Infiltration anesthesia can be so superficial as to include only the skin. It also can include deeper structures, including intra-abdominal organs, when these too are infiltrated.

The duration of infiltration anesthesia can be approximately doubled by the addition of epinephrine (5 μg/mL) to the injection solution. *Epinephrine-containing solutions should not, however, be injected into tissues supplied by end arteries (e.g., fingers and toes, ears, the nose, and the penis). The resulting vasoconstriction may cause gangrene.* The local anesthetics used most frequently for infiltration anesthesia are lidocaine (0.5-1%), procaine (0.5-1%), and bupivacaine (0.125-0.25%). When used without epinephrine, up to 4.5 mg/kg of lidocaine, 7 mg/kg of procaine, or 2 mg/kg of bupivacaine can be employed in adults. When epinephrine is added, these amounts can be increased by one-third. The advantage of infiltration anesthesia and other regional anesthetic techniques is that it can provide satisfactory anesthesia without disrupting normal bodily functions. The chief disadvantage of infiltration anesthesia is that relatively large amounts of drug must be used to anesthetize relatively small areas. The amount of anesthetic required to anesthetize an area can be reduced significantly and the duration of anesthesia increased markedly by specifically blocking the nerves that innervate the area of interest.

FIELD BLOCK ANESTHESIA

Field block anesthesia is produced by subcutaneous injection of a solution of local anesthetic in order to anesthetize the region distal to the injection. For example, subcutaneous infiltration of the proximal portion of the volar surface of the forearm results in an extensive area of cutaneous anesthesia that starts 2-3 cm distal to the site of injection. The drugs, concentrations, and doses recommended are the same as for infiltration anesthesia. The advantage of field block anesthesia is that less drug can be used to provide a greater area of anesthesia than when infiltration anesthesia is used. Knowledge of the relevant neuroanatomy obviously is essential for successful field block anesthesia.

NERVE BLOCK ANESTHESIA

Injection of a solution of a local anesthetic into or about peripheral nerves or nerve plexuses produces greater areas of anesthesia than do the techniques already described. Blockade of mixed peripheral nerves and nerve plexuses also usually anesthetizes somatic motor nerves, producing skeletal muscle relaxation, which is essential for some surgical procedures. The areas of sensory and motor block usually start several centimeters distal to the site of injection.

Brachial plexus blocks are particularly useful for procedures on the upper extremity and shoulder. Intercostal nerve blocks are effective for anesthesia and relaxation of the anterior abdominal wall. Cervical plexus block is appropriate for surgery of the neck. Sciatic and femoral nerve blocks are useful for surgery distal to the knee. Other useful nerve blocks prior to surgical procedures include blocks of individual nerves at the wrist and at the ankle, blocks of individual nerves such as the median or ulnar at the elbow, and blocks of sensory cranial nerves.

Major determinants of the onset of sensory anesthesia following injection near a nerve are:

- Proximity of the injection to the nerve
- Concentration and volume of drug
- Degree of ionization of the drug
- Time

Local anesthetic is never intentionally injected into the nerve, as this would be painful and could cause nerve damage. Instead, the anesthetic agent is deposited as close to the nerve as possible. Thus, the local anesthetic must diffuse into the nerve where it acts. The rate of diffusion is determined by the concentration of the drug, its degree of ionization (ionized local anesthetic diffuses more slowly), its hydrophobicity, and the physical characteristics of the tissue surrounding the nerve. Higher concentrations of local anesthetic will provide a more rapid onset of peripheral nerve block. The utility of higher concentrations, however, is limited by systemic toxicity and by direct neural toxicity of concentrated local anesthetic solutions. Local anesthetics with lower pK_a values tend to have a more rapid onset of action because more drug is uncharged at neutral pH. Increased hydrophobicity might be expected to speed onset by increased penetration into nerve tissue. However, it also will increase binding in tissue lipids. The amount of connective tissue that must be penetrated can slow or even prevent adequate diffusion of local anesthetic to the nerve fibers.

Duration of nerve block anesthesia depends on the physical characteristics of the local anesthetic used and the presence or absence of vasoconstrictors. It is useful to think of 3 categories:

- Those with a short (20-45 min) duration of action in mixed peripheral nerves, such as procaine
- Those with an intermediate (60-120 min) duration of action, such as lidocaine and mepivacaine
- Those with a long (400-450 min) duration of action, such as bupivacaine, ropivacaine, and tetracaine

Block duration of the intermediate-acting local anesthetics such as lidocaine can be prolonged by the addition of epinephrine (5 μg/mL).

The types of nerve fibers that are blocked when a local anesthetic is injected about a mixed peripheral nerve depend on the concentration of drug used, nerve-fiber size, internodal distance, and frequency and pattern of nerve-impulse transmission. Anatomical factors are similarly important. Nerves in the outer mantle of the mixed nerve are blocked first. These fibers usually are distributed to more proximal anatomical structures than are those situated near the core of the mixed nerve and often are motor. If the volume and concentration of local anesthetic solution deposited about the nerve are adequate, the local anesthetic eventually will diffuse inward in amounts adequate to block even the most centrally located fibers. Lesser amounts of drug will block only nerves in the mantle and the smaller and more sensitive central fibers. Furthermore, since removal of local anesthetics occurs primarily in the core of a mixed nerve or nerve trunk, where the vascular supply is located, the duration of blockade of centrally located nerves is shorter than that of more peripherally situated fibers.

The choice of local anesthetic and the amount and concentration administered are determined by the nerves and the types of fibers to be blocked, the required duration of anesthesia, and the size and health of the patient. For blocks of 2-4 h, lidocaine (1-1.5%) can be used in the amounts recommended earlier. Mepivacaine (up to 7 mg/kg of a 1-2% solution) provides anesthesia that lasts about as long as that from lidocaine. Bupivacaine (2-3 mg/kg of a 0.25-0.375% solution) can be used when a longer duration of action is required. The amount of local anesthetic that can be injected must be adjusted according to the anatomical site of the nerve(s) to be blocked to minimize untoward effects.

INTRAVENOUS REGIONAL ANESTHESIA (BIER BLOCK)

This technique relies on using the vasculature to bring the local anesthetic solution to the nerve trunks and endings. In this technique, an extremity is exsanguinated with an Esmarch (elastic) bandage, and a proximally located tourniquet is inflated to 100-150 mm Hg above the systolic blood pressure. The Esmarch bandage is removed, and the local anesthetic is injected into a previously cannulated vein. Typically, complete anesthesia of the limb ensues within 5-10 min. Pain from the tourniquet and the potential for ischemic nerve injury limits tourniquet inflation to 2 h or less. However, the tourniquet should remain inflated for at least 15-30 min to prevent toxic amounts of local anesthetic from entering the circulation following deflation. Lidocaine, 40-50 mL (0.5 mL/kg in children) of a 0.5% solution without epinephrine is the drug of choice for this technique. For intravenous regional anesthesia in adults using a 0.5% solution without epinephrine, the dose administered should not exceed 4 mg/kg. A few clinicians prefer prilocaine (0.5%) over lidocaine because of its higher therapeutic index. The attractiveness of this technique lies in its simplicity. Its primary disadvantages are that it can be used only for a few anatomical regions, sensation (pain) returns quickly after tourniquet deflation, and premature release or failure of the tourniquet can produce toxic levels of local anesthetic (e.g., 50 mL of 0.5% lidocaine contains 250 mg of lidocaine). The more cardiotoxic local anesthetic, bupivacaine, is not recommended for this technique. Intravenous regional anesthesia is used most often for surgery of the forearm and hand, but can be adapted for the foot and distal leg.

SPINAL ANESTHESIA

Spinal anesthesia follows the injection of local anesthetic into the cerebrospinal fluid (CSF) in the lumbar space. For a number of reasons, including the ability to produce anesthesia of a considerable fraction of the body with a dose of local anesthetic that produces negligible plasma levels, spinal anesthesia is popular. In most adults, the spinal cord terminates above the second lumbar vertebra; between that point and the termination of the thecal sac in the sacrum, the lumbar and sacral roots are bathed in CSF. Thus, in this region there is a relatively large volume of CSF within which to inject drug, thereby minimizing the potential for direct nerve trauma.

Most of the physiological side effects of spinal anesthesia are a consequence of the sympathetic blockade produced by local anesthetic block of the sympathetic fibers in the spinal nerve roots. The consequences of sympathetic blockade vary among patients as a function of age, physical conditioning, and disease state. Interestingly, sympathetic blockade during spinal anesthesia appears to be minimal in healthy children. The most important effects of sympathetic blockade during spinal anesthesia are on the cardiovascular system. At all but the lowest levels of spinal blockade, some vasodilation will occur. This reduction in circulating blood volume is well tolerated at low levels of spinal anesthesia in healthy patients. As the level of spinal block ascends, the rate of cardiovascular compromise can accelerate if not carefully observed and treated. Treatment of hypotension usually is warranted when the blood pressure decreases to ~30% of *resting* values. Therapy is aimed at maintaining brain and cardiac perfusion and oxygenation. Because the usual cause of hypotension is decreased venous return, possibly complicated by decreased heart rate, drugs with preferential venoconstrictive and chronotropic properties are preferred. For this reason, ephedrine, 5-10 mg intravenously, often is the drug of choice. In addition, direct-acting α_1 adrenergic receptor agonists such as phenylephrine (*see* Chapter 12) can be administered either by bolus or continuous infusion.

PHARMACOLOGY OF SPINAL ANESTHESIA. In the U.S., lidocaine, tetracaine, and bupivacaine are most commonly used in spinal anesthesia. Procaine occasionally is used for diagnostic blocks when a short duration of action is desired. General guidelines are to use lidocaine for short procedures, bupivacaine for intermediate to long procedures, and tetracaine for long procedures.

The factors contributing to the distribution of local anesthetics in the CSF determine the height of block. The most important pharmacological factors include the amount, and possibly the volume, of drug injected and its baricity. For a given preparation of local anesthetic, administration of increasing amounts leads to a fairly predictable increase in the level of block attained. For example, 100 mg of lidocaine, 20 mg of bupivacaine, or 12 mg of tetracaine usually will result in a T4 sensory block. Vasoconstrictors may prolong spinal anesthesia by decreasing spinal cord blood flow and thus decreasing clearance of local anesthetic from the CSF. Epinephrine and other α adrenergic agonists decrease nociceptive transmission in the spinal cord, an effect that may involve activation of α_{2A} adrenergic receptors. Such actions may contribute to the beneficial effects of epinephrine, clonidine, and dexmedetomidine when these agents are added to spinal local anesthetics.

DRUG BARICITY AND PATIENT POSITION. The baricity of the local anesthetic injected will determine the direction of migration within the dural sac. Hyperbaric solutions will tend to settle in the dependent portions of the sac, while hypobaric solutions will tend to migrate in the opposite direction. Isobaric solutions usually will stay in the vicinity where they were injected, diffusing slowly in all directions. Consideration of the patient position during and after the performance of the block and the choice of a local anesthetic of the appropriate baricity is crucial for a successful block during some surgical procedures.

COMPLICATIONS OF SPINAL ANESTHESIA. Persistent neurological deficits following spinal anesthesia are extremely rare. Possible causes include introduction of foreign substances into the subarachnoid space, infection, hematoma, or direct mechanical trauma. Aside from drainage of an abscess or hematoma, treatment usually is ineffective. High concentrations of local anesthetic can cause irreversible block. After administration, local anesthetic solutions are diluted rapidly, quickly reaching nontoxic concentrations. It is prudent to avoid spinal anesthesia in patients with progressive diseases of the spinal cord. However, spinal anesthesia may be very useful in patients with fixed, chronic spinal cord injury. A more common sequela following any lumbar puncture, including spinal anesthesia, is a postural headache with classic features. The incidence of headache decreases with increasing age of the patient and decreasing needle diameter. Headache following lumbar puncture must be evaluated to exclude serious complications such as meningitis. Treatment usually is with bed rest and analgesics. If this approach fails, an epidural blood patch with the injection of autologous blood can be performed.

EVALUATION OF SPINAL ANESTHESIA. Spinal anesthesia is a safe and effective technique, especially during surgery involving the lower abdomen, the lower extremities, and the perineum. The physiological perturbations associated with low spinal anesthesia often have less potential harm than those associated with general anesthesia. The same does not apply for high spinal anesthesia. Equally satisfactory and safer operating conditions can be realized by combining the spinal anesthetic with a "light" general anesthetic or by the administration of a general anesthetic and a neuromuscular blocking agent.

EPIDURAL ANESTHESIA

Epidural anesthesia is administered by injecting local anesthetic into the epidural space—the space bounded by the ligamentum flavum posteriorly, the spinal periosteum laterally, and the dura anteriorly. Its current popularity arises from the development of catheters that can be placed into the epidural space, allowing either continuous infusions or repeated bolus administration of local anesthetics. The primary site of action is on the spinal nerve roots. However, epidurally administered local anesthetics also may act on the spinal cord and on the paravertebral nerves.

The choice of drugs to be used during epidural anesthesia is dictated primarily by the duration of anesthesia desired. However, when an epidural catheter is placed, short-acting drugs can be administered repeatedly, providing more control over the duration of block. Bupivacaine, 0.5-0.75%, is used when a long duration of surgical block is desired. Lower concentrations—0.25%, 0.125%, or 0.0625%—of bupivacaine, often with 2 μg/mL of fentanyl added, frequently are used to provide analgesia during labor. Lidocaine 2% is the most frequently used intermediate-acting epidural local anesthetic. Addition of epinephrine prolongs duration of action, decreases systemic toxicity, and also makes inadvertent intravascular injection easier to detect and modifies the effect of sympathetic blockade during epidural anesthesia. The concentration of local anesthetic used determines the type of nerve fibers blocked. The highest concentrations are used when sympathetic, somatic sensory, and somatic motor blockade are required. Intermediate concentrations allow somatic sensory anesthesia without muscle relaxation. Low concentrations will block only preganglionic sympathetic fibers.

A significant difference between epidural and spinal anesthesia is that the dose of local anesthetic used can produce high concentrations in blood following absorption from the epidural space. Peak blood concentrations are a function of the total dose of drug administered rather than the concentration or volume of solution following epidural injection. The risk of inadvertent intravascular injection is increased in epidural anesthesia, as the epidural space contains a rich venous plexus.

Another major difference between epidural and spinal anesthesia is that there is no zone of differential sympathetic blockade with epidural anesthesia; thus, the level of sympathetic block is close to the level of sensory block. Cardiovascular responses to epidural anesthesia might be expected to be less prominent; however, in practice the potential advantage of epidural anesthesia is offset by the cardiovascular responses to the high concentration of anesthetic in blood that occurs during epidural anesthesia. This is most apparent when epinephrine is added to the epidural injection. The resulting concentration of epinephrine in blood is sufficient to produce significant β_2 adrenergic receptor-mediated vasodilation. As a consequence, blood pressure decreases, even though cardiac output increases due to the positive inotropic and chronotropic effects of epinephrine (*see* Chapter 12).

High concentrations of local anesthetics in blood during epidural anesthesia are especially important when this technique is used to control pain during labor and delivery. Local anesthetics cross the placenta, enter the fetal circulation, and at high concentrations may cause depression of the neonate. These concerns have been lessened by the trend toward using more dilute solutions of bupivacaine for labor analgesia.

EPIDURAL AND INTRATHECAL OPIATE ANALGESIA. Small quantities of opioid injected intrathecally or epidurally produce segmental analgesia. The analgesia is confined to sensory nerves that enter the spinal cord dorsal horn in the vicinity of the injection.

Presynaptic opioid receptors inhibit the release of substance P and other neurotransmitters from primary afferents, while postsynaptic opioid receptors decrease the activity of certain dorsal horn neurons in the spinothalamic tracts (*see* Chapter 18). Because conduction in autonomic, sensory, and motor nerves is not affected by the opioids, blood pressure, motor function, and non-nociceptive sensory perception typically are not influenced by spinal opioids. Side effects include urinary retention, pruritus, nausea, and vomiting.

Spinally administered opioids by themselves do not provide satisfactory anesthesia for surgical procedures but are used during surgical procedures and for the relief of postoperative and chronic pain. In selected patients, spinal or epidural opioids can provide excellent analgesia following thoracic, abdominal, pelvic, or lower extremity surgery without the side effects associated with high doses of systemically administered opioids. For cancer pain, repeated doses of epidural opioids can provide analgesia of several months' duration. Unfortunately, as with systemic opioids, tolerance will develop to the analgesic effects of epidural opioids.

For a complete Bibliographical Listing see Goodman & Gilman's ***The Pharmacological Basis of Therapeutics***, 12th ed., or Goodman & Gilman Online at www.AccessMedicine.com.

Pharmacotherapy of the Epilepsies

Epileptic seizures often cause transient impairment of consciousness, leaving the individual at risk of bodily harm and often interfering with education and employment. Therapy is symptomatic: Available drugs inhibit seizures, but neither effective prophylaxis nor cure is available. The mechanisms of action of antiseizure drugs fall into 3 major categories:

1. Limiting the sustained, repetitive firing of neurons, an effect mediated by promoting the inactivated state of voltage-activated Na^+ channels
2. Enhancing synaptic inhibition mediated γ-aminobutyric acid (GABA), a drug effect that may occur via presynaptic or postsynaptic action
3. Inhibition of voltage-activated Ca^{2+} channels responsible for T-type Ca^{2+} currents

Drugs effective against the most common forms of epileptic seizures, *partial and secondarily generalized tonic-clonic seizures*, appear to work by one of the first two mechanisms. Drugs effective against the less common *absence seizure* work by the third mechanism.

TERMINOLOGY AND EPILEPTIC SEIZURE CLASSIFICATION

The term *seizure* refers to a transient alteration of behavior due to the disordered, synchronous, and rhythmic firing of populations of brain neurons. The term *epilepsy* refers to a disorder of brain function characterized by the periodic and unpredictable occurrence of seizures. Seizures are thought to arise from the cerebral cortex, not from other CNS structures. Epileptic seizures are classified as *partial* seizures, those beginning focally in a cortical site, and *generalized* seizures, those that involve both hemispheres widely from the outset. The behavioral manifestations of a seizure are determined by the functions normally served by the cortical site at which the seizure arises. For example, a seizure involving motor cortex is associated with clonic jerking of the body part controlled by this region of cortex. A *simple* partial seizure is associated with preservation of consciousness. A *complex* partial seizure is associated with impairment of consciousness. The majority of complex partial seizures originate from the temporal lobe. Examples of generalized seizures include absence, myoclonic, and tonic-clonic. The type of epileptic seizure is one determinant of the drug selected for therapy. Table 21–1 presents more detailed information on the classification of seizures and available medications.

More than 50 distinct epileptic syndromes have been identified and categorized into partial versus generalized epilepsies. The partial epilepsies account for roughly 60% of all epilepsies. The etiology commonly consists of a lesion in some part of the cortex, such as a tumor, developmental malformation, or damage due to trauma or stroke. The generalized epilepsies account for ~40% of all epilepsies and the etiology is usually genetic. The most common generalized epilepsy, referred to as juvenile myoclonic epilepsy, accounts for ~10% of all epileptic syndromes. Like most of the generalized-onset epilepsies, juvenile myoclonic epilepsy is a complex genetic disorder that is probably due to inheritance of multiple susceptibility genes.

NATURE AND MECHANISMS OF SEIZURES AND ANTISEIZURE DRUGS

PARTIAL EPILEPSIES

Either reduction of inhibitory synaptic activity or enhancement of excitatory synaptic activity might be expected to trigger a seizure; pharmacological studies of seizures support this notion. The neurotransmitters mediating the bulk of synaptic transmission in the mammalian brain are amino acids, with GABA and glutamate being the principal inhibitory and excitatory neurotransmitters, respectively (*see* Chapter 14). *Antagonists* of the $GABA_A$ receptor or *agonists* of different glutamate-receptor subtypes (NMDA, AMPA, or kainic acid) trigger seizures in experimental animals in vivo. Conversely, drugs that enhance GABA-mediated synaptic inhibition or glutamate-receptor antagonists inhibit seizures in diverse models.

Table 21–1

Classification of Epileptic Seizures

SEIZURE TYPE	FEATURES	CONVENTIONAL ANTISEIZURE DRUGS	RECENTLY DEVELOPED ANTISEIZURE DRUGS
Partial Seizures			
Simple partial	Diverse manifestations determined by the region of cortex activated by the seizure (e.g., if motor cortex representing left thumb, clonic jerking of left thumb results; if somatosensory cortex representing left thumb, paresthesia of left thumb results), lasting approximating 20-60 seconds. *Key feature is preservation of consciousness.*	Carbamazepine, phenytoin, valproate (simple partial and complex partial)	Gabapentin, lacosamide, lamotrigine, levetiracetam, rufinamide, tiagabine, topiramate, zonisamide (all partial seizures)
Complex partial	Impaired consciousness lasting 30 seconds to 2 minutes, often associated with purposeless movements such as lip smacking or hand wringing.		
Partial with secondarily generalized tonic-clonic seizure	Simple or complex partial seizure evolves into a tonic-clonic seizure with loss of consciousness and sustained contractions (tonic) of muscles throughout the body followed by periods of muscle contraction alternating with periods of relaxation (clonic), typically lasting 1-2 minutes.	Carbamazepine, phenobarbital, phenytoin, primidone, valproate	
Generalized Seizures			
Absence seizure	Abrupt onset of impaired consciousness associated with staring and cessation of ongoing activities typically lasting less than 30 seconds.	Ethosuximide, valproate, clonazepam	Lamotrigine
Myoclonic seizure	A brief (perhaps a second), shocklike contraction of muscles that may be restricted to part of one extremity or may be generalized.	Valproate, clonazepam	Levetiracetam
Tonic-clonic seizure	As described above for partial with secondarily generalized tonic-clonic seizures, except that it is not preceded by a partial seizure.	Carbamazepine, phenobarbital, phenytoin, primidone, valproate	Lamotrigine, levetiracetam, topiramate

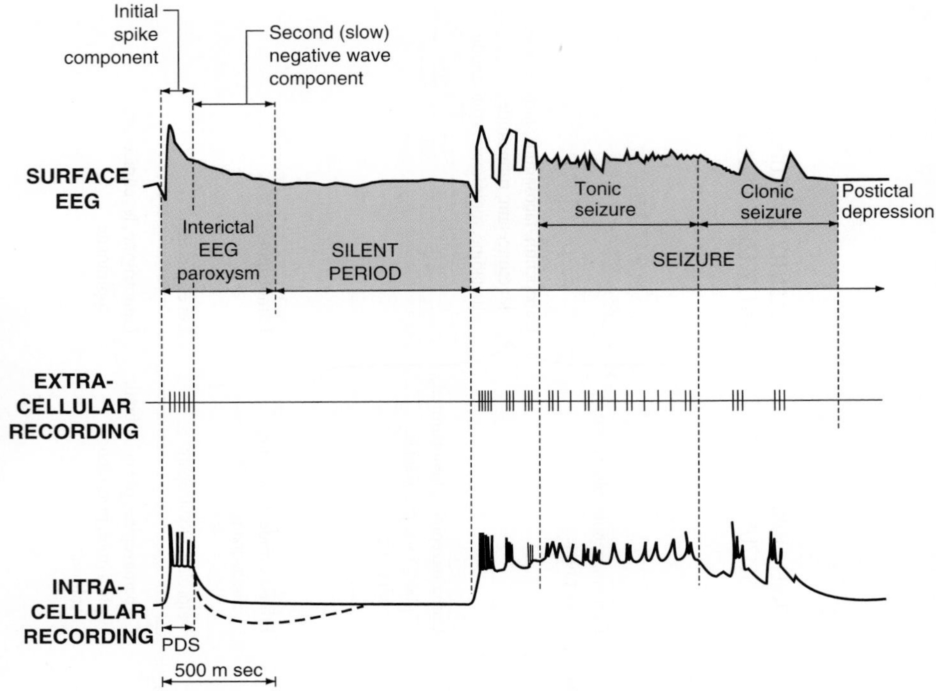

Figure 21–1 *Cortical EEG, extracellular, and intracellular recordings in a seizure focus induced by local application of a convulsant agent to mammalian cortex.* The extracellular recording was made through a high-pass filter. Note the high-frequency firing of the neuron evident in both extracellular and intracellular recording during the paroxysmal depolarization shift (PDS). (Modified with permission from Ayala GF, Dichter M, Gumnit RJ, et al. Genesis of epileptic interictal spikes. New knowledge of cortical feedback systems suggests a neurophysiological explanation of brief paroxysms. *Brain Res*, 1973;52:1–17. Copyright © Elsevier.)

Electrophysiological analyses of individual neurons during a partial seizure demonstrate that the neurons undergo depolarization and fire action potentials at high frequencies (Figure 21–1). This pattern of neuronal firing is characteristic of a seizure and is uncommon during physiological neuronal activity. Thus, selective inhibition of this pattern of firing would be expected to reduce seizures with minimal unwanted effects. Inhibition of the high-frequency firing may be mediated by reducing the ability of Na^+ channels to recover from inactivation (Figure 21–2). Depolarization-triggered opening of the Na^+ channels in the axonal membrane of

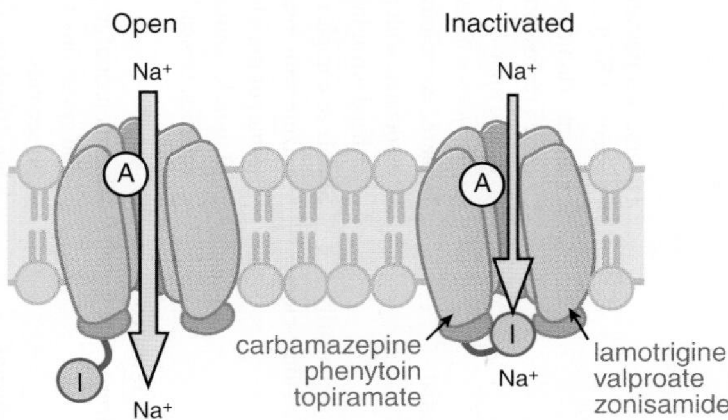

Figure 21–2 *Antiseizure drug-enhanced Na^+ channel inactivation.* Some antiseizure drugs (shown in *blue text*) prolong the inactivation of the Na^+ channels, thereby reducing the ability of neurons to fire at high frequencies. Note that the inactivated channel itself appears to remain open, but is blocked by the inactivation gate **I. A**, activation gate.

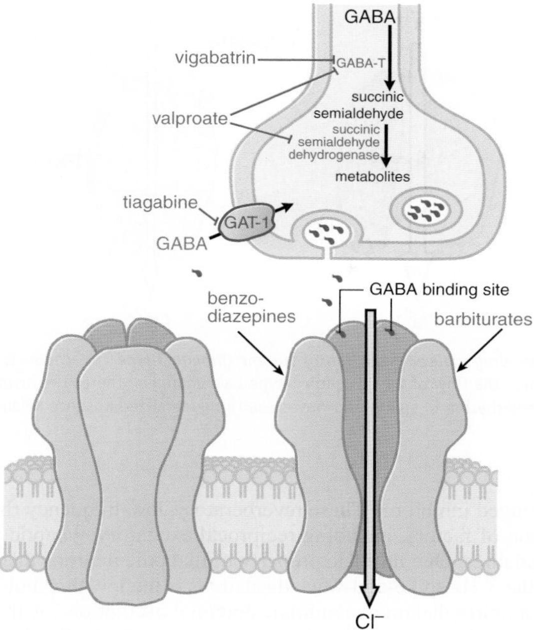

Figure 21–3 *Enhanced GABA synaptic transmission.* In the presence of GABA, the $GABA_A$ receptor (*structure on left*) is opened, allowing an influx of Cl^-, which in turn increases membrane polarization. Some antiseizure drugs (show in larger *blue text*) act by reducing the metabolism of GABA. Others act at the $GABA_A$ receptor, enhancing Cl^- influx in response to GABA. As outlined in the text, gabapentin acts presynaptically to promote GABA release; its molecular target is currently under investigation. GABA molecules; GABA-T, GABA transaminase; GAT-1, GABA transporter.

a neuron is required for an action potential; after opening, the channels spontaneously close, a process termed *inactivation*. This inactivation is thought to cause the refractory period during which it is not possible to evoke another action potential. Because firing at a slow rate permits sufficient time for Na^+ channels to recover from inactivation, inactivation has little or no effect on low-frequency firing. However, reducing the rate of recovery of Na^+ channels from inactivation would limit the ability of a neuron to fire at high frequencies, an effect that likely underlies the effects of carbamazepine, lamotrigine, phenytoin, topiramate, valproic acid, and zonisamide against partial seizures.

Enhancing GABA-mediated synaptic inhibition would reduce neuronal excitability and raise the seizure threshold. Several drugs are thought to inhibit seizures by regulating GABA-mediated synaptic inhibition through an action at distinct sites of the synapse. The principal postsynaptic receptor of synaptically released GABA is termed the $GABA_A$ receptor (*see* Chapters 14 and 17). Activation of the $GABA_A$ receptor inhibits the postsynaptic cell by increasing the inflow of Cl^- ions into the cell, which tends to hyperpolarize the neuron. Clinically relevant concentrations of both benzodiazepines and barbiturates enhance $GABA_A$ receptor–mediated inhibition through distinct actions on the $GABA_A$ receptor (Figure 21–3), and this enhanced inhibition probably underlies the effectiveness of these compounds against partial and tonic-clonic seizures in humans. At higher concentrations, such as might be used for status epilepticus, these drugs also can inhibit high-frequency firing of action potentials. A second mechanism of enhancing GABA-mediated synaptic inhibition is thought to underlie the antiseizure mechanism of tiagabine; tiagabine inhibits the GABA transporter, GAT-1, and reduces neuronal and glial uptake of GABA.

GENERALIZED-ONSET EPILEPSIES: ABSENCE SEIZURES

In contrast to partial seizures, which arise from localized regions of the cerebral cortex, generalized-onset seizures arise from the reciprocal firing of the thalamus and cerebral cortex. Among the diverse forms of generalized seizures, absence seizures have been studied most intensively. The EEG hallmark of an absence seizure is generalized spike-and-wave discharges at a frequency of 3 per second (3 Hz). EEG spikes are associated with the firing of action potentials and the following

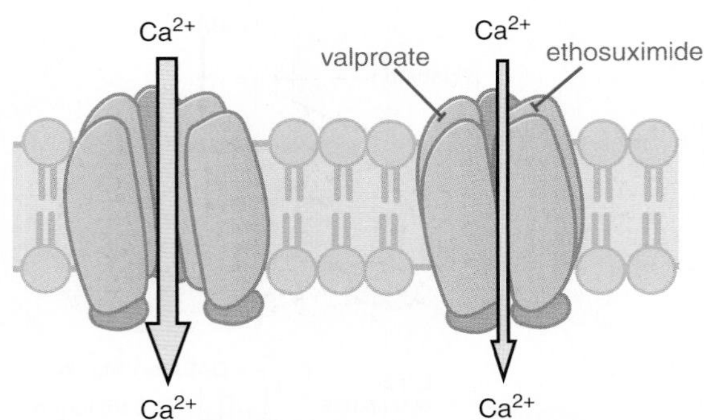

Figure 21–4 *Antiseizure drug-induced reduction of current through T-type Ca^{2+} channels.* Some antiseizure drugs (shown in *blue text*) reduce the flow of Ca^{2+} through T-type Ca^{2+} channels, thereby reducing the pacemaker current that underlies the thalamic rhythm in spikes and waves seen in generalized absence seizures.

slow wave with prolonged inhibition. These reverberatory, low-frequency rhythms are made possible by a combination of factors, including reciprocal excitatory synaptic connections between the neocortex and thalamus. One intrinsic property of thalamic neurons that is pivotally involved in the generation of the 3-Hz spike-and-wave discharges is the low threshold ("T-type") Ca^{2+} current. T-type currents amplify thalamic membrane potential oscillations, with one oscillation being the 3-Hz spike-and-wave discharge of the absence seizure. Importantly, the principal mechanism by which anti–absence-seizure drugs (ethosuximide, valproic acid) are thought to act is by inhibition of the T-type Ca^{2+} channels (Figure 21–4). Thus, inhibiting voltage-gated ion channels is a common mechanism of action among antiseizure drugs, with anti–partial-seizure drugs inhibiting voltage-activated Na^+ channels and anti–absence-seizure drugs inhibiting voltage-activated Ca^{2+} channels.

GENETIC APPROACHES TO THE EPILEPSIES. Genetic causes are solely responsible for rare epileptic forms inherited in an autosomal dominant or autosomal recessive manner. Genetic causes also are mainly responsible for more common forms such as juvenile myoclonic epilepsy (JME) or childhood absence epilepsy (CAE), the majority of which are likely due to inheritance of 2 or more susceptibility genes. Genetic determinants also may contribute some degree of risk to epilepsies caused by injury of the cerebral cortex. Because most patients with epilepsy are neurologically normal, elucidating the mutant genes underlying familial epilepsy in otherwise normal individuals is of particular interest. This has led to the identification of 25 distinct genes implicated in distinct idiopathic epilepsy syndromes that account for <1% of all of the human epilepsies. Almost all of the mutant genes encode voltage- or ligand-gated ion channels. Mutations have been identified in Na^+, K^+, Ca^{2+}, and Cl^- channels, in channels gated by GABA and acetylcholine, and most recently, in intracellular Ca^{2+} release channels (RyR2) activated by Ca^{2+}. The genotype-phenotype correlations of these genetic syndromes are complex. The cellular electrophysiological consequences of these mutations help describe the mechanisms of seizures and antiseizure drugs. For example, generalized epilepsy with febrile seizures ($GEFS^+$) is caused by a point mutation in the β subunit of a voltage-gated Na^+ channel (*SCN1B*). The phenotype of the mutated Na^+ channel appears to involve defective inactivation.

ANTISEIZURE DRUGS: GENERAL CONSIDERATIONS

Table 21–2 presents proposed mechanisms of action of antiseizure drugs, classified according to likely molecular target and activity. It is important to select the appropriate drug or combination of drugs that best controls seizures in an individual patient at an acceptable level of untoward effects. As a general rule, complete control of seizures can be achieved in up to 50% of patients, while another 25% can be improved significantly. The degree of success varies as a function of seizure type, cause, and other factors. Drugs used currently frequently cause unwanted effects that range in severity from minimal impairment of the CNS to ideation and attempt of suicide to death from aplastic anemia or hepatic failure. To minimize toxicity, treatment with a single drug is preferred. If seizures are not controlled with the initial agent at adequate plasma concentrations, substitution of a second drug is preferred to the concurrent administration of another agent.

Table 21–2

Proposed Mechanisms of Action of Antiseizure Drugs

MOLECULAR TARGET AND ACTIVITY	DRUG	CONSEQUENCES OF ACTION
Na^+ channel modulators that: *enhance fast inactivation*	PHT, CBZ, LTG, FBM, OxCBZ, TPM, VPA	• block action potential propagation • stabilize neuronal membranes • ↓ neurotransmitter release, focal firing, and seizure spread
enhance slow inactivation	LCM	• ↑ spike frequency adaptation • ↓ AP bursts, focal firing, and seizure spread • stabilize neuronal membrane
Ca^{2+} channel blockers	ESM, VPA, LTG	• ↓ neurotransmitter release (N- & P-types) • ↓ slow-depolarization (T-type) and spike-wave discharges
α2δ ligands	GBP, PGB	• modulate neurotransmitter release
$GABA_A$ receptor allosteric modulators	BZDs, PB, FBM, TPM, CBZ, OxCBZ	• ↑ membrane hyperpolarization and seizure threshold • ↓ focal firing BZDs—attenuate spike-wave discharges PB, CBZ, OxCBZ—aggravate spike-wave discharges
GABA uptake inhibitors/ GABA-transaminase inhibitors	TGB, VGB	• ↑ extrasynaptic GABA levels and membrane hyperpolarization • ↓ focal firing • aggravate spike-wave discharges
NMDA receptor antagonists	FBM	• ↓ slow excitatory neurotransmission • ↓ excitatory amino acid neurotoxicity • delay epileptogenesis
AMPA/kainate receptor antagonists	PB, TPM	• ↓ fast excitatory neurotransmission and focal firing
Enhancers of HCN channel activity	LTG	• buffers large hyperpolarizing and depolarizing inputs • suppresses action potential initiation by dendritic inputs
SV2A protein ligand	LEV	• unknown; may decrease transmitter release
Inhibitors of brain carbonic anhydrase	ACZ, TPM, ZNS	• ↑ HCN-mediated currents • ↓ NMDA-mediated currents • ↑ GABA-mediated inhibition

ACZ, acetazolamide; BZDs, benzodiazepines; CBZ, carbamazepine; ESM, ethosuximide; FBM, felbamate; GBP, gabapentin; LCM, lacosamide; LEV, levetiracetam; LTG, Lamotrigine; OxCBZ, oxcarbazepine; PB, phenobarbital; PGB, pregagalin; PHT, phenytoin; TGB, tiagabine; TPM, topiramate; VGB, vigaba-trin; VPA, valproic acid; ZNA, zonisamide. Modified with permission from Leppik IE, Kelly KM, deToledo-Morrell L, et al. Basic research in epilepsy and aging. Epilepsy Res, 2006, 68 (Suppl 1): 21. Copyright © Elsevier.

However, multiple-drug therapy may be required, especially when 2 or more types of seizure occur in the same patient. Measurement of drug concentrations in plasma facilitates optimizing antiseizure medication. However, clinical effects of some drugs do not correlate well with their concentrations in plasma. The ultimate therapeutic regimen must be determined by clinical assessment of effect and toxicity. Many of these agents interact noticeably with other medications via induction or inhibition of hepatic CYPs and UGTs that are responsible for drug metabolism (Table 21–3).

Table 21–3

Interactions of Antiseizure Drugs with Hepatic Microsomal Enzymes

	INDUCES		INHIBITS		METABOLIZED BY	
DRUG	CYP	UGT	CYP	UGT	CYP	UGT
Carbamazepine	2C9/3A	Yes			1A2/2C8 2C9/3A4	No
Ethosuximide	No	No	No	No	?	?
Gabapentin	No	No	No	No	No	No
Lacosamide	No	No	No	No	2C19	?
Lamotrigine	No	Yes	No	No	No	Yes
Levetiracetam	No	No	No	No	No	No
Oxcarbazepine	3A4/5	Yes	2C19	Weak	No	Yes
Phenobarbital	2C/3A	Yes	Yes	No	2C9/19	No
Phenytoin	2C/3A	Yes	Yes	No	2C9/19	No
Pregabalin	No	No	No	No	No	No
Primidone	2C/3A	Yes	Yes	No	2C9/19	No
Rufinamide	3A4	2C9/19	No	?	No	Yes
Tiagabine	No	No	No	No	3A4	No
Topiramate	No	No	2C19	No		
Valproate	No	No	2C9	Yes	2C9/19	Yes
Vigabatrin	No	No	No	No	No	No
Zonisamide	No	No	No	No	3A4	Yes

CYP, cytochrome P450; UGT, uridine diphosphate-glucuronosyltransferase.

HYDANTOINS

PHENYTOIN

Phenytoin (DILANTIN) is effective against all types of partial and tonic-clonic seizures but not absence seizures.

PHARMACOLOGICAL EFFECTS. Phenytoin exerts antiseizure activity without causing general depression of the CNS. In toxic doses, it may produce excitatory signs and at lethal levels a type of decerebrate rigidity. Phenytoin limits the repetitive firing of action potentials evoked by a sustained depolarization. This effect is mediated by a slowing of the rate of recovery of voltage-activated Na^+ channels from inactivation, an action that is both voltage- (greater effect if membrane is depolarized) and use-dependent. At therapeutic concentrations, the effects on Na^+ channels are selective, and no changes of spontaneous activity or responses to iontophoretically applied GABA or glutamate are detected. At concentrations 5- to 10-fold higher, multiple effects of phenytoin are evident, including reduction of spontaneous activity and enhancement of responses to GABA; these effects may underlie some of the unwanted toxicity associated with high levels of phenytoin.

PHARMACOKINETIC PROPERTIES. Phenytoin is available in 2 types of oral formulations that differ in their pharmacokinetics: rapid-release and extended-release forms. Once-daily dosing is possible only with the extended-release formulations, and due to differences in dissolution and other formulation-dependent factors, the plasma phenytoin level may change when converting from 1 formulation to another. Comparable doses can be approximated by considering "phenytoin equivalents," but serum-level monitoring is necessary to assure therapeutic safety. Phenytoin is extensively bound (~90%) to serum proteins, mainly albumin. Increased proportions of free drug are evident in the neonate, in patients with hypoalbuminemia, and in uremic patients. Some agents can compete with phenytoin for binding sites on plasma proteins and increase free phenytoin. Valproate competes for protein binding sites *and* inhibits phenytoin metabolism, resulting in marked and sustained increases in free phenytoin. Measurement of free rather than total phenytoin permits direct assessment of this potential problem in patient management.

The plasma $t_{1/2}$ of phenytoin (6 to 24 h at plasma concentrations < 10 μg/mL) increases with higher concentrations; as a result, plasma drug concentration increases disproportionately as dosage is increased, even with small adjustments for levels near the therapeutic range. The majority (95%) of phenytoin is metabolized by hepatic CYP2C9/10 and to a lesser extent CYP2C19 (*see* Table 21–3). Other drugs that are metabolized by these enzymes can inhibit the metabolism of phenytoin and increase its plasma concentration. Conversely, the degradation rate of other drugs that are substrates for these enzymes can be inhibited by phenytoin; one such drug is warfarin, and addition of phenytoin to a patient receiving warfarin can lead to bleeding disorders (*see* Chapter 30). Phenytoin has the capacity to induce CYPs (*see* Chapter 6); coadministration of phenytoin and medications metabolized by CYPs can lead to an increased degradation of such medications. For example, treatment with phenytoin can enhance the metabolism of oral contraceptives and lead to unplanned pregnancy. Phenytoin also has potential teratogenic effects. Carbamazepine, oxcarbazepine, phenobarbital, and primidone also can induce CYP3A4 and likewise might increase degradation of oral contraceptives.

The low water solubility of phenytoin hindered its intravenous use and led to production of fosphenytoin, a water-soluble prodrug. *Fosphenytoin* (CEREBYX, others) is converted into phenytoin by phosphatases in liver and red blood cells with a $t_{1/2}$ of 8-15 min. Fosphenytoin is extensively bound (95-99%) to human plasma proteins, primarily albumin. Fosphenytoin is useful for adults with partial or generalized seizures when IV or intramuscular administration is indicated.

TOXICITY. The toxic effects of phenytoin depend on the route of administration, the duration of exposure, and the dosage. When fosphenytoin, the water-soluble prodrug, is administered intravenously at an excessive rate in the emergency treatment of status epilepticus, the most notable toxic signs are cardiac arrhythmias with or without hypotension, and/or CNS depression. Cardiac toxicity occurs more frequently in older patients and in those with known cardiac disease than young, healthy patients. These complications can be minimized by administering fosphenytoin at a rate of $<$ 150 mg of phenytoin sodium equivalents per minute. Acute oral overdosage results primarily in signs referable to the cerebellum and vestibular system; high doses have been associated with marked cerebellar atrophy. Toxic effects associated with chronic treatment also are primarily dose-related cerebellar-vestibular effects but also include other CNS effects, behavioral changes, increased frequency of seizures, GI symptoms, gingival hyperplasia, osteomalacia, and megaloblastic anemia. Hirsutism is an annoying untoward effect in young females. Usually, these phenomena can be diminished by adjustment of dosage. Serious adverse effects, including those on the skin, bone marrow, and liver, probably are manifestations of rare drug allergy and necessitate withdrawal of the drug. Moderate elevation of the plasma concentrations of hepatic transaminases sometimes are observed.

Gingival hyperplasia occurs in ~20% of all patients during chronic therapy. The condition can be minimized by good oral hygiene. Inhibition of release of antidiuretic hormone (ADH) has been observed. Hyperglycemia and glycosuria appear to be due to inhibition of insulin secretion. Osteomalacia, with hypocalcemia and elevated alkaline phosphatase activity, has been attributed to both altered metabolism of vitamin D and the attendant inhibition of intestinal absorption of Ca^{2+}. Phenytoin also increases the metabolism of vitamin K and reduces the concentration of vitamin K–dependent proteins that are important for normal Ca^{2+} metabolism in bone. Hypersensitivity reactions include morbilliform rash in 2-5% of patients and occasionally more serious skin reactions, including Stevens-Johnson syndrome and toxic epidermal necrolysis. Hematological reactions include neutropenia and leukopenia. A few cases of red-cell aplasia, agranulocytosis, and mild thrombocytopenia also have been reported. Lymphadenopathy, resembling Hodgkin disease and malignant lymphoma, is associated with reduced immunoglobulin A (IgA) production. Hypoprothrombinemia and hemorrhage have occurred in the newborns of mothers who received phenytoin during pregnancy; vitamin K is effective treatment or prophylaxis.

PLASMA DRUG CONCENTRATIONS. A good correlation usually is observed between the total concentration of phenytoin in plasma and its clinical effect. Control of seizures generally is obtained with total concentrations $>$ 10 μg/mL: toxic effects such as nystagmus develop at total concentrations ~20 μg/mL. Control of seizures generally is obtained with free phenytoin concentrations of 0.75-1.25 μg/mL.

DRUG INTERACTIONS. Drugs metabolized by CYP2C9 or CYP2C10 can increase the plasma concentration of phenytoin by decreasing its rate of metabolism. Carbamazepine, which may enhance the metabolism of phenytoin, causes a decrease in phenytoin concentration. Conversely, phenytoin reduces the concentration of carbamazepine.

THERAPEUTIC USES

Epilepsy. Phenytoin is one of the more widely used antiseizure agents, and it is effective against partial and tonic-clonic but not absence seizures. Phenytoin preparations differ significantly in bioavailability and rate of absorption. In general, patients should consistently be treated with the same drug from a single manufacturer. However, if it becomes necessary to switch between products, care should be taken to select a therapeutically equivalent product and patients should be monitored for loss of seizure control or onset of new toxicities.

Other Uses. Trigeminal and related neuralgias occasionally respond to phenytoin, but carbamazepine may be preferable.

ANTISEIZURE BARBITURATES

The pharmacology of the barbiturates as a class is described in Chapter 17; discussion in this chapter is limited to phenobarbital.

PHENOBARBITAL

Phenobarbital (LUMINAL, others) was of the more effective organic antiseizure agent. It has relatively low toxicity, and is inexpensive.

MECHANISM OF ACTION. Phenobarbital likely inhibits seizures by potentiation of synaptic inhibition through an action on the $GABA_A$ receptor. At therapeutic concentrations, phenobarbital increases the $GABA_A$ receptor–mediated current by increasing the duration of bursts of $GABA_A$ receptor–mediated currents without changing the frequency of bursts. At levels exceeding therapeutic concentrations, phenobarbital also limits sustained repetitive firing; this may underlie some of the antiseizure effects of higher concentrations of phenobarbital achieved during therapy of status epilepticus.

PHARMACOKINETIC PROPERTIES. Oral absorption of phenobarbital is complete but somewhat slow; peak concentrations in plasma occur several hours after a single dose. Phenobarbital is 40-60% bound to plasma and tissue proteins. Up to 25% of a dose is eliminated by pH-dependent renal excretion of the unchanged drug; the remainder is inactivated by hepatic CYPs. Phenobarbital induces UGTs as well as the CYP2C and CYP3A subfamilies, thereby stimulating degradation of drugs cleared by these mechanisms (oral contraceptives are metabolized by CYP3A4).

TOXICITY. Sedation, the most frequent undesired effect of phenobarbital, is apparent upon initiation of therapy, but tolerance develops during chronic medication. Nystagmus and ataxia occur at excessive dosage. Phenobarbital can produce irritability and hyperactivity in children, and agitation and confusion in the elderly. Scarlatiniform or morbilliform rash, possibly with other manifestations of drug allergy, occurs in 1-2% of patients. Exfoliative dermatitis is rare. Hypoprothrombinemia with hemorrhage has been observed in the newborns of mothers who have received phenobarbital during pregnancy; vitamin K is effective for treatment or prophylaxis. As with phenytoin, megaloblastic anemia that responds to folate and osteomalacia that responds to high doses of vitamin D occur during chronic phenobarbital therapy. Other adverse effects of phenobarbital are discussed in Chapter 17.

PLASMA DRUG CONCENTRATIONS. During long-term therapy, the plasma concentration of phenobarbital averages 10 μg/mL per daily dose of 1 mg/kg in adults and 5-7 μg/mL per 1 mg/kg in children. Plasma concentrations of 10-35 μg/mL are usually recommended for control of seizures. Sedation, nystagmus, and ataxia usually are absent at concentrations < 30 μg/mL during long-term therapy, but adverse effects may be apparent for several days at lower concentrations when therapy is initiated or whenever the dosage is increased. Concentrations > 60 μg/mL may be associated with marked intoxication in the nontolerant individual. The plasma phenobarbital concentration should be increased above 30-40 μg/mL only if the increment is adequately tolerated and only if it contributes significantly to control of seizures.

DRUG INTERACTIONS. Interactions between phenobarbital and other drugs usually involve induction of the hepatic CYPs by phenobarbital (*see* Table 21–3). The interaction between phenytoin and phenobarbital is variable. Concentrations of phenobarbital in plasma may be elevated by as much as 40% during concurrent administration of valproic acid.

THERAPEUTIC USES. Phenobarbital is an effective agent for generalized tonic-clonic and partial seizures. Its efficacy, low toxicity, and low cost make it an important agent for these types of epilepsy. However, its sedative effects and its tendency to disturb behavior in children have reduced its use as a primary agent.

IMINOSTILBENES

CARBAMAZEPINE

Carbamazepine (TEGRETOL, CARBATROL, others) is considered to be a primary drug for the treatment of partial and tonic-clonic seizures.

MECHANISM OF ACTION. Like phenytoin, carbamazepine limits the repetitive firing of action potentials evoked by a sustained depolarization by slowing the rate of recovery of voltage-activated Na^+ channels from inactivation. At therapeutic drug levels, the effects of carbamazepine are selective in that there are no effects on spontaneous activity or on responses to iontophoretically applied GABA or glutamate. The carbamazepine metabolite, 10,11-epoxycarbamazepine, also limits sustained repetitive firing at therapeutically relevant concentrations, suggesting that this metabolite may contribute to the antiseizure efficacy of carbamazepine.

PHARMACOKINETIC PROPERTIES. The pharmacokinetics of carbamazepine are complex. They are influenced by its limited aqueous solubility and by the capacity of carbamazepine to increase its conversion to active metabolites by hepatic CYPs (*see* Table 21–3). Carbamazepine is absorbed slowly and erratically after oral administration. Peak concentrations in plasma usually are observed 4-8 h after oral ingestion, but may be delayed by as much as 24 h, especially following the administration of a large dose. The drug distributes rapidly into all tissues. Approximately 75% of carbamazepine binds to plasma proteins and concentrations in the CSF appear to correspond to the concentration of free drug in plasma. Hepatic CYP3A4 is primarily responsible for biotransformation of carbamazepine to the 10, 11-epoxide. This metabolite is as active as the parent compound; its concentrations in plasma and brain may reach 50% of those of carbamazepine, especially during the concurrent administration of phenytoin or phenobarbital. The 10, 11-epoxide is metabolized further to inactive compounds that are excreted in the urine. Carbamazepine induces CYPs, and UGTs.

TOXICITY. Acute intoxication with carbamazepine can result in stupor or coma, hyperirritability, convulsions, and respiratory depression. During long-term therapy, the more frequent untoward effects of the drug include drowsiness, vertigo, ataxia, diplopia, and blurred vision. The frequency of seizures may increase, especially with overdosage. Other adverse effects include nausea, vomiting, serious hematological toxicity (aplastic anemia, agranulocytosis), and hypersensitivity reactions (dangerous skin reactions, eosinophilia, lymphadenopathy, splenomegaly). A late complication of therapy with carbamazepine is retention of water, with decreased osmolality and concentration of Na^+ in plasma, especially in elderly patients with cardiac disease. Some tolerance develops to the neurotoxic effects of carbamazepine, and they can be minimized by gradual increase in dosage or adjustment of maintenance dosage. Various hepatic or pancreatic abnormalities have been reported during therapy with carbamazepine, most commonly a transient elevation of hepatic transaminases in plasma in 5-10% of patients. A transient, mild leukopenia occurs in ~10% of patients during initiation of therapy and usually resolves within the first 4 months of continued treatment; transient thrombocytopenia also has been noted. A persistent leukopenia may develop that requires withdrawal of the drug. Aplastic anemia occurs in ~1 in 200,000 patients. Possible teratogenic effects are discussed later in the chapter.

PLASMA DRUG CONCENTRATIONS. There is no simple relationship between the dose of carbamazepine and concentrations of the drug in plasma. Therapeutic concentrations are reported to be 6-12 μg/mL, although considerable variation occurs. Side effects referable to the CNS are frequent at concentrations > 9 μg/mL.

DRUG INTERACTIONS. Phenobarbital, phenytoin, and valproate may increase the metabolism of carbamazepine by inducing CYP3A4; carbamazepine may enhance the biotransformation of phenytoin. Concurrent administration of carbamazepine may lower concentrations of valproate, lamotrigine, tiagabine, and topiramate. Carbamazepine reduces both the plasma concentration and therapeutic effect of haloperidol. The metabolism of carbamazepine may be inhibited by propoxyphene, erythromycin, cimetidine, fluoxetine, and isoniazid.

THERAPEUTIC USES. Carbamazepine is useful in patients with generalized tonic-clonic and both simple and complex partial seizures (*see* Table 21–1). When it is used, renal and hepatic function and hematological parameters should be monitored. Carbamazepine is the primary agent for treatment of trigeminal and glossopharyngeal neuralgias. It is also effective for lightning-type ("tabetic") pain associated with bodily wasting. About 70% of patients with neuralgia obtain continuing relief. Adverse effects require discontinuation of medication in 5-20% of patients. Carbamazepine is also used in the treatment of bipolar affective disorders (*see* Chapter 16).

OXCARBAZEPINE

Oxcarbazepine (TRILEPTAL, others) is a keto analog of carbamazepine. Oxcarbazepine is a prodrug that is almost immediately converted to its main active metabolite, a 10-monohydroxy derivative, which is inactivated by glucuronide conjugation and eliminated by renal excretion. Its mechanism of action is similar to that of carbamazepine. Oxcarbazepine is a less potent enzyme inducer than carbamazepine. Substitution of oxcarbazepine for carbamazepine is associated with increased levels of phenytoin and valproic acid, presumably because of reduced induction of hepatic enzymes. Oxcarbazepine does not induce the hepatic enzymes involved in its own degradation. Although oxcarbazepine does not appear to reduce the anticoagulant effect of warfarin, it does induce CYP3A and thus reduces plasma levels of steroid oral contraceptives. It is approved for monotherapy or adjunct therapy for partial seizures in adults, as monotherapy for partial seizures in children ages 4-16, and as adjunctive therapy in children 2 years of age and older with epilepsy.

ETHOSUXIMIDE

Ethosuximide (ZARONTIN, others) is a primary agent for the treatment of absence seizures. Ethosuximide reduces low threshold Ca^{2+} currents (T-type currents) in thalamic neurons. At therapeutic concentrations, ethosuximide inhibits the T-type current without modifying the voltage dependence of steady-state inactivation or the time course of recovery from inactivation. Ethosuximide does not inhibit sustained repetitive firing or enhance GABA responses at clinically relevant concentrations.

PHARMACOKINETIC PROPERTIES. Absorption of ethosuximide is complete, with peak plasma concentrations occurring ~3 h after a single oral dose. Ethosuximide is not significantly bound to plasma proteins; during long-term therapy, its concentration in the CSF is similar to that in plasma. About 25% of the drug is excreted unchanged in the urine; the remainder is metabolized by hepatic enzymes. The plasma $t_{1/2}$ is 40-50 h in adults and ~30 h in children.

TOXICITY. The most common dose-related side effects are GI complaints (nausea, vomiting, and anorexia) and CNS effects (drowsiness, lethargy, euphoria, dizziness, headache, and hiccough) to which some tolerance develops. Parkinson-like symptoms and photophobia also have been reported. Restlessness, agitation, anxiety, aggressiveness, inability to concentrate, and other behavioral effects have occurred primarily in patients with a prior history of psychiatric disturbance. Urticaria and other skin reactions, including Stevens-Johnson syndrome, as well as systemic lupus erythematosus, eosinophilia, leukopenia, thrombocytopenia, pancytopenia, and aplastic anemia also have been attributed to the drug.

THERAPEUTIC USES AND PLASMA DRUG CONCENTRATIONS. Ethosuximide is effective against absence seizures but not tonic-clonic seizures. An initial daily dose of 250 mg in children (3-6 years old) and 500 mg in older children and adults is increased by 250-mg increments at weekly intervals until seizures are adequately controlled or toxicity intervenes. Divided dosage is required occasionally to prevent nausea or drowsiness associated with once-daily dosing. The usual maintenance dose is 20 mg/kg per day. Increased caution is required if the daily dose exceeds 1500 mg in adults or 750-1000 mg in children. The plasma concentration of ethosuximide averages ~2 μg/mL per daily dose of 1 mg/kg. A plasma concentration of 40-100 μg/mL usually is required for satisfactory control of absence seizures.

VALPROIC ACID

Valproic acid (DEPAKENE, others) produces effects on isolated neurons similar to those of phenytoin and ethosuximide (*see* Table 21–2). At therapeutically relevant concentrations, valproate inhibits sustained repetitive firing induced by depolarization of cortical or spinal cord neurons. The action appears to be mediated by a prolonged recovery of voltage-activated Na^+ channels from inactivation. Valproate also produces small reductions of T-type Ca^{2+} currents. These actions of limiting sustained repetitive firing and reducing T-type currents may contribute to the effectiveness of valproic acid against partial and tonic-clonic seizures and absence seizures, respectively. In vitro, valproate can stimulate GABA synthesis and inhibit GABA degradation.

PHARMACOKINETIC PROPERTIES. Valproic acid is absorbed rapidly and completely after oral administration. Peak concentration in plasma is observed in 1-4 h (delayed by several hours if the drug is ingested with food or taken as enteric-coated tablets). Its extent of binding to plasma proteins is ~90%, but the fraction bound is reduced as the total concentration of valproate is increased through the therapeutic range. The majority of valproate (95%) is cleared by hepatic metabolism, mainly by UGTs and β-oxidation. Two of the drug's metabolites, 2-propyl-2-pentenoic acid and 2-propyl-4-pentenoic acid, are nearly as potent antiseizure agents as the parent molecule. The $t_{1/2}$ of valproate is ~15 h but is reduced in patients taking other antiepileptic drugs.

TOXICITY. The most common side effects are transient GI symptoms, including anorexia, nausea, and vomiting in ~16% of patients. Effects on the CNS include sedation, ataxia, and tremor; these symptoms occur infrequently and usually respond to a decrease in dosage. Rash, alopecia, and stimulation of appetite have been observed occasionally; weight gain has been seen with chronic valproic acid treatment in some patients. Elevation of hepatic transaminases in plasma is observed in up to 40% of patients. A rare complication is a fulminant hepatitis that is frequently fatal. Children < 2 years of age with other medical conditions who were given multiple antiseizure agents were especially likely to suffer fatal hepatic injury. Acute pancreatitis and hyperammonemia also have been frequently associated with the use of valproic acid. Valproic acid can also produce teratogenic effects.

DRUG INTERACTIONS. Valproate inhibits the metabolism of drugs that are substrates for CYP2C9, including phenytoin and phenobarbital. Valproate also inhibits UGT and thus inhibits the metabolism of lamotrigine and lorazepam. A high proportion of valproate is bound to albumin, and the high molar concentrations of valproate result in valproate's displacing phenytoin and other drugs from albumin.

THERAPEUTIC USES AND PLASMA DRUG CONCENTRATIONS. Valproate is a broad-spectrum antiseizure drug effective in the treatment of absence, myoclonic, partial, and tonic-clonic seizures. The initial daily dose usually is 15 mg/kg, increased at weekly intervals by 5-10 mg/kg/day to a maximum daily dose of 60 mg/kg. Plasma concentrations associated with therapeutic effects are ~30-100 μg/mL, with a threshold at ~30-50 μg/mL. However, there is a poor correlation between the plasma concentration and efficacy.

BENZODIAZEPINES

The benzodiazepines are used primarily as sedative-antianxiety drugs; their pharmacology is described in Chapters 14 and 17. A large number of benzodiazepines have broad antiseizure properties, but only clonazepam (KLONOPIN, others) and clorazepate (TRANXENE, others) have been approved in the U.S. for the long-term treatment of certain seizures. Midazolam was designated an orphan drug for intermittent treatment of bouts of increased seizure activity in refractory patients with epilepsy who are on stable regimens of antiseizure drugs. Diazepam (VALIUM, DIASTAT; others) and lorazepam (ATIVAN, others) have well-defined roles in the management of status epilepticus.

MECHANISM OF ACTION. The antiseizure actions of the benzodiazepines result in large part from their ability to enhance GABA-mediated synaptic inhibition. The benzodiazepine receptor is an integral part of the $GABA_A$ receptor (*see* Figure 14–6). Benzodiazepines act at subsets of $GABA_A$ receptors and increase the frequency, but not duration, of openings at GABA-activated Cl^- channels. At high concentrations, diazepam and many other benzodiazepines can reduce sustained high-frequency firing of neurons, similar to the effects of phenytoin, carbamazepine, and valproate. Although these concentrations correspond to concentrations achieved in patients during treatment of status epilepticus with diazepam, they are considerably higher than those associated with antiseizure or anxiolytic effects in ambulatory patients.

PHARMACOKINETIC PROPERTIES. Benzodiazepines are well absorbed after oral administration. Concentrations in plasma peak within 1-4 h. After intravenous administration, central effects develop promptly but wane rapidly as the drugs redistribute to other tissues. Diazepam has a $t_{1/2}$ of redistribution of ~1 h. The extent of binding of benzodiazepines to plasma proteins correlates with lipid solubility, ranging from ~99% for diazepam to ~85% for clonazepam. The major metabolite of diazepam, N-desmethyl-diazepam, is somewhat less active than the parent drug and may behave as a partial agonist. The $t_{1/2}$ of diazepam in plasma is between 1 and 2 days, while that of N-desmethyl-diazepam is ~60 h. Clonazepam is metabolized to produce inactive 7 amino derivatives. Less than 1% of the drug is recovered unchanged in the urine. The $t_{1/2}$ of clonazepam in plasma is ~23 h. Lorazepam is metabolized chiefly by conjugation with glucuronic acid; its $t_{1/2}$ in plasma is ~14 h.

TOXICITY. The principal side effects of long-term oral therapy with clonazepam are drowsiness and lethargy. These occur in ~50% of patients initially, but tolerance often develops with continued administration. Muscular incoordination and ataxia are less frequent. Although these symptoms usually can be kept to tolerable levels by reducing the dosage or the rate at which it is increased, they sometimes force drug discontinuation. Other side effects include hypotonia, dysarthria, and dizziness. Behavioral disturbances, especially in children, may include aggression, hyperactivity, irritability, and difficulty in concentration. Both anorexia and hyperphagia have been reported. Increased salivary and bronchial secretions may cause difficulties in children. Seizures are sometimes exacerbated, and status epilepticus may be precipitated if the drug is discontinued abruptly. Cardiovascular and respiratory depression may occur after the intravenous administration of diazepam, clonazepam, or lorazepam, particularly if administered after other antiseizure agents or central depressants.

PLASMA DRUG CONCENTRATIONS. Because tolerance affects the relationship between drug concentration and drug antiseizure effect, plasma concentrations of benzodiazepines are of limited value.

THERAPEUTIC USES. Clonazepam is useful in the therapy of absence seizures as well as myoclonic seizures in children. Tolerance to its antiseizure effects usually develops after 1-6 months of administration, after which some patients will no longer respond to clonazepam at any dosage. The initial dose of clonazepam for adults should not exceed 1.5 mg per day and for children 0.01-0.03 mg/kg per day. The dose-dependent side effects are reduced if 2 or 3 divided doses are given each day. The dose may be increased every 3 days in amounts of 0.25-0.5 mg per day in children and 0.5-1 mg per day in adults. The maximal recommended dose is 20 mg per day for adults and 0.2 mg/kg per day for children. Clonazepam intranasal spray is designated as an orphan drug for recurrent acute repetitive seizures.

While diazepam is an effective agent for treatment of status epilepticus, its short duration of action is a disadvantage, leading to the more frequent use of lorazepam. Clorazepate is effective in combination with certain other drugs in the treatment of partial seizures. The maximal initial dose of clorazepate is 22.5 mg per day in 3 portions for adults and children > 12 years and 15 mg per day in 2 divided doses in children 9-12 years of age. Clorazepate is not recommended for children < 9 years. Clobazam (ONFI, others) is recently FDA-approved for the adjunctive treatment of seizures associated with Lennox-Gastaut syndrome in children > 2 years of age. Starting dose is 5 mg in children < 30 kg in body weight, maximal dose is 20 mg. Starting dose for > 30 kg body weight is 10 mg and maximal dose is 40 mg.

OTHER ANTISEIZURE DRUGS

GABAPENTIN AND PREGABALIN

Gabapentin (NEURONTIN, others) and pregabalin (LYRICA) are antiseizure drugs that consist of a GABA molecule covalently bound to a lipophilic cyclohexane ring or isobutane, respectively. Gabapentin was designed to be a centrally active GABA agonist, with its high lipid solubility aimed at facilitating its transfer across the blood-brain barrier.

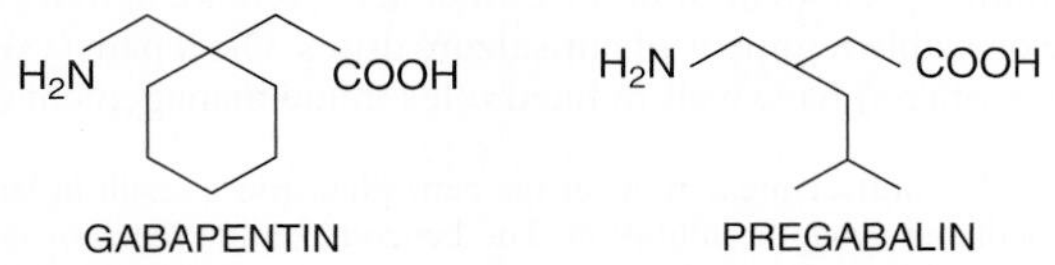

H_2N COOH H_2N COOH

GABAPENTIN PREGABALIN

MECHANISMS OF ACTION. Gabapentin inhibits tonic hind-limb extension in the electroshock seizure model and clonic seizures induced by pentylenetetrazol. Its efficacy in both these tests parallels that of valproic acid and distinguishes it from phenytoin and carbamazepine. Despite their design as GABA agonists, neither gabapentin nor pregabalin mimics GABA when applied to neurons in primary culture. These compounds bind with high affinity to a protein in cortical membranes with an amino acid sequence identical to that of the Ca^{2+} channel subunit α2δ-1 but their molecular mechanism of action remains unknown, providing job security for researchers in this area. These compounds also have analgesic properties; the analgesic efficacy of pregabalin is eliminated in mice carrying a mutation in the α2δ-1 protein.

PHARMACOKINETICS. Gabapentin and pregabalin are absorbed after oral administration and are not metabolized in humans. These compounds are not bound to plasma proteins and are excreted unchanged in the urine. Their half-lives approximate 6 h. These compounds have no known interactions with other antiseizure drugs.

THERAPEUTIC USES AND TOXICITY. Gabapentin and pregabalin are effective for partial seizures, with and without secondary generalization, when used in addition to other antiseizure drugs. Pregabalin is approved for treatment of neuropathic pain associated with spinal cord injury. Gabapentin also is used for the treatment of migraine, chronic pain, bipolar disorder, and restless leg syndrome. Gabapentin usually is effective in doses of 900-1800 mg daily in 3 doses, although 3600 mg may be required in some patients. Therapy usually is begun with a low dose (300 mg/day), which is increased by 300 mg /day until an effective dose is reached. Gabapentin is well tolerated. Common adverse effects include mild to moderate somnolence, dizziness, ataxia, and fatigue that resolve within 2 weeks of onset during continued treatment. Gabapentin and pregabalin are listed in pregnancy category C.

LAMOTRIGINE

Lamotrigine (LAMICTAL, others) is a phenyltriazine derivative initially developed as an antifolate agent but the drug's effectiveness as an antiseizure medication is unrelated to its antifolate properties.

MECHANISMS OF ACTION. Lamotrigine blocks sustained repetitive firing of mouse spinal cord neurons and delays the recovery from inactivation of recombinant Na^+ channels, mechanisms similar to those of phenytoin and carbamazepine. Lamotrigine is effective against a broader spectrum of seizures than phenytoin and carbamazepine, suggesting that lamotrigine may have actions in addition to regulating recovery from inactivation of Na^+ channels. The mechanisms underlying its broad spectrum of actions may involve inhibiting synaptic release of glutamate.

PHARMACOKINETICS. Lamotrigine is completely absorbed from the GI tract and is metabolized primarily by glucuronidation. The plasma $t_{1/2}$ of a single dose is 24-30 h. Administration of phenytoin, carbamazepine, or phenobarbital reduces the $t_{1/2}$ and plasma concentrations of lamotrigine. Addition of valproate markedly increases plasma concentrations of lamotrigine, likely by inhibiting glucuronidation. Addition of lamotrigine to valproic acid produces a reduction of valproate concentrations by ~25% over a few weeks. Concurrent use of lamotrigine and carbamazepine is associated with increases of the 10,11-epoxide of carbamazepine and clinical toxicity.

THERAPEUTIC USE. Lamotrigine is useful for monotherapy and add-on therapy of partial and secondarily generalized tonic-clonic seizures in adults and Lennox-Gastaut syndrome in both children and adults. Patients already taking a hepatic enzyme–inducing antiseizure drug (such as carbamazepine, phenytoin, phenobarbital, or primidone, but not valproate) should be given lamotrigine initially at 50 mg/day for 2 weeks. The dose is increased to 50 mg twice per day for 2 weeks and then increased in increments of 100 mg/day each week up to a maintenance dose of 300-500 mg/day divided into 2 doses. For patients taking valproate in addition to an enzyme-inducing antiseizure drug, the initial dose should be 25 mg every other day for 2 weeks, followed by an increase to 25 mg/day for 2 weeks; the dose then can be increased by 25-50 mg/day every 1-2 weeks up to a maintenance dose of 100-150 mg/day divided into 2 doses.

TOXICITY. The most common adverse effects are dizziness, ataxia, blurred or double vision, nausea, vomiting, and rash when lamotrigine was added to another antiseizure drug. A few cases of Stevens-Johnson syndrome and disseminated intravascular coagulation have been reported. The incidence of serious rash in pediatric patients (~0.8%) is higher than in the adult population (0.3%).

LEVETIRACETAM

Levetiracetam (KEPPRA, others) is FDA-approved for adjunctive therapy for myoclonic, partial-onset, and primary generalized tonic-clonic seizures in adults and children as young as 4 years old. The mechanism by which levetiracetam exerts these antiseizure effects is unknown.

PHARMACOKINETICS. Levetiracetam is rapidly and almost completely absorbed after oral administration and is not bound to plasma proteins. Ninety-five percent of the drug and its inactive metabolite are excreted in the urine, 65% as unchanged drug; the main metabolite results from hydrolysis of the acetamide group. Levetiracetam is devoid of known interactions with other antiseizure drugs, oral contraceptives, or anticoagulants.

THERAPEUTIC USE AND TOXICITY. In clinical trials, levetiracetam given in addition to other antiseizure medications in adults with either refractory partial seizures or uncontrolled generalized tonic-clonic seizures was superior to placebo. Levetiracetam also has efficacy as adjunctive therapy for refractory generalized myoclonic seizures. Insufficient evidence is available about its use as monotherapy for partial or generalized epilepsy. Levetiracetam is well tolerated. Adverse effects include somnolence, asthenia, and dizziness.

TIAGABINE

Tiagabine (GABITRIL) is used for partial seizures in adults. Tiagabine inhibits the GABA transporter, GAT-1, and thereby reduces GABA uptake into neurons and glia, thereby prolonging the dwell time of GABA at inhibitory synapses.

PHARMACOKINETICS. Tiagabine is rapidly absorbed after oral administration, extensively bound to serum or plasma proteins, and metabolized mainly by hepatic CYP3A. Its $t_{1/2}$ of ~8 h is shortened by 2-3 h when coadministered with hepatic enzyme–inducing drugs such as phenobarbital, phenytoin, or carbamazepine.

THERAPEUTIC USE AND TOXICITY. Tiagabine is effective as add-on therapy of refractory partial seizures with or without secondary generalization. Its efficacy as monotherapy for newly diagnosed or refractory partial and generalized epilepsy has not been established. Adverse effects include dizziness, somnolence, and tremor that are mild to moderate in severity and appear shortly after initiation of therapy. Tiagabine-enhanced effects of synaptically released GABA can facilitate spike-and-wave discharges in animal models of absence seizures. Case reports suggest that tiagabine treatment of patients with a history of spike-and-wave discharges causes exacerbations of their EEG abnormalities. Thus, tiagabine may be contraindicated in patients with generalized absence epilepsy. Paradoxically, tiagabine has been associated with the occurrence of seizures in patients without epilepsy and off-label use of the drug is discouraged.

TOPIRAMATE

Topiramate (TOPAMAX, others) is FDA-approved as initial monotherapy (in patients at least 10 years old) and as adjunctive therapy (for patients as young as 2 years of age) for partial-onset or primary generalized tonic-clonic seizures, for Lennox-Gastaut syndrome in patients 2 years of age and older, and for migraine headache prophylaxis in adults.

MECHANISMS OF ACTION. Topiramate reduces voltage-gated Na^+ currents in cerebellar granule cells and may act on the inactivated state of the channel similar to phenytoin. In addition, topiramate activates a hyperpolarizing K^+ current, enhances postsynaptic $GABA_A$ receptor currents, and limits activation of

AMPA-kainate receptors (*see* Table 14–1 and Figures 14–6, 14–7, and 14–8). Topiramate is a weak carbonic anhydrase inhibitor.

PHARMACOKINETICS. Topiramate is rapidly absorbed after oral administration, exhibits little (10-20%) binding to plasma proteins, and is mainly excreted unchanged in the urine. The remainder undergoes metabolism by hydroxylation, hydrolysis, and glucuronidation with no single metabolite accounting for > 5% of an oral dose. Its $t_{1/2}$ is ~1 day. Reduced estradiol plasma concentrations occur with concurrent topiramate, suggesting the need for higher doses of oral contraceptives when coadministered with topiramate.

THERAPEUTIC USE AND TOXICITY. Topiramate is equivalent to valproate and carbamazepine in children and adults with newly diagnosed partial and primary generalized epilepsy. It is effective as monotherapy for refractory partial epilepsy and refractory generalized tonic-clonic seizures. Topiramate is also effective as adjunctive therapy (against both drop attacks and tonic-clonic seizures in patients with Lennox-Gastaut syndrome, and for migraine headache prophylaxis in adults). Topiramate is well tolerated. Common adverse effects are somnolence, fatigue, weight loss, and nervousness. It can precipitate renal calculi, which is most likely due to inhibition of carbonic anhydrase. Topiramate has been associated with cognitive impairment and patients may complain about a change in the taste of carbonated beverages.

ZONISAMIDE

Zonisamide (ZONEGRAN, others) is a sulfonamide derivative used as adjunctive therapy of partial seizures in adults. Zonisamide inhibits the T-type Ca^{2+} currents. In addition, zonisamide inhibits the sustained, repetitive firing of spinal cord neurons, presumably by prolonging the inactivated state of voltage-gated Na^+ channels in a manner similar to actions of phenytoin and carbamazepine.

PHARMACOKINETICS. Zonisamide is almost completely absorbed after oral administration, has a long $t_{1/2}$ (~63 h), and is ~40% bound to plasma protein. Approximately 85% of an oral dose is excreted in the urine, principally as unmetabolized zonisamide and a glucuronide of a metabolite formed by CYP3A4. Phenobarbital, phenytoin, and carbamazepine decrease the plasma concentration/dose ratio of zonisamide, whereas lamotrigine increases this ratio. Zonisamide has little effect on the plasma concentrations of other antiseizure drugs.

THERAPEUTIC USE AND TOXICITY. In clinical trials, the addition of zonisamide to other drugs in patients with refractory partial seizures was superior to placebo. There is insufficient evidence for its efficacy as monotherapy for newly diagnosed or refractory epilepsy. Zonisamide is well tolerated. Common adverse effects include somnolence, ataxia, anorexia, nervousness, and fatigue. Approximately 1% of individuals develop renal calculi, which may relate to its ability to inhibit carbonic anhydrase. Zonisamide can cause metabolic acidosis, which is more frequent in younger patients. Patients with predisposing conditions (e.g., renal disease, severe respiratory disorders, diarrhea, surgery, ketogenic diet) may be at greater risk. Measurement of serum bicarbonate prior to initiating therapy and periodically thereafter is recommended.

LACOSAMIDE

Lacosamide (VIMPAT) is approved as adjunctive therapy for partial-onset seizures in patients 17 years of age and older.

Lacosamide enhances slow inactivation of voltage-gated Na^+ channels and limits sustained repetitive firing, the neuronal firing pattern characteristic of partial seizures. Lacosamide also binds collapsin response mediator protein 2 (crmp-2), a phosphoprotein involved in neuronal differentiation and axon outgrowth. Its antiseizure mechanism of action is more likely mediated by its enhancing slow inactivation of Na^+ channels. Clinical studies of adults with refractory partial seizures demonstrated that addition of lacosamide to other drugs was superior to placebo.

RUFINAMIDE

Rufinamide (BANZEL) is a triazole derivative approved for adjunctive treatment of seizures associated with Lennox-Gastaut syndrome. Rufinamide enhances slow inactivation of voltage-gated Na^+ channels and limits sustained repetitive firing, the firing pattern characteristic of partial seizures. Whether this is the mechanism by which rufinamide suppresses seizures is presently unclear.

VIGABATRIN

Vigabatrin (SABRIL) is used as adjunctive therapy of refractory partial complex seizures in adults. In addition, vigabatrin is designated as an orphan drug for treatment of infantile spasms. Due to progressive and permanent bilateral vision loss, vigabatrin must be reserved for patients who have failed several alternative therapies.

Vigabatrin is a structural analog of GABA that irreversibly inhibits GABA degradation, thereby leading to increased concentrations of GABA in the brain. A 2-week, randomized, clinical trial of vigabatrin for infantile spasms in children < 2 years old revealed time- and dose-dependent increases in responders, evident as freedom from spasms for 7 consecutive days. The subset of children in whom infantile spasms were caused by tuberous sclerosis was particularly responsive to vigabatrin.

EZOGABINE

Ezogabine (POTIGA) is a carbamate ethyl ester and K^+- channel activator approved by the FDA for the treatment of partial-onset seizures.

Ezogabine is administered orally. Starting dose is 100 mg 3 times daily that is increased gradually to a maximal dose of 1200 mg/day. Ezogabine is metabolized primarily via glucuronidation and eliminated mainly through renal excretion. Its $t_{1/2}$ is ~8-11 h. Serious adverse effects are dose related and include difficulty in urination, hallucination, suicidal thoughts, and QT prolongation. Less serious side effects include drowsiness, dizziness, fatigue, blurred vision, tremor, memory impairment, asthenia, gait disturbance and balance disorder, and slurred speech.

PERAMPANEL

Perampanel (FYCOMPA) is a selective noncompetitive antagonist of the AMPA glutamate receptor. It is approved for the treatment of partial-onset seizures with or without secondarily generalized seizures.

Recommended starting oral dose is 2 mg once daily titrated to a maximal dose of 4-12 mg once daily taken at bedtime. The drug is rapidly absorbed after oral administration. The $t_{1/2}$ is ~105 h. It is 95% bound to plasma protein, mainly albumin. It is metabolized by oxidation followed by glucuronidation. Adverse effects include aggressive behavior, suicidal thoughts, sleepiness, vertigo, dizziness, nausea, problems with walking and muscle coordination, and weight gain.

ACETAZOLAMIDE

Acetazolamide, the prototype for the carbonic anhydrase inhibitors (*see* Chapter 25), is sometimes effective against absence seizures but its usefulness is limited by the rapid development of tolerance.

FELBAMATE

Felbamate (FELBATOL) is a dicarbamate. An association between felbamate and aplastic anemia resulted in the withdrawal of most patients from treatment with this drug. Postmarketing experience revealed an association between felbamate exposure and liver failure.

GENERAL PRINCIPLES AND CHOICE OF DRUGS FOR THE THERAPY OF THE EPILEPSIES

Early diagnosis and treatment of seizure disorders with a single appropriate agent offers the best prospect of achieving prolonged seizure-free periods with the lowest risk of toxicity. An attempt should be made to determine the cause of the epilepsy with the hope of discovering a correctable lesion, either structural or metabolic. The drugs commonly used for distinct seizure types are listed in Table 21–1. The efficacy combined with the unwanted effects of a given drug determine which particular drug is optimal for a given patient.

In the absence of extenuating circumstances such as status epilepticus, only monotherapy should be initiated. Initial dosing should be low and should target steady-state plasma drug concentrations within the lower range associated with clinical efficacy. Dosage is increased and monitored at appropriate intervals as required for control of seizures or as limited by toxicity. Compliance with a properly selected, single drug in maximal tolerated dosage results in complete control of seizures in ~50% of patients. If compliance has been confirmed yet seizures persist, another drug should be substituted. Unless serious adverse effects of the drug dictate otherwise, dosage always should be reduced gradually to minimize risk of seizure recurrence. The literature suggests that among previously untreated patients, 47% become seizure-free with the first drug and an additional 14% become seizure-free with a second or third agent. If therapy with a second single drug is inadequate, combination therapy is warranted; the decision to use combination therapy should not be made lightly, because most patients obtain optimal seizure control *with fewest unwanted effects* when taking a single drug. In choosing a combination, it seems wise to select 2 drugs that act by distinct mechanisms (e.g., one that promotes Na^+ channel inactivation and another that enhances GABA-mediated synaptic inhibition) (*see* Table 21–2). Side effects of each drug and the potential drug interactions also should be considered.

DURATION OF THERAPY

Antiseizure drugs are typically continued for at least 2 years. Tapering and discontinuing therapy should be considered, if the patient is seizure-free after 2 years. Factors associated with high risk for recurrent seizures following discontinuation of therapy include EEG abnormalities, known structural lesions, abnormalities on neurological exam, and history of frequent seizures or medically refractory seizures prior to control. Conversely, factors associated with low risk for recurrent seizures include idiopathic epilepsy, normal EEG, onset in childhood, and seizures easily controlled with a single drug. Typically, 80% of recurrences will occur within 4 months of discontinuing therapy. Clinician and patient must weigh the risk of recurrent seizure and the associated potential deleterious consequences (e.g., loss of driving privileges) against the various implications of continuing medication including cost, unwanted effects, implications of diagnosis of epilepsy, etc. Medications should be tapered slowly over a period of several months.

SIMPLE AND COMPLEX PARTIAL AND SECONDARILY GENERALIZED TONIC-CLONIC SEIZURES

The efficacy and toxicity of carbamazepine, phenobarbital, and phenytoin for treatment of partial and secondarily generalized *tonic-clonic seizures* in adults have been compared. Carbamazepine and phenytoin were the most effective agents.

ABSENCE SEIZURES

Ethosuximide and valproate are considered equally effective in the treatment of absence seizures. Between 50% and 75% of newly diagnosed patients are free of seizures following therapy with either drug. If tonic-clonic seizures are present or emerge during therapy, valproate is the agent of first choice. Lamotrigine is also effective for newly diagnosed absence epilepsy although it is not FDA-approved for this indication.

MYOCLONIC SEIZURES

Valproic acid is the drug of choice for myoclonic seizures in the syndrome of juvenile myoclonic epilepsy, in which myoclonic seizures often coexist with tonic-clonic and absence seizures. Levetiracetam also has demonstrated efficacy as adjunctive therapy for refractory generalized myoclonic seizures.

FEBRILE CONVULSIONS

Two to 4% of children experience a convulsion associated with a febrile illness. From 25-33% of these children will have another febrile convulsion. Only 2-3% become epileptic in later years. Several factors are associated with an increased risk of developing epilepsy: preexisting neurological disorder or developmental delay, a family history of epilepsy, or a complicated febrile seizure (i.e., the febrile seizure lasted > 15 min, was one-sided, or was followed by a second seizure in the same day). If all of these risk factors are present, the risk of developing epilepsy is ~10%. Uncertainties regarding the efficacy of prophylaxis for reducing epilepsy combined with substantial side effects of phenobarbital prophylaxis argue against the use of chronic therapy for prophylactic purposes in these cases. For children at high risk of developing recurrent febrile seizures and epilepsy, rectally administered diazepam at the time of fever may prevent recurrent seizures and avoid side effects of chronic therapy.

SEIZURES IN INFANTS AND YOUNG CHILDREN

Infantile spasms with *hypsarrhythmia* are refractory to the usual antiseizure agents. Corticotropin or glucocorticoids are commonly used. Vigabatrin (γ-vinyl GABA; SABRIL) is efficacious in comparison to placebo. The potential for progressive and permanent vision loss has resulted in vigabatrin being labeled with a black box warning and marketed under a restrictive distribution program. The drug has an orphan drug status for the treatment of infantile spasms. Lennox-Gastaut syndrome is a severe form of epilepsy, which usually begins in childhood and is characterized by cognitive impairments and multiple types of seizures including tonic-clonic, tonic, atonic, myoclonic, and atypical absence seizures. Lamotrigine is an effective and well-tolerated additive drug for this treatment-resistant form of epilepsy. Felbamate also is effective for seizures in this syndrome, but the occasional occurrence of aplastic anemia and hepatic failure have limited its use. Topiramate has also been demonstrated to be effective.

STATUS EPILEPTICUS AND OTHER CONVULSIVE EMERGENCIES

Status epilepticus is a neurological emergency. Mortality for adults approximates 20%. The goal of treatment is rapid termination of behavioral and electrical seizure activity due to the risk of permanent brain damage. Prompt treatment is essential with effective drugs in adequate doses, and attention to hypoventilation and hypotension. Because hypoventilation may result from high doses of drugs used, it may be necessary to assist respiration temporarily. Drugs should be administered by the IV route only. Four IV treatments: diazepam followed by phenytoin; lorazepam; phenobarbital; and phenytoin alone seem to have similar efficacies, with success rates ranging from 44-65%. Lorazepam alone was found to be significantly better than phenytoin alone. No significant differences were found with respect to recurrences or adverse reactions.

ANTISEIZURE THERAPY AND PREGNANCY

The effectiveness of oral contraceptives appears to be reduced by concomitant use of antiseizure drugs. This may be caused by the increased rate of oral contraceptive metabolism by antiseizure drugs that induce CYPs (*see* Table 21–3). Antiseizure drugs that induce CYPs have been associated with vitamin K deficiency in the newborn, which can result in a coagulopathy and intracerebral hemorrhage. Treatment with vitamin K_1, 10 mg/day during the last month of gestation, has been recommended for prophylaxis.

TERATOGENICITY. Antiseizure drugs have teratogenic effects. The malformations include congenital heart defects, neural tube defects, cleft lip, cleft palate, and others. Phenytoin, carbamazepine, valproate, lamotrigine, and phenobarbital all have been associated with teratogenic effects. One consideration for a woman with epilepsy who wishes to become pregnant is a trial free of antiseizure drug; monotherapy with careful attention to drug levels is another alternative. Polytherapy with toxic levels should be avoided. Folate supplementation (0.4 mg/day) is recommended for all women of childbearing age to reduce the likelihood of neural tube defects.

For a complete Bibliographical Listing see Goodman & Gilman's ***The Pharmacological Basis of Therapeutics***, 12th ed., or Goodman & Gilman Online at www.AccessMedicine.com.

Treatment of Central Nervous System Degenerative Disorders

Neurodegenerative disorders are characterized by progressive and irreversible loss of neurons from specific regions of the brain. Prototypical neurodegenerative disorders include Parkinson disease (PD) and Huntington disease (HD), where loss of neurons from structures of the basal ganglia results in abnormalities in the control of movement; Alzheimer disease (AD), where the loss of hippocampal and cortical neurons leads to impairment of memory and cognitive ability; and amyotrophic lateral sclerosis (ALS), where muscular weakness results from the degeneration of spinal, bulbar, and cortical motor neurons. Currently available therapies for neurodegenerative disorders alleviate the disease symptoms but do not alter the underlying neurodegenerative process.

SELECTIVE VULNERABILITY AND NEUROPROTECTIVE STRATEGIES

SELECTIVE VULNERABILITY. A striking feature of neurodegenerative disorders is the exquisite specificity of the disease processes for particular types of neurons. For example, in PD there is extensive destruction of the dopaminergic neurons of the substantia nigra, whereas neurons in the cortex and many other areas of the brain are unaffected. In contrast, neural injury in AD is most severe in the hippocampus and neocortex, and even within the cortex, the loss of neurons is not uniform but varies dramatically in different functional regions. In HD the mutant gene responsible for the disorder is expressed throughout the brain and in many other organs, yet the pathological changes are most prominent in the neostriatum. In ALS, there is loss of spinal motor neurons and the cortical neurons that provide their descending input. The diversity of these patterns of neural degeneration suggests that the process of neural injury results from the interaction of genetic and environmental influences.

GENETICS AND ENVIRONMENT. Each of the major neurodegenerative disorders may be familial in nature. HD is exclusively familial; it is transmitted by autosomal dominant inheritance, and the molecular mechanism of the genetic defect has been defined. Nevertheless, environmental factors importantly influence the age of onset and rate of progression of HD symptoms. PD, AD, and ALS are mostly sporadic without clear pattern of inheritance. But for each there are well-recognized genetic forms. For example, there are both dominant (*α-synuclein, LRRK2*) and recessive (*parkin, DJ-1, PINK1*) gene mutations that may give rise to PD. In AD, mutations in the genes coding for the amyloid precursor protein (APP) and proteins known as the presenilins (involved in APP processing) lead to inherited forms of the disease. Mutations in the gene coding for copper-zinc superoxide dismutase (*SOD1*) account for about 2% of the cases of adult-onset ALS. There are also genetic risk factors that influence the probability of disease onset and modify the phenotype. For example, the apolipoprotein E (apoE) genotype constitutes an important risk factor for AD. Three distinct isoforms of this protein exist. Although all isoforms carry out their primary role in lipid metabolism equally well, individuals who are homozygous for the apoE4 allele ("4/4") have a much higher lifetime risk of AD than do those homozygous for the apoE2 allele ("2/2").

Environmental factors including infectious agents, environmental toxins, and acquired brain injury have been proposed in the etiology of neurodegenerative disorders. Traumatic brain injury has been suggested as a trigger for neurodegenerative disorders. At least one toxin, *N*-methyl-4-phenyl-1,2,3,6-tetrahydropyridine (MPTP), can induce a condition closely resembling PD. More recently, evidence has linked pesticide exposure with PD. Exposure of soldiers to neurotoxic chemicals has been implicated in ALS (as part of "Gulf War syndrome").

COMMON CELLULAR MECHANISMS OF NEURODEGENERATION. Despite their varied phenotypes, the neurodegenerative disorders share some common features. For example, misfolded and aggregated proteins are found in every major neurodegenerative disorder: alpha-synuclein, in PD; amyloid-β (Aβ) and tau in AD; huntingtin in HD; and SOD and TDP-43 in ALS. The accumulation of misfolded proteins may result from either genetic mutations producing abnormal structure, or from impaired cellular clearance.

The term *excitotoxicity* describes the neural injury that results from the presence of excess glutamate in the brain. Glutamate is used as a neurotransmitter to mediate most excitatory synaptic transmission in the mammalian brain (*see* Table 14–1). The presence of excessive amounts of glutamate can lead to excitotoxic cell death (*see* Figure 14–8). The destructive effects of glutamate are mediated by glutamate receptors, particularly those of the *N*-methyl-D-aspartate (NMDA) type. Excitotoxic injury contributes to the neuronal death that occurs in acute processes such as stroke and head trauma. The role of excitotoxicity is less certain in the chronic neurodegenerative disorders; nevertheless, regional and cellular differences in susceptibility to excitotoxic injury, conveyed, e.g., by differences in types of glutamate receptors, may contribute to selective vulnerability. This has led to the development of glutamate antagonists as neuroprotective therapies, with 2 such agents (memantine and riluzole, described later) currently in clinical use.

Aging is associated with a progressive impairment in the capacity of neurons for oxidative metabolism with consequent production of reactive compounds such as hydrogen peroxide and oxygen radicals. These reactive species can lead to DNA damage, peroxidation of membrane lipids, and neuronal death. This has led to pursuit of drugs that can enhance cellular metabolism (such as the mitochondrial cofactor coenzyme Q_{10}) and antioxidant strategies as treatments to prevent or retard degenerative diseases.

PARKINSON DISEASE (PD)

CLINICAL OVERVIEW. Parkinsonism is a clinical syndrome with 4 cardinal features:

- Bradykinesia (slowness and poverty of movement)
- Muscular rigidity
- Resting tremor (which usually abates during voluntary movement)
- An impairment of postural balance leading to disturbances of gait and to falling

The most common form of parkinsonism is idiopathic PD, first described by James Parkinson in 1817 as *paralysis agitans,* or the "shaking palsy." The pathological hallmark of PD is the loss of the pigmented, dopaminergic neurons of the substantia nigra pars compacta, with the appearance of intracellular inclusions known as *Lewy bodies*. A loss of 70-80% of these dopamine-containing neurons accompanies symptomatic PD.

Without treatment, PD progresses over 5-10 years to a rigid, akinetic state in which patients are incapable of caring for themselves. Death frequently results from complications of immobility, including aspiration pneumonia or pulmonary embolism. The availability of effective pharmacological treatment has radically altered the prognosis of PD; in most cases, good functional mobility can be maintained for many years. Life expectancy of adequately treated patients is increased substantially, but overall mortality remains higher than that of the general population. In addition, while DA neuron loss is the most prominent feature of the disease, the disorder affects a wide range of other brain structures, including the brainstem, hippocampus, and cerebral cortex. This pathology is likely responsible for the "non-motor" features of PD, which include sleep disorders, depression, and memory impairment.

Several disorders other than idiopathic PD also may produce parkinsonism, including some relatively rare neurodegenerative disorders, stroke, and intoxication with DA-receptor antagonists. Drugs that may cause parkinsonism include antipsychotics such as haloperidol and chlorpromazine (*see* Chapter 16) and antiemetics such as prochlorperazine and metoclopramide (*see* Chapter 46). The distinction between idiopathic PD and other causes of parkinsonism is important because parkinsonism arising from other causes usually is refractory to all forms of treatment.

PATHOPHYSIOLOGY. The dopaminergic deficit in PD arises from a loss of the neurons in the substantia nigra pars compacta that provide innervation to the striatum (caudate and putamen). The current understanding of the pathophysiology of PD is based on the finding that the striatal DA content is reduced in excess of 80%, with a parallel loss of neurons from the substantia nigra, suggesting that replacement of DA could restore function. We now have a model of the function of the basal ganglia that, while incomplete, is still useful.

DOPAMINE SYNTHESIS, METABOLISM, AND RECEPTORS. DA, a catecholamine, is synthesized in the terminals of dopaminergic neurons from tyrosine and stored, released, reaccumulated, and metabolized by processes described in Chapter 13 and summarized in Figure 22–1. The actions of DA in the brain are mediated by DA receptor, of which there are 2 broad classes. D1 and D2, with 5 distinct subtypes, D_1-D_5 (*see* Figure 13–6). All the DA receptors are G protein–coupled receptors (GPCRs). Receptors of the D1 group (D_1 and D_5 subtypes) couple to G_s and thence to activation of the cyclic AMP pathway. The D2 group (D_2, D_3, and D_4 receptors) couple to G_i to reduce the adenylyl cyclase activity and voltage-gated Ca^{2+} currents while activating K^+ currents (*see* Chapters 3 and 13 for details). Each of the 5 DA receptors has a distinct anatomical pattern of expression in the brain (*see* Figure 13–6). D_1 and D_2 proteins are abundant in the striatum and are the most important receptor sites with regard to the causes and treatment of PD. The D_4 and D_5 proteins are largely extrastriatal,

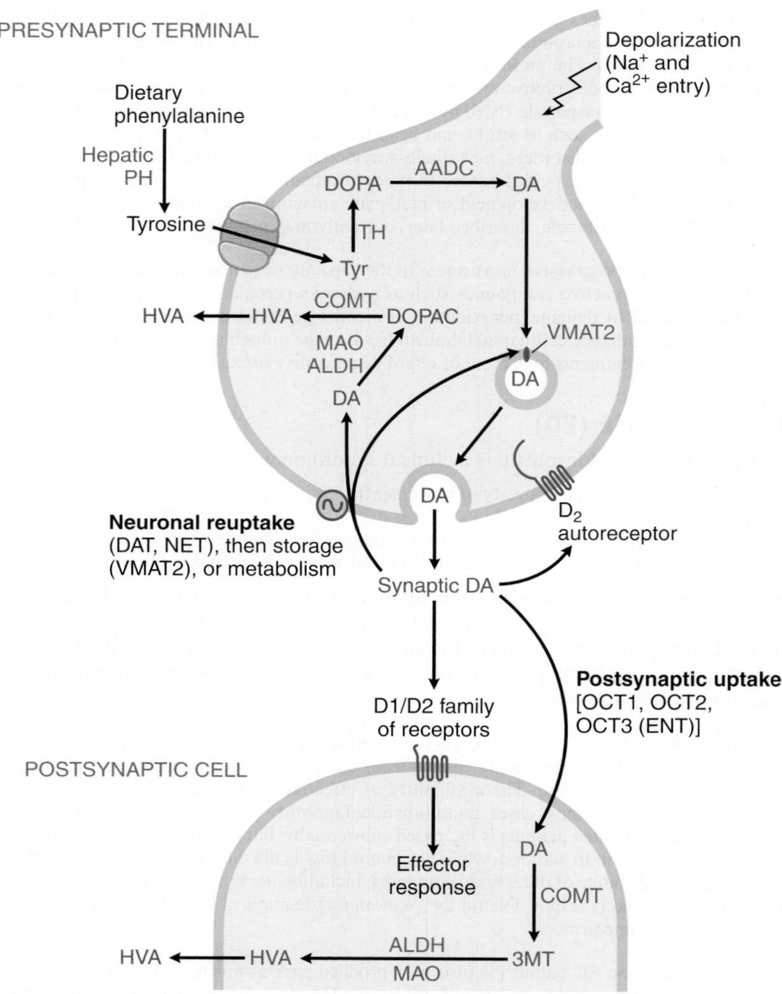

Figure 22–1 *Dopaminergic nerve terminal.* Dopamine (DA) is synthesized from tyrosine in the nerve terminal by the sequential actions of tyrosine hydrolase (TH) and aromatic amino acid decarboxylase (AADC). DA is sequestered by VMAT2 in storage granules and released by exocytosis. Synaptic DA activates presynaptic autoreceptors and postsynaptic D1 and D2 receptors. Synaptic DA may be taken up into the neuron via the DA and NE transporters (DAT, NET), or removed by postsynaptic uptake via OCT3 transporters. Cytosolic DA is subject to degradation by monoamine oxidase (MAO) and aldehyde dehydrogenase (ALDH) in the neuron, and by catechol-*O*-methyl transferase (COMT) and MAO/ALDH in non-neuronal cells; the final metabolic product is homovanillic acid (HVA). See structures in Figure 22–4. PH, phenylalanine hydroxylase.

whereas D_3 expression is low in the caudate and putamen but more abundant in the nucleus accumbens and olfactory tubercle.

NEURAL MECHANISM OF PARKINSONISM: A MODEL OF BASAL GANGLIA FUNCTION. Considerable effort has been devoted to understanding how the loss of dopaminergic input to the neurons of the neostriatum gives rise to the clinical features of PD. The basal ganglia can be viewed as a modulatory side loop that regulates the flow of information from the cerebral cortex to the motor neurons of the spinal cord (Figure 22–2).

The neostriatum is the principal input structure of the basal ganglia and receives excitatory glutamatergic input from many areas of the cortex. Most neurons within the striatum are projection neurons that innervate

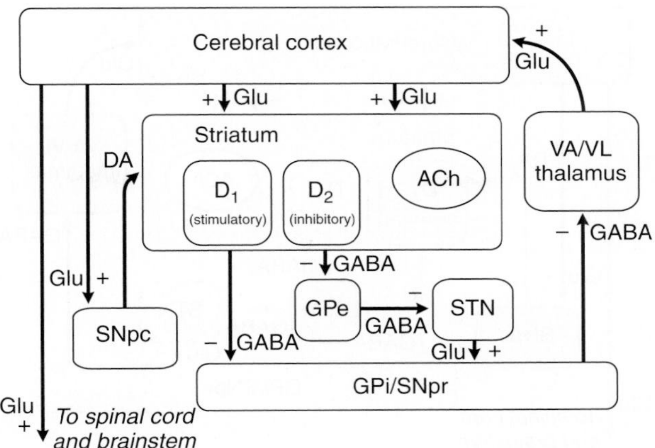

Figure 22–2 *Schematic wiring diagram of the basal ganglia.* The striatum is the principal input structure of the basal ganglia and receives excitatory glutamatergic input from many areas of cerebral cortex. The striatum contains projection neurons expressing predominantly D_1 or D_2 dopamine receptors, as well as interneurons that use ACh as a neurotransmitter. Outflow from the striatum proceeds along 2 routes. The direct pathway, from the striatum to the substantia nigra pars reticulata (SNpr) and globus pallidus interna (GPi), uses the inhibitory transmitter GABA. The indirect pathway, from the striatum through the globus pallidus externa (GPe) and the subthalamic nucleus (STN) to the SNpr and GPi, consists of 2 inhibitory GABA-ergic links and 1 excitatory glutamatergic projection (Glu). The substantia nigra pars compacta (SNpc) provides dopaminergic innervation to the striatal neurons, giving rise to both the direct and indirect pathways, and regulates the relative activity of these 2 paths. The SNpr and GPi are the output structures of the basal ganglia and provide feedback to the cerebral cortex through the ventroanterior and ventrolateral nuclei of the thalamus (VA/VL).

other basal ganglia structures. A small but important subgroup of striatal neurons consists of interneurons that connect neurons within the striatum but do not project beyond its borders. Acetylcholine (ACh) and neuropeptides are used as transmitters by these striatal interneurons.

The outflow of the striatum proceeds along 2 distinct routes, termed the *direct* and *indirect pathways.* The direct pathway is formed by neurons in the striatum that project directly to the output stages of the basal ganglia, the substantia nigra pars reticulata (SNpr) and the globus pallidus interna (GPi); these, in turn, relay to the ventroanterior and ventrolateral thalamus, which provides excitatory input to the cortex. The neurotransmitter of both links of the direct pathway is γ-aminobutyric acid (GABA), which is inhibitory, so that *the net effect of stimulation of the direct pathway at the level of the striatum is to increase the excitatory outflow from the thalamus to the cortex.*

The indirect pathway is composed of striatal neurons that project to the globus pallidus externa (GPe). This structure, in turn, innervates the subthalamic nucleus (STN), which provides outflow to the SNpr and GPi output stage. The first 2 links—the projections from striatum to GPe and GPe to STN—use the inhibitory transmitter GABA; however, the final link—the projection from STN to SNpr and GPi—is an excitatory glutamatergic pathway. Thus, *the net effect of stimulating the indirect pathway at the level of the striatum is to reduce the excitatory outflow from the thalamus to the cerebral cortex.* The key feature of this model of basal ganglia function, which accounts for the symptoms observed in PD as a result of loss of dopaminergic neurons, is the differential effect of DA on the direct and indirect pathways (Figure 22–3).

The dopaminergic neurons of the substantia nigra pars compacta (SNpc) innervate all parts of the striatum; however, the target striatal neurons express distinct types of DA receptors. The striatal neurons giving rise to the direct pathway express primarily the *excitatory* D_1 dopamine receptor protein, whereas the striatal neurons forming the indirect pathway express primarily the *inhibitory* D_2 type. Thus, DA released in the striatum tends to increase the activity of the direct pathway and reduce the activity of the indirect pathway, whereas the depletion that occurs in PD has the opposite effect. The net effect of the reduced dopaminergic input in PD is to increase markedly the inhibitory outflow from the SNpr and GPi to the thalamus and reduce excitation of the motor cortex. There are several limitations of this model of basal ganglia function. The anatomical connections are considerably more complex and many of the pathways involved use several neurotransmitters. Nevertheless, the model is useful and has important implications for the rational design and use of pharmacological agents in PD.

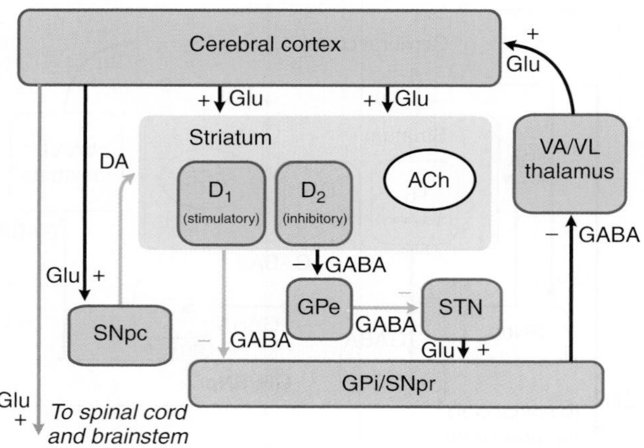

Figure 22–3 *The basal ganglia in Parkinson disease.* The primary defect is destruction of the dopaminergic neurons of the SNpc. The striatal neurons that form the direct pathway from the striatum to the SNpr and GPi express primarily the *excitatory* D_1 DA receptor, whereas the striatal neurons that project to the GPe and form the indirect pathway express the *inhibitory* D_2 dopamine receptor. Thus, loss of the dopaminergic input to the striatum has a differential effect on the 2 outflow pathways; the direct pathway to the SNpr and GPi is less active (*structures in purple*), whereas the activity in the indirect pathway is increased (*structures in red*). The net effect is that neurons in the SNpr and GPi become more active. This leads to increased inhibition of the VA/VL thalamus and reduced excitatory input to the cortex. *Light blue lines* indicate primary pathways with reduced activity. (See legend to Figure 22–2 for definitions of anatomical abbreviations.)

TREATMENT OF PARKINSON DISEASE

Table 22–1 summarizes commonly used medications for the treatment of PD.

LEVODOPA. Levodopa (L-dopa, LARODOPA, L-3,4-dihydroxyphenylalanine), the metabolic precursor of DA, is the single most effective agent in the treatment of PD.

The effects of levodopa result from its decarboxylation to DA. When administered orally, levodopa is absorbed rapidly from the small bowel by the transport system for aromatic amino acids. Concentrations of the drug in plasma usually peak between 0.5 and 2 h after an oral dose. The $t_{1/2}$ in plasma is short (1-3 h). The rate and extent of absorption of levodopa depends on the rate of gastric emptying, the pH of gastric juice, and the length of time the drug is exposed to the degradative enzymes of the gastric and intestinal mucosa. Administration of levodopa with high-protein meals delays absorption and reduces peak plasma concentrations. Entry of the drug into the CNS across the blood-brain barrier is mediated by a membrane transporter for aromatic amino acids. In the brain, levodopa is converted to DA by decarboxylation primarily within the presynaptic terminals of dopaminergic neurons in the striatum. The DA produced is responsible for the therapeutic effectiveness of the drug in PD; after release, it is either transported back into dopaminergic terminals by the presynaptic uptake mechanism or metabolized by the actions of MAO and catechol-*O*-methyltransferase (COMT) (Figure 22–4).

In clinical practice, levodopa is almost always administered in combination with a peripherally acting inhibitor of aromatic L-amino acid decarboxylase, such as carbidopa or benserazide (available outside the U.S.), drugs that do not penetrate well into the CNS. If levodopa is administered alone, the drug is largely decarboxylated by enzymes in the intestinal mucosa and other peripheral sites so that relatively little unchanged drug reaches the cerebral circulation and probably < 1% penetrates the CNS. In addition, DA release into the circulation by peripheral conversion of levodopa produces undesirable effects, particularly nausea. Inhibition of peripheral decarboxylase markedly increases the fraction of administered levodopa that remains unmetabolized and available to cross the blood-brain barrier (Figure 22–5) and reduces the incidence of GI side effects.

A daily dose of 75 mg carbidopa is generally sufficient to prevent the development of nausea. For this reason, the most commonly prescribed form of carbidopa/levodopa (SINEMET, ATAMET, others) is the 25/100 form, containing 25 mg carbidopa and 100 mg levodopa. With this formulation, dosage schedules of 3 or more tablets daily provide acceptable inhibition of decarboxylase in most individuals.

Levodopa therapy can have a dramatic effect on all the signs and symptoms of PD. Early in the course of the disease, the degree of improvement in tremor, rigidity, and bradykinesia may

Table 22–1

Commonly Used Medications for the Treatment of Parkinson Disease

AGENT	TYPICAL INITIAL DOSE	DAILY DOSE RANGE	COMMENTS
Levodopa Formulations			
Carbidopa/levodopa	25 mg carbidopa + 100 mg levodopa ("25/100" tablet), 2-3x daily	200-1200 mg levodopa	
Carbidopa/levodopa sustained-release	50 mg carbidopa + 200 mg levodopa ("50/200 sustained-release" tablet) 2x daily	200-1200 mg levodopa	Bioavailability 75% of immediate-release form
Carbidopa-levodopa orally disintegrating tablets (PARCOPA)	25 mg carbidopa + 100 mg levodopa ("25/100" tablet), 2-3x daily	200-1200 mg levodopa	
COMT Inhibitors			
Entacapone	200 mg with each dose of levodopa/carbidopa	600-2000 mg	
Tolcapone	100 mg with carbidopa/ levodopa	100-300 mg	May be hepatotoxic. Use only in patients not responding satisfactorily to other treatments. Monitor liver function
Carbidopa/levodopa/ entacapone	12.5 mg carbidopa + 50 mg levodopa + 200 mg entacapone (STALEVO 50), 3x daily	150-1200 mg levodopa	
DA Agonists			
Apomorphine	2 mg subcutaneous	6-18 mg subcutaneous	Trimethobenzamide is used to reduce nausea when initiating therapy
Bromocriptine	1.25 mg	2.5-15 mg daily	Ergot; long-term use is associated with cardiac valve fibrosis
Pramipexole	0.125 mg 3x daily	1.5-4.5 mg	
Ropinirole	0.25 mg 3x daily	1.5-24 mg	
Ropinirole sustained-release	2 mg per day	2-24 mg	
MAO Inhibitors			
Rasagiline	1 mg daily	0.5-1 mg	
Selegiline	5 mg 2x daily	2.5-10 mg	
Other Medications			
Trihexyphenidyl HCl	1 mg 2x daily	2-15 mg	
Amantadine	100 mg 2x daily	100-200 mg	

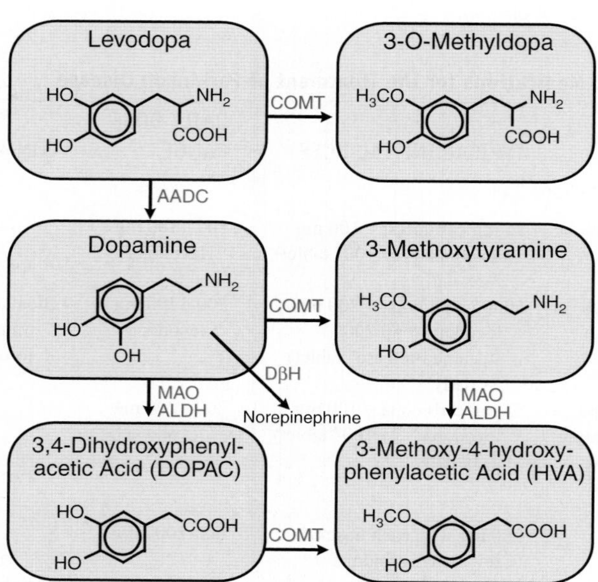

Figure 22–4 *Metabolism of levodopa (L-dopa).* AADC, aromatic L-amino acid decarboxylase; ALDH, aldehyde dehydrogenase; COMT, catechol-*O*-methyltransferase; DβH, dopamine-β-hydroxylase; MAO, monoamine oxidase.

be nearly complete. With long-term levodopa therapy, the "buffering" capacity is lost, and the patient's motor state may fluctuate dramatically with each dose of levodopa, producing the *motor complications* of levodopa.

A common problem is the development of the "wearing off" phenomenon: Each dose of levodopa effectively improves mobility for a period of time, perhaps 1-2 h, but rigidity and akinesia return rapidly at the end of the dosing interval. Increasing the dose and frequency of administration can improve this situation, but this often is limited by the development of dyskinesias, excessive and abnormal involuntary movements. In the later stages of PD, patients may fluctuate rapidly between being "off," having no beneficial effects from their medications, and being "on" but with disabling dyskinesias (the *on/off phenomenon*). A sustained-release formulation consisting of carbidopa/levodopa in an erodable wax matrix (SINEMET CR) is helpful in some cases, but absorption of the sustained-release formulation is not entirely predictable.

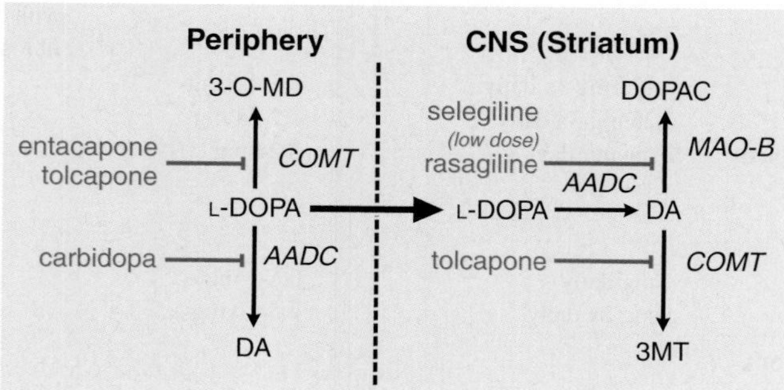

Figure 22–5 *Pharmacological preservation of L-DOPA and striatal dopamine.* The principal site of action of inhibitors of COMT (e.g., tolcapone and entacapone) is in the peripheral circulation. They block the *O*-methylation of L-dopa and increase the fraction of the drug available for delivery to the brain. Tolcapone also has effects in the CNS. Inhibitors of MAO-B, such as low-dose selegiline and rasagiline, will act within the CNS to reduce oxidative deamination of DA, thereby enhancing vesicular stores. AADC, aromatic L-amino acid decarboxylase; DA, dopamine; DOPAC, 3,4-dihydroxyphenylacetic acid; MAO, monoamine oxidase; 3MT, 3-methoxyltyramine; 3-OMD, 3-O-methyl DOPA.

Does levodopa alter the course of the underlying disease or merely modify the symptoms? A recent randomized trial has provided evidence that levodopa does not have an adverse effect on the course of the underlying disease, but has also confirmed that high doses of levodopa are associated with early onset of dyskinesias. Most practitioners have adopted a pragmatic approach, using levodopa only when the symptoms of PD cause functional impairment and other treatments are inadequate or not well tolerated.

A frequent and troubling adverse effect is the induction of hallucinations and confusion, especially in elderly patients or in patients with preexisting cognitive dysfunction. Conventional antipsychotic agents, such as the phenothiazines, are effective against levodopa-induced psychosis but may cause marked worsening of parkinsonism, probably through actions at the D_2 DA receptor. An alternative approach has been to use "atypical" antipsychotic agents (*see* Chapter 16). The 2 drugs that are most effective and best tolerated in patients with advanced PD are clozapine and quetiapine. Peripheral decarboxylation of levodopa and release of DA into the circulation may activate vascular DA receptors and produce orthostatic hypotension. Administration of levodopa with nonspecific inhibitors of MAO accentuates the actions of levodopa and may precipitate life-threatening hypertensive crisis and hyperpyrexia; nonspecific MAO inhibitors always should be discontinued at least 14 days before levodopa is administered [note that this prohibition does not include the MAO-B subtype-specific inhibitors selegiline and rasagiline (AZILECT)]. Abrupt withdrawal of levodopa or other dopaminergic medications may precipitate the *neuroleptic malignant syndrome* of confusion, rigidity, and hyperthermia, a potentially lethal adverse effect.

DOPAMINE RECEPTOR AGONISTS. The DA receptor agonists in clinical use have durations of action substantially longer than that of levodopa; they are often used in the management of dose-related fluctuations in motor state, and may be helpful in preventing motor complications. It has been suggested that DA receptor agonists may have the potential to modify the course of PD by reducing endogenous release of DA as well as the need for exogenous levodopa, thereby reducing free radical formation.

Two orally administered DA receptor agonists are commonly used for treatment of PD: ropinirole (REQUIP) and pramipexole (MIRAPEX). Ropinirole and pramipexole have selective activity at D_2 class sites (specifically at the D_2 and D_3 receptor) and little or no activity at D_1 class sites. Both are well absorbed orally and have similar therapeutic actions. Like levodopa, they can relieve the clinical symptoms of PD. The duration of action of the DA agonists (8-24 h) often is longer than that of levodopa (6-8 h), and they are particularly effective in the treatment of patients who have developed on/off phenomena. Ropinirole is also available in a once-daily sustained-release formulation (REQUIP XL), which is more convenient and may reduce adverse effects related to intermittent dosing. Both pramipexole and ropinirole may produce hallucinosis or confusion, similar to that observed with levodopa, and may cause nausea and orthostatic hypotension. They should be initiated at low dose and titrated slowly to minimize these effects. The DA agonists, as well as levodopa itself, are also associated with fatigue and somnolence. Practitioners prefer a DA agonist as initial therapy in younger patients in order to reduce the occurrence of motor complications. In older patients or those with substantial comorbidity, levodopa/carbidopa is generally better tolerated.

APOMORPHINE. Apomorphine (APOKYN) is a dopaminergic agonist that can be administered by subcutaneous injection. It has high affinity for D_4 receptors; moderate affinity for D_2, D_3, D_5, and adrenergic α_{1D}, α_{2B}, and α_{2C} receptors; and low affinity for D_1 receptors. Apomorphine is FDA-approved as a "rescue therapy" for the acute intermittent treatment of "off" episodes in patients with a fluctuating response to dopaminergic therapy.

Apomorphine has the same side effects as the oral DA agonists. Apomorphine is highly emetogenic and requires pre- and posttreatment antiemetic therapy. Oral trimethobenzamide (TIGAN), at a dose of 300 mg 3 times daily, should be started 3 days prior to the initial dose of apomorphine and continued at least during the first 2 months of therapy. Profound hypotension and loss of consciousness have occurred when apomorphine was administered with ondansetron; hence, the concomitant use of apomorphine with antiemetic drugs of the 5-HT_3 antagonist class is contraindicated. Other potentially serious side effects of apomorphine include QT prolongation, injection-site reactions, and the development of a pattern of abuse characterized by increasingly frequent dosing leading to hallucinations, dyskinesia, and abnormal behavior. Because of these potential adverse effects, use of apomorphine is appropriate only when other measures, such as oral DA agonists or COMT inhibitors, have failed to control the "off" episodes. Apomorphine therapy should be initiated with a 2-mg test dose in a setting where the patient can be monitored carefully. If tolerated, it can be titrated slowly up to a maximum dosage of 6 mg. For effective control of symptoms, patients may require 3 or more injections daily.

CATECHOL-*O*-METHYLTRANSFERASE INHIBITORS. When levodopa is administered orally, most is converted by aromatic L-amino acid decarboxylase (AADC) to DA (*see* Figure 22–5), which causes nausea and hypotension. Addition of an AADC inhibitor such as carbidopa reduces the formation of DA but increases the fraction of levodopa that is methylated by COMT. COMT inhibitors block this peripheral conversion of levodopa to 3-*O*-methyl DOPA, increasing both the plasma $t_{1/2}$ of levodopa as well as the fraction of each dose that reaches the CNS.

The COMT inhibitors tolcapone (TASMAR) and entacapone (COMTAN) reportedly reduce significantly the "wearing off" symptoms in patients treated with levodopa/carbidopa. The 2 drugs differ only in their pharmacokinetic properties and adverse effects: tolcapone has a relatively long duration of action, and appears to act by both central and peripheral inhibition of COMT. Entacapone has a short duration of action (2 h) and principally inhibits peripheral COMT. Common adverse effects of these agents include nausea, orthostatic hypotension, vivid dreams, confusion, and hallucinations. An important adverse effect associated with tolcapone is hepatotoxicity. At least 3 fatal cases of fulminant hepatic failure in patients taking tolcapone have been observed, leading to addition of a black box warning to the label. Tolcapone should be used only in patients who have not responded to other therapies and with appropriate monitoring for hepatic injury. Entacapone has not been associated with hepatotoxicity. Entacapone also is available in fixed-dose combinations with levodopa/carbidopa (STALEVO).

SELECTIVE MAO-B INHIBITORS. Two isoenzymes of MAO oxidize catecholamines: MAO-A and MAO-B. MAO-B is the predominant form in the striatum and is responsible for most of the oxidative metabolism of DA in the brain. Selective MAO-B inhibitors are used for the treatment of PD: selegiline (ELDEPRYL, EMSAM, ZELAPAR) and rasagiline (AZILECT). These agents selectively and irreversibly inactivate MAO-B. Both agents exert modest beneficial effects on the symptoms of PD. The basis of this efficacy is, presumably, inhibition of breakdown of DA in the striatum.

Selective MAO-B inhibitors do not substantially inhibit the peripheral metabolism of catecholamines and can be taken safely with levodopa. These agents also do not exhibit the "cheese effect," the potentially lethal potentiation of catecholamine action observed when patients on nonspecific MAO inhibitors ingest indirectly acting sympathomimetic amines such as the tyramine found in certain cheeses and wine.

Selegiline is generally well tolerated in younger patients for symptomatic treatment of early or mild PD. In patients with more advanced PD or underlying cognitive impairment, selegiline may accentuate the adverse motor and cognitive effects of levodopa therapy. Metabolites of selegiline include amphetamine and methamphetamine, which may cause anxiety, insomnia, and other adverse symptoms. Selegiline has become available in an orally disintegrating tablet (ZELAPAR) as well as a transdermal patch (EMSAM). Both of these delivery routes are intended to reduce hepatic first-pass metabolism and limit the formation of the amphetamine metabolites.

Unlike selegiline, rasagiline does not give rise to undesirable amphetamine metabolites. Rasagiline monotherapy is effective in early PD. Adjunctive therapy with rasagiline significantly reduces levodopa-related "wearing off" symptoms in advanced PD. Although selective MAO-B inhibitors are generally well tolerated, drug interactions can be troublesome. Similar to the nonspecific MAO inhibitors, selegiline can lead to the development of stupor, rigidity, agitation, and hyperthermia when administered with the analgesic meperidine. Although the mechanics of this interaction is uncertain, selegiline or rasagiline should not be given in combination with meperidine. Adverse effects, although uncommon, have been reported from coadministration of MAO-B inhibitors with tricyclic antidepressants or with serotonin-reuptake inhibitors.

MUSCARINIC RECEPTOR ANTAGONISTS. Antimuscarinic drugs currently used in the treatment of PD include trihexyphenidyl and benztropine mesylate, as well as the antihistaminic diphenhydramine hydrochloride, which also interacts at central muscarinic receptors. The biological basis for the therapeutic actions of muscarinic antagonists is not completely understood. They may act within the neostriatum through the receptors that normally mediate the response to intrinsic cholinergic innervation of this structure, which arises primarily from cholinergic striatal interneurons.

These drugs have relatively modest antiparkinsonian activity and are used only in the treatment of early PD or as an adjunct to dopamimetic therapy. Adverse effects result from their anticholinergic properties. Most troublesome are sedation and mental confusion. All anticholinergic drugs must be used with caution in patients with narrow-angle glaucoma (*see* Chapter 64). The pharmacology and signaling mechanisms of muscarinic receptors are thoroughly covered in Chapter 9.

AMANTADINE. Amantadine (SYMMETREL), an antiviral agent used for the prophylaxis and treatment of influenza A (*see* Chapter 58), has antiparkinsonian activity. Amantadine appears to alter DA release in the striatum, has anticholinergic properties, and blocks NMDA glutamate receptors. It is used as initial therapy of mild PD. It also may be helpful as an adjunct in patients on levodopa with dose-related fluctuations and dyskinesias. Amantadine is usually administered at a dose of

100 mg twice a day and is well tolerated. Dizziness, lethargy, anticholinergic effects, and sleep disturbance, as well as nausea and vomiting, these effects are mild and reversible.

NEUROPROTECTIVE TREATMENTS FOR PARKINSON DISEASE. Inhibition of MAO-B in the brain reduces the overall catabolism of DA, which may decrease the formation of potentially toxic-free radicals and consequently the rate of neurodegeneration in PD. In a recent study, rasagiline has been reported to have a neuroprotective effect. Another strategy under study is the use of compounds that augment cellular energy metabolism such coenzyme Q10, a cofactor required for the mitochondrial electron-transport chain. A small study has demonstrated that this drug is well tolerated in PD and has suggested that coenzyme Q10 may slow the course of the disease.

CLINICAL SUMMARY. Pharmacological treatment of PD should be tailored to the individual patient. Drug therapy is not obligatory in early PD; many patients can be managed for a time with exercise and lifestyle interventions. For patients with mild symptoms, MAO-B inhibitors, amantadine, or (in younger patients) anticholinergics are reasonable choices. In most patients, treatment with a dopaminergic drug, either levodopa or a DA agonist, is eventually required. Practitioners prefer DA agonist as initial therapy in younger patients in order to reduce the occurrence of motor complications. In older patients or those with substantial comorbidity, levodopa/carbidopa is generally better tolerated.

ALZHEIMER DISEASE (AD)

CLINICAL OVERVIEW. The brain region most vulnerable to neuronal dysfunction and cell loss in AD is the medial temporal lobe, including entorhinal cortex and hippocampus. Typical early AD symptoms are due to dysfunction of these structures resulting in anterograde episodic memory loss: repeated questions, misplaced items, missed appointments, and forgotten details of daily life. A typical patient presents with memory dysfunction that is noticeable but not severe enough to impair daily function. Because current diagnostic criteria for AD require the presence of dementia (i.e., cognitive impairments sufficient to reduce function), these patients are generally given a diagnosis of mild cognitive impairment (MCI). Patients with MCI progress at a rate of about 10% per year to AD, although not all MCI patients will develop AD. Gradual but relentless progression in AD involves other cognitive domains including visuospatial and executive function. The later stages of the disease are characterized by increasing dependence and progression toward the akinetic-mute state that typifies end-stage neurologic disease. Death, most often from a complication of immobility such as pneumonia or pulmonary embolism, usually ensues within 6-12 years of onset.

GENETICS. Mutations in 3 genes have been identified as causes of autosomal dominant, early onset AD: *APP*, which encodes amyloid-β precursor protein, and *PSEN1* and *PSEN2,* encoding presenilin 1 and 2. All 3 genes are involved in the production of amyloid-β peptides (Aβ). Aβ is generated by sequential proteolytic cleavage of APP by 2 enzymes, β-secretase and γ-secretase; the presenilins form the catalytic core of γ -secretase. The genetic evidence, combined with the fact that Aβ accumulates in the brain in the form of soluble oligomers and amyloid plaques, and is toxic when applied to neurons, forms the basis for the amyloid hypothesis of AD pathogenesis. Many genes have been identified as having alleles that increase AD risk. By far the most important of these is *APOE*, which encodes the lipid carrier protein apoE. Individuals inheriting the ε4 allele of *APOE* have a more than 3-fold higher risk of developing AD. While they make up less than one-fourth of the population, they account for more than half of all AD cases.

PATHOPHYSIOLOGY. The pathological hallmarks of AD are amyloid plaques, which are extracellular accumulations of Aβ, and intracellular neurofibrillary tangles composed of the microtubule-associated protein tau. While the development of amyloid plaques is an early and invariant feature of AD, tangle burden accrues over time in a manner that correlates more closely with the development of cognitive impairment. In autosomal dominant AD, Aβ accumulates due to mutations that cause its overproduction. Aggregation of Aβ is an important event in AD pathogenesis. While plaques consist of highly ordered fibrils of Aβ, it appears that soluble Aβ oligomers, perhaps as small as dimers, are more highly pathogenic. Tau also aggregates to form the paired helical filaments that make up neurofibrillary tangles. Posttranslational modifications of tau including phosphorylation, proteolysis, and other changes cause loss of tau's normal functions and increase its propensity to aggregate. Mechanisms by which Aβ and tau induce neuronal dysfunction and death may include direct impairment of synaptic transmission and plasticity, excitotoxicity, oxidative stress, and neuroinflammation.

NEUROCHEMISTRY. The most striking neurochemical disturbance in AD is a deficiency of acetylcholine. The anatomical basis of the cholinergic deficit is atrophy and degeneration of subcortical cholinergic neurons. The selective deficiency of ACh in AD and the observation that central cholinergic antagonists (e.g., atropine) can induce a confusional state resembling the dementia of AD, have given rise to the "*cholinergic hypothesis*" that a deficiency of ACh is critical in the genesis of the AD symptoms. AD, however, is complex and also involves multiple neurotransmitter systems, including glutamate, 5-HT, and neuropeptides, and there is destruction of not only cholinergic neurons but also the cortical and hippocampal targets that receive cholinergic input.

TREATMENT OF ALZHEIMER DISEASE

At present, no disease-modifying therapy for AD is available; current treatment is aimed at alleviating symptoms.

TREATMENT OF COGNITIVE SYMPTOMS. Augmentation of the cholinergic transmission is currently the mainstay of AD treatment. Three drugs, donepezil, rivastigmine, and galantamine, are widely used for this purpose; a fourth, tacrine, is rarely used now because of its extensive side effects compared to the newer agents (Table 22–2). All 4 agents are reversible antagonists of cholinesterases (*see* Chapter 10). Cholinesterase inhibitors are the usual first-line therapy for symptomatic treatment of cognitive impairments in mild or moderate AD. They are also widely used to treat other neurodegenerative diseases with cholinergic deficits, including dementia with Lewy bodies and vascular dementia. The drugs are usually well tolerated, with the most common side effects being GI distress, muscle cramping, and abnormal dreams. They should be use with caution in patients with bradycardia or syncope.

Memantine (NAMENDA) is used either as an adjunct or an alternative to cholinesterase inhibitors in AD, and is also commonly used to treat other neurodegenerative dementias. Memantine is a noncompetitive antagonist of the NMDA-type glutamate receptor. Memantine significantly reduces the rate of clinical deterioration in patients with moderate to severe AD. Adverse effects of memantine include mild headache or dizziness. The drug is excreted by the kidneys, and dosage should be reduced in patients with severe renal impairment.

TREATMENT OF BEHAVIORAL SYMPTOMS. In addition to cognitive decline, behavioral and psychiatric symptoms in dementia (BPSD) are common, particularly in middle stages of the disease. These symptoms include irritability and agitation, paranoia and delusional thinking, wandering, anxiety, and depression. Treatment can be difficult, and nonpharmacological approaches should generally be first-line.

A variety of pharmacological options are also available. Both cholinesterase inhibitors and memantine reduce some BPSD. However, their effects are modest, and they do not treat some of the most troublesome symptoms, such as agitation. Atypical antipsychotics, such as risperidone, olanzapine, and quetiapine (*see* Chapter 16),

Table 22–2

Cholinesterase Inhibitors Used for the Treatment of Alzheimer Disease

	DONEPEZIL	RIVASTIGMINE	GALANTAMINE	TACRINE[a]
Target[b]	AChE	AChE, BuChE	AChE	AChE, BuChE
Mechanism	Noncompetitive	Noncompetitive	Competitive	Noncompetitive
Typical maintenance dose[c]	10 mg once daily	9.5 mg/24h (transdermal) 3-6 mg 2x daily (oral)	8-12 mg 2x daily (immediate-release) 16-24 mg/day (extended-release)	20 mg 4x daily
FDA-approved indications	Mild-severe AD	Mild-moderate AD Mild-moderate PDD[d]	Mild-moderate AD	Mild-moderate AD
Metabolism[e]	CYP2D6, 3A4	Esterases	CYP2D6, 3A4	CYP1A2

[a]*Tacrine is now rarely used because of hepatotoxicity and adverse effects.*
[b]*AChE (acetylcholinesterase) is the major cholinesterase in the brain; BuChE (butyrylcholinesterase) is a serum and hepatic cholinesterase that is upregulated in AD brain.*
[c]*Typical starting doses are one-half of the maintenance dose and are given for the first month of therapy.*
[d]*PDD, Parkinson disease dementia.*
[e]*Drugs metabolized by CYP2D6 and CYP3A4 are subject to increased serum levels when coadministered with drugs known to inhibit these enzymes, such as ketoconazole and paroxetine. CYP1A2 inhibitors theophylline, cimetidine, and fluvoxamine will increase tacrine levels.*

are the most efficacious therapy for agitation and psychosis in AD. Risperidone and olanzapine are effective, but their use is often limited by adverse effects, including parkinsonism, sedation, and falls. In addition, the use of atypical antipsychotics in elderly patients with dementia-related psychosis has been associated with a higher risk of stroke and overall mortality. Benzodiazepines (*see* Chapter 17) can be used for occasional control of acute agitation, but are not recommended for long-term management because of their adverse effects on cognition and other risks in the elderly population. The typical antipsychotic haloperidol (*see* Chapter 16) may be useful for aggression, but sedation and extrapyramidal symptoms limit its use to control of acute episodes. Antidepressants (*see* Chapter 15) can be useful for BPSD, particularly when depression or anxiety contribute. Trazodone has modest benefits, but for the most part, selective serotonin reuptake inhibitors (SSRIs) are the preferred class of drugs.

CLINICAL SUMMARY. The typical AD patient presenting in early stages of disease should probably be treated with a cholinesterase inhibitor. Patients and families should be counseled that a realistic goal of therapy is to induce a temporary reprieve from progression, or at least a reduction in the rate of decline, rather than long-term recovery of cognition. As the disease progresses, memantine can be added to the regimen. Behavioral symptoms are often treated with a serotonergic antidepressant or, if they are severe enough to warrant the risk of higher mortality, an atypical antipsychotic. Eliminating drugs likely to aggravate cognitive impairments, particularly anticholinergics, benzodiazepines, and other sedative/hypnotics, from the patient's regimen is another important aspect of AD pharmacotherapy.

HUNTINGTON DISEASE (HD)

HD is a dominantly inherited disorder characterized by the gradual onset of motor incoordination and cognitive decline in midlife. Symptoms develop insidiously, either as a movement disorder manifest by brief, jerk-like movements of the extremities, trunk, face, and neck (chorea) or as personality changes or both. Fine-motor incoordination and impairment of rapid eye movements are early features. As the disorder progresses, the involuntary movements become more severe, dysarthria and dysphagia develop, and balance is impaired. The cognitive disorder manifests first as slowness of mental processing and difficulty in organizing complex tasks. Memory is impaired, but affected persons rarely lose their memory of family, friends, and the immediate situation. Such persons often become irritable, anxious, and depressed. The outcome of HD is invariably fatal; over a course of 15-30 years, the affected person becomes totally disabled and unable to communicate, requiring full-time care; death ensues from the complications of immobility.

PATHOLOGY AND PATHOPHYSIOLOGY. HD is characterized by prominent neuronal loss in the striatum (caudate/putamen) of the brain. Atrophy of these structures proceeds in an orderly fashion, first affecting the tail of the caudate nucleus and then proceeding anteriorly from mediodorsal to ventrolateral. Other areas of the brain also are affected. Interneurons and afferent terminals are largely spared, whereas the striatal projection neurons (the medium spiny neurons) are severely affected. This leads to large decreases in striatal GABA concentrations, whereas somatostatin and DA concentrations are relatively preserved.

Selective vulnerability also appears to underlie the development of chorea. In most adult-onset cases, the medium spiny neurons that project to the GPi and SNpr (the indirect pathway) appear to be affected earlier than those projecting to the GPe (the direct pathway; *see* Figure 22–2). The disproportionate impairment of the indirect pathway increases excitatory drive to the neocortex, producing involuntary choreiform movements (Figure 22–6). In some individuals, rigidity rather than chorea is the predominant clinical feature; this is especially common in juvenile-onset cases. Here, the striatal neurons giving rise to both the direct and indirect pathways are impaired to a comparable degree.

GENETICS. HD is an autosomal dominant disorder with nearly complete penetrance. The average age of onset is between 35 and 45 years, but the range varies from as early as age 2 to as late as the middle 80s. Although the disease is inherited equally from mother and father, more than 80% of those developing symptoms before age 20 inherit the defect from the father. Known homozygotes for HD show clinical characteristics identical to the typical HD heterozygote, indicating that the unaffected chromosome does not attenuate the disease symptomatology.

A region near the end of the short arm of chromosome 4 contains a polymorphic $(CAG)_n$ trinucleotide repeat that is significantly expanded in all individuals with HD. The expansion of this trinucleotide repeat is the genetic alteration responsible for HD. The range of CAG repeat length in normal individuals is between 9 and 34 triplets, with a median repeat length on normal chromosomes of 19. The repeat length in HD varies from 40 to over 100. Repeat length is correlated inversely with age of onset of HD. The younger the age of onset, the higher the probability of a large repeat number. The mechanism by which the expanded trinucleotide repeat leads to the clinical and pathological features of HD is unknown. The HD mutation lies within a large gene

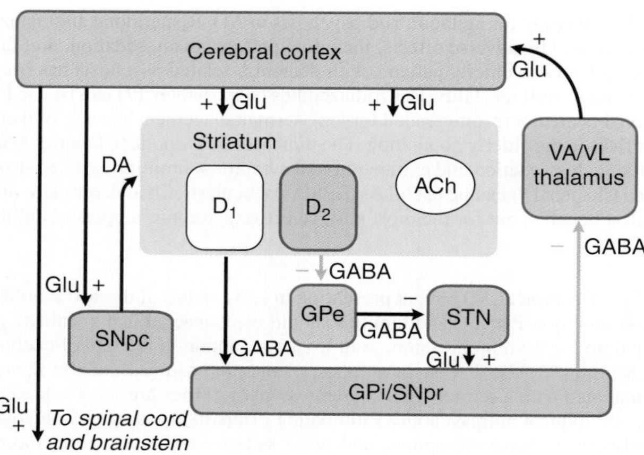

Figure 22–6 *The basal ganglia in Huntington disease.* HD is characterized by loss of neurons from the striatum. The neurons that project from the striatum to the GPe and form the indirect pathway are affected earlier in the course of the disease than those that project to the GPi. This leads to a loss of inhibition of the GPe. The increased activity in this structure, in turn, inhibits the STN, SNpr, and GPi, resulting in a loss of inhibition to the VA/VL thalamus and increased thalamocortical excitatory drive. *Structures in purple* have reduced activity in HD, whereas structures in *red* have increased activity. *Light blue lines* indicate primary pathways of reduced activity. (See legend to Figure 22–2 for definitions of anatomical abbreviations.)

(10 kilobases) designated *IT15*. It encodes a protein of ~348,000 Da. The trinucleotide repeat, which encodes the amino acid glutamine, occurs at the 5′ end of *IT15* and is followed directly by a second, shorter repeat of $(CCG)_n$ that encodes proline. The protein, *huntingtin*, does not resemble any other known protein, and the normal function of the protein has not been identified.

TREATMENT OF HUNTINGTON DISEASE

SYMPTOMATIC TREATMENT. None of the currently available medications slows the progression of the disease.

Symptomatic treatment is needed for patients who are depressed, irritable, paranoid, excessively anxious, or psychotic. Depression can be treated effectively with standard antidepressant drugs with the caveat that drugs with substantial anticholinergic profiles can exacerbate chorea. Fluoxetine (*see* Chapter 15) is effective treatment for both the depression and the irritability manifest in symptomatic HD. Carbamazepine (*see* Chapter 21) also has been found to be effective for depression. Paranoia, delusional states, and psychosis are treated with antipsychotic drugs, but usually at lower doses than those used in primary psychiatric disorders (*see* Chapter 16). These agents also reduce cognitive function and impair mobility and thus should be used in the lowest doses possible and should be discontinued when the psychiatric symptoms resolve. In individuals with predominantly rigid HD, clozapine, quetiapine (*see* Chapter 16), or carbamazepine may be more effective for treatment of paranoia and psychosis.

Tetrabenazine (XENAZINE, NITOMAN) is available for the treatment of large-amplitude chorea associated with HD. Tetrabenazine, and the related drug reserpine, are inhibitors of the vesicular monoamine transporter 2 (VMAT2), and cause presynaptic depletion of catecholamines. Tetrabenazine is a reversible inhibitor; inhibition by reserpine is irreversible and may lead to long-lasting effects. Both drugs may cause hypotension and depression with suicidality; the shorter duration of effect of tetrabenazine greatly simplifies the clinical management. Many HD patients exhibit worsening of involuntary movements as a result of anxiety or stress. In these situations, judicious use of sedative or anxiolytic benzodiazepines can be very helpful. In juvenile-onset cases where rigidity rather than chorea predominates, DA agonists have had variable success in the improvement of rigidity. These individuals also occasionally develop myoclonus and seizures that can be responsive to clonazepam, valproic acid, and other anticonvulsants (*see* Chapter 21).

AMYOTROPHIC LATERAL SCLEROSIS (ALS)

ALS (or Lou Gehrig disease) is a disorder of the motor neurons of the ventral horn of the spinal cord (lower motor neurons) and the cortical neurons that provide their afferent input (upper motor neurons). The disorder is characterized by rapidly progressive weakness, muscle atrophy and fasciculations, spasticity, dysarthria, dysphagia, and respiratory compromise. Many ALS patients exhibit behavioral changes and cognitive dysfunction, and there is clinical, genetic, and neuropathological overlap between ALS and frontotemporal dementia spectrum disorders. ALS usually is progressive and fatal. Most patients die of respiratory compromise and pneumonia after 2-3 years, although some survive for many years.

ETIOLOGY. About 10% of ALS cases are familial (FALS), usually with an autosomal dominant pattern of inheritance. An important subset of FALS patients are families with a mutation in the gene for the enzyme SOD1. Mutations in this protein account for about 20% of cases of FALS. Mutations in the *TARDBP* gene encoding TAR DNA-binding protein (TDP-43) and in the *FUS/TLS* gene have been identified as causes of FALS. Both TDP-43 and FUS/TLS bind DNA and RNA, and regulate transcription and alternative splicing. More than 90% of ALS cases are sporadic. Of these, a few are caused by de novo mutations in *SOD1*, *TDP-43*, *FUS/TLS*, or other genes, but for the majority of sporadic cases the etiology remains unclear. There is evidence that glutamate reuptake may be abnormal in the disease, leading to accumulation of glutamate and excitotoxic injury. The only currently approved therapy for ALS, riluzole, is based on these observations.

TREATMENT OF ALS

RILUZOLE. Riluzole (2-amino-6-[trifluoromethoxy] benzothiazole; RILUTEK) is an agent with complex actions in the nervous system.

Riluzole is absorbed orally and is highly protein bound. It undergoes extensive metabolism in the liver by both CYP–mediated hydroxylation and glucuronidation. Its $t_{1/2}$ is ~12 h. In vitro studies have shown that riluzole has both presynaptic and postsynaptic effects. It inhibits glutamate release, but it also blocks postsynaptic NMDA- and kainate-type glutamate receptors and inhibits voltage-dependent Na^+ channels. The recommended dose is 50 mg twice daily, taken 1 h before or 2 h after a meal. Riluzole usually is well tolerated, although nausea or diarrhea may occur. Rarely, riluzole may produce hepatic injury with elevations of serum transaminases, and periodic monitoring of these is recommended. Meta-analyses of the available clinical trials indicate that riluzole extends survival by 2-3 months. Although the magnitude of the effect of riluzole on ALS is small, it represents a significant therapeutic milestone in the treatment of a disease refractory to all previous treatments.

SYMPTOMATIC THERAPY OF ALS: SPASTICITY. Spasticity is an important component of the clinical features of ALS and the feature most amenable to present forms of treatment. *Spasticity* is defined as an increase in muscle tone characterized by an initial resistance to passive displacement of a limb at a joint, followed by a sudden relaxation (the so-called clasped-knife phenomenon). Spasticity results from loss of descending inputs to the spinal motor neurons, and the character of the spasticity depends on which nervous system pathways are affected.

Baclofen. The best agent for the symptomatic treatment of spasticity in ALS is baclofen (LIORESAL), a $GABA_B$ receptor agonist. Initial doses of 5-10 mg/day are recommended, which can be increased to as much as 200 mg/day if necessary. Alternatively, baclofen can be delivered directly into the space around the spinal cord using a surgically implanted pump and an intrathecal catheter. This approach minimizes the adverse effects of the drug, especially sedation, but it carries the risk of potentially life-threatening CNS depression.

Tizanidine. Tizanidine (ZANAFLEX) is an agonist of α_2 adrenergic receptors in the CNS. It reduces muscle spasticity, probably by increasing presynaptic inhibition of motor neurons. Tizanidine is primarily used in the treatment of spasticity in multiple sclerosis or after stroke, but it also may be effective in patients with ALS. Treatment should be initiated at a low dose of 2-4 mg at bedtime and titrated upward gradually. Drowsiness, asthenia, and dizziness may limit the dose that can be administered.

Other Agents. Benzodiazepines (*see* Chapter 17) such as clonazepam (KLONOPIN) are effective antispasticity agents, but they may contribute to respiratory depression in patients with advanced ALS.

Dantrolene (DANTRIUM), approved in the U.S. for the treatment of muscle spasm, is not used in ALS because it can exacerbate muscular weakness. Dantrolene acts directly on skeletal muscle fibers, impairing Ca^{2+} release from the sarcoplasmic reticulum. It is effective in treating spasticity associated with stroke or spinal cord injury and in treating malignant hyperthermia (*see* Chapter 11). Dantrolene may cause hepatotoxicity, so it is important to monitor liver associated enzymes before and during therapy with the drug.

For a complete Bibliographical Listing see Goodman & Gilman's ***The Pharmacological Basis of Therapeutics***, 12th ed., or Goodman & Gilman Online at www.AccessMedicine.com.

23 chapter Ethanol and Methanol

The 2-carbon alcohol ethanol (CH_3CH_2OH), or beverage alcohol, is one of the most versatile drugs known to man, with multiple direct effects on a diverse range of neurochemical systems. Produced in nature, rewarding in its effects, and easy to manufacture, it has been taken by humans since the beginning of recorded history, is consumed by a large majority of people in the Western world, and is likely to contribute to more morbidity, mortality, and public health costs than all of the illicit drugs combined.

ETHANOL CONSUMPTION. Compared with other drugs, surprisingly large amounts of alcohol are required for physiological effects, resulting in its consumption more as a food than a drug. The alcohol content of beverages typically ranges from 4-6% (volume/volume) for beer, 10-15% for wine, and 40% and higher for distilled spirits (the "proof" of an alcoholic beverage is twice its percentage of alcohol; e.g., 40% alcohol is 80 proof). A glass of beer or wine, a mixed drink, or a shot of spirits contains ~14 g alcohol, or ~0.3 mol ethanol. Thus, alcohol is consumed in gram quantities, whereas most other drugs are taken in milligram or microgram doses.

Because the ratio of ethanol in end-expiratory alveolar air and ethanol in the blood is relatively consistent, blood ethanol concentrations (BECs) in humans can be estimated readily by the measurement of alcohol levels in expired air; the partition coefficient for ethanol between blood and alveolar air is approximately 2000:1. Because of the causal relationship between excessive alcohol consumption and vehicular accidents, there has been a near-universal adoption of laws attempting to limit the operation of vehicles while under the influence of alcohol. Legally allowed BECs in the U.S. typically are set at or below 80 mg% (80 mg ethanol per 100 mL blood; 0.08% w/v), which is equivalent to a concentration of 17 mM ethanol in blood. A 12-oz bottle of beer, a 5-oz glass of wine, and a 1.5-oz "shot" of 40% liquor each contains approximately 14 g ethanol, and the consumption of 1 of these beverages by a 70-kg person would produce a BEC of ~30 mg%. However, it is important to note that this is approximate because the BEC is determined by a number of factors, including the rate of drinking, gender, body weight and water percentage, and the rates of metabolism and stomach emptying (see "Acute Ethanol Intoxication" later in the chapter).

PHARMACOLOGICAL PROPERTIES

ETHANOL

ABSORPTION. After oral administration, ethanol is absorbed rapidly into the bloodstream from the stomach and small intestine and distributes into total-body water (0.5-0.7 L/kg). Peak blood levels occur about 30 min after ingestion of ethanol when the stomach is empty. Because absorption occurs more rapidly from the small intestine than from the stomach, delays in gastric emptying (owing, e.g., to the presence of food) slow ethanol absorption. Because of first-pass metabolism by gastric and liver alcohol dehydrogenase (ADH), oral ingestion of ethanol leads to lower BECs than would be obtained if the same quantity were administered intravenously. Gastric metabolism of ethanol is lower in women than in men, which may contribute to the greater susceptibility of women to ethanol. *Aspirin* increases ethanol bioavailability by inhibiting gastric ADH.

METABOLISM. Ethanol is metabolized largely (90-98%) by sequential hepatic oxidation, first to acetaldehyde by ADH and then to acetic acid by aldehyde dehydrogenase (ALDH) (Figure 23–1). Each metabolic step requires NAD^+; this greatly exceeds the supply of NAD^+ in the liver and NAD^+ availability limits ethanol metabolism to ~8 g or 10 mL (~170 mmol) per hour in a 70-kg adult, or ~120 mg/kg/h. Thus, hepatic ethanol metabolism functionally saturates at relatively low blood levels compared with the high BECs achieved, and ethanol metabolism is a zero-order process (constant amount per unit time). Small amounts of ethanol are excreted in urine, sweat, and breath.

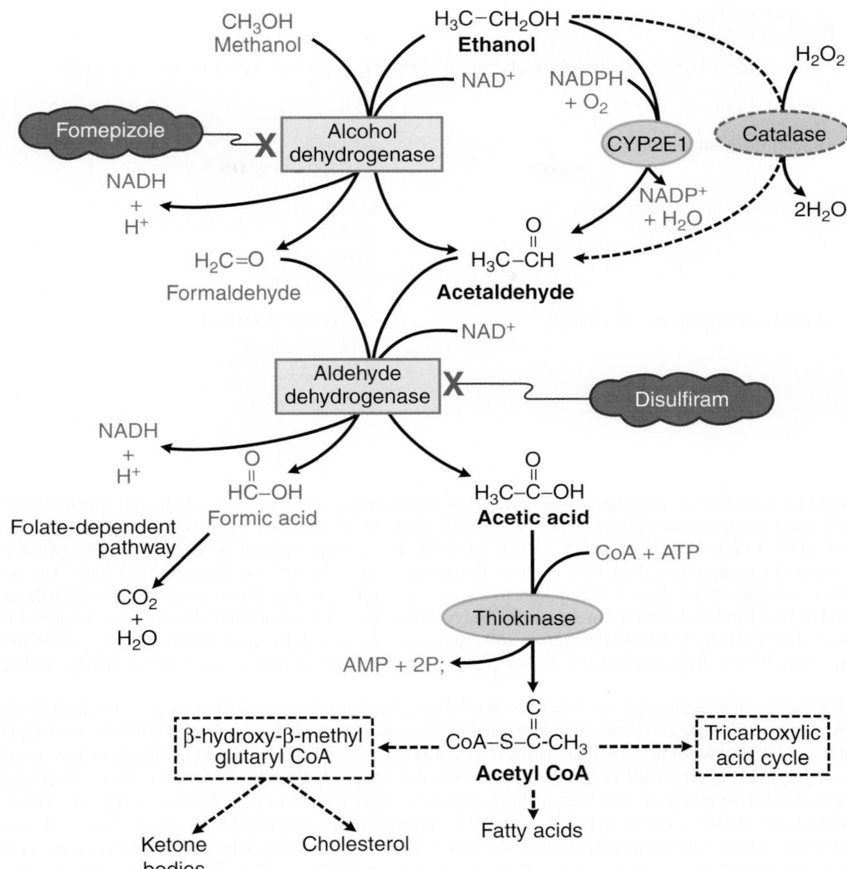

Figure 23–1 *Metabolism of ethanol and methanol.*

CYP2E1 also can contribute, especially at higher ethanol concentrations. CYP2E1 is induced by chronic consumption of ethanol, increasing the clearance of its substrates and the activation of certain toxins such as CCl_4. There can be decreased clearance of the same drugs, however, after acute consumption of ethanol because ethanol competes with them for oxidation by the enzyme system (e.g., phenytoin and warfarin).

The large increase in the hepatic NADH:NAD^+ ratio during ethanol oxidation has profound consequences in addition to limiting the rate of ethanol metabolism. Enzymes requiring NAD^+ are inhibited; thus, lactate accumulates, activity of the tricarboxylic acid cycle is reduced, and acetyl coenzyme A (acetyl CoA) accumulates (and it is produced in quantity from ethanol-derived acetic acid; *see* Figure 23–1). The combination of increased NADH and elevated–acetyl CoA supports fatty acid synthesis and the storage and accumulation of triacylglycerides; ketone bodies accrue, exacerbating lactic acidosis. Ethanol metabolism by the CYP2E1 pathway produces elevated $NADP^+$, limiting the availability of NADPH for the regeneration of reduced glutathione (GSH), thereby enhancing oxidative stress.

Genetic Variation in Ethanol Metabolism. The enzymes involved in ethanol metabolism are mainly ADH and ALDH, and secondarily, catalase and CYP2E1. CYPs 1A2 and 3A4 may also participate. Several of these enzymes have genetic variants that alter alcohol metabolism and susceptibility to its effects.

The genetics of the ADH isoforms are important for understanding risk factors for severe repetitive ethanol problems. The 3 relevant forms are ADH1A, 1B, and 1C. These class I ADHs have K_m <34 mmol (0.15 g/dL) and are responsible for 70% of the ethanol metabolizing capacity at BECs of 22 mM (i.e., ~0.10 g/dL). These ADH forms are the rate-limiting step in ethanol metabolism, reducing the BECs by ~4-5 mM (0.015-0.020 g/dL) per hour, the approximate levels of alcohol resulting from the consumption of 1 standard drink.

Table 23–1

Genes for Intermediate Phenotypes Affecting Risk for Alcohol Use Disorder

PHENOTYPE	GENES
Facial flush after drinking	ALDH2 ADH1B, ADH1C
Impulsivity and disinhibition	GABRA2 ADH4 CHRM2 DRD2, DRD4
Low level of response to ethanol	GABRA1, GABRA6 5HTT promoter KCNMA1 CHRN cluster

The ADH1A gene has no polymorphisms known to significantly affect the rate of alcohol metabolism. The ADH1B gene has a polymorphism, ADH1B*2, with arginine 47 replaced by histidine to produce a variant form of ADH with a 40-fold higher V_{max} than ADH1B. This polymorphism is seen in 30-45% of Chinese, Japanese, and Koreans, less than 10% of most Europeans, but in 50-90% of Russians and Jews. The potential faster metabolism of ethanol may result in a transient slightly higher blood level of acetaldehyde and is reported to be associated with a lower risk for heavy drinking and ethanol-related problems. A second polymorphism for ADH1B, ADH1B*3 (arginine 269 replaced by cysteine), has a 30-fold higher V_{max}. ADHlB*3 is seen in about 30% of Africans and also is associated with lower risk of heavy drinking and ethanol problems.

Acetaldehyde is produced from the breakdown of ethanol at the rate of approximately 1 standard drink per hour. As shown in Figure 23–1, the acetaldehyde is then rapidly broken down through the actions of ALDH2, primarily in the mitochondria of liver cells. The actions of ALDH2 are important because low levels of acetaldehyde may be perceived as rewarding and stimulating, while high blood levels of this substance produce severe adverse reactions that can include vomiting, diarrhea, and unstable blood pressure. There is a mutation in the ALDH2 gene (12q24), ALDH2*2 (resulting from a substitution of glycine 487 with lysine). Homozygotes with a nonfunctional ALDH2*2 occur in 5-10% of Japanese, Chinese, and Korean individuals, for whom severe adverse reactions occur after consumption of 1 drink or less. This reaction operates through the same mechanism that occurs with drinking after taking the ALDH2 inhibitor, disulfiram. Heterozygotes for this polymorphism (ALDH2*2, 2*1) make up 30-40% of Asian individuals who, after consuming ethanol experience a facial flush and an enhanced sensitivity to beverage alcohol, but who do not necessarily report an overall adverse response to the drug. A number of these polymorphisms affect risk for alcohol use disorder (Table 23–1).

METHANOL

Methanol (CH_3OH), is also known as methyl and wood alcohol. It is an important industrial reagent and solvent found in products such as paint removers, shellac, and antifreeze; methanol is added to industrial-use ethanol to mark it unsafe for human consumption.

Absorption and Metabolism. Methanol is rapidly absorbed via the oral route, inhalation, and through the skin, with the latter 2 routes most relevant to industrial settings. Methanol is metabolized by ADH and ALDH. Competition between methanol and ethanol for ADH forms the basis of the use of ethanol in methanol poisoning. Several drugs inhibit alcohol metabolism, including fomepizole (4-methylpyrazole), an ADH inhibitor useful in ethylene glycol poisoning, and *disulfiram,* an ALDH inhibitor used in treating alcoholism.

Feelings of intoxication from methanol, while similar in many ways to those with ethanol, are less intense, and often delayed by 8 or more hours from ingestion, progressing even more slowly if methanol is taken along with ethanol. As little as 15 mL of methanol can produce toxicity, including blindness, with doses in excess of 70 mL capable of producing death. Methanol poisoning consists of headache, GI distress, and pain (partially related to pancreatic injury), difficulty breathing, restlessness, and blurred vision associated with hyperemic optic disks. Severe metabolic acidosis can develop due to the accumulation of formic acid, and the respiratory depression can be severe, especially in the context of coma. The visual disturbances occur as a consequence of injury to ganglion cells of the retina by the metabolite, formic acid, with subsequent inflammation, atrophy, and potential bilateral blindness. The clinical picture can also include necrosis of the pancreas.

William Shakespeare described the acute pharmacological effects of imbibing ethanol in the Porter scene (act 2, scene 3) of *Macbeth*. The Porter, awakened from an alcohol-induced sleep by Macduff, explains three effects of alcohol and then wrestles with a fourth effect that combines the contradictory aspects of soaring overconfidence with physical impairment:

> **Porter:** . . . and drink, sir, is a great provoker of three things.
> **Macduff:** What three things does drink especially provoke?
> **Porter:** Marry, sir, nose-painting [*cutaneous vasodilation*], sleep [*CNS depression*], and urine [*a consequence of the inhibition of antidiuretic hormone (vasopressin) secretion, exacerbated by volume loading*]. Lechery, sir, it provokes and unprovokes: it provokes the desire but it takes away the performance. Therefore much drink may be said to be an equivocator with lechery: it makes him and it mars him; it sets him on and it takes him off; it persuades him and disheartens him, makes him stand to and not stand to [*the imagination desires what the corpus cavernosum cannot deliver*]; in conclusion, equivocates him in a sleep, and, giving him the lie, leaves him.

More recent research has added details to Shakespeare's enumeration—see the bracketed additions to the Porter's words in the preceding paragraph and the section on organ systems later in the chapter—but the most noticeable consequences of the recreational use of ethanol still are well summarized by the gregarious and garrulous Porter, whose delighted and devilish demeanor demonstrates frequently observed influences of modest concentrations of ethanol on the CNS.

CENTRAL NERVOUS SYSTEM

Although the public often views alcoholic drinks as stimulating, ethanol primarily is a CNS depressant. Ingestion of moderate amounts of ethanol, like that of other depressants such as barbiturates and benzodiazepines, can have antianxiety actions and produce behavioral disinhibition at a wide range of dosages. Individual signs of intoxication vary from expansive and vivacious affect to uncontrolled mood swings and emotional outbursts that may have violent components. With more severe intoxication, CNS function generally is impaired, and a condition of general anesthesia ultimately prevails. However, there is little margin between the anesthetic actions and lethal effects (usually owing to respiratory depression).

Chronic alcohol abuse is accompanied by tolerance, dependence, and craving for the drug. Alcoholism is characterized by compulsive use despite clearly deleterious social and medical consequences. Alcoholism is a progressive illness, and brain damage from chronic alcohol abuse contributes to the deficits in cognitive functioning and judgment seen in alcoholics. Alcoholism is a leading cause of dementia in the U.S. Chronic alcohol abuse results in shrinkage of the brain owing to loss of both white and gray matter. In addition to loss of brain tissue, alcohol abuse also reduces brain metabolism, and this hypometabolic state rebounds to a level of increased metabolism during detoxification. The magnitude of decrease in metabolic state is determined by the number of years of alcohol use and the age of the patients.

Actions of Ethanol on Neurochemical Pathways and Signaling. Ethanol affects almost all brain systems. The changes across neural pathways occur simultaneously and the alterations often interact. An additional complication in describing CNS effects is the rapid adaptation to ethanol observed in the brain, with the result that the acute effects of the first dose of ethanol are often the opposite of the neurochemical consequences from repeated administration and those observed during falling blood ethanol levels and withdrawal syndromes. Alcohol perturbs the balance between excitatory and inhibitory influences in the brain, resulting in anxiolysis, ataxia, and sedation. This is accomplished by either enhancing inhibitory or antagonizing excitatory neurotransmission. The 12th edition of the parent text summarizes research supporting effects of ethanol on a number of ion channels and neurotransmitter signal transducing systems that alter neuronal excitability within the CNS.

Ethanol Consumption and CNS Function. Large doses of ethanol can interfere with encoding of memories, producing anterograde amnesias, commonly referred to as *alcoholic blackouts*; affected individuals are unable to recall all or part of experiences during the period of heavy intake. Perhaps reflecting the effect of ethanol on respirations as well as the muscle-relaxant effects of this drug, heavier drinking can be associated with sleep apnea, especially in older alcohol-dependent subjects. The transient CNS effects of heavy ethanol consumption that produce a hangover—the "next morning" syndrome of headache, thirst, nausea, and cognitive impairment—may reflect mechanisms similar to mild alcohol withdrawal, dehydration, and/or mild acidosis.

Chronic heavy drinking reportedly increases the probability of developing *alcoholic dementia*. The signs of cognitive deficits and brain atrophy observed soon after a heavy drinking period often reverse over the subsequent several weeks to months following abstinence. The thiamine depletion that can accompany heavy ethanol consumption contributes to Wernicke-Korsakoff syndromes. Perhaps 3% of alcohol-dependent men and women report experiencing temporary auditory hallucinations and paranoid delusions that resemble schizophrenia beginning during periods of heavy intoxication; all of these psychiatric syndromes are likely to markedly improve within several days to a month of abstinence.

CARDIOVASCULAR SYSTEM

Ethanol intake greater than 3 standard drinks per day elevates the risk for heart attacks and bleeding-related strokes. The risk includes a 6-fold increased risk for coronary artery disease, a heightened risk for cardiac arrhythmias, and an elevated rate of congestive heart failure. The causes are complex and observations are complicated by certain positive effects of small amounts of ethanol.

Serum Lipoproteins and Cardiovascular Effects. In France, the risk of mortality due to coronary heart disease (CHD) is relatively low despite the consumption of high quantities of saturated fats (the "French paradox"). Epidemiological studies suggest that widespread wine consumption (20-30 g ethanol per day) is 1 of the factors conferring a cardioprotective effect, resulting in a 10-40% decreased risk of coronary heart disease compared with abstainers. In contrast, daily consumption of greater amounts of alcohol leads to an increased incidence of non-coronary causes of cardiovascular failure, such as arrhythmias, cardiomyopathy, and hemorrhagic stroke, offsetting the beneficial effects of alcohol on coronary arteries.

One possible mechanism by which alcohol could reduce the risk of CHD is through its effects on blood lipids. Changes in plasma lipoprotein levels, particularly increases in high-density lipoprotein (HDL; *see* Chapter 31), have been associated with the protective effects of ethanol. HDL binds cholesterol and returns it to the liver for elimination or reprocessing, decreasing tissue cholesterol levels. Ethanol-induced increases in HDL-cholesterol thus could antagonize cholesterol accumulation in arterial walls, lessening the risk of infarction. HDL is found as 2 subfractions, named HDL_2 and HDL_3. Increased levels of HDL_2 (and possibly also HDL_3) are associated with reduced risk of myocardial infarction. Levels of both subfractions are increased following alcohol consumption and decrease when alcohol consumption ceases. Apolipoproteins A-I and A-II are constituents of HDL. Increased levels of both apolipoproteins A-I and A-II are associated with individuals who are daily heavy drinkers. In contrast, there are reports of decreased serum apolipoprotein(a) levels following acute alcohol consumption. Elevated apolipoprotein(a) levels have been associated with an increased risk for the development of atherosclerosis.

All forms of alcoholic beverages confer cardio-protection. The flavonoids found in red wine (and purple grape juice) may have an additional anti-atherogenic role by protecting low-density lipoprotein (LDL) from oxidative damage. Alcohol consumption also is linked to elevated levels of tissue plasminogen activator (a clot-dissolving enzyme), decreased fibrinogen concentrations, and inhibition of platelet activation.

Hypertension. Heavy alcohol use can raise diastolic and systolic blood pressure. Consumption >30 g alcohol per day (>2 standard drinks) is associated with a 1.5-2.3 mm Hg rise in diastolic and systolic blood pressure.

Cardiac Arrhythmias. Alcohol prolongs the QT interval, prolongs ventricular repolarization, and enhances sympathetic stimulation. Atrial arrhythmias associated with chronic alcohol use include supraventricular tachycardia, atrial fibrillation, and atrial flutter. Some 15-20% of idiopathic cases of atrial fibrillation may be induced by chronic ethanol use.

Cardiomyopathy. Alcohol can depress cardiac contractility and lead to cardiomyopathy. Echocardiography demonstrates global hypokinesis. Approximately half of all patients with idiopathic cardiomyopathy are alcohol-dependent. Alcohol-induced cardiomyopathy has a better prognosis if patients are able to stop drinking. Women are at greater risk of alcohol-induced cardiomyopathy than are men.

Stroke. Clinical studies indicate an increased incidence of hemorrhagic and ischemic stroke in persons who drink >40-60 g alcohol per day. Proposed etiological factors include:

- Alcohol-induced cardiac arrhythmias and associated thrombus formation
- High blood pressure from chronic alcohol consumption and subsequent cerebral artery degeneration
- Acute increases in systolic blood pressure and alterations in cerebral artery tone
- Head trauma

SKELETAL MUSCLE

Chronic, heavy, daily alcohol consumption is associated with decreased muscle strength, even when adjusted for other factors such as age, nicotine use, and chronic illness. Heavy doses of alcohol also can cause irreversible damage to muscle, reflected by a marked increase in the activity of creatine kinase in plasma. Muscle biopsies from heavy drinkers also reveal decreased glycogen stores and reduced pyruvate kinase activity. Approximately 50% of chronic heavy drinkers have evidence of type II fiber atrophy. Most patients with chronic alcoholism show evidence of a skeletal myopathy similar to alcoholic cardiomyopathy.

BODY TEMPERATURE

Ingestion of ethanol causes a feeling of warmth because alcohol enhances cutaneous and gastric blood flow. Increased sweating also may occur. Heat, therefore, is lost more rapidly, and the internal body temperature falls. After consumption of large amounts of ethanol, the central temperature-regulating mechanism becomes depressed, and the fall in body temperature may become pronounced. The action of alcohol in lowering body temperature is greater and more dangerous when the ambient environmental temperature is low. Studies of deaths from hypothermia suggest that alcohol is a major risk factor in these events.

DIURESIS

Alcohol inhibits the release of vasopressin (antidiuretic hormone) from the posterior pituitary gland, resulting in enhanced diuresis. Alcoholics withdrawing from alcohol exhibit increased vasopressin release and a consequent retention of water, as well as dilutional hyponatremia.

GI SYSTEM

Esophagus. Alcohol is 1 of multiple factors associated with esophageal dysfunction. Ethanol also is associated with the development of esophageal reflux, Barrett esophagus, traumatic rupture of the esophagus, Mallory-Weiss tears, and esophageal cancer. Compared with nonalcoholic nonsmokers, alcohol-dependent patients who smoke have a 10-fold increased risk of developing cancer of the esophagus. There is little change in esophageal function at low blood alcohol concentrations, but at higher blood alcohol concentrations, a decrease in peristalsis and decreased lower esophageal sphincter pressure occur. Patients with chronic reflux esophagitis may respond to proton pump inhibitors and abstinence from alcohol.

Stomach. Heavy alcohol use can disrupt the gastric mucosal barrier and cause acute and chronic gastritis. Ethanol appears to stimulate gastric secretions by exciting sensory nerves in the buccal and gastric mucosa and promoting the release of gastrin and histamine. Beverages containing more than 40% alcohol also have a direct toxic effect on gastric mucosa. Clinical symptoms include acute epigastric pain that is relieved with antacids or histamine H_2 receptor antagonists. Alcohol exacerbates the clinical course and severity of ulcer symptoms. It appears to act synergistically with *Helicobacter pylori* to delay healing.

Intestines. Many alcoholics have chronic diarrhea as a result of malabsorption in the small intestine. The rectal fissures and *pruritus ani* that frequently are associated with heavy drinking probably are related to chronic diarrhea. The diarrhea is caused by structural and functional changes in the small intestine; the intestinal mucosa has flattened villi, and digestive enzyme levels often are decreased. These changes frequently are reversible after a period of abstinence.

Pancreas. Heavy alcohol use is the most common cause of both acute and chronic pancreatitis in the U.S. Acute alcoholic pancreatitis is characterized by the abrupt onset of abdominal pain, nausea, vomiting, and increased levels of serum or urine pancreatic enzymes. Management usually involves intravenous fluid replacement—often with nasogastric suction—and opioid pain medication. The etiology of acute pancreatitis probably is related to a direct toxic metabolic effect of alcohol on pancreatic acinar cells. Chronic pancreatitis is treated by replacing the endocrine and exocrine deficiencies that result from pancreatic insufficiency. The development of hyperglycemia often requires insulin for control of blood-sugar levels (*see* Chapter 43). Pancreatic enzyme capsules containing lipase, amylase, and proteases may be necessary to treat malabsorption (*see* Chapter 46).

Liver. Ethanol produces dose-related deleterious effects in the liver that include fatty infiltration of the liver, hepatitis, and cirrhosis. The accumulation of fat in the liver is an early event and can occur in normal individuals after the ingestion of relatively small amounts of ethanol. This accumulation results from inhibition of both the tricarboxylic acid cycle and the oxidation of fat, in part owing to the generation of excess NADH produced by the actions of ADH and ALDH (*see* Figure 23–1). Fibrosis, resulting from tissue necrosis and chronic inflammation, is the underlying cause of alcoholic cirrhosis. Alcohol can affect stellate cells in the liver directly; chronic alcohol use is associated with transformation of stellate cells into collagen-producing, myofibroblast-like cells, resulting in deposition of collagen around terminal hepatic venules. The histological hallmark of alcoholic cirrhosis is the formation of Mallory bodies, which are thought to be related to an altered intermediate cytoskeleton. Acetaminophen-induced hepatic toxicity (*see* Chapters 4, 6, and 34) has been associated with alcoholic cirrhosis as a result of alcohol-induced increases in microsomal production of toxic acetaminophen metabolites.

VITAMINS AND MINERALS

Alcoholics often present with nutritional deficiencies owing to decreased intake, decreased absorption, or impaired utilization of nutrients. The peripheral neuropathy, Korsakoff psychosis, and Wernicke encephalopathy seen in alcoholics probably are caused by deficiencies of the B complex of vitamins (particularly thiamine). Retinol and ethanol compete for metabolism by ADH; vitamin A supplementation therefore should be monitored carefully in alcoholics when they are consuming alcohol to avoid retinol-induced hepatotoxicity. The chronic consumption of alcohol inflicts an oxidative stress on the liver owing to the generation of free radicals, contributing to ethanol-induced liver injury. The antioxidant effects of α-tocopherol (vitamin E) may ameliorate some of this ethanol-induced toxicity in the liver. Chronic alcohol consumption has been implicated in osteoporosis. Acute administration of ethanol produces an initial reduction in serum parathyroid hormone (PTH) and Ca^{2+} levels, followed by a rebound increase in PTH that does not restore Ca^{2+} levels to normal.

SEXUAL FUNCTION

Despite the widespread belief that alcohol can enhance sexual activities, the opposite effect is generally noted. Many drugs of abuse, including alcohol, have disinhibiting effects that may lead initially to increased libido. Both acute and chronic alcohol use can lead to impotence in men. Increased blood ethanol concentrations lead to decreased sexual arousal, increased ejaculatory latency, and decreased orgasmic pleasure. The incidence of impotence may be as high as 50% in patients with chronic alcoholism. Additionally, many chronic alcoholics develop testicular atrophy and decreased fertility. Gynecomastia is associated with alcoholic liver disease and is related to increased cellular response to estrogen and to accelerated metabolism of testosterone. Many female alcoholics complain of decreased libido, decreased vaginal lubrication, and menstrual cycle abnormalities. Their ovaries often are small and without follicular development. Some data suggest that fertility rates are lower for alcoholic women.

HEMATOLOGICAL AND IMMUNOLOGICAL EFFECTS

Chronic alcohol use is associated with a number of anemias including microcytic anemias, macrocytic anemias, normochromic anemias, and alcohol-induced sideroblastic anemia. Alcohol-induced sideroblastic anemia may respond to vitamin B_6 replacement. Alcohol use also is associated with reversible thrombocytopenia, although platelet counts $<20,000/mm^3$ are rare. Alcohol also affects granulocytes and lymphocytes. Effects include leukopenia, alteration of lymphocyte subsets, decreased T-cell mitogenesis, and changes in immunoglobulin production. In some patients, depressed leukocyte migration into inflamed areas may account in part for the poor resistance of alcoholics to some types of infection (e.g., *Klebsiella* pneumonia, listeriosis, and tuberculosis). In vitro studies with human lymphocytes suggest that alcohol can suppress CD4 T-lymphocyte function.

ACUTE ETHANOL INTOXICATION

Signs of intoxication typical of CNS depression are seen in most people following 2-3 drinks, with the most prominent effect seen at the times of peak BEC, ~30-60 min following consumption on an empty stomach. These symptoms include an initial feeling of stimulation (perhaps due to inhibition of CNS inhibitory systems), giddiness, muscle relaxation, and impaired judgment. Higher blood levels (~80 mg/dL or ~17 mM) are associated with slurred speech, incoordination, unsteady gait, and potential impairments of attention; levels between 80 and 200 mg/dL (~17-43 mM) are associated with more intense mood lability, and greater cognitive deficits, potentially accompanied by aggressiveness, and anterograde amnesia (an alcoholic blackout). Blood ethanol levels >200 mg/dL can produce nystagmus and unwanted falling asleep; levels of 300 mg/dL (~65 mM) and higher can produce failing vital signs, coma, and death. All of these symptoms are likely to be exacerbated and occur at a lower BEC when ethanol is taken along with other CNS depressants (e.g., diazepam or similar benzodiazepines), or with any drug or medication for which sleepiness and uncoordination are likely.

Many factors, such as body weight and composition and the rate of absorption from the GI tract, determine the concentration of ethanol in the blood after ingestion of a given amount of ethanol. On average, the ingestion of 3 standard drinks (42 g ethanol) on an empty stomach results in a maximum blood concentration of 67-92 mg/dL in men. After a mixed meal, the maximal blood concentration from 3 drinks is 30-53 mg/dL in men. For individuals with normal hepatic function, ethanol is metabolized at a rate of 1 standard drink every 60-90 min. In women with smaller body size and a lower leaner body mass (lower volume of distribution for ethanol), the equivalent consumption could produce levels about 30-50% higher, on average.

Diabetic coma, drug intoxication, cardiovascular accidents, and skull fractures may be confused with alcohol intoxication. Breath odor in a case of suspected intoxication can be misleading because there can be other causes of breath odor similar to that after alcohol consumption. Blood alcohol levels are necessary to confirm the presence or absence of alcohol intoxication.

The treatment of acute alcohol intoxication is based on the severity of respiratory and CNS depression. Patients with evidence of respiratory depression should be intubated to protect the airway and to provide ventilatory assistance. The stomach may be lavaged. Because ethanol is freely miscible with water, ethanol can be removed from blood by hemodialysis. Acute alcohol intoxication is not always associated with coma, and careful observation is the primary treatment. Usual care involves observing the patient in the emergency room for 4-6 h while the patient metabolizes the ingested ethanol. Blood ethanol levels will be reduced by

~15 mg/dL/h. Great care must be taken, however, when using sedatives to treat patients who have ingested an excessive amount of another CNS depressant, such as, ethanol, because of synergistic effects.

CLINICAL USES OF ETHANOL

Systemically administered ethanol is confined to the treatment of poisoning by methyl alcohol and ethylene glycol. Methanol ingestion results in formation of methanol's metabolites, formaldehyde and formic acid (*see* Figure 23–1). Formic acid causes nerve damage; its effects on the retina and optic nerve can cause blindness. Treatment consists of sodium bicarbonate to combat acidosis, hemodialysis, and the administration of ethanol, which slows formate production by competing with methanol for metabolism by alcohol dehydrogenase.

Dehydrated alcohol may be injected in close proximity to nerves or sympathetic ganglia to relieve the long-lasting pain related to trigeminal neuralgia, inoperable carcinoma, and other conditions. Epidural, subarachnoid, and lumbar paravertebral injections of ethanol also have been employed for inoperable pain. For example, lumbar paravertebral injections of ethanol may destroy sympathetic ganglia and thereby produce vasodilation, relieve pain, and promote healing of lesions in patients with vascular disease of the lower extremities.

TOLERANCE, DEPENDENCE, AND CHRONIC ETHANOL USE

Tolerance is defined as a reduced behavioral or physiological response to the same dose of ethanol (*see* Chapter 24). There is a marked acute tolerance that is detectable soon after administration of ethanol. Acute tolerance can be demonstrated by measuring behavioral impairment at the same BECs on the ascending limb of the absorption phase of the BEC–time curve (minutes after ingestion of alcohol) and on the descending limb of the curve as BECs are lowered by metabolism (1 or more hours after ingestion). Behavioral impairment and subjective feelings of intoxication are much greater at a given BEC on the ascending than on the descending limb. There also is a chronic tolerance that develops in the long-term heavy drinker. In contrast to acute tolerance, chronic tolerance often has a metabolic component owing to induction of alcohol-metabolizing enzymes.

Physical dependence is demonstrated by the elicitation of a withdrawal syndrome when alcohol consumption is terminated. The symptoms and severity are determined by the amount and duration of alcohol consumption and include sleep disruption, autonomic nervous system (sympathetic) activation, tremors, and in severe cases, seizures. In addition, 2 or more days after withdrawal, some individuals experience *delirium tremens,* characterized by hallucinations, delirium, fever, and tachycardia. Another aspect of dependence is craving and drug-seeking behavior, often termed *psychological dependence*.

ETIOLOGY OF ALCOHOL USE DISORDERS AND THE ROLE OF GENES

Environmental and cultural factors that contribute to alcohol use include stress, drinking patterns within one's culture and peer group, availability of alcohol, and attitudes toward drunkenness. These nonbiological forces contribute to perhaps 70-80% of the initial decision to drink and at least 40% of the transition from drinking to alcohol-related problems and alcohol use disorders. Correspondingly, ~60% of the susceptibility to alcohol use disorders results from heritable factors (*see* Table 23–1).

Polymorphisms in the enzymes of ethanol metabolism seem to explain why some populations (mainly Asian) are protected from alcoholism. This has been attributed to genetic differences in alcohol- and aldehyde-metabolizing enzymes. Specifically, genetic variants of ADH that exhibit high activity and variants of ALDH that exhibit low activity protect against heavy drinking, probably because alcohol consumption by individuals who have these variants results in accumulation of acetaldehyde, which produces a variety of unpleasant effects. In contrast to these protective genetic variants, there are few consistent data about genes responsible for increased risk for alcoholism. A genetic mechanism associated with an enhanced risk for both alcohol and other drug use disorders operates through the intermediate characteristic (or phenotype) of impulsivity and disinhibition. The identified polymorphisms include 2 variations of the $GABA_A$ receptors, a variation in ADH4 hypothesized to be related to personality characteristics, and a muscarinic cholinergic receptor gene, CHRM2.

Another phenotype is associated with a low level of response to ethanol. Genetic contributions to the level of response have been tentatively identified for 2 $GABA_A$ subunits, a polymorphism in the promoter region of the 5HT transporter that is associated with lower levels of 5HT in the synaptic space, a polymorphism of the α subunit of K^+ channel KCNMA1, and a variant nicotinic ACh receptor that is also related to an increased risk for heavy smoking and related consequences. Antisocial alcoholism has been linked with polymorphisms of several 5HT receptors.

TERATOGENIC EFFECTS: FETAL ALCOHOL SYNDROME

Children born to alcoholic mothers display a common pattern of distinct dysmorphology known as *fetal alcohol syndrome* (FAS). The diagnosis of FAS typically is based on the observance of a triad of abnormalities in the newborn, including:

- A cluster of craniofacial abnormalities
- CNS dysfunction
- Pre- and/or postnatal stunting of growth

Hearing, language, and speech disorders also may become evident as the child ages. Children who do not meet all the criteria for a diagnosis of FAS still may show physical and mental deficits consistent with a partial phenotype, termed *fetal alcohol effects* (FAEs) or *alcohol-related neurodevelopmental disorders*. FAS is seen in offspring born to ~5% of heavy-drinking females. The incidence of FAS is believed to be in the range of 0.5-1 per 1000 live births in the general U.S. population, with rates as high as 2-3 per 1000 in African American and Native American populations.

Craniofacial abnormalities commonly observed in the diagnosis of FAS consist of a pattern of microcephaly, a long and smooth philtrum, shortened palpebral fissures, a flat midface, and epicanthal folds. Magnetic resonance imaging studies demonstrate decreased volumes in the basal ganglia, corpus callosum, cerebrum, and cerebellum. Maternal drinking in the first trimester has been associated with craniofacial abnormalities. CNS dysfunction following in utero exposure to alcohol manifests in the form of hyperactivity, attention deficits, mental retardation, and learning disabilities. FAS is the most common cause of preventable mental retardation in the Western world, with afflicted children consistently scoring lower than their peers on a variety of IQ tests. Although the evidence is not conclusive, there is a suggestion that even moderate alcohol consumption (2 drinks per day) in the second trimester of pregnancy is correlated with impaired academic performance of offspring at age 6. Maternal age also may be a factor. Pregnant women over age 30 who drink alcohol create greater risks to their children than do younger women who consume similar amounts of alcohol. Apart from the risk of FAS or FAEs to the child, the intake of high amounts of alcohol by a pregnant woman, particularly during the first trimester, greatly increases the chances of spontaneous abortion.

PHARMACOTHERAPY OF ALCOHOLISM

Currently, 3 drugs are approved in the U.S. for treatment of alcoholism: disulfiram (ANTABUSE), naltrexone (REVIA), and acamprosate (Table 23–2). Disulfiram has a long history of use but has fallen into disfavor because of its side effects and problems with patient adherence to therapy. Naltrexone and acamprosate were introduced more recently. The goal of these medications is to assist the patient in maintaining abstinence.

NALTREXONE

Naltrexone, a μ-opioid receptor antagonist, is chemically related to the highly selective opioid-receptor antagonist naloxone (NARCAN) but has higher oral bioavailability and a longer duration of action. These drugs were used initially in the treatment of opioid overdose and dependence because of their ability to antagonize all the actions of opioids (*see* Chapters 18 and 24). There is evidence that naltrexone blocks activation by alcohol of dopaminergic pathways in the brain that are thought to be critical to reward.

Table 23–2

Oral Medications for Treating Alcohol Abuse

MEDICATION	USUAL DOSE	MECHANISM/EFFECT
Disulfiram	250 mg/day (range 125-500 mg/day)	Inhibits ALDH with resulting ↑ acetaldehyde after drinking. Abstinence is reinforced to avoid the resulting adverse reaction.
Naltrexone	50 mg/day	μ opioid receptor antagonist; felt to ↓ drinking through ↓ feelings of reward with alcohol and/or ↓ craving.
Acamprosate	666 mg three times daily	Weak antagonist of NMDA receptors, activator of $GABA_A$ receptors; may ↓ mild protracted abstinence syndromes with ↓ feelings of a "need" for alcohol.

Naltrexone helps to maintain abstinence by reducing the urge to drink and increasing control when a "slip" occurs. It is not a "cure" for alcoholism and does not prevent relapse in all patients. Naltrexone works best when used in conjunction with some form of psychosocial therapy, such as cognitive behavioral therapy. It typically is administered after detoxification and given at a dose of 50 mg/day for several months. Adherence to the regimen is important to ensure the therapeutic value of naltrexone and has proven to be a problem for some patients. The most common side effect of naltrexone is nausea, which is more common in women than in men and subsides if the patients abstain from alcohol. When given in excessive doses, naltrexone can cause liver damage. It is contraindicated in patients with liver failure or acute hepatitis and should be used only after careful consideration in patients with active liver disease. **Nalmefene** (REVEX) is another opioid antagonist that has a number of advantages over naltrexone, including greater oral bioavailability, longer duration of action, and lack of dose-dependent liver toxicity.

ACAMPROSATE

Acamprosate (*N*-acetylhomotaurine; CAMPRAL) is an analogue of GABA.

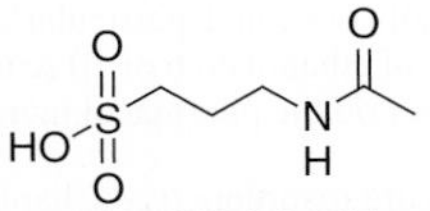

ACAMPROSATE

A number of double-blind, placebo-controlled studies have demonstrated that acamprosate (1.3-2 g/day) decreases drinking frequency and reduces relapse drinking in abstinent alcoholics and appears to have efficacy similar to that of naltrexone. Acamprosate generally is well tolerated by patients, with diarrhea being the main side effect. The drug undergoes minimal metabolism in the liver, is excreted primarily by the kidneys, and has an elimination $t_{1/2}$ of 18 h after oral administration. Concomitant use of disulfiram appears to increase the effectiveness of acamprosate, without any adverse drug interactions being noted.

DISULFIRAM

Disulfiram (tetraethylthiuram disulfide; ANTABUSE), given alone, is a relatively nontoxic substance, but it inhibits ALDH activity and causes the blood acetaldehyde concentration to rise to 5-10 times above the level achieved when ethanol is given to an individual not pretreated with disulfiram.

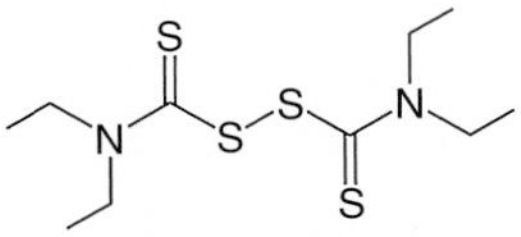

DISULFIRAM

Following the administration of disulfiram, both cytosolic and mitochondrial forms of ALDH are irreversibly inactivated to varying degrees, and the concentration of acetaldehyde rises. It is unlikely that disulfiram itself is responsible for the enzyme inactivation in vivo; several active metabolites of the drug, especially diethylthiomethylcarbamate, behave as suicide-substrate inhibitors of ALDH in vitro. These metabolites reach significant concentrations in plasma following the administration of disulfiram.

The ingestion of alcohol by individuals previously treated with disulfiram gives rise to marked signs and symptoms of acetaldehyde poisoning. Within 5-10 min, the face feels hot and soon afterward becomes flushed and scarlet in appearance. As the vasodilation spreads over the whole body, intense throbbing is felt in the head and neck, and a pulsating headache may develop. Respiratory difficulties, nausea, copious vomiting, sweating, thirst, chest pain, considerable hypotension, orthostatic syncope, marked uneasiness, weakness, vertigo, blurred vision, and confusion are observed. The facial flush is replaced by pallor; the blood pressure may fall to shock levels. Alarming reactions may result from the ingestion of even small amounts of alcohol in persons being treated with disulfiram. The use of disulfiram as a therapeutic agent thus is not without danger, and it should be attempted only under careful medical and nursing supervision. Patients must learn to avoid disguised forms of alcohol, as in sauces, fermented vinegar, cough syrups, and even aftershave lotions and back rub lotions.

Disulfiram never should be administered until the patient has abstained from alcohol for at least 12 h. In the initial phase of treatment, a maximal daily dose of 500 mg is given for 1-2 weeks. Maintenance dosage then ranges from 125-500 mg daily depending on tolerance to side effects. Unless sedation is prominent, the daily dose should be taken in the morning, the time when the resolve not to drink may be strongest. Sensitization to alcohol may last as long as 14 days after the last ingestion of disulfiram because of the slow rate of restoration of ALDH.

Disulfiram and/or its metabolites can inhibit many enzymes with crucial sulfhydryl groups, and it thus has a wide spectrum of biological effects. It inhibits hepatic CYPs and thereby interferes with the metabolism of phenytoin, chlordiazepoxide, barbiturates, warfarin, and other drugs. Disulfiram by itself usually is innocuous, but it may cause acne-form eruptions, urticaria, lassitude, tremor, restlessness, headache, dizziness, a garlic-like or metallic taste, and mild GI disturbances. Peripheral neuropathies, psychosis, and ketosis also have been reported.

OTHER AGENTS

Ondansetron, a $5HT_3$-receptor antagonist and antiemetic drug (*see* Chapters 13 and 46), reduces alcohol consumption in laboratory animals and currently is being tested in humans. Preliminary findings suggest that ondansetron is effective in the treatment of early onset alcoholics, who respond poorly to psychosocial treatment alone, although the drug does not appear to work well in other types of alcoholics. Ondansetron administration lowers the amount of alcohol consumed, particularly by drinkers who consume <10 drinks per day. It also decreases the subjective effects of ethanol on 6 of 10 scales measured, including the desire to drink, while at the same time not having any effect on the pharmacokinetics of ethanol.

Topiramate, a drug used for treating seizure disorders (*see* Chapter 21), appears useful for treating alcohol dependence. Compared with the placebo group, patients taking topiramate achieved more abstinent days and a lower craving for alcohol. The mechanism of action of topiramate is not well understood but is distinct from that of other drugs used for the treatment of dependence (e.g., opioid antagonists), suggesting that it may provide a new and unique approach to pharmacotherapy of alcoholism.

For a complete Bibliographical Listing see Goodman & Gilman's ***The Pharmacological Basis of Therapeutics***, 12th ed., or Goodman & Gilman Online at www.AccessMedicine.com.

Drug Addiction

The terminology used in discussing drug dependence, abuse, and addiction has long been confusing. Confusion stems from the fact that repeated use of certain prescribed medications can produce neuroplastic changes resulting in 2 distinctly abnormal states. The first is *dependence*, or "physical" dependence, produced when there is progressive pharmacological adaptation to the drug resulting in tolerance. In the tolerant state, repeating the same dose of drug produces a smaller effect. If the drug is abruptly stopped, a withdrawal syndrome ensues in which the adaptive responses are now unopposed by the drug. The appearance of withdrawal symptoms is the cardinal sign of "physical" dependence. *Addiction*, the second abnormal state produced by repeated drug use, occurs in only a minority of those who initiate drug use; addiction leads progressively to compulsive, out-of-control drug use.

Addiction can be defined fundamentally as a form of maladaptive memory. It begins with the administration of substances (e.g., cocaine) or behaviors (e.g., the thrill of gambling) that directly and intensely activate brain reward circuits. Activation of these circuits motivates normal behavior and most humans simply enjoy the experience without being compelled to repeat it. For some (~16% of those who try cocaine) the experience produces strong conditioned associations to environmental cues that signal the availability of the drug or the behavior. The individual becomes drawn into compulsive repetition of the experience focusing on the immediate pleasure despite negative long-term consequences and neglect of important social responsibilities. The distinction between dependence and addiction is important because patients with pain sometimes are deprived of adequate opioid medication simply because they have shown evidence of tolerance or they exhibit withdrawal symptoms if the analgesic medication is stopped or reduced abruptly.

ORIGINS OF SUBSTANCE DEPENDENCE

Most of those who initiate drug use do not progress to become addicts. Many variables operate simultaneously to influence the likelihood that a beginning drug user will lose control and develop an addiction. These variables can be organized into 3 categories: agent (drug), host (user), and environment (Table 24–1).

AGENT (DRUG) VARIABLES. *Reinforcement* refers to the capacity of drugs to produce effects that make the user wish to take them again. The more strongly reinforcing a drug is, the greater is the likelihood that the drug will be abused. Reinforcing properties of drugs are associated with their capacity to increase neuronal activity in critical brain areas (*see* Chapter 14). Cocaine, amphetamine, ethanol, opiates, cannabinoids, and nicotine all reliably increase extracellular fluid dopamine (DA) levels in the ventral striatum, specifically the nucleus accumbens region. In contrast, drugs that block DA receptors generally produce bad feelings, i.e., *dysphoric effects*. Despite strong correlative findings, a causal relationship between DA and euphoria/dysphoria has not been established, and other findings emphasize additional roles of serotonin (5HT), glutamate, norepinephrine (NE), endogenous opioids, and γ-aminobutyric acid (GABA) in mediating the reinforcing effects of drugs.

The *abuse liability* of a drug is enhanced by rapidity of onset. When coca leaves are chewed, cocaine is absorbed slowly and this produces low cocaine levels in the blood and few, if any, behavior problems. Crack, sold illegally and at a low price ($1-3 per dose), is alkaloidal cocaine (free base) that can be readily vaporized by heating. Simply inhaling the vapors produces blood levels comparable to those resulting from intravenous cocaine owing to the large surface area for absorption into the pulmonary circulation following inhalation. Thus, inhalation of crack cocaine is much more addictive than chewing, drinking, or sniffing cocaine. The risk for developing addiction among those who try nicotine is about twice that for those who try cocaine (Table 24–2). This does not imply that the pharmacological addiction liability of nicotine is twice that of cocaine. Rather, there are other variables listed in the categories of host factors and environmental conditions that influence the development of addiction.

HOST (USER) VARIABLES. Effects of drugs vary among individuals. Polymorphism of genes that encode enzymes involved in absorption, metabolism, and excretion and in receptor-mediated responses may contribute to the different degrees of reinforcement or euphoria observed among individuals (*see* Chapters 6 and 7).

Table 24–1

Multiple Simultaneous Variables Affecting Onset and Continuation of Drug Abuse and Addiction

Agent (drug)

Availability
Cost
Purity/potency
Mode of administration
  Chewing (absorption *via* oral mucous membranes)
  Gastrointestinal
  Intranasal
  Subcutaneous and intramuscular
  Intravenous
  Inhalation
Speed of onset and termination of effects (pharmacokinetics: combination of agent and host)

Host (user)

Heredity
  Innate tolerance
  Speed of developing acquired tolerance
  Likelihood of experiencing intoxication as pleasure
Metabolism of the drug (nicotine and alcohol data already available)
Psychiatric symptoms
Prior experiences/expectations
Propensity for risk-taking behavior

Environment

Social setting
Community attitudes
  Peer influence, role models
Availability of other reinforcers (sources of pleasure or recreation)
Employment or educational opportunities
Conditioned stimuli: environmental cues become associated with drugs after repeated use in the same environment

Table 24–2

Dependence among Users 1990–1992

AGENT	EVER USED[a] (%)	ADDICTION (%)	RISK OF ADDICTION (%)
Tobacco	75.6	24.1	31.9
Alcohol	91.5	14.1	15.4
Illicit drugs	51.0	7.5	14.7
Cannabis	46.3	4.2	9.1
Cocaine	16.2	2.7	16.7
Stimulants	15.3	1.7	11.2
Anxiolytics	12.7	1.2	9.2
Analgesics	9.7	0.7	7.5
Psychedelics	10.6	0.5	4.9
Heroin	1.5	0.4	23.1
Inhalants	6.8	0.3	3.7

[a]*The ever-used and addiction percentages are those of the general population. The risk of addiction is specific to the drug indicated and refers to the percentage who met criteria for addiction among those who reported having used the agent at least once (i.e., each value in column 4 was obtained by expressing the number in column 3 as a percentage of the number in column 2, subject to errors of rounding).*

Source: Anthony JC et al. Comparative epidemiology of dependence on tobacco, alcohol, controlled substances and the inhalants: Basic findings from the National Comorbidity Survey. Exp Clin Psychopharmacol, 1994, 2:244–268.

Innate tolerance to alcohol may represent a biological trait that contributes to the development of alcoholism (*see* Chapter 23). While innate tolerance increases vulnerability to alcoholism, impaired metabolism may *protect* against it (*see* Chapter 23). Similarly, individuals who inherit a gene associated with slow nicotine metabolism may experience unpleasant effects when beginning to smoke and reportedly have a lower probability of becoming nicotine dependent.

Psychiatric disorders constitute another category of host variables. People with anxiety, depression, insomnia, or even shyness may find that certain drugs give them relief. However, the apparent beneficial effects are transient, and repeated use of the drug may lead to tolerance and eventually compulsive, uncontrolled drug use. While psychiatric symptoms are seen commonly in drug abusers presenting for treatment, most of these symptoms begin *after* the person starts abusing drugs. Thus, drugs of abuse appear to produce more psychiatric symptoms than they relieve.

ENVIRONMENTAL VARIABLES. Initiating and continuing illegal drug use is influenced significantly by societal norms and peer pressure.

PHARMACOLOGICAL PHENOMENA

TOLERANCE. Tolerance, the most common response to repetitive use of the same drug, can be defined as the reduction in response to the drug after repeated administrations. Figure 24–1 shows an idealized dose-response curve for an administered drug. As the dose of the drug increases, the observed effect of the drug increases. With repeated use of the drug, however, the curve shifts to the right (tolerance). There are many forms of tolerance likely arising through multiple mechanisms.

Tolerance to some drug effects develops much more rapidly than to other effects of the same drug. For example, tolerance develops rapidly to the euphoria produced by opioids such as heroin, and addicts tend to increase their dose in order to reexperience that elusive "high." In contrast, tolerance to the GI effects of opioids develops more slowly. The discrepancy between tolerance to euphorigenic effects (rapid) and tolerance to effects on vital functions (slow), such as respiration and blood pressure, can lead to potentially fatal overdoses.

Innate tolerance refers to genetically determined lack of sensitivity to a drug that is observed the first time that the drug is administered. ***Acquired tolerance*** can be divided into 3 major types: pharmacokinetic, pharmacodynamic, and learned tolerance, and includes acute, reverse, and cross-tolerance. ***Pharmacokinetic* or *dispositional tolerance*** refers to changes in the distribution or metabolism of a drug after repeated administrations such that a given dose produces a lower blood concentration than the same dose did on initial exposure. The most common mechanism is an increase in the rate of metabolism of the drug. For example, barbiturates stimulate the production of higher levels of hepatic CYPs, causing more rapid removal and breakdown of barbiturates from the circulation.

Pharmacodynamic tolerance refers to adaptive changes that have taken place within systems affected by the drug so that response to a given concentration of the drug is reduced. Examples include drug-induced changes in receptor density or efficiency of receptor coupling to signal-transduction pathways (*see* Chapter 3).

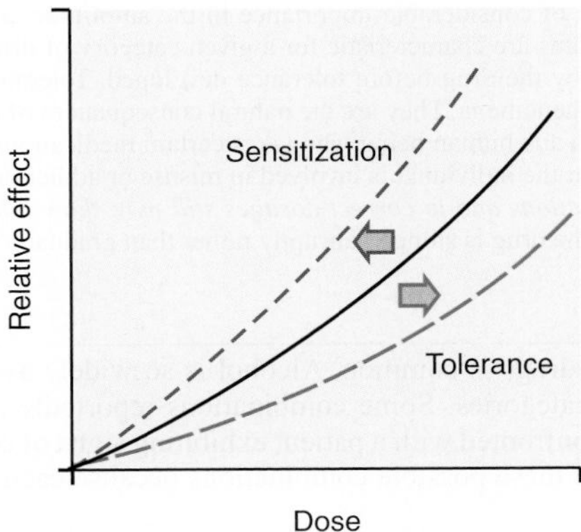

Figure 24–1 *Shifts in a dose-response curve with tolerance and sensitization.* With tolerance, there is a shift of the curve to the right such that doses higher than initial doses are required to achieve the same effects. With sensitization, there is a leftward shift of the curve such that for a given dose, there is a greater effect than seen after the initial dose.

Learned tolerance refers to a reduction in the effects of a drug due to compensatory mechanisms that are acquired by past experiences. One type of learned tolerance is called *behavioral tolerance.* A common example is learning to walk a straight line despite the motor impairment produced by alcohol intoxication. At higher levels of intoxication, behavioral tolerance is overcome, and the deficits are obvious.

Conditioned tolerance (situation-specific tolerance) develops when environmental cues or situations consistently are paired with the administration of a drug. When a drug affects homeostatic balance by producing sedation and changes in blood pressure, pulse rate, gut activity, and so on, there is usually a reflexive counteraction or adaptation in the direction of maintaining the status quo. If a drug always is taken in the presence of specific environmental cues (e.g., smell of drug preparation and sight of syringe), these cues begin to predict the effects of the drug, and the adaptations begin to occur, which will prevent the full manifestation of the drug's effects (i.e., cause tolerance). This mechanism follows classical (pavlovian) principles of learning and results in drug tolerance under circumstances where the drug is "expected."

Acute tolerance refers to rapid tolerance developing with repeated use on a single occasion, such as in a "binge." For example, repeated doses of cocaine over several hours produce a decrease in response to subsequent doses of cocaine during the binge. This is the opposite of *sensitization*, observed with an intermittent dosing schedule. ***Sensitization* or *reverse tolerance*** refers to an increase in response with repetition of the same dose of the drug. Sensitization results in a shift to the left of the dose-response curve (*see* Figure 24–1). Sensitization, in contrast to acute tolerance during a binge, requires a longer interval between doses, usually ~1 day. Sensitization can occur with stimulants such as cocaine or amphetamine. ***Cross-tolerance*** occurs when repeated use of a drug in a given category confers tolerance not only to that drug but also to other drugs in the same structural and mechanistic category. Understanding cross-tolerance is important in the medical management of persons dependent on any drug.

Detoxification is a form of treatment for drug dependence that involves giving gradually decreasing doses of the drug to prevent withdrawal symptoms, thereby weaning the patient from the drug of dependence. Detoxification can be accomplished with any medication in the same category as the initial drug of dependence. For example, users of heroin also are tolerant to other opioids. Thus, the detoxification of heroin-dependent patients can be accomplished with any medication that activates opioid receptors.

PHYSICAL DEPENDENCE. Physical dependence is a state that develops as a result of the adaptation (tolerance) produced by a resetting of homeostatic mechanisms in response to repeated drug use. A person in this adapted or physically dependent state requires continued administration of the drug to maintain normal function. If administration of the drug is stopped abruptly, there is another imbalance, and the affected systems must readjust to a new equilibrium without the drug.

WITHDRAWAL SYNDROME. The appearance of a withdrawal syndrome when administration of the drug is terminated is the only actual evidence of physical dependence. Withdrawal signs and symptoms occur when drug administration in a physically dependent person is terminated abruptly. Withdrawal symptoms have at least 2 origins:

- Removal of the drug of dependence
- CNS hyperarousal owing to readaptation to the absence of the drug of dependence

Pharmacokinetic variables are of considerable importance in the amplitude and duration of the withdrawal syndrome. Withdrawal symptoms are characteristic for a given category of drugs and tend to be opposite to the original effects produced by the drug before tolerance developed. Tolerance, physical dependence, and withdrawal are all biological phenomena. They are the natural consequences of drug use and can be produced in experimental animals and in any human being who takes certain medications repeatedly. These symptoms in themselves do not imply that the individual is involved in misuse or addiction. *Patients who take medicine for appropriate medical indications and in correct dosages still may show tolerance, physical dependence, and withdrawal* symptoms if the drug is stopped abruptly rather than gradually.

CLINICAL ISSUES

Abuse of combinations of drugs is common. Alcohol is so widely available that it is combined with practically all other categories. Some combinations reportedly are taken because of their interactive effects. When confronted with a patient exhibiting signs of overdose or withdrawal, the physician must be aware of these possible combinations because each drug may require specific treatment.

CNS DEPRESSANTS

ETHANOL. More than 90% of American adults report experience with ethanol (commonly called "alcohol"). Ethanol is classified as a depressant because it produces sedation and sleep. However, the initial effects of alcohol, particularly at lower doses, often are perceived as stimulation owing to a suppression of inhibitory systems (*see* Chapter 23). Heavy use of ethanol causes development of tolerance and physical dependence sufficient to define an alcohol withdrawal syndrome (Table 24–3).

Tolerance, Physical Dependence, and Withdrawal. The symptoms of mild intoxication by alcohol vary among individuals. Some experience motor incoordination and sleepiness. Others initially become stimulated. As the blood level increases, the sedating effects increase, with eventual coma and death occurring at high alcohol levels. The innate tolerance to alcohol varies greatly among individuals and is related to family history of alcoholism. Experience with alcohol can produce greater tolerance (acquired tolerance) such that extremely high blood levels (300-400 mg/dL) can be found in alcoholics who do not appear grossly sedated. In these cases, the lethal dose does not increase proportionately to the sedating dose, and thus the margin of safety (therapeutic index) is decreased.

Heavy consumers of alcohol acquire tolerance and also develop a state of physical dependence. This often leads to drinking in the morning to restore blood alcohol levels diminished during the night. The alcohol-withdrawal syndrome generally depends on the size of the average daily dose and usually is "treated" by resumption of alcohol ingestion. Withdrawal symptoms are experienced frequently but usually are not severe or life-threatening until they occur in conjunction with other problems, such as infection, trauma, malnutrition, or electrolyte imbalance. In the setting of such complications, the syndrome of *delirium tremens* becomes likely.

Alcohol addiction produces cross-tolerance to other sedatives such as benzodiazepines. This tolerance is operative in abstinent alcoholics, but while the alcoholic is drinking, the sedating effects of alcohol add to those of other sedatives. This is particularly true for benzodiazepines, which are relatively safe in overdose when given alone but potentially are lethal in combination with alcohol. The chronic use of alcohol and other sedatives is associated with the development of depression and the risk of suicide. Cognitive deficits have been reported in alcoholics tested while sober. These deficits usually improve with abstinence. More severe recent memory impairment is associated with specific brain damage caused by nutritional deficiencies common in alcoholics (e.g., thiamine deficiency). Medical complications of alcohol abuse and dependence include liver disease, cardiovascular disease, endocrine and GI effects, and malnutrition, in addition to the CNS dysfunctions outlined earlier. Ethanol readily crosses the placental barrier, producing the fetal alcohol syndrome, a major cause of mental retardation (*see* Chapter 23).

PHARMACOLOGICAL INTERVENTIONS

Detoxification. Although most mild cases of alcohol withdrawal never come to medical attention, severe cases require general evaluation; attention to hydration and electrolytes; vitamins, especially high-dose thiamine; and a sedating medication that has cross-tolerance with alcohol. To block or diminish the symptoms described in Table 24–3, a short-acting benzodiazepine such as oxazepam can be used at a dose of 15-30 mg every 6-8 h according to the stage and severity of withdrawal; some authorities recommend a long-acting benzodiazepine unless there is demonstrated liver impairment. Anticonvulsants such as carbamazepine have been shown to be effective in alcohol withdrawal, but not as well as benzodiazepines.

Pharmacotherapy. Detoxification is the first step of treatment. Complete abstinence is the objective of long-term treatment, and this is accomplished mainly by behavioral approaches. Disulfiram (ANTABUSE; *see* Chapter 23) has been useful in some programs that focus behavioral efforts on ingestion of the medication. Disulfiram blocks aldehyde dehydrogenase, resulting in the accumulation of acetaldehyde, which produces an unpleasant flushing reaction when alcohol is ingested. Knowledge of this unpleasant reaction helps the patient to resist taking a drink. However, disulfiram has not been found to be effective in controlled clinical trials because so many patients failed to take it.

Naltrexone (REVIA; *see* Chapter 23) is an opioid receptor antagonist that blocks the reinforcing properties of alcohol. Chronic administration of naltrexone was found to decrease the rate of relapse to alcohol drinking. It works best in combination with behavioral treatment programs that encourage adherence to medication and abstinence from alcohol. A depot preparation with a duration of 30 days (VIVITROL) is now available; it greatly improves medication adherence. Acamprosate (CAMPRAL) is a competitive inhibitor of the *N*-methyl-D-aspartate (NMDA)–type glutamate receptor (*see* Table 23–2). The drug appears to normalize the dysregulated neurotransmission associated with chronic ethanol intake and thereby to attenuate one of the mechanisms that lead to relapse (*see* Chapter 23).

BENZODIAZEPINES. Benzodiazepines are used mainly for the treatment of anxiety disorders and insomnia (*see* Chapters 15 and 17). Considering their widespread use, intentional abuse of prescription benzodiazepines is relatively uncommon. The proportion of patients who become tolerant increases after several months of use and reducing the dose or stopping the medication produces withdrawal symptoms (Table 24–4).

Table 24–3

Alcohol Withdrawal Syndrome

Alcohol craving
Tremor, irritability
Nausea
Sleep disturbance
Tachycardia
Hypertension
Sweating
Perceptual distortion
Seizures (6-48 h after last drink)
Visual (and occasionally auditory or tactile) hallucinations (12-48 h after last drink)
Delirium tremens (48-96 h after last drink; rare in uncomplicated withdrawal)
Severe agitation, confusion
Fever, profuse sweating
Tachycardia, dilated pupils
Nausea, diarrhea

Table 24–4

Benzodiazepine Withdrawal Symptoms

Following moderate dose usage
Anxiety, agitation
Increased sensitivity to light and sound
Paresthesias, strange sensations
Muscle cramps
Myoclonic jerks
Sleep disturbance
Dizziness
Following high-dose usage
Seizures
Delirium

It can be difficult to distinguish withdrawal symptoms from the reappearance of the anxiety symptoms for which the benzodiazepine was prescribed initially. Some patients may increase their dose over time because tolerance definitely develops to the sedative effects. Antianxiety benefits, however, seem to continue to occur long after tolerance to the sedating effects. Moreover, these patients continue to take the medication for years according to medical directions without increasing their dose and are able to function very effectively as long as they take the benzodiazepine. Patients with a history of alcohol- or other drug-abuse problems have an increased risk for the development of benzodiazepine abuse and should rarely, if ever, be treated with benzodiazepines on a chronic basis.

Pharmacological Interventions. If patients receiving long-term benzodiazepine treatment by prescription wish to stop their medication, the process may take months of gradual dose reduction. Withdrawal symptoms may occur during this outpatient detoxification, but in most cases the symptoms are mild. If anxiety symptoms return, a non-benzodiazepine such as buspirone may be prescribed. Some authorities recommend transferring the patient to a long $t_{1/2}$ benzodiazepine during detoxification; others recommend the anticonvulsants carbamazepine and phenobarbital. Patients who have been on low doses of benzodiazepines for years usually have no adverse effects. The specific benzodiazepine receptor antagonist flumazenil is useful in the treatment of overdose and in reversing the effects of long-acting benzodiazepines used in anesthesia.

Abusers of high doses of benzodiazepines usually require inpatient detoxification. Frequently, benzodiazepine abuse is part of a combined dependence involving alcohol, opioids, and cocaine. Detoxification can be a complex clinical pharmacological problem requiring knowledge of the pharmacokinetics of each drug. One approach to complex detoxification is to focus on the CNS-depressant drug and temporarily hold the opioid component constant with a low dose of methadone. A long-acting benzodiazepine such as diazepam or clorazepate (TRANXENE, others) or a long-acting barbiturate such as phenobarbital can be used to block the sedative withdrawal symptoms. After detoxification, the prevention of relapse requires a long-term outpatient rehabilitation program similar to the treatment of alcoholism. No specific medications have been found to be useful in the rehabilitation of sedative abusers but specific psychiatric disorders such as depression or schizophrenia, if present, require appropriate medications.

BARBITURATES. Abuse problems with barbiturates resemble those seen with benzodiazepines in many ways.

Treatment of abuse and addiction to barbiturates should be handled similarly to interventions for the abuse of alcohol and benzodiazepines. Because drugs in this category frequently are prescribed as hypnotics for patients complaining of insomnia, physicians should be aware of the problems that can develop when the hypnotic agent is withdrawn and of possible causes for insomnia that are treatable by other means. Insomnia often is a symptom of an underlying chronic problem, such as depression or respiratory dysfunction. Prescription of sedative medications can change the physiology of sleep with subsequent tolerance to these medication effects. When the sedative is stopped, there is a rebound effect with worsened insomnia. This medication-induced insomnia requires detoxification by gradual dose reduction.

Table 24–5

Nicotine Withdrawal Symptoms
Irritability, impatience, hostility
Anxiety
Dysphoric or depressed mood
Difficulty concentrating
Restlessness
Decreased heart rate
Increased appetite or weight gain

NICOTINE

Nicotine and agents for smoking cessation are discussed in Chapter 11. Because nicotine provides the reinforcement for cigarette smoking, the most common cause of preventable death and disease in the U.S., it is arguably the most dangerous dependence-producing drug. Although >80% of smokers express a desire to quit, only 35% try to stop each year, and fewer than 5% are successful in unaided attempts to quit.

Cigarette (nicotine) addiction is influenced by multiple variables. Nicotine itself produces reinforcement; users compare nicotine to stimulants such as cocaine or amphetamine, although its effects are of lower magnitude. While there are many casual users of alcohol and cocaine, few individuals who smoke cigarettes smoke a small enough quantity (≤5 cigarettes per day) to avoid dependence. Nicotine is absorbed readily through the skin, mucous membranes, and lungs. The pulmonary route produces discernible CNS effects in as little as 7 seconds. Thus, each puff produces some discrete reinforcement. With 10 puffs per cigarette, the 1-pack-per-day smoker reinforces the habit 200 times daily.

Negative reinforcement refers to the benefits obtained from the termination of an unpleasant state. In dependent smokers, the urge to smoke correlates with a low blood nicotine level, as though smoking were a means to achieve a certain nicotine level and thus avoid nicotine withdrawal symptoms (Table 24–5). Depressed mood (dysthymic disorder, affective disorder) is associated with nicotine dependence, but it is not known whether depression can predispose one to begin smoking or depression develops during the course of nicotine dependence.

PHARMACOLOGICAL INTERVENTIONS. The nicotine withdrawal syndrome can be alleviated by nicotine-replacement therapy, available with a prescription (e.g., NICOTROL inhaler and nasal spray) or without (e.g., NICORETTE gum and others; COMMIT lozenges and others; and NICODERM CQ transdermal patch and others). Different methods of nicotine delivery provide different blood nicotine levels over varying time courses (Figure 24–2). These methods suppress the symptoms of nicotine withdrawal. Although this results in more smokers achieving abstinence, most resume smoking over the ensuing weeks or months. A sustained-release preparation of the antidepressant bupropion (ZYBAN; *see* Chapter 15) improves abstinence rates among smokers and remains a useful option. The cannabinoid CB_1 receptor inverse agonist rimonabant improves abstinence rates and reduces the weight gain seen frequently in ex-smokers but is linked to depressive and neurologic symptoms. Varenicline, a partial agonist at the $\alpha_4\beta_2$ subtype of the nicotinic acetylcholine receptor, improves abstinence rates but has also been linked to risk of developing suicidal ideation. *See* Chapter 11 for the pharmacology of varenicline.

OPIOIDS

Opioid drugs are used primarily for the treatment of pain (*see* Chapter 18). Some of the CNS mechanisms that reduce the perception of pain also produce a state of well-being or euphoria. Thus, opioid drugs also are taken outside medical channels for the purpose of obtaining the effects on mood.

Heroin is the most frequently abused opiate. There is no legal supply of heroin for clinical use in the U.S.; however, heroin is widely available on the illicit market. The purity of street heroin in the U.S. has increased from ~4 mg heroin per 100 mg bag (range: 0-8 mg; the rest was filler such as quinine) to reach 45-75% purity in many large cities, with some samples testing as high as 90%. This increase in purity has led to increased levels of physical dependence among heroin addicts. Users who interrupt regular dosing develop more severe withdrawal symptoms. The more potent supplies can be smoked or administered nasally (snorted), making the initiation of heroin use accessible to people who would not insert a needle into their veins.

TOLERANCE, DEPENDENCE, AND WITHDRAWAL. Injection of a heroin solution produces a variety of sensations described as warmth, taste, or high and intense pleasure ("rush") often compared with sexual orgasm. There are some differences among the opioids in their acute effects, with morphine producing more of a histamine-releasing effect and meperidine producing more excitation or confusion. Even experienced opioid

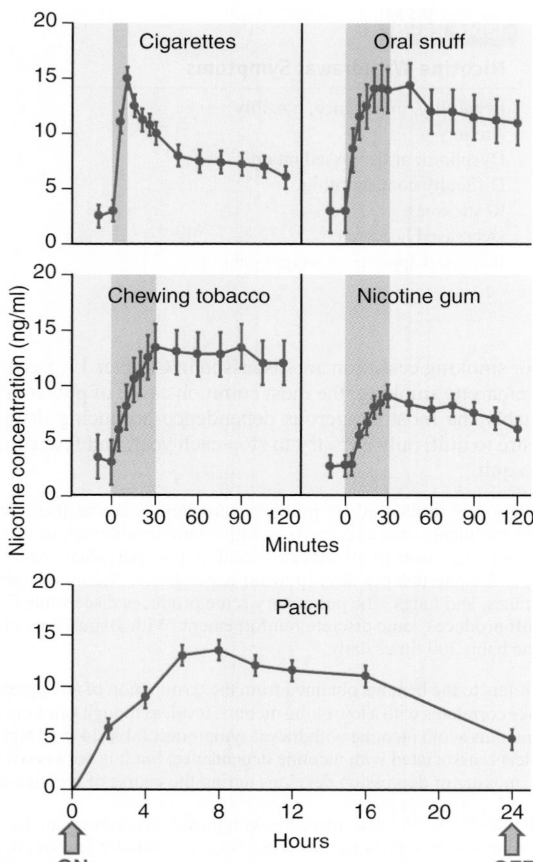

Figure 24–2 *Nicotine concentrations in blood resulting from 5 different nicotine delivery systems. Shaded areas* (upper panel) indicate the periods of nicotine delivery. *Arrows* (lower panel) indicate when the nicotine patch was put on and taken off. (With permission from Benowitz NL, Porchet H, Sheiner L, Jacob P III. Nicotine absorption and cardiovascular effects with smokeless tobacco use: Comparison with cigarettes and nicotine gum. *Clin Pharmacol Ther*, 1988, 44:23–28 © Macmillan Publishers Ltd. and Srivastava ED, Russell MA, Feyerabend C, et al. Sensitivity and tolerance to nicotine in smokers and nonsmokers. *Psychopharmacology*, 1991, 105:63–68 © Springer Science and Business Media.)

addicts, however, cannot distinguish between heroin and hydromorphone in double-blind tests. The popularity of heroin may be due to its availability on the illicit market and its rapid onset. After intravenous injection, the effects begin in less than a minute. Heroin has high lipid solubility, crosses the blood-brain barrier quickly, and is deacetylated to the active metabolites 6-monoacetyl morphine and morphine. After the intense euphoria, which lasts from 45 seconds to several minutes, there is a period of sedation and tranquility ("on the nod") lasting up to an hour. The effects of heroin wear off in 3-5 h, depending on the dose. Experienced users may inject 2 to 4 times per day. Thus, the heroin addict is constantly oscillating between being "high" and feeling the sickness of early withdrawal (Figure 24–3). This produces many problems in the homeostatic systems regulated at least in part by endogenous opioids.

Based on patient reports, tolerance develops early to the euphoria-producing effects of opioids. There also is tolerance to the respiratory depressant, analgesic, sedative, and emetic properties. Heroin users tend to increase their daily dose, depending on their financial resources and the availability of the drug. Overdose is likely to occur when potency of the street sample is unexpectedly high or when the heroin is mixed with a far more potent opioid, such as fentanyl (SUBLIMAZE, others).

Addiction to heroin or other short-acting opioids produces behavioral disruptions and usually becomes incompatible with a productive life. Apart from the behavioral changes and the risk of overdose, chronic use of opioids is relatively nontoxic in and of itself. Nonetheless, the mortality rate for street heroin users is

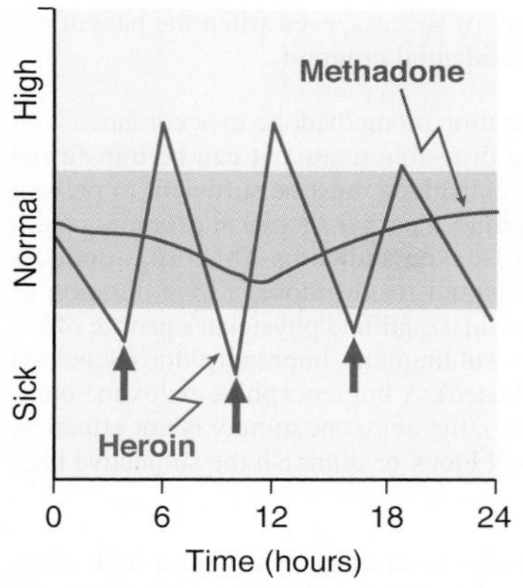

Figure 24–3 *Comparative responses to heroin and methadone.* A person who injects heroin (↑) several times per day oscillates (red line) between being sick and being high. In contrast, the a methadone patient (purple line) remains in the "normal" range (blue band) with little fluctuation after dosing once per day. Ordinate values represent the subject's mental and physical state, not plasma levels of the drug.

Table 24–6

Characteristics of Opioid Withdrawal

SYMPTOMS	SIGNS
Regular withdrawal	
Craving for opioids	Pupillary dilation
Restlessness, irritability	Sweating
Increased sensitivity to pain	Piloerection ("gooseflesh")
Nausea, cramps	Tachycardia
Muscle aches	Vomiting, diarrhea
Dysphoric mood	Increased blood pressure
Insomnia, anxiety	Yawning
	Fever
Protracted withdrawal	
Anxiety	Cyclic changes in weight, pupil size, respiratory center sensitivity
Insomnia	
Drug craving	

very high. Heroin users commonly acquire bacterial infections producing skin abscesses; endocarditis; pulmonary infections, especially tuberculosis; and viral infections producing hepatitis C and acquired immune deficiency syndrome (AIDS).

Opioids frequently are used in combinations with other drugs. A common combination is heroin and cocaine ("speedball"). Users report an improved euphoria because of the combination, and there is evidence of an interaction, because cocaine reduces the signs of opiate withdrawal, and heroin may reduce the irritability seen in chronic cocaine users.

The first stage of treatment addresses physical dependence and consists of detoxification. The opioid-withdrawal syndrome (Table 24–6) is very unpleasant but not life-threatening. It begins within 6-12 h after the last dose of a short-acting opioid and as long as 72-84 h after a very long-acting opioid medication. The duration and intensity of the syndrome are related to the clearance of the individual drug. Heroin withdrawal is brief (5-10 days) and intense. Methadone withdrawal is slower in onset and lasts longer.

PHARMACOLOGICAL INTERVENTIONS. Opioid withdrawal signs and symptoms can be treated by 3 different approaches. *The first and most commonly used approach* consists of transfer to a prescription opioid medication and then gradual dose reduction. It is convenient to change the patient from a short-acting opioid such as heroin to a long-acting one such as methadone. The initial dose of methadone is typically 20-30 mg. The first day's total dose then can be calculated depending on the response and then reduced by 20% per day during the course of detoxification.

A second approach to detoxification involves the use of oral clonidine (CATAPRES, others), an α_2 adrenergic agonist that decreases adrenergic neurotransmission from the locus ceruleus. Many of the autonomic symptoms of opioid withdrawal result from the loss of opioid suppression of the locus ceruleus system during the abstinence syndrome. Clonidine can alleviate many of the symptoms of opioid withdrawal but not the generalized aches and opioid craving. When using clonidine to treat withdrawal, the dose must be titrated according to the stage and severity of withdrawal; postural hypotension is commonly a side effect. *A third method* of treating opioid withdrawal involves activation of the endogenous opioid system without medication. The techniques proposed include acupuncture and several methods of CNS activation using transcutaneous electrical stimulation. While attractive theoretically, this has not yet been found to be practical.

LONG-TERM MANAGEMENT. If patients are simply discharged from the hospital after withdrawal from opioids, there is a high probability of a quick return to compulsive opioid use. Numerous factors influence relapse. The withdrawal syndrome does not end in 5-7 days; a *protracted withdrawal syndrome* (*see* Table 24–6) persists for up to 6 months. Physiological measures tend to oscillate as though a new set point were being established;

during this phase, outpatient drug-free treatment has a low probability of success, even when the patient has received intensive prior treatment while protected from relapse in a residential program.

The most successful treatment for heroin addiction consists of stabilization on methadone in accordance with state and federal regulations. Patients who relapse repeatedly during drug-free treatment can be transferred directly to methadone without requiring detoxification. The dose of methadone must be sufficient to prevent withdrawal symptoms for at least 24 h. The introduction of buprenorphine, a partial agonist at μ-opioid receptors (*see* Chapter 18), represents a major change in the treatment of opiate addiction. This drug produces minimal withdrawal symptoms when discontinued and has a low potential for overdose, a long duration of action, and the ability to block heroin effects. Treatment can take place in a qualified physician's private office rather than in a special center, as required for methadone. When taken sublingually, buprenorphine (SUBUTEX) is active, but it also has the potential to be dissolved and injected (abused). A buprenorphine-naloxone combination (SUBOXONE) is also available. When taken orally (sublingually), the naloxone moiety is not effective, but if the patient abuses the medication by injecting, the naloxone will block or diminish the subjective high that could be produced by buprenorphine alone.

ANTAGONIST TREATMENT. Naltrexone (REVIA, others; *see* Chapter 18) is an antagonist with a high affinity for the μ-opioid receptor; it will competitively block the effects of heroin or other μ-receptor agonists. Naltrexone will not satisfy craving or relieve protracted withdrawal symptoms, but it can be used after detoxification for patients with high motivation to remain opioid-free.

COCAINE AND OTHER PSYCHOSTIMULANTS

COCAINE. The number of frequent users (at least weekly) of cocaine in the U.S. has remained steady since 1991 at ~600,000. Not all users become addicts. A key factor is the widespread availability of relatively inexpensive cocaine in the alkaloidal form (free base, "crack") suitable for smoking and in the hydrochloride powder form suitable for nasal or intravenous use. Drug abuse occurs about twice as frequently in men as in women.

The reinforcing effects of cocaine and cocaine analogs correlate best with their effectiveness in blocking the transporter that recovers DA from the synapse. This leads to increased DA concentrations at critical brain sites. However, cocaine also blocks both NE and 5HT reuptake, and chronic use of cocaine leads to changes in these neurotransmitter systems. The general pharmacology and medicinal use of cocaine as a local anesthetic are discussed in Chapter 20. Cocaine produces a dose-dependent increase in heart rate and blood pressure accompanied by increased arousal, improved performance on tasks of vigilance and alertness, and a sense of self-confidence and well-being. Higher doses produce euphoria, which has a brief duration and often is followed by a desire for more drug. Repeated doses may lead to involuntary motor activity, stereotyped behavior, and paranoia. Irritability and increased risk of violence are found among heavy chronic users. The $t_{1/2}$ of cocaine in plasma is ~50 min, but inhalant (crack) users typically desire more cocaine after 10-30 min.

The major route for cocaine metabolism involves hydrolysis of each of its 2 ester groups. Benzoylecgonine, produced on loss of the methyl group, represents the major urinary metabolite and can be found in the urine for 2-5 days after a binge. As a result, the benzoylecgonine test is a valid method for detecting cocaine use; the metabolite remains detectable in the urine of heavy users for up to 10 days. Ethanol is frequently abused with cocaine, as it reduces the irritability induced by cocaine. Dual addiction to alcohol and cocaine is common. When cocaine and alcohol are taken concurrently, cocaine may be transesterified to cocaethylene, which is equipotent to cocaine in blocking DA reuptake.

Addiction is the most common complication of cocaine abuse. In general, stimulants tend to be abused much more irregularly than opioids, nicotine, and alcohol. Binge use is very common, and a binge may last hours to days, terminating only when supplies of the drug are exhausted.

Toxicity. Other risks of cocaine, beyond the potential for addiction, include cardiac arrhythmias, myocardial ischemia, myocarditis, aortic dissection, cerebral vasoconstriction, and seizures. Death from trauma also is associated with cocaine use. Cocaine may induce premature labor and abruptio placentae. Cocaine has been reported to produce a prolonged and intense orgasm if taken prior to intercourse, and users often indulge in compulsive and promiscuous sexual activity. However, chronic cocaine use reduces sexual drive. Chronic use is also associated with psychiatric disorders, including anxiety, depression, and psychosis.

Tolerance, Dependence, and Withdrawal. In intermittent users of cocaine, the euphoric effect typically is not subject to sensitization. On the contrary, most experienced users become desensitized and, over time, require more cocaine to obtain euphoria, i.e., tolerance develops. Because cocaine typically is used intermittently, even heavy users go through frequent periods of withdrawal or "crash." The symptoms of withdrawal seen in users admitted to hospitals are listed in Table 24–7. Careful studies of cocaine users during withdrawal show gradual diminution of these symptoms over 1-3 weeks. Residual depression, often seen after cocaine withdrawal, should be treated with antidepressant agents if it persists (*see* Chapter 15).

Table 24–7

Cocaine Withdrawal Symptoms and Signs

Dysphoria, depression
Sleepiness, fatigue
Cocaine craving
Bradycardia

Pharmacological Interventions. Because cocaine withdrawal is generally mild, treatment of withdrawal symptoms usually is not required. The major problem in treatment is not detoxification but helping the patient to resist the urge to resume compulsive cocaine use. Rehabilitation programs involving individual and group psychotherapy based on the principles of Alcoholics Anonymous, and behavioral treatments based on reinforcing cocaine-free urine tests, result in significant improvement in the majority of cocaine users. Nonetheless, there is great interest in finding a medication that can aid in the rehabilitation of cocaine addicts.

AMPHETAMINE AND RELATED AGENTS. Subjective effects similar to those of cocaine are produced by *amphetamine*, *dextroamphetamine*, *methamphetamine*, *phenmetrazine*, *methylphenidate*, and *diethylpropion*.

Amphetamines increase synaptic DA, NE, and 5HT primarily by stimulating pre-synaptic release rather than by blockade of reuptake, as is the case with cocaine. Intravenous or smoked methamphetamine produces an abuse/dependence syndrome similar to that of cocaine, although clinical deterioration may progress more rapidly. Methamphetamine addiction has become a major public health problem in the U.S. Behavioral and medical treatments for methamphetamine addiction are similar to those used for cocaine.

CAFFEINE. Caffeine, a mild stimulant, is the most widely used psychoactive drug in the world. It is present in soft drinks, coffee, tea, cocoa, chocolate, and numerous prescription and over-the-counter drugs.

Caffeine mildly increases NE and DA release and enhances neural activity in numerous brain areas. Caffeine is absorbed from the digestive tract, is distributed rapidly throughout all tissues, and easily crosses the placental barrier. Many of caffeine's effects are believed to occur by means of competitive antagonism at adenosine receptors. Adenosine is a neuromodulator (*see* Chapter 14) that resembles caffeine structurally. The mild sedating effects that occur when adenosine activates particular adenosine-receptor subtypes can be antagonized by caffeine. Tolerance occurs rapidly to the stimulating effects of caffeine. Thus, a mild withdrawal syndrome has been produced in controlled studies by abruptly discontinuing the intake of as little as 1 to 2 cups of coffee per day. Caffeine withdrawal consists of feelings of fatigue and sedation. With higher doses, headaches and nausea have been reported during withdrawal; vomiting is rare.

CANNABINOIDS (MARIJUANA)

The cannabis plant has been cultivated for centuries for its presumed medicinal and psychoactive properties. The smoke from burning cannabis contains many chemicals, including 61 different cannabinoids that have been identified. One of these, Δ-9-tetrahydrocannabinol (Δ-9-THC), produces most of the characteristic pharmacological effects of smoked marijuana. Marijuana is the most commonly used illegal drug in the U.S. The human cannabinoid endogenous ligand/receptor/signaling systems are described in Chapter 14.

The pharmacological effects of Δ-9-THC vary with the dose, route of administration, experience of the user, vulnerability to psychoactive effects, and setting of use. Intoxication with marijuana produces changes in mood, perception, and motivation, but the effect most frequently sought is the "high" and "mellowing out." This effect is described as different from the high produced by a stimulant or opiate. Effects vary with dose, but typically last ~2 h. During the high, cognitive functions, perception, reaction time, learning, and memory are impaired. Coordination and tracking behavior may be impaired for several hours beyond the perception of the high. Marijuana also produces complex behavioral changes such as giddiness and increased hunger. Unpleasant reactions such as panic or hallucinations and even acute psychosis may occur. These reactions are seen commonly with higher doses and with oral ingestion rather than smoked marijuana. Numerous clinical reports suggest that marijuana use may precipitate a recurrence of psychosis in people with a history of schizophrenia. One of the most controversial of the reputed effects of marijuana is the production of an "amotivational syndrome." This syndrome is not an official diagnosis, but it has been used to describe young people who drop out of social activities and show little interest in school, work, or other goal-directed activity. There is no evidence that marijuana damages brain cells or produces any permanent functional changes.

Table 24–8

Marijuana Withdrawal Syndrome

Restlessness
Irritability
Mild agitation
Insomnia
Sleep EEG disturbance
Nausea, cramping

Marijuana has medicinal effects, including antiemetic properties that relieve side effects of anticancer chemotherapy. It also has muscle-relaxing effects, anticonvulsant properties, and the capacity to reduce the elevated intraocular pressure of glaucoma. These medical benefits come at the cost of the psychoactive effects that often impair normal activities. Thus, there is no clear advantage of marijuana over conventional treatments for any of these indications.

TOLERANCE, DEPENDENCE, AND WITHDRAWAL. Tolerance to most of the effects of marijuana can develop rapidly after only a few doses, but also disappears rapidly. Withdrawal symptoms are not seen in clinical populations. Human subjects develop a withdrawal syndrome when they receive regular oral doses of the agent (Table 24–8). This syndrome, however, is only seen clinically in persons who use marijuana on a daily basis and then suddenly stop. Marijuana abuse and addiction have no specific treatments. Heavy users may suffer from accompanying depression and thus may respond to antidepressant medication.

PSYCHEDELIC AGENTS

There are 2 main categories of psychedelic compounds, indoleamines and phenethylamines. The indoleamine hallucinogens include LSD, N,N-dimethyltryptamine (DMT), and psilocybin. The phenethylamines include mescaline, dimethoxymethylamphetamine (DOM), methylenedioxyamphetamine (MDA), and MDMA. Both groups have a relatively high affinity for $5HT_2$ receptors (*see* Chapter 13), but they differ in their affinity for other subtypes of 5HT receptors. There is a good correlation between the relative affinity of these compounds for $5HT_2$ receptors and their potency as hallucinogens in humans. However, LSD interacts with many receptor subtypes at nanomolar concentrations, and it is not possible to attribute the psychedelic effects to any single 5HT receptor subtype.

LSD. LSD is the most potent hallucinogenic drug and produces significant psychedelic effects with a total dose of as little as 25-50 μg. This drug is >3000 times more potent than mescaline. LSD is sold on the illicit market in a variety of forms. A popular contemporary system involves postage stamp-sized papers impregnated with varying doses of LSD (50-300 μg or more).

The effects of hallucinogenic drugs are variable, even in the same individual on different occasions. LSD is absorbed rapidly after oral administration, with effects beginning at 40-60 min, peaking at 2-4 h, and gradually returning to baseline over 6-8 h. At a dose of 100 μg, LSD produces perceptual distortions and sometimes hallucinations; mood changes, including elation, paranoia, or depression; intense arousal; and sometimes a feeling of panic. Signs of LSD ingestion include pupillary dilation, increased blood pressure and pulse, flushing, salivation, lacrimation, and hyperreflexia. Visual effects are prominent. Colors seem more intense, and shapes may appear altered. The subject may focus attention on unusual items such as the pattern of hairs on the back of the hand. A "bad trip" usually consists of severe anxiety, although at times it is marked by intense depression and suicidal thoughts. Visual disturbances usually are prominent. There are no documented toxic fatalities from LSD use, but fatal accidents and suicides have occurred during or shortly after intoxication. Prolonged psychotic reactions lasting 2 days or more may occur after the ingestion of a hallucinogen. Schizophrenic episodes may be precipitated in susceptible individuals, and there is some evidence that chronic use of these drugs is associated with the development of persistent psychotic disorders. Claims about the potential of psychedelic drugs for enhancing psychotherapy and for treating addictions and other mental disorders are not supported by controlled studies; there is no current indication for these drugs as medications.

Tolerance, Physical Dependence, and Withdrawal. Frequent, repeated use of psychedelic drugs is unusual, and thus tolerance is not commonly seen. Tolerance does develop to the behavioral effects of LSD after 3 or 4 daily doses, but no withdrawal syndrome has been observed.

Pharmacological Intervention. Because of the unpredictability of psychedelic drug effects, any use carries some risk. Users may require medical attention because of "bad trips." Severe agitation may respond to diazepam (20 mg orally). "Talking down" by reassurance also is effective and is the management of first choice. Antipsychotic medications (*see* Chapter 16) may intensify the experience and thus are not indicated. A particularly troubling aftereffect of the use of LSD and similar drugs is the occasional occurrence of episodic visual disturbances. These originally were called "flashbacks" and resembled the experiences of prior LSD trips. Flashbacks belong to an official diagnostic category called the *hallucinogen persisting perception disorder*. The symptoms include false fleeting perceptions in the peripheral fields, flashes of color, geometric pseudohallucinations, and positive afterimages. The visual disorder appears stable in half the cases and represents an apparently permanent alteration of the visual system. Precipitants include stress, fatigue, emergence into a dark environment, marijuana, antipsychotic agents, and anxiety states.

MDMA ("ECSTASY") AND MDA. MDMA and MDA are phenylethylamines that have stimulant as well as psychedelic effects.

Acute effects are dose-dependent and include feelings of energy, altered sense of time, and pleasant sensory experiences with enhanced perception. Negative effects include tachycardia, dry mouth, jaw clenching, and muscle aches. At higher doses, visual hallucinations, agitation, hyperthermia, and panic attacks have been reported. A typical oral dose is 1 or 2 100-mg tablets and lasts 3-6 h, although dosage and potency of street samples are variable (~100 mg per tablet).

PHENCYCLIDINE (PCP). PCP was developed originally as an anesthetic in the 1950s and later was abandoned because of a high frequency of postoperative delirium with hallucinations. It was classified as a dissociative anesthetic because, in the anesthetized state, the patient remains conscious with staring gaze, flat facies, and rigid muscles. PCP became a drug of abuse in the 1970s, first in an oral form and then in a smoked version enabling a better regulation of the dose.

As little as 50 μg/kg produces emotional withdrawal, concrete thinking, and bizarre responses to projective testing. Catatonic posturing also is produced and resembles that of schizophrenia. Abusers taking higher doses may appear to be reacting to hallucinations and may exhibit hostile or assaultive behavior. Anesthetic effects increase with dosage; stupor or coma may occur with muscular rigidity, rhabdomyolysis, and hyperthermia. Intoxicated patients in the emergency room may progress from aggressive behavior to coma, with elevated blood pressure and enlarged nonreactive pupils. PCP binds with high affinity to sites located in the cortex and limbic structures, resulting in blocking of NMDA–type glutamate receptors (*see* Chapter 14). LSD and other psychedelics do not bind to NMDA receptors. There is evidence that NMDA receptors are involved in ischemic neuronal death caused by high levels of excitatory amino acids; as a result, there is interest in PCP analogs that block NMDA receptors but with fewer psychoactive effects. Both PCP and ketamine ("Special K"), another "club drug," produce similar effects by altering the distribution of the neurotransmitter glutamate.

Pharmacological Intervention. Overdose must be treated by life support because there is no antagonist of PCP effects and no proven way to enhance excretion, although acidification of the urine has been proposed. PCP coma may last 7-10 days. The agitated or psychotic state produced by PCP can be treated with diazepam. Prolonged psychotic behavior requires antipsychotic medication. Because of the anticholinergic activity of PCP, antipsychotic agents with significant anticholinergic effects such as chlorpromazine should be avoided.

For a complete Bibliographical Listing see Goodman & Gilman's ***The Pharmacological Basis of Therapeutics***, 12th ed., or Goodman & Gilman Online at www.AccessMedicine.com.

Section III Modulation of Cardiovascular Function

Chapter 25 Regulation of Renal Function and Vascular Volume

RENAL ANATOMY AND PHYSIOLOGY

The basic urine-forming unit of the kidney is the nephron, which consists of a filtering apparatus, the glomerulus, connected to a long tubular portion that reabsorbs and conditions the glomerular ultrafiltrate. Each human kidney is composed of ~1 million nephrons. Figure 25–1 illustrates subdivisions of the nephron.

GLOMERULAR FILTRATION. In the glomerular capillaries, a portion of plasma water is forced through a filter that has 3 basic components: the fenestrated capillary endothelial cells, a basement membrane lying just beneath the endothelial cells, and the filtration slit diaphragms formed by epithelial cells that cover the basement membrane on its urinary space side. Solutes of small size flow with filtered water (solvent drag) into the urinary (Bowman's) space, whereas formed elements and macromolecules are retained by the filtration barrier.

OVERVIEW OF NEPHRON FUNCTION. The kidney filters large quantities of plasma, reabsorbs substances that the body must conserve, and leaves behind or secretes substances that must be eliminated. The changing architecture and cellular differentiation along the length of a nephron is crucial to these functions (*see* Figure 25–1). The 2 kidneys in humans produce together ~120 mL of ultrafiltrate per minute, yet only 1 mL/min of urine is produced. Therefore, >99% of the glomerular ultrafiltrate is reabsorbed at a staggering energy cost. The kidneys consume 7% of total-body oxygen intake despite the fact that the kidneys make up only 0.5% of body weight.

The proximal tubule is contiguous with Bowman's capsule and takes a tortuous path until finally forming a straight portion that dives into the renal medulla. Normally, ~65% of filtered Na^+ is reabsorbed in the proximal tubule, and since this part of the tubule is highly permeable to water, reabsorption is essentially isotonic. Between the outer and inner strips of the outer medulla, the tubule abruptly changes morphology to become the descending thin limb (DTL), which penetrates the inner medulla, makes a hairpin turn, and then forms the ascending thin limb (ATL). At the juncture between the inner and outer medulla, the tubule once again changes morphology and becomes the thick ascending limb (TAL, with 3 segments noted in Figure 25–1). Together the proximal straight tubule, DTL, ATL, and TAL segments are known as the *loop of Henle*.

The DTL is highly permeable to water, yet its permeability to NaCl and urea is low. In contrast, the ATL is permeable to NaCl and urea but is impermeable to water. The TAL actively reabsorbs NaCl but is impermeable to water and urea. Approximately 25% of filtered Na^+ is reabsorbed in the loop of Henle, mostly in the TAL, which has a large reabsorptive capacity. The TAL passes between the afferent and efferent arterioles and makes contact with the afferent arteriole by means of a cluster of specialized columnar epithelial cells known as the *macula densa*. The macula densa is strategically located to sense concentrations of NaCl leaving the loop of Henle. If the concentration of NaCl is too high, the macula densa sends a chemical signal (perhaps adenosine or ATP) to the afferent arteriole of the same nephron, causing it to constrict, thereby reducing the glomerular filtration rate (GFR). This homeostatic mechanism, known as *tubuloglomerular feedback* (TGF), protects the organism from salt and volume wasting. The macula densa also regulates renin release from the adjacent juxtaglomerular cells in the wall of the afferent arteriole.

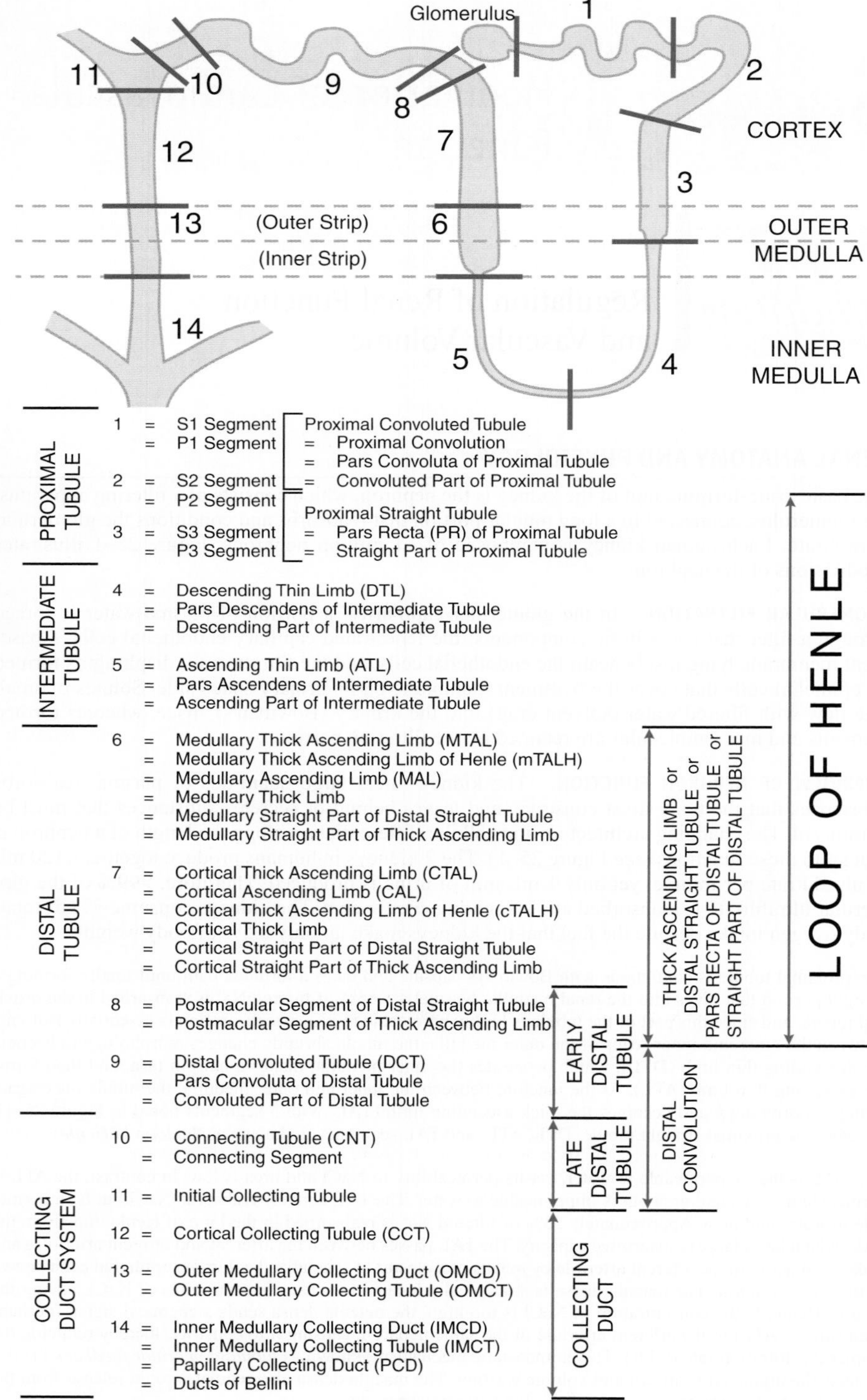

Figure 25–1 *Anatomy and nomenclature of the nephron.*

Approximately 0.2 mm past the macula densa, the tubule changes morphology once again to become the distal convoluted tubule (DCT). Like the TAL, the DCT actively transports NaCl and is impermeable to water. Because these characteristics impart the ability to produce a dilute urine, the TAL and the DCT are collectively called the *diluting segment of the nephron*, and the tubular fluid in the DCT is hypotonic regardless of hydration status. However, unlike the TAL, the DCT does not contribute to the countercurrent-induced hypertonicity of the medullary interstitium (described below).

The collecting duct system (segments 10–14 in Figure 25–1) is an area of fine control of ultrafiltrate composition and volume. It is here that final adjustments in electrolyte composition are made, a process modulated by the adrenal steroid aldosterone. In addition, vasopressin (also called antidiuretic hormone [ADH]) modulates water permeability of this part of the nephron. The more distal portions of the collecting duct pass through the renal medulla, where the interstitial fluid is markedly hypertonic. In the absence of ADH, the collecting duct system is impermeable to water, and a dilute urine is excreted. In the presence of ADH, the collecting duct system is permeable to water, so water is reabsorbed. The movement of water out of the tubule is driven by the steep concentration gradient that exists between tubular fluid and medullary interstitium.

The hypertonicity of the medullary interstitium plays a vital role in the ability of mammals and birds to concentrate urine, which is accomplished by a combination of the unique topography of the loop of Henle and the specialized permeability features of the loop's subsegments. The "passive countercurrent multiplier hypothesis" proposes that active transport in the TAL concentrates NaCl in the interstitium of the outer medulla. Because this segment of the nephron is impermeable to water, active transport in the ascending limb dilutes the tubular fluid. As the dilute fluid passes into the collecting-duct system, water is extracted if, and only if, ADH is present. Since the cortical and outer medullary collecting ducts have a low permeability to urea, urea is concentrated in the tubular fluid. The inner medullary collecting duct, however, is permeable to urea, so urea diffuses into the inner medulla, where it is trapped by countercurrent exchange in the vasa recta. Because the DTL is impermeable to salt and urea, the high urea concentration in the inner medulla extracts water from the DTL and concentrates NaCl in the tubular fluid of the DTL. As the tubular fluid enters the ATL, NaCl diffuses out of the salt-permeable ATL, thus contributing to the hypertonicity of the medullary interstitium.

GENERAL MECHANISM OF RENAL EPITHELIAL TRANSPORT. There are multiple mechanisms by which solutes may cross cell membranes (*see* Figure 5–4). The kinds of transport achieved in a nephron segment depend mainly on which transporters are present and whether they are embedded in the luminal or basolateral membrane. Figure 25–2 presents a general model of renal tubular transport that be summarized as follows:

1. Na^+, K^+-ATPase (sodium pump) in the basolateral membrane transports Na^+ into the intercellular and interstitial spaces and K^+ into the cell, establishing an electrochemical gradient for Na^+ across the cell membrane directed inward.
2. Na^+ can diffuse down this Na^+ gradient across the luminal membrane via Na^+ channels and via membrane symporters that use the energy stored in the Na^+ gradient to transport solutes out of the tubular lumen and into the cell (e.g., Na^+-glucose, Na^+-$H_2PO_4^-$, and Na^+-amino acid) and antiporters (e.g., Na^+-H^+) that move solutes into the lumen as Na^+ moves out of the tubular lumen and into the cell.
3. Na^+ exits the basolateral membrane into intercellular and interstitial spaces via the Na^+ pump.
4. The action of Na^+-linked symporters in the luminal membrane causes the concentration of substrates for these symporters to rise in the epithelial cell. These substrate/solute gradients then permit simple diffusion or mediated transport (e.g., symporters, antiporters, uniporters, and channels) of solutes into the intercellular and interstitial spaces.
5. Accumulation of Na^+ and other solutes in the intercellular space creates a small osmotic pressure differential across the epithelial cell. In water-permeable epithelium, water moves into the intercellular spaces driven by the osmotic pressure differential. Water moves through aqueous pores in both the luminal and the basolateral cell membranes, as well as through tight junctions (paracellular pathway). Bulk water flow carries some solutes into the intercellular space by solvent drag.
6. Movement of water into the intercellular space concentrates other solutes in the tubular fluid, resulting in an electrochemical gradient for these substances across the epithelium. Membrane-permeable solutes then move down their electrochemical gradients into the intercellular space by both the transcellular (e.g., simple diffusion, symporters, antiporters, uniporters, and channels) and paracellular pathways. Membrane-impermeable solutes remain in the tubular lumen and are excreted in the urine with an obligatory amount of water.
7. As water and solutes accumulate in the intercellular space, hydrostatic pressure increases, thus providing a driving force for bulk water flow. Bulk water flow carries solute out of the intercellular space into the interstitial space and, finally, into the peritubular capillaries.

ORGANIC ACID AND ORGANIC BASE SECRETION

The kidney is a major organ involved in the elimination of organic chemicals from the body. Organic molecules may enter the renal tubules by glomerular filtration or may be actively secreted directly into tubules. The

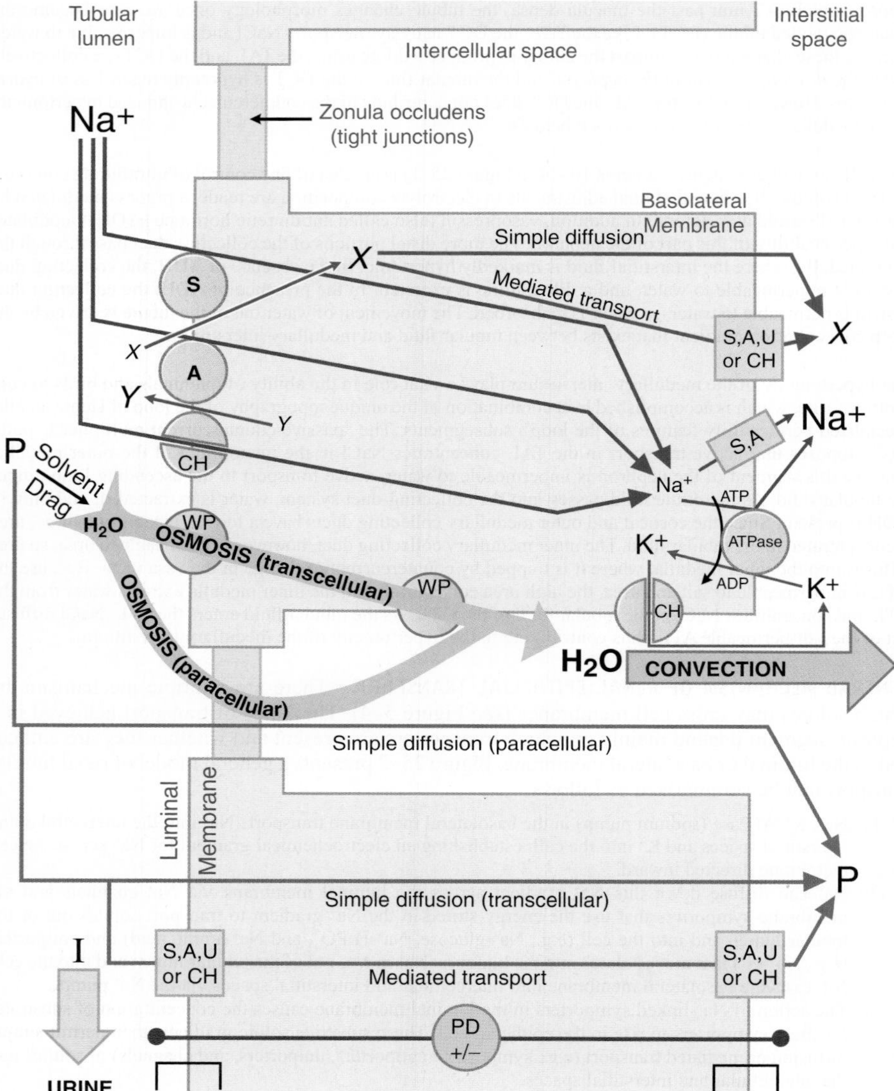

Figure 25–2 *Generic mechanism of renal epithelial cell transport (see text for details).* S, symporter; A, antiporter; CH, ion channel; WP, water pore; U, uniporter; ATPase, Na^+,K^+-ATPase (sodium pump); *X* and *Y*, transported solutes; *P*, membrane-permeable (reabsorbable) solutes; *I*, membrane-impermeable (nonreabsorbable) solutes; PD, potential difference across indicated membrane or cell.

proximal tubule has a highly efficient transport system for organic acids and an equally efficient but separate transport system for organic bases. Current models for these secretory systems are illustrated in Figure 25–3. Both systems are powered by the sodium pump in the basolateral membrane, involve secondary and tertiary active transport, and use a facilitated-diffusion step. There are at least 9 different organic acid and 5 different organic base transporters (*see* Chapter 5). A family of organic anion transporters (OATs) links countertransport of organic anions with dicarboxylates (Figure 25–3A).

RENAL HANDLING OF SPECIFIC ANIONS AND CATIONS

Reabsorption of Cl^- generally follows reabsorption of Na^+. In segments of the tubule with low-resistance tight junctions (i.e., "leaky" epithelium), such as the proximal tubule and TAL, Cl^- movement can occur

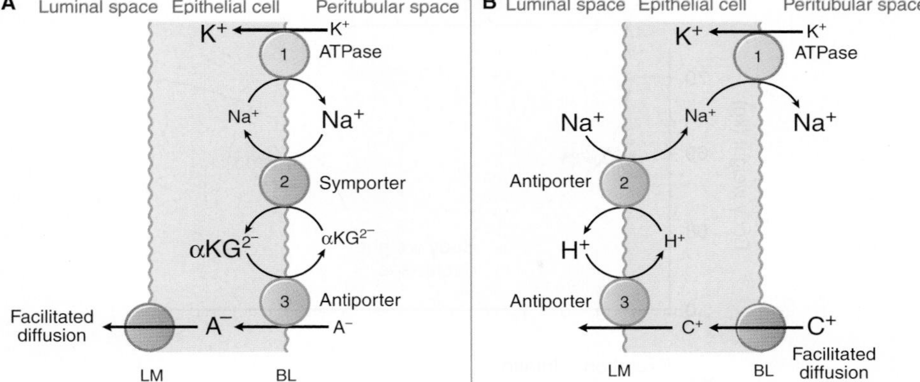

Figure 25–3 *Mechanisms of organic acid (A) and organic base (B) secretion in the proximal tubule.* The numbers 1, 2, and 3 refer to primary, secondary, and tertiary active transport. A^-, organic acid [anion]; C^+, organic base [cation]; αKG^{2-}, α-ketoglutarate but also other dicarboxylates. BL and LM indicate basolateral and luminal membranes, respectively.

paracellularly. Cl^- crosses the luminal membrane by antiport with formate and oxalate (proximal tubule), symport with Na^+/K^+ (TAL), symport with Na^+ (DCT), and antiport with HCO_3^- (collecting-duct system). Cl^- crosses the basolateral membrane by symport with K^+ (proximal tubule and TAL), antiport with Na^+/HCO_3^- (proximal tubule), and Cl^- channels (TAL, DCT, collecting-duct system).

Eighty to ninety percent of filtered K^+ is reabsorbed in the proximal tubule (diffusion and solvent drag) and TAL (diffusion), largely through the paracellular pathway. The DCT and collecting-duct system secrete variable amounts of K^+ by a channel-mediated pathway. Modulation of the rate of K^+ secretion in the collecting-duct system, particularly by aldosterone, allows urinary K^+ excretion to be matched with dietary intake. The transepithelial potential difference (V_T), lumen-positive in the TAL and lumen-negative in the collecting-duct system, drives K^+ reabsorption and secretion, respectively.

Most of the filtered Ca^{2+} (~70%) is reabsorbed by the proximal tubule by passive diffusion through a paracellular route. Another 25% of filtered Ca^{2+} is reabsorbed by the TAL in part by a paracellular route driven by the lumen-positive V_T and in part by active transcellular Ca^{2+} reabsorption modulated by parathyroid hormone (PTH; *see* Chapter 44). Most of the remaining Ca^{2+} is reabsorbed in DCT by a transcellular pathway. The transcellular pathway in the TAL and DCT involves passive Ca^{2+} influx across the luminal membrane through Ca^{2+} channels (TRPV5), followed by Ca^{2+} extrusion across the basolateral membrane by a Ca^{2+}-ATPase. Also, in DCT and CNT, Ca^{2+} crosses the basolateral membrane by Na^+-Ca^{2+} exchanger (antiport). Inorganic phosphate (P_i) is largely reabsorbed (80% of filtered load) by the proximal tubule. The Na^+-P_i symporter uses the free energy of the Na^+ electrochemical gradient to transport P_i into the cell. The Na^+-P_i symporter is inhibited by PTH.

The renal tubules reabsorb HCO_3^- and secrete protons (tubular acidification), thereby participating in acid–base balance. These processes are described in the section on carbonic anhydrase inhibitors.

PRINCIPLES OF DIURETIC ACTION

Diuretics are drugs that increase the rate of urine flow; clinically useful diuretics also increase the rate of Na^+ excretion (natriuresis) and of an accompanying anion, usually Cl^-. Most clinical applications of diuretics are directed toward reducing extracellular fluid volume by decreasing total-body NaCl content.

Although continued diuretic administration causes a sustained net deficit in total-body Na^+, the time course of natriuresis is finite because renal compensatory mechanisms bring Na^+ excretion in line with Na^+ intake, a phenomenon known as *diuretic braking*. These compensatory mechanisms include activation of the sympathetic nervous system, activation of the renin–angiotensin–aldosterone axis, decreased arterial blood pressure (which reduces pressure natriuresis), renal epithelial cell hypertrophy, increased renal epithelial transporter expression, and perhaps alterations in natriuretic hormones such as atrial natriuretic peptide. The net effects on extracellular volume and body weight are shown in Figure 25–4.

Diuretics may modify renal handling of other cations (e.g., K^+, H^+, Ca^{2+}, and Mg^{2+}), anions (e.g., Cl^-, HCO_3^-, and $H_2PO_4^-$), and uric acid. In addition, diuretics may alter renal hemodynamics indirectly. Table 25–1 gives a comparison of the general effects of the major diuretic classes.

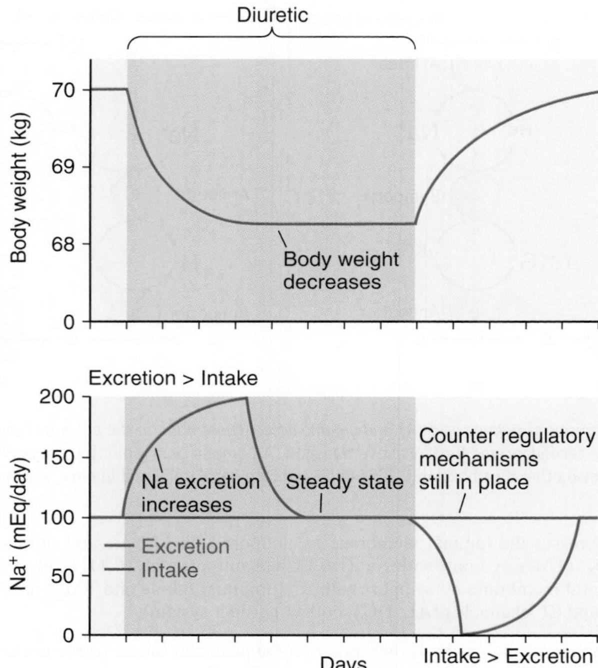

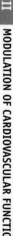

Figure 25–4 *Changes in extracellular fluid volume and weight with diuretic therapy.* The period of diuretic administration is shown in the shaded box along with its effects on body weight in the upper part of the figure and Na^+ excretion in the lower half of the figure. Initially, when Na^+ excretion exceeds intake, body weight and extracellular fluid volume (ECFV) decrease. Subsequently, a new steady state is achieved where Na^+ intake and excretion are equal but at a lower ECFV and body weight. This results from activation of the renin-angiotensin-aldosterone system (RAAS) and sympathetic nervous system (SNS), "the braking phenomenon." When the diuretic is discontinued, body weight and ECFV rise during a period where Na^+ intake exceeds excretion. A new steady state is then reached as stimulation of the RAAS and SNS wane.

INHIBITORS OF CARBONIC ANHYDRASE

There are 3 orally administered carbonic anhydrase inhibitors—acetazolamide, dichlorphenamide (not marketed in the U.S.), and methazolamide (Table 25–2).

MECHANISM AND SITE OF ACTION. Proximal tubular epithelial cells are richly endowed with the zinc metalloenzyme carbonic anhydrase, which is found in the luminal and basolateral membranes (type IV carbonic anhydrase), as well as in the cytoplasm (type II carbonic anhydrase) (Figure 25–5). Carbonic anhydrase plays a role in $NaHCO_3$ reabsorption and acid secretion.

In the proximal tubule, the free energy in the Na^+ gradient established by the basolateral Na^+ pump is used by a Na^+-H^+ antiporter (a.k.a. Na^+-H^+ exchanger [NHE]) in the luminal membrane to transport H^+ into the tubular lumen in exchange for Na^+. In the lumen, H^+ reacts with filtered HCO_3^- to form H_2CO_3, which decomposes rapidly to CO_2 and water in the presence of carbonic anhydrase in the brush border. Carbonic anhydrase reversibly accelerates this reaction several thousand fold. CO_2 is lipophilic and rapidly diffuses across the luminal membrane into the epithelial cell, where it reacts with water to form H_2CO_3, a reaction catalyzed by cytoplasmic carbonic anhydrase. Continued operation of the Na^+-H^+ antiporter maintains a low proton concentration in the cell, so H_2CO_3 ionizes spontaneously to form H^+ and HCO_3^-, creating an electrochemical gradient for HCO_3^- across the basolateral membrane. The electrochemical gradient for HCO_3^- is used by a Na^+-HCO_3^- symporter (a.k.a. the Na^+-HCO_3^- co-transporter [NBC]) in the basolateral membrane to transport $NaHCO_3$ into the interstitial space. The net effect of this process is transport of $NaHCO_3$ from the tubular lumen to the interstitial space, followed by movement of water (isotonic reabsorption). Removal of water concentrates Cl^- in the tubular lumen, and consequently, Cl^- diffuses down its concentration gradient into the interstitium by the paracellular pathway.

Carbonic anhydrase inhibitors potently inhibit both the membrane-bound and cytoplasmic forms of carbonic anhydrase, resulting in nearly complete abolition of $NaHCO_3$ reabsorption in the proximal tubule. Because

Table 25–1

Excretory and Renal Hemodynamic Effects of Diuretics[a]

Diuretic Mechanism	CATIONS					ANIONS			URIC ACID		RENAL HEMODYNAMICS			
(Primary site of action)	Na^+	K^+	H^+[b]	Ca^{2+}	Mg^{2+}	Cl^-	HCO_3^-	$H_2PO_4^-$	*Acute*	*Chronic*	RBF	GFR	FF	TGF
Inhibitors of CA (proximal tubule)	+	++	–	NC	V	(+)	++	++	I	–	–	–	NC	+
Osmotic diuretics (loop of Henle)	++	+	I	+	++	+	+	+	+	I	+	NC	–	I
Inhibitors of Na^+-K^+-$2Cl^-$ symport (thick ascending limb)	++	++	+	++	++	++	+[c]	+[c]	+	–	V(+)	NC	V(–)	–
Inhibitors of Na^+-Cl^- symport (distal convoluted tubule)	+	++	+	V(–)	V(+)	+	+[c]	+[c]	+	–	NC	V(–)	V(–)	NC
Inhibitors of renal epithelial Na^+ channels (late distal tubule, collecting duct)	+	–	–	–	–	+	(+)	NC	I	–	NC	NC	NC	NC
Antagonists of mineralocorticoid receptors (late distal tubule, collecting duct)	+	–	–	I	–	+	(+)	I	I	–	NC	NC	NC	NC

RBF, renal blood flow; GFR, glomerular filtration rate; FF, filtration fraction; TGF, tubuloglomerular feedback; CA, carbonic anhydrase.

[a]*Except for uric acid, changes are for acute effects of diuretics in the absence of significant volume depletion, which would trigger complex physiological adjustments.*

[b]*H^+, titratable acid and NH_4^+.*

[c]*In general, these effects are restricted to those individual agents that inhibit carbonic anhydrase. However, there are notable exceptions in which symport inhibitors increase bicarbonate and phosphate (e.g., metolazone, bumetanide). ++, +, (+),–, NC, V, V(+), V(–) and I indicate marked increase, mild to moderate increase, slight increase, decrease, no change, variable effect, variable increase, variable decrease, and insufficient data, respectively. For cations and anions, the indicated effects refer to absolute changes in fractional excretion.*

Table 25–2

Inhibitors of Carbonic Anhydrase

DRUG	RELATIVE POTENCY	ORAL AVAILABILITY	$t_{1/2}$ (hours)	ROUTE OF ELIMINATION
Acetazolamide (DIAMOX)	1	~100%	6-9	R
Dichlorphenamide (DARAMIDE)	30	ID	ID	ID
Methazolamide (GLAUCTABS)	>1; <10	~100%	~14	~25%, ~75% M

R, renal excretion of intact drug; M, metabolism; ID, insufficient data.

of the large excess of carbonic anhydrase in proximal tubules, a high percentage of enzyme activity must be inhibited before an effect on electrolyte excretion is observed. Although the proximal tubule is the major site of action of carbonic anhydrase inhibitors, carbonic anhydrase also is involved in secretion of titratable acid in the collecting duct system, which is a secondary site of action for this class of drugs.

EFFECTS ON URINARY EXCRETION. Inhibition of carbonic anhydrase is associated with a rapid rise in urinary HCO_3^- excretion to ~35% of filtered load. This, along with inhibition of titratable acid and NH_4^+ secretion in the collecting-duct system, results in an increase in urinary pH to ~8 and development of a metabolic acidosis. However, even with a high degree of inhibition of carbonic anhydrase, 65% of HCO_3^- is rescued from excretion. The loop of Henle has a large reabsorptive capacity and captures most of the Cl^- and a portion of the Na^+. Thus, only a small increase in Cl^- excretion occurs, HCO_3^- being the major anion excreted along with the cations Na^+ and K^+. The fractional excretion of Na^+ may be as much as 5%, and the fractional excretion of

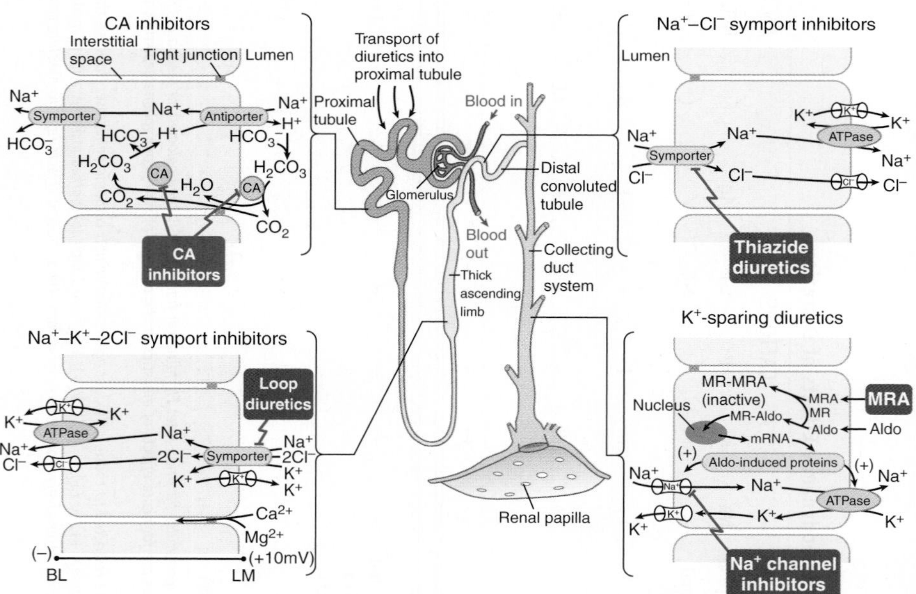

Figure 25–5 *Sites and mechanisms of action of diuretics.* Three important features are noteworthy:

1. Transport of solute across epithelial cells in all nephron segments involves highly specialized proteins, which for the most part are apical and basolateral membrane integral proteins.
2. Diuretics target and block the action of epithelial proteins involved in solute transport.
3. The site and mechanism of action of a given class of diuretics are determined by the specific protein inhibited by the diuretic.

CA, carbonic anhydrase; MR, mineralocorticoid receptor; MRA, mineralocorticoid receptor antagonist; Aldo, aldosterone; BL, basolateral membrane; LM, luminal membrane.

K^+ can be as much as 70%. The increased excretion of K^+ is in part secondary to increased delivery of Na^+ to the distal nephron, as described in the section on inhibitors of Na^+ channels. The effects of carbonic anhydrase inhibitors on renal excretion are self-limiting, probably because the resulting metabolic acidosis decreases the filtered load of HCO_3^- to the point that the uncatalyzed reaction between CO_2 and water is sufficient to achieve HCO_3^- reabsorption.

EFFECTS ON RENAL HEMODYNAMICS. By inhibiting proximal reabsorption, carbonic anhydrase inhibitors increase delivery of solutes to the macula densa. This triggers TGF, which increases afferent arteriolar resistance and reduces renal blood flow (RBF) and GFR.

OTHER ACTIONS. These agents have extrarenal sites of action. Carbonic anhydrase in the ciliary processes of the eye mediates formation of HCO_3^- in aqueous humor. Inhibition of carbonic anhydrase decreases the rate of formation of aqueous humor and consequently reduces intraocular pressure. Acetazolamide frequently causes paresthesias and somnolence, suggesting an action of carbonic anhydrase inhibitors in the CNS. The efficacy of acetazolamide in epilepsy is due in part to the production of metabolic acidosis; however, direct actions of acetazolamide in the CNS also contribute to its anticonvulsant action. Owing to interference with carbonic anhydrase activity in erythrocytes, carbonic anhydrase inhibitors increase CO_2 levels in peripheral tissues and decrease CO_2 levels in expired gas. Acetazolamide causes vasodilation by opening vascular Ca^{2+}-activated K^+ channels; however, the clinical significance of this effect is unclear.

ABSORPTION AND ELIMINATION. *See* Table 25–2 for pharmacokinetic data.

TOXICITY, ADVERSE EFFECTS, CONTRAINDICATIONS, DRUG INTERACTIONS. Serious toxic reactions to carbonic anhydrase inhibitors are infrequent; however, these drugs are sulfonamide derivatives and, like other sulfonamides, may cause bone marrow depression, skin toxicity, sulfonamide-like renal lesions, and allergic reactions. With large doses, many patients exhibit drowsiness and paresthesias. Most adverse effects, contraindications, and drug interactions are secondary to urinary alkalinization or metabolic acidosis, including: (1) diversion of ammonia of renal origin from urine into the systemic circulation, a process that may induce or worsen hepatic encephalopathy (the drugs are contraindicated in patients with hepatic cirrhosis); (2) calculus formation and ureteral colic owing to precipitation of calcium phosphate salts in an alkaline urine; (3) worsening of metabolic or respiratory acidosis (the drugs are contraindicated in patients with hyperchloremic acidosis or severe chronic obstructive pulmonary disease); (4) reduction of the urinary excretion rate of weak organic bases.

THERAPEUTIC USES. The efficacy of carbonic anhydrase inhibitors as single agents is low. The combination of acetazolamide with diuretics that block Na^+ reabsorption at more distal sites in the nephron causes a marked natriuretic response in patients with low basal fractional excretion of Na^+ (<0.2%) who are resistant to diuretic monotherapy. Even so, the long-term usefulness of carbonic anhydrase inhibitors often is compromised by the development of metabolic acidosis. The major indication for carbonic anhydrase inhibitors is open-angle glaucoma. Two products developed specifically for this use are dorzolamide (TRUSOPT, others) and brinzolamide (AZOPT), which are available only as ophthalmic drops. Carbonic anhydrase inhibitors also may be employed for secondary glaucoma and preoperatively in acute angle-closure glaucoma to lower intraocular pressure before surgery (*see* Chapter 64). Acetazolamide also is used for the treatment of epilepsy (*see* Chapter 21). Acetazolamide can provide symptomatic relief in patients with *high-altitude illness* or *mountain sickness*. Acetazolamide also is useful in patients with familial periodic paralysis. The mechanism for the beneficial effects of acetazolamide in altitude sickness and familial periodic paralysis may be related to the induction of a metabolic acidosis. Finally, carbonic anhydrase inhibitors can be useful for correcting a metabolic alkalosis, especially one caused by diuretic-induced increases in H^+ excretion.

OSMOTIC DIURETICS

Osmotic diuretics are freely filtered at the glomerulus, undergo limited reabsorption by the renal tubule, and are relatively inert pharmacologically. Osmotic diuretics are administered in doses large enough to increase significantly the osmolality of plasma and tubular fluid. Table 25–3 lists 4 osmotic diuretics—glycerin (OSMOGLYN), isosorbide, mannitol (OSMITROL, others), and urea (currently not available in the U.S.).

MECHANISM AND SITE OF ACTION. Osmotic diuretics act both in proximal tubule and loop of Henle, with the latter being the primary site of action. By extracting water from intracellular compartments, osmotic diuretics expand extracellular fluid volume, decrease blood viscosity, and inhibit renin release. These effects increase RBF, and the increase in renal medullary blood flow removes NaCl and urea from the renal medulla, thus reducing medullary tonicity. A reduction in medullary tonicity causes a decrease in the extraction of water from the DTL, which in turn limits the concentration of NaCl in the tubular fluid entering the ATL. This latter effect diminishes the passive reabsorption of NaCl in the ATL. In addition osmotic diuretics inhibit Mg^{2+} reabsorption in the TAL.

Table 25–3

Osmotic Diuretics

DRUG	ORAL AVAILABILITY	$t_{1/2}$ (hours)	ROUTE OF ELIMINATION
Glycerin	Orally active	0.5-0.75	~80% M ~20% U
Isosorbide	Orally active	5-9.5	R
Mannitol	Negligible	0.25-1.7[a]	~80% R ~20% M + B
Urea	Negligible	ID	R

R, renal excretion of intact drug; M, metabolism; B, excretion of intact drug into bile; U, unknown pathway of elimination; ID, insufficient data.

[a]In renal failure, 6–36.

EFFECTS ON URINARY EXCRETION. Osmotic diuretics increase urinary excretion of nearly all electrolytes, including Na^+, K^+, Ca^{2+}, Mg^{2+}, Cl^-, HCO_3^-, and phosphate.

EFFECTS ON RENAL HEMODYNAMICS. Osmotic diuretics increase RBF by a variety of mechanisms, but total GFR is little changed.

ABSORPTION AND ELIMINATION. Pharmacokinetic data on the osmotic diuretics are gathered in Table 25–3. Glycerin and isosorbide can be given orally, whereas mannitol and urea must be administered intravenously.

TOXICITY, ADVERSE EFFECTS, CONTRAINDICATIONS, AND DRUG INTERACTIONS. Osmotic diuretics are distributed in the extracellular fluid and contribute to the extracellular osmolality. Thus, water is extracted from intracellular compartments, and the extracellular fluid volume becomes expanded. In patients with heart failure or pulmonary congestion, this may cause frank pulmonary edema. Extraction of water also causes hyponatremia, which may explain the common adverse effects, including headache, nausea, and vomiting. Conversely, loss of water in excess of electrolytes can cause hypernatremia and dehydration. Osmotic diuretics are contraindicated in patients who are anuric owing to severe renal disease. Urea may cause thrombosis or pain if extravasation occurs, and it should not be administered to patients with impaired liver function because of the risk of elevation of blood ammonia levels. Both mannitol and urea are contraindicated in patients with active cranial bleeding. Glycerin is metabolized and can cause hyperglycemia.

THERAPEUTIC USES. One use for mannitol is in the treatment of dialysis disequilibrium syndrome. Overly removing solutes from the extracellular fluid by hemodialysis results in a reduction in the osmolality of extracellular fluid. Consequently, water moves from the extracellular compartment into the intracellular compartment, causing hypotension and CNS symptoms (headache, nausea, muscle cramps, restlessness, CNS depression, and convulsions). Osmotic diuretics increase the osmolality of the extracellular fluid compartment and thereby shift water back into the extracellular compartment. By increasing the osmotic pressure of plasma, osmotic diuretics extract water from the eye and brain. All osmotic diuretics are used to control intraocular pressure during acute attacks of glaucoma and for short-term reductions in intraocular pressure both preoperatively and postoperatively in patients who require ocular surgery. Also, mannitol and urea are used to reduce cerebral edema and brain mass before and after neurosurgery.

INHIBITORS OF Na^+-K^+-$2Cl^-$ SYMPORT (LOOP DIURETICS, HIGH-CEILING DIURETICS)

These diuretics inhibit activity of the Na^+-K^+-$2Cl^-$ symporter in the TAL of the loop of Henle, hence the moniker *loop diuretics*. Although the proximal tubule reabsorbs ~65% of filtered Na^+, diuretics acting only in the proximal tubule have limited efficacy because the TAL has the capacity to reabsorb most of the rejectate from the proximal tubule. In contrast, inhibitors of Na^+-K^+-$2Cl^-$ symport in the TAL, sometimes called *high-ceiling diuretics*, are highly efficacious because (1) ~25% of the filtered Na^+ load normally is reabsorbed by the TAL, and (2) nephron segments past the TAL do not possess the resorptive capacity to rescue the flood of rejectate exiting the TAL.

Of the inhibitors of Na^+-K^+-$2Cl^-$ symport (Table 25–4), only furosemide (LASIX), bumetanide (BUMEX), ethacrynic acid (EDECRIN), and torsemide (DEMADEX) are available currently in the U.S. Furosemide and bumetanide contain a sulfonamide moiety. Ethacrynic acid is a phenoxyacetic acid derivative; torsemide is a sulfonylurea. All loop diuretics except torsemide are available as oral and injectable formulations.

Table 25–4

Inhibitors of Na^+–K^+–$2Cl^-$ Symport (Loop Diuretics, High-Ceiling Diuretics)

DRUG	RELATIVE POTENCY	ORAL AVAILABILITY	$t_{1/2}$ (hours)	ROUTE OF ELIMINATION
Furosemide	1	~60%	~1.5	~65% R, ~35% M[b]
Bumetanide	40	~80%	~0.8	~62% R, ~38% M
Ethacrynic acid	0.7	~100%	~1	~67% R, ~33% M
Torsemide	3	~80%	~3.5	~20% R, ~80% M
Axosemide[a]	1	~12%	~2.5	~27% R, 63% M
Piretanide[a]	3	~80%	0.6-1.5	~50% R, ~50% M
Tripamide[a]	ID	ID	ID	ID

R, renal excretion of intact drug; M, metabolism; ID, insufficient data.
[a]Not available in the United States.
[b]For furosemide, metabolism occurs predominantly in the kidney.

MECHANISM AND SITE OF ACTION. These agents act primarily in the TAL, where the flux of Na^+, K^+, and Cl^- from the lumen into epithelial cells is mediated by a Na^+-K^+-$2Cl^-$ symporter (Figure 25–5). Inhibitors of Na^+-K^+-$2Cl^-$ symport block its function, bringing salt transport in this segment of the nephron to a virtual standstill. Evidence suggests that these drugs attach to the Cl^- binding site located in the symporter's transmembrane domain. Inhibitors of Na^+K^+-$2Cl^-$ symport also inhibit Ca^{2+} and Mg^{2+} reabsorption in the TAL by abolishing the transepithelial potential difference that is the dominant driving force for reabsorption of these cations. Na^+-K^+-$2Cl^-$ symporters are found in many secretory and absorbing epithelia. The Na^+-K^+-$2Cl^-$ symporters are of 2 varieties. The "absorptive" symporter (called *ENCC2, NKCC2*, or *BSCl*) is expressed only in the kidney, is localized to the apical membrane and subapical intracellular vesicles of the TAL, and is regulated by cyclic AMP/PKA. The "secretory" symporter (called *ENCC3, NKCCl*, or *BSC2*) is a "housekeeping" protein that is expressed widely and, in epithelial cells, is localized to the basolateral membrane. The affinity of loop diuretics for the secretory symporter is somewhat less than for the absorptive symporter (e.g., 4-fold difference for bumetanide).

EFFECTS ON URINARY EXCRETION. Loop diuretics increase urinary Na^+ and Cl^- excretion profoundly (i.e., up to 25% of the filtered Na^+ load) and markedly increase Ca^{2+} and Mg^{2+} excretion. Furosemide has weak carbonic anhydrase–inhibiting activity and thus increases urinary excretion of HCO_3^- and phosphate. All inhibitors of Na^+-K^+-$2Cl^-$ symport increase urinary K^+ and titratable acid excretion. This effect is due in part to increased Na^+ delivery to the distal tubule (the mechanism by which increased distal Na^+ delivery enhances K^+ and H^+ excretion is discussed in the section on Na^+ channel inhibitors). Other mechanisms contributing to enhanced K^+ and H^+ excretion include flow-dependent enhancement of ion secretion by the collecting duct, nonosmotic vasopressin release, and activation of the renin–angiotensin–aldosterone axis.

Acutely, loop diuretics increase uric acid excretion; their chronic administration results in reduced uric acid excretion. Chronic effects of loop diuretics on uric acid excretion may be due to enhanced proximal tubule transport or secondary to volume depletion or to competition between diuretic and uric acid for the organic acid secretory mechanism in proximal tubule. Asymptomatic hyperuricemia is a common consequence of loop diuretics, but painful episodes of gout are rarely reported. By blocking active NaCl reabsorption in the TAL, inhibitors of Na^+-K^+-$2Cl^-$ symport interfere with a critical step in the mechanism that produces a hypertonic medullary interstitium. Therefore, loop diuretics block the kidney's ability to concentrate urine. Also, because the TAL is part of the diluting segment, inhibitors of Na^+-K^+-$2Cl^-$ symport markedly impair the kidney's ability to excrete a dilute urine during water diuresis.

EFFECTS ON RENAL HEMODYNAMICS. If volume depletion is prevented by replacing fluid losses, inhibitors of Na^+-K^+-$2Cl^-$ symport generally increase total RBF and redistribute RBF to the midcortex. The mechanism of the increase in RBF is not known, but may involve prostaglandins: nonsteroidal anti-inflammatory drugs (NSAIDs) attenuate the diuretic response to loop diuretics in part by preventing prostaglandin-mediated increases in RBF. Loop diuretics block TGF by inhibiting salt transport into the macula densa so that the macula densa no longer can detect NaCl concentrations in the tubular fluid. Therefore, unlike carbonic anhydrase inhibitors, loop diuretics do not decrease GFR by activating TGF. Loop diuretics are powerful stimulators of renin release. This effect is due to interference with NaCl transport by the macula densa and, if volume depletion occurs, to reflex activation of the sympathetic nervous system and stimulation of the intrarenal baroreceptor mechanism.

OTHER ACTIONS. Loop diuretics, particularly furosemide, acutely increase systemic venous capacitance and thereby decrease left ventricular filling pressure. This effect, which may be mediated by prostaglandins and requires intact kidneys, benefits patients with pulmonary edema even before diuresis ensues. High doses of inhibitors of Na^+-K^+-$2Cl^-$ symport can inhibit electrolyte transport in many tissues, but this effect is clinically important only in the inner ear.

ABSORPTION AND ELIMINATION. Table 25–4 presents some pharmacokinetic properties of the agents. Because these drugs are bound extensively to plasma proteins, delivery of these drugs to the tubules by filtration is limited. However, they are secreted efficiently by the organic acid transport system in the proximal tubule, and thereby gain access to the Na^+-K^+-$2Cl^-$ symporter in the luminal membrane of the TAL. Approximately 65% of furosemide is excreted unchanged in urine, and the remainder is conjugated to glucuronic acid in the kidney. Thus, in patients with renal disease, the elimination $t_{1/2}$ of furosemide is prolonged. Bumetanide and torsemide have significant hepatic metabolism, so liver disease can prolong the elimination $t_{1/2}$ of these loop diuretics. Oral bioavailability of furosemide varies (10-100%). In contrast, oral availabilities of bumetanide and torsemide are reliably high. Heart failure patients have fewer hospitalizations and better quality of life with torsemide than with furosemide, perhaps because of its more reliable absorption.

As a class, loop diuretics have short elimination half lives; prolonged-release preparations are not available. Consequently, often the dosing interval is too short to maintain adequate levels of loop diuretics in the tubular lumen. Note that torsemide has a longer $t_{1/2}$ than other agents available in the U.S. As the concentration of loop diuretic in the tubular lumen declines, nephrons begin to avidly reabsorb Na^+, which often nullifies the overall effect of the loop diuretic on total-body Na^+. This phenomenon of "postdiuretic Na^+ retention" can be overcome by restricting dietary Na^+ intake or by more frequent administration of the loop diuretic.

TOXICITY, ADVERSE EFFECTS, CONTRAINDICATIONS, DRUG INTERACTIONS. Most adverse effects are due to abnormalities of fluid and electrolyte balance. Overzealous use of loop diuretics can cause serious depletion of total-body Na^+. This may manifest as hyponatremia and/or extracellular fluid volume depletion associated with hypotension, reduced GFR, circulatory collapse, thromboembolic episodes, and in patients with liver disease, hepatic encephalopathy. Increased Na^+ delivery to the distal tubule, particularly when combined with activation of the renin–angiotensin system, leads to increased urinary K^+ and H^+ excretion, causing a hypochloremic alkalosis. If dietary K^+ intake is not sufficient, hypokalemia may develop, and this may induce cardiac arrhythmias, particularly in patients taking cardiac glycosides. Increased Mg^{2+} and Ca^{2+} excretion may result in hypomagnesemia (a risk factor for cardiac arrhythmias) and hypocalcemia (rarely leading to tetany). Loop diuretics should be avoided in postmenopausal osteopenic women, in whom increased Ca^{2+} excretion may have deleterious effects on bone metabolism.

Loop diuretics can cause ototoxicity that manifests as tinnitus, hearing impairment, deafness, vertigo, and a sense of fullness in the ears. Hearing impairment and deafness are usually, but not always, reversible. Ototoxicity occurs most frequently with rapid intravenous administration and least frequently with oral administration. Ethacrynic acid appears to induce ototoxicity more often than do other loop diuretics and should be reserved for use only in patients who cannot tolerate other loop diuretics. Loop diuretics also can cause hyperuricemia (occasionally leading to gout) and hyperglycemia (infrequently precipitating diabetes mellitus) and can increase plasma levels of LDL cholesterol and triglycerides while decreasing plasma levels of HDL cholesterol. Other adverse effects include skin rashes, photosensitivity, paresthesias, bone marrow depression, and GI disturbances. Contraindications to the use of loop diuretics include severe Na^+ and volume depletion, hypersensitivity to sulfonamides (for sulfonamide-based loop diuretics), and anuria unresponsive to a trial dose of loop diuretic.

Drug interactions may occur when loop diuretics are coadministered with:

- Aminoglycosides, carboplatin, paclitaxel, and others (synergism of ototoxicity)
- Anticoagulants (increased anticoagulant activity)
- Digitalis glycosides (increased digitalis-induced arrhythmias)
- Lithium (increased plasma levels of lithium)
- Propranolol (increased plasma levels of propranolol)
- Sulfonylureas (hyperglycemia)
- Cisplatin (increased risk of diuretic-induced ototoxicity)
- NSAIDs (blunted diuretic response and salicylate toxicity with high doses of salicylates)
- Probenecid (blunted diuretic response)
- Thiazide diuretics (synergism of diuretic activity of both drugs leading to profound diuresis)
- Amphotericin B (increased potential for nephrotoxicity and intensification of electrolyte imbalance)

THERAPEUTIC USES. A major use of loop diuretics is in the treatment of acute pulmonary edema. A rapid increase in venous capacitance in conjunction with a brisk natriuresis reduces left ventricular filling pressures and thereby rapidly relieves pulmonary edema. Loop diuretics also are used widely for treatment of chronic congestive heart failure when diminution of extracellular fluid volume is desirable to minimize venous and pulmonary congestion (*see* Chapter 28). Diuretics cause a significant reduction in mortality and the risk of worsening heart failure, as well as an improvement in exercise capacity. Diuretics are used widely for treatment of hypertension (*see* Chapter 28). Na^+-K^+-$2Cl^-$ symport inhibitors appear to lower blood pressure as effectively as Na^+-Cl^- symport inhibitors while causing smaller perturbations in the lipid profile. However, the relative potency and short elimination half-lives of loop diuretics render them less useful for hypertension than thiazide-type diuretics.

The edema of nephrotic syndrome often is refractory to less potent diuretics, and loop diuretics often are the only drugs capable of reducing the massive edema associated with this renal disease. Loop diuretics also are employed in the treatment of edema and ascites of liver cirrhosis; however, care must be taken not to induce volume contraction. In patients with a drug overdose, loop diuretics can be used to induce a forced diuresis to facilitate more rapid renal elimination of the offending drug. Loop diuretics, combined with isotonic saline administration to prevent volume depletion, are used to treat hypercalcemia. Loop diuretics interfere with the kidney's capacity to produce a concentrated urine. Consequently, loop diuretics combined with hypertonic saline are useful for the treatment of life-threatening hyponatremia. Loop diuretics also are used to treat edema associated with chronic kidney disease, in which the dose-response curve may be right-shifted, requiring higher doses of the loop diuretic (*see* Figure 25–8 in the 12th edition of the parent text).

INHIBITORS OF Na^+-Cl^- SYMPORT (THIAZIDE AND THIAZIDE-LIKE DIURETICS)

The term *thiazide diuretics* generally refers to all inhibitors of Na^+-Cl^- symport (Table 25–5), so named because the original inhibitors of Na^+-Cl^- symport were benzothiadiazine derivatives. The class now includes drugs that are pharmacologically similar to thiazide diuretics but differ structurally (*thiazide-like diuretics*).

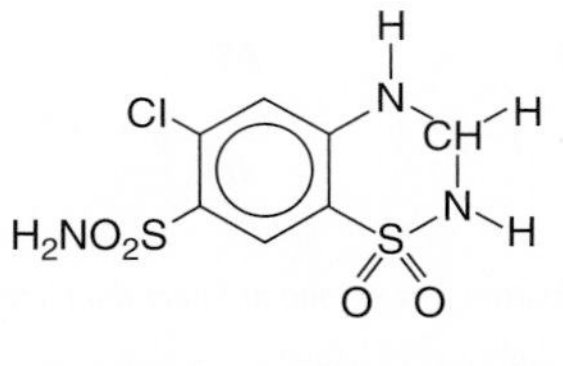

HYDROCHLOROTHIAZIDE

MECHANISM AND SITE OF ACTION. Thiazide diuretics inhibit NaCl transport in DCT; the proximal tubule may represent a secondary site of action.

Figure 25–5 illustrates the current model of electrolyte transport in DCT. Transport is powered by a Na^+ pump in the basolateral membrane. Free energy in the electrochemical gradient for Na^+ is harnessed by a Na^+-Cl^- symporter in the luminal membrane that moves Cl^- into the epithelial cell against its electrochemical gradient. Cl^- then exits the basolateral membrane passively by a Cl^- channel. Thiazide diuretics inhibit the Na^+-Cl^- symporter (called *ENCCl* or *TSC*) that is expressed predominantly in kidney and localized to the apical membrane of DCT epithelial cells. Expression of the symporter is regulated by aldosterone. Mutations in the Na^+-Cl^- symporter cause a form of inherited hypokalemic alkalosis called Gitelman syndrome.

EFFECTS ON URINARY EXCRETION. Inhibitors of Na^+-Cl^- symport increase Na^+ and Cl^- excretion. However, thiazides are only moderately efficacious (i.e., maximum excretion of filtered Na^+ load is only 5%) because ~90% of the filtered Na^+ load is reabsorbed before reaching the DCT. Some thiazide diuretics also are weak inhibitors of carbonic anhydrase, an effect that increases HCO_3^- and phosphate excretion and probably accounts for their weak proximal tubular effects. Inhibitors of Na^+-Cl^- symport increase K^+ and titratable acid excretion by the same mechanisms discussed for loop diuresis. Acute thiazide administration increases uric acid excretion. However, uric acid excretion is reduced following chronic administration by the same mechanisms discussed for loop diuretics. Acute effects of inhibitors of Na^+-Cl^- symport on Ca^{2+} excretion are variable; when administered chronically, thiazide diuretics decrease Ca^{2+} excretion. The mechanism involves increased proximal reabsorption owing to volume depletion, as well as direct effects of thiazides to increase Ca^{2+} reabsorption in the DCT. Thiazide diuretics may cause a mild magnesuria; long-term use of thiazide diuretics may cause magnesium deficiency, particularly in the elderly. Because inhibitors of Na^+-Cl^- symport inhibit transport in the cortical diluting segment, thiazide diuretics attenuate the kidney's ability to excrete dilute urine during water diuresis. However, since the DCT is not involved in the mechanism that generates a hypertonic medullary interstitium, thiazide diuretics do not alter the kidney's ability to concentrate urine

Table 25–5

Inhibitors of Na^+-Cl^- Symport (Thiazide and Thiazide-like Diuretics)

DRUG	RELATIVE POTENCY	ORAL AVAILABILITY	$t_{1/2}$ (hours)	ROUTE OF ELIMINATION
Bendroflumethiazide (NATURETIN)	10	~100%	3–3.9	~30% R, ~70% M
Chlorothiazide (DIURIL)	0.1	9–56% (dose-dependent)	~1.5	R
Hydrochlorothiazide (HYDRODIURIL)	1	~70%	~2.5	R
Hydroflumethiazide (SALURON)	1	~50%	~17	40-80% R, 20-60% M
Methyclothiazide (ENDURON)	10	ID	ID	M
Polythiazide (RENESE)	25	~100%	~25	~25% R, ~75% U
Trichlormethiazide (NAQUA)	25	ID	2.3–7.3	R
Chlorthalidone (HYGROTON)	1	~65%	~47	~65% R, ~10% B, ~25% U
Indapamide (LOZOL)	20	~93%	~14	M
Metolazone (MYKROX, ZAROXOLYN)	10	~65%	ID	~80% R, ~10% B, ~10% M
Quinethazone (HYDROMOX)	1	ID	ID	ID

R, renal excretion of intact drug; M, metabolism; B, excretion of intact drug into bile; U, unknown pathway of elimination; ID, insufficient data.

during hydropenia. In general, inhibitors of Na^+-Cl^- symport do not affect RBF and only variably reduce GFR owing to increases in intratubular pressure. Thiazides have little or no influence on TGF.

ABSORPTION AND ELIMINATION. Table 25–5 lists pharmacokinetic parameters of Na^+-Cl^- symport inhibitors. Note the wide range of half-lives for these drugs. Sulfonamides, as organic acids, are secreted into the proximal tubule by the organic acid secretory pathway. Because thiazides must gain access to the tubular lumen to inhibit the Na^+-Cl^- symporter, drugs such as probenecid can attenuate the diuretic response to thiazides by competing for transport into proximal tubule. However, plasma protein binding varies considerably among thiazide diuretics, and this parameter determines the contribution that filtration makes to tubular delivery of a specific thiazide.

TOXICITY, ADVERSE EFFECTS, CONTRAINDICATIONS, DRUG INTERACTIONS. Thiazide diuretics rarely cause CNS (e.g., vertigo, headache), GI, hematological, and dermatological (e.g., photosensitivity and skin rashes) disorders. The incidence of erectile dysfunction is greater with Na^+-Cl^- symport inhibitors than with several other antihypertensive agents, but usually is tolerable. As with loop diuretics, most serious adverse effects of thiazides are related to abnormalities of fluid and electrolyte balance. These adverse effects include extracellular volume depletion, hypotension, hypokalemia, hyponatremia, hypochloremia, metabolic alkalosis, hypomagnesemia, hypercalcemia, and hyperuricemia. Thiazide diuretics have caused fatal or near-fatal hyponatremia, and some patients are at recurrent risk of hyponatremia when rechallenged with thiazides.

Thiazide diuretics also decrease glucose tolerance, and latent diabetes mellitus. The mechanism of impaired glucose tolerance appears to involve reduced insulin secretion and alterations in glucose metabolism. Hyperglycemia is reduced when K^+ is given along with the diuretic. Thiazide-induced hypokalemia also impairs the antihypertensive effect and cardiovascular protection afforded by thiazides in patients with hypertension. Thiazide diuretics also may increase plasma levels of LDL cholesterol, total cholesterol, and total triglycerides. Thiazide diuretics are contraindicated in individuals who are hypersensitive to sulfonamides. Thiazide diuretics may diminish the effects of anticoagulants, uricosuric agents used to treat gout, sulfonylureas, and insulin and may increase the effects of anesthetics, diazoxide, digitalis glycosides, lithium, loop diuretics, and vitamin D. The effectiveness of thiazide diuretics may be reduced by NSAIDs, nonselective or selective COX-2 inhibitors, and bile acid sequestrants (reduced absorption of thiazides). Amphotericin B and corticosteroids increase the risk of hypokalemia induced by thiazide diuretics.

A potentially lethal drug interaction warranting special emphasis is that involving thiazide diuretics and quinidine. Prolongation of the QT interval by quinidine can lead to the development of polymorphic ventricular tachycardia (torsade de pointes; *see* Chapter 29). Torsade de pointes may deteriorate into fatal ventricular fibrillation. Hypokalemia increases the risk of quinidine-induced torsade de pointes, and thiazide diuretic–induced K^+ depletion may account for many cases of quinidine-induced torsade de pointes.

THERAPEUTIC USES. Thiazide diuretics are used for the treatment of edema associated with diseases of the heart (congestive heart failure), liver (hepatic cirrhosis), and kidney (nephrotic syndrome, chronic renal failure, and acute glomerulonephritis). With the possible exceptions of metolazone and indapamide, most thiazide diuretics are ineffective when the GFR is <30-40 mL/min. Thiazide diuretics decrease blood pressure in hypertensive patients and are used widely for the treatment of hypertension either alone or in combination with other antihypertensive drugs (*see* Chapter 27). Thiazide diuretics are inexpensive, as efficacious as other classes of antihypertensive agents, and well tolerated. Thiazides can be administered once daily, do not require dose titration, and have few contraindications. Moreover, thiazides have additive or synergistic effects when combined with other classes of antihypertensive agents.

Thiazide diuretics, which reduce urinary Ca^{2+} excretion, sometimes are employed to treat Ca^{2+} nephrolithiasis and may be useful for treatment of osteoporosis (*see* Chapter 44). Thiazide diuretics also are the mainstay for treatment of nephrogenic diabetes insipidus, reducing urine volume by up to 50%. Although it may seem counterintuitive to treat a disorder of increased urine volume with a diuretic, thiazides reduce the kidney's ability to excrete free water: They increase proximal tubular water reabsorption (secondary to volume contraction) and block the ability of the DCT to form dilute urine. This latter effect results in an increase in urine osmolality. Because other halides are excreted by renal processes similar to those for Cl^-, thiazide diuretics may be useful for the management of Br^- intoxication.

INHIBITORS OF RENAL EPITHELIAL Na^+ CHANNELS (K^+-SPARING DIURETICS)

Triamterene (DYRENIUM) and amiloride (MIDAMOR) are the only 2 drugs of this class in clinical use. Both drugs cause small increases in NaCl excretion and usually are employed for their antikaliuretic actions to offset the effects of other diuretics that increase K^+ excretion. Consequently, triamterene and amiloride, along with spironolactone (described in the next section), often are classified as *potassium* (K^+)*-sparing diuretics*.

Both drugs are organic bases and are transported by the organic base secretory mechanism in proximal tubule and have similar mechanisms of action (Figure 25–5). Principal cells in the late distal tubule and collecting duct have, in their luminal membranes, epithelial Na^+ channels that provide a conductive pathway for Na^+ entry into the cell down the electrochemical gradient created by the basolateral Na^+ pump. The higher permeability of the luminal membrane for Na^+ depolarizes the luminal membrane but not the basolateral membrane, creating a lumen-negative transepithelial potential difference. This transepithelial voltage provides an important driving force for the secretion of K^+ into the lumen by K^+ channels (ROMK) in the luminal membrane. Carbonic anhydrase inhibitors, loop diuretics, and thiazide diuretics increase Na^+ delivery to the late distal tubule and collecting duct, a situation that often is associated with increased K^+ and H^+ excretion.

Amiloride blocks epithelial Na^+ channels in the luminal membrane of principal cells in late distal tubule and collecting duct. The amiloride-sensitive Na^+ channel (called *ENaC*) consists of 3 subunits (α, β, and γ). Although the α subunit is sufficient for channel activity, maximal Na^+ permeability is induced when all 3 subunits are coexpressed in the same cell, probably forming a tetrameric structure consisting of 2 α subunits, 1 β subunit, and 1 γ subunit. Liddle syndrome is an autosomal dominant form of low-renin, volume-expanded hypertension that is due to mutations in the β or γ subunits, leading to increased basal ENaC activity.

EFFECTS ON URINARY EXCRETION. The late distal tubule and collecting duct have a limited capacity to reabsorb solutes, thus, Na^+ channel blockade in this part of the nephron increases Na^+ and Cl^- excretion rates only mildly (~2% of filtered load). Blockade of Na^+ channels hyperpolarizes the luminal membrane, reducing the lumen-negative transepithelial voltage. Because the lumen-negative potential difference normally opposes cation reabsorption and facilitates cation secretion, attenuation of the lumen-negative voltage decreases K^+, H^+, Ca^{2+}, and Mg^{2+} excretion rates. Volume contraction may increase reabsorption of uric acid in the proximal tubule; hence chronic administration of amiloride and triamterene may decrease uric acid excretion. Amiloride and triamterene have little or no effect on renal hemodynamics and do not alter TGF.

ABSORPTION AND ELIMINATION. Table 25–6 lists pharmacokinetic data for amiloride and triamterene. Amiloride is eliminated predominantly by urinary excretion of intact drug. Triamterene is metabolized in the

Table 25–6

Inhibitors of Renal Epithelial Na^+ Channels (K^+-Sparing Diuretics)

DRUG	RELATIVE POTENCY	ORAL BIOAVAILABILITY	$t_{1/2}$ (hours)	ROUTE OF ELIMINATION
Amiloride	1	15–25%	~21	R
Triamterene	0.1	~50%	~4	M

R, renal excretion of intact drug; M, metabolism; however, triamterene is transformed into an active metabolite that is excreted in the urine.

liver to an active metabolite, 4-hydroxytriamterene sulfate, and this metabolite is excreted in urine. Therefore, triamterene toxicity may be enhanced in both hepatic disease and renal failure.

TOXICITY, ADVERSE EFFECTS, CONTRAINDICATIONS, DRUG INTERACTIONS. The most dangerous adverse effect of renal Na^+-channel inhibitors is hyperkalemia, which can be life threatening. Consequently, amiloride and triamterene are contraindicated in patients with hyperkalemia, as well as in patients at increased risk of developing hyperkalemia (e.g., patients with renal failure, patients receiving other K^+-sparing diuretics, patients taking angiotensin-converting enzyme inhibitors, or patients taking K^+ supplements). Even NSAIDs can increase the likelihood of hyperkalemia in patients receiving Na^+-channel inhibitors. Routine monitoring of the serum K^+ level is essential in patients receiving K^+-sparing diuretics. Cirrhotic patients are prone to megaloblastosis because of folic acid deficiency, and triamterene, a weak folic acid antagonist, may increase the likelihood of this adverse event. Triamterene also can reduce glucose tolerance and induce photosensitization and has been associated with interstitial nephritis and renal stones. Both drugs can cause CNS, GI, musculoskeletal, dermatological, and hematological adverse effects. The most common adverse effects of amiloride are nausea, vomiting, diarrhea, and headache; those of triamterene are nausea, vomiting, leg cramps, and dizziness.

THERAPEUTIC USES. Because of the mild natriuresis induced by Na^+-channel inhibitors, these drugs seldom are used as sole agents in treatment of edema or hypertension; their major utility is in combination with other diuretics. Coadministration of a Na^+-channel inhibitor augments the diuretic and antihypertensive response to thiazide and loop diuretics. More important, the ability of Na^+-channel inhibitors to reduce K^+ excretion tends to offset the kaliuretic effects of thiazide and loop diuretics and to result in normal plasma K^+ values.

Liddle syndrome can be treated effectively with Na^+-channel inhibitors. Aerosolized amiloride has been shown to improve mucociliary clearance in patients with cystic fibrosis. By inhibiting Na^+ absorption from the surfaces of airway epithelial cells, amiloride augments hydration of respiratory secretions and thereby improves mucociliary clearance. Amiloride also is useful for lithium-induced nephrogenic diabetes insipidus because it blocks Li^+ transport into collecting tubule cells.

ANTAGONISTS OF MINERALOCORTICOID RECEPTORS (ALDOSTERONE ANTAGONISTS, K^+-SPARING DIURETICS)

Mineralocorticoids cause salt and water retention and increase K^+ and H^+ excretion by binding to specific mineralocorticoid receptors (MRs). Two MR antagonists are available in the U.S., spironolactone and eplerenone (Table 25–7).

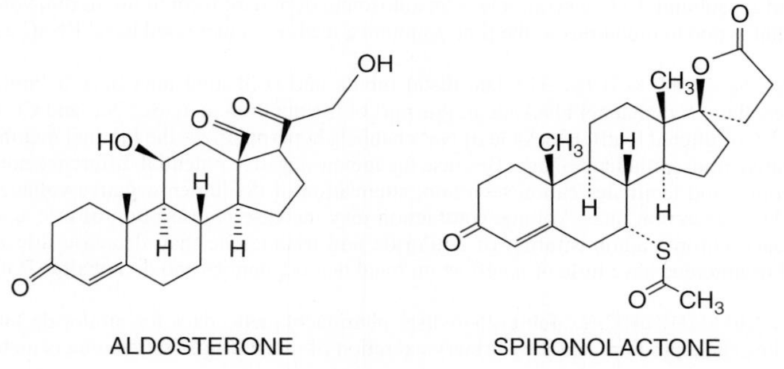

ALDOSTERONE

SPIRONOLACTONE

Table 25–7

Mineralocorticoid Receptor Antagonists (Aldosterone Antagonists, K^+-Sparing Diuretics)

DRUG	ORAL AVAILABILITY	$t_{1/2}$ (hours)	ROUTE OF ELIMINATION
Spironolactone	~65%	~1.6	M
Canrenone[a]	ID	~16.5	M
Potassium canrenoate[a]	ID	ID	M
Eplerenone	ID	~5	M

M, metabolism; ID, insufficient data.
[a]Not available in United States.

MECHANISM AND SITE OF ACTION (FIGURE 25–6). Epithelial cells in late distal tubule and collecting duct contain cytosolic MRs with a high aldosterone affinity. When aldosterone binds to MRs, the MR-aldosterone complex translocates to the nucleus, where regulates the expression of multiple gene products called *aldosterone-induced proteins* (AIPs). Consequently, transepithelial NaCl transport is enhanced, and the lumen-negative transepithelial voltage is increased. The latter effect increases the driving force for K^+ and H^+ secretion into the tubular lumen.

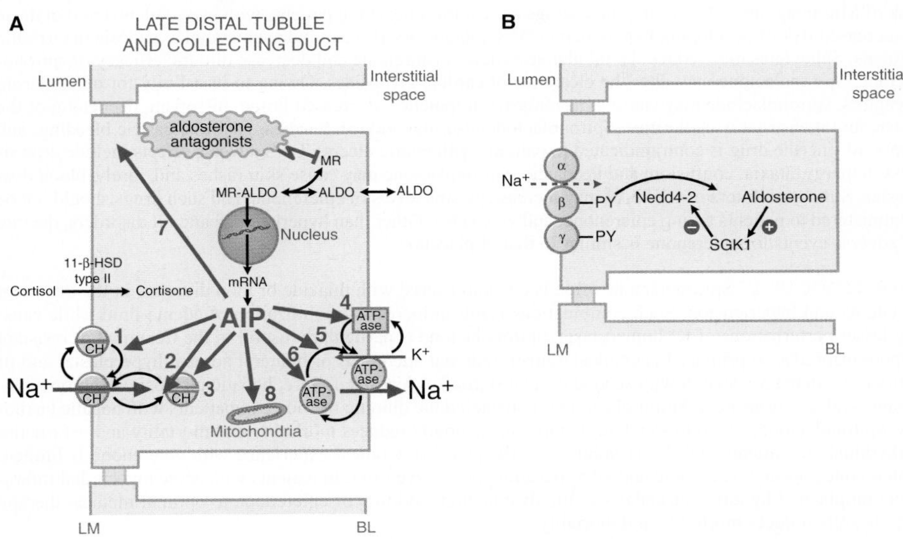

Figure 25–6 *Effects of aldosterone on late distal tubule and collecting duct and diuretic mechanism of aldosterone antagonists.* **A.** Cortisol also has affinity for the mineralocorticoid receptor (MR), but is inactivated in the cell by 11-β-hydroxysteroid dehydrogenase (HSD) type II. **B.** Serum and glucorticoid-regulated kinase (SGK)-1 is upregulated by aldosterone. SGK-1 phosphorylates and inactivates Nedd4-2, a ubiquitin-protein ligase that acts on ENaC, leading to its degradation. Phosphorylated Nedd4-2 no longer interacts with the PY motif of ENaC; as a result, the protein is not ubiquitinated and remains in the membrane, leading to increased Na^+ entry into the cell.

1. Activation of membrane-bound Na^+ channels
2. Na^+ channel (ENaC) removal from the membrane inhibited
3. *De novo* synthesis of Na^+ channels
4. Activation of membrane-bound Na^+,K^+-ATPase
5. Redistribution of Na^+,K^+-ATPase from cytosol to membrane
6. *De novo* synthesis of Na^+,K^+-ATPase
7. Changes in permeability of tight junctions
8. Increased mitochondrial production of ATP

AIP, aldosterone-induced proteins; ALDO, aldosterone; CH, ion channel; BL, basolateral membrane; LM, luminal membrane.

Drugs such as spironolactone and eplerenone competitively inhibit the binding of aldosterone to the MR. Unlike the MR-aldosterone complex, the MR-spironolactone complex is not able to induce the synthesis of AIPs. Since spironolactone and eplerenone block biological effects of aldosterone, these agents also are referred to as *aldosterone antagonists*. MR antagonists are the only diuretics that do not require access to the tubular lumen to induce diuresis.

EFFECTS ON URINARY EXCRETION. The effects of MR antagonists on urinary excretion are very similar to those induced by renal epithelial Na^+-channel inhibitors. However, unlike Na^+-channel inhibitors, the clinical efficacy of MR antagonists is a function of endogenous aldosterone levels. The higher the endogenous aldosterone level, the greater the effects of MR antagonists on urinary excretion. MR antagonists have little or no effect on renal hemodynamics and do not alter TGF.

OTHER ACTIONS. Spironolactone has some affinity toward progesterone and androgen receptors and thereby induces side effects such as gynecomastia, impotence, and menstrual irregularities. Owing to its 9,11-epoxide group, eplerenone has very low affinity for progesterone and androgen receptors (<1% and <0.1%, respectively) compared with spironolactone. High spironolactone concentrations can interfere with steroid biosynthesis by inhibiting steroid hydroxylases; these effects have limited clinical relevance.

ABSORPTION AND ELIMINATION. Spironolactone is absorbed partially (~65%), is metabolized extensively (even during its first passage through the liver), undergoes enterohepatic recirculation, is highly protein bound, and has a short $t_{1/2}$ (~1.6 h). The $t_{1/2}$ is prolonged to 9 h in patients with cirrhosis. Eplerenone has good oral availability and is eliminated primarily by metabolism by CYP3A4 to inactive metabolites, with a $t_{1/2}$ of ~5 h. Canrenone and K^+ canrenoate also are in clinical use. Canrenoate is not active but is converted to canrenone.

TOXICITY, ADVERSE EFFECTS, CONTRAINDICATIONS, DRUG INTERACTIONS. Hyperkalemia is the principal risk of MR antagonists. Therefore, these drugs are contraindicated in patients with hyperkalemia and in those at increased risk of developing hyperkalemia. MR antagonists also can induce metabolic acidosis in cirrhotic patients. Salicylates may reduce the tubular secretion of canrenone and decrease diuretic efficacy of spironolactone. Spironolactone may alter the clearance of cardiac glycosides. Owing to its affinity for other steroid receptors, spironolactone may cause gynecomastia, impotence, decreased libido, hirsutism, deepening of the voice, and menstrual irregularities. Spironolactone also may induce diarrhea, gastritis, gastric bleeding, and peptic ulcers (the drug is contraindicated in patients with peptic ulcers). CNS adverse effects include drowsiness, lethargy, ataxia, confusion, and headache. Spironolactone may cause skin rashes and, rarely, blood dyscrasias. Strong inhibitors of CYP3A4 may increase plasma levels of eplerenone, and such drugs should not be administered to patients taking eplerenone, and vice versa. Other than hyperkalemia and GI disorders, the rate of adverse events for eplerenone is similar to that of placebo.

THERAPEUTIC USES. Spironolactone often is coadministered with thiazide or loop diuretics in the treatment of edema and hypertension. Such combinations result in increased mobilization of edema fluid while causing lesser perturbations of K^+ homeostasis. Spironolactone is particularly useful in the treatment of resistant hypertension due to primary hyperaldosteronism (adrenal adenomas or bilateral adrenal hyperplasia) and of refractory edema associated with secondary aldosteronism (cardiac failure, hepatic cirrhosis, nephrotic syndrome, and severe ascites). Spironolactone is considered the diuretic of choice in patients with hepatic cirrhosis. Spironolactone, added to standard therapy, substantially reduces morbidity and mortality and ventricular arrhythmias in patients with heart failure (*see* Chapter 28). Clinical experience with eplerenone is limited. Eplerenone appears to be a safe and effective antihypertensive drug. In patients with acute myocardial infarction complicated by left ventricular systolic dysfunction, addition of eplerenone to optimal medical therapy significantly reduces morbidity and mortality.

INHIBITORS OF THE NONSPECIFIC CATION CHANNEL: ATRIAL NATRIURETIC PEPTIDES

Four natriuretic peptides are relevant with respect to human physiology: atrial natriuretic peptide (ANP), brain natriuretic peptide (BNP), C-type natriuretic peptide (CNP), and urodilatin. The inner medullary collecting duct (IMCD) is a major site of action of natriuretic peptides.

Three natriuretic peptides (NPs)—ANP, BNP, and CNP—share a common homologous 17-member amino acid ring formed by a disulfide bridge between cysteine residues, although they are products of different genes. Urodilatin, also structurally similar, arises from altered processing of the same precursor molecule as ANP and has 4 additional amino acids at the N terminus. ANP and BNP are produced by the heart in response to wall stretch, CNP is of endothelial and renal cell origin; urodilatin is found in the kidney and urine. NP receptors (NPRs), classified as types A, B and C, are membrane monospans. NPRA (binds ANP and BNP) and NPRB (binds CNP) have intracellular domains with guanylate cyclase activity and a protein kinase element. NPRC (binds all NPs) has a truncated intracellular domain and may help with NP clearance. The various NPs

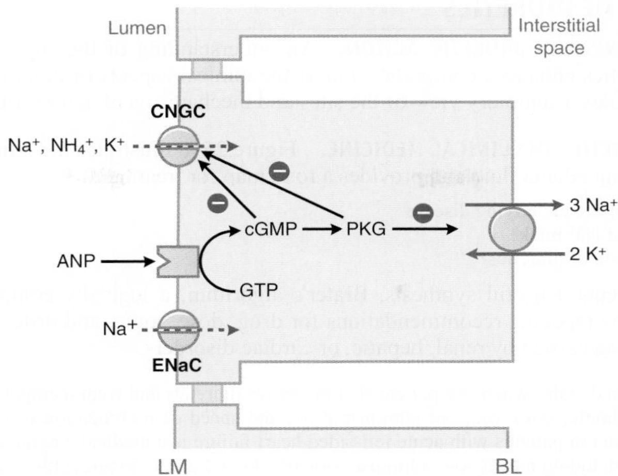

Figure 25–7 *Inner medullary collecting duct (IMCD) Na^+ transport and its regulation.* Na^+ enters the IMCD cell in one of two ways: via epithelial Na^+ channel (ENaC), and through a cyclic nucleotide gated nonspecific cation channel (CNGC) that transports Na^+, K^+, and NH_4^+ and is gated by cyclic GMP. Na^+ then exits the cell via the Na^+, K^+-ATPase. The CNGC is the primary pathway for Na^+ entry, and is inhibited by natriuretic peptides. Atrial natriuretic peptides (ANP) bind to surface receptors (natriuretic peptide receptors A, B, and C). The A and B receptors are isoforms of particulate guanylyl cyclase that synthesize cyclic GMP. Cyclic GMP inhibits the CNGC directly, and indirectly through PKG. PKG activation also inhibits Na^+ exit via the Na^+, K^+-ATPase.

have somewhat overlapping effects, causing natriuresis, inhibition of production of renin and aldosterone, and vasodilation (the result of cyclic GMP elevation in vascular smooth muscle).

MECHANISM AND SITE OF ACTION. The IMCD is the final site along the nephron where Na^+ is reabsorbed. Up to 5% of the filtered Na^+ load can be reabsorbed here. The effects of NPs are mediated via effects of cyclic GMP on Na^+ transporters (Figure 25–7). Two types of Na^+ channels are expressed in IMCD. The first is an amiloride-sensitive, 28pS, nonselective, cyclic nucleotide gated cation (CNG) channel. This channel is inhibited by cGMP and by ANPs via their capacity to stimulate membrane-bound guanylyl cyclase activity and elevate cellular cGMP. The second type of Na^+ channel expressed in the IMCD is the low-conductance 4 pS highly selective Na^+ channel ENaC. The majority of Na^+ reabsorption in the IMCD is mediated via the CNG channel.

EFFECTS ON URINARY EXCRETION AND RENAL HEMODYNAMICS. Nesiritide (human recombinant BNP) inhibits Na^+ transport in both the proximal and distal nephron but its primary effect is in the IMCD. Urinary Na^+ excretion increases with nesiritide but the effect may be attenuated by upregulation of Na^+ reabsorption in upstream segments of the nephron. GFR increases in response to nesiritide in normal subjects, but in treated patients with congestive heart failure GFR may increase, decrease, or remain unchanged.

OTHER ACTIONS. Administration of nesiritide decreases systemic and pulmonary resistances and left ventricular filling pressure, and induces a secondary increase in cardiac output.

ELIMINATION. Natriuretic peptides are administered intravenously. Nesiritide has a distribution $t_{1/2}$ of 2 min and a mean terminal $t_{1/2}$ of 18 min. There is no need to adjust the dose for renal insufficiency.

TOXICITY, ADVERSE EFFECTS, CONTRAINDICATIONS, DRUG INTERACTIONS. There are concerns about adverse renal effects and reports of increased short-term mortality in patients treated with nesiritide. Increases in serum creatinine concentration may be related to decreases in extracellular fluid volume, higher doses of diuretics used, decreases in blood pressure, and activation of the renin–angiotensin–aldosterone system. The *Vasodilation in the Management of Acute CHF* (VAMC) trial showed no increased risk with low or moderate doses of diuretics but an increased risk with high-dose diuretics (>160 mg furosemide), rising with increasing doses. Oral ACE inhibitors may increase the risk of hypotension with nesiritide. There are no data to suggest that nesiritide reduces mortality in the short term or long term in patients with acute decompensated CHF.

THERAPEUTIC USES. Human recombinant ANP (carperitide, available only in Japan) and BNP (nesiritide [NATRECOR]) are the available therapeutic agents of this class. Urodilatin (ularitide) is in development. Use of nesiritide should be limited to patients with acutely decompensated CHF with shortness of breath at rest; the drug should not be used in place of diuretics. Nesiritide reduces symptoms and improves hemodynamic parameters in those with dyspnea at rest who are not hypotensive.

SITE AND MECHANISM OF DIURETIC ACTION. An understanding of the sites and mechanisms of action of diuretics enhances comprehension of the clinical aspects of diuretic pharmacology. Figure 25–5 provides a summary view of the sites and mechanisms of actions of diuretics.

THE ROLE OF DIURETICS IN CLINICAL MEDICINE. Figure 25–8 illustrates the 3 fundamental strategies for mobilizing edema fluid and provides a road map for treatment:

- Correction of the underlying disease
- Restriction of Na^+ intake
- Administration of diuretics

Figure 25–9 presents a useful synthesis, Brater's algorithm, a logically compelling algorithm for diuretic therapy (specific recommendations for drug, dose, route, and drug combinations) in patients with edema caused by renal, hepatic, or cardiac disorders.

The clinical situation dictates whether a patient should receive diuretics and what therapeutic regimen should be used (type of diuretic, dose, route of administration, and speed of mobilization of edema fluid). Massive pulmonary edema in patients with acute left-sided heart failure is a medical emergency requiring rapid, aggressive therapy including intravenous administration of a loop diuretic. In this setting, use of oral diuretics is inappropriate. Conversely, mild pulmonary and venous congestion associated with chronic heart failure is best treated with an oral loop or thiazide diuretic, the dosage of which should be titrated carefully to maximize the benefit-to-risk ratio. Loop and thiazide diuretics decrease morbidity and mortality in heart failure patients: MR antagonists also demonstrate reduced morbidity and mortality in heart failure patients receiving optimal therapy with other drugs.

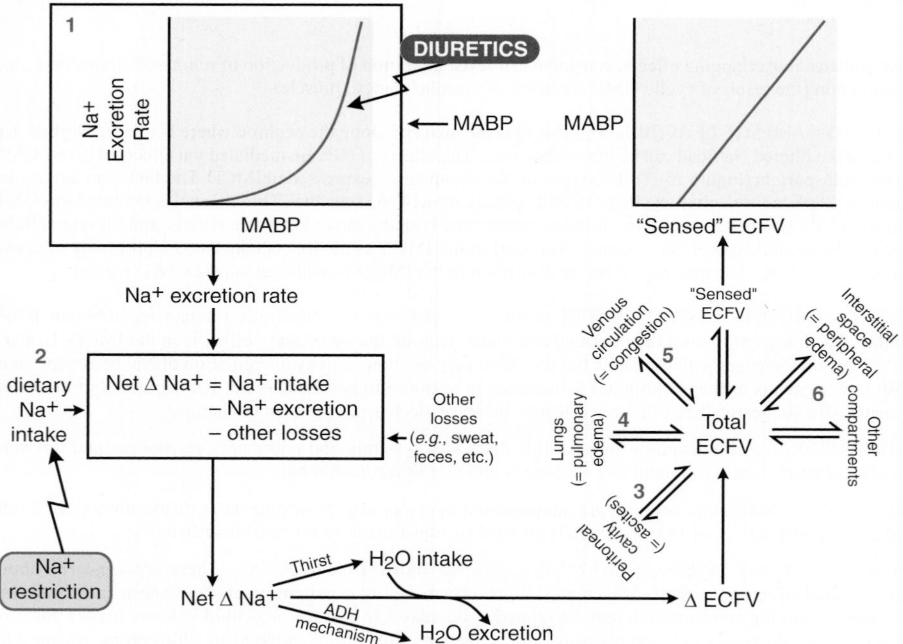

Figure 25–8 *Interrelationships among renal function, Na^+ intake, water homeostasis, distribution of extracellular fluid volume, and mean arterial blood pressure.* Pathophysiological mechanisms of edema formation. 1. Rightward shift of renal pressure natriuresis curve. 2. Excessive dietary Na^+ intake. 3. Increased distribution of extracellular fluid volume (ECFV) to peritoneal cavity (e.g., liver cirrhosis with increased hepatic sinusoidal hydrostatic pressure) leading to ascites formation. 4. Increased distribution of ECFV to lungs (e.g., left-sided heart failure with increased pulmonary capillary hydrostatic pressure) leading to pulmonary edema. 5. Increased distribution of ECFV to venous circulation (e.g., right-sided heart failure) leading to venous congestion. 6. Peripheral edema caused by altered Starling forces causing increased distribution of ECFV to interstitial space (e.g., diminished plasma proteins in nephrotic syndrome, severe burns, and liver disease).

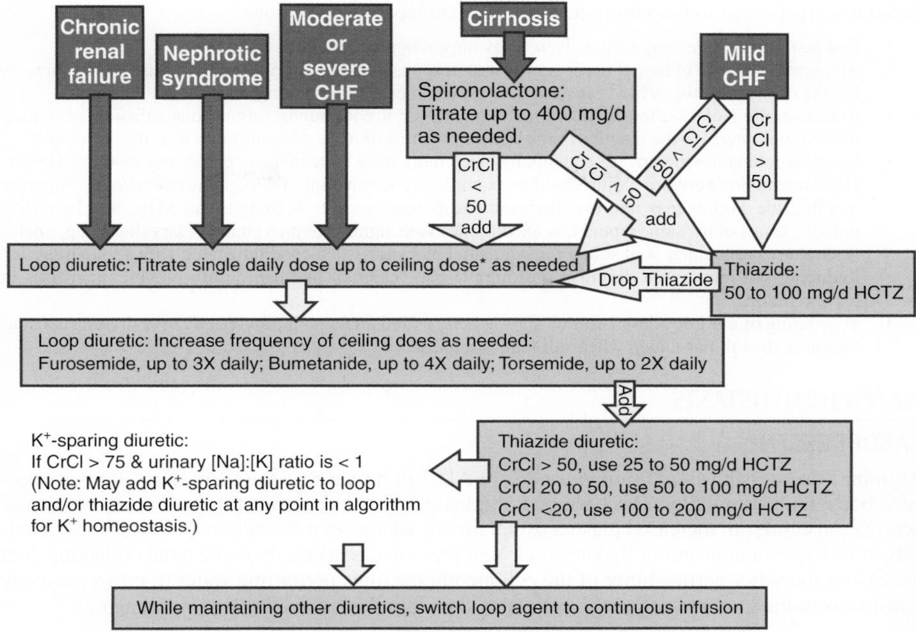

Figure 25–9 *"Brater's algorithm" for diuretic therapy of chronic renal failure, nephrotic syndrome, congestive heart failure, and cirrhosis.* Follow algorithm until adequate response is achieved. If adequate response is not obtained, advance to the next step. For illustrative purposes, the thiazide diuretic used is hydrochlorothiazide (HCTZ). An alternative thiazide-type diuretic may be substituted with dosage adjusted to be pharmacologically equivalent to the recommended dose of HCTZ. *Do not combine 2 K^+-sparing diuretics due to the risk of hyperkalemia.* CrCl indicates creatinine clearance in mL/min, and ceiling dose refers to the smallest dose of diuretic that produces a near-maximal effect. Ceiling doses of loop diuretics and dosing regimens for continuous intravenous infusions of loop diuretics are disease-state-specific. Doses are for adults only.

Periodic administration of diuretics to cirrhotic patients with ascites may eliminate the necessity for or reduce the interval between paracenteses, adding to patient comfort and sparing protein reserves that are lost during the paracenteses. Although diuretics can reduce edema associated with chronic renal failure, increased doses of more powerful loop diuretics usually are required. In nephrotic syndrome, diuretic response often is disappointing. In chronic renal failure and cirrhosis, edema will not pose an immediate health risk, but can greatly reduce quality of life. In such cases, only partial removal of edema fluid should be attempted, and fluid should be mobilized slowly using a diuretic regimen that accomplishes the task with minimal perturbation of normal physiology.

Diuretic resistance refers to edema that is or has become refractory to a given diuretic. If diuretic resistance develops against a less efficacious diuretic, a more efficacious diuretic should be substituted, such as a loop diuretic for a thiazide. However, resistance to loop diuretics can be due to several causes. NSAID coadministration is a common preventable cause of diuretic resistance. Prostaglandin production, especially PGE_2, is an important counterregulatory mechanism in states of reduced renal perfusion such as volume contraction, congestive heart failure, and cirrhosis characterized by activation of the renin–angiotensin–aldosterone (RAA) and sympathetic nervous systems. NSAID administration can block these prostaglandin-mediated effects that counterbalance the RAA and sympathetic nervous system, resulting in salt and water retention. Diuretic resistance also occurs with COX-2-selective inhibitors.

In chronic renal failure, a reduction in RBF decreases delivery of diuretics to the kidney, and accumulation of endogenous organic acids competes with loop diuretics for transport at the proximal tubule. Consequently, diuretic concentration at the active site in the tubular lumen is diminished. In nephrotic syndrome, binding of diuretics to luminal albumin was postulated to limit response; however, the validity of this concept has been challenged. In hepatic cirrhosis, nephrotic syndrome, and heart failure, nephrons may have diminished diuretic responsiveness because of increased proximal tubular Na^+ reabsorption, leading to diminished Na^+ delivery to distal nephron.

Faced with resistance to loop diuretics, the clinician has several options:

- Bed rest may restore drug responsiveness by improving the renal circulation.
- An increase in dose of loop diuretic may restore responsiveness; however, nothing is gained by increasing the dose above that which causes a near-maximal effect (the ceiling dose) of the diuretic.
- Administration of smaller doses more frequently or a continuous intravenous infusion of a loop diuretic will increase the length of time that an effective diuretic concentration is at the active site.
- Use of combination therapy to sequentially block more than 1 site in the nephron may result in a synergistic interaction between 2 diuretics. For example, a combination of a loop diuretic with a K^+-sparing or a thiazide diuretic may improve therapeutic response; however, nothing is gained by the administration of 2 drugs of the same type. Thiazide diuretics with significant proximal tubular effects (e.g., metolazone) are particularly well suited for sequential blockade when coadministered with a loop diuretic.
- Reducing salt intake will diminish postdiuretic Na^+ retention that can nullify previous increases in Na^+ excretion.
- Scheduling of diuretic administration shortly before food intake will provide effective diuretic concentration in the tubular lumen when salt load is highest.

WATER HOMEOSTASIS

VASOPRESSIN

Arginine vasopressin (*antidiuretic hormone* or ADH in humans) is the main hormone that regulates body fluid osmolality. The hormone is released by the posterior pituitary whenever water deprivation causes an increased plasma osmolality or whenever the cardiovascular system is challenged by hypovolemia and/or hypotension. Vasopressin acts primarily in the renal collecting duct increasing the water permeability of the cell membrane, thus permitting water to move passively down an osmotic gradient across the collecting duct into the extracellular compartment.

Vasopressin is a potent vasopressor/vasoconstrictor. It is also a neurotransmitter; among its actions in the CNS are apparent roles in the secretion of adrenocorticotropic hormone (ACTH) and in regulation of the cardiovascular system, temperature, and other visceral functions. Vasopressin also promotes release of coagulation factors by vascular endothelium and increases platelet aggregability.

PHYSIOLOGY

ANATOMY. The antidiuretic mechanism in mammals involves 2 anatomical components: a CNS component for synthesis, transport, storage, and release of vasopressin and a renal collecting-duct system composed of epithelial cells that respond to vasopressin by increasing their water permeability. The CNS component of the antidiuretic mechanism is called the *hypothalamo-neurohypophyseal system* and consists of neurosecretory neurons with perikarya located predominantly in 2 specific hypothalamic nuclei, the supraoptic nucleus (SON) and paraventricular nucleus (PVN). Long axons of magnocellular neurons in SON and PVN terminate in the neural lobe of the posterior pituitary (neurohypophysis), where they release vasopressin and oxytocin (*see* Figure 38–1).

SYNTHESIS. Vasopressin and oxytocin are synthesized mainly in the perikarya of magnocellular neurons in the SON and PVN. Parvicellular neurons in the PVN also synthesize vasopressin. Vasopressin synthesis appears to be regulated solely at the transcriptional level. In humans, a 168-amino acid preprohormone (Figure 25–10) is synthesized and then packaged into membrane-associated granules. The prohormone contains 3 domains: vasopressin (residues 1-9), vasopressin (VP)-neurophysin (residues 13-105), and VP-glycopeptide (residues 107-145). The vasopressin domain is linked to the VP-neurophysin domain through a GLY-LYS-ARG-processing signal, and the VP-neurophysin is linked to the VP-glycopeptide domain by an ARG-processing signal. In secretory granules, an endopeptidase, exopeptidase, monooxygenase, and lyase act sequentially on the prohormone to produce vasopressin, VP-neurophysin (sometimes referred to as neurophysin II), and VP-glycopeptide. The synthesis and transport of vasopressin depend on the preprohormone conformation. In particular, VP-neurophysin binds vasopressin and is critical to correct processing, transport, and storage of vasopressin. Genetic mutations in either the signal peptide or VP-neurophysin give rise to central diabetes insipidus.

VASOPRESSIN SYNTHESIS OUTSIDE THE CNS. Vasopressin also is synthesized by heart and adrenal gland. In the heart, elevated wall stress increases vasopressin synthesis several fold.

REGULATION OF VASOPRESSIN SECRETION. An increase in plasma osmolality is the principal physiological stimulus for vasopressin secretion by the posterior pituitary. Severe hypovolemia/hypotension also is a powerful stimulus for vasopressin release. In addition, pain, nausea, and hypoxia can stimulate vasopressin secretion, and several endogenous hormones and pharmacological agents can modify vasopressin release.

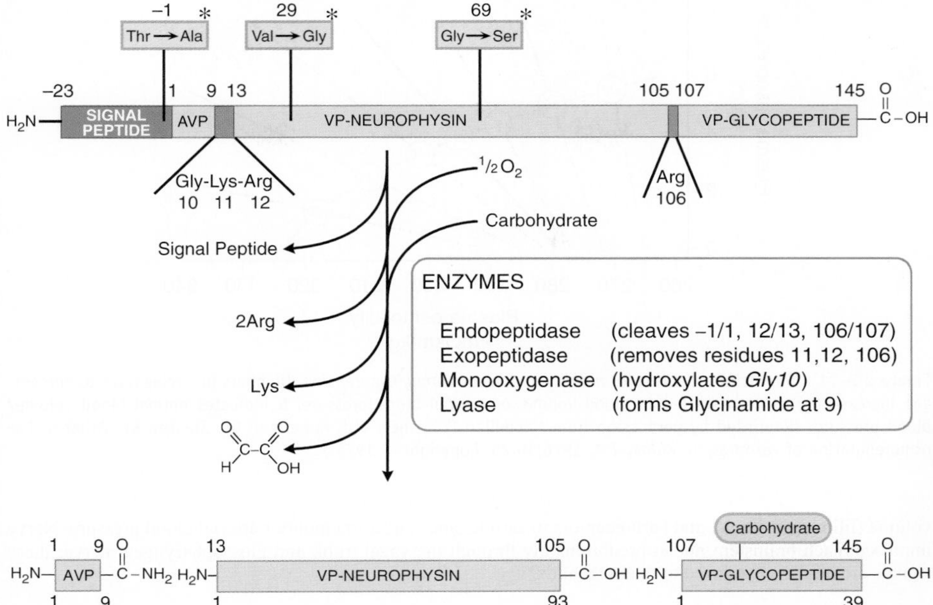

Figure 25–10 *Processing of human arginine vasopressin (AVP) preprohormone.* More than 40 mutations in the single gene on chromosome 20 that encodes AVP preprohormone give rise to central diabetes insipidus. *Boxes indicate mutations leading to central diabetes insipidus.

HYPEROSMOLALITY. The osmolality threshold for secretion is ~280 mOsm/kg. Below the threshold, vasopressin is barely detectable in plasma, and above the threshold, vasopressin levels are a steep and relatively linear function of plasma osmolality. Indeed, a 2% elevation in plasma osmolality causes a 2- to 3-fold increase in plasma vasopressin levels, which in turn causes increased solute-free water reabsorption, with an increase in urine osmolality. Increases in plasma osmolality above 290 mOsm/kg lead to an intense desire for water (thirst). Thus, the vasopressin system affords the organism longer thirst-free periods and, in the event that water is unavailable, allows the organism to survive longer periods of water deprivation. Above a plasma osmolality of ~290 mOsm/kg, plasma vasopressin levels exceed 5 p*M*. Since urinary concentration is maximal (~1200 mOsm/kg) when vasopressin levels exceed 5 p*M*, further defense against hypertonicity depends entirely on water intake rather than on decreases in water loss. *See* Figure 25–17 in the 12th edition of the parent text for more details.

HEPATIC PORTAL OSMORECEPTORS. An oral salt load activates hepatic portal osmoreceptors leading to increased vasopressin release. This mechanism augments plasma vasopressin levels even before the oral salt load increases plasma osmolality.

HYPOVOLEMIA AND HYPOTENSION. Vasopressin secretion is regulated hemodynamically by changes in effective blood volume and/or arterial blood pressure. Regardless of the cause (e.g., hemorrhage, Na^+ depletion, diuretics, heart failure, hepatic cirrhosis with ascites, adrenal insufficiency, or hypotensive drugs), reductions in effective blood volume and/or arterial blood pressure are associated with high circulating vasopressin concentrations. However, unlike osmoregulation, hemodynamic regulation of vasopressin secretion is exponential; i.e., small decreases (5%) in blood volume and/or pressure have little effect on vasopressin secretion, whereas larger decreases (20-30%) can increase vasopressin levels to 20-30 times normal (exceeding the vasopressin concentration required to induce maximal antidiuresis). Vasopressin is one of the most potent vasoconstrictors known, and the vasopressin response to hypovolemia or hypotension serves as a mechanism to stave off cardiovascular collapse during periods of severe blood loss and/or hypotension. Hemodynamic regulation of vasopressin secretion does not disrupt osmotic regulation; rather, hypovolemia/hypotension alters the set point and slope of the plasma osmolality-plasma vasopressin relationship (Figure 25–11).

Neuronal pathways that mediate hemodynamic regulation of vasopressin release are different from those involved in osmoregulation. Baroreceptors in left atrium, left ventricle, and pulmonary veins sense blood

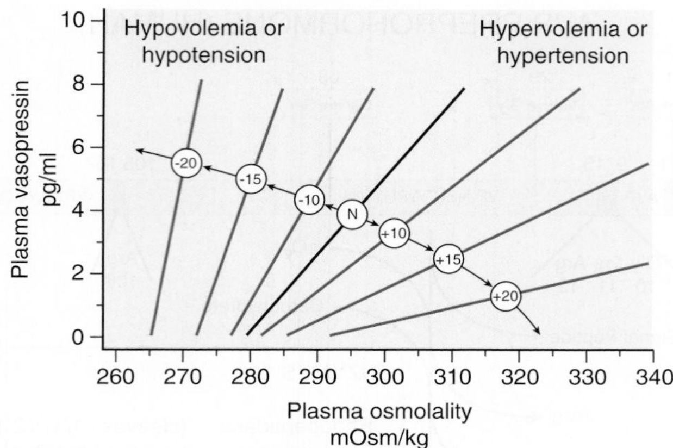

Figure 25–11 *Interactions between osmolality and hypovolemia/hypotension.* Numbers in circles refer to percentage increase (+) or decrease (–) in blood volume or arterial blood pressure. N indicates normal blood volume/blood pressure. (Reprinted by permission from Macmillan Publishers Ltd: Robertson GL, Shelton RL, Athar S, The osmoregulation of vasopressin. *Kidney Int,* 1976;10:25, Copyright © 1976.)

volume (filling pressures), and baroreceptors in carotid sinus and aorta monitor arterial blood pressure. Nerve impulses reach brainstem nuclei predominantly through the vagal trunk and glossopharyngeal nerve; these signals are ultimately relayed to the SON and PVN.

HORMONES AND NEUROTRANSMITTERS. Vasopressin-synthesizing magnocellular neurons have a large array of receptors on both perikarya and nerve terminals; therefore, vasopressin release can be accentuated or attenuated by chemical agents acting at both ends of the magnocellular neuron. Also, hormones and neurotransmitters can modulate vasopressin secretion by stimulating or inhibiting neurons in nuclei that project, either directly or indirectly, to the SON and PVN. Because of these complexities, modulation of vasopressin secretion by most hormones or neurotransmitters is unclear. Several agents stimulate vasopressin secretion, including acetylcholine (by nicotinic receptors), histamine (by H_1 receptors), dopamine (by both D_1 and D_2 receptors), glutamine, aspartate, cholecystokinin, neuropeptide Y, substance P, vasoactive intestinal polypeptide, prostaglandins, and angiotensin II (AngII). Inhibitors of vasopressin secretion include ANP, γ-aminobutyric acid, and opioids (particularly dynorphin *via* κ receptors). The affects of AngII have received the most attention. AngII synthesized in the brain and circulating AngII may stimulate vasopressin release. Inhibition of the conversion of AngII to AngIII blocks AngII-induced vasopressin release, suggesting that AngIII is the main effector peptide of the brain renin–angiotensin system controlling vasopressin release.

PHARMACOLOGICAL AGENTS. A number of drugs alter urine osmolality by stimulating or inhibiting vasopressin secretion. In most cases the mechanism is not known. Stimulators of vasopressin secretion include vincristine, cyclophosphamide, tricyclic antidepressants, nicotine, epinephrine, and high doses of morphine. Lithium, which inhibits the renal effects of vasopressin, also enhances vasopressin secretion. Inhibitors of vasopressin secretion include ethanol, phenytoin, low doses of morphine, glucocorticoids, fluphenazine, haloperidol, promethazine, oxilorphan, and butorphanol. Carbamazepine has a renal action to produce antidiuresis in patients with central diabetes insipidus but actually inhibits vasopressin secretion by a central action.

BASIC PHARMACOLOGY

VASOPRESSIN RECEPTORS. Cellular vasopressin effects are mediated mainly by interactions of the hormone with the 3 types of receptors, V_{1a}, V_{1b}, and V_2. All are GPCRs.

The V_{1a} receptor is the most widespread subtype of vasopressin receptor; it is found in vascular smooth muscle, adrenal gland, myometrium, bladder, adipocytes, hepatocytes, platelets, renal medullary interstitial cells, vasa recta in the renal microcirculation, epithelial cells in the renal cortical collecting-duct, spleen, testis, and many CNS structures. V_{1b} receptors have a more limited distribution and are found in the anterior pituitary, several brain regions, pancreas, and adrenal medulla. V_2 receptors are located predominantly in principal cells of the renal collecting-duct system but also are present on epithelial cells in TAL and on vascular endothelial cells.

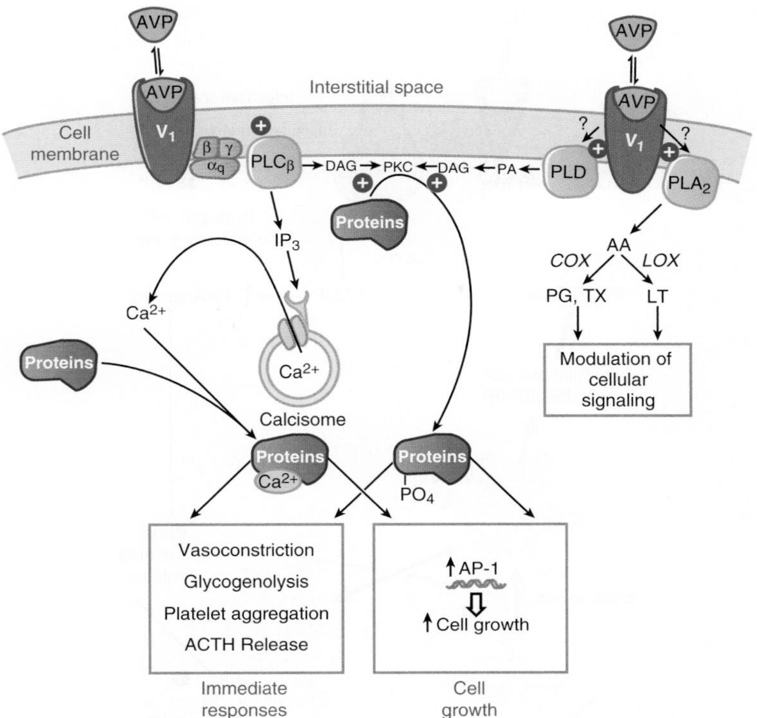

Figure 25–12 *Mechanism of V_1 receptor-effector coupling.* Binding of AVP to V_1 vasopressin receptors (V_1) stimulates membrane-bound phospholipases. Stimulation of the G_q activates the PLCβ-IP_3/DAG-Ca^{2+}-PKC pathway. Activation of V_1 receptors also causes influx of extracellular Ca^{2+} by an unknown mechanism. PKC and Ca^{2+}/calmodulin-activated protein kinases phosphorylate cell-type-specific proteins leading to cellular responses. A further component of the AVP response derives from the production of eicosanoids secondary to the activation of PLA_2; the resulting mobilization of arachidonic acid (AA) provides substrate for eicosanoid synthesis by the cyclooxygenase (COX) and lipoxygenase (LOX) pathways, leading to local production of prostaglandins (PG), thromboxanes (TX), and leukotrienes (LT), which may activate myriad signaling pathways, including those linked to G_s and G_q.

V_1 RECEPTOR-EFFECTOR COUPLING. Figure 25–12 summarizes the current model of V_1 receptor-effector coupling. Vasopressin binding to V_1 receptors activates the G_q-PLC-IP_3 pathway, thereby mobilizing intracellular Ca^{2+} and activating PKC, ultimately causing biological effects that include immediate responses (e.g., vasoconstriction, glycogenolysis, platelet aggregation, and ACTH release) and growth responses in smooth muscle cells.

V_2 RECEPTOR-EFFECTOR COUPLING. Principal cells in renal collecting duct have V_2 receptors on their basolateral membranes that couple to G_S to stimulate adenylyl cyclase activity (Figure 25–13). When vasopressin binds to V_2 receptors, the resulting activation of the cyclic AMP/PKA pathway triggers an increased rate of insertion of water channel-containing vesicles (WCVs) into the apical membrane and a decreased rate of endocytosis of WCVs from the apical membrane. Because WCVs contain preformed functional water channels (aquaporin 2), their net shift into apical membranes in response to V_2 receptor stimulation greatly increases water permeability of the apical membrane (*see* Figures 25–13 and 25–14).

V_2-receptor activation also increases urea permeability by 400% in the terminal portions of the IMCD. V_2 receptors increase urea permeability by activating a vasopressin-regulated urea transporter (termed *VRUT*, *UT1*, or *UTA1*), most likely by PKA-induced phosphorylation. Kinetics of vasopressin-induced water and urea permeability differ, and vasopressin-induced regulation of VRUT does not entail vesicular trafficking to the plasma membrane.

V_2-receptor activation also increases Na^+ transport in TAL and collecting duct. Increased Na^+ transport in TAL is mediated by 3 mechanisms that affect the Na^+-K^+-$2Cl^-$ symporter: rapid phosphorylation of the symporter,

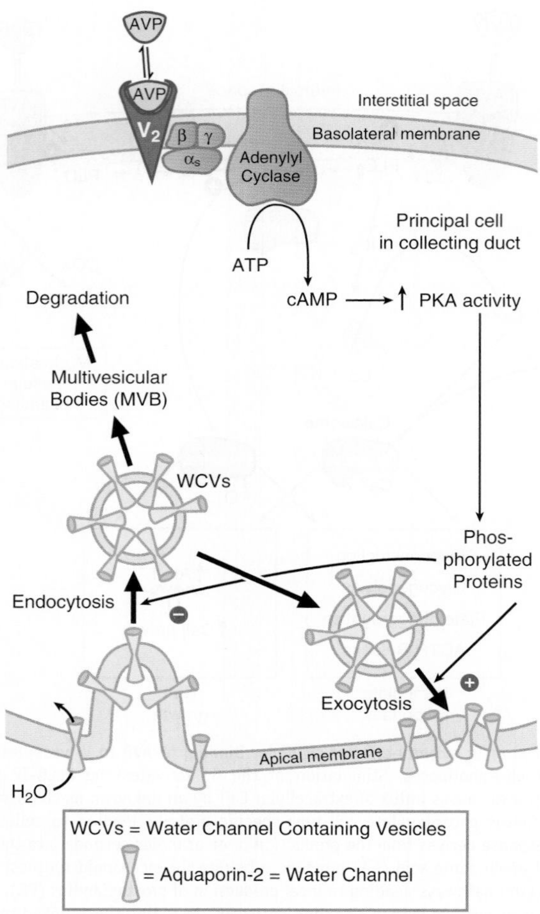

Figure 25–13 *Mechanism of V_2 receptor-effector coupling.* Binding of vasopressin (AVP) to the V_2 receptor activates the G_s-adenylyl cyclase-cAMP-PKA pathway and shifts the balance of aquaporin 2 trafficking toward the apical membrane of the principal cell of the collecting duct, thus enhancing water permeability. Although phosphorylation of *Ser256* of aquaporin 2 is involved in V_2 receptor signaling, other proteins located both in the water channel-containing vesicles and the apical membrane of the cytoplasm also may be involved.

translocation of the symporter into the luminal membrane, and increased expression of symporter protein. Enhanced Na^+ transport in collecting duct is mediated by increased expression of subunits of the epithelial Na^+ channel. The multiple mechanisms by which vasopressin increases water reabsorption are summarized in Figure 25–15.

RENAL ACTIONS OF VASOPRESSIN. Several sites of vasopressin action in kidney involve both V_1 and V_2 receptors (*see* Figure 25–15).

V_1 receptors mediate contraction of mesangial cells in the glomerulus and contraction of vascular smooth muscle cells in vasa recta and efferent arteriole. V_1-receptor-mediated reduction of inner medullary blood flow contributes to the maximum concentrating capacity of the kidney. V_1 receptors also stimulate prostaglandin synthesis by medullary interstitial cells. Since PGE_2 inhibits adenylyl cyclase in collecting duct, stimulation of prostaglandin synthesis by V_1 receptors may counterbalance V_2-receptor-mediated antidiuresis. V_1 receptors on principal cells in cortical collecting duct may inhibit V_2-receptor-mediated water flux by activation of PKC. V_2 receptors mediate the most prominent response to vasopressin, which is increased water permeability of the collecting duct at concentrations as low as 50 fM. Thus, V_2-receptor-mediated effects of vasopressin occur at concentrations far lower than are required to engage V_1-receptor-mediated actions. Other renal actions mediated by V_2 receptors include increased urea transport in IMCD and increased Na^+ transport in

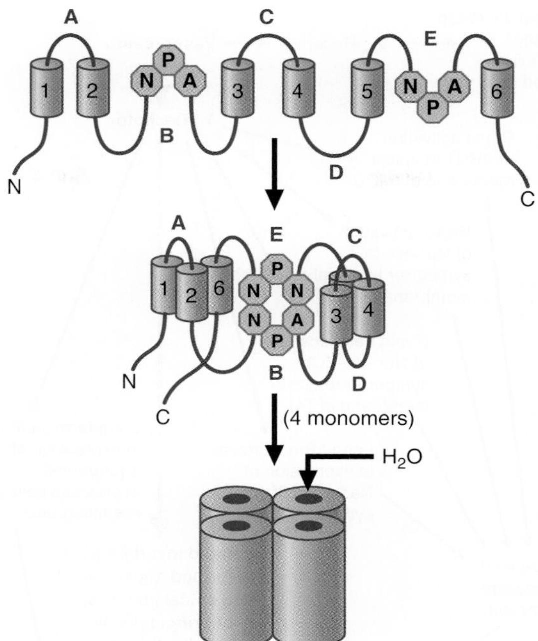

Figure 25–14 *Structure of aquaporins.* Aquaporins have 6 transmembrane domains, and the NH_2 and COOH termini are intracellular. Loops B and E each contain an asparagine-proline-alanine (NPA) sequence. Aquaporins fold with transmembrane domains 1, 2, and 6 in close proximity and transmembrane domains 3, 4 and 5 in juxtaposition. The long B and E loops dip into the membrane, and the NPA sequences align to create a pore through which water can diffuse. Most likely aquaporins form a tetrameric oligomer. At least 7 aquaporins are expressed at distinct sites in the kidney. Aquaporin 1, abundant in the proximal tubule and descending thin limb, is essential for concentration of urine. Aquaporin 2, exclusively expressed in the principal cells of the connecting tubule and collecting duct, is the major vasopressin-regulated water channel. Aquaporin 3 and aquaporin 4 are expressed in the basolateral membranes of collecting-duct principal cells and provide exit pathways for water reabsorbed apically by aquaporin 2. Aquaporin 7 is in the apical brush border of the straight proximal tubule. Aquaporins 6-8 are also expressed in kidney; their functions remain to be clarified. Vasopressin regulates water permeability of the collecting duct by influencing the trafficking of aquaporin 2 from intracellular vesicles to the apical plasma membrane (Figure 25–13). AVP-induced activation of the cAMP-PKA pathway also enhances expression of aquaporin 2 mRNA and protein; chronic dehydration thus causes upregulation of aquaporin 2 and water transport in the collecting duct.

TAL; both effects contribute to the urine-concentrating ability of the kidney. V_2 receptors also increase Na^+ transport in cortical collecting duct, and this may synergize with aldosterone to enhance Na^+ reabsorption during hypovolemia.

PHARMACOLOGICAL MODIFICATION OF THE ANTIDIURETIC RESPONSE TO VASOPRESSIN. NSAIDs, particularly indomethacin, enhance the antidiuretic response to vasopressin. Because prostaglandins attenuate antidiuretic responses to vasopressin and NSAIDs inhibit prostaglandin synthesis, reduced prostaglandin production probably accounts for potentiation of vasopressin's antidiuretic response. Carbamazepine and chlorpropamide also enhance antidiuretic effects of vasopressin by unknown mechanisms. In rare instances, chlorpropamide can induce water intoxication. A number of drugs inhibit the antidiuretic actions of vasopressin. Lithium is of particular importance because of its use in the treatment of manic-depressive disorders. Acutely, Li^+ appears to reduce V_2-receptor-mediated stimulation of adenylyl cyclase. Also, Li^+ increases plasma levels of PTH, a partial antagonist to vasopressin. In most patients, the antibiotic demeclocycline attenuates the antidiuretic effects of vasopressin, probably owing to decreased accumulation and action of cyclic AMP.

NONRENAL ACTIONS OF VASOPRESSIN

Cardiovascular System. The cardiovascular effects of vasopressin are complex. Vasopressin is a potent vasoconstrictor (V_1 receptor-mediated), and resistance vessels throughout the circulation may be affected. Vascular smooth muscle in the skin, skeletal muscle, fat, pancreas, and thyroid gland appears most sensitive, with

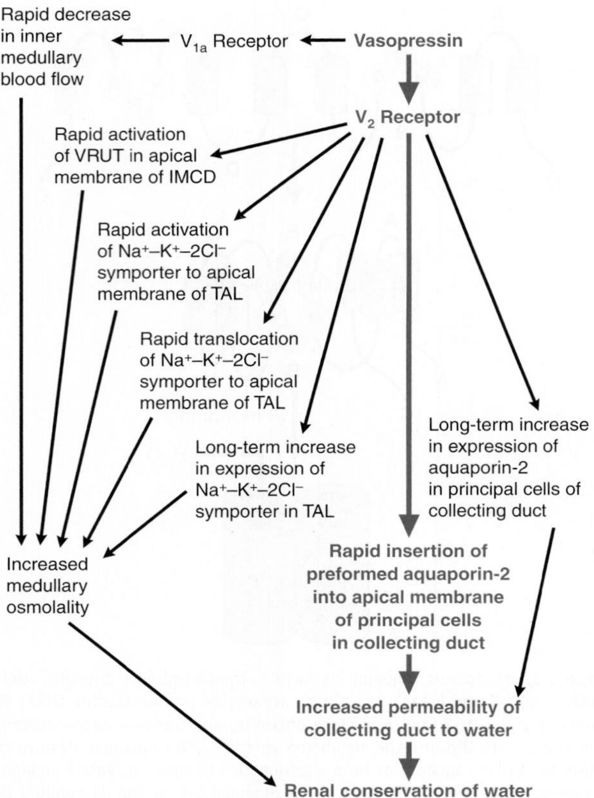

Figure 25–15 *Mechanisms by which vasopressin increases the renal conservation of water.* Red and black arrows denote major and minor pathways, respectively. IMCD, inner medullary collecting duct; TAL, thick ascending limb; VRUT, vasopressin-regulated urea transporter.

significant vasoconstriction also occurring in GI tract, coronary vessels, and brain. Despite the potency of vasopressin as a direct vasoconstrictor, vasopressin-induced pressor responses in vivo are minimal and occur only with vasopressin concentrations significantly higher than those required for maximal antidiuresis. To a large extent, this is due to circulating vasopressin actions on V_1 receptors to inhibit sympathetic efferents and potentiate baroreflexes. In addition, V_2 receptors cause vasodilation in some blood vessels.

Vasopressin helps to maintain arterial blood pressure during episodes of severe hypovolemia/hypotension. The effects of vasopressin on heart (reduced cardiac output and heart rate) are largely indirect and result from coronary vasoconstriction, decreased coronary blood flow, and alterations in vagal and sympathetic tone. Some patients with coronary insufficiency experience angina even in response to the relatively small amounts of vasopressin required to control diabetes insipidus, and vasopressin-induced myocardial ischemia has led to severe reactions and even death.

CNS. Vasopressin likely plays a role as a neurotransmitter and/or neuromodulator. Although vasopressin can modulate CNS autonomic systems controlling heart rate, arterial blood pressure, respiration rate, and sleep patterns, the physiological significance of these actions is unclear. While vasopressin is not the principal corticotropin-releasing factor, vasopressin may provide for sustained activation of the hypothalamic-pituitary-adrenal axis during chronic stress. CNS effects of vasopressin appear to be mediated predominantly by V_1 receptors.

Blood Coagulation. Activation of V_2 receptors by desmopressin or vasopressin increases circulating levels of procoagulant factor VIII and of von Willebrand factor. These effects are mediated by extrarenal V_2 receptors. Presumably, vasopressin stimulates secretion of von Willebrand factor and of factor VIII from storage sites in vascular endothelium. However, since release of von Willebrand factor does not occur when desmopressin is applied directly to cultured endothelial cells or to isolated blood vessels, intermediate factors are likely to be involved.

Other Nonrenal Effects of Vasopressin. At high concentrations, vasopressin stimulates smooth muscle contraction in uterus (by oxytocin receptors) and GI tract (by V_1 receptors). Vasopressin is stored in platelets, and activation of V_1 receptors stimulates platelet aggregation. Also, activation of V_1 receptors on hepatocytes stimulates glycogenolysis.

VASOPRESSIN RECEPTOR AGONISTS AND ANTAGONISTS

A number of vasopressin-like peptides occur naturally across the animal kingdom (Table 25–8); all are nonapeptides. In all mammals except swine, the neurohypophyseal peptide is 8-arginine vasopressin, and the terms vasopressin, arginine vasopressin (AVP), and ADH are used interchangeably. There are also a number of synthetic peptides with receptor-subtype specificity, and 1 non-peptide agonist.

Table 25–8

Vasopressin Receptor Agonists

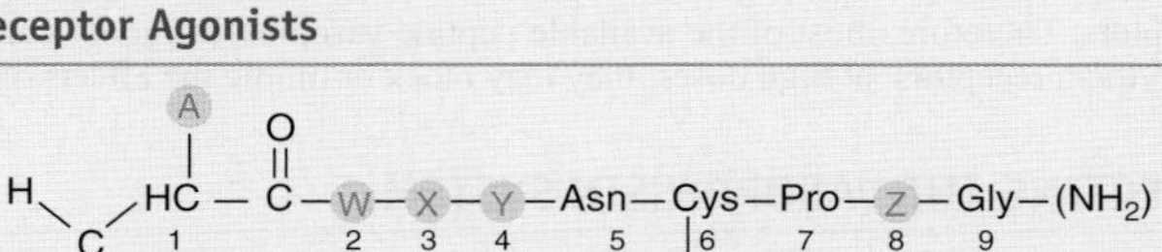

$$\mathrm{H_2C}(\mathrm{S})\text{—}\underset{1}{\overset{A}{\mathrm{HC}}}\text{—}\mathrm{C(=O)}\text{—}\underset{2}{W}\text{—}\underset{3}{X}\text{—}\underset{4}{Y}\text{—}\underset{5}{\mathrm{Asn}}\text{—}\underset{6}{\mathrm{Cys(S)}}\text{—}\underset{7}{\mathrm{Pro}}\text{—}\underset{8}{Z}\text{—}\underset{9}{\mathrm{Gly}}\text{—}(\mathrm{NH_2})$$

(S of residue 1 linked by disulfide bond to S of Cys 6)

	A	W	X	Y	Z
I. NATURALLY OCCURRING VASOPRESSIN-LIKE PEPTIDES					
A. *Vertebrates*					
1. Mammals					
Arginine vasopressin[a] (AVP) (humans and other mammals)	NH_2	Tyr	Phe	Gln	Arg
Lypressin[a] (pigs, marsupials)	NH_2	Tyr	Phe	Gln	Lys
Phenypressin (macropodids)	NH_2	Phe	Phe	Gln	Arg
2. Nonmammalian vertebrates					
Vasotocin	NH_2	Tyr	Ile	Gln	Arg
B. *Invertebrates*					
1. Arginine conopressin (*Conus striatus*)	NH_2	Ile	Ile	Arg	Arg
2. Lysine conopressin (*Conus geographicus*)	NH_2	Phe	Ile	Arg	Lys
3. Locust subesophageal ganglia peptide	NH_2	Leu	Ile	Thr	Arg
II. SYNTHETIC VASOPRESSIN PEPTIDES					
A. *V_1-selective agonists*					
1. V_{1a}-selective: [Phe[2], Ile[3], Orn[8]] AVP	NH_2	Phe	Ile	Gln	Orn
2. V_{1b}-selective: Deamino [D-3-(3′-pyridyl)-Ala[2]]AVP	H	D-3-(3′-pyridyl)-Ala[2]	Phe	Gln	Arg
B. *V_2-selective agonists*					
1. Desmopressin[a] (DDAVP)	H	Tyr	Phe	Gln	D-Arg
2. Deamino[Val[4], D-Arg[8]]AVP	H	Tyr	Phe	Val	D-Arg
III. NONPEPTIDE AGONIST					
A. *OPC-51803*					

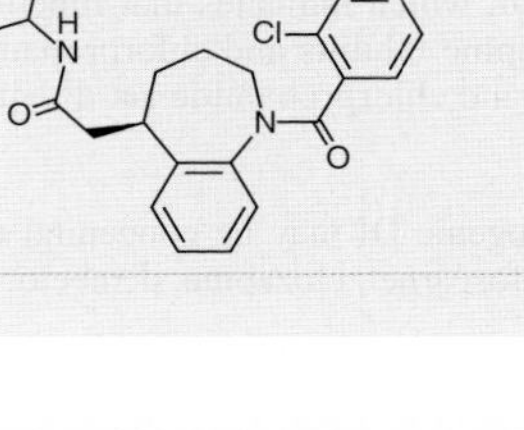

[a]*Available for clinical use.*

Many vasopressin analogs were synthesized with the goal of increasing duration of action and selectivity for vasopressin receptor subtypes (V_1 versus V_2 receptors, which mediate pressor responses and antidiuretic responses, respectively). Thus, the antidiuretic-to-vasopressor ratio for the V_2–selective agonist, 1-deamino-8-D-arginine vasopressin, also called desmopressin (DDAVP, MINIRIN, STIMATE), is ~3000 times greater than that for vasopressin, and is the preferred drug for the treatment of central diabetes insipidus. Substitution of valine for glutamine in position 4 further increases the antidiuretic selectivity, and the antidiuretic to vasopressor ratio for deamino [Val^4, D-Arg^8]AVP is ~11,000 times greater than that for vasopressin.

Increasing V_1 selectivity has proved more difficult than increasing V_2 selectivity. Vasopressin receptors in the adenohypophysis that mediate vasopressin-induced ACTH release are neither classical V_1 nor V_2 receptors. Because vasopressin receptors in the adenohypophysis appear to share a common signal-transduction mechanism with classical V_1 receptors, and since many vasopressin analogs with vasoconstrictor activity release ACTH, V_1 receptors have been subclassified into V_{1a} (vascular/hepatic) and V_{1b} (pituitary) receptors (also called V_3 receptors). There are selective agonists for V_{1a} and V_{1b} receptors.

The chemical structure of oxytocin is closely related to that of vasopressin: oxytocin is [Ile^3, Leu^8]AVP. With such structural similarities, it is not surprising that vasopressin and oxytocin agonists and antagonists can bind to each other's receptors. Therefore, most of the available peptide vasopressin agonists and antagonists have some affinity for oxytocin receptors; at high doses, they may block or mimic the effects of oxytocin.

DISEASES AFFECTING THE VASOPRESSIN SYSTEM

DIABETES INSIPIDUS (DI). DI is a disease of impaired renal water conservation owing either to inadequate vasopressin secretion from the neurohypophysis (central DI) or to insufficient renal vasopressin response (nephrogenic DI). Very rarely, DI can be caused by an abnormally high degradation rate of vasopressin by circulating vasopressinases. Pregnancy may accentuate or reveal central and/or nephrogenic DI by increasing plasma levels of vasopressinase and by reducing renal sensitivity to vasopressin. Patients with DI excrete large volumes (>30 mL/kg per day) of dilute (<200 mOsm/kg) urine and, if their thirst mechanism is functioning normally, are polydipsic. Central DI can be distinguished from nephrogenic DI by administration of desmopressin, which will increase urine osmolality in patients with central DI but have little or no effect in patients with nephrogenic DI. DI can be differentiated from primary polydipsia by measuring plasma osmolality, which will be low to low-normal in patients with primary polydipsia and high to high-normal in patients with DI.

CENTRAL DI. Head injury, either surgical or traumatic, in the region of the pituitary and/or hypothalamus may cause central DI. Postoperative central DI may be transient, permanent, or triphasic (recovery followed by permanent relapse). Other causes include hypothalamic or pituitary tumors, cerebral aneurysms, CNS ischemia, and brain infiltrations and infections. Central DI may also be idiopathic or familial. Familial central DI usually is autosomal dominant (chromosome 20), and vasopressin deficiency occurs several months or years after birth and worsens gradually. Autosomal dominant central DI is linked to mutations in the vasopressin preprohormone gene that cause the prohormone to misfold and oligomerize improperly. Accumulation of mutant vasopressin precursor causes neuronal death, hence the dominant mode of inheritance. Rarely, familial central DI is autosomal recessive owing to a mutation in the vasopressin peptide itself that gives rise to an inactive vasopressin mutant.

Antidiuretic peptides are the primary treatment for central DI, with desmopressin being the peptide of choice. For patients with central DI who cannot tolerate antidiuretic peptides because of side effects or allergic reactions, other treatment options are available. Chlorpropamide, an oral sulfonylurea, potentiates the action of small or residual amounts of circulating vasopressin and will reduce urine volume in more than half of all patients with central DI. Doses of 125-500 mg daily appear effective in patients with partial central DI. If polyuria is not controlled satisfactorily with chlorpropamide alone, addition of a thiazide diuretic to the regimen usually results in an adequate reduction in urine volume. Carbamazepine (800-1000 mg daily in divided doses) also reduces urine volume in patients with central DI. Long-term use may induce serious adverse effects; therefore, carbamazepine is used rarely to treat central DI. These agents are not effective in nephrogenic DI, which indicates that functional V_2 receptors are required for the antidiuretic effect. Because carbamazepine inhibits and chlorpropamide has little effect on vasopressin secretion, it is likely that carbamazepine and chlorpropamide act directly on the kidney to enhance V_2-receptor-mediated antidiuresis.

NEPHROGENIC DI. Nephrogenic DI may be congenital or acquired. Hypercalcemia, hypokalemia, postobstructive renal failure, Li^+, foscarnet, clozapine, demeclocycline, and other drugs can induce nephrogenic DI.

As many as 1 in 3 patients treated with Li^+ may develop nephrogenic DI. X-linked nephrogenic DI is caused by mutations in the gene encoding the V_2 receptor, which maps to Xq28. Mutations in the V_2-receptor gene may cause impaired routing of the V_2 receptor to the cell surface, defective coupling of the receptor to G proteins, or decreased receptor affinity for vasopressin. Autosomal recessive and dominant nephrogenic DI result from inactivating mutations in aquaporin 2. These findings indicate that aquaporin 2 is essential for the antidiuretic effect of vasopressin in humans.

Although the mainstay of treatment of nephrogenic DI is assurance of an adequate water intake, drugs also can be used to reduce polyuria. Amiloride blocks Li^+ uptake by the Na^+ channel in the collecting-duct system and may be effective in patients with mild to moderate concentrating defects. Thiazide *diuretics* reduce the polyuria of patients with DI and often are used to treat nephrogenic DI. In infants with nephrogenic DI, use of thiazides may be crucial because uncontrolled polyuria may exceed the child's capacity to imbibe and absorb fluids. It is possible that the natriuretic action of thiazides and resulting extracellular fluid volume depletion play an important role in thiazide-induced antidiuresis. The antidiuretic effects appear to parallel the thiazide's ability to cause natriuresis, and the drugs are given in doses similar to those used to mobilize edema fluid. In patients with DI, a 50% reduction of urine volume is a good response to thiazides. Moderate restriction of Na^+ intake can enhance the antidiuretic effectiveness of thiazides.

A number of case reports describe the effectiveness of indomethacin in the treatment of nephrogenic DI; however, other prostaglandin synthase inhibitors (e.g., ibuprofen) appear to be less effective. The mechanism of the effect may involve a decrease in GFR, an increase in medullary solute concentration, and/or enhanced proximal fluid reabsorption. Also, because prostaglandins attenuate vasopressin-induced antidiuresis in patients with at least a partially intact V_2-receptor system, some of the antidiuretic response to indomethacin may be due to diminution of the prostaglandin effect and enhancement of vasopressin effects on the principal cells of collecting duct.

SYNDROME OF INAPPROPRIATE SECRETION OF ANTIDIURETIC HORMONE (SIADH). SIADH is a disease of impaired water excretion with accompanying hyponatremia and hypoosmolality caused by the *inappropriate* secretion of vasopressin. Clinical manifestations of plasma hypotonicity resulting from SIADH may include lethargy, anorexia, nausea and vomiting, muscle cramps, coma, convulsions, and death. A multitude of disorders can induce SIADH, including malignancies, pulmonary diseases, CNS injuries/diseases (e.g., head trauma, infections, and tumors), and general surgery.

Three drug classes are commonly implicated in drug-induced SIADH: psychotropic medications (e.g., selective serotonin reuptake inhibitors, haloperidol, and tricyclic antidepressants), sulfonylureas (e.g., chlorpropamide), and vinca alkaloids (e.g., vincristine and vinblastine). Other drugs strongly associated with SIADH include clonidine, cyclophosphamide, enalapril, felbamate, ifosfamide, and methyldopa, pentamidine, and vinorelbine. In a normal individual, an elevation in plasma vasopressin per se does not induce plasma hypotonicity because the person simply stops drinking owing to an osmotically induced aversion to fluids. Therefore, plasma hypotonicity only occurs when excessive fluid intake (oral or intravenous) accompanies inappropriate secretion of vasopressin. Treatment of hypotonicity in the setting of SIADH includes water restriction, intravenous administration of hypertonic saline, loop diuretics (which interfere with kidney's concentrating ability), and drugs that inhibit the effect of vasopressin to increase water permeability in collecting ducts. To inhibit vasopressin's action in collecting ducts, demeclocycline, a tetracycline, has been the preferred drug, but tolvaptan and conivaptan, V_2 receptor antagonists, are now available (*see* next section and Table 25–9).

Although Li^+ can inhibit the renal actions of vasopressin, it is effective in only a minority of patients, may induce irreversible renal damage when used chronically, and has a low therapeutic index. Therefore, Li^+ should be considered for use only in patients with symptomatic SIADH who cannot be controlled by other means or in whom tetracyclines are contraindicated (e.g., patients with liver disease). It is important to stress that the majority of patients with SIADH do not require therapy because plasma Na^+ stabilizes in the range of 125-132 m*M*; such patients usually are asymptomatic. Only when symptomatic hypotonicity ensues, generally when plasma Na^+ levels drop below 120 m*M*, should therapy with demeclocycline be initiated. Since hypotonicity, which causes an influx of water into cells with resulting cerebral swelling, is the cause of symptoms, the goal of therapy is simply to increase plasma osmolality toward normal.

OTHER WATER-RETAINING STATES. In patients with congestive heart failure, cirrhosis, or nephrotic syndrome, *effective* blood volume often is reduced, and hypovolemia frequently is exacerbated by the liberal use of diuretics. Because hypovolemia stimulates vasopressin release, patients may become hyponatremic owing to vasopressin-mediated retention of water. The development of potent orally active V_2 receptor antagonists and specific inhibitors of water channels in the collecting duct has provided a new therapeutic strategy not only in patients with SIADH but also in the more common setting of hyponatremia in patients with heart failure, liver cirrhosis, and nephrotic syndrome.

AGONISTS

Two antidiuretic peptides are available for clinical use in the U.S.:

- *Vasopressin* (synthetic 8-L-arginine vasopressin; PITRESSIN, others) is available as a sterile aqueous solution; it may be administered subcutaneously, intramuscularly, or intranasally.
- *Desmopressin acetate* (synthetic 1-deamino-8-D-arginine vasopressin; DDAVP, others) is available as a sterile aqueous solution packaged for intravenous or subcutaneous injection, in a solution for intranasal administration with either a nasal spray pump or rhinal tube delivery system, and in tablets for oral administration.

THERAPEUTIC USES. The therapeutic uses of vasopressin and its congeners can be divided into 2 main categories according to the vasopressin receptor involved.

V_1 receptor-mediated therapeutic applications are based on the rationale that V_1 receptors cause GI and vascular smooth muscle contraction. Vasopressin is the main agent used.

V_1 receptor-mediated GI smooth muscle contraction has been used to treat postoperative ileus and abdominal distension and to dispel intestinal gas before abdominal roentgenography to avoid interfering gas shadows. V_1 receptor-mediated vasoconstriction of the splanchnic arterial vessels reduces blood flow to the portal system and, thereby, attenuates pressure and bleeding in esophageal varices. Although endoscopic variceal banding ligation is the treatment of choice for bleeding esophageal varices, V_1 receptor agonists have been used in an emergency setting until endoscopy can be performed. Simultaneous administration of nitroglycerin with V_1 receptor agonists may attenuate the cardiotoxic effects of V_1 agonists while enhancing their beneficial splanchnic effects. Also, V_1 receptor agonists have been used during abdominal surgery in patients with portal hypertension to diminish the risk of hemorrhage during the procedure. Finally, V_1 receptor-mediated vasoconstriction has been used to reduce bleeding during acute hemorrhagic gastritis, burn wound excision, cyclophosphamide-induced hemorrhagic cystitis, liver transplant, cesarean section, and uterine myoma resection.

The applications of V_1 receptor agonists can be accomplished with vasopressin; however, the use of vasopressin for all these indications is no longer recommended because of significant adverse reactions. Terlipressin (LUCASSIN) is preferred for bleeding esophageal varices because of increased safety compared with vasopressin and is designated as an orphan drug for this use. Moreover, terlipressin is effective in patients with hepatorenal syndrome, particularly when combined with albumin. Terlipressin has been granted priority review, orphan drug status, and fast-track designation by the FDA for type I hepatorenal syndrome. Vasopressin levels in patients with vasodilatory shock are inappropriately low, and such patients are extraordinarily sensitive to the pressor actions of vasopressin. The combination of vasopressin and norepinephrine is superior to norepinephrine alone in the management of catecholamine-resistant vasodilatory shock. However, recent clinical trials show that, in comparison to catecholamines alone, addition of vasopressin does not improve outcomes in either cardiac arrest or septic shock.

V_2 receptor-mediated therapeutic applications are based on the rationale that V_2 receptors cause water conservation and release of blood coagulation factors. Desmopressin is the standard drug of choice.

Central but not nephrogenic DI can be treated with V_2 receptor agonists, and polyuria and polydipsia usually are well controlled by these agents. Some patients experience transient DI (e.g., in head injury or surgery in the area of the pituitary); however, therapy for most patients with DI is lifelong. Desmopressin is the drug of choice for the vast majority of patients. The duration of effect from a single intranasal dose is from 6-20 h; twice-daily administration is effective in most patients. The usual intranasal dosage in adults is 10-40 μg daily either as a single dose or divided into 2 or 3 doses. In view of the high cost of the drug and the importance of avoiding water intoxication, the schedule of administration should be adjusted to the minimal amount required. In some patients, chronic allergic rhinitis or other nasal pathology may preclude reliable peptide absorption following nasal administration. Oral administration of desmopressin in doses 10-20 times the intranasal dose provides adequate desmopressin blood levels to control polyuria. Subcutaneous administration of 1-2 μg daily of desmopressin also is effective in central DI.

Vasopressin has little, if any, place in the long-term therapy of DI because of its short duration of action and V_1 receptor-mediated side effects. Vasopressin can be used as an alternative to desmopressin in the initial diagnostic evaluation of patients with suspected DI and to control polyuria in patients with DI who recently have undergone surgery or experienced head trauma. Under these circumstances, polyuria may be transient, and long-acting agents may produce water intoxication.

Desmopressin is used in bleeding disorders. In most patients with type I von Willebrand disease (vWD) and in some with type IIn vWD, desmopressin will elevate von Willebrand factor and shorten bleeding time. However, desmopressin generally is ineffective in patients with types IIa, IIb, and III vWD. Desmopressin may cause a marked transient thrombocytopenia in individuals with type IIb vWD and is contraindicated in such patients. Desmopressin also increases factor VIII levels in patients with mild to moderate hemophilia A. Desmopressin is not indicated in patients with severe hemophilia A, those with hemophilia B, or those with factor VIII antibodies. In patients with renal insufficiency, desmopressin shortens bleeding time and increases circulating levels of factor VIII coagulant activity, factor VIII-related antigen, and ristocetin cofactor. It also induces the appearance of larger von Willebrand factor multimers. Desmopressin is effective in some patients with liver cirrhosis- or drug-induced (e.g., heparin, hirudin, and antiplatelet agents) bleeding disorders. Desmopressin, given intravenously at a dose of 0.3 μg/kg, increases factor VIII and von Willebrand factor for >6 h. Desmopressin can be given at intervals of 12-24 h depending on the clinical response and severity of bleeding. Tachyphylaxis to desmopressin usually occurs after several days (owing to depletion of factor VIII and von Willebrand factor storage sites) and limits its usefulness to preoperative preparation, postoperative bleeding, excessive menstrual bleeding, and emergency situations.

Another V_2 receptor-mediated therapeutic application is the use of desmopressin for primary nocturnal enuresis. Bedtime administration of desmopressin intranasal spray or tablets provides a high response rate that is sustained with long-term use, that is safe, and that accelerates the cure rate. Desmopressin also relieves post-lumbar puncture headache, probably by causing water retention and thereby facilitating rapid fluid equilibration in the CNS.

PHARMACOKINETICS. When vasopressin and desmopressin are given orally, they are inactivated quickly by trypsin. Inactivation by peptidases in various tissues (particularly liver and kidney) results in a plasma $t_{1/2}$ of vasopressin of 17-35 min. Following intramuscular or subcutaneous injection, antidiuretic effects of vasopressin last 2-8 h.

TOXICITY, ADVERSE EFFECTS, CONTRAINDICATIONS, DRUG INTERACTIONS. Most adverse effects are mediated through V_1 receptor activation on vascular and GI smooth muscle; such adverse effects are much less common and less severe with desmopressin than with vasopressin. After injection of large doses of vasopressin, marked facial pallor owing to cutaneous vasoconstriction is observed commonly. Increased intestinal activity is likely to cause nausea, belching, cramps, and an urge to defecate. Vasopressin should be administered with extreme caution in individuals suffering from vascular disease, especially coronary artery disease. Other cardiac complications include arrhythmia and decreased cardiac output. Peripheral vasoconstriction and gangrene were encountered in patients receiving large doses of vasopressin.

The major V_2 receptor-mediated adverse effect is water intoxication. Many drugs, including carbamazepine, chlorpropamide, morphine, tricyclic antidepressants, and NSAIDs, can potentiate the antidiuretic effects of these peptides. Several drugs such as Li^+, demeclocycline, and ethanol can attenuate the antidiuretic response to desmopressin. Desmopressin and vasopressin should be used cautiously in disease states in which a rapid increase in extracellular water may impose risks (e.g., in angina, hypertension, and heart failure) and should not be used in patients with acute renal failure. Patients receiving desmopressin to maintain hemostasis should be advised to reduce fluid intake. Also, it is imperative that these peptides not be administered to patients with primary or psychogenic polydipsia because severe hypotonic hyponatremia will ensue. Mild facial flushing and headache are the most common adverse effects. Allergic reactions ranging from urticaria to anaphylaxis may occur with desmopressin or vasopressin. Intranasal administration may cause local adverse effects in the nasal passages, such as edema, rhinorrhea, congestion, irritation, pruritus, and ulceration.

VASOPRESSIN RECEPTOR ANTAGONISTS

Table 25–9 summarizes selectivity of vasopressin receptor antagonists.

THERAPEUTIC USES. When the kidney perceives the arterial blood volume to be low (as in the disease states of CHF, cirrhosis, and nephrosis), AVP perpetuates a state of total body salt and water excess. V_2 receptor (V_2R) antagonists or "aquaretics" may have a therapeutic role in these conditions, especially in patients with concomitant hyponatremia. They are also effective in hyponatremia associated with SIADH. Aquaretics increase renal free water excretion with little or no change in electrolyte excretion. Since they do not affect Na^+ reabsorption they do not stimulate the TGF mechanism with its associated consequence of reducing GFR.

AVAILABLE AGENTS

Mozavaptan. Mozavaptan causes a dose-dependent increase in free water excretion with only slight increases in urinary Na^+ and K^+ excretion. Mozavaptan is available in 30-mg tablets. Its peak effects occur 60-90 min after an oral dose. Mozavaptan's major side effects are dry mouth and abnormal liver function tests.

Tolvaptan. Tolvaptan (SAMSCA) is a selective oral V_2R antagonist. Tolvaptan is approved for clinically significant hypervolemic and euvolemic hyponatremia. The drug is labeled with a black box warning against

Table 25–9

Vasopressin Receptor Antagonists

I. PEPTIDE ANTAGONISTS

```
                                 O
                                 ||
      CH2—CH2         CH2 —C —(X)—Phe—(Y)—Asn—Cys—Pro—Arg—(Z)
H2C           C              1     2     3    4     5    |6     7     8     9
      CH2—CH2         S ———————————————————————————————— S
```

	X	Y	Z
A. *V_1-selective antagonists*			
V_{1a}-selective antagonist $d(CH_2)_5[Tyr(Me)^2]AVP$	Tyr—OMe	Gln	Gly (NH_2)
V_{1b}-selective antagonist dP $[Tyr(Me)^2]AVP$[a,b]	Tyr—OMe	Gln	Gly (NH_2)
B. *V_2-selective antagonists*[a]			
1. des Gly-NH_2^9-$d(CH_2)_5$[D-Ile^2, Ile^4]AVP	D-Ile	Ile	—
2. $d(CH_2)_5$[D-Ile^2, Ile^4, Ala-NH_2^9]AVP	D-Ile	Ile	Ala(NH_2)

II. NONPEPTIDE ANTAGONISTS

A. *V_{1a}-selective antagonists*
- OPC-21268
- SR 49059 (relcovaptan)

B. *V_{1b}-selective antagonists*
- SSR 149415

C. *V_2-selective antagonists*
- SR 121463A
- VPA-985 (lixivaptan)
- OPC-31260 (mozavaptan)[c]
- OPC-41061 (tolvaptan)[c]

D. *V_{1a}-/V_2-selective antagonists*
- YM-471
- YM 087 (conivaptan)[c]
- JTV-605
- CL-385004

[a]*Also blocks V_{1a} receptor.*

[b] $(H_3C)_2C$ *rather than* $H_2C(CH_2—CH_2)_2C$ *V_2 antagonistic activity in rats; however, antagonistic activity may be less or nonexistent in other species. Also, with prolonged infusion may exhibit significant agonist activity.*

[c]*Available for clinical use.*

too rapid correction of hyponatremia (can have serious and fatal consequences) and the recommendation to initiate therapy in a hospital setting capable of close monitoring of serum Na^+. Tolvaptan is contraindicated in patients receiving drugs that inhibit CYP3A4.

Tolvaptan is available in 15 and 30 mg tablets. Tolvaptan is 29 times more selective for the V_2R than the $V_{1a}R$. Tolvaptan has a $t_{1/2}$ of 6-8 h and <1% is excreted in the urine. Tolvaptan is a substrate and inhibitor of P-glycoprotein and is eliminated entirely by CYP3A metabolism. Plasma concentrations of the drug are increased by ketoconazole. Adverse effects include GI effects, hyperglycemia, and pyrexia. Less common are cerebrovascular accident, deep vein thrombosis, disseminated intravascular coagulation, intracardiac thrombus, ventricular fibrillation, urethral hemorrhage, vaginal hemorrhage, pulmonary embolism, respiratory failure, diabetic ketoacidosis, ischemic colitis, increase in prothrombin time, and rhabdomyolysis.

Conivaptan. Conivaptan (VAPRISOL) is a nonselective $V_{1a}R/V_2R$ antagonist that is FDA-approved for the treatment of hospitalized patients with euvolemic hyponatremia and hypervolemic hyponatremia. The drug is available only for intravenous infusion. In CHF patients, conivaptan increases renal free water excretion without a change in systemic vascular resistance.

Conivaptan is highly protein bound, has a terminal elimination $t_{1/2}$ of 5-12 h, is metabolized via CYP3A4, and is partially excreted by the kidney. Caution should be exercised in those with hepatic and renal disease. At higher doses clearance may be reduced in the elderly. Conivaptan should not be administered in patients receiving ketoconazole, itraconazole, ritonavir, indinavir, clarithromycin, or other strong CYP3A4 inhibitors. Conivaptan increases levels of simvastatin, digoxin, amlodipine, and midazolam. The most common adverse effect of conivaptan is an infusion site reaction. Other adverse effects include headache, hypertension, hypotension, hypokalemia, and pyrexia.

For a complete Bibliographical Listing see Goodman & Gilman's ***The Pharmacological Basis of Therapeutics***, 12th ed., or Goodman & Gilman Online at www.AccessMedicine.com.

Renin and Angiotensin

The renin–angiotensin system (RAS) participates significantly in the pathophysiology of hypertension, congestive heart failure, myocardial infarction, and diabetic nephropathy.

COMPONENTS OF THE RENIN–ANGIOTENSIN SYSTEM

Angiotensin II (AngII), the most vasoactive angiotensin peptide, participates in blood pressure regulation, aldosterone release, Na^+ reabsorption from renal tubules, and electrolyte and fluid homeostasis. AngII is derived from angiotensinogen in two 2 proteolytic steps (Figure 26–1). First, renin, an enzyme released from the juxtaglomerular cells of the kidneys, cleaves the decapeptide angiotensin I (AngI) from the amino terminus of angiotensinogen (renin substrate). Then, angiotensin-converting enzyme (ACE) removes the carboxy-terminal dipeptide of AngI to produce the octapeptide AngII. AngII is an agonist ligand for 2 GPCRs, AT_1 and AT_2. The RAS includes local (tissue) RAS, alternative pathways for AngII synthesis (ACE-independent), formation of other biologically active angiotensin peptides (AngIII, AngIV, Ang[1–7]), and additional angiotensin-binding receptors (AT_1, AT_2, AT_4, Mas) that participate in cell growth differentiation, hypertrophy, inflammation, fibrosis, and apoptosis.

RENIN AND THE PRORENIN/RENIN RECEPTOR. Renin is the major determinant of the rate of AngII production. It is synthesized, stored, and secreted by exocytosis into the renal arterial circulation by the granular juxtaglomerular cells (Figure 26–2) located in the walls of the afferent arterioles that enter the glomeruli. Renin is an aspartyl protease that cleaves the bond between residues 10 and 11 at the amino terminus of angiotensinogen to generate AngI. The active form of renin is a large glycoprotein that is synthesized as a preproenzyme and processed to prorenin. Prorenin may be activated in 2 ways: proteolytically, by proconvertase 1 or cathepsin B that remove 43 amino acids (propeptide) from prorenin's amino terminus to uncover the active site of renin (Figure 26–3); and nonproteolytically, when prorenin binds to the prorenin/renin receptor (PRR), resulting in conformational changes that unfold the propeptide and expose the active catalytic site of the enzyme. Both renin and prorenin are stored in the juxtaglomerular cells. The concentration of plasma prorenin is ~10x that of the active enzyme. The $t_{1/2}$ of circulating renin is ~15 min.

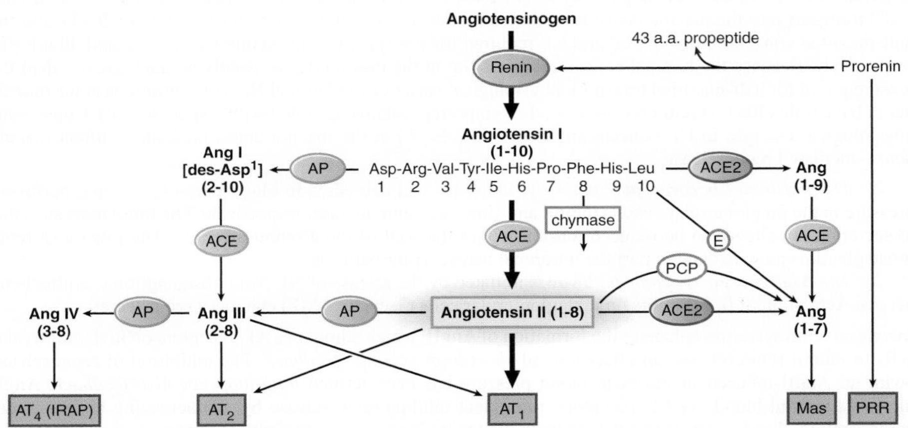

Figure 26–1 *Components of the RAS.* The heavy arrows show the classical pathway, and the light arrows indicate alternative pathways. ACE, angiotensin-converting enzyme; Ang, angiotensin; AP, aminopeptidase; E, endopeptidases; IRAP, insulin-regulated aminopeptidases; PCP, prolylcarboxylpeptidase; PRR, (pro)renin receptor. Receptors involved: AT_1, AT_2, Mas, AT_4, and PRR. *Exposure of the active site of renin can also occur nonproteolytically; *see* text and Figure 26–4.

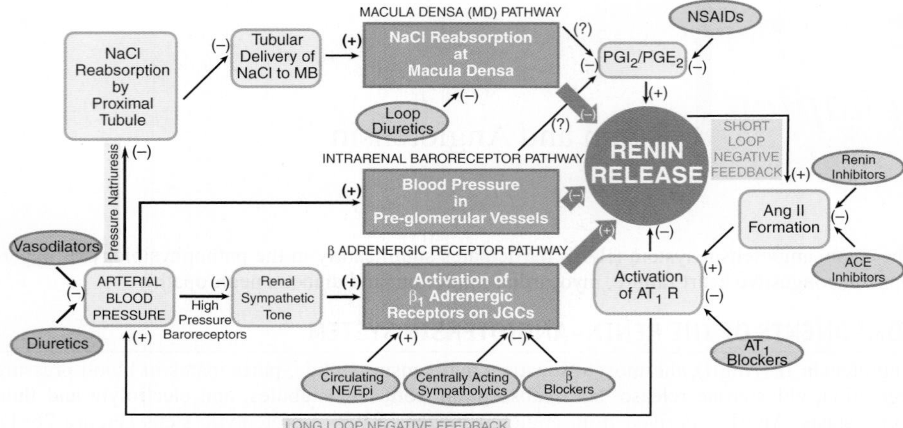

Figure 26–2 *Physiological pathways, feedback loops, and pharmacological regulation of the renin-angiotensin system.* Schematic portrayal of the three major physiological pathways regulating renin release. *See* text for details. MD, macula densa; PGI_2/PGE_2 prostaglandins I_2 and E_2; NSAIDs, nonsteroidal anti-inflamatory drugs; Ang II, angiotensin II: ACE, angiotensin-converting enzyme. AT_1 R, angiotensin subtype 1 receptor; NE/Epi, norepinephrine/epinephrine; JGCs, juxtaglomerular cells.

CONTROL OF RENIN SECRETION. The secretion of renin from juxtaglomerular cells is controlled predominantly by 3 pathways (*see* Figure 26–2):

1. *The macula densa pathway*. The macula densa lies adjacent to the juxtaglomerular cells and is composed of specialized columnar epithelial cells in the wall of the cortical thick ascending limb that passes between the afferent and efferent arterioles of the glomerulus. A change in NaCl reabsorption by the macula densa results in the transmission to nearby juxtaglomerular cells of chemical signals that modify renin release. Increases in NaCl flux across the macula densa inhibit renin release, whereas decreases in NaCl flux stimulate renin release.

ATP, adenosine, and prostaglandins modulate the macula densa pathway (Figure 26–3). ATP and adenosine are released when NaCl transport increases: ATP acts on P2Y receptors and adenosine acts via the A_1 adenosine receptor to inhibit renin release. Prostaglandins (PGE_2, PGI_2) are released when NaCl transport decreases, and stimulate renin release through enhancing cyclic AMP formation. Prostaglandin production is stimulated by inducible COX-2 and neuronal NO synthase.

Regulation of the macula densa pathway is more dependent on the luminal concentration of Cl^- than Na^+. NaCl transport into the macula densa is mediated by the Na^+–K^+–$2Cl^-$ symporter (*see* Figure 26–3), and the half-maximal concentrations of Na^+ and Cl^- required for transport via this symporter are 2-3 and 40 mEq/L, respectively. Because the luminal concentration of Na^+ at the macula densa usually is much greater than the level required for half-maximal transport, physiological variations in luminal Na^+ concentrations at the macula densa have little effect on renin release (i.e., the symporter remains saturated with respect to Na^+). Conversely, physiological changes in Cl^- concentrations (20-60 mEq/L) at the macula densa profoundly affect macula densa–mediated renin release.

2. *The intrarenal baroreceptor pathway*. Increases and decreases in blood pressure or renal perfusion pressure in the preglomerular vessels inhibit and stimulate renin release, respectively. The immediate stimulus to secretion is believed to be reduced tension within the wall of the afferent arteriole. The release of renal prostaglandins may mediate in part the intrarenal baroreceptor pathway.

3. *The β adrenergic receptor pathway* is initiated by the release of NE from postganglionic sympathetic nerves. Activation of $β_1$ receptors on juxtaglomerular cells (↑ cyclic AMP) enhances renin secretion.

Increased renin secretion enhances the formation of AngII, which stimulates AT_1 receptors on juxtaglomerular cells to inhibit renin release, an effect termed *short-loop negative feedback*. The inhibition of renin release owing to AngII-induced increases in blood pressure has been termed *long-loop negative feedback*. AngII increases arterial blood via AT_1 receptors; this effect inhibits renin release by: (1) activating high-pressure baroreceptors, thereby reducing renal sympathetic tone; (2) increasing pressure in the preglomerular vessels; and (3) reducing NaCl reabsorption in the proximal tubule (pressure natriuresis), which increases tubular delivery of NaCl to the macula densa.

Renin release is regulated by arterial blood pressure, dietary salt intake, and a number of pharmacological agents (*see* Figure 26–2). Loop diuretics stimulate renin release by decreasing arterial blood pressure and by blocking

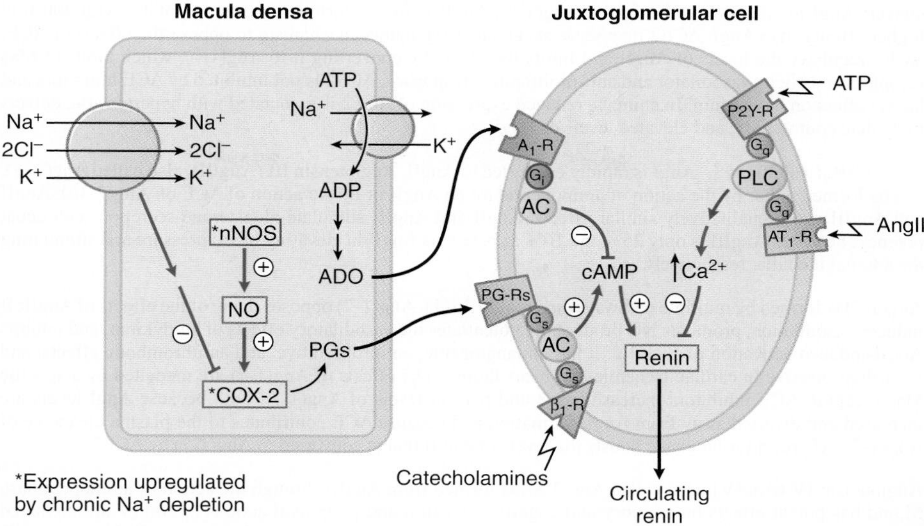

Figure 26–3 *Regulation of J-G cell renin release by the macula densa.* Mechanisms by which the macula densa regulates renin release. Changes in tubular delivery of NaCl to the macula densa cause appropriate signals to be conveyed to the juxtaglomerular cells. Sodium depletion upregulates nNOS and COX-2 in the macula densa to enhance production of prostaglandins (PGs). PGs and catecholamines stimulate cyclic AMP production and thence renin release from the juxtaglomerular cells. Increased NaCl transport depletes ATP and increases adenosine (ADO) levels. Adenosine diffuses to the juxtaglomerular cells and inhibits cyclic AMP production and renin release via G_i-coupled A_1 receptors. Increased NaCl transport in the macula densa augments the efflux of ATP, which may inhibit renin release directly by binding to P2Y receptors and activating the G_q-PLC-IP_3-Ca^{2+} pathway in juxtaglomerular cells. Circulating AngII also inhibits renin release on juxtaglomerular cells via G_q- coupled AT_1 receptors.

the reabsorption of NaCl at the macula densa. *Nonsteroidal anti-inflammatory drugs* (NSAIDs) inhibit prostaglandin synthesis and thereby decrease renin release. ACE inhibitors, angiotensin receptor blockers (ARBs), and renin inhibitors interrupt both the short- and long-loop negative feedback mechanisms and therefore increase renin release. Centrally acting sympatholytic drugs, as well as β adrenergic receptor antagonists, decrease renin secretion by reducing activation of β_1 adrenergic receptors on juxtaglomerular cells.

ANGIOTENSINOGEN. AngI is cleaved by renin from the amino terminus of angiotensinogen, an abundant globular protein synthesized mainly by the liver. Angiotensinogen transcripts also are abundant in fat, certain regions of the CNS, and the kidneys. Angiotensinogen synthesis is stimulated by inflammation, insulin, estrogens, glucocorticoids, thyroid hormone, and AngII. During pregnancy, plasma levels of angiotensinogen increase several-fold owing to increased estrogen. Circulating levels of angiotensinogen are approximately equal to the K_m of renin for its substrate (~1 μM). Consequently, the rate of AngII synthesis, and therefore blood pressure, can be influenced by changes in angiotensinogen levels. Oral contraceptives containing estrogen increase circulating levels of angiotensinogen and can induce hypertension.

ANGIOTENSIN-CONVERTING ENZYME (ACE, KININASE II, DIPEPTIDYL CARBOXYPEPTIDASE). ACE is an ectoenzyme and glycoprotein that contains 2 homologous domains, each with a catalytic site and a Zn^{2+}-binding region. ACE is rather nonspecific and cleaves dipeptide units from substrates with diverse amino acid sequences. Preferred substrates have only 1 free carboxyl group in the carboxyl-terminal amino acid, and proline must not be the penultimate amino acid; thus, the enzyme does not degrade AngII. ACE is identical to kininase II, the enzyme that inactivates bradykinin and other potent vasodilator peptides. Although slow conversion of AngI to AngII occurs in plasma, the very rapid metabolism that occurs in vivo is due largely to the activity of membrane-bound ACE present on the luminal surface of endothelial cells throughout the vascular system.

The *ACE* gene contains an insertion/deletion polymorphism in intron 16 that explains 47% of the phenotypic variance in serum ACE levels. The deletion allele, associated with higher levels of serum ACE and increased metabolism of bradykinin, may confer an increased risk of hypertension, cardiac hypertrophy, atherosclerosis, and diabetic nephropathy.

ANGIOTENSIN-CONVERTING ENZYME 2 (ACE2). Human ACE2 contains a single catalytic domain that is 42% identical to the 2 catalytic domains of ACE. ACE2 cleaves 1 amino acid from the carboxyl terminal to convert AngI to Ang(1-9) and AngII to Ang(1-7). AngII is the preferred substrate for ACE2 with 400-fold higher affinity than AngI. ACE2 may serve as a counterregulatory mechanism to oppose the effects of ACE. ACE2 regulates the levels of AngII and limits its effects by converting it to Ang(1-7), which binds to Mas receptors and elicits vasodilator and anti-proliferative responses. ACE2 is not inhibited by ACE inhibitors and has no effect on bradykinin. In animals, reduced expression of ACE2 is associated with hypertension, defects in cardiac contractility, and elevated levels of AngII.

ANGIOTENSIN PEPTIDES. AngI is rapidly converted to AngII. Angiotensin III (AngIII), also called Ang(2–8), can be formed either by the action of aminopeptidase on AngII or by the action of ACE on Ang(2-10). AngII and AngIII cause qualitatively similar effects. AngII and AngIII stimulate aldosterone secretion with equal potency; however, AngIII is only 25% and 10% as potent as AngII in elevating blood pressure and stimulating the adrenal medulla, respectively.

Ang(1-7) is formed by multiple pathways (*see* Figure 26–1). Ang(1-7) opposes many of the effects of AngII: It induces vasodilation, promotes NO production, potentiates the vasodilatory effects of bradykinin, and inhibits AngII-induced activation of ERK1/2; it has antiangiogenic, antiproliferative, and antithrombotic effects; and is cardioprotective in cardiac ischemia and heart failure. The effects of Ang(1-7) are mediated by a specific Mas receptor. ACE inhibitors increase tissue and plasma levels of Ang(1-7), both because AngI levels are increased and diverted away from AngII formation and because ACE contributes to the plasma clearance of Ang(1-7). AT_1 receptor blockade boosts the levels of AngII that is converted to Ang(1-7) by ACE2.

Angiotensin IV (AngIV), also called Ang(3-8), is formed from AngIII through the action of aminopeptidase M and has potent effects on memory and cognition. Central and peripheral actions of AngIV are mediated through specific AT_4 receptors identified as insulin-regulated aminopeptidases (IRAPs). AngIV binding to AT_4 receptors inhibits the catalytic activity of IRAPs and enables accumulation of various neuropeptides linked to memory potentiation. Other actions include renal vasodilation, natriuresis, neuronal differentiation, hypertrophy, inflammation, and extracellular matrix remodeling. Analogs of angiotensin IV are being developed for their therapeutic potential in cognition in Alzheimer disease or head injury.

LOCAL (TISSUE) RENIN–ANGIOTENSIN SYSTEMS. Many tissues—including the brain, pituitary, blood vessels, heart, kidney, and adrenal gland—express mRNAs for renin, angiotensinogen, and/or ACE, and various cells cultured from these tissues produce renin, angiotensinogen, ACE, and angiotensins I, II, and III. Thus, it appears that local RASs exist independently of the renal/hepatic-based system and may influence vascular, cardiac, and renal function and structure. Activation of (tissue) RAS and local AngII production require the binding of renin or prorenin to the specific (pro)renin receptor (PRR), located on cell surfaces.

The (Pro)Renin Receptor. The PRR is the functional cell surface receptor that binds prorenin and renin with high affinity (K_D ~6 and 20 nM, respectively) and specificity. Binding of (pro)renin to PRR enhances the catalytic activity of renin by 4- to 5-fold and induces non-proteolytic activation of prorenin (Figure 26–4). Bound, activated (pro)renin catalyzes the conversion of angiotensinogen to AngI, which can be converted to AngII by ACE located on the cell surface. AngII binds to AT_1 receptors and activates intracellular signaling events that regulate cell growth, collagen deposition, fibrosis, inflammation, and apoptosis.

The binding of (pro)renin to PRR also induces *AngII-independent* signaling events that include activation of ERK1/2, p38, tyrosine kinases, TGF-β gene expression, and plasminogen activator inhibitor type 1 (PAI-1). These signaling pathways are not blocked by ACE inhibitors or AT_1 receptor antagonists and are reported to

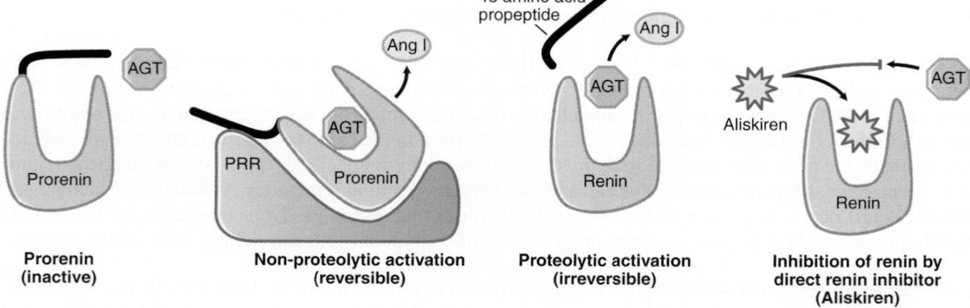

Figure 26–4 *Biological activation of prorenin and pharmacological inhibition of renin.* Prorenin is inactive; accessibility of angiotensinogen (AGT) to the catalytic site is blocked by the propeptide (black segment). The blocked catalytic site can be activated non-proteolytically by the binding of prorenin to the (pro)renin receptor (PRR) or by proteolytic removal of the propeptide. The competitive renin inhibitor, aliskiren, has a higher affinity (~0.1 μm) for the active site of renin than does AGT (~1 μm).

contribute to fibrosis, nephrosis, and organ damage. PRR is abundant in the heart, brain, eye, adrenals, placenta, adipose tissue, liver, and kidneys.

Prorenin is no longer considered the inactive precursor of renin, as it is capable of activating local RAS and AngII-independent events that may contribute to organ damage. Circulating plasma concentrations of prorenin are 10-fold higher than renin in healthy subjects but are elevated to 100-fold in diabetic patients and are associated with increased risk of nephropathy, renal fibrosis, and retinopathy. The interaction of prorenin with PRR has become a target for therapeutic interventions.

Prorenin and renin also bind to the mannose-6-phosphate receptor (M6P), an insulin-like growth factor II receptor that functions as a clearance receptor. Knockout of the PRR gene is lethal. In humans, mutations in the PRR gene are associated with mental retardation and epilepsy, suggesting an important role in cognition, brain development, and survival.

ALTERNATIVE PATHWAYS FOR ANGIOTENSIN BIOSYNTHESIS. Angiotensinogen may be converted to AngI or directly to AngII by cathepsin G and tonin. Other enzymes that convert AngI to AngII include cathepsin G, chymostatin-sensitive AngII-generating enzyme, and heart chymase.

ANGIOTENSIN RECEPTORS. AngII and AngIII bind to specific GPCRs designated AT_1 and AT_2. Most of the known biological effects of AngII are mediated by the AT_1 receptor. The AT_1 receptor gene contains a polymorphism (A-to-C transversion in position 1166) associated with hypertension, hypertrophic cardiomyopathy, and coronary artery vasoconstriction. Preeclampsia is associated with the development of agonistic auto-antibodies against the AT_1 receptor.

The functional role of the AT_2 receptor is less defined, but may counterbalance many of the effects of the AT_1 receptor by having antiproliferative, proapoptotic, vasodilatory, natriuretic, and antihypertensive effects. The AT_2 receptor is distributed widely in fetal tissues, but its distribution is more restricted in adults. Expression of AT_2 receptor is upregulated in cardiovascular diseases, including heart failure, cardiac fibrosis, and ischemic heart disease; however, the significance of increased AT_2 receptor expression is unclear.

The Mas receptor mediates the effects of Ang(1-7), which include vasodilation and antiproliferation. Deletion of the *Mas* gene in transgenic mice reveals cardiac dysfunction.

The AT_4 receptor mediates the effects of AngIV. This receptor is a single transmembrane protein (1025 amino acids) that co-localizes with the glucose transporter GLUT4. AT_4 receptors are detectable in a number of tissues, such as heart, vasculature, adrenal cortex, and brain regions processing sensory and motor functions.

ANGIOTENSIN RECEPTOR–EFFECTOR COUPLING. AT_1 receptors activate a large array of signal-transduction systems to produce effects that vary with cell type and that are a combination of primary and secondary responses. AT_1 receptors couple to several heterotrimeric G proteins, including G_q, $G_{12/13}$, and G_i. In most cell types, AT_1 receptors couple to G_q to activate the PLCβ–IP_3–Ca^{2+} pathway. Secondary to G_q activation, activation of PKC, PLA_2, and PLD and eicosanoid production, as well as activation of Ca^{2+}-dependent and MAP kinases and the Ca^{2+}–calmodulin–dependent activation of NOS may occur. Activation of G_i may occur and will reduce the activity of adenylyl cyclase, lowering cellular cyclic AMP content. The βγ subunits of G_i and activation of $G_{12/13}$ lead to activation of tyrosine kinases and small G proteins such as Rho. Ultimately, the JAK/STAT pathway may be activated and a variety of transcriptional regulatory factors induced. AT_1 receptors also stimulate the activity of a membrane-bound NADH/NADPH oxidase that generates reactive oxygen species (ROS). ROS may contribute to biochemical effects (activation of MAP kinase, tyrosine kinase, and phosphatases; inactivation of NO; and expression of monocyte chemoattractant protein-1) and physiological effects (acute effects on renal function, chronic effects on blood pressure, and vascular hypertrophy and inflammation). The presence of other receptors may alter the response to AT_1 receptor activation. For example, AT_1 receptors heterodimerize with bradykinin B_2 receptors, a process that enhances AngII sensitivity in preeclampsia.

Signaling from AT_2 receptors is mediated by G protein-dependent and independent pathways. Stimulation of AT_2 receptor activates phosphoprotein phosphatases, K^+ channels, synthesis of NO and cyclic GMP, bradykinin production, and inhibition of Ca^{2+} channel functions. AT_2 receptors may possess constitutive activity: overexpression of AT_2 receptors can induce NO production in vascular smooth muscle cells and hypertrophy in cardiac myocytes through an intrinsic activity of the AT_2 receptor independent of AngII binding.

FUNCTIONS AND EFFECTS OF THE RENIN–ANGIOTENSIN SYSTEM

AngII increases total peripheral resistance (TPR) and alters renal function and cardiovascular structure through direct and indirect mechanisms (Figure 26–5).

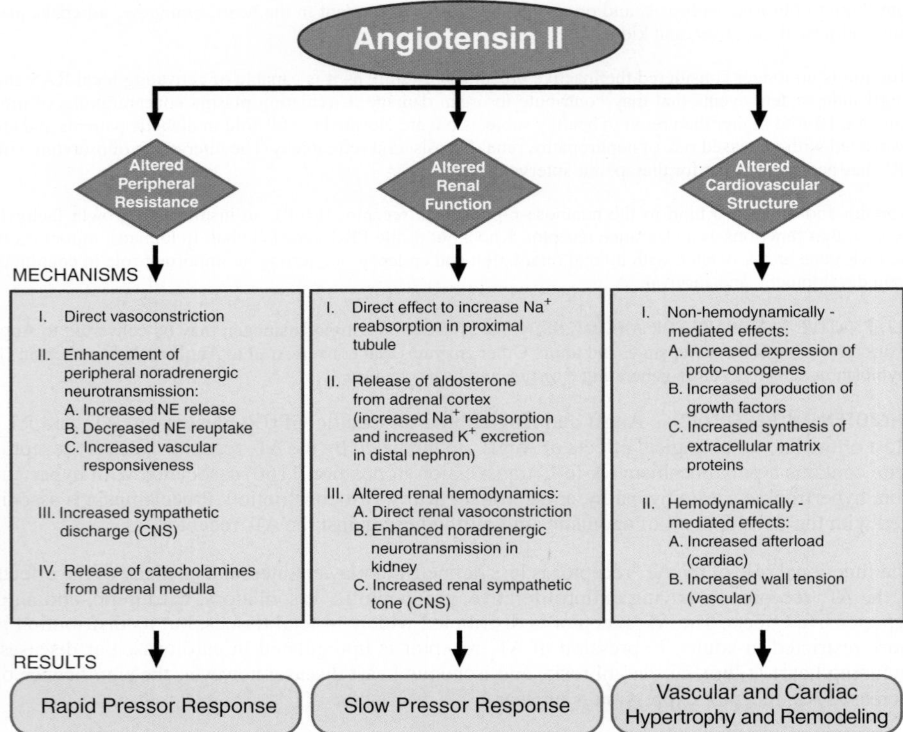

Figure 26–5 *Major effects of AngII.* NE, norepinephrine.

EFFECTS ON TPR

Direct Vasoconstriction. AngII constricts precapillary arterioles and, to a lesser extent, postcapillary venules by activating AT_1 receptors located on vascular smooth muscle cells and stimulating the G_q–PLC–IP_3–Ca^{2+} pathway. AngII has differential effects on vascular beds. Direct vasoconstriction is strongest in the kidneys (*see* Figure 26–5) and the splanchnic vascular bed. AngII-induced vasoconstriction is much less in vessels of the brain, lungs, and skeletal muscle. Nevertheless, high circulating concentrations of AngII may decrease cerebral and coronary blood flow.

Enhancement of Peripheral Noradrenergic Neurotransmission. AngII augments NE release from sympathetic nerve terminals by inhibiting the reuptake of NE into nerve terminals and by enhancing the vascular response to NE.

Effects on the CNS. AngII increases sympathetic tone. Small amounts of AngII infused into the vertebral arteries cause an increase in arterial blood pressure. This response reflects effects of the hormone on circumventricular nuclei that are not protected by a blood-brain barrier. Circulating AngII also attenuates baroreceptor-mediated reductions in sympathetic discharge, thereby increasing arterial pressure. The CNS is affected both by blood-borne AngII and by AngII formed within the brain. The brain contains all components of the RAS. AngII also causes a centrally mediated dipsogenic (thirst) effect and enhances the release of vasopressin from the neurohypophysis.

Release of Catecholamines from the Adrenal Medulla. AngII stimulates the release of catecholamines from the adrenal medulla by depolarizing chromaffin cells.

EFFECTS ON RENAL FUNCTION

Alteration of Renal Function. AngII has pronounced effects on renal function, reducing the urinary excretion of Na^+ and water while increasing the excretion of K^+. The overall effect of AngII on the kidneys is to shift the renal pressure–natriuresis curve to the right (Figure 26–6).

Direct Effects of Angiotensin II on Na^+ Reabsorption in the Renal Tubules. Very low concentrations of AngII stimulate Na^+/H^+ exchange in the proximal tubule—an effect that increases Na^+, Cl^-, and bicarbonate reabsorption. Approximately 20-30% of the bicarbonate handled by the nephron may be affected by this mechanism. AngII

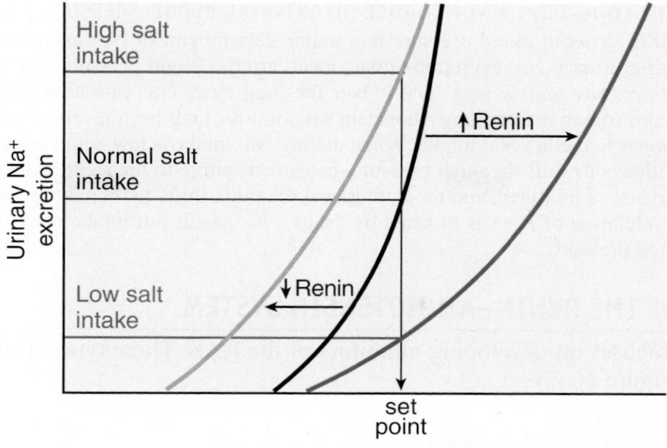

Figure 26–6 *Pressure-natriuresis curve: effects of Na⁺ intake on renin release (AngII formation) and arterial blood pressure.* Inhibition of the renin-angiotensin system will cause a large drop in blood pressure in Na^+-depleted individuals. (Modified with permission from Jackson EK, Branch RA, et al: Physiological functions of the renal prostaglandin, renin, and kallikrein systems, in Seldin DW, Giebisch GH, eds: *The Kidney: Physiology and Pathophysiology*, Vol 1. Philadelphia: Lippincott Williams & Wilkins, 1985, p 624.)

also increases the expression of the Na^+–glucose symporter in the proximal tubule. Paradoxically, at high concentrations, AngII may inhibit Na^+ transport in the proximal tubule. AngII also directly stimulates the Na^+–K^+–$2Cl^-$ symporter in the thick ascending limb.

Release of Aldosterone from the Adrenal Cortex. AngII stimulates the zona glomerulosa of the adrenal cortex to increase the synthesis and secretion of aldosterone, and augments responses to other stimuli (e.g., adrenocorticotropic hormone, K^+). Increased output of aldosterone is elicited by concentrations of AngII that have little or no acute effect on blood pressure. Aldosterone acts on the distal and collecting tubules to cause retention of Na^+ and excretion of K^+ and H^+. The stimulant effect of AngII on aldosterone synthesis and release is enhanced under conditions of hyponatremia or hyperkalemia and is reduced when concentrations of Na^+ and K^+ in plasma are altered in the opposite directions.

Altered Renal Hemodynamics. AngII reduces renal blood flow and renal excretory function by directly constricting the renal vascular smooth muscle, by enhancing renal sympathetic tone (a CNS effect), and by facilitating renal adrenergic transmission (an intrarenal effect). AngII-induced vasoconstriction of preglomerular microvessels is enhanced by endogenous adenosine owing to signal-transduction systems activated by AT_1 and the adenosine A_1 receptor. AngII influences glomerular filtration rate (GFR) by means of several mechanisms:

- Constriction of the afferent arterioles, which reduces intraglomerular pressure and tends to reduce GFR
- Contraction of mesangial cells, which decreases the capillary surface area within the glomerulus available for filtration and also tends to decrease GFR
- Constriction of efferent arterioles, which increases intraglomerular pressure and tends to increase GFR

Normally, GFR is slightly reduced by AngII; however, during renal artery hypotension, the effects of AngII on the efferent arteriole predominate so that AngII increases GFR. Thus, blockade of the RAS may cause acute renal failure in patients with bilateral renal artery stenosis or in patients with unilateral stenosis who have only a single kidney.

EFFECTS ON CARDIOVASCULAR STRUCTURE. Pathological alterations involving cardiac hypertrophy and remodeling increase morbidity and mortality. The cells involved include vascular smooth muscle cells, cardiac myocytes, and fibroblasts. AngII stimulates the migration, proliferation, and hypertrophy of vascular smooth muscle cells; causes hypertrophy of cardiac myocytes; and increases extracellular matrix production by cardiac fibroblasts. AngII alters extracellular matrix formation and degradation indirectly by increasing aldosterone. In addition to the direct cellular effects of AngII on cardiovascular structure, changes in cardiac preload (volume expansion owing to Na^+ retention) and afterload (increased arterial blood pressure) probably contribute to cardiac hypertrophy and remodeling. Arterial hypertension also contributes to hypertrophy and remodeling of blood vessels.

ROLE OF THE RAS IN LONG-TERM MAINTENANCE OF ARTERIAL BLOOD PRESSURE DESPITE EXTREMES IN DIETARY NA⁺ INTAKE. Arterial blood pressure is a major determinant of Na^+ excretion. This is illustrated graphically by plotting urinary Na^+ excretion versus mean arterial blood pressure (*see* Figure 26–6), a plot known as the *renal pressure–natriuresis curve*. Over the long term, Na^+ excretion must equal Na^+ intake. The RAS plays a major role in maintaining a constant set point for long-term levels of arterial blood pressure despite extreme changes in dietary Na^+ intake. When dietary Na^+ intake is low, renin release is stimulated, and AngII acts on the kidneys to shift the renal pressure–natriuresis curve to the right. Conversely, when dietary Na^+ is high, renin release is inhibited, and the withdrawal of AngII shifts the renal pressure–natriuresis curve to the left. When modulation of RAS is blocked by drugs, changes in salt intake markedly affect long-term levels of arterial blood pressure.

INHIBITORS OF THE RENIN–ANGIOTENSIN SYSTEM

Clinical interest focuses on developing inhibitors of the RAS. Three types of inhibitors are used therapeutically (Figure 26–7):

- ACE inhibitors (ACEIs)
- Angiotensin receptor blockers (ARBs)
- Direct renin inhibitors (DRIs)

While all of these classes of agents will reduce the actions of AngII and lower blood pressure, they have different effects on the individual components of the RAS (Table 26–1).

ANGIOTENSIN-CONVERTING ENZYME INHIBITORS

PHARMACOLOGICAL EFFECTS. The effect of ACE inhibitors on the RAS is to inhibit the conversion of AngI to the active AngII. Inhibition of AngII production will lower blood pressure and enhance natriuresis. ACE is an enzyme with many substrates; thus, there are other consequences of its inhibition, including inhibition of bradykinin degradation. ACE inhibitors increase by 5-fold the circulating levels of the natural stem cell regulator *N*-acetyl-seryl-aspartyl-lysyl-proline, which may contribute to the cardioprotective effects of ACE inhibitors. In addition, ACE inhibitors will increase renin release and the rate of formation of AngI by interfering with both short- and long-loop negative feedbacks on renin release (*see* Figure 26–2). Accumulating AngI is directed down alternative metabolic routes that increase production of vasodilator peptides such as Ang(1-7).

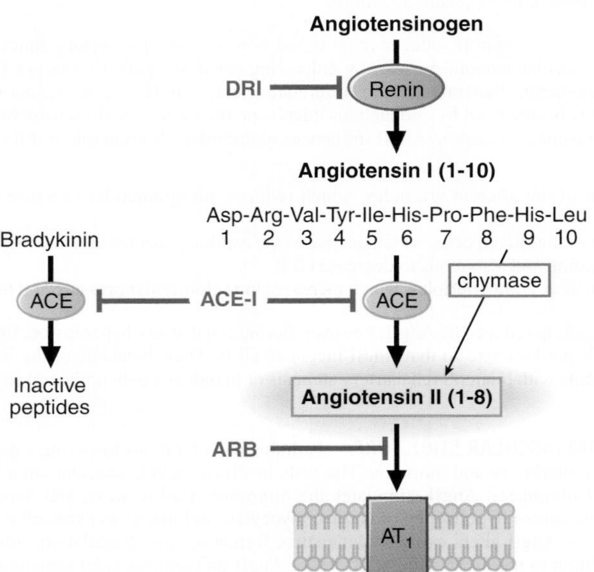

Figure 26–7 *Inhibitors of the RAS.* ACE-I, angiotensin-converting enzyme inhibitor; ARB, angiotensin receptor blocker; DRI, direct renin inhibitor.

Clinical Pharmacology. ACE inhibitors can be classified into 3 broad groups based on chemical structure: (1) sulfhydryl-containing ACE inhibitors structurally related to captopril; (2) dicarboxyl-containing ACE inhibitors structurally related to enalapril (e.g., lisinopril, benazepril, quinapril, moexipril, ramipril, trandolapril, perindopril); and (3) phosphorus-containing ACE inhibitors structurally related to fosinopril. Many ACE inhibitors are ester-containing prodrugs that are 100-1000 times less potent but have a better oral bioavailability than the active molecules. With the exceptions of fosinopril and spirapril (which display balanced elimination by the liver and kidneys), ACE inhibitors are cleared predominantly by the kidneys. Impaired renal function significantly diminishes the plasma clearance of most ACE inhibitors, and dosages of these drugs should be reduced in patients with renal impairment.

All ACE inhibitors block the conversion of AngI to AngII and have similar therapeutic indications, adverse-effect profiles, and contraindications. Because hypertension usually requires lifelong treatment, quality-of-life issues are an important consideration in comparing antihypertensive drugs. ACE inhibitors differ markedly in tissue distribution, and it is possible that this difference could be exploited to inhibit some local (tissue) RAS while leaving others relatively intact.

Captopril (CAPOTEN, others). Captopril is a potent ACE inhibitor with a K_i of 1.7 nM. Given orally, captopril is absorbed rapidly and has a bioavailability ~75%. Bioavailability is reduced by 25-30% with food. Peak concentrations in plasma occur within an hour, and the drug is cleared rapidly with a $t_{1/2}$ ~2 h. Most of the drug is eliminated in urine, 40-50% as captopril and the rest as captopril disulfide dimers and captopril–cysteine disulfide. The oral dose of captopril ranges from 6.25-150 mg 2-3 times daily, with 6.25 mg 3 times daily or 25 mg twice daily being appropriate for the initiation of therapy for heart failure or hypertension, respectively.

Enalapril (VASOTEC, others). Enalapril maleate is a prodrug that is hydrolyzed by esterases in the liver to enalaprilat. Enalaprilat is a potent inhibitor of ACE with a K_i of 0.2 nM. Enalapril is absorbed rapidly and has an oral bioavailability of ~60% (not reduced by food). Although peak concentrations of enalapril in plasma occur within an hour, enalaprilat concentrations peak only after 3-4 h. Enalapril has a $t_{1/2}$ ~1.3 h, but enalaprilat, because of tight binding to ACE, has a plasma $t_{1/2}$ of ~11 h. Elimination is by the kidneys as either intact enalapril or enalaprilat. The oral dosage of enalapril ranges from 2.5-40 mg daily, with 2.5 and 5 mg daily being appropriate for the initiation of therapy for heart failure and hypertension, respectively.

Enalaprilat (VASOTEC INJECTION, others). Enalaprilat is not absorbed orally but is available for intravenous administration when oral therapy is not appropriate. For hypertensive patients, the dosage is 0.625 to 1.25 mg given intravenously over 5 min. This dosage may be repeated every 6 h.

Lisinopril (PRINIVIL, ZESTRIL, others). Lisinopril is the lysine analog of enalaprilat; unlike enalapril, lisinopril itself is active. Lisinopril is absorbed slowly, and incompletely (~30%) after oral administration (not reduced by food); peak concentrations in plasma are achieved in ~7 h. It is cleared as the intact compound by the kidney, and its $t_{1/2}$ in plasma is ~12 h. Lisinopril does not accumulate in tissues. The oral dosage of lisinopril ranges from 5–40 mg daily (single or divided dose), with 5 and 10 mg daily being appropriate for the initiation of therapy for heart failure and hypertension, respectively. A daily dose of 2.5 mg and close medical supervision is recommended for patients with heart failure who are hyponatremic or have renal impairment.

Benazepril (LOTENSIN, others). Hepatic esterases transforms benazepril, a prodrug, into benazeprilat. Benazepril is absorbed rapidly but incompletely (37%) after oral administration (only slightly reduced by food). Benazepril is metabolized to benazeprilat and to the glucuronide conjugates of benazepril and benazeprilat, which are excreted into both the urine and bile; peak concentrations of benazepril and benazeprilat in plasma are achieved in 0.5-1 h and 1-2 h, respectively. Benazeprilat has a plasma $t_{1/2}$ of 10-11 h. With the exception of the lungs, benazeprilat does not accumulate in tissues. The oral dosage of benazepril ranges from 5-80 mg daily (single or divided dose).

Fosinopril (MONOPRIL, others). Cleavage of the ester moiety by hepatic esterases transforms fosinopril into fosinoprilat. Fosinopril is absorbed slowly and incompletely (36%) after oral administration (rate but not extent reduced by food). Fosinopril is largely metabolized to fosinoprilat (75%) and to the glucuronide conjugate of fosinoprilat. These are excreted in both the urine and bile; peak concentrations of fosinoprilat in plasma are achieved in ~3 h. Fosinoprilat has an effective plasma $t_{1/2}$ of ~11.5 h; its clearance is not significantly altered by renal impairment. The oral dosage of fosinopril ranges from 10-80 mg daily (single or divided dose). The initial dose is reduced to 5 mg daily in patients with Na^+ or water depletion or renal failure.

Trandolapril (MAVIK, others). An oral dose of trandolapril is absorbed without reduction by food and produces plasma levels of trandolapril (10% bioavailability) and trandolaprilat (70% bioavailability). Trandolaprilat is ~8 times more potent than trandolapril as an ACE inhibitor. Trandolapril is metabolized to trandolaprilat and to inactive metabolites that are recovered in the urine (33%, mostly trandolaprilat) and feces (66%). Trandolaprilat displays biphasic elimination kinetics with an initial $t_{1/2}$ of ~10 h (the major component of elimination), followed by a more prolonged $t_{1/2}$ (owing to slow dissociation of trandolaprilat from tissue ACE).

Plasma clearance of trandolaprilat is reduced by both renal and hepatic insufficiency. The oral dosage ranges from 1 to 8 mg daily (single or divided dose). The initial dose is 0.5 mg in patients who are taking a diuretic or who have renal impairment, and 2 mg for African Americans.

Quinapril (ACCUPRIL, others). Cleavage of the ester moiety by hepatic esterases transforms quinapril, a prodrug, into quinaprilat. Quinapril is absorbed rapidly (peak concentrations are achieved in 1 h), and the rate, but not extent, of oral absorption (60%) may be reduced by food (delayed peak). Quinaprilat and other minor metabolites of quinapril are excreted in the urine (61%) and feces (37%). Conversion of quinapril to quinaprilat is reduced in patients with diminished liver function. The initial $t_{1/2}$ of quinaprilat is ~2 h; a prolonged terminal $t_{1/2}$ ≈25 h may be due to high-affinity binding of the drug to tissue ACE. The oral dosage range of quinapril is 5-80 mg daily.

Ramipril (ALTACE, others). Cleavage of the ester moiety by hepatic esterases transforms ramipril into ramiprilat, an ACE inhibitor that in vitro is about as potent as benazeprilat and quinaprilat. Ramipril is absorbed rapidly (peak concentrations are achieved in 1 h), and the rate but not extent of its oral absorption (50-60%) is reduced by food. Ramipril is metabolized to ramiprilat and to inactive metabolites that are excreted predominantly by the kidneys. Ramiprilat displays triphasic elimination kinetics with half-lives of 2-4 h, 9-18 h, and >50 h. This triphasic elimination is due to extensive distribution to all tissues (initial $t_{1/2}$), clearance of free ramiprilat from plasma (intermediate $t_{1/2}$), and dissociation of ramiprilat from tissue ACE (long terminal $t_{1/2}$). The oral dosage range of ramipril is 1.25-20 mg daily (single or divided dose).

Moexipril (UNIVASC, others). Moexipril's antihypertensive activity is due to its de-esterified metabolite, moexiprilat. Moexipril is absorbed incompletely, with bioavailability as moexiprilat of ~13%. Bioavailability is markedly decreased by food. The elimination $t_{1/2}$ varies between 2 and 12 h. The recommended dosage range is 7.5-30 mg daily (single or divided doses). The dosage range is halved in patients who are taking diuretics or who have renal impairment.

Perindopril (ACEON). Perindopril erbumine is a prodrug, and 30-50% of systemically available perindopril is transformed to perindoprilat by hepatic esterases. Although the oral bioavailability of perindopril (75%) is not affected by food, the bioavailability of perindoprilat is reduced by ~35%. Perindopril is metabolized to perindoprilat and to inactive metabolites that are excreted predominantly by the kidneys. Perindoprilat displays biphasic elimination kinetics with half-lives of 3-10 h (the major component of elimination) and 30-120 h (owing to slow dissociation of perindoprilat from tissue ACE). The oral dosage range is 2-16 mg daily (single or divided dose).

THERAPEUTIC USES OF ACE INHIBITORS. Drugs that interfere with RAS play a prominent role in the treatment of cardiovascular disease, the major cause of mortality in modern Western societies.

ACE Inhibitors in Hypertension. Inhibition of ACE lowers systemic vascular resistance and mean, diastolic, and systolic blood pressures in various hypertensive states except when high blood pressure is due to primary aldosteronism (*see* Chapter 27). The initial change in blood pressure tends to be positively correlated with plasma renin activity (PRA) and AngII plasma levels prior to treatment. The long-term decrease in systemic blood pressure observed in hypertensive individuals treated with ACE inhibitors is accompanied by a leftward shift in the renal pressure–natriuresis curve (*see* Figure 26–6) and a reduction in total peripheral resistance in which there is variable participation by different vascular beds. The kidney is a notable exception: because the renal vessels are extremely sensitive to the vasoconstrictor actions of AngII, ACE inhibitors increase renal blood flow via vasodilation of the afferent and efferent arterioles. Increased renal blood flow occurs without an increase in GFR; thus, the filtration fraction is reduced.

ACE inhibitors cause systemic arteriolar dilation and increase the compliance of large arteries, which contributes to a reduction of systolic pressure. Cardiac function in patients with uncomplicated hypertension generally is little changed, although stroke volume and cardiac output may increase slightly with sustained treatment. Baroreceptor function and cardiovascular reflexes are not compromised, and responses to postural changes and exercise are little impaired. Even when a substantial lowering of blood pressure is achieved, heart rate and concentrations of catecholamines in plasma generally increase only slightly, if at all. This perhaps reflects an alteration of baroreceptor function with increased arterial compliance and the loss of the normal tonic influence of AngII on the sympathetic nervous system.

Aldosterone secretion is reduced, but not seriously impaired, by ACE inhibitors. Aldosterone secretion is maintained at adequate levels by other steroidogenic stimuli, such as ACTH and K^+. Excessive retention of K^+ is encountered in patients taking supplemental K^+, in patients with renal impairment, or in patients taking other medications that reduce K^+ excretion.

ACE inhibitors alone normalize blood pressure in ~50% of patients with mild to moderate hypertension. Ninety percent of patients with mild to moderate hypertension will be controlled by the combination of an ACE inhibitor and either a Ca^{2+} channel blocker, a β adrenergic receptor blocker, or a diuretic. Several ACE inhibitors are marketed in fixed-dose combinations with a thiazide diuretic or Ca^{2+} channel blocker for the management of hypertension.

ACE Inhibitors in Left Ventricular Systolic Dysfunction. Unless contraindicated, ACE inhibitors should be given to patients with impaired left ventricular systolic function whether or not they have symptoms of overt heart failure (*see* Chapter 28). Inhibition of ACE in patients with systolic dysfunction prevents or delays the progression of heart failure, decreases the incidence of sudden death and myocardial infarction, decreases hospitalization, and improves quality of life. Inhibition of ACE commonly reduces afterload and systolic wall stress, and both cardiac output and cardiac index increase. In systolic dysfunction, AngII decreases arterial compliance, and this is reversed by ACE inhibition. Heart rate generally is reduced. Systemic blood pressure falls, sometimes steeply at the outset, but tends to return toward initial levels. Renovascular resistance falls sharply, and renal blood flow increases. Natriuresis occurs as a result of the improved renal hemodynamics, the reduced stimulus to the secretion of aldosterone by AngII, and the diminished direct effects of AngII on the kidney. The excess volume of body fluids contracts, which reduces venous return to the right side of the heart. A further reduction results from venodilation and an increased capacity of the venous bed.

The response to ACE inhibitors also involves reductions of pulmonary arterial pressure, pulmonary capillary wedge pressure, and left atrial and left ventricular filling volumes and pressures. The better hemodynamic performance results in increased exercise tolerance and suppression of the sympathetic nervous system. Cerebral and coronary blood flows usually are well maintained, even when systemic blood pressure is reduced. In heart failure, ACE inhibitors reduce ventricular dilation and tend to restore the heart to its normal elliptical shape. ACE inhibitors may reverse ventricular remodeling via changes in preload/afterload, by preventing the growth effects of AngII on myocytes, and by attenuating cardiac fibrosis induced by AngII and aldosterone.

ACE Inhibitors in Acute Myocardial Infarction. The beneficial effects of ACE inhibitors in acute myocardial infarction are particularly large in hypertensive and diabetic patients (*see* Chapter 27). Unless contraindicated (e.g., cardiogenic shock or severe hypotension), ACE inhibitors should be started immediately during the acute phase of myocardial infarction and can be administered along with thrombolytics, aspirin, and β adrenergic receptor antagonists. In high-risk patients (e.g., large infarct, systolic ventricular dysfunction), ACE inhibition should be continued long term.

ACE Inhibitors in Patients Who Are at High Risk of Cardiovascular Events. Patients at high risk of cardiovascular events benefit considerably from treatment with ACE inhibitors. ACE inhibition significantly decreases the rates of myocardial infarction, stroke, and death. In patients with coronary artery disease but without heart failure, ACE inhibition reduces cardiovascular disease death and myocardial infarction.

ACE Inhibitors in Diabetes Mellitus and Renal Failure. Diabetes mellitus is the leading cause of renal disease. In patients with type 1 diabetes mellitus and diabetic nephropathy, captopril prevents or delays the progression of renal disease. Renoprotection in type 1 diabetes, as defined by changes in albumin excretion, also is observed with lisinopril. The renoprotective effects of ACE inhibitors in type 1 diabetes are in part independent of blood pressure reduction. In addition, ACE inhibitors may decrease retinopathy progression in type 1 diabetics and attenuate the progression of renal insufficiency in patients with a variety of non-diabetic nephropathies.

Several mechanisms participate in the renal protection afforded by ACE inhibitors. Increased glomerular capillary pressure induces glomerular injury, and ACE inhibitors reduce this parameter both by decreasing arterial blood pressure and by dilating renal efferent arterioles. ACE inhibitors increase the permeability selectivity of the filtering membrane, thereby diminishing exposure of the mesangium to peptide and protein factors that may stimulate mesangial cell proliferation and matrix production, 2 processes that contribute to expansion of the mesangium in diabetic nephropathy. Because AngII is a growth factor, reductions in the intrarenal levels of AngII may further attenuate mesangial cell growth and matrix production.

ADVERSE EFFECTS OF ACE INHIBITORS

In general, ACE inhibitors are well tolerated. The drugs do not alter plasma concentrations of uric acid or Ca^{2+} and may improve insulin sensitivity in patients with insulin resistance and decrease cholesterol and lipoprotein (a) levels in proteinuric renal disease.

Hypotension. A steep fall in blood pressure may occur following the first dose of an ACE inhibitor in patients with elevated PRA. Care should be exercised in patients who are salt depleted, are on multiple antihypertensive drugs, or who have congestive heart failure.

Cough. In 5-20% of patients, ACE inhibitors induce a bothersome, dry cough mediated by the accumulation in the lungs of bradykinin, substance P, and/or prostaglandins. Thromboxane antagonism, aspirin, and iron supplementation reduce cough induced by ACE inhibitors. ACE dose reduction or switching to an ARB is sometimes effective. Once ACE inhibitors are stopped, the cough disappears, usually within 4 days.

Hyperkalemia. ACE inhibitors may cause hyperkalemia in patients with renal insufficiency or diabetes or in patients taking K^+-sparing diuretics, K^+ supplements, β receptor blockers, or NSAIDs.

Acute Renal Failure. Inhibition of ACE can induce acute renal insufficiency in patients with bilateral renal artery stenosis, stenosis of the artery to a single remaining kidney, heart failure, or volume depletion owing to diarrhea or diuretics.

Fetopathic Potential. The fetopathic effects may be due in part to fetal hypotension. Once pregnancy is diagnosed, use of ACE inhibitors must be discontinued immediately.

Skin Rash. ACE inhibitors occasionally cause a maculopapular rash that may itch, but that may resolve spontaneously or with antihistamines.

Angioedema. In 0.1-0.5% of patients, ACE inhibitors induce a rapid swelling in the nose, throat, mouth, glottis, larynx, lips, and/or tongue. Once ACE inhibitors are stopped, angioedema disappears within hours; meanwhile, the patient's airway should be protected, and if necessary, epinephrine, an antihistamine, and/or a glucocorticoid should be administered. Although rare, angioedema of the intestine (visceral angioedema) characterized by emesis, watery diarrhea, and abdominal pain also has been reported.

Other Side Effects. Extremely rare but reversible side effects include *dysgeusia* (an alteration in or loss of taste), *neutropenia* (symptoms include sore throat and fever), *glycosuria* (spillage of glucose into the urine in the absence of hyperglycemia), and *hepatotoxicity*.

Drug Interactions. Antacids may reduce the bioavailability of ACE inhibitors; capsaicin may worsen ACE inhibitor–induced cough; NSAIDs, including aspirin, may reduce the antihypertensive response to ACE inhibitors; and K^+-sparing diuretics and K^+ supplements may exacerbate ACE inhibitor–induced hyperkalemia. ACE inhibitors may increase plasma levels of digoxin and lithium and may increase hypersensitivity reactions to allopurinol.

NON-PEPTIDE ANGIOTENSIN II RECEPTOR ANTAGONISTS

PHARMACOLOGICAL EFFECTS. The AngII receptor blockers bind to the AT_1 receptor with high affinity and show >10,000-fold selectivity for the AT_1 receptor over the AT_2 receptor. Although binding of ARBs to the AT_1 receptor is competitive, the inhibition by ARBs of biological responses to AngII often is insurmountable (the maximal response to AngII cannot be restored in the presence of the ARB regardless of the concentration of AngII added to the experimental preparation).

ARBs inhibit most of the biological effects of AngII which include AngII–induced: (1) contraction of vascular smooth muscle, (2) rapid pressor responses, (3) slow pressor responses, (4) thirst, (5) vasopressin release, (6) aldosterone secretion, (7) release of adrenal catecholamines, (8) enhancement of noradrenergic neurotransmission, (9) increases in sympathetic tone, (10) changes in renal function, and (11) cellular hypertrophy and hyperplasia.

Do ARBs have therapeutic efficacy equivalent to that of ACE inhibitors? Although both classes of drugs block the RAS, they differ in several important aspects:

- *ARBs reduce activation of AT_1 receptors more effectively than do ACE inhibitors.* ACE inhibitors do not inhibit alternative non-ACE AngII-generating pathways. ARBs block the actions of AngII via the AT_1 receptor regardless of the biochemical pathway leading to AngII formation.
- *ARBs permit activation of AT_2 receptors.* Both ACE inhibitors and ARBs stimulate renin release; however, with ARBs, this translates into a several-fold increase in circulating levels of AngII. Because ARBs block AT_1 receptors, this increased level of AngII is available to activate AT_2 receptors.
- *ACE inhibitors may increase Ang(1-7) levels more than do ARBs.* ACE is involved in the clearance of Ang(1-7), so inhibition of ACE may increase Ang(1-7) levels more so than do ARBs.
- *ACE inhibitors increase the levels of a number of ACE substrates, including bradykinin and Ac-SDKP.*

Whether the pharmacological differences between ARBs and ACE inhibitors result in significant differences in therapeutic outcomes is an open question.

CLINICAL PHARMACOLOGY

Oral bioavailability of ARBs generally is modest (<50%, except for irbesartan, 70%), and protein binding is high (>90%).

Candesartan Cilexetil (ATACAND). Candesartan cilexetil is an inactive ester prodrug that is completely hydrolyzed to the active form, candesartan, during absorption from the GI tract. Plasma $t_{1/2}$ is ~9 h. Plasma clearance of candesartan is due to renal elimination (33%) and biliary excretion (67%). The plasma clearance of candesartan is affected by renal insufficiency but not by mild-to-moderate hepatic insufficiency. Candesartan cilexetil should be administered orally once or twice daily for a total daily dose of 4-32 mg.

Eprosartan (TEVETEN). Peak plasma levels are obtained 1-2 h after oral administration, and the plasma $t_{1/2}$ is 5-9 h. Eprosartan is metabolized in part to the glucuronide conjugate. Clearance is by renal elimination and biliary excretion. The plasma clearance of eprosartan is affected by both renal insufficiency and hepatic insufficiency. The recommended dosage of eprosartan is 400-800 mg/day in 1 or 2 doses.

Irbesartan (AVAPRO). The plasma $t_{1/2}$ is 11-15 h. Irbesartan is metabolized in part to the glucuronide conjugate; the parent compound and its glucuronide conjugate are cleared by renal elimination (20%) and biliary excretion (80%). The plasma clearance of irbesartan is unaffected by either renal or mild-to-moderate hepatic insufficiency. The oral dosage of irbesartan is 150-300 mg once daily.

Losartan (COZAAR). Approximately 14% of an oral dose of losartan is converted by CYP2C9 and CYP3A4 to the 5-carboxylic acid metabolite EXP 3174, which is more potent than losartan as an AT_1 receptor antagonist. Plasma half-lives of losartan and EXP 3174 are 2.5 and 6-9 h, respectively. The plasma clearances of losartan and EXP 3174 are due to renal clearance and hepatic clearance (metabolism and biliary excretion) and are affected by hepatic but not renal insufficiency. Losartan should be administered orally once or twice daily for a total daily dose of 25-00 mg. Losartan is a competitive antagonist of the thromboxane A_2 receptor and attenuates platelet aggregation. Also, EXP 3179, a metabolite of losartan without angiotensin receptor effects, reduces COX-2 mRNA upregulation and COX-dependent prostaglandin generation.

Olmesartan Medoxomil (BENICAR). Olmesartan medoxomil is an inactive ester prodrug that is completely hydrolyzed to the active form, olmesartan, during absorption from the gastrointestinal tract. The plasma $t_{1/2}$ is 10-15 h. Plasma clearance of olmesartan is due to both renal elimination and biliary excretion. Although renal impairment and hepatic disease decrease the plasma clearance of olmesartan, no dose adjustment is required in patients with mild-to-moderate renal or hepatic impairment. The oral dosage of olmesartan medoxomil is 20-40 mg once daily.

Telmisartan (MICARDIS). The plasma $t_{1/2}$ is ~24 h. Telmisartan is cleared from the circulation mainly by biliary secretion of intact drug. The plasma clearance of telmisartan is affected by hepatic but not renal insufficiency. The recommended oral dosage of telmisartan is 40-80 mg once daily.

Valsartan (DIOVAN). The plasma $t_{1/2}$ is ~9 h. Food markedly decreases absorption. Valsartan is cleared from the circulation by the liver (~70% of total clearance). The plasma clearance of valsartan is affected by hepatic but not renal insufficiency. The oral dosage of valsartan is 80-320 mg once daily.

Azilsartan Medoxomil (EDARBI) is a prodrug that is hydrolyzed in the GI tract to the active drug azilsartan. The drug is available in 40 mg and 80 mg once-daily doses. The bioavailability of azilsartan is ~60% and is not affected by food. The elimination $t_{1/2}$ is ~11 h. Azilsartan is metabolized mostly by CYP2C9 into inactive metabolites. Elimination of the drug is 55% in feces and 42% in urine. No dose adjustments are necessary for elderly patients or patients with renal impairment or mild to moderate hepatic impairment. The recommended dose is 80 mg once a day. Fixed–doses of azilsartan medoxomil with the diuretic chlorthalidone (EDARBYCLOR) are available as 40/12.5 mg and 40/25 mg once-daily single tablets.

Therapeutic Uses of AngII Receptor Antagonists. All ARBs are approved for the treatment of hypertension. In addition, irbesartan and losartan are approved for diabetic nephropathy, losartan is approved for stroke prophylaxis, and valsartan is approved for heart failure and to reduce cardiovascular mortality in clinically stable patients with left ventricular failure or left ventricular dysfunction following myocardial infarction. The efficacy of ARBs in lowering blood pressure is comparable with that of ACE inhibitors and other established antihypertensive drugs, with a favorable adverse-effect profile. ARBs also are available as fixed-dose combinations with hydrochlorothiazide or amlodipine (*see* Chapters 27 and 28).

Current recommendations are to use ACE inhibitors as first-line agents for the treatment of heart failure and to reserve ARBs for treatment of heart failure in patients who cannot tolerate or have an unsatisfactory response to ACE inhibitors. There is conflicting evidence regarding the advisability of combining an ARB and an ACE inhibitor in heart failure patients.

ARBs are renoprotective in type 2 diabetes mellitus, in part via blood pressure–independent mechanisms. Many experts now consider them the drugs of choice for renoprotection in diabetic patients.

Adverse Effects. ARBs are well tolerated. The incidence of angioedema and cough with ARBs is less than that with ACE inhibitors. ARBs have teratogenic potential and should be discontinued in pregnancy. In patients whose arterial blood pressure or renal function is highly dependent on the RAS (e.g., renal artery stenosis), ARBs can cause hypotension, oliguria, progressive azotemia, or acute renal failure. ARBs may cause hyperkalemia in patients with renal disease or in patients taking K^+ supplements or K^+-sparing diuretics. There are rare reports of anaphylaxis, abnormal hepatic function, hepatitis, neutropenia, leukopenia, agranulocytosis, pruritus, urticaria, hyponatremia, alopecia, and vasculitis, including Henoch-Schönlein purpura.

DIRECT RENIN INHIBITORS

DRIs are a new class of antihypertensive drugs that inhibit the RAS at the level of the rate limiting step, renin. Angiotensinogen is the only specific substrate for renin, and its conversion to AngI presents a rate-limiting step for the generation of angiotensin peptides. Aliskiren hemifumarate (TEKTURNA) is the only DRI approved for clinical use.

Pharmacological Effects. Aliskiren is a low-molecular-weight non-peptide that is a potent competitive inhibitor of renin. It binds the active site of renin to block conversion of angiotensinogen to AngI, thus reducing the consequent production of AngII (*see* Figure 26–4). Aliskiren has a 10,000-fold higher affinity to renin (IC_{50} ~0.6 nM) than to any other aspartic peptidases. In healthy volunteers, aliskiren (40-640 mg/day) induces a dose-dependent decrease in blood pressure, reduces PRA and AngI and AngII levels, but increases plasma renin *concentration* by 16- to 34-fold due to the loss of the short-loop negative feedback by AngII. Aliskiren also decreases plasma and urinary aldosterone levels and enhances natriuresis.

Clinical Pharmacology. Aliskiren is recommended as a single oral dose of 150 or 300 mg/day. Bioavailability is low (~2.5%), but its high affinity and potency compensate for the low bioavailability. Peak plasma concentrations are reached within 3-6 h. The $t_{1/2}$ is 20-45 h; steady-state plasma level is achieved in 5-8 days. Aliskiren is a substrate for P-glycoprotein (Pgp), which accounts for low absorption. Fatty meals significantly decrease the absorption of aliskiren. Elimination is mostly as unchanged drug in feces. About 25% of the absorbed dose appears in the urine as parent drug. Aliskiren is well tolerated in the elderly population, in patients with hepatic disease and renal insufficiency, and in patients with type 2 diabetes.

Therapeutic Uses of Aliskiren in Hypertension. Aliskiren is an effective antihypertensive agent that induces significant dose-dependent (75-300 mg) reductions in blood pressure. Aliskiren is as effective as ACE inhibitors (ramipril), ARBs (losartan, irbesartan, valsartan), and hydrochlorothiazide (HCTZ) in lowering blood pressure in patients with mild-to-moderate hypertension. Aliskiren also is as effective as lisinopril in lowering blood pressure in patients with severe hypertension. The long $t_{1/2}$ of aliskiren allows its antihypertensive effects to be sustained for several days following termination of therapy.

Several studies indicate that the effect of aliskiren in combination with ACE inhibitors, ARBs, and HCTZ is additive in lowering systolic and diastolic blood pressure than any of the drugs alone. PRA is inhibited by aliskiren but significantly elevated with ramipril, irbesartan, and HCTZ (*see* Table 26–1). Coadministration of aliskiren with ramipril, irbesartan, or HCTZ neutralizes the increase in PRA to baseline levels. Because plasma renin levels correlate with the capacity to generate AngII, the ability of aliskiren to neutralize plasma renin in combination therapy may contribute to better control of blood pressure than monotherapy. Combination therapy of aliskiren with ACE inhibitors or ARBs is contraindicated in patients with diabetes or kidney impairment. Fixed-dose combinations of aliskiren/HCTZ (TEKTURNA HCT), aliskiren and the Ca^{++} channel blocker amlodipine besylate (TEKAMLO) and aliskiren/HCTZ/ amlodipine besylate (AMTURNIDE) are available for antihypertensive therapy.

Aliskiren is an effective antihypertensive agent that is well tolerated in monotherapy and combination therapy. It has cardioprotective and renoprotective effects in combination therapy The ability of aliskiren to inhibit the increased PRA caused by ACE inhibitors and ARBs theoretically provides a more comprehensive blockade of the RAS and may limit activation of the local (tissue) RAS (*see* Table 26–1). Studies are ongoing to address whether aliskiren provides long-term advantages against end-organ damage in cardiovascular disease.

Aliskiren is currently recommended in patients who are intolerant to other antihypertensive therapies or for use in combination with other drugs for further blood pressure control.

Adverse Events. Aliskiren is well tolerated, and adverse events are mild or comparable to placebo with no gender difference. Adverse effects include mild gastrointestinal symptoms such as diarrhea observed at high doses (600 mg daily), abdominal pain, dyspepsia, and gastroesophageal reflux; headache; nasopharyngitis; dizziness; fatigue; upper respiratory tract infection; back pain; angioedema; and cough (much less common than with ACE inhibitors). Other adverse effects reported for aliskiren that were slightly increased compared with placebo include rash, hypotension, hyperkalemia in diabetics on combination therapy, elevated uric acid, renal stones, and gout. Like other RAS inhibitors, aliskiren is not recommended in pregnancy.

Drug Interactions. Aliskiren does not interact with drugs that interact with CYPs. Aliskiren reduces absorption of furosemide by 50%. Irbesartan reduces the C_{max} of aliskiren by 50%. Aliskiren plasma levels are increased by drugs, such as ketoconazole, atorvastatin, and cyclosporine, that inhibit P-glycoprotein.

Table 26–1

Effects of Antihypertensive Agents on Components of the RAS

	DIRECT RENIN INHIBITORS	ACE-INHIBITORS	ARBs	DIURETICS	Ca^{2+} CHANNEL BLOCKERS	β BLOCKERS
PRC	↑	↑	↑	↑	↔ or ↑	↓
PRA	↓	↑	↑	↑	↔	↓
AngI	↓	↑	↑	↑	↔	↓
AngII	↓	↓	↑	↑	↔	↓
ACE	↔	↓	↔			
Bradykinin	↔	↑	↔			
AT_1 receptors	↔	↔	inhibition			
AT_2 receptors	↔	↔	stimulation			

PRC, plasma renin concentration; PRA, plasma renin activity; ACE, angiotensin-converting enzyme; ARB, angiotensin receptor blocker.

PHARMACOLOGICAL LOWERING OF BLOOD PRESSURES ALTERS COMPONENTS OF THE RAS

The RAS responds to alterations in blood pressure with compensatory changes (*see* Figure 26–2). Thus, pharmacological agents that lower blood pressure will alter the feedback loops that regulate the RAS and cause changes in the levels and activities of the system's components. These changes are summarized in Table 26–1.

For a complete Bibliographical Listing see Goodman & Gilman's ***The Pharmacological Basis of Therapeutics***, 12th ed., or Goodman & Gilman Online at www.AccessMedicine.com.

Treatment of Myocardial Ischemia and Hypertension

PATHOPHYSIOLOGY OF ISCHEMIC HEART DISEASE

Angina pectoris, the primary symptom of ischemic heart disease, is caused by transient episodes of myocardial ischemia that are due to an imbalance in the myocardial oxygen supply–demand relationship that may be caused by an increase in myocardial oxygen demand or by a decrease in myocardial oxygen supply or sometimes by both (Figure 27–1). Typical angina is experienced as a heavy, pressing substernal discomfort (rarely described as a "pain"), often radiating to the left shoulder, flexor aspect of the left arm, jaw, or epigastrium. However, a significant minority of patients note discomfort in a different location or of a different character. Myocardial ischemia also may be *silent*, with electrocardiographic, echocardiographic, or radionuclide evidence of ischemia appearing in the absence of symptoms.

This section describes the principal pharmacological agents used in the treatment of angina: nitrovasodilators, β adrenergic receptor antagonists, and Ca^{2+} channel antagonists. These anti-anginal agents improve the balance of myocardial O_2 supply and O_2 demand, increasing supply by dilating the coronary vasculature and/or decreasing demand by reducing cardiac work (*see* Figure 27–1).

Drugs used in typical angina function principally by reducing myocardial O_2 demand by decreasing heart rate, myocardial contractility, and/or ventricular wall stress. By contrast, the principal therapeutic goal in unstable angina is to increase myocardial blood flow; strategies include the use of antiplatelet agents and *heparin* to reduce intracoronary thrombosis, often accompanied by efforts to restore flow by mechanical means, including percutaneous coronary interventions using coronary stents, or (less commonly) emergency coronary bypass surgery. The principal therapeutic aim in variant or Prinzmetal angina is to prevent coronary vasospasm.

ORGANIC NITRATES

These agents are prodrugs that are sources of nitric oxide (NO) (Table 27–1).

Organic nitrates are polyol esters of nitric acid, whereas organic nitrites are esters of nitrous acid. Nitrate esters (—C—O—NO_2) and nitrite esters (—C—O—NO) are characterized by the sequence of carbon–oxygen–nitrogen. Organic nitrates of low molecular mass (such as nitroglycerin) are moderately volatile, oily liquids, whereas the high-molecular-mass nitrate esters (e.g., erythrityl tetranitrate, isosorbide dinitrate, and isosorbide mononitrate) are solids. The organic nitrates and nitrites, collectively termed *nitrovasodilators*, must be metabolized (reduced) to produce gaseous NO, the active principle of this class of compounds. NO gas also may be administered by inhalation.

PHARMACOLOGICAL PROPERTIES

Mechanism of Action. Nitrites, organic nitrates, nitroso compounds, and a variety of other nitrogen oxide–containing substances (including *nitroprusside*) are basically exogenous sources of NO. NO can activate guanylyl cyclase and thereby increase the cellular level of cyclic GMP, which activates PKG and can modulate the activities of cyclic nucleotide phosphodiesterases (PDEs 2, 3, and 5) in a variety of cell types. In smooth muscle, the net result is phosphorylative activation of myosin light chain phosphatase, reduced phosphorylation of myosin light chain, reduced Ca^{2+} concentration in the cytosol, and relaxation. The pharmacological and biochemical effects of the nitrovasodilators appear to be identical to those of EDRF (endothelium-derived relaxing factor), now known to be NO. This NO-mediated pathway leads to relaxation of smooth muscle in the vasculature, bronchi, and GI tract, and inhibition of platelet aggregation. Chapter 3 presents details of NO biosynthesis and action.

Cardiovascular Effects; Hemodynamic Effects. Low concentrations of nitroglycerin preferentially dilate veins more than arterioles. This venodilation decreases venous return, leading to a fall in left and right ventricular chamber size and end-diastolic pressures, but usually results in little change in systemic vascular resistance. Systemic arterial pressure may fall slightly; heart rate is unchanged or may increase slightly in response to a

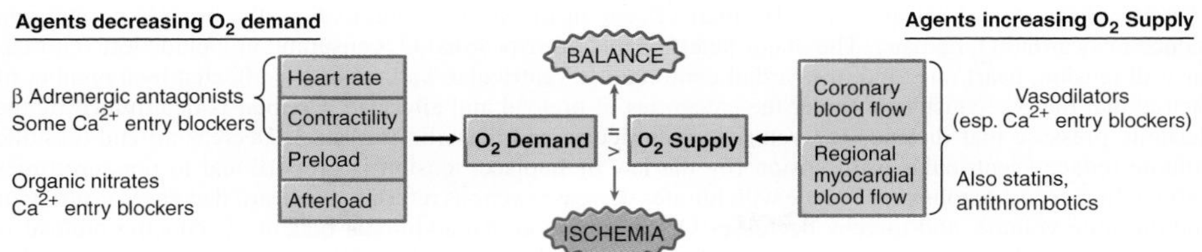

Figure 27–1 *Pharmacological modification of the major determinants of myocardial O_2 supply.* When myocardial O_2 requirements exceed O_2 supply, an ischemic episode results. This figure shows the primary hemodynamic sites of actions of pharmacological agents that can reduce O_2 demand (*left side*) or enhance O_2 supply (*right side*). Some classes of agents have multiple effects. Stents, angioplasty, and coronary bypass surgery are mechanical interventions that increase O_2 supply. Both pharmacotherapy and mechanotherapy attempt to restore a dynamic balance between O_2 demand and O_2 supply.

decrease in blood pressure. Pulmonary vascular resistance and cardiac output are slightly reduced. Doses of nitroglycerin that do not alter systemic arterial pressure may still produce arteriolar dilation in the face and neck, resulting in a facial flush, or dilation of meningeal arterial vessels, causing headache.

Higher doses of organic nitrates cause further venous pooling and may decrease arteriolar resistance as well, thereby decreasing systolic and diastolic blood pressure and cardiac output and causing pallor, weakness, dizziness, and activation of compensatory sympathetic reflexes. The reflex tachycardia and peripheral arteriolar vasoconstriction tend to restore systemic vascular resistance; this is superimposed on sustained venous pooling. Coronary blood flow may increase transiently as a result of coronary vasodilation but may decrease subsequently if cardiac output and blood pressure decrease sufficiently. In patients with autonomic dysfunction and an inability to increase sympathetic outflow, the physiological means to compensate for this fall in blood pressure are absent. In these clinical contexts, nitrates may reduce arterial pressure and coronary perfusion pressure significantly, producing potentially life-threatening hypotension and even aggravating angina. The appropriate therapy in patients with orthostatic angina and normal coronary arteries is to correct the orthostatic hypotension by expanding volume (*fludrocortisone* and a high-sodium diet), to prevent venous pooling with fitted support garments, and to carefully titrate use of oral vasopressors. Because patients with autonomic dysfunction occasionally may have coexisting coronary artery disease, the coronary anatomy should be defined before therapy is undertaken.

Effects on Coronary Blood Flow. Myocardial ischemia is a powerful stimulus to coronary vasodilation, and regional blood flow is adjusted by autoregulatory mechanisms. In the presence of atherosclerotic coronary artery narrowing, ischemia distal to the lesion stimulates vasodilation; if the stenosis is severe, much of the capacity to dilate is used to maintain resting blood flow and further dilation may not be possible when demand increases. Significant coronary stenoses disproportionately reduce blood flow to the subendocardial regions of the heart, which are subjected to the greatest extravascular compression during systole; organic nitrates tend to restore blood flow in these regions toward normal. The hemodynamic mechanisms responsible for these effects are likely the capacity of organic nitrates to cause dilation and prevent vasoconstriction of large epicardial vessels without impairing autoregulation in the small vessels. An important indirect mechanism for a preferential increase in subendocardial blood flow is the nitroglycerin-induced reduction in intracavitary systolic and diastolic pressures that oppose blood flow to the subendocardium (*see* below).

Table 27–1

Organic Nitrates

AGENT	PREPARATIONS, DOSES, ADMINISTRATION[a]	
Nitroglycerin (glyceryl trinitrate)	T: 0.3-0.6 mg as needed S: 0.4 mg per spray as needed C: 2.5-9 mg 2-4 times daily B: 1 mg every 3-5 h	O: 2.5-5 cm, topically every 4-8 h D: 1 disc (2.5-15 mg) for 12-16 h/day IV: 10-20 μg/min; ↑ 10 μg/min to max of 400 μg/min
Isosorbide dinitrate	T: 2.5-10 mg every 2-3 h T(C): 5-10 mg every 2-3 h	T(O): 5-40 mg every 8 h C: 40-80 mg every 12 h
Isosorbide-5-mononitrate	T: 10-40 mg twice daily	C: 60-120 mg daily

[a]*B, buccal (transmucosal) tablet; C, sustained-release capsule or tablet; D, transdermal disc or patch; IV, intravenous injection; O, ointment; S, lingual spray; T, tablet for sublingual use; T(C), chewable tablet; T(O), oral tablet or capsule.*

Effects on Myocardial O_2 Requirements. By their effects on the systemic circulation, the organic nitrates can reduce myocardial O_2 demand. The major determinants of myocardial O_2 consumption include left ventricular wall tension, heart rate, and myocardial contractility. Ventricular wall tension is affected by a number of factors that may be considered under the categories of preload and afterload. *Preload* is determined by the diastolic pressure that distends the ventricle (ventricular end-diastolic pressure). Decreasing end-diastolic volume reduces ventricular wall tension (by the law of Laplace, tension is proportional to pressure times radius). Increasing venous capacitance with nitrates decreases venous return to the heart, decreases ventricular end-diastolic volume, and thereby decreases O_2 consumption. An additional benefit of reducing preload is that it increases the pressure gradient for perfusion across the ventricular wall, which favors subendocardial perfusion. *Afterload* is the impedance against which the ventricle must eject. In the absence of aortic valvular disease, afterload is related to peripheral resistance. Decreasing peripheral arteriolar resistance reduces afterload and thus myocardial work and O_2 consumption.

Organic nitrates decrease both preload and afterload as a result of respective dilation of venous capacitance and arteriolar resistance vessels. They do not directly alter the inotropic or chronotropic state of the heart. Since nitrates reduce the primary determinants of myocardial O_2 demand, their net effect usually is to decrease myocardial O_2 consumption. The effect of nitrovasodilators to inhibit platelet function may contribute to their anti-anginal efficacy, this effect appears to be modest.

Mechanism of Relief of Symptoms of Angina Pectoris. The capacity of nitrates to dilate epicardial coronary arteries, even in areas of atherosclerotic stenosis, is modest, and the preponderance of evidence continues to favor a reduction in myocardial work, and thus in myocardial O_2 demand, as their primary effect in chronic stable angina. Paradoxically, high doses of organic nitrates may reduce blood pressure to such an extent that coronary flow is compromised; reflex tachycardia and adrenergic enhancement of contractility also occur. These effects may override the beneficial action of the drugs on myocardial O_2 demand and can aggravate ischemia. Additionally, sublingual nitroglycerin administration may produce bradycardia and hypotension, probably owing to activation of the Bezold-Jarisch reflex.

OTHER EFFECTS. The nitrovasodilators act on almost all smooth muscle tissues. Bronchial smooth muscle is relaxed irrespective of the preexisting tone. The muscles of the biliary tract, including those of the gallbladder, biliary ducts, and sphincter of Oddi, are effectively relaxed. Smooth muscle of the GI tract, including that of the esophagus, can be relaxed and its spontaneous motility decreased by nitrates both in vivo and in vitro. The effect may be transient and incomplete in vivo, but abnormal "spasm" frequently is reduced. Indeed, many incidences of atypical chest pain and "angina" are due to biliary or esophageal spasm, and these too can be relieved by nitrates. Similarly, nitrates can relax ureteral and uterine smooth muscle, but these responses are of uncertain clinical significance.

ADME AND PREPARATIONS

Nitroglycerin. In humans, peak concentrations of nitroglycerin are found in plasma within 4 min of sublingual administration; the drug has a $t_{1/2}$ of 1-3 min. The onset of action of nitroglycerin may be even more rapid if it is delivered as a sublingual spray rather than as a sublingual tablet. Glyceryl dinitrate metabolites, which have about one-tenth the vasodilator potency, appear to have half-lives of ~40 min.

Isosorbide Dinitrate. The major route of metabolism of isosorbide dinitrate in humans appears to be by enzymatic denitration followed by glucuronide conjugation. Sublingual administration produces maximal plasma concentrations of the drug by 6 min, and the fall in concentration is rapid ($t_{1/2}$ of ~45 min). The primary initial metabolites, isosorbide-2-mononitrate and isosorbide-5-mononitrate, have longer half-lives (3-6 h) and presumably contribute to the therapeutic efficacy of the drug.

Isosorbide-5-Mononitrate. This agent is available in tablet form. It does not undergo significant first-pass metabolism and so has excellent bioavailability after oral administration. The mononitrate has a significantly longer $t_{1/2}$ than does isosorbide dinitrate and has been formulated as a plain tablet and as a sustained-release preparation; both preparations have longer durations of action than the corresponding dosage forms of isosorbide dinitrate.

Inhaled NO. Nitric oxide gas administered by inhalation appears to exert most of its therapeutic effects on the pulmonary vasculature; systemically, it rapidly interacts with heme groups in hemoglobin in the blood. Inhaled NO is used to treat pulmonary hypertension in hypoxemic neonates, where inhaled NO reduces morbidity and mortality.

TOLERANCE

Sublingual organic nitrates should be taken at the time of an anginal attack or in anticipation of exercise or stress. Such intermittent treatment provides reproducible cardiovascular effects. However, frequently repeated or continuous exposure to high doses of organic nitrates leads to a marked attenuation in the magnitude of most of their pharmacological effects. The magnitude of tolerance is a function of dosage and frequency of use. Tolerance may result from a reduced capacity of the vascular smooth muscle to convert nitroglycerin to NO, *true vascular tolerance*, or to the activation of mechanisms extraneous to the vessel wall, *pseudotolerance*. Multiple mechanisms have been proposed to account for nitrate tolerance, including volume expansion, neurohumoral activation, cellular depletion of sulfhydryl groups, and the generation of free radicals. Inactivation of mitochondrial aldehyde dehydrogenase, an enzyme implicated in biotransformation of nitroglycerin, is seen in models of nitrate tolerance, potentially associated with oxidative stress. A reactive intermediate formed during the generation of NO from organic nitrates may itself damage and inactivate the enzymes of the activation pathway; tolerance could involve endothelium-derived reactive oxygen species.

An effective approach to restoring responsiveness is to interrupt therapy for 8-12 h each day, which allows the return of efficacy. It is usually most convenient to omit dosing at night in patients with exertional angina either by adjusting dosing intervals of oral or buccal preparations or by removing cutaneous nitroglycerin. However, patients whose anginal pattern suggests its precipitation by increased left ventricular filling pressures (i.e., occurring in association with orthopnea or paroxysmal nocturnal dyspnea) may benefit from continuing nitrates at night and omitting them during a quiet period of the day. Tolerance also has been seen with isosorbide-5-mononitrate; an eccentric twice-daily dosing schedule appears to maintain efficacy. Some patients develop an increased frequency of nocturnal angina when a nitrate-free interval is employed using nitroglycerin patches; such patients may require another class of anti-anginal agent during this period. Tolerance is not universal, and some patients develop only partial tolerance. The problem of anginal rebound during nitrate-free intervals is especially problematic in the treatment of unstable angina with intravenous nitroglycerin. As tolerance develops, increasing doses are required to achieve the same therapeutic effects; eventually, despite dose escalation, the drug loses efficacy.

A special form of nitroglycerin tolerance is observed in individuals exposed to nitroglycerin in the manufacture of explosives. If protection is inadequate, workers may experience severe headaches, dizziness, and postural weakness during the first several days of employment. Tolerance then develops, but headache and other symptoms may reappear after a few days away from the job—the "Monday disease." The most serious effect of chronic exposure is a form of organic nitrate dependence. Workers without demonstrable organic vascular disease have been reported to have an increase in the incidence of acute coronary syndromes during the 24-72-h periods away from the work environment. Because of the potential problem of nitrate dependence, it seems prudent not to withdraw nitrates abruptly from a patient who has received such therapy chronically.

TOXICITY AND UNTOWARD RESPONSES. Untoward responses to the therapeutic use of organic nitrates are almost all secondary to actions on the cardiovascular system. Headache is common and can be severe. It usually decreases over a few days if treatment is continued and often can be controlled by decreasing the dose. Transient episodes of dizziness, weakness, and other manifestations associated with postural hypotension may develop, particularly if the patient is standing immobile, and may progress occasionally to loss of consciousness, a reaction that appears to be accentuated by alcohol. It also may be seen with very low doses of nitrates in patients with autonomic dysfunction. Even in severe nitrate syncope, positioning and other measures that facilitate venous return are the only therapeutic measures required. All the organic nitrates occasionally can produce drug rash.

INTERACTION OF NITRATES WITH PDE5 INHIBITORS. Erectile dysfunction is a frequently encountered problem whose risk factors parallel those of coronary artery disease. Thus, many men desiring therapy for erectile dysfunction already may be receiving (or may require, especially if they increase physical activity) anti-anginal therapy. The combination of sildenafil and other phosphodiesterase 5 (PDE5) inhibitors with organic nitrate vasodilators can cause extreme hypotension.

Cells in the corpus cavernosum produce NO during sexual arousal in response to nonadrenergic, noncholinergic neurotransmission. NO stimulates the formation of cyclic GMP, which leads to relaxation of smooth muscle of the corpus cavernosum and penile arteries, engorgement of the corpus cavernosum, and erection. The accumulation of cyclic GMP can be enhanced by inhibition of the cyclic GMP–specific PDE5 family. Sildenafil (VIAGRA, REVATIO) and congeners inhibit PDE5 and have been demonstrated to improve erectile function in patients with erectile dysfunction. Not surprisingly, PDE5 inhibitors have assumed the status of widely used recreational drugs. Since the introduction of sildenafil, 3 additional PDE5 inhibitors have been developed for use in therapy of erectile dysfunction. Tadalafil (CIALIS, ADCIRCA), vardenafil (LEVITRA), and avanafil (STENDRA) share similar therapeutic efficacy and side-effect profiles with sildenafil; tadalafil has a longer time to onset of action and a longer therapeutic $t_{1/2}$ than the other PDE5 inhibitors. Sildenafil has been the most thoroughly characterized of these compounds, but all 3 PDE5 inhibitors are contraindicated for patients taking organic nitrate vasodilators, and the PDE5 inhibitors should be used with caution in patients taking α or β adrenergic receptor antagonists (*see* Chapter 12).

The side effects of sildenafil and other PDE5 inhibitors are largely predictable on the basis of their effects on PDE5. Headache, flushing, and rhinitis may be observed, as well as dyspepsia owing to relaxation of the lower esophageal sphincter. Sildenafil and vardenafil also weakly inhibit PDE6, the enzyme involved in photoreceptor signal transduction (*see* Chapters 3 and 64), and can produce visual disturbances, most notably changes in the perception of color hue or brightness. In addition to visual disturbances, sudden one-sided hearing loss has also been reported. Tadalafil inhibits PDE11, a widely distributed PDE isoform, but the clinical importance of this effect is not clear. The most important toxicity of all these PDE5 inhibitors is hemodynamic. When given alone to men with severe coronary artery disease, these drugs have modest effects on blood pressure, producing >10% fall in systolic, diastolic, and mean systemic pressures and in pulmonary artery systolic and mean pressures. However, sildenafil, tadalafil, and vardenafil all have a significant and potentially dangerous interaction with organic nitrates, which act therapeutically via enhancing cyclic GMP production in smooth muscle. In the presence of a PDE5 inhibitor, nitrates cause profound increases in cyclic GMP and can produce dramatic reductions in blood pressure. This drug class toxicity is the basis for the warning that PDE5 inhibitors should not be prescribed to patients receiving any form of nitrate and dictates that patients should be warned about the prior use of PDE5 inhibitors within 24 h of administration of nitrates. A period of longer than 24 h may be needed following administration of a PDE5 inhibitor for safe use of nitrates, especially with tadalafil because of its prolonged $t_{1/2}$. In the event that patients develop significant hypotension following combined administration of sildenafil and a nitrate, fluids and α adrenergic receptor agonists, if needed, should be used for support. These same hemodynamic responses to PDE5 inhibition also may underlie the efficacy of sildenafil in the treatment of patients with primary pulmonary hypertension, in whom chronic treatment with the drug appears to result in enhanced exercise capacity associated with a decrease in pulmonary vascular resistance. PDE5 inhibitors also are being studied in patients with congestive heart failure and cardiac hypertrophy (*see* Chapter 28).

Sildenafil, tadalafil, vardenafil, and avanafil are metabolized via CYP3A4, and their toxicity may be enhanced in patients who receive other substrates of this enzyme, including macrolide and imidazole antibiotics, some statins, and antiretroviral agents (*see* individual chapters and Chapter 6). PDE5 inhibitors also may prolong cardiac repolarization by blocking the I_{Kr}. In patients with coronary artery disease whose exercise capacity indicates that sexual activity is unlikely to precipitate angina and who are not currently taking nitrates, the use of PDE5 inhibitors can be considered. Such therapy needs to be individualized, and appropriate warnings must be given about the risk of toxicity if nitrates are taken subsequently for angina. Alternative non-nitrate anti-anginal therapy, such as β adrenergic receptor antagonists, should be used during these time periods.

THERAPEUTIC USES

ANGINA. Diseases that predispose to angina should be treated as part of a comprehensive therapeutic program with the primary goal being to prolong life. Conditions such as hypertension, anemia, thyrotoxicosis, obesity, heart failure, cardiac arrhythmias, and acute anxiety can precipitate anginal symptoms in many patients. Patients should be counseled to stop smoking, lose weight, and maintain a low-fat, high-fiber diet; hypertension and hyperlipidemia should be corrected; and daily aspirin (or clopidogrel if aspirin is not tolerated) (*see* Chapter 30) should be prescribed. Exposure to sympathomimetic agents (e.g., those in nasal decongestants and other sources) probably should be avoided. The use of drugs that modify the perception of pain is a poor approach to the treatment of angina because the underlying myocardial ischemia is not relieved. Table 27–1 lists the preparations and dosages of the nitrites and organic nitrates.

Sublingual Administration. Because of its rapid action, long-established efficacy, and low cost, nitroglycerin is the most useful drug of the organic nitrates given sublingually. The onset of action is within 1-2 min, but the effects are undetectable by 1 h after administration.

Oral Administration. Oral nitrates often are used to provide prophylaxis against anginal episodes. Higher doses of either isosorbide dinitrate (e.g., 20 mg or more orally every 4 h) or sustained-release preparations of nitroglycerin decrease the frequency of anginal attacks and improve exercise tolerance. Effects peak at 60-90 min and last for 3-6 h. Administration of isosorbide mononitrate (typically starting at 20 mg) once or twice daily (in the latter case, with the doses administered 7 h apart) is efficacious in the treatment of chronic angina, and once-daily dosing or an eccentric twice-daily dosing schedule can minimize the development of tolerance.

Cutaneous Administration. Nitroglycerin ointment (2%) is applied to the skin (2.5-5 cm); the dosage must be adjusted for each patient. Effects are apparent within 30-60 min (although absorption is variable) and last for 4-6 h. The ointment is particularly useful for controlling nocturnal angina, which commonly develops within 3 h after the patient goes to sleep. To avoid tolerance, therapy should be interrupted for at least 8 h each day.

Transmucosal or Buccal Nitroglycerin. This formulation is inserted under the upper lip above the incisors, where it adheres to the gingiva and dissolves gradually in a uniform manner. Hemodynamic effects are seen within 2-5 min, and it is therefore useful for short-term prophylaxis of angina.

CONGESTIVE HEART FAILURE. The utility of nitrovasodilators to relieve pulmonary congestion and to increase cardiac output in congestive heart failure is addressed in Chapter 28.

UNSTABLE ANGINA PECTORIS AND NON-ST-SEGMENT–ELEVATION MYOCARDIAL INFARCTION. The term *unstable angina pectoris* has been used to describe a broad spectrum of clinical entities characterized by an acute or subacute worsening in a patient's anginal symptoms. The variable prognosis of unstable angina reflects the broad range of clinical entities subsumed by the term. Efforts have been directed toward identifying patients with unstable angina on the basis of their risks for subsequent adverse outcomes such as MI or death. The term *acute coronary syndrome* has been useful in this context: Common to most clinical presentations of acute coronary syndrome is disruption of a coronary plaque, leading to local platelet aggregation and thrombosis at the arterial wall, with subsequent partial or total occlusion of the vessel. There is some variability in the pathogenesis of unstable angina, with gradually progressive atherosclerosis accounting for some cases of new-onset exertional angina. Less commonly, vasospasm in minimally atherosclerotic coronary vessels may account for some cases where rest angina has not been preceded by symptoms of exertional angina. For the most part, the pathophysiological principles that underlie therapy for exertional angina—which are directed at decreasing myocardial oxygen *demand*—have limited efficacy in the treatment of acute coronary syndromes characterized by an insufficiency of myocardial oxygen (blood) *supply*.

OTHER AGENTS; DRUG COMBINATIONS. Drugs that reduce myocardial O_2 consumption by reducing ventricular preload (nitrates) or by reducing heart rate and ventricular contractility (β adrenergic receptor antagonists) are efficacious, but additional therapies are directed at an atherosclerotic plaque and the consequences (or prevention) of its rupture. These therapies include combinations of:

- Antiplatelet agents, including aspirin and thioenopyridines such as clopidogrel or prasugrel
- Antithrombin agents such as heparin and the thrombolytics anti-integrin therapies that directly inhibit platelet aggregation mediated by glycoprotein (GP)IIb/IIIa mechano-pharmacological approaches with percutaneously deployed intracoronary stents
- Coronary bypass surgery for selected patients

Along with nitrates and β adrenergic receptor antagonists, antiplatelet agents represent the cornerstone of therapy for acute coronary syndrome. Aspirin inhibits platelet aggregation and improves survival. Heparin (either unfractionated or low-molecular-weight) also appears to reduce angina and prevent infarction. These and related agents are discussed in detail in Chapters 30 and 34. Anti-integrin agents directed against the platelet integrin GPIIb/IIIa (including abciximab, tirofiban, and eptifibatide) are effective in combination with heparin, as discussed later. Nitrates are useful both in reducing vasospasm and in reducing myocardial O_2 consumption by decreasing ventricular wall stress. Intravenous administration of nitroglycerin allows high concentrations of drug to be attained rapidly. Because nitroglycerin is degraded rapidly, the dose can be titrated quickly and safely using intravenous administration. If coronary vasospasm is present, intravenous nitroglycerin is likely to be effective, although the addition of a Ca^{2+} channel blocker may be required to achieve complete control.

ACUTE MYOCARDIAL INFARCTION. Therapeutic maneuvers in MI are directed at reducing the size of the infarct, preserving or retrieving viable tissue by reducing the O_2 demand of the myocardium, and preventing ventricular remodeling that could lead to heart failure.

Nitroglycerin is commonly administered to relieve ischemic pain in patients presenting with MI, but evidence that nitrates improve mortality in MI is sparse. Because they reduce ventricular preload through vasodilation, nitrates are effective in relief of pulmonary congestion. A decreased ventricular preload should be avoided in patients with right ventricular infarction because higher right-sided heart filling pressures are needed in this clinical context. Nitrates are relatively contraindicated in patients with systemic hypotension. According to the American Heart Association/American College of Cardiology (AHA/ACC) guidelines, "nitrates should not be used if hypotension limits the administration of β blockers, which have more powerful salutary effects." Because the proximate cause of MI is intracoronary thrombosis, reperfusion therapies are critically important, employing, when possible, direct percutaneous coronary interventions (PCIs) for acute MI, usually using drug-eluting intracoronary stents. Thrombolytic agents are administered at hospitals where emergency PCI is not performed, but outcomes are better with direct PCI than with thrombolytic therapy.

VARIANT (PRINZMETAL) ANGINA. The large coronary arteries normally contribute little to coronary resistance. However, in variant angina, coronary constriction results in reduced blood flow and ischemic pain. Whereas long-acting nitrates alone are occasionally efficacious in abolishing episodes of variant angina, additional therapy with Ca^{2+} channel blockers usually is required.

Ca^{2+} CHANNEL ANTAGONISTS

Voltage-sensitive Ca^{2+} channels (L-type or slow channels) mediate the entry of extracellular Ca^{2+} (~1.25 mM) into smooth muscle and cardiac myocytes and sinoatrial (SA) and atrioventricular (AV) nodal cells (cytosolic concentration in resting cell, ~100 nM) in response to electrical

Table 27–2

Comparative CV Effects[a] of Ca^{2+} Channel Blockers

DRUG CLASS Example	VASODILATION	↓ CARDIAC CONTRACTILITY	↓ AUTOMATICITY (SA NODE)	↓ CONDUCTION (AV NODE)
Phenylalkylamine Verapamil	4	4	5	5
Benzothiazepine Diltiazem	3	2	5	4
Dihydropyridine[b] Nifedipine	5	1	1	0

[a]*Relative effects are ranked from no effect (0) to prominent (5). NR, not ranked.*
[b]*See text for individual characteristic of the numerous dihydropyridines.*

depolarization. In both smooth muscle and cardiac myocytes, Ca^{2+} is a trigger for contraction, albeit by different mechanisms. Ca^{2+} channel antagonists, also called *Ca^{2+} entry blockers*, inhibit Ca^{2+} channel function. In vascular smooth muscle, this leads to relaxation, especially in arterial beds. In the heart, these drugs can produce negative inotropic and chronotropic effects.

Clinically used Ca^{2+} channel antagonists include the phenylalkylamine compound verapamil, the benzothiazepine diltiazem, and numerous dihydropyridines, including nifedipine, amlodipine, felodipine, isradipine, nicardipine, nisoldipine, and nimodipine. The specificities of several of these drugs are shown in Table 27–2. Although these drugs are commonly grouped together as "Ca^{2+} channel blockers," there are fundamental differences among verapamil, diltiazem, and the dihydropyridines, especially with respect to pharmacological characteristics, drug interactions, and toxicities.

Mechanisms of Action. An increased concentration of cytosolic Ca^{2+} causes increased contraction in both cardiac and vascular smooth muscle cells. The entry of extracellular Ca^{2+} initiates contraction of cardiac myocytes (Ca^{2+}-induced Ca^{2+} release, where the bulk of contractile Ca^{2+} is from the sarcoplasmic reticulum) and provides a major source of contractile Ca^{2+} in smooth muscle (in which the release of Ca^{2+} from IP_3-sensitive intracellular storage vesicles and Ca^{2+} entry via receptor-operated channels can also contribute to contraction, particularly in some vascular beds). The Ca^{2+} channel antagonists produce their effects by binding to the α_1 subunit of the L-type Ca^{2+} channels and reducing Ca^{2+} flux through the channel. The vascular and cardiac effects of some of the Ca^{2+} channel blockers are summarized in the next section and in Table 27–2.

PHARMACOLOGICAL PROPERTIES

CARDIOVASCULAR EFFECTS

Vascular Tissue. At least 3 distinct mechanisms may be responsible for contraction of vascular smooth muscle cells. First, voltage-sensitive Ca^{2+} channels open in response to depolarization of the membrane, and extracellular Ca^{2+} moves down its electrochemical gradient into the cell. Second, agonist-induced contractions that occur without depolarization of the membrane result from stimulation of the G_q–PLC–IP_3 pathway, resulting in the release of intracellular Ca^{2+} from the sarcoplasmic reticulum (*see* Chapter 3). Third, receptor-operated Ca^{2+} channels allow the entry of extracellular Ca^{2+} in response to receptor occupancy.

Ca^{2+} channel antagonists inhibit the voltage-dependent Ca^{2+} channels in vascular smooth muscle at significantly lower concentrations than are required to interfere with the release of intracellular Ca^{2+} or to block receptor-operated Ca^{2+} channels. All Ca^{2+} channel blockers relax arterial smooth muscle, but they have a less pronounced effect on most venous beds and hence do not affect cardiac preload significantly.

Cardiac Cells. In the SA and AV nodes, depolarization largely depends on the movement of Ca^{2+} through the slow channel. The effect of a Ca^{2+} channel blocker on AV conduction and on the rate of the sinus node pacemaker depends on whether or not the agent delays the recovery of the slow channel. Although nifedipine reduces the slow inward current in a dose-dependent manner, it does not affect the rate of recovery of the slow Ca^{2+} channel. The channel blockade caused by nifedipine and related dihydropyridines also shows little dependence on the frequency of stimulation. At doses used clinically, nifedipine does not affect conduction through the AV node. In contrast, verapamil not only reduces the magnitude of the Ca^{2+} current through the slow channel but also decreases the rate of recovery of the channel. In addition, channel blockade caused by verapamil (and to a lesser extent by diltiazem) is enhanced as the frequency of stimulation increases, a phenomenon known as *frequency dependence* or *use dependence*. Verapamil and diltiazem depress the rate of the sinus node pacemaker and slow AV conduction; the latter effect is the basis for their use in the treatment of supraventricular tachyarrhythmias (*see* Chapter 29). Bepridil, like verapamil, inhibits both slow inward Ca^{2+} current and fast inward Na^{+} current. It has a direct negative inotropic effect. Its electrophysiological properties lead to slowing of the heart rate, prolongation of the AV nodal effective refractory period, and importantly, prolongation of the QTc interval. Particularly in the setting of hypokalemia, the last effect can be associated with *torsade de pointes*, a potentially lethal ventricular arrhythmia (*see* Chapter 29).

In cardiac myocytes, initiation of Ca^{2+}-induced Ca^{2+} release relies on entry Ca^{2+} of through the L-type channel in response to depolarization. By reducing this entry, Ca^{2+} channel blockers can produce a negative inotropic effect.

Hemodynamic Effects. All the Ca^{2+} channel blockers approved for clinical use decrease coronary vascular resistance and can lead to an increase in coronary blood flow. The dihydropyridines are more potent vasodilator than verapamil, which is more potent than diltiazem. The hemodynamic effects of these agents vary depending on the route of administration and the extent of left ventricular dysfunction. Drugs that significantly lower mean pressure will elicit a baroreceptor reflex response.

Nifedipine, the prototypical dihydropyridine, selectively dilates arterial resistance vessels. The decrease in arterial blood pressure elicits sympathetic reflexes, with resulting tachycardia and positive inotropy. Nifedipine has direct negative inotropic effects in vitro but relaxes vascular smooth muscle at significantly lower concentrations than those required for prominent direct effects on the heart. Thus, arteriolar resistance and blood pressure are lowered, contractility and segmental ventricular function are improved, and heart rate and cardiac output are increased modestly. After oral administration of nifedipine, arterial dilation increases peripheral blood flow; venous tone does not change. The other dihydropyridines—amlodipine, felodipine, isradipine, nicardipine, nisoldipine, nimodipine, and clevidipine—share many of the cardiovascular effects of nifedipine.

Amlodipine has a slow absorption and a prolonged effect. Amlodipine produces both peripheral arterial vasodilation and coronary dilation. There is less reflex tachycardia with amlodipine than with nifedipine, possibly because the long $t_{1/2}$ (35-50 h) produces minimal peaks and troughs in plasma concentrations. Felodipine may have even greater vascular specificity than does nifedipine or amlodipine. At concentrations producing vasodilation, there is no negative inotropic effect. Nicardipine has anti-anginal properties similar to those of nifedipine and may have selectivity for coronary vessels. Isradipine also produces the typical peripheral vasodilation seen with other dihydropyridines, but because of its inhibitory effect on the SA node, little or no rise in heart rate is seen. Despite the negative chronotropic effect, isradipine appears to have little effect on the AV node, so it may be used in patients with AV block or combined with a β adrenergic receptor antagonist. In general, because of their lack of myocardial depression and, to a greater or lesser extent, lack of negative chronotropic effect, dihydropyridines are less effective as monotherapy in stable angina than are verapamil, diltiazem, or a β adrenergic receptor antagonist. Nisoldipine is more than 1000 times more potent in preventing contraction of human vascular smooth muscle than in preventing contraction of human cardiac muscle in vitro, suggesting a high degree of vascular selectivity. Although nisoldipine has a short elimination $t_{1/2}$, a sustained-release preparation that is efficacious as an anti-anginal agent has been developed. Nimodipine has high lipid solubility and is effective in inhibiting cerebral vasospasm and has been used primarily to treat patients with neurological defects associated with cerebral vasospasm after subarachnoid hemorrhage.

Clevidipine is a novel dihydropyridine L-type Ca^{2+} channel blocker—available for intravenous administration—that has a very rapid ($t_{1/2}$ ~2 min) onset and offset of action. It is metabolized by esterases in blood, similar to the fate of esmolol. Clevidipine preferentially affects arterial smooth muscle compared to targeting veins or the heart. Infusions are typically started at a rate of 1-2 μg/kg/min and titrated to the desired effect on blood pressure.

Verapamil is a less potent vasodilator the dihydropyridines. Like dihydropyridines, verapamil causes little effect on venous resistance vessels at concentrations that produce arteriolar dilation. With doses of verapamil sufficient to produce peripheral arterial vasodilation, there are more direct negative chronotropic, dromotropic, and inotropic effects than with the dihydropyridines. Intravenous verapamil causes a decrease in arterial blood pressure owing to a decrease in vascular resistance, but the reflex tachycardia is blunted or abolished by the direct negative chronotropic effect of the drug. This intrinsic negative inotropic effect is partially offset by both a decrease in afterload and the reflex increase in adrenergic tone. Thus, in patients without congestive heart failure, ventricular performance is not impaired and actually may improve, especially if ischemia limits performance. In contrast, in patients with congestive heart failure, intravenous verapamil can cause a marked decrease in contractility and left ventricular function. Oral administration of verapamil reduces peripheral vascular resistance and blood pressure, often with minimal changes in heart rate. The relief of pacing-induced angina seen with verapamil is due primarily to a reduction in myocardial oxygen demand.

Intravenous administration of diltiazem can result initially in a marked decrease in peripheral vascular resistance and arterial blood pressure, which elicits a reflex increase in heart rate and cardiac output. Heart rate then falls below initial levels because of the direct negative chronotropic effect of the agent. Oral administration of diltiazem decreases both heart rate and mean arterial blood pressure. While diltiazem and verapamil produce similar effects on the SA and AV nodes, the negative inotropic effect of diltiazem is more modest.

ADME. Although the absorption of these agents is nearly complete after oral administration, their bioavailability is reduced, in some cases markedly, by first-pass hepatic metabolism. The effects of these drugs are evident within 30-60 min of an oral dose, with the exception of the more slowly absorbed and longer-acting agents amlodipine, isradipine, and felodipine. These agents all are bound extensively to plasma proteins (70-98%); their elimination half-lives vary widely, from 1.3 to 64 h. During repeated oral administration, bioavailability and $t_{1/2}$ may increase because of saturation of hepatic metabolism. The bioavailability of some of these drugs may be increased by grapefruit juice, likely through inhibition of enzyme CYP3A4. A major metabolite of diltiazem is desacetyldiltiazem, which has about one-half of diltiazem's potency as a vasodilator. *N*-Demethylation of verapamil results in production of norverapamil, which is biologically active but much less potent than the parent compound. The $t_{1/2}$ of norverapamil is ~10 h. The metabolites of the dihydropyridines are inactive or weakly active. In patients with hepatic cirrhosis, the bioavailabilities and half-lives of the Ca^{2+} channel blockers may be increased, and dosage should be adjusted. The half-lives of these agents also may be longer in older patients. Except for diltiazem and nifedipine, all the Ca^{2+} channel blockers are administered as racemic mixtures.

Toxicity and Untoward Responses. The profile of adverse reactions to the Ca^{2+} channel blockers varies among the drugs in this class. Patients receiving immediate-release capsules of nifedipine develop headache, flushing, dizziness, and peripheral edema. Dizziness and flushing are much less of a problem with the sustained-release formulations and with the dihydropyridines having a long $t_{1/2}$ and relatively constant concentrations of drug in plasma. Peripheral edema may occur in some patients with Ca^{2+} channel blockers; it most likely results from increased hydrostatic pressure in the lower extremities owing to precapillary dilation and reflex postcapillary constriction. Some other adverse effects of these drugs are due to actions in nonvascular smooth muscle. Contraction of the lower esophageal sphincter is inhibited by the Ca^{2+} channel blockers. Ca^{2+} channel blockers can cause or aggravate gastroesophageal reflux. Constipation is a common side effect of verapamil, but it occurs less frequently with other Ca^{2+} channel blockers. Uncommon adverse effects include urinary retention, rash, and elevations of liver enzymes.

Worsened myocardial ischemia has been observed with nifedipine from excessive hypotension and decreased coronary perfusion, selective coronary vasodilation in nonischemic regions of the myocardium in a setting where vessels perfusing ischemic regions were already maximally dilated (i.e., coronary steal), or an increase in O_2 demand owing to increased sympathetic tone and excessive tachycardia. Although bradycardia, transient asystole, and exacerbation of heart failure have been reported with verapamil, these responses usually have occurred after intravenous administration of verapamil in patients with disease of the SA node or AV nodal conduction disturbances or in the presence of β blockade. The use of intravenous verapamil with an intravenous β adrenergic receptor antagonist is contraindicated because of the increased propensity for AV block and/or severe depression of ventricular function. Patients with ventricular dysfunction, SA or AV nodal conduction disturbances, and systolic blood pressures <90 mm Hg should not be treated with verapamil or diltiazem, particularly intravenously. Some Ca^{2+} channel antagonists such as verapamil can cause an increase in the concentration of digoxin in plasma; resulting toxicity from the cardiac glycoside rarely develops, but the use of verapamil to treat digitalis toxicity thus is contraindicated; AV nodal conduction disturbances may be exacerbated.

Drug Interactions. Verapamil blocks the P-glycoprotein drug transporter. Both the renal and hepatic disposition of digoxin occurs via this transporter. Accordingly, verapamil inhibits the elimination of digoxin and other drugs that are cleared from the body by the P-glycoprotein (*see* Chapter 5). When used with quinidine, Ca^{2+} channel blockers may cause excessive hypotension, particularly in patients with idiopathic hypertrophic subaortic stenosis.

THERAPEUTIC USES

VARIANT ANGINA. Variant angina results from reduced blood flow rather than increased oxygen demand. Ca^{2+} channel blocking agents have proven efficacy for the treatment of variant angina. These drugs can attenuate ergonovine-induced vasospasm in patients with variant angina, which suggests that protection in variant angina is due to coronary dilation rather than to alterations in peripheral hemodynamics.

EXERTIONAL ANGINA. Ca^{2+} channel antagonists also are effective in the treatment of exertional, or exercise-induced, angina. Their utility may result from an increase in blood flow owing to coronary arterial dilation, from a decrease in myocardial oxygen demand (secondary to a decrease in arterial blood pressure, heart rate, or contractility), or both. These drugs decrease the number of anginal attacks and attenuate exercise-induced ST-segment depression.

Ca^{2+} channel antagonists, particularly the dihydropyridines, may aggravate anginal symptoms in some patients when used without a β adrenergic receptor antagonist. This adverse effect is not prominent with verapamil or diltiazem because of their limited ability to induce marked peripheral vasodilation and reflex tachycardia. Concurrent therapy with nifedipine and the β receptor antagonist propranolol or with amlodipine and any of several β receptor antagonists has proven more effective than either agent given alone in exertional angina, presumably because the β antagonist suppresses reflex tachycardia. This concurrent drug therapy is particularly attractive because the dihydropyridines, unlike verapamil and diltiazem, do not delay AV conduction and will not enhance the negative dromotropic effects associated with β receptor blockade. Although concurrent administration of verapamil or diltiazem with a β receptor antagonist also may reduce angina, the potential for AV block, severe bradycardia, and decreased left ventricular function requires that these combinations be used judiciously, especially if left ventricular function is compromised prior to therapy. Amlodipine produces less reflex tachycardia than does nifedipine probably because of a flatter plasma concentration profile. Isradipine, approximately equivalent to nifedipine in enhancing exercise tolerance, also produces less rise in heart rate, possibly because of its slower onset of action.

Unstable Angina. Medical therapy for unstable angina involves the administration of aspirin, which reduces mortality, nitrates, β adrenergic receptor blocking agents, and heparin. Because vasospasm occurs in some patients with unstable angina, Ca^{2+} channel blockers may offer an additional approach to this condition.

Myocardial Infarction. There is no evidence that Ca^{2+} channel antagonists are of benefit in the early treatment or secondary prevention of acute MI. Diltiazem and verapamil may reduce the incidence of reinfarction in patients with MI who are not candidates for a β adrenergic receptor antagonist, but β adrenergic receptor antagonists remain the drugs of first choice.

Other Uses. Ca^{2+} channel antagonists are also used as anti-arrhythmic agents, for the treatment of hypertension, and for the treatment of heart failure. Verapamil has been demonstrated to improve left ventricular outflow obstruction and symptoms in patients with hypertrophic cardiomyopathy. Verapamil also has been used in the prophylaxis of migraine headaches. While several studies suggest that dihydropyridines may suppress the progression of mild atherosclerosis, there is no evidence that this alters mortality or reduces the incidence of ischemic events. Nimodipine has been approved for use in patients with neurological deficits secondary to cerebral vasospasm after the rupture of a congenital intracranial aneurysm. Nifedipine, diltiazem, amlodipine, and felodipine appear to provide symptomatic relief in Raynaud disease. The Ca^{2+} channel antagonists cause relaxation of the myometrium *in vitro* and may be effective in stopping preterm uterine contractions in preterm labor (*see* Chapter 66).

β ADRENERGIC RECEPTOR ANTAGONISTS

β Adrenergic receptor antagonists are effective in reducing the severity and frequency of attacks of exertional angina and in improving survival in patients who have had an MI. In contrast, these agents are not useful for vasospastic angina and, if used in isolation, may worsen the condition. *Timolol*, metoprolol, *atenolol*, and propranolol exert cardioprotective effects. The effectiveness of β adrenergic receptor antagonists in the treatment of exertional angina is attributable primarily to a fall in myocardial O_2 consumption at rest and during exertion; there also is some tendency for increased flow toward ischemic regions. The decrease in myocardial O_2 consumption is due to a negative chronotropic effect (particularly during exercise), a negative inotropic effect, and a reduction in arterial blood pressure (particularly systolic pressure) during exercise.

Not all actions of β adrenergic receptor antagonists are beneficial in all patients. The decreases in heart rate and contractility cause increases in the systolic ejection period and left ventricular end-diastolic volume; these alterations tend to increase O_2 consumption. However, the net effect of β receptor blockade usually is to decrease myocardial O_2 consumption, particularly during exercise. In patients with limited cardiac reserve who are critically dependent on adrenergic stimulation, β receptor blockade can result in profound decreases in left ventricular function. Despite this, several β adrenergic receptor antagonists have been shown to reduce mortality in patients with congestive heart failure (*see* Chapters 12 and 28). Numerous β receptor antagonists are approved for clinical use in the U.S. (*see* Chapter 12).

THERAPEUTIC USES

UNSTABLE ANGINA. β Adrenergic receptor antagonists are effective in reducing recurrent episodes of ischemia and the risk of progression to acute MI. Clinical trials have lacked sufficient statistical power to demonstrate beneficial effects of β receptor antagonists on mortality. If the underlying pathophysiology is coronary vasospasm, nitrates and Ca^{2+} channel blockers may be effective, and β receptor antagonists should be used with caution. In some patients, there is a combination of severe fixed disease and superimposed vasospasm; if adequate antiplatelet therapy and vasodilation have been provided by other agents and angina continues, the addition of a β receptor antagonist may be helpful.

MYOCARDIAL INFARCTION. β Adrenergic receptor antagonists that do not have intrinsic sympathomimetic activity improve mortality in MI. They should be given early and continued indefinitely in patients who can tolerate them.

COMPARISON OF ANTI-ANGINAL THERAPEUTIC STRATEGIES

In evaluating trials in which different forms of anti-anginal therapy are compared, one must pay careful attention to the patient population studied and to the pathophysiology and stage of the disease. An important placebo effect may be seen in these trials. The efficacy of anti-anginal treatment will depend on the severity of angina, the presence of coronary vasospasm, and myocardial O_2 demand. Optimally, the dose of each agent should be titrated to maximum benefit.

Task forces from the ACC and the AHA have published guidelines that are useful in the selection of appropriate initial therapy for patients with chronic stable angina pectoris. Patients with coronary artery disease should be treated with aspirin and a β receptor blocking drug (particularly if there is a history of prior MI). The guidelines also note that solid data support the use of ACE inhibitors in patients with coronary artery disease who also have left ventricular dysfunction and/or diabetes. Therapy of hypercholesterolemia also is indicated. Nitrates, for treatment of angina symptoms, and Ca^{2+} antagonists also may be used. Table 27–3 summarizes the issues that the ACC/AHA task force considered to be relevant in choosing between β receptor antagonists and Ca^{2+} channel blockers in patients with angina and other medical conditions. Comparison of β adrenergic receptor antagonists with Ca^{2+} channel blockers showed that β receptor antagonists are associated with fewer episodes of angina per week and a lower rate of withdrawal because of adverse events. However, there were no differences in time to ischemia during exercise or in the frequency of adverse events when Ca^{2+} channel blockers other than nifedipine were compared with β adrenergic receptor antagonists. There were no significant differences in outcome between the studies comparing long-acting nitrates and Ca^{2+} channel blockers and the studies comparing long-acting nitrates with β receptor antagonists.

COMBINATION THERAPY AND NEW ANTI-ANGINAL DRUGS. Because the different categories of anti-anginal agents have different mechanisms of action, it has been suggested that combinations of these agents would allow the use of lower doses, increasing effectiveness and reducing the incidence of side effects. Despite the predicted advantages, combination therapy rarely achieves this potential and may be accompanied by serious side effects. The new anti-anginal agent ranolazine elicits its therapeutic effects by different and incompletely understood mechanisms that distinguish this new drug from the "classical" classes of anti-anginal drugs (organic nitrates, β adrenergic blockers and Ca^{2+} channel blockers). Ranolazine may have additional efficacy in combination with other anti-anginal agents, and the effects of ranolazine on cardiac arrhythmias and glucose metabolism may identify indications for this drug independent of its role as an anti-anginal agent. Table 27–3 shows some of the important indications and contraindications for use of anti-anginal agents in the context of other disease states.

Nitrates and β Adrenergic Receptor Antagonists. The concurrent use of organic nitrates and β adrenergic receptor antagonists can be very effective in the treatment of typical exertional angina. The additive efficacy primarily is a result of the blockade by one drug of a reflex effect elicited by the other. β Adrenergic receptor antagonists can block the baroreceptor-mediated reflex tachycardia and positive inotropic effects that are sometimes associated with nitrates, whereas nitrates, by increasing venous capacitance, can attenuate the increase in left ventricular end-diastolic volume associated with β receptor blockade. Concurrent administration of nitrates also can alleviate the increase in coronary vascular resistance associated with blockade of β adrenergic receptors.

Ca^{2+} Channel Blockers and β Receptor Antagonists. Because there is a proven mortality benefit from the use of β adrenergic receptor antagonists in patients with heart disease, this class of drugs represents the first line of therapy. However, when angina is not controlled adequately by a β receptor antagonist plus nitrates, additional improvement sometimes can be achieved by the addition of a Ca^{2+} channel blocker, especially if there is a component of coronary vasospasm. The differences among the chemical classes of Ca^{2+} channel blockers can lead to important adverse or salutary drug interactions with β receptor antagonists. If the patient already is being treated with maximal doses of verapamil or diltiazem, it is difficult to demonstrate any additional benefit of β receptor blockade, and excessive bradycardia, heart block, or heart failure may ensue. However, in patients treated with a dihydropyridine such as nifedipine or with nitrates, substantial reflex tachycardia often limits the effectiveness of these agents. A β receptor antagonist may be a helpful addition in this situation, resulting in a lower heart rate and blood pressure with exercise.

Relative contraindications to the use of β receptor antagonists for treatment of angina—bronchospasm, Raynaud syndrome, or Prinzmetal angina—may lead to a choice to initiate therapy with a Ca^{2+} channel blocker. Fluctuations in coronary tone are important determinants of variant angina. It is likely that episodes of

Table 27–3

Recommended Drug Therapy for Angina in Patients with Other Medical Conditions

CONDITION	RECOMMENDED TREATMENT (AND ALTERNATIVES) FOR ANGINA	DRUGS TO AVOID
Medical Conditions		
Systemic hypertension	β receptor antagonists (Ca^{2+} channel antagonists)	
Migraine or vascular headaches	β receptor antagonists (Ca^{2+} channel antagonists)	
Asthma or chronic obstructive pulmonary disease with bronchospasm	Verapamil or diltiazem	β receptor antagonists
Hyperthyroidism	β receptor antagonists	
Raynaud's syndrome	Long-acting, slow-release Ca^{2+} antagonists	β receptor antagonists
Insulin-dependent diabetes mellitus	β receptor antagonists (particularly if prior MI) or long-acting, slow-release Ca^{2+} channel antagonists	
Non-insulin-dependent diabetes mellitus	β receptor antagonists or long-acting, slow-release Ca^{2+} channel antagonists	
Depression	Long-acting, slow-release Ca^{2+} channel antagonists	β receptor antagonists
Mild peripheral vascular disease	β receptor antagonists or Ca^{2+} channel antanogists	
Severe peripheral vascular disease with rest ischemia	Ca^{2+} channel antagonists	β receptor antagonists
Cardiac Arrhythmias and Conduction Abnormalities		
Sinus bradycardia	Dihydropyridine Ca^{2+} channel antagonists	β receptor antagonists, diltiazem, verapamil
Sinus tachycardia (not due to heart failure)	β receptor antagonists	
Supraventricular tachycardia	Verapamil, diltiazem, or β receptor antagonists	
Atrioventricular block	Dihydropyridine Ca^{2+} channel antagonists	β receptor antagonists, diltiazem, verapamil
Rapid atrial fibrillation (with digitalis)	Verapamil, diltiazem, or β receptor antagonists	
Ventricular arrhythmias	β receptor antagonists	
Left Ventricular Dysfunction		
Congestive heart failure		
Mild (LVEF ≥40%)	β receptor antagonists	
Moderate to severe (LVEF <40%)	Amlodipine or felodipine (nitrates)	
Left-sided valvular heart disease		
Mild aortic stenosis	β receptor antagonists	
Aortic insufficiency	Long-acting, slow-release dihydropyridines	
Mitral regurgitation	Long-acting, slow-release dihydropyridines	
Mitral stenosis	β receptor antagonists	
Hypertrophic cardiomyopathy	β receptor antagonists, non-dihydropyridine Ca^{2+} channel antagonists	Nitrates, dihydropyridine Ca^{2+} channel antagonists

MI, myocardial infarction; LVEF, left ventricular ejection fraction. (Gibbons RJ, et al. ACC/AHA/ACP-ASIM. Guidelines for the management of patients with chronic stable angina. J Am Coll Cardiol, 1999;33:2092–197. Copyright © 1999 by the American College of Cardiology Foundation.)

increased tone, such as those precipitated by cold and by emotion, superimposed on fixed disease have a role in the variable anginal threshold seen in some patients with otherwise chronic stable angina. Increased coronary tone also may be important in the anginal episodes occurring early after MI and after coronary angioplasty, and it probably accounts for those patients with unstable angina who respond to dihydropyridines. Atherosclerotic arteries have abnormal vasomotor responses to a number of stimuli, including exercise, other forms of sympathetic activation, and cholinergic agonists; in such vessels, stenotic segments actually may become more severely stenosed during exertion. This implies that the normal exercise-induced increase in coronary flow is lost in atherosclerosis. Similar exaggerated vascular contractile responses are seen in hyperlipidemia, even before anatomical evidence of atherosclerosis develops. Because of this, coronary vasodilators (nitrates and/or Ca^{2+} channel blockers) are an important part of the therapeutic program in the majority of patients with ischemic heart disease.

Ca^{2+} Channel Blockers and Nitrates. In severe exertional or vasospastic angina, the combination of a nitrate and a Ca^{2+} channel blocker may provide additional relief over that obtained with either type of agent alone. Because nitrates primarily reduce preload, whereas Ca^{2+} channel blockers reduce afterload, the net effect on reduction of O_2 demand should be additive. However, excessive vasodilation and hypotension can occur. The concurrent administration of a nitrate and nifedipine has been advocated in particular for patients with exertional angina with heart failure, the sick-sinus syndrome, or AV nodal conduction disturbances, but excessive tachycardia may be seen.

Ca^{2+} Channel Blockers, β Receptor Antagonists, and Nitrates. In patients with exertional angina that is not controlled by the administration of 2 types of anti-anginal agents, the use of all 3 may provide improvement, although the incidence of side effects increases significantly. The dihydropyridines and nitrates dilate epicardial coronary arteries, the dihydropyridines decrease afterload, the nitrates decrease preload, and the β receptor antagonists decrease heart rate and myocardial contractility. Combining verapamil or diltiazem with a β receptor antagonist greatly increases the risk of conduction system and left ventricular dysfunction–related side effects and should be undertaken only with extreme caution.

ANTIPLATELET, ANTI-INTEGRIN, AND ANTITHROMBOTIC AGENTS

Aspirin reduces the incidence of MI and death in patients with unstable angina. In addition, low doses of aspirin appear to reduce the incidence of MI in patients with chronic stable angina. Aspirin, given in doses of 160-325 mg at the onset of treatment of MI, reduces mortality in patients presenting with unstable angina. The addition of the clopidogrel to aspirin therapy reduces mortality in patients with acute coronary syndromes; a related thienopyridine, prasugrel, has been approved for treatment of acute coronary syndromes. Heparin, in its unfractionated form and as low-molecular-weight heparin, also reduces symptoms and prevents infarction in unstable angina. Thrombin inhibitors, such as hirudin or bivalirudin, directly inhibit even clot-bound thrombin, are not affected by circulating inhibitors, and function independently of antithrombin III. Thrombolytic agents, on the other hand, are of no benefit in unstable angina. Intravenous inhibitors of the platelet GPIIb/IIIa receptor (abciximab, tirofiban, and eptifibatide) are effective in preventing the complications of PCIs and in the treatment of some patients presenting with acute coronary syndromes.

TREATMENT OF CLAUDICATION AND PERIPHERAL VASCULAR DISEASE

Most patients with peripheral vascular disease also have coronary artery disease, and the therapeutic approaches for peripheral and coronary arterial diseases overlap. Mortality in patients with peripheral vascular disease is most commonly due to cardiovascular disease, and treatment of coronary disease remains the central focus of therapy. Many patients with advanced peripheral arterial disease are more limited by the consequences of peripheral ischemia than by myocardial ischemia. In the cerebral circulation, arterial disease may be manifest as stroke or transient ischemic attacks. The painful symptoms of peripheral arterial disease in the lower extremities (claudication) typically are provoked by exertion, with increases in skeletal muscle O_2 demand exceeding blood flow impaired by proximal stenoses. When flow to the extremities becomes critically limiting, peripheral ulcers and rest pain from tissue ischemia can become debilitating.

Most of the therapies that are efficacious for treatment of coronary artery disease also have a salutary effect on progression of peripheral artery disease. Reductions in cardiovascular morbidity and mortality in patients with peripheral arterial disease have been documented with antiplatelet therapy using aspirin, clopidogrel, ticlopidine, ACE inhibitors, and treatment of hyperlipidemia. Interestingly, neither intensive treatment of diabetes mellitus nor antihypertensive therapy appears to alter the progression of symptoms of claudication. Other risk factor and lifestyle modifications remain cornerstones of therapy for patients with claudication: physical exercise, rehabilitation, and smoking cessation have proven efficacy.

Drugs used specifically in the treatment of lower-extremity claudication include pentoxifylline and cilostazol. Pentoxifylline is a methylxanthine derivative that is called a *rheologic modifier* for its effects on increasing the deformability of red blood cells. The effects of pentoxifylline on lower-extremity claudication appear to be modest. Cilostazol is an inhibitor of PDE3 and promotes accumulation of intracellular cyclic AMP in many cells, including blood platelets. Cilostazol-mediated increases in cyclic AMP inhibit platelet aggregation and promote vasodilation. The drug is metabolized by CYP3A4 and has important drug interactions with other drugs metabolized via this pathway (*see* Chapter 6). Cilostazol treatment improves symptoms of claudication but has no effect on cardiovascular mortality. As a PDE3 inhibitor, cilostazol is in the same drug class as milrinone, which had been used orally as an inotropic agent for patients with heart failure. Milrinone therapy was associated with an increase in sudden cardiac death, and the oral form of the drug was withdrawn from the market. Concerns about several other inhibitors of PDE3 (inamrinone, flosequinan) followed. Cilostazol, therefore, is labeled as being contraindicated in patients with heart failure, although it is not clear that cilostazol itself leads to increased mortality in such patients. Cilostazol has been reported to increase nonsustained ventricular tachycardia; headache is the most common side effect. Other treatments for claudication, including naftidrofuryl, propionyl levocarnitine, and prostaglandins, may also be efficacious.

MECHANO-PHARMACOLOGY: DRUG-ELUTING ENDOVASCULAR STENTS

Intracoronary stents can ameliorate angina and reduce adverse events in patients with acute coronary syndromes. However, the long-term efficacy of intracoronary stents is limited by subacute luminal restenosis within the stent, which occurs in a substantial minority of patients. The pathways that lead to "in-stent restenosis" are complex, but smooth muscle proliferation within the lumen of the stented artery is a common pathological finding.

Two drugs are currently being used on intravascular stents as localized anti-proliferative therapy: paclitaxel and sirolimus. Paclitaxel is a tricyclic diterpene that inhibits cellular proliferation by binding to and stabilizing polymerized microtubules. Sirolimus is a hydrophobic macrolide that binds to the cytosolic immunophilin FKBP12; the FKBP12–sirolimus complex inhibits the mammalian kinase target of rapamycin (mTOR), thereby inhibiting cell-cycle progression (*see* Chapter 62). Stent-induced damage to the vascular endothelial cell layer can lead to thrombosis; patients typically are treated with antiplatelet agents, including clopidogrel (for up to 6 months) and aspirin (indefinitely), sometimes in conjunction with intravenous heparin and/or GPIIb/IIIa inhibitors. The inhibition of cellular proliferation by paclitaxel and sirolimus not only affects vascular smooth muscle cell proliferation but also attenuates the formation of an intact endothelial layer within the stented artery. Therefore, antiplatelet therapy is continued for several months after intracoronary stenting with drug-eluting stents. The rate of restenosis with drug-eluting stents is reduced markedly compared with "bare metal" stents. Stent thrombosis can occur even many months after placement of the stent, sometimes temporally associated with discontinuation of antiplatelet therapy.

THERAPY OF HYPERTENSION

Hypertension is the most common cardiovascular disease; its prevalence increases with advancing age. Elevated arterial pressure causes pathological changes in the vasculature and hypertrophy of the left ventricle. Hypertension is the principal cause of stroke, a major risk factor for coronary artery disease and its complications, and a major contributor to cardiac failure, renal insufficiency, and dissecting aneurysm of the aorta.

Hypertension is defined conventionally as a sustained increase in blood pressure ≥140/90 mm Hg, a criterion that characterizes a group of patients whose risk of hypertension-related cardiovascular disease is high enough to merit medical attention. Actually, the risk of both fatal and nonfatal cardiovascular disease in adults is lowest with systolic blood pressures of <120 mm Hg and diastolic BP <80 mm Hg; these risks increase progressively with higher systolic and diastolic blood pressures (Table 27–4). Isolated systolic hypertension (sometimes defined as systolic BP >140-160 mm Hg with diastolic BP <90 mm Hg) is largely confined to people older than 60 years of age. At very high blood pressures (systolic ≥210 mm Hg and/or diastolic ≥120 mm Hg), a subset of patients develops fulminant arteriopathy characterized by endothelial injury and a marked proliferation of cells in the intima, leading to intimal thickening and ultimately to arteriolar occlusion. This is associated with rapidly progressive microvascular occlusive disease in the kidney (with renal failure), brain (hypertensive encephalopathy), congestive heart failure, and pulmonary edema. These patients typically require in-hospital management on an emergency basis for prompt lowering of blood pressure. Pharmacological treatment of patients with hypertension decreases morbidity and mortality from cardiovascular disease.

PRINCIPLES OF ANTIHYPERTENSIVE THERAPY. Nonpharmacological therapy is an important component of treatment of all patients with hypertension. In some stage 1 hypertensives, blood pressure may be adequately controlled by a combination of weight loss (in overweight individuals), restricting sodium intake, increasing aerobic exercise, and moderating consumption of alcohol. These lifestyle changes may facilitate pharmacological control of blood pressure.

Table 27–4

Criteria for Hypertension in Adults

CLASSIFICATION	BLOOD PRESSURE (mm Hg) SYSTOLIC	DIASTOLIC
Normal	<120	and <80
Prehypertension	120-139	or 80-89
Hypertension, stage 1	140-159	or 90-99
Hypertension, stage 2	≥160	or ≥100

Antihypertensive drugs can be classified according to their sites or mechanisms of action (Table 27–5). Drugs lower blood pressure by actions on peripheral resistance, cardiac output, or both (recall that arterial pressure is the product of cardiac output and peripheral vascular resistance). Drugs may decrease the cardiac output by inhibiting myocardial contractility or by decreasing ventricular filling pressure. Reduction in ventricular filling pressure may be achieved by actions on the venous tone or on blood volume via renal effects. Drugs can decrease peripheral resistance by acting on smooth muscle to cause relaxation of resistance vessels or by interfering with the activity of systems that produce constriction of resistance vessels. In patients with isolated systolic hypertension, complex hemodynamics in a rigid arterial system contribute to increased blood pressure; drug effects may be mediated by changes in peripheral resistance but also via effects on large artery stiffness.

The concurrent use of drugs from different classes is a strategy for achieving effective control of blood pressure while minimizing dose-related adverse effects. Hemodynamic consequences of longterm antihypertensive therapy provide a rationale for multidrug therapy (Table 27–6).

Table 27–5

Classification of Antihypertensive Drugs by Primary Site or Mechanism of Action

Diuretics (Chapter 25)

1. Thiazides and related agents (hydrochlorothiazide, chlorthalidone, chlorothiazide, indapamide, methylclothiazide, metolazone)
2. Loop diuretics (furosemide, bumetanide, torsemide, ethacrynic acid)
3. K^+-sparing diuretics (amiloride, triamterene, spironolactone)

Sympatholytic drugs (Chapter 12)

1. β receptor antagonists (metoprolol, atenolol, betaxolol, bisoprolol, carteolol, esmolol, nadolol, nebivolol, penbutolol, pindolol, propranolol, timolol)
2. α receptor antagonists (prazosin, terazosin, doxazosin, phenoxybenzamine, phentolamine)
3. Mixed α-β receptor antagonists (labetalol, carvedilol)
4. Centrally acting adrenergic agents (methyldopa, clonidine, guanabenz, guanfacine)
5. Adrenergic neuron blocking agents (guanadrel, reserpine)

Ca^{2+} channel blockers (verapamil, diltiazem, nisoldipine, felodipine, nicardipine, isradipine, amlodipine, clevidipine, nifedipine[a])

Angiotensin-converting enzyme inhibitors (Chapter 26; captopril, enalapril, lisinopril, quinapril, ramipril, benazepril, fosinopril, moexipril, perindopril, trandolapril)

AngII receptor antagonists (Chapter 26; losartan, candesartan, irbesartan, valsartan, telmisartan, eprosartan, olmesartan)

Direct Renin Inhibitor (Chapter 26; aliskiren)

Vasodilators

1. Arterial (hydralazine, minoxidil, diazoxide, fenoldopam)
2. Arterial and venous (nitroprusside)

[a] *Extended-release nifedipine is approved for hypertension.*

Table 27–6

Hemodynamic Effects of Long-Term Administration of Antihypertensive Agents

	HEART RATE	CARDIAC OUTPUT	TOTAL PERIPHERAL RESISTANCE	PLASMA VOLUME	PLASMA RENIN ACTIVITY
Diuretics	↔	↔	↓	–↓	↑
Sympatholytic agents					
Centrally acting	–↓	–↓	↓	–↑	–↓
Adrenergic neuron blockers	–↓	↓	↓	↑	–↑
α receptor antagonists	–↑	–↑	↓	–↑	↔
β receptor antagonists					
No IAA	↓	↓	–↓	–↑	↓
IAA	↔	↔	↓	–↑	–↓
Arteriolar vasodilators	↑	↑	↓	↑	↑
Ca^{2+} channel blockers	↓ or ↑	↓ or ↓	↓	–↑	–↑
ACE inhibitors	↔	↔	↓	↔	↑
AT_1 receptor antagonists	↔	↔	↓	↔	↑
Renin inhibitor	↔	↔	↓	↔	↓ (but [renin] ↑)

↑, increased; ↓, decreased; –↑, increased or no change; –↓, decreased or no change; ↔, unchanged. ACE, angiotensin-converting enzyme; AT_1, the type 1 receptor for angiotensin II; IAA, intrinsic agonist activity.

DIURETICS

Diuretic agents (*see* Chapter 25) have antihypertensive effects when used alone, and they enhance the efficacy of virtually all other antihypertensive drugs.

The exact mechanism for reduction of arterial blood pressure by diuretics is not certain. The drugs decrease extracellular volume by inhibiting the NaCl co-transporter (NCC) in the distal convoluted tubule, enhancing Na^+ excretion in the urine, and leading to a fall in cardiac output. However, the hypotensive effect is maintained during long-term therapy due to decreased vascular resistance; cardiac output returns to pretreatment values and extracellular volume returns almost to normal due to compensatory responses such as activation of the RAS. *Hydrochlorothiazide* may open Ca^{2+}-activated K^+ channels, leading to hyperpolarization of vascular smooth muscle cells, which leads in turn to closing of L-type Ca^{2+} channels and lower probability of opening, resulting in decreased Ca^{2+} entry and reduced vasoconstriction.

BENZOTHIADIAZIDES AND RELATED COMPOUNDS. Benzothiadiazides ("thiazides") and related diuretics are the most frequently used class of antihypertensive agents in the U.S. Following the discovery of *chlorothiazide*, a number of oral diuretics were developed that have an arylsulfonamide structure and block the NaCl co-transporter. Some of these are not benzothiadiazines but have structural features and molecular functions that are similar to the original benzothiadiazine compounds; consequently, they are designated as members of the thiazide class of diuretics. For example, chlorthalidone, one of the non-benzothiadiazines, is widely used in the treatment of hypertension, as is indapamide.

Regimen for Administration of the Thiazide-Class Diuretics in Hypertension. Antihypertensive effects can be achieved in many patients with as little as 12.5 mg daily of chlorthalidone or hydrochlorothiazide. Furthermore, when used as monotherapy, the maximal daily dose of thiazide-class diuretics usually should not exceed 25 mg of hydrochlorothiazide or chlorthalidone (or equivalent). Higher doses are not generally more efficacious in lowering blood pressure in patients with normal renal function. Urinary K^+ loss can be a problem with thiazides. ACE inhibitors and angiotensin receptor antagonists will attenuate diuretic-induced loss of K^+ to some degree, and this is a consideration if a second drug is required to achieve further blood pressure reduction beyond that attained with the diuretic alone. Because the diuretic and hypotensive effects of these drugs are greatly enhanced when they are given in combination, care should be taken to initiate combination therapy with low doses of each of these drugs. Administration of ACE inhibitors or angiotensin receptor antagonists together with other K^+-sparing agents or with K^+ supplements requires great caution; combining K^+-sparing agents with each other or with K^+ supplementation can cause potentially dangerous hyperkalemia in some patients.

Treatment of severe hypertension that is unresponsive to 3 or more drugs may require larger doses of the thiazide-class diuretics. Hypertensive patients may become refractory to drugs that block the sympathetic nervous system or to vasodilator drugs, because these drugs engender a state in which the blood pressure is very volume-dependent. Therefore, it is appropriate to consider the use of thiazide-class diuretics in doses of 50 mg of daily hydrochlorothiazide equivalent when treatment with appropriate combinations and doses of 3 or more drugs fails to yield adequate control of the blood pressure. Alternatively, there may be a need to use higher-capacity diuretics such as furosemide, especially if renal function is not normal, in some of these patients. Dietary Na^+ restriction is a valuable adjunct to the management of such refractory patients and will minimize the dose of diuretic that is required. Because the degree of K^+ loss relates to the amount of Na^+ delivered to the distal tubule, such restriction of Na^+ can minimize the development of hypokalemia and alkalosis. The effectiveness of thiazides as diuretics or antihypertensive agents is progressively diminished when the glomerular filtration rate falls below 30 mL/min. One exception is metolazone, which retains efficacy in patients with this degree of renal insufficiency.

Most patients will respond to thiazide diuretics with a reduction in blood pressure within about 4-6 weeks. Therefore, doses should not be increased more often than every 4-6 weeks. Because the effect of thiazide diuretics is additive with that of other antihypertensive drugs, combination regimens that include these diuretics are common and rational. A wide range of fixed-dose combination products containing a thiazide are marketed for this purpose. Diuretics also have the advantage of minimizing the retention of salt and water that is commonly caused by vasodilators and some sympatholytic drugs. Omitting or underutilizing a diuretic is a frequent cause of "resistant hypertension."

Adverse Effects and Precautions. The adverse effects of diuretics are discussed in Chapter 25. Erectile dysfunction is a troublesome adverse effect of the thiazide-class diuretics. Gout may be a consequence of the hyperuricemia induced by these diuretics. Precipitation of acute gout is relatively uncommon with low doses of diuretics. Hydrochlorothiazide may cause rapidly developing, severe hyponatremia in some patients. Thiazides inhibit renal Ca^{2+} excretion, occasionally leading to hypercalcemia; although generally mild, this can be more severe in patients with primary hyperparathyroidism. The thiazide-induced decreased Ca^{2+} excretion may be used therapeutically in patients with osteoporosis or hypercalciuria.

Two types of ventricular arrhythmias may be enhanced by K^+ depletion. One of these is polymorphic ventricular tachycardia (*torsade de pointes*), which is induced by a number of drugs, including quinidine. Because K^+ currents normally mediate repolarization, drugs that produce K^+ depletion potentiate polymorphic ventricular tachycardia. The second is ischemic ventricular fibrillation, the leading cause of sudden cardiac death and a major contributor to cardiovascular mortality in treated hypertensive patients. There is a positive correlation between diuretic dose and sudden cardiac death, and an inverse correlation between the use of adjunctive K^+-sparing agents and sudden cardiac death. All of the thiazide-like drugs cross the placenta but they have not been shown to have direct adverse effects on the fetus. If administration of a thiazide is begun during pregnancy, there is a risk of transient volume depletion that may result in placental hypoperfusion. Because the thiazides appear in breast milk, they should be avoided by nursing mothers.

OTHER DIURETIC ANTIHYPERTENSIVE AGENTS. The thiazide diuretics are more effective antihypertensive agents than are the loop diuretics, such as furosemide and bumetanide in patients who have normal renal function. This differential effect likely relates to the short duration of action of loop diuretics, such that a single daily dose does not cause a significant net loss of Na^+ for an entire 24-h period. Indeed, loop diuretics are frequently and inappropriately prescribed as a once-daily medication in the treatment of hypertension, congestive heart failure, and ascites. The spectacular efficacy of the loop diuretics in producing a rapid and profound natriuresis can be detrimental for the treatment of hypertension. When a loop diuretic is given twice daily, the acute diuresis can be excessive and lead to more side effects than with a slower-acting, milder thiazide diuretic. Loop diuretics may be particularly useful in patients with azotemia or with severe edema associated with a vasodilator such as minoxidil.

Amiloride is a K^+-sparing diuretic that has some efficacy in lowering blood pressure in patients with hypertension. Spironolactone lowers blood pressure but has some significant adverse effects, especially in men (e.g., erectile dysfunction, gynecomastia, benign prostatic hyperplasia). Eplerenone is a newer aldosterone receptor antagonist that does not have the sexually related adverse effects. Triamterene is a K^+-sparing diuretic that decreases the risk of hypokalemia in patients treated with a thiazide diuretic but does not have efficacy in lowering blood pressure by itself. These agents should be used cautiously with frequent measurements of K^+ concentrations in plasma in patients predisposed to hyperkalemia. Patients should be cautioned regarding the concurrent use of K^+-containing salt substitutes. Renal insufficiency is a relative contraindication to the use of K^+-sparing diuretics. *Concomitant use of an ACE inhibitor or an angiotensin receptor antagonist magnifies the risk of hyperkalemia with these agents.*

DIURETIC-ASSOCIATED DRUG INTERACTIONS. The K^+- and Mg^{2+}-depleting effects of the thiazides and loop diuretics can potentiate arrhythmias that arise from digitalis toxicity. Corticosteroids can amplify the hypokalemia produced by the diuretics. All diuretics can decrease the clearance of Li^+, resulting in increased plasma concentrations of Li^+ and potential toxicity. NSAIDs (*see* Chapter 34), including selective COX-2 inhibitors, that inhibit the synthesis of prostaglandins reduce the antihypertensive effects of diuretics. NSAIDs, β receptor antagonists, and ACE inhibitors reduce plasma concentrations of aldosterone and can potentiate the hyperkalemic effects of a K^+-sparing diuretic.

SYMPATHOLYTIC AGENTS

Antagonists of α and β adrenergic receptors are mainstays of antihypertensive therapy (*see* Table 27–5).

β ADRENERGIC RECEPTOR ANTAGONISTS

β Adrenergic receptor antagonists have antihypertensive effects. Antagonism of β adrenergic receptors affects the regulation of the circulation through a number of mechanisms, including a reduction in myocardial contractility, heart rate, and cardiac output. An important consequence is blockade of the β_1 receptors of the juxtaglomerular complex, reducing renin secretion and thereby diminishing production of circulating AngII. Some β receptor antagonists may lower blood pressure by other mechanisms. For example, labetalol is also an α_1 receptor antagonist, and nebivolol promotes endothelium-dependent vasodilation via activation of the NO pathway.

Pharmacological Effects. The β adrenergic blockers vary in their selectivity for the β_1 receptor subtype, presence of partial agonist or intrinsic sympathomimetic activity, and vasodilating capacity. These differences do influence the clinical pharmacokinetics and spectrum of adverse effects of the various drugs. Drugs without intrinsic sympathomimetic activity produce an initial reduction in cardiac output and a reflex-induced rise in peripheral resistance, generally with no net change in arterial pressure. Persistently reduced cardiac output and possibly decreased peripheral resistance accounts for the reduction in arterial pressure. Drugs with intrinsic sympathomimetic activity produce lesser decreases in resting heart rate and cardiac output; the fall in arterial pressure correlates with a fall in vascular resistance below pretreatment levels, possibly because of stimulation of vascular β_2 receptors that mediate vasodilation.

Adverse Effects and Precautions. The adverse effects of β adrenergic blocking agents are discussed in Chapter 12. These drugs should be avoided in patients with asthma or with SA or AV nodal dysfunction or in combination with other drugs that inhibit AV conduction, such as verapamil. The risk of hypoglycemic reactions may be increased in diabetics taking insulin. β Receptor antagonists without intrinsic sympathomimetic activity increase concentrations of triglycerides in plasma and lower those of HDL cholesterol without changing total cholesterol concentrations. β receptor blocking agents with intrinsic sympathomimetic activity have little or no effect on blood lipids or increase HDL cholesterol.

Sudden discontinuation of β adrenergic blockers can produce a withdrawal syndrome that is likely due to upregulation of β receptors causing enhanced tissue sensitivity to endogenous catecholamines; this can exacerbate the symptoms of coronary artery disease or cause rebound hypertension. Thus, β adrenergic blockers should be tapered gradually over 10-14 days.

NSAIDs such as *indomethacin* can blunt the antihypertensive effect of propranolol and probably other β receptor antagonists. This effect may be related to inhibition of vascular synthesis of prostacyclin, as well as to retention of Na^+.

Epinephrine can produce severe hypertension and bradycardia when a nonselective β antagonist is present due to the unopposed stimulation of α adrenergic receptors when vascular β_2 receptors are blocked. The bradycardia is the result of reflex vagal stimulation. Such hypertensive responses to β receptor antagonists have been observed in patients with hypoglycemia or pheochromocytoma, during withdrawal from *clonidine*, following administration of epinephrine as a therapeutic agent, or in association with the illicit use of cocaine.

Therapeutic Uses. The β receptor antagonists provide effective therapy for all grades of hypertension. The antihypertensive effect of all the β blockers is of sufficient duration to permit once- or twice-daily administration. Populations that tend to have a lesser antihypertensive response to β blocking agents include the elderly and African Americans. However, intra-individual differences in antihypertensive efficacy are generally much larger than differences between racial or age-related groups. The β receptor antagonists usually do not cause retention of salt and water, but do have additive antihypertensive effects when combined with diuretics. β receptor antagonists are preferred drugs for hypertensive patients with conditions such as MI, ischemic heart disease, or congestive heart failure.

α_1 ADRENERGIC RECEPTOR ANTAGONISTS

Drugs that selectively block α_1 adrenergic receptors without affecting α_2 adrenergic receptors are used in hypertension. Prazosin, terazosin, and doxazosin are the agents that are available for the treatment of hypertension.

Pharmacological Effects. Initially, α_1 adrenergic receptor antagonists reduce arteriolar resistance and increase venous capacitance; this causes a sympathetically mediated reflex increase in heart rate and plasma renin activity. During long-term therapy, vasodilation persists, but cardiac output, heart rate, and plasma renin activity return to normal. Renal blood flow is unchanged during therapy. The α_1 adrenergic blockers cause a variable amount of postural hypotension, depending on the plasma volume. Retention of salt and water occurs in many patients during continued administration, and this attenuates the postural hypotension. α_1 Receptor antagonists reduce plasma concentrations of triglycerides and total LDL cholesterol and increase HDL cholesterol. These potentially favorable effects on lipids persist when a thiazide-type diuretic is given concurrently. The long-term consequences of these small, drug-induced changes in lipids are unknown.

Adverse Effects. The use of doxazosin as monotherapy for hypertension increases the risk for developing congestive heart failure. This may be an adverse effect of all of the α_1 receptor antagonists. A major precaution regarding the use of the α_1 receptor antagonists for hypertension is the so-called first-dose phenomenon, in which symptomatic orthostatic hypotension occurs within 30-90 min (or longer) of the initial dose of the drug or after a dosage increase. This effect may occur in up to 50% of patients, especially in patients who are already receiving a diuretic or an α receptor antagonist. After the first few doses, patients develop a tolerance to this marked hypotensive response.

Therapeutic Uses. α_1 Receptor antagonists are not recommended as monotherapy for hypertensive patients but are used primarily in conjunction with diuretics, β blockers, and other antihypertensive agents. β Receptor antagonists enhance the efficacy of the α_1 blockers. α_1 Receptor antagonists are not the drugs of choice in patients with pheochromocytoma, because a vasoconstrictor response to epinephrine can still result from activation of unblocked vascular α_2 adrenergic receptors. α_1 Receptor antagonists improve urinary symptoms in hypertensive patients with benign prostatic hyperplasia.

COMBINED α_1 AND β ADRENERGIC RECEPTOR ANTAGONISTS

Labetalol (*see* Chapter 12) is an equimolar mixture of 4 stereoisomers. One isomer is an α_1 antagonist (like prazosin), another is a nonselective β antagonist with partial agonist activity (like pindolol), and the other 2 isomers are inactive. Because of its capacity to block α_1 adrenergic receptors, labetalol given intravenously can reduce blood pressure sufficiently rapidly to be useful for the treatment of hypertensive emergencies. Labetalol has efficacy and adverse effects that would be expected with any combination of β and α_1 receptor antagonists.

Carvedilol (*see* Chapter 12) is a β receptor antagonist with α_1 receptor antagonist activity. The drug has been approved for the treatment of hypertension and symptomatic heart failure. The ratio of α_1 to β receptor antagonist potency for carvedilol is approximately 1:10. Carvedilol is oxidized by hepatic CYP2D6 and then glucuronidated. Carvedilol reduces mortality in patients with congestive heart failure associated with systolic dysfunction when used as an adjunct to therapy with diuretics and ACE inhibitors. It should not be given to those patients with decompensated heart failure who are dependent on sympathetic stimulation. As with labetalol, the side effects of carvedilol in hypertension are predictable based on its properties as a β and α_1 adrenergic receptor antagonist.

Nebivolol is a β_1-selective adrenergic antagonist that also promotes vasodilatation; nebivolol augments arterial smooth muscle relaxation via NO, and has agonist activity at β_3 receptors, although the clinical significance of this effect is not known.

METHYLDOPA

Methyldopa is a centrally acting antihypertensive agent. It is a prodrug that exerts its antihypertensive action via an active metabolite. Methyldopa's significant adverse effects limit its current use largely to treatment of hypertension in pregnancy, where it has a record for safety.

Methyldopa is metabolized by the L-aromatic amino acid decarboxylase in adrenergic neurons to α-methyldopamine, which then is converted to α-methylnorepinephrine (α-CH_3-NE). α-CH_3-NE is stored in the secretory vesicles of adrenergic neurons, substituting for NE. Thus, when the adrenergic neuron discharges its neurotransmitter, α-CH_3-NE is released instead of NE. α-CH_3-NE acts in the CNS to inhibit adrenergic neuronal outflow from the brainstem and probably acts as an agonist at presynaptic α_2 adrenergic receptors in the brainstem, attenuating NE release and thereby reducing the output of vasoconstrictor adrenergic signals to the peripheral sympathetic nervous system.

ADME. Because methyldopa is a prodrug that is metabolized in the brain to the active form, its concentration in plasma has less relevance for its effects than that for many other drugs. Peak concentrations in plasma occur after 2-3 h. The drug is eliminated with a $t_{1/2}$ of ~2 h but is prolonged to 4-6 h in patients with renal failure. The peak effect of methyldopa is delayed for 6-8 h, even after intravenous administration, and the duration of action of a single dose is usually about 24 h; this permits once- or twice-daily dosing. The discrepancy between the effects of methyldopa and the measured concentrations of the drug in plasma is most likely related to the time required for transport into the CNS, conversion to the active metabolite, storage of α-CH_3-NE and its subsequent release at relevant α_2 receptors in the CNS.

Adverse Effects and Precautions. Methyldopa produces sedation that is largely transient; depression occurs occasionally. Methyldopa may produce dryness of the mouth, diminished libido, parkinsonian signs, and hyperprolactinemia that may become sufficiently pronounced to cause gynecomastia and galactorrhea. Methyldopa may precipitate severe bradycardia and sinus arrest. Hepatotoxicity, sometimes associated with fever, is an uncommon but potentially serious toxic effect of methyldopa. At least 20% of patients who receive methyldopa for a year develop a positive Coombs test (antiglobulin test) that is due to autoantibodies directed against the Rh antigen on erythrocytes; 1-5% of these patients will develop a hemolytic anemia that requires prompt discontinuation of the drug. The Coombs test may remain positive for as long as a year after discontinuation of methyldopa, but the hemolytic anemia usually resolves within a matter of weeks. Severe hemolysis may be attenuated by treatment with glucocorticoids. Rarer adverse effects include leukopenia, thrombocytopenia, red cell aplasia, lupus erythematosus–like syndrome, lichenoid and granulomatous skin eruptions, myocarditis, retroperitoneal fibrosis, pancreatitis, diarrhea, and malabsorption.

Therapeutic Uses. Methyldopa is a preferred drug for treatment of hypertension during pregnancy based on its effectiveness and safety for both mother and fetus. The usual initial dose of methyldopa is 250 mg twice daily, and there is little additional effect with doses >2 g/day.

CLONIDINE, GUANABENZ, AND GUANFACINE

The detailed pharmacology of the α_2 adrenergic agonists clonidine, *guanabenz*, and *guanfacine* is discussed in Chapter 12. These drugs stimulate the α_{2A} subtype of α_2 adrenergic receptors in the brainstem, resulting in a reduction in sympathetic outflow from the CNS. Patients who have had a spinal cord transection above the level of the sympathetic outflow tracts do not display a hypotensive response to clonidine. At doses higher than those required to stimulate central α_{2A} receptors, these drugs can activate α_2 receptors of the α_{2B} subtype on vascular smooth muscle cells. This effect accounts for the initial vasoconstriction that is seen when overdoses of these drugs are taken, and may be responsible for the loss of therapeutic effect that is observed with high doses.

Pharmacological Effects. The α_2 adrenergic agonists lower arterial pressure by an effect on both cardiac output and peripheral resistance. In the supine position, when the sympathetic tone to the vasculature is low, the major effect is to reduce both heart rate and stroke volume; however, in the upright position, when sympathetic outflow to the vasculature is normally increased, these drugs reduce vascular resistance and may lead to postural hypotension. The decrease in cardiac sympathetic tone leads to a reduction in myocardial contractility and heart rate that could promote congestive heart failure in susceptible patients.

Adverse Effects and Precautions. Sedation and xerostomia are prominent adverse effects. The xerostomia may be accompanied by dry nasal mucosa, dry eyes, and parotid gland swelling and pain. Postural hypotension and erectile dysfunction may be prominent in some patients. Clonidine may produce a lower incidence of dry mouth and sedation when given transdermally. Less common CNS side effects include sleep disturbances with vivid dreams or nightmares, restlessness, and depression. Cardiac effects related to the sympatholytic action of these drugs include symptomatic bradycardia and sinus arrest in patients with dysfunction of the SA node and AV block in patients with AV nodal disease or in patients taking other drugs that depress AV conduction. Some 15-20% of patients who receive transdermal clonidine may develop contact dermatitis.

Sudden discontinuation of clonidine and related α_2 adrenergic agonists may cause a withdrawal syndrome consisting of headache, apprehension, tremors, abdominal pain, sweating, and tachycardia. The arterial blood pressure may rise to levels above those that were present prior to treatment. Symptoms typically occur 18-36 h after the drug is stopped and are associated with increased sympathetic discharge. The withdrawal syndrome is likely dose related and more dangerous in patients with poorly controlled hypertension. In the absence of life-threatening target organ damage, patients can be treated by restoring the use of clonidine. If a more rapid effect is required, *sodium nitroprusside* or a combination of an α and β adrenergic blocker is appropriate. β Adrenergic blocking agents should not be used alone in this setting, because they may accentuate the hypertension by allowing unopposed α adrenergic vasoconstriction caused by activation of the sympathetic nervous system.

Surgical patients who are being treated with an α_2 adrenergic agonist either should be switched to another drug prior to elective surgery or should receive their morning dose and/or transdermal clonidine prior to the procedure. All patients who receive one of these drugs should be warned of the potential danger of discontinuing the drug abruptly, and patients suspected of being noncompliant with medications should not be given α_2

adrenergic agonists for hypertension. Adverse drug interactions with α_2 adrenergic agonists are rare. Diuretics predictably potentiate the hypotensive effect of these drugs. Tricyclic antidepressants may inhibit the antihypertensive effect of clonidine, but the mechanism of this interaction is not known.

Therapeutic Uses. The CNS effects are such that this class of drugs is not a leading option for monotherapy of hypertension. They effectively lower blood pressure in some patients who have not responded adequately to combinations of other agents.

GUANADREL

Guanadrel specifically inhibits the function of peripheral postganglionic adrenergic neurons. It is an exogenous false neurotransmitter that is accumulated, stored, and released like NE but is inactive at adrenergic receptors. In the neuron, guanadrel is concentrated within the adrenergic storage vesicle, where it replaces NE. Because guanadrel can promote NE release from pheochromocytomas, it is contraindicated in those patients.

Pharmacological Effects. The antihypertensive effect is achieved by a reduction in peripheral vascular resistance that results from inhibition of α receptor–mediated vasoconstriction. Arterial pressure is reduced modestly in the supine position when sympathetic activity is usually low, but the pressure can fall to a greater extent during situations in which reflex sympathetic activation is an important mechanism for maintaining arterial pressure, particularly when standing.

ADME. The maximum effect on blood pressure is not seen until 4-5 h. The $t_{1/2}$ of the pharmacological effect of guanadrel is determined by the drug's persistence in this neuronal pool and is at least 10 h.

Adverse Effects. Guanadrel produces undesirable effects that are related to sympathetic blockade such as symptomatic hypotension during standing, exercise, ingestion of alcohol, or in hot weather. A general feeling of fatigue and lassitude is partially related to postural hypotension. Sexual dysfunction usually presents as delayed or retrograde ejaculation. Diarrhea also may occur. Drugs that block or compete for the catecholamine transporter on the presynaptic membrane (e.g., tricyclic antidepressants *cocaine*, *chlorpromazine*, *ephedrine*, *phenylpropanolamine*, and *amphetamine; see* Chapter 8) also will inhibit the effect of guanadrel.

Therapeutic Uses. Because of the availability of a number of drugs that lower blood pressure without producing similar adverse effects, guanadrel is used very rarely; the drug is no longer marketed in the U.S.

RESERPINE

Reserpine is an alkaloid extracted from the root of *Rauwolfia serpentina*. Reserpine inhibits the vesicular catecholamine transporter, VMAT2, so that nerve endings lose their capacity to concentrate and store NE and dopamine. Catecholamines leak into the cytoplasm, where they are metabolized. Consequently, little or no active transmitter is released from nerve endings, resulting in a pharmacological sympathectomy. Recovery of sympathetic function requires synthesis of new storage vesicles, which takes days to weeks after discontinuation of the drug. Reserpine depletes amines in the CNS as well as in the peripheral adrenergic neuron and its antihypertensive effects may be related to both central and peripheral actions.

Pharmacological Effects. Both cardiac output and peripheral vascular resistance are reduced during long-term therapy with reserpine.

ADME. Data available on the pharmacokinetic properties of reserpine are limited because of the lack of an assay capable of detecting low concentrations of the drug or its metabolites. Since reserpine binding is irreversible, the amount of drug in plasma is unlikely to bear any consistent relationship to drug concentration at the site of action. Free reserpine is entirely metabolized.

Toxicity and Precautions. Most adverse effects of reserpine are due to its effect on the CNS. Sedation and inability to concentrate or perform complex tasks are the most common adverse effects. More serious is the occasional psychotic depression that can lead to suicide. Reserpine must be discontinued at the first sign of depression; reserpine-induced depression may last several months after the drug is discontinued. The risk of depression is likely dose related and is uncommon with doses of 0.25 mg/day or less. Other adverse effects include nasal stuffiness and exacerbation of peptic ulcer disease, which is uncommon with small oral doses.

Therapeutic Uses. The use of reserpine has diminished because of its CNS side effects. Reserpine is used once daily with a diuretic, and several weeks are necessary to achieve a maximum effect. The daily dose should be limited to 0.25 mg or less, and as little as 0.05 mg/day may be efficacious when a diuretic is also used.

METYROSINE

Metyrosine (DEMSER), α-methyl-L-tyrosine, inhibits tyrosine hydroxylase, the enzyme that catalyzes the conversion of tyrosine to DOPA and the rate-limiting step in catecholamine biosynthesis (*see* Chapter 8).

At a dose of 1-4 g/day, metyrosine decreases catecholamine biosynthesis by 35-80% in patients with pheochromocytoma. The maximal decrease in synthesis occurs only after several days and may be assessed by measurements of urinary catecholamines and their metabolites. Metyrosine is used as an adjuvant to phenoxybenzamine and other α adrenergic blocking agents for the management of pheochromocytoma and in the preoperative preparation of patients for resection of pheochromocytoma. Metyrosine carries a risk of crystalluria, which can be minimized by maintaining a daily urine volume of >2 L. Other adverse effects include orthostatic hypotension, sedation, extrapyramidal signs, diarrhea, anxiety, and psychic disturbances. Doses must be titrated carefully to minimize these side effects.

Ca^{2+} CHANNEL ANTAGONISTS

Ca^{2+} channel blocking agents are important drugs for the treatment of hypertension. The pharmacology of these drugs is presented earlier in this chapter. Because contraction of vascular smooth muscle is dependent on the free intracellular concentration of Ca^{2+}, inhibition of transmembrane movement of Ca^{2+} through voltage-sensitive Ca^{2+} channels can decrease the total amount of Ca^{2+} that reaches intracellular sites. Ca^{2+} channel blockers lower blood pressure by relaxing arteriolar smooth muscle and decreasing peripheral vascular resistance; however, this evokes a baroreceptor-mediated sympathetic discharge. With dihydropyridines, tachycardia may occur from the adrenergic stimulation of the SA node. Tachycardia is typically minimal to absent with verapamil and diltiazem because of the direct negative chronotropic effect of these 2 drugs. Indeed, the concurrent use of a β receptor antagonist drug may magnify negative chronotropic effects of these drugs or cause heart block in susceptible patients.

Ca^{2+} channel blockers are effective when used alone or in combination with other drugs for the treatment of hypertension. However, there is no place in the treatment of hypertension for the use of nifedipine or other dihydropyridine Ca^{2+} channel blockers with short half-lives, administered in a standard (immediate-release) formulation, because of the oscillation in blood pressure and concurrent surges in sympathetic reflex activity within each dosage interval. Parenteral administration of the dihydropyridine clevidipine may be useful in treating severe or perioperative hypertension. Compared with other classes of antihypertensive agents, there may be a greater frequency of achieving blood pressure control with Ca^{2+} channel blockers as monotherapy in elderly subjects and in African Americans, population groups in which the low renin status is more prevalent. Ca^{2+} channel blockers are effective in lowering blood pressure and decreasing cardiovascular events in the elderly with isolated systolic hypertension.

ANGIOTENSIN-CONVERTING ENZYME INHIBITORS

Angiotensin II is an important regulator of cardiovascular function (*see* Chapter 26). ACE inhibitors include captopril, enalapril, lisinopril, quinapril, ramipril, benazepril, moexipril, fosinopril, trandolapril, and perindopril. Chapter 26 presents the pharmacology of ACE inhibitors in detail. The ACE inhibitors appear to confer a special advantage in the treatment of patients with diabetes, slowing the development and progression of diabetic glomerulopathy. They also are effective in slowing the progression of other forms of chronic renal disease, such as glomerulosclerosis; many of these patients also have hypertension. An ACE inhibitor is the preferred initial agent in these patients. Patients with hypertension and ischemic heart disease are candidates for treatment with ACE inhibitors; administration of ACE inhibitors in the immediate post-MI period has been shown to improve ventricular function and reduce morbidity and mortality (*see* Chapter 28).

Because ACE inhibitors blunt the rise in aldosterone concentrations in response to Na^+ loss, the normal role of aldosterone to oppose diuretic-induced natriuresis is diminished. Consequently, ACE inhibitors tend to enhance the efficacy of diuretic drugs. Thus, even very small doses of diuretics may substantially improve the antihypertensive efficacy of ACE inhibitors; conversely, the use of high doses of diuretics together with ACE inhibitors may lead to excessive reduction in blood pressure and Na^+ loss. The attenuation of aldosterone production by ACE inhibitors also influences K^+ homeostasis; substantial retention of K^+ can occur in some patients with renal insufficiency. Furthermore, the potential for developing hyperkalemia should be considered when ACE inhibitors are used with other drugs that can cause K^+ retention, including the K^+-sparing diuretics (amiloride, triamterene, and spironolactone), NSAIDs, K^+ supplements, and β receptor antagonists. Patients with diabetic nephropathy may be at greater risk of hyperkalemia. Angioedema is a rare but serious and potentially fatal adverse effect of the ACE inhibitors. ACE inhibitors are contraindicated during pregnancy.

In most patients, there is no appreciable change in glomerular filtration rate following the administration of ACE inhibitors. However, in renovascular hypertension, the glomerular filtration rate is generally maintained as the result of increased resistance in the postglomerular arteriole caused by AngII. Accordingly, in patients with bilateral renal artery stenosis or stenosis in a sole kidney, the administration of an ACE inhibitor will reduce the filtration fraction and cause a substantial reduction in glomerular filtration rate.

ACE inhibitors lower the blood pressure to some extent in most patients with hypertension. Following the initial dose of an ACE inhibitor, there may be a considerable fall in blood pressure in some patients; this response to the initial dose is a function of plasma renin activity prior to treatment. The potential for a large initial drop in blood pressure is the reason for using a low dose to initiate therapy, especially in patients who may have a very active RAS supporting blood pressure, such as patients with diuretic-induced volume contraction or congestive heart failure. With continuing treatment, there usually is a progressive fall in blood pressure that in most patients does not reach a maximum for several weeks. The blood pressure seen during chronic treatment is not strongly correlated with the pretreatment plasma renin activity. While most ACE inhibitors are approved for once-daily dosing for hypertension, a significant fraction of patients has a response that lasts <24 h and may require twice-daily dosing for adequate control of blood pressure.

AT_1 RECEPTOR ANTAGONISTS

Nonpeptide antagonists of the AT_1 AngII receptor approved for treatment of hypertension include losartan, candesartan, irbesartan, valsartan, telmisartan, olmesartan, eprosartan, and azilsartan. The pharmacology of AT_1 receptor antagonists is presented in detail in Chapter 26. By antagonizing the effects of AngII, these agents permit relaxation of smooth muscle and vasodilation, increase renal salt and water excretion, reduce plasma volume, and decrease cellular hypertrophy.

There are 2 distinct subtypes of AngII receptors, AT_1 and AT_2. Because the AT_1 receptor mediates feedback inhibition of renin release, renin and AngII concentrations are increased during AT_1 receptor antagonism. The clinical consequences of increased AngII effects on an uninhibited AT_2 receptor are unknown; however, emerging data suggest that the AT_2 receptor may elicit antigrowth and antiproliferative responses.

Adverse Effects and Precautions. Adverse effects of ACE inhibitors that result from inhibiting AngII-related functions (*see* above and Chapter 26) also occur with AT_1 receptor antagonists. These include hypotension, hyperkalemia, and reduced renal function, including that associated with bilateral renal artery stenosis and stenosis in the artery of a solitary kidney. Cough, an adverse effect of ACE inhibitors, is less frequent with AT_1 receptor antagonists. Angioedema occurs very rarely.

Therapeutic Uses. When given in adequate doses, the AT_1 receptor antagonists appear to be as effective as ACE inhibitors in the treatment of hypertension. The full effect of AT_1 receptor antagonists on blood pressure typically is not observed until about 4 weeks after the initiation of therapy. If blood pressure is not controlled by an AT_1 receptor antagonist alone, a second drug acting by a different mechanism (e.g., a diuretic or Ca^{2+} channel blocker) may be added. The combination of an ACE inhibitor and an AT_1 receptor antagonist is not recommended.

DIRECT RENIN INHIBITORS

Aliskiren is an orally effective direct renin inhibitor that lowers blood pressure in patients with hypertension. The detailed pharmacology of aliskiren is covered in Chapter 26.

Pharmacological Effects. Aliskiren directly and competitively inhibits the catalytic activity of renin, which leads to diminished production of AngI—and ultimately AngII and aldosterone—with a resulting fall in blood pressure. Aliskiren along with ACE inhibitors and AT_1 receptor antagonists lead to an adaptive increase in the plasma concentrations of renin; however, because aliskiren inhibits renin activity, plasma renin activity does not increase as occurs with these other classes of drugs (*see* Table 26–1).

Absorption, Metabolism, and Excretion. Aliskiren is poorly absorbed; bioavailability is <3%. High-fat meal may substantially decrease plasma concentrations of the drug. The $t_{1/2}$ is at least 24 h. Elimination of the drug may be primarily through hepatobiliary excretion with limited metabolism via CYP3A4.

Therapeutic Uses. Aliskiren (TEKTURNA) is effective as monotherapy in treating patients with hypertension with dose-dependent increasing efficacy at 150-300 mg/day. The combination of aliskiren with hydrochlorothiazide has a greater lowering effect on blood pressure than either drug alone. Aliskiren appears to have greater efficacy when added to other agents in the treatment of hypertension, including ACE inhibitors, AT_1 receptor antagonists, and Ca^{2+} channel blockers. Combination therapy of aliskiren with ACE inhibitors or ARBs is contraindicated in patients with diabetes or kidney impairment due to increased risk of hyperkalemia, hypotension, and renal complications. Overall, aliskiren appears to be well tolerated.

VASODILATORS

HYDRALAZINE

Hydralazine directly relaxes arteriolar smooth muscle. The molecular mechanisms mediating this action are not clear but may ultimately involve a fall in intracellular Ca^{2+} concentrations. The drug does not relax venous smooth muscle. Hydralazine-induced vasodilation is associated with powerful stimulation of the sympathetic nervous system, likely due to baroreceptor-mediated reflexes, which results in increased heart rate and contractility, and increased plasma renin activity; all of these effects tend to counteract the antihypertensive effect of hydralazine.

The decrease in blood pressure after administration of hydralazine is associated with a selective decrease in vascular resistance in the coronary, cerebral, and renal circulations, with a smaller effect in skin and muscle. Because of preferential dilation of arterioles over veins, postural hypotension is not a common problem; hydralazine lowers blood pressure similarly in the supine and upright positions.

Absorption, Metabolism, and Excretion. Hydralazine is well absorbed through the GI tract, but the systemic bioavailability is low (16% in fast acetylators and 35% in slow acetylators). Hydralazine is *N*-acetylated in the bowel and/or the liver. Although its $t_{1/2}$ in plasma is ~1 h, the duration of the hypotensive effect of hydralazine can last up to 12 h. Systemic clearance of the drug is ~50 mL/kg/min. The rate of acetylation is genetically determined; about half of the U.S. population acetylates rapidly, and half do so slowly. The acetylated compound is inactive; thus, the dose necessary to produce a systemic effect is larger in fast acetylators (acetylation rate is genetically determined; *see* Figure 56–4). The peak concentration of hydralazine in plasma and the peak hypotensive effect of the drug occur within 30-120 min of ingestion.

Toxicity and Precautions. Adverse effects of the drug, include headache, nausea, flushing, hypotension, palpitations, tachycardia, dizziness, and angina pectoris. Myocardial ischemia can occur on account of increased O_2 demand induced by the baroreceptor reflex-induced stimulation of the sympathetic nervous system. Following parenteral administration to patients with coronary artery disease, the myocardial ischemia may be sufficiently severe and protracted to cause frank MI. For this reason, parenteral administration of hydralazine is not advisable in hypertensive patients with coronary artery disease, hypertensive patients with multiple cardiovascular risk factors, or older patients. In addition, if the drug is used alone, there may be salt retention with development of high-output congestive heart failure. When combined with a β adrenergic receptor blocker and a diuretic, hydralazine is better tolerated.

Other adverse effects are caused by immunological reactions, of which the drug-induced lupus syndrome is the most common. Hydralazine also can result in an illness that resembles serum sickness, hemolytic anemia, vasculitis, and rapidly progressive glomerulonephritis. The mechanism of these autoimmune reactions is unknown. The drug-induced lupus syndrome usually occurs after at least 6 months of continuous treatment with hydralazine, and its incidence is related to dose, sex, acetylator phenotype, and race. Discontinuation of the drug is all that is necessary for most patients with the hydralazine-induced lupus syndrome, but symptoms may persist in a few patients, and administration of corticosteroids may be necessary. Hydralazine also can produce a pyridoxine-responsive polyneuropathy. The mechanism appears to be related to the ability of hydralazine to combine with pyridoxine to form a hydrazone. This side effect is very unusual with doses ≤200 mg/day.

Therapeutic Uses. Due to its relatively unfavorable adverse-effect profile, hydralazine is no longer a first-line drug in the treatment of hypertension. The drug is marketed as a combination pill containing isosorbide dinitrate (BiDil) that is used for the treatment of heart failure (*see* Chapter 28). Hydralazine may have utility in the treatment of some patients with congestive heart failure (in combination with nitrates for patients who cannot tolerate ACE inhibitors or AT_1 receptor antagonists), and may be useful in the treatment of hypertensive emergencies in pregnant women (especially preeclampsia). Hydralazine should be used with the great caution in elderly patients and in hypertensive patients with coronary artery disease because of the possibility of precipitation of myocardial ischemia due to reflex tachycardia. The usual oral dosage of hydralazine is 25-100 mg twice daily. The maximum recommended dose of hydralazine is 200 mg/day to minimize the risk of drug-induced lupus syndrome.

K_{ATP} CHANNEL OPENERS: MINOXIDIL

Minoxidil is efficacious in patients with the most severe and drug-resistant forms of hypertension. Minoxidil is metabolized by hepatic sulfotransferase to the active molecule, minoxidil *N-O* sulfate. Minoxidil sulfate activates the ATP-modulated K^+ channel. By opening K^+ channels in smooth muscle and thereby permitting K^+ efflux, it causes hyperpolarization and relaxation of smooth muscle. Minoxidil produces arteriolar vasodilation with essentially no effect on the capacitance vessels.

Minoxidil increases blood flow to skin, skeletal muscle, the gastrointestinal tract, and the heart. The disproportionate increase in blood flow to the heart may have a metabolic basis, in that administration of minoxidil is associated with a reflex increase in myocardial contractility and in cardiac output. The cardiac output can increase markedly, as much as 3- to 4-fold. The increased venous return probably results from enhancement of flow in the regional vascular beds, with a fast time constant for venous return to the heart. The adrenergic increase in myocardial contractility contributes to the increased cardiac output but is not the predominant causal factor. Minoxidil is a renal artery vasodilator, but systemic hypotension produced by the drug occasionally can decrease renal blood flow. Renal function usually improves in patients who take minoxidil for the treatment of hypertension, especially if renal dysfunction is secondary to hypertension. Minoxidil is a very potent stimulator of renin secretion; this effect is mediated by a renal sympathetic stimulation and activation of the intrinsic renal mechanisms for regulation of renin release.

ADME. Minoxidil is well absorbed from the GI tract. Although peak concentrations of minoxidil in blood occur 1 h after oral administration, the maximal hypotensive effect of the drug occurs later, possibly because formation of the active metabolite is delayed. The bulk of the absorbed drug is eliminated by hepatic metabolism; ~20% is excreted unchanged in the urine. Minoxidil has a plasma $t_{1/2}$ of 3-4 h, but its duration of action is 24 h or longer.

Adverse Effects and Precautions. The adverse effects of minoxidil can be severe and are divided into 3 major categories: fluid and salt retention, cardiovascular effects, and hypertrichosis.

Retention of salt and water results from increased proximal renal tubular reabsorption, which is in turn secondary to reduced renal perfusion pressure and to reflex stimulation of renal tubular α adrenergic receptors. Similar antinatriuretic effects can be observed with the other arteriolar dilators (e.g., diazoxide and hydralazine). Although administration of minoxidil causes increased secretion of renin and aldosterone, this is not an important mechanism for retention of salt and water in this case. Fluid retention usually can be controlled by the administration of a diuretic. However, thiazides may not be sufficiently efficacious, and it may be necessary to use a loop diuretic, especially if the patient has any degree of renal dysfunction.

The cardiac consequences of the baroreceptor-mediated activation of the sympathetic nervous system during minoxidil therapy include increases in heart rate, myocardial contractility, and myocardial O_2 consumption. Thus, myocardial ischemia can be induced by minoxidil in patients with coronary artery disease. The cardiac sympathetic responses are attenuated by concurrent administration of a β adrenergic blocker. The adrenergically-induced increase in renin secretion also can be ameliorated by a β receptor antagonist or an ACE inhibitor.

Minoxidil has particularly adverse consequences in those hypertensive patients who have left ventricular hypertrophy and diastolic dysfunction. Such poorly compliant ventricles respond suboptimally to increased volume loads, with a resulting increase in left ventricular filling pressure. This likely contributes to the increased pulmonary artery pressure seen with minoxidil therapy in hypertensive patients and is compounded by the retention of salt and water. Cardiac failure can result from minoxidil therapy in such patients; the potential for this complication can be reduced but not prevented by effective diuretic therapy. Pericardial effusion is an uncommon but serious complication of minoxidil. Although more commonly described in patients with cardiac and renal failure, pericardial effusion can occur in patients with normal cardiovascular and renal function. Mild and asymptomatic pericardial effusion is not an indication for discontinuing minoxidil, but the situation should be monitored closely to avoid progression to tamponade. Effusions usually clear when the drug is discontinued but can recur if treatment with minoxidil is resumed.

Flattened and inverted T waves frequently are observed in the electrocardiogram following the initiation of minoxidil treatment. These are not ischemic in origin and are seen with other drugs that activate K^+ channels. Openers of the ATP-modulated K^+ channel accelerate myocardial repolarization, shorten the refractory period, and one of them, *pinacidil*, lowers the ventricular fibrillation threshold and increases spontaneous ventricular fibrillation in the setting of myocardial ischemia. Hypertrichosis occurs in patients who receive minoxidil for an extended period and is probably a consequence of K^+ channel activation. Growth of hair occurs on the face, back, arms, and legs and is particularly offensive to women. Topical minoxidil (ROGAINE) is used for male pattern baldness: It may have cardiovascular effects in some individuals. Other side effects of the drug are rare and include rashes, Stevens-Johnson syndrome, glucose intolerance, serosanguineous bullae, formation of antinuclear antibodies, and thrombocytopenia.

Therapeutic Uses. Systemic minoxidil is best reserved for the treatment of severe hypertension that responds poorly to other antihypertensive medications, especially in male patients with renal insufficiency. Minoxidil should be given concurrently with a diuretic to avoid fluid retention and with a sympatholytic drug (usually a β receptor antagonist) to control reflex cardiovascular effects. The initial daily dose of minoxidil may be as little as 1.25 mg, which can be increased gradually to 40 mg in 1 or 2 daily doses.

SODIUM NITROPRUSSIDE

Nitroprusside is a nitrovasodilator that acts by releasing NO that stimulates the guanylyl cyclase–cyclic GMP–PKG pathway, leading to vasodilation. Tolerance develops to *nitroglycerin* but not to nitroprusside. Nitroprusside dilates both arterioles and venules, and the hemodynamic response to its administration results from a combination of venous pooling and reduced arterial impedance.

In subjects with normal left ventricular function, venous pooling affects cardiac output more than does the reduction of afterload; cardiac output tends to fall. In contrast, in patients with severely impaired left ventricular function and diastolic ventricular distention, the reduction of arterial impedance is the predominant effect, leading to a rise in cardiac output (*see* Chapter 28).

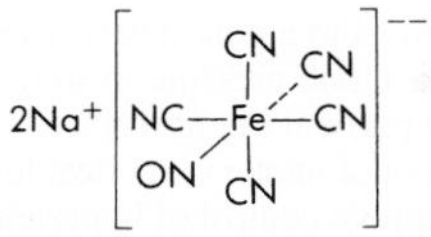

SODIUM NITROPRUSSIDE

Sodium nitroprusside is a nonselective vasodilator, and regional distribution of blood flow is little affected by the drug. In general, renal blood flow and glomerular filtration are maintained, and plasma renin activity increases. Sodium nitroprusside usually causes only a modest increase in heart rate and an overall reduction in myocardial O_2 demand.

Absorption, Metabolism, and Excretion. Sodium nitroprusside is an unstable molecule that must be protected from light and given by continuous intravenous infusion to be effective. Its onset of action is within 30 sec; the peak hypotensive effect occurs within 2 min, and the effect disappears within 3 min after infusion is stopped. The metabolism of nitroprusside by smooth muscle is initiated by its reduction, which is followed by the release of cyanide and then NO. Cyanide is further metabolized by liver rhodanese to form thiocyanate, which is eliminated almost entirely in the urine. The mean elimination $t_{1/2}$ for thiocyanate is 3 days in patients with normal renal function, and it can be much longer in patients with renal insufficiency.

Therapeutic Uses. Sodium nitroprusside is used primarily to treat hypertensive emergencies but also can be used in many situations when short-term reduction of cardiac preload and/or afterload is desired. Nitroprusside has been used to lower blood pressure during acute aortic dissection; improve cardiac output in congestive heart failure, especially in hypertensive patients with pulmonary edema that does not respond to other treatment (*see* Chapter 28); and decrease myocardial oxygen demand after acute MI. In addition, nitroprusside is used to induce controlled hypotension during anesthesia in order to reduce bleeding in surgical procedures. In the treatment of acute aortic dissection, it is important to administer a β adrenergic receptor antagonist with nitroprusside, because reduction of blood pressure with nitroprusside alone can increase the rate of rise in pressure in the aorta as a result of increased myocardial contractility, thereby enhancing propagation of the dissection.

Sodium nitroprusside is available in vials that contain 50 mg. The contents of the vial should be dissolved in 2-3 mL of 5% dextrose in water. Addition of this solution to 250-1000 mL of 5% dextrose in water produces a concentration of 50-200 μg/mL. Because the compound decomposes in light, only fresh solutions should be used, and the bottle should be covered with an opaque wrapping. The drug must be administered as a controlled continuous infusion, and the patient must be closely observed. Most hypertensive patients respond to an infusion of 0.25-1.5 μg/kg/min. Higher rates of infusion are necessary to produce controlled hypotension in normotensive patients under surgical anesthesia. Patients who are receiving other antihypertensive medications usually require less nitroprusside to lower blood pressure. If infusion rates of 10 μg/kg/min do not produce adequate reduction of blood pressure within 10 min, the rate of administration of nitroprusside should be reduced to minimize potential toxicity.

Toxicity and Precautions. The short-term adverse effects of nitroprusside are due to excessive vasodilation. Close monitoring of blood pressure and the use of a continuous variable-rate infusion pump will prevent an excessive hemodynamic response to the drug. Less commonly, toxicity may result from conversion of nitroprusside to cyanide and thiocyanate. Toxic accumulation of cyanide leading to severe lactic acidosis usually occurs when sodium nitroprusside is infused at a rate >5 μg/kg/min but also can occur in some patients receiving doses ~2 μg/kg/min for a prolonged period. The concomitant administration of sodium thiosulfate can prevent accumulation of cyanide in patients who are receiving higher-than-usual doses of sodium nitroprusside. The risk of thiocyanate toxicity increases when sodium nitroprusside is infused for more than 24-48 h, especially if renal function is impaired. Signs and symptoms of thiocyanate toxicity include anorexia, nausea, fatigue, disorientation, and toxic psychosis. The plasma concentration of thiocyanate should be monitored during prolonged infusions of nitroprusside and should not be allowed to exceed 0.1 mg/mL. Rarely, excessive concentrations of thiocyanate may cause hypothyroidism by inhibiting iodine uptake by the thyroid gland. In patients with renal failure, thiocyanate can be removed readily by hemodialysis.

Nitroprusside can worsen arterial hypoxemia in patients with chronic obstructive pulmonary disease because the drug interferes with hypoxic pulmonary vasoconstriction and therefore promotes mismatching of ventilation with perfusion.

NONPHARMACOLOGICAL THERAPY OF HYPERTENSION

Nonpharmacological approaches to the treatment of hypertension may be sufficient in patients with modestly elevated blood pressure and can augment the effects of antihypertensive drugs in patients with more marked initial elevations in blood pressure.

- Reduction in body weight for people who are modestly overweight or frankly obese may be useful.
- Restricting Na^+ consumption lowers blood pressure in some patients. The Dietary Approaches to Stop Hypertension (DASH) diet may be particularly useful.
- For some patients, restriction of ethanol intake to modest levels may lower blood pressure.
- Increased physical activity may improve control of hypertension.

SELECTION OF ANTIHYPERTENSIVE DRUGS IN INDIVIDUAL PATIENTS

National guidelines recommend diuretics as preferred initial therapy for most patients with uncomplicated stage 1 hypertension (*see* Table 27–4) who are unresponsive to nonpharmacological measures. Patients also are commonly treated with other drugs: β receptor antagonists, ACE inhibitors/AT_1 receptor antagonists, and Ca^{2+} channel blockers. Patients with uncomplicated stage 2 hypertension will likely require the early introduction of a diuretic and another drug from a different class. Subsequently, doses can be titrated upward and additional drugs added to achieve goal blood pressures (blood pressure <140/90 mm Hg in uncomplicated patients).

An important and high-risk group of patients with hypertension are those with compelling indications for specific drugs on account of other underlying serious cardiovascular disease (heart failure, post-MI, or with high risk for coronary artery disease), chronic kidney disease, or diabetes. For example, a hypertensive patient with congestive heart failure ideally should be treated with a diuretic, β receptor antagonist, ACE inhibitor/ AT_1 receptor antagonist, and (in selected patients) spironolactone because of the benefit of these drugs in congestive heart failure, even in the absence of hypertension (*see* Chapter 28). Similarly, ACE inhibitors/ AT_1 receptor antagonists should be first-line drugs in the treatment of diabetics with hypertension in view of these drugs' well-established benefits in diabetic nephropathy.

Other patients may have less serious underlying diseases that could influence choice of antihypertensive drugs. For example, a hypertensive patient with symptomatic benign prostatic hyperplasia might benefit from having an α_1 receptor antagonist as part of his or her therapeutic program, because α_1 antagonists are efficacious in both diseases. Similarly, a patient with recurrent migraine attacks might particularly benefit from use of a β receptor antagonist because a number of drugs in this class are efficacious in preventing migraine attacks. Patients with isolated systolic hypertension benefit particularly from diuretics and also from Ca^{2+} channel blockers and ACE inhibitors. These should be first-line drugs in these patients in terms of efficacy, but compelling indications as noted earlier need to be taken into account.

For a complete Bibliographical Listing see Goodman & Gilman's ***The Pharmacological Basis of Therapeutics***, 12th ed., or Goodman & Gilman Online at www.AccessMedicine.com.

Pharmacotherapy of Congestive Heart Failure

Congestive heart failure (CHF) is responsible for more than half a million deaths annually in the U.S., carries a 1-year mortality rate of more than 50% in patients with advanced forms of the condition. Substantive advances in CHF pharmacotherapy have altered clinical practice by shifting the paradigm of its management from exclusively symptom palliation to modification of disease progression and prolonged survival.

DEFINING CONGESTIVE HEART FAILURE. The onset and progression of clinically evident CHF from left ventricular (LV) systolic dysfunction follows a pathophysiologic sequence in response to an initial insult to myocardial dysfunction. A reduction in forward cardiac output leads to expanded activation of the sympathetic nervous system and the renin–angiotensin–aldosterone axis that, together, maintain perfusion of vital organs by increasing LV preload, stimulating myocardial contractility, and increasing arterial tone. Acutely, these mechanisms sustain cardiac output by allowing the heart to operate at elevated end-diastolic volumes, while peripheral vasoconstriction promotes regional redistribution of the cardiac output to the CNS, coronary, and renal vascular beds.

Unfortunately, these compensatory mechanisms over time propagate disease progression. Intravascular volume expansion increases diastolic and systolic wall stress that disrupts myocardial energetics and causes pathologic LV hypertrophy. By increasing LV afterload, peripheral arterial vasoconstriction also adversely affects diastolic ventricular wall stress, thereby increasing myocardial O_2 demand. Finally, neurohumoral effectors such as NE and AngII are associated with myocyte apoptosis, abnormal myocyte gene expression, and pathologic changes in the extracellular matrix that increase LV stiffness.

Clinically, the term CHF describes a final common pathway for the expression of myocardial dysfunction. While some emphasize the clinical distinction between systolic versus diastolic heart failure, many patients demonstrate dysfunction in both contractile performance and ventricular relaxation/filling. Indeed, these physiologic processes are interrelated; for example, the rate and duration of LV diastolic filling are directly influenced by impairment in systolic contractile performance. The following definitions are useful for establishing a conceptual framework to describe this clinical syndrome:

Congestive heart failure is the pathophysiologic state in which the heart is unable to pump blood at a rate commensurate with the requirements of metabolizing tissues, or can do so only from an elevated filling pressure.

Heart failure is a complex of symptoms—fatigue, shortness of breath, and congestion—that are related to the inadequate perfusion of tissue during exertion and often to the retention of fluid. Its primary cause is an impairment of the heart's ability to fill or empty the left ventricle properly.

One may consider CHF as a condition in which failure of the heart to provide adequate forward output at normal end-diastolic filling pressures results in a clinical syndrome of decreased exercise tolerance with pulmonary and systemic venous congestion. Numerous cardiovascular comorbidities are associated with CHF, including coronary artery disease, MI, and sudden cardiac death.

PHARMACOLOGIC TREATMENT OF HEART FAILURE

The abnormalities of myocardial structure and function that characterize CHF are often irreversible. These changes narrow the end-diastolic volume range that is compatible with normal cardiac function. Although CHF is predominately a chronic disease, subtle changes to an individual's hemodynamic status (e.g., increased circulating volume from high dietary sodium intake, increased systemic blood pressure from medication nonadherence) often provoke an acute clinical decompensation.

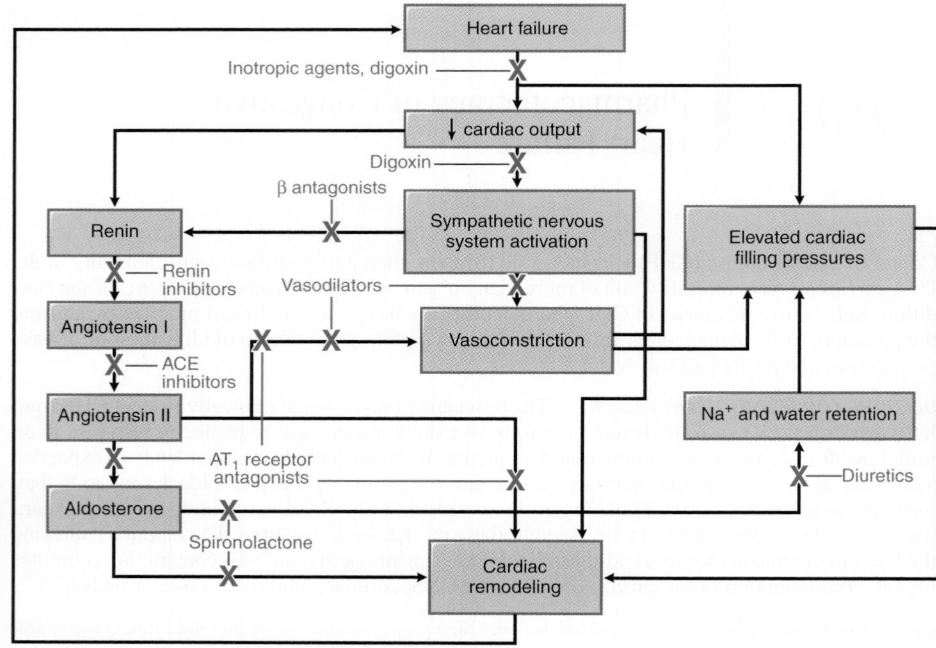

Figure 28–1 *Pathophysiologic mechanisms of heart failure and major sites of drug action.* Congestive heart failure is accompanied by compensatory neurohormonal responses, including activation of the sympathetic nervous and renin–angiotensin–aldosterone axis. Increased ventricular afterload, due to systemic vasoconstriction and chamber dilation, causes depression in systolic function. In addition, increased afterload and the direct effects of angiotensin and norepinephrine on the ventricular myocardium cause pathologic remodeling characterized by progressive chamber dilation and loss of contractile function. Key congestive heart failure medications and their targets of action are presented. ACE, angiotensin-converting enzyme; AT_1 receptor, type 1 angiotensin receptor.

Not surprisingly, therefore, CHF therapy has for many years used diuretics to control volume overload and subsequent worsening in LV function. Other proven pharmacotherapies target ventricular wall stress, the renin–angiotensin–aldosterone axis, and the sympathetic nervous system to decrease pathologic ventricular remodeling, attenuate disease progression, and improve survival in selected patients with severe CHF and low LV ejection fraction. Figure 28–1 provides an overview of the sites of action for major drug classes commonly used to improve cardiac hemodynamics and function through preload reduction, afterload reduction, and enhancement of inotropy (i.e., myocardial contractility).

DIURETICS

Diuretics reduce extracellular fluid volume and ventricular filling pressure (or "preload"). Because CHF patients often operate on a "plateau" phase of the *Frank-Starling* curve (Figure 28–2), incremental preload reduction occurs under these conditions without a reduction in cardiac output. Sustained natriuresis and/or a rapid decline in intravascular volume, however, may "push" one's profile leftward on the Frank-Starling curve, resulting in an unwanted decrease in cardiac output. In this way, excessive diuresis is counterproductive secondary to reciprocal neurohormonal *overactivation* from volume depletion. Thus, it is preferable to avoid diuretics in patients with asymptomatic LV dysfunction and to only administer the minimal dose required to maintain euvolemia in those patients symptomatic from hypervolemia. Despite the efficacy of loop or thiazide diuretics in controlling congestive symptoms and improving exercise capacity, their use is not associated with a reduction in CHF mortality.

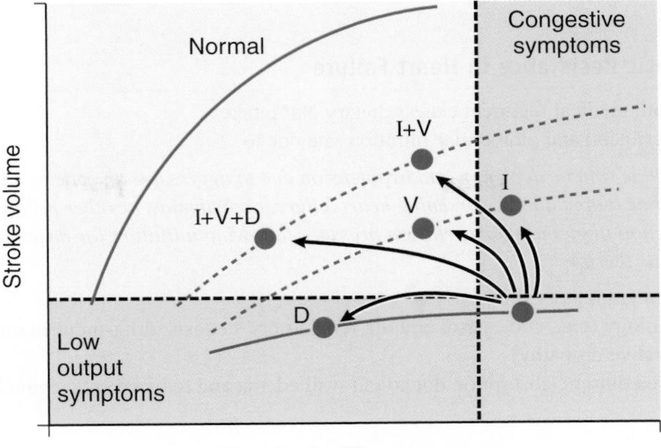

Figure 28–2 *Hemodynamic responses to pharmacologic interventions in heart failure.* The relationships between diastolic filling pressure (preload) and stroke volume (ventricular performance) are illustrated for a normal heart (*green line*; the Frank-Starling relationship) and for a patient with heart failure due to predominant systolic dysfunction (*red line*). Note that positive inotropic agents (I), such as cardiac glycosides or dobutamine, move patients to a higher ventricular function curve (*lower dashed line*), resulting in greater cardiac work for a given level of ventricular filling pressure. Vasodilators (V), such as angiotensin-converting enzyme (ACE) inhibitors or nitroprusside, also move patients to improved ventricular function curves while reducing cardiac filling pressures. Diuretics (D) improve symptoms of congestive heart failure by moving patients to lower cardiac filling pressures along the same ventricular function curve.

Dietary Na^+ Restriction. All patients with clinically significant LV dysfunction, regardless of symptom status, should be advised to limit dietary sodium intake to 2-3 g/day. More stringent salt restriction is seldom necessary and may be counterproductive, as it can lead to hyponatremia, hypokalemia, and hypochloremic metabolic alkalosis when combined with loop diuretic.

Loop Diuretics. Furosemide (LASIX, others), bumetanide (BUMEX, others), and torsemide (DEMADEX, others) are widely used in the treatment of CHF. Due to the increased risk of ototoxicity, ethacrynic acid (EDECRIN) is recommended only for patients with sulfonamides allergies or who are intolerant to alternative options. Loop diuretics inhibit a specific ion transport protein, the Na^+-K^+-$2Cl^-$ symporter on the apical membrane of renal epithelial cells in the ascending limb of the loop of Henle to increase Na^+ and fluid delivery to distal nephron segments (*see* Chapter 25). These drugs also enhance K^+ secretion, particularly in the presence of elevated aldosterone levels, as is typical in CHF.

The bioavailability of orally administered furosemide ranges from 40-70%. High drug concentrations often are required to initiate diuresis in patients with worsening symptoms or in those with impaired gastrointestinal absorption, as may occur in severely hypervolemic patients with CHF-induced gut edema. In contrast, the oral bioavailabilities of bumetanide and torsemide are >80%, and as a result, these agents are more consistently absorbed but are financially more costly. Furosemide and bumetanide are short-acting drugs, and rebound Na^+ retention that occurs with sub-steady state drug levels make ≥2/day dosing an acceptable treatment strategy when using these agents, provided adequate monitoring of daily body weight and blood electrolyte level monitoring is possible.

Thiazide Diuretics. Monotherapy with thiazide diuretics (DIURIL, HYDRODIURIL, others) has a limited role in CHF. However, combination therapy with loop diuretics is often effective in those refractory to loop diuretics alone. Thiazide diuretics act on the Na^+ Cl^- co-transporter in the distal convoluted tubule (*see* Chapter 25) and are associated with a greater degree K^+ wasting per fluid volume reduction when compared to loop diuretics.

K^+-Sparing Diuretics. K^+-sparing diuretics (*see* Chapter 25) inhibit apical membrane Na^+-conductance channels in renal epithelial cells (e.g., amiloride, triamterene) or are mineralocorticoid (e.g., aldosterone) receptor antagonists (e.g., canrenone [not commercially available in the U.S.], spironolactone, and eplerenone). Collectively, these agents are weak diuretics, but have been used to achieve volume reduction with limited K^+ and Mg^{2+} wasting.

Table 28–1

Causes of Diuretic Resistance in Heart Failure

Noncompliance with medical regimen; excess dietary Na^+ intake
Decreased renal perfusion and glomerular filtration rate due to:
Excessive vascular volume depletion and hypotension due to aggressive diuretic or vasodilator therapy
Decline in cardiac output due to worsening heart failure, arrhythmias, or other primary cardiac causes
Selective reduction in glomerular perfusion pressure following initiation (or dose increase) of ACE-inhibitor therapy
Nonsteroidal anti-inflammatory drugs
Primary renal pathology (e.g., cholesterol emboli, renal artery stenosis, drug-induced interstitial nephritis, obstructive uropathy)
Reduced or impaired diuretic absorption due to gut wall edema and reduced splanchnic blood flow

Diuretics in Clinical Practice. The majority of CHF patients will require chronic administration of a loop diuretic to maintain euvolemia. In patients with clinically evident fluid retention, furosemide typically is started at a dose of 40 mg once or twice daily, and the dosage is increased until an adequate diuresis is achieved. A larger initial dose may be necessary in patients with advanced CHF and azotemia. Serum electrolytes and renal function are monitored frequently. If present, hypokalemia from therapy may be corrected by oral or intravenous K^+ supplementation or by the addition of a K^+-sparing diuretic.

Diuretics in the Decompensated Patient. In patients with decompensated CHF warranting hospital admission, repetitive intravenously administered boluses or a constant infusion titrated to achieve a desired response may be needed to provide expeditious diuresis. A typical continuous furosemide infusion is initiated with a 40-mg bolus injection followed by a constant rate of 10 mg/h, with uptitration as necessary. If renal perfusion is reduced, drug efficacy may be enhanced by coadministration of drugs that increase cardiac output (e.g., *dobutamine*).

Diuretic Resistance. (Table 28–1). A compensatory increase in renal tubular Na^+ reabsorption may prevent effective diuresis when dosed daily; as a result, reduction of diuretic dosing intervals may be warranted. In advanced CHF, invasive assessment of intracardiac filling pressures and cardiac output may be required to distinguish between low intravascular volume from aggressive diuresis versus low cardiac output states. Other factors can contribute to diuretic resistance (*see* Table 28–1).

Metabolic Consequences of Diuretic Therapy. With regard to diuretic use in CHF, the most important adverse sequelae of diuretics are electrolyte abnormalities, including hyponatremia, hypokalemia, and hypochloremic metabolic alkalosis.

Adenosine A_1 Receptor Antagonists. Adenosine A_1 receptor antagonists may provide a renal protective therapeutic strategy for enhanced volume loss in decompensated CHF. Adenosine is secreted from the macula densa in the renal arteriole in response to diuretic-induced increases in Na^+ and Cl^- tubular flow concentrations. This results in increased Na^+ resorption, a volume-loss counterregulatory mechanism (*see* Chapter 26). Na^+ reabsorption, in addition to adenosine-induced renal arteriole vasoconstriction, appears responsible (in part) for the development of complications common to the use of diuretics in decompensated CHF patients, particularly prerenal azotemia. The role of adenosine in the macula densa and juxtaglomerular (granular) cells suggests other effects of A_1 antagonists on the renin-angiotensin system (*see* Figure 26–3). Administration of A_1 antagonists *KW-3902* (ROLOFYLLINE) or *BG9179* (NAXIFYLLINE), to patients with decompensated CHF already treated with loop diuretics, has been associated with increased volume reduction, improved renal function, and lower diuretic dosing, however, a clinical trial failed to show significant benefits of rolofylline in patients with CHF and clinical development of the drug was stopped in 2009. No A_1 antagonists are currently marketed in the U.S.

ALDOSTERONE ANTAGONISTS AND CLINICAL OUTCOME

LV systolic dysfunction decreases renal blood flow and results in overactivation of the renin–angiotensin–aldosterone axis and may increase circulating plasma aldosterone levels in CHF to 20-fold above normal. The pathophysiologic effects of hyperaldosteronemia are diverse (Table 28–2) and extend beyond Na^+ and fluid retention; however, the precise mechanism by which aldosterone receptor blockade improves outcome in CHF remains unresolved.

Aldosterone-receptor antagonists in combination with ACE inhibitor therapy have provided beneficial effects in clinical trials. In CHF patients with low LV ejection fraction, *spironolactone* (25 mg/day) decreased

Table 28–2

Potential Roles of Aldosterone in the Pathophysiology of Heart Failure

MECHANISM	PATHOPHYSIOLOGIC EFFECT
Increased Na^+ and water retention	Edema, elevated cardiac filling pressures
K^+ and Mg^{2+} loss	Arrhythmogenesis and risk of sudden cardiac death
Reduced myocardial NE uptake	Potentiation of NE affects: myocardial remodeling and arrhythmogenesis
Reduced baroreceptor sensitivity	Reduced parasympathetic activity and risk of sudden cardiac death
Myocardial fibrosis, fibroblast proliferation	Remodeling and ventricular dysfunction
Alterations in Na^+ channel expression	Increased excitability and contractility of cardiac myocytes

mortality by ~30% (from progressive heart failure or sudden cardiac death), and patients had fewer CHF-related hospitalizations compared with the placebo group. Treatment was well tolerated; however, 10% of men reported gynecomastia and 2% of all patients developed severe hyperkalemia (>6.0 mEq/L).

ORAL VASODILATORS

Although numerous vasodilators have been developed that improve CHF symptoms, only the *hydralazine–isosorbide dinitrate* combination, ACE inhibitors, and AT_1 receptor blockers (ARBs) demonstrably improve survival. The therapeutic use of vasodilators in the treatment of hypertension and myocardial ischemia is considered in detail in Chapter 27. This chapter focuses on the uses for some of these same vasodilator drugs in the treatment of CHF, mainly through their capacity to reduce preload and afterload (Table 28–3).

NITROVASODILATORS. Nitrovasodilators are *nitric oxide (NO) donors* that activate soluble guanylate cyclase in vascular smooth muscle cells, leading to vasodilation. Unlike *nitroprusside*, which is converted to NO• by cellular reducing agents such as glutathione, *nitroglycerin* and other organic nitrates undergo a more complex enzymatic biotransformation to NO• or bioactive *S*-nitrosothiols. The activities of specific enzyme(s) and cofactor(s) required for this biotransformation appear to differ by target organ and even by different vasculature beds within a particular organ.

Organic Nitrates. Organic nitrates are available in a number of formulations that include rapid-acting *nitroglycerin* tablets or spray for sublingual administration, short-acting oral agents such as *isosorbide dinitrate* (ISORDIL, others), long-acting oral agents such as *isosorbide mononitrate* (ISMO, others), topical preparations such as nitroglycerin ointment and transdermal patches, and intravenous nitroglycerin. The principal action of these preparations in CHF is reducing LV filling pressure. This occurs, in part, by augmentation of peripheral venous capacitance that results in preload reduction. Additional effects of organic nitrates include pulmonary and systemic vascular resistance reduction, and coronary artery vasodilation for which systolic and diastolic ventricular function is enhanced by increased coronary blood flow. These beneficial physiologic effects translate into improved exercise capacity and CHF-symptom reduction. However, these drugs do not substantially influence systemic vascular resistance, and *pharmacologic tolerance* limits their utility over time. Organic nitrates are commonly used with other vasodilators (e.g., *hydralazine)* to increase the clinical effectiveness.

Nitrate Tolerance. *Nitrate tolerance may limit the long-term effectiveness of these drugs in the treatment of CHF. Blood nitrate levels may be permitted to fall to negligible levels for at least 6-8 h each day* (see Chapter 27). Patients with recurrent orthopnea or paroxysmal nocturnal dyspnea, e.g., might benefit from nighttime nitrate use. Likewise, co-treatment with hydralazine may decrease nitrate tolerance by an antioxidant effect that attenuates superoxide formation, thereby increasing the bioavailable NO levels.

PARENTERAL VASODILATORS

Sodium Nitroprusside. Sodium nitroprusside (NITRO-PRESS, others) is a direct NO donor and potent vasodilator that is effective in reducing both ventricular filling pressure and systemic vascular resistance (Figure 28–3). Onset to action is rapid (2-5 min) as the drug is quickly metabolized to NO. Nitroprusside is effective in treating critically ill patients with CHF who have elevated systemic vascular resistance or mechanical

Table 28–3

Vasodilator Drugs Used to Treat Heart Failure

DRUG CLASS	EXAMPLES	MECHANISM OF VASODILATING ACTION	PRELOAD REDUCTION	AFTERLOAD REDUCTION
Organic nitrates	Nitroglycerin, isosorbide dinitrate	NO-mediated vasodilation	+++	+
NO donors	Nitroprusside	NO-mediated vasodilation	+++	+++
ACE inhibitors	Captopril, enalapril, lisinopril	Inhibition of AngII generation, ↓ BK degradation	++	++
Ang II receptor blockers	Losartan, candesartan	AT_1 receptors blockade	++	++
PDE inhibitors	Milrinone, inamrinone	Inhibition of cyclic AMP degradation	++	++
K^+ channel agonist	Hydralazine	Unknown	+	+++
	Minoxidil	Hyperpolarization of vascular smooth muscle cells	+	+++
α_1 antagonists	Doxazosin, prazosin	Selective α_1 adrenergic receptor blockade	+++	++
Nonselective α antagonists	Phentolamine	Nonselective α adrenergic receptor blockade	+++	+++
β/α_1 antagonists	Carvedilol, labetalol	Selective α_1 adrenergic receptor blockade	++	++
Ca^{2+} channel blockers	Amlodipine, nifedipine, felodipine	Inhibition of L-type Ca^{2+} channels	+	+++
β agonists	Isoproterenol	Stimulation of vascular β_2 adrenergic receptors	+	++

Ang II, angiotensin II; AT_1 type 1 angiotensin II receptor; NO, nitric oxide; ACE, angiotensin-converting enzyme; PDE, cyclic nucleotide phosphodiesterase; BK, bradykinin.

complications that follow acute MI (e.g., mitral regurgitation or ventricular septal defect-induced left-to-right shunts). It increases cardiac output and renal blood flow, improving both glomerular filtration and diuretic effectiveness. The most common adverse side effect of nitroprusside is hypotension. Excessive reduction of systemic arterial pressure may limit or prevent an increase in renal blood flow in patients with more severe LV contractile dysfunction.

Cyanide produced during the biotransformation of nitroprusside is rapidly metabolized by the liver to thiocyanate, which is then renally excreted. Thiocyanate and/or cyanide toxicity is uncommon but may occur in the setting of hepatic or renal failure, or following prolonged periods of high-dose drug infusion (*see* Chapter 27 for details). Typical symptoms include unexplained abdominal pain, mental status changes, convulsions, and lactic acidosis. Methemoglobinemia is another unusual complication and is due to the oxidation of hemoglobin by NO•.

Intravenous Nitroglycerin. Intravenous nitroglycerin is a vasoactive NO donor that is used in the intensive care unit setting. Unlike nitroprusside, nitroglycerin is relatively selective for venous capacitance vessels, particularly at low infusion rates. In CHF, intravenous nitroglycerin is most commonly used in the treatment of LV dysfunction due to an acute myocardial ischemia. Parenteral nitroglycerin also is used in the treatment of non-ischemic cardiomyopathy when expeditious LV filling pressure reduction is desired. At higher infusion rates, this drug also may decrease systemic arterial resistance. Nitroglycerin therapy may be limited by headache and nitrate tolerance; tolerance may be partially offset by increasing the dosage.

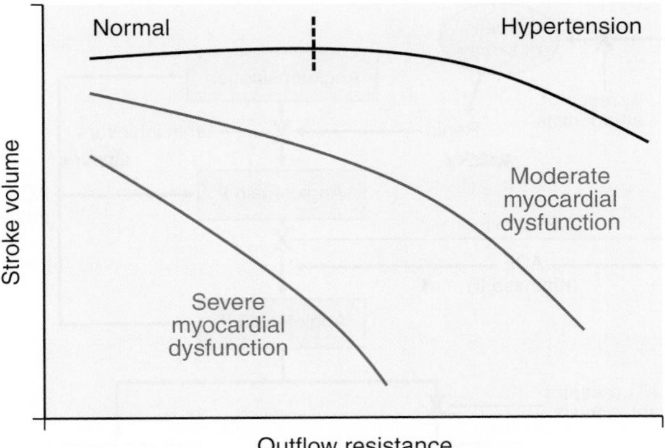

Figure 28–3 *Relationship between ventricular outflow resistance and stroke volume in patients with systolic ventricular dysfunction*. An increase in ventricular outflow resistance, a principal determinant of afterload, has little effect on stroke volume in normal hearts, as illustrated by the relatively flat curve. In contrast, in patients with systolic ventricular dysfunction, an increase in outflow resistance often is accompanied by a sharp decline in stroke volume. With more severe ventricular dysfunction, this curve becomes steeper. Because of this relationship, a reduction in systemic vascular resistance (1 component of outflow resistance) in response to an arterial vasodilator may markedly increase stroke volume in patients with severe myocardial dysfunction. The resultant increase in stroke volume may be sufficient to offset the decrease in systemic vascular resistance, thereby preventing a fall in systemic arterial pressure. (Adapted from Cohn and Franciosa, 1977.)

Hydralazine. Hydralazine is a direct vasodilator whose mechanism of action is poorly understood. Hydralazine is an effective antihypertensive drug (*see* Chapter 27), particularly when combined with agents that blunt compensatory increases in sympathetic tone and salt and water retention. In CHF, hydralazine reduces right and LV afterload by reducing pulmonary and systemic vascular resistance. This results in an augmentation of forward stroke volume and a reduction in ventricular wall stress in systole. Hydralazine also appears to have moderate "direct" positive inotropic activity in cardiac muscle independent of its afterload-reducing effects. Hydralazine is effective in reducing renal vascular resistance and in increasing renal blood flow. Hydralazine often is used in CHF patients with renal dysfunction intolerant of ACE-inhibitor therapy. Combination therapy with isosorbide dinitrate and hydralazine reduces CHF mortality in patients with systolic dysfunction. Hydralazine provides additional hemodynamic improvement for patients with advanced CHF (with or without nitrates) already treated with conventional doses of an ACE inhibitor, digoxin, and diuretics.

The oral bioavailability and pharmacokinetics of hydralazine are not altered significantly in CHF, unless severe hepatic congestion or hypoperfusion is present. Hydralazine is typically started at a dose of 10-25 mg 3 or 4 times per day and uptitrated to a maximum of 100 mg 3 or 4 times daily, as tolerated. At total daily doses >200 mg, hydralazine is associated with an increased risk of lupus-like effects.

There are several important considerations for hydralazine use. First, ACE inhibitors appear to be superior to hydralazine for mortality reduction in severe CHF. Second, side effects requiring dose adjustment of hydralazine withdrawal are common. The lupus-like side effects associated with hydralazine are relatively uncommon and may be more likely to occur in selected patients with the "slow-acetylator" phenotype (*see* Chapter 27). Finally, hydralazine is a medication taken 3 or 4 times daily, and adherence may be difficult for CHF patients, who are prescribed multiple medications concurrently.

TARGETING NEUROHORMONAL REGULATION: THE RENIN–ANGIOTENSIN–ALDOSTERONE AXIS AND VASOPRESSIN ANTAGONISTS

RENIN–ANGIOTENSIN–ALDOSTERONE AXIS ANTAGONISTS. The renin–angiotensin–aldosterone axis plays a central role in the pathophysiology of CHF (Figure 28–4).

AngII is a potent arterial vasoconstrictor and an important mediator of Na^+ and water retention through its effects on glomerular filtration pressure and aldosterone secretion. AngII also modulates neural and adrenal

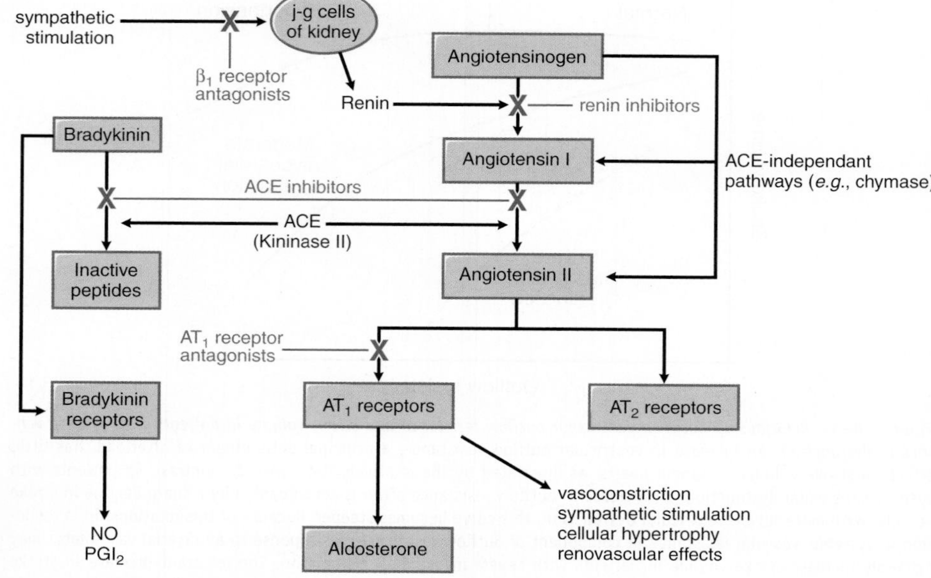

Figure 28–4 *The renin–angiotensin–aldosterone axis*. Renin, excreted in response to β adrenergic stimulation of the juxtaglomerular (j-g) or granular cells of the kidney, cleaves plasma angiotensinogen to produce angiotensin I. Angiotensin-converting enzyme (ACE) catalyzes the conversion of angiotensin I to angiotensin II (AngII). Most of the known biologic effects of AngII are mediated by the type 1 angiotensin (AT_1) receptor. In general, the AT_2 receptor appears to counteract the effects of AngII that are mediated by activation of the AT_1 pathway. AngII also may be formed through ACE-independent pathways. These pathways, and possibly incomplete inhibition of tissue ACE, may account for persistence of AngII in patients treated with ACE inhibitors. ACE inhibition decreases bradykinin degradation, thus enhancing its levels and biologic effects, including the production of NO and PGI_2. Bradykinin may mediate some of the biological effects of ACE inhibitors.

medulla catecholamine release, is arrhythmogenic, promotes vascular hyperplasia and myocardial hypertrophy, and induces myocyte death. Consequently, reduction of the effects of AngII constitutes a cornerstone of CHF management.

ACE inhibitors suppress AngII (and aldosterone) production, decrease sympathetic nervous system activity, and potentiate the effects of diuretics in CHF. However, AngII levels frequently return to baseline values following chronic treatment with ACE inhibitors (*see* Chapter 26), due in part to AngII production via ACE-independent enzymes. This AngII "escape" suggests that alternate mechanisms contribute to the clinical benefits of ACE inhibitors in CHF. ACE is identical to kininase II, which degrades bradykinin and other kinins that stimulate production of NO, cyclic GMP, and vasoactive eicosanoids. These oppose AngII-induced vascular smooth muscle cell and cardiac fibroblasts proliferation and inhibit unfavorable extracellular matrix deposition.

ACE inhibitors are preferential arterial vasodilators. ACE-inhibitor–mediated decreases in LV afterload result in increased stroke volume and cardiac output. Heart rate typically is unchanged with treatment, often despite decreases in systemic arterial pressure, a response that probably is a consequence of decreased sympathetic nervous system activity from ACE inhibition. Most clinical actions of AngII are mediated through the AT_1 angiotensin receptor, whereas AT_2 receptor activation appears to counterbalance the downstream biologic effects of AT_1 receptor stimulation. Owing to enhanced target specificity, AT_1 receptor antagonists more efficiently block the effects of AngII than do ACE inhibitors. In addition, the elevated level of circulating AngII that occurs secondary to AT_1 receptor blockade results in a relative increase in AT_2 receptor activation. Unlike ACE inhibitors, AT_1 blockers do not influence bradykinin metabolism (see the next section).

ANGIOTENSIN-CONVERTING ENZYME INHIBITORS. The ACE inhibitors captopril, enalapril, ramipril, lisinopril, quinapril, trandolapril, and fosinopril (*see* Chapter 26) are FDA-approved for the treatment of CHF. Data from numerous clinical trials support ACE inhibition in the management of CHF of any severity, including those with asymptomatic LV dysfunction.

ACE-inhibitor therapy typically is initiated at a low dose (e.g., 6.25 mg of captopril, 5 mg of lisinopril) to avoid iatrogenic hypotension. ACE-inhibitor doses customarily are increased over several days in hospitalized patients or over weeks in ambulatory patients, with monitoring of blood pressure, serum electrolytes, and creatinine levels. In CHF patients with decreased renal blood flow, ACE inhibitors impair autoregulation of glomerular perfusion pressure, reflecting their selective effect on efferent (over afferent) arteriolar tone. In the event of acute renal failure or a decrease in the glomerular filtration rate by >20%, ACE-inhibitor dosing should be reduced or the drug discontinued.

ACE-Inhibitor Side Effects. Elevated bradykinin levels from ACE inhibition are associated with angioedema, a potentially life-threatening drug side effect. If this occurs, immediate and permanent cessation of *all* ACE inhibitors is indicated. A characteristic, dry cough from the same mechanism is common; in this case, substitution of an AT_1 receptor antagonist for the ACE inhibitor often is curative. A small rise in serum K^+ levels is common with ACE-inhibitor use. This increase may be substantial in patients with renal impairment or in diabetic patients with type IV renal tubular acidosis. Mild hyperkalemia is best managed by institution of a low-potassium diet or dose adjustment.

ACE Inhibitors and Survival in CHF. When compared with other vasodilators, ACE inhibitors appear superior in reducing mortality in CHF. ACE inhibitors improve survival in patients with CHF due to systolic dysfunction. ACE inhibitors also prevent the development of clinically significant LV dysfunction after acute MI. ACE inhibitors appear to confer these benefits by preventing postinfarction-associated adverse ventricular remodeling. In asymptomatic patients with LV dysfunction, ACE inhibitors slow the development of symptomatic CHF.

AT_1 RECEPTOR ANTAGONISTS. AT_1 receptor antagonism obviates AngII "escape" and decreases the probability of developing bradykinin-mediated side effects associated with ACE inhibition. Although rare, angioedema has been reported with AT_1 receptor antagonist use. AT_1 receptor blockers (ARBs) are effective antihypertensives, and their influence on mortality in acute or chronic CHF from systolic dysfunction after acute MI is akin to that of ACE-inhibitor therapy. Owing to their favorable side-effect profile, ARBs are an excellent alternative in CHF patients intolerant of ACE inhibitors. In the elderly, there is an increased probability of developing clinically significant hypotension, renal dysfunction, and hyperkalemia.

The role of combination ACE-inhibitor and ARB therapy in the treatment of CHF remains unresolved. Based on the hypothesis that ARB efficacy is at least in part a consequence of reduced circulating aldosterone levels, combined. Combined ARB treatment with aldosterone receptor inhibition has also been explored. Combination therapy is associated with a significant increase in LV ejection fraction and quality of life scores in patients with CHF from systolic dysfunction treated for 1 year with candesartan (8 mg daily) and spironolactone (25 mg daily) compared to those treated with candesartan alone. Data regarding mortality benefit attendant to combination therapy are not available at present.

DIRECT RENIN INHIBITORS. Maximal pharmacologic ACE inhibition alone may be insufficient for optimal attenuation of AngII-induced cardiovascular dysfunction in patients with CHF. Several molecular mechanisms may contribute:

- ACE-independent pathways that facilitate AngI → AngII conversion
- Suppression of the negative feedback exerted by AngII on renin secretion in the kidney

Thus, inhibition of renin to further suppress AngII synthesis in CHF has gained popularity. Renin-mediated conversion of angiotensinogen to AngI is the first and rate-limiting step in the biochemical cascade that generates AngII and aldosterone (*see* Figures 26–1 and 28–4).

Aliskiren (TEKTURNA, RASILEZ) is the first orally administered direct renin inhibitor to obtain FDA approval for use in clinical practice. The pharmacokinetic advantages of aliskiren over earlier direct renin inhibitor prototypes include an increased bioavailability (2.7%) and a long plasma $t_{1/2}$ (~23 h). Aliskiren induces a concentration-dependent decrease in plasma renin activity and AngI and AngII levels that are associated with a decrease in systemic blood pressure without significant reflex tachycardia (*see* Chapter 26).

Aliskiren is as effective as an ARB for monotherapy of mild-to-moderate hypertension. Aliskiren also appears to exert beneficial effects on myocardial remodeling by decreasing LV mass in hypertensive patients, suggesting that direct renin inhibition may attenuate hypertension-induced end-organ damage. Collectively, these observations provide evidence that aliskiren-mediated reductions in plasma renin activity and circulating levels of AngII may have salutary effects on the cardiovascular system in hypertension. Combining aliskiren (150 mg/day) with a β receptor antagonist and an ACE inhibitor or ARB did not produce a significant increase in hypotension or hyperkalemia in a cohort that mainly included symptomatic CHF patients with a low LV ejection fraction (~30%). Results from this trial also demonstrated that aliskiren significantly decreased plasma *N*-terminal-proBNP levels, a clinically useful neurohumoral biomarker of active CHF. These findings affirm that inhibition of renin activity is an important potential target for improving symptoms and functional capacity in CHF.

VASOPRESSIN RECEPTOR ANTAGONISTS. Neurohumoral dysregulation in CHF includes abnormal arginine vasopressin (AVP) secretion, resulting in the perturbation of fluid balance. AVP is secreted into the systemic circulation in response to: (1) serum hypertonicity-induced activation of anterior pituitary osmoreceptors, and (2) a perceived drop in blood pressure detected by baroreceptors in the carotid artery, aortic arch, and left atrium (*see* Chapter 25).

The active form of AVP is a 9–amino acid peptide that interacts with 3 receptor subtypes: V_{1a}, V_{1b}, and V_2. The AVP-V_2 receptor interaction on the basolateral membrane of the renal collecting ducts stimulates de novo synthesis of aquaporin-2 water channels that mediate free water reabsorption, thereby impairing diuresis and, ultimately, correcting plasma hypertonicity. Additional cell signaling pathways important in the pathophysiology of CHF include vasoconstriction, cell hypertrophy, and increased platelet aggregation mediated by activation of V_{1a} receptors in vascular smooth muscle cells and cardiac myocytes. In addition, AngII-mediated activation of centrally located AT_1 receptors is associated with increased AVP levels in CHF and may represent 1 mechanism by which the use of AT_1-receptor antagonists are effective in the clinical management of these patients.

AVP levels are nearly 2-fold above normal in CHF patients. This dysregulation of AVP synthesis in CHF may involve impaired atrial stretch receptor sensitivity, normally a counterregulatory mechanism for AVP secretion, and increased adrenergic tone. However, elevated levels of AVP have been observed in *asymptomatic* patients with significantly decreased LV function. CHF may have a component of *abnormal responsiveness to vasopressin* rather than one of excessive vasopressin production alone. Vasopressin infusion in CHF patients decreases cardiac output and stroke volume and causes an exaggerated increase in systemic vascular resistance and pulmonary capillary wedge pressure. In turn, V_2 antagonists attenuate the adverse pathophysiologic effects of hypervasopressinemia by decreasing capillary wedge pressure, right atrial pressure, and pulmonary artery systolic blood pressure. These agents also restore and maintain normal serum sodium levels in decompensated CHF patients, but their long-term use has not yet been convincingly linked to a decrease in CHF-associated symptoms or mortality.

Tolvaptan (SAMSCA), which preferentially binds the V_2 receptor over the V_{1a} receptor (receptor selectivity ~29:1), is perhaps the most widely tested vasopressin receptor antagonist in patients with CHF and also is approved for hyponatremia. Due to the risk of overly rapid correction of hyponatremia causing osmotic demyelination, tolvaptan should be started only in a hospital setting where Na^+ levels can be monitored closely and possible drug interactions mediated by CYP and P-gp can be considered (black box warning). Conivaptan, used mainly for the treatment of hyponatremia rather than for CHF per se, differs from tolvaptan in that it may be intravenously administered, has high affinity for both V_2 and V_{1a} receptors, and has a $t_{1/2}$ nearly twice as long.

β ADRENERGIC RECEPTOR ANTAGONISTS

Long-term sympathomimetic use is associated with increased CHF mortality rates, whereas a survival benefit is associated with chronic administration of β receptor antagonists. β antagonists (e.g., *metoprolol*) improve symptoms, exercise tolerance, and are measures of LV function over several months in idiopathic dilated cardiomyopathy patients with CHF. Serial echocardiographic measurements in CHF patients indicate that a decrease in systolic function occurs immediately after initiation of a β antagonist treatment, but this recovers and improves beyond baseline over the ensuing 2-4 months.

Mechanism of Action. The mechanisms by which β receptor antagonists influence outcome in CHF patients are not fully delineated. By preventing myocardial ischemia without significantly influencing serum electrolytes, β receptor antagonists probably influence mortality, in part, by decreasing the frequency of unstable tachyarrhythmias to which CHF patients are particularly prone. In addition, these agents may influence survival by favorably affecting LV geometry, specifically by decreasing LV chamber size and increasing LV ejection fraction. Through inhibition of sustained sympathetic nervous system activation, these agents prevent or delay progression of myocardial contractile dysfunction by inhibiting maladaptive proliferative cell signaling in the myocardium, reducing catecholamine-induced cardiomyocyte toxicity, and decreasing myocyte apoptosis. β Receptor antagonists may also induce positive LV remodeling by decreasing oxidative stress in the myocardium.

Metoprolol. Metoprolol (LOPRESSOR, TOPROL XL, others) is a β_1-selective receptor antagonist. The short-acting form of this drug has a $t_{1/2}$ of ~6 h. The extended-release formulation is sufficiently dosed once daily. A number of clinical trials have demonstrated the beneficial effects of β-antagonist therapy in CHF.

Carvedilol. Carvedilol (COREG, others) is a nonselective β receptor antagonist and α_1-selective antagonist that is FDA approved for the management of mild-to-severe CHF. In clinical trials, carvedilol (25 mg twice daily) was associated with a 65% reduction in all-cause mortality that was independent of age, sex, CHF etiology, or LV ejection fraction. The mortality benefit and improvement in LV ejection fraction was carvedilol concentration dependent. Exercise capacity (e.g., 6-min walk test) did not improve with carvedilol, but therapy did appear to slow the progression of CHF in a subgroup of patients with good exercise capacity and mild symptoms at baseline.

CLINICAL USE OF β ADRENERGIC RECEPTOR ANTAGONISTS IN CHF

Data from patients with mild-to-moderate chronic CHF establish that β receptor antagonists improve disease-associated symptoms, hospitalization, and mortality. Accordingly, β antagonists are recommended for use in patients with an LV ejection fraction <35% and NYHA class II or III symptoms in conjunction with an ACE inhibitor or AT_1 receptor antagonist, and diuretics as required to palliate symptoms.

The role of β receptor antagonists in severe CHF or under circumstances of an acute clinical decompensation is not yet clear. Likewise, the utility of β blockade in patients with asymptomatic LV dysfunction has not been systematically evaluated. The marked heterogeneous pharmacologic characteristics (e.g., receptor selectivity, pharmacokinetics) of specific agents play a key role in predicting the overall efficacy of a particular β receptor antagonist. β receptor antagonist therapy is customarily initiated at very low doses, generally less than one-tenth of the final target dose, and titrated upward.

CARDIAC GLYCOSIDES

The benefits of cardiac glycosides in CHF are generally attributed to:

- Inhibition of the plasma membrane Na^+, K^+-ATPase in myocytes
- A positive inotropic effect on the failing myocardium
- Suppression of rapid ventricular rate response in CHF-associated atrial fibrillation
- Regulation of downstream deleterious effects of sympathetic nervous system overactivation

Mechanism of the Positive Inotropic Effect. With cardiac myocyte depolarization (Figure 28–5), Ca^{2+} enters the cell via the L-type Ca^{2+} channel and triggers the release of stored Ca^{2+} from the sarcoplasmic reticulum via the ryanodine receptor (RyR). This Ca^{2+}-induced Ca^{2+} release increases the level of cytosolic Ca^{2+} available for interaction with myocyte contractile proteins, ultimately increasing myocardial contraction force. During myocyte repolarization and relaxation, cellular Ca^{2+} is re-sequestered by the sarcoplasmic reticular Ca^{2+}-ATPase and is removed from the cell by the Na^+ Ca^{2+} exchanger and by the sarcolemmal Ca^{2+}-ATPase.

Cardiac glycosides bind and inhibit the phosphorylated α subunit of the sarcolemmal Na^+,K^+-ATPase and thereby decreasing Na^+ extrusion and increasing cytosolic [Na^+]. This decreases the transmembrane Na^+ gradient that drives Na^+–Ca^{2+} exchange during myocyte repolarization. As a consequence, less Ca^{2+} is removed from the cell and more Ca^{2+} is accumulated in the sarcoplasmic reticulum (SR) by SERCA2. This increase in releasable Ca^{2+} (from the SR) is the mechanism by which cardiac glycosides enhance myocardial contractility. Elevated extracellular K^+ levels (i.e., hyperkalemia) cause dephosphorylation of the ATPase α subunit, altering the site of action of the most commonly used cardiac glycoside, *digoxin*, and thereby reducing the drug's effect.

Electrophysiologic Actions. At therapeutic plasma concentrations (i.e., 1-2 ng/mL), digoxin decreases automaticity and increases the maximal diastolic resting membrane potential in atrial and atrioventricular (AV) nodal tissues. This occurs via increases in vagal tone and sympathetic nervous system activity inhibition. In addition, digoxin prolongs the effective refractory period and decreases conduction velocity in AV nodal tissue. Collectively, these may contribute to sinus bradycardia, sinus arrest, prolongation of AV conduction, or high-grade AV block. At higher concentrations, cardiac glycosides may increase sympathetic nervous system activity that influences cardiac tissue automaticity, change associated with atrial and ventricular arrhythmias. Increased intracellular Ca^{2+} loading and sympathetic tone increases the spontaneous (phase 4) rate of diastolic depolarization as well as promoting delayed after depolarization; together, these decrease the threshold for generation of a propagated action potential and predisposes to malignant ventricular arrhythmias (*see* Chapter 29).

Regulation of Sympathetic Nervous System Activity. Sympathetic nervous system overactivation in CHF occurs, in part, from aberrant arterial baroreflex responses to low cardiac output. Specifically, a decline in baroreflex response to blood pressure results in a decline in baroreflex-mediated tonic suppression of CNS-directed sympathetic activity. This cascade contributes to the sustained elevation in plasma NE, renin, and vasopressin. Cardiac glycosides favorably influence carotid baroreflex responsiveness to changes in carotid sinus pressure. In patients with moderate-to-advanced CHF, cardiac glycoside infusion increases forearm blood flow and cardiac index and decreased heart rate. Digoxin also decreases centrally mediated sympathetic nervous system tone, although the mechanism to explain this is unresolved.

Pharmacokinetics. The elimination $t_{1/2}$ for digoxin is 36-48 h permitting once-daily dosing. Steady-state blood levels are achieved ~7 days after initiation of maintenance therapy. Digoxin is excreted by the kidney, and

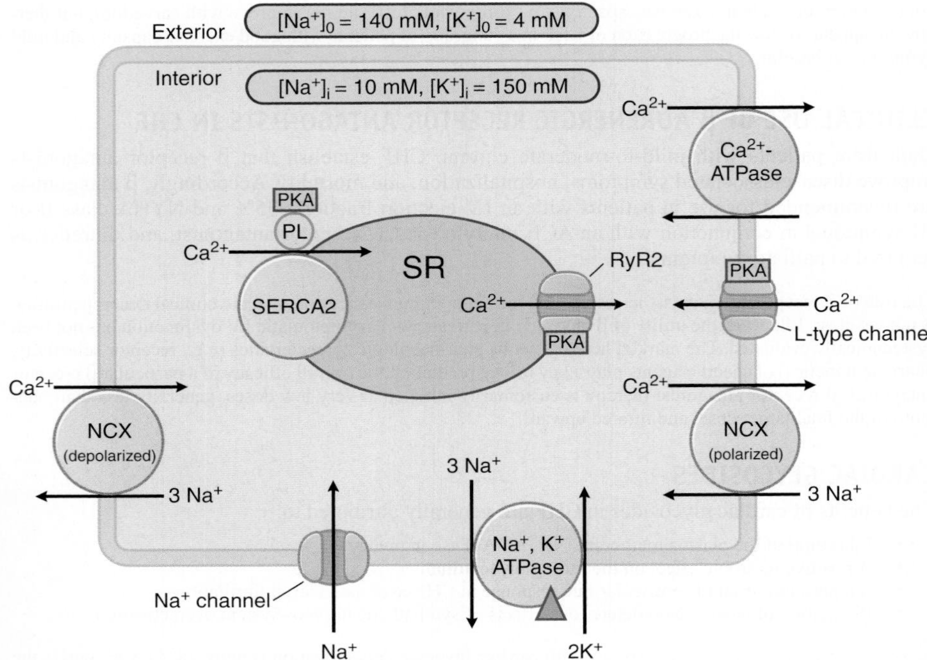

Figure 28–5 *Sarcolemmal exchange of Na^+ and Ca^{2+} during cell depolarization and repolarization.* Na^+ and Ca^{2+} enter the cardiac myocyte via the Na^+ channel and the L-type Ca^{2+} channel during each cycle of membrane depolarization, triggering the release, through the ryanodine receptor (RyR), of larger amounts of Ca^{2+} from internal stores in the sarcoplasmic reticulum (SR). The resulting increase in intracellular Ca^{2+} interacts with troponin C and activates interactions between actin and myosin that result in sarcomere shortening. The electrochemical gradient for Na^+ across the sarcolemma is maintained by active transport of Na^+ out of the cell by the sarcolemmal Na^+,K^+-ATPase. The bulk of cytosolic Ca^{2+} is pumped back into the SR by a Ca^{2+}-ATPase, SERCA2. The remainder is removed from the cell by either a sarcolemmal Ca^{2+}-ATPase or a high-capacity Na^+-Ca^{2+} exchanger, NCX. NCX exchanges 3 Na^+ for a Ca^{2+}, using the electrochemical potential of Na^+ to drive Ca^{2+} extrusion. The direction of Na^+-Ca^{2+} exchange may reverse briefly during depolarization, when the electrical gradient across the sarcolemma is transiently reversed. β adrenergic agonists and PDE inhibitors, by increasing intracellular cyclic AMP levels, activate PKA, which phosphorylates phospholamban (PL), the α subunit of the L-type Ca^{2+} channel, and regulatory components of the RyR, as well as TnI, the inhibitory subunit of troponin (not shown). As a result, the probabilities of opening of the L-type Ca^{2+} channel and the RyR2 Ca^{2+} channel are doubled; SERCA2 is uninhibited and accumulates Ca^{2+} into the SR faster, more avidly, and to a higher concentration; and relaxation occurs at slightly higher $[Ca^{2+}]_i$ due to slightly reduced sensitivity of the troponin complex to Ca^{2+}. The net effect of these phosphorylations is a positive inotropic effect: *a faster rate of tension development to a higher level of tension, followed by a faster rate of relaxation*. ▲ indicates site of cardiac glycoside binding. See the text for the mechanism of positive inotropic effect of cardiac glycosides.

increases in cardiac output or renal blood flow from vasodilator therapy or sympathomimetic agents may increase renal digoxin clearance, necessitating adjustment of daily maintenance doses. The volume of distribution and drug clearance rate are both decreased in elderly patients. Digoxin is not removed effectively by hemodialysis due to the drug's large (4-7 L/kg) volume of distribution. The principal tissue reservoir is skeletal muscle and dosing should be based on estimated lean body mass. Liquid-filled capsules of digoxin (LANOXICAPS) have a higher bioavailability than do tablets (LANOXIN). Digoxin is available for intravenous administration.

Chronic renal failure decreases the volume of distribution of digoxin and therefore requires a decrease in maintenance dosage of the drug. Drug interactions that may influence circulating serum digoxin levels include several commonly used cardiovascular medications such as verapamil, amiodarone, propafenone, and spironolactone. The rapid administration of Ca^{2+} increases the risk of inducing malignant arrhythmias in patients already treated with digoxin. Electrolyte disturbances, especially hypokalemia, acid–base imbalances, and one's form of underlying heart disease also may alter a patient's susceptibility to digoxin side effects. Maximal increase in LV contractility becomes apparent at serum digoxin levels ~1.4 ng/mL (1.8 nmol). Higher serum concentrations are not associated with incrementally increased clinical benefit. The risk of death is greater with increasing serum concentrations and it is recommended to maintain digoxin levels <1 ng/mL.

Clinical Use of Digoxin in Heart Failure. Overall, digoxin use usually is limited to CHF patients with LV systolic dysfunction in atrial fibrillation or to patients in sinus rhythm who remain symptomatic despite maximal therapy with ACE inhibitors and β adrenergic receptor antagonists. The latter agents are viewed as first-line therapies because of their proven mortality benefit.

Digoxin Toxicity. The incidence and severity of digoxin toxicity have declined substantially in the past 2 decades as a consequence of alternative drugs available for the treatment of supraventricular arrhythmias in CHF and increased understanding of digoxin pharmacokinetics. Common electrophysiologic manifestations of digoxin toxicity are ectopic beats originating from the AV junction or ventricle, first-degree AV block, abnormally slow ventricular rate response to atrial fibrillation, or an accelerated AV junctional pacemaker. Lidocaine or phenytoin, which have minimal effects on AV conduction, may be used for the treatment of digoxin-induced ventricular arrhythmias that threaten hemodynamic compromise (*see* Chapter 29). Electrical cardioversion carries an increased risk of inducing severe rhythm disturbances in patients with overt digitalis toxicity. Inhibition of the Na^+,K^+-ATPase activity of skeletal muscle can cause hyperkalemia. An effective antidote for digoxin toxicity is anti-digoxin immunotherapy. Purified Fab fragments from ovine anti-digoxin antisera (DIGIBIND) are usually dosed by the estimated total dose of digoxin ingested in order to achieve a fully neutralizing effect.

β ADRENERGIC AND DOPAMINERGIC AGONISTS

In decompensated CHF from reduced cardiac output, the principal focus of initial therapy is to increase myocardial contractility. Dopamine and dobutamine are positive inotropic agents most often used to accomplish this. These drugs stimulate cardiac myocyte dopamine (D_1) and β adrenergic receptors that stimulate the G_s-adenylyl cyclase-cyclic AMP–PKA pathway. PDE inhibitors slow degradation of cyclic AMP, thereby raising the steady-state level of cyclic AMP in cells. The catalytic subunit of PKA phosphorylates a number of substrates that enhance Ca^{2+}-dependent myocardial contraction and accelerate relaxation (*see* Figure 28–5). Isoproterenol, Epi, and NE have little role in routine CHF management. Indeed, inotropic agents that elevate cardiac cell cyclic AMP are consistently associated with increased risks of hospitalization and death. At the cellular level, enhanced cyclic AMP levels have been associated with apoptosis (*see* Chapter 12).

Dopamine (DA). The pharmacologic and hemodynamic effects of DA are concentration dependent. *Low doses* (≤2 μg/kg lean body mass/min) induces cyclic AMP–dependent vascular smooth muscle vasodilation. Activation of D_2 receptors on sympathetic nerves in the peripheral circulation at these concentrations also inhibits NE release and reduces α adrenergic stimulation of vascular smooth muscle, particularly in splanchnic and renal arterial beds. Low-dose DA infusion often is used to increase renal blood flow and thereby maintain an adequate glomerular filtration rate in hospitalized CHF patients with impaired renal function refractory to diuretics. DA also exhibits a pro-diuretic effect directly on renal tubular epithelial cells that contributes to volume reduction. *At intermediate infusion rates* (2-5 μg/kg/min), dopamine directly stimulates cardiac β receptors and vascular sympathetic neurons that enhance myocardial contractility and neural NE release. At *higher infusion rates* (5-15 μg/kg/min), α adrenergic receptor stimulation–mediated peripheral arterial and venous constriction occurs. This may be desirable in patients with critically reduced arterial pressure or in those with circulatory failure from severe vasodilation (e.g., sepsis, anaphylaxis), but has little role in the treatment of patients with primary cardiac contractile dysfunction. Tachycardia, which is more pronounced with DA than with dobutamine, may provoke ischemia in patients with coronary artery disease.

Dobutamine. Dobutamine is the β agonist of choice for the management of CHF patients with systolic dysfunction. For clinical use, dobutamine is available as a racemic mixture that stimulates both β_1 and β_2 receptor subtypes. In addition, the (–) enantiomer is an agonist for α adrenergic receptors, whereas the (+) enantiomer is a weak, partial agonist. At infusion rates that result in a positive inotropic effect in humans, the β_1 adrenergic effect in the myocardium predominates. In the vasculature, the α adrenergic agonist effect of the (–) enantiomer appears to be offset by the (+) enantiomer and vasodilating effects of β_2 receptor stimulation. Thus, the principal hemodynamic effect of dobutamine is an increase in stroke volume from positive inotropy, although β_2 receptor activation may cause a decrease in systemic vascular resistance and, therefore, mean arterial pressure. Despite increases in cardiac output, there is relatively little chronotropic effect. Continuous dobutamine infusions are typically initiated at 2-3 μg/kg/min and uptitrated until the desired hemodynamic response is achieved. Pharmacologic tolerance may limit infusion efficacy beyond 4 days, and, therefore, addition or substitution with a class III PDE inhibitor may be necessary to maintain adequate circulatory support. The major side effects of dobutamine are tachycardia and supraventricular or ventricular arrhythmias, which may require a reduction in dosage. Recent β receptor antagonist use is a common cause of blunted clinical responsiveness to dobutamine.

PHOSPHODIESTERASE INHIBITORS

The cyclic AMP–PDE inhibitors decrease cellular cyclic AMP degradation, resulting in elevated levels of cyclic AMP. The physiologic effects are positive myocardial inotropism and dilation of resistance and capacitance vessels. Collectively, PDE inhibition improves cardiac output through inotropy and by decreasing preload and afterload (thus giving rise to the term *inodilator*).

Inamrinone and Milrinone. Parenteral formulations of *inamrinone* (previously named amrinone) and *milrinone* are approved for short-term circulation support in advanced CHF. Both drugs are selective inhibitors of PDE3, the cyclic GMP–inhibited cyclic AMP PDE. By elevating cellular cyclic AMP levels, these drugs stimulate myocardial contractility and accelerate myocardial relaxation. In addition, they cause balanced arterial and venous dilation with a consequent fall in systemic and pulmonary vascular resistances and left and right-heart filling pressure. As a result of its effect on LV contractility, the increase in cardiac output from milrinone is superior to that from nitroprusside. Conversely, the arterial and venodilatory effects of milrinone are greater than those of dobutamine at concentrations that produce similar increases in cardiac output.

For inamrinone, a 0.75-mg/kg bolus injection administered over 2-3 min is typically followed by a 2-20-μg/kg/min infusion. The loading dose of milrinone is ordinarily 50 μg/kg, and the continuous infusion rate ranges from 0.25-1 μg/kg/min. The elimination half-lives of inamrinone and milrinone in normal individuals are 2-3 h and 0.5-1 h, respectively, but are nearly doubled in patients with severe CHF. Clinically significant thrombocytopenia occurs in ~10% of those receiving inamrinone but is rare with milrinone. Because of enhanced selectivity for PDE3, short $t_{1/2}$, and favorable side-effect profile, milrinone is the agent of choice among currently available PDE inhibitors for *short-term*, parenteral inotropic support.

Sildenafil. In contrast to inamrinone and milrinone, sildenafil (REVATIO) inhibits PDE5, which is the most common PDE isoform in lung tissue. This characteristic of PDE5 likely accounts for the enhanced pulmonary artery specificity observed with sildenafil use. In fact, until recently, the primary clinical application of sildenafil in CHF has mainly been limited to those with isolated right ventricular systolic failure from pulmonary artery hypertension. However, recently published reports suggest that sildenafil favorably influences exercise capacity and right-heart hemodynamics in patients with pulmonary hypertension from LV systolic dysfunction as well. The pharmacology of PDE5 inhibitors is presented in Chapter 27.

CHRONIC POSITIVE INOTROPIC THERAPY

Although improvements in CHF symptoms, functional status, and hemodynamic profile have been reported, the effect of long-term therapy on mortality is disappointing. In fact, the dopaminergic agonist ibopamine; PDE inhibitors milrinone, inamrinone, and vesnarinone; and pimobendan are associated with increased mortality. At present, digoxin remains the only oral inotropic agent available for CHF patient use.

DIASTOLIC HEART FAILURE

Up to 40% of CHF patients have preserved LV systolic function. The pathogenesis of diastolic CHF includes structural and functional abnormalities of the ventricle(s) that are associated with impaired ventricular relaxation and LV distensibility. These abnormalities are reflected in the LV pressure–volume relationship during diastole, which is shifted upward and to the left relative to normal subjects (Figure 28–6). Diastolic CHF is diagnosed when the LV is unable to maintain adequate cardiac output without filling at an abnormally elevated end-diastolic filling pressure.

In patients with *primary* diastolic dysfunction, the myocardial abnormality that accounts for abnormal filling is intrinsic to the myocardium; e.g., by infiltrative disorders including cardiac amyloidosis, hemochromatosis, sarcoidosis, and rarer conditions such as endomyocardial fibrosis and Fabry disease. Although not a disease of myocardium infiltration, CHF may occur despite intact LV systolic function in familial hypertrophic cardiomyopathy. *Secondary* diastolic dysfunction occurs as a consequence of excessive preload (e.g., renal failure), excessive afterload (e.g., systemic hypertension), or changes in LV geometry that occur in response to chronically abnormal loading conditions. Diastolic CHF also is observed in patients with long-standing epicardial coronary artery or pericardial disease. The prevalence of secondary diastolic dysfunction is higher in women

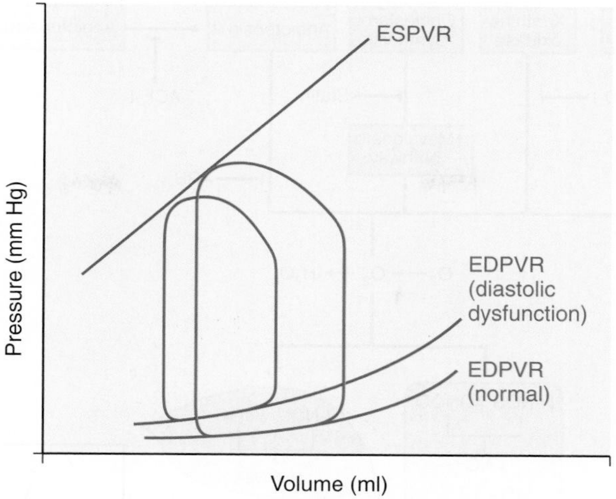

Figure 28–6 *Pressure–volume relationships in normal heart and heart with diastolic dysfunction.* Normal P-V loop (*green*) based on normal end-diastolic pressure–volume relationship (EDPVR). P-V loop with diastolic dysfunction is shown in red. ESPVR, end-systolic pressure–volume relationship.

and with advanced age. Reported annual mortality rates for diastolic CHF are 5-8%, likely represents an underestimation.

Patients with diastolic CHF are typically dependent on preload to maintain adequate cardiac output. Although hypervolemic patients generally benefit from careful intravascular volume reduction, this must be accomplished gradually with frequent reassessment of treatment goals. Maintaining synchronous atrial contraction (or at least ventricular rate response control) helps to maintain adequate LV filling during the latter phase of diastole and is therefore a paramount goal in the management of CHF from diastolic dysfunction. Treatment of predisposing conditions to impaired diastolic function, such as myocardial ischemia and poorly controlled systemic hypertension, are fundamental to the overall pharmacotherapeutic strategy of this complex form of CHF.

TARGETING VASCULAR DYSFUNCTION IN CHF

Vascular dysfunction is an established component of the CHF syndrome associated with poorer clinical outcome and has evolved into a novel pharmacotherapeutic target (Figure 28–7). Elevated levels of oxidant, nitrosative, and other forms of inflammatory stress observed in patients with CHF may impair vascular reactivity by disruption of cell signaling pathways that lead to vasodilation.

Xanthine Oxidase and Vascular Dysfunction. Xanthine oxidase (XO) is necessary for normal purine metabolism and catalyzes the oxidation of hypoxanthine to xanthine and xanthine to uric acid in a reaction that generates superoxide. Elevated levels of uric acid are associated with clinically evident CHF. Epidemiologic data support a positive, graded association between impaired exercise capacity and circulating uric acid levels. The myocardium and vascular endothelial cells contain high concentrations of XO. This lead to the hypothesis that increased XO-generated superoxide impairs vascular reactivity in CHF patients.

Allopurinol (300 mg/day), an XO inhibitor, effectively decreases generation of free oxygen radicals and improves peripheral arterial vasodilation and blood flow in hyperuricemic patients with mild-to-moderate CHF from systolic dysfunction. Interestingly, *probenecid*, which decreases circulating urate levels by enhancing its elimination rather than by inhibiting XO activity, has not been shown to influence vascular reactivity. In patients with advanced CHF, allopurinol-induced serum uric acid level reduction (over 24 weeks) is associated with functional class improvement, but only in those with baseline serum uric acid levels >9.5 mg/dL.

Statins and Vascular Dysfunction. HMG-CoA (3-hydroxy-3-methyl-glutaryl–coenzyme A) reductase catalyzes the formation of L-mevalonic acid, a key biochemical precursor in the cholesterol synthesis pathway. Current evidence suggests a role of crosstalk between mevalonate metabolism and cell signaling pathways involved in inflammation and oxidant stress. Intermediate by-products of mevalonate metabolism (i.e., isopenylated

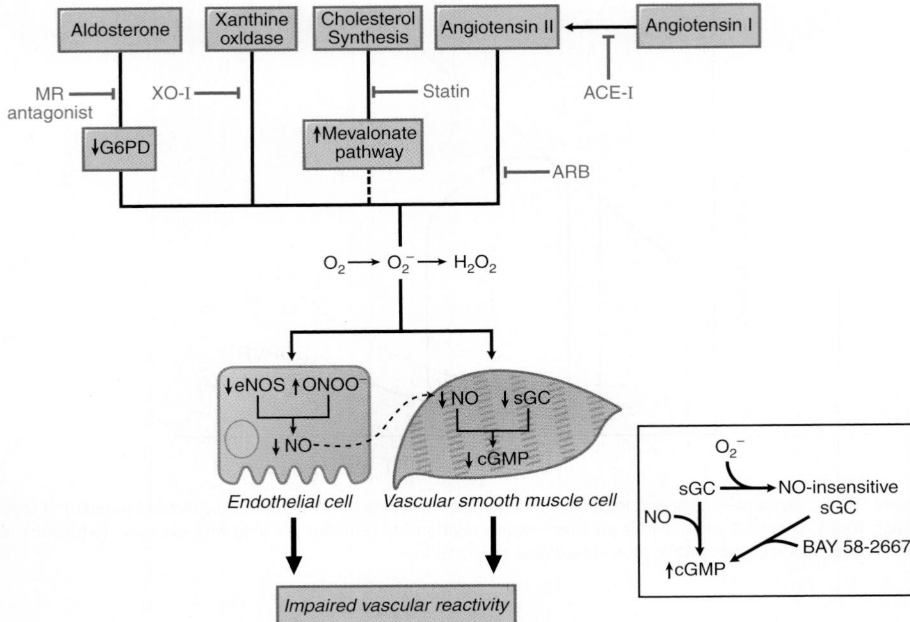

Figure 28–7 *Preserving normal vascular reactivity is a target of evolving priority in the treatment of patients with chronic CHF.* Increased levels of reactive oxygen species (ROS, e.g., superoxide [O_2^-] and hydrogen peroxide [H_2O_2]) that are generated in endothelial cells (EC) and vascular smooth muscle cells (VSMC) impair key signaling pathways necessary for normal vascular function. For example, excessive aldosterone can cause a reduction in antioxidant enzyme activity in EC, such as glucose-6-phosphate dehydrogenase (G6PD), resulting in increased ROS formation. Likewise, increased xanthine oxidase (XO) activity, AT_1 receptor activation, and upregulation of signaling pathways associated with cholesterol metabolism favor ROS formation. In EC, elevated levels of ROS impair vascular reactivity, in part, by decreasing endothelial nitric oxide synthase (eNOS) activity and increasing peroxynitrite ($ONOO^-$) formation (which will decrease bioavailable NO). In VSMC, oxidant stress decreases NO levels and impairs sensitivity of soluble guanylyl cyclase (sGC) to NO, reducing cyclic GMP-dependent VSMC relaxation. Mineralocorticoid (MR)-receptor antagonists, XO inhibitors (XO-I), HMG-CoA-reductase inhibitors (statin), AT_1 receptor blockers (ARBs), and angiotensin-converting enzyme inhibitors (ACE-I) block various cellular reactions associated with elevated levels of ROS and impaired vascular reactivity. The BAY compounds (e.g., BAY 58-2667; *figure inset*), are a novel group of direct sGC activators that increase enzyme activity despite oxidant stress-induced sGC modifications that convert the enzyme to an NO-insensitive state.

proteins that upregulate activation of Rho, RAS, and other G proteins) are linked to impaired vascular function by increasing levels of oxidant stress and decreasing bioavailable NO levels. Statins inhibit these intermediary pathways and appear to restore endothelium-dependent and endothelium-independent vascular function. A large number of population studies have demonstrated a favorable effect of statin therapy on outcome in CHF.

Direct Activators of Soluble Guanylyl Cyclase. Soluble guanylyl cyclase (sGC) is an enzyme that catalyzes the conversion of GTP to cyclic GMP, a second messenger necessary for normal vascular smooth muscle cell relaxation. Under physiologic conditions, NO is the primary biologically active stimulator of sGC. Elevated levels of oxidant stress deactivate sGC through various molecular mechanisms. Organic nitrates, which promote sGC activation by increasing bioavailable NO levels, are subject to pharmacologic tolerance that complicates long-term drug use, dosing, and administration frequency (*see* Chapter 27). BAY compounds (e.g., BAY 58-2667 [cinaciguat]) activate sGC by an NO-independent mechanism, thereby promoting normal sGC function despite conditions of oxidant stress. In healthy humans, BAY compound administration has not been associated with severe side effects, but hypotension and headaches have been reported. The utility of BAY 58-2667 in the clinical management of patients with CHF is a topic of ongoing investigation.

PROGESSION OF DISEASE AND THERAPY IN CHF

CHF is a chronic and usually progressive illness. Therapy also needs to be progressive in response to the disease:

Stage 1. *Patient at risk but asymptomatic:*

- Identify and reduce risk factors, educate patient and family
- Manage measurable risk factors; treat hypertension, diabetes, dyslipidemias

Stage 2. *With structural remodeling but few symptoms:*

- Reduce effects of AngII (ACEI or AT_1 blocker); add β_1 blocker as appropriate

Stage 3. *Structural disease, symptoms of failure:*

- Add ACEI or AT_1 blocker and β_1 blocker
- Reduce dietary Na^+ intake; add diuretics, digoxin
- Treat bundle-branch block (resynchronize), if needed
- Revascularize, replace mitral valve, as appropriate
- Add aldosterone antagonist

Stage 4. *Symptoms refractory to treatment:*

- Use inotropic agents
- Employ surgical interventions (ventricular assist device; heart transplant)

A few new treatments are advancing through clinical trials. The hormone relaxin, which acts via four GPCRs, has a complex physiology but appears to be useful in heart failure. In the near future, we may have treatments that correct some of the molecular contributors of heart failure, such as a SERCA2 transgene that enhances uptake, storage, and release of Ca^{2+} in cardiac myocytes (*see* Figure 28–5).

For a complete Bibliographical Listing see Goodman & Gilman's ***The Pharmacological Basis of Therapeutics***, 12th ed., or Goodman & Gilman Online at www.AccessMedicine.com.

Anti-Arrhythmic Drugs

Cardiac cells undergo depolarization and repolarization to form cardiac action potentials ~60 times/min. The shape and duration of each action potential are determined by the activity of ion channel protein complexes in the membranes of individual cells, and the genes encoding most of these proteins now have been identified.

Arrhythmias can range from incidental, asymptomatic clinical findings to life-threatening abnormalities. In some human arrhythmias, precise mechanisms are known, and treatment can be targeted specifically against those mechanisms. In other cases, mechanisms can be only inferred, and the choice of drugs is based largely on the results of prior experience. Anti-arrhythmic drug therapy can have 2 goals: termination of an ongoing arrhythmia or prevention of an arrhythmia. Unfortunately, anti-arrhythmic drugs not only help to control arrhythmias but also can cause them, especially during long-term therapy. Thus, prescribing anti-arrhythmic drugs requires that precipitating factors be excluded or minimized, that a precise diagnosis of the type of arrhythmia be made, and that the risks of drug therapy can be minimized.

PRINCIPLES OF CARDIAC ELECTROPHYSIOLOGY

The flow of ions across cell membranes generates the currents that make up cardiac action potentials. Most anti-arrhythmic drugs affect more than one ion current, and many exert ancillary effects such as modification of cardiac contractility or autonomic nervous system function. Thus, anti-arrhythmic drugs usually exert multiple actions and can be beneficial or harmful in individual patients.

THE CARDIAC CELL AT REST: A K^+-PERMEABLE MEMBRANE

The normal cardiac cell at rest maintains a transmembrane potential ~80-90 mV negative to the exterior; this gradient is established by pumps, especially the Na^+,K^+-ATPase, and fixed anionic charges within cells. There are both an electrical and a concentration gradient that would move Na^+ ions into resting cells (Figure 29–1). However, Na^+ channels, which allow Na^+ to move along this gradient, are closed at negative transmembrane potentials, so Na^+ does not enter normal resting cardiac cells. In contrast, a specific type of K^+ channel protein (the inward rectifier channel) is in an open conformation at negative potentials. Hence, K^+ can move through these channels across the cell membrane at negative potentials in response to either electrical or concentration gradients.

For each individual ion, there is an equilibrium potential E_x at which there is no net driving force for the ion to move across the membrane. E_x can be calculated using the Nernst equation:

$$E_x = -(RT/FZ_x)\ \ln([x]_i/[x]_0)$$

where Z_x is the valence of the ion, T is the absolute temperature, R is the gas constant, F is Faraday's constant, $[x]_o$ is the extracellular concentration of the ion, and $[x]_i$ is the intracellular concentration. For K^+, $[K]_o = 4$ mM and $[K]_i = 140$ mM, the calculated K^+ equilibrium potential E_K is –94 mV. There is thus no net force driving K^+ ions into or out of a cell when the transmembrane potential is –94 mV, close to the resting potential. Thus, at rest, the normal cardiac cell is permeable to K^+ (because inward rectifier channels are open) and $[K]_o$ is the major determinant of resting potential. If $[K]_o$ is elevated to 10 mM, as might occur in diseases such as renal failure or myocardial ischemia, the calculated E_K rises to –70 mV.

THE CARDIAC ACTION POTENTIAL

Na^+ channels have a life cycle of openings and closings that help to regulate membrane excitability (Figure 29–2). To initiate an action potential, a cardiac myocyte at rest is depolarized above a threshold potential, usually via gap junctions by a neighboring myocyte. Upon membrane depolarization, Na^+ channel proteins change from the "closed" (resting) state to the "open" (conducting) state, allowing up to 10^7 Na^+ ions/sec to enter each cell and moving the transmembrane potential toward E_{Na} (+65 mV). This surge of Na^+ ions lasts only about a millisecond, after which the Na^+ channel protein rapidly moves to an "inactivated," nonconducting

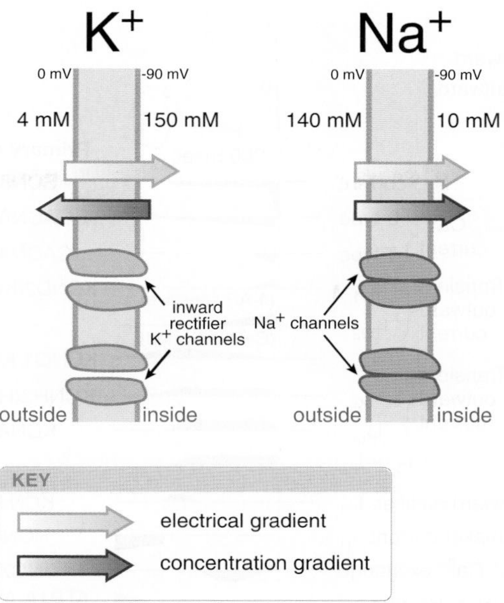

Figure 29–1 *Electrical and chemical gradients for K^+ and Na^+ in a resting cardiac cell.* Inward rectifier K^+ channels are open (*left*), allowing K^+ ions to move across the membrane and the transmembrane potential to approach E_K. In contrast, Na^+ does not enter the cell despite a large net driving force because Na^+ channel proteins are in the closed conformation (*right*) in resting cells.

state. The maximum upstroke slope of phase 0 (dV/dt_{max}, or V_{max}) of the action potential (Figure 29–3) is largely governed by Na^+ current and plays a role in the conduction velocity of a propagating action potential. Under normal conditions, Na^+ channels, once inactivated, cannot reopen until they reassume the closed conformation.

A small population of Na^+ channels may continue to open during the action potential plateau in some cells, providing further inward current. Certain mutations in the cardiac isoform of the Na^+ channel can further increase the number of channels that do not properly inactivate, thereby prolonging the action potential, and cause a form of the congenital long QT syndrome. In general, however, as the cell membrane repolarizes, the negative membrane potential moves Na^+ channel proteins from inactivated to "closed" conformations. The relationship between Na^+ channel availability and transmembrane potential is an important determinant of conduction and refractoriness in many cells.

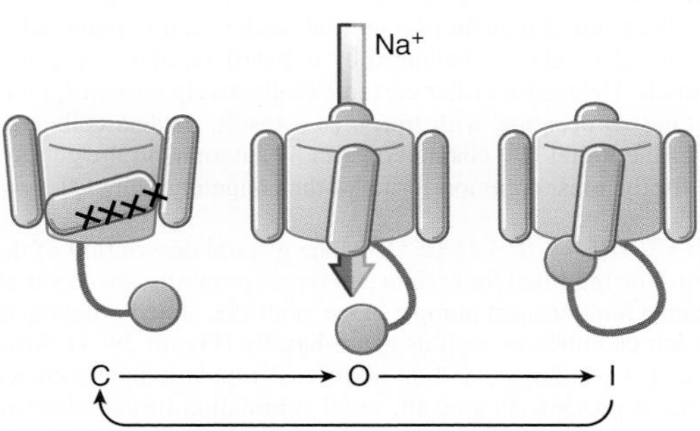

Figure 29–2 *Life cycle of a voltage-sensitive channel.* Voltage-dependent conformational changes determine current flow through Na^+ channels. At hyperpolarized potentials, the channel is in a closed conformation (**C**) and no current flows. As depolarization begins, the pore opens (**O**), allowing conduction. As depolarization is maintained, a nearby region of a channel subunit moves to block current flow, putting the channel into an inactivated, nonconducting state (**I**). Restoration of the normal resting E_m restores the conformation to the closed state (**C**). *See* Figure 20–2 for structural details.

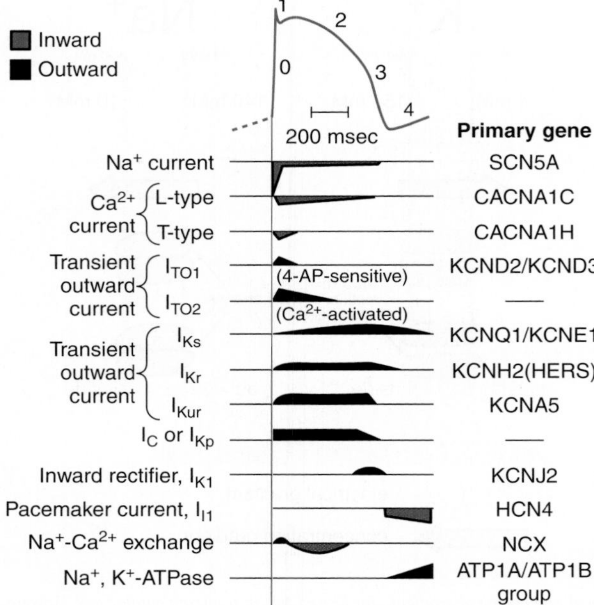

Figure 29–3 *The relationship between an action potential from the conducting system and the currents that generate it.* The current magnitudes are not to scale; the Na^+ current is ordinarily 50 times larger than any other current, although the portion that persists into the plateau (phase 2) is small. Multiple types of Ca^{2+} current, transient outward current (I_{TO}), and delayed rectifier (I_K) have been identified. Each represents a different channel protein, usually associated with ancillary (function-modifying) subunits. 4-AP (4-aminopyridine) is a widely used in vitro blocker of K^+ channels. I_{TO2} may be a Cl^- current in some species. Components of I_K have been separated on the basis of how rapidly they activate: slowly (I_{Ks}), rapidly (I_{Kr}), or ultra-rapidly (I_{Kur}). The voltage-activated, time-independent current may be carried by Cl^- (I_{Cl}) or K^+ (I_{Kp}, p for plateau). The genes encoding the major pore-forming proteins have been cloned for most of the channels shown here and are included in the right-hand column. The right-hand column lists the primary genes coding for the various ion channels and transporters.

The changes in transmembrane potential generated by the inward Na^+ current produce a series of openings (and in some cases subsequent inactivation) of other channels (*see* Figure 29–3). For example, when a cell is depolarized by the Na^+ current, "transient outward" K^+ channels quickly enter an open, or conducting, state; because the transmembrane potential at the end of phase 0 is positive to E_K, the opening of transient outward channels results in an outward, or repolarizing, K^+ current (termed I_{TO}), which contributes to the phase 1 "notch" seen in action potentials from these tissues. Transient outward K^+ channels, like Na^+ channels, inactivate rapidly. During the phase 2 plateau of a normal cardiac action potential, inward, depolarizing currents, primarily through Ca^{2+} channels, are balanced by outward, repolarizing currents primarily through K^+ ("delayed-rectifier") channels. Delayed-rectifier currents (collectively termed I_K) increase with time, whereas Ca^{2+} currents inactivate (and so decrease with time); as a result, cardiac cells repolarize (phase 3) several hundred milliseconds after the initial Na^+ channel opening. Mutations in the genes encoding repolarizing K^+ channels are responsible for the most common forms of the congenital long QT syndrome.

ACTION POTENTIAL HETEROGENEITY IN THE HEART. The general description of the action potential and the currents that underlie it must be modified for certain cell types, primarily due to variability in the expression of ion channels and electrogenic ion transport pumps. In the ventricle, action potential duration (APD) and shape vary across the wall of each chamber, as well as apico-basally (Figure 29–4). Atrial cells have short action potentials, probably because I_{TO} is larger, and an additional repolarizing K^+ current, activated by the neurotransmitter acetylcholine, is present. As a result, vagal stimulation further shortens atrial action potentials. Cells of the sinus and atrioventricular (AV) nodes lack substantial Na^+ currents. In addition, these cells, as well as cells from the conducting system, normally display the phenomenon of spontaneous diastolic, or phase 4 depolarization and thus spontaneously reach threshold for regeneration of action potentials. The rate of spontaneous firing usually is fastest in sinus node cells, which therefore serve as the natural pacemaker of the heart.

One of the pacemaking currents responsible for this automaticity is generated via specialized K^+ channels, the hyperpolarization-activated, cyclic nucleotide-gated (HCN) channels that are permeable to both potassium

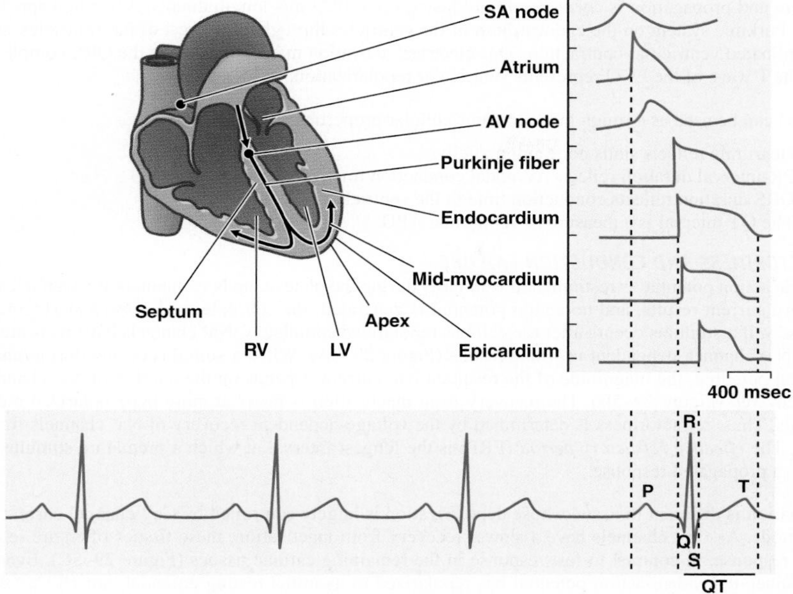

Figure 29–4 *Normal impulse propagation.* A schematic of the human heart with example action potentials from different regions of the heart (*top*) for a normal beat and their corresponding contributions to the macroscopic ECG (*bottom*). AV, atrioventricular; LV, left ventricle; RV, right ventricle; SA, sinoatrial. (Used with permission from The Am Physiol Soc. Nerbonne JM, Kass RS. *Physiol Rev,* 2005;85:1205-1253.)

and sodium. Another mechanism responsible for automaticity is the repetitive spontaneous Ca^{2+} release from the sarcoplasmic reticulum (SR). The rise in cytosolic Ca^{2+} causes membrane depolarizations when Ca^{2+} is extruded from the cell via the electrogenic Na-Ca exchanger (NCX). In addition, sinus node cells lack *inward rectifier K^+ currents* that are primarily responsible for protecting working myocardium against spontaneous membrane depolarizations.

MAINTENANCE OF INTRACELLULAR ION HOMEOSTASIS

With each action potential, the cell interior gains Na^+ ions and loses K^+ ions. The Na^+,K^+-ATPase (Na^+ pump) is activated in most cells to maintain intracellular homeostasis, extruding 3 Na^+ ions for every 2 K^+ ions shuttled from the exterior of the cell to the interior; as a result, the act of pumping itself generates a net outward (repolarizing) current.

Normally, basal intracellular Ca^{2+} is maintained at very low levels (<100 nM). In cardiac myocytes, the entry of Ca^{2+} during each action potential through L-type Ca^{2+} channels is a signal to the SR to release its Ca^{2+} stores. The efflux of Ca^{2+} from the SR occurs through ryanodine-receptor (RyR2) Ca^{2+} release channels, and the resulting increase in intracellular Ca^{2+} subsequently triggers Ca^{2+}-dependent contractile processes (= excitation-contraction coupling). Removal of intracellular Ca^{2+} occurs by both Ca^{2+}-ATPase (which moves Ca^{2+} ions back into the SR) and NCX, which exchanges 3 Na^+ ions from the exterior for each Ca^{2+} ion extruded (*see* Figure 28–5). Abnormal regulation of intracellular Ca^{2+} is increasingly well described in heart failure and contributes to arrhythmias in this setting. Furthermore, mutations that disrupt the normal activity of the RyR2 channels and the cardiac isoform of calsequestrin have been linked to catecholaminergic polymorphic ventricular tachycardia (CPVT), thereby demonstrating a direct link between spontaneous SR Ca^{2+} release and cardiac arrhythmias.

IMPULSE PROPAGATION AND THE ELECTROCARDIOGRAM

Normal cardiac impulses originate in the sinus node. Once impulses leave the sinus node, they propagate rapidly throughout the atria, resulting in atrial systole and the P wave of the surface electrocardiogram (ECG; *see* Figure 29–4). Propagation slows markedly through the AV node, where the inward current (through Ca^{2+} channels) is much smaller than the Na^+ current in atria, ventricles, or the subendocardial conducting system. This conduction delay allows the atrial contraction to propel blood into the ventricle, thereby optimizing cardiac output. Once impulses exit the AV node, they enter the conducting system, where Na^+ currents are larger than elsewhere and propagation is correspondingly faster, up to 0.75 m/s longitudinally. Activation spreads from the His–Purkinje system on the endocardium of the ventricles throughout the rest of the ventricles, stimulating coordinated ventricular contraction. This electrical activation manifests itself as the QRS complex on the ECG. The T wave of the ECG represents ventricular repolarization.

The ECG can be used as a rough guide to some cellular properties of cardiac tissue:

- Heart rate reflects sinus node automaticity.
- PR-interval duration reflects AV nodal conduction time.
- QRS duration reflects conduction time in the ventricle.
- The QT interval is a measure of ventricular APD.

REFRACTORINESS AND CONDUCTION FAILURE

If a single action potential is restimulated very early during the plateau, no Na^+ channels are available to open, no inward current results, and no action potential is generated: the cell is termed *refractory* (Figure 29–5). Conversely, if a stimulus occurs after the cell has repolarized completely, Na^+ channels have recovered, and a normal Na^+ channel–dependent upstroke results (Figure 29–5A). When a stimulus occurs during phase 3 of the action potential, the magnitude of the resultant Na^+ current depends on the number of Na^+ channels that have recovered (Figure 29–5B). The recovery from inactivation is faster at more hyperpolarized membrane potentials. Thus, refractoriness is determined by the voltage-dependent recovery of Na^+ channels from inactivation. The *effective refractory period* (ERP) is the longest interval at which a premature stimulus fails to generate a propagated response.

The situation is different in tissue whose depolarization is largely controlled by Ca^{2+} channel current such as the AV node. As Ca^{2+} channels have a slower recovery from inactivation, these tissues often are referred to as slow response, in contrast to fast response in the remaining cardiac tissues (Figure 29–5C). Even after a Ca^{2+} channel–dependent action potential has repolarized to its initial resting potential, not all Ca^{2+} channels are available for re-excitation. Therefore, an extra stimulus applied shortly after repolarization is complete and generates a reduced Ca^{2+} current, which may propagate slowly to adjacent cells prior to extinction. An extra stimulus applied later will result in a larger Ca^{2+} current and faster propagation. Thus, in Ca^{2+} channel–dependent tissues, which include not only the AV node but also tissues whose underlying characteristics have been altered by factors such as myocardial ischemia, refractoriness is prolonged and propagation occurs

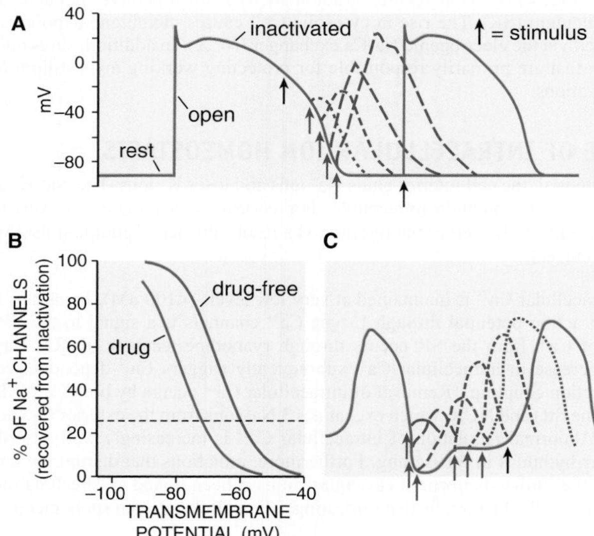

Figure 29–5 *Qualitative differences in responses of nodal and conducting tissues to premature stimuli.* **A.** With a very early premature stimulus (*black arrow*) in ventricular myocardium, all Na^+ channels still are in the inactivated state, and no upstroke results. As the action potential repolarizes, Na^+ channels recover from the inactivated to the resting state, from which opening can occur. The phase 0 upstroke slope of the premature action potentials (*purple*) are greater with later stimuli because recovery from inactivation is voltage dependent. **B.** The relationship between transmembrane potential and degree of recovery of Na^+ channels from inactivation. The *dotted line* indicates 25% recovery. Most Na^+ channel–blocking drugs shift this relationship to the left. **C.** In nodal tissues, premature stimuli delivered even after full repolarization of the action potential are depressed; recovery from inactivation is time dependent.

slowly. Slow conduction in the heart, a critical factor in the genesis of reentrant arrhythmias (see next section), also can occur when Na^+ currents are depressed by disease or membrane depolarization (e.g., elevated $[K]_o$), resulting in decreased steady-state Na^+ channel availability (*see* Figure 29–5B).

MECHANISMS OF CARDIAC ARRHYTHMIAS

When the normal sequence of impulse initiation and propagation is perturbed, an arrhythmia occurs. Failure of impulse initiation, in the sinus node, may result in slow heart rates (bradyarrhythmias), whereas failure in the normal propagation of action potentials from atrium to ventricle results in dropped beats (commonly referred to as heart block) that usually reflect an abnormality in either the AV node or the His–Purkinje system. These abnormalities may be caused by drugs (Table 29–1) or by structural heart disease; in the latter case, permanent cardiac pacing may be required.

Abnormally rapid heart rhythms (tachyarrhythmias) are common clinical problems that may be treated with anti-arrhythmic drugs. Three major underlying mechanisms have been identified: enhanced automaticity, triggered automaticity, and reentry. These often are interrelated mechanisms, as the first 2 often serve to initiate reentry.

Table 29–1

Drug-Induced Cardiac Arrhythmias

ARRHYTHMIA	DRUG	LIKELY MECHANISM	TREATMENT[a]	CLINICAL FEATURES
Sinus bradycardia AV block	Digoxin	↑Vagal tone	Antidigoxin antibodies Temporary pacing	Atrial tachycardia may also be present
Sinus bradycardia AV block	Verapamil Diltiazem	Ca^{2+} channel block	Ca^{2+} Temporary pacing	
Sinus bradycardia AV block	β Blockers Clonidine Methyldopa	Sympatholytic	Isoproterenol Temporary pacing	
Sinus tachycardia Any other tachycardia	β Blocker withdrawal	Upregulation of β receptors with chronic therapy; β blocker withdrawal ⇒ ↑ β effects	β Blockade	Hypertension, angina also possible
↑ Ventricular rate in atrial flutter	Quinidine Flecainide Propafenone	Conduction slowing in atrium, with enhanced (quinidine) or unaltered AV conduction	AV nodal blockers	QRS complexes often widened at fast rates
↑ Ventricular rate in atrial fibrillation in patients with WPW syndrome	Digoxin Verapamil	↓ accessory pathway refractoriness	IV procainamide DC cardioversion	Ventricular rate can exceed 300 beats/min
Multifocal atrial tachycardia	Theophylline	↑ intracellular Ca^{2+} and DADs	Withdraw theophylline ?Verapamil	Often in advanced lung disease

(continued)

Table 29–1

Drug-Induced Cardiac Arrhythmias (*Continued*)

ARRHYTHMIA	DRUG	LIKELY MECHANISM	TREATMENT[a]	CLINICAL FEATURES
Polymorphic VT with ↑ QT interval (torsades de pointes)	Quinidine Sotalol Procainamide Disopyramide Dofetilide Ibutilide "Noncardioactive" drugs (see text) Amiodarone (rare)	EAD-related triggered activity	Cardiac pacing Isoproterenol Magnesium	Hypokalemia, bradycardia frequent Related to ↑ plasma concentrations, except for quinidine
Frequent or difficult to terminate VT ("incessant" VT)	Flecainide Propafenone Quinidine (rarer)	Conduction slowing in reentrant circuits	Na^+ bolus reported effective in some cases	Most often in patients with advanced myocardial scarring
Atrial tachycardia with AV block; ventricular bigeminy, others	Digoxin	DAD-related triggered activity (± ↑ vagal tone)	Antidigoxin antibodies	Coexistence of abnormal impulses with abnormal sinus or AV nodal function
Ventricular fibrillation	Inappropriate use of IV verapamil	Severe hypotension and/or myocardial ischemia	Cardiac resuscitation (DC cardioversion)	Misdiagnosis of VT as PSVT and inappropriate use of verapamil

AV, atrioventricular; DAD, delayed afterdepolarization; DC, direct current; EAD, early afterdepolarization; IV, intravenous; PSVT, paroxysmal supraventricular tachycardia; VT, ventricular tachycardia; WPW, Wolff–Parkinson–White supraventricular tachycardia; ↑, increase; ↓, decrease; ?, unclear.

[a]In each of these cases, recognition and withdrawal of the offending drug(s) are mandatory.

ENHANCED AUTOMATICITY. Enhanced automaticity may occur in cells that normally display spontaneous diastolic depolarization—the sinus and AV nodes and the His–Purkinje system. β Adrenergic stimulation, hypokalemia, and mechanical stretch of cardiac muscle cells increase phase 4 slope and accelerate pacemaker rate; acetylcholine reduces pacemaker rate both by decreasing phase 4 slope and through hyperpolarization (making the maximum diastolic potential more negative). Automatic behavior may also occur in sites that ordinarily lack spontaneous pacemaker activity; e.g., depolarization of ventricular cells (e.g., by ischemia) may produce "abnormal" automaticity. When impulses propagate from a region of enhanced normal or abnormal automaticity to excite the rest of the heart, more complex arrhythmias may result from the induction of functional reentry.

AFTERDEPOLARIZATIONS AND TRIGGERED AUTOMATICITY. Under some pathophysiologic conditions, a normal cardiac action potential may be interrupted or followed by an abnormal depolarization (Figure 29–6). If this abnormal depolarization reaches threshold, it may give rise to secondary upstrokes that can propagate and create abnormal rhythms. These abnormal secondary upstrokes occur only after an initial normal, or "triggering," upstroke and are termed *triggered rhythms*.

In the first form of triggered rhythm, under conditions of intracellular or SR Ca^{2+} overload (e.g., myocardial ischemia, adrenergic stress, digitalis intoxication, heart failure), a normal action potential may be followed by a *delayed afterdepolarization* (DAD; Figure 29–6A). If this afterdepolarization reaches threshold, a secondary triggered beat or beats may occur. In the second type of triggered activity, the key abnormality is marked prolongation of the cardiac action potential. When this occurs, phase 3 repolarization may be interrupted by an *early afterdepolarization* (EAD; Figure 29–6B). EAD-mediated triggering in vitro and

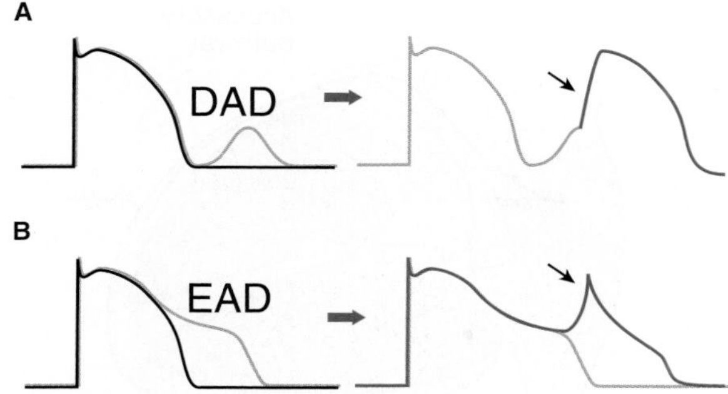

Figure 29–6 *Afterdepolarizations and triggered activity.* **A.** Delayed afterdepolarization (DAD) arising after full repolarization. DADs are typically caused by spontaneous Ca^{2+} release from the sarcoplasmic reticulum under conditions of Ca^{2+} overload. The extra cytosolic Ca^{2+} is removed from the cytosol by the electrogenic Na-Ca exchanger (NCX), which produces Na^+ influx and causes a cell membrane depolarization in the form of a DAD. A DAD that reaches threshold results in a triggered upstroke (*black arrow, right*). **B.** Early afterdepolarization (EAD) interrupting phase 3 repolarization. Multiple ion channels and transporters can contribute to EADs (e.g., Na^+ channel, L-type Ca^{2+} channel, NCX). Under some conditions, triggered beat(s) can arise from an EAD (*black arrow, right*).

clinical arrhythmias are most common when the underlying heart rate is slow, extracellular K^+ is low, and certain drugs that prolong APD are present. EAD-related triggered upstrokes probably reflect inward current through Na^+ or Ca^{2+} channels. EADs are induced much more readily in Purkinje cells than in epicardial or endocardial cells. When cardiac repolarization is markedly prolonged, polymorphic ventricular tachycardia with a long QT interval, known as the *torsade de pointes* syndrome, may occur. This arrhythmia is thought to be caused by EADs, which trigger functional reentry owing to heterogeneity of APDs across the ventricular wall. Congenital long QT syndrome, a disease in which *torsade de pointes* is common, can most often be caused by mutations in the genes encoding the Na^+ channels or the channels underlying the repolarizing currents I_{Kr} and I_{Ks}.

REENTRY. Reentry occurs when a cardiac impulse travels in a path such as to return to its original site and reactivate the original site and self-perpetuate rapid activation independent of the normal sinus node conduction. This abnormal activation path (or reentrant circuit) requires an isotropic conduction slowing (or failure) due to either an anatomic or functional barrier.

ANATOMICALLY DEFINED REENTRY. Reentry can occur when impulses propagate by more than 1 pathway between 2 points in the heart, and those pathways have heterogeneous electrophysiologic properties. Patients with Wolff–Parkinson–White (WPW) syndrome have accessory connections between the atrium and ventricle (Figure 29–7). With each sinus node depolarization, impulses can excite the ventricle via the normal structures (AV node) or the accessory pathway. However, the electrophysiologic properties of the AV node and accessory pathways are different: Accessory pathways usually consist of nonnodal tissue and consequently vastly differ in refractoriness with the AV node. Thus, with a premature atrial beat, conduction may fail in the accessory pathway but continue, albeit slowly, in the AV node and then through the His–Purkinje system; there, the propagating impulse may encounter the ventricular end of the accessory pathway when it is no longer refractory. The likelihood that the accessory pathway is no longer refractory increases as AV nodal conduction slows. When the impulse reenters the atrium, it then can reenter the ventricle via the AV node, reenter the atrium via the accessory pathway, and so on. Reentry of this type, referred to as *AV reentrant tachycardia*, is determined by:

- The presence of an anatomically defined circuit
- Heterogeneity in refractoriness among regions in the circuit
- Slow conduction in one part of the circuit

Similar "anatomically defined" reentry commonly occurs in the region of the AV node (*AV nodal reentrant tachycardia*) and in the atrium (*atrial flutter*). The term *paroxysmal supraventricular tachycardia* (PSVT) includes both AV reentry and AV nodal reentry, which share many clinical features. It now is sometimes possible to identify and ablate critical segments of reentrant pathway (or automatic foci), thus curing the patient and obviating the need for long-term drug therapy.

FUNCTIONALLY DEFINED REENTRY. Reentry also may occur in the absence of a distinct, anatomically defined pathway (Figure 29–8). If ischemia or other electrophysiologic perturbations result in an area of sufficiently slow conduction in the ventricle, the impulses exiting from that area find the rest of the myocardium

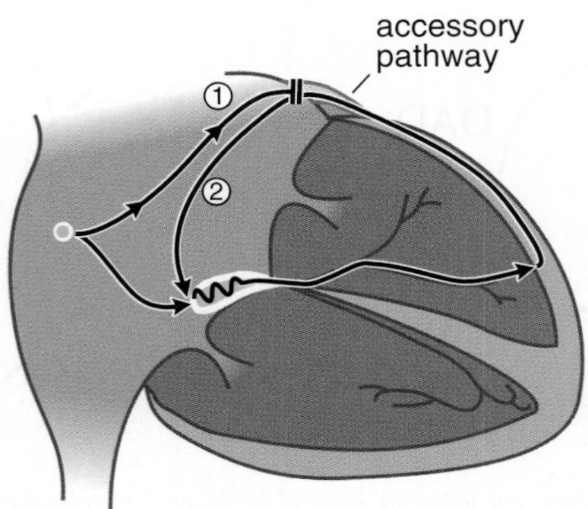

Figure 29–7 *Atrioventricular reentrant tachycardia in the Wolff–Parkinson–White syndrome.* In these patients, an accessory atrioventricular (AV) connection is present (*light blue*). A premature atrial impulse blocks in the accessory pathway (1) and propagates slowly through the AV node and conducting system. On reaching the accessory pathway (by now no longer refractory), the impulse reenters the atrium (2), where it then can reenter the ventricle via the AV node and become self-sustaining (*see* Figure 29–9C). AV nodal blocking drugs readily terminate this tachycardia. Recurrences can be prevented by drugs that prevent atrial premature beats, by drugs that alter the electrophysiologic characteristics of tissue in the circuit (e.g., they prolong AV nodal refractoriness), and by nonpharmacologic techniques that section the accessory pathway.

re-excitable and reentry may ensue. Atrial or ventricular fibrillation (VF) is an extreme example of "functionally defined" (or "leading circle") reentry. Cells are re-excited as soon as they are repolarized sufficiently to allow enough Na^+ channels to recover from inactivation. In this setting, neither organized activation patterns nor coordinated contractile activity is present.

COMMON ARRHYTHMIAS AND THEIR MECHANISMS

Table 29–2 lists common arrhythmias, their likely mechanisms, and approaches that should be considered for their acute termination and for long-term therapy to prevent recurrence.

MECHANISMS OF ANTI-ARRHYTHMIC DRUG ACTION

Anti-arrhythmic drugs almost invariably have multiple effects in patients, and their effects on arrhythmias can be complex. A drug can modulate additional targets in addition to its primary mode of action. A single arrhythmia may result from multiple underlying mechanisms. Drugs may be anti-arrhythmic by suppressing the initiating mechanism or by altering the reentrant circuit. In some cases, drugs may suppress the initiator but nonetheless promote reentry.

Drugs may slow automatic rhythms by altering any of the 4 determinants of spontaneous pacemaker discharge (Figure 29–9):

- Decrease phase 4 slope
- Increase threshold potential
- Increase maximum diastolic potential
- Increase APD

Adenosine and *acetylcholine* may increase maximum diastolic potential, and β *receptor antagonists* may decrease phase 4 slope. Blockade of Na^+ or Ca^{2+} channels usually results in altered threshold, and blockade of cardiac K^+ channels prolongs the action potential.

Anti-arrhythmic drugs may block arrhythmias owing to DADs or EADs by 2 major mechanisms:

- Inhibition of the development of afterdepolarizations
- Interference with the inward current (usually through Na^+ or Ca^{2+} channels), which is responsible for the upstroke

Thus, arrhythmias owing to digitalis-induced DADs may be inhibited by *verapamil* (which blocks the development of DAD by reducing Ca^{2+} influx and subsequent storage/release) or by *quinidine* (which blocks Na^+ channels, thereby elevating the threshold required to produce the abnormal upstroke). Similarly, 2 approaches

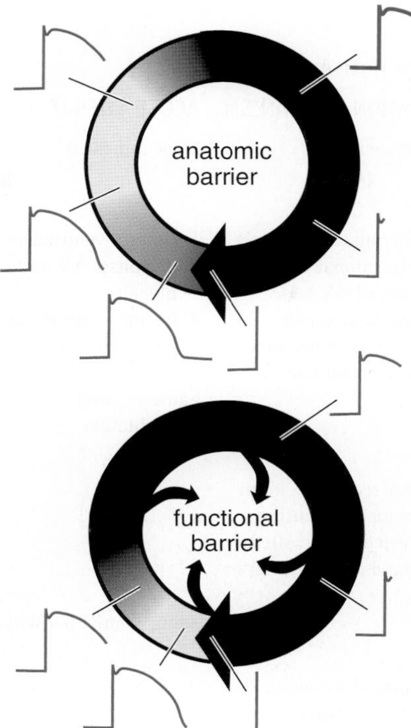

Figure 29–8 *Two types of reentry*. The border of a propagating wavefront is denoted by a heavy black arrowhead. In anatomically defined reentry (*top*), a fixed pathway is present (e.g., Figure 29–7). The *black area* denotes tissue in the reentrant circuit that is completely refractory because of the recent passage of the propagating wavefront; the *gray area* denotes tissue in which depressed upstrokes can be elicited (*see* Figure 29–5A), and the *red area* represents tissue in which restimulation would result in action potentials with normal upstrokes. The red area is termed an *excitable gap*. In functionally defined, or "leading circle," reentry (*bottom*), there is no anatomic pathway and no excitable gap. Rather, the circulating wavefront creates an area of inexcitable tissue at its core. In this type of reentry, the circuit does not necessarily remain in the same anatomic position during consecutive beats, and multiple such "rotors" may be present.

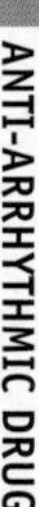

are used in arrhythmias related to EAD-triggered beats (*see* Tables 29–1 and 29–2). EADs can be inhibited by shortening APD; in practice, heart rate is accelerated by *isoproterenol* infusion or by pacing. Triggered beats arising from EADs can be inhibited by Mg^{2+}, without normalizing repolarization in vitro or QT interval. In patients with a congenitally prolonged QT interval, *torsade de pointes* often occurs with adrenergic stress; therapy includes β adrenergic blockade (which does not shorten the QT interval) as well as pacing.

In anatomically determined reentry, drugs may terminate the arrhythmia by blocking propagation of the action potential. In the example of the WPW-related arrhythmia, drugs that prolong AV nodal refractoriness and slow AV nodal conduction, such as Ca^{2+} channel blockers, β adrenergic receptor antagonists, or digitalis glycosides, are likely to be effective. Conversely, slowing conduction in functionally determined reentrant circuits may change the pathway without extinguishing the circuit. Slow conduction generally promotes the development of reentrant arrhythmias, whereas the most likely approach for terminating functionally determined reentry is prolongation of refractoriness. In atrial and ventricular myocytes, refractoriness can be prolonged by delaying the recovery of Na^+ channels from inactivation. Drugs blocking Na^+ channels generally shift the voltage dependence of recovery from block (*see* Figure 29–5B) and so prolong refractoriness (Figure 29–10). Drugs that increase APD without direct action on Na^+ channels (e.g., by blocking delayed-rectifier currents) also will prolong refractoriness. In sinoatrial or AV nodal tissues, Ca^{2+} channel blockade prolongs refractoriness.

STATE-DEPENDENT ION CHANNEL BLOCK

A key concept is that ion channel–blocking drugs bind to specific sites on the ion channel proteins to modify function (e.g., decrease current) and that the affinity of the ion channel protein for the drug on its target site will vary as the ion channel protein shuttles among functional states (*see* Figure 29–2). Most useful agents of

Table 29–2

A Mechanistic Approach to Anti-Arrhythmic Therapy

ARRHYTHMIA	COMMON MECHANISM	ACUTE THERAPY[a]	CHRONIC THERAPY[a]
Premature atrial, nodal, or ventricular depolarizations	Unknown	None indicated	None indicated
Atrial fibrillation	Disorganized "functional" reentry Continual AV node stimulation and irregular, often rapid, ventricular rate	1. Control ventricular response: AV node block[b] 2. Restore sinus rhythm: DC cardioversion Same as atrial fibrillation	1. Control ventricular response: AV nodal block[b] 2. Maintain normal rhythm: K^+ channel block, Na^+ channel block, Na^+ channel block with $\tau_{recovery}$ >1 second
Atrial flutter	Stable reentrant circuit in the right atrium Ventricular rate often rapid and irregular	Same as atrial fibrillation	Same as atrial fibrillation AV nodal blocking drugs especially desirable to avoid ↑ ventricular rate Ablation in selected cases[c]
Atrial tachycardia	Enhanced automaticity, DAD-related automaticity, or reentry in atrium	*Adenosine	Same as atrial fibrillation Ablation of tachycardia "focus"[c]
AV nodal reentrant tachycardia (PSVT)	Reentrant circuit within or near AV node	AV nodal block Less commonly: ↑ vagal tone (digitalis, edrophonium, phenylephrine)	*AV nodal block Flecainide Propafenone *Ablation[c]
Arrhythmias associated with WPW syndrome: 1. AV reentry (PSVT)	Reentry (Figure 29–7)	Same as AV nodal reentry	K^+ channel block Na^+ channel block with $\tau_{recovery}$ >1 second *Ablation[c]
2. Atrial fibrillation with atrioventricular conduction via accessory pathway	Very rapid rate due to nondecremental properties of accessory pathway	*DC cardioversion *Procainamide Lidocaine	K^+ channel block Na^+ channel block with $\tau_{recovery}$ >1 second (AV nodal blockers can be harmful)
VT in patients with remote myocardial infarction	Reentry near the rim of the healed myocardial infarction	Amiodarone Procainamide DC cardioversion Adenosine[e]	*ICD[d] Amiodarone K^+ channel block Na^+ channel block
VT in patients without structural heart disease	DADs triggered by ↑ sympathetic tone	Verapamil[e] β Blockers[e] DC cardioversion *DC cardioversion	Verapamil[e] β Blockers[e]

(*continued*)

Table 29–2

A Mechanistic Approach to Anti-Arrhythmic Therapy (*Continued*)

ARRHYTHMIA	COMMON MECHANISM	ACUTE THERAPY[a]	CHRONIC THERAPY[a]
VF	Disorganized reentry	Lidocaine Amiodarone Procainamide Pacing	*ICD[d] Amiodarone K^+ channel block Na^+ channel block
Torsades de pointes, congenital or acquired; (often drug related)	EAD-related triggered activity	Magnesium Isoproterenol	β Blockade Pacing

*Indicates treatment of choice.

[a]*Acute drug therapy is administered intravenously; chronic therapy implies long-term oral use.*

[b]*AV nodal block can be achieved clinically by adenosine, Ca^{2+} channel block, β adrenergic receptor blockade, or increased vagal tone (a major anti-arrhythmic effect of digitalis glycosides).*

[c]*Ablation is a procedure in which tissue responsible for the maintenance of a tachycardia is identified by specialized recording techniques and then selectively destroyed, usually by high-frequency radio waves delivered through a catheter placed in the heart.*

[d]*ICD, implanted cardioverter–defibrillator: a device that can sense VT or VF and deliver pacing and/or cardioverting shocks to restore normal rhythm.*

[e]*These may be harmful in reentrant VT and so should be used for acute therapy only if the diagnosis is secure. DAD, delayed afterdepolarization; EAD, early afterdepolarization; WPW, Wolff–Parkinson–White syndrome; PSVT, paroxysmal supraventricular tachycardia; VT, ventricular tachycardia; VF, ventricular fibrillation.*

this type block open and/or inactivated Na^+ channels and have very little affinity for channels in the resting state. Thus, with each action potential, drugs bind to Na^+ channels and block them, and with each diastolic interval, drugs dissociate, and the block is released. When heart rate increases, the time available for dissociation decreases, and steady-state Na^+ channel block increases. The rate of recovery from block also slows as cells are depolarized, as in ischemia. This explains the finding that Na^+ channel blockers depress Na^+ current, and hence conduction, to a greater extent in ischemic tissues than in normal tissues. Open versus inactivated-state block also may be important in determining the effects of some drugs. Increased APD, which results in a relative increase in time spent in the inactivated state, may increase block by drugs that bind to inactivated channels, such as lidocaine or amiodarone.

The rate of recovery from block often is expressed as a time constant ($\tau_{recovery}$, the time required for ~63% of an exponentially determined process to be complete). In the case of drugs such as lidocaine, $\tau_{recovery}$ is so short (<<1 s) that recovery from block is very rapid, and substantial Na^+ channel block occurs only in rapidly driven tissues, particularly in ischemia. Conversely, drugs such as flecainide have such long $\tau_{recovery}$ values (>10 s) that roughly the same number of Na^+ channels is blocked during systole and diastole. As a result, marked slowing of conduction occurs even in normal tissues at normal rates.

CLASSIFYING ANTI-ARRHYTHMIC DRUGS

To the extent that the clinical actions of drugs can be predicted, classifying drugs by their basic electrophysiologic properties is useful. However, differences in pharmacologic effects occur even among drugs that share the same classification, some of which may be responsible for the observed clinical differences in responses to drugs of the same broad "class" (Table 29–3). Another way of approaching therapy is to classify arrhythmia mechanisms and then to target drug therapy to the electrophysiologic mechanism most likely to terminate or prevent the arrhythmia (*see* Table 29–2).

Na^+ Channel Block. The extent of Na^+ channel block depends critically on heart rate and membrane potential, as well as on drug-specific physicochemical characteristics that determine $\tau_{recovery}$ (Figure 29–11). When Na^+ channels are blocked, excitability is decreased (i.e., greater membrane depolarization is required to bring Na^+ channels from the resting to open state). This change in the threshold of excitability probably contributes to the clinical findings that Na^+ channel blockers tend to increase both pacing threshold and the energy required for defibrillation.

These deleterious effects may be important if anti-arrhythmic drugs are used in patients with pacemakers or implanted defibrillators. Na^+ channel block decreases conduction velocity in nonnodal tissue and increases

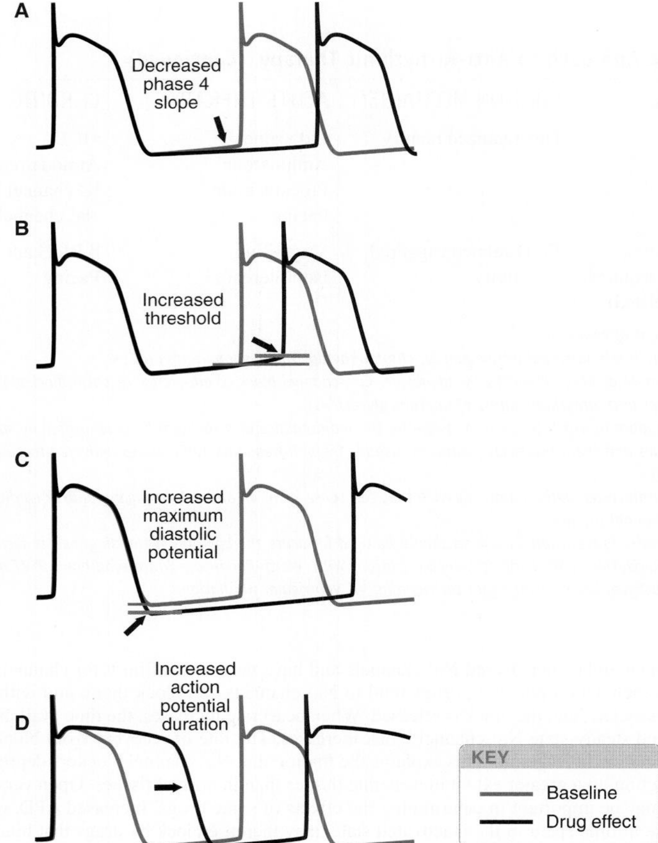

Figure 29–9 *Four ways to reduce the rate of spontaneous discharge.* The blue horizontal line represents threshold potential.

QRS duration. Usual doses of flecainide prolong QRS intervals by 25% or more during normal rhythm, whereas lidocaine increases QRS intervals only at very fast heart rates. Drugs with $\tau_{recovery}$ values greater than 10 s (e.g., flecainide) also tend to prolong the PR interval; it is not known whether this represents additional Ca^{2+} channel block (see below) or block of fast-response tissue in the region of the AV node. Drug effects on the PR interval also are highly modified by autonomic effects. For example, quinidine actually tends to shorten the PR interval largely as a result of its vagolytic properties. Action potential duration either is unaffected or shortened by Na^+ channel block; some Na^+ channel–blocking drugs do prolong cardiac action potentials but by other mechanisms, usually K^+ channel block (*see* Table 29–3).

Na^+ channel block decreases automaticity (Figure 29–9B) and can inhibit triggered activity arising from DADs or EADs. Many Na^+ channel blockers also decrease phase 4 slope (Figure 29–9A). In anatomically defined reentry, Na^+ channel blockers may decrease conduction sufficiently to extinguish the propagating reentrant wavefront. However, conduction slowing owing to Na^+ channel block may exacerbate reentry. Thus, whether a given drug exacerbates or suppresses reentrant arrhythmias depends on the balance between its effects on refractoriness and on conduction in a particular reentrant circuit. *Lidocaine* and *mexiletine* have short $\tau_{recovery}$ values and are not useful in atrial fibrillation or flutter, whereas *quinidine, flecainide, propafenone*, and similar agents are effective in some patients. Many of these agents owe part of their anti-arrhythmic activity to blockade of K^+ channels.

Late Na^+ Channel Current Block. The long QT syndrome variant 3 (LQT3) is characterized by late inward Na^+ current caused by defects in the inactivation of the cardiac isoform of the Na^+ channel. This late current prolongs the APD and predisposes to arrhythmia. Many drugs with local anesthetic effects, including *mexiletine*, preferentially block this late current and can be used to successfully treat LQT3 patients.

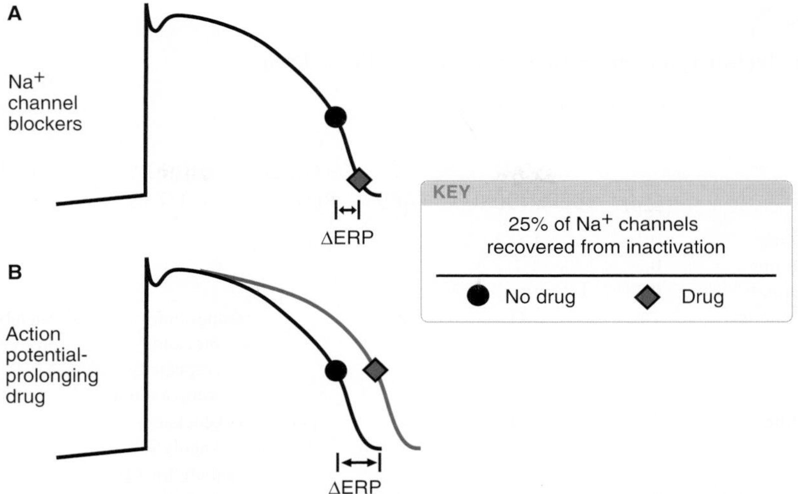

Figure 29–10 *Two ways to increase refractoriness.* The *black dot* indicates the point at which a sufficient number of Na^+ channels (an arbitrary 25%; *see* Figure 29–5B) have recovered from inactivation to allow a premature stimulus to produce a propagated response in the absence of a drug. Block of Na^+ channels (**A**) shifts voltage dependence of recovery (Figure 29–5B) and delays the point at which 25% of channels have recovered (*red diamond*), prolonging refractoriness. If the drug also dissociates slowly from the channel (*see* Figure 29–11), refractoriness in fast-response tissues actually can extend beyond full repolarization ("postrepolarization refractoriness"). Drugs that prolong the action potential (**B**) also will extend the point at which an arbitrary percentage of Na^+ channels have recovered from inactivation, even without directly interacting with Na^+ channels. ERP, effective refractory period.

Na^+ Channel–Blocker Toxicity. Conduction slowing in potential reentrant circuits can account for toxicity of drugs that block the Na^+ channel (*see* Table 29–1). For example, Na^+ channel block decreases conduction velocity and hence slows atrial flutter rate. Normal AV nodal function permits a greater number of impulses to penetrate the ventricle, and heart rate actually may increase (*see* Figure 29–9). Thus, atrial flutter rate may drop from 300/min, with 2:1 or 4:1 AV conduction (i.e., a heart rate of 150 or 75 beats/min), to 220/min, but with 1:1 transmission to the ventricle (i.e., a heart rate of 220 beats/min), with potentially disastrous consequences. This form of drug-induced arrhythmia is especially common during treatment with quinidine because the drug also increases AV nodal conduction through its vagolytic properties; flecainide and propafenone also have been implicated. Therapy with Na^+ channel blockers in patients with reentrant ventricular tachycardia after a myocardial infarction (MI) can increase the frequency and severity of arrhythmic episodes. Slowed conduction allows the reentrant wavefront to persist within the tachycardia circuit. Such drug-exacerbated arrhythmia can be very difficult to manage, and deaths owing to intractable drug-induced ventricular tachycardia have been reported. In this setting, Na^+ infusion may be beneficial.

Action Potential Prolongation. Most drugs that prolong the action potential do so by blocking K^+ channels, although enhanced inward Na^+ current also can cause prolongation. Enhanced inward current may underlie QT prolongation (and arrhythmia suppression) by *ibutilide*. Block of cardiac K^+ channels increases APD and reduces normal automaticity (Figure 29–9D). Increased APD, seen as an increase in QT interval, increases refractoriness (*see* Figure 29–10) and therefore should be an effective way of treating reentry. Experimentally, K^+ channel block produces a series of desirable effects: reduced defibrillation energy requirement, inhibition of VF owing to acute ischemia, and increased contractility. Most K^+ channel–blocking drugs also interact with β adrenergic receptors (*sotalol*) or other channels (e.g., amiodarone, quinidine) (*see* Table 29–3). Amiodarone and sotalol appear to be at least as effective as drugs with predominant Na^+ channel–blocking properties in both atrial and ventricular arrhythmias. "Pure" action potential–prolonging drugs (e.g., *dofetilide, ibutilide*) also are available.

Toxicity of Drugs That Prolong QT Interval. Most of these agents disproportionately prolong cardiac action potentials when underlying heart rate is slow and can cause *torsade de pointes* (*see* Table 29–1). While this effect usually is seen with QT-prolonging anti-arrhythmic drugs, it can occur more rarely with drugs that are used for noncardiac indications. For such agents, the risk of *torsade de pointes* may become apparent only after widespread use postmarketing. Sex hormones modify cardiac ion channels and may account for the clinically observed increased incidence of drug-induced *torsade de pointes* in women.

Table 29–3

Major Electrophysiologic Actions of Anti-Arrhythmic Drugs

DRUG	Na⁺ CHANNEL BLOCK: $\tau_{RECOVERY}$[c] (sec)	Na⁺ CHANNEL BLOCK: STATE DEPENDENCE[c]	↑ APD	Ca^{2+} CHANNEL BLOCK	AUTONOMIC EFFECTS	OTHER EFFECTS
Lidocaine	0.1	I > O				
Phenytoin	0.2	I				
Mexiletine[a]	0.3					
Procainamide	1.8	O	✓		Ganglionic blockade (especially intravenous)	✓: Metabolite prolongs APD
Quinidine	3	O	✓	(x)	α Blockade, vagolytic Anticholinergic	
Disopyramide[b]	9	O	✓		Anticholinergic	
Propafenone[b]	11	O ≈ I	✓		β Blockade (variable clinical effect)	
Flecainide[a]	11	O	(x)	(x)		
β Blockers: Propanolol[b]					β Blockade	Na⁺ channel block in vitro
Sotalol[b]			✓		β Blockade	
Amiodarone, dronedarone	1.6	I	✓	(x)	Noncompetitive β blockade	Antithyroid action
Dofetilide			✓			
Ibutilide			✓			
Verapamil[a]				✓		
Diltiazem[a]				✓		
Digoxin					✓: Vagal stimulation	✓: Inhibition of Na⁺, K⁺-ATPase
Adenosine				✓	✓: Adenosine receptor activation	✓: Activation of outward K⁺ current
Magnesium				? ✓		Mechanism not well understood

✓Indicates an effect that is important in mediating the clinical action of a drug. (x)Indicates a demonstrable effect whose relationship to drug action in patients is less well established.

[a]Indicates drugs prescribed as racemates, and the enantiomers are thought to exert similar electrophysiologic effects.

[b]Indicates racemates for which clinically relevant differences in the electrophysiologic properties of individual enantiomers have been reported (see text). One approach to classifying drugs is:

Class	Major action
I	*Na⁺ channel block*
II	*β blockade*
III	*action potential prolongation (usually by K⁺ channel block)*
IV	*Ca^{2+} channel block*

Drugs are listed here according to this scheme. It is important to bear in mind, however, that many drugs exert multiple effects that contribute to their clinical actions. It is occasionally clinically useful to subclassify Na⁺ channel blockers by their rates of recovery from drug-induced block ($\tau_{recovery}$) under physiologic conditions. Because this is a continuous variable and can be modulated by factors such as depolarization of the resting potential, these distinctions can become blurred: class Ib, $\tau_{recovery}$ <1 s; class Ia, $\tau_{recovery}$ 1–10 s; class Ic, $\tau_{recovery}$ >10 s. These class and subclass effects are associated with distinctive ECG changes, characteristic "class" toxicities, and efficacy in specific arrhythmia syndromes (see text).

[c]These data are dependent on experimental conditions, including species and temperature. The $\tau_{recovery}$ values cited here are from Courtney (1987). O, open-state blocker; I, inactivated-state blocker; APD, action potential duration.

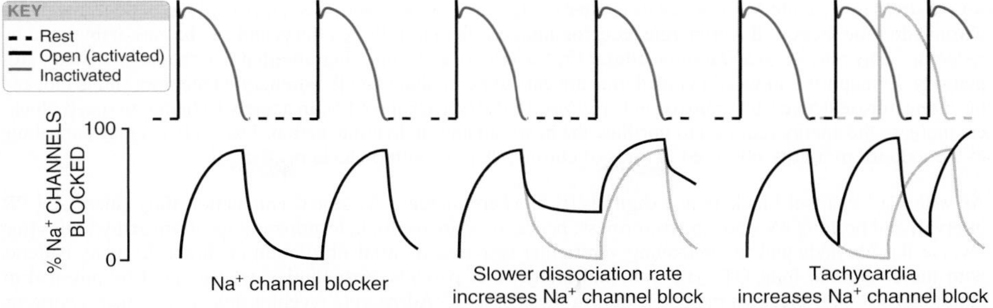

Figure 29–11 *Recovery from block of Na^+ channels during diastole.* This recovery is the critical factor determining extent of steady-state Na^+ channel block. Na^+ channel blockers bind to (and block) Na^+ channels in the open and/or inactivated states, resulting in phasic changes in the extent of block during the action potential. In the *middle* panel, a decrease in the rate of recovery from block increases the extent of block. Different drugs have different rates of recovery, and depolarization reduces the rate of recovery. Increasing heart rate, which results in relatively less time spent in the resting state, also increases the extent of block (*right* panel). (Modified from Roden DM, Echt DS, Lee JT, Murray KT. Clinical pharmacology of antiarrhythmic agents. In: Josephson ME, ed. *Sudden Cardiac Death*. London: Blackwell Scientific; 1993:182–185, with permission from Wiley-Blackwell Publishing.)

Ca^{2+} Channel Block. The major electrophysiologic effects resulting from block of cardiac Ca^{2+} channels are in nodal tissues. Dihydropyridines, such as *nifedipine*, which are used commonly in angina and hypertension, preferentially block Ca^{2+} channels in vascular smooth muscle; their cardiac electrophysiologic effects, such as heart rate acceleration, result principally from reflex sympathetic activation secondary to peripheral vasodilation. Only *verapamil*, *diltiazem*, and *bepridil* block Ca^{2+} channels in cardiac cells at clinically used doses. These drugs generally slow heart rate (Figure 29–9A), although hypotension, if marked, can cause reflex sympathetic activation and tachycardia. The velocity of AV nodal conduction decreases, so the PR interval increases. AV nodal block occurs as a result of *decremental* conduction, as well as increased AV nodal refractoriness. These latter effects form the basis of the anti-arrhythmic actions of Ca^{2+} channel blockers in reentrant arrhythmias whose circuit involves the AV node, such as AV reentrant tachycardia (*see* Figure 29–7).

Another important indication for anti-arrhythmic therapy is to reduce ventricular rate in atrial flutter or fibrillation. Rare forms of ventricular tachycardia appear to be DAD-mediated and respond to verapamil. Parenteral verapamil and diltiazem are approved for rapid conversion of PSVTs to sinus rhythm and for temporary control of rapid ventricular rate in atrial flutter or fibrillation. Oral verapamil may be used in conjunction with digoxin to control ventricular rate in chronic atrial flutter or fibrillation and for prophylaxis of repetitive PSVT. Unlike β adrenergic receptor antagonists, Ca^{2+} channel blockers have not been shown to reduce mortality after MI.

Verapamil and Diltiazem. The major adverse effect of intravenous verapamil or diltiazem is hypotension, particularly with bolus administration. This is a particular problem if the drugs are used mistakenly in patients with ventricular tachycardia (in whom Ca^{2+} channel blockers usually are not effective) misdiagnosed as AV nodal reentrant tachycardia. Hypotension also is frequent in patients receiving other vasodilators, including quinidine, and in patients with underlying left ventricular dysfunction, which the drugs can exacerbate. Severe sinus bradycardia or AV block occurs, especially in patients also receiving β blockers. With oral therapy, these adverse effects tend to be less severe.

Verapamil (CALAN, ISOPTIN, VERELAN, COVERA-HS, and others) is supplied as a racemate. L-Verapamil is a more potent calcium channel blocker than is D-verapamil. However, with oral therapy, the L-enantiomer undergoes more extensive first-pass hepatic metabolism. For this reason, a given concentration of verapamil prolongs the PR interval to a greater extent when administered intravenously (where concentrations of the L- and D-enantiomers are equivalent) than when administered orally. *Diltiazem* (CARDIZEM, TIAZAC, DILACOR XR, and others) also undergoes extensive first-pass hepatic metabolism, and both drugs have metabolites that exert Ca^{2+} channel–blocking actions. Adverse effects during therapy with verapamil or diltiazem are determined largely by underlying heart disease and concomitant therapy; plasma concentrations of these agents are not measured routinely. Both drugs can increase serum digoxin concentration, although the magnitude of this effect is variable; excess slowing of ventricular response may occur in patients with atrial fibrillation. Constipation can occur with oral verapamil.

Blockade of β Adrenergic Receptors. β Adrenergic stimulation increases the magnitude of the Ca^{2+} current and slows its inactivation, increases the magnitude of repolarizing K^+ and Cl^- currents, increases pacemaker current (thereby increasing sinus rate), increases the Ca^{2+} stored in the SR, and under pathophysiologic conditions, can increase both DAD- and EAD-mediated arrhythmias. The increases in plasma epinephrine associated with severe stress (e.g., acute MI, resuscitation after cardiac arrest) lower serum K^+, especially in patients receiving chronic diuretic therapy. β Adrenergic receptor antagonists inhibit these effects and can be anti-arrhythmic by reducing heart rate, decreasing intracellular Ca^{2+} overload, and inhibiting afterdepolarization-mediated automaticity. Epinephrine-induced hypokalemia appears to be mediated by β_2 adrenergic receptors and is blocked by "noncardioselective" antagonists such as *propranolol* (*see* Chapter 12). In acutely ischemic tissue, β blockers increase the energy required to fibrillate the heart, an anti-arrhythmic action. These effects may contribute to the reduced mortality observed in trials of chronic therapy with β blockers after MI.

As with Ca^{2+} channel blockers and digitalis, β blockers increase AV nodal conduction time (increased PR interval) and prolong AV nodal refractoriness; hence, they are useful in terminating reentrant arrhythmias that involve the AV node and in controlling ventricular response in atrial fibrillation or flutter. In many patients with the congenital long QT syndrome and many other patients, arrhythmias are triggered by physical or emotional stress; β blockers may be useful in these cases. β Adrenergic receptor antagonists also reportedly are effective in controlling arrhythmias Na^+ channel blockers; this effect may be due in part to slowing of the heart rate, which then decreases the extent of rate-dependent conduction slowing by Na^+ channel block. Adverse effects of β blockade include fatigue, bronchospasm, hypotension, impotence, depression, worsening of symptoms owing to peripheral vascular disease, and masking of the symptoms of hypoglycemia in diabetic patients (*see* Chapter 12). In patients with arrhythmias owing to excess sympathetic stimulation (e.g., pheochromocytoma, *clonidine* withdrawal), β blockers can result in unopposed α adrenergic stimulation, with resulting severe hypertension and/or α adrenergic–mediated arrhythmias. In such patients, arrhythmias should be treated with both α and β adrenergic antagonists or with a drug such as *labetalol* that combines α and β blocking properties. Abrupt discontinuation of chronic β blocker therapy can lead to "rebound" symptoms; thus, β receptor antagonists are tapered over 2 weeks.

Selected β Adrenergic Receptor Blockers. It is likely that most β adrenergic antagonists share anti-arrhythmic properties. Some, such as propranolol, also exert Na^+ channel–blocking effects at high concentrations. Acebutolol is as effective as quinidine in suppressing ventricular ectopic beats, an arrhythmia that many clinicians no longer treat. Sotalol is more effective for many arrhythmias than other β blockers, probably because of its K^+ channel–blocking actions. Esmolol is a β_1-selective agent that has a very short elimination $t_{1/2}$. Intravenous esmolol is useful in clinical situations in which immediate β adrenergic blockade is desired.

PRINCIPLES IN THE CLINICAL USE OF ANTI-ARRHYTHMIC DRUGS

Drugs that modify cardiac electrophysiology often have a small therapeutic index. Moreover, anti-arrhythmic drugs can induce new arrhythmias with possibly fatal consequences. Nonpharmacologic treatments, such as cardiac pacing, electrical defibrillation, or ablation of targeted regions, are indicated for some arrhythmias; in other cases, no therapy is required, even though an arrhythmia is detected. The fundamental principles of therapeutics described here must be applied to optimize anti-arrhythmic therapy.

1. IDENTIFY AND REMOVE PRECIPITATING FACTORS

Factors that commonly precipitate cardiac arrhythmias include hypoxia, electrolyte disturbances (especially hypokalemia), myocardial ischemia, and certain drugs.

For example, theophylline can cause multifocal atrial tachycardia, while *torsade de pointes* can arise not only during therapy with action potential–prolonging anti-arrhythmics but also with other drugs not ordinarily classified as having effects on ion channels, including erythromycin (*see* Chapter 55); the antiprotozoal pentamidine (*see* Chapter 50); some antipsychotics, notably thioridazine (*see* Chapter 16); some analgesics, notably methadone and celecoxib; some antiemetics (e.g., droperidol, dolasetron); antihistamines such as diphenhydramine; azole antifungals such as voriconazole and fluconazole; bronchodilators such as albuterol, formoterol, and salmeterol; prednisone; cisapride; famotidine; tacrolimus; some selective serotonin reuptake inhibitors (including citalopram, fluoxetine, paroxetine sertraline, and venlafaxine); haloperidol; trazodone; some serotonin $5HT_1$ agonists (e.g., sumatriptan, zolmitriptan); some antiretrovirals (e.g., efavirenz); most quinolone antibiotics (e.g., levofloxacin); tizanidine; and certain tricyclic antidepressants (*see* Chapter 15).

2. ESTABLISH THE GOALS OF TREATMENT

SOME ARRHYTHMIAS SHOULD NOT BE TREATED. The mere detection of an abnormality does not equate with the need for therapy. In the Cardiac Arrhythmia Suppression Trial (CAST), patients whose ventricular ectopic beats were suppressed by the potent Na^+ channel blockers *encainide* (no longer marketed) or *flecainide* were randomly assigned to receive those drugs or placebo. Unexpectedly, the mortality rate was 2- to 3-fold higher among patients treated with the drugs than those treated with placebo. This pivotal clinical trial reemphasizes the concept that therapy should be initiated only when a clear benefit to the patient can be identified. When symptoms are obviously attributable to an ongoing arrhythmia, there usually is little doubt that termination of the arrhythmia will be beneficial; when chronic therapy is used to prevent recurrence of an arrhythmia, the risks may be greater. *Among the anti-arrhythmic drugs discussed here, only β adrenergic blockers and, to a lesser extent, amiodarone have been shown to reduce mortality during long-term therapy.*

SYMPTOMS DUE TO ARRHYTHMIAS. If patients with an arrhythmia are asymptomatic, establishing any benefit from treatment will be difficult. Some patients may present with presyncope, syncope, or even cardiac arrest, which may be due to brady- or tachyarrhythmias. The sensation of irregular heartbeats (i.e., palpitations) can be minimally symptomatic in some individuals and incapacitating in others. The irregular heartbeats may be due to intermittent premature contractions or to sustained arrhythmias such as atrial fibrillation (which results in an irregular ventricular rate). Finally, patients may present with symptoms owing to decreased cardiac output. The most common symptom is breathlessness either at rest or on exertion. Rarely, sustained tachycardias may produce no "arrhythmia" symptoms (such as palpitations) but will depress contractile function; these patients may present with congestive heart failure that can be controlled by treating the arrhythmia.

CHOOSING AMONG THERAPEUTIC APPROACHES. In selecting therapy, establish clear therapeutic goals. For example, 3 options are available in patients with atrial fibrillation: (1) reduce the ventricular response using AV nodal blocking agents such as digitalis, verapamil, diltiazem, or β adrenergic antagonists (*see* Table 29–1); (2) restore and maintain normal rhythm using drugs such as quinidine, flecainide, or amiodarone; or (3) decide not to implement anti-arrhythmic therapy, especially if the patient truly is asymptomatic. Most patients with atrial fibrillation also benefit from anticoagulation to reduce stroke incidence regardless of symptoms. Factors that contribute to choice of therapy include not only symptoms but also the type and extent of structural heart disease, the QT interval prior to drug therapy, the coexistence of conduction system disease, and the presence of noncardiac diseases (Table 29–4). In the rare patient with the WPW syndrome and atrial fibrillation, the ventricular response can be extremely rapid and can be accelerated paradoxically by AV nodal blocking drugs such as digitalis or Ca^{2+} channel blockers; deaths owing to drug therapy have been reported.

The frequency and reproducibility of arrhythmia should be established prior to initiating therapy because inherent variability in the occurrence of arrhythmias can be confused with a beneficial or adverse drug effect. Techniques for this assessment include recording cardiac rhythm for prolonged periods or evaluating the response of the heart to artificially induced premature beats. It is important to recognize that drug therapy may be only partially effective. A marked decrease in the duration of paroxysms of atrial fibrillation may be sufficient to render a patient asymptomatic.

Table 29–4

Patient-Specific Anti-Arrhythmic Drug Contraindications

CONDITION	EXCLUDE/USE WITH CAUTION
Cardiac	
Heart failure	Disopyramide, flecainide
Sinus or AV node dysfunction	Digoxin, verapamil, diltiazem, β receptor antagonists, amiodarone
Wolff–Parkinson–White syndrome (risk of extremely rapid rate if atrial fibrillation develops)	Digoxin, verapamil, diltiazem
Infranodal conduction disease	Na^+ channel blockers, amiodarone
Aortic/subaortic stenosis	Bretylium
History of myocardial infarction	Flecainide
Prolonged QT interval	Quinidine, procainamide, disopyramide, sotalol, dofetilide, ibutilide, amiodarone
Cardiac transplant	Adenosine
Noncardiac	
Diarrhea	Quinidine
Prostatism, glaucoma	Disopyramide
Arthritis	Chronic procainamide
Lung disease	Amiodarone
Tremor	Mexiletine
Constipation	Verapamil
Asthma, peripheral vascular disease, hypoglycemia	β blockers, propafenone

3. MINIMIZE RISKS

ANTI-ARRHYTHMIC DRUGS CAN CAUSE ARRHYTHMIAS. One risk of anti-arrhythmic therapy is the provoking of new arrhythmias, with potentially life-threatening consequences. Anti-arrhythmic drugs can provoke arrhythmias by different mechanisms (*see* Table 29–1). These drug-provoked arrhythmias must be recognized because further treatment with anti-arrhythmic drugs often exacerbates the problem. Targeting therapies at underlying mechanisms of the arrhythmias may be required.

MONITORING OF PLASMA CONCENTRATION. Some adverse effects of anti-arrhythmic drugs result from excessive plasma drug concentrations. Measuring plasma concentration and adjusting the dose to maintain the concentration within a prescribed therapeutic range may minimize some adverse effects. In many patients, serious adverse reactions relate to interactions involving anti-arrhythmic drugs (often at usual plasma concentrations), transient factors such as electrolyte disturbances or myocardial ischemia, and the type and extent of the underlying heart disease.

PATIENT-SPECIFIC CONTRAINDICATIONS. Another way to minimize the adverse effects of anti-arrhythmic drugs is to avoid certain drugs in certain patient subsets altogether. For example, patients with a history of congestive heart failure are particularly prone to develop heart failure during disopyramide therapy. In other cases, adverse effects of drugs may be difficult to distinguish from exacerbations of underlying disease. Amiodarone may cause interstitial lung disease; its use therefore is undesirable in a patient with advanced pulmonary disease in whom the development of this potentially fatal adverse effect would be difficult to detect. Specific diseases that constitute relative or absolute contraindications to specific drugs are listed in Table 29–4.

4. CONSIDER THE ELECTROPHYSIOLOGY OF THE HEART AS A "MOVING TARGET"

Cardiac electrophysiology varies dynamically in response to external influences such as changing autonomic tone, myocardial ischemia, and myocardial stretch. For example, in response to myocardial ischemia, a normal heart may display changes in resting potential, conduction velocity, intracellular Ca^{2+} concentrations, and repolarization, any one of which then may create arrhythmias or alter response to anti-arrhythmic therapy.

ANTI-ARRHYTHMIC DRUGS

Summaries of important electrophysiologic and pharmacokinetic features of the drugs considered here are presented in Tables 29–3 and 29–5, respectively. Ca^{2+} channel blockers and β adrenergic antagonists are discussed in Chapters 12, 27, and 28. The drugs are presented in alphabetical order.

ADENOSINE. Adenosine (ADENOCARD, others) is a naturally occurring nucleoside that is administered as a rapid intravenous bolus for the acute termination of reentrant supraventricular arrhythmias. Adenosine also has been used to produce controlled hypotension during some surgical procedures and in the diagnosis of coronary artery disease. Intravenous ATP appears to produce effects similar to those of adenosine.

Pharmacologic Effects. The effects of adenosine are mediated by its interaction with specific GPCRs. Adenosine activates acetylcholine-sensitive K^+ current in the atrium and sinus and AV nodes, resulting in shortening of APD, hyperpolarization, and slowing of normal automaticity (Figure 29–9C). Adenosine also inhibits the electrophysiologic effects of increased intracellular cyclic AMP that occur with sympathetic stimulation. Because adenosine thereby reduces Ca^{2+} currents, it can be anti-arrhythmic by increasing AV nodal refractoriness and by inhibiting DADs elicited by sympathetic stimulation. Administration of an intravenous bolus of adenosine to humans transiently slows sinus rate and AV nodal conduction velocity and increases AV nodal refractoriness. A bolus of adenosine can produce transient sympathetic activation by interacting with carotid baroreceptors; a continuous infusion can cause hypotension.

Adverse Effects. A major advantage of adenosine therapy is that adverse effects are short lived because the drug is transported into cells and deaminated so rapidly. Transient asystole is common but usually lasts less than 5 sec and is in fact the therapeutic goal. Most patients feel a sense of chest fullness and dyspnea when therapeutic doses (6-12 mg) of adenosine are administered. Rarely, an adenosine bolus can precipitate bronchospasm or atrial fibrillation.

Clinical Pharmacokinetics. Adenosine is eliminated with a $t_{1/2}$ of seconds by carrier-mediated uptake and subsequent metabolism by adenosine deaminase. Adenosine probably is the only drug whose efficacy requires a rapid bolus dose, preferably through a large central intravenous line; slow administration results in elimination of the drug prior to its arrival at the heart. The effects of adenosine are potentiated in patients receiving *dipyridamole*, an adenosine uptake inhibitor, and in patients with cardiac transplants owing to denervation

Table 29–5

Pharmacokinetic Characteristics and Doses of Anti-Arrhythmic Drugs

DRUG	BIOAVAILABILITY	PROTEIN BINDING	ELIMINATION			ELIMINATION	ACTIVE	EFFECTIVE[b] C_p	USUAL DOSES[c]	
	Reduced First-Pass Metabolism	>80%	Renal	Hepatic	Other	$t_{1/2}$*	METABOLITE(S)		Loading Doses	Maintenance Doses
Adenosine[d]					✓	<10 s	✓		6-12 mg (IV only)	
Amiodarone		✓		✓		wk	✓	0.5-2 μg/mL	800-1600 mg/d × 1-3 wk (IV: 1000 mg over 24 h)	400 mg/day (IV: 0.5 mg/min)
Digoxin	–80%		✓			36 h		0.5-2.0 ng/mL	0.6-1 mg over 12-24 h	0.0625-0.5 mg/24 h
Diltiazem	✓			✓		4 h	(x)		0.25 mg/kg over 10 min (IV)	5-15 mg/h (IV); 180-360 mg/d in 3-4 divided doses (immediate release); 120-180 mg/24 h (extended release)[e]
Disopyramide	>80%		✓	✓		4-10 h	(x)	2-5 μg/mL		150 mg/6 h (immediate release); 300 mg (controlled release)[f]
Dofetilide	>80%		✓	(x)		7-10 h				0.5 mg/12 h
Dronedarone	✓	>98 %	✓			13-19 h	✓			400 mg/12 h
Esmolol					✓	5-10 min			0.5 mg/kg over 1 min (IV)	0.05-0.3 mg/kg/min for 4 min (IV)

(*continued*)

Table 29–5

Pharmacokinetic Characteristics and Doses of Anti-Arrhythmic Drugs (*Continued*)

DRUG	BIOAVAILABILITY	PROTEIN BINDING	ELIMINATION			ELIMINATION	ACTIVE		USUAL DOSES[c]	
	Reduced First-Pass Metabolism	>80%	Renal	Hepatic	Other	$t_{1/2}$*	METABOLITE(S)	EFFECTIVE[b] C_p	Loading Doses	Maintenance Doses
Flecainide	>80%			✓		10-18 h		0.2-1 μg/mL		50-100 mg/12 h
Ibutilide	✓			✓		6 h			1 mg (IV) over 10 min; may repeat once 10 min later	
Lidocaine	✓	✓		✓		120 min	(x)	1.5-5 μg/mL	50-100 mg administered at a rate of 25-50 mg/min (IV)	1-4 mg/min (IV)
Mexiletine	>80%			✓		9-15 h		0.5-2 μg/mL	400 mg	200 mg/8 h
Procainamide	>80%		✓	✓		3-4 h	✓	4-8 μg/mL	500-600 mg (IV), given at 20 mg/min	2-6 mg/min (IV); 250 mg q3h; 500-1000 mg q6h
(*N*-Acetyl procainamide)	(>80%)		(✓)			(6-10 h)		(10-20 μg/mL)		
Propafenone	✓			✓		2-32 h	✓	<1 μg/mL		150 mg/8h (immediate release); 225 mg/12h (extended release)

Propranolol	✓	✓	✓			4 h			1-3 mg administered no faster than 1 mg/min, may repeat[e] after 2 min (IV)	10-30 mg q6-8h (immediate release)
Quinidine	>80%	–80%	(x)	✓		4-10 h	✓	2-5 μg/mL		648 mg (gluconate) every 8h
Sotalol	>80%		✓			8 h		<5 μg/mL (?)		80-160 mg/12h
Verapamil	✓	✓		✓		3-7 h	✓		5-10 mg given over 2 min or more (IV)	40-120 mg/6-8h (immediate release)

✓ Indicates an effect that affects the clinical action of the drug. (x): metabolite or route of elimination probably of minor clinical importance.

[a]*The elimination $t_{1/2}$ is one, but not the only, determinant of how frequently a drug must be administered to maintain a therapeutic effect and avoid toxicity (Chapter 2). For some drugs with short elimination half-lives, infrequent dosing is nevertheless possible, e.g., verapamil. Formulations that allow slow release into the GI tract of a rapidly eliminated compound (available for many drugs, including procainamide, disopyramide, verapamil, diltiazem, and propranolol) also allow infrequent dosing.*

[b]*The therapeutic range is bounded by a plasma concentration below which no therapeutic effect is likely, and an upper concentration above which the risk of adverse effects increases. Many serious adverse reactions to anti-arrhythmic drugs can occur at "therapeutic" concentrations in susceptible individuals. When only an upper limit is cited, a lower limit has not been well defined. Variable generation of active metabolites may further complicate the interpretation of plasma concentration data (Chapter 2).*

[c]*Oral doses are presented unless otherwise indicated. Doses are presented as suggested ranges in adults of average build; lower doses are less likely to produce toxicity. Lower maintenance dosages may be required in patients with renal or hepatic disease. Loading doses are only indicated when a therapeutic effect is desired before maintenance therapy would bring drug concentrations into a therapeutic range—that is, for acute therapy (e.g., lidocaine, verapamil, adenosine) or when the elimination $t_{1/2}$ is extremely long (amiodarone).*

[d]*Bioavailability reduced by incomplete absorption.*

[e]*Indicates suggested dosage using slow-release formulation.*

[f]*This drug is available only in a restricted distribution system (see text). IV, intravenous.*

hypersensitivity. Methylxanthines such as theophylline and caffeine block adenosine receptors; therefore, larger than usual doses are required to produce an anti-arrhythmic effect in patients who have consumed these agents in coffee and sodas or as therapy.

AMIODARONE. Amiodarone (CORDARONE, PACERONE, others) exerts myriad pharmacologic effects, none of which is clearly linked to its arrhythmia-suppressing properties. Amiodarone is a structural analog of thyroid hormone, and some of its anti-arrhythmic actions and its toxicity are due to interaction with thyroid hormone receptors.

Amiodarone is highly lipophilic, is concentrated in many tissues, and is eliminated extremely slowly; consequently, adverse effects may resolve very slowly. In the U.S., the drug is indicated for oral therapy in patients with recurrent ventricular tachycardia or fibrillation resistant to other drugs. Oral amiodarone also is effective in maintaining sinus rhythm in patients with atrial fibrillation. An intravenous form is indicated for acute termination of ventricular tachycardia or fibrillation and is supplanting lidocaine as first-line therapy for out-of-hospital cardiac arrest. Despite uncertainties about its mechanisms of action and the potential for serious toxicity, amiodarone now is used very widely in the treatment of common arrhythmias such as atrial fibrillation.

Pharmacologic Effects. Amiodarone blocks inactivated Na^+ channels and has a relatively rapid rate of recovery (time constant ~1.6 s) from block. It also decreases Ca^{2+} current and transient outward delayed-rectifier and inward rectifier K^+ currents and exerts a noncompetitive adrenergic blocking effect. Amiodarone potently inhibits abnormal automaticity and, in most tissues, prolongs APD. Amiodarone decreases conduction velocity by Na^+ channel block and by a poorly understood effect on cell–cell coupling that may be especially important in diseased tissue. Prolongations of the PR, QRS, and QT intervals and sinus bradycardia are frequent during chronic therapy. Amiodarone prolongs refractoriness in all cardiac tissues; Na^+ channel block, delayed repolarization owing to K^+ channel block, and inhibition of cell–cell coupling all may contribute to this effect.

Adverse Effects. Hypotension owing to vasodilation and depressed myocardial performance are frequent with the intravenous form of amiodarone. Although depressed contractility can occur during long-term oral therapy, it is unusual. Despite administration of high doses that would cause serious toxicity if continued long term, adverse effects are unusual during oral drug-loading regimens, which typically require several weeks. Occasionally during the loading phase, patients develop nausea, which responds to a decrease in daily dose.

Adverse effects during long-term therapy reflect both the size of daily maintenance doses and the cumulative dose, suggesting that tissue accumulation may be responsible. The most serious adverse effect during chronic amiodarone therapy is pulmonary fibrosis, which can be rapidly progressive and fatal. Underlying lung disease, doses of 400 mg/day or more, and recent pulmonary insults such as pneumonia appear to be risk factors. Serial chest X-rays or pulmonary function studies may detect early amiodarone toxicity; monitoring plasma concentrations has not been useful. With low doses, such as 200 mg/day or less used in atrial fibrillation, pulmonary toxicity is unusual. Other adverse effects during long-term therapy include corneal microdeposits (which often are asymptomatic), hepatic dysfunction, neuromuscular symptoms (peripheral neuropathy or proximal muscle weakness), photosensitivity, and hypo- or hyperthyroidism. Treatment consists of withdrawal of the drug and supportive measures, including corticosteroids. Dose reduction may be sufficient if the drug is deemed necessary and the adverse effect is not life-threatening. Despite the marked QT prolongation and bradycardia typical of chronic amiodarone therapy, *torsade de pointes* and other drug-induced tachyarrhythmias are unusual.

Clinical Pharmacokinetics. Amiodarone's oral bioavailability is ~30%, which is important in calculating equivalent dosing regimens when converting from intravenous to oral therapy. After the initiation of amiodarone therapy, increases in refractoriness, a marker of pharmacologic effect, require several weeks to develop. Amiodarone undergoes hepatic metabolism by CYP3A4 to desethyl-amiodarone, a metabolite with pharmacologic effects similar to those of the parent drug. When amiodarone therapy is withdrawn from a patient who has been receiving therapy for several years, plasma concentrations decline with a $t_{1/2}$ of weeks to months. The mechanism whereby amiodarone and desethyl-amiodarone are eliminated is not well established.

A therapeutic plasma amiodarone concentration range of 0.5-2 μg/mL has been proposed. However, efficacy apparently depends as much on duration of therapy as on plasma concentration, and elevated plasma concentrations do not predict toxicity. Because of amiodarone's slow accumulation in tissue, a high-dose oral loading regimen (e.g., 800-1600 mg/day) usually is administered for several weeks before maintenance therapy is started. If the presenting arrhythmia is life-threatening, dosages of >300 mg/day normally are used unless unequivocal toxicity occurs. On the other hand, maintenance doses of ≤200 mg/day are used if recurrence of an arrhythmia would be tolerated, as in patients with atrial fibrillation. Because of its very slow elimination, amiodarone is administered once daily, and omission of 1 or 2 doses during chronic therapy rarely results in recurrence of arrhythmia. Dosage adjustments are not required in hepatic, renal, or cardiac dysfunction. Amiodarone potently inhibits the hepatic metabolism or renal elimination of many compounds. Mechanisms identified to date include inhibition of CYP3A4, CYP2C9, and P-glycoprotein (*see* Chapters 5 and 6). Dosages of warfarin, other anti-arrhythmics (e.g., flecainide, procainamide, quinidine), or digoxin usually require reduction during amiodarone therapy.

DIGOXIN. Digitalis glycosides exert positive inotropic effects and are used in heart failure (*see* Chapter 28). Their inotropic action results from increased intracellular Ca^{2+} (Figure 28–5), which also forms the basis for arrhythmias related to cardiac glycoside intoxication.

Pharmacologic Effects. Cardiac glycosides increase phase 4 slope (i.e., increase the rate of automaticity), especially if $[K]_o$ is low. They also exert prominent vagotonic actions, resulting in inhibition of Ca^{2+} currents in the AV node and activation of acetylcholine-mediated K^+ currents in the atrium. Thus, the major "indirect" electrophysiologic effects of cardiac glycosides are hyperpolarization, shortening of atrial action potentials, and increases in AV nodal refractoriness. The latter action accounts for the utility of digoxin in terminating reentrant arrhythmias involving the AV node and in controlling ventricular response in patients with atrial fibrillation.

Cardiac glycosides may be especially useful in atrial fibrillation because many such patients have heart failure, which can be exacerbated by other AV nodal blocking drugs such as Ca^{2+} channel blockers or β adrenergic receptor antagonists. However, sympathetic drive is increased markedly in many patients with advanced heart failure, so digitalis is not very effective in decreasing the rate; however, even a modest decrease in rate can ameliorate heart failure. Similarly, in other conditions in which high sympathetic tone drives rapid AV conduction (e.g., chronic lung disease, thyrotoxicosis), digitalis therapy may be only marginally effective in slowing the rate. In heart transplant patients, in whom innervation has been ablated, cardiac glycosides are ineffective for rate control. Increased sympathetic activity and hypoxia can potentiate digitalis-induced changes in automaticity and DADs, thus increasing the risk of digitalis toxicity. A further complicating feature in thyrotoxicosis is increased digoxin clearance. The major ECG effects of cardiac glycosides are PR prolongation and a nonspecific alteration in ventricular repolarization (manifested by depression of the ST segment), whose underlying mechanism is not well understood.

Adverse Effects. Because of the low therapeutic index of cardiac glycosides, their toxicity is a common clinical problem (*see* Chapter 28). Arrhythmias, nausea, disturbances of cognitive function, and blurred or yellow vision are the usual manifestations. Elevated serum concentrations of digitalis, hypoxia, and electrolyte abnormalities (e.g., hypokalemia, hypomagnesemia, hypercalcemia) predispose patients to digitalis-induced arrhythmias. Although digitalis intoxication can cause virtually any arrhythmia, certain types of arrhythmias that should raise a strong suspicion of digitalis intoxication are those in which DAD-related tachycardias occur along with impairment of sinus node or AV nodal function. Atrial tachycardia with AV block is classic, but ventricular bigeminy (sinus beats alternating with beats of ventricular origin), "bidirectional" ventricular tachycardia (a very rare entity), AV junctional tachycardias, and various degrees of AV block also can occur. With severe intoxication (e.g., with suicidal ingestion), severe hyperkalemia owing to poisoning of Na^+,K^+-ATPase and profound bradyarrhythmias are seen. In patients with elevated serum digitalis levels, the risk of precipitating VF by DC cardioversion probably is increased; in those with therapeutic blood levels, DC cardioversion can be used safely.

Minor forms of cardiac glycoside intoxication may require no specific therapy beyond monitoring cardiac rhythm until symptoms and signs of toxicity resolve. Sinus bradycardia and AV block often respond to intravenous atropine. Mg^{2+} has been used successfully in some cases of digitalis-induced tachycardia. Any serious arrhythmia should be treated with antidigoxin Fab fragments (DIGIBIND, DIGIFAB), which are highly effective in binding digoxin and digitoxin and greatly enhance their renal excretion (*see* Chapter 28). Temporary cardiac pacing may be required for advanced sinus node or AV node dysfunction. Digitalis exerts direct arterial vasoconstrictor effects, which can be deleterious in patients with advanced atherosclerosis who receive intravenous drug.

Clinical Pharmacokinetics. The only digitalis glycoside used in the U.S. is digoxin (LANOXIN). Digitoxin also is used for chronic oral therapy outside the U.S. Digoxin tablets are ~75% bioavailable. In some patients, intestinal microflora may metabolize digoxin, markedly reducing bioavailability. In these patients, higher than usual doses are required for clinical efficacy; toxicity is a serious risk if antibiotics that destroy intestinal microflora are administered. Inhibition of P-glycoprotein also may play a role in cases of toxicity. Digoxin is 20-30% protein bound. The anti-arrhythmic effects of digoxin can be achieved with intravenous or oral therapy. However, digoxin undergoes relatively slow distribution to effector site(s); therefore, even with intravenous therapy, there is a lag of several hours between drug administration and the development of measurable anti-arrhythmic effects such as PR-interval prolongation or slowing of the ventricular rate in atrial fibrillation. To avoid intoxication, a loading dose of ~0.6-1 mg digoxin is administered over 24 h. Measurement of postdistribution serum digoxin concentration and adjustment of the daily dose (0.0625-0.5 mg) to maintain concentrations of 0.5-2 ng/mL are useful during chronic digoxin therapy (*see* Table 29–5). Some patients may require and tolerate higher concentrations but with an increased risk of adverse effects.

Digoxin is largely excreted unchanged by the kidney with an elimination $t_{1/2}$ ~36 h, so maintenance doses are administered once daily. Digoxin doses should be reduced (or dosing interval increased) and serum concentrations monitored closely in patients with impaired excretion owing to renal failure or in patients who are hypothyroid. Digitoxin undergoes primarily hepatic metabolism and may be useful in patients with fluctuating or advanced renal dysfunction. Digitoxin's elimination $t_{1/2}$ is even longer than that of digoxin (~7 days); it is highly protein bound, and its therapeutic range is 10-30 ng/mL. Digitoxin metabolism is accelerated by drugs such as phenytoin and rifampin that induce hepatic metabolism. Amiodarone, quinidine, verapamil, diltiazem, cyclosporine, itraconazole, propafenone, and flecainide decrease digoxin clearance, likely by inhibiting P-glycoprotein, the major route of digoxin elimination. New steady-state digoxin concentrations are approached in about a week. Digitalis toxicity results so often with quinidine or amiodarone that it is routine to decrease the dose of digoxin if these drugs are started. In all cases, digoxin concentrations should be measured regularly and the dose adjusted if necessary. Hypokalemia will potentiate digitalis-induced arrhythmias.

DISOPYRAMIDE. Disopyramide (NORPACE, others) exerts electrophysiologic effects very similar to those of quinidine, but the drugs produce different adverse effects. Disopyramide is used to maintain sinus rhythm in patients with atrial flutter or atrial fibrillation and to prevent recurrence of ventricular tachycardia or VF.

Pharmacologic Actions and Adverse Effects. The in vitro electrophysiologic actions of *S*-(+)-disopyramide are similar to those of quinidine. The *R*-(−)-enantiomer produces similar Na^+ channel block but does not prolong cardiac action potentials. Unlike quinidine, racemic disopyramide is not an α adrenergic receptor antagonist, but it does exert prominent anticholinergic actions that account for many of its adverse effects. These include precipitation of glaucoma, constipation, dry mouth, and urinary retention. Disopyramide commonly depresses contractility, which can precipitate heart failure and also can cause *torsade de pointes*.

Clinical Pharmacokinetics. Disopyramide is well absorbed. Binding to plasma proteins is concentration dependent, so a small increase in total concentration may represent a disproportionately larger increase in free drug concentration. Disopyramide is eliminated by both hepatic metabolism (to a weakly active metabolite) and renal excretion of unchanged drug. The dose should be reduced in patients with renal dysfunction. Higher than usual dosages may be required in patients receiving drugs that induce hepatic metabolism, such as phenytoin.

DOFETILIDE. Dofetilide (TIKOSYN) is a potent and "pure" I_{Kr} blocker that has virtually no extracardiac effects. Dofetilide is effective in maintaining sinus rhythm in patients with atrial fibrillation. Dofetilide is available through a restricted distribution system that includes only physicians, hospitals, and other institutions that have received special educational programs covering proper dosing and in-hospital treatment initiation.

Adverse Effects. Torsade de pointes occurred in 1-3% of patients in clinical trials where strict exclusion criteria (e.g., hypokalemia) were applied and continuous ECG monitoring was used to detect marked QT prolongation in the hospital. The incidence of this adverse effect during more widespread use of the drug postmarketing is unknown.

Clinical Pharmacokinetics. Most of a dose of dofetilide is excreted unchanged by the kidneys. In patients with mild to moderate renal failure, decreases in dosage based on creatinine clearance are required to minimize the risk of *torsade de pointes*. The drug should not be used in patients with advanced renal failure or with inhibitors of renal cation transport. Dofetilide also undergoes minor hepatic metabolism.

DRONEDARONE. Dronedarone (MULTAQ) is a derivative of amiodarone approved for the treatment of atrial fibrillation and atrial flutter. Compared to amiodarone, dronedarone treatment is associated with significantly fewer adverse events, but it also is significantly less effective in maintaining sinus rhythm. Dronedarone reduces morbidity and mortality in patients with high-risk atrial fibrillation. However, dronedarone *increases* mortality in patients with severe heart failure and is contraindicated in patients with NYHA class 4 heart failure and in patients with a recent decompensation of heart failure requiring hospitalization.

Pharmacologic Effects. Similar to amiodarone, dronedarone is a potent blocker of multiple ion currents, including the rapidly activating delayed-rectifier K^+ current (I_{Kr}), the slowly activating delayed-rectifier K^+ current (I_{Ks}), the inward rectifier K^+ current (I_{K1}), the acetylcholine activated K^+ current, the peak Na^+ current, and the L-type Ca^{2+} current. It has stronger anti-adrenergic effects than amiodarone.

Adverse Effects and Drug Interactions. The most common adverse reactions are diarrhea, nausea, abdominal pain, vomiting, and asthenia. Dronedarone causes dose-dependent prolongation of QT interval, but *torsade de pointes* is rare. Dronedarone is metabolized by CYP3A and is a moderate inhibitor of CYP3A, CYP2D6, and P-glycoprotein. A potent CYP3A4 inhibitor such as ketoconazole may increase dronedarone exposure by as much as 25-fold. Dronedarone should not be coadministered with potent CYP3A4 inhibitors. Coadministration with other drugs metabolized by CYP2D6 (e.g., metoprolol) or transported by P-glycoprotein (e.g., digoxin) may result in increased drug concentrations.

ESMOLOL. (BREVIBLOC, others) is a β_1-selective agent that is metabolized by erythrocyte esterases and so has a very short elimination $t_{1/2}$ (9 min). Intravenous esmolol is useful in clinical situations in which immediate β adrenergic blockade is desired (e.g., for rate control of rapidly conducted atrial fibrillation).

FLECAINIDE. The effects of flecainide (TAMBOCOR, others) are likely attributable to the drug's very long $\tau_{recovery}$ from Na^+ channel block. It is approved for the maintenance of sinus rhythm in patients with supraventricular arrhythmias, including atrial fibrillation, in whom structural heart disease is absent.

Pharmacologic Effects. Flecainide blocks Na^+ current, delayed-rectifier K^+ current (I_{Kr}) and Ca^{2+} currents. APD is shortened in Purkinje cells, probably owing to block of late-opening Na^+ channels, but prolonged in ventricular cells, probably owing to block of delayed-rectifier current. Flecainide does not cause EADs in vitro but has been associated with rare cases of *torsade de pointes*. In atrial tissue, flecainide disproportionately prolongs action potentials at fast rates, an especially desirable anti-arrhythmic drug effect; this effect contrasts with that of quinidine, which prolongs atrial action potentials to a greater extent at slower rates. Flecainide prolongs the duration of PR, QRS, and QT intervals even at normal heart rates. Flecainide also is an open channel blocker of RyR2 Ca^{2+} release channels and prevents arrhythmogenic Ca^{2+} release from the SR in isolated myocytes. The blockade of the RyR2 channel by flecainide targets directly the underlying molecular defect in patients with mutations in the ryanodine receptor and cardiac calsequestrin, which may explain why flecainide suppresses ventricular arrhythmias in CPVT patients refractory to standard drug therapy.

Adverse Effects. Dose-related blurred vision is the most common noncardiac adverse effect. It can exacerbate congestive heart failure in patients with depressed left ventricular performance. The most serious adverse effects are provocation or exacerbation of potentially lethal arrhythmias. These include acceleration of ventricular rate in patients with atrial flutter, increased frequency of episodes of reentrant ventricular tachycardia, and increased mortality in patients convalescing from MI. These may be attributed to Na^+ channel block. Flecainide also can cause heart block in patients with conduction system disease.

Clinical Pharmacokinetics. Flecainide is well absorbed. Elimination occurs by both renal excretion of unchanged drug and hepatic metabolism by CYP2D6 to inactive metabolites. However, in patients who lack this pathway due to genetic polymorphism or inhibition by other drugs (i.e., quinidine, fluoxetine), renal excretion ordinarily is sufficient to prevent drug accumulation. In the rare patient with renal dysfunction and lack of active CYP2D6, flecainide may accumulate to toxic plasma concentrations. Some reports suggest that plasma flecainide concentrations greater than 1 μg/mL should be avoided to minimize the risk of flecainide toxicity; but the adverse electrophysiologic effects of flecainide therapy can occur at therapeutic plasma concentrations.

IBUTILIDE. Ibutilide (CORVERT) is an I_{Kr} blocker that in some systems also activates an inward Na^+ current. The action potential–prolonging effect of the drug may arise from either mechanism.

Ibutilide is administered as a rapid infusion (1 mg over 10 min) for the immediate conversion of atrial fibrillation or flutter to sinus rhythm. The drug's efficacy rate is higher in patients with atrial flutter (50-70%) than in those with atrial fibrillation (30-50%). In atrial fibrillation, the conversion rate is lower in those in whom the arrhythmia has been present for weeks or months compared with those in whom it has been present for days. The major toxicity with ibutilide is *torsade de pointes*, which occurs in up to 6% of patients and requires immediate cardioversion in up to one-third of these. The drug undergoes extensive first-pass metabolism and so is not used orally. It is eliminated by hepatic metabolism with a $t_{1/2}$ of 2-12 h.

LIDOCAINE. Lidocaine (XYLOCAINE, others) is a local anesthetic that also is useful in the acute intravenous therapy of ventricular arrhythmias. Its pharmacology is presented in Chapter 20. See also *mexiletine*, below.

Pharmacologic Effects. Lidocaine blocks both open and inactivated cardiac Na^+ channels. Recovery from block is very rapid, so lidocaine exerts greater effects in depolarized (e.g., ischemic) and/or rapidly driven tissues. Lidocaine is not useful in atrial arrhythmias possibly because atrial action potentials are so short that the Na^+ channel is in the inactivated state only briefly compared with long diastolic (recovery) times. Lidocaine can hyperpolarize Purkinje fibers depolarized by low $[K]_o$ or stretch; the resulting increased conduction velocity may be anti-arrhythmic in reentry. Lidocaine decreases automaticity by reducing the slope of phase 4 and altering the threshold for excitability. APD usually is unaffected or is shortened; such shortening may be due to block of the few Na^+ channels that inactivate late during the cardiac action potential. Lidocaine usually exerts no significant effect on PR or QRS duration; QT is unaltered or slightly shortened. The drug exerts little effect on hemodynamic function, although rare cases of lidocaine-associated exacerbations of heart failure have been reported in patients with very poor left ventricular function.

Adverse Effects. When a large intravenous dose of lidocaine is administered rapidly, seizures can occur. When plasma concentrations of the drug rise slowly above the therapeutic range, as may occur during maintenance therapy, tremor, dysarthria, and altered levels of consciousness are more common. Nystagmus is an early sign of lidocaine toxicity.

Clinical Pharmacokinetics. Lidocaine is well absorbed but undergoes extensive though variable first-pass hepatic metabolism; thus, oral use is inappropriate and the intravenous route is preferred (*see* Table 29–5). Lidocaine's metabolites, glycine xylidide (GX) and monoethyl GX, are less potent as Na^+ channel blockers than the parent drug. GX and lidocaine appear to compete for access to the Na^+ channel, suggesting that with infusions during which GX accumulates, lidocaine's efficacy may be diminished. With infusions lasting longer than 24 h, the clearance of lidocaine falls—an effect that has been attributed to competition between parent drug and metabolites for access to hepatic drug-metabolizing enzymes.

The initial drop in plasma lidocaine following intravenous administration occurs rapidly, with a $t_{1/2}$ of ~8 min, and represents distribution from the central compartment to peripheral tissues. The terminal elimination $t_{1/2}$, usually ~110 min, represents drug elimination by hepatic metabolism. Lidocaine's efficacy depends on maintenance of therapeutic plasma concentrations in the central compartment. Therefore, the administration of a single bolus dose of lidocaine can result in transient arrhythmia suppression that dissipates rapidly as the drug is distributed and concentrations in the central compartment fall. To avoid this distribution-related loss of efficacy, a loading regimen of 3-4 mg/kg over 20-30 min is used—e.g., an initial 100 mg followed by 50 mg every 8 min for 3 doses. Subsequently, stable concentrations can be maintained in plasma with an infusion of 1-4 mg/min, which replaces drug removed by hepatic metabolism. The time to steady-state lidocaine concentrations is ~8-10 h. Routine measurement of plasma lidocaine concentration at the time of expected steady state is useful in adjusting the maintenance infusion rate to avoid toxicities (therapeutic range, 1.5-5 μg/mL). In heart failure, the central volume of distribution is decreased, so the total loading dose should be decreased. Lidocaine clearance also is reduced in hepatic disease, during treatment with *cimetidine* or β blockers, and during prolonged infusions. Lidocaine is bound to the acute-phase reactant α-1-acid glycoprotein. Diseases such as acute MI are associated with increases in α-1-acid glycoprotein and protein binding and hence a decreased proportion of free drug. These findings may explain why some patients require and tolerate higher than usual total plasma lidocaine concentrations to maintain anti-arrhythmic efficacy.

MAGNESIUM. The intravenous administration of 1-2 g $MgSO_4$ reportedly is effective in preventing recurrent episodes of *torsade de pointes*, even if the serum Mg^{2+} concentration is normal. However, controlled studies of this effect have not been performed.

The mechanism of action is unknown because the QT interval is not shortened; an effect on the inward current, possibly a Ca^{2+} current, responsible for the triggered upstroke arising from EADs (*black arrow*, Figure 29–6B) is possible. Intravenous Mg^{2+} also has been used successfully in arrhythmias related to digitalis intoxication.

MEXILETINE. Mexiletine (MEXITIL, others) is an analog of lidocaine that has been modified to reduce first-pass hepatic metabolism and permit chronic oral therapy. The electrophysiologic actions are similar to those of lidocaine. Tremor and nausea, the major dose-related adverse effects, can be minimized by taking the drugs with food.

Mexiletine undergoes hepatic metabolism, which is inducible by drugs such as phenytoin. Mexiletine is approved for treating ventricular arrhythmias; combinations of mexiletine with quinidine or sotalol may increase efficacy while reducing adverse effects. In vitro studies and clinical case reports suggest a role for mexiletine (or flecainide) in correcting the aberrant late inward Na^+ current in congenital LQT3.

PROCAINAMIDE. Procainamide (PROCAN SR, others) is an analog of the local anesthetic procaine (*see* Chapter 20). It exerts electrophysiologic effects similar to those of quinidine but lacks quinidine's vagolytic and α adrenergic blocking activity. Procainamide is better tolerated than quinidine when given intravenously. Loading and maintenance intravenous infusions are used in the acute therapy of many supraventricular and ventricular arrhythmias; long-term oral treatment is poorly tolerated and often is stopped owing to adverse effects.

Pharmacologic Effects. Procainamide is a blocker of open Na^+ channels with an intermediate $\tau_{recovery}$ from block. It also prolongs cardiac action potentials, probably by blocking outward K^+ current(s). Procainamide decreases automaticity, increases refractory periods, and slows conduction. Its major metabolite, *N*-acetyl procainamide, lacks the Na^+ channel-blocking activity of the parent drug but is equipotent in prolonging action potentials. Because the plasma concentrations of *N*-acetyl procainamide often exceed those of procainamide, increased refractoriness and QT prolongation during chronic procainamide therapy may be partly attributable to the metabolite. However, it is the parent drug that slows conduction and produces QRS-interval prolongation. Hypotension may occur at high plasma concentrations, this effect is attributable to ganglionic blockade rather than to any negative inotropic effect.

Adverse Effects. Hypotension and marked slowing of conduction are major adverse effects of high concentrations (>10 μg/mL) of procainamide, especially during intravenous use. Dose-related nausea is frequent during oral therapy and may be attributable in part to high plasma concentrations of *N*-acetyl procainamide. *Torsade de pointes* can occur, particularly when plasma concentrations of *N*-acetyl procainamide rise to >30 μg/mL. Procainamide produces potentially fatal bone marrow aplasia in 0.2% of patients. During long-term therapy, most patients will develop biochemical evidence of the drug-induced lupus syndrome, such as circulating antinuclear antibodies. Therapy need not be interrupted merely because of the presence of antinuclear antibodies. However, 25-50% of patients eventually develop symptoms of the lupus syndrome; common early symptoms are rash and small-joint arthralgias. Other symptoms of lupus, including pericarditis with tamponade, can occur, although renal involvement is unusual. The lupuslike symptoms resolve on cessation of therapy or during treatment with *N*-acetyl procainamide (see below).

Clinical Pharmacokinetics. Procainamide is eliminated rapidly ($t_{1/2}$ = 3-4 h) by both renal excretion of unchanged drug and hepatic metabolism. The major pathway for hepatic metabolism is conjugation by *N*-acetyl transferase, to form *N*-acetyl procainamide. *N*-Acetyl procainamide is eliminated by renal excretion ($t_{1/2}$ = 6-10 h). Oral procainamide usually is administered as a slow-release formulation. In patients with renal failure reduction dose and dosing frequency and monitoring of plasma concentrations of both compounds are required. Because the parent drug and metabolite exert different pharmacologic effects, the past practice of using the sum of their concentrations to guide therapy is inappropriate. In individuals who are "slow acetylators," the procainamide-induced lupus syndrome develops more often and earlier during treatment than among rapid acetylators. In addition, the symptoms of procainamide-induced lupus resolve during treatment with *N*-acetyl procainamide. Both these findings suggest that it is chronic exposure to the parent drug (or an oxidative metabolite) that results in the lupus syndrome.

PROPAFENONE. Propafenone (RYTHMOL, others) is a Na^+ channel blocker with a relatively slow time constant for recovery from block. Like flecainide, propafenone also blocks K^+ channels. Its major electrophysiologic effect is to slow conduction in fast-response tissues.

The drug is prescribed as a racemate; although the enantiomers do not differ in their Na^+ channel–blocking properties, *S*-(+)-propafenone is a β receptor antagonist. Propafenone prolongs PR and QRS durations. Chronic therapy with oral propafenone is used to maintain sinus rhythm in patients with supraventricular tachycardias, including atrial fibrillation. It also can be used in ventricular arrhythmias, but with only modest efficacy.

Adverse Effects. Adverse effects during propafenone therapy include acceleration of ventricular response in patients with atrial flutter, increased frequency or severity of episodes of reentrant ventricular tachycardia, exacerbation of heart failure, and the adverse effects of β adrenergic blockade, such as sinus bradycardia and bronchospasm.

Clinical Pharmacokinetics. Propafenone is well absorbed and is eliminated by both hepatic and renal routes. The activity of CYP2D6 is a major determinant of plasma propafenone concentration. In most subjects ("extensive metabolizers"), propafenone undergoes extensive first-pass hepatic metabolism to 5-hydroxy propafenone, a metabolite equipotent to propafenone as a Na^+ channel blocker but much less potent as a β adrenergic receptor antagonist. A second metabolite, *N*-desalkyl propafenone, is formed by non–CYP2D6-mediated metabolism and is a less potent blocker of Na^+ channels and β adrenergic receptors. CYP2D6-mediated metabolism of propafenone is saturable, so small increases in dose can increase plasma propafenone concentration disproportionately. In "poor metabolizer" subjects lacking functional CYP2D6, plasma propafenone concentrations will be much higher after an equal dose. The incidence of adverse effects of propafenone therapy is higher in poor metabolizers.

CYP2D6 activity can be inhibited markedly by a number of drugs, including quinidine and fluoxetine. In extensive metabolizer subjects receiving such drugs or in poor metabolizer subjects, plasma propafenone concentrations of more than 1 μg/mL are associated with clinical effects of β receptor blockade, such as reduction of exercise heart rate. Patients with moderate to severe liver disease should be reduced to ~20-30% of the usual dose, with careful monitoring. Slow-release formulation allows twice-daily dosing.

QUINIDINE. Quinidine, a diastereomer of the antimalarial quinine, is used to maintain sinus rhythm in patients with atrial flutter or atrial fibrillation and to prevent recurrence of ventricular tachycardia or VF.

Pharmacologic Effects. Quinidine blocks Na^+ current and multiple cardiac K^+ currents. It is an open-state blocker of Na^+ channels, with a $\tau_{recovery}$ in the intermediate (~3 s) range; as a consequence, QRS duration increases modestly, usually by 10-20%, at therapeutic dosages. At therapeutic concentrations, quinidine commonly prolongs the QT interval up to 25%, but the effect is highly variable. At concentrations as low as 1 μM, quinidine blocks Na^+ current and the rapid component of delayed rectifier (I_{Kr}); higher concentrations block the slow component of delayed rectifier, inward rectifier, transient outward current, and L-type Ca^{2+} current.

Quinidine's Na^+ channel–blocking properties result in an increased threshold for excitability and decreased automaticity. Due to K^+ channel–blocking actions, quinidine prolongs action potentials in most cardiac cells, most prominently at slow heart rates. In some cells, such as midmyocardial cells and Purkinje cells, quinidine consistently elicits EADs at slow heart rates, particularly when $[K]_o$ is low. Quinidine prolongs refractoriness in most tissues, probably as a result of both prolongation of APD and Na^+ channel blockade.

Quinidine also produces β receptor blockade and vagal inhibition. Thus, the intravenous use of quinidine is associated with marked hypotension and sinus tachycardia. Quinidine's vagolytic effects tend to inhibit its direct depressant effect on AV nodal conduction, so the effect of drug on the PR interval is variable. Moreover, quinidine's vagolytic effect can result in increased AV nodal transmission of atrial tachycardias such as atrial flutter (*see* Table 29–1).

Adverse Effects—Noncardiac. Diarrhea is the most common adverse effect during quinidine therapy, occurring in 30-50% of patients, usually within the first several days of quinidine therapy but can occur later. Diarrhea-induced hypokalemia may potentiate *torsade de pointes* due to quinidine. A number of immunologic reactions can occur during quinidine therapy. The most common is thrombocytopenia, which can be severe but resolves rapidly with drug discontinuation. Hepatitis, bone marrow depression, and lupus syndrome occur rarely. None of these effects is related to elevated plasma quinidine concentrations. Quinidine also can produce cinchonism, a syndrome that includes headache and tinnitus. In contrast to other adverse responses to quinidine therapy, cinchonism usually is related to elevated plasma quinidine concentrations and can be managed by dose reduction.

Adverse Effects—Cardiac. Between 2-8% will develop marked QT-interval prolongation and *torsade de pointes*. In contrast to effects of sotalol, *N*-acetyl procainamide, and many other drugs, quinidine-associated *torsade de pointes* generally occurs at therapeutic or even subtherapeutic plasma concentrations. The reasons for individual susceptibility are not known. At high plasma concentrations of quinidine, marked Na^+ channel block can occur, with resulting ventricular tachycardia. Quinidine can exacerbate heart failure or conduction system disease. However, in most patients with congestive heart failure, quinidine is well tolerated, perhaps because of its vasodilating actions.

Clinical Pharmacokinetics. Quinidine is well absorbed and is 80% bound to plasma proteins, including albumin and α-1-acid glycoprotein. As with lidocaine, greater than usual doses (and total plasma quinidine concentrations) may be required to maintain therapeutic concentrations of free quinidine in high-stress states such as acute MI. Quinidine undergoes extensive hepatic oxidative metabolism, and ~20% is excreted unchanged by the kidneys. One metabolite, 3-hydroxyquinidine, is nearly as potent as quinidine in blocking cardiac Na^+ channels and prolonging cardiac action potentials. Concentrations of unbound 3-hydroxyquinidine equal to or exceeding those of quinidine are tolerated by some patients. There is substantial individual variability in the range of dosages required to achieve therapeutic plasma concentrations of 2-5 μg/mL. In patients with advanced renal disease or congestive heart failure, quinidine clearance is decreased only modestly. Thus, dosage requirements in these patients are similar to those in other patients.

Drug Interactions. Quinidine is a potent inhibitor of CYP2D6. Drugs that undergo extensive CYP2D6-mediated metabolism may result in altered drug effects. For example, inhibition of CYP2D6-mediated metabolism of *codeine* to its active metabolite *morphine* results in decreased analgesia. Conversely, inhibition of CYP2D6-mediated metabolism of propafenone results in elevated plasma propafenone concentrations and increased β adrenergic receptor blockade. Quinidine reduces the clearance of digoxin; inhibition of P-glycoprotein–mediated digoxin transport has been implicated. Quinidine metabolism is induced by drugs such as *phenobarbital* and phenytoin. In patients receiving these agents, very high doses of quinidine may be required to achieve therapeutic concentrations. Cimetidine and verapamil also elevate plasma quinidine concentrations, but these effects usually are modest.

SOTALOL. Sotalol (BETAPACE, BETAPACE AF) is a nonselective β adrenergic receptor antagonist that also prolongs cardiac action potentials by inhibiting delayed-rectifier and possibly other K^+ currents.

Sotalol is prescribed as a racemate; the L-enantiomer is a much more potent β adrenergic receptor antagonist than the D-enantiomer, but the 2 are equipotent as K^+ channel blockers. In the U.S., sotalol is an orphan drug approved for use in patients with both ventricular tachyarrhythmias (BETAPACE) and atrial fibrillation or flutter (BETAPACE AF). It is at least as effective as most Na^+ channel blockers in ventricular arrhythmias. Sotalol prolongs QT interval, decreases automaticity, slows AV nodal conduction, and prolongs AV refractoriness by blocking both K^+ channels and β adrenergic receptors; but it exerts no effect on conduction velocity in fast-response tissue. Sotalol causes EADs and triggered activity in vitro and can cause *torsade de pointes*, especially when the serum K^+ concentration is low. The incidence of *torsade de pointes* seems to depend on the dose of sotalol. Occasional cases occur at low dosages, often in patients with renal dysfunction, because sotalol is eliminated by renal excretion. For adverse effects associated with β receptor blockade (*see* Chapter 12).

For a complete Bibliographical Listing see Goodman & Gilman's ***The Pharmacological Basis of Therapeutics***, 12th ed., or Goodman & Gilman Online at www.AccessMedicine.com.

Blood Coagulation and Anticoagulant, Fibrinolytic, and Antiplatelet Drugs

Blood must remain fluid within the vasculature and yet clot quickly when exposed to subendothelial surfaces at sites of vascular injury. Under normal circumstances, a delicate balance between coagulation and fibrinolysis prevents both thrombosis and hemorrhages. Alteration of this balance in favor of coagulation results in thrombosis. Thrombi, composed of platelet aggregates, fibrin, and trapped red blood cells, can form in arteries or veins. Antithrombotic drugs used to treat thrombosis include antiplatelet drugs, which inhibit platelet activation or aggregation; anticoagulants, which attenuate fibrin formation; and fibrinolytic agents, which degrade fibrin. All antithrombotic drugs increase the risk of bleeding.

This chapter reviews the agents commonly used for controlling blood fluidity, including:

- The parenteral anticoagulant heparin and its derivatives, which activate a natural inhibitor of coagulant proteases
- The coumarin anticoagulants, which block multiple steps in the coagulation cascade
- Fibrinolytic agents, which degrade thrombi
- Antiplatelet agents, including aspirin, thienopyridines, and glycoprotein (GP) IIb/IIIa inhibitors

OVERVIEW OF HEMOSTASIS: PLATELET FUNCTION, BLOOD COAGULATION, AND FIBRINOLYSIS

Hemostasis is the cessation of blood loss from a damaged vessel. Platelets first adhere to macromolecules in the subendothelial regions of the injured blood vessel, where they become activated. Adherent platelets release substances that activate nearby platelets, thereby recruiting them to the site of injury. Activated platelets then aggregate to form the primary hemostatic plug.

Vessel wall injury also exposes *tissue factor (TF)*, which initiates the coagulation system. Platelets enhance activation of the coagulation system by providing a surface onto which clotting factors assemble and by releasing stored clotting factors. This results in a burst of *thrombin (factor IIa)* generation. Thrombin then converts fibrinogen to fibrin and amplifies platelet activation and aggregation.

Later, as wound healing occurs, the platelet aggregates and fibrin clots are degraded. The processes of platelet aggregation and blood coagulation are summarized in Figures 30–1 and 30–2 (see also the animation on the Goodman & Gilman website). The pathway of clot removal, fibrinolysis, is shown in Figure 30–3, along with sites of action of fibrinolytic agents. Coagulation involves a series of zymogen activation reactions, as shown in Figure 30–2. At each stage, a precursor protein, or *zymogen,* is converted to an active protease by cleavage of 1 or more peptide bonds in the precursor molecule. The final protease generated is thrombin.

CONVERSION OF FIBRINOGEN TO FIBRIN. Fibrinogen, a 340,000-Da protein, is a dimer, each half of which consists of 3 pairs of polypeptide chains (designated Aα, Bβ, and γ). Disulfide bonds covalently link the chains and the 2 halves of the molecule together. Thrombin converts fibrinogen to fibrin monomers by releasing fibrinopeptide A (a 16–amino acid fragment) and fibrinopeptide B (a 14–amino acid fragment) from the amino termini of the Aα and Bβ chains, respectively. Removal of the fibrinopeptides creates new amino termini, which fit into preformed holes on other fibrin monomers to form a fibrin gel, which is the end point of in vitro tests of coagulation (see "Coagulation in vitro"). Initially, the fibrin monomers are bound to each other noncovalently. Subsequently, factor XIII, a transglutaminase that is activated by thrombin, catalyzes interchain covalent cross-links between adjacent fibrin monomers, which enhance the strength of the clot.

STRUCTURE OF COAGULATION FACTORS. In addition to factor XIII, the coagulation factors include factors II (prothrombin), VII, IX, X, XI, XII, and prekallikrein. A stretch of ~200 amino acid residues at the

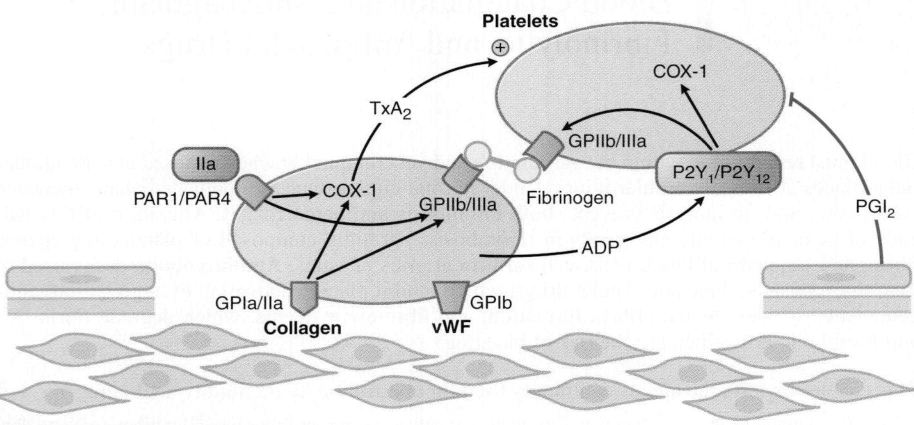

Figure 30–1 *Platelet adhesion and aggregation.* GPIa/IIa and GPIb are platelet receptors that bind to collagen and von Willebrand factor (vWF), causing platelets to adhere to the subendothelium of a damaged blood vessel. PAR1 and PAR4 are protease-activated receptors that respond to thrombin (IIa); $P2Y_1$ and $P2Y_{12}$ are receptors for ADP; when stimulated by agonists, these receptors activate the fibrinogen-binding protein GPIIb/IIIa and cyclooxygenase-1 (COX-1) to promote platelet aggregation and secretion. Thromboxane A_2 (TxA_2) is the major product of COX-1 involved in platelet activation. Prostaglandin I_2 (prostacyclin, PGI_2), synthesized by endothelial cells, inhibits platelet activation.

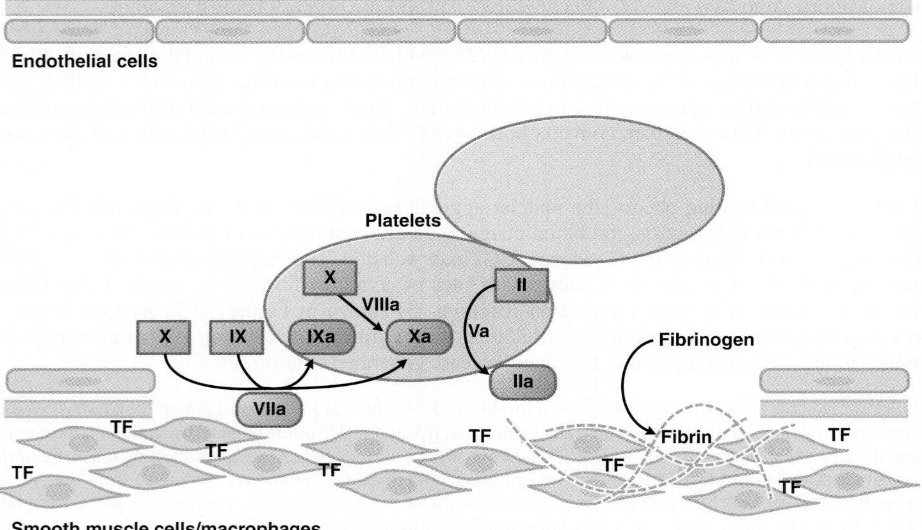

Figure 30–2 *Major reactions of blood coagulation.* Shown are interactions among proteins of the "extrinsic" (tissue factor and factor VII), "intrinsic" (factors IX and VIII), and "common" (factors X, V, and II) coagulation pathways that are important in vivo. Boxes enclose the coagulation factor zymogens (indicated by Roman numerals); the rounded boxes represent the active proteases. TF, tissue factor. Activated coagulation factors are followed by the letter "a": II, prothrombin; IIa, thrombin.

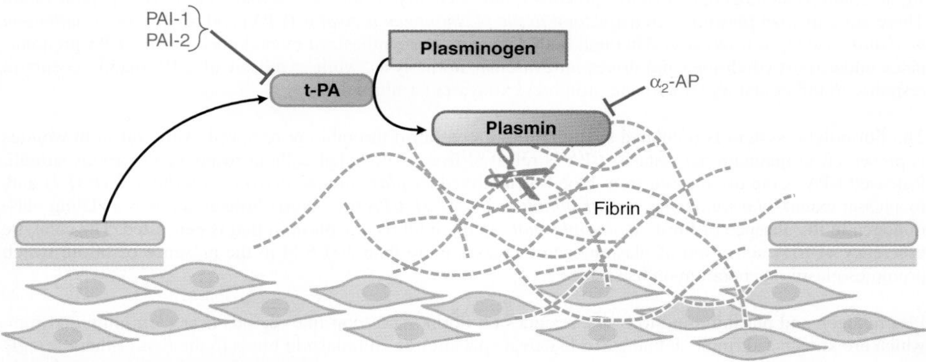

Figure 30–3 *Fibrinolysis.* Endothelial cells secrete tissue plasminogen activator (t-PA) at sites of injury. t-PA binds to fibrin and converts plasminogen to plasmin, which digests fibrin. Plasminogen activator inhibitors-1 and -2 (PAI-1, PAI-2) inactivate t-PA; α_2-antiplasmin (α_2-AP) inactivates plasmin.

carboxyl-termini of each of these zymogens exhibits homology to trypsin and contains the active site of the proteases. In addition, 9-12 glutamate residues near the amino termini of factors II, VII, IX, and X are converted to γ-carboxyglutamate (Gla) residues that bind Ca^{2+} and are necessary for the coagulant activities of these proteins.

NONENZYMATIC PROTEIN COFACTORS. Factors V and VIII serve as cofactors. Factor VIII circulates in plasma bound to *von Willebrand factor*. Factor V circulates in plasma, is stored in platelets in a partially activated form, and is released when platelets are activated. Thrombin cleaves factors V and VIII to yield activated cofactors (factors Va and VIIIa).

Factors Va and VIIIa serve as cofactors by binding to the surface of activated platelets and acting as receptors for factors Xa and IXa, respectively. The activated cofactors also help localize prothrombin and factor X, the respective substrates for these enzymes, on the activated platelet surface. These coagulation factor complexes increase the catalytic efficiency of factors Xa and IXa by ~10^9-fold.

TF is a nonenzymatic lipoprotein cofactor; it initiates coagulation by enhancing the catalytic efficiency of factor VIIa. Not normally present on blood-contacting cells, TF is constitutively expressed on the surface of subendothelial smooth muscle cells and fibroblasts, which are exposed when the vessel wall is damaged. Another plasma protein, high-molecular-weight kininogen, also serves as a cofactor.

ACTIVATION OF PROTHROMBIN. By cleaving 2 peptide bonds on prothrombin, factor Xa converts it to thrombin. In the presence of factor Va, a negatively charged phospholipid surface, and Ca^{2+}, factor Xa activates prothrombin with 10^9-fold greater efficiency. The maximal rate of activation only occurs when prothrombin and factor Xa contain Gla residues, which endow them with the capacity to bind to phospholipids.

Initiation of Coagulation. TF exposed at sites of vessel wall injury initiates coagulation via the *extrinsic pathway*. The small amount of factor VIIa circulating in plasma binds subendothelial TF and the TF-factor VIIa complex, then activates factors X and IX (*see* Figure 30–2). TF, in the presence of phospholipids and Ca^{2+}, increases the activity of factor VIIa by 30,000-fold.

The *intrinsic pathway* is initiated in vitro when factor XII, prekallikrein, and high-molecular-weight kininogen interact with kaolin, glass, or another surface to generate small amounts of factor XIIa. Activation of factor XI to factor XIa and factor IX to factor IXa follows. Factor IXa then activates factor X in a reaction accelerated by factor VIIIa, anionic phospholipids, and Ca^{2+}. Optimal thrombin generation depends on the formation of this factor IXa complex because it activates factor X more efficiently than the TF-factor VIIa complex.

Activation of factor XII is not essential for hemostasis, as evidenced by the fact that patients deficient in factor XII, prekallikrein, or high-molecular-weight kininogen do not have excessive bleeding. Factor XI deficiency is associated with a variable and usually mild bleeding disorder.

Fibrinolysis. The pathway of fibrinolysis is summarized in Figure 30–3. The fibrinolytic system dissolves intravascular *fibrin* through the action of *plasmin*. To initiate fibrinolysis, plasminogen activators first convert single-chain plasminogen, an inactive precursor, into 2-chain *plasmin* by cleavage of a specific peptide bond. There are 2 distinct plasminogen activators: *tissue plasminogen activator* (t-PA) and *urokinase plasminogen activator* (u-PA), or urokinase. Although both activators are synthesized by endothelial cells, t-PA predominates under most conditions and drives intravascular fibrinolysis, while synthesis of u-PA mainly occurs in response to inflammatory stimuli and promotes extravascular fibrinolysis.

The fibrinolytic system is regulated such that unwanted fibrin thrombi are removed, while fibrin in wounds is preserved to maintain hemostasis. t-PA is released from endothelial cells in response to various stimuli. Released t-PA is rapidly cleared from blood or inhibited by *plasminogen activator inhibitor-1 (PAI-1)* and, to a lesser extent, *plasminogen activator inhibitor-2 (PAI-2)*; t-PA thus exerts little effect on circulating plasminogen in the absence of fibrin. α_2*-antiplasmin* rapidly inhibits any plasmin that is generated. The catalytic efficiency of t-PA activation of plasminogen increases more than 300-fold in the presence of fibrin, which promotes plasmin generation on its surface.

Plasminogen and plasmin bind to lysine residues on fibrin via 5 loop-like regions near their amino termini, which are known as kringle domains. To inactivate plasmin, α_2-antiplasmin binds to the first of these kringle domains and then blocks the active site of plasmin. Because the kringle domains are occupied when plasmin binds to fibrin, plasmin on the fibrin surface is protected from inhibition by α_2-antiplasmin and can digest the fibrin. Once the fibrin clot undergoes degradation, α_2-antiplasmin rapidly inhibits any plasmin that escapes from this local milieu. To prevent premature clot lysis, factor XIIIa mediates the covalent cross-linking of small amounts of α_2-antiplasmin onto fibrin.

When thrombi occlude major arteries or veins, therapeutic doses of plasminogen activators sometimes are administered to degrade the fibrin and rapidly restore blood flow. In high doses, these plasminogen activators promote the generation of so much plasmin that the inhibitory controls are overwhelmed. Plasmin is a relatively nonspecific protease; it also degrades several coagulation factors. Reduction in the levels of these coagulation proteins impairs the capacity for thrombin generation, which can contribute to bleeding. In addition, unopposed plasmin tends to dissolve fibrin in hemostatic plugs as well as that in pathological thrombi, a phenomenon that also increases the risk of bleeding. Therefore, fibrinolytic drugs can be toxic, producing hemorrhage as their major side effect.

Coagulation in vitro. Whole blood normally clots in 4-8 min when placed in a glass tube. Clotting is prevented if a chelating agent such as ethylenediaminetetraacetic acid (EDTA) or citrate is added to bind Ca^{2+}. Recalcified plasma normally clots in 2-4 min. The clotting time after recalcification is shortened to 26-33 seconds by the addition of negatively charged phospholipids and a particulate substance, such as kaolin (aluminum silicate) or celite (diatomaceous earth), which activates factor XII; the measurement of this is termed the *activated partial thromboplastin time* (aPTT). Alternatively, recalcified plasma clots in 12-14 seconds after addition of "thromboplastin" (a mixture of TF and phospholipids); the measurement of this is termed the *prothrombin time* (PT).

Natural Anticoagulant Mechanisms. Platelet activation and coagulation do not normally occur within an intact blood vessel. Thrombosis is prevented by several regulatory mechanisms that require a healthy vascular endothelium. NO and PGI_2, synthesized by endothelial cells, inhibit platelet activation (*see* Chapter 33).

Antithrombin is a plasma protein that inhibits coagulation enzymes of the intrinsic and common pathways. Heparan sulfate proteoglycans synthesized by endothelial cells enhance the activity of antithrombin by ~1000-fold. Another regulatory system involves protein C, a plasma zymogen that is homologous to factors II, VII, IX, and X; its activity depends on the binding of Ca^{2+} to Gla residues within its amino-terminal domain. Protein C binds to endothelial protein C receptor (EPCR), which presents protein C to the thrombin–thrombomodulin complex for activation. Activated protein C then dissociates from EPCR and, in combination with protein S, its nonenzymatic Gla-containing cofactor, activated protein C degrades factors Va and VIIIa. Without these activated cofactors, the rates of activation of prothrombin and factor X are greatly diminished. Deficiency of protein C or protein S is associated with an increased risk of pathological thrombus formation.

Tissue factor pathway inhibitor (TFPI), is a natural anticoagulant found in the lipoprotein fraction of plasma. TFPI first binds and inhibits factor Xa, and this binary complex then inhibits factor VIIa. By this mechanism, factor Xa regulates its own generation.

HEPARIN AND ITS DERIVATIVES

Heparin, a glycosaminoglycan found in the secretory granules of mast cells, is synthesized from UDP-sugar precursors as a polymer of alternating D-glucuronic acid and *N*-acetyl-D-glucosamine residues.

Heparin is commonly extracted from porcine intestinal mucosa, which is rich in mast cells, and preparations may contain small amounts of other glycosaminoglycans. The biological activities among different commercial preparations of heparin are similar (~150 USP units/mg). A USP unit reflects the quantity of heparin that prevents 1 mL of citrated sheep plasma from clotting for 1 h after the addition of 0.2 mL of 1% $CaCl_2$. European manufacturers measure potency with an antifactor Xa assay. To determine heparin potency, residual factor Xa activity in the sample is compared with that detected in controls containing known concentrations of an international heparin standard. When assessed this way, heparin potency is expressed in international units per mg. Effective October 1, 2009, the new USP unit dose has been harmonized to the international unit dose. As a result, the new USP unit dose is less potent than the old USP unit dose by ~10%, and heparin doses using the new USP units will have to increase slightly to achieve the same level of anticoagulation.

HEPARIN DERIVATIVES. Derivatives of heparin in current use include low-molecular-weight heparins (LMWHs) and fondaparinux (see their comparison in Table 30–1).

Mechanism of Action. Heparin, LMWHs, and fondaparinux have no intrinsic anticoagulant activity; rather, these agents bind to antithrombin and accelerate the rate at which it inhibits various coagulation proteases. Synthesized in the liver, antithrombin circulates in plasma at an approximate concentration of 2.6 μM. Antithrombin inhibits activated coagulation factors involved in the intrinsic and common pathways but has relatively little activity against factor VIIa. Antithrombin is a "suicide substrate" for these proteases; inhibition occurs when the protease attacks a specific Arg–Ser peptide bond in the reactive center loop of antithrombin and becomes trapped as a stable 1:1 complex. Heparin binds to antithrombin via a specific pentasaccharide sequence that contains a 3-*O*-sulfated glucosamine residue (Figure 30–4). Pentasaccharide binding to antithrombin induces a conformational change in antithrombin that renders its reactive site more accessible to the target protease (Figure 30–5). This conformational change accelerates the rate of factor Xa inhibition by at least 2 orders of magnitude but has no effect on the rate of thrombin inhibition. To enhance the rate of thrombin inhibition by antithrombin, heparin serves as a catalytic template to which both the inhibitor and the protease bind. Only heparin molecules composed of 18 or more saccharide units (molecular weight >5400 Da) are of sufficient length to bridge antithrombin and thrombin together. Consequently, by definition, heparin catalyzes the rates of factor Xa and thrombin to a similar extent, as expressed by an antifactor Xa to antifactor IIa (thrombin) ratio of 1:1. In contrast, at least half of LMWH molecules (mean molecular weight of 5000 Da, ~17 saccharide units) are too short to provide this bridging function and have no effect on the rate of thrombin inhibition by antithrombin. Because these shorter molecules still induce the conformational change in antithrombin that accelerates inhibition of factor Xa, LMWHs have greater antifactor Xa activity than antifactor IIa activity, and the ratio ranges from 3:1 to 2:1 depending on the preparation. Fondaparinux, an analog of the pentasaccharide sequence in heparin or LMWHs that mediates their interaction with antithrombin, has only antifactor Xa activity because it is too short to bridge antithrombin to thrombin (*see* Figure 30–5).

Table 30–1

Comparison of Heparin, LMWH, and Fondaparinux

FEATURES	HEPARIN	LMWH	FONDAPARINUX
Source	Biological	Biological	Synthetic
Molecular weight (Da)	15,000	5000	1500
Target	Xa and IIa	Xa and IIa	Xa
Bioavailability (%)	30	90	100
$t_{1/2}$ *(h)*	1	4	17
Renal excretion	No	Yes	Yes
Antidote effect	Complete	Partial	None
Thrombocytopenia	<5%	<1%	<1%

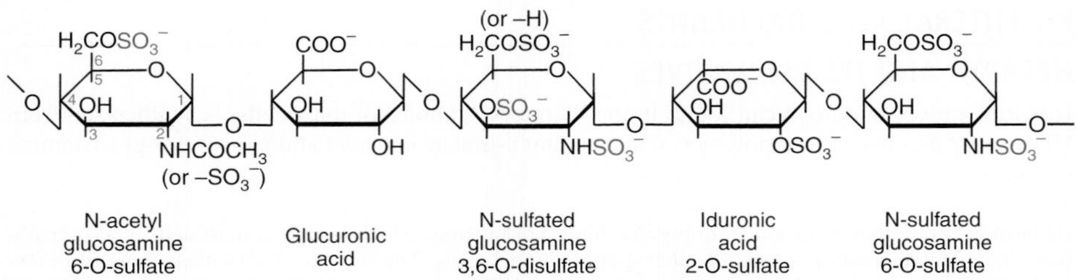

Figure 30–4 *The antithrombin-binding pentasaccharide structure of heparin.* Sulfate groups required for binding to antithrombin are indicated in red.

Heparin, LMWHs, and fondaparinux act in a catalytic fashion. After binding to antithrombin and promoting the formation of covalent complexes between antithrombin and target proteases, the heparin, LMWH, or fondaparinux dissociates from the complex and can then catalyze other antithrombin molecules.

Platelet factor 4, a cationic protein released from the α granules during platelet activation, binds heparin and prevents it from interacting with antithrombin. This phenomenon may limit the activity of heparin in the vicinity of platelet-rich thrombi. Because LMWH and fondaparinux have a lower affinity for platelet factor 4, these agents may retain their activity in the vicinity of such thrombi to a greater extent than heparin.

Miscellaneous Pharmacological Effects. High doses of heparin can interfere with platelet aggregation and prolong bleeding time. In contrast, LMWHs and fondaparinux have little effect on platelets. Heparin "clears" lipemic plasma in vivo by causing the release of lipoprotein lipase into the circulation. Lipoprotein lipase hydrolyzes triglycerides to glycerol and free fatty acids. The clearing of lipemic plasma may occur at concentrations of heparin below those necessary to produce an anticoagulant effect.

Clinical Use. Heparin, LMWH, and fondaparinux can be used to initiate treatment of venous thrombosis and pulmonary embolism because of their rapid onset of action. An oral vitamin K antagonist, such as warfarin, usually is started concurrently, and the heparin or heparin derivative is continued for at least 5 days to allow warfarin to achieve its full therapeutic effect. Heparin, LMWH, or fondaparinux also can be used in the initial management of patients with unstable angina or acute myocardial infarction. For most of these indications, LMWHs and fondaparinux have replaced continuous heparin infusions because of their pharmacokinetic advantages, which permit subcutaneous administration once or twice daily in fixed or weight-adjusted doses without coagulation monitoring. Thus, LMWHs or fondaparinux can be used for out-of-hospital management of patients with venous thrombosis or pulmonary embolism.

Heparin and LMWH are used during coronary balloon angioplasty with or without stent placement to prevent thrombosis. Fondaparinux is not used in this setting because of the risk of catheter thrombosis, a complication caused by catheter-induced activation of factor XII; longer heparin molecules are better than shorter ones for blocking this process. Cardiopulmonary bypass circuits also activate factor XII, which can cause clotting of the oxygenator. Heparin remains the agent of choice for surgery requiring cardiopulmonary bypass. Heparin also is used to treat selected patients with disseminated intravascular coagulation. Subcutaneous administration of low-dose heparin remains the recommended regimen for the prevention of postoperative deep venous thrombosis (DVT) and pulmonary embolism in patients undergoing major abdominothoracic surgery or who are at risk of developing thromboembolic disease.

Unlike warfarin, heparin, LMWH, and fondaparinux do not cross the placenta and have not been associated with fetal malformations, making them the drugs of choice for anticoagulation during pregnancy. Heparin, LMWH, and fondaparinux do not appear to increase fetal mortality or prematurity. If possible, the drugs should be discontinued 24 h before delivery to minimize the risk of postpartum bleeding.

ADME. Heparin, LMWHs, and fondaparinux are not absorbed through the GI mucosa and must be given parenterally. Heparin is given by continuous intravenous infusion, intermittent infusion every 4-6 h, or subcutaneous injection every 8-12 h. Heparin has an immediate onset of action when given intravenously. In contrast, there is considerable variation in the bioavailability of heparin given subcutaneously, and the onset of action is delayed 1-2 h. LMWH and fondaparinux are absorbed more uniformly after subcutaneous injection. The $t_{1/2}$ of heparin in plasma depends on the dose administered. When doses of 100, 400, or 800 units/kg of heparin are injected intravenously, the half-lives of the anticoagulant activities are ~1, 2.5, and 5 h. Heparin appears to be cleared and degraded primarily by the reticuloendothelial system; a small amount of undegraded heparin appears in the urine.

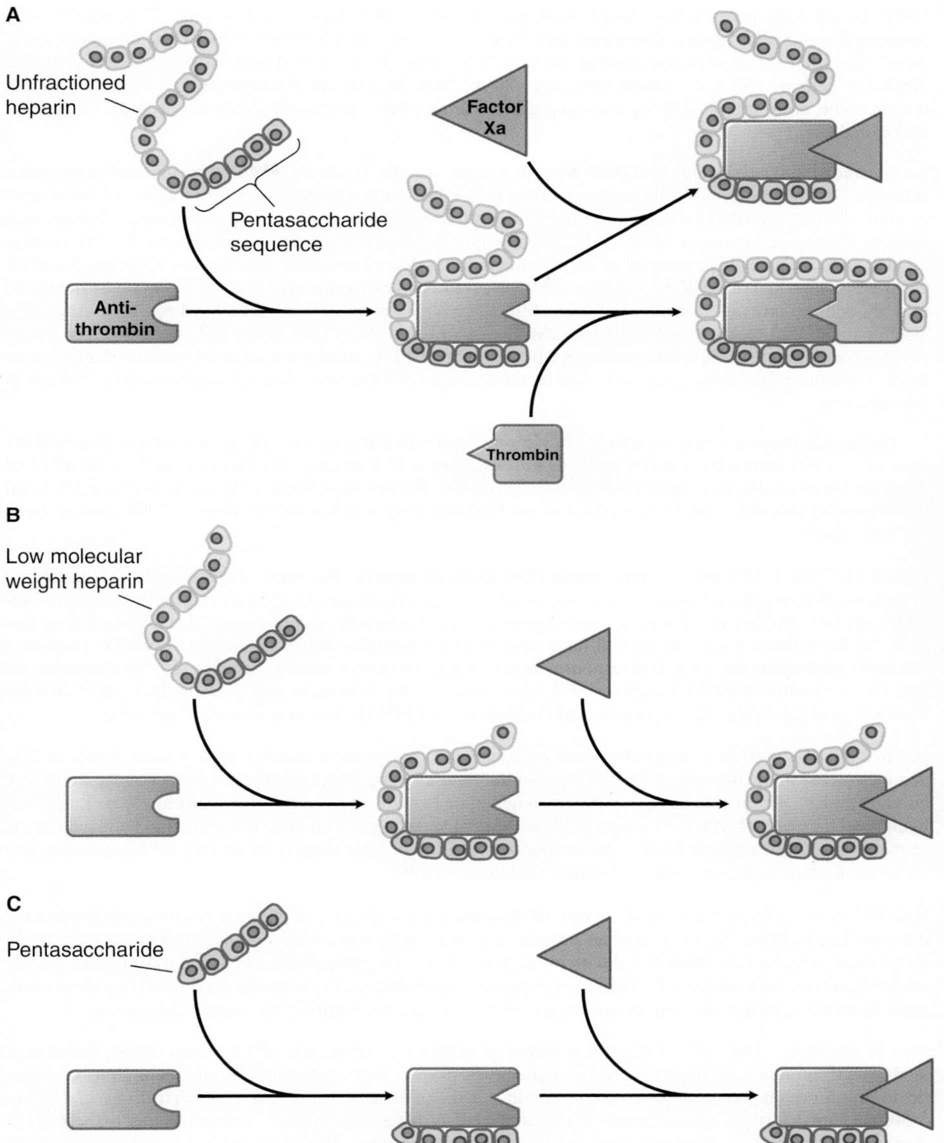

Figure 30–5 *Mechanism of action of heparin, low-molecular-weight heparin (LMWH), and fondaparinux, a synthetic pentasaccharide.* **A.** Heparin binds to antithrombin via its pentasaccharide sequence. This induces a conformational change in the reactive center loop of antithrombin that accelerates its interaction with factor Xa. To potentiate thrombin inhibition, heparin must simultaneously bind to antithrombin and thrombin. Only heparin chains composed of at least 18 saccharide units (MW ~5,400 Da) are of sufficient length to perform this bridging function. With a mean MW ~15,000 Da, virtually all of the heparin chains are long enough to do this. **B.** LMWH has greater capacity to potentiate factor Xa inhibition by antithrombin than thrombin because at least half of the LMWH chains (mean MW ~4,500-5,000 Da) are too short to bridge antithrombin to thrombin. **C.** The pentasaccharide accelerates only factor Xa inhibition by antithrombin; the pentasaccharide is too short to bridge antithrombin to thrombin.

LMWHs and fondaparinux have longer biological half-lives than heparin, 4-6 h and ~17 h, respectively. Because these smaller heparin fragments are cleared almost exclusively by the kidneys, the drugs can accumulate in patients with renal impairment and lead to bleeding. Both LMWH and fondaparinux are contraindicated in patients with a creatinine clearance <30 mL/min. In addition, fondaparinux is contraindicated in patients with body weight <50 kg undergoing hip fracture, hip replacement, knee replacement surgery, or abdominal surgery.

Administration and Monitoring. Full-dose heparin therapy usually is administered by continuous intravenous infusion. Treatment of venous thromboembolism is initiated with a fixed-dose bolus injection of 5000 units or with a weight-adjusted bolus, followed by 800-1600 units/h delivered by an infusion pump. Therapy routinely is monitored by measuring the aPTT. The therapeutic range for heparin is considered to be that which is equivalent to a plasma heparin level of 0.3-0.7 units/mL, as determined with an antifactor Xa assay. An aPTT 2-3 times the normal mean aPTT value generally is assumed to be therapeutic. The aPTT should be measured initially and the infusion rate adjusted every 6 h. Once a steady dosage schedule has been established in a stable patient, daily laboratory monitoring usually is sufficient. Very high doses of heparin are required to prevent coagulation during cardiopulmonary bypass. The aPTT is infinitely prolonged over the dosage range used. A less sensitive coagulation test, such as the activated clotting time, is employed to monitor therapy in this situation.

For therapeutic purposes, heparin also can be administered subcutaneously on a twice-daily basis. A total daily dose of ~35,000 units administered as divided doses every 8-12 h usually is sufficient to achieve an aPTT of twice the control value (measured midway between doses). For low-dose heparin therapy (to prevent DVT and thromboembolism in hospitalized medical or surgical patients), a subcutaneous dose of 5000 units is given 2-3 times daily.

LMWH PREPARATIONS include Enoxaparin (LOVENOX), dalteparin (FRAGMIN), tinzaparin (INNOHEP, others), ardeparin (NORMIFLO), nadroparin (FRAXIPARINE, others), and reviparin (CLIVARINE) (the latter 3 are not currently available in the United States). These agents differ considerably; do not assume that 2 preparations that have similar antifactor Xa activity will have equivalent antithrombotic effects. Because LMWHs produce a relatively predictable anticoagulant response, monitoring is not done routinely. Patients with renal impairment may require monitoring with an antifactor Xa assay because this condition may prolong the $t_{1/2}$ and slow the elimination of LMWHs. Obese patients and children given LMWHs also may require monitoring.

FONDAPARINUX (ARIXTRA) is administered by subcutaneous injection, reaches peak plasma levels in 2 h, and is excreted in the urine ($t_{1/2}$ ~17 h). It should not be used in patients with renal failure. Fondaparinux can be given once a day at a fixed dose without coagulation monitoring. Fondaparinux appears to be much less likely than heparin or LMWH to trigger the syndrome of heparin-induced thrombocytopenia. Fondaparinux is approved for thromboprophylaxis in patients undergoing hip or knee surgery or surgery for hip fracture, and for initial therapy in patients with pulmonary embolism or DVT.

IDRAPARINUX, a hypermethylated version of fondaparinux with a $t_{1/2}$ of 80 h; it is given subcutaneously once-weekly. To overcome the lack of an antidote, a biotin moiety was added to idraparinux to generate idrabiotaparinux, which can be neutralized with intravenous avidin. Ongoing phase III clinical trials are comparing idrabiotaparinux with warfarin for treatment of pulmonary embolism or for stroke prevention in patients with atrial fibrillation. Idraparinux, idrabiotaparinux, and avidin are not available for routine clinical use.

Heparin Resistance. The dose of heparin required to produce a therapeutic aPTT varies due to differences in the concentrations of heparin-binding proteins in plasma that competitively inhibit binding of heparin to antithrombin. Some patients do not achieve a therapeutic aPTT unless very high doses of heparin (>50,000 units/day) are administered. Such patients may have "therapeutic" concentrations of heparin in plasma at the usual dose when measured using an antifactor Xa assay. This "pseudo" heparin resistance occurs because these patients have short aPTT values prior to treatment, as a result of increased concentrations of factor VIII. Other patients may require large doses of heparin because of accelerated clearance of the drug, as may occur with massive pulmonary embolism. Patients with inherited antithrombin deficiency ordinarily have 40-60% of the usual plasma concentration of this inhibitor and respond normally to intravenous heparin. However, acquired antithrombin deficiency, where concentrations may be <25% of normal, may occur in patients with hepatic cirrhosis, nephrotic syndrome, or disseminated intravascular coagulation; large doses of heparin may not prolong the aPTT in these individuals.

Because LMWHs and fondaparinux exhibit reduced binding to plasma proteins other than antithrombin, heparin resistance rarely occurs with these agents. For this reason, routine coagulation monitoring is unnecessary.

TOXICITY AND ADVERSE EVENTS

BLEEDING. Bleeding is the primary untoward effect of heparin. Major bleeding occurs in 1-5% of patients treated with intravenous heparin for venous thromboembolism. The incidence of bleeding is somewhat less in patients treated with LMWH for this indication. Often an underlying cause for bleeding is present, such as recent surgery, trauma, peptic ulcer disease, or platelet dysfunction.

The anticoagulant effect of heparin disappears within hours of discontinuation of the drug. Mild bleeding due to heparin usually can be controlled without the administration of an antagonist. If life-threatening hemorrhage occurs, the effect of heparin can be reversed quickly by the intravenous infusion of *protamine sulfate* (a mixture of basic polypeptides isolated from salmon sperm) that binds tightly to heparin and neutralizes its anticoagulant effect. Protamine also interacts with platelets, fibrinogen, and other plasma proteins and may cause an anticoagulant effect of its own. Therefore, one should give the minimal amount of protamine required to neutralize the heparin present in the plasma. This amount is ~1 mg of protamine for every 100 units of heparin remaining in the patient; protamine (up to a maximum of 50 mg) is given intravenously at a slow rate (over 10 min). Protamine binds only long heparin molecules. Therefore, protamine only partially reverses the anticoagulant activity of LMWHs and has no effect on that of fondaparinux.

Heparin-Induced Thrombocytopenia. Heparin-induced thrombocytopenia (platelet count <150,000/mL or a 50% decrease from the pretreatment value) occurs in ~0.5% of medical patients 5-10 days after initiation of therapy with heparin. Although the incidence may be lower, thrombocytopenia also occurs with LMWHs and fondaparinux, and platelet counts should be monitored. Thrombotic complications that can be life-threatening or lead to amputation occur in about one-half of the affected heparin-treated patients and may precede the onset of thrombocytopenia. Women are twice as likely as men to develop this condition.

Venous thromboembolism occurs most commonly, but arterial thromboses causing limb ischemia, myocardial infarction, and stroke also occur. Bilateral adrenal hemorrhage, skin lesions at the site of subcutaneous heparin injection, and a variety of systemic reactions may accompany heparin-induced thrombocytopenia. The development of IgG antibodies against complexes of heparin with platelet factor 4 (or, rarely, other chemokines) appears to cause all of these reactions.

Heparin, LMWH, and fondaparinux should be discontinued immediately if unexplained thrombocytopenia or any of the clinical manifestations mentioned above occur 5 or more days after beginning therapy, regardless of the dose or route of administration. The diagnosis of heparin-induced thrombocytopenia can be confirmed by a heparin-dependent platelet activation assay or an assay for antibodies that react with heparin/platelet factor IV complexes. Because thrombotic complications may occur after cessation of therapy, an alternative anticoagulant such as lepirudin, argatroban (see the next section), or fondaparinux should be administered to patients with heparin-induced thrombocytopenia. LMWH preparations should be avoided, because these drugs often cross-react with heparin. Warfarin may precipitate venous limb gangrene or multicentric skin necrosis in patients with heparin-induced thrombocytopenia and should not be used.

Other Toxicities. Abnormalities of hepatic function tests occur frequently in patients who are receiving heparin or LMWHs. Osteoporosis resulting in spontaneous vertebral fractures can occur, albeit infrequently, in patients who have received therapeutic doses of heparin (>20,000 units/day) for extended periods (e.g., 3-6 months). Risk of osteoporosis is lower with LMWHs or fondaparinux than it is with heparin. Heparin can inhibit the synthesis of aldosterone by the adrenal glands and occasionally causes hyperkalemia. Allergic reactions to heparin are rare.

OTHER PARENTERAL ANTICOAGULANTS

LEPIRUDIN. Lepirudin (REFLUDAN) is a recombinant derivative of hirudin, a direct thrombin inhibitor present in the salivary glands of the medicinal leech. Lepirudin is a 65–amino acid polypeptide that binds tightly to both the catalytic site and the extended substrate recognition site of thrombin. Lepirudin is approved in the U.S. for treatment of patients with heparin-induced thrombocytopenia.

Lepirudin is administered intravenously at a dose adjusted to maintain the aPTT at 1.5-2.5 times the median of the laboratory's normal range for aPTT. The drug is excreted by the kidneys and has a $t_{1/2}$ of ~1.3 h. Lepirudin should be used cautiously in patients with renal failure. Patients may develop antibodies against hirudin that occasionally prolong the $t_{1/2}$ and cause a paradoxical increase in the aPTT; therefore, daily monitoring of the aPTT is recommended. There is no antidote for lepirudin.

DESIRUDIN. Desirudin (IPRIVASK) is a recombinant derivative of hirudin that differs only by the lack of a sulfate group on Tyr^{63}.

Desirudin is indicated for the prophylaxis of DVT in patients undergoing elective hip replacement surgery. The recommended dose is 15 mg every 12 h by subcutaneous injection. It is eliminated by the kidney; the $t_{1/2}$ is ~2 h following subcutaneous administration. The drug should be used cautiously in patients with decreased renal function, and serum creatinine and aPTT should be monitored daily.

BIVALIRUDIN. Bivalirudin (ANGIOMAX) is a synthetic 20–amino acid polypeptide that directly inhibits thrombin by a mechanism similar to that of lepirudin.

Bivalirudin is administered intravenously and is used as an alternative to heparin in patients undergoing coronary angioplasty or cardiopulmonary bypass surgery. Patients with heparin-induced thrombocytopenia or a history of this disorder also can be given bivalirudin instead of heparin during coronary angioplasty. The $t_{1/2}$ of bivalirudin is 25 min; dosage reductions are recommended for patients with renal impairment.

ARGATROBAN. Argatroban, a synthetic compound based on the structure of l-arginine, binds reversibly to the catalytic site of thrombin.

Argatroban is administered intravenously. Its $t_{1/2}$ is 40-50 min. It is metabolized by hepatic CYPs and is excreted in the bile. Dosage reduction is required for patients with hepatic insufficiency. Argatroban can be used as an alternative to lepirudin for prophylaxis or treatment of patients with, or at risk of developing, heparin-induced thrombocytopenia. In addition to prolonging the aPTT, argatroban also prolongs the PT, which can complicate the transitioning of patients from argatroban to warfarin. A chromogenic factor X assay can be used instead of the PT to monitor warfarin in these patients.

ANTITHROMBIN. Antithrombin (ATRYN) is a recombinant form of human antithrombin produced from the milk of genetically modified goats. It is approved as an anticoagulant for patients with hereditary antithrombin deficiency undergoing surgical procedures.

DROTRECOGIN ALFA. Drotrecogin alfa (XIGRIS) is a recombinant form of human-activated protein C that inhibits coagulation by proteolytic inactivation of factors Va and VIIIa. It also has anti-inflammatory effects. Xigris was withdrawn from the U.S. market in October, 2011, after a major clinical study showed no improvement in 28-day survival in adult patients with sepsis.

ORAL ANTICOAGULANTS

WARFARIN

Investigating a hemorrhagic disorder in cattle resulting from ingestion of spoiled sweet clover silage, Campbell and Link, in 1939, identified the hemorrhagic agent as bishydroxycoumarin (dicoumarol). Subsequently, a more potent synthetic congener was introduced as a rodenticide; the compound was named *warfarin* after the patent holder, Wisconsin Alumni Research Foundation (WARF). These anticoagulants have become mainstays for prevention of thromboembolic disease.

MECHANISM OF ACTION. The oral anticoagulants are antagonists of vitamin K. Coagulation factors II, VII, IX, and X and the anticoagulant proteins C and S are synthesized mainly in the liver and are biologically inactive unless 9-13 of the amino-terminal glutamate residues are carboxylated to form the Ca^{2+}-binding Gla residues. This reaction of the decarboxy precursor protein requires CO_2, O_2, and reduced vitamin K and is catalyzed by γ-glutamyl carboxylase (Figure 30–6). Carboxylation is coupled to the oxidation of vitamin K to its corresponding epoxide. Reduced vitamin K must be regenerated from the epoxide for sustained carboxylation and synthesis of biologically competent proteins. The enzyme that catalyzes this, vitamin K epoxide reductase (VKOR), is inhibited by therapeutic doses of warfarin.

Therapeutic doses of warfarin decrease by 30-50% the total amount of each vitamin K-dependent coagulation factor made by the liver; in addition, the secreted molecules are under-carboxylated, resulting in diminished biological activity (10-40% of normal). Congenital deficiencies of the procoagulant proteins to these levels cause mild bleeding disorders. Vitamin K antagonists have no effect on the activity of fully carboxylated molecules in the circulation. The approximate $t_{1/2}$ (in hours) are as follows: factor VII, 6; factor IX, 24; factor X, 36; factor II, 50; protein C, 8; and protein S, 30. Because of the long $t_{1/2}$ of some of the coagulation factors, in particular factor II, the full antithrombotic effect of warfarin is not achieved for several days, even though the PT may be prolonged soon after administration due to the more rapid reduction of factors with a shorter $t_{1/2}$, in particular factor VII.

DOSAGE. The usual adult dosage of warfarin is 2-5 mg/day for 2-4 days, followed by 1-10 mg/day as indicated by measurements of the international normalized ratio (INR), a value derived from the patient's PT (see the functional definition of INR in the section on "Laboratory Monitoring"). As presented later, common genetic polymorphisms render patients more or less sensitive to warfarin. A lower initial dose should be given to patients with an increased risk of bleeding, including the elderly. Warfarin usually is administered orally. Warfarin also can be given intravenously without modification of the dose. Intramuscular injection is not recommended.

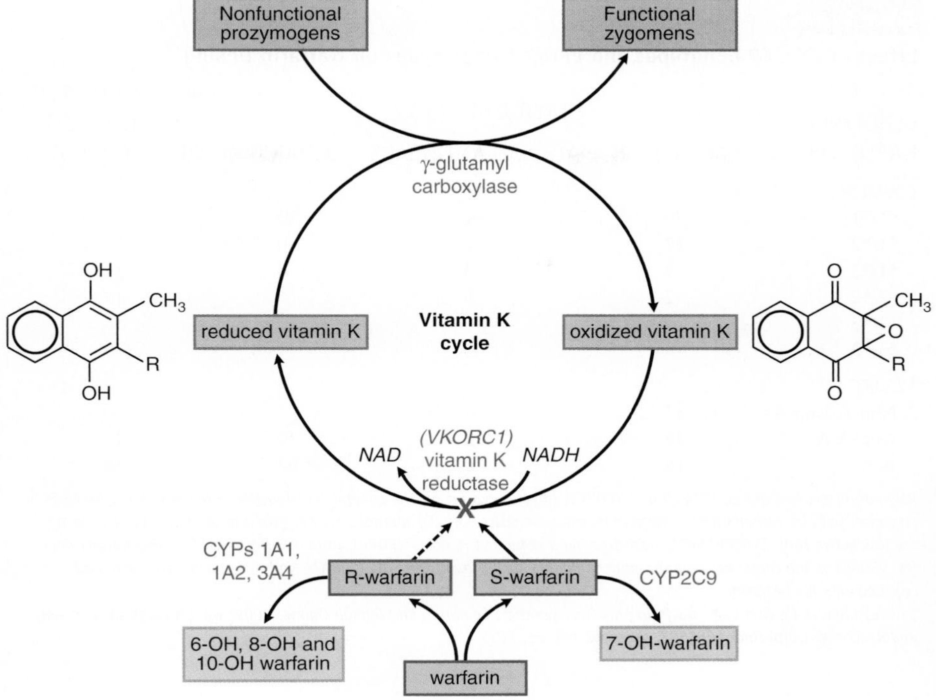

Figure 30–6 *The vitamin K cycle and mechanism of action of warfarin.* In the racemic mixture of S- and R-enantiomers, S-warfarin is more active. By blocking vitamin K epoxide reductase encoded by the *VKORC1* gene, warfarin inhibits the conversion of oxidized vitamin K epoxide into its reduced form, vitamin K hydroquinone. This inhibits vitamin K-dependent γ-carboxylation of factors II, VII, IX, and X because reduced vitamin K serves as a cofactor for a γ-glutamyl carboxylase that catalyzes the γ-carboxylation process whereby prozymogens are converted to zymogens capable of binding Ca^{2+} and interacting with anionic phospholipids. S-warfarin is metabolized by *CYP2C9;* common genetic polymorphisms in this enzyme increase warfarin metabolism. Polymorphisms in the C1 subunit of vitamin K reductase (VKORC1) increase the susceptibility of the enzyme to warfarin-induced inhibition. Thus, patients expressing polymorphisms in these 2 enzymes require reduction of warfarin dosage (*see* Table 30–2).

ADME. The bioavailability of warfarin is nearly complete when the drug is administered orally, intravenously, or rectally. Different commercial preparations of warfarin tablets vary in their rate of dissolution, and this causes some variation in the rate and extent of absorption. Food in the GI tract also can decrease the rate of absorption. Plasma concentrations peak in 2-8 h. Warfarin is administered as a racemic mixture of S- and R-warfarin. S-warfarin is 3- to 5-fold more potent than R-warfarin and is metabolized principally by CYP2C9. Inactive metabolites of warfarin are excreted in urine and stool. The $t_{1/2}$ varies (25-60 h); the duration of action of warfarin is 2-5 days.

Table 30–2 summarizes the effects of known genetic factors on warfarin dose requirements. Polymorphisms in 2 genes, *CYP2C9* and *VKORC1* (vitamin K epoxide reductase complex, subunit 1) account for most of the genetic contribution to variability in warfarin response. *CYP2C9* variants affect warfarin pharmacokinetics, whereas *VKORC1* variants affect warfarin pharmacodynamics. Common variations in the *CYP2C9* gene (designated *CYP2C9*2* and **3*), encode an enzyme with decreased activity, and thus are associated with higher drug concentrations and reduced warfarin dose requirements. *VKORC1* is the target of coumarin anticoagulants such as warfarin (*see* Figure 30–6). *VKORC1* variants are more prevalent than those of *CYP2C9*. The prevalence of *VKORC1* genetic variants is higher in Asians, followed by European Americans and African Americans. The warfarin dose requirement is decreased in these variants. Based on evidence that genetic variations affect warfarin dose requirements and responses to therapy, the FDA amended the prescribing information for warfarin to indicate that lower warfarin initiation doses be considered for patients with *CYP2C9* and *VKORC1* genetic variations. Efforts to facilitate the rational incorporation of genetic information into patient care include the development of a warfarin-dosing algorithm and point-of-care methods for *CYP2C9* and *VKORC1* genotyping.

Table 30–2

Effect of *CYP2C9* Genotypes and *VKORC1* Haplotypes on Warfarin Dosing

GENOTYPE/ HAPLOTYPE	FREQUENCY (%) CAUCASIANS	AFRICAN AMERICANS	ASIANS	DOSE REDUCTION COMPARED WITH WILD-TYPE (%)
CYP2C9				
*1/*1	70	90	95	—
*1/*2	17	2	0	22
*1/*3	9	3	4	34
*2/*2	2	0	0	43
*2/*3	1	0	0	53
*3/*3	0	0	1	76
VKORC1				
Non-A/Non-A	37	82	7	—
Non-A/A	45	12	30	26
A/A	18	6	63	50

Polymorphisms in 2 genes, CYP2C9 *and* VKORC1, *largely account for the genetic contribution to the variability in warfarin response.* CYP2C9 *variants affect warfarin pharmacokinetics.* CYP2C9 *metabolizes warfarin and the non-*1/*1 variants are less active than* CYP2C9*1/*1, *necessitating a reduction in dose.* VKORC1 *variants affect warfarin pharmacodynamics. VKORC1 is the target of coumarin anticoagulants such as warfarin. The non-A/A and A/A forms have decreased requirements for warfarin.*

Source: Ghimire LV, Stein CM. Warfarin pharmacogenetics, Goodman and Gilman Online, 2009; www.AccessMedicine.com/updatesContent.aspx?aid=1001507, accessed July 26, 2013.

DRUG AND OTHER INTERACTIONS WITH ORAL ANTICOAGULANTS. Any substance or condition is potentially dangerous if it alters:

- The uptake or metabolism of the oral anticoagulant or vitamin K
- The synthesis, function, or clearance of any factor or cell involved in hemostasis or fibrinolysis
- The integrity of any epithelial surface

Patients must be educated to report the addition or deletion of any medication, including nonprescription drugs and food supplements. Some of the more commonly described factors that cause a decreased effect of oral anticoagulants include:

- Reduced absorption of drug caused by binding to cholestyramine in the GI tract
- Increased volume of distribution and a short $t_{1/2}$ secondary to hypoproteinemia, as in nephrotic syndrome
- Increased metabolic clearance of drug secondary to induction of hepatic enzymes, especially *CYP2C9*, by barbiturates, carbamazepine, or rifampin
- Ingestion of large amounts of vitamin K-rich foods or supplements
- Increased levels of coagulation factors during pregnancy

The PT can be shortened in any of these cases.

Frequently cited interactions that enhance the risk of hemorrhage in patients taking oral anticoagulants include decreased metabolism due to *CYP2C9* inhibition by amiodarone, azole antifungals, cimetidine, clopidogrel, cotrimoxazole, disulfiram, fluoxetine, isoniazid, metronidazole, sulfinpyrazone, tolcapone, or zafirlukast, and displacement from protein-binding sites caused by loop diuretics or valproate. Relative deficiency of vitamin K may result from inadequate diet (e.g., postoperative patients on parenteral fluids), especially when coupled with the elimination of intestinal flora by antimicrobial agents. Gut bacteria synthesize vitamin K and are an important source of this vitamin. Consequently, antibiotics can cause excessive PT prolongation in patients adequately controlled on warfarin. Low concentrations of coagulation factors may result from impaired hepatic function, congestive heart failure, or hypermetabolic states, such as hyperthyroidism; generally, these conditions increase the prolongation of the PT. Serious interactions that do not alter the PT include inhibition of platelet function by agents such as *aspirin* and gastritis or frank ulceration induced by anti-inflammatory drugs. Agents may have more than 1 effect; e.g., clofibrate increases the rate of turnover of coagulation factors and inhibits platelet function.

SENSITIVITY TO WARFARIN. ~10% of patients require <1.5 mg/day of warfarin to achieve an INR of 2-3. These patients often possess variant alleles of *CYP2C9* or variant *VKORC1* haplotypes, which affect the pharmacokinetics or pharmacodynamics of warfarin, respectively.

TOXICITIES

BLEEDING. Bleeding is the major toxicity of warfarin. The risk of bleeding increases with the intensity and duration of anticoagulant therapy, the use of other medications that interfere with hemostasis, and the presence of a potential anatomical source of bleeding. The incidence of major bleeding episodes is generally <3% per year in patients treated with a target INR of 2-3. The risk of intracranial hemorrhage increases dramatically with an INR >4.

If the INR is above the therapeutic range but <5 and the patient is not bleeding or in need of a surgical procedure, warfarin can be discontinued temporarily and restarted at a lower dose once the INR is within the therapeutic range. If the INR is ≥5, vitamin K_1 (phytonadione, MEPHYTON, AQUAMEPHYTON) can be given orally at a dose of 1-2.5 mg (for 5≤ INR ≤9) or 3-5 mg (for INR >9). These doses of oral vitamin K_1 generally cause the INR to fall substantially within 24-48 h without rendering the patient resistant to further warfarin therapy. Higher doses or parenteral administration may be required if more rapid correction of the INR is necessary. The effect of vitamin K_1 is delayed for at least several hours because reversal of anticoagulation requires synthesis of fully carboxylated coagulation factors. If immediate hemostatic competence is necessary because of serious bleeding or profound warfarin overdosage (INR >20), adequate concentrations of vitamin K-dependent coagulation factors can be restored by transfusion of fresh frozen plasma (10-20 mL/kg), supplemented with 10 mg of vitamin K_1, given by slow intravenous infusion. Transfusion of plasma may need to be repeated because the transfused factors (particularly factor VII) are cleared from the circulation more rapidly than the residual oral anticoagulant. Vitamin K_1 administered intravenously carries the risk of anaphylactoid reactions and therefore should be used cautiously. Patients who receive high doses of vitamin K_1 may become unresponsive to warfarin for several days, but heparin can be used if continued anticoagulation is required.

Birth Defects. Administration of warfarin during pregnancy causes birth defects and abortion. CNS abnormalities have been reported following exposure during the second and third trimesters. Fetal or neonatal hemorrhage and intrauterine death may occur, even when maternal PT values are in the therapeutic range. Vitamin K antagonists should not be used during pregnancy, but heparin, LMWH, or fondaparinux can be used safely in this circumstance.

Skin Necrosis. Warfarin-induced skin necrosis is a rare complication characterized by the appearance of skin lesions 3-10 days after treatment is initiated. The lesions typically are on the extremities, but adipose tissue, the penis, and the female breast also may be involved.

Other Toxicities. A reversible, sometimes painful, blue-tinged discoloration of the plantar surfaces and sides of the toes that blanches with pressure and fades with elevation of the legs (purple toe syndrome) may develop 3-8 weeks after initiation of therapy with warfarin; cholesterol emboli released from atheromatous plaques have been implicated as the cause. Other infrequent reactions include alopecia, urticaria, dermatitis, fever, nausea, diarrhea, abdominal cramps, and anorexia.

CLINICAL USE. Vitamin K antagonists are used to prevent the progression or recurrence of acute DVT or pulmonary embolism following an initial course of heparin. They also are effective in preventing venous thromboembolism in patients undergoing orthopedic or gynecological surgery, recurrent coronary ischemia in patients with acute myocardial infarction, and systemic embolization in patients with prosthetic heart valves or chronic atrial fibrillation.

Prior to initiation of therapy, laboratory tests are used in conjunction with the history and physical examination to uncover hemostatic defects that might make the use of vitamin K antagonists more dangerous (e.g., congenital coagulation factor deficiency, thrombocytopenia, hepatic or renal insufficiency, vascular abnormalities). Thereafter, the INR calculated from the patient's PT is used to monitor the extent of anticoagulation and compliance. Therapeutic INR ranges for various clinical indications have been established empirically and reflect dosages that reduce the morbidity from thromboembolic disease while minimally increasing the risk of serious hemorrhage. For most indications, the target INR is 2-3. A higher target INR (e.g., 2.5-3.5) generally is recommended for patients with high-risk mechanical prosthetic heart valves.

For treatment of acute venous thromboembolism, heparin, LMWH, or fondaparinux usually is continued for at least 5 days after warfarin therapy is begun and until the INR is in the therapeutic range on 2 consecutive days. This overlap allows for adequate depletion of the vitamin K-dependent coagulation factors with long $t_{1/2}$, especially factor II. Frequent INR measurements are indicated at the onset of therapy to guard against excessive anticoagulation in the unusually sensitive patient.

PHENPROCOUMON AND ACENOCOUMAROL. These agents generally are not available in the U.S. but are prescribed in the E.U. and elsewhere. Phenprocoumon (MARCUMAR) has a longer plasma $t_{1/2}$ (5 days) than warfarin, as well as a somewhat slower onset of action and a longer duration of action (7-14 days). It is administered in daily maintenance doses of 0.75-6 mg. Acenocoumarol (SINTHROME) has a shorter $t_{1/2}$ (10-24 h), a more rapid effect on the PT, and a shorter duration of action (2 days). The maintenance dose is 1-8 mg daily.

INDANDIONE DERIVATIVES. Anisindione (MIRADON) is available for clinical use in some countries. It is similar to warfarin in its kinetics of action but offers no clear advantages and may have a higher frequency of untoward effects. Phenindione (DINDEVAN) still is available in some countries. Serious hypersensitivity reactions, occasionally fatal, can occur within a few weeks of starting therapy with this drug.

RODENTICIDES. Bromadoline, brodifacoum, diphenadione, chlorophacinone, and pindone are long-acting agents (prolongation of the PT may persist for weeks). They are of interest because they sometimes are agents of accidental or intentional poisoning. In this setting, reversal of the coagulopathy can require very large doses of vitamin K (i.e., >100 mg/day) for weeks or months.

NEW ORAL ANTICOAGULANTS

DABIGATRAN ETEXILATE (PRADAXA, PRADAX). Dabigatran etexilate is a prodrug that is rapidly converted to dabigatran, which reversibly blocks the active site of thrombin.

The drug has oral bioavailability of ~6%, a peak onset of action in 2 h, and a plasma $t_{1/2}$ of 12-14 h. When given in fixed doses, dabigatran etexilate produces such a predictable anticoagulant response that routine coagulation monitoring is unnecessary. Dabigatran etexilate is approved for stroke prevention in patients with atrial fibrillation.

RIVAROXABAN (XARELTO). Rivaroxaban is an oral factor Xa inhibitor.

It has 80% oral bioavailability, a peak onset of action in 3 h, and a plasma $t_{1/2}$ of 7-11 h. About one-third of the drug is excreted unchanged in the urine, the remainder is metabolized by the liver, and inactive metabolites are excreted in the urine or feces. This drug is given in fixed doses and does not require coagulation monitoring. Rivaroxaban is approved for prophylaxis of venous thromboembolism in patients undergoing hip or knee replacement surgery and for stroke prevention in patients with non-valvular atrial fibrillation.

APIXABAN (ELIQUIS). Apixaban is an oral factor Xa inhibitor.

Apixaban is indicated for the prevention of stroke and embolism in patients with nonvalvular fibrillation. The recommended oral dose is 5 mg taken twice daily, and half that in patients ≥80 years old, ≤60 kg, or whose serum creatinine ≥1.5mg/dL. Apixaban has 50% oral bioavailability, peak onset 3-4 h, and an apparent $t_{1/2}$ of 12 h due to prolonged absorption from the GI tract. The drug is metabolized mainly by *CYP3A4* and is a substrate for P-gp. Thus, coadministration with other inhibitors/substrates of these enzymes (e.g., ketoconazole, itraconazole, ritonavir, clarithromycin) requires halving the dose rate for apixaban.

FIBRINOLYTIC DRUGS

The fibrinolytic pathway is summarized by Figure 30–3. The action of fibrinolytic agents is best understood in conjunction with an understanding of the characteristics of its components.

PLASMINOGEN. Plasminogen is a single-chain glycoprotein that is converted to the active protease plasmin by proteolytic cleavage.

Plasminogen's 5 kringle domains mediate the binding of plasminogen (or plasmin) to carboxyl-terminal lysine residues in partially degraded fibrin; this enhances fibrinolysis. A plasma carboxypeptidase termed *thrombin-activatable fibrinolysis inhibitor* (TAFI) can remove these lysine residues and thereby attenuate fibrinolysis. The lysine-binding kringle domains of plasminogen also promote formation of complexes of plasmin with α_2-antiplasmin, the major physiological plasmin inhibitor. A degraded form of plasminogen termed *lys-plasminogen* binds to fibrin with higher affinity than intact plasminogen.

α_2-ANTIPLASMIN. α_2-Antiplasmin, a glycoprotein, forms a stable complex with plasmin, thereby inactivating it.

Plasma concentrations of α_2-antiplasmin (1 μM) are sufficient to inhibit about 50% of potential plasmin. When massive activation of plasminogen occurs, the inhibitor is depleted, and free plasmin causes a "systemic lytic state" in which hemostasis is impaired. In this state, fibrinogen is degraded and fibrinogen degradation products impair fibrin polymerization and therefore increase bleeding from wounds. α_2-Antiplasmin inactivates plasmin nearly instantaneously, as long as the first kringle domain on plasmin is unoccupied by fibrin or other antagonists, such as *aminocaproic acid* (see "Inhibitors of Fibrinolysis" section).

TISSUE PLASMINOGEN ACTIVATOR. t-PA is a serine protease and a poor plasminogen activator in the absence of fibrin. t-PA binds to fibrin and activates fibrin-bound plasminogen several hundred-fold more rapidly than it activates plasminogen in the circulation.

Because it has little activity except in the presence of fibrin, physiological t-PA concentrations of 5-10 ng/mL do not induce systemic plasmin generation. During therapeutic infusions of t-PA, however, when concentrations rise to 300-3000 ng/mL, a systemic lytic state can occur. Clearance of t-PA primarily occurs by hepatic metabolism, and its $t_{1/2}$ is ~5 min. t-PA is effective in lysing thrombi during treatment of acute myocardial infarction or acute ischemic stroke.

t-PA (alteplase, ACTIVASE) is produced by recombinant DNA technology. The currently recommended ("accelerated") regimen for coronary thrombolysis is a 15-mg intravenous bolus, followed by 0.75 mg/kg of body weight over 30 min (not to exceed 50 mg) and 0.5 mg/kg (up to 35 mg accumulated dose) over the following hour. Recombinant variants of t-PA now are available (reteplase, RETAVASE and tenecteplase, TNKASE). They differ from native t-PA by having longer plasma half-lives that allow convenient bolus dosing. They also are relatively resistant to inhibition by PAI-1. Despite these apparent advantages, these agents are similar to t-PA in efficacy and toxicity.

STREPTOKINASE. Streptokinase (STREPTASE) is a 47,000-Da protein produced by β-hemolytic streptococci.

It has no intrinsic enzymatic activity but forms a stable, noncovalent 1:1 complex with plasminogen. This produces a conformational change that exposes the active site on plasminogen and facilitates the formation of plasmin. Streptokinase is rarely used clinically for fibrinolysis.

HEMORRHAGIC TOXICITY OF THROMBOLYTIC THERAPY. The major toxicity of all thrombolytic agents is hemorrhage, which results from 2 factors:

1. The lysis of fibrin in hemostatic plugs at sites of vascular injury
2. The systemic lytic state that results from systemic plasmin generation, which produces fibrinogenolysis and degradation of other coagulation factors (especially factors V and VIII)

The contraindications to fibrinolytic therapy are listed in Table 30–3. Patients with these conditions should not receive such treatment.

Table 30–3

Absolute and Relative Contraindications to Fibrinolytic Therapy

Absolute Contraindications

- Prior intracranial hemorrhage
- Known structural cerebral vascular lesion
- Known malignant intracranial neoplasm
- Ischemic stroke within 3 months
- Suspected aortic dissection
- Active bleeding or bleeding diathesis (excluding menses)
- Significant closed-head trauma or facial trauma within 3 months

Relative Contraindications

- Uncontrolled hypertension (systolic blood pressure >180 mm Hg or diastolic blood pressure >110 mm Hg)
- Traumatic or prolonged CPR or major surgery within 3 weeks
- Recent (within 2-4 weeks) internal bleeding
- Noncompressible vascular punctures
- For streptokinase: prior exposure (more than 5 days ago) or prior allergic reaction to streptokinase
- Pregnancy
- Active peptic ulcer
- Current use of warfarin and INR >1.7

CPR, cardiopulmonary resuscitation; INR, international normalized ratio.

If heparin is used concurrently with t-PA, serious hemorrhage will occur in 2-4% of patients. Intracranial hemorrhage is by far the most serious problem. Hemorrhagic stroke occurs with all regimens and is more common when heparin is used. The efficacies of t-PA and streptokinase in treating myocardial infarction are essentially identical. Both agents reduce death and reinfarction by ~30% in regimens containing aspirin.

INHIBITORS OF FIBRINOLYSIS

AMINOCAPROIC ACID. Aminocaproic acid (AMICAR) is a lysine analog that competes for lysine binding sites on plasminogen and plasmin, blocking the interaction of plasmin with fibrin. Aminocaproic acid is thereby a potent inhibitor of fibrinolysis and can reverse states that are associated with excessive fibrinolysis.

The main problem with its use is that thrombi that form during treatment with the drug are not lysed. For example, in patients with hematuria, ureteral obstruction by clots may lead to renal failure after treatment with aminocaproic acid. Aminocaproic acid has been used to reduce bleeding after prostatic surgery or after tooth extractions in hemophiliacs. Aminocaproic acid is absorbed rapidly after oral administration, and 50% is excreted unchanged in the urine within 12 h. For intravenous use, a loading dose of 4-5 g is given over 1 h, followed by an infusion of 1-1.25 g/h until bleeding is controlled. No more than 30 g should be given in a 24-h period. Rarely, the drug causes myopathy and muscle necrosis.

TRANEXAMIC ACID. Tranexamic acid (CYKLOKAPRON, LYSTEDA) is a lysine analog that competes for lysine binding sites on plasminogen and plasmin, thus blocking their interaction with fibrin.

Tranexamic acid is used for the same indications as aminocaproic acid and given intravenously or orally. Tranexamic acid is excreted in the urine; dose reductions are necessary in patients with renal impairment. Oral tranexamic acid is approved for treatment of heavy menstrual bleeding, usually given at a dose of 1 g 4 times a day for 4 days.

ANTIPLATELET DRUGS

Platelets provide the initial hemostatic plug at sites of vascular injury. They also participate in pathological thromboses that lead to myocardial infarction, stroke, and peripheral vascular thromboses. Potent inhibitors of platelet function have been developed in recent years. These drugs act by discrete mechanisms (Figure 30–7); thus, in combination, their effects are additive or even synergistic.

ASPIRIN. In platelets, the major cyclooxygenase product is TxA_2, a labile inducer of platelet aggregation and a potent vasoconstrictor. Aspirin blocks production of TxA_2 by acetylating a serine residue near the active site of platelet cyclooxygenase-1 (COX-1). Because platelets do not synthesize new proteins, the action of aspirin on platelet COX-1 is permanent, lasting for the life of the platelet (7-10 days). Thus, repeated doses of aspirin produce a cumulative effect on platelet function.

Complete inactivation of platelet COX-1 is achieved with a daily aspirin dose of 75 mg. Therefore, aspirin is maximally effective as an antithrombotic agent at doses much lower than those required for other actions of the drug. Numerous trials indicate that aspirin, when used as an antithrombotic drug, is maximally effective at doses of 50-320 mg/day. Higher doses do not improve efficacy and potentially are less efficacious because of inhibition of prostacyclin production, which can be largely spared by using lower doses of aspirin. Higher doses also increase toxicity, especially bleeding. Other NSAIDs that are reversible inhibitors of COX-1 have not been shown to have antithrombotic efficacy and in fact may even interfere with low-dose aspirin regimens (*see* Chapters 33 and 34).

DIPYRIDAMOLE. Dipyridamole (PERSANTINE) interferes with platelet function by increasing the cellular concentration of cyclic AMP.

This effect is mediated by inhibition of cyclic nucleotide phosphodiesterases and/or by blockade of uptake of adenosine, thereby increasing the dwell time of adenosine at cell surface adenosine A_2 receptors that link to the stimulation of platelet adenylyl cyclase. Dipyridamole is a vasodilator that, in combination with warfarin, inhibits embolization from prosthetic heart valves.

TICLOPIDINE (TICLID, OTHERS). Ticlopidine is a thienopyridine prodrug that inhibits the $P2Y_{12}$ receptor.

Platelets contain 2 purinergic receptors, $P2Y_1$ and $P2Y_{12}$; both are GPCRs for ADP. The ADP-activated platelet $P2Y_1$ receptor couples to the G_q–PLC–IP_3–Ca^{2+} pathway and induces a shape change and aggregation. The $P2Y_{12}$ receptor couples to G_i and, when activated by ADP, inhibits adenylyl cyclase, resulting in lower levels

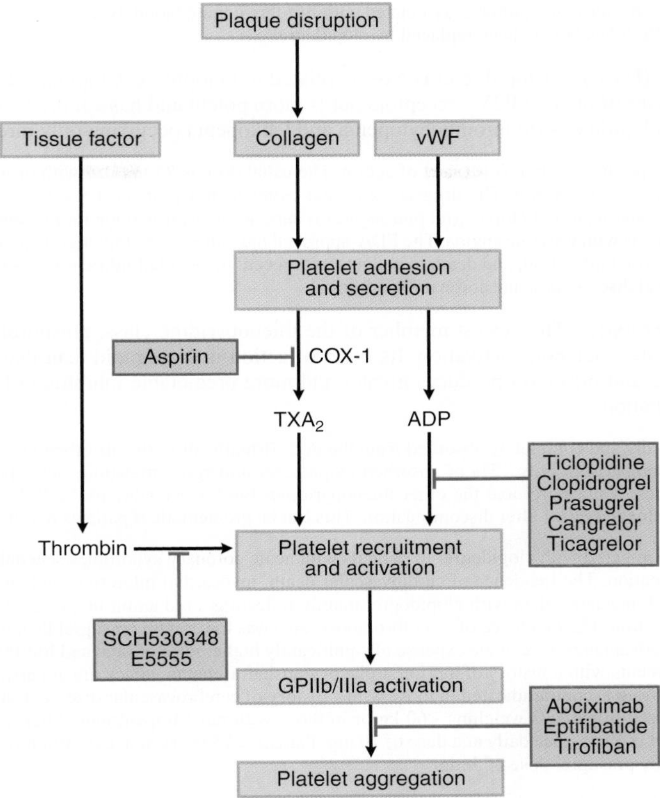

Figure 30–7 *Sites of action of antiplatelet drugs.* Aspirin inhibits thromboxane A_2 (TxA_2) synthesis by irreversibly acetylating cyclooxygenase-1 (COX-1). Reduced TxA_2 release attenuates platelet activation and recruitment to the site of vascular injury. Ticlopidine, clopidogrel, and prasugrel irreversibly block $P2Y_{12}$, a key ADP receptor on the platelet surface; cangrelor and ticagrelor are reversible inhibitors of $P2Y_{12}$. Abciximab, eptifibatide, and tirofiban inhibit the final common pathway of platelet aggregation by blocking fibrinogen and von Willebrand factor (vWF) from binding to activated glycoprotein (GP) IIb/IIIa. SCH530348 and E5555 inhibit thrombin-mediated platelet activation by targeting protease-activated receptor-1 (PAR-1), the major thrombin receptor on platelets.

of cyclic AMP and thereby less cyclic AMP–dependent inhibition of platelet activation. Both receptors must be stimulated to result in platelet activation.

Ticlopidine is converted to the active thiol metabolite by a hepatic CYP. It is rapidly absorbed and highly bioavailable. It permanently inhibits the $P2Y_{12}$ receptor by forming a disulfide bridge between the thiol on the drug and a free cysteine residue in the extracellular region of the receptor; thus the effect is prolonged effect, even though the free drug has a short $t_{1/2}$. Maximal inhibition of platelet aggregation is not seen until 8-11 days after starting therapy. The usual dose is 250 mg twice daily. Loading doses of 500 mg sometimes are given to achieve a more rapid onset of action. Inhibition of platelet aggregation persists for a few days after the drug is stopped.

Adverse Effects. The most common side effects are nausea, vomiting, and diarrhea. The most serious is severe neutropenia (absolute neutrophil count <500/μL), which occurred in 2.4% of stroke patients given the drug during premarketing clinical trials. Fatal agranulocytosis with thrombopenia has occurred within the first 3 months of therapy; therefore, frequent blood counts should be obtained during the first few months of therapy, with immediate discontinuation of therapy should cell counts decline. Platelet counts also should be monitored, as thrombocytopenia has been reported. Rare cases of thrombotic thrombocytopenic purpura hemolytic uremic syndrome (TTP-HUS) have been associated with ticlopidine, with high incidence (1 in 1600-4800 patients) when the drug is used after cardiac stenting and high mortality among those affected. Remission of TTP-HUS has been reported when the drug is stopped.

Therapeutic Uses. Because ticlopidine is associated with life-threatening blood dyscrasias and a relatively high rate of TTP-HUS, it has largely been replaced by clopidogrel.

CLOPIDOGREL (PLAVIX). Clopidogrel is closely related to ticlopidine. Clopidogrel also is an irreversible inhibitor of platelet $P2Y_{12}$ receptors but is more potent and has a more favorable toxicity profile than ticlopidine, with thrombocytopenia and leukopenia occurring only rarely.

Clopidogrel is a prodrug with a slow onset of action. The usual dose is 75 mg/day with or without an initial loading dose of 300 or 600 mg. The drug is somewhat better than aspirin in the secondary prevention of stroke, and the combination of clopidogrel plus aspirin is superior to aspirin alone for prevention of recurrent ischemia in patients with unstable angina. The FDA-approved indications for clopidogrel are to reduce the rate of stroke, myocardial infarction, and death in patients with recent myocardial infarction or stroke, established peripheral arterial disease, or acute coronary syndrome.

PRASUGREL (EFFIENT). The newest member of the thienopyridine class, prasugrel also is a prodrug that requires metabolic activation. Its onset of action is more rapid than that of ticlopidine or clopidogrel, and prasugrel produces greater and more predictable inhibition of ADP-induced platelet aggregation.

Prasugrel is rapidly and completely absorbed from the gut. Virtually all of the absorbed prasugrel undergoes activation; by comparison, only 15% of absorbed clopidogrel undergoes metabolic activation. Because the active metabolites of prasugrel and the other thienopyridines bind irreversibly to the $P2Y_{12}$ receptor, these drugs have a prolonged effect after discontinuation. This can be problematic if patients require urgent surgery.

Prasugrel was compared with clopidogrel in patients with acute coronary syndromes scheduled to undergo a coronary intervention. The incidence of cardiovascular death, myocardial infarction, and stroke was significantly lower with prasugrel than with clopidogrel mainly reflecting a reduction in the incidence of nonfatal myocardial infarction. The incidence of stent thrombosis also was lower with prasugrel than with clopidogrel. However, these advantages were at the expense of significantly higher rates of fatal and life-threatening bleeding. Because patients with a history of a prior stroke or transient ischemic attack are at particularly high risk of bleeding, the drug is contraindicated in those with a history of cerebrovascular disease. Caution is required if prasugrel is used in patients weighing <60 kg or in those with renal impairment. After a loading dose of 60 mg, prasugrel is given once daily at a dose of 10 mg. Patients >75 years of age or weighing <60 kg may do better with a daily prasugrel dose of 5 mg.

GLYCOPROTEIN IIB/IIIA INHIBITORS. Glycoprotein IIb/IIIa is a platelet-surface integrin, designated $\alpha_{IIb}\beta_3$ by the integrin nomenclature. This dimeric glycoprotein undergoes a conformational transformation when platelets are activated to serve as a receptor for fibrinogen and von Willebrand factor, which anchor platelets to foreign surfaces and to each other, thereby mediating aggregation. Thus, inhibitors of this receptor are potent antiplatelet agents that act by a mechanism distinct from that of aspirin or the thienopyridine platelet inhibitors. Three agents are approved for use at present; their features are highlighted in Table 30–4.

ABCIXIMAB. Abciximab (REOPRO) is the Fab fragment of a humanized monoclonal antibody directed against the $\alpha_{IIb}\beta_3$ receptor. It also binds to the vitronectin receptor on platelets, vascular endothelial cells, and smooth muscle cells.

Table 30–4

Features of GPIIb/IIIa Antagonists

FEATURE	ABCIXIMAB	EPTIFIBATIDE	TIROFIBAN
Description	Fab fragment of humanized mouse monoclonal antibody	Cyclical KGD-containing heptapeptide	Nonpeptidic RGD-mimetic
Specific for GPIIb/IIIa	No	Yes	Yes
Plasma $t_{1/2}$	Short (min)	Long (2.5 h)	Long (2.0 h)
Platelet-bound $t_{1/2}$	Long (days)	Short (sec)	Short (sec)
Renal clearance	No	Yes	Yes

KGD, Lysine - Glycine - Aspartate; RGD, Arginine - Glycine - Aspartate.

The antibody is administered to patients undergoing percutaneous angioplasty for coronary thromboses, and when used in conjunction with aspirin and heparin, has been shown to prevent restenosis, recurrent myocardial infarction, and death. The $t_{1/2}$ of the unbound antibody is ~30 min, but antibody remains bound to the $\alpha_{IIb}\beta_3$ receptor and inhibits platelet aggregation as measured in vitro for 18-24 h after infusion. It is given as a 0.25 to mg/kg bolus followed by 0.125 μg/kg/min for 12 h or longer.

Adverse Effects. The major side effect of abciximab is bleeding, and the contraindications to its use are similar to those for the fibrinolytic agents listed in Table 30–3. The frequency of major hemorrhage in clinical trials varies from 1-10%, depending on the intensity of anticoagulation with heparin. Thrombocytopenia with a platelet count <50,000 occurs in about 2% of patients and may be due to development of neo-epitopes induced by bound antibody. Since the duration of action is long, if major bleeding or emergent surgery occurs, platelet transfusions can reverse the aggregation defect because free antibody concentrations fall rapidly after cessation of infusion. Readministration of antibody has been performed in a small number of patients without evidence of decreased efficacy or allergic reactions. The expense of the antibody limits its use.

EPTIFIBATIDE. Eptifibatide (INTEGRILIN) is a cyclic peptide inhibitor of the fibrinogen binding site on $\alpha_{IIb}\beta_3$. It is administered intravenously and blocks platelet aggregation.

Eptifibatide is given as a bolus of 180 μg/kg followed by 2 μg/kg/min for up to 96 h. It is used to treat acute coronary syndrome and for angioplastic coronary interventions (myocardial infarction and death have been reduced by ~20%). The benefit of the drug is somewhat less than that obtained with abciximab, perhaps because eptifibatide is specific for $\alpha_{IIb}\beta_3$ and does not react with the vitronectin receptor. Platelet aggregation is restored within 6-12 h after cessation of infusion. Eptifibatide generally is administered in conjunction with aspirin and heparin.

Adverse Effects. The major side effect is bleeding, as is the case with abciximab. The frequency of major bleeding in trials was about 10%, compared with ~9% in a placebo group, which included heparin. Thrombocytopenia has been seen in 0.5-1% of patients.

TIROFIBAN. *Tirofiban* (AGGRASTAT) is a nonpeptide, small-molecule inhibitor of $\alpha_{IIb}\beta_3$ that appears to have a mechanism of action similar to eptifibatide.

Tirofiban has a short duration of action and has efficacy in non-Q-wave myocardial infarction and unstable angina. Reductions in death and myocardial infarction have been ~20% compared to placebo. Side effects also are similar to those of eptifibatide. The agent is specific to $\alpha_{IIb}\beta_3$ and does not react with the vitronectin receptor. Meta-analysis of trials using $\alpha_{IIb}\beta_3$ inhibitors suggests that their value in antiplatelet therapy after acute myocardial infarction is limited. Tirofiban is administered intravenously at an initial rate of 0.4 μg/kg/min for 30 min, and then continued at 0.1 μg/kg/min for 12-24 h after angioplasty or atherectomy. It is used in conjunction with heparin.

NEWER ANTIPLATELET AGENTS

TICAGRELOR (BRILINTA). Ticagrelor is an orally active, reversible inhibitor of $P2Y_{12}$. The drug is given twice daily and not only has a more rapid onset and offset of action than clopidogrel, but also produces greater and more predictable inhibition of ADP-induced platelet aggregation. Ticagrelor is FDA approved for the prevention of thrombotic events. It is the first new antiplatelet drug to demonstrate a reduction in cardiovascular death compared with clopidogrel in patients with acute coronary syndromes.

Other new agents in advanced stages of development include cangrelor, reversible $P2Y_{12}$ antagonist, and SCH530348 and E5555, orally effective inhibitors of the protease-activated receptor-1 (PAR-1), the major thrombin receptor on platelets.

THE ROLE OF VITAMIN K

Green plants are a nutritional source of vitamin K for humans, in whom vitamin K is an essential cofactor in the γ-carboxylation of multiple glutamate residues of several clotting factors and anticoagulant proteins. The vitamin K-dependent formation of Gla residues permits the appropriate interactions of clotting factors, Ca^{2+}, and membrane phospholipids and modulator proteins (*see* Figures 30–1, 30–2, and 30–3). Vitamin K antagonists (coumarin derivatives) block Gla (γ-carboxyglutamate) formation and thereby inhibit clotting; excess vitamin K_1 can reverse the effects.

Vitamin K activity is associated with at least 2 distinct natural substances, designated as vitamin K_1 and vitamin K_2. Vitamin K_1, or *phytonadione* (also referred to as *phylloquinone*), is 2-methyl-3-phytyl-1, 4-naphthoquinone; it is found in plants and is the only natural vitamin K available for therapeutic use. Vitamin K_2 actually is a series of compounds (the *menaquinones*) in which the phytyl side chain of phytonadione has been replaced by a side chain built up of 2-13 prenyl units. Considerable synthesis of menaquinones occurs in gram-positive bacteria; indeed, intestinal flora synthesize the large amounts of vitamin K contained in human and animal feces. Menadione is at least as active on a molar basis as phytonadione.

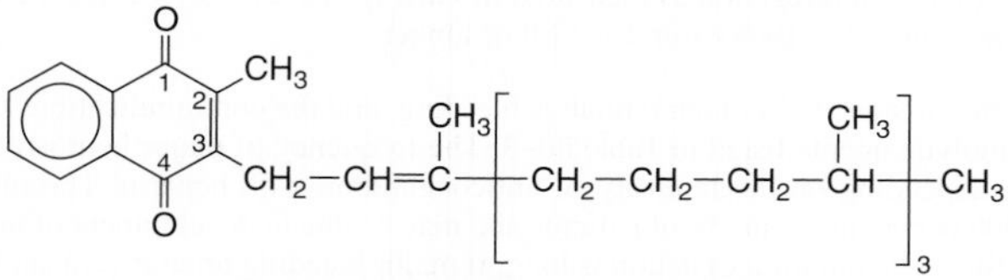

PHYTONADIONE (vitamin K_1, phylloquinone)

PHYSIOLOGICAL FUNCTIONS AND PHARMACOLOGICAL ACTIONS. Phytonadione and menaquinones promote the biosynthesis of:

- The Gla forms of factors II (prothrombin), VII, IX, and X
- Anticoagulant proteins C and S; protein Z (a cofactor to the inhibitor of Xa)
- The bone Gla protein osteocalcin
- The matrix Gla protein
- The growth arrest–specific protein 6 (Gas6)
- Four transmembrane monospans of unknown function

Figure 30–6 summarizes the coupling of the vitamin K cycle with glutamate carboxylation. The γ-glutamyl carboxylase and epoxide reductase are integral membrane proteins of the endoplasmic reticulum and function as a multicomponent complex. With respect to proteins affecting blood coagulation, these reactions occur in the liver, but γ-carboxylation of glutamate also occurs in lung, bone, and other cell types. Two natural mutations in γ-glutamyl carboxylase lead to bleeding disorders.

HUMAN REQUIREMENTS. In patients made vitamin K deficient by a starvation diet and antibiotic therapy for 3-4 weeks, the minimum daily requirement is estimated to be 0.03 μg/kg of body weight and possibly as high as 1 μg/kg, which is approximately the recommended intake for adults (70 μg/day).

SYMPTOMS OF DEFICIENCY. The chief clinical manifestation of vitamin K deficiency is an increased tendency to bleed. Ecchymoses, epistaxis, hematuria, GI bleeding, and postoperative hemorrhage are common; intracranial hemorrhage may occur. Hemoptysis is uncommon. The discovery of a vitamin K-dependent protein in bone suggests that the fetal bone abnormalities associated with the administration of oral anticoagulants during the first trimester of pregnancy ("fetal warfarin syndrome") may be related to a deficiency of the vitamin. Vitamin K plays a role in adult skeletal maintenance and the prevention of osteoporosis. Low concentrations of the vitamin are associated with deficits in bone mineral density and fractures; vitamin K supplementation increases the carboxylation state of osteocalcin and also improves bone mineral density, but the relationship of these 2 effects is unclear. Bone mineral density in adults is not changed by therapeutic use of vitamin K antagonists, but new bone formation may be affected.

TOXICITY. Phytonadione and the menaquinones are nontoxic. Menadione and its derivatives (synthetic forms of vitamin K) have been implicated in producing hemolytic anemia and kernicterus in neonates, and should not be used as a therapeutic form of vitamin K.

ADME. The mechanism of intestinal absorption of compounds with vitamin K activity varies with their solubility. In the presence of bile salts, phytonadione and the menaquinones are adequately absorbed from the intestine, phytonadione by an energy-dependent, saturable process in proximal portions of the small intestine, menaquinones by diffusion in the distal portions of the small intestine and in the colon. Following absorption, phytonadione is incorporated into chylomicrons in close association with triglycerides and lipoproteins. The extremely low phytonadione levels in newborns may be partly related to very low plasma lipoprotein concentrations at birth and may lead to an underestimation of vitamin K tissue stores. After absorption, phytonadione and menaquinones are concentrated in the liver, but the concentration of phytonadione declines rapidly. Menaquinones, produced in the lower bowel, are less biologically active due to their long side chain. Very little vitamin K accumulates in other tissues. There is only modest storage of vitamin K in the body: under circumstances in which lack of bile interferes with absorption of vitamin K, hypoprothrombinemia develops slowly over several weeks.

THERAPEUTIC USES. Vitamin K is used therapeutically to correct the bleeding tendency or hemorrhage associated with its deficiency. Vitamin K deficiency can result from inadequate intake, absorption, or utilization of the vitamin, or as a consequence of the action of a vitamin K antagonist.

Phytonadione (AQUAMEPHYTON, KONAKION, MEPHYTON) is available as tablets and in a dispersion with buffered polysorbate and propylene glycol (KONAKION) or polyoxyethylated fatty acid derivatives and dextrose

(AQUAMEPHYTON). KONAKION is administered only intramuscularly. AQUAMEPHYTON may be given by any route; however, oral or subcutaneous injection is preferred because severe reactions resembling anaphylaxis have followed its intravenous administration.

Inadequate Intake. After infancy, hypoprothrombinemia due to dietary deficiency of vitamin K is extremely rare. The vitamin is present in many foods and is synthesized by intestinal bacteria. Occasionally, the use of a broad-spectrum antibiotic may itself produce a hypoprothrombinemia that responds readily to small doses of vitamin K and reestablishment of normal bowel flora. Hypoprothrombinemia can occur in patients receiving prolonged intravenous alimentation. It is recommended to give 1 mg of phytonadione per week (the equivalent of about 150 μg/day) to patients on total parenteral nutrition.

HYPOPROTHROMBINEMIA OF THE NEWBORN

Healthy newborn infants show decreased plasma concentrations of vitamin K-dependent clotting factors for a few days after birth, the time required to obtain an adequate dietary intake of the vitamin and to establish a normal intestinal flora. Measurements of non-γ-carboxylated prothrombin suggest that vitamin K deficiency occurs in about 3% of live births.

Hemorrhagic disease of the newborn has been associated with breast-feeding; human milk has low concentrations of vitamin K. In addition, the intestinal flora of breast-fed infants may lack microorganisms that synthesize the vitamin. Commercial infant formulas are supplemented with vitamin K. In the neonate with hemorrhagic disease of the newborn, the administration of vitamin K raises the concentration of these clotting factors to the level normal for the newborn infant and controls the bleeding tendency within about 6 h. The routine administration of 1 mg phytonadione intramuscularly at birth is required by law in the U.S. This dose may have to be increased or repeated if the mother has received anticoagulant or anticonvulsant drug therapy or if the infant develops bleeding tendencies. Alternatively, some clinicians treat mothers who are receiving anticonvulsants with oral vitamin K prior to delivery (20 mg/day for 2 weeks).

Inadequate Absorption. Vitamin K is poorly absorbed in the absence of bile. Thus, hypoprothrombinemia may be associated with either intrahepatic or extrahepatic biliary obstruction or a severe defect in the intestinal absorption of fat from other causes.

BILIARY OBSTRUCTION OR FISTULA

Bleeding that accompanies obstructive jaundice or biliary fistula responds promptly to the administration of vitamin K. Oral phytonadione administered with bile salts is both safe and effective and should be used in the care of the jaundiced patient, both preoperatively and postoperatively. In the absence of significant hepatocellular disease, the prothrombin activity of the blood rapidly returns to normal. If oral administration is not feasible, a parenteral preparation should be used. The usual dose is 10 mg/day of vitamin K.

MALABSORPTION SYNDROMES

Among the disorders that result in inadequate absorption of vitamin K from the intestinal tract are cystic fibrosis, sprue, Crohn disease and enterocolitis, ulcerative colitis, dysentery, and extensive resection of bowel. Because drugs that greatly reduce the bacterial population of the bowel are used frequently in many of these disorders, the availability of the vitamin may be further reduced. For immediate correction of the deficiency, parenteral therapy should be used.

Inadequate Utilization. Hepatocellular disease may be accompanied or followed by hypoprothrombinemia. Hepatocellular damage also may be secondary to long-lasting biliary obstruction. If an inadequate secretion of bile salts is contributing to the syndrome, some benefit may be obtained from the parenteral administration of 10 mg of phytonadione daily. Paradoxically, the administration of large doses of vitamin K or its analogs in an attempt to correct the hypoprothrombinemia associated with severe hepatitis or cirrhosis actually may result in a further depression of the concentration of prothrombin.

Drug- and Venom-Induced Hypoprothrombinemia. Anticoagulant drugs such as warfarin and its congeners act as competitive antagonists of vitamin K and interfere with the hepatic biosynthesis of Gla-containing clotting factors. The treatment of bleeding caused by oral anticoagulants is above. Vitamin K may be of help in combating the bleeding and hypoprothrombinemia that follow the bite of the tropical American pit viper or other species whose venom destroys or inactivates prothrombin.

For a complete Bibliographical Listing see Goodman & Gilman's ***The Pharmacological Basis of Therapeutics***, 12th ed., or Goodman & Gilman Online at www.AccessMedicine.com.

Drug Therapy for Hypercholesterolemia and Dyslipidemia

Hyperlipidemia is a major cause of atherosclerosis and atherosclerosis-induced conditions, such as coronary heart disease (CHD), ischemic cerebrovascular disease, and peripheral vascular disease. These conditions cause morbidity or mortality in a majority of middle-aged or older adults. Dyslipidemias, including hyperlipidemia (hypercholesterolemia) and low levels of high-density-lipoprotein cholesterol (HDL-C), are major causes of increased atherogenic risk; both genetic disorders and lifestyle contribute to the dyslipidemias seen in countries around the world.

Classes of drugs that modify cholesterol levels include:

- Statins, inhibitors of 3-hydroxy-3-methylglutaryl–coenzyme A (HMG-CoA) reductase
- Bile acid–binding resins
- Nicotinic acid (*niacin*)
- Fibric acid derivatives
- *Ezetimibe*, an inhibitor of cholesterol absorption

These drugs provide benefit in patients across the entire spectrum of cholesterol levels, primarily by reducing levels of low-density-lipoprotein cholesterol (LDL-C). Drug regimens that reduce LDL-C levels moderately (30-40%) can reduce fatal and nonfatal CHD events and strokes by as much as 30-40%. In patients with low HDL-C and average LDL-C levels, appropriate drug therapy reduces CHD endpoint events by 20-35%. Because two-thirds of patients with CHD in the U.S. have low HDL-C levels (<40 mg/dL in men, <50 mg/dL in women), low-HDL-C patients should be treated for dyslipidemia, even if their LDL-C levels are in the normal range.

Severe hypertriglyceridemia (i.e., triglyceride levels of >1000 mg/dL) requires therapy to prevent pancreatitis. Moderately elevated triglyceride levels (150-400 mg/dL) are of concern because they often occur as part of the metabolic syndrome, which includes insulin resistance, obesity, hypertension, low HDL-C levels, a procoagulant state, and substantially increased risk of CVD. Atherogenic dyslipidemia in patients with metabolic syndrome also is characterized by lipid-depleted LDL (sometimes referred to as "small, dense LDL"). Metabolic syndrome affects ~25% of adults and is common in CVD patients; hence, identification of moderate hypertriglyceridemia in a patient, even if the total cholesterol level is normal, should trigger an evaluation to identify insulin-resistant patients with this disorder.

PLASMA LIPOPROTEIN METABOLISM

Lipoproteins are macromolecular assemblies that contain lipids and proteins. The lipid constituents include free and esterified cholesterol, triglycerides, and phospholipids. The protein components, known as *apolipoproteins* or *apoproteins*, provide structural stability to the lipoproteins and also may function as ligands in lipoprotein–receptor interactions or as cofactors in enzymatic processes that regulate lipoprotein metabolism. The major classes of lipoproteins and their properties are summarized in Table 31–1. Apoproteins have well-defined roles in plasma lipoprotein metabolism (Table 31–2).

In all spherical lipoproteins, the most water-insoluble lipids (cholesteryl esters and triglycerides) are core components, and the more polar, water-soluble components (apoproteins, phospholipids, and unesterified cholesterol) are located on the surface. Except for apo(a), the lipid-binding regions of all apoproteins contain amphipathic helices that interact with the polar, hydrophilic lipids (such as surface phospholipids) and with the aqueous plasma environment in which the lipoproteins circulate. Differences in the non–lipid-binding regions determine the functional specificities of the apolipoproteins.

Figure 31–1 summarizes the pathways involved in the uptake and transport of dietary fat and cholesterol, pathways that involve the lipoprotein structures described below.

CHYLOMICRONS. Chylomicrons are synthesized from the fatty acids of dietary triglycerides and cholesterol absorbed by epithelial cells in the small intestine. Chylomicrons are the largest and

Table 31–1

Characteristics of Plasma Lipoproteins

LIPOPROTEIN CLASS	DENSITY (g/mL)	MAJOR LIPID CONSTITUENT	TG:CHOL	SIGNIFICANT APOPROTEINS	SITE OF SYNTHESIS	CATABOLIC PATHWAY
Chylomicrons and remnants	<<1.006	Dietary triglycerides and cholesterol	10:1	B-48, E, A-I, A-IV, C-I, C-II, C-III	Intestine	Triglyceride hydrolysis by LPL, apoE-mediated remnant uptake by liver
VLDL	<1.006	"Endogenous" or hepatic triglycerides	5:1	B-100, E, C-I, C-II, C-III	Liver	Triglyceride hydrolysis by LPL
IDL	1.006-1.019	Cholesteryl esters and "endogenous" triglycerides	1:1	B-100, E, C-II, C-III	Product of VLDL catabolism	50% converted to LDL mediated by HL; 50% apoE-mediated uptake by liver
LDL	1.019-1.063	Cholesteryl esters	NS	B-100	Product of VLDL catabolism	ApoB-100-mediated uptake by LDL receptor (~75% in liver)
HDL	1.063-1.21	Phospholipids, cholesteryl esters	NS	A-I, A-II, E, C-I, C-II, C-III	Intestine, liver, plasma	Complex: transfer of cholesteryl ester to VLDL and LDL; uptake of HDL cholesterol by hepatocytes
Lp(a)	1.05-1.09	Cholesteryl esters	NS	B-100, apo(a)	Liver	Unknown

Apo, apolipoprotein; CHOL, cholesterol; HDL, high-density lipoproteins; IDL, intermediate-density lipoproteins; Lp(a), lipoprotein(a); LDL, low-density lipoproteins; NS, not significant (triglyceride is <5% of LDL and HDL); TG, triglyceride; VLDL, very-low-density lipoproteins; HL, hepatic lipase; LPL, lipoprotein lipase.

Table 31–2

Apolipoproteins

APOLIPOPROTEIN (MW in kDa)	AVERAGE CONCENTRATION (mg/dL)	SITES OF SYNTHESIS	FUNCTIONS
ApoA-I (~29)	130	Liver, intestine	Structural in HDL; LCAT cofactor; ligand of ABCA1 receptor; reverse cholesterol transport
ApoA-II (~17)	40	Liver	Forms -*S*-*S*-complex with apoE-2 and E-3, which inhibits E-2 and E-3 binding to lipoprotein receptors
ApoA-V (~40)	<1	Liver	Modulates triglyceride incorporation into hepatic VLDL; activates LPL
ApoB-100 (~513)	85	Liver	Structural protein of VLDL, IDL, LDL; LDL receptor ligand
ApoB-48 (~241)	Fluctuates according to dietary fat intake	Intestine	Structural protein of chylomicrons
ApoC-I (~6.6)	6	Liver	LCAT activator; modulates receptor binding of remnants
ApoC-II (8.9)	3	Liver	Lipoprotein lipase cofactor
ApoC-III (8.8)	12	Liver	Modulates receptor binding of remnants
ApoE (34)	5	Liver, brain, skin, gonads, spleen	Ligand for LDL receptor and receptors binding remnants; reverse cholesterol transport (HDL with apoE)
Apo(a) (Variable)	Variable (under genetic control)	Liver	Modulator of fibrinolysis

Apo, apolipoprotein; HDL, high-density lipoproteins; IDL, intermediate-density lipoproteins; LCAT, lecithin-cholesterol acyltransferase; LDL, low-density lipoproteins; LPL, lipoprotein lipase; VLDL, very-low-density lipoproteins.

lowest density plasma lipoproteins. In normolipidemic individuals, chylomicrons are present in plasma for 3-6 h after a fat-containing meal has been ingested. Intestinal cholesterol absorption is mediated by Niemann-Pick C1–Like 1 protein (NPC1L1), which appears to be the target of *ezetimibe*, a cholesterol absorption inhibitor.

After their synthesis in the endoplasmic reticulum, triglycerides are transferred by *microsomal triglyceride transfer protein* (MTP) to the site where newly synthesized apoB-48 is available to form chylomicrons. ApoB-48, synthesized only by intestinal epithelial cells, is unique to chylomicrons and functions primarily as a structural component of chylomicrons. Dietary cholesterol is esterified by the type 2 isozyme of acyl coenzyme A:cholesterol acyltransferase (ACAT-2). ACAT-2 is found in the intestine and in the liver, where cellular free cholesterol is esterified before triglyceride-rich lipoproteins (chylomicrons and very-low-density lipoproteins [VLDL]) are assembled.

After entering the circulation via the thoracic duct, chylomicrons are metabolized initially at the capillary luminal surface of tissues that synthesize *lipoprotein lipase* (LPL), (*see* Figure 31–1), including adipose tissue, skeletal and cardiac muscle, and breast tissue of lactating women. The resulting free fatty acids are taken up and used by the adjacent tissues. The interaction of chylomicrons and LPL requires apoC-II as a cofactor.

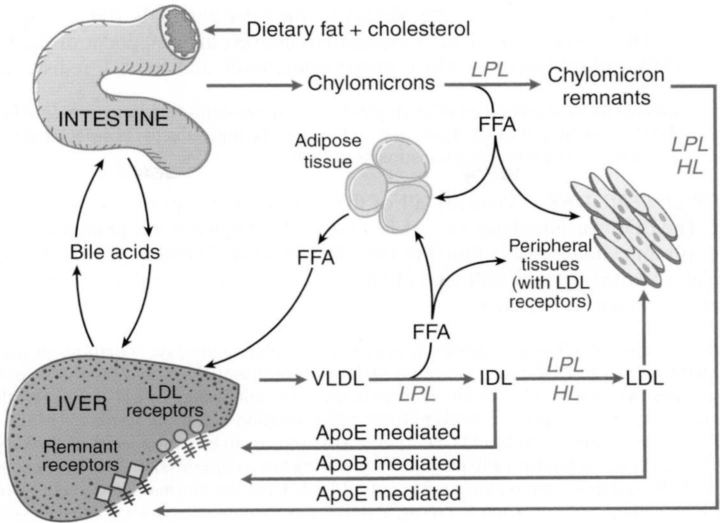

Figure 31–1 *The major pathways involved in the metabolism of chylomicrons synthesized by the intestine and VLDL synthesized by the liver.* Chylomicrons are converted to chylomicron remnants by the hydrolysis of their triglycerides by LPL. Chylomicron remnants are rapidly cleared from the plasma by the liver. "Remnant receptors" include the LDL receptor–related protein (LRP), LDL receptors, and perhaps other receptors. Free fatty acid (FFA) released by LPL is used by muscle tissue as an energy source or taken up and stored by adipose tissue. HL, hepatic lipase; IDL, intermediate-density lipoproteins; LDL, low-density lipoproteins; LPL, lipoprotein lipase; VLDL, very-low-density lipoproteins.

CHYLOMICRON REMNANTS. After LPL-mediated removal of much of the dietary triglycerides, the *chylomicron remnants*, with all of the dietary cholesterol, detach from the capillary surface and within minutes are removed from the circulation by the liver (*see* Figure 31–1). First, the remnants are sequestered by the interaction of apoE with heparan sulfate proteoglycans on the surface of hepatocytes and are processed by *hepatic lipase* (HL), further reducing the remnant triglyceride content. Next, apoE mediates remnant uptake by interacting with the hepatic LDL receptor or the *LDL receptor–related protein* (LRP).

During the initial hydrolysis of chylomicron triglycerides by LPL, apoA-I and phospholipids are shed from the surface of chylomicrons and remain in the plasma. This is one mechanism by which nascent (precursor) HDL are generated. Chylomicron remnants are not precursors of LDL, but the dietary cholesterol delivered to the liver by remnants increases plasma LDL levels by reducing LDL receptor–mediated catabolism of LDL by the liver.

VERY-LOW-DENSITY LIPOPROTEINS. VLDL are produced in the liver when triglyceride production is stimulated by an increased flux of free fatty acids or by increased de novo synthesis of fatty acids by the liver.

ApoB-100, apoE, and apoC-I, C-II, and C-III are synthesized constitutively by the liver and incorporated into VLDL (*see* Table 31–2). Triglycerides are synthesized in the endoplasmic reticulum, and along with other lipid constituents, are transferred by MTP to the site in the endoplasmic reticulum where newly synthesized apoB-100 is available to form nascent (precursor) VLDL. Small amounts of apoE and the C apoproteins are incorporated into nascent particles within the liver before secretion, but most of these apoproteins are acquired from plasma HDL after the VLDL are secreted by the liver. Mutations of MTP that result in the inability of triglycerides to be transferred to either apoB-100 in the liver or apoB-48 in the intestine prevent VLDL and chylomicron production and cause the genetic disorder *abetalipoproteinemia*.

Plasma VLDL is catabolized by LPL in the capillary beds in a process similar to the lipolytic processing of chylomicrons (*see* Figure 31–1). When triglyceride hydrolysis is nearly complete, the VLDL remnants, usually termed *IDL*, are released from the capillary endothelium and reenter the circulation. ApoB-100 containing small VLDL and IDL, which have a $t_{1/2}$ <30 min, have 2 potential fates. About 40-60% are cleared from the plasma by the liver via apoB-100 and apoE-mediated interaction with LDL receptors and LRP. LPL and HL convert the remainder of the IDL to LDL by removal of additional triglycerides. The C apoproteins, apoE, and apoA-V redistribute to HDL.

ApoE plays a major role in the metabolism of triglyceride-rich lipoproteins (chylomicrons, chylomicron remnants, VLDL, and IDL). About half of the apoE in the plasma of fasting subjects is associated with triglyceride-rich lipoproteins, and the other half is a constituent of HDL.

LOW-DENSITY LIPOPROTEINS. Virtually all of the LDL particles in the circulation are derived from VLDL. The LDL particles have a $t_{1/2}$ of 1.5-2 days. In subjects without hypertriglyceridemia, two-thirds of plasma cholesterol is found in the LDL. Plasma clearance of LDL is mediated primarily by LDL receptors (ApoB-100 binds LDL to its receptor); a small component is mediated by nonreceptor clearance mechanisms.

The most common cause of autosomal dominant hypercholesterolemia involves mutations of the LDL receptor gene. Defective or absent LDL receptors cause high levels of plasma LDL and familial hypercholesterolemia. LDL becomes atherogenic when modified by oxidation, a required step for LDL uptake by the scavenger receptors of macrophages. This process leads to foam-cell formation in arterial lesions. At least 2 scavenger receptors (SRs) are involved (SR-AI/II and CD36). SR-AI/II appears to be expressed more in early atherogenesis, and CD36 expression is greater as foam cells form during lesion progression. The liver expresses a large complement of LDL receptors and removes ~75% of all LDL from the plasma. Consequently, manipulation of hepatic LDL receptor gene expression is a most effective way to modulate plasma LDL-C levels. Thyroxine and estrogen enhance LDL receptor gene expression, which explains their LDL-C–lowering effects. *The most effective dietary alteration (decreased consumption of saturated fat and cholesterol) and pharmacological treatment (statins) for hypercholesterolemia act by enhancing hepatic LDL receptor expression.*

HIGH-DENSITY LIPOPROTEINS. HDL are protective lipoproteins that decrease the risk of CHD; thus, high levels of HDL are desirable. This protective effect may result from the participation of HDL in reverse cholesterol transport, the process by which excess cholesterol is acquired from cells and transferred to the liver for excretion. HDL effects also include putative anti-inflammatory, anti-oxidative, platelet anti-aggregatory, anticoagulant, and profibrinolytic activities. ApoA-I is the major HDL apoprotein, and its plasma concentration is a more powerful inverse predictor of CHD risk than is the HDL-C level. ApoA-I synthesis is required for normal production of HDL.

Mutations in the apoA-I gene that cause HDL deficiency often are associated with accelerated atherogenesis. In addition, 2 major subclasses of mature HDL particles in the plasma can be differentiated by their content of the major HDL apoproteins, apoA-I and apoA-II. Epidemiologic evidence in humans suggests that apoA-II may be atheroprotective.

The membrane transporter ABCA1 facilitates the transfer of free cholesterol from cells to HDL. After free cholesterol is acquired by the pre-β1 HDL, it is esterified by lecithin:cholesterol acyltransferase. The newly esterified and nonpolar cholesterol moves into the core of the particle, which becomes progressively more spherical, larger, and less dense with continued cholesterol acquisition and esterification. As the cholesteryl ester content of the particle (now called HDL_2) increases, the cholesteryl esters of these particles begin to be exchanged for triglycerides derived from any of the triglyceride-containing lipoproteins (chylomicrons, VLDL, remnant lipoproteins, and LDL). This exchange, mediated by the cholesteryl ester transfer protein (CETP), accounts for the removal of about two-thirds of the cholesterol associated with HDL in humans. The transferred cholesterol subsequently is metabolized as part of the lipoprotein into which it was transferred.

Treatments that target CETP and the ABC transporters have yielded equivocal results in humans. While CETP inhibitors effectively reduce LDL, they also paradoxically increase the frequency of adverse cardiovascular events (angina, revascularization, myocardial infarction, heart failure, and death).

The triglyceride that is transferred into HDL_2 is hydrolyzed in the liver by HL, a process that regenerates smaller, spherical HDL_3 particles that recirculate and acquire additional free cholesterol from tissues containing excess free cholesterol.

HL activity is regulated and modulates HDL-C levels. Androgens increase HL gene expression/activity, which accounts for the lower HDL-C values observed in men than in women. Estrogens reduce HL activity, but their impact on HDL-C levels in women is substantially less than that of androgens on HDL-C levels in men. HL appears to have a pivotal role in regulating HDL-C levels, as HL activity is increased in many patients with low HDL-C levels.

LIPOPROTEIN (a). Lipoprotein(a) [Lp(a)] is composed of an LDL particle that has a second apoprotein, apo(a), in addition to apoB-100. Apo(a) of Lp(a) is structurally related to plasminogen and appears to be atherogenic.

HYPERLIPIDEMIA AND ATHEROSCLEROSIS

The major conventional risk factors for CVD are elevated LDL-C, reduced HDL-C, cigarette smoking, hypertension, type 2 diabetes mellitus, advancing age, and a family history of premature CHD events (men <55 years; women <65 years) in a first-degree relative (Table 31–3). When total cholesterol levels are below 160 mg/dL, CHD risk is markedly attenuated, even in the presence of additional risk factors. This pivotal role of hypercholesterolemia in atherogenesis gave rise to the almost universally accepted cholesterol-diet-CHD hypothesis: elevated plasma cholesterol levels cause CHD, diets rich in saturated (animal) fat and cholesterol raise cholesterol levels, and lowering cholesterol levels reduces CHD risk.

Modest reductions in total cholesterol and LDL-C are associated with reductions in fatal and nonfatal CHD events but not total mortality. Patients benefit regardless of gender, age, baseline lipid values, or whether they have a prior history of vascular disease or type 2 diabetes mellitus. Statin therapy is effective in preventing first and subsequent atherothrombotic strokes. Moderate doses of statins that lower LDL-C levels by about 40% reduce cardiovascular events by about one-third. More intensive regimens that lower LDL-C by 45-50% reduce CVD events by as much as 50%.

MANAGING PATIENTS WITH DYSLIPIDEMIA: NATIONAL CHOLESTEROL EDUCATION PROGRAM (NCEP) GUIDELINES

Primary prevention involves management of risk factors to prevent a first-ever CHD event. Secondary prevention is aimed at patients who have had a prior CHD event and whose risk factors must be treated aggressively. Recently, the concept of primordial prevention has been applied to CHD. This is a population-based approach to prevention (rather than treatment) that targets smoking, weight management, physical activity, healthy eating habits, cholesterol and glucose levels, and blood pressure.

The patient-based approach to manage dyslipidemia is designed for primary and secondary prevention, requires a risk assessment, and focuses on lowering LDL-C and non-HDL-C (*see* ranges in Table 31–4). Before drug therapy is initiated, secondary causes of hyperlipidemia (Table 31–5) should be excluded. Treatment of the disorder causing secondary dyslipidemia may preclude the necessity of treatment with hypolipidemic drugs. Table 31–6 summarizes current risk category-treatment guidelines based on LDL-C levels.

Table 31–3

Risk Factors for Coronary Heart Disease
Age Male >45 years of age or female >55 years of age
Family history of premature CHD A first-degree relative (male <55 years of age or female <65 years of age when the first CHD clinical event occurs)
Current cigarette smoking Defined as smoking within the preceding 30 days
Hypertension Blood pressure ≥140/90 or use of antihypertensive medication, irrespective of blood pressure
Low HDL-C <40 mg/dL (consider <50 mg/dL as "low" for women)
Obesity Body mass index >25 kg/m^2 and waist circumference >40 inches (men) or >35 inches (women)
Type 2 diabetes mellitus
From The Expert Panel, 2002.

Table 31–4

Classification of Plasma Lipid Levels (mg/dL)

Total cholesterol	
<200	Desirable
200-239	Borderline high
≥240	High
HDL-C	
<40	Low (consider <50 mg/dL as low for women)
>60	High
LDL-C	
<70	Optimal for very high risk (minimal goal for CHD equivalent patients)
<100	Optimal
100-129	Near optimal
130-159	Borderline high
160-189	High
≥190	Very high
Triglycerides	
<150	Normal
150-199	Borderline high
200-499	High
≥500	Very high

HDL-C, high-density-lipoprotein cholesterol; LDL-C, low-density-lipoprotein cholesterol.
From The Expert Panel, 2002.

WHOM AND WHEN TO TREAT?

Large-scale trials with statins have provided new insights into which patients with dyslipidemia should be treated and when treatment should be initiated.

Gender. Both men and women benefit from lipid-lowering therapy. Statins are the recommended first-line drug therapy for lowering lipids and preventing CHD events in postmenopausal women.

Age. Age >45 years in men and >55 years in women is considered to be a CHD risk factor. The statin trials have shown that patients >65 years of age benefit from therapy as much as do younger patients. Old age per se is not a reason to refrain from initiating drug therapy in an otherwise healthy person.

Cerebrovascular Disease Patients. Plasma cholesterol levels correlate positively with the risk of ischemic stroke and statins reduce stroke and transient ischemic attacks in patients with and without CHD.

Peripheral Vascular Disease Patients. Statins are beneficial in patients with peripheral vascular disease.

Table 31–5

Secondary Causes of Dyslipidemia

DISORDER	MAJOR LIPID EFFECT
Diabetes mellitus	Triglycerides > cholesterol; low HDL-C
Nephrotic syndrome	Triglycerides usually > cholesterol
Alcohol use	Triglycerides > cholesterol
Contraceptive use	Triglycerides > cholesterol
Estrogen use	Triglycerides > cholesterol
Glucocorticoid excess	Triglycerides > cholesterol
Hypothyroidism	Cholesterol > triglycerides
Obstructive liver disease	Cholesterol > triglycerides

HDL-C, high-density-lipoprotein cholesterol.

Table 31–6

Treatment Based on LDL-C Levels (2004 Revision of NCEP Adult Treatment Panel III Guidelines)

RISK CATEGORY	LDL-C GOAL (mg/dL)	Non-HDL-C GOAL (mg/dL)	THERAPEUTIC LIFESTYLE CHANGE	THRESHOLD FOR DRUG THERAPY (mg/dL)
Very high risk Atherosclerosis-induced CHD plus one of: • multiple risk factors • diabetes mellitus • a poorly controlled single factor • acute coronary syndrome • metabolic syndrome	<70[a]	<100	No threshold (initiate change)	No threshold (initiate therapy)
High risk CHD or CHD equivalent	<100[a]	<130	No threshold	No threshold
Moderately high risk 2+ risk factors 10-year risk: <10-20%	<130 (or <100)	<160	No threshold	≥130 (100-129)[b]
Moderate risk 2+ risk factors 10-year risk <10%	<130	<160	No threshold	>160
0-1 risk factor	<160	<160	No threshold	≥190 (optional: 160-189)[c]

After attaining the LDL-C goal, additional therapy may be necessary to reach the non-HDL-C goal.

CHD, coronary heart disease; CHD equivalent, peripheral vascular disease, abdominal aortic aneurysm, symptomatic carotid artery disease, >20% 10-year CHD risk, or diabetes mellitus; HDL-C, high-density-lipoprotein cholesterol; LDL-C, low-density-lipoprotein cholesterol; NCEP, National Cholesterol Education Program.

[a]If pretreatment LDL-C is near or below LDL-C goal value, then a statin dose sufficient to lower LDL-C by 30-40% should be prescribed.

[b]Patients in this category include those with a 10-year risk of 10-20% and one of the following: age >60 years, three or more risk factors, a severe risk factor, triglycerides >200 mg/dL and HDL-C <40 mg/dL, metabolic syndrome, highly sensitive C-reactive protein (CRP) >3 mg/L, and coronary calcium score (age/gender adjusted) >75th percentile.

[c]Patients include those with any severe single risk factor, multiple major risk factors, 10-year risk >8%.

Hypertensive Patients and Smokers. The risk reduction for coronary events in statin trials of hypertensive patients and smokers is similar to that in subjects without hypertension.

Type 2 Diabetes Mellitus. Patients with type 2 diabetes benefit very significantly from aggressive lipid lowering (see below).

Post–Myocardial Infarction or Revascularization Patients. As soon as CHD is diagnosed, it is essential to begin lipid-lowering therapy (NCEP guidelines: LDL-C goal <70 mg/dL for very high-risk patients). Statin therapy also improves the long-term outcome after bypass surgery.

TREATMENT OF TYPE 2 DIABETES PATIENTS

Diabetes mellitus is an independent predictor of high risk for CHD. Glucose control is essential but provides only minimal benefit with respect to CHD prevention. Aggressive treatment of diabetic dyslipidemia through diet, weight control, and drugs is critical in reducing risk. Diabetic dyslipidemia

Table 31–7

Clinical Identification of the Metabolic Syndrome

RISK FACTOR	DEFINING LEVEL
Abdominal obesity	Waist circumference
Men	>102 cm (>40 in)
Women	>88 cm (>35 in)
Triglycerides	≥150 mg/dL
HDL-C	
Men	<40 mg/dL
Women	<50 mg/dL
Blood pressure	≥130/≥85 mm Hg
Fasting glucose	>100 mg/dL

The 2001 National Cholesterol Education Program (NCEP) guidelines define the metabolic syndrome as the presence of three or more of these risk factors.
From The Expert Panel, 2002.

usually is characterized by high triglycerides, low HDL-C, and moderate elevations of total cholesterol and LDL-C. Diabetics without diagnosed CHD have the same level of risk as nondiabetics with established CHD. Thus, the dyslipidemia treatment guidelines for diabetic patients are the same as for patients with CHD, irrespective of whether the diabetic patient has had a CHD event.

METABOLIC SYNDROME

There is an increased CHD risk associated with the insulin-resistant, prediabetic state described under the rubric of "metabolic syndrome." This syndrome consists of a constellation of 5 CHD risk factors: abdominal obesity, hypertension, insulin-resistance, hypertriglyceridemia, and low HDL (Table 31–7). Treatment should focus on weight loss and increased physical activity. Specific treatment of lipid abnormalities should also be undertaken.

TREATMENT OF HYPERTRIGLYCERIDEMIA

There is increased CHD risk associated with the presence of triglyceride levels >150 mg/dL. Three categories of hypertriglyceridemia are recognized (*see* Table 31–4), and treatment is recommended based on the degree of elevation. Weight loss, increased exercise, and alcohol restriction are important for all hypertriglyceridemic patients. If triglycerides remain >200 mg/dL after the LDL-C goal is reached (*see* Table 31–6), further reduction in triglycerides may be achieved by increasing the dose of a statin or of niacin. Combination therapy (statin plus niacin or statin plus fibrate) may be required, but caution is necessary with these combinations to avoid myopathy (see below).

TREATMENT OF LOW HDL-C

The most frequent risk factor for premature CHD is low HDL-C.

In patients with low HDL-C, the total cholesterol:HDL-C ratio is a particularly useful predictor of CHD risk. Observational studies suggest that a ratio >4.5 is associated with increased risk (Table 31–8). The treatment of low HDL-C patients focuses on lowering LDL-C to the target level based on the patient's risk factor or CHD status (*see* Table 31–6) *and* a reduction of VLDL cholesterol to <30 mg/dL to reach the target for non-HDL-C. Satisfactory treatment results are a ratio of total cholesterol: HDL-C ≤3.5.

DRUG THERAPY OF DYSLIPIDEMIA

STATINS

The statins are the most effective and best-tolerated agents for treating dyslipidemia. These drugs are competitive inhibitors of HMG-CoA reductase, which catalyzes an early, rate-limiting step in cholesterol biosynthesis. Higher doses of the more potent statins (e.g., atorvastatin, simvastatin, and rosuvastatin) also can reduce triglyceride levels caused by elevated VLDL levels. Some statins also are indicated for raising HDL-C levels, although the clinical significance of these effects on HDL-C remains to be proven. Figure 31–2 shows a representative statin structure and the reaction catalyzed by HMG-CoA reductase.

Table 31–8

Guidelines Based on LDL-C and Total Cholesterol:HDL-C Ratio for Treatment of Low HDL-C Patients[a]

RISK CATEGORY	GOALS			LIFESTYLE CHANGE INITIATED FOR			DRUG THERAPY INITIATED FOR		
	LDL-C		TC:HDL-C	LDL-C		TC:HDL-C	LDL-C		TC:HDL-C
CHD or equivalent	<100	and	<3.5	≥100	or	≥3.5	≥100	or	≥3.5
2+ risk factors	<130	and	<4.5	≥130	or	≥4.5	≥130	or	≥6.0
0.1 risk factor	<160	and	<5.5	≥160	or	≥5.5	≥160	or	≥7.0

CHD, coronary heart disease; HDL-C, high-density-lipoprotein cholesterol; LDL-C, low-density-lipoprotein cholesterol; TC, total cholesterol.
[a]Units for LDL-C: mg/dL.

MECHANISM OF ACTION

Statins exert their major effect—reduction of LDL levels—through a mevalonic acid–like moiety that competitively inhibits HMG-CoA reductase. By reducing the conversion of HMG-CoA to mevalonate, statins inhibit an early and rate-limiting step in cholesterol biosynthesis. Statins affect blood cholesterol levels by inhibiting hepatic cholesterol synthesis, which results in increased expression of the LDL receptor gene. Some studies suggest that statins also can reduce LDL levels by enhancing the removal of LDL precursors (VLDL and IDL) and by decreasing hepatic VLDL production. The reduction in hepatic VLDL production induced by statins is thought to be mediated by reduced synthesis of cholesterol, a required component of VLDL.

THERAPEUTIC EFFECTS

Triglyceride Reduction by Statins. Triglyceride levels >250 mg/dL are reduced substantially by statins, and the percent reduction achieved is similar to the percent reduction in LDL-C.

Effect of Statins on HDL-C Levels. Most studies of patients treated with statins have systematically excluded patients with low HDL-C levels. In studies of patients with elevated LDL-C levels and gender-appropriate HDL-C levels (40-50 mg/dL for men; 50-60 mg/dL for women), an increase in HDL-C of 5-10% was observed, irrespective of the dose or statin employed. However, in patients with reduced HDL-C levels (<35 mg/dL), statins may differ in their effects on HDL-C levels. More studies are needed to ascertain whether the effects of statins on HDL-C in patients with low HDL-C levels are clinically significant.

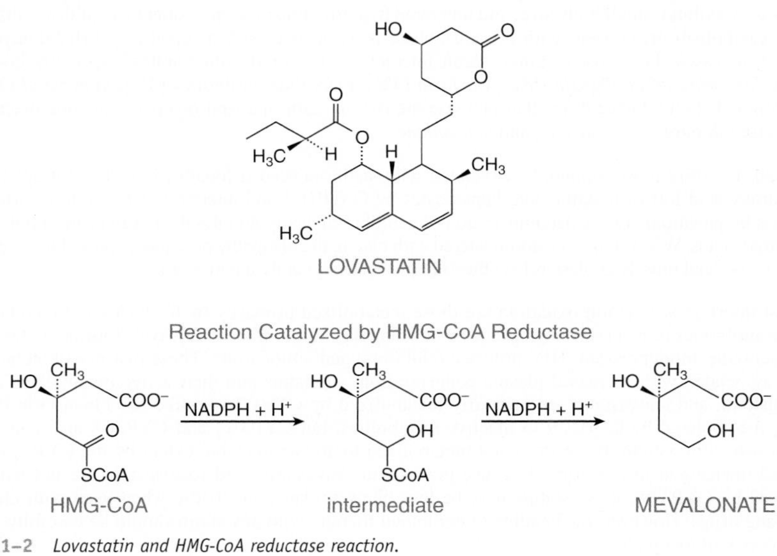

Figure 31–2 *Lovastatin and HMG-CoA reductase reaction.*

Effects of Statins on LDL-C Levels. Dose-response relationships for all statins demonstrate that the efficacy of LDL-C lowering is log-linear; LDL-C is reduced by ~6% (from baseline) with each doubling of the dose. Maximal effects on plasma cholesterol levels are achieved within 7-10 days. The statins are effective in almost all patients with high LDL-C levels. The exception is patients with homozygous familial hypercholesterolemia, who have very attenuated responses to the usual doses of statins because both alleles of the LDL receptor gene code for dysfunctional LDL receptors. Statin therapy does not reduce Lp(a) levels.

Potential Cardioprotective Effects Other Than LDL Lowering. Although the statins clearly exert their major effects on CHD by lowering LDL-C and improving the lipid profile as reflected in plasma cholesterol levels, a multitude of potentially cardioprotective effects are being ascribed to these drugs. However, it is not known whether these potential pleiotropic effects represent a class-action effect, differ among statins, or are biologically or clinically relevant.

ADME

After oral administration, intestinal absorption of the statins is variable (30-85%). All the statins, except simvastatin and lovastatin, are administered in the β-hydroxy acid form, which is the form that inhibits HMG-CoA reductase. Simvastatin and lovastatin are administered as inactive lactones that must be transformed in the liver to their respective β-hydroxy acids, simvastatin acid (SVA) and lovastatin acid (LVA). There is extensive first-pass hepatic uptake of all statins, mediated primarily by the organic anion transporter OATP1B1 (*see* Chapter 5).

Due to extensive first-pass hepatic uptake, systemic bioavailability of the statins and their hepatic metabolites varies between 5% and 30% of administered doses. The metabolites of all statins, except fluvastatin and pravastatin, have some HMG-CoA reductase inhibitory activity. Under steady-state conditions, small amounts of the parent drug and its metabolites produced in the liver can be found in the systemic circulation. In the plasma, >95% of statins and their metabolites are protein bound, with the exception of pravastatin and its metabolites, which are only 50% bound. Peak plasma concentrations of statins are achieved in 1-4 h. The $t_{1/2}$ of the parent compounds are 1-4 h, except in the case of atorvastatin and rosuvastatin, which have half-lives of ~20 h, and simvastatin with a $t_{1/2}$ ~12 h. The longer $t_{1/2}$ of atorvastatin and rosuvastatin may contribute to their greater cholesterol-lowering efficacy. The liver biotransforms all statins, and more than 70% of statin metabolites are excreted by the liver, with subsequent elimination in the feces.

ADVERSE EFFECTS AND DRUG INTERACTIONS

Hepatotoxicity. Although serious hepatotoxicity is rare, a rate of about 1 case per million person-years of use; it is reasonable to measure alanine aminotransferase (ALT) at baseline and thereafter when clinically indicated.

Myopathy. The major adverse effect associated with statin use is myopathy. The risk of myopathy and rhabdomyolysis increases in proportion to statin dose and plasma concentrations. Consequently, factors inhibiting statin catabolism are associated with increased myopathy risk, including advanced age (especially >80 years of age), hepatic or renal dysfunction, perioperative periods, multisystem disease (especially in association with diabetes mellitus), small body size, and untreated hypothyroidism. Concomitant use of drugs that diminish statin catabolism or interfere with hepatic uptake is associated with myopathy and rhabdomyolysis in 50-60% of all cases. The most common statin interactions occurred with fibrates, especially *gemfibrozil* (38%), *cyclosporine* (4%), *digoxin* (5%), *warfarin* (4%), macrolide antibiotics (3%), *mibefradil* (2%), and azole antifungals (1%). Other drugs that increase the risk of statin-induced myopathy include niacin (rare), HIV protease inhibitors, *amiodarone*, and *nefazodone*.

Gemfibrozil, the drug most commonly associated with statin-induced myopathy, inhibits both uptake of the active hydroxy acid forms of statins into hepatocytes by OATP1B1 and interferes with the transformation of most statins by glucuronidases. Coadministration of gemfibrozil nearly doubles the plasma concentration of the statin hydroxy acids. When statins are administered with niacin, the myopathy probably is caused by an enhanced inhibition of skeletal muscle cholesterol synthesis (a pharmacodynamic interaction).

Drugs that interfere with statin oxidation are those metabolized primarily by CYP3A4 and include certain macrolide antibiotics (e.g., *erythromycin*); azole antifungals (e.g., *itraconazole*); cyclosporine; nefazodone, a phenylpiperazine antidepressant; HIV protease inhibitors; and amiodarone. These pharmacokinetic interactions are associated with increased plasma concentrations of statins and their active metabolites. Atorvastatin, lovastatin, and simvastatin are primarily metabolized by CYPs 3A4 and 3A5. Fluvastatin is mostly (50-80%) metabolized by CYP2C9 to inactive metabolites, but CYP3A4 and CYP2C8 also contribute to its metabolism. Pravastatin, however, is not metabolized to any appreciable extent by the CYP system and is excreted unchanged in the urine. Because pravastatin, fluvastatin, and rosuvastatin are not extensively metabolized by CYP3A4, these statins may be less likely to cause myopathy when used with one of the predisposing drugs. However, the benefits of combined therapy with any statin should be carefully weighed against the risk of myopathy.

Table 31–9

Statin Doses (mg) Required for Reductions in LDL-C

	LDL-C REDUCTIONS FROM BASELINE (%)					
	20-25%	26-30%	31-35%	36-40%	41-50%	51-55%
STATIN						
Atorvastatin	—	—	10	20	40	80
Fluvastatin	20	40	80			
Lovastatin	10	20	40	80		
Pitavastatin		1	2	4		
Pravastatin	10	20	40			
Rosuvastatin	—	—	—	5	10	20, 40
Simvastatin	—	10	20	40	80	

THERAPEUTIC USES. *Hepatic cholesterol synthesis is maximal between midnight and 2:00* A.M. *Thus, statins with $t_{1/2}$ ≤4 h (all but atorvastatin and rosuvastatin) should be taken in the evening.* Each statin has a low recommended starting dose that reduces LDL-C by 20-30% (Table 31–9).

The initial recommended dose of **lovastatin** (MEVACOR) is 20 mg and is slightly more effective if taken with the evening meal than if it is taken at bedtime. The dose of lovastatin may be increased every 3-6 weeks up to a maximum of 80 mg/day. The 80-mg dose is slightly (2-3%) more effective if given as 40 mg twice daily. Lovastatin, at 20 mg, is marketed in combination with 500, 750, or 1000 mg of extended-release niacin (ADVICOR). Few patients are appropriate candidates for this fixed-dose combination (*see* next section on "Nicotinic Acid").

The usual starting dose of **simvastatin** (ZOCOR) for most patients is 20 mg at bedtime. The maximal dose is 80 mg. In patients taking cyclosporine, fibrates, or niacin, the daily dose should not exceed 20 mg. Simvastatin, 20 mg, is marketed in combination with 500, 750, or 1000 mg of extended-release niacin (SIMCOR).

Pravastatin (PRAVACHOL) therapy is initiated with a 20- or 40-mg dose that may be increased to 80 mg. This drug should be taken at bedtime. Because pravastatin is a hydroxy acid, bile-acid sequestrants will bind it and reduce its absorption. Pravastatin also is marketed in combination with buffered aspirin (PRAVIGARD). The small advantage of combining these 2 drugs should be weighed against the disadvantages inherent in fixed-dose combinations.

For **fluvastatin** (LESCOL), the starting dose is 20 or 40 mg, and the maximum is 80 mg/day. Like pravastatin, it is administered as a hydroxy acid and should be taken at bedtime, several hours after ingesting a bile-acid sequestrant (if the combination is used).

Atorvastatin (LIPITOR) has a long $t_{1/2}$, which allows administration of this statin at any time of the day. The starting dose is 10 mg, and the maximum is 80 mg/day. Atorvastatin is marketed in combination with the Ca^{2+}-channel blocker amlodipine (CADUET) for patients with hypertension or angina as well as hypercholesterolemia.

Rosuvastatin (CRESTOR) is available in doses ranging between 5 and 40 mg. It has a $t_{1/2}$ of 20-30 h and may be taken at any time of day. If the combination of gemfibrozil with rosuvastatin is used, the dose of rosuvastatin should not exceed 10 mg.

Pitavastatin (LIVALO) is available in doses of 1, 2, and 4 mg. Gemfibrozil reduces clearance of pitavastatin and raises blood concentrations; consequently, gemfibrozil should be used cautiously, if at all, in combination with pitavastatin.

The choice of statins should be based on efficacy (reduction of LDL-C) and cost. Three drugs (lovastatin, simvastatin, and pravastatin) have been used safely in clinical trials. Baseline determinations of ALT and repeat testing at 3-6 months are recommended. If ALT is normal after the initial 3-6 months, then it need not be repeated more than once every 6-12 months. Measurements of CK are not routinely necessary unless the patient also is taking a drug that enhances the risk of myopathy.

Statins in Combination with Other Lipid-Lowering Drugs. Statins, in combination with the bile acid–binding resins *cholestyramine* and *colestipol*, produce 20-30% greater reductions in LDL-C than can be achieved with statins alone. Preliminary data indicate that *colesevelam hydrochloride* plus a statin lowers LDL-C by 8-16% more than statins alone. Niacin also can enhance the effect of statins, but the occurrence of myopathy increases when statin doses >25% of maximum (e.g., 20 mg of simvastatin or atorvastatin) are used with niacin. The combination of a fibrate (*clofibrate*, gemfibrozil, or fenofibrate) with a statin is particularly useful in patients with hypertriglyceridemia and high LDL-C levels. This combination increases the risk of myopathy but usually is safe with a fibrate at its usual maximal dose and a statin at no more than 25% of its maximal dose. Triple therapy with resins, niacin, and statins can reduce LDL-C by up to 70%. VYTORIN, a fixed-dose combination of simvastatin (10, 20, 40, or 80 mg) and ezetimibe (10 mg), decreased LDL-C levels by up to 60% at 24 weeks.

Statin Use by Children. Some statins have been approved for use in children with heterozygous familial hypercholesterolemia. Atorvastatin, lovastatin, and simvastatin are indicated for children ≥11 years. Pravastatin is approved for children ≥8 years.

Pregnancy. The safety of statins during pregnancy has not been established.

BILE-ACID SEQUESTRANTS

CHOLESTYRAMINE, COLESTIPOL, COLESEVELAM. The bile-acid sequestrants cholestyramine and colestipol are among the oldest of the hypolipidemic drugs and are probably the safest, because they are not absorbed from the intestine. These resins also are recommended for patients 11-20 years of age. Because statins are so effective as monotherapy, the resins are most often used as second agents if statin therapy does not lower LDL-C levels sufficiently. When used with a statin, cholestyramine and colestipol usually are prescribed at submaximal doses. Maximal doses can reduce LDL-C by up to 25% but are associated with unacceptable GI side effects (bloating and constipation). Colesevelam, a newer bile-acid sequestrant, lowers LDL-C by 18% at its maximum dose.

MECHANISM OF ACTION. The bile-acid sequestrants are highly positively charged and bind negatively charged bile acids. Because of their large size, the resins are not absorbed, and the bound bile acids are excreted in the stool. Because more than 95% of bile acids are normally reabsorbed, interruption of this process depletes the pool of bile acids, and hepatic bile-acid synthesis increases. As a result, hepatic cholesterol content declines, stimulating the production of LDL receptors, an effect similar to that of statins. The increase in hepatic LDL receptors increases LDL clearance and lowers LDL-C levels, but this effect is partially offset by the enhanced cholesterol synthesis caused by upregulation of HMG-CoA reductase. Inhibition of reductase activity by a statin substantially increases the effectiveness of the resins. The resin-induced increase in bile-acid production is accompanied by an increase in hepatic triglyceride synthesis, which is of consequence in patients with significant hypertriglyceridemia (baseline triglyceride level >250 mg/dL). Use of colesevelam to lower LDL-C levels in hypertriglyceridemic patients should be accompanied by frequent (every 1-2 weeks) monitoring of fasting triglyceride levels.

EFFECTS ON LIPOPROTEIN LEVELS. The reduction in LDL-C by resins is dose dependent. Doses of 8-12 g of cholestyramine or 10-15 g of colestipol are associated with 12-18% reductions in LDL-C. Maximal doses (24 g of cholestyramine, 30 g of colestipol) may reduce LDL-C by as much as 25% but will cause GI side effects. One to 2 weeks is sufficient to attain maximal LDL-C reduction by a given resin dose. In patients with normal triglyceride levels, triglycerides may increase transiently and then return to baseline. HDL-C levels increase 4-5%. Statins plus resins or niacin plus resins can reduce LDL-C by 40-60%. Colesevelam, in doses of 3-3.75 g, reduces LDL-C levels by 9-19%.

ADVERSE EFFECTS AND DRUG INTERACTIONS. The resins are generally safe, as they are not systemically absorbed. Because they are administered as chloride salts, rare instances of hyperchloremic acidosis have been reported. Severe hypertriglyceridemia is a contraindication to the use of cholestyramine and colestipol because these resins increase triglyceride levels. At present, there are insufficient data on the effect of colesevelam on triglyceride levels.

Cholestyramine and colestipol both are available as a powder that must be mixed with water and drunk as a slurry. The gritty sensation is unpleasant but generally tolerated. Colestipol is available in a tablet form. Colesevelam is available as a hard capsule that absorbs water and creates a soft, gelatinous material that allegedly minimizes the potential for GI irritation. Patients taking cholestyramine and colestipol complain of bloating and dyspepsia. These symptoms can be substantially reduced if the drug is completely suspended in liquid several hours before ingestion. Constipation may occur but sometimes can be prevented by adequate daily water intake and psyllium. Colesevelam may be less likely to cause the dyspepsia, bloating, and constipation.

Cholestyramine and colestipol bind and interfere with the absorption of many drugs, including some thiazides, *furosemide*, *propranolol*, L-*thyroxine*, digoxin, warfarin, and some of the statins. The effect of cholestyramine and colestipol on the absorption of most drugs has not been studied. For this reason, it is wise to administer all drugs either 1 h before or 3-4 h after a dose of cholestyramine or colestipol. Colesevelam does not appear to interfere with the absorption of fat-soluble vitamins or of drugs such as digoxin, lovastatin, warfarin, *metoprolol*, *quinidine*, and *valproic acid*. Colesevelam reduces the maximum concentration and the AUC of sustained-release *verapamil* by 31% and 11%, respectively. In the absence of information to the contrary, prudence suggests that patients take other medications 1 h before or 3-4 h after a dose of colesevelam. The safety and efficacy of colesevelam have not been studied in pediatric patients or pregnant women.

PREPARATIONS AND USE. The powdered forms of cholestyramine (QUESTRAN, others, 4 g/dose) and colestipol (COLESTID, others, 5 g/dose) are either mixed with a fluid (water or juice) and drunk as a slurry or mixed with crushed ice in a blender. Ideally, patients should take the resins before breakfast and before supper, starting with 1 scoop or packet twice daily, and increasing the dosage after several weeks or longer as needed and as tolerated. Patients generally will not take more than 2 doses (scoops or packets) twice daily. Colesevelam hydrochloride (WELCHOL) is available as a solid tablet containing 0.625 g of colesevelam and as a powder in packets of 3.75 g or 1.875 g. The starting dose is either 3 tablets taken twice daily with meals or all 6 tablets taken with a meal. The tablets should be taken with a liquid. The maximum daily dose is 7 tablets (4.375 g).

NIACIN (*NICOTINIC ACID*)

Niacin is a water-soluble B-complex vitamin that functions as a vitamin only after conversion to NAD or NADP, in which it occurs as an amide. Both niacin and its amide may be given orally as a source of niacin for its functions as a vitamin, but only niacin affects lipid levels. The hypolipidemic effects of niacin require larger doses than are required for its vitamin effects.

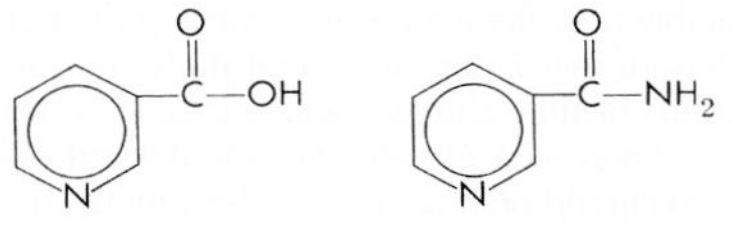

NICOTINIC ACID NICOTINAMIDE

MECHANISM OF ACTION. In adipose tissue, niacin inhibits the lipolysis of triglycerides by hormone-sensitive lipase, which reduces transport of free fatty acids to the liver and decreases hepatic triglyceride synthesis. Niacin may exert its effects on lipolysis by stimulating a GPCR (GPR109A) that couples to G_i and inhibits cyclic AMP production in adipocytes. In the liver, niacin reduces triglyceride synthesis by inhibiting both the synthesis and esterification of fatty acids, effects that increase apoB degradation. Reduction of triglyceride synthesis reduces hepatic VLDL production, which accounts for the reduced LDL levels. Niacin also enhances LPL activity, which promotes the clearance of chylomicrons and VLDL triglycerides. Niacin raises HDL-C levels by decreasing the fractional clearance of apoA-I in HDL rather than by enhancing HDL synthesis.

EFFECTS ON PLASMA LIPOPROTEIN LEVELS. Regular or crystalline niacin in doses of 2-6 g/day reduces triglycerides by 35-50% (as effectively as fibrates and statins); the maximal effect occurs within 4-7 days. Reductions of 25% in LDL-C levels are possible with doses of 4.5-6 g/day; 3-6 weeks are required for maximal effect. Niacin is the best agent available for increasing HDL-C (30-40%), but the effect is less in patients with HDL-C levels <35 mg/dL. Niacin also is the only lipid-lowering drug that reduces Lp(a) levels significantly. Despite salutary effect on lipids, niacin's side effects limit its use (see "Adverse Effects").

ADME. The doses of regular (crystalline) niacin used to treat dyslipidemia are almost completely absorbed, and peak plasma concentrations (up to 0.24 mmol) are achieved within 30-60 min. The $t_{1/2}$ is about 60 min, which necessitates dosing 2 to 3 times daily. At lower doses, most niacin is taken up by the liver; only the major metabolite, nicotinuric acid, is found in the urine. At higher doses, a greater proportion of the drug is excreted in the urine as unchanged nicotinic acid.

ADVERSE EFFECTS. Two of niacin's side effects, flushing and dyspepsia, limit patient compliance. The cutaneous effects include flushing and pruritus of the face and upper trunk, skin rashes, and acanthosis nigricans. Flushing and associated pruritus are prostaglandin mediated. Taking an aspirin each day alleviates the flushing in many patients. Flushing is worse when therapy is initiated or the dosage is increased but ceases in most patients after 1-2 weeks of a stable dose. Flushing is more likely to occur when niacin is consumed with hot beverages or with alcohol. Flushing is minimized if therapy is initiated with low doses (100-250 mg twice daily) and if the drug is taken after a meal. Dry skin, a frequent complaint, can be dealt with by using skin moisturizers, and acanthosis nigricans can be dealt with by using lotions containing *salicylic acid*. Dyspepsia and rarer episodes of nausea, vomiting, and diarrhea are less likely to occur if the drug is taken after a meal. Patients with any history of peptic ulcer disease should not take niacin.

The most common, medically serious side effects are hepatotoxicity, manifested as elevated serum transaminases, and hyperglycemia. Both regular (crystalline) niacin and sustained-release niacin, which was developed to reduce flushing and itching, have been reported to cause severe liver toxicity. An extended-release niacin (NIASPAN) appears to be less likely to cause severe hepatotoxicity, perhaps simply because it is administered once daily. The incidence of flushing and pruritus with this preparation is not substantially different from that with regular niacin. Severe hepatotoxicity is more likely to occur when patients take more than 2 g of sustained-release, over-the-counter preparations. Affected patients experience flu-like fatigue and weakness. Usually, aspartate transaminase and ALT are elevated, serum albumin levels decline, and total cholesterol and LDL-C levels decline substantially.

In patients with diabetes mellitus, niacin should be used cautiously because niacin-induced insulin resistance can cause severe hyperglycemia. If niacin is prescribed for patients with known or suspected diabetes, blood glucose levels should be monitored at least weekly until proven to be stable. Niacin also elevates uric acid levels and may reactivate gout. A history of gout is a relative contraindication for niacin use. Rarer reversible side effects include toxic amblyopia and toxic maculopathy. Atrial tachyarrhythmias and atrial fibrillation have been reported, more commonly in elderly patients. *Niacin, at doses used in humans, has been associated with birth defects in experimental animals and should not be taken by pregnant women.*

THERAPEUTIC USE. Niacin is indicated for hypertriglyceridemia and elevated LDL-C; it is especially useful in patients with both hypertriglyceridemia and low HDL-C levels. There are 2 commonly available forms of niacin. Crystalline niacin (immediate-release or regular) refers to niacin tablets that dissolve quickly after ingestion. Sustained-release niacin refers to preparations that continuously release niacin for 6-8 h after ingestion. NIASPAN is the only preparation of niacin that is FDA-approved for treating dyslipidemia and that requires a prescription.

Crystalline niacin tablets are available over the counter in a variety of strengths from 50- to 500-mg tablets. The dose may be increased stepwise every 7 days to a total daily dose of 1.5-2 g. After 2-4 weeks at this dose, transaminases, serum albumin, fasting glucose, and uric acid levels should be measured. Lipid levels should be checked and the dose increased further until the desired effect on plasma lipids is achieved. After a stable dose is attained, blood should be drawn every 3-6 months to monitor for the various toxicities. Over-the-counter, sustained-release niacin preparations and NIASPAN are effective up to a total daily dose of 2 g. All doses of sustained-release niacin, but particularly doses above 2 g/day, have been reported to cause hepatotoxicity, which may occur soon after beginning therapy or after several years of use. The potential for severe liver damage should preclude use of OTC preparations in most patients. NIASPAN may be less likely to cause hepatotoxicity.

Because concurrent use of niacin and a statin can cause myopathy, the statin should be administered at no more than 25% of its maximal dose. Patients also should be instructed to discontinue therapy if flu-like muscle aches occur. Routine measurement of CK in patients taking niacin and statins does not assure that severe myopathy will be detected before onset of symptoms.

FIBRIC ACID DERIVATIVES: PPAR ACTIVATORS

Clofibrate is a halogenated fibric acid derivative. Gemfibrozil is a nonhalogenated acid that is distinct from the halogenated fibrates. A number of fibric acid analogs (e.g., fenofibrate, *bezafibrate*, *ciprofibrate*) have been developed and are used in Europe and elsewhere.

MECHANISM OF ACTION. The mechanisms by which fibrates lower lipoprotein levels, or raise HDL levels, remain unclear. Many of the effects of these compounds on blood lipids are mediated by their interaction with peroxisome proliferator-activated receptors (PPARs), which regulate gene transcription. Fibrates bind to PPARα and reduce triglycerides through PPARα-mediated stimulation of fatty acid oxidation, increased LPL synthesis, and reduced expression of apoC-III. Increased LPL synthesis would enhance the clearance of triglyceride-rich lipoproteins. Reduced hepatic production of apoC-III, which serves as an inhibitor of lipolysis and receptor-mediated clearance, would enhance the clearance of VLDL. Fibrate-mediated increases in HDL-C are due to PPARα stimulation of apoA-I and apoA-II expression, which increases HDL levels. Fenofibrate is more effective than gemfibrozil at increasing HDL levels. Most fibrates have potential anti-thrombotic effects, including inhibition of coagulation and enhancement of fibrinolysis.

EFFECTS ON LIPOPROTEIN LEVELS. Effects of fibric acid agents on lipoprotein levels differ widely, depending on the starting lipoprotein profile, the presence or absence of a genetic hyperlipoproteinemia, the associated environmental influences, and the specific fibrate used. Patients with type III hyperlipoproteinemia (dysbetalipoproteinemia) are among the most sensitive responders to fibrates. Elevated triglyceride and cholesterol levels are dramatically lowered, and tuberoeruptive and palmar xanthomas may regress completely. Angina and intermittent claudication also improve.

In patients with mild hypertriglyceridemia (e.g., triglycerides <400 mg/dL), fibrate treatment decreases triglyceride levels by up to 50% and increases HDL-C concentrations by about 15%; LDL-C levels may be unchanged or increase. Normotriglyceridemic patients with heterozygous familial hypercholesterolemia usually experience little change in LDL levels with gemfibrozil; with the other fibric acid agents, reductions as great as 20% may occur in some patients. Fibrates usually are the drugs of choice for treating severe hypertriglyceridemia and the chylomicronemia syndrome. While the primary therapy is to remove alcohol and lower dietary fat intake as much as possible, fibrates assist by increasing triglyceride clearance and decreasing hepatic triglyceride synthesis. In patients with chylomicronemia syndrome, fibrate maintenance therapy and a low-fat diet keep triglyceride levels well below 1000 mg/dL and thus prevent episodes of pancreatitis.

ADME. Fibrates are absorbed rapidly and efficiently (>90%) when given with a meal but less efficiently when taken on an empty stomach. Peak plasma concentrations are attained within 1-4 h. More than 95% of these drugs in plasma are bound to protein, nearly exclusively to albumin. The $t_{1/2}$ of fibrates range from 1.1 h (gemfibrozil) to 20 h (fenofibrate). The drugs are widely distributed throughout the body, and concentrations in liver, kidney, and intestine exceed the plasma level. Gemfibrozil is transferred across the placenta. The fibrate drugs are excreted predominantly as glucuronide conjugates (60-90%) in the urine, with smaller amounts appearing in the feces. Excretion of these drugs is impaired in renal failure.

ADVERSE EFFECTS AND DRUG INTERACTIONS. Fibric acid compounds usually are well tolerated. GI side effects occur in up to 5% of patients. Infrequent side effects include rash, urticaria, hair loss, myalgias, fatigue, headache, impotence, and anemia. Minor increases in liver transaminases and alkaline phosphatase have been reported. Clofibrate, bezafibrate, and fenofibrate reportedly potentiate the action of oral anticoagulants, in part by displacing them from binding sites on albumin. Careful monitoring of the prothrombin time and reduction in dosage of the anticoagulant may be appropriate.

A myopathy syndrome occasionally occurs in subjects taking clofibrate, gemfibrozil, or fenofibrate and may occur in up to 5% of patients treated with a combination of gemfibrozil and higher doses of statins. Statin doses should be reduced when combination therapy is employed. Gemfibrozil inhibits hepatic uptake of statins by OATP1B1, and competes for the same glucuronosyl transferases that metabolize most statins. Thus, levels of both drugs may be elevated when they are coadministered. Patients taking this combination should be followed at 3-month intervals with careful history and determination of CK values until a stable pattern is established. Patients taking fibrates with rosuvastatin should be followed especially closely even if low doses (5-10 mg) of rosuvastatin are employed. Fenofibrate is glucuronidated by enzymes that are not involved in statin glucuronidation; thus, fenofibrate-statin combinations are less likely to cause myopathy than combination therapy with gemfibrozil and statins.

All of the fibrates increase the lithogenicity of bile. Clofibrate use has been associated with increased risk of gallstone formation. Renal failure is a relative contraindication to the use of fibric acid agents, as is hepatic dysfunction. *Fibrates should not be used by children or pregnant women.*

THERAPEUTIC USE. Clofibrate is available for oral administration and may be useful in patients who do not tolerate gemfibrozil or fenofibrate. The usual dose is 2 g/day in divided doses. Gemfibrozil (LOPID) usually is administered as a 600-mg dose taken twice daily, 30 min before the morning and evening meals. The TRICOR brand of fenofibrate is available in tablets of 48 and 145 mg. The usual daily dose is 145 mg. Generic fenofibrate (LOFIBRA) is available in capsules containing 67, 134, and 200 mg. The choline salt of fenofibric acid (TRILIPIX) is available in capsules of 135 and 45 mg. TRILIPIX, 135 mg, is equivalent to TRICOR, 145 mg, and LOFIBRA, 200 mg. Fibrates are the drugs of choice for treating hyperlipidemic subjects with type III hyperlipoproteinemia as well as subjects with severe hypertriglyceridemia (triglycerides >1000 mg/dL) who are at risk for pancreatitis. Fibrates appear to have an important role in subjects with high triglycerides and low HDL-C levels associated with the metabolic syndrome or type 2 diabetes mellitus. In these patients, the LDL levels need to be monitored; if LDL levels rise, the addition of a low dose of a statin may be needed. Many experts now treat such patients first with a statin and then add a fibrate, based on the reported benefit of gemfibrozil therapy.

EZETIMIBE AND THE INHIBITION OF DIETARY CHOLESTEROL UPTAKE

Ezetimibe is the first compound approved for lowering total and LDL-C levels that inhibits cholesterol absorption by enterocytes in the small intestine. It lowers LDL-C levels by ~20% and is used primarily as adjunctive therapy with statins.

MECHANISM OF ACTION. Ezetimibe inhibits luminal cholesterol uptake by jejunal enterocytes, by inhibiting the transport protein NPC1L1. In human subjects, ezetimibe reduces cholesterol absorption by 54%, precipitating a compensatory increase in cholesterol synthesis that can be inhibited with a cholesterol synthesis inhibitor (e.g., a statin). The consequence of inhibiting intestinal cholesterol absorption is a reduction in the incorporation of cholesterol into chylomicrons; this diminishes the delivery of cholesterol to the liver by chylomicron remnants. The diminished remnant cholesterol content may decrease atherogenesis directly, as chylomicron remnants are very atherogenic lipoproteins. Reduced delivery of intestinal cholesterol to the liver by chylomicron remnants stimulates expression of the hepatic genes regulating LDL receptor expression and cholesterol biosynthesis. The greater expression of hepatic LDL receptors enhances LDL-C clearance from the plasma. Ezetimibe reduces LDL-C levels by 15-20%.

ADME. Ezetimibe is highly water insoluble, precluding studies of its bioavailability. After ingestion, it is glucuronidated in the intestinal epithelium and absorbed and then enters an enterohepatic recirculation. Pharmacokinetic studies indicate that about 70% is excreted in the feces and about 10% in the urine (as a glucuronide conjugate). Bile-acid sequestrants inhibit absorption of ezetimibe, and the 2 agents should not be administered together.

ADVERSE EFFECTS AND DRUG INTERACTIONS. Other than rare allergic reactions, specific adverse effects have not been observed in patients taking ezetimibe. *Since all statins are contraindicated in pregnant and nursing women, combination products containing ezetimibe and a statin should not be used by women in childbearing years in the absence of contraception.*

THERAPEUTIC USE. Ezetimibe (ZETIA) is available as a 10-mg tablet that may be taken at any time during the day, with or without food. Ezetimibe may be taken with any medication other than bile-acid sequestrants, which inhibit its absorption.

The role of ezetimibe as monotherapy of patients with elevated LDL-C levels is limited to the small group of statin-intolerant patients. The actions of are complementary to those of statins. Dual therapy with these 2 classes of drugs prevents both the enhanced cholesterol synthesis induced by ezetimibe and the increase in cholesterol absorption induced by statins, providing additive reductions in LDL-C levels. A combination tablet containing ezetimibe, 10 mg, and various doses of simvastatin (10, 20, 40, and 80 mg) has been approved (VYTORIN). At the highest simvastatin dose (80 mg), plus ezetimibe (10 mg), average LDL-C reduction was 60%.

RECENTLY APPROVED ADJUNCT MEDICATIONS

ICOSAPENT ETHYL. Icosapent ethyl (VASCEPA) is an ethyl ester derivative of the omega-3 fatty acid eicosapentaenoic acid (EPA). EPA reduces VLDL triglycerides and is used as an adjunct to diet for treatment of adult patients with severe hypertriglyceridemia (≥500 mg/dL). Recommended daily oral dose is 4 g/day administered with food. Adverse effects may include arthralgia. Since omega-3-fatty acids may prolong bleeding time, patients taking anticoagulants should be monitored.

LOMITAPIDE. Lomitapide mesylate (JUXTAPID) acts by inhibiting MTP, which is essential for formation of VLDL. Lomitapide is used as an adjunct to diet for lowering LDL-C, total cholesterol, apoB, and non-HDL-C in patients with homozygous familial hypercholesterolemia. The recommended starting oral dose (5 mg/day) is titrated upwards to a maximum dose of 60 mg daily. The drug is metabolized by CYP3A4 and is contraindicated with inhibitors of CYP3A4. Reported adverse effects include diarrhea, vomiting, abdominal pain, and hepatotoxicity. The agent is used under an FDA risk evaluation and mitigation strategy.

MIPOMERSEN SODIUM. Mipomersen (KYNAMRO), an antisense oligonucleotide, inhibits the synthesis of apoB-100. The drug is approved as an addition to lipid-lowering medications and diet for patients with homozygous familial hypercholesterolemia. The recommended dose is 1 mL of 200 mg/mL solution, injected subcutaneously, once a week. Common adverse effects include injection site reactions, flu-like symptoms, headache, and elevation of liver enzymes. The agent is used under an FDA risk evaluation and mitigation strategy.

For a complete Bibliographical Listing see Goodman & Gilman's ***The Pharmacological Basis of Therapeutics***, 12th ed., or Goodman & Gilman Online at www.AccessMedicine.com.

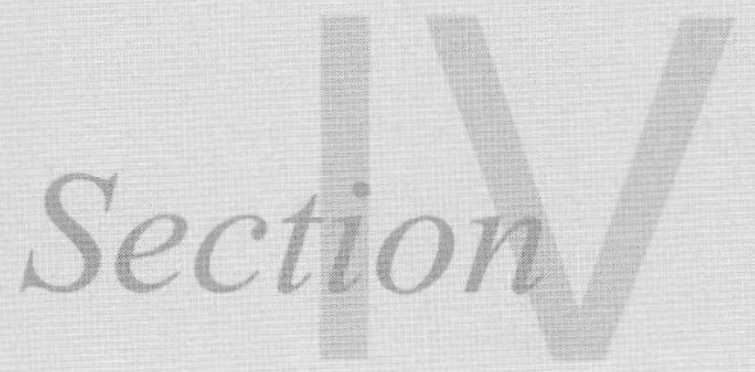

Section IV Inflammation, Immunomodulation, and Hematopoiesis

chapter 32 Histamine, Bradykinin, and Their Antagonists

Histamine is a major mediator of inflammation, anaphylaxis, and gastric acid secretion; in addition, histamine plays a role in neurotransmission. Our understanding of the physiological and pathophysiological roles of histamine has been enhanced by the development of subtype-specific receptor antagonists and by the cloning of 4 receptors for histamine. Competitive antagonists of H_1 receptors are used therapeutically in treating allergies, urticaria, anaphylactic reactions, nausea, motion sickness, insomnia, and some symptoms of asthma. Antagonists of the H_2 receptor are effective in reducing gastric acid secretion. The peptide, bradykinin, has cardiovascular effects similar to those of histamine and plays prominent roles in inflammation and nociception.

HISTAMINE

Histamine is a hydrophilic molecule consisting of an imidazole ring and an amino group connected by an ethylene group, biosynthesized from histidine by decarboxylation (Figure 32–1). The 4 histamine receptors, all GPCRs, can be differentially activated by analogs of histamine and inhibited by specific antagonists (Table 32–1).

DISTRIBUTION AND BIOSYNTHESIS

DISTRIBUTION. Almost all mammalian tissues contain histamine in amounts ranging from <1 to >100 μg/g. Concentrations in plasma and other body fluids generally are very low, but human cerebrospinal fluid (CSF) contains significant amounts. The concentration of histamine is particularly high in tissues that contain large numbers of mast cells, such as skin, bronchial mucosa, and intestinal mucosa.

SYNTHESIS, STORAGE, AND METABOLISM. Histamine is formed by the decarboxylation of the amino acid histidine by the enzyme L-histidine decarboxylase (*see* Figure 32–1). Mast cells and basophils synthesize histamine and store it in secretory granules. At the secretory granule pH of ~5.5, histamine is positively charged and ionically complexed with negatively charged acidic groups on other granule constituents, primarily proteases and heparin or chondroitin sulfate proteoglycans. The turnover rate of histamine in secretory granules is slow. Non–mast cell sites of histamine formation include the epidermis, the gastric mucosa, neurons within the CNS, and cells in regenerating or rapidly growing tissues. Turnover is rapid at these non–mast cell sites because the histamine is released continuously rather than stored. Non–mast cell sites of histamine production contribute significantly to the daily excretion of histamine metabolites in the urine. Because L-histidine decarboxylase is an inducible enzyme, the histamine-forming capacity at such sites is subject to regulation. Histamine that is ingested is rapidly metabolized, and the metabolites are eliminated in the urine.

RELEASE AND FUNCTIONS OF ENDOGENOUS HISTAMINE

Histamine is released from storage granules as a result of the interaction of antigen with immunoglobulin E (IgE) antibodies on the mast cell surface. Histamine plays a central role in immediate hypersensitivity and allergic responses. The actions of histamine on bronchial smooth muscle and blood vessels account for many of the symptoms of the allergic response. In addition, some drugs act directly on mast cells to release histamine, causing untoward effects. Histamine has a major role in regulating gastric acid secretion and also modulates neurotransmitter release.

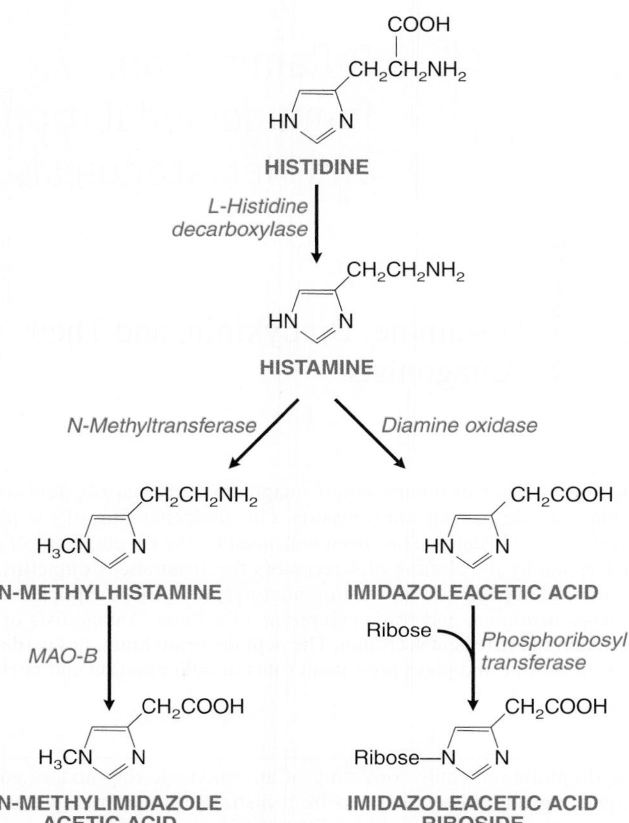

Figure 32–1 *Histamine synthesis and metabolism in humans.* Histamine is synthesized from histidine by decarboxylation. Histamine is metabolized via 2 pathways, predominantly by methylation of the ring followed by oxidative deamination (*left side of figure*), and secondarily by oxidative deamination and then conjugation with ribose. These metabolites have little or no activity and are excreted in the urine. Measurement of urinary *N*-methylhistamine affords a reliable index of histamine production. Artifactually elevated levels of histamine in urine arise from genitourinary tract bacteria that can decarboxylate histidine. MAO, monoamine oxidase.

ROLE IN ALLERGIC RESPONSES. The principal target cells of immediate hypersensitivity reactions are mast cells and basophils. As part of the allergic response to an antigen, IgE antibodies are generated and bind to the surfaces of mast cells and basophils via specific high-affinity F_c receptors. This receptor, FcεRI, consists of α, β, and 2 γ chains (*see* Chapter 35). Antigen bridges the IgE molecules and via FcεRI activates signaling pathways in mast cells or basophils involving tyrosine kinases and subsequent phosphorylation of multiple protein substrates within 5-15 sec of contact with antigen. These events trigger the exocytosis of the contents of secretory granules.

RELEASE OF OTHER AUTACOIDS. Stimulation of IgE receptors also activates phospholipase A_2 (PLA_2), leading to the production of a host of mediators, including platelet-activating factor (PAF) and metabolites of arachidonic acid such as leukotrienes C_4 and D_4, which contract the smooth muscles of the bronchial tree.

HISTAMINE RELEASE BY DRUGS, PEPTIDES, VENOMS, AND OTHER AGENTS. Many compounds, including a large number of therapeutic agents, stimulate the release of histamine from mast cells directly and without prior sensitization. Responses of this sort are most likely to occur following intravenous injections of certain categories of substances. Tubocurarine, succinylcholine, morphine, some antibiotics, radiocontrast media, and certain carbohydrate plasma expanders also may elicit the response. The phenomenon is one of clinical concern, and may account for unexpected anaphylactoid reactions. Basic polypeptides often are effective histamine releasers, and over a limited range, their potency generally increases with the number of basic groups. For example, bradykinin is a poor histamine releaser, whereas kallidin (Lys-bradykinin) and substance P, with more positively charged amino acids, are more active. Some venoms, such as that of the wasp, contain potent

Table 32–1

Characteristics of Histamine Receptors

	H_1	H_2	H_3	H_4
G protein coupling (2nd messengers)	$G_{q/11}$ (↑ Ca^{2+}; ↑ NO and ↑ cGMP)	G_s (↑ cAMP)	$G_{i/o}$ (↓ cAMP; ↑ MAPK)	$G_{i/o}$ (↓ cAMP; ↑ Ca^{2+})
Distribution	Smooth muscle, endothelial cells, CNS	Gastric parietal cells, cardiac muscle, mast cells, CNS	CNS: presynaptic	Cells of hematopoietic origin
Representative agonist	2-CH_3-histamine	Amthamine	(*R*)-α-CH_3-histamine	4-CH_3-histamine
Representative antagonist	Chlorpheniramine	Ranitidine	Tiprolisant	JNJ7777120

cAMP, cyclic AMP; cGMP, cyclic GMP; CNS, central nervous system; MAPK, MAP kinase; NO, nitric oxide.

histamine-releasing peptides. Basic polypeptides released upon tissue injury constitute pathophysiological stimuli to secretion for mast cells and basophils.

Within seconds of the intravenous injection of a histamine liberator, human subjects experience a burning, itching sensation. This effect, most marked in the palms of the hand and in the face, scalp, and ears, is soon followed by a feeling of intense warmth. The skin reddens, and the color rapidly spreads over the trunk. Blood pressure falls, the heart rate accelerates, and the subject usually complains of headache. After a few minutes, blood pressure recovers, and crops of hives usually appear on the skin. Colic, nausea, hypersecretion of acid, and moderate bronchospasm also frequently occur. Histamine liberators do not deplete tissues of non–mast cell histamine.

INCREASED PROLIFERATION OF MAST CELLS AND BASOPHILS AND GASTRIC CARCINOID TUMORS. In urticaria pigmentosa (cutaneous mastocytosis), mast cells aggregate in the upper corium and give rise to pigmented cutaneous lesions that sting when stroked. In systemic mastocytosis, overproliferation of mast cells also is found in other organs. Patients with these syndromes suffer a constellation of signs and symptoms attributable to excessive histamine release, including urticaria, dermographism, pruritus, headache, weakness, hypotension, flushing of the face, and a variety of GI effects, such as diarrhea or peptic ulceration. Gastric carcinoid tumors secrete histamine, which is responsible for episodes of vasodilation as part of the patchy "geographical" flush.

GASTRIC ACID SECRETION. Histamine acting at H_2 receptors is a powerful gastric secretagogue, evoking a copious secretion of acid from parietal cells (*see* Figure 45–1); it also increases the output of pepsin and intrinsic factor. The secretion of gastric acid from parietal cells also is caused by stimulation of the vagus nerve and by the enteric hormone gastrin. However, histamine undoubtedly is the dominant physiological mediator of acid secretion; blockade of H_2 receptors not only antagonizes acid secretion in response to histamine but also inhibits responses to gastrin and vagal stimulation (*see* Chapter 45).

CNS. Histamine-containing neurons control both homeostatic and higher brain functions, including regulation of the sleep-wake cycle, circadian and feeding rhythms, immunity, learning, memory, drinking, and body temperature. However, no human disease has yet been directly linked to dysfunction of the brain histamine system. Histamine, histidine decarboxylase, enzymes that metabolize histamine, and H_1, H_2, and H_3 receptors are distributed widely but non-uniformly in the CNS. H_1 receptors are associated with both neuronal and non-neuronal cells and are concentrated in regions that control neuroendocrine function, behavior, and nutritional state. Distribution of H_2 receptors is more consistent with histaminergic projections than H_1 receptors, suggesting that they mediate many of the postsynaptic actions of histamine. H_3 receptors also are concentrated in areas known to receive histaminergic projections, consistent with their function as presynaptic autoreceptors. Histamine inhibits appetite and increases wakefulness via H_1 receptors.

PHARMACOLOGICAL EFFECTS

RECEPTOR–EFFECTOR COUPLING AND MECHANISMS OF ACTION. Histamine receptors are GPCRs, coupling to second messenger systems and producing effects as noted in Table 32–1.

H_3 and H_4 receptors have a much higher affinity for histamine than do H_1 and H_2 receptors. Activation of H_3 receptors also can activate MAP kinase and inhibit the Na^+/H^+ exchanger; activation of H_4 receptors mobilizes stored Ca^{2+} in some cells. Activation of H_1 receptors on vascular endothelium stimulates eNOS to produce nitric oxide (NO), which diffuses to nearby smooth muscle cells to increase cyclic GMP and cause relaxation. Stimulation of H_1 receptors on smooth muscle will mobilize Ca^{2+} and cause contraction, whereas activation of H_2 receptors on the same smooth muscle cell will link via G_s to enhanced cyclic AMP accumulation, activation of PKA, and thence to relaxation. Pharmacological definition of H_1, H_2, and H_3 receptors is clear because relatively specific agonists and antagonists are available. However, the H_4 receptor exhibits 35-40% homology to isoforms of the H_3 receptor, and the 2 were harder to distinguish pharmacologically. Several non-imidazole compounds that are more selective H_3 antagonists have been developed, and there are now several selective H_4 antagonists. 4-Methylhistamine and dimaprit, previously identified as specific H_2 agonists, are actually more potent H_4 agonists.

H_1 AND H_2 RECEPTORS. H_1 and H_2 receptors are distributed widely in the periphery and in the CNS. Histamine causes itching and stimulates secretion from nasal mucosa. It contracts many smooth muscles, such as those of the bronchi and gut, but markedly relaxes others, including those in small blood vessels. Histamine also is a potent stimulus of gastric acid secretion. Other, less prominent effects include formation of edema and stimulation of sensory nerve endings. Bronchoconstriction and contraction of the gut are mediated by H_1 receptors. Gastric secretion results from the activation of H_2 receptors. Some responses, such as vascular dilation, are mediated by both H_1 and H_2 receptor stimulation.

H_3 AND H_4 RECEPTORS. H_3 receptors are expressed mainly in the CNS, especially in the basal ganglia, hippocampus, and cortex. H_3 receptors function as autoreceptors on histaminergic neurons, inhibiting histamine release and modulating the release of other neurotransmitters. H_3 receptors have high constitutive activity and histamine release is tonically inhibited. Inverse agonists thus reduce receptor activation and increase histamine release from histaminergic neurons. H_3 agonists promote sleep; thus, H_3 antagonists promote wakefulness. H_4 receptors primarily are found in eosinophils, dendritic cells, mast cells, monocytes, basophils, and T cells but have also been detected in the GI tract, dermal fibroblasts, CNS, and primary sensory afferent neurons. Activation of H_4 receptors has been associated with induction of cellular shape change, chemotaxis, secretion of cytokines, and upregulation of adhesion molecules, suggesting that H_4 antagonists may be useful inhibitors of allergic and inflammatory responses.

FEEDBACK REGULATION OF RELEASE. H_2 receptor stimulation increases cyclic AMP and leads to feedback inhibition of histamine release from mast cells and basophils, whereas activation of H_3 and H_4 receptors has the opposite effect by decreasing cellular cyclic AMP. Activation of presynaptic H_3 receptors also inhibits histamine release from histaminergic neurons.

CARDIOVASCULAR SYSTEM. Histamine dilates resistance vessels, increases capillary permeability, and lowers systemic blood pressure. In some vascular beds, histamine constricts veins, contributing to the extravasation of fluid and edema formation upstream in capillaries and post-capillary venules.

Vasodilation. This is the most important vascular effect of histamine in humans. H_1 receptors have a higher affinity for histamine and cause Ca^{2+}-dependent activation of eNOS in endothelial cells; NO diffuses to vascular smooth muscle, increasing cyclic GMP (*see* Table 32–1) and causing rapid and short-lived vasodilation. By contrast, activation of H_2 receptors on vascular smooth muscle stimulates the cyclic AMP–PKA pathway, causing dilation that develops more slowly and is more sustained. As a result, H_1 antagonists effectively counter small dilator responses to low concentrations of histamine but only blunt the initial phase of larger responses to higher concentrations of the amine.

Increased "Capillary" Permeability. Histamine's effect on small vessels results in efflux of plasma protein and fluid into the extracellular spaces and an increase lymph flow, causing edema. H_1 receptors on endothelial cells are the major mediators of this response; the role of H_2 receptors is uncertain.

Triple Response of Lewis. If histamine is injected intradermally, it elicits a characteristic phenomenon known as the *triple response*. This consists of:

- A localized "reddening" around the injection site, appearing within a few seconds, maximal ~1 min
- A "flare" or red flushing extending ~1 cm beyond the original red spot and developing more slowly
- A "wheal" or swelling that is discernible in 1-2 min at the injection site

The initial red spot (a few mm) results from the direct vasodilating effect of histamine (H_1 receptor–mediated NO production), the flare is due to histamine-induced stimulation of axon reflexes that cause vasodilation indirectly, and the wheal reflects histamine's capacity to increase capillary permeability (edema formation).

Heart. Histamine affects both cardiac contractility and electrical events directly. It increases the force of contraction of both atrial and ventricular muscle by promoting the influx of Ca^{2+}, and it speeds heart rate by hastening diastolic depolarization in the sinoatrial (SA) node. It also directly slows atrioventricular (AV) conduction to increase automaticity and, in high doses, can elicit arrhythmias. The slowed AV conduction involves mainly H_1 receptors, while the other effects are largely attributable to H_2 receptors and cyclic AMP accumulation. The direct cardiac effects of histamine given intravenously are overshadowed by baroreceptor reflexes due to reduced blood pressure.

EXTRAVASCULAR SMOOTH MUSCLE. Histamine directly contracts or, more rarely, relaxes various extravascular smooth muscles. Contraction is due to activation of H_1 receptors on smooth muscle to increase intracellular Ca^{2+}, and relaxation is mainly due to activation of H_2 receptors. Although the spasmogenic influence of H_1 receptors is dominant in human bronchial muscle, H_2 receptors with dilator function also are present. Thus, histamine-induced bronchospasm in vitro is potentiated slightly by H_2 blockade.

PERIPHERAL NERVE ENDINGS. Histamine stimulates various nerve endings and sensory effects. In the epidermis, it causes itch; in the dermis, it evokes pain, sometimes accompanied by itching.

HISTAMINE SHOCK. Histamine given in large doses or released during systemic anaphylaxis causes a profound and progressive fall in blood pressure. As the small blood vessels dilate, they trap large amounts of blood, their permeability increases, and plasma escapes from the circulation. Resembling surgical or traumatic shock, these effects diminish effective blood volume, reduce venous return, and greatly lower cardiac output.

HISTAMINE TOXICITY FROM INGESTION. Histamine is the toxin in food poisoning from spoiled scombroid fish such as tuna. Symptoms include severe nausea, vomiting, headache, flushing, and sweating. Histamine toxicity also can follow red wine consumption in persons with a diminished ability to degrade histamine. The symptoms of histamine poisoning can be suppressed by H_1 antagonists.

H_1 RECEPTOR ANTAGONISTS

PHARMACOLOGICAL PROPERTIES

All the available H_1 receptor "antagonists" are actually inverse agonists (*see* Chapter 3) that reduce constitutive activity of the receptor and compete with histamine. At the tissue level, the effect is proportional to receptor occupancy by the antihistamine. Most H_1 antagonists have similar pharmacological actions and therapeutic applications. Their effects are largely predictable from knowledge of the consequences of the activation of H_1 receptors by histamine.

Like histamine, many H_1 antagonists contain a substituted ethylamine moiety.

$$-\overset{|}{\underset{|}{C}}-\overset{|}{\underset{|}{C}}-N\langle$$

Unlike histamine, which has a primary amino group and a single aromatic ring, most H_1 antagonists have a tertiary amino group linked by a 2- or 3-atom chain to 2 aromatic substituents and conform to the general formula

$$\begin{matrix} Ar_1 \\ Ar_2 \end{matrix}\rangle X-\overset{|}{\underset{|}{C}}-\overset{|}{\underset{|}{C}}-N\langle$$

where Ar is aryl and X is a nitrogen or carbon atom or a —C—O— ether linkage to the β-aminoethyl side chain. Sometimes the 2 aromatic rings are bridged, as in the tricyclic derivatives, or the ethylamine may be part of a ring structure.

EFFECTS ON PHYSIOLOGICAL SYSTEMS

Smooth Muscle. H_1 antagonists inhibit both the vasoconstrictor effects of histamine and, to a degree, the more rapid vasodilator effects mediated by activation of H_1 receptors on endothelial cells (synthesis/release of NO and other mediators).

Capillary Permeability. H_1 antagonists strongly block the increased capillary permeability and formation of edema and wheal caused by histamine.

Flare and Itch. H_1 antagonists suppress the action of histamine on nerve endings, including the flare component of the triple response and the itching caused by intradermal injection.

Exocrine Glands. H_1 antagonists do not suppress gastric secretion. However, the antimuscarinic properties of many H_1 antagonists may contribute to lessened secretion in cholinergically innervated glands and reduce ongoing secretion in, e.g., the respiratory tree.

Immediate Hypersensitivity Reactions: Anaphylaxis and Allergy. During hypersensitivity reactions, histamine is one of the many potent autacoids released and its relative contribution to the ensuing symptoms varies widely with species and tissue. The protection afforded by H_1 antagonists thus also varies accordingly. In humans, edema formation and itch are effectively suppressed. Other effects, such as hypotension, are less well antagonized.

CNS. The first-generation H_1 antagonists can both stimulate and depress the CNS. Stimulation occasionally is encountered in patients given conventional doses; they become restless, nervous, and unable to sleep. Central excitation also is a striking feature of overdose, which commonly results in convulsions, particularly in infants. Central depression, on the other hand, usually accompanies therapeutic doses of the older H_1 antagonists. Diminished alertness, slowed reaction times, and somnolence are common manifestations. Patients vary in their susceptibility and responses to individual drugs. The ethanolamines (e.g., diphenhydramine) are particularly prone to causing sedation. Because of the sedation that occurs with first-generation antihistamines, these drugs cannot be tolerated or used safely by many patients except at bedtime. Even then, patients may experience an antihistamine "hangover" in the morning, resulting in sedation with or without psychomotor impairment. Second-generation "nonsedating" H_1 antagonists do not cross the blood-brain barrier appreciably; their sedative effects are similar to those of placebo.

Many antipsychotic agents are H_1 and H_2 receptor antagonists, but it is unclear whether this property plays a role in the antipsychotic effects of these agents. The atypical antipsychotic agent *clozapine* is an effective H_1 antagonist and a weak H_3 antagonist but an H_4 receptor agonist in the rat. The H_1 antagonist activity of typical and atypical antipsychotic drugs is responsible for the effect of these agents to cause weight gain.

Anticholinergic Effects. Many of the first-generation H_1 antagonists tend to inhibit responses to ACh that are mediated by muscarinic receptors and may be manifest during clinical use. Some H_1 antagonists also can be used to treat motion sickness (*see* Chapters 9 and 46), probably as a result of their anticholinergic properties. Indeed, promethazine has perhaps the strongest muscarinic-blocking activity among these agents and is the most effective H_1 antagonist in combating motion sickness. The second-generation H_1 antagonists have no effect on muscarinic receptors.

Local Anesthetic Effect. Some H_1 antagonists have local anesthetic activity, and a few are more potent than procaine. Promethazine (PHENERGAN) is especially active. However, the concentrations required for this effect are much higher than those that antagonize histamine's interactions with its receptors.

ADME. The H_1 antagonists are well absorbed from the GI tract. Following oral administration, peak plasma concentrations are achieved in 2-3 h, and effects usually last 4-6 h; however, some of the drugs are much longer acting (Table 32–2). Diphenhydramine, given orally, reaches a maximal concentration in the blood in ~2 h, remains there for another 2 h, then falls exponentially with a plasma elimination $t_{1/2}$ of ~4-8 h. The drug is distributed widely throughout the body, including the CNS. Little, if any, is excreted unchanged in the urine; most appears there as metabolites. Peak concentrations of these drugs in the skin may persist after plasma levels have declined. Thus, inhibition of "wheal and flare" responses to the intradermal injection of histamine or allergen can persist for ≥36 h after treatment, even when the concentration in plasma is low. Like other extensively metabolized drugs, H_1 antagonists are eliminated more rapidly by children than by adults and more slowly in those with severe liver disease. H_1 receptor antagonists also induce hepatic CYPs and thus may facilitate their own metabolism.

The second-generation H_1 antagonist loratadine is absorbed rapidly from the GI tract and metabolized in the liver to an active metabolite by CYPs. Consequently, metabolism of loratadine can be affected by other drugs that compete CYPs. Two other second-generation H_1 antagonists that were marketed previously, *terfenadine* and *astemizole*, also were converted by CYPs to active metabolites. Both of these drugs were found in rare cases to induce a potentially fatal arrhythmia, *torsade de pointes*, when their metabolism was impaired, such as by liver disease or drugs that inhibit the CYP3A family (*see* Chapter 29). This led to the withdrawal of terfenadine and astemizole from the market. The active metabolite of terfenadine, fexofenadine, is its replacement. Fexofenadine lacks the toxic side effects of terfenadine, is not sedating, and retains the anti-allergic properties of the parent compound. Another antihistamine developed using this strategy is *desloratadine*, an active metabolite of loratadine. Cetirizine, loratadine, and fexofenadine are all well absorbed and are excreted mainly in the unmetabolized form. Cetirizine and loratadine are excreted primarily into the urine, whereas fexofenadine is excreted primarily in the feces. Levocetirizine represents the active enantiomer of cetirizine.

THERAPEUTIC USES

H_1 antagonists are used for treatment of various immediate hypersensitivity reactions. The central properties of some of the drugs also are of therapeutic value for suppressing motion sickness or for sedation.

ALLERGIC DISEASES. H_1 antagonists are useful in acute types of allergy that present with symptoms of rhinitis, urticaria, and conjunctivitis. Their effect is confined to the suppression of symptoms attributable to the histamine released by the antigen-antibody reaction. In bronchial asthma, histamine antagonists have limited efficacy and are not used as sole therapy (*see* Chapter 36). In the treatment of systemic anaphylaxis, where autacoids other than histamine are important, the mainstay of therapy is *epinephrine;* histamine antagonists have only a subordinate and adjuvant role. The same is true for severe angioedema, in which laryngeal swelling constitutes a threat to life.

Certain allergic dermatoses respond favorably to H_1 antagonists. The benefit is most striking in acute urticaria. Angioedema also responds to treatment with H_1 antagonists, but the paramount importance of epinephrine in the severe attack must be reemphasized, especially in life-threatening laryngeal edema (*see* Chapter 12). H_1 antagonists have a place in the treatment of pruritus. Some relief may be obtained in many patients with atopic and contact dermatitis (although topical corticosteroids are more effective) and in such diverse conditions as insect bites and poison ivy. The urticarial and edematous lesions of serum sickness respond to H_1 antagonists, but fever and arthralgia often do not.

COMMON COLD. H_1 antagonists are without value in combating the common cold. The weak anticholinergic effects of the older agents may tend to lessen rhinorrhea, but this drying effect may do more harm than good, as may their tendency to induce somnolence.

MOTION SICKNESS, VERTIGO, AND SEDATION. Scopolamine, the muscarinic antagonist, given orally, parenterally, or transdermally, is the most effective drug for the prophylaxis and treatment of motion sickness.

Table 32–2

Preparations and Dosage of Representative H_1 Receptor Antagonists[a]

CLASS and GENERIC NAME	DURATION OF ACTION, (h)[b]	PREPARATIONS[c]	SINGLE DOSE (adult)
First Generation Agents			
Tricyclic Dibenzoxepins			
Doxepin HCl	6-24	O, L, T	10-150 mg
Ethanolamines			
Carbinoxamine maleate	3-6	O, L	4-8 mg
Clemastine fumarate	12	O, L	1.34-2.68 mg
Diphenhydramine HCl	12	O, L, I, T	25-50 mg
Dimenhydrinate[e]	4-6	O, L, I	50-100 mg
Ethylenediamines			
Pyrilamine maleate	4-6	O, L, T	25-50 mg
Tripelennamine HCl	4-6	O	25-50 mg, 100 mg (SR)
Tripelennamine citrate	4-6	L	37.5-75 mg
Alkylamines			
Chlorpheniramine maleate	24	O, L, I	4 mg, 5-20 mg (I) 8-12 mg (SR)
Brompheniramine maleate	4-6	O, L, I	4 mg, 5-20 mg (I) 8-12 mg (SR)
Piperazines			
Hydroxyzine HCl	6-24	O, L, I	25-100 mg
Hydroxyzine pamoate	6-24	O, L	25-100 mg
Cyclizine HCl	4-6	O	50 mg
Cyclizine lactate	4-6	I	50 mg
Meclizine HCl	12-24	O	12.5-50 mg
Phenothiazines			
Promethazine HCl	4-6	O, L, I, S	12.5-50 mg
Piperidines			
Cyproheptadine HCl[f]	4-6	O, L	4 mg
Phenindamine tartrate	4-6	O	25 mg

(*continued*)

Table 32–2

Preparations and Dosage of Representative H_1 Receptor Antagonists[a] (*Continued*)

CLASS and GENERIC NAME	DURATION OF ACTION, (h)[b]	PREPARATIONS[c]	SINGLE DOSE (adult)
Second Generation Agents			
Tricyclic			
Dibenzoxepins	6-8	T	1 drop/eye
Olopatadine HCl	6-8	T	2 sprays/nostril
Alkylamines			
Acrivastine[d]	6-8	O	8 mg
Piperazines			
Cetirizine HCl[d]	12-24	O	5-10 mg
Levocetirizine HCl	12-24	O	2.5-5 mg
Phthalazinones			
Azelastine HCl[d]	12-24	T	2 sprays/nostril
Piperidines			
Levocabastine HCl	6-12	T	1 drop/eye
Ketotifen fumarate	8-12	T	1 drop/eye
Loratadine	24	O, L	10 mg
Desloratadine	24	O	5 mg
Ebastine	24	O	10-20 mg
Mizolastine	24	O	10 mg
Fexofenadine HCl	12-24	O	60-180 mg

[a]*For a discussion of phenothiazines, see Chapter 16.*
[b]*Duration of action of H_1 antihistamines by objective assessment of suppression of histamine- or allergen-induced symptoms is longer than expected from measurement of plasma concentrations or terminal elimination $t_{1/2}$ values.*
[c]*Preparations are designated as follows: O, oral solids; L, oral liquids; I, injection; S, suppository; SR, sustained release; T, topical. Many H_1 receptor antagonists also are available in preparations that contain multiple drugs.*
[d]*Has mild sedating effects.*
[e]*Dimenhydrinate is a combination of diphenhydramine and 8-chlorotheophylline in equal molecular proportions.*
[f]*Also has anti-serotonin properties.*

Some H_1 antagonists are useful for milder cases and have fewer adverse effects. These drugs include dimenhydrinate and the piperazines (e.g., cyclizine, meclizine). Promethazine, a phenothiazine, is more potent and more effective; its additional antiemetic properties may be of value in reducing vomiting, but its pronounced sedative action usually is disadvantageous. Whenever possible, the various drugs should be administered ~1 h before the anticipated motion. Treatment after the onset of nausea and vomiting rarely is beneficial. Some H_1 antagonists, notably dimenhydrinate and meclizine, often are of benefit in vestibular disturbances such as Meniere disease and in other types of true vertigo. Only promethazine is useful in treating the nausea and vomiting subsequent to chemotherapy or radiation therapy for malignancies; however, other, more effective antiemetic drugs (e.g., $5HT_3$ antagonists) are available (*see* Chapter 46). Diphenhydramine can reverse the extrapyramidal side effects caused by phenothiazines (*see* Chapter 16). The tendency of some H_1 receptor antagonists to produce somnolence has led to their use as hypnotics. H_1 antagonists, principally diphenhydramine, often are present in various proprietary over-the-counter remedies for insomnia. The sedative and mild antianxiety activities of hydroxyzine contribute to its use as a weak anxiolytic.

ADVERSE EFFECTS. The most frequent side effect in first-generation H_1 antagonists is sedation. Concurrent ingestion of alcohol or other CNS depressants produces an additive effect that impairs motor skills. Other untoward central actions include dizziness, tinnitus, lassitude, incoordination, fatigue, blurred vision, diplopia, euphoria, nervousness, insomnia, and tremors. Other side effects include loss of appetite, nausea, vomiting, epigastric distress, and constipation or diarrhea. Taking the drug with meals may reduce their incidence. H_1 antagonists such as cyproheptadine may increase appetite and cause weight gain. Other side effects, owing to the antimuscarinic actions of some first-generation H_1 antagonists, include dryness of the mouth and respiratory passages (sometimes inducing cough), urinary retention or frequency, and dysuria. These effects are not observed with second-generation H_1 antagonists.

Allergic dermatitis is not uncommon; other hypersensitivity reactions include drug fever and photosensitization. Hematological complications, such as leukopenia, agranulocytosis, and hemolytic anemia, are very rare. Because H_1 antihistamines cross the placenta, caution is advised for women who are or may become pregnant. Several antihistamines (e.g., azelastine, hydroxyzine, fexofenadine) had teratogenic effects in animal studies, whereas others (e.g., chlorpheniramine, diphenhydramine, cetirizine, loratadine) did not. Antihistamines can be excreted in small amounts in breast milk, and first-generation antihistamines taken by lactating mothers may cause symptoms such as irritability, drowsiness, or respiratory depression in the nursing infant.

In acute poisoning with H_1 antagonists, their central excitatory effects constitute the greatest danger. The syndrome includes hallucinations, excitement, ataxia, incoordination, athetosis, and convulsions. Fixed, dilated pupils with a flushed face, together with sinus tachycardia, urinary retention, dry mouth, and fever, lend the syndrome a remarkable similarity to that of atropine poisoning. Terminally, there is deepening coma with cardiorespiratory collapse and death usually within 2-18 h. Treatment is along general symptomatic and supportive lines.

Pediatric and Geriatric Indications and Problems. Although little clinical testing has been done, second-generation antihistamines are recommended for elderly patients (>65 years of age), especially those with impaired cognitive function, because of the sedative and anticholinergic effects of first-generation drugs. First-generation antihistamines are not recommended for use in children because their sedative effects can impair learning and school performance. The second-generation drugs have been approved by the FDA for use in children and are available in appropriate lower-dose formulations (e.g., chewable or rapidly dissolving tablets, syrup). Use of over-the-counter cough and cold medicines (containing mixtures of antihistamines, decongestants, antitussives, expectorants) in young children has been associated with serious side effects and deaths. In 2008, the FDA recommended that they not be used in children <2 years of age, and drug manufacturers affiliated with the Consumer Healthcare Products Association voluntarily relabeled products "do not use" for children <4 years of age.

AVAILABLE H_1 ANTAGONISTS. Summarized below are the therapeutic side effects of a number of H_1 antagonists, grouped by their chemical structures. Representative preparations are listed in Table 32–2.

Dibenzoxepin Tricyclics (Doxepin). Doxepin, the only drug in this class, is marketed as a tricyclic antidepressant (*see* Chapter 16). It also is one of the most potent H_1 antagonists and has significant H_2 antagonist activity, but this does not translate into greater clinical effectiveness. It can cause drowsiness and is associated with anticholinergic effects. Doxepin is better tolerated by patients with depression than those who are not depressed, where even small doses (e.g., 20 mg) may cause disorientation and confusion.

Ethanolamines (Prototype: Diphenhydramine). These drugs possess significant antimuscarinic activity and have a pronounced tendency to induce sedation. About half of those treated acutely with conventional doses experience somnolence. The incidence of GI side effects, however, is low with this group.

Ethylenediamines (Prototype: Pyrilamine). These include some of the most specific H_1 antagonists. Although their central effects are relatively feeble, somnolence occurs in a fair proportion of patients. GI side effects are quite common.

Alkylamines (Prototype: Chlorpheniramine). These are among the most potent H_1 antagonists. The drugs are less prone to produce drowsiness and are more suitable for daytime use, but a significant proportion of patients do experience sedation. Side effects involving CNS stimulation are more common than with other groups.

First-Generation Piperazines. The oldest member of this group, chlorcyclizine, has a more prolonged action and produces a comparatively low incidence of drowsiness. Hydroxyzine is a long-acting compound that is used widely for skin allergies; its considerable CNS-depressant activity may contribute to its prominent anti-pruritic action. Cyclizine and meclizine have been used primarily to counter motion sickness, although promethazine and diphenhydramine are more effective (as is the antimuscarinic scopolamine).

Second-Generation Piperazines (Cetirizine). Cetirizine is the only drug in this class. It has minimal anticholinergic effects. It also has negligible penetration into the brain but is associated with a somewhat higher incidence of drowsiness than the other second-generation H_1 antagonists. The active enantiomer levocetirizine has slightly greater potency and may be used at half the dose with less resultant sedation.

Phenothiazines (Prototype: Promethazine). Most drugs of this class are H_1 antagonists and also possess considerable anticholinergic activity. Promethazine, which has prominent sedative effects, and its many congeners are used primarily for their antiemetic effects (*see* Chapter 46).

First-Generation Piperidines (Cyproheptadine, Phenindamine). Cyproheptadine uniquely has both antihistamine and anti-serotonin activity. Cyproheptadine and phenindamine cause drowsiness and also have significant anticholinergic effects and can increase appetite.

Second-Generation Piperidines (Prototype: Terfenadine). Terfenadine and astemizole were withdrawn from the market. Current drugs in this class include loratadine, desloratadine, and fexofenadine. These agents are highly selective for H_1 receptors, lack significant anticholinergic actions, and penetrate poorly into the CNS. Taken together, these properties appear to account for the low incidence of side effects of piperidine antihistamines.

H_2 RECEPTOR ANTAGONISTS

The pharmacology and clinical utility of H_2 antagonists to inhibit gastric acid secretion are described in Chapter 45.

H_3 RECEPTOR AND LIGANDS

H_3 receptors are presynaptic autoreceptors on histaminergic neurons that originate in the tuberomammillary nucleus in the hypothalamus and project throughout the CNS, most prominently to the hippocampus, amygdala, nucleus accumbens, globus pallidus, striatum, hypothalamus, and cortex. The activated H_3 receptor depresses neuronal firing at the level of cell bodies/dendrites and decreases histamine release from depolarized terminals. Thus, H_3 agonists decrease histaminergic transmission, and antagonists increase it.

H_3 receptors also are presynaptic heteroreceptors on a variety of neurons in brain and peripheral tissues, and their activation inhibits release from noradrenergic, serotoninergic, GABA-ergic, cholinergic, and glutamatergic neurons, as well as pain-sensitive C fibers. H_3 receptors in the brain have significant constitutive activity in the absence of agonist; consequently, inverse agonists will activate these neurons.

H_3 antagonists/inverse agonists have a wide range of central effects; for example, they promote wakefulness, improve cognitive function (e.g., enhance memory, learning, and attention), and reduce food intake. As a result, there is considerable interest in developing H_3 antagonists for possible treatment of sleeping disorders, attention deficit hyperactivity disorder (ADHD), epilepsy, cognitive impairment, schizophrenia, obesity, neuropathic pain, and Alzheimer disease. Thioperamide was the first "specific" H_3 antagonist/inverse agonist available experimentally, but was equally effective at the H_4 receptor. A number of other imidazole derivatives have been developed as H_3 antagonists, including clobenpropit, ciproxifan, and proxyfan. More selective non-imidazole H_3 antagonists/inverse agonists are in phase II clinical trials.

H_4 RECEPTOR AND LIGANDS

H_4 receptors are expressed on cells with inflammatory or immune functions and can mediate histamine-induced chemotaxis, induction of cell shape change, secretion of cytokines, and upregulation of adhesion molecules. The H_4 receptors also have a role in pruritus and neuropathic pain. Because of the unique localization and function of H_4 receptors, H_4 antagonists are promising candidates to treat these conditions. No H_4 antagonists have yet been tested in clinical trials.

The H_4 receptor has the highest homology with the H_3 receptor and binds many H_3 ligands, especially those with imidazole rings, although sometimes with different effects. For example, thioperamide is an effective inverse agonist at both H_3 and H_4 receptors, whereas H_3 inverse agonist clobenpropit is a partial agonist of the H_4 receptor; impentamine (an H_3 agonist) and iodophenpropit (an H_3 inverse agonist) are both neutral H_4 antagonists.

BRADYKININ, KALLIDIN, AND THEIR ANTAGONISTS

Tissue damage, allergic reactions, viral infections, and other inflammatory events activate a series of proteolytic reactions that generate bradykinin and kallidin in tissues. These peptides contribute to inflammatory responses as autacoids that act locally to produce pain, vasodilation, and increased vascular permeability but can also have beneficial effects, for example in the heart, kidney, and circulation. Much of their activity is due to stimulation of the release of potent mediators such as prostaglandins, NO, or endothelium-derived hyperpolarizing factor (EDHF).

THE ENDOGENOUS KALLIKREIN–KININOGEN–KININ SYSTEM

Bradykinin is a nonapeptide. Kallidin is a decapeptide containing an additional N-terminal lysine, is sometimes referred to as *lysyl-bradykinin* (Table 32–3). The 2 peptides are cleaved from α_2 globulins termed *kininogens* (Figure 32–2). There are 2 kininogens: high-molecular-weight (HMW) kininogen and low-molecular-weight (LMW) kininogen. A number of serine proteases will generate kinins, but the highly specific proteases that release bradykinin and kallidin from the kininogens are termed *kallikreins*.

Table 32–3

Structure of Kinin Agonists and Antagonists

NAME	STRUCTURE	FUNCTION
Bradykinin	Arg-Pro-Pro-Gly-Phe-Ser-Pro-Phe-Arg	Agonist, B_2
Kallidin	Lys-Arg-Pro-Pro-Gly-Phe-Ser-Pro-Phe-Arg	Agonist, B_2
[des-Arg^9]-bradykinin	Arg-Pro-Pro-Gly-Phe-Ser-Pro-Phe	Agonist, B_1
[des-Arg^{10}]-kallidin	Lys-Arg-Pro-Pro-Gly-Phe-Ser-Pro-Phe	Agonist, B_1
des-Arg^{10}-[Leu^9]-kallidin	Lys-Arg-Pro-Pro-Gly-Phe-Ser-Pro-Leu	Antagonist, B_1
NPC-349	[D-Arg]-Arg-Pro-Hyp-Gly-Thi-Ser-D-Phe-Thi-Arg	Antagonist, B_2
HOE-140	[D-Arg]-Arg-Pro-Hyp-Gly-Thi-Ser-Tic-Oic-Arg	Antagonist, B_2
[des-Arg^{10}]-HOE-140	[D-Arg]-Arg-Pro-Hyp-Gly-Thi-Ser-Tic-Oic	Antagonist, B_1
FR173657	*see* Figure 32–3 of the 12th edition of the parent text	Antagonist, B_2
FR190997		Agonist, B_2
SSR240612		Antagonist, B_1

Hyp, trans-4-hydroxy-Pro; Thi, β-(2-thienyl)-Ala; Tic, [D]-1,2,3,4-tetrahydroisoquinolin-3-yl-carbonyl; Oic, (3as,7as)-octahy-droindol-2-yl-carbonyl.

KALLIKREINS. Bradykinin and kallidin are cleaved from HMW or LMW kininogens by plasma and tissue kallikrein, respectively (*see* Figure 32–2). Plasma kallikrein and tissue kallikrein are distinct enzymes that are activated by different mechanisms. Plasma prekallikrein is an inactive protein of ~88,000 Da that complexes with its substrate, HMW kininogen. The ensuing proteolytic cascade is restrained by the protease inhibitors present in plasma. Among the most important of these are the inhibitor of the activated first component of complement (C1-INH) and α_2 macroglobulin. Under experimental conditions, the kallikrein–kinin system is activated by the binding of factor XII, also known as *Hageman factor*, to negatively charged surfaces. Factor XII, a protease that is common to both the kinin and the intrinsic coagulation cascades (*see* Chapter 30), undergoes autoactivation and, in turn, activates prekallikrein. Importantly, kallikrein further activates factor XII, thereby exerting a positive feedback on the system. Tissue kallikrein (29,000 Da) is synthesized as a preproprotein in the epithelial cells or secretory cells in several tissues, including salivary glands, pancreas, prostate, and distal nephron. Tissue kallikrein also is expressed in human neutrophils. It acts locally near its sites of origin. The synthesis of tissue prokallikrein is controlled by a number of factors, including aldosterone in the kidney and salivary gland and androgens in certain other glands. The activation of tissue prokallikrein to kallikrein requires proteolytic cleavage to remove a 7–amino acid propeptide.

KININOGENS. The 2 substrates for the kallikreins, HMW kininogen and LMW kininogen, are derived from a single gene by alternative splicing. HMW kininogen is cleaved by plasma and tissue kallikrein to yield bradykinin and kallidin, respectively. LMW kininogen is a substrate only of tissue kallikrein, and the product is kallidin.

METABOLISM OF KININS. The decapeptide kallidin is about as active as the nonapeptide bradykinin, even without conversion to bradykinin, which occurs when the N-terminal lysine residue is removed by an aminopeptidase (*see* Figure 32–2). The $t_{1/2}$ of kinins in plasma is only ~15 sec; 80-90% of the kinins may be destroyed in a single passage through the pulmonary vascular bed. Plasma concentrations of bradykinin are difficult to measure because inadequate inhibition of kininogenases or kininases in the blood can lead to artifactual formation or degradation of bradykinin during blood collection. When care is taken to inhibit these processes, the reported physiological concentrations of bradykinin in blood are in the picomolar range.

The principal catabolizing enzyme in the lung and other vascular beds is kininase II, or ACE (*see* Chapter 26). Removal of the C-terminal dipeptide by ACE or neutral endopeptidase 24.11 (neprilysin) inactivates kinins (Figure 32–3). A slower-acting enzyme, carboxypeptidase N (lysine carboxypeptidase, kininase I), releases the C-terminal arginine residue, producing [desArg^9]-bradykinin or [des-Arg^{10}]-kallidin (*see* Table 32–3 and Figures 32–2 and 32–3), which are potent B_1 receptor agonists. Carboxypeptidase N is expressed constitutively in blood plasma. A familial carboxypeptidase N deficiency is associated with angioedema or urticaria. Carboxypeptidase M, which also cleaves basic C-terminal amino acids, is a widely distributed plasma membrane–bound enzyme. Finally, aminopeptidase P can cleave the N-terminal arginine, rendering bradykinin inactive and susceptible to cleavage by dipeptidyl peptidase IV.

KININ RECEPTORS. The B_1 and B_2 kinin receptors are GPCRs.

The bradykinin B_2 receptor is expressed in most normal tissues, where it selectively binds intact bradykinin and kallidin (*see* Table 32–3 and *see* Figure 32–2). The B_2 receptor mediates most of bradykinin's effects

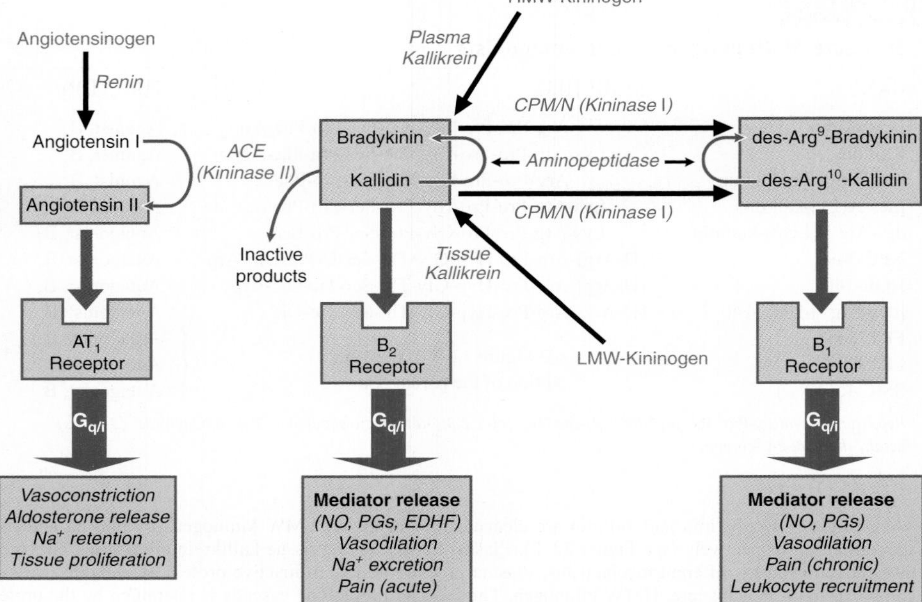

Figure 32–2 *Synthesis and signaling in the kallikrein-kinin and renin-angiotensin systems.* Bradykinin is generated by the action of *plasma* kallikrein on high-molecular-weight (HMW) kininogen and kallidin is released by the hydrolysis of low-molecular-weight (LMW) kininogen by *tissue* kallikrein. Kallidin and bradykinin are the natural ligands of the B_2 receptor but can be converted to corresponding agonists of the B_1 receptor by removal of the C-terminal Arg by kininase I–type enzymes: the plasma membrane–bound carboxypeptidase M (CPM) or soluble plasma carboxypeptidase N (CPN). Kallidin or [des-Arg^{10}]-kallidin can be converted to the active peptides bradykinin or to [des-Arg^9]-bradykinin by aminopeptidase cleavage of the N-terminal Lys residue. In a parallel fashion, angiotensin I is generated by the action of renin on angiotensinogen. Angiotensin I is then converted by angiotensin-converting enzyme (ACE) to the active peptide angiotensin II (AngII). These 2 systems have opposing effects. Bradykinin is a vasodilator that stimulates Na^+ excretion by activating the B_2 receptor. AngII is a potent vasoconstrictor that also causes aldosterone release and Na^+ retention via activation of the AT_1 receptor. ACE simultaneously generates active AngII and inactivates bradykinin and kallidin; thus, its effects are prohypertensive, and ACE inhibitors are effective antihypertensive agents.

under normal circumstances, whereas synthesis of the B_1 receptor is induced by inflammatory mediators in inflammatory conditions. Both B_1 and B_2 receptors couple through G_q to activate PLC and increase intracellular Ca^{2+}; the physiological response depends on receptor distribution on particular cell types and occupancy by agonist peptides. For example, on endothelial cells, activation of B_2 receptors results in Ca^{2+}–calmodulin–dependent activation of eNOS and generation of NO, which causes cyclic GMP accumulation and relaxation in neighboring smooth muscle cells. However, in endothelial cells under inflammatory conditions, B_1 receptor stimulation results in prolonged NO production via G_i and MAP kinase-dependent activation of iNOS expression. On smooth muscle cells, activation of kinin receptors coupling through G_q results in an increased $[Ca^{2+}]_i$ and contraction. Bradykinin activates the pro-inflammatory transcription factor NF-κB through $G\alpha_q$ and $\beta\gamma$ subunits and also activates the MAP kinase pathway. B_1 and B_2 receptors also can couple through G_i to activate PLA_2, causing the release of arachidonic acid and the local generation of a variety of metabolites, including inflammatory mediators and vasodilator epoxyeicosatrienoic acids (EETs) and prostacyclin such as EDHF. Kallikrein also plays a role in the intrinsic blood coagulation pathway.

The B_1 receptor is activated by the des-Arg metabolites of bradykinin and kallidin produced by the actions of carboxypeptidases N and M (*see* Table 32–3). Interestingly, carboxypeptidase M and the B_1 receptor interact on the cell surface to form an efficient signaling complex. B_1 receptors are normally absent or expressed at low levels in most tissues. B_1 receptor expression is upregulated by tissue injury and inflammation and by cytokines, endotoxins, and growth factors. Carboxypeptidase M expression also is increased by cytokines, to such a degree that B_1 receptor effects may predominate over B_2 effects. The B_1 and B_2 receptors differ in their time courses of downregulation; the B_2 receptor response is rapidly desensitized, whereas the B_1 response is not. This likely is due to modification at a Ser/Thr-rich cluster present in the C-terminal tail of the B_2 receptor that is not conserved in the B_1 receptor sequence.

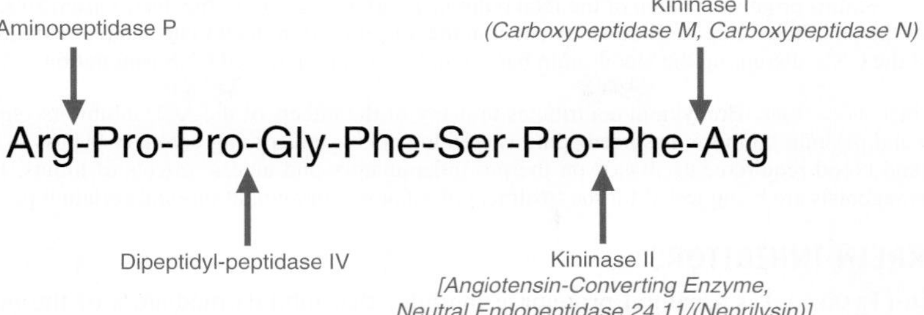

Figure 32–3 *Degradation of bradykinin.*

FUNCTIONS AND PHARMACOLOGY OF KALLIKREINS AND KININS

The utility of specific kinin-receptor antagonists currently is being investigated in diverse areas such as pain, inflammation, chronic inflammatory diseases, and the cardiovascular system. That the beneficial effects of ACE inhibitor therapy rests in part on enhancing bradykinin activity (e.g., on the heart, kidney, blood pressure; *see* Chapter 26) demonstrates the complexities in interpreting bradykinin's actions.

Pain. The kinins are powerful algesic agents that cause an intense burning pain when applied to the exposed base of a blister. Bradykinin excites primary sensory neurons and provokes the release of neuropeptides such as substance P, neurokinin A, and calcitonin gene–related peptide. Although there is overlap, B_2 receptors generally mediate acute bradykinin algesia, whereas the pain of chronic inflammation appears to involve increased numbers and activation of B_1 receptors.

Inflammation. Kinins participate in a variety of inflammatory conditions. Plasma kinins increase permeability in the microcirculation, acting on the small venules to cause disruption of the inter-endothelial junctions. This, together with an increased hydrostatic pressure gradient, causes edema. Edema, coupled with stimulation of nerve endings, results in a "wheal and flare" response to intradermal injection. In hereditary angioedema, bradykinin is formed, and there is depletion of the upstream components of the kinin cascade during episodes of swelling, laryngeal edema, and abdominal pain. B_1 receptors on inflammatory cells (e.g., macrophages) can elicit production of the inflammatory mediators IL-1 and TNF-α. Kinin levels are increased in a number of chronic inflammatory diseases and may be significant in gout, disseminated intravascular coagulation, inflammatory bowel disease, rheumatoid arthritis, or asthma. Kinins also may contribute to the skeletal changes seen in chronic inflammatory states. Kinins stimulate bone resorption through B_1 and possibly B_2 receptors, perhaps by osteoblast-mediated osteoclast activation (*see* Chapter 44).

Respiratory Disease. The kinins have been implicated in allergic airway disorders such as asthma and rhinitis. Inhalation or intravenous injection of kinins causes bronchospasm in asthmatic patients but not in normal individuals. This bradykinin-induced bronchoconstriction is blocked by anticholinergic agents but not by antihistamines or cyclooxygenase inhibitors. Similarly, nasal challenge with bradykinin is followed by sneezing and glandular secretions in patients with allergic rhinitis.

Cardiovascular System. Infusion of bradykinin causes vasodilation and lowers blood pressure. Bradykinin causes vasodilation by activating its B_2 receptor on endothelial cells, resulting in the generation of NO, prostacyclin, and a hyperpolarizing EET that is a CYP-derived metabolite of arachidonic acid. The endogenous kallikrein–kinin system plays a minor role in the regulation of normal blood pressure, but it may be important in hypertensive states. Urinary kallikrein concentrations are decreased in individuals with high blood pressure.

The kallikrein–kinin system is cardioprotective. Many of the beneficial effects of ACE inhibitors on heart function are attributable to enhancement of bradykinin effects, such as their antiproliferative activity or ability to increase glucose uptake in tissue. Bradykinin contributes to the beneficial effect of preconditioning to protect the heart against ischemia and reperfusion injury. Bradykinin also stimulates tissue plasminogen activator (tPA) release from the vascular endothelium and may contribute to the endogenous defense against some cardiovascular events, such as myocardial infarction and stroke.

Kidney. Renal kinins act in a paracrine manner to regulate urine volume and composition. Kallikrein is synthesized and secreted by the connecting cells of the distal nephron. Tissue kininogen and kinin receptors are present in the cells of the collecting duct. Like other vasodilators, kinins increase renal blood flow. Bradykinin also causes natriuresis by inhibiting sodium reabsorption at the cortical collecting duct. Treatment with mineralocorticoids, ACE inhibitors, and neutral endopeptidase (neprilysin) inhibitors increases renal kallikrein.

Other Effects. Kinins promote dilation of the fetal pulmonary artery, closure of the ductus arteriosus, and constriction of the umbilical vessels, all of which occur in the transition from fetal to neonatal circulation. Kinins also affect the CNS, disrupting the blood-brain barrier and allowing increased CNS penetration.

Potential Therapeutic Uses. Bradykinin contributes to many of the effects of the ACE inhibitors. *Aprotinin*, a kallikrein and plasmin inhibitor, has been administered to patients undergoing coronary bypass to minimize bleeding and blood requirements. Based on the pro-inflammatory and algesic effects of kinins, B_1 and B_2 receptor antagonists are being tested for the treatment of inflammatory conditions and certain types of pain.

KALLIKREIN INHIBITORS

Aprotinin (TRASYLOL) is a natural proteinase inhibitor that inhibits mediators of the inflammatory response, fibrinolysis, and thrombin generation following cardiopulmonary bypass surgery, including kallikrein and plasmin. Aprotinin has been employed clinically to reduce blood loss in patients undergoing coronary artery bypass surgery, but unfavorable survival statistics in retrospective and prospective studies have resulted in its discontinuation. Ecallantide (DX-88), a synthetic plasma kallikrein inhibitor, inhibits acute episodes of angioedema in patients with hereditary angioedema.

BRADYKININ AND THE EFFECTS OF ACE INHIBITORS. ACE inhibitors, widely used in the treatment of hypertension, congestive heart failure, and diabetic nephropathy, block the conversion of AngI to AngII and also block the degradation of bradykinin by ACE (*see* Figure 32–2 and Chapter 26). Numerous studies demonstrate that bradykinin contributes to many of the protective effects of ACE inhibitors. The search is on to find a suitable stable B_2 agonist for clinical evaluation that provides cardiovascular benefit without pro-inflammatory effects.

A rare side effect of ACE inhibitors is angioedema, which may be connected to the inhibition of kinin metabolism by ACE. A common side effect of ACE inhibitors is a chronic, nonproductive cough that dissipates when the drug is stopped. Bradykinin may contribute to the effects of the AT_1-receptor antagonists. During AT_1 receptor blockade, AngII concentrations increase, which enhances signaling through the unopposed AT_2 subtype receptor, causing an increase in renal bradykinin concentrations.

KININ RECEPTOR ANTAGONISTS. The selective B_2 receptor antagonist HOE-140 (*icatibant*; FIRAZYR) has been approved in the E.U. and recently in the U.S. for treatment of acute episodes of swelling in patients with hereditary angioedema. It is administered by subcutaneous injection.

For a complete Bibliographical Listing see Goodman & Gilman's ***The Pharmacological Basis of Therapeutics***, 12th ed., or Goodman & Gilman Online at www.AccessMedicine.com.

33 chapter Lipid-Derived Autacoids: Eicosanoids and Platelet-Activating Factor

Membrane lipids supply the substrate for the synthesis of *eicosanoids* and *platelet-activating factor* (PAF). Eicosanoids—arachidonate metabolites, including *prostaglandins* (PGs), *prostacyclin* (PGI_2), *thromboxane A_2* (TxA_2), *leukotrienes* (LTs), *lipoxins*, and *hepoxilins*—are not stored but are produced by most cells when a variety of physical, chemical, and hormonal stimuli activate acyl hydrolases that make arachidonate available. Membrane glycerophosphocholine derivatives can be modified enzymatically to produce PAF. PAF is formed by a smaller number of cell types, principally leukocytes, platelets, and endothelial cells. Eicosanoids and PAF lipids contribute to inflammation, smooth muscle tone, hemostasis, thrombosis, parturition, and gastrointestinal secretion. Several classes of drugs, most notably aspirin, the traditional nonsteroidal anti-inflammatory agents (tNSAIDs), and the specific inhibitors of cyclooxygenase-2 (COX-2), such as the coxibs, owe their principal therapeutic effects to blockade of eicosanoid formation.

EICOSANOIDS

PGs, LTs, and related compounds are called *eicosanoids*, from the Greek *eikosi* ("twenty"). Precursor essential fatty acids contain 20 carbons and 3, 4, or 5 double bonds. Arachidonic acid (AA; 5,8,11,14-eicosatetraenoic acid) is the most abundant precursor, derived from dietary linoleic acid (9,12-octadecadienoic acid) or ingested directly as a dietary constituent.

BIOSYNTHESIS. Biosynthesis of eicosanoids is limited by the availability of AA and depends primarily on the removal of esterified AA from membrane phospholipids or other complex lipids by acyl hydrolases, notably phospholipase A_2 (PLA_2). Once liberated, AA is metabolized rapidly to oxygenated products by *cyclooxygenases* (COXs), *lipoxygenases* (LOXs), and CYPs (Figure 33–1).

Chemical and physical stimuli activate the Ca^{2+}-dependent translocation of group IV_A cytosolic PLA_2 ($cPLA_2$) to the membrane, where it hydrolyzes the *sn*-2 ester bond of membrane phosphatidylcholine and phosphatidylethanolamine, releasing AA. Multiple additional PLA_2 isoforms (secretory [s] and Ca^{2+}-independent [i] forms) have been characterized. Under basal conditions, AA liberated by $iPLA_2$ is reincorporated into cell membranes. The inducible $sPLA_2$ contributes to AA release under conditions of sustained or intense stimulation of AA production.

PRODUCTS OF PROSTAGLANDIN G/H SYNTHASES (CYCLOOXYGENASES). PG endoperoxide G/H synthase also is called *cyclooxygenase* or *COX*. Products of this pathway are PGs, prostacyclin (PGI_2), and thromboxanes (TX_2), collectively termed *prostanoids*. The pathway is well described by Figure 33–1 and its legend.

Prostanoids are distinguished by substitutions on their cyclopentane rings the number of double bonds in their side chains, as indicated by numerical subscripts (dihomo-γ-linolenic acid is the precursor of *series*$_1$, AA for *series*$_2$, and EPA for *series*$_3$). Prostanoids derived from AA carry the subscript 2 and are the major series in mammals.

There are 2 distinct COX isoforms, COX-1 and COX-2. COX-1, expressed constitutively in most cells, is the dominant source of prostanoids for housekeeping functions. COX-2, in contrast, is upregulated by cytokines, shear stress, and growth factors and is the principal source of prostanoid formation in inflammation and cancer. However, this distinction is not absolute; both enzymes may contribute to the generation of prostanoids of some physiologic and pathophysiologic processes. These enzymes are expressed in a relatively cell-specific fashion. For example, COX-1-derived TxA_2 is the dominant product in platelets, whereas COX-2-derived PGE_2 and TxA_2 dominate in activated macrophages. Prostanoids are released from cells predominantly by facilitated transport through the PG transporter and possibly other transporters.

LIPOXYGENASE (LOX) PRODUCTS. Products of the LOX pathways are hydroxy fatty acid derivatives (HETEs), LTs, and lipoxins (LXs) (Figure 33–2). LTs play a major role in the development and persistence of the inflammatory response.

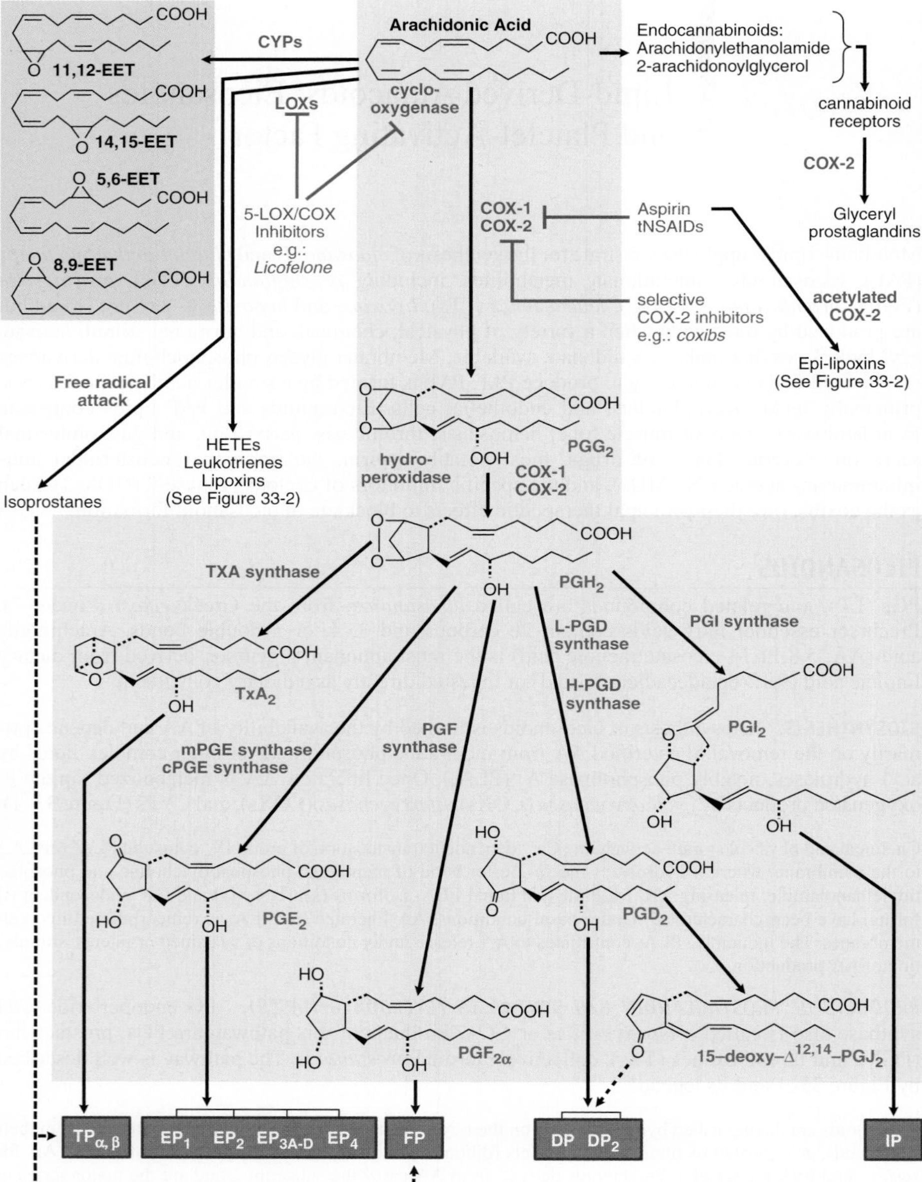

Figure 33–1 *Metabolism of arachidonic acid (AA)*. The cyclooxygenase (COX) pathway is highlighted in *gray*. The lipoxygenase (LOX) pathways are expanded in Figure 33–2. Major degradation pathways are shown in Figure 33–3. Cyclic endoperoxides (PGG_2 and PGH_2) arise from the sequential cyclooxygenase and hydroperoxidase actions of COX-1 or COX-2 on AA released from membrane phospholipids. Subsequent products are generated by tissue-specific synthases and transduce their effects via membrane-bound receptors (*blue boxes*). Dashed lines indicate putative ligand-receptor interactions. Epoxyeicosatrienoic acids (EETs; *shaded in blue*) and isoprostanes are generated via CYP activity and non-enzymatic free radical attack, respectively. COX-2 can use modified arachidonoylglycerol, an endocannabinoid, to generate the glyceryl prostaglandins. Aspirin and tNSAIDs are nonselective inhibitors of COX-1 and COX-2 but do not affect LOX activity. Epilipoxins are generated by COX-2 following its acetylation by aspirin (*see* Figure 33–2). Dual 5-LOX-COX inhibitors interfere with both pathways. See the text for other abbreviations.

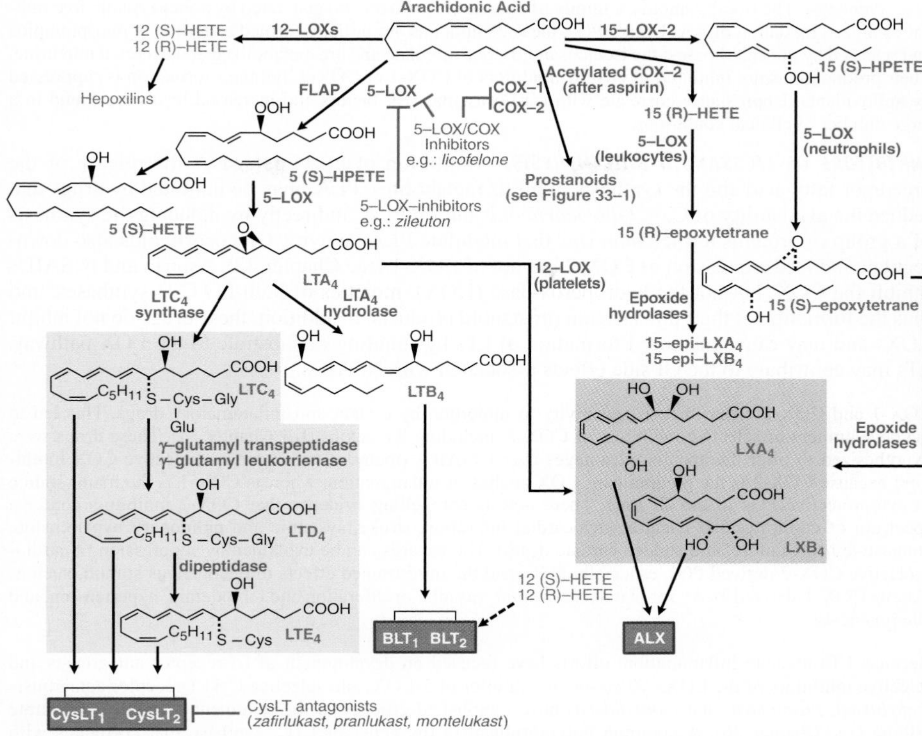

Figure 33–2 *Lipoxygenase pathways of arachidonic acid metabolism.* 5-LOX-activating protein (FLAP) presents arachidonic acid to 5-LOX, leading to the generation of the LTs. CysLTs are shaded in *gray*. Lipoxins (*shaded in orange*) are products of cellular interaction via a 5-LOX-12-LOX pathway or via a 15-LOX-5-LOX pathway. Biological effects are transduced via membrane-bound receptors (*blue boxes*). The *dashed line* indicates putative ligand–receptor interactions. Zileuton inhibits 5-LOX but not the COX pathways (expanded in Figure 33–1). Dual 5-LOX-COX inhibitors interfere with both pathways. CysLT antagonists prevent activation of the CysLT1 receptor. See the text for abbreviations.

LOXs are a family of non-heme iron–containing enzymes that catalyze the oxygenation of polyenic fatty acids to corresponding lipid hydroperoxides. The enzymes require a fatty acid substrate with 2 cis double bonds separated by a methylene group. AA is metabolized to hydroperoxy eicosatetraenoic acids (HPETEs). HPETEs are converted to HETEs and leukotrienes.

The 5-LOX pathway leads to the synthesis of the LTs. When eosinophils, mast cells, polymorphonuclear leukocytes, or monocytes are activated, 5-LOX translocates to the nuclear membrane and associates with 5-LOX-activating protein (FLAP), an integral membrane protein that facilitates AA to 5-LOX interaction. Drugs that inhibit FLAP block LT production. A 2-step reaction is catalyzed by 5-LOX: oxygenation of AA to form 5-HPETE, followed by dehydration of 5-HPETE to an unstable epoxide, LTA_4. LTA_4 is transformed by LTA_4 hydrolase to LTB_4; or is conjugated with GSH by LTC_4 synthase to form LTC_4. Extracellular metabolism of the peptide moiety of LTC_4 and the removal of glutamic acid and subsequent cleavage of glycine generates LTD_4 and LTE_4, respectively. LTC_4, LTD_4, and LTE_4 are the *cysteinyl leukotrienes* (CysLTs). LTB_4 and LTC_4 are actively transported out of the cell. LTA_4, the primary product of the 5-LOX pathway, is metabolized by 12-LOX to form the *lipoxins* LXA_4 and LXB_4. These mediators also can arise through 5-LOX metabolism of 15-HETE.

PRODUCTS OF CYPs. AA is metabolized to epoxyeicosatrienoic acids (EETs) by CYP epoxygenases, primarily CYP2C and CYP2J. EETs are synthesized in endothelial cells, where they function as endothelium-derived hyperpolarizing factors (EDHFs), particularly in the coronary circulation. EETs biosynthesis can be altered by pharmacological, nutritional, and genetic factors that affect CYP expression.

Other Pathways. The isoeicosanoids, a family of eicosanoid isomers, are generated by nonenzymatic free radical catalyzed oxidation of AA. Unlike PGs, these compounds are initially formed esterified in phospholipids and released by phospholipases; the isoeicosanoids then circulate and are metabolized and excreted into urine. Their production is not inhibited in vivo by inhibitors of COX-1 or COX-2, but their formation is suppressed by antioxidants. Isoprostanes correlate with cardiovascular risk factors and increased levels are found in a large number of clinical conditions.

INHIBITORS OF EICOSANOID BIOSYNTHESIS. Inhibition of PLA_2 decreases the release of the precursor fatty acid and the synthesis of all its metabolites. PLA_2 may be inhibited by drugs that reduce the availability of Ca^{2+}. *Glucocorticoids* inhibit PLA_2 indirectly by inducing the synthesis of a group of proteins termed *annexins* that modulate PLA_2 activity. Glucocorticoids also down-regulate induced expression of COX-2 but not of COX-1 (*see* Chapter 42). Aspirin and tNSAIDs inhibit the COX, but not the hydroperoxidase (HOX), moieties of both PG G/H synthases, and thus the formation of their downstream prostanoid products. In addition, these drugs do not inhibit LOXs and may cause increased formation of LTs by shunting of substrate to the LOX pathway. LTs may contribute to the GI side effects associated with NSAIDs.

COX-1 and COX-2 differ in their sensitivity to inhibition by certain anti-inflammatory drugs. This led to the development of selective inhibitors of COX-2, including the coxibs (*see* Chapter 34). These drugs were hypothesized to offer therapeutic advantages over tNSAIDs (many of which are nonselective COX inhibitors) because COX-2 is the predominant COX at sites of inflammation, whereas COX-1 is the major source of cytoprotective PGs in the GI tract. There now is compelling evidence that COX-2 inhibitors confer a spectrum of cardiovascular hazards (myocardial infarction, stroke, systemic and pulmonary hypertension, congestive heart failure, and sudden cardiac death). The hazards can be explained by suppression of cardioprotective COX-2-derived PGs, especially PGI_2, and the unrestrained effects of endogenous stimuli, such as platelet COX-1-derived TxA_2, for platelet activation, vascular proliferation and remodeling, hypertension, and atherogenesis.

Because LTs mediate inflammation, efforts have focused on development of LT-receptor antagonists and selective inhibitors of the LOXs. *Zileuton*, an inhibitor of 5-LOX, and selective CysLT-receptor antagonists (*zafirlukast, pranlukast*, and *montelukast*) have established efficacy in the treatment of mild to moderate asthma (*see* Chapter 36). A common polymorphism in the gene for LTC_4 synthase that correlates with increased LTC_4 generation is associated with aspirin-intolerant asthma and with the efficacy of anti-LT therapy. Interestingly, although polymorphisms in the genes encoding 5-LOX or FLAP do not appear to be linked to asthma, studies have demonstrated an association of these genes with myocardial infarction, stroke, and atherosclerosis; thus, inhibition of LT biosynthesis may be useful in the prevention of cardiovascular disease.

EICOSANOID DEGRADATION (FIGURE 33–3). Most eicosanoids are efficiently and rapidly inactivated. The enzymatic catabolic reactions are of 2 types: a rapid initial step, catalyzed by widely distributed PG-specific enzymes, wherein PGs lose most of their biological activity; and a second step in which these metabolites are oxidized, probably by enzymes identical to those responsible for the β and ω oxidation of fatty acids. The lung, kidney, and liver play prominent roles in the enzymatically catalyzed reactions. PGI_2 and TxA_2 undergo spontaneous hydrolysis as a first degradative step.

PHARMACOLOGICAL PROPERTIES

The eicosanoids function through activation of specific GPCRs that couple to intracellular second-messenger systems to modulate cellular activity (Table 33–1 and Figure 33–4).

Prostaglandin Receptors. PGs activate membrane receptors locally near their sites of formation. Eicosanoid receptors interact with G_s, G_i, and G_q to modulate the activities of adenylyl cyclase and phospholipase C (*see* Chapter 3). Single gene products have been identified for the receptors for PGI_2 (the IP), $PGF_{2\alpha}$ (the FP), and TxA_2 (the TP). Four distinct PGE_2 receptors ($EP_{1\text{-}4}$) and 2 PGD_2 receptors (DP_1 and DP_2—also known as $CRTH_2$) have been cloned. Additional isoforms of the TP (α and β), FP (A and B), and EP_3 (I-VI, e, f) receptors can arise through differential mRNA splicing.

The prostanoid receptors appear to derive from an ancestral EP receptor and share high homology. Phylogenetic comparison of this receptor family reveals 3 subclusters:

- The relaxant receptors EP_2, EP_4, IP, and DP_1, which increase cellular cyclic AMP generation
- The contractile receptors EP_1, FP, and TP, which increase cytosolic levels of Ca^{2+}
- EP_3, which can couple to both elevation of cytosolic $[Ca^{2+}]$ and inhibition of adenylyl cyclase

The DP_2 receptor is an exception and is unrelated to the other prostanoid receptors; rather, it is a member of the formyl-methionyl-leucyl-phenylalanine (fMLP)-receptor superfamily.

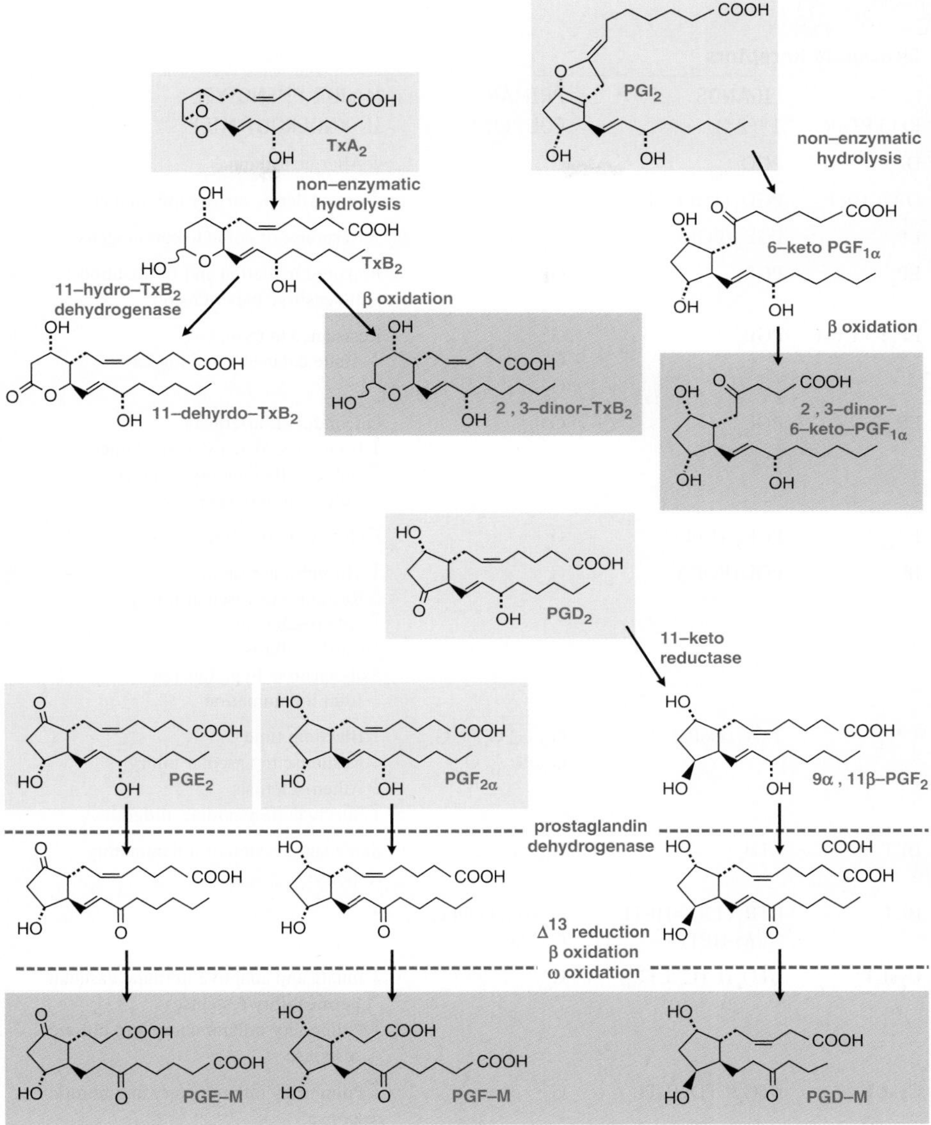

Figure 33–3 *Major pathways of prostanoid degradation.* Active metabolites are shaded in *gray*. Major urinary metabolites are shaded in *orange*. The *red dashed lines* indicate reactions that use common enzymatic processes. M, metabolite. See the text for other abbreviations.

Leukotriene and Lipoxin Receptors. Two receptors exist for both LTB_4 (BLT_1 and BLT_2) and the cysteinyl leukotrienes ($CysLT_1$ and $CysLT_2$). A receptor that binds lipoxin, ALX, is identical to the fMLP-1 receptor; the nomenclature now reflects LXA_4 as a natural and potent ligand. All are GPCRs and couple with G_q and other G proteins, depending on the cellular context. BLT_1 is expressed predominantly in leukocytes, thymus, and spleen, whereas BLT_2, the low-affinity receptor for LTB_4, is found in spleen, leukocytes, ovary, liver, and intestine. $CysLT_1$ binds LTD_4 with higher affinity than LTC_4, while $CysLT_2$ shows equal affinity for both LTs. Both receptors bind LTE_4 with low affinity. $CysLT_1$ is expressed in lung and intestinal smooth muscle, spleen, and peripheral blood leukocytes, whereas $CysLT_2$ is found in heart, spleen, peripheral blood leukocytes, adrenal medulla, and brain. Responses to ALX-receptor activation vary with cell type. The ALX receptor is expressed in lung, peripheral blood leukocytes, and spleen.

Table 33–1

Eicosanoid Receptors

RECEPTOR	LIGANDS 1°(2°)	PRIMARY COUPLING	MAJOR PHENOTYPE IN KNOCKOUT MICE
DP_1	PGD_2	G_s	↓ Allergic asthma
DP_2/$CHRT_2$	PGD_2 (15d-PGJ_2)	G_i	↑ or ↓ Allergic airway inflammation
EP_1	PGE_2 (PGI_2)	G_q	↓ Response of colon to carcinogens
EP_2	PGE_2	G_s	Impaired ovulation and fertilization Salt-sensitive hypertension
EP_3 I-VI, e, f	PGE_2	G_i; G_s; G_q	Resistance to pyrogens ↓ Acute cutaneous inflammation
EP_4	PGE_2	G_s	Patent ductus arteriosus ↓ Bone mass/density in aged mice ↑ Bowel inflammatory response ↓ Colon carcinogenesis
$FP_{A,B}$	$PGF_{2\alpha}$ (IsoPs)	G_q	Failure of parturition
IP	PGI_2 (PGE_2)	G_s	↑ Thrombotic response ↓ Response to vascular injury ↑ Atherosclerosis ↑ Cardiac fibrosis Salt-sensitive hypertension ↓ Joint inflammation
$TP_{\alpha,\beta}$	TxA_2 (IsoPs)	G_q, G_i, $G_{12/13}$, G_{16}; G_q, $G_{12/13}$, G_{16}	↑ Bleeding time ↓ Response to vascular injury ↓ Atherosclerosis ↑ Survival after cardiac allograft
BLT_1	LTB_4	G_{16}, G_i	Some suppression of inflammatory response
BLT_2	LTB_4 (12(*S*)-HETE, 12(*R*)-HETE)	G_q-like, G_i-like, G_z-like	?
$CysLT_1$	LTD_4 (LTC_4/LTE_4)	G_q	↓ Innate and adaptive immune vascular permeability response ↑ Pulmonary inflammatory and fibrotic response
$CysLT_2$	LTC_4/LTD_4 (LTE_4)	G_q	↓ Pulmonary inflammatory and fibrotic response

This table lists the major classes of eicosanoid receptors and their signaling characteristics. Splice variants for EP_3, TP, and FP are indicated. IsoPs, isoprostanes; 15d-PGJ_2, 15-deoxy-$\Delta^{12,14}$-PGJ_2; DP_2 is a member of the fMLP-receptor superfamily; fMLP, formyl-methionyl-leucyl-phenylalanine.

Other Agents. Other AA metabolites (e.g., isoprostanes, epoxyeicosatrienoic acids, hepoxilins) have potent biological activities, and there is evidence for distinct receptors for some of these substances. Specific receptors for the HETEs and EETs have been proposed but not yet isolated.

PHARMACOLOGICAL EFFECTS

CARDIOVASCULAR SYSTEM. In most vascular beds, PGE_2, PGI_2, and PGD_2 elicit vasodilation and a drop in blood pressure; physiologically, these responses are quite local, since endogenous prostanoids are paracrine mediators that do not circulate. Responses to $PGF_{2\alpha}$ vary with vascular bed; it is a potent constrictor of both pulmonary arteries and veins; however, it does not alter blood pressure in humans. TxA_2 is a potent vasoconstrictor and a mitogen in smooth muscle cells.

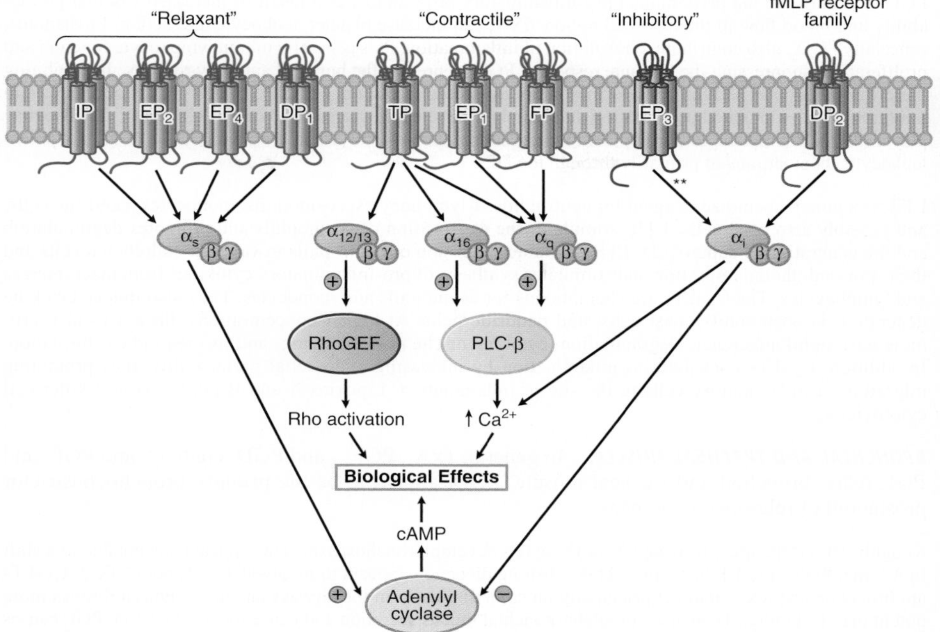

Figure 33–4 *Prostanoid receptors and their primary signaling pathways.* Prostanoid receptors are heptaspanning GPCRs. The terms "relaxant," "contractile," and "inhibitory" refer to the phylogenetic characterization of their primary effects. **All EP_3 isoforms couple through G_i; some can also activate G_s or $G_{12/13}$ pathways. See the text for additional details.

PGE_2 can cause vasoconstriction through activation of the EP_1 and EP_3 receptors. Infusion of PGD_2 in humans results in flushing, nasal stuffiness, and hypotension. Local subcutaneous release of PGD_2 contributes to dilation of the vasculature in the skin, which causes facial flushing associated with niacin treatment in humans. Subsequent formation of F-ring metabolites from PGD_2 may result in hypertension. PGI_2 relaxes vascular smooth muscle, causing hypotension and reflex tachycardia on intravenous administration. LTC_4 and LTD_4 can constrict or relax isolated vascular smooth muscle preparations, depending on the concentrations used and the vascular bed. The renal vasculature is resistant to this constrictor action, but the mesenteric vasculature is not. LTC_4 and LTD_4 act in the microvasculature to increase permeability of postcapillary venules; they are ~1,000-fold more potent than histamine in this regard. At higher concentrations, LTC_4 and LTD_4 can constrict arterioles and reduce exudation of plasma. EETs cause vasodilation in a number of vascular beds by activating the large conductance Ca^{2+}-activated K^+ channels of smooth muscle cells, thereby hyperpolarizing the smooth muscle and causing relaxation. EETs likely also function as EDHFs. Isoprostanes usually are vasoconstrictors, although there are examples of vasodilation in preconstricted vessels.

PLATELETS. Mature platelets express only COX-1. TxA_2, the major product of COX-1 in platelets, induces platelet aggregation and amplifies the signal for other, more potent platelet agonists, such as thrombin and ADP. Low concentrations of PGE_2, via the EP_3, enhance platelet aggregation. In contrast, higher concentrations of PGE_2, acting via the IP or possibly EP_2 or EP_4 receptors, inhibit platelet aggregation. Both PGI_2 and PGD_2 inhibit the aggregation of platelets. PGI_2 limits platelet activation by TxA_2, and disaggregates preformed clumps.

TxA_2 induces platelet shape change, through G_{12}/G_{13}-mediated Rho/Rho-kinase-dependent regulation of myosin light-chain phosphorylation, and aggregation through G_q-dependent activation of PKC. The actions of TxA_2 on platelets are restrained by its short $t_{1/2}$ (~30 sec), by rapid TP desensitization, and by endogenous inhibitors of platelet function, including NO and PGI_2.

INFLAMMATION AND IMMUNITY. Eicosanoids play a major role in the inflammatory and immune responses. LTs generally are pro-inflammatory and lipoxins anti-inflammatory. Prostanoids can exert both kinds of activity. COX-2 is the major source of prostanoids formed during and after an inflammatory response.

PGE_2 and PGI_2 are the predominant pro-inflammatory prostanoids, as a result of increased vascular permeability and blood flow in the inflamed region. TxA_2 can increase platelet–leukocyte interaction. Prostanoids, especially PGD_2, also contribute to resolution of inflammation. PGs generally inhibit lymphocyte function and proliferation, suppressing the immune response. PGE_2 depresses the humoral antibody response by inhibiting the differentiation of B lymphocytes into antibody-secreting plasma cells. PGE_2 acts on T lymphocytes to inhibit mitogen-stimulated proliferation and lymphokine release by sensitized cells. PGE_2 and TxA_2 also may play a role in T lymphocyte development by regulating apoptosis of immature thymocytes. PGD_2 is a potent leukocyte chemoattractant primarily through the DP_2.

LTB_4 is a potent chemotactic agent for neutrophils, T lymphocytes, eosinophils, monocytes, dendritic cells, and possibly also mast cells. LTB_4 stimulates the aggregation of eosinophils and promotes degranulation and the generation of superoxide. LTB_4 promotes adhesion of neutrophils to vascular endothelial cells and their transendothelial migration and stimulates synthesis of pro-inflammatory cytokines from macrophages and lymphocytes. The CysLTs are chemotaxins for eosinophils and monocytes. They also induce cytokine generation in eosinophils, mast cells, and dendritic cells. At higher concentrations, these LTs also promote eosinophil adherence, degranulation, cytokine or chemokine release, and oxygen radical formation. In addition, CysLTs contribute to inflammation by increasing endothelial permeability, thus promoting migration of inflammatory cells to the site of inflammation. Lipoxins A and B inhibit natural killer cell cytotoxicity.

BRONCHIAL AND TRACHEAL MUSCLE. In general, TxA_2, $PGF_{2\alpha}$, and PGD_2 contract, and PGE_2 and PGI_2 relax, bronchial and tracheal muscle. PGD_2 appear to be the primary bronchoconstrictor prostanoid of relevance in humans.

Roughly 10% of people given aspirin or tNSAIDs develop bronchospasm. This appears attributable to a shift in AA metabolism to LT formation. This substrate diversion appears to involve COX-1, not COX-2. CysLTs are bronchoconstrictors that act principally on smooth muscle in the airways and are a thousand times more potent than histamine. They also stimulate bronchial mucus secretion and cause mucosal edema. PGI_2 causes bronchodilation in most species; human bronchial tissue is particularly sensitive, and PGI_2 antagonizes bronchoconstriction induced by other agents.

UTERUS. Strips of nonpregnant human uterus are contracted by $PGF_{2\alpha}$ and TxA_2 but are relaxed by PGEs. PGE_2, together with oxytocin, is essential for the onset of parturition. PGI_2 and high concentrations of PGE_2 produce relaxation. The intravenous infusion of low concentrations of PGE_2 or $PGF_{2\alpha}$ to pregnant women produces a dose-dependent increase in uterine tone and in the frequency and intensity of rhythmic uterine contractions. PGEs and PGFs are used to terminate pregnancy.

GI SMOOTH MUSCLE. PGEs and PGFs stimulate contraction of the main longitudinal muscle from stomach to colon. Circular muscle generally relaxes in response to PGE_2 and contracts in response to $PGF_{2\alpha}$. The LTs have potent contractile effects. Diarrhea, cramps, and reflux of bile have been noted in response to oral PGE. PGEs and PGFs stimulate the movement of water and electrolytes into the intestinal lumen. PGE_2 appears to contribute to the water and electrolyte loss in cholera, a disease that is somewhat responsive to therapy with tNSAIDs.

GASTRIC AND INTESTINAL SECRETIONS. In the stomach, PGE_2 and PGI_2 contribute to increased mucus secretion (*cytoprotection*), reduced acid secretion, and reduced pepsin content. PGE_2 and its analogs also inhibit gastric damage caused by a variety of ulcerogenic agents and promote healing of duodenal and gastric ulcers (*see* Chapter 45). CysLTs, by constricting gastric blood vessels and enhancing production of pro-inflammatory cytokines, may contribute to the gastric damage.

KIDNEY. COX-2-derived PGE_2 and PGI_2 increase medullary blood flow and inhibit tubular sodium reabsorption. Expression of medullary COX-2 is increased during high salt intake. COX-1-derived products promote salt excretion in the collecting ducts. Cortical COX-2-derived PGE_2 and PGI_2 increase renal blood flow and glomerular filtration through their local vasodilating effects. There is an added layer of complexity: low dietary salt intake increases expression of cortical COX-2 expression. Through the action of PGE_2, and also possibly PGI_2, this results in increased renin release, leading to sodium retention and elevated blood pressure.

TxA_2, generated at low levels in the normal kidney, has potent vasoconstrictor effects that reduce renal blood flow and glomerular filtration rate. Infusion of $PGF_{2\alpha}$ causes both natriuresis and diuresis. Conversely, $PGF_{2\alpha}$ may activate the renin–angiotensin system, contributing to elevated blood pressure. There is substantial evidence for a role of the CYP epoxygenase products in regulating renal function, although their exact role in the human kidney remains unclear. Both 20-HETE and the EETs are generated in renal tissue. 20-HETE constricts the renal arteries, while EETs mediate vasodilation and natriuresis.

EYE. $PGF_{2\alpha}$ induces constriction of the iris sphincter muscle, but its overall effect in the eye is to decrease intraocular pressure (IOP) by increasing the aqueous humor outflow. A variety of FP receptor agonists have proven effective in the treatment of open-angle glaucoma, a condition associated with the loss of COX-2 expression in the pigmented epithelium of the ciliary body (*see* Chapter 64).

CNS. PGE_2 induces fever.

The hypothalamus regulates the body temperature set point, which is elevated by endogenous pyrogens. The response is mediated by coordinate induction of COX-2 and mPGE synthase-1 in the endothelium of blood vessels in the preoptic hypothalamic area to form PGE_2. PGE_2 acts on EP_3, and perhaps EP_1, on thermosensitive neurons. This triggers the hypothalamus to elevate body temperature. Exogenous $PGF_{2\alpha}$ and PGI_2 induce fever but do not contribute to the pyretic response. PGD_2 and TxA_2 do not induce fever. PGD_2 also appears to act on arachnoid trabecular cells in the basal forebrain to mediate an increase in extracellular adenosine that, in turn, facilitates induction of sleep. COX-2-derived prostanoids also have been implicated in several CNS degenerative disorders (e.g., Alzheimer disease, Parkinson disease; *see* Chapter 22).

PAIN. Inflammatory mediators, including LTs and PGs, increase the sensitivity of nociceptors and potentiate pain perception.

Centrally, both COX-1 and COX-2 are expressed in the spinal cord under basal conditions and release PGs in response to peripheral pain stimuli. PGE_2, and perhaps PGD_2, PGI_2, and $PGF_{2\alpha}$, can increase excitability in pain transmission neuronal pathways in the spinal cord, causing hyperalgesia and allodynia. Hyperalgesia also is produced by LTB_4. The role of PGE_2 and PGI_2 in inflammatory pain is discussed in more detail in Chapter 34.

ENDOCRINE SYSTEM. The systemic administration of PGE_2 increases circulating concentrations of adrenocorticotropic hormone (ACTH), growth hormone, prolactin, and gonadotropins. Other effects include stimulation of steroid production by the adrenals, stimulation of insulin release, and thyrotropin-like effects on the thyroid. The critical role of $PGF_{2\alpha}$ in parturition relies on its ability to induce an oxytocin-dependent decline in progesterone levels. PGE_2 works as part of a positive-feedback loop to induce oocyte maturation required for fertilization during and after ovulation. LOX metabolites also have endocrine effects. 12-HETE stimulates the release of aldosterone from the adrenal cortex and mediates a portion of the aldosterone release stimulated by AngII, but not that which occurs in response to ACTH.

BONE. PGs are strong modulators of bone metabolism. COX-1 is expressed in normal bone, while COX-2 is upregulated in settings such as inflammation and during mechanical stress. PGE_2 stimulates bone formation by increasing osteoblastogenesis and bone resorption via activation of osteoclasts.

THERAPEUTIC USES

INHIBITORS AND ANTAGONISTS. The nonselective tNSAIDs, and those with selective COX-2 inhibition, are used widely as anti-inflammatory drugs, whereas low-dose aspirin is employed frequently for cardioprotection. LT antagonists are useful clinically in the treatment of asthma, and FP agonists are used in the treatment of open-angle glaucoma (*see* Chapter 64). EP agonists are used to induce labor and to ameliorate gastric irritation owing to tNSAIDs. DP_1 antagonists may be useful in offsetting the facial flushing associated with niacin. Orally active antagonists of LTC_4 and D_4, which block the $CysLT_1$ receptor, are used in the treatment of mild to moderately severe asthma (*see* Chapter 36). Their effectiveness in patients with aspirin-induced asthma also has been shown. Prostanoids have a short $t_{1/2}$ in the circulation and their systemic administration produces significant adverse effects. Nonetheless, several prostanoids are of clinical utility in the following situations.

Therapeutic Abortion. PGEs, PGFs, and their analogs, are used to induce labor and terminate pregnancy at any stage by promoting uterine contractions. Dinoprostone, a synthetic preparation of PGE_2, is approved for inducing abortion in the second trimester of pregnancy, for missed abortion, for cervical ripening prior to induction of labor, and for managing benign hydatidiform moles. Systemic or intravaginal administration of the PGE_1 analog misoprostol in combination with mifepristone (RU486) or methotrexate is highly effective in the termination of early pregnancy. An analog of $PGF_{2\alpha}$, carboprost tromethamine, is used to induce second-trimester abortions and to control postpartum hemorrhage that is not responding to conventional methods.

Gastric Cytoprotection. Several PG analogs are used to suppress gastric ulceration. Misoprostol (CYTOTEC), a PGE_1 analog, is approved for prevention of NSAID-induced gastric ulcers.

Impotence. PGE_1 (alprostadil), given as an intracavernous injection (CAVERJECT, EDEX) or urethral suppository (MUSE) is a second-line treatment of erectile dysfunction, PDE5 inhibitors being preferred (*see* Chapters 27 and 28).

Maintenance of Patent Ductus Arteriosus. The ductus arteriosus in neonates is highly sensitive to vasodilation by PGE_1. PGE_1 (alprostadil, PROSTIN VR PEDIATRIC) is highly effective for palliative therapy to maintain temporary patency until surgery can be performed.

Pulmonary Hypertension. Long-term therapy with PGI_2 (prostacyclin; epoprostenol, FLOLAN), via continuous intravenous infusion, improves symptoms and can delay or preclude the need for lung or heart-lung transplantation in a number of patients. Several PGI_2 analogs with longer $t_{1/2}$ have been used clinically. Iloprost can be inhaled (VENTAVIS) or delivered by intravenous administration (not available in the U.S.). Treprostinil (REMODULIN) ($t_{1/2}$ ~4 h) may be delivered by continuous subcutaneous or intravenous infusion.

Glaucoma. Latanoprost, a $PGF_{2\alpha}$ derivative, was the first prostanoid used for glaucoma. Similar prostanoids with ocular hypotensive effects include bimatoprost and travoprost. These drugs act as agonists at the FP receptor and are administered as ophthalmic drops (*see* Chapter 64).

PLATELET-ACTIVATING FACTOR

PAF is 1-*O*-alkyl-2-acetyl-*sn*-glycero-3-phosphocholine. PAF represents a family of phospholipids because the alkyl group at position 1 can vary in length from 12-18 carbon atoms. In human neutrophils, PAF consists predominantly of a mixture of the 16- and 18-carbon ethers, but its composition may change when cells are stimulated. PAF is not stored in cells but is synthesized from an acyl precursor in response to stimulation by a 2-step process (Figure 33–5).

PAF is synthesized by platelets, neutrophils, monocytes, mast cells, eosinophils, renal mesangial cells, renal medullary cells, and vascular endothelial cells. Depending on cell type, PAF can either remain cell-associated or be secreted. For example, PAF is released from monocytes but retained by leukocytes and endothelial cells. In endothelial cells, PAF is displayed on the surface for juxtacrine signaling and stimulates adherent leukocytes. PAF-like molecules can be formed from the oxidative fragmentation of membrane phospholipids (oxPLs). These compounds are increased in settings of oxidant stress, such as cigarette smoking, and differ structurally from PAF in that they contain a fatty acid at the *sn*-1 position of glycerol joined through an ester bond and various short-chain acyl groups at the *sn*-2 position. oxPLs mimic the structure of PAF closely enough to bind to its receptor and elicit the same responses. Increased levels of plasma PAF acyl hydrolase (PAF-AH) have been associated with colon cancer, cardiovascular disease, and stroke.

MECHANISM OF ACTION OF PAF. Extracellular PAF exerts its actions by stimulating a specific GPCR. The PAF receptor couples to G_q (to activate the PLC-IP_3–Ca^{2+} pathway) and to G_i (to inhibit adenylyl cyclase). Consequent activation of phospholipases A_2, C, and D gives rise to myriad messengers, including AA-derived PGs, TxA_2, or LTs, which may function as mediators of the effects of PAF.

In addition, p38 MAP kinase is activated downstream of the PAF-receptor- G_q interaction, while ERK activation can occur via interaction of activated PAF receptor with G_q, G_o, or $G_{\beta\gamma}$, or via transactivation of the EGF receptor, leading to NF-κB activation. PAF exerts many of its important pro-inflammatory actions without leaving its cell of origin. For example, PAF is synthesized in a regulated fashion by endothelial cells stimulated by inflammatory mediators. This PAF is presented on the surface of the endothelium, where it activates the PAF receptor on juxtaposed cells, including platelets, polymorphonuclear leukocytes, and monocytes, and acts cooperatively with P selectin to promote adhesion. This function of PAF is important for orchestrating the interaction of platelets and circulating inflammatory cells with the inflamed endothelium.

PHYSIOLOGICAL AND PATHOLOGICAL FUNCTIONS OF PAF

Inflammatory and Allergic Responses. The administration of PAF reproduces many of the signs and symptoms in anaphylactic shock. However, the effects of PAF antagonists in the treatment of inflammatory and allergic disorders have been disappointing. In patients with asthma, PAF antagonists partially inhibit the bronchoconstriction induced by antigen challenge but not by challenges by methacholine, exercise, or inhalation of cold air.

Cardiovascular System. PAF is a potent vasodilator in most vascular beds; when administered intravenously, it causes hypotension. PAF-induced vasodilation is independent of effects on sympathetic innervation, the renin–angiotensin system, or AA metabolism and likely results from a combination of direct and indirect actions. PAF may, alternatively, induce vasoconstriction depending on the concentration, vascular bed, and involvement of platelets or leukocytes. Intradermal injection of PAF causes an initial vasoconstriction followed by a typical wheal and flare. PAF increases vascular permeability and edema in the same manner as

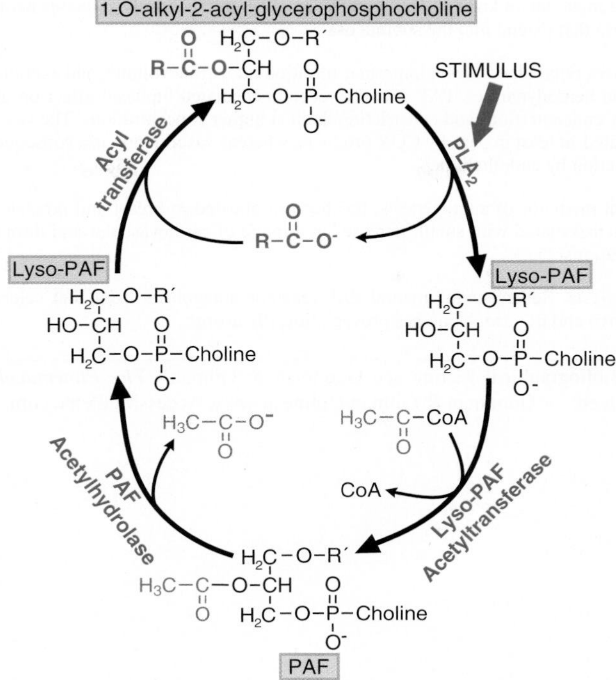

Figure 33–5 *Synthesis and degradation of platelet-activating factor (PAF).* PAF synthesis occurs in 2 steps. In the first step, activated PLA_2 cleaves membrane 1-*O*-alkyl-2-acyl-glycerophosphocholine to form lyso-PAF and a free fatty acid (usually AA that may be metabolized to eicosanoids). In the rate-limiting second step, PAF is formed from lyso-PAF by an acetyl CoA-lyso-PAF acetyltransferase. The synthesis of PAF may be stimulated during antigen–antibody reactions or by a variety of agents, including chemotactic peptides, thrombin, collagen, and other autacoids; PAF also can stimulate its own formation. PAF synthesis is regulated by the availability of Ca^{2+}. PAF is degraded by the reversal of the synthetic steps, de-acetylation by acetylhydrolases (AHs) followed by acylation at the 2 position to regenerate a 1-*O*-alkyl-2-acyl-glycerophosphocholine. PAF synthesis also can occur *de novo*: a phosphocholine substituent is transferred to alkyl acetyl glycerol by a distinct lyso-glycerophosphate acetyl-CoA transferase. CoA, coenzyme A.

histamine and bradykinin. The increase in permeability is due to contraction of venular endothelial cells, but PAF is more potent than histamine or bradykinin by 3 orders of magnitude.

Platelets. The PAF receptor is constitutively expressed on the surface of platelets. PAF potently stimulates platelet aggregation in vitro and in vivo. Although this is accompanied by the release of TxA_2 and the granular contents of the platelet, PAF does not require the presence of TxA_2 or other aggregating agents to produce this effect. The intravenous injection of PAF causes formation of intravascular platelet aggregates and thrombocytopenia.

Leukocytes. PAF is a potent and common activator of inflammatory cells. PAF stimulates a variety of responses in polymorphonuclear leukocytes (eosinophils, neutrophils, and basophils). PAF stimulates PMNs to aggregate, degranulate, and generate free radicals and LTs. PAF is a potent chemotactic for eosinophils, neutrophils, and monocytes and promotes PMN-endothelial adhesion contributing, along with other adhesion molecular systems, to leukocyte rolling, tight adhesion, and migration through the endothelial monolayer. PAF also stimulates basophils to release histamine, activates mast cells, and induces cytokine release from monocytes. In addition, PAF promotes aggregation of monocytes and degranulation of eosinophils.

Smooth Muscle. PAF contracts GI, uterine, and pulmonary smooth muscle. PAF enhances the amplitude of spontaneous uterine contractions; these contractions are inhibited by inhibitors of PG synthesis. PAF does not affect tracheal smooth muscle but contracts airway smooth muscle. When given by aerosol, PAF increases airway resistance as well as the responsiveness to other bronchoconstrictors. PAF also increases mucus secretion and the permeability of pulmonary microvessels.

Stomach. PAF is the most potent known ulcerogen. When given intravenously, it causes hemorrhagic erosions of the gastric mucosa that extend into the submucosa.

Kidney. PAF decreases renal blood flow, glomerular filtration rate, urine volume, and excretion of Na^+ without changes in systemic hemodynamics. PAF exerts a receptor-mediated biphasic effect on afferent arterioles, dilating them at low concentrations and constricting them at higher concentrations. The vasoconstrictor effect appears to be mediated, at least in part, by COX products, whereas vasodilation is a consequence of the stimulation of NO production by endothelium.

Other. PAF, a potent mediator of angiogenesis, has been implicated in breast and prostate cancer. PAF-AH deficiency has been associated with small increases in a range of cardiovascular and thrombotic diseases in some human populations.

PAF Receptor Antagonists. Several experimental PAF-receptor antagonists exist that selectively inhibit the actions of PAF in vivo and in vitro. None has proven clinically useful.

For a complete Bibliographical Listing see Goodman & Gilman's ***The Pharmacological Basis of Therapeutics***, 12th ed., or Goodman & Gilman Online at www.AccessMedicine.com.

Pharmacotherapy of Inflammation, Fever, Pain, and Gout

The chapter describes the nonsteroidal anti-inflammatory drugs (NSAIDs) used to treat inflammation, pain, and fever and the drugs used for hyperuricemia and gout. The NSAIDS are first considered by class, then by groups of chemically similar agents described in more detail. Many of the basic properties of these drugs are summarized in Tables 34–2, 34–3, and 34–4. Most currently available traditional NSAIDs (tNSAIDs) act by inhibiting the prostaglandin (PG) G/H synthase enzymes, colloquially known as the cyclooxygenases (COXs; *see* Chapter 33). The inhibition of cyclooxygenase-2 (COX-2) is thought to mediate, in large part, the antipyretic, analgesic, and anti-inflammatory actions of tNSAIDs, while the simultaneous inhibition of cyclooxygenase-1 (COX-1) largely but not exclusively accounts for unwanted adverse effects in the GI tract. Selective inhibitors of COX-2 (celecoxib, etoricoxib, lumiracoxib) are a subclass of NSAIDs. Aspirin irreversibly acetylates COX; several structural subclasses of tNSAIDs, including propionic acid derivatives (ibuprofen, naproxen), acetic acid derivatives (indomethacin), and enolic acids (piroxicam) compete in a reversible manner with arachidonic acid (AA) at the active site of COX-1 and COX-2. Acetaminophen (paracetamol) is effective as an antipyretic and analgesic agent at typical doses that partly inhibit COXs, has only weak anti-inflammatory activity, and exhibits fewer GI side effects than the tNSAIDs.

INFLAMMATION, PAIN, AND FEVER

INFLAMMATION. The inflammatory process is the response to an injurious stimulus. It can be evoked by noxious agents, infections, antibodies, physical injuries. The ability to mount an inflammatory response is essential for survival in the face of environmental pathogens and injury; in some situations and diseases, the inflammatory response may be exaggerated and sustained without apparent benefit and even with severe adverse consequences. The inflammatory response is characterized mechanistically by:

- Transient local vasodilation and increased capillary permeability
- Infiltration of leukocytes and phagocytic cells
- Tissue degeneration and fibrosis

Many molecules are involved in the promotion and resolution of the inflammatory process. Histamine, bradykinin, 5-HT, prostanoids, leukotrienes (LTs), and platelet-activating factor are important mediators of inflammation (*see* Chapter 33).

Prostanoid biosynthesis is significantly increased in inflamed tissue. Inhibitors of the COXs, which depress prostanoid formation, are effective and widely used anti-inflammatory agents. Prostaglandin E_2 (PGE_2) and prostacyclin (PGI_2) are the primary prostanoids that mediate inflammation. They increase local blood flow, vascular permeability, and leukocyte infiltration through activation of their respective receptors, EP_2 and IP. PGD_2, a major product of mast cells, contributes to inflammation in allergic responses, particularly in the lung.

Activation of endothelial cells plays a key role in "targeting" circulating cells to inflammatory sites. Endothelial activation results in leukocyte adhesion as the leukocytes recognize newly expressed L- and P-selectin and E-selectin with sialylated Lewis X and other glycoproteins on the leukocyte surface and endothelial intercellular adhesion molecule-1 (ICAM-1) with leukocyte integrins.

The recruitment of inflammatory cells to sites of injury also involves the concerted interactions of several types of soluble mediators. These include the complement factor C5a, PAF, and the eicosanoid LTB_4 (*see* Chapter 33). All can act as chemotactic agonists. Several cytokines also play essential roles in orchestrating the inflammatory process, especially tumor necrosis factor (TNF) and interleukin-1 (IL-1). Other cytokines and growth factors (e.g., IL-2, IL-6, IL-8, GM-CSF) contribute to manifestations of the inflammatory response. The concentrations of many of these factors are increased in the synovia of patients with inflammatory arthritis. Glucocorticoids interfere with the synthesis and actions of cytokines, such as

IL-1 or TNF-α (*see* Chapter 35). Although some of the actions of these cytokines are accompanied by the release of PGs and thromboxane A_2 (TxA_2), cyclooxygenase (COX) inhibitors appear to block only their pyrogenic effects.

PAIN. Inflammatory mediators released from nonneuronal cells during tissue injury increase the sensitivity of nociceptors and potentiate pain perception. Among these mediators are bradykinin, H^+, 5-HT, ATP, neurotrophins (nerve growth factor), LTs, and PGs. PGE_2 and PGI_2 reduce the threshold to stimulation of nociceptors, causing *peripheral sensitization*. Centrally active PGE_2 and perhaps also PGD_2, PGI_2, and $PGF_{2\alpha}$ contribute to *central sensitization*, an increase in excitability of spinal dorsal horn neurons that causes hyperalgesia and allodynia in part by disinhibition of glycinergic pathways.

FEVER. The hypothalamus regulates the set point at which body temperature is maintained. This set point is elevated in fever, reflecting an infection, or resulting from tissue damage, inflammation, graft rejection, or malignancy. These conditions all enhance formation of cytokines such as IL-1β, IL-6, TNF-α, and interferons, which act as endogenous pyrogens. The initial phase of the thermoregulatory response to such pyrogens may be mediated by ceramide release in neurons of the preoptic area in the anterior hypothalamus. A late response is mediated by coordinate induction of COX-2 and formation of PGE_2. PGE_2 can cross the blood-brain barrier and acts on EP_3 and perhaps EP_1 receptors on thermosensitive neurons. This triggers the hypothalamus to elevate body temperature by promoting an increase in heat generation and a decrease in heat loss. NSAIDs suppress this response by inhibiting PGE_2 synthesis.

NONSTEROIDAL ANTI-INFLAMMATORY DRUGS

NSAIDs are classified as *tNSAIDs*, which inhibit both COX-1 and COX-2, and *COX-2–selective NSAIDs*. Most NSAIDs are competitive, reversible, active site inhibitors of the COX enzymes. However, aspirin (acetyl salicylic acid, ASA) acetylates the isozymes and inhibits them irreversibly; thus, aspirin often is distinguished from the tNSAIDs. Similarly, acetaminophen, which is antipyretic and analgesic but largely devoid of anti-inflammatory activity, also is conventionally segregated from the group.

The vast majority of tNSAID compounds are organic acids with relatively low pK_a values (Figure 34–1). Even the nonacidic parent drug nabumetone is converted to an active acetic acid derivative in vivo. As organic acids, the compounds generally are well absorbed orally, highly bound to plasma proteins, and excreted either by glomerular filtration or by tubular secretion. They also accumulate in sites of inflammation, where the pH is lower, potentially confounding the relationship between plasma concentrations and duration of drug effect. Most COX-2–selective NSAIDs are diaryl heterocyclic compounds with a relatively bulky side group, which aligns with a large side pocket in the AA binding channel of COX-2 but hinders its optimal orientation in the smaller binding channel of COX-1. Both tNSAIDs and the COX-2–selective NSAIDs generally are hydrophobic drugs, a feature that allows them to access the hydrophobic arachidonate binding channel and results in shared pharmacokinetic characteristics. Again, aspirin and acetaminophen are exceptions to this rule.

MECHANISM OF ACTION

CYCLOOXYGENASE INHIBITION. The principal therapeutic effects of NSAIDs derive from their ability to inhibit PG production. The first enzyme in the PG synthetic pathway is COX, also known as PG G/H synthase. This enzyme converts AA to the unstable intermediates PGG_2 and PGH_2 and leads to the production of the prostanoids, TxA_2, and a variety of PGs (*see* Chapter 33). There are 2 forms of COX, COX-1 and COX-2. COX-1, expressed constitutively in most cells, is the dominant source of prostanoids for housekeeping functions. Conversely, COX-2, induced by cytokines, shear stress, and tumor promoters, is the more important source of prostanoid formation in inflammation and perhaps in cancer (*see* Chapter 33). COX-1 is the dominant isoform in gastric epithelial cells and is thought to be the major source of cytoprotective PG formation. Inhibition of COX-1 accounts for the gastric adverse events that complicate therapy with tNSAIDs.

Aspirin and NSAIDs inhibit the COX enzymes and PG production; they do not inhibit the lipoxygenase (LOX) pathways of AA metabolism and hence do not suppress LT formation (*see* Chapter 33).

IRREVERSIBLE CYCLOOXYGENASE INHIBITION BY ASPIRIN. Aspirin covalently modifies COX-1 and COX-2, irreversibly inhibiting COX activity. This is an important distinction from all the

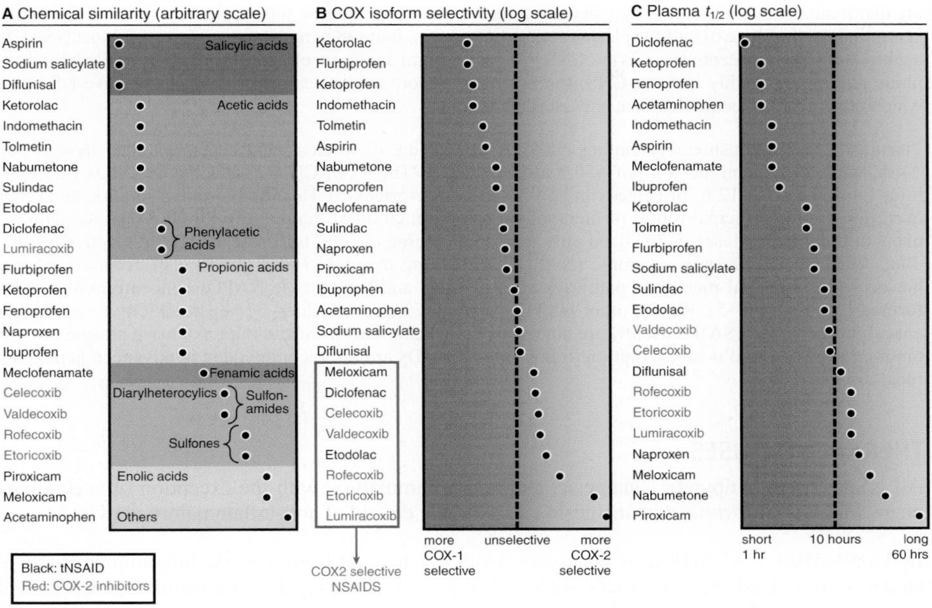

Figure 34–1 *Classification of NSAIDs by chemical similarity (panel A), cyclooxygenase (COX) isoform selectivity (panel B), and plasma* $t_{1/2}$ (panel C). The COX selectivity chart is plotted from data published in Warner et al., 1999, and FitzGerald and Patrono, 2001. tNSAIDs, traditional nonsteroidal anti-inflammatory drugs.

NSAIDs because the duration of aspirin's effects is related to the turnover rate of COXs in different target tissues.

The importance of enzyme turnover in recovery from aspirin action is most notable in platelets, which, being anucleate, have a markedly limited capacity for protein synthesis. Thus, the consequences of inhibition of platelet COX-1 last for the lifetime of the platelet. Inhibition of platelet COX-1–dependent TxA_2 formation therefore is cumulative with repeated doses of aspirin (at least as low as 30 mg/day) and takes ~8-12 days (the platelet turnover time) to recover fully once therapy has been stopped. The unique sensitivity of platelets to inhibition by such low doses of aspirin is related to their presystemic inhibition in the portal circulation before aspirin is deacetylated to salicylate on first pass through the liver. In contrast to aspirin, salicylic acid has no acetylating capacity. It is a weak, reversible, competitive inhibitor of COX.

SELECTIVE INHIBITION OF CYCLOOXYGENASE-2. The therapeutic use of the tNSAIDs is limited by their poor GI tolerability. Since COX-1 was the predominant source of cytoprotective PGs formed by the GI epithelium, selective inhibitors of COX-2 were developed to afford efficacy similar to tNSAIDs with better GI tolerability. Six COX-2 inhibitors, the coxibs, were initially approved for use: celecoxib, rofecoxib, valdecoxib and its prodrug parecoxib, etoricoxib, and lumiracoxib. Most coxibs have been either restricted in their use or withdrawn from the market in view of their adverse event profile. Celecoxib (CELEBREX) currently is the only COX-2 inhibitor licensed for use in the U.S.

ADME

NSAIDs are rapidly absorbed following oral ingestion, and peak plasma concentrations are reached within 2-3 h. Food intake may delay absorption and systemic availability (i.e., fenoprofen, sulindac). Antacids, commonly prescribed to patients on NSAID therapy, variably delay, absorption. Some compounds (e.g., diclofenac, nabumetone) undergo first-pass or presystemic elimination. Aspirin begins to acetylate platelets within minutes of reaching the presystemic circulation.

Most NSAIDs are extensively bound to plasma proteins (95-99%), usually albumin. Highly protein bound NSAIDs have the potential to displace other drugs, if they compete for the same binding sites. Most NSAIDs are distributed widely throughout the body and readily penetrate arthritic joints, yielding synovial fluid concentrations in the range of half the plasma concentration (i.e., ibuprofen, naproxen, piroxicam). Most NSAIDs achieve sufficient concentrations in the CNS to have a central analgesic effect. Celecoxib is particularly lipophilic and moves readily into the CNS. Lumiracoxib is more acidic than other COX-2–selective NSAIDs, which may favor its accumulation at sites of inflammation.

Plasma $t_{1/2}$ varies considerably among NSAIDs. Ibuprofen, diclofenac, and acetaminophen have $t_{1/2}$ of 1-4 h, while piroxicam has a $t_{1/2}$ of ~50 h at steady state. The $t_{1/2}$ of COX-2–selective NSAIDs vary (2-6 h for lumiracoxib, 6-12 h for celecoxib, and 20-26 h for etoricoxib). Hepatic biotransformation and renal excretion are the principal routes of metabolism and elimination of the majority of NSAIDs. Acetaminophen, at therapeutic doses, is oxidized only to a small degree to form traces of the highly reactive metabolite, *N*-acetyl-*p*-benzoquinone imine (NAPQI). Following overdose (usually >10 g of acetaminophen), however, the principal metabolic pathways are saturated, and hepatotoxic NAPQI concentrations can be formed (*see* Figure 4–5). Rarely, other NSAIDs also may be complicated by hepatotoxicity (e.g., diclofenac, lumiracoxib). NSAIDs usually are not removed by hemodialysis due to their extensive plasma protein binding; salicylic acid is an exemption to this rule. NSAIDs are not recommended in advanced hepatic or renal disease.

THERAPEUTIC USES

All NSAIDs are antipyretic, analgesic, and anti-inflammatory, with the exception of acetaminophen, which is antipyretic and analgesic but is largely devoid of anti-inflammatory activity.

INFLAMMATION. NSAIDs provide mostly symptomatic relief from pain and inflammation associated with musculoskeletal disorders, such as rheumatoid arthritis and osteoarthritis. Some NSAIDs are approved for the treatment of ankylosing spondylitis and gout.

PAIN. NSAIDs are effective only against pain of low to moderate intensity. Although their maximal efficacy is much less than the opioids, NSAIDs lack the unwanted adverse effects of opiates. Coadministration of NSAIDs can reduce the opioid dose needed for sufficient pain control and reduce the likelihood of adverse opioid effects. NSAIDs are particularly effective when inflammation has caused peripheral and/or central sensitization of pain perception. An exception to this is menstrual pain. The release of PGs by the endometrium during menstruation may cause severe cramps and other symptoms of primary dysmenorrhea; treatment of this condition with NSAIDs has met with considerable success. NSAIDs are commonly used to treat migraine attacks and can be combined with drugs such as the triptans (e.g., TREXIMET, a fixed-dose combination of naproxen and sumatriptan) or with antiemetics to aid relief of the associated nausea. NSAIDs lack efficacy in neuropathic pain.

FEVER. Antipyretic therapy is reserved for patients in whom fever in itself may be deleterious and for those who experience considerable relief when fever is lowered. NSAIDs reduce fever in most situations, but not the circadian variation in temperature or the rise in response to exercise or increased ambient temperature. COX-2 is the dominant source of PGs that mediate the rise in temperature evoked by bacterial lipopolysaccharide (LPS) administration.

FETAL CIRCULATORY SYSTEM. PGs are implicated in the maintenance of patency of the ductus arteriosus, and indomethacin, ibuprofen, and other tNSAIDs have been used in neonates to close the inappropriately patent ductus.

CARDIOPROTECTION. Ingestion of aspirin prolongs bleeding time. This effect is due to irreversible acetylation of platelet COX and the consequent inhibition of platelet function. It is the permanent suppression of platelet TxA_2 formation that is thought to underlie the cardioprotective effect of aspirin.

Aspirin reduces the risk of serious vascular events in high-risk patients (e.g., those with previous myocardial infarction) by 20-25%. Low-dose (<100 mg/day) aspirin is relatively selective for COX-1 and is associated with a lower risk for GI adverse events. However, low-dose aspirin increases the incidence of serious GI bleeds. It also increases the incidence of intracranial bleeds. The benefit from aspirin outweighs these risks in the case of secondary prevention of cardiovascular disease. Given their relatively short $t_{1/2}$ and reversible COX inhibition, most other tNSAIDs are not thought to afford cardioprotection. Data suggest that cardioprotection is lost when combining low-dose aspirin with ibuprofen. COX-2–selective NSAIDs are devoid of antiplatelet activity, as mature platelets do not express COX-2.

OTHER CLINICAL USES

Systemic Mastocytosis. Systemic mastocytosis is a condition in which there are excessive mast cells in the bone marrow, reticuloendothelial system, GI system, bones, and skin. In patients with systemic mastocytosis, PGD_2, released from mast cells is the major mediator of severe episodes of flushing, vasodilation, and hypotension. The addition of aspirin or ketoprofen has provided relief. However, aspirin and tNSAIDs can cause degranulation of mast cells, so blockade with H_1 and H_2 histamine receptor antagonists should be established before NSAIDs are initiated.

Niacin Tolerability. Large doses of niacin (nicotinic acid) effectively lower serum cholesterol levels, reduce low-density lipoprotein, and raise high-density lipoprotein (*see* Chapter 31). However, niacin induces intense facial flushing mediated largely by release of PGD_2 from the skin, which can be inhibited by treatment with aspirin.

Cancer Chemoprevention. Epidemiological studies suggested that frequent use of aspirin is associated with as much as a 50% decrease in the risk of colon cancer. Similar observations have been made with NSAID use in this and other cancers.

ADVERSE EFFECTS OF NSAID THERAPY

Common adverse events of aspirin and NSAIDs are outlined in Table 34–1.

GASTROINTESTINAL. The most common symptoms associated with these drugs are GI, including anorexia, nausea, dyspepsia, abdominal pain, and diarrhea. These symptoms may be related to the induction of gastric or intestinal ulcers, which is estimated to occur in 15-30% of regular users. Ulceration may be complicated by bleeding, perforation, or obstruction. The risk is further increased in those with *Helicobacter pylori* infection, heavy alcohol consumption, or other risk factors for mucosal injury, including the concurrent use of glucocorticoids. All selective COX-2 inhibitors are less prone to induce gastric ulcers than equally efficacious doses of tNSAIDs.

CARDIOVASCULAR. COX-2–selective NSAIDs were developed to improve the GI safety. However, clinical trials—with celecoxib, valdecoxib (withdrawn), and rofecoxib (withdrawn)—revealed an increase in the incidence of myocardial infarction, stroke, and thrombosis. COX-2-inhibitors depress formation of PGI_2 but do not inhibit COX-1 catalyzed formation of platelet thromboxane TxA_2. PGI_2 inhibits platelet aggregation and constrains the effect of prothrombotic and atherogenic stimuli by TxA_2.

BLOOD PRESSURE, RENAL, AND RENOVASCULAR ADVERSE EVENTS. NSAIDs and COX-2 inhibitors have been associated with renal and renovascular adverse events. In patients with congestive heart failure, hepatic cirrhosis, chronic kidney disease, hypovolemia, and other states of activation of the sympathoadrenal or

Table 34–1

Common and Shared Side Effects of NSAIDs

SYSTEM	MANIFESTATIONS
GI	Abdominal pain, nausea, diarrhea, anorexia, gastric erosions/ulcers[a]
	Anemia[a], GI hemorrhage[a], perforation/obstruction[a]
Platelets	Inhibited platelet activation[a], propensity for bruising[a]
	Increased risk of hemorrhage[a]
Renal	Salt and water retention, ↓ urate excretion (especially with aspirin)
	Edema, worsening of renal function in renal/cardiac and cirrhotic patients
	↓ effectiveness of antihypertensive meds
	↓ effectiveness of diuretics, hyperkalemia
Cardiovascular	Closure of ductus arteriosus, MI[b], stroke[b], thrombosis[b]
CNS	Headache, vertigo, dizziness, confusion, hyperventilation (salicylates)
Uterus	Prolongation of gestation, inhibition of labor
Hypersensitivity	Vasomotor rhinitis, angioneurotic edema, asthma
	Urticaria, flushing, hypotension, shock

MI, myocardial infarction.
[a]Side effects decreased with COX-2-selective NSAIDs.
[b]With the exception of low-dose aspirin.

renin–angiotensin systems, PG formation becomes crucial. NSAIDs are associated with loss of the PG-induced inhibition of both the reabsorption of Cl^- and the action of antidiuretic hormone, leading to the retention of salt and water. Epidemiological studies suggest hypertensive complications occur more commonly in patients treated with coxibs than with tNSAIDs.

ANALGESIC NEPHROPATHY. Analgesic nephropathy is a condition of slowly progressive renal failure, decreased concentrating capacity of the renal tubule, and sterile pyuria. Risk factors are the chronic use of high doses of combinations of NSAIDs and frequent urinary tract infections.

PREGNANCY AND LACTATION. Myometrial COX-2 expression and levels of PGE_2 and $PGF_{2\alpha}$ increase markedly in the myometrium during labor. Prolongation of gestation by NSAIDs has been demonstrated in humans. Some NSAIDs, particularly indomethacin, have been used off-label to terminate preterm labor. However, this use is associated with closure of the ductus arteriosus and impaired fetal circulation in utero, particularly in fetuses older than 32 weeks' gestation. COX-2–selective inhibitors have been used off-label as tocolytic agents; this use has been associated with stenosis of the ductus arteriosus and oligohydramnios. Finally, the use of NSAIDs and aspirin late in pregnancy may increase the risk of postpartum hemorrhage. Therefore, pregnancy, especially close to term, is a relative contraindication to the use of all NSAIDs. In addition, their use must be weighed against potential fetal risk, even in cases of premature labor, and especially in cases of pregnancy-induced hypertension.

HYPERSENSITIVITY. Hypersensitivity symptoms to aspirin and NSAIDs range from vasomotor rhinitis, generalized urticaria, and bronchial asthma to laryngeal edema, bronchoconstriction, flushing, hypotension, and shock. Aspirin intolerance is a contraindication to therapy with any other NSAID because cross-sensitivity. Treatment of aspirin hypersensitivity is similar to that of other severe hypersensitivity reactions, with support of vital organ function and administration of epinephrine.

ASPIRIN RESISTANCE. All forms of treatment failure with aspirin have been collectively called *aspirin resistance*. Genetic variants of COX-1 that cosegregate with resistance have been described, but the relation to clinical outcome is not clear.

REYE SYNDROME. Due to the possible association with Reye syndrome, aspirin and other salicylates are contraindicated in children and young adults < 20 years of age with viral illness–associated fever. Reye syndrome, a severe and often fatal disease, is characterized by the acute onset of encephalopathy, liver dysfunction, and fatty infiltration of the liver and other viscera. Although a mechanistic understanding is lacking, the epidemiologic association between aspirin use and Reye syndrome is sufficiently strong that aspirin and bismuth subsalicylate labels now must indicate the risk. As the use of aspirin in children has declined dramatically, so has the incidence of Reye syndrome. Acetaminophen has not been implicated in Reye syndrome and is the drug of choice for antipyresis in children and young adults.

CONCOMITANT NSAIDS AND LOW-DOSE ASPIRIN. Many patients combine either tNSAIDs or COX-2 inhibitors with low-dose aspirin for "cardioprotection." Epidemiological studies suggest that this combination therapy increases significantly the likelihood of GI adverse events over either class of NSAID alone.

DRUG INTERACTIONS

Angiotensin-converting enzyme (ACE) inhibitors act, at least partly, by preventing the breakdown of kinins that stimulate PG production (*see* Figure 32–2). Thus, it is logical that NSAIDs might attenuate the effectiveness of ACE inhibitors by blocking the production of vasodilator and natriuretic PGs. Due to hyperkalemia, the combination of NSAIDs and ACE inhibitors also can produce marked bradycardia leading to syncope, especially in the elderly and in patients with hypertension, diabetes mellitus, or ischemic heart disease. Corticosteroids and SSRIs may increase the frequency or severity of GI complications when combined with NSAIDs. NSAIDs may augment the risk of bleeding in patients receiving warfarin both because almost all tNSAIDs suppress normal platelet function temporarily during the dosing interval and because some NSAIDs also increase warfarin levels by interfering with its metabolism. Many NSAIDs are highly bound to plasma proteins and thus may displace other drugs from their binding sites. Such interactions can occur in patients given salicylates or other NSAIDs together with warfarin, sulfonylurea hypoglycemic agents, or methotrexate; the dosage of such agents may require adjustment to prevent toxicity. Patients taking lithium should be monitored because certain NSAIDs (e.g., piroxicam) can reduce the renal excretion of this drug and lead to toxicity, while others can decrease lithium levels (e.g., sulindac).

PEDIATRIC AND GERIATRIC USE

THERAPEUTIC USES IN CHILDREN. Therapeutic indications for NSAID use in children include fever, mild pain, postoperative pain, and inflammatory disorders, such as juvenile arthritis and Kawasaki disease. Only drugs that have been extensively tested in children should be used (acetaminophen, ibuprofen, and naproxen).

PHARMACOKINETICS IN CHILDREN. NSAID dosing recommendations frequently are based on extrapolation of pharmacokinetic data from adults or children >2 years, and there is often insufficient data for dose selection in younger infants. For example, the pharmacokinetics of the most commonly used NSAID in children, acetaminophen, differ substantially between the neonatal period and older children or adults. The systemic bioavailability of rectal acetaminophen formulations in neonates and preterm babies is higher than in older patients. Acetaminophen clearance is reduced in preterm neonates probably due to their immature glucuronide conjugation system (sulfation is the principal route of biotransformation at this age). Therefore, acetaminophen dosing intervals need to be extended (8-12 h) or daily doses reduced to avoid accumulation and liver toxicity. Aspirin elimination also is delayed in neonates and young infants compared to adults bearing the risk of accumulation. Disease also may affect NSAID disposition in children. For example, ibuprofen plasma concentrations are reduced and clearance increased (~80%) in children with cystic fibrosis. This probably is related to the GI and hepatic pathologies associated with this disease. Aspirin's kinetics are markedly altered during the febrile phase of rheumatic fever or Kawasaki vasculitis. The reduction in serum albumin associated with these conditions causes an elevation of the free salicylate concentration, which may saturate renal excretion and result in salicylate accumulation to toxic levels. In addition to dose reduction, monitoring of the free drug may be warranted in these situations.

PHARMACOKINETICS IN THE ELDERLY. The clearance of many NSAIDs is reduced in the elderly due to changes in hepatic metabolism. NSAIDs with a long $t_{1/2}$ and primarily oxidative metabolism (i.e., piroxicam, tenoxicam, celecoxib) have elevated plasma concentrations in elderly patients. For example, plasma concentrations after the same dose of celecoxib may rise up to 2-fold higher in patients >65 years than in patients <50 years of age, warranting dose adjustment. The capacity of plasma albumin to bind drugs is diminished in older patients and may result in higher concentrations of unbound NSAIDs. The higher susceptibility of older patients to GI complications may be due to a reduction in gastric mucosal defense and to elevated total and/or free NSAID concentrations. Generally, it is advisable to start most NSAIDs at a low dosage in the elderly and increase the dosage only if the therapeutic efficacy is insufficient.

SPECIFIC PROPERTIES OF INDIVIDUAL NSAIDS

General properties shared by NSAIDs were considered in the preceding section, "Nonsteroidal Anti-Inflammatory Drugs." In this section, important characteristics of individual substances are discussed. NSAIDs are grouped by their chemical similarity, as in Figure 34–1.

ASPIRIN AND OTHER SALICYLATES

The salicylates include, aspirin, salicylic acid, methyl salicylate, diflunisal, salsalate, olsalazine, and sulfasalazine. Aspirin is the most widely consumed analgesic, antipyretic, and anti-inflammatory agent. Because aspirin is so available, the possibility of misuse and serious toxicity is underappreciated.

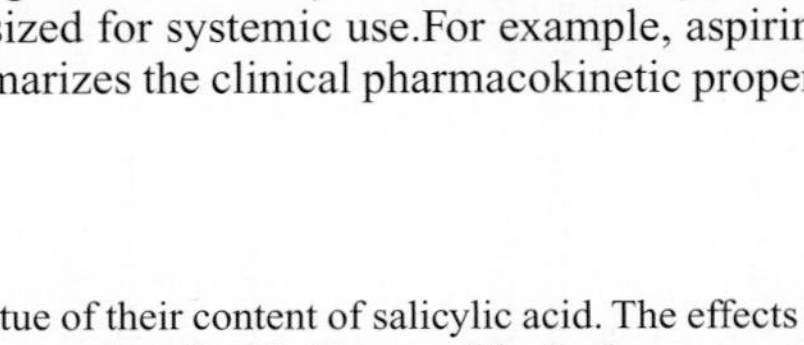

COOH, OH — SALICYLIC ACID

COOH, $OCOCH_3$ — ASPIRIN

Salicylic acid is so irritating that it can only be used externally; therefore various derivatives of this acid have been synthesized for systemic use.For example, aspirin is the acetate ester of salicylic acid. Table 34–2 summarizes the clinical pharmacokinetic properties of 2 salicylates, aspirin and diflunisal.

MECHANISM OF ACTION

Salicylates generally act by virtue of their content of salicylic acid. The effects of aspirin are largely caused by its capacity to acetylate proteins, as described in "Irreversible Cyclooxygenase Inhibition by Aspirin," above.

ADME

ABSORPTION. Orally ingested salicylates are absorbed rapidly, partly from the stomach but mostly from the upper small intestine. Appreciable concentrations are found in plasma in <30 min; after a single dose, the peak plasma level is reached in ~1 h and then declines gradually. The rate of absorption is determined by disintegration and dissolution rates of the tablets administered, the pH at the mucosal surface, and gastric emptying time. The presence of food delays absorption of salicylates. Rectal absorption of salicylate usually is slower than oral absorption and is incomplete and inconsistent.

Table 34–2

Comparison of NSAIDS: Salicylates, Acetaminophen, and Acetic Acid Derivatives

CLASS/Drug	PHARMACOKINETICS		DOSING[d]		COMMENTS	COMPARED TO ASPIRIN
Salicylates						
Aspirin	Peak C_p[a] Protein binding Metabolites[b] $t_{1/2}$[c], therapeutic $t_{1/2}$, toxic dose	1 h 80-90% Salicyluric acid 2-3 h 15-30 h	Antiplatelet Pain/fever Rheumatic fever Children	40-80 mg/day 325-650 mg/ 4-6 h 1 g/4-6 h 10 mg/kg/4-6 h	Permanent platelet COX-1 inhibition Main side effects: GI, increased bleeding time, hypersensitivity Avoid in children with acute febrile illness	
Diflunisal	Peak C_p Protein binding Metabolites $t_{1/2}$	2-3 h 99% Glucuronide 8-12 h	250-500 mg every 8-12 h		Not metabolized to salicylate Competitive COX inhibitor Excreted into breast milk	Analgesic and anti-inflammatory, 4-5× more potent Antipyretic, weaker Fewer platelet and GI side effects
Para-aminophenol derivative						
Acetaminophen	Peak C_p Protein binding Metabolites $t_{1/2}$	30-60 min 20-50% Glucuronides (60%); sulfates (35%) 2 h	10-15 mg/kg every 4 h (maximum of 5 doses/24 h)		Weak nonspecific inhibitor at common doses Potency may be modulated by peroxides Overdose ⇒ toxic metabolite, liver necrosis	Analgesic/antipyretic, equivalent Anti-inflammatory, GI, and platelet effects < aspirin at 1000 mg/day
Acetic acid derivatives						
Indomethacin	Peak C_p Protein binding Metabolites $t_{1/2}$	1-2 h 90% *O*-demethyl (50%); unchanged (20%) 2.5 h	25 mg 2-3 times/day; 75-100 mg at night		Side effects (3-50%): frontal headache, neutropenia, thrombocytopenia; 20% discontinue	10-40× more potent; intolerance limits dose

Sulindac (sulfoxide prodrug)	Peak C_p	1-2 h; active sulfide metabolite 8 h; extensive enterohepatic circulation	150-200 mg twice/day	20%, GI side effects; 10%, CNS side effects	Efficacy comparable
	Metabolites	Sulfone/conjugates (30%); sulindac/conjugates (25%)			
	$t_{1/2}$	7 h; 18 h for active metabolite			
Etodolac	Peak C_p	1 h	200-400 mg 3-4 times/day	Some COX-2 selectivity in vitro	100 mg etodolac efficacy ≈ 650 mg of aspirin, may be better tolerated
	Protein binding	99%			
	Metabolites	Hepatic metabolites			
	$t_{1/2}$	7 h			
Tolmetin	Peak C_p	20-60 min	Adults: 400-600 mg 3 times/day Children >2 years: 20 mg/kg/day in 3-4 divided doses	Food delays and decreases peak absorption May persist in synovial fluid ⇒ biological efficacy > its plasma $t_{1/2}$	Efficacy similar; 25-40% develop side effects; 5-10% discontinue drug
	Protein binding	99%			
	Metabolites	Carboxylate conjugates			
	$t_{1/2}$	5 h			
Ketorolac	Peak C_p	30-60 min	<65 y: 20 mg orally, then 10 mg/4-6 h (max: 40 mg/24 h); >65 y: 10 mg/4-6 h (max: 40 mg/24 h)	Parenterally (60 mg IM, then 30 mg every 6 h, or 30 mg IV every 6 h) Available as ocular prep	Potent analgesic, poor anti-inflammatory
	Protein binding	99%			
	Metabolites	Glucuronide (90%)			
	$t_{1/2}$	4-6 h			
Diclofenac	Peak C_p	2-3 h	50 mg 3 times/day or 75 mg twice/day	As topical gel, ocular solution, oral tablets combined with misoprostol First-pass effect; oral bioavailability, 50%	More potent; 20%, side effects; 2% discontinue; 15%, elevated liver enzymes
	Protein binding	99%			
	Metabolites	Glucuronide and sulfide (renal 65%, bile 35%)			
	$t_{1/2}$	1-2 h			

For explanation of nomenclature and abbreviations, see legend to Table 34–4.

Salicylic acid is absorbed rapidly from the intact skin, especially when applied in oily liniments or ointments, and systemic poisoning has occurred from its application to large areas of skin. Methyl salicylate likewise is speedily absorbed when applied cutaneously; however, its GI absorption may be delayed many hours, making gastric lavage effective for removal even in poisonings that present late after oral ingestion.

DISTRIBUTION. After absorption, salicylates are distributed throughout most body tissues and transcellular fluids, primarily by pH-dependent passive processes. Salicylates are transported actively out of the CSF across the choroid plexus. The drugs readily cross the placental barrier. Ingested aspirin mainly is absorbed as such, but some enters the systemic circulation as salicylic acid after hydrolysis by esterases in the GI mucosa and liver. Roughly 80-90% of the salicylate in plasma is bound to proteins, especially albumin; the proportion of the total that is bound declines as plasma concentrations increase. Hypoalbuminemia, as may occur in rheumatoid arthritis, is associated with a proportionately higher level of free salicylate in the plasma. Salicylate competes with a variety of compounds for plasma protein binding sites; these include thyroxine, triiodothyronine, penicillin, phenytoin, sulfinpyrazone, bilirubin, uric acid, and other NSAIDs such as naproxen. Aspirin is bound to a more limited extent; however, it acetylates human plasma albumin in vivo by reaction with the ε-amino group of lysine and may change the binding of other drugs to albumin. Aspirin also acetylates hormones, DNA, and hemoglobin and other proteins.

METABOLISM AND ELIMINATION. The 3 chief metabolic products are salicyluric acid (the glycine conjugate), the ether or phenolic glucuronide, and the ester or acyl glucuronide. Salicylates and their metabolites are excreted in the urine The excretion of free salicylates is variable and depends on the dose and the urinary pH. For example, the clearance of salicylate is about 4 times as great at pH 8 as at pH 6, and it is well above the glomerular filtration rate at pH 8. High rates of urine flow decrease tubular reabsorption, whereas the opposite is true in oliguria. The plasma $t_{1/2}$ for aspirin is ~20 min, and for salicylate is 2-3 h at antiplatelet doses, rising to 12 h at usual anti-inflammatory doses. The $t_{1/2}$ of salicylate may rise to 15-30 h at high therapeutic doses or when there is intoxication. This dose-dependent elimination is the result of the limited capacity of the liver to form salicyluric acid and the phenolic glucuronide, resulting in a larger proportion of unchanged drug being excreted in the urine at higher doses. Salicylate clearance is reduced and salicylate exposure is significantly increased in the elderly. The plasma concentration of salicylate is increased by conditions that decrease glomerular filtration rate or reduce proximal tubule secretion, such as renal disease or the presence of inhibitors that compete for the transport system (e.g., probenecid).

THERAPEUTIC USES

SYSTEMIC USES. The *analgesic–antipyretic* dose of aspirin for adults is 324-1000 mg orally every 4-6 h. The anti-inflammatory doses of aspirin recommended for *arthritis, spondyloarthropathies, and systemic lupus erythematosus* (SLE) range from 3-4 g/day in divided doses. The maximum recommended daily dose of aspirin for adults and children >12 years or older is 4 g. The rectal administration of aspirin suppositories may be preferred in infants or when the oral route is unavailable. Salicylates suppress clinical signs and improve tissue inflammation in acute rheumatic fever. Other salicylates available for systemic use include salsalate (salicylsalicylic acid), magnesium salicylate, and a combination of choline salicylate and magnesium salicylate (choline magnesium–trisalicylate).

Diflunisal is a difluorophenyl derivative of salicylic acid that is not converted to salicylic acid in vivo. Diflunisal is a competitive inhibitor of COX, it is a potent anti-inflammatory but is largely devoid of antipyretic effects, perhaps because of poor penetration into the CNS. The drug has been used as an analgesic in the treatment of *osteoarthritis* and musculoskeletal strains or sprains; in these circumstances, it is 3-4 times more potent than aspirin. The usual initial dose is 1000 mg, followed by 500 mg every 8-12 h. Diflunisal produces fewer auditory side effects (see "Ototoxic Effects") and appears to cause fewer GI and antiplatelet effects than does aspirin.

LOCAL USES. Mesalamine (5-aminosalicylic acid) is a salicylate that is used for its local effects in the treatment of *inflammatory bowel disease* (*see* Figure 47–4). Oral formulations that deliver drug to the lower intestine are efficacious in the treatment of inflammatory bowel disease (in particular, ulcerative colitis). These preparations rely on pH-sensitive coatings and other delayed release mechanisms, such as linkage to another moiety to create a poorly absorbed parent compound that must be cleaved by bacteria in the colon to form the active drug. Some over-the-counter medications to relieve indigestion and diarrhea agents contain bismuth subsalicylate (PEPTO-BISMOL, others) and have the potential to cause salicylate intoxication, particularly in children.

The keratolytic action of free salicylic acid is employed for the local treatment of warts, corns, fungal infections, and certain types of eczematous dermatitis. After treatment with salicylic acid, tissue cells swell, soften, and desquamate. Methyl salicylate (oil of wintergreen) is a common ingredient of ointments and deep-heating liniments used in the management of musculoskeletal pain. The cutaneous application of methyl salicylate can result in pharmacologically active, and even toxic, systemic salicylate concentrations and has been reported to increase prothrombin time in patients receiving warfarin.

ADVERSE EFFECTS

RESPIRATION. Salicylates increase O_2 consumption and CO_2 production (especially in skeletal muscle) at anti-inflammatory doses, a result of uncoupling oxidative phosphorylation. The increased production of CO_2 stimulates respiration. Salicylates also stimulate the respiratory center directly in the medulla. Respiratory rate and depth increases, the Pco_2 falls, and primary respiratory alkalosis ensues.

ACID–BASE AND ELECTROLYTE BALANCE AND RENAL EFFECTS. Therapeutic doses of salicylate produce definite changes in the acid–base balance and electrolyte pattern. Compensation for the initial event, respiratory alkalosis, is achieved by increased renal excretion of bicarbonate, which is accompanied by increased Na^+ and K^+ excretion; plasma bicarbonate is thus lowered, and blood pH returns toward normal. This is the stage of compensatory renal acidosis. This stage is most often seen in adults given intensive salicylate therapy and seldom proceeds further unless toxicity ensues (see "Salicylate Intoxication"). Salicylates can cause retention of salt and water, as well as acute reduction of renal function in patients with congestive heart failure, renal disease, or hypovolemia. Although long-term use of salicylates alone rarely is associated with nephrotoxicity, the prolonged and excessive ingestion of analgesic mixtures containing salicylates in combination with other NSAIDs can produce papillary necrosis and interstitial nephritis (see "Analgesic Nephropathy").

CARDIOVASCULAR EFFECTS. Low doses of aspirin (≤100 mg daily) are used widely for their cardioprotective effects. At high therapeutic doses (≥3 g daily), as might be given for acute rheumatic fever, salt and water retention can lead to an increase (≤20%) in circulating plasma volume and decreased hematocrit (via a dilutional effect). There is a tendency for the peripheral vessels to dilate because of a direct effect on vascular smooth muscle. Cardiac output and work are increased. Those with carditis or compromised cardiac function may not have sufficient cardiac reserve to meet the increased demands, and congestive cardiac failure and pulmonary edema can occur. High doses of salicylates can produce noncardiogenic pulmonary edema, particularly in older patients who ingest salicylates regularly over a prolonged period.

GI EFFECTS. Ingestion of salicylates may result in epigastric distress, nausea, and vomiting. Salicylates also may cause gastric ulceration, exacerbation of peptic ulcer symptoms (heartburn, dyspepsia), GI hemorrhage, and erosive gastritis. These effects occur primarily with acetylated salicylates (i.e., aspirin). Because nonacetylated salicylates lack the capacity to acetylate COX and irreversibly inhibit its activity, they are weaker inhibitors than aspirin.

HEPATIC EFFECTS. Salicylates can cause hepatic injury, usually after high doses of salicylates that result in plasma concentrations of >150 μg/mL. The injury is not an acute effect; rather, the onset characteristically occurs after several months of treatment. The majority of cases occur in patients with connective tissue disorders. There usually are no symptoms, simply an increase in serum levels of hepatic transaminases, but some patients note right upper quadrant abdominal discomfort and tenderness. Overt jaundice is uncommon. The injury usually is reversible upon discontinuation of salicylates. However, the use of salicylates is contraindicated in patients with chronic liver disease. Considerable evidence implicates the use of salicylates as an important factor in the severe hepatic injury and encephalopathy observed in Reye syndrome. Large doses of salicylates may cause hyperglycemia and glycosuria and deplete liver and muscle glycogen.

URICOSURIC EFFECTS. The effects of salicylates on uric acid excretion are markedly dependent on dose. Low doses (1 or 2 g/day) may decrease urate excretion and elevate plasma urate concentrations; intermediate doses (2 or 3 g/day) usually do not alter urate excretion. Large doses (>5 g/day) induce uricosuria and lower plasma urate levels; however, such large doses are tolerated poorly. Even small doses of salicylate can block the effects of probenecid and other uricosuric agents that decrease tubular reabsorption of uric acid.

HEMATOLOGIC EFFECTS. Irreversible inhibition of platelet function underlies the cardioprotective effect of aspirin. If possible, aspirin therapy should be stopped at least 1 week before surgery; however, preoperative aspirin often is recommended prior to carotid artery stenting, carotid endarterectomy, infrainguinal arterial bypass, and PCI (percutaneous coronary intervention) procedures. Patients with severe hepatic damage, hypoprothrombinemia, vitamin K deficiency, or hemophilia should avoid aspirin because the inhibition of platelet hemostasis can result in hemorrhage. Aspirin is used widely for the prophylaxis of thromboembolic disease.

OTOTOXIC EFFECTS. Hearing impairment, alterations of perceived sounds, and tinnitus commonly occur during high-dose salicylate therapy. Ototoxic symptoms sometimes are observed at low doses. Symptoms usually resolve within 2 or 3 days after withdrawal of the drug. As most competitive COX inhibitors are not associated with hearing loss or tinnitus, a direct effect of salicylic acid rather than suppression of PG synthesis is likely.

SALICYLATES AND PREGNANCY. Infants born to women who ingest salicylates for long periods may have significantly reduced birth weights. When administered during the third trimester, there also is an increase in perinatal mortality, anemia, and complicated deliveries; thus, its use during this period should be avoided. NSAIDs during the third trimester of pregnancy also can cause premature closure of the ductus arteriosus.

DRUG INTERACTIONS. The plasma concentration of salicylates generally is little affected by other drugs, but concurrent administration of aspirin lowers the concentrations of indomethacin, naproxen, ketoprofen, and fenoprofen, at least in part by displacement from plasma proteins. Important adverse interactions of aspirin with warfarin, sulfonylureas, and methotrexate are mentioned above (in "Drug Interactions"). Other interactions of aspirin include the antagonism of spironolactone-induced natriuresis and the blockade of the active transport of penicillin from CSF to blood. Magnesium-aluminum hydroxide antacids can alkalize the urine enough to increase salicylic acid clearance significantly and reduce steady-state concentrations. Conversely, discontinuation of antacid therapy can increase plasma concentrations to toxic levels.

SALICYLATE INTOXICATION

Salicylate poisoning or serious intoxication often occurs in children and sometimes is fatal. CNS effects, intense hyperpnea, and hyperpyrexia are prominent symptoms. Death has followed use of 10-30 g of sodium salicylate or aspirin in adults, but much larger amounts (130 g of aspirin in 1 case) have been ingested without a fatal outcome. The lethal dose of methyl salicylate (also known as oil of wintergreen, sweet birch oil, gaultheria oil, betula oil) is considerably less than that of sodium salicylate. As little as a 4 mL (4.7 g) of methyl salicylate may cause severe systemic toxicity in children. Mild chronic salicylate intoxication is called *salicylism*. When fully developed, the syndrome includes headache, dizziness, tinnitus, difficulty hearing, dimness of vision, mental confusion, lassitude, drowsiness, sweating, thirst, hyperventilation, nausea, vomiting, and occasionally diarrhea.

NEUROLOGICAL EFFECTS. In high doses, salicylates have toxic effects on the CNS, consisting of stimulation (including convulsions) followed by depression. Confusion, dizziness, tinnitus, high-tone deafness, delirium, psychosis, stupor, and coma may occur. Salicylates induce nausea and vomiting, which result from stimulation of sites that are accessible from the CSF, probably in the medullary chemoreceptor trigger zone.

RESPIRATION. The respiratory effects of salicylates contribute to the serious acid–base balance disturbances that characterize poisoning by this class of compounds. Salicylates stimulate respiration indirectly by uncoupling of oxidative phosphorylation and directly by stimulation of the respiratory center in the medulla (described above). Uncoupling of oxidative phosphorylation also leads to excessive heat production, and salicylate toxicity is associated with hyperthermia, particularly in children. Prolonged exposure to high doses of salicylates leads to depression of the medulla, with central respiratory depression and circulatory collapse, secondary to vasomotor depression. Because enhanced CO_2 production continues, respiratory acidosis ensues. Respiratory failure is the usual cause of death in fatal cases of salicylate poisoning.

ACID–BASE BALANCE AND ELECTROLYTES. High therapeutic doses of salicylate are associated with a primary respiratory alkalosis and compensatory renal acidosis. The phase of primary respiratory alkalosis rarely is recognized in children with salicylate toxicity. They usually present in a state of mixed respiratory and renal acidosis, characterized by a decrease in blood pH, a low plasma bicarbonate concentration, and normal or nearly normal plasma Pco_2. Direct salicylate-induced depression of respiration prevents adequate respiratory hyperventilation to match the increased peripheral production of CO_2. Consequently, plasma Pco_2 increases and blood pH decreases. Because the concentration of bicarbonate in plasma already is low due to increased renal bicarbonate excretion, the acid–base status at this stage essentially is an uncompensated respiratory acidosis. Superimposed, however, is a true metabolic acidosis caused by accumulation of acids as a result of 3 processes. *First*, toxic concentrations of salicylates displace ~2-3 mEq/L of plasma bicarbonate. *Second*, vasomotor depression caused by toxic doses of salicylates impairs renal function, with consequent accumulation of sulfuric and phosphoric acids; renal failure can ensue. *Third*, salicylates in toxic doses may decrease aerobic metabolism as a result of inhibition of various enzymes. This derangement of carbohydrate metabolism leads to the accumulation of organic acids, especially pyruvic, lactic, and acetoacetic acids.

The low plasma Pco_2 leads to decreased renal tubular reabsorption of bicarbonate and increased renal excretion of Na^+, K^+, and water. Dehydration, which can be profound, particularly in children, rapidly occurs. Because more water than electrolyte is lost through the lungs and by sweating, the dehydration is associated with hypernatremia.

MANAGEMENT OF SALICYLATE OVERDOSE. Salicylate poisoning represents an acute medical emergency, and death may result despite heroic efforts. Monitoring of salicylate levels is a useful guide to therapy but must be used in conjunction with an assessment of the patient's overall clinical condition, acid–base balance, formulation of salicylate ingested, timing, and dose. There is no specific antidote for salicylate poisoning. Management begins with a rapid assessment followed by the ABCD approach to medical emergencies: A (airway), B (breathing), C (circulation), D (decontamination).

ACETAMINOPHEN

Acetaminophen (paracetamol; TYLENOL, others) is the active metabolite of phenacetin.

ACETAMINOPHEN

Acetaminophen is available without a prescription and is used as a common household analgesic. It also is available in fixed-dose combinations containing narcotic and nonnarcotic analgesics (including aspirin and other salicylates), barbiturates, caffeine, vascular headache remedies, sleep aids, toothache remedies, antihistamines, antitussives, decongestants, expectorants, cold and flu preparations, and sore throat treatments. Acetaminophen is well tolerated and has a low incidence of GI side effects. However, acute overdosage can cause severe hepatic damage (*see* Figure 4–4), and the number of poisonings with acetaminophen continues to grow.

MECHANISM OF ACTION

Acetaminophen has analgesic and antipyretic effects similar to those of aspirin, but only weak anti-inflammatory effects. Acetaminophen is postulated to have a poor ability to inhibit COX isoforms in the presence of high concentrations of peroxides, as occur at sites of inflammation. COX inhibition might be disproportionately pronounced in the brain, explaining its antipyretic efficacy.

ADME

Oral acetaminophen has excellent bioavailability. Peak plasma concentrations occur within 30-60 min, and the $t_{1/2}$ in plasma is ~2 h. Binding of the drug to plasma proteins is variable but less than with other NSAIDs; only 20-50% is bound at the concentrations encountered during acute intoxication. Some 90-100% of drug may be recovered in the urine within the first day at therapeutic dosing, primarily after hepatic conjugation with glucuronic acid (*see* Table 34–2). Children have less capacity for glucuronidation of the drug than do adults. A small proportion of acetaminophen undergoes CYP-mediated *N*-hydroxylation to form NAPQI, a highly reactive intermediate.

THERAPEUTIC USES

Acetaminophen is suitable for analgesic or antipyretic uses; it is particularly valuable for patients in whom aspirin is contraindicated (e.g., those with peptic ulcer, aspirin hypersensitivity, children with a febrile illness). The conventional oral dose of acetaminophen is 325-650 mg every 4-6 h; total daily doses should not exceed 4000 mg (2000 mg/day for chronic alcoholics). Single doses for children 2-11 years old range from 160-480 mg, depending on age and weight; no more than 5 doses should be administered in 24 h. A dose of 10 mg/kg also may be used. An injectable preparation is now available (see recent review on the Goodman & Gilman website at AccessMedicine.com).

ADVERSE EFFECTS AND TOXICITY

Acetaminophen usually is well tolerated. Rash and other allergic reactions occur occasionally, but sometimes it is more serious and may be accompanied by drug fever and mucosal lesions. Patients who show hypersensitivity reactions to the salicylates only rarely exhibit sensitivity to acetaminophen. The most serious acute adverse effect of overdosage of acetaminophen is a potentially fatal hepatic necrosis. Hepatic injury with acetaminophen involves its conversion to the toxic metabolite, NAPQI. The glucuronide and sulfate conjugation pathways become saturated, and increasing amounts undergo CYP-mediated *N*-hydroxylation to form NAPQI. This is eliminated rapidly by conjugation with GSH and then further metabolized to a mercapturic acid and excreted into the urine. In the setting of acetaminophen overdose, hepatocellular levels of GSH become depleted. The highly reactive NAPQI metabolite binds covalently to cell macromolecules, leading to dysfunction of enzymatic systems and structural and metabolic disarray. Furthermore, depletion of intracellular GSH renders the hepatocytes highly susceptible to oxidative stress and apoptosis (*see* Figure 4–4). Renal tubular necrosis and hypoglycemic coma also may occur.

MANAGEMENT OF ACETAMINOPHEN OVERDOSE. Severe liver damage occurs in 90% of patients with plasma concentrations of acetaminophen >300 μg/mL at 4 h or 45 μg/mL at 15 h after the ingestion of the drug. Activated charcoal, if given within 4 h of ingestion, decreases acetaminophen absorption by 50-90% and is the preferred method of gastric decontamination. Gastric lavage generally is not recommended.

N-acetylcysteine (NAC) (MUCOMYST, ACETADOTE) is indicated for those at risk of hepatic injury. NAC functions by detoxifying NAPQI. It both repletes GSH stores and may conjugate directly with NAPQI by serving as a GSH substitute. In addition to NAC therapy, aggressive supportive care is warranted. This includes management of hepatic and renal failure if they occur and intubation if the patient becomes obtunded. Hypoglycemia can result from liver failure, and plasma glucose should be monitored closely. Fulminant hepatic failure is an indication for liver transplantation, and a liver transplant center should be contacted early in the course of treatment of patients who develop severe liver injury despite NAC therapy.

ACETIC ACID DERIVATIVES

INDOMETHACIN

Indomethacin (INDOCIN, others) is indicated for the treatment of moderate to severe rheumatoid arthritis, osteoarthritis, and acute gouty arthritis; ankylosing spondylitis; and acute painful shoulder. Indomethacin is a more potent nonselective inhibitor of the COXs than is aspirin; it also inhibits the motility of polymorphonuclear leukocytes, depresses the biosynthesis of mucopolysaccharides, and may have a direct, COX-independent vasoconstrictor effect. Indomethacin has prominent anti-inflammatory and analgesic–antipyretic properties similar to those of the salicylates. The ADME data for indomethacin are summarized in Table 34–2.

THERAPEUTIC USES. Indomethacin is estimated to be ~20 times more potent than aspirin. A high rate of intolerance limits the long-term analgesic use of indomethacin. Indomethacin is approved for closure of persistent patent ductus arteriosus in premature infants who weigh between 500 and 1750 g, who have a hemodynamically significant patent ductus arteriosus, and in whom other supportive maneuvers have been attempted. Successful closure can be expected in >70% of neonates treated. The principal limitation of treating neonates is renal toxicity, and therapy is interrupted if the output of urine falls to <0.6 mL/kg/h.

ADVERSE EFFECTS AND DRUG INTERACTIONS. A very high percentage (35%-50%) of patients receiving indomethacin experience untoward symptoms. GI adverse events are common and can be fatal; elderly patients are at significantly greater risk. Diarrhea may occur and sometimes is associated with ulcerative lesions of the bowel. Acute pancreatitis has been reported, as have rare, but potentially fatal, cases of hepatitis. The most frequent CNS effect is severe frontal headache. Dizziness, vertigo, light-headedness, and mental confusion may occur. Seizures have been reported, as have severe depression, psychosis, hallucinations, and suicide. Caution is advised when administering indomethacin to elderly patients or to those with underlying epilepsy, psychiatric disorders, or Parkinson's disease, because they are at greater risk for the development of serious CNS adverse effects. Hematopoietic reactions include neutropenia, thrombocytopenia, and rarely aplastic anemia.

SULINDAC

Sulindac (CLINORIL, others) is a congener of indomethacin. Sulindac, which is less than half as potent as indomethacin, is a prodrug whose anti-inflammatory activity resides in its sulfide metabolite (which is >500 times more potent than sulindac as an inhibitor of COX but less than half as potent as indomethacin). ADME data are summarized in Table 34–2. *The same precautions that apply to other NSAIDs regarding patients at risk for GI toxicity, cardiovascular risk, and renal impairment also apply to sulindac.*

THERAPEUTIC USES. Sulindac is used for the treatment of rheumatoid arthritis, osteoarthritis, ankylosing spondylitis, tendonitis, bursitis, and the pain of acute gout. Its analgesic and anti-inflammatory effects are comparable to those achieved with aspirin. The most common dosage for adults is 150-200 mg twice a day.

ADVERSE EFFECTS. Although the incidence of toxicity is lower than with indomethacin, untoward reactions to sulindac are common. The typical NSAID GI side effects are seen in nearly 20% of patients. CNS side effects as described above for indomethacin are seen in ≤10% of patients. Rash and pruritus occur in 5% of patients. Transient elevations of hepatic transaminases in plasma are less common.

ETODOLAC

Etodolac is an acetic acid derivative with some degree of COX-2 selectivity (*see* Table 34–2). At anti-inflammatory doses, the frequency of gastric irritation may be less than with other tNSAIDs. A single oral dose (200-400 mg) of etodolac provides postoperative analgesia that lasts for 6-8 h. Etodolac also is effective in the treatment of osteoarthritis, rheumatoid arthritis, and mild to moderate pain, and the drug appears to be uricosuric. Sustained-release preparations are available. Etodolac is relatively well tolerated. About 5% of patients who have taken the drug for ≤1 year discontinue treatment because of GI side effects, rashes, and CNS effects.

TOLMETIN

Tolmetin (TOLECTIN, others) is approved for the treatment of osteoarthritis, rheumatoid arthritis, and juvenile rheumatoid arthritis; and has been used in the treatment of ankylosing spondylitis. ADME and comparison to aspirin are in Table 34–2. Tolmetin recommended doses (200-600 mg 3 times/day) typically given with meals, milk, or antacids to lessen abdominal discomfort. However, peak plasma concentrations and bioavailability are reduced when the drug is taken with food. Side effects occur in 25-40% of patients who take tolmetin. GI side effects are the most common (15%), and gastric ulceration has been observed. CNS side effects similar to those seen with indomethacin and aspirin occur, but they are less common and less severe.

KETOROLAC

Ketorolac is a potent analgesic but only a moderately effective anti-inflammatory drug. The use of ketorolac is limited to ≤5 days for acute pain requiring opioid-level analgesia and can be administered intramuscularly, intravenously, or orally. Typical doses are 30-60 mg (intramuscular), 15-30 mg (intravenous), and 10-20 mg (oral). Ketorolac has a rapid onset of action and a short duration of action (*see* Table 34–2). It is widely used in postoperative patients, but it should not be used for routine obstetric analgesia. Topical (ophthalmic) ketorolac (ACULAR, others) is approved for the treatment of seasonal allergic conjunctivitis and postoperative ocular inflammation. Side effects include somnolence, dizziness, headache, GI pain, dyspepsia, nausea, and pain at the site of injection. The black box warning for ketorolac stresses the possibility of serious adverse GI, renal, bleeding, and hypersensitivity reactions. Patients receiving greater than recommended doses or concomitant NSAID therapy and the elderly appear to be particularly at risk.

NABUMETONE

Nabumetone is the prodrug of 6-methoxy-2-naphthylacetic acid. Nabumetone is an anti-inflammatory agent with substantial efficacy in the treatment of rheumatoid arthritis and osteoarthritis. Its comparative pharmacokinetic properties are summarized in Table 34–2. Nabumetone is associated with crampy lower abdominal pain and diarrhea, but the incidence of GI ulceration appears to be lower than with other tNSAIDs. Other side effects include rash, headache, dizziness, heartburn, tinnitus, and pruritus.

DICLOFENAC

Diclofenac, a phenylacetic acid derivative, is among the most commonly used NSAID in the E.U. Diclofenac has analgesic, antipyretic, and anti-inflammatory activities. Its potency is substantially greater than that of indomethacin, naproxen, or several other tNSAIDs. The selectivity of diclofenac for COX-2 resembles that of celecoxib. Diclofenac displays rapid absorption, extensive protein binding, and a $t_{1/2}$ of 1-2 h (*see* Table 34–2). The short $t_{1/2}$ makes it necessary to dose diclofenac considerably higher than would be required to inhibit COX-2 fully at peak plasma concentrations to afford inhibition throughout the dosing interval. There is a substantial first-pass effect, such that only ~50% of diclofenac is available systemically. The drug accumulates in synovial fluid after oral administration, which may explain why its duration of therapeutic effect is considerably longer than its plasma $t_{1/2}$.

THERAPEUTIC USES. Diclofenac is approved in the U.S. for the long-term symptomatic treatment of rheumatoid arthritis, osteoarthritis, ankylosing spondylitis, pain, primary dysmenorrhea, and acute migraine. Myriad oral formulations are available to provide a range of release times; the usual daily oral dosage is 100-200 mg, given in several divided doses. For migraine, a powdered form is available for dissolution in water; a gel and a transdermal patch are also available. Diclofenac also is available in combination with misoprostol, a PGE_1 analog (ARTHROTEC); this combination retains the efficacy of diclofenac while reducing the frequency of GI ulcers and erosions. In addition, an ophthalmic solution of diclofenac (VOLTAREN, others) is available for treatment of postoperative inflammation following cataract extraction.

ADVERSE EFFECTS. Diclofenac produces side effects (particularly GI) in ~20% of patients. The incidence of GI adverse effects are similar to the COX-2–selective inhibitors celecoxib and etoricoxib. Hypersensitivity reactions have occurred following topical application. Modest reversible elevation of hepatic transaminases in plasma occurs in 5-15% of patients. Transaminases should be monitored during the first 8 weeks of therapy with diclofenac. Other untoward responses to diclofenac include CNS effects, rashes, allergic reactions, fluid retention, edema, and renal function impairment. The drug is not recommended for children, nursing mothers, or pregnant women. Unlike ibuprofen, diclofenac does not interfere with the antiplatelet effect of aspirin.

PROPIONIC ACID DERIVATIVES

The propionic acid derivatives **ibuprofen, naproxen, flurbiprofen, fenoprofen, ketoprofen**, and **oxaprozin**, are available in the U.S. (Table 34–3). Ibuprofen is the most commonly used tNSAID in the U.S. and is available without a prescription. Naproxen, also available without prescription, has a longer but variable $t_{1/2}$. Oxaprozin also has a long $t_{1/2}$ and may be given once daily.

Table 34–3

Comparison of NSAIDS: Fenamates and Propionic Acid Derivatives

CLASS/Drug	PHARMACOKINETICS		DOSING[d]	COMMENTS	COMPARED TO ASPIRIN
Fenamates					
Mefenamic acid	Peak C_p	2-4 h	500-mg load, then 250 mg/6 h	Isolated cases of hemolytic anemia	Efficacy similar; GI side effects (25%)
	Protein binding	High		May have some central action	
	Metabolites	Conjugates of 3–OH and 3–C=O			
	$t_{1/2}$	3-4 h			
Meclofenamate	Peak C_p	0.5-2 h	50-100 mg 4-6/day (max of 400 mg/day)		Efficacy similar; GI side effects (25%)
	Protein binding	99%			
	Metabolites	Hepatic; fecal and renal excretion			
	$t_{1/2}$	2-3 h			
Flufenamic acid	*Not available in the U.S.*				
Propionic acid derivatives (Intolerance of one does not preclude use of another propionate derivative. Usually better tolerated than aspirin.)					
Ibuprofen	Peak C_p	15-30 min	Analgesia: 200-400 mg/4-6 h	10-15% discontinue	Equipotent
	Protein binding	99%	Anti-inflammatory: 300 mg/6-8 h or 400-800 mg 3-4 ×/day	Children's dosing	
	Metabolites	Conjugates of –OH and $–COO^-$ metabolites		Fever: 5-10 mg/kg/6 h (max: 40 mg/kg/day); inflammation: 20-40 mg/kg/day in 3-4 divided doses	
	$t_{1/2}$	2-4 h			
Naproxen	Peak C_p	1 h	250 mg 4 ×/day or 500 mg 2 ×/day	Peak anti-inflammatory effects after 2-4 weeks;	Usually better tolerated; variably prolonged $t_{1/2}$ may afford cardioprotection
	Protein binding	99% (less in elderly)	Children, anti-inflammatory: 5 mg/kg/day	↓ protein binding and ↓ excretion ⇒↑ risk of toxicity in elderly	
	Metabolites	6-demethyl and other metabolites			
	$t_{1/2}$	14 h			

Fenoprofen	Peak C_p	2 h	200 mg 4-6 times/day; 300-600 mg 3-4 times/day		15% experience side effects; few discontinue use
	Protein binding	99%			
	Metabolites	Glucuronide, 4-OH metabolite			
	$t_{1/2}$	2 h			
Ketoprofen	Peak C_p	1-2 h	Analgesia, 25 mg, 3-4/day		30% develop side effects (usually GI, usually mild)
	Protein binding	98%	Anti-inflammatory, 50-75 mg, 3-4/day		
	Metabolites	Glucuronide conjugates			
	$t_{1/2}$	2 h			
Flurbiprofen	Peak C_p	1-2 h	200-300 mg/day in 2-4 divided doses	Available as ophthalmic solution	
	Protein binding	99%			
	Metabolites	−OH and conjugates			
	$t_{1/2}$	6 h			
Oxaprozin	Peak C_p	3-4 h	600-1800 mg/day	Long $t_{1/2}$ permits daily dosing slow onset; not for fever/ acute analgesia	
	Protein binding	99%			
	Major metabolites	Oxidates and glucuronides			
	$t_{1/2}$	40-60 h			

CNS, central nervous system; COX, cyclooxygenase; GI, gastrointestinal; h, hours; IM, intramuscularly; IV, intravenously; min, minutes.

[a] *Time to peak plasma drug concentration (C_p) after a single dose. In general, food delays absorption but does not decrease peak concentration.*

[b] *The majority of NSAIDs undergo hepatic metabolism, and the metabolites are excreted in the urine. Major metabolites or disposal pathways are listed.*

[c] *Typical $t_{1/2}$ is listed for therapeutic doses; if $t_{1/2}$ is much different with the toxic dose, this is also given.*

[d] *Limited dosing information given. For additional information, refer to the text and product information literature.*

MECHANISM OF ACTION

Propionic acid derivatives are nonselective COX inhibitors with the effects and side effects common to other tNSAIDs. Some of the propionic acid derivatives, particularly naproxen, have prominent inhibitory effects on leukocyte function, and some data suggest that naproxen may have slightly better efficacy with regard to analgesia and relief of morning stiffness. This suggestion of benefit accords with the clinical pharmacology of naproxen that suggests that some but not all individuals dosed with 500 mg twice daily sustain platelet inhibition throughout the dosing interval.

THERAPEUTIC USES

Propionic acid derivatives are approved for use in the symptomatic treatment of rheumatoid arthritis and osteoarthritis. Some also are approved for pain, ankylosing spondylitis, acute gouty arthritis, tendinitis, bursitis, and migraine and for primary dysmenorrhea. These agents may be comparable in efficacy to aspirin for the control of the signs and symptoms of rheumatoid arthritis and osteoarthritis.

DRUG INTERACTIONS

Ibuprofen has been shown to interfere with the antiplatelet effects of aspirin. There also is evidence for a similar interaction between aspirin and naproxen. Propionic acid derivatives have not been shown to alter the pharmacokinetics of the oral hypoglycemic drugs or warfarin.

IBUPROFEN

Table 34–3 summarizes the comparative pharmacokinetics of ibuprofen.

THERAPEUTIC USES. Ibuprofen [ADVIL, MOTRIN IB, BRUFEN, others] is supplied as tablets, capsules, caplets, and gelcaps containing 50-800 mg; as oral drops; and as an oral suspension. Dosage forms containing ≤200 mg are available without a prescription. Ibuprofen is licensed for marketing in fixed-dose combinations with antihistamines, decongestants, oxycodone (COMBUNOX, others), and hydrocodone (REPREXAIN, IBUDONE, VICOPROFEN, others). The usual dose for mild to moderate pain is 400 mg every 4-6 h as needed.

ADVERSE EFFECTS. Ibuprofen is thought to be better tolerated than aspirin, and indomethacin and has been used in patients with a history of GI intolerance to other NSAIDs. Nevertheless, 5-15% of patients experience GI side effects. Less frequent adverse effects of ibuprofen include rashes, thrombocytopenia, rashes, headache, dizziness, blurred vision, and in a few cases, toxic amblyopia, fluid retention, and edema. Patients who develop ocular disturbances should discontinue the use of ibuprofen. Ibuprofen can be used occasionally by pregnant women; however, the concerns apply regarding third-trimester effects, including delay of parturition. Excretion into breast milk is thought to be minimal, so ibuprofen also can be used with caution by women who are breastfeeding.

NAPROXEN

Naproxen (ALEVE, NAPROSYN, others) is supplied as tablets, delayed-release tablets, controlled-release tablets, gelcaps, and caplets containing 200 -750 mg of naproxen or naproxen sodium and as an oral suspension. Dosage forms containing ≤200 mg are available without a prescription. Naproxen is licensed for marketing in fixed-dose combinations with pseudoephedrine (ALEVE-D SINUS & COLD, others) and sumatriptan (TREXIMET) and is copackaged with lansoprazole (PREVACID NAPRAPAC). Naproxen is indicated for juvenile and rheumatoid arthritis, osteoarthritis, ankylosing spondylitis, pain, primary dysmenorrhea, tendonitis, bursitis, and acute gout.

Naproxen is absorbed fully after oral administration. The $t_{1/2}$ of naproxen in plasma is variable; from 14 h in the young, it may increase ~2-fold in the elderly because of age-related decline in renal function (*see* Table 34–3). Naproxen crosses the placenta and appears in the milk of lactating women at ~1% of the maternal plasma concentration.

ADVERSE EFFECTS. The relative risk of myocardial infarction may be reduced by ~10% by naproxen, compared to a reduction of 20-25% by aspirin. However, increased rates of cardiovascular events also have been reported. GI adverse effects with naproxen occur at approximately the same frequency as with indomethacin and other tNSAIDs but perhaps with less severity. CNS side effects range from drowsiness, headache, dizziness, and sweating to fatigue, depression, and ototoxicity. Less common reactions include pruritus and a variety of dermatological problems. A few instances of jaundice, impairment of renal function, angioedema, thrombocytopenia, and agranulocytosis have been reported.

THE FENAMATES

The fenamates include mefenamic, meclofenamic, and flufenamic acids. The pharmacological properties of the fenamates are those of typical tNSAIDs, and therapeutically, they have no clear advantages over others in the class. *See* Table 34–3. Mefenamic acid [PONSTEL, PONSTAN (U.K.), DYSMAN (U.K.)] and meclofenamate sodium are used in the short-term treatment of pain in soft-tissue injuries, dysmenorrhea, and rheumatoid and osteoarthritis. These drugs are not recommended for use in children or pregnant women. Approximately 25% of users develop GI side effects at therapeutic doses. Roughly 5% of patients develop a reversible elevation of hepatic transaminases. Diarrhea, which may be severe and associated with steatorrhea and inflammation of the bowel, also is relatively common. Autoimmune hemolytic anemia is a potentially serious but rare side effect.

ENOLIC ACIDS (OXICAMS)

The oxicam derivatives are enolic acids that inhibit COX-1 and COX-2 and have anti-inflammatory, analgesic, and antipyretic activity. These agents are similar in efficacy to aspirin, indomethacin, or naproxen for the long-term treatment of rheumatoid arthritis or osteoarthritis. The main advantage suggested for these compounds is their long $t_{1/2}$, which permits once-a-day dosing (*see* comparative pharmacokinetic and dosing data in Table 34–4).

PIROXICAM

Piroxicam can inhibit activation of neutrophils, apparently independently of its ability to inhibit COX; hence, additional modes of anti-inflammatory action have been proposed, including inhibition of proteoglycanase and collagenase in cartilage. Piroxicam is approved for the treatment of rheumatoid arthritis and osteoarthritis. Due to its slow onset of action and delayed attainment of steady state, it is less suited for acute analgesia but has been used to treat acute gout. The usual daily dose is 20 mg, steady-state blood levels are reached in 7-12 days. Approximately 20% of patients experience side effects with piroxicam, and ~5% of patients discontinue use because of these effects. Piroxicam may be with more GI and serious skin reactions than other nonselective NSAIDs. The European Medicines Agency no longer considers piroxicam a first-line agent.

MELOXICAM

Meloxicam (MOBIC, others) is approved for use in osteoarthritis. The recommended dose for meloxicam is 7.5-15 mg once daily. Meloxicam demonstrates some COX-2 selectivity, however, a clinical advantage or hazard has yet to be established. There is significantly less gastric injury compared to piroxicam (20 mg/day) in subjects treated with 7.5 mg/day of meloxicam, but the advantage is lost with a dosage of 15 mg/day.

COX-2–SELECTIVE NSAIDS

Celecoxib, a diaryl heterocyclic coxib, is the only such compound still approved in the U.S. (*see* its clinical pharmacokinetic properties and precautions in Table 34–4).

Etoricoxib is approved in several countries; rofecoxib (VIOXX) and valdecoxib were withdrawn worldwide. Lumiracoxib, a derivative diclofenac, has been discussed earlier. Selective inhibitors of COX-2 are used for relief of dental pain and relief from inflammation in osteoarthritis and rheumatoid arthritis.

CELECOXIB

ADME. The bioavailability of oral celecoxib (CELEBREX) is not known, peak plasma levels occur at 2-4 h after administration. The elderly (≥65 years of age) may have up to 2-fold higher peak concentrations and AUC values than younger patients (≤55 years of age). Celecoxib is bound extensively to plasma proteins. Most is excreted as carboxylic acid and glucuronide metabolites in the urine and feces. The elimination $t_{1/2}$ is ~11 h. The drug commonly is given once or twice daily during chronic treatment. Celecoxib has not been studied in patients with severe renal insufficiency. Plasma concentrations are increased in patients with mild and moderate hepatic impairment, requiring reduction in dose. Celecoxib is metabolized predominantly by CYP2C9 and inhibits CYP2D6. Clinical vigilance is necessary during coadministration of drugs that are known to inhibit CYP2C9 and drugs that are metabolized by CYP2D6.

THERAPEUTIC USES. Celecoxib is used for the management of acute pain for the treatment of osteoarthritis, rheumatoid arthritis, juvenile rheumatoid arthritis, ankylosing spondylitis, and primary dysmenorrhea. The recommended dose for treating osteoarthritis is 200 mg/day as a single dose or divided as 2 doses. In the treatment of rheumatoid arthritis, the recommended dose is 100-200 mg twice daily. Due to cardiovascular hazard, physicians are advised to use the lowest possible dose for the shortest possible time. Celecoxib also is approved for the chemoprevention of polyposis coli.

ADVERSE EFFECTS. Celecoxib confers a risk of myocardial infarction and stroke and this appears to relate to dose and the underlying risk of cardiovascular disease. Effects attributed to inhibition of PG production in the kidney—hypertension and edema—occur with nonselective COX inhibitors and also with celecoxib. None of the coxibs has established superior efficacy over tNSAIDs. Selective COX-2 inhibitors lose their GI advantage over a tNSAID alone when used in conjunction with aspirin.

Table 34–4

Comparison of NSAIDS: Enolic Acid Derivatives and Coxibs

CLASS/Drug	PHARMACOKINETICS		DOSING[d]	COMMENTS	COMPARED TO ASPIRIN
Enolic acid derivatives					
Piroxicam	Peak C_p Protein binding Metabolites $t_{1/2}$	3-5 h 99% Hydroxylated, then conjugated 45-50 h	20 mg/day	May inhibit activation of neutrophils, activity of proteoglycanase, collagenases	Equipotent; perhaps better tolerated 20% side effects; 5% discontinue
Meloxicam	Peak C_p Protein binding Metabolites, $t_{1/2}$	5-10 h 99% Hydroxylation 15-20 h	7.5-15 mg/day		Some COX-2 selectivity, especially at lower doses
Nabumetone (naphthyl alkanone)	Peak C_p Protein binding Major metabolites $t_{1/2}$	3-6 h 99% *O*-demethyl conjugate 24 h	500-1000 mg 1-2 times/day	A prodrug, rapidly metabolized to 6-methoxy- 2-naphthyl acetic acid; pharmacokinetics reflect active compound	Shows some COX-2 selectivity (active metabolite does not) Fewer GI side effects than many NSAIDs
Diaryl heterocyclic NSAIDs (*COX-2 selective*)				Evidence for cardiovascular adverse events	Decrease in GI side effects and in platelet effects
Celecoxib	Peak C_p Protein binding Metabolites $t_{1/2}$	2-4 h 97% Carboxylate, glucuronide 6-12 h	100 mg 1-2 times/day	Substrate for CYP2C9; inhibitor of CYP2D6 Coadminister with CYP2C9 inhibitors or CYP2D6 substrates cautiously	See the text for an overview of COX-inhibitors
Parecoxib Etoricoxib Lumaricoxib	*Not approved for use in the U.S.*				

For explanation of nomenclature and abbreviations, see legend to Table 34–3.

PARECOXIB

Parecoxib is the only COX-2–selective NSAID administered by injection and has been shown to be an effective analgesic for the perioperative period when patients are unable to take oral medication. It is not widely available, and clinical experience is limited.

ETORICOXIB

Etoricoxib (ARCOXIA) is a COX-2–selective inhibitor with selectivity second only to that of lumiracoxib. Etoricoxib is incompletely (~80%) absorbed and has a long $t_{1/2}$ of ~20-26 h. It is extensively metabolized before excretion. Patients with hepatic impairment are prone to drug accumulation. Renal insufficiency does not affect drug clearance. Etoricoxib is approved for symptomatic relief in the treatment of osteoarthritis, rheumatoid arthritis, and acute gouty arthritis, as well as for the short-term treatment of musculoskeletal pain, postoperative pain, and primary dysmenorrhea. The drug is associated with increased the risk of heart attack and stroke.

OTHER NSAIDS

APAZONE (AZAPROPAZONE). Apazone is a tNSAID that has anti-inflammatory, analgesic, and antipyretic activity and is a potent uricosuric agent. Some of its efficacy may arise from its capacity to inhibit neutrophil migration, degranulation, and superoxide production.

Apazone has been used for the treatment of rheumatoid arthritis, osteoarthritis, ankylosing spondylitis, and gout but usually is restricted to cases where other tNSAIDs have failed. Typical doses are 600 mg 3 times per day for acute gout. Once symptoms have abated, or for non-gout indications, typical dosage is 300 mg 3 to 4 times per day. Clinical experience to date suggests that apazone is well tolerated. Mild GI side effects (nausea, epigastric pain, dyspepsia) and rashes occur in ~3% of patients, while CNS effects (headache, vertigo) are reported less frequently. Precautions appropriate to other nonselective COX inhibitors also apply to apazone.

NIMESULIDE. Nimesulide is a sulfonanilide compound available in Europe that demonstrates COX-2 selectivity similar to celecoxib in whole-blood assays. Additional effects include inhibition of neutrophil activation, decrease in cytokine production, decrease in degradative enzyme production, and possibly activation of glucocorticoid receptors. Nimesulide is administered orally in doses ≤100 mg twice daily as an anti-inflammatory, analgesic, and antipyretic. Its use in the E.U. is limited to ≤15 days due to the risk of hepatotoxicity.

DISEASE-MODIFYING ANTIRHEUMATIC DRUGS

Rheumatoid arthritis is an autoimmune disease that affects ~1% of the population. The pharmacological management of rheumatoid arthritis includes symptomatic relief through the use of NSAIDs. However, although they have anti-inflammatory effects, NSAIDs have minimal, if any effect on progression of joint deformity. Disease-modifying antirheumatic drugs (DMARDs), on the other hand, reduce the disease activity of rheumatoid arthritis and retard the progression of arthritic tissue destruction. DMARDs include a diverse group of small molecule nonbiological and biological agents (mainly antibodies or binding proteins), as summarized in Table 34–5.

Biological DMARDs remain reserved for patients with persistent moderate or high disease activity and indicators of poor prognosis. Therapy is tailored to the individual patient, and the use of these agents must be weighed against their potentially serious adverse effects. The combination of NSAIDs with these agents is common.

PHARMACOTHERAPY OF GOUT

Gout results from the precipitation of urate crystals in the tissues and the subsequent inflammatory response. Acute gout usually causes painful distal monoarthritis and also can cause joint destruction, subcutaneous deposits (tophi), and renal calculi and damage. Gout affects ~0.5-1% of the population of Western countries.

The pathophysiology of gout is incompletely understood. Hyperuricemia, while a prerequisite, does not inevitably lead to gout. Uric acid, the end product of purine metabolism, is relatively insoluble compared to its hypoxanthine and xanthine precursors, and normal serum urate levels (~5 mg/dL, or 0.3 mM) approach the limit of solubility. In most patients with gout, hyperuricemia arises from underexcretion rather than overproduction of urate. Mutations of one of the renal urate transporters, URAT-1, are associated with hypouricemia. Urate tends to crystallize as monosodium urate in colder or more acidic conditions. Monosodium urate crystals activate monocytes/macrophages via the toll-like receptor pathway mounting an innate immune response. This results in the secretion of cytokines, including IL-1β and TNF-α; endothelial activation; and attraction of neutrophils to the site of inflammation. Neutrophils secrete inflammatory mediators that lower the local pH and lead to further urate precipitation.

Table 34–5

Disease-Modifying Anti-Rheumatic Drugs

DRUG	CLASS OR ACTION	CHAPTER NUMBER
Small molecules		
Methotrexate	Anti-folate	61
Leflunomide	Pyrimidine synthase inhibitor	61
Hydroxychloroquine	Anti-malarial	49
Minocycline	5-lipoxygenase inhibitor, tetracycline antibiotic	33, 55
Sulfasalazine	Salicylate	34, 47
Azathioprine	Purine synthase inhibitor	61
Cyclosporine	Calcineurin inhibitor	35
Cyclophosphamide	Alkylating agent	61
Biologicals		
Adalimumab	Ab, TNF-α antagonist	35
Golimumab	Ab, TNF-α antagonist	35
Infliximab	IgG-TNF receptor fusion protein (anti-TNF)	35
Certolizumab	Fab fragment toward TNF-α	35
Abatacept	T-cell costimulation inhibitor (binds B7 protein on antigen-presenting cell)	35
Rituximab	Ab toward CD20 (cytotoxic toward B cells)	62
Anakinra	IL-1-receptor antagonist	35, 62

IL, interleukin; TNF, tumor necrosis factor.

The aims of treatment are to:

- *Decrease the symptoms of an acute attack.*
- *Decrease the risk of recurrent attacks.*
- *Lower serum urate levels.*

The substances available for these purposes are:

- *Drugs that relieve inflammation and pain (NSAIDs, colchicine, glucocorticoids)*
- *Drugs that prevent inflammatory responses to crystals (colchicine and NSAIDs)*
- *Drugs that act by inhibition of urate formation (allopurinol, febuxostat) or to augment urate excretion (probenecid)*

NSAIDs have been discussed earlier. Glucocorticoids are discussed in Chapter 42. This section focuses on colchicine, allopurinol, febuxostat, and the uricosuric agents probenecid and benzbromarone.

COLCHICINE

Colchicine is one of the oldest available therapies for acute gout. Colchicine is considered second-line therapy because it has a narrow therapeutic window and a high rate of side effects, particularly at higher doses.

MECHANISM OF ACTION. Colchicine exerts a variety of pharmacological effects, but how these relate to its activity in gout is not well understood. It has antimitotic effects, arresting cell division in G_1 by interfering with microtubule and spindle formation (an effect shared with vinca alkaloids). This effect is greatest on cells with rapid turnover (e.g., neutrophils, GI epithelium). Colchicine may alter neutrophil motility and decreases the secretion of chemotactic factors and superoxide anions by activated neutrophils. Colchicine inhibits the release of histamine-containing granules from mast cells, the secretion of insulin from pancreatic β cells, and the movement of melanin granules in melanophores. Colchicine also exhibits a variety of other pharmacological effects. It lowers body temperature, increases the sensitivity to central depressants, depresses the respiratory center, enhances the response to sympathomimetic agents, constricts blood vessels, and induces hypertension by central vasomotor stimulation. It enhances GI activity by neurogenic stimulation but depresses it by a direct effect, and alters neuromuscular function.

ADME. Absorption of oral colchicine is rapid but variable. Peak plasma concentrations occur 0.5-2 h after dosing. In plasma, 50% of colchicine is protein bound. There is significant enterohepatic circulation. The exact metabolism of colchicine in humans is unknown, but in vitro studies indicate that it may undergo oxidative demethylation by CYP3A4. Only 10-20% is excreted in the urine, although this increases in patients with liver disease. The kidney, liver, and spleen also contain high concentrations of colchicine, but it apparently is largely excluded from heart, skeletal muscle, and brain. The plasma $t_{1/2}$ of colchicine is ~9 h.

THERAPEUTIC USES. A minimum of 3 days, but preferably 7-14 days, should elapse between courses of gout treatment with colchicine to avoid cumulative toxicity. Patients with hepatic or renal disease and dialysis patients should receive reduced doses and/or less frequent therapy. For elderly patients, adjust the dose for renal function.

Acute Gout. Colchicine dramatically relieves acute attacks of gout. It is effective in roughly two-thirds of patients if given within 24 h of attack onset. Pain, swelling, and redness abate within 12 h and are completely gone within 48-72 h. The regimen approved for adults recommends a total of 2 doses taken 1 h apart: 1.2 mg (2 tablets) at the first sign of a gout flare followed by 0.6 mg (1 tablet) 1 h later.

Prevention of Acute Gout. The main off-label indication for colchicine is in the prevention of recurrent gout, particularly in the early stages of antihyperuricemic therapy. The typical dose for prophylaxis is 0.6 mg taken orally 3 or 4 days/wk for patients who have <1 attack per year, 0.6 mg daily for patients who have >1 attack per year, and 0.6 mg 2-3 times daily for patients who have severe attacks. The dose must be decreased for patients with impaired renal function.

ADVERSE EFFECTS. Exposure of the GI tract to large amounts of colchicine and its metabolites via enterohepatic circulation and the rapid rate of turnover of the GI mucosa may explain why the GI tract is particularly susceptible to colchicine toxicity. Nausea, vomiting, diarrhea, and abdominal pain are the most common untoward effects and the earliest signs of impending colchicine toxicity. Drug administration should be discontinued as soon as these symptoms occur. There is a latent period, which is not altered by dose or route of administration, of several hours or more between the administration of the drug and the onset of symptoms. A dosing study demonstrated that 1 dose initially and a single additional dose after 1 h was much less toxic than traditional hourly dosing for acute gout flares. Acute intoxication causes hemorrhagic gastropathy. Other serious side effects of colchicine therapy include myelosuppression, leukopenia, granulocytopenia, thrombopenia, aplastic anemia, and rhabdomyolysis. Life-threatening toxicities are associated with administration of concomitant therapy with *P*-glycoprotein or CYP3A4 inhibitors. The FDA suspended the U.S. marketing of all injectable dosage forms of colchicine in 2008.

ALLOPURINOL

Allopurinol inhibits xanthine oxidase (XO) and prevents the synthesis of urate from hypoxanthine and xanthine. Allopurinol is used to treat hyperuricemia in patients with gout and to prevent it in those with hematological malignancies about to undergo chemotherapy (acute tumor lysis syndrome). Even though underexcretion rather than overproduction is the underlying defect in most gout patients, allopurinol remains effective therapy.

Allopurinol is an analog of hypoxanthine. Its active metabolite, oxypurinol, is an analog of xanthine.

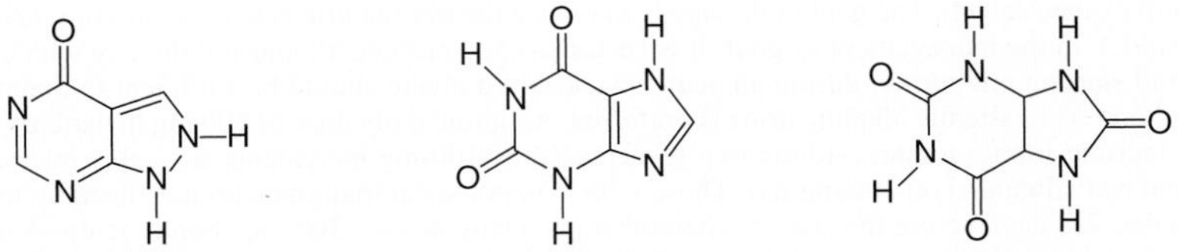

ALLOPURINOL

XANTHINE

URIC ACID

MECHANISM OF ACTION. Both allopurinol and its primary metabolite, oxypurinol (alloxanthine), reduce urate production by inhibiting XO, which converts xanthine to uric acid. Allopurinol competitively inhibits XO at low concentrations and is a noncompetitive inhibitor at high concentrations. Allopurinol also is a substrate for XO; the product of this reaction, oxypurinol, also is a noncompetitive inhibitor of the enzyme. The formation of oxypurinol, together with its long persistence in tissues, is responsible for much of the pharmacological activity of allopurinol.

In the absence of allopurinol, the dominant urinary purine is uric acid. During allopurinol treatment, the urinary purines include hypoxanthine, xanthine, and uric acid. Because each has its independent solubility, the concentration of uric acid in plasma is reduced and purine excretion increased, without exposing the urinary tract to an excessive load of uric acid. Despite their increased concentrations during allopurinol therapy, hypoxanthine and xanthine are efficiently excreted, and tissue deposition does not occur. There is a small risk of xanthine stones in patients with a very high urate load before allopurinol therapy, which can be minimized by liberal fluid intake and alkalization.

Allopurinol facilitates the dissolution of tophi and prevents the development or progression of chronic gouty arthritis by lowering the uric acid concentration in plasma below the limit of its solubility. The formation of uric acid stones virtually disappears with therapy, which prevents the development of nephropathy. Once significant renal injury has occurred, allopurinol cannot restore renal function but may delay disease progression. The incidence of acute attacks of gouty arthritis may increase during the early months of allopurinol therapy as a consequence of mobilization of tissue stores of uric acid. Coadministration of colchicine helps suppress such acute attacks. In some patients, the allopurinol-induced increase in excretion of oxypurines is less than the reduction in uric acid excretion; this disparity primarily is a result of reutilization of oxypurines and feedback inhibition of de novo purine biosynthesis.

ADME. Allopurinol is absorbed relatively rapidly after oral ingestion, and peak plasma concentrations are reached within 60-90 min. About 20% is excreted in the feces in 48-72 h, presumably as unabsorbed drug, and 10-30% is excreted unchanged in the urine. The remainder undergoes metabolism, mostly to oxypurinol. Oxypurinol is excreted slowly in the urine by glomerular filtration, counterbalanced by some tubular reabsorption. The plasma $t_{1/2}$ of allopurinol and oxypurinol is ~1-2 h and ~18-30 h (longer in those with renal impairment), respectively. This allows for once-daily dosing and makes allopurinol the most commonly used antihyperuricemic agent. Allopurinol and its active metabolite oxypurinol are distributed in total tissue water, with the exception of brain, where their concentrations are about one-third of those in other tissues. Neither compound is bound to plasma proteins. The plasma concentrations of the 2 compounds do not correlate well with therapeutic or toxic effects.

DRUG INTERACTIONS. Allopurinol increases the $t_{1/2}$ of probenecid and enhances its uricosuric effect, while probenecid increases the clearance of oxypurinol, thereby increasing dose requirements of allopurinol. Allopurinol inhibits the enzymatic inactivation of mercaptopurine and its derivative azathioprine by XO. Thus, when allopurinol is used concomitantly with oral mercaptopurine or azathioprine, dosage of the antineoplastic agent must be reduced to 25-33% of the usual dose (*see* Chapters 35 and 61). This is of importance when treating gout in the transplant recipient. The risk of bone marrow suppression also is increased when allopurinol is administered with cytotoxic agents that are not metabolized by XO, particularly cyclophosphamide. Allopurinol also may interfere with the hepatic inactivation of other drugs, including warfarin. Although the effect is variable, increased monitoring of prothrombin activity is recommended in patients receiving both medications.

It remains to be established whether the increased incidence of rash in patients receiving concurrent allopurinol and ampicillin should be ascribed to allopurinol or to hyperuricemia. Hypersensitivity reactions have been reported in patients with compromised renal function, especially those who are receiving a combination of allopurinol and a thiazide diuretic. The concomitant administration of allopurinol and theophylline leads to increased accumulation of an active metabolite of theophylline, 1-methylxanthine; the concentration of theophylline in plasma also may be increased (*see* Chapter 36).

THERAPEUTIC USES. Allopurinol (ZYLOPRIM, ALOPRIM, others) is available for oral and intravenous use. Oral therapy provides effective therapy for primary and secondary gout, hyperuricemia secondary to malignancies, and calcium oxalate calculi. The goal of therapy is to reduce the plasma uric acid concentration to <6 mg/dL (<360 μmol/L). In the management of gout, it is customary to antecede allopurinol therapy with colchicine and to avoid starting allopurinol during an acute attack. Fluid intake should be sufficient to maintain daily urinary volume >2 L; slightly alkaline urine is preferred. An initial daily dose of 100 mg in patients with estimated glomerular filtration rates >40 mg/min is increased by 100-mg increments at weekly intervals. Most patients can be maintained on 300 mg/day. Those with hematological malignancies may need up to 800 mg/day beginning 2-3 days before the start of chemotherapy. Daily doses >300 mg should be divided. Dosage must be reduced in patients in proportion to the reduction in glomerular filtration.

The usual daily dose in children with secondary hyperuricemia associated with malignancies is 150-300 mg, depending on age. Allopurinol also is useful in lowering the high plasma concentrations of uric acid in patients with Lesch-Nyhan syndrome and thereby prevents the complications resulting from hyperuricemia; there is no evidence that it alters the progressive neurological and behavioral abnormalities that are characteristic of the disease.

ADVERSE EFFECTS. Allopurinol generally is well tolerated. The most common adverse effects are hypersensitivity reactions that may manifest after months or years of therapy. Serious hypersensitivity reactions preclude further use of the drug. The cutaneous reaction caused by allopurinol is predominantly a pruritic, erythematous, or maculopapular eruption, but occasionally the lesion is urticarial or purpuric. Rarely, toxic epidermal necrolysis or Stevens-Johnson syndrome occurs, which can be fatal. The risk for Stevens-Johnson syndrome is limited primarily to the first 2 months of treatment. Because the rash may precede severe hypersensitivity reactions, patients who develop a rash should discontinue allopurinol. If indicated, desensitization to allopurinol can be carried out starting at 10-25 μg/day, with the drug diluted in oral suspension and doubled every 3-14 days until the desired dose is reached. This is successful in approximately half of patients. Oxypurinol has orphan drug status and is available for compassionate use in the U.S. for patients intolerant of allopurinol. Fever, malaise, and myalgias also may occur in ~3% of patients, more frequently in those with renal impairment. Transient leukopenia or leukocytosis and eosinophilia are rare reactions that may require cessation of therapy. Hepatomegaly and elevated levels of transaminases in plasma and progressive renal insufficiency also may occur.

Allopurinol is contraindicated in patients who have exhibited serious adverse effects or hypersensitivity reactions to the medication and in nursing mothers and children, except those with malignancy or certain inborn errors of purine metabolism (e.g., Lesch-Nyhan syndrome). Allopurinol generally is used in patients with hyperuricemia post-transplantation. It can be used in conjunction with a uricosuric agent.

FEBUXOSTAT

Febuxostat is an XO inhibitor approved for treatment of hyperuricemia in patients with gout.

MECHANISM OF ACTION. Febuxostat is a nonpurine inhibitor of XO. Unlike oxypurinol, the active metabolite of allopurinol, which inhibits the reduced form of XO, febuxostat forms a stable complex with both the reduced and oxidized enzymes and inhibits catalytic function in both states.

ADME. Febuxostat is rapidly absorbed with maximum plasma concentrations at 1-1.5 h postdose. The absolute bioavailability is unknown. Magnesium hydroxide and aluminum hydroxide delay absorption by ~1 h. Food reduces absorption slightly. Febuxostat, $t_{1/2}$ of 5-8 h, is extensively metabolized by oxidation by CYPs 1A2, 2C8, and 2C9 and non-CYP enzymes and is eliminated by both hepatic and renal pathways. Mild to moderate renal or hepatic impairment does not affect its elimination kinetics relevantly.

THERAPEUTIC USE. Febuxostat (ULORIC; ADENURIC) is approved for hyperuric patients with gout attacks, but not recommended for treatment of asymptomatic hyperuricemia. It is available in 40- and 80-mg oral tablets. A dose of 40 mg/day febuxostat lowered serum uric acid to similar levels as 300 mg/day allopurinol. More patients reached the target concentration of 6.0 mg/dL (360 μmol/L) on 80 mg/day febuxostat than on 300 mg/day allopurinol. Thus, therapy should be initiated with 40 mg/day and the dose increased if the target serum uric acid concentration is not reached within 2 weeks.

ADVERSE EVENTS. The most common adverse reactions in clinical studies were liver function abnormalities, nausea, joint pain, and rash. Liver function should be monitored periodically. An increase in gout flares was frequently observed after initiation of therapy, due to reduction in serum uric acid levels resulting in mobilization of urate from tissue deposits. Concurrent prophylactic treatment with an NSAID or colchicine is usually required. There was a higher rate of myocardial infarction and stroke in patients on febuxostat than on allopurinol. Whether there is a causal relationship between the cardiovascular events and febuxostat therapy or whether these were due to chance is not clear. Meanwhile patients should be monitored for cardiovascular complications.

DRUG INTERACTIONS. Plasma levels of drugs metabolized by XO (e.g., theophylline, mercaptopurine, azathioprine) will increase when administered concurrently with febuxostat. Thus, febuxostat is contraindicated in patients on azathioprine, mercaptopurine, or theophylline.

RASBURICASE

Rasburicase (ELITEK) is a recombinant urate oxidase that catalyzes the enzymatic oxidation of uric acid into the soluble and inactive metabolite allantoin. It has been shown to lower urate levels more effectively than allopurinol. It is indicated for the initial management of elevated plasma uric acid levels in pediatric patients with leukemia, lymphoma, and solid tumor malignancies who are receiving anticancer therapy expected to result in tumor lysis and significant hyperuricemia.

Rasburicase is produced by a genetically modified *Saccharomyces cerevisiae* strain. The drug's efficacy may be hampered by the production of antibodies against the drug. Hemolysis G6PD-deficient patients, methemoglobinemia, acute renal failure, and anaphylaxis have been associated with the use of rasburicase. Other frequently observed adverse reactions include vomiting, fever, nausea, headache, abdominal pain, constipation, diarrhea, and mucositis. Rasburicase causes enzymatic degradation of the uric acid in blood samples, and special handling is required to prevent spuriously low values for plasma uric acid in patients receiving the drug. The recommended dose of rasburicase is 0.15 mg/kg or 0.2 mg/kg as a single daily dose for 5 days, with chemotherapy initiated 4-24 h after infusion of the first rasburicase dose.

URICOSURIC AGENTS

Uricosuric agents increase the rate of excretion of uric acid. In humans, urate is filtered, secreted, and reabsorbed by the kidneys. Reabsorption is robust, such that the net the amount excreted usually is ~10% of that filtered. Reabsorption is mediated by an organic anion transporter family member, URAT-1, which can be inhibited.

URAT-1 exchanges urate for either an organic anion such as lactate or nicotinate or less potently for an inorganic anion such as chloride. Uricosuric drugs such as probenecid, sulfinpyrazone, benzbromarone, and losartan compete with urate for the transporter, thereby inhibiting its reabsorption via the urate–anion exchanger system. However, transport is bidirectional, and depending on dosage, a drug may either decrease or increase the excretion of uric acid. There are 2 mechanisms by which 1 drug may nullify the uricosuric action of another. First, the drug may inhibit the secretion of the uricosuric agent, thereby denying it access to its site of action, the luminal aspect of the brush border. Second, the inhibition of urate secretion by 1 drug may counterbalance the inhibition of urate reabsorption by the other.

PROBENECID. Probenecid is a highly lipid-soluble benzoic acid derivative (pK_a 3.4).

$(CH_3CH_2CH_2)_2NSO_2-C_6H_4-COOH$

PROBENECID

MECHANISM OF ACTION

Inhibition of Organic Acid Transport. The actions of probenecid are confined largely to inhibition of the transport of organic acids across epithelial barriers. Probenecid inhibits the reabsorption of uric acid by organic anion transporters, principally URAT-1. Uric acid is the only important endogenous compound whose excretion is known to be increased by probenecid. The uricosuric action of probenecid is blunted by the coadministration of salicylates.

Inhibition of Transport of Miscellaneous Substances. Probenecid inhibits the tubular secretion of a number of drugs, such as methotrexate and the active metabolite of clofibrate. It inhibits renal secretion of the inactive glucuronide metabolites of NSAIDs such as naproxen, ketoprofen, and indomethacin, and thereby can increase their plasma concentrations. Probenecid inhibits the transport of 5-hydroxyindoleacetic acid (5-HIAA) and other acidic metabolites of cerebral monoamines from the CSF to the plasma. The transport of drugs such as penicillin G also may be affected. Probenecid depresses the biliary secretion of certain compounds, including the diagnostic agents indocyanine green and bromosulfophthalein (BSP). It also decreases the biliary secretion of rifampin, leading to higher plasma concentrations.

ADME. Probenecid is absorbed completely after oral administration. Peak plasma concentrations are reached in 2-4 h. The $t_{1/2}$ of the drug in plasma is dose-dependent and varies from <5 h to >8 h. Between 85% and 95% of the drug is bound to plasma albumin; the 5% to 15% of unbound drug is cleared by glomerular filtration and active secretion by the proximal tubule. A small amount of probenecid glucuronide appears in the urine. It also is hydroxylated to metabolites that retain their carboxyl function and have uricosuric activity.

THERAPEUTIC USES (GOUT). Probenecid [PROBALAN, BENURYL] is marketed for oral administration. The starting dose is 250 mg twice daily, increasing over 1-2 weeks to 500-1000 mg twice daily. Probenecid increases urinary urate levels. Liberal fluid intake therefore should be maintained throughout therapy to minimize the risk of renal stones. Probenecid should not be used in gouty patients with nephrolithiasis or with overproduction of uric acid. Concomitant colchicine or NSAIDs are indicated early in the course of therapy to avoid precipitating an attack of gout, which may occur in ≤20% of gouty patients treated with probenecid alone.

Combination with Penicillin. Higher doses of probenecid are used as an adjuvant to prolong the dwell-time of penicillin in the body. This dosing method usually is confined to those being treated for gonorrhea or neurosyphilis infections or penicillin resistance (*see* Chapter 53).

ADVERSE EFFECTS. Probenecid is well tolerated. Approximately 2% of patients develop mild GI irritation. The risk is increased at higher doses. It is ineffective in patients with renal insufficiency and should be avoided in those with creatinine clearance of <50 mL/min. Hypersensitivity reactions usually are mild and occur in 2-4% of patients. Substantial overdosage with probenecid results in CNS stimulation, convulsions, and death from respiratory failure.

BENZBROMARONE

Benzbromarone is a potent uricosuric agent that is used in Europe. It is a reversible inhibitor of the urate–anion exchanger in the proximal tubule. Hepatotoxicity has been reported in conjunction with its use. The drug is absorbed readily after oral ingestion; peak plasma levels are achieved in ~4 h. It is metabolized to monobrominated and dehalogenated derivatives, both of which have uricosuric activity, and is excreted primarily in the bile.

As the micronized powder, it is effective in a single daily dose of 40-80 mg. It is effective in patients with renal insufficiency and may be prescribed to patients who are either allergic or refractory to other drugs used for the treatment of gout. Preparations that combine allopurinol and benzbromarone are more effective than either drug alone in lowering serum uric acid levels, in spite of the fact that benzbromarone lowers plasma levels of oxypurinol, the active metabolite of allopurinol. The uricosuric action is blunted by aspirin or sulfinpyrazone.

For a complete Bibliographical Listing, see Goodman & Gilman's ***The Pharmacological Basis of Therapeutics***, 12th ed., or Goodman & Gilman Online at www.AccessMedicine.com.

Immunosuppressants, Tolerogens, and Immunostimulants

This chapter reviews the components of the immune response and drugs that modulate immunity in 3 ways: immunosuppression, tolerance, and immunostimulation. Four major classes of immunosuppressive drugs are discussed: glucocorticoids (*see* Chapter 42), calcineurin inhibitors, antiproliferative and antimetabolic agents (*see* Chapter 61), and antibodies. The chapter ends with a brief case study of immunotherapy for MS.

THE IMMUNE RESPONSE

The immune system evolved to discriminate self from nonself. *Innate immunity* (natural immunity) is primitive, does not require priming, and is of relatively low affinity, but is broadly reactive. *Adaptive immunity* (learned immunity) is antigen specific, depends on antigen exposure or priming, and can be of very high affinity. The 2 arms of immunity work closely together, with the innate immune system being most active early in an immune response and adaptive immunity becoming progressively dominant over time.

The major effectors of *innate immunity* are complement, granulocytes, monocytes/macrophages, natural killer cells, mast cells, and basophils. The major effectors of *adaptive immunity* are B and T lymphocytes. B lymphocytes make antibodies; T lymphocytes function as helper, cytolytic, and regulatory (suppressor) cells. These cells are important in the normal immune response to infection and tumors but also mediate transplant rejection and autoimmunity.

Immunoglobulins (antibodies) on the *B-lymphocyte* surface are receptors for a large variety of specific structural conformations. In contrast, *T lymphocytes* recognize antigens as peptide fragments in the context of self major histocompatibility complex (MHC) antigens (called human leukocyte antigens [HLAs] in humans) on the surface of antigen-presenting cells, such as dendritic cells, macrophages, and other cell types expressing MHC class I and class II antigens. Once activated by specific antigen recognition, both B and T lymphocytes are triggered to differentiate and divide, leading to release of soluble mediators (cytokines, lymphokines) that perform as effectors and regulators of the immune response.

IMMUNOSUPPRESSION

Immunosuppressive drugs are used to dampen the immune response in organ transplantation and autoimmune disease. In transplantation, the major classes of immunosuppressive drugs used today are:

- Glucocorticoids
- Calcineurin inhibitors
- Antiproliferative/antimetabolic agents
- Biologicals (antibodies)

Table 35–1 summarizes the sites of action of representative immunosuppressants on T-cell activation.

These drugs are used in treating conditions such as acute immune rejection of organ transplants and severe auto-immune diseases. However, such therapies require lifelong use and nonspecifically suppress the entire immune system, exposing patients to considerably higher risks of infection and cancer. The calcineurin inhibitors and glucocorticoids, in particular, are nephrotoxic and diabetogenic, respectively, thus restricting their usefulness in a variety of clinical settings. Monoclonal and polyclonal antibody preparations directed at reactive T cells are important adjunct therapies and provide a unique opportunity to target specifically immune-reactive cells. Finally, newer small molecules and antibodies have expanded the arsenal of immunosuppressives. In particular, mammalian target of rapamycin (mTOR) inhibitors (sirolimus, everolimus) and *anti-CD25* (interleukin-2 receptor [IL-2R]) antibodies (basiliximab, daclizumab) target growth-factor pathways, substantially limiting clonal expansion and thus potentially promoting tolerance.

Table 35–1

Sites of Action of Selected Immunosuppressive Agents on T-Cell Activation

DRUG	SITE OF ACTION
Glucocorticoids	Glucocorticoid response elements in DNA (regulate gene transcription)
Muromonab-CD3	T-cell receptor complex (blocks antigen recognition)
Cyclosporine	Calcineurin (inhibits phosphatase activity)
Tacrolimus	Calcineurin (inhibits phosphatase activity)
Azathioprine	DNA (false nucleotide incorporation)
Mycophenolate mofetil	Inosine monophosphate dehydrogenase (inhibits activity)
Daclizumab, basiliximab	IL-2 receptor (block IL-2-mediated T-cell activation)
Sirolimus	Protein kinase involved in cell-cycle progression (mTOR) (inhibits activity)

IL, interleukin; mTOR, mammalian target of rapamycin.

GENERAL APPROACH TO ORGAN TRANSPLANTATION THERAPY. Organ transplantation therapy is organized around 5 general principles.

- Carefully prepare patient and select the best available ABO blood type–compatible HLA match for organ donation.
- Employ multitiered immunosuppressive therapy; simultaneously use several agents, each of which is directed at a different molecular target within the allograft response. Synergistic effects permit use of the various agents at relatively low doses, thereby limiting specific toxicities while maximizing the immunosuppressive effect.
- Employ intensive induction and lower-dose maintenance drug protocols; greater immunosuppression is required to gain early engraftment and/or to treat established rejection than to maintain long-term immunosuppression.
- Investigation of each episode of transplant dysfunction is required, including evaluation for rejection, drug toxicity, and infection.
- Reduce dosage or withdraw a drug if its toxicity exceeds its benefit.

BIOLOGICAL INDUCTION THERAPY. Induction therapy with polyclonal and monoclonal antibodies (mAbs) has been an important component of immunosuppression since the 1960s, when Starzl and colleagues demonstrated the beneficial effect of antilymphocyte globulin (ALG) in the prophylaxis of rejection. Two preparations are FDA-approved for use in transplantation: lymphocyte immune globulin (ATGAM) and antithymocyte globulin (ATG; THYMOGLOBULIN). ATG is the most frequently used depleting agent. Alemtuzumab, a humanized anti-CD52 monoclonal antibody that produces prolonged lymphocyte depletion, is approved for use in chronic lymphocytic leukemia but is increasingly used off label as induction therapy in transplantation.

In many transplant centers, induction therapy with biological agents is used to delay the use of the nephrotoxic calcineurin inhibitors or to intensify the initial immunosuppressive therapy in patients at high risk of rejection (i.e., repeat transplants, broadly presensitized patients, African American patients, or pediatric patients). Most of the limitations of murine-based mAbs generally were overcome by the introduction of chimeric or humanized mAbs that lack antigenicity and have a prolonged serum $t_{1/2}$. Antibodies derived from transgenic mice carrying human antibody genes are labeled "humanized" (90-95% human) or "fully human" (100% human); antibodies derived from human cells are labeled "human." However, all 3 types of antibodies probably are of equal efficacy and safety. Chimeric antibodies generally contain ~33% mouse protein and 67% human protein and can still produce an antibody response, resulting in reduced efficacy and shorter $t_{1/2}$ compared to humanized antibodies.

Biological agents for induction therapy in the prophylaxis of rejection currently are used in ~70% of de novo transplant patients. Biological agents for induction can be divided into 2 groups: the *depleting agents* and the *immune modulators*. The depleting agents consist of lymphocyte immune globulin, ATG, and muromonab-CD3 mAb; their efficacy derives from their ability to deplete the recipient's CD3-positive cells at the time of transplantation and antigen presentation. The second group of biological agents, the anti–IL-2R mAbs, do not deplete T lymphocytes, with the possible exception of T regulatory cells, but rather block IL-2–mediated T-cell activation by binding to the α chain of IL-2R. For patients with high levels of anti-HLA antibodies and humoral rejection, more aggressive therapies include plasmapheresis, intravenous immunoglobulin, and rituximab, a chimeric anti-CD20 monoclonal antibody.

MAINTENANCE IMMUNOTHERAPY. Basic immunosuppressive therapy uses multiple drugs simultaneously, typically a calcineurin inhibitor, glucocorticoids, and mycophenolate (a purine metabolism inhibitor), each directed at a discrete site in T-cell activation. Glucocorticoids, azathioprine, cyclosporine, tacrolimus, mycophenolate, sirolimus, and various monoclonal and polyclonal antibodies all are approved for use in transplantation.

THERAPY FOR ESTABLISHED REJECTION. Low doses of prednisone, calcineurin inhibitors, purine metabolism inhibitors, or sirolimus are effective in preventing acute cellular rejection; they are less effective in blocking activated T lymphocytes and thus are not very effective against established, acute rejection or for the total prevention of chronic rejection. Therefore, treatment of established rejection requires the use of agents directed against activated T cells. These include glucocorticoids in high doses (pulse therapy), polyclonal antilymphocyte antibodies, or muromonab-CD3.

GLUCOCORTICOIDS

The glucocorticoids are described in Chapter 42. Prednisone, prednisolone, and other glucocorticoids are used alone and in combination with other immunosuppressive agents for treatment of transplant rejection and autoimmune disorders.

Mechanism of Action. Glucocorticoids have broad anti-inflammatory effects on multiple components of cellular immunity, but relatively little effect on humoral immunity. Glucocorticoids bind to receptors inside cells and regulate the transcription of numerous other genes (*see* Chapter 42). Glucocorticoids also curtail activation of NF-κB, suppress formation of pro-inflammatory cytokines such as IL-1 and IL-6, inhibit T cells from making IL-2 and proliferating, and inhibit the activation of cytotoxic T lymphocytes. In addition, neutrophils and monocytes display poor chemotaxis and decreased lysosomal enzyme release.

Therapeutic Uses. Glucocorticoids commonly are combined with other immunosuppressive agents to prevent and treat transplant rejection. Glucocorticoids also are efficacious for treatment of graft-versus-host disease in bone-marrow transplantation. Glucocorticoids are routinely used to treat autoimmune disorders such as rheumatoid and other arthritides, systemic lupus erythematosus, systemic dermatomyositis, psoriasis and other skin conditions, asthma and other allergic disorders, inflammatory bowel disease, inflammatory ophthalmic diseases, auto-immune hematological disorders, and acute exacerbations of MS (see "Multiple Sclerosis," below). In addition, glucocorticoids limit allergic reactions that occur with other immunosuppressive agents and are used in transplant recipients to block first-dose cytokine storm caused by treatment with muromonab-CD3 and to a lesser extent ATG (see "Antithymocyte Globulin").

Toxicity. Extensive steroid use often results in disabling and life-threatening adverse effects described in Chapter 42. The advent of combined glucocorticoid/calcineurin inhibitor regimens has allowed reduced doses or rapid withdrawal of steroids, resulting in lower steroid-induced morbidities.

CALCINEURIN INHIBITORS

The most effective immunosuppressive drugs in routine use are the calcineurin inhibitors, cyclosporine and tacrolimus, which target intracellular signaling pathways induced as a consequence of T-cell–receptor activation (Figure 35–1). Cyclosporine and tacrolimus bind to an immunophilin (cyclophilin for cyclosporine, or FKBP-12 for tacrolimus), resulting in subsequent interaction with calcineurin to block its phosphatase activity. Calcineurin-catalyzed dephosphorylation is required for movement of a component of the nuclear factor of activated T lymphocytes (NFAT) into the nucleus. NFAT, in turn, is required to induce a number of cytokine genes, including that for IL-2, a prototypic T-cell growth and differentiation factor.

TACROLIMUS. Tacrolimus (PROGRAF, FK506) is a macrolide antibiotic produced by *Streptomyces tsukubaensis*. Because of perceived slightly greater efficacy and ease of blood level monitoring, tacrolimus has become the preferred calcineurin inhibitor in most transplant centers.

Mechanism of Action. Like cyclosporine, tacrolimus inhibits T-cell activation by inhibiting calcineurin. Tacrolimus binds to an intracellular protein, FK506-binding protein–12 (FKBP-12), an immunophilin structurally related to cyclophilin. A complex of tacrolimus-FKBP-12, Ca^{2+}, calmodulin, and calcineurin then forms, and calcineurin phosphatase activity is inhibited (*see* Figure 35–1). Inhibition of phosphatase activity prevents dephosphorylation and nuclear translocation of NFAT and inhibits T-cell activation. Thus, although the intracellular receptors differ, cyclosporine and tacrolimus target the same pathway for immunosuppression.

ADME. Tacrolimus is available for oral administration as capsules (0.5, 1, and 5 mg) and as a solution for injection (5 mg/mL). Because of intersubject variability in pharmacokinetics, individualized dosing is required for

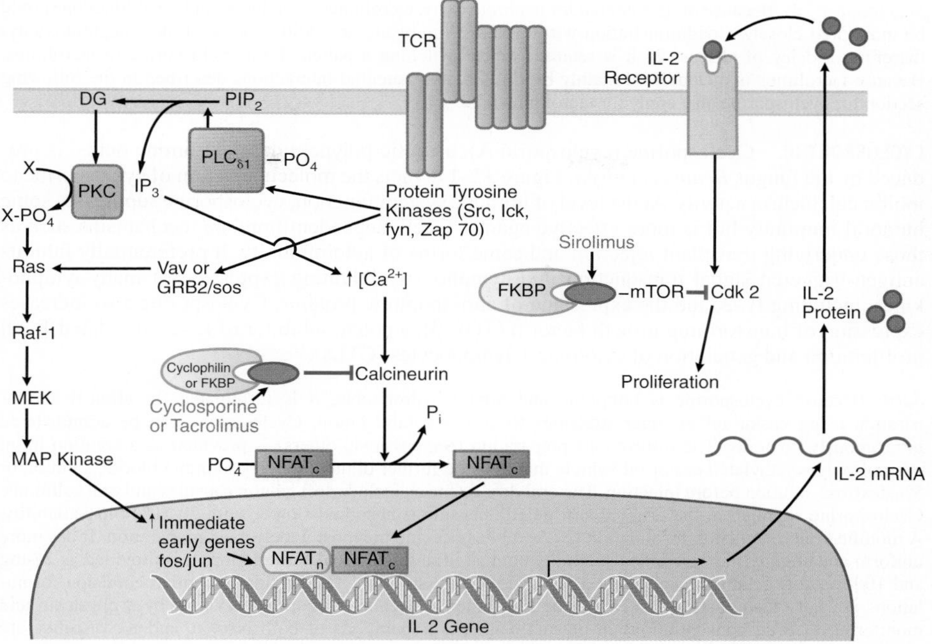

Figure 35–1 *Mechanisms of action of cyclosporine, tacrolimus, and sirolimus on T cells.* Cyclosporine and tacrolimus bind to immunophilins (cyclophilin and FK506-binding protein [FKBP], respectively), forming a complex that inhibits the phosphatase calcineurin and the calcineurin-catalyzed dephosphorylation that permits translocation of nuclear factor of activated T cells (NFAT) into the nucleus. NFAT is required for transcription of interleukin-2 (IL-2) and other growth and differentiation–associated cytokines (lymphokines). Sirolimus (rapamycin) works downstream of the IL-2 receptor, binding to FKBP; the FKBP-sirolimus complex binds to and inhibits the mammalian target of rapamycin (mTOR), a kinase involved in cell-cycle progression (proliferation). TCR, the T-cell receptor that recognizes antigens bound to the major histocompatibility complex. (Reproduced with permission from Clayberger C, Krensky AM. Mechanisms of allograft rejection. In Neilson EG, Couser WG, eds, *Immunologic Renal Diseases*, 2nd ed. Philadelphia: Lippincott Williams & Wilkins, 2001, pp 321–346. http://lww.com.)

optimal therapy. For tacrolimus, whole blood seems to be the best sampling compartment; the trough drug level in whole blood seems to correlate better with clinical events for tacrolimus than for cyclosporine. Target concentrations are 10-15 ng/mL in the early preoperative period and 100-200 ng/mL 3 months after transplantation. GI absorption is incomplete and variable. Food decreases the rate and extent of absorption. Plasma protein binding of tacrolimus is 75-99%, involving primarily albumin and α1-acid glycoprotein. The $t_{1/2}$ of tacrolimus is ~12 h. Tacrolimus is extensively metabolized in the liver by CYP3A; some of the metabolites are active. The bulk of excretion of the parent drug and metabolites is in the feces.

Therapeutic Uses. Tacrolimus is indicated for the prophylaxis of solid-organ allograft rejection in a manner similar to cyclosporine (see "Cyclosporine") and is used off label as rescue therapy in patients with rejection episodes despite "therapeutic" levels of cyclosporine. Recommended initial oral doses are 0.2 mg/kg/day for adult kidney transplant patients, 0.1-0.15 mg/kg/day for adult liver transplant patients, 0.075 mg/kg/day for adult heart transplant patients, and 0.15-0.2 mg/kg/day for pediatric liver transplant patients in 2 divided doses 12 h apart. These dosages are intended to achieve typical blood trough levels in the 5- to 20-ng/mL range.

Toxicity. Nephrotoxicity, neurotoxicity (e.g., tremor, headache, motor disturbances, seizures), GI complaints, hypertension, hyperkalemia, hyperglycemia, and diabetes all are associated with tacrolimus use. Tacrolimus has a negative effect on pancreatic islet β cells, and glucose intolerance and diabetes mellitus are well-recognized complications of tacrolimus-based immunosuppression. As with other immunosuppressive agents, there is an increased risk of secondary tumors and opportunistic infections. Notably, tacrolimus does not adversely affect uric acid or LDL cholesterol. Diarrhea and alopecia are common in patients on concomitant mycophenolate therapy.

Drug Interactions. Because of its potential for nephrotoxicity, tacrolimus blood levels and renal function should be monitored closely. Coadministration with cyclosporine results in additive or synergistic nephrotoxicity; therefore, a delay of at least 24 h is required when switching a patient from cyclosporine to tacrolimus. Because tacrolimus is metabolized mainly by CYP3A, the potential interactions described in the following section for cyclosporine also apply for tacrolimus.

CYCLOSPORINE. Cyclosporine (cyclosporin A), a cyclic polypeptide of 11 amino acids, is produced by the fungus *Beauveria nivea*. Figure 35–1 depicts the molecular action of cyclosporine to inhibit calcineurin activity. At the level of immune system function, cyclosporine suppresses some humoral immunity but is more effective against T cell–dependent immune mechanisms such as those underlying transplant rejection and some forms of autoimmunity. It preferentially inhibits antigen-triggered signal transduction in T lymphocytes, blunting expression of many lymphokines, including IL-2, and the expression of anti-apoptotic proteins. Cyclosporine also increases expression of transforming growth factor β (TGF-β), a potent inhibitor of IL-2–stimulated T-cell proliferation and generation of cytotoxic T lymphocytes (CTLs).

ADME. Because cyclosporine is lipophilic and highly hydrophobic, it is formulated for clinical administration using castor oil or other strategies to ensure solubilization. Cyclosporine can be administered intravenously or orally. The intravenous preparation (SANDIMMUNE, others) is provided as a solution in an ethanol-polyoxyethylated castor oil vehicle that must be further diluted in 0.9% sodium chloride solution or 5% dextrose solution before injection. The oral dosage forms include soft gelatin capsules and oral solutions. Cyclosporine supplied in the original soft gelatin capsule is absorbed slowly, with 20-50% bioavailability. A modified microemulsion formulation (NEORAL) has become the most widely used preparation. It has more uniform and slightly increased bioavailability compared to the original formulation. It is provided as 25-mg and 100-mg soft gelatin capsules and a 100-mg/mL oral solution. The original and microemulsion formulations are not bioequivalent and cannot be used interchangeably without supervision by a physician and monitoring of drug concentrations in plasma. Generic preparations of both NEORAL and SANDIMMUNE are bioequivalent by FDA criteria. Transplant units need to educate patients that SANDIMMUNE and its generics are not the same as NEORAL and its generics, such that one preparation cannot be substituted for another without risk of inadequate immunosuppression or increased toxicity.

Blood levels taken 2 h after a dose administration (so-called C_2 levels) may correlate better with the AUC than other single points, but no single time point can simulate the exposure better than more frequent drug sampling. In practice, if a patient has clinical signs or symptoms of toxicity, or if there is unexplained rejection or renal dysfunction, a pharmacokinetic profile can be used to estimate that person's exposure to the drug.

Cyclosporine absorption is incomplete following oral administration and varies with the individual patient and the formulation used. The elimination of cyclosporine from the blood generally is biphasic, with a terminal $t_{1/2}$ of 5-18 h. After intravenous infusion, clearance is ~5-7 mL/min/kg in adult recipients of renal transplants, but results differ by age and patient populations. For example, clearance is slower in cardiac transplant patients and more rapid in children. Thus, the intersubject variability is so large that individual monitoring is required. After oral administration of cyclosporine (as NEORAL), the time to peak blood concentrations is 1.5-2 h. Administration with food delays and decreases absorption. High- and low-fat meals consumed within 30 min of administration decrease the AUC by ~13% and the maximum concentration by 33%. This makes it imperative to individualize dosage regimens for outpatients. Cyclosporine is extensively metabolized by hepatic CYP3A and to a lesser degree by the GI tract and kidneys. Cyclosporine and its metabolites are excreted principally through the bile into the feces, with ~6% excreted in the urine. Cyclosporine also is excreted in human milk. In the presence of hepatic dysfunction, dosage adjustments are required. No adjustments generally are necessary for dialysis or renal failure patients.

Therapeutic Uses. Clinical indications for cyclosporine are kidney, liver, heart, and other organ transplantation; rheumatoid arthritis; and psoriasis. Its use in dermatology is discussed in Chapter 65. Cyclosporine usually is combined with other agents, especially glucocorticoids and either azathioprine or mycophenolate and, most recently, sirolimus. The dose of cyclosporine varies, depending on the organ transplanted and the other drugs used in the specific treatment protocol(s). The initial dose generally is not given before the transplant because of the concern about nephrotoxicity. Dosing is guided by signs of rejection (too low a dose), renal or other toxicity (too high a dose), and close monitoring of blood levels. Great care must be taken to differentiate renal toxicity from rejection in kidney transplant patients. Ultrasound-guided allograft biopsy is the best way to assess the reason for renal dysfunction. Because adverse reactions have been ascribed more frequently to the intravenous formulation, this route of administration is discontinued as soon as the patient can take the drug orally.

In rheumatoid arthritis, cyclosporine is used in severe cases that have not responded to methotrexate. Cyclosporine can be combined with methotrexate, but the levels of both drugs must be monitored closely. In psoriasis, cyclosporine is indicated for treatment of adult immunocompetent patients with severe and disabling disease for whom other systemic therapies have failed. Because of its mechanism of action, there is a theoretical basis for the use of cyclosporine in a variety of other T cell–mediated diseases. Cyclosporine reportedly is effective in Behçet's acute ocular syndrome, endogenous uveitis, atopic dermatitis, inflammatory bowel disease, and nephrotic syndrome, even when standard therapies have failed.

Toxicity. The principal adverse reactions to cyclosporine therapy are renal dysfunction and hypertension; tremor, hirsutism, hyperlipidemia, and gum hyperplasia also are frequently encountered. Hypertension occurs in ~50% of renal transplant and almost all cardiac transplant patients. Hyperuricemia may lead to worsening of gout, increased P-glycoprotein activity, and hypercholesterolemia. Nephrotoxicity occurs in the majority of patients and is the major reason for cessation or modification of therapy. Combined use of calcineurin inhibitors and glucocorticoids is particularly diabetogenic. Especially at risk are obese patients, African American or Hispanic transplant recipients, or those with a family history of type II diabetes or obesity. Cyclosporine, as opposed to tacrolimus, is more likely to produce elevations in LDL cholesterol.

Drug Interactions. Any drug that affects CYPs, especially CYP3A, may impact cyclosporine blood concentrations. Substances that inhibit this enzyme can decrease cyclosporine metabolism and increase blood concentrations. These include Ca^{2+} channel blockers (e.g., *verapamil, nicardipine*), antifungal agents (e.g., *fluconazole, ketoconazole*), antibiotics (e.g., *erythromycin*), glucocorticoids (e.g., *methylprednisolone*), HIV-protease inhibitors (e.g., *indinavir*), and other drugs (e.g., *allopurinol, metoclopramide*). Grapefruit juice inhibits CYP3A and the P-glycoprotein multidrug efflux pump and thereby can increase cyclosporine blood concentrations. In contrast, drugs that induce CYP3A activity can increase cyclosporine metabolism and decrease blood concentrations. Such drugs include antibiotics (e.g., *nafcillin, rifampin*), anticonvulsants (e.g., *phenobarbital, phenytoin*), and others (e.g., *octreotide, ticlopidine*).

Interactions between cyclosporine and sirolimus require that administration of the 2 drugs be separated by time. Sirolimus aggravates cyclosporine-induced renal dysfunction, while cyclosporine increases sirolimus-induced hyperlipidemia and myelosuppression. Additive nephrotoxicity may occur when cyclosporine is coadministered with *NSAIDs* and other drugs that cause renal dysfunction; elevation of methotrexate levels when the 2 drugs are coadministered; and reduced clearance of other drugs, including *prednisolone, digoxin*, and statins.

ANTIPROLIFERATIVE AND ANTIMETABOLIC DRUGS

SIROLIMUS

Sirolimus (rapamycin; RAPAMUNE) is a macrocyclic lactone produced by *Streptomyces hygroscopicus*. Sirolimus inhibits T-lymphocyte activation and proliferation downstream of the IL-2 and other T-cell growth factor receptors (*see* Figure 35–1). Like cyclosporine and tacrolimus, therapeutic action of sirolimus requires formation of a complex with an immunophilin, in this case *FKBP-12*. The *sirolimus–FKBP-12 complex* does not affect calcineurin activity; rather, it binds to and inhibits the protein kinase *mTOR*, which is a key enzyme in cell-cycle progression. Inhibition of mTOR blocks cell-cycle progression at the $G_1 \rightarrow S$ phase transition.

ADME. After oral administration, sirolimus is absorbed rapidly and reaches a peak blood concentration within ~1 h after a single dose in healthy subjects and within ~2 h after multiple oral doses in renal transplant patients. Systemic availability is ~15%, and blood concentrations are proportional to dose between 3 and 12 mg/m². A high-fat meal decreases peak blood concentration by 34%; sirolimus therefore should be taken consistently either with or without food, and blood levels should be monitored closely. About 40% of sirolimus in plasma is protein bound, especially to albumin. The drug partitions into formed elements of blood (blood-to-plasma ratio = 38 in renal transplant patients). Sirolimus is extensively metabolized by CYP3A4 and is transported by P-glycoprotein. Although some of its metabolites are active, sirolimus itself is the major active component in whole blood and contributes > 90% of the immunosuppressive effect. The blood $t_{1/2}$ after multiple doses in stable renal transplant patients is 62 h. A loading dose of 3 times the maintenance dose will provide nearly steady-state concentrations within 1 day in most patients.

Therapeutic Uses. Sirolimus is indicated for prophylaxis of organ transplant rejection usually in combination with a reduced dose of calcineurin inhibitor and glucocorticoids. Sirolimus has been used with glucocorticoids and mycophenolate to avoid permanent renal damage. Sirolimus dosing regimens are relatively complex with blood levels generally targeted between 5 and 15 ng/mL. It is recommended that the daily maintenance dose be reduced by approximately one-third in patients with hepatic impairment. Sirolimus also has been incorporated into stents to inhibit local cell proliferation and blood vessel occlusion.

Toxicity. The use of sirolimus in renal transplant patients is associated with a dose-dependent increase in serum cholesterol and triglycerides that may require treatment. Although immunotherapy with sirolimus per se is not nephrotoxic, patients treated with cyclosporine plus sirolimus have impaired renal function compared to patients treated with cyclosporine alone. Sirolimus also may prolong delayed graft function in deceased-donor kidney transplants, presumably because of its antiproliferative action. Renal function therefore must be monitored closely in such patients. Lymphocele, a known surgical complication associated with renal transplantation, is increased in a dose-dependent fashion by sirolimus, requiring close postoperative follow-up.

Other adverse effects include anemia, leukopenia, thrombocytopenia, mouth ulcer, hypokalemia, proteinuria, and GI effects. Delayed wound healing may occur with sirolimus use. As with other immunosuppressive agents, there is an increased risk of neoplasms, especially lymphomas, and infections.

Drug Interactions. Because sirolimus is a substrate for CYP3A4 and is transported by P-glycoprotein, close attention to interactions with other drugs that are metabolized or transported by these proteins is required. Dose adjustment may be required when sirolimus is coadministered with diltiazem or rifampin.

EVEROLIMUS

Everolimus [40-*O*-(2-hydroxyethyl)-rapamycin] is closely related to sirolimus but has distinct pharmacokinetics. The main difference is a shorter $t_{1/2}$ and thus a shorter time to achieve steady-state concentrations of the drug. Dosage on a milligram per kilogram basis is similar to that of sirolimus. As with sirolimus, the combination of a calcineurin inhibitor and an mTOR inhibitor produces worse renal function at 1 year than does calcineurin inhibitor therapy alone. The toxicity of everolimus and the drug interactions seem to be the same as with sirolimus.

AZATHIOPRINE

Azathioprine (IMURAN, others) is a purine antimetabolite. It is an imidazolyl derivative of 6-mercaptopurine, metabolites of which can inhibit purine synthesis.

Mechanism of Action. Following exposure to nucleophiles such as glutathione, azathioprine is cleaved to 6-mercaptopurine, which in turn is converted to additional metabolites that inhibit de novo purine synthesis (*see* Chapter 61). A fraudulent nucleotide, 6-thio-IMP, is converted to 6-thio-GMP and finally to 6-thio-GTP, which is incorporated into DNA. Cell proliferation thereby is inhibited, impairing a variety of lymphocyte functions. Azathioprine appears to be a more potent immunosuppressive agent than 6-mercaptopurine.

Disposition and Pharmacokinetics. Azathioprine is well absorbed orally and reaches maximum blood levels within 1-2 h after administration. The $t_{1/2}$ of azathioprine is ~10 min, and $t_{1/2}$ of 6-mercaptopurine is ~1 h. Blood levels have limited predictive value because of extensive metabolism, significant activity of many different metabolites, and high tissue levels attained. Azathioprine and mercaptopurine are moderately bound to plasma proteins and are partially dialyzable. Both are rapidly removed from the blood by oxidation or methylation in the liver and/or erythrocytes.

Therapeutic Uses. Azathioprine is indicated as an adjunct for prevention of organ transplant rejection and in severe rheumatoid arthritis. The usual starting dose of azathioprine is 3-5 mg/kg/day. Lower initial doses (1 mg/kg/day) are used in treating rheumatoid arthritis. Complete blood count and liver function tests should be monitored.

Toxicity. The major side effect of azathioprine is bone marrow suppression, including leukopenia (common), thrombocytopenia (less common), and/or anemia (uncommon). Other important adverse effects include increased susceptibility to infections (especially varicella and herpes simplex viruses), hepatotoxicity, alopecia, GI toxicity, pancreatitis, and increased risk of neoplasia.

Drug Interactions. Xanthine oxidase, an enzyme of major importance in the catabolism of azathioprine metabolites, is blocked by allopurinol. Adverse effects resulting from coadministration of azathioprine with other myelosuppressive agents or angiotensin-converting enzyme inhibitors include leukopenia, thrombocytopenia, and anemia as a result of myelosuppression.

MYCOPHENOLATE MOFETIL

Mycophenolate mofetil (MMF; CELLCEPT) is the 2-morpholinoethyl ester of mycophenolic acid (MPA). MMF is a prodrug that is rapidly hydrolyzed to the active drug, MPA, a selective, noncompetitive, reversible inhibitor of inosine monophosphate dehydrogenase (IMPDH), an important enzyme in the de novo pathway of guanine nucleotide synthesis. B and T lymphocytes are highly dependent on this pathway for cell proliferation; MPA thus selectively inhibits lymphocyte proliferation and functions, including antibody formation, cellular adhesion, and migration.

Disposition and Pharmacokinetics. MMF undergoes rapid and complete metabolism to MPA after oral or intravenous administration. MPA is then metabolized to the inactive glucuronide MPAG. The $t_{1/2}$ of MPA is ~16 h. Most (87%) is excreted in the urine as MPAG. Plasma concentrations of MPA and MPAG are increased in patients with renal insufficiency.

Therapeutic Uses. MMF is indicated for prophylaxis of transplant rejection, and it typically is used in combination with glucocorticoids and a calcineurin inhibitor but not with azathioprine. Combined treatment with sirolimus is possible, although potential drug interactions necessitate careful monitoring of drug levels. For renal transplants, 1 g is administered orally or intravenously (over 2 h) twice daily (2 g/day). A higher dose, 1.5 g twice daily (3 g/day), may be recommended for African American renal transplant patients and all liver and cardiac transplant patients. MMF is increasingly used off label in systemic lupus. A delayed-release formulation of MPA (MYFORTIC) is available. It does not release MPA under acidic conditions (pH < 5), as in the stomach, but is soluble in neutral pH, as in the intestine. The enteric coating results in a delay in the time to reach maximum MPA concentrations.

Toxicity. The principal toxicities of MMF are GI and hematologic: leukopenia, pure red cell aplasia, diarrhea, and vomiting. There also is an increased incidence of some infections, especially sepsis associated with cytomegalovirus. Tacrolimus in combination with MMF has been associated with activation of polyoma viruses such as BK virus, which can cause interstitial nephritis. The use of mycophenolate in pregnancy is associated with congenital anomalies and increased risk of pregnancy loss.

Drug Interactions. Tacrolimus delays elimination of MMF by impairing the conversion of MPA to MPAG. This may enhance GI toxicity. Coadministration with antacids containing aluminum or magnesium hydroxide leads to decreased absorption of MMF; thus, these drugs should not be administered simultaneously. MMF should not be administered with cholestyramine or other drugs that affect enterohepatic circulation. Such agents decrease plasma MPA concentrations, probably by binding free MPA in the intestines. Acyclovir and ganciclovir may compete with MPAG for tubular secretion, possibly resulting in increased concentrations of both MPAG and the antiviral agents in the blood, an effect that may be compounded in patients with renal insufficiency.

OTHER ANTIPROLIFERATIVE AND CYTOTOXIC AGENTS

Many of the cytotoxic and antimetabolic agents used in cancer chemotherapy (*see* Chapter 61) are immunosuppressive due to their action on lymphocytes and other cells of the immune system. Other cytotoxic drugs that have been used off label as immunosuppressive agents include methotrexate, cyclophosphamide, thalidomide (THALOMID), and chlorambucil (LEUKERAN). Methotrexate is used for treatment of graft-versus-host disease, rheumatoid arthritis, psoriasis, and some cancers. Cyclophosphamide and chlorambucil are used in leukemia and lymphomas and a variety of other malignancies. Cyclophosphamide also is FDA-approved for childhood nephrotic syndrome and is used widely for treatment of severe systemic lupus erythematosus and other vasculitides such as Wegener granulomatosis. Leflunomide (ARAVA, others) is a pyrimidine-synthesis inhibitor indicated for the treatment of adults with rheumatoid arthritis. This drug has found increasing empirical use in the treatment of polyomavirus nephropathy seen in immunosuppressed renal transplant recipients. There are no controlled studies showing efficacy compared with control patients treated with only withdrawal or reduction of immunosuppression alone in BK virus nephropathy. The drug inhibits dihydroorotate dehydrogenase in the de novo pathway of pyrimidine synthesis. It is hepatotoxic and can cause fetal injury when administered to pregnant women.

FINGOLIMOD (FTY720). This is the first agent in a new class of small molecules, sphingosine-1-phosphate receptor (S1P-R) agonists. This S1P receptor prodrug reduces recirculation of lymphocytes from the lymphatic system to the blood and peripheral tissues, thereby shunting lymphocytes away from inflammatory lesions and organ grafts.

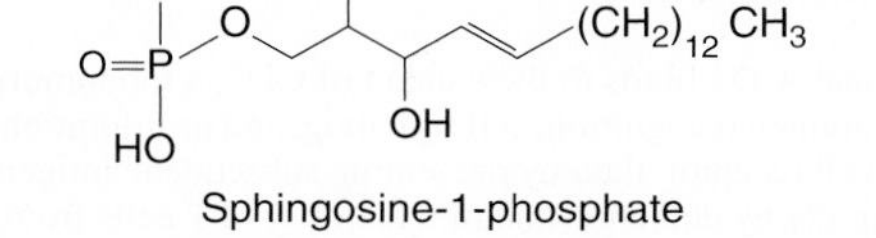

HO NH2 HO

FTY720 (Fingolimod)

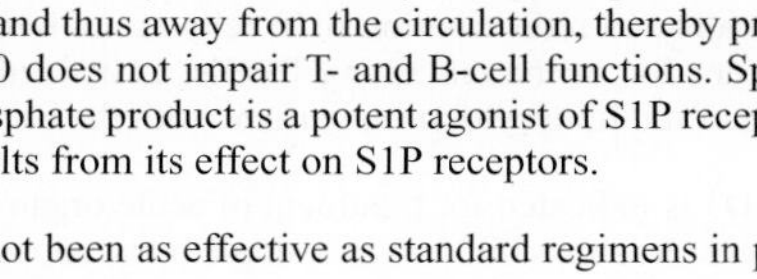

HO O=P HO O $\overset{+}{N}H_3$ OH $(CH_2)_{12}CH_3$

Sphingosine-1-phosphate

Mechanism of Action. FTY720 specifically and reversibly causes sequestration of host lymphocytes into the lymph nodes and Peyer patches and thus away from the circulation, thereby protecting lesions and grafts from T cell–mediated attack. FTY720 does not impair T- and B-cell functions. Sphingosine kinase-2 phosphorylates FTY720; the FTY720-phosphate product is a potent agonist of S1P receptors. Altered lymphocyte traffic induced by FTY720 clearly results from its effect on S1P receptors.

Therapeutic Uses. The drug has not been as effective as standard regimens in phase III trials, and further drug development has been limited.

Toxicity. Lymphopenia, the predictable and most common side effect of FTY720, reverses upon discontinuation of the drug. Of greater concern is the negative chronotropic effect of FTY720 on the heart, which has been observed with the first dose in up to 30% of patients.

IMMUNOSUPPRESSION ANTIBODIES AND FUSION RECEPTOR PROTEIN

Polyclonal and monoclonal antibodies against lymphocyte cell-surface antigens are widely used for prevention and treatment of organ transplant rejection. Polyclonal antisera are generated by repeated injections of human thymocytes (ATG) or lymphocytes (ALG) into animals and then purifying the serum immunoglobulin fraction. These preparations vary in efficacy and toxicity from batch to batch. The capacity to produce monoclonal antibodies has overcome the problems of variability in efficacy and toxicity seen with the polyclonal products, but monoclonal Abs are more limited in their target specificity.

Another class of biological agents being developed for both autoimmunity and transplantation are fusion receptor proteins. These agents consist of the ligand-binding domains of receptors bound to the Fc region of an immunoglobulin (usually IgG_1) to provide a longer $t_{1/2}$.

ANTITHYMOCYTE GLOBULIN

ATG is a purified gamma globulin from the serum of rabbits immunized with human thymocytes.

MECHANISM OF ACTION. ATG contains cytotoxic antibodies that bind to CD2, CD3, CD4, CD8, CD11a, CD18, CD25, CD44, CD45, and HLA class I and II molecules on the surface of human T lymphocytes. The antibodies deplete circulating lymphocytes by direct cytotoxicity (both complement and cell mediated) and block lymphocyte function by binding to cell surface molecules involved in the regulation of cell function.

Therapeutic Uses. ATG is used for induction immunosuppression, although the only approved indication is in the treatment of acute renal transplant rejection in combination with other immunosuppressive agents. Antilymphocyte-depleting agents (THYMOGLOBULIN, ATGAM, and OKT3) are not registered for use as induction immunosuppression. A course of antithymocyte-globulin often is given to renal transplant patients with delayed graft function to avoid early treatment with the nephrotoxic calcineurin inhibitors, thereby aiding in recovery from ischemic reperfusion injury. The recommended dose for acute rejection of renal grafts is 1.5 mg/kg/day (over 4-6 h) for 7-14 days. Mean T-cell counts fall by day 2 of therapy. ATG also is used for acute rejection of other types of organ transplants and for prophylaxis of rejection.

Toxicity. Polyclonal antibodies are xenogeneic proteins that can elicit major side effects, including fever and chills with the potential for hypotension. Premedication with corticosteroids, acetaminophen, and/or an antihistamine and administration of the antiserum by slow infusion (over 4-6 h) into a large-diameter vessel minimize such reactions. Serum sickness and glomerulonephritis can occur; anaphylaxis is rare. Hematologic complications include leukopenia and thrombocytopenia. As with other immunosuppressive agents, there is an increased risk of infection and malignancy, especially when multiple immunosuppressive agents are combined.

MONOCLONAL ANTIBODIES

ANTI-CD3 MONOCLONAL ANTIBODIES. Antibodies directed at the ε chain of CD3, a trimeric molecule adjacent to the T-cell receptor on the surface of human T lymphocytes, have been used with considerable efficacy in human transplantation. The original mouse IgG_{2a} antihuman CD3 monoclonal antibody, muromonab-CD3 (OKT3, ORTHOCLONE OKT3), still is used to reverse glucocorticoid-resistant rejection episodes.

Mechanism of Action. Muromonab-CD3 binds to the ε chain of CD3, a monomorphic component of the T-cell receptor complex involved in antigen recognition, cell signaling, and proliferation. Antibody treatment induces rapid internalization of the T-cell receptor, thereby preventing subsequent antigen recognition. Administration of the antibody is followed rapidly by depletion and of a majority of T cells from the bloodstream and peripheral lymphoid organs such as lymph nodes and spleen. This absence of detectable T cells from the usual lymphoid regions is secondary both to complement activation-induced cell death and to margination of T cells onto vascular endothelial walls and redistribution of T cells to nonlymphoid organs such as the lungs. Muromonab-CD3 also reduces function of the remaining T cells, as defined by lack of IL-2 production and great reduction in the production of multiple cytokines, perhaps with the exception of IL-4 and IL-10.

Therapeutic Uses. Muromonab-CD3 is indicated for treatment of acute organ transplant rejection. The recommended dose is 5 mg/day (in adults; less for children) in a single intravenous bolus (< 1 min) for 10-14 days. Circulating T cells disappear from the blood within minutes of administration and return within ~1 week after termination of therapy. Repeated use of muromonab-CD3 results in the immunization of the patient against the mouse determinants of the antibody and generally is contraindicated. Administration of glucocorticoids before the injection of muromonab-CD3 is standard; it prevents the release of cytokines and reduces first-dose reactions considerably, and now is a standard procedure. Volume status of patients also must be monitored carefully before therapy; a fully competent resuscitation facility must be immediately available for patients receiving their first several doses of this therapy.

Toxicity. The major side effect of anti-CD3 therapy is the "cytokine release syndrome." The syndrome typically begins 30 min after infusion of the antibody (but can occur later) and may persist for h. The syndrome is associated with increased serum levels of cytokines (including tumor necrosis factor-α [TNF-α], IL-2, IL-6, and interferon-γ [IFN-γ]) released by activated T cells and/or monocytes. Clinical manifestations include high fever, chills/rigor, headache, tremor, nausea, vomiting, diarrhea, abdominal pain, malaise, myalgias, arthralgias, and generalized weakness. Less common complaints include skin reactions and cardiorespiratory and CNS disorders. Potentially fatal pulmonary edema, acute respiratory distress syndrome, cardiovascular collapse, cardiac arrest, and arrhythmias have been described. Other toxicities associated with anti-CD3 therapy include anaphylaxis and the usual infections and neoplasms associated with immunosuppressive therapy. "Rebound" rejection has been observed when muromonab-CD3 treatment is stopped. Anti-CD3 therapies may be limited by anti-idiotypic or antimurine antibodies in the recipient. Muromonab-CD3 rarely is used in transplantation. It has been replaced by ATG and alemtuzumab.

NEW-GENERATION ANTI-CD3 ANTIBODIES. Recently, genetically altered anti-CD3 monoclonal antibodies have been developed that are "humanized" to minimize the occurrence of anti-antibody responses and mutated to prevent binding to Fc receptors. In initial clinical trials, a humanized anti-CD3 monoclonal antibody that does not bind to Fc receptors reversed acute renal allograft rejection without causing the first-dose cytokine-release syndrome.

ANTI-IL-2 RECEPTOR (ANTI-CD25) ANTIBODIES. **Daclizumab** (ZENAPAX) is a humanized murine complementarity-determining region (CDR)/human IgG_1 chimeric monoclonal antibody. **Basiliximab** (SIMULECT) is a murine-human chimeric monoclonal antibody.

Mechanism of Action. The anti-CD25 mAbs bind to the IL-2 receptor on the surface of activated T cells. Significant depletion of T cells does not appear to play a major role in the mechanism of action of these mAbs. Therapy with the anti IL-2R mAbs results in a relative decrease of the expression of the α chain epitope of the IL-2R on activated lymphocytes. The β chain may be downregulated by the anti-CD25 antibody. Daclizumab has a somewhat lower affinity but a longer $t_{1/2}$ (20 days) than basiliximab.

Therapeutic Uses. Anti–IL-2-receptor monoclonal antibodies are used for prophylaxis of acute organ rejection in adult patients.

Clinical trials indicate that the $t_{1/2}$ of daclizumab is 20 days, resulting in saturation of the IL-2Rα on circulating lymphocytes for up to 120 days after transplantation. Daclizumab was administered in 5 doses (1 mg/kg given intravenously over 15 min in 50-100 mL of normal saline) starting immediately preoperatively, and subsequently at biweekly intervals. Daclizumab was used with maintenance immunosuppressive regimens (cyclosporine, azathioprine, and steroids; cyclosporine and steroids).

The $t_{1/2}$ of basiliximab is 7 days. In trials, basiliximab was administered in a fixed dose of 20 mg preoperatively and on days 0 and 4 after transplantation. This regimen of basiliximab saturated IL-2R on circulating lymphocytes for 25-35 days after transplantation. Basiliximab was used with a maintenance regimen consisting of cyclosporine and prednisone and was found to be safe and effective when used in a maintenance regimen consisting of cyclosporine, MMF, and prednisone.

Toxicity. No cytokine-release syndrome has been noted, but anaphylactic reactions and rare lymphoproliferative disorders and opportunistic infections may occur. No drug interactions have been described.

Alemtuzumab. Alemtuzumab (CAMPATH) is a humanized mAb approved for use in chronic lymphocytic leukemia. The antibody targets CD52, a glycoprotein expressed on lymphocytes, monocytes, macrophages, and natural killer cells; the drug causes lympholysis by inducing apoptosis of targeted cells. It has achieved some use in renal transplantation because it produces prolonged T- and B-cell depletion and allows drug minimization.

ANTI-TNF REAGENTS. TNF-α is a proinflammatory cytokine that has been implicated in the pathogenesis of several immune-mediated intestinal, skin, and joint diseases. Several diseases (rheumatoid arthritis, Crohn disease) are associated with elevated levels of TNF-α. As a result, a number of anti-TNF agents have been developed as treatments.

Infliximab (REMICADE) is a chimeric IgG_1 monoclonal antibody containing a human constant (Fc) region and a murine variable region. It binds with high affinity to TNF-α and prevents the cytokine from binding to its receptors. Infliximab is approved in the U.S. for treating the symptoms of rheumatoid arthritis and is typically used in combination with methotrexate in patients who do not respond to methotrexate alone. Infliximab also is approved for treatment of symptoms of Crohn disease, ankylosing spondylitis, plaque psoriasis, psoriatic arthritis, and ulcerative colitis. About 1 of 6 patients receiving infliximab experiences an infusion reaction characterized by fever, urticaria, hypotension, and dyspnea within 1-2 h after antibody administration. The development of antinuclear antibodies, and rarely a lupus-like syndrome, has been reported after treatment with infliximab.

Etanercept (ENBREL) is a fusion protein that targets TNF-α. Etanercept contains the ligand-binding portion of a human TNF-α receptor fused to the Fc portion of human IgG_1, and binds to TNF-α and prevents it from interacting with its receptors. It is approved for treatment of the symptoms of rheumatoid arthritis, ankylosing spondylitis, plaque psoriasis, polyarticular juvenile idiopathic arthritis, and psoriatic arthritis. Etanercept can be used in combination with methotrexate in patients who have not responded adequately to methotrexate alone. Injection-site reactions (i.e., erythema, itching, pain, or swelling) have occurred.

Adalimumab (HUMIRA) is another anti-TNF product for intravenous use. This recombinant human IgG_1 monoclonal antibody is approved for use in rheumatoid arthritis, ankylosing spondylitis, Crohn disease, juvenile idiopathic arthritis, plaque psoriasis, psoriatic arthritis, and ulcerative colitis.

Toxicity. All anti-TNF agents (i.e., infliximab, etanercept, adalimumab) increase the risk for serious infections, lymphomas, and other malignancies. For example, fatal hepatosplenic T-cell lymphomas have been reported in adolescent and young adult patients with Crohn disease treated with infliximab in conjunction with azathioprine or 6-mercaptopurine.

IL-1 INHIBITION

Plasma IL-1 levels are increased in patients with active inflammation (*see* Chapter 34). In addition to the naturally occurring IL-1 receptor antagonist (IL-1RA), several IL-1 receptor antagonists are in development and a few have been approved for clinical use. **Anakinra** is an FDA-approved recombinant, nonglycosylated form of human IL-1RA for the management of joint disease in rheumatoid arthritis. It can be used alone or in combination with anti-TNF agents such as etanercept, infliximab, or adalimumab. **Canakinumab** (ILARIS) is an IL-1β monoclonal antibody that is FDA-approved for Cryopyrin-associated periodic syndromes (CAPS), a group of rare inherited inflammatory diseases associated with overproduction of IL-1 that includes familial cold autoinflammatory and Muckle-Wells syndromes. Canakinumab is also being evaluated for use in chronic obstructive pulmonary disease. **Rilonacept** (IL-1 TRAP) is another IL-1 blocker (a fusion protein that binds IL-1) that is being evaluated for gout; IL-1 is an inflammatory mediator of joint pain associated with elevated uric acid crystals.

LYMPHOCYTE FUNCTION–ASSOCIATED ANTIGEN-1 (LFA-1) INHIBITION

Efalizumab (RAPTIVA) is a humanized IgG_1 mAb targeting the CD11a chain of lymphocyte function–associated antigen-1 (LFA-1). Efalizumab binds to LFA-1 on lymphocytes and prevents the LFA-1 interaction with intercellular adhesion molecule (ICAM) thereby inhibiting T-cell adhesion, trafficking, and activation. Efalizumab is approved for use in patients with psoriasis.

Alefacept (AMEVIVE) is a human LFA-3-IgG_1 fusion protein. The LFA-3 portion of alefacept binds to CD2 on T lymphocytes, blocking the interaction between LFA-3 and CD2 and interfering with T-cell activation. Alefacept is approved for use in psoriasis. Treatment with alefacept has been shown to produce a dose-dependent reduction in T-effector memory cells (CD45, RO+) but not in naïve cells (CD45, RA+).

TARGETING B CELLS

Most of the advances in transplantation can be attributed to drugs designed to inhibit T-cell responses. As a result, T cell–mediated acute rejection has been become much less of a problem, while B cell–mediated responses such as antibody-mediated rejection and other effects of donor-specific antibodies have become more evident. Both biologicals and small molecules with B-cell specific effects now are in development for transplantation, including humanized monoclonal antibodies to CD20 and inhibitors of the 2 B cell–activation factors BLYS and APRIL and their respective receptors. Belimumab (BENLYSTA), a monoclonal antibody that targets BLYS, was recently approved for use in patients with systemic lupus erythromatosus.

TOLERANCE

Immunosuppression has concomitant risks of opportunistic infections and secondary tumors. Therefore, the ultimate goal of research on organ transplantation and autoimmune diseases is to induce and maintain immunological tolerance, the active state of antigen-specific nonresponsiveness. Tolerance, if attainable, would represent a true cure for conditions discussed earlier in this section without the side effects of the various immunosuppressive therapies. The calcineurin inhibitors prevent tolerance induction in some, but not all, preclinical models. In these same model systems, sirolimus does not prevent tolerance and may even promote tolerance.

CO-STIMULATORY BLOCKADE. Induction of specific immune responses by T lymphocytes requires 2 signals: an antigen-specific signal via the T-cell receptor and a co-stimulatory signal provided by the interaction of molecules such as CD28 on the T lymphocyte and CD80 and CD86 on the antigen-presenting cell (Figure 35–2). Inhibition of the co-stimulatory signal has been shown to induce tolerance.

Abatacept (CTLA4-Ig) is a fusion protein that contains the binding region of cytotoxic T-lymphocyte-associated antigen 4 (CTLA4), which is a CD28 homolog, and the Fc region of the human IgG_1. CTLA4-Ig competitively inhibits CD28 binding to CD80 and CD86 and thus activation of T-cells. CTLA4-Ig is effective in the treatment of rheumatoid arthritis in patients resistant to other drugs.

Belatacept (NULOJIX, LEA29Y) is a second-generation CTLA4-Ig with 2 amino acid substitutions. Belatacept has higher affinity for CD80 (2-fold) and CD86 (4-fold), yielding a 10-fold increase in potency in vitro as compared to CTLA4-Ig. Preclinical renal transplant studies in nonhuman primates showed that belatacept did not induce tolerance but did prolong graft survival. Because of the risk of post-transplant lymphoproliferative disease (PTLD), EBV negative patients should not be treated with belatacept. Belatacept is approved as an immunosuppressant to prevent organ rejection in renal transplantation.

A second co-stimulatory pathway involves the interaction of CD40 on activated T cells with CD40 ligand (CD154) on B cells, endothelium, and/or antigen-presenting cells (*see* Figure 35–2). Among the purported

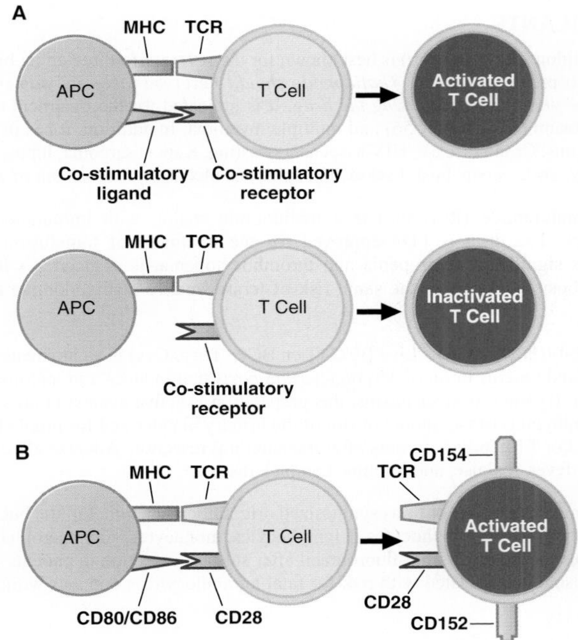

Figure 35–2 *Co-stimulation.* **A.** Two signals are required for T-cell activation. Signal 1 is *via* the T-cell receptor (TCR) and signal 2 is *via* a co-stimulatory receptor-ligand pair. Signal 1 in the absence of signal 2 results in an inactivated T cell. **B.** One important co-stimulatory pathway involves CD28 on the T cell and B7-1 (CD80) and B7-2 (CD86) on the antigen-presenting cell (APC). After a T cell is activated, it expresses additional co-stimulatory molecules. CD152 is CD40 ligand, which interacts with CD40 as a co-stimulatory pair. CD154 (CTLA4) interacts with CD80 and CD86 to dampen or downregulate an immune response. Antibodies against CD80, CD86, and CD152 are being evaluated as potential therapeutic agents. CTLA4-Ig, a chimeric protein consisting of part of an immunoglobulin molecule and part of CD154, also has been tested as a therapeutic agent. (Adapted with permission from Clayberger C, Krensky AM. Mechanisms of allograft rejection. In Neilson EG, Couser WG, eds, *Immunologic Renal Diseases*, 2nd ed. Philadelphia: Lippincott Williams & Wilkins, 2001, pp 321–346. http://lww.com.)

activities of anti-CD154 antibody treatment is the blockade of B7 expression induced by immune activation. Two humanized anti-CD154 monoclonal antibodies have been used in clinical trials in renal transplantation and autoimmune diseases. The development of these antibodies, however, is on hold because of associated thromboembolic events. An alternative approach to block the CD154-CD40 pathway is to target CD40 with monoclonal antibodies. These antibodies are undergoing trials in non-Hodgkin lymphoma but are also likely to be developed for autoimmunity and transplantation.

DONOR CELL CHIMERISM. A promising approach is induction of chimerism (coexistence of cells from 2 genetic lineages in a single individual) by first dampening or eliminating immune function in the recipient with ionizing radiation, drugs such as cyclophosphamide, and/or antibody treatment, and then providing a new source of immune function by adoptive transfer (transfusion) of bone marrow or hematopoietic stem cells. Upon reconstitution of immune function, the recipient no longer recognizes new antigens provided during a critical period as "nonself." Such tolerance is long lived and less likely to be complicated by the use of calcineurin inhibitors.

ANTIGENS. Specific antigens induce immunological tolerance in preclinical models of diabetes mellitus, arthritis, and MS. In vitro and preclinical in vivo studies demonstrate that one can selectively inhibit immune responses to specific antigens without the associated toxicity of immunosuppressive therapies. With these insights comes the promise of specific immune therapies to treat an array of immune disorders from autoimmunity to transplant rejection.

IMMUNOSTIMULATION

In contrast to immunosuppressive agents that inhibit the immune response in transplant rejection and autoimmunity, a few immunostimulatory drugs have been developed with applicability to infection, immunodeficiency, and cancer.

IMMUNOSTIMULANTS

THALIDOMIDE. Thalidomide (THALOMID) is best known for the severe, life-threatening birth defects it caused when administered to pregnant women. *Thalidomide should never be taken by women who are pregnant or who could become pregnant while taking the drug.* It is indicated for the treatment of patients with erythema nodosum leprosum (*see* Chapter 56) and multiple myeloma. In addition, it has orphan drug status for mycobacterial infections, Crohn disease, HIV-associated wasting, Kaposi sarcoma, lupus, myelofibrosis, brain malignancies, leprosy, graft-versus-host disease, and aphthous ulcers. Its mechanism of action is unclear.

LENALIDOMIDE. Lenalidomide (REVLIMID) is a thalidomide analog with immunomodulatory and antiangiogenic properties. The drug is FDA-approved for the treatment of transfusion-dependent anemia. Lenalidomide causes significant neutropenia and thrombocytopenia, is associated with a significant risk for deep vein thrombosis, and carries the same risk of teratogenicity as thalidomide (pregnancy must be avoided).

BACILLUS CALMETTE-GUÉRIN (BCG). Live BCG (TICE BCG, THERACYS) is an attenuated, live culture of the bacillus of Calmette and Guérin strain of *Mycobacterium bovis* that induces a granulomatous reaction at the site of administration. By unclear mechanisms, this preparation is active against tumors and is indicated for the treatment and prophylaxis of carcinoma in situ of the urinary bladder and for prophylaxis of primary and recurrent stage Ta and/or T1 papillary tumors after transurethral resection. Adverse effects include hypersensitivity, shock, chills, fever, malaise, and immune complex disease.

LEVAMISOLE. Levamisole (ERGAMISOL) was synthesized originally as an anthelmintic but appears to "restore" depressed immune function of B lymphocytes, T lymphocytes, monocytes, and macrophages. Its only clinical indication was as adjuvant therapy with 5-fluorouracil after surgical resection in patients with Dukes' stage C colon cancer. Levamisole is associated with risk for fatal agranulocytosis and was withdrawn from the U.S. market.

RECOMBINANT CYTOKINES

INTERFERONS. Although interferons (α, β, and γ) initially were identified by their antiviral activity, these agents also have important immunomodulatory activities. The interferons bind to specific cell-surface receptors that initiate a series of intracellular events: induction of certain enzymes, inhibition of cell proliferation, and enhancement of immune activities, including increased phagocytosis by macrophages and augmentation of specific cytotoxicity by T lymphocytes.

Recombinant IFN-α-2b (INTRON A) is obtained from *Escherichia coli* by recombinant expression. It is a member of a family of naturally occurring small proteins (15-27 KDa), produced and secreted by cells in response to viral infections and other inducers. IFN-α-2b is indicated in the treatment of myriad tumors (e.g., hairy cell leukemia, malignant melanoma, follicular lymphoma, and AIDS-related Kaposi sarcoma) and for infectious diseases, chronic hepatitis B, and condylomata acuminata. IFN-α-2b is supplied in combination with ribavirin (REBETRON) for treatment of chronic hepatitis C in patients with compensated liver function not treated previously with IFN-α-2b or who have relapsed after IFN-α-2b therapy. Flu-like symptoms are the most common adverse effects after IFN-α-2b administration. Adverse cardiovascular effects (e.g., hypotension, arrhythmias, cardiomyopathy, and myocardial infarction) and CNS effects (e.g., depression, confusion) are less frequent. All α interferons carry a black-box warning regarding development of pulmonary hypertension.

IFN-γ-1b (ACTIMMUNE) is a recombinant polypeptide that activates phagocytes and induces their generation of oxygen metabolites that are toxic to a number of microorganisms. It is indicated to reduce the frequency and severity of serious infections associated with chronic granulomatous disease and to delay the time to progression in severe malignant osteopetrosis. Adverse reactions include fever, headache, rash, fatigue, GI distress, anorexia, weight loss, myalgia, and depression.

IFN-β-1a (AVONEX, REBIF), a 166–amino acid recombinant glycoprotein, and IFN-β-1b (BETASERON), a 165–amino acid recombinant protein, have antiviral and immunomodulatory properties. They are FDA-approved for the treatment of relapsing MS to reduce the frequency of clinical exacerbations (see below). The mechanism of their action in MS is unclear. Flu-like symptoms (e.g., fever, chills, myalgia) and injection-site reactions are common adverse effects.

INTERLEUKIN-2. Human recombinant IL-2 (aldesleukin, PROLEUKIN; des-alanyl-1, serine-125 human IL-2) differs from native IL-2 in that it is not glycosylated, has no amino-terminal alanine, and has a serine substituted for the cysteine at amino acid 125. Aldesleukin activates cellular immunity, with lymphocytosis, eosinophilia, thrombocytopenia, and release of multiple cytokines (e.g., TNF, IL-1, IFN-γ). Aldesleukin is indicated for the treatment of adults with metastatic renal cell carcinoma and melanoma.

The potency of the preparation is represented in International Units in a lymphocyte proliferation assay such that 1.1 mg of recombinant IL-2 protein equals 18 million IU. Administration of aldesleukin has been associated with serious cardiovascular toxicity resulting from capillary leak syndrome, which involves loss of vascular tone and leak of plasma proteins and fluid into the extravascular space. Hypotension, reduced organ perfusion, and death may occur. An increased risk of disseminated infection due to impaired neutrophil function also has been associated with aldesleukin treatment.

IMMUNIZATION

Active immunization involves stimulation with an antigen to develop immunological defenses against a future exposure. *Passive immunization* involves administration of pre-formed antibodies to an individual who is already exposed or is about to be exposed to an antigen.

VACCINES. Active immunization, vaccination, involves administration of an antigen as a whole, killed (inactivated) organism; attenuated (live) organism; or a specific protein or peptide constituent of an organism. Booster doses often are required, especially when killed organisms are used as the immunogen. In the U.S., vaccination has sharply curtailed or practically eliminated a variety of major infections, including diphtheria, measles, mumps, pertussis, rubella, tetanus, *Haemophilus influenzae* type b, and pneumococcus.

Although most vaccines have targeted infectious diseases, a new generation of vaccines may provide complete or limited protection from specific cancers or autoimmune diseases. Because T cells optimally are activated by peptides and co-stimulatory ligands that are present on antigen-presenting cells (APCs), one approach for vaccination has consisted of immunizing patients with APCs expressing a tumor antigen. Multiple studies have demonstrated the efficacy of DNA vaccines in small- and large-animal models of infectious diseases and cancer. Compared to peptide immunization, DNA immunization has the advantage of permitting generation of entire proteins, enabling determinant selection to occur in the host without having to restrict immunization to patients bearing specific HLA alleles. However, a safety concern about this technique is the potential for integration of the plasmid DNA into the host genome, possibly disrupting important genes and thereby leading to phenotypic mutations or carcinogenicity. A final approach to generate or enhance immune responses against specific antigens consists of infecting cells with recombinant viruses that encode the protein antigen of interest.

IMMUNE GLOBULIN. Passive immunization is indicated when an individual is deficient in antibodies because of a congenital or acquired immunodeficiency, when an individual with a high degree of risk is exposed to an agent and there is inadequate time for active immunization (e.g., measles, rabies, hepatitis B), or when a disease is already present but can be ameliorated by

Table 35–2

Selected Immune Globulin Preparations

GENERIC NAME	COMMON SYNONYMS	ORIGIN
Antithymocyte globulin	ATG	Rabbit
Botulism immune globulin intravenous	BIG-IV	Human
Cytomegalovirus immune globulin intravenous	CMV-IGIV	Human
Hepatitis B immune globulin	HBIG	Human
Immune globulin intramuscular	Gamma globulin, IgG, IGIM	Human
Immune globulin intravenous	IVIG	Human
Immune globulin subcutaneous	IGSC	Human
Lymphocyte immune globulin	ALG, antithymocyte globulin (equine), ATG (equine)	Equine
Rabies immune globulin	RIG	Human
Rho(D) immune globulin intramuscular	Rho[D] IGIM	Human
Rho(D) immune globulin intravenous	Rho[D] IGIV	Human
Rho(D) immune globulin microdose	Rho[D] IG microdose	Human
Tetanus immune globulin	TIG	Human
Vaccinia immune globulin intravenous	VIGIV	Human

passive antibodies (e.g., botulism, diphtheria, tetanus). Passive immunization may be provided by several different products (Table 35–2).

Nonspecific immunoglobulins or highly specific immunoglobulins may be provided based on the indication. The protection provided usually lasts 1-3 months. Immune globulin is derived from pooled plasma of adults by an alcohol-fractionation procedure. It contains largely IgG (95%) and is indicated for antibody-deficiency disorders, exposure to infections such as hepatitis A and measles, and specific immunological diseases such as immune thrombocytopenic purpura and Guillain-Barré syndrome. In contrast, specific immune globulins ("hyperimmune") differ from other immune globulin preparations in that donors are selected for high titers of the desired antibodies. Specific immune globulin preparations are available for hepatitis B, rabies, tetanus, varicella-zoster, cytomegalovirus, botulism, and respiratory syncytial virus. Rho(D) immune globulin is a specific hyperimmune globulin for prophylaxis against hemolytic disease of the newborn due to Rh incompatibility between mother and fetus. All such plasma-derived products carry the theoretical risk of transmission of infectious disease.

RHO(D) IMMUNE GLOBULIN. The commercial forms of Rho(D) immune globulin (*see* Table 35–2) consist of IgG containing a high titer of antibodies against the Rh(D) antigen on the surface of red blood cells. All donors are carefully screened to reduce the risk of transmitting infectious diseases. Fractionation of the plasma is performed by precipitation with cold alcohol followed by passage through a viral clearance system. Rho(D) immune globulin binds Rho antigens, preventing sensitization. Rh-negative women may be sensitized to the "foreign" Rh antigen on red blood cells via the fetus at the time of birth, miscarriage, ectopic pregnancy, or any transplacental hemorrhage. If the women go on to have a primary immune response, they will make antibodies to Rh antigen that can cross the placenta and damage subsequent fetuses by lysing red blood cells. This syndrome, called hemolytic disease of the newborn, is life threatening but is largely preventable by Rho(D) immune globulin. Rho(D) immune globulin is indicated whenever fetal red blood cells are suspected to have entered the circulation of an Rh-negative mother unless the fetus is known to be Rh negative. The drug is given intramuscularly. The $t_{1/2}$ of circulating immunoglobulin is ~21-29 days. Systemic reactions are extremely rare; myalgia, lethargy, and anaphylactic shock have been reported.

INTRAVENOUS IMMUNOGLOBULIN (IVIG). Indications for the use of IVIG have expanded beyond replacement therapy for agammaglobulinemia and other immunodeficiencies to include a variety of bacterial and viral infections, and an array of autoimmune and inflammatory diseases as diverse as thrombocytopenic purpura, Kawasaki disease, and autoimmune skin, neuromuscular, and neurological diseases. The mechanism of action of IVIG in immune modulation remains largely unknown.

IMMUNOTHERAPY FOR MULTIPLE SCLEROSIS

CLINICAL FEATURES AND PATHOLOGY. MS is a demyelinating inflammatory disease of the CNS white matter that displays a triad of pathogenic symptoms: mononuclear cell infiltration, demyelination, and scarring (gliosis). The peripheral nervous system is uninvolved. MS may be episodic or progressive, and occurs with prevalence increasing from late adolescence to 35 years of age and then declining. MS is roughly 3-fold more common in females than in males and occurs mainly in higher latitudes of the temperate climates. Epidemiologic studies suggest a role for environmental factors in the pathogenesis of MS; despite many suggestions, associations with infectious agents have proven inconclusive. A stronger linkage is the genetic one: people of northern European ancestry have a higher susceptibility to MS, and studies in twins and siblings suggest a strong genetic component.

MS is a complex genetic disease in which multiple allelic variants lead to disease susceptibility. HLA-DR2 clearly is associated with risk of developing MS. There also is substantial evidence of an autoimmune component to MS: In MS patients, there are activated T cells that are reactive to different myelin antigens, including myelin basic protein (MBP). In addition, there is evidence for the presence of auto-antibodies to myelin oligodendrocyte glycoprotein (MOG) and to MBP that can be eluted from the CNS plaque tissue. These antibodies may act with pathogenic T cells to produce some of the cellular pathology of MS. The neurophysiological result is altered conduction (both positive and negative) in myelinated fibers within the CNS (cerebral white matter, brain stem, cerebellar tracts, optic nerves, spinal cord); some alterations appear to result from exposure of voltage-dependent K^+ channels that normally are covered by myelin.

Attacks are classified by type and severity and likely correspond to specific degrees of CNS damage and pathological processes. Thus, physicians refer to relapsing-remitting MS (the form in 85% of younger patients), secondary progressive MS (progressive neurological deterioration following a long period of relapsing-remitting disease), and primary progressive MS (~15% of patients, wherein deterioration with relatively little inflammation is apparent at onset).

PHARMACOTHERAPY FOR MS. Table 35–3 summarizes current immunomodulatory therapies for MS. Specific therapies are aimed at resolving acute attacks, reducing recurrences and exacerbations, and slowing the progression of disability. Nonspecific therapies focus on maintaining function and quality of life. For acute attacks, pulse glucocorticoids often are employed (typically, 1 g/day of methylprednisolone administered intravenously for 3-5 days). For relapsing-remitting attacks, immunomodulatory therapies are approved: β-1 interferons [IFN-β-1a, IFN-β-1b], and glatiramer acetate (COPAXONE).

Random polymers that contain amino acids commonly used as MHC anchors and T cell–receptor contact residues have been proposed as possible "universal APLs (altered peptide ligands)." ***Glatiramer acetate*** (GA), a random-sequence polypeptide consisting of 4 amino acids [alanine (A), lysine (K), glutamate (E), and tyrosine (Y)] with an average length of 40-100 amino acids, binds efficiently to MHC class II DR molecules, but does not bind MHC class II DQ or MHC class I molecules in vitro. In clinical trials, GA, administered subcutaneously to patients with relapsing-remitting MS, decreased the rate of exacerbations by ~30%. In vivo administration of GA induces highly cross-reactive $CD4^+$ T cells that are immune deviated to secrete Th2 cytokines and prevents the appearance of new lesions detectable by magnetic resonance imaging. This represents one of the first successful uses of an agent that ameliorates autoimmune disease by altering signals through the T cell–receptor complex.

For relapsing-remitting attacks and for secondary progressive MS, the alkylating agent cyclophosphamide and **mitoxantrone** (NOVANTRONE, others) currently are used in patients refractory to other immunomodulators. These agents, primarily used for cancer chemotherapy, have significant toxicities (*see* Chapter 61). Mitoxantrone generally is tolerated only up to an accumulated dose of 100-140 mg/m^2. However, the FDA recommends that left ventricular ejection fraction (LVEF) be evaluated before initiating therapy, prior to each dose, and annually after patients have finished treatment to detect late-occurring cardiac toxicity.

The monoclonal antibody, **natalizumab** (TYSABRI), directed against the adhesion molecule α_4 integrin, antagonizes interactions with integrin heterodimers containing α_4 integrin, such as $\alpha_4\beta_1$ integrin that is expressed on the surface of activated lymphocytes and monocytes. An interaction of $\alpha_4\beta_1$ integrin with vascular-cellular adhesion molecule (VCAM)-1 seems critical for T-cell trafficking from the periphery into the CNS; blocking this interaction would hypothetically inhibit disease exacerbations. Use of natalizumab has been associated with the development of progressive multifocal leukoencephalopathy, and availability is limited to a special distribution program (TOUCH) administered by the manufacturer. Monoclonal antibodies directed against the IL-2 receptor and against CD52 (**alemtuzumab**; CAMPATH) are in phase III clinical trials.

Each of the agents mentioned has side effects and contraindications that may be limiting: infections (for glucocorticoids), hypersensitivity and pregnancy (for immunomodulators), and prior anthracycline/anthracenedione use, mediastinal irradiation, or cardiac disease (mitoxantrone). With all of these agents, the earlier they are used, the more effective they are in preventing disease relapses. What is not clear is whether any of these agents will prevent or diminish the later onset of secondary progressive disease, which causes the more severe disability.

Table 35–3

Pharmacotherapy of Multiple Sclerosis

THERAPEUTIC AGENT	BRAND NAME (Regimen)	INDICATIONS	RESULTS	MECHANISM OF ACTION
IFN-β-1a	AVONEX (30 μg, IM, weekly) REBIFF (22 or 44 μg, SC, 3 ×/week)	Treatment of RRMS	↓ relapses by 33% ↓ new MRI T2 lesions and volume of enlarging T2 lesions ↓ number and volume of Gd-enhancing lesions Slowing of brain atrophy	Acts on BBB to interfere with T-cell adhesion to the endothelium (binds VLA-4 on T cells or inhibits T-cell expression of MMP) ↓ T cell activation by interfering with HLA class II and co-stimulators B7/CD28 and CD40:CD40L Immune deviation of Th2 over Th1 cytokine profile
IFN-β-1b	BETASERON (0.25 mg, SC, every other day after 6-week titration)	Treatment of RRMS	Same as IFN-β-1a, above	Same as IFN-β-1a, above
Glatiramer acetate	COPAXONE (20 mg, SC, daily)	Treatment of RRMS	↓ relapses by 33% ↓ number and volume of Gd-enhancing lesions	Induces T-helper type 2 cells that enter the CNS; mediates bystander suppression at sites of inflammation
Mitoxantrone	NOVANTRONE, generic (12 mg/m^2, as 5-15 min IV infusion every 90 days)	Worsening forms of RRMS SPMS	↓ relapses by 67% Slows progression on EDSS, ambulation index, and MRI disease activity	Intercalates DNA (*see* Chapter 61) ↓ cellular and humoral immune response

BBB, blood-brain barrier; EDSS, Expanded Disability Status Scale, a neurologic assessment scale; Gd, gadolinium, used in Gd-enhanced MRI to assess the number and size of inflammatory brain lesions; IFN, interferon; IM, intramuscular; IV, intravenous; MMP, matrix metalloprotease; MS, multiple sclerosis; RRMS, relapsing-remitting MS; SC, subcutaneous; SPMS, secondary progressive MS; MRI, magnetic resonance imaging; ↓, reduction.

For a complete Bibliographical Listing see Goodman & Gilman's ***The Pharmacological Basis of Therapeutics***, 12th ed., or Goodman & Gilman Online at www.AccessMedicine.com.

Pulmonary Pharmacology

This chapter discusses the pharmacotherapy of obstructive airways disease, particularly bronchodilators, which act mainly by reversing airway smooth muscle contraction, and anti-inflammatory drugs, which suppress the inflammatory response in the airways. The chapter focuses on the pulmonary pharmacology of β_2 agonists and corticosteroids; their basic pharmacology is presented elsewhere (*see* Chapters 12 and 42). This chapter also discusses other drugs used to treat obstructive airway diseases, such as mucolytics and respiratory stimulants, and covers the drug therapy of cough, the most common respiratory symptom, as well as drugs used to treat pulmonary hypertension. Drugs used in the treatment of lung infections, including tuberculosis (*see* Chapter 56), are covered elsewhere.

MECHANISMS OF ASTHMA

Asthma is a chronic inflammatory disease of the airways that is characterized by activation of *mast cells* (generally present in increased numbers), infiltration of *eosinophils*, and *T helper 2 (T_H2) lymphocytes* (Figure 36–1). Mast cell activation by allergens and physical stimuli releases bronchoconstrictor mediators, such as histamine, leukotriene D_4, and PGD_2, which cause bronchoconstriction, microvascular leakage, and plasma exudation (*see* Chapters 32 and 33). Many of the symptoms of asthma are due to airway smooth muscle contraction; thus, bronchodilators are important as symptom relievers. Whether airway smooth muscle is intrinsically abnormal in asthma is not clear, but increased contractility of airway smooth muscle may contribute to airway hyperresponsiveness, the physiological hallmark of asthma. The mechanism of chronic inflammation in asthma is still not well understood. It may initially be driven by allergen exposure, but it appears to become autonomous so that asthma is essentially incurable. The inflammation may be orchestrated by dendritic cells that regulate T_H2 cells that drive eosinophilic inflammation and IgE formation by B lymphocytes. Airway epithelium plays an important role through the release of myriad inflammatory mediators and through the release of growth factors in an attempt to repair the damage caused by inflammation.

Chronic inflammation may lead to structural changes in the airways, including an increase in the number and size of airway smooth muscle cells, blood vessels, and mucus-secreting cells. A characteristic histological feature of asthma is collagen deposition (fibrosis) below the basement membrane of the airway epithelium (*see* Figure 36–1).

MECHANISMS OF COPD

COPD involves inflammation of the respiratory tract with a pattern that differs from that of asthma. In COPD, there is a predominance of *neutrophils, macrophages*, and *cytotoxic T-lymphocytes* (Tc1 cells). The inflammation predominantly affects *small airways*, resulting in progressive small airway narrowing and fibrosis (chronic obstructive bronchiolitis) and destruction of the lung parenchyma with destruction of the alveolar walls (emphysema) (Figure 36–2). These pathological changes result in airway closure on expiration, leading to air trapping and hyperinflation, particularly on exercise. This accounts for shortness of breath on exertion and exercise limitation that are characteristic symptoms of COPD.

Bronchodilators reduce air trapping by dilating peripheral airways and are the mainstay of treatment in COPD. In contrast to asthma, the airflow obstruction of COPD tends to be progressive. A discrete pattern of inflammatory mediators and cytokines mediates the inflammation in the peripheral lung of COPD patients. In contrast to asthma, the inflammation of COPD is largely corticosteroid-resistant, and there are currently no effective anti-inflammatory treatments. Many patients with COPD have systemic manifestations (skeletal muscle wasting, weight loss, depression, osteoporosis, anemia) and comorbid diseases (ischemic heart disease, hypertension, congestive heart failure, diabetes). Whether these are due to spillover of inflammatory mediators from

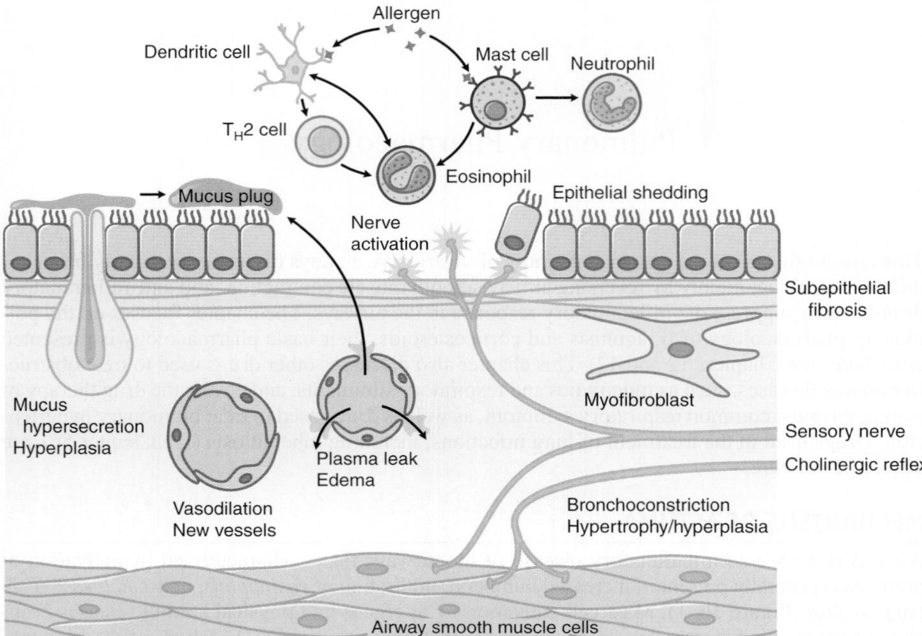

Figure 36–1 *Cellular mechanisms of asthma.* Myriad inflammatory cells are recruited and activated in the airways, where they release multiple inflammatory mediators, which can also arise from structural cells. These mediators lead to bronchoconstriction, plasma exudation and edema, vasodilation, mucus hypersecretion, and activation of sensory nerves. Chronic inflammation leads to structural changes, including subepithelial fibrosis (basement membrane thickening), airway smooth muscle hypertrophy and hyperplasia, angiogenesis, and hyperplasia of mucus-secreting cells.

the lung or due to common causal mechanisms (such as smoking) is not yet clear, but it may be important to treat the systemic components in the overall management of COPD.

ROUTES OF DRUG DELIVERY TO THE LUNGS

INHALED ROUTE

Inhalation (Figure 36–3) is the preferred mode of delivery of many drugs with a direct effect on airways, particularly for asthma and COPD. The major advantage of inhalation is the delivery of drug to the airways in doses that are effective with a much lower risk of systemic side effects. This is particularly important with the use of inhaled corticosteroids (ICS), which largely avoids systemic side effects. In addition, inhaled bronchodilators have a more rapid onset of action than when taken orally.

PARTICLE SIZE. The size of particles for inhalation is of critical importance in determining the site of deposition in the respiratory tract. The optimum size for particles to settle in the airways is 2-5 μm mass median aerodynamic diameter (MMAD). Larger particles settle out in the upper airways, whereas smaller particles remain suspended and are therefore exhaled. There is increasing interest in delivering drugs to small airways, particularly in COPD and severe asthma. This involves delivering drug particles of ~1 μm MMAD, which is now possible using drugs formulated in hydrofluoroalkane (HFA) propellant.

PHARMACOKINETICS. Of the total drug delivered, only 10-20% enters the lower airways with a conventional pressurized metered-dose inhaler. Drugs are absorbed from the airway lumen and have direct effects on target cells of the airway. Drugs may also be absorbed into the bronchial circulation and then distributed to more peripheral airways. Drugs with higher molecular weights tend to be retained to a greater extent in the airways. Nevertheless, several drugs have greater therapeutic efficacy when given by the inhaled route. More extensive pulmonary distribution of a drug with a smaller MMAD increases alveolar deposition and thus is likely to increase absorption from the lungs into the general circulation resulting in more systemic side effects.

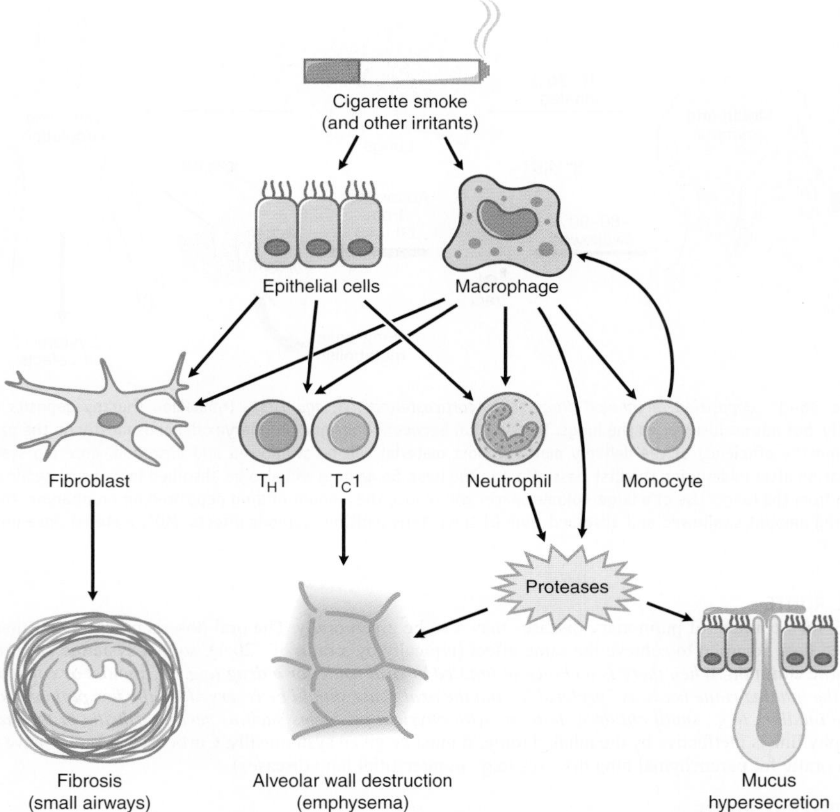

Figure 36–2 *Cellular mechanisms in chronic obstructive pulmonary disease.* Cigarette smoke and other irritants activate epithelial cells and macrophages in the lung to release mediators that attract circulating inflammatory cells, including monocytes (which differentiate to macrophages within the lung), neutrophils, and T lymphocytes (T_H1 and T_C1 cells). Fibrogenic factors released from epithelial cells and macrophages lead to fibrosis of small airways. Release of proteases results in alveolar wall destruction (emphysema) and mucus hypersecretion (chronic bronchitis).

DELIVERY DEVICES

Pressurized Metered-Dose Inhalers (pMDIs). Drugs are propelled from a canister with the aid of a propellant, previously with a chlorofluorocarbon (Freon) but now replaced by an *HFA* that is "ozone friendly." These devices are convenient, portable, and typically deliver 100-400 doses of drug.

Spacer Chambers. Large-volume spacer devices between the pMDI and the patient reduce the velocity of particles entering the upper airways and the size of the particles by allowing evaporation of liquid propellant. This reduces the amount of drug that impinges on the oropharynx and gets swallowed, and increases the proportion of drug inhaled into the lower airways. Application of spacer chambers is useful in the reduction of the oropharyngeal deposition of ICS and the consequent reduction in the local and systemic side effects of these drugs. Spacer devices are also useful in delivering inhaled drugs to small children who are not able to use a pMDI.

Dry Powder Inhalers. Drugs may also be delivered as a dry powder using devices that scatter a fine powder dispersed by air turbulence on inhalation. Children <7 years of age find it difficult to use a dry powder inhaler (DPI). DPIs have been developed to deliver peptides and proteins, such as insulin (e.g., EXUBERA, AFRESA), systemically.

Nebulizers. Two types of nebulizer are available. *Jet nebulizers* are driven by a stream of gas (air or oxygen), whereas *ultrasonic nebulizers* use a rapidly vibrating piezo-electric crystal and thus do not require a source of compressed gas. The nebulized drug is inspired during tidal breathing, and it is possible to deliver much higher doses of drug compared with pMDI. Nebulizers are useful in treating acute exacerbations of asthma and COPD, for delivering inhaled drugs to infants and small children, and for giving drugs such as antibiotics when relatively high doses must be delivered.

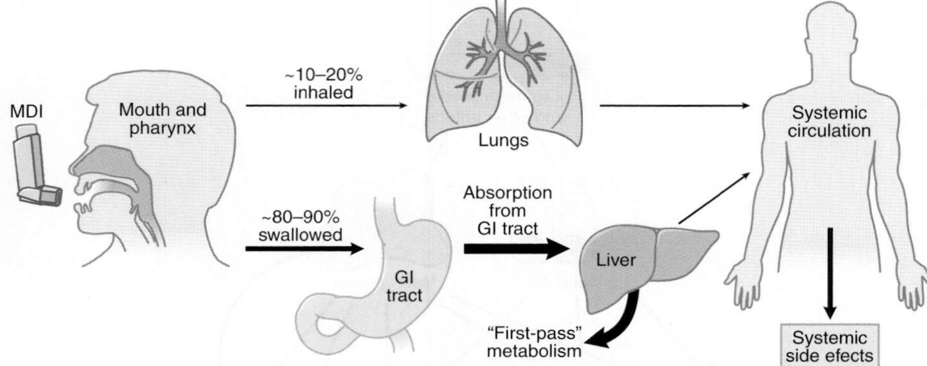

Figure 36–3 *Deposition of inhaled drugs (e.g., corticosteroids, β_2 agonists).* Inhalation therapy deposits drugs directly, but not exclusively, in the lungs. Distribution between lungs and oropharynx depends mostly on the particle size and the efficiency of the delivery method. Most material will be swallowed and absorbed, entering systemic circulation after undergoing the first-pass effect in the liver. Some drug will also be absorbed into the systemic circulation from the lungs. Use of a large-volume spacer will reduce the amount of drug deposited on oropharynx, thereby reducing amount swallowed and absorbed from GI tract, thus limiting systemic effects. MDI, metered-dose inhaler.

ORAL ROUTE

Drugs for treatment of pulmonary diseases may also be given orally. The oral dose is much higher than the inhaled dose required to achieve the same effect (typically by a ratio of ~20:1), so that systemic side effects are more common. *When there is a choice of inhaled or oral route for a drug (e.g., β_2 agonist or corticosteroid), the inhaled route is always preferable, and the oral route should be reserved for the few patients unable to use inhalers (e.g., small children, patients with physical problems such as severe arthritis of the hands).* Theophylline is ineffective by the inhaled route; it must be given systemically. Corticosteroids may have to be given orally for parenchymal lung diseases (e.g., in interstitial lung diseases).

PARENTERAL ROUTE

The intravenous route should be reserved for delivery of drugs in the severely ill patient who is unable to absorb drugs from the GI tract. Side effects are generally frequent due to the high plasma concentrations.

BRONCHODILATORS

Bronchodilator drugs relax constricted airway smooth muscle in vitro and cause immediate reversal of airway obstruction in asthma in vivo. They also prevent bronchoconstriction (and thereby provide bronchoprotection). Three main classes of bronchodilator are in current clinical use:

- *β_2 Adrenergic agonists (sympathomimetics)*
- *Theophylline (a methylxanthine)*
- *Anticholinergic agents (muscarinic receptor antagonists)*

Drugs such as cromolyn sodium, which prevent bronchoconstriction, have no direct bronchodilator action and are ineffective once bronchoconstriction has occurred. Anti-leukotrienes (leukotriene receptor antagonists and 5′-lipoxygenase inhibitors) have a small bronchodilator effect in some asthmatic patients and appear to prevent bronchoconstriction. Corticosteroids, although gradually improving airway obstruction, have no direct effect on contraction of airway smooth muscle and are not therefore considered to be bronchodilators.

β_2 ADRENERGIC AGONISTS

Inhaled β_2 agonists are the bronchodilator treatment of choice in asthma because they are the most effective bronchodilators and have minimal side effects when used correctly. The basic pharmacology of these agents (albuterol, terbutaline, salmeterol, formoterol, indacaterol, and related compounds) is presented in Chapters 8 and 12.

MODE OF ACTION

Agonist stimulation of β_2 receptors in airway smooth muscle results in the activation of the G_s-adenylyl cyclase-cAMP-PKA pathway and consequent phosphorylative events leading to

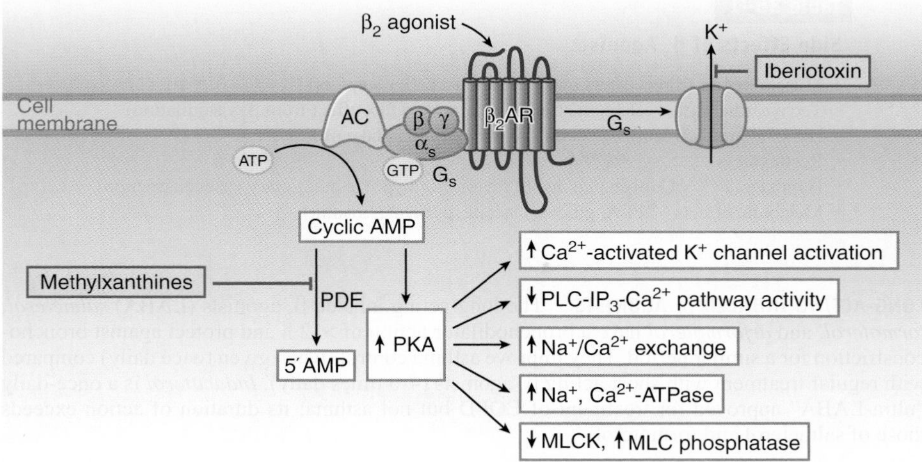

Figure 36–4 *Molecular actions of β_2 agonists to induce relaxation of airway smooth muscle cells.* A rise in $[Ca^{2+}]_i$ initiates contraction by activating myosin light-chain kinase (MLCK), thereby enhancing the level of phosphorylation of myosin light chains and increasing the contractile interaction of actin and myosin. Stimulation of β_2 receptors activates cyclic AMP-PKA pathway and reverses the contractile process by reducing $[Ca^{2+}]_i$, reducing MLCK activation, and promoting dephosphorylation of light chains. PKA phosphorylates a variety of target substrates, resulting in: opening of Ca^{2+}-activated K^+ channels (K_{Ca}) [which facilitates hyperpolarization], decreased phosphoinositide (PI) hydrolysis, increased Na^+/Ca^{2+} exchange, increased Na^+,Ca^{2+}-ATPase activity, decreased MLCK activity, and increased MLC phosphatase activity. β_2 Receptors may also couple to K_{Ca} via G_s. PDE, cyclic nucleotide phosphodiesterase.

bronchial smooth muscle relaxation (Figure 36–4), effectively reversing the Ca^{2+}-stimulated events that initiate contraction.

β_2 agonists may cause bronchodilation in vivo not only via a direct action on airways smooth muscle, but also *indirectly* by inhibiting the release of bronchoconstrictor mediators from inflammatory cells and of bronchoconstrictor neurotransmitters from airway nerves. These mechanisms include:

- Prevention of mediator release from isolated human lung mast cells (via β_2 receptors)
- Prevention of microvascular leakage and thus the development of bronchial mucosal edema after exposure to mediators, such as histamine and leukotriene D_4
- Increase in *mucus secretion* from submucosal glands and *ion transport* across airway epithelium (may enhance mucociliary clearance, reversing defective clearance found in asthma)
- Reduction in *neurotransmission* in human airway cholinergic nerves by an action at presynaptic β_2 receptors to inhibit acetylcholine release

β_2 agonists do not appear to have a significant inhibitory effect on the *chronic* inflammation of asthmatic airways, which is suppressed by corticosteroids. This may be related to the fact that effects of β_2 agonists on macrophages, eosinophils, and lymphocytes are rapidly desensitized.

CLINICAL USE

SHORT-ACTING β_2 AGONISTS. Inhaled short-acting β_2 agonists are the most widely used and effective bronchodilators in the treatment of asthma due to their functional antagonism of bronchoconstriction. These agents also are effective in protecting against various challenges, such as exercise, cold air, and allergens. Inhalation is preferable to the oral administration because inhalation may be more effective and systemic side effects are less. *Short-acting inhaled β_2 agonists, such as albuterol, should be used "as required" by symptoms and not on a regular basis in the treatment of mild asthma; increased use indicates the need for more anti-*inflammatory *therapy.*

Slow-release preparations (e.g., slow-release albuterol and bambuterol) may be indicated in nocturnal asthma; however, these agents have an increased risk of side effects. All short-acting β_2 agonists currently available are usable by inhalation and orally, have a similar duration of action (~3-4 h; less in severe asthma), and similar side effects. Drugs in clinical use include *albuterol (salbutamol)*, *levalbuterol*, *metaproterenol*, *terbutaline* (in the U.S.), *fenoterol*, *tulobuterol*, *rimiterol*, and *pirbuterol* (in other countries).

Table 36–1

Side Effects of β_2 Agonists

- Muscle tremor (direct effect on skeletal muscle β_2 receptors)
- Tachycardia (direct effect on atrial β_2 receptors, reflex effect from β_2 vasodilation)
- Hypokalemia (direct β_2 effect on skeletal muscle uptake of K^+)
- Restlessness
- Hypoxemia (↑ $\dot{V}/\dot{Q}$ mismatch due to reversal of hypoxic pulmonary vasoconstriction)
- Metabolic effects (↑ FFA, glucose, lactate, pyruvate, insulin)

LONG-ACTING INHALED β_2 AGONISTS. The long-acting inhaled β_2 agonists (LABA) *salmeterol*, *formoterol*, and *arformoterol* have a bronchodilator action of >12 h and protect against bronchoconstriction for a similar period. They improve asthma control (when given twice daily) compared with regular treatment with short-acting β_2 agonists (4-6 times daily). *Indacaterol* is a once-daily "ultra-LABA" approved for treatment of COPD but not asthma; its duration of action exceeds those of salmeterol and formoterol.

In COPD, LABA are effective bronchodilators that may be used alone or in combination with anticholinergics or ICS. LABA improve symptoms and exercise tolerance by reducing both air trapping and exacerbations. In asthma patients, LABA should never be used alone because they do not treat the underlying chronic inflammation; rather, LABA should always be used in combination with ICS (preferably in a fixed-dose combination inhaler). LABA are an effective add-on therapy to ICS and are more effective than increasing the dose of ICS when asthma is not controlled at low doses. Tolerance to the bronchodilator effect of formoterol and the bronchoprotective effects of formoterol and salmeterol has been demonstrated but is of doubtful clinical significance. No significant clinical differences between salmeterol and formoterol have been found in the treatment of patients with severe asthma.

COMBINATION INHALERS. Combination inhalers that contain a LABA and a corticosteroid (e.g., fluticasone/salmeterol [ADVAIR], budesonide/formoterol [SYMBICORT]) are now widely used in the treatment of asthma and COPD. Combining LABA with a corticosteroid offers complementary synergistic actions. The combination inhaler is more convenient for patients, simplifies therapy, and improves compliance. These combination inhalers are also more effective in COPD patients than LABA and ICS alone.

SIDE EFFECTS. Unwanted effects are dose related and due to stimulation of extrapulmonary β receptors (Table 36–1 and Chapter 12). Side effects are not common with inhaled therapy but quite common with oral or intravenous administration, usually only after large systemic doses. Short-acting inhaled β_2 agonists should only be used on demand for symptom control, and with an ICS if they are required more than 3 times weekly. LABA should only be used when ICS are also prescribed. All LABA approved in the U.S. carry a black box warning cautioning against overuse. There are less safety concerns with LABA use in COPD.

METHYLXANTHINES

The methylxanthine, theophylline, is still widely used in developing countries because it is inexpensive. However, the frequency of side effects and the relative low efficacy of theophylline have led to reduced use because inhaled β_2 agonists are far more effective as bronchodilators and ICS have a greater anti-inflammatory effect. In patients with severe asthma and COPD, theophylline remains a very useful drug.

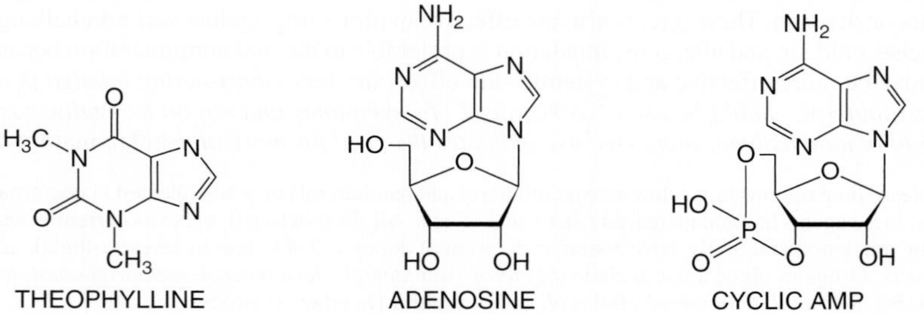

THEOPHYLLINE

ADENOSINE

CYCLIC AMP

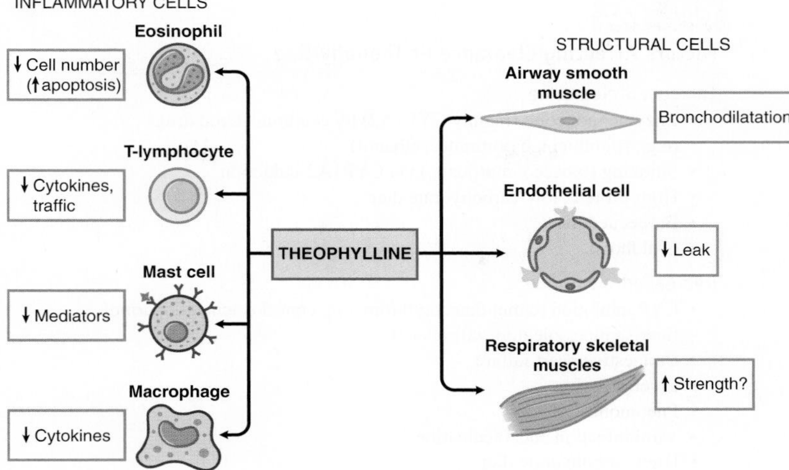

Figure 36–5 *Theophylline affects multiple cell types in the airway.*

MECHANISM OF ACTION. The mechanisms of action of theophylline are still uncertain. In addition to its bronchodilator action, theophylline has many nonbronchodilator effects that may be relevant to its effects in asthma and COPD (Figure 36–5). Several molecular mechanisms of action have been proposed:

- *Inhibition of cyclic nucleotide phosphodiesterases.* Theophylline is a nonselective PDE inhibitor. PDE inhibition and the concomitant elevation of cellular cyclic AMP and cyclic GMP likely account for the bronchodilator action of theophylline (*see* Figure 36–4). The PDE isoenzymes recognized in smooth muscle relaxation include PDE3, PDE4, and PDE5.
- *Adenosine receptor antagonism.* Theophylline antagonizes adenosine receptors at therapeutic concentrations. Adenosine causes bronchoconstriction in airways from asthmatic patients by releasing histamine and leukotrienes. Antagonism of A_1 receptors may be responsible for serious side effects, including cardiac arrhythmias and seizures.
- *Interleukin-10 release.* IL-10 has a broad spectrum of anti-inflammatory effects, and there is evidence that its secretion is reduced in asthma. IL-10 release is increased by theophylline, and this effect may be mediated via inhibition of PDE activities.
- *Effects on gene transcription.* Theophylline prevents the translocation of the pro-inflammatory transcription factor NF-κB into the nucleus, potentially reducing the expression of inflammatory genes in asthma and COPD. However, these effects are seen at high concentrations and may be mediated by inhibition of PDE.
- *Effects on apoptosis.* Prolonged survival of granulocytes due to a reduction in apoptosis may be important in perpetuating chronic inflammation in asthma (eosinophils) and COPD (neutrophils). Theophylline promotes apoptosis in eosinophils and neutrophils in vitro. This effect may be mediated by antagonism of adenosine A_{2A} receptors. Theophylline also induces apoptosis in T lymphocytes via PDE inhibition.
- *Histone deacetylase activation.* Recruitment of histone deacetylase-2 (HDAC2) by glucocorticoid receptors switches off inflammatory genes. Therapeutic concentrations of theophylline activate HDAC, thereby enhancing the anti-inflammatory effects of corticosteroids. This mechanism appears to be mediated by inhibition of PI3-kinase-δ, which is activated by oxidative stress.

NONBRONCHODILATOR EFFECTS. There is increasing evidence that theophylline has anti-inflammatory effects in asthma. For example, chronic oral treatment with theophylline inhibits the late response to inhaled allergen and reduces infiltration of eosinophils and $CD4^+$ lymphocytes into the airways after allergen challenge. In patients with COPD, theophylline reduces the total number and proportion of neutrophils in induced sputum, the concentration of IL-8, and neutrophil chemotactic responses. Theophylline withdrawal in COPD patients results in worsening of disease. In vitro theophylline is able to increase responsiveness to corticosteroids and to reverse corticosteroid resistance in cells from COPD subjects.

Table 36–2

Factors Affecting Clearance of Theophylline

Increased clearance

- Enzyme induction (mainly CYP1A2) by coadministered drugs (e.g., rifampicin, barbiturates, ethanol)
- Smoking (tobacco, marijuana) via CYP1A2 induction
- High-protein, low-carbohydrate diet
- Barbecued meat
- Childhood

Decreased clearance

- CYP inhibition (cimetidine, erythromycin, ciprofloxacin, allopurinol, fluvoxamine, zileuton, zafirlukast)
- Congestive heart failure
- Liver disease
- Pneumonia
- Viral infection and vaccination
- High-carbohydrate diet
- Old age

PHARMACOKINETICS AND METABOLISM. Theophylline has anti-asthma effects other than bronchodilation below 10 mg/L, so the therapeutic range is now taken as 5-15 mg/L. The dose of theophylline required to give these therapeutic concentrations varies among subjects, largely because of differences in clearance of the drug. In addition, there may be differences in bronchodilator response to theophylline; furthermore, with acute bronchoconstriction, higher concentrations may be required to produce bronchodilation. Theophylline is rapidly and completely absorbed, but there are large interindividual variations in clearance, due to differences in hepatic metabolism. Theophylline is metabolized in the liver, mainly by CYP1A2; myriad factors influence metabolism and clearance of theophylline (Table 36–2). Because of these variations in clearance, individualization of theophylline dosage is required and plasma concentrations should be measured 4 h after the last dose with slow-release preparations when steady state has been achieved.

PREPARATIONS AND ROUTES OF ADMINISTRATION. *Intravenous* aminophylline (the ethylenediamine salt of theophylline, with better solubility at neutral pH) is used in the treatment of acute severe asthma, at a recommended dose of 6 mg/kg over 20-30 min, followed by a maintenance dose of 0.5 mg/kg/h. If the patient is already taking theophylline, or has decreased clearance, these doses should be halved and the plasma level checked more frequently. *Oral* immediate-release theophylline tablets or elixir, which are rapidly absorbed, give wide fluctuations in plasma levels, and are not recommended. Sustained-release preparations provide steady plasma concentrations over a 12- to 24-h period. Both slow-release aminophylline and theophylline are equally effective. For continuous treatment twice daily therapy (~8 mg/kg twice daily) is needed.

CLINICAL USE. In patients with acute asthma, intravenous aminophylline is less effective than nebulized β_2 agonists and should therefore be reserved for those patients who fail to respond to, or are intolerant of, β agonists. Addition of low-dose theophylline to either a high or low dose of ICS in patients who are not adequately controlled provides better symptom control and lung function than doubling the dose of inhaled steroid. Although theophylline is less effective than a β_2 agonist and corticosteroids, a minority of asthmatic patients appears to derive unexpected benefit; even patients on oral steroids may show a deterioration in lung function when theophylline is withdrawn. Although LABA are more effective as an add-on therapy, theophylline is considerably less expensive when the costs of medication are limiting.

Theophylline is still used as a bronchodilator in COPD, but inhaled anticholinergics and β_2 agonists are preferred. Theophylline tends to be added to these inhaled bronchodilators in more severe patients and has been shown to give additional clinical improvement when added to a long-acting β_2 agonist.

SIDE EFFECTS. Unwanted effects of theophylline are usually related to plasma concentration and tend to occur at $C_p > 15$ mg/L. The most common side effects are headache, nausea, and vomiting, abdominal discomfort, and restlessness (Table 36–3). There may also be increased acid secretion and diuresis. Theophylline may lead to behavioral disturbance and learning difficulties in schoolchildren. At high concentrations, cardiac arrhythmias and seizures may occur. Using low doses of theophylline to achieve plasma concentrations of 5-10 mg/L largely avoids side effects and drug interactions.

Table 36–3

Side Effects of Theophylline and Mechanisms

SIDE EFFECT	PROPOSED MECHANISM
Nausea and vomiting	PDE4 inhibition
Headaches	PDE4 inhibition
Gastric discomfort	PDE4 inhibition
Diuresis	Adenosine A_1 receptor antagonism
Behavioral disturbance (?)	?
Cardiac arrhythmias	PDE3 inhibition, A_1 receptor antagonism
Epileptic seizures	Adenosine A_1 receptor antagonism

MUSCARINIC CHOLINERGIC ANTAGONISTS

MODE OF ACTION

As competitive antagonists of endogenous ACh at muscarinic receptors, these agents inhibit the direct constrictor effect on bronchial smooth muscle mediated via the M_3-G_q-PLC-IP_3-Ca^{2+} pathway (*see* Chapters 3 and 9). Their efficacy stems from the role of the parasympathetic nervous system in regulating bronchomotor tone. The effects of ACh on the respiratory system include not only bronchoconstriction but also increased tracheobronchial secretion and stimulation of the chemoreceptors of the carotid and aortic bodies. However, the myriad inflammatory mediators involved in the pathogenesis of asthma and COPD may also induce components of muscarinic responsiveness, such as $G\alpha_q$ and rho, and contribute to hyperresponsiveness of the airway. Thus, the contractility of bronchial smooth muscle and antagonism of muscarinic responsiveness could be moving targets in asthma and COPD.

CLINICAL USE. In asthmatic patients, anticholinergic drugs are less effective as bronchodilators than β_2 agonists and offer less efficient protection against bronchial challenges. Anticholinergics are currently used as an additional bronchodilator in asthmatic patients not controlled on an LABA. In the acute and chronic treatment of asthma, anticholinergic drugs may have an additive effect with β_2 agonists and should be considered when control of asthma is not adequate with nebulized β_2 agonists. In COPD, anticholinergic drugs may be as effective as or even superior to β_2 agonists. Their relatively greater effect in COPD than in asthma may be explained by an inhibitory effect on vagal tone (Figure 36–6).

THERAPEUTIC CHOICES. *Ipratropium bromide* (ATROVENT, others) is available as a pMDI and nebulized preparation. The onset of bronchodilation is relatively slow and is usually maximal 30-60 min after inhalation, but may persist for 6-8 h. It is usually given by MDI 3 to 4 times daily on a regular basis, rather than intermittently for symptom relief, in view of its slow onset of action. *Oxitropium bromide* (not available in the U.S.) is a quaternary anticholinergic bronchodilator that is similar to ipratropium bromide. It is available in higher doses by inhalation and may therefore have a more prolonged effect.

Combination inhalers of an anticholinergic and β_2 agonist, such as ipratropium/albuterol (COMBIVENT, DUONEB, others), are popular, particularly among patients with COPD. The additive effects of these 2 drugs may provide an advantage over increasing the dose of β_2 agonist in patients who have side effects.

Tiotropium bromide is a long-acting anticholinergic drug that is suitable for once-daily dosing as a DPI (SPIRIVA) or via a soft mist mini-nebulizer device (not available in the U.S.). Tiotropium binds to all muscarinic receptor subtypes but dissociates very slowly from M_3 and M_1 receptors, giving it a degree of kinetic receptor selectivity for these receptors compared with M_2 receptors, from which it dissociates more rapidly. Thus, compared with ipratropium, tiotropium is less likely to antagonize M_2-mediated inhibition of ACh release. It is an effective bronchodilator in patients with COPD and is more effective than ipratropium 4 times daily without any loss of efficacy over a 1-year treatment period. Over a 4-year period, tiotropium improves lung function and health status and reduces exacerbations and all-cause mortality, although there is no effect on disease progression. As a result, tiotropium is becoming the bronchodilator of choice for COPD patients.

Aclidinium bromide (TUDORZA Pressair) is a long-acting, anticholinergic inhalation powder approved for long-term maintenance treatment of COPD.

ADVERSE EFFECTS. Systemic side effects after ipratropium bromide and tiotropium bromide are uncommon because there is little systemic absorption. A significant unwanted effect is the unpleasant *bitter taste* of inhaled

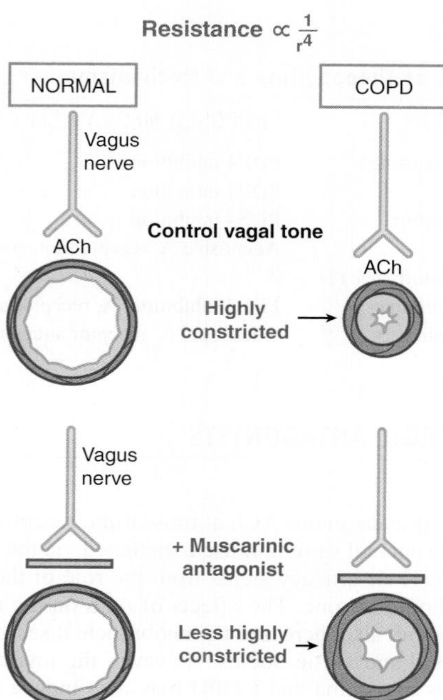

Figure 36–6 *Anticholinergic drugs inhibit vagally mediated airway tone, thereby producing bronchodilation.* This effect is small in normal airways but is greater in airways of patients with chronic obstructive pulmonary disease (COPD), which are structurally narrowed and have higher resistance to airflow because airway resistance is inversely related to the fourth power of the radius (r). ACh, acetylcholine.

ipratropium, which may reduce compliance. Nebulized ipratropium bromide may precipitate *glaucoma* in elderly patients due to a direct effect of the nebulized drug on the eye. This may be prevented by nebulization with a mouthpiece rather than a face mask. Occasionally, bronchoconstriction may occur with ipratropium bromide given by MDI. Tiotropium causes dryness of the mouth in 10-15% of patients, but this usually disappears during continued therapy. Urinary retention is occasionally seen in elderly patients.

CORTICOSTEROIDS

The introduction of ICS, has revolutionized the treatment of chronic asthma. Because asthma is a chronic inflammatory disease, ICS are considered as first-line therapy in all but the mildest of patients. In marked contrast, ICS are much less effective in COPD and should only be used in patients with severe disease who have frequent exacerbations. Oral corticosteroids remain the mainstay of treatment of several other pulmonary diseases, such as sarcoidosis, interstitial lung diseases, and pulmonary eosinophilic syndromes (*see* Chapter 42).

MECHANISM OF ACTION. Probably the most important action of ICS in suppressing asthmatic inflammation is the inhibition of expression of multiple inflammatory genes in airway epithelial cells. Corticosteroids reverse the activating effect of pro-inflammatory transcription factors on histone acetylation by recruiting HDAC2 to inflammatory genes that have been activated through acetylation of associated histones (see molecular details in Figure 36–7). Steroids have inhibitory effects on many inflammatory and structural cells that are activated in asthma and prevent the recruitment of inflammatory cells into the airways (Figure 36–8). Steroids potently inhibit the formation of cytokines (e.g., IL-1, IL-3, IL-4, IL-5, IL-9, IL-13, TNF-α, and granulocyte-macrophage colony-stimulating factor, GM-CSF) that are secreted in asthma by T-lymphocytes, macrophages, and mast cells.

Corticosteroids have no direct effect on contractile responses of airway smooth muscle; improvement in lung function after ICS is presumably due to an effect on the chronic airway inflammation and airway hyperresponsiveness. A single dose of ICS has no effect on the early response to allergen (reflecting their lack of effect on mast cell mediator release) but inhibits the late response (which may be due to an effect on macrophages, eosinophils, and airway wall edema) and also inhibits the increase in airway hyperresponsiveness.

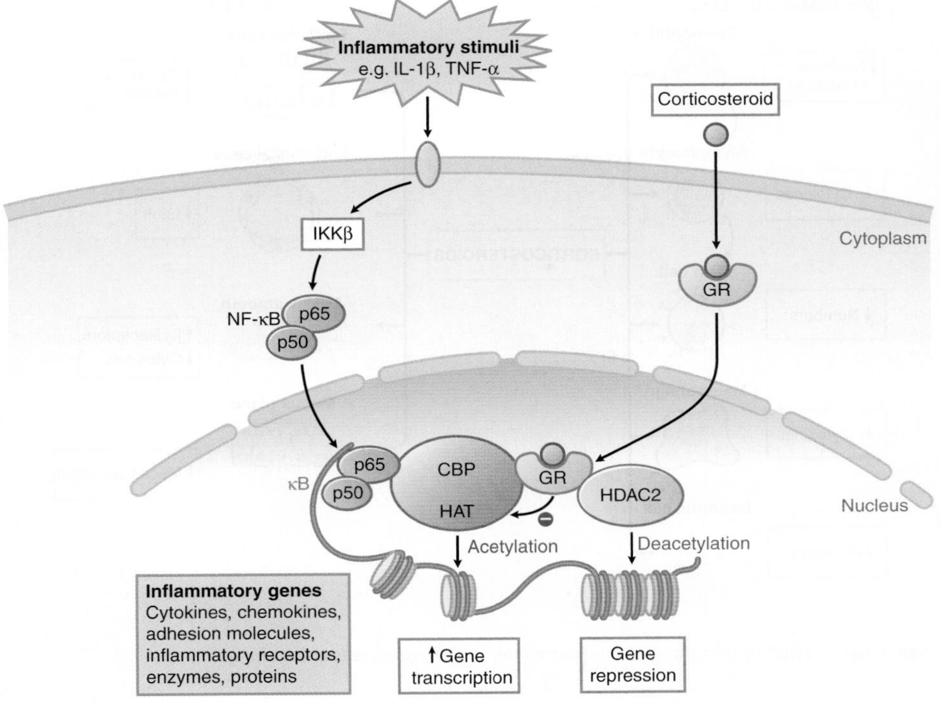

Figure 36–7 *Mechanism of anti-inflammatory action of corticosteroids in asthma.* Inflammatory stimuli activate the NF-κB pathway, leading to increased histone acetyltransferase (HAT) activity, resulting in acetylation of core histones and increased expression of genes encoding multiple inflammatory proteins. Corticosteroids, acting via cytosolic glucocorticoid receptors (GR), antagonize HAT activity in two ways: directly and, more importantly, by recruiting histone deacetylase-2 (HDAC2), which reverses histone acetylation, leading to the suppression of activated inflammatory genes. CBP, CREB binding protein.

Corticosteroids *suppress* inflammation in the airways but do not cure the underlying disease. When steroids are withdrawn, there is a recurrence of the same degree of airway hyperresponsiveness, although in patients with mild asthma it may take several months to return.

RECIPROCAL SYNERGISTIC EFFECTS OF β_2 AGONISTS AND CORTICOSTEROIDS. Steroids potentiate the effects of β agonists on bronchial smooth muscle and prevent and reverse β receptor desensitization in airways. At a molecular level, corticosteroids increase the transcription of the β_2 receptor gene in human lung in vitro and in the respiratory mucosa in vivo and increase the stability of its messenger RNA. They also prevent or reverse uncoupling of β_2 receptors from G_s. In animal systems, corticosteroids prevent downregulation of β_2 receptors. β_2 Agonists also increase the association of liganded glucocorticoid receptors (GR) with DNA, an effect demonstrated in sputum macrophages of asthmatic patients after an ICS and inhaled LABA, suggesting that β_2 agonists and corticosteroids enhance each other's beneficial effects in asthma therapy.

PHARMACOKINETICS. The pharmacokinetics of oral corticosteroids are described in Chapter 42. The pharmacokinetics of ICS are important in relation to systemic effects. The fraction of steroid that is inhaled into the lungs acts locally on the airway mucosa but may be absorbed from the airway and alveolar surface and reaches the systemic circulation. Furthermore, the fraction of inhaled steroid that is deposited in the oropharynx is swallowed and absorbed from the gut. The absorbed fraction may be metabolized in the liver (first-pass metabolism) before reaching the systemic circulation (*see* Figure 36–3). The use of a spacer chamber reduces oropharyngeal deposition and therefore reduces systemic absorption of ICS. Beclomethasone dipropionate and ciclesonide are prodrugs that release the active corticosteroid after the ester group is cleaved by esterases in the lung. Ciclesonide is available as an MDI (ALVESCO) for asthma and as a nasal spray for allergic rhinitis (OMNARIS). Budesonide and fluticasone propionate have a greater first-pass metabolism than beclomethasone dipropionate and are therefore less likely to produce systemic effects at high inhaled doses.

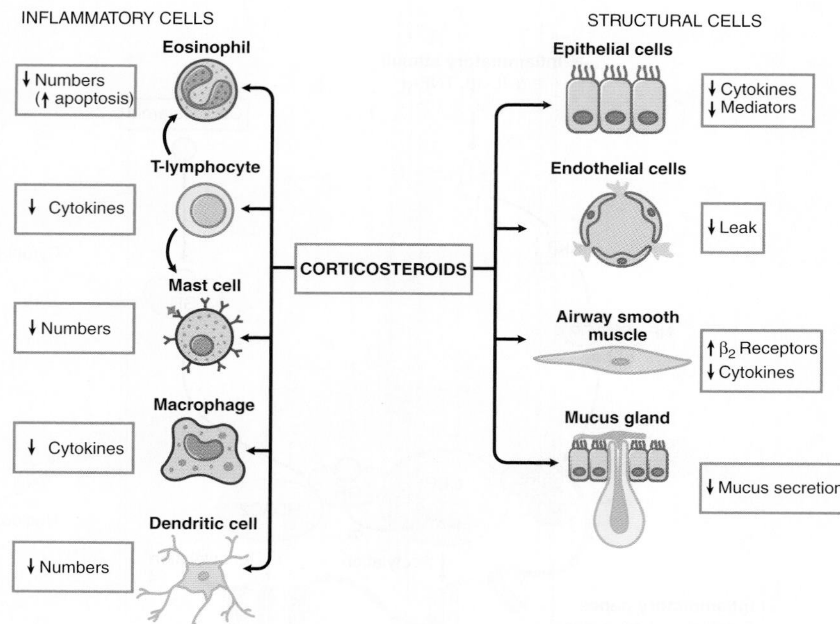

Figure 36–8 *Effect of corticosteroids on inflammatory and structural cells in the airways.*

ROUTES OF ADMINISTRATION AND DOSING

INHALED CORTICOSTEROIDS IN ASTHMA. Inhaled corticosteroids are recommended as first-line therapy for all patients with persistent asthma. They should be started in any patient who needs to use a β_2 agonist inhaler for symptom control more than twice weekly.

Most of the benefit may be obtained from doses <400 μg beclomethasone dipropionate or equivalent. However, some patients (with relative corticosteroid resistance) may benefit from higher doses (up to 2000 μg/day). For most patients, ICS should be used twice daily, a regimen that improves compliance once control of asthma has been achieved (which may require 4-times daily dosing initially or a course of oral steroids if symptoms are severe). Administration once daily of some steroids (e.g., budesonide, mometasone, and ciclesonide) is effective when doses ≤400 μg are needed. If a dose >800 μg daily via pMDI is used, a spacer device should be employed to reduce the risk of oropharyngeal side effects. ICS may be used in children in the same way as in adults.

INHALED CORTICOSTEROIDS IN CHRONIC OBSTRUCTIVE PULMONARY DISEASE

Patients with COPD occasionally respond to steroids, and these patients are likely to have concomitant asthma. Corticosteroids do not appear to have any significant anti-inflammatory effect in COPD; there appears to be an active resistance mechanism, which may be explained by impaired activity of HDAC2 as a result of oxidative stress. Patients with cystic fibrosis, which involves inflammation of the airways, are also resistant to high doses of ICS.

SYSTEMIC STEROIDS. Intravenous steroids are indicated in acute asthma if lung function is <30% predicted and in patients who show no significant improvement with nebulized β_2 agonist. Hydrocortisone is the steroid of choice because it has the most rapid onset (5-6 h after administration), compared with 8 h with prednisolone.

It is common to give hydrocortisone 4 mg/kg initially, followed by a maintenance dose of 3 mg/kg every 6 h. Oral prednisolone (40-60 mg) has a similar effect to intravenous hydrocortisone. Prednisolone and prednisone are the most commonly used oral steroids. The usual maintenance dose is ~10-15 mg/day. Oral steroids are usually given as a single dose in the morning because this coincides with the normal diurnal increase in plasma cortisol and produces less adrenal suppression than if given in divided doses or at night.

Adverse Effects. Corticosteroids inhibit ACTH and cortisol secretion by a negative feedback effect on the pituitary gland (*see* Chapter 42). Hypothalamic-pituitary-adrenal (HPA) axis suppression depends on dose

Table 36–4

Side Effects of Inhaled Corticosteroids

Local side effects
Dysphonia, oropharyngeal candidiasis, cough
Systemic side effects
Adrenal suppression and insufficiency, growth suppression
Bruising, osteoporosis, cataracts, glaucoma, pneumonia
Metabolic abnormalities (glucose, insulin, triglycerides)
Psychiatric disturbances (euphoria, depression)

and usually only occurs with doses of prednisone >7.5-10 mg/day. Significant suppression after short courses of corticosteroid therapy is not usually a problem. *Steroid doses after prolonged oral therapy must be reduced slowly.* Symptoms of "steroid withdrawal syndrome" include lassitude, musculoskeletal pains, and, occasionally, fever. HPA suppression with inhaled steroids is usually seen only when the daily inhaled dose exceeds 2000 μg beclomethasone dipropionate or its equivalent daily.

Side effects of long-term oral corticosteroid therapy include fluid retention, increased appetite, weight gain, osteoporosis, capillary fragility, hypertension, peptic ulceration, diabetes, cataracts, and psychosis. Their frequency tends to increase with age. Very occasionally adverse reactions (such as anaphylaxis) to intravenous hydrocortisone have been described, particularly in aspirin-sensitive asthmatic patients.

ICS may have *local side effects* due to the deposition of inhaled steroid in the oropharynx. The most common problem is hoarseness and weakness of the voice (dysphonia) due to atrophy of the vocal cords following laryngeal deposition of steroid; it may occur in up to 40% of patients and is noticed particularly by patients who need to use their voices during their work (lecturers, teachers, and singers). Throat irritation and coughing after inhalation are common with MDI and appear to be due to additives since these problems are not usually seen if the patient switches to a DPI. Oropharyngeal candidiasis occurs in ~5% of patients. Growing evidence suggests that high doses of ICS increase the risk of pneumonia in patients with COPD using high doses of fluticasone propionate. The incidence of *systemic side effects* after ICS is an important consideration, particularly in children (Table 36–4). Adrenal suppression can occur with inhaled doses >1500-2000 μg/day, possibly less. It is important to reduce the likelihood of systemic effects by using the lowest dose of inhaled steroid needed to control the asthma, and by use of a large-volume spacer to reduce oropharyngeal deposition.

Therapeutic Choices. Numerous ICS are now available including beclomethasone dipropionate (QVAR), triamcinolone, flunisolide (AEROBID), budesonide (PULMICORT, *others*), fluticasone *hemihydrate* (AEROSPAN), fluticasone propionate (FLOVENT), mometasone furoate (ASMANEX), and ciclesonide (ALVESCO). All are equally effective as anti-asthma drugs, but there are differences in their pharmacokinetics: Budesonide, fluticasone, mometasone, and ciclesonide have a lower oral bioavailability than beclomethasone dipropionate because they are subject to greater first-pass hepatic metabolism; this results in reduced systemic absorption and thus reduced adverse effects. Ciclesonide is another choice; it is a prodrug that is converted to the active metabolite by esterases in the lung, giving it a low oral bioavailability and a high therapeutic index.

CROMONES

Cromolyn sodium (sodium cromoglycate) is a derivative of khellin, an Egyptian herbal remedy. A structurally related drug, *nedocromil* sodium, was subsequently developed. The use of cromolyn has sharply declined with the widespread use of the more effective ICS.

MEDIATOR ANTAGONISTS

Both H_1 antihistamines and antileukptrienes have been applied to airway disease, but their added benefit over β_2 agonists and corticosteroids is slight.

ANTIHISTAMINES. Histamine mimics many of the features of asthma and is released from mast cells in acute asthmatic responses, suggesting that antihistamines may be useful in asthma therapy. There is little evidence that histamine H_1 receptor antagonists provide any useful clinical benefit, as demonstrated by a meta-analysis. Newer antihistamines, including cetirizine and azelastine, have some beneficial effects, but this may be unrelated to H_1 receptor antagonism.

ANTILEUKOTRIENES. There is considerable evidence that cysteinyl-leukotrienes (LTs) are produced in asthma and that they have potent effects on airway function, inducing bronchoconstriction, airway hyperresponsiveness, plasma exudation, mucus secretion, and eosinophilic inflammation (Figure 36–9; also *see* Chapter 33). These data motivated the development of 5′-lipoxygenase (5-LO) enzyme inhibitors (of which zileuton [ZYFLO] is

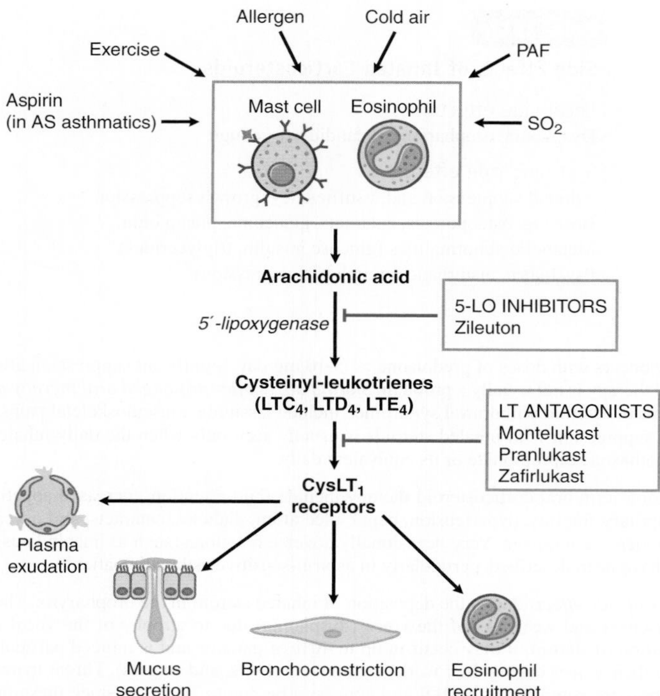

Figure 36–9 *Effects of cysteinyl-leukotrienes on the airways and their inhibition by antileukotrienes.* AS, aspirin sensitive; 5-LO, 5′-lipoxygenase; LT, leukotriene; PAF, platelet-activating factor.

the only drug marketed) and several antagonists of the cys-LT_1 receptor, including montelukast (SINGULAIR), zafirlukast (ACCOLATE), and pranlukast.

Clinical Studies. In patients with mild to moderate asthma, antileukotrienes cause a significant improvement in lung function and asthma symptoms, with a reduction in the use of rescue inhaled β_2 agonists. However, antileukotrienes are considerably less effective than ICS in the treatment of mild asthma and cannot be considered the treatment of first choice. Antileukotrienes are indicated as an add-on therapy in patients who are not well controlled on ICS. The added benefit is small and less effective than adding an LABA.

Antileukotrienes are effective in preventing exercise-induced asthma, with efficacy similar to that of LABA. Antileukotrienes appear to act mainly as antibronchoconstrictor drugs, and they are clearly less broadly effective than β_2 agonists because they antagonize only one of several bronchoconstrictor mediators. Cys-LT1 receptor antagonists have no role in the therapy of COPD.

Adverse Effects. Zileuton, zafirlukast, and montelukast are all associated with rare cases of hepatic dysfunction; thus, liver-associated enzymes should be monitored. Several cases of Churg-Strauss syndrome have been associated with the use of zafirlukast and montelukast.

IMMUNOMODULATORY THERAPIES

IMMUNOSUPPRESSIVE THERAPY

Immunosuppressive therapies (e.g., methotrexate, cyclosporine A, gold, intravenous immunoglobulin) have been considered in asthma when other treatments have been unsuccessful or to reduce the dose of oral steroids required. However, immunosuppressive treatments are less effective and have a greater propensity for side effects than oral corticosteroids.

ANTI-IgE RECEPTOR THERAPY

Omalizumab is a humanized monoclonal antibody that blocks the binding of IgE to high-affinity IgE receptors (FcεRI) on mast cells and thus prevents their activation by allergens (Figure 36–10).

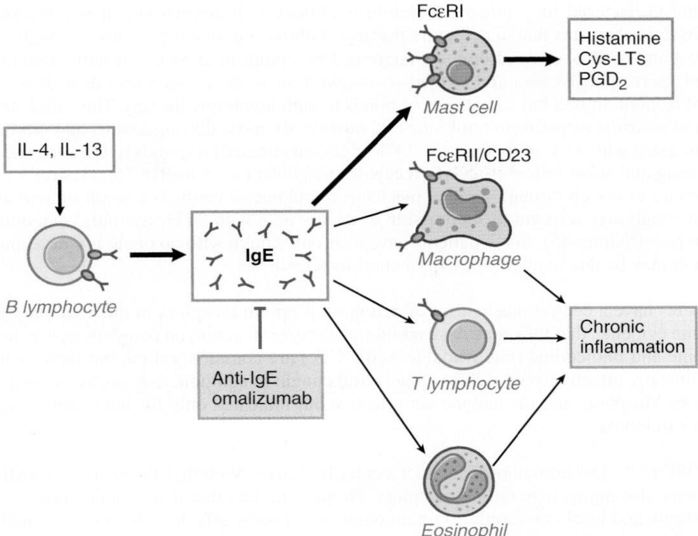

Figure 36–10 *Immunoglobulin (Ig) E plays a central role in allergic diseases.* Blocking IgE using an antibody, such as omalizumab, is a rational therapeutic approach. IgE may activate high-affinity receptors (FcεRI) on mast cells as well as low-affinity receptors (FcεRII, CD23) on other inflammatory cells. Omalizumab prevents these interactions and the resulting inflammation. cys-LT, cysteinyl-leukotriene; IL, interleukin; PG, prostaglandin.

It also blocks binding on IgE to low-affinity IgE receptors (FcεRII, CD23) on other inflammatory cells, including T and B lymphocytes, macrophages, and possibly eosinophils, to inhibit chronic inflammation. Omalizumab also reduces levels of circulating IgE.

Clinical Use. Omalizumab is used for the treatment of patients with severe asthma. The antibody is administered by subcutaneous injection every 2-4 weeks, and the dose is determined by the titer of circulating IgE. Omalizumab reduces the requirement for oral and ICS and markedly reduces asthma exacerbations. Because of its very high cost, this treatment is generally used only in patients with very severe asthma who are poorly controlled even on oral corticosteroids and in patients with very severe concomitant allergic rhinitis. The major side effect of omalizumab is an anaphylactic response, which is uncommon (<0.1%).

MUCOREGULATORS

Mucus hypersecretion occurs in chronic bronchitis, COPD, cystic fibrosis, and asthma. In chronic bronchitis, mucus hypersecretion is related to chronic irritation by cigarette smoke and may involve neural mechanisms and the activation of neutrophils to release enzymes such as neutrophil elastase and proteinase-3 that have powerful stimulatory effects on mucus secretion. Mast cell–derived chymase is also a potent mucus secretagogue. Systemic anticholinergic drugs appear to reduce mucociliary clearance, but this is not observed with either ipratropium bromide or tiotropium bromide, presumably reflecting their poor absorption from the respiratory tract. β_2 Agonists increase mucus production and mucociliary clearance. Because inflammation leads to mucus hypersecretion, anti-inflammatory treatments should reduce mucus hypersecretion; ICS are very effective in reducing increased mucus production in asthma.

Sensory nerves and neuropeptides are important in the secretory activities of the submucosal gland and goblet cell (more notable in peripheral airways). Opioids and K^+ channel openers inhibit mucus secretion mediated via sensory neuropeptide release; peripherally acting opioids may be developed to control mucus hypersecretion due to irritants in the future.

ANTITUSSIVES

Whenever possible, treat the underlying cause, not the cough.

Viral infections of the upper respiratory tract are the most common cause of cough; postviral cough is usually self-limiting and commonly patient-medicated. Because cough is a defensive reflex, its suppression may be inappropriate in bacterial lung infection. Before treatment with antitussives, it is important to identify underlying causal mechanisms that may require therapy. Asthma commonly presents as cough, and the cough will usually respond to ICS. A syndrome characterized by cough in association with sputum eosinophilia but no airway hyperresponsiveness and termed *eosinophilic bronchitis* also responds to ICS. Nonasthmatic cough does not respond to ICS but sometimes responds to anticholinergic therapy. The cough associated with postnasal drip of sinusitis responds to antibiotics (if warranted), nasal decongestants, and intranasal steroids. The cough associated with ACE inhibitors (in ~15% of patients treated) responds to lowering the dose or withdrawal of the drug and substitution of an AT_1 receptor antagonist (*see* Chapter 26). Gastroesophageal reflux is a common cause of cough through a reflex mechanism and occasionally as a result of acid aspiration into the lungs. This cough may respond to suppression of gastric acid with an H_2 receptor antagonist or a proton pump inhibitor (*see* Chapter 45). Some patients have a chronic cough with no obvious cause, and this chronic idiopathic cough may be due to airway sensory neural hyperesthesia.

OPIATES. Opiates have a central mechanism of action on μ opioid receptors in the medullary cough center, but there is some evidence that they may have additional peripheral action on cough receptors in the proximal airways. Codeine and pholcodine (not available in the U.S.) are commonly used, but there is little evidence that they are clinically effective, particularly on postviral cough; in addition, they are associated with sedation and constipation. Morphine and methadone are effective but indicated only for intractable cough associated with bronchial carcinoma.

DEXTROMETHORPHAN. Dextromethorphan is a centrally active *N*-methyl-D-aspartate (NMDA) receptor antagonist. It may also antagonize opioid receptors. Despite the fact that it is in numerous over-the-counter cough suppressants and used commonly to treat cough, it is poorly effective. It can cause hallucinations at higher doses and has significant abuse potential.

BENZONATATE. (TESSALON, others), a local anesthetic, acts peripherally by anesthetizing the stretch receptors located in the respiratory passages, lungs, and pleura. By dampening the activity of these receptors, benzonatate may reduce the cough reflex at its source. The recommended dose is 100 mg, three times daily, and up to 600 mg/day, if needed. Side effects include dizziness and dysphagia. Seizures and cardiac arrest have occurred following an acute ingestion. Severe allergic reactions have been reported in patients allergic to para-aminobenzoic acid, a metabolite of benzonatate.

OTHER DRUGS. Several other drugs reportedly have small benefits in reducing cough in pulmonary diseases. These drugs include ***moguisteine*** (not available in the U.S.), which acts peripherally and appears to open ATP-sensitive K^+ channels; ***baclofen***, a $GABA_B$-selective agonist; and ***theobromine***, a naturally occurring methylxanthine.

DRUGS FOR DYSPNEA AND VENTILATORY CONTROL

DRUGS FOR DYSPNEA

Bronchodilators should reduce breathlessness in patients with airway obstruction. Chronic oxygen may have a beneficial effect, but in a few patients dyspnea may be extreme. Drugs that reduce breathlessness may also depress ventilation and may therefore be dangerous. Some patients show a beneficial response to dihydrocodeine and diazepam; however, these drugs must be used with great caution because of the risk of ventilatory depression. Slow-release morphine tablets may also be helpful in COPD patients with extreme dyspnea. Nebulized morphine may also reduce breathlessness in COPD and could act in part on opioid receptors in the lung.

VENTILATORY STIMULANTS

Selective respiratory stimulants are indicated if ventilation is impaired as a result of overdose with sedatives, in post-anesthetic respiratory depression, and in idiopathic hypoventilation. Respiratory stimulants are rarely indicated in COPD because respiratory drive is already maximal and further stimulation of ventilation may be counterproductive because of the increase in energy expenditure caused by the drugs.

DOXAPRAM. (DOPRAM, others). At low doses (0.5 mg/kg IV), doxapram stimulates carotid chemoreceptors; at higher doses it stimulates medullary respiratory centers. Its effect is transient; thus, intravenous infusion (0.3-3 mg/kg/min) is needed for sustained effect. Unwanted effects include nausea, sweating, anxiety, and hallucinations. At higher doses, increased pulmonary and systemic pressures may occur. Both the kidney and the liver participate in the clearance of doxapram, which should be used with caution if hepatic or renal function is impaired. In COPD, the infusion of doxapram is restricted to 2 h. The use of doxapram to treat ventilatory failure in COPD has now largely been replaced by noninvasive ventilation.

ALMITRINE. Almitrine bismesylate is a piperazine derivative that appears to selectively stimulate peripheral chemoreceptors and is without central actions. Almitrine stimulates ventilation only when there is hypoxia. Long-term use of almitrine is associated with peripheral neuropathy, limiting its availability in most countries.

ACETAZOLAMIDE. The carbonic anhydrase inhibitor acetazolamide (*see* Chapter 25) induces metabolic acidosis and thereby stimulates ventilation, but it is not widely used because the metabolic imbalance it produces may be detrimental in the face of respiratory acidosis. It has a very small beneficial effect in respiratory failure in COPD patients. The drug has proved useful in prevention of high altitude sickness.

NALOXONE. Naloxone is a competitive opioid antagonist that is indicated only if ventilatory depression is due to overdose of opioids.

FLUMAZENIL. Flumazenil is a benzodiazepine receptor antagonist that can reverse respiratory depression due to overdose of benzodiazepines.

PHARMACOTHERAPY OF PULMONARY ARTERIAL HYPERTENSION

Pulmonary arterial hypertension (PAH) is characterized by vascular proliferation and remodeling of small pulmonary arteries, resulting in a progressive increase in pulmonary vascular resistance that may lead to right heart failure and death. PAH involves dysfunction of pulmonary vascular endothelial and smooth muscle cells and their interplay and results from an imbalance in vasoconstrictor and vasodilator mediators. Vasodilators are the mainstay of drug therapy for PAH. However, the vasodilators used to treat systemic hypertension lower systemic blood pressure, which may result in reduced pulmonary perfusion. Calcium channel blockers, such as nifedipine, are poorly effective, but a few patients may benefit. In PAH, there is an increase in the vasoconstrictor mediators ET-1, TxA_2, and 5HT, and a decrease in the vasodilating mediators prostacyclin (PGI_2), NO, and VIP. Therapies aim at antagonizing the vasoconstrictive mediators and enhancing vasodilation (Figure 36–11).

Most cases of pulmonary hypertension are associated with connective tissue disorders, such as systemic sclerosis, or they are secondary to hypoxic lung diseases, such as interstitial lung disease and COPD, where chronic hypoxia leads to hypoxic pulmonary vasoconstriction. In secondary pulmonary hypertension due to chronic hypoxia, the initial treatment is correction of hypoxia using supplementary O_2 therapy. Right heart failure is treated initially with diuretics. Anticoagulants are indicated for the treatment of pulmonary hypertension secondary to chronic thromboembolic disease, but they may also be indicated for patients with severe pulmonary hypertension who have an increased risk of venous thrombosis.

PROSTACYCLIN

Prostacyclin (PGI_2; epoprostenol) is produced by endothelial cells in the pulmonary circulation and directly relaxes pulmonary vascular smooth muscle cells by increasing intracellular cyclic AMP concentrations (*see* Chapter 33). Reduced prostacyclin production in PAH has led to the therapeutic use of epoprostenol and other stable prostacyclin derivatives. Functionally, PGI_2 opposes the effects of TXA_2.

Intravenous epoprostenol (FLOLAN, others) is effective in lowering pulmonary arterial pressures, improving exercise performance, and prolonging survival in primary PAH (PPAH). Because of its short plasma $t_{1/2}$, prostacyclin must be administered by continuous intravenous infusion using an infusion pump. Common side effects are headache, flushing, diarrhea, nausea, and jaw pain. Continuous intravenous infusion is inconvenient and very expensive. This has led to the development of more stable prostacyclin analogs. Treprostinil (REMODULIN) is given by continuous subcutaneous infusion or as an inhalation (TYVASO), consisting of 4 daily treatment sessions with 9 breaths per session. Iloprost (VENTAVIS) is a stable analog that is given by inhalation, but it needs to be given by nebulizer 6 to 9 times daily. It is associated with the vasodilator side effects of prostacyclin, including syncope. It may also cause cough and bronchoconstriction because it sensitizes airway sensory nerves.

ENDOTHELIN RECEPTOR ANTAGONISTS

Endothelin-1 (ET-1) is a potent pulmonary vasoconstrictor that is produced in increased amounts in PAH. ET-1 contracts vascular smooth muscle cells and causes proliferation mainly via ET_A receptors. ET_B receptors mediate the release of prostacyclin and NO from endothelial cells. Several endothelin antagonists are now on the market for the treatment of PPAH.

Bosentan (TRACLEER) is an ET_A/ET_B receptor antagonist. Bosentan is effective in reducing symptoms and improving mortality in PPAH. Starting dose is 62.5 mg twice daily for 4 weeks, and maintenance dose is 125 mg twice daily. The drug is generally well tolerated. Adverse effects include abnormal liver function tests, anemia, headaches, peripheral edema, and nasal congestion. Liver aminotransferases should be monitored monthly. A class effect is a risk of testicular atrophy and infertility; bosentan is potentially teratogenic.

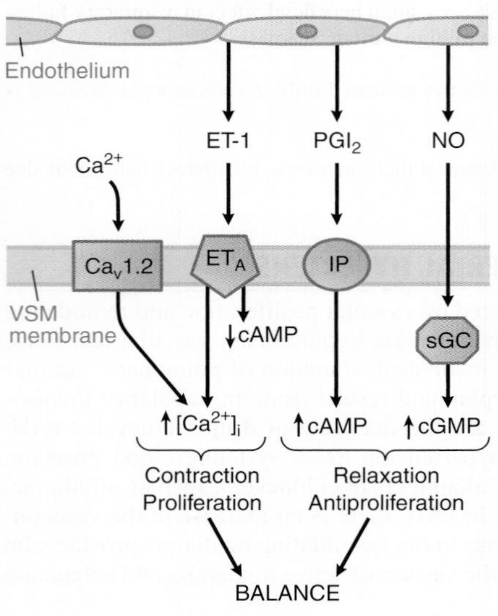

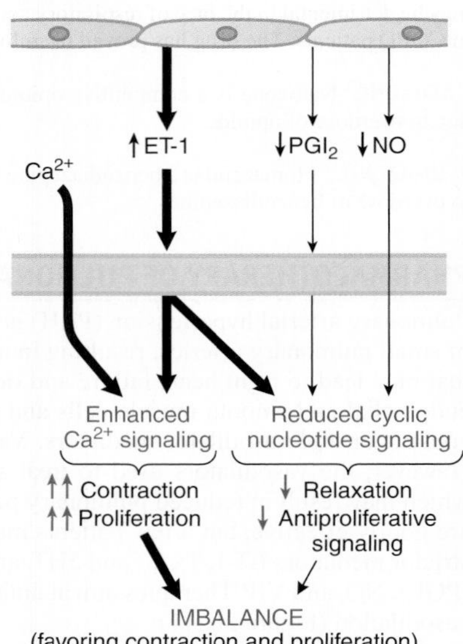

Figure 36–11 *Interactions of endothelium and vascular smooth muscle in pulmonary artery hypertension (PAH).* **A.** In normal pulmonary artery, there is a balance between constrictor and relaxant influences that may be viewed as competition between Ca^{2+} signaling pathways and cyclic nucleotide signaling pathways in vascular smooth muscle (VSM). Endothelin (ET-1) binds to the ET_A receptor on VSM cells and activates the G_q-PLC-IP_3 pathway to increase cytosolic Ca^{2+}; ET-1 may also couple to G_i to inhibit cyclic AMP (cAMP) production. In depolarizing VSM cells, Ca^{2+} may enter via the L-type Ca^{2+} channel (Ca_v1.2). Endothelial cells also produce relaxant factors, prostacyclin (PGI_2) and NO. NO stimulates the soluble guanylyl cyclase (cGC), causing accumulation of cyclic GMP (cGMP) in VSM cells; PGI_2 binds to the IP receptor and stimulates cAMP production; elevation of these cyclic nucleotides promotes VSM relaxation (*see* Figures 36–4 and 3–11). **B.** In PAH, ET-1 production is enhanced, production of PGI_2 and NO is reduced, and the balance is shifted toward constriction and proliferation of vascular smooth muscle.

Ambrisentan (LETAIRIS) is a selective ET_A receptor antagonist. It is given orally once daily at a dose of 5-10 mg with clinical efficacy and adverse effects similar to that of bosentan. Use of ambrisentan also requires monthly monitoring of liver aminotransferases. *Sitaxsentan* (THELIN, not available in the U.S.) is a selective ET_A receptor antagonist that was withdrawn from the market because of post-marketing reports of fatal liver complications in patients with PAH related to its use.

PDE5 INHIBITORS

Nitric oxide activates soluble guanylate cyclase to increase cyclic GMP, which is hydrolyzed to 5′GMP by PDE5 (*see* Chapter 27). Elevation of cGMP in smooth muscle causes relaxation (*see* Chapter 3), which the inhibition of PDE5 prolongs and accentuates. In the pulmonary bed, inhibition of PDE5 induces vasodilation.

SILDENAFIL. Sildenafil (REVATIO) is a selective PDE5 inhibitor that is given at a dose (20 mg 3 time daily orally) that is lower than used for erectile dysfunction (100 mg; *see* Chapter 27). It is effective in lowering pulmonary resistance and improving exercise tolerance in patients with PAH. Side effects include headache, flushing, dyspepsia, and visual disturbances.

TADALAFIL. Tadalafil (ADCIRCA) has a longer duration of action than sildenafil so may be suitable for once-daily dosing.

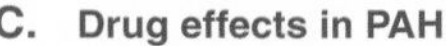

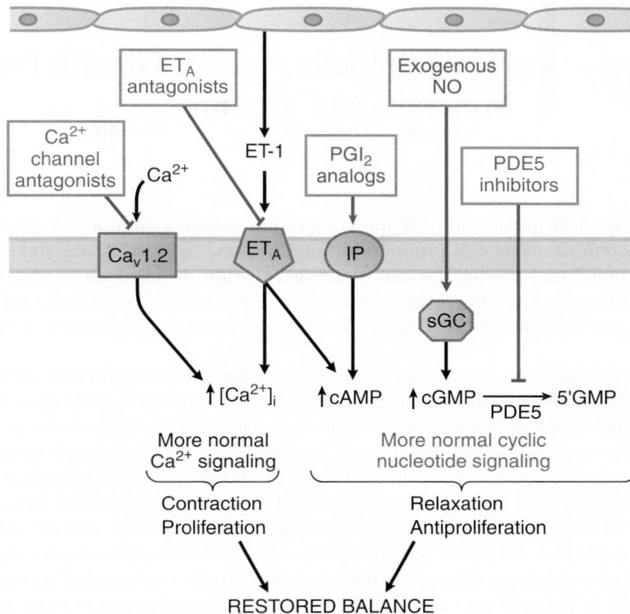

Figure 36–11 *Continued* **C.** In treating PAH, ET$_A$ receptor antagonists can reduce the constrictor effects of ET-1, and Ca^{2+} channel antagonists can further reduce Ca^{2+}-dependent contraction. Exogenous PGI$_2$ and NO can be supplied to promote vasodilation (relaxation of VSM); inhibition of PDE5 can enhance the relaxant effect of NO by inhibiting the degradation of cGMP. Thus, these drugs can reduce Ca^{2+} signaling and enhance cyclic nucleotide signaling, restoring the balance between the forces of contraction/proliferation and relaxation/antiproliferation. Remodeling and deposition of extracellular matrix by adjacent fibroblasts is influenced positively and negatively by the same contractile and relaxant signaling pathways, respectively.

PDE4 INHIBITORS

Roflumilast. Roflumilast (DALIRESP) and its active metabolite (roflumilast N-oxide) selectively inhibit PDE4, have anti-inflammtory effects, and are used to decrease exacerbations of severe COPD. Roflumilast is metabolized by CYPs to roflumilast N-oxide and then to conjugates that are mostly excreted in urine. Adverse effects include diarrhea, weight loss, nausea, headache, and can be dose-limiting. Some patients may experience anxiety, depression, and suicidal thoughts.

For a complete Bibliographical Listing see Goodman & Gilman's ***The Pharmacological Basis of Therapeutics***, 12th ed., or Goodman & Gilman Online at www.AccessMedicine.com.

37 chapter Hematopoietic Agents: Growth Factors, Minerals, and Vitamins

The finite life span of most mature blood cells requires their continuous replacement, a process termed *hematopoiesis*. New cell production must respond to basal needs and states of increased demand. Red blood cell production can increase >20-fold in response to anemia or hypoxemia, white blood cell production increases dramatically in response to a systemic infection, and platelet production can increase 10- to 20-fold when platelet consumption results in thrombocytopenia.

The regulation of blood cell production is complex. Hematopoietic stem cells are rare bone marrow cells that manifest self-renewal and lineage commitment, resulting in cells destined to differentiate into the 9 distinct blood-cell lineages. For the most part, this process occurs in the marrow cavities of the skull, vertebral bodies, pelvis, and proximal long bones; it involves interactions among hematopoietic stem and progenitor cells and the cells and complex macromolecules of the marrow stroma, and is influenced by a number of soluble and membrane-bound hematopoietic growth factors. Some of these hormones and cytokines have been identified and cloned, permitting their production in quantities sufficient for therapeutic use. Clinical applications range from the treatment of primary hematologic diseases to use as adjuncts in the treatment of severe infections and in the management of patients who are undergoing cancer chemotherapy or marrow transplantation.

Hematopoiesis also requires an adequate supply of minerals (e.g., iron, cobalt, and copper) and vitamins (e.g., folic acid, vitamin B_{12}, pyridoxine, ascorbic acid, and riboflavin); deficiencies generally result in characteristic anemias or, less frequently, a general failure of hematopoiesis. Therapeutic correction of a specific deficiency state depends on the accurate diagnosis of the anemic state, and on knowledge about the correct dose, the use of these agents in appropriate combinations, and the expected response.

Hematopoietic Growth Factors

GROWTH FACTOR PHYSIOLOGY. Steady-state hematopoiesis encompasses the production of >400 billion blood cells each day. This production is tightly regulated and can be increased several-fold with increased demand. The hematopoietic organ also is unique in adult physiology in that several mature cell types are derived from a much smaller number of multipotent progenitors, which develop from a more limited number of pluripotent hematopoietic stem cells. Such cells are capable of maintaining their own number and differentiating under the influence of cellular and humoral factors to produce the large and diverse number of mature blood cells.

Stem cell differentiation can be described as a series of steps that produce so-called burst-forming units (BFUs) and colony-forming units (CFUs) for each of the major cell lines. These early progenitors (BFU and CFU) are capable of further proliferation and differentiation, increasing their number by some 30-fold. Subsequently, colonies of morphologically distinct cells form under the control of an overlapping set of additional growth factors (granulocyte colony-stimulating factor [G-CSF], macrophage colony-stimulating factor [M-CSF], erythropoietin, and thrombopoietin). Proliferation and maturation of the CFU for each cell line can amplify the resulting mature cell product by another 30-fold or more, generating >1000 mature cells from each committed stem cell.

Hematopoietic and lymphopoietic growth factors are glycoproteins produced by a number of marrow cells and peripheral tissues. They are active at very low concentrations and typically affect more than 1 committed cell lineage. Most interact synergistically with other factors and also stimulate production of additional growth factors, a process called *networking*. Growth factors generally exert actions at several points in the processes of cell proliferation and differentiation and in mature cell function. However, the network of growth factors that contributes to any given cell lineage depends absolutely on a nonredundant, lineage-specific factor, such that absence of factors that stimulate developmentally early progenitors is compensated for by redundant cytokines, but loss of the lineage-specific factor leads to a specific cytopenia.

Some of the overlapping and nonredundant effects of the more important hematopoietic growth factors are illustrated in Figure 37–1 and Table 37–1.

ERYTHROPOIESIS-STIMULATING AGENTS

Erythropoiesis-stimulating agent (ESA) is the term given to a pharmacological substance that stimulates red blood cell production.

Erythropoietin is the most important regulator of the proliferation of committed erythroid progenitors (CFU-E) and their immediate progeny. In its absence, severe anemia is invariably present, commonly seen in patients with renal failure. Erythropoiesis is controlled by a feedback system in which a sensor in the kidney detects changes in oxygen delivery to modulate the erythropoietin secretion. The sensor mechanism is now understood at the molecular level.

Hypoxia-inducible factor (HIF-1), a heterodimeric (HIF-1α and HIF-1β) transcription factor, enhances expression of multiple hypoxia-inducible genes, such as vascular endothelial growth factor and erythropoietin. HIF-1α is labile due to its prolyl hydroxylation and subsequent polyubiquitination and degradation, aided by the *von Hippel-Lindau* (VHL) *protein*. During states of hypoxia, the prolyl hydroxylase is inactive,

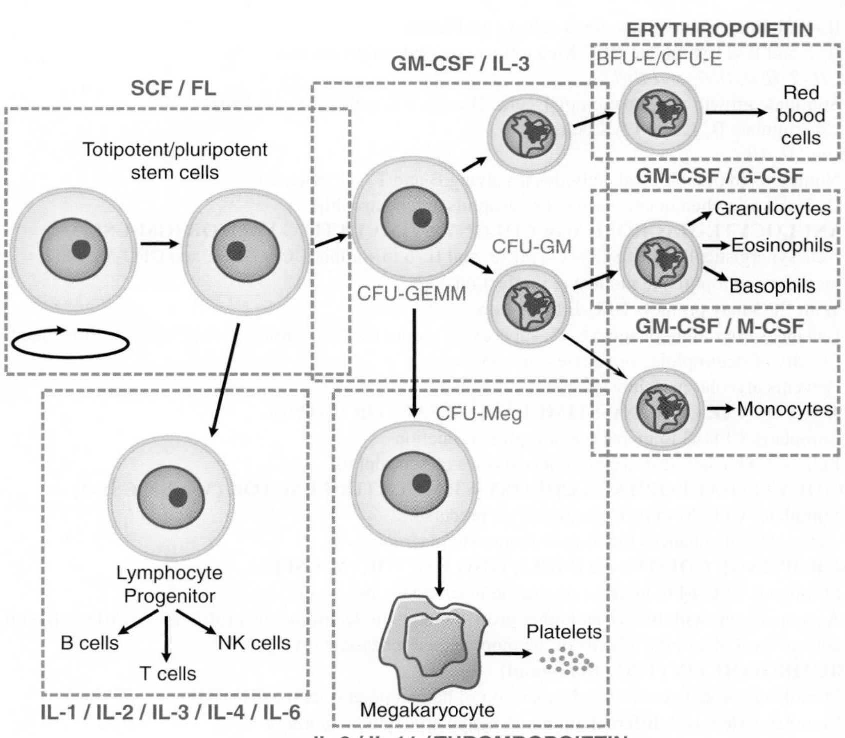

Figure 37–1 *Sites of action of hematopoietic growth factors in the differentiation and maturation of marrow cell lines.* A self-sustaining pool of marrow stem cells differentiates under the influence of specific hematopoietic growth factors to form a variety of hematopoietic and lymphopoietic cells. Stem cell factor (SCF), ligand (FL), interleukin-3 (IL-3), and granulocyte-macrophage colony-stimulating factor (GM-CSF), together with cell–cell interactions in the marrow, stimulate stem cells to form a series of burst-forming units (BFU) and colony-forming units (CFU): CFU-GEMM (granulocyte, erythrocyte, monocyte and megakaryocyte), CFU-GM (granulocyte and macrophage), CFU-Meg (megakaryocyte), BFU-E (erythrocyte), and CFU-E (erythrocyte). After considerable proliferation, further differentiation is stimulated by synergistic interactions with growth factors for each of the major cell lines—granulocyte colony-stimulating factor (G-CSF), monocyte/macrophage-stimulating factor (M-CSF), thrombopoietin, and erythropoietin. Each of these factors also influences the proliferation, maturation, and in some cases the function of the derivative cell line (Table 37–1).

Table 37–1

Hematopoietic Growth Factors

ERYTHROPOIETIN (EPO)

- Stimulates proliferation and maturation of committed erythroid progenitors to increase red cell production

STEM CELL FACTOR (SCF, c-kit ligand, Steel factor) and FLT-3 LIGAND (FL)

- Act synergistically with a wide range of other colony-stimulating factors and interleukins to stimulate pluripotent and committed stem cells
- FL also stimulates both dendritic and NK cells (antitumor response)
- SCF also stimulates mast cells and melanocytes

INTERLEUKINS

IL-1, IL-3, IL-5, IL-6, IL-9, and IL-11

- Act synergistically with each other and SCF, GM-CSF, G-CSF, and EPO to stimulate BFU-E, CFU-GEMM, CFU-GM, CFU-E, and CFU-Meg growth
- Numerous immunologic roles, including stimulation of B cell and T cell growth

IL-5

- Controls eosinophil survival and differentiation

IL-6

- IL-6 stimulates human myeloma cells to proliferate
- IL-6 and IL-11 stimulate BFU-Meg to increase platelet production

IL-1, IL-2, IL-4, IL-7, and IL-12

- Stimulate growth and function of T cells, B cells, NK cells, and monocytes
- Co-stimulate B, T, and LAK cells

IL-8 and IL-10

- Numerous immunological activities involving B and T cell functions
- IL-8 acts as a chemotactic factor for basophils and neutrophils

GRANULOCYTE-MACROPHAGE COLONY-STIMULATING FACTOR (GM-CSF)

- Acts synergistically with SCF, IL-1, IL-3, and IL-6 to stimulate CFU-GM, and CFU-Meg to increase neutrophil and monocyte production
- With EPO may promote BFU-E formation
- Enhances migration, phagocytosis, superoxide production, and antibody-dependent cell-mediated toxicity of neutrophils, monocytes, and eosinophils
- Prevents alveolar proteinosis

GRANULOCYTE COLONY-STIMULATING FACTOR (G-CSF)

- Stimulates CFU-G to increase neutrophil production
- Enhances phagocytic and cytotoxic activities of neutrophils

MONOCYTE/MACROPHAGE COLONY-STIMULATING FACTOR (M-CSF, CSF-1)

- Stimulates CFU-M to increase monocyte precursors
- Activates and enhances function of monocyte/macrophages

MACROPHAGE COLONY-STIMULATING FACTOR (M-CSF)

- Stimulates CFU-M to increase monocyte/macrophage precursors
- Acts in concert with tissues and other growth factors to determine the proliferation, differentiation, and survival of a range of cells of the mononuclear phagocyte system

THROMBOPOIETIN (TPO, *Mpl* ligand)

- Stimulates the self-renewal and expansion of hematopoietic stem cells
- Stimulates stem cell differentiation into megakaryocyte progenitors
- Selectively stimulates megakaryocytopoiesis to increase platelet production
- Acts synergistically with other growth factors, especially IL-6 and IL-11

BFU, burst-forming unit; CFU, colony-forming unit; E, erythrocyte; G, granulocyte; M, macrophage; Meg, megakaryocyte; NK cells, natural killer cells; LAK cells, lymphokine-activated killer cells.

allowing the accumulation of HIF-1α and activating erythropoietin expression, which in turn stimulates a rapid expansion of erythroid progenitors. Specific alteration of VHL leads to an oxygen-sensing defect, characterized by constitutively elevated levels of HIF-1α and erythropoietin, with a resultant polycythemia.

Erythropoietin is expressed primarily in peritubular interstitial cells of the kidney. Erythropoietin contains 193 amino acids, of which the first 27 are cleaved during secretion. The final hormone is heavily glycosylated and has a molecular mass of ~30 kDa. After secretion, erythropoietin binds to a receptor on the surface of committed erythroid progenitors in the marrow and is internalized. With anemia or hypoxemia, synthesis rapidly increases by 100-fold or more, serum erythropoietin levels rise, and marrow progenitor cell survival, proliferation, and maturation are dramatically stimulated. This finely tuned feedback loop can be disrupted by kidney disease, marrow damage, or a deficiency in iron or an essential vitamin. With an infection or an inflammatory state, erythropoietin secretion, iron delivery, and progenitor proliferation all are suppressed by inflammatory cytokines, but this accounts for only part of the resultant anemia; interference with iron metabolism also is an effect of inflammatory mediator effects on the hepatic protein *hepcidin*.

PREPARATIONS. Available preparations of recombinant human erythropoietin (*epoetin alfa*) include EPOGEN, PROCRIT, and EPREX, supplied in single-use vials containing 2000-40,000 units/mL for intravenous or subcutaneous administration. When injected intravenously, epoetin alfa is cleared from plasma with a $t_{1/2}$ of 4-8 h. However, the effect on marrow progenitors lasts much longer, and once-weekly dosing can be sufficient to achieve an adequate response. A novel erythropoiesis-stimulating protein, darbepoetin alfa (ARANESP), has been approved for clinical use in patients with indications similar to those for epoetin alfa. It is a genetically modified form of erythropoietin in which 4 amino acids have been mutated such that additional carbohydrate side chains are added during its synthesis, prolonging the circulatory survival of the drug to 24-26 h. Another erythropoiesis-stimulating peptide, Peginesatide (OMONTYS), was approved in 2012 for the treatment of anemia due to chronic kidney disease. Postmarketing reports of serious hypersensitivity reactions and anaphylaxis have necessitated a recall.

Recombinant human erythropoietin (*epoetin alfa*) is nearly identical to the endogenous hormone. The carbohydrate modification pattern of epoetin alfa differs slightly from the native protein, but this difference apparently does not alter kinetics, potency, or immunoreactivity of the drug. Modern assays can detect these differences and thereby identify athletes who use the recombinant product for "blood doping."

THERAPEUTIC USES, MONITORING, AND ADVERSE EFFECTS. Recombinant erythropoietin therapy, in conjunction with adequate iron intake, can be highly effective in a number of anemias, especially those associated with a poor erythropoietic response. Epoetin alfa is effective in the treatment of anemias associated with surgery, AIDS, cancer chemotherapy, prematurity, and certain chronic inflammatory conditions. Darbepoetin alfa also has been approved for use in patients with anemia associated with chronic kidney disease.

During erythropoietin therapy, absolute or functional iron deficiency may develop. Functional iron deficiency (i.e., normal ferritin levels but low transferrin saturation) presumably results from the inability to mobilize iron stores rapidly enough to support the increased erythropoiesis. Supplemental iron therapy is recommended for all patients whose serum ferritin is <100 μg/L or whose serum transferrin saturation is <20%. During initial therapy and after any dosage adjustment, the hematocrit is determined once a week (HIV-infected and cancer patients) or twice a week (renal failure patients) until it has stabilized in the target range and the maintenance dose has been established; the hematocrit then is monitored at regular intervals. If the hematocrit increases by >4 points in any 2-week period, the dose should be decreased. Due to the time required for erythropoiesis and the erythrocyte half-life, hematocrit changes lag behind dosage adjustments by 2-6 weeks. The dose of darbepoetin should be decreased if the hemoglobin increase exceeds 1 g/dL in any 2-week period because of the association of excessive rate of rise of hemoglobin with adverse cardiovascular events.

During hemodialysis, patients receiving epoetin alfa or darbepoetin may require increased anticoagulation. The risk of thrombotic events is higher in adults with ischemic heart disease or congestive heart failure receiving epoetin alfa therapy with the goal of reaching a normal hematocrit (42%) than in those with a lower target hematocrit of 30%. ESA use is associated with increased rates of cancer recurrence and decreased on-study survival in patients in whom the drugs are administered for cancer-induced or for chemotherapy-induced anemia. The most common side effect of epoetin alfa therapy is aggravation of hypertension, which occurs in 20-30% of patients and most often is associated with a rapid rise in hematocrit. ESAs should not be used in patients with preexisting uncontrolled hypertension. Patients may require initiation of, or increases in, antihypertensive therapy. Hypertensive encephalopathy and seizures have occurred in chronic renal failure patients treated with epoetin alfa. Headache, tachycardia, edema, shortness of breath, nausea, vomiting, diarrhea, injection site stinging, and flu-like symptoms (e.g., arthralgias and myalgias) also have been reported in conjunction with epoetin alfa therapy.

Anemia of Chronic Renal Failure. Patients with anemia secondary to chronic kidney disease are ideal candidates for epoetin alfa therapy. The response in predialysis, peritoneal dialysis, and hemodialysis patients depends on the severity of the renal failure, the erythropoietin dose and route of administration, and iron availability. The subcutaneous route of administration is preferred over the intravenous route because absorption is slower and the amount of drug required is reduced by 20-40%. The dose of epoetin alfa should be adjusted to obtain a gradual rise in the hematocrit over a 2- to 4-month period to a final hematocrit of 33-36%. Treatment to hematocrit levels >36% is not recommended.

Patients are started on doses of 80-120 units/kg of epoetin alfa, given subcutaneously, 3 times a week. The final maintenance dose of epoetin alfa can vary from 10 units/kg to >300 units/kg, with an average dose of

75 units/kg, 3 times a week. Children <5 years of age generally require a higher dose. Resistance to therapy is common in patients who develop an inflammatory illness or become iron deficient, so close monitoring of general health and iron status is essential. Less common causes of resistance include occult blood loss, folic acid deficiency, carnitine deficiency, inadequate dialysis, aluminum toxicity, and osteitis fibrosa cystica secondary to hyperparathyroidism. Darbepoetin alfa is approved for use in patients who are anemic secondary to chronic kidney disease. The recommended starting dose is 0.45 μg/kg administered intravenously or subcutaneously once weekly, with dose adjustments depending on the response. Like epoetin alfa, side effects tend to occur when patients experience a rapid rise in hemoglobin concentration; a rise of <1 g/dL every 2 weeks generally is considered safe.

Anemia in AIDS Patients. Epoetin alfa therapy has been approved for the treatment of HIV-infected patients, especially those on zidovudine therapy. Excellent responses to doses of 100-300 units/kg, given subcutaneously 3 times a week, generally are seen in patients with zidovudine-induced anemia.

Cancer-Related Anemias. Epoetin alfa therapy, 150 units/kg 3 times a week or 450-600 units/kg once a week, can reduce the transfusion requirement in cancer patients undergoing chemotherapy. Therapeutic guidelines recommend the use of epoetin alfa in patients with chemotherapy-associated anemia when hemoglobin levels fall below 10 g/dL, basing the decision to treat less severe anemia (Hb, 10-12 g/dL) on clinical circumstances. For anemia associated with hematologic malignancies, the guidelines support the use of recombinant erythropoietin in patients with low-grade myelodysplastic syndrome. A baseline serum erythropoietin level may help to predict the response; most patients with blood levels >500 IU/L are unlikely to respond to any dose of the drug. Most patients treated with epoetin alfa experience an improvement in their anemia and their sense of well-being.

Recent case reports suggest a direct effect of both epoetin alfa and darbepoetin alfa in stimulation of tumor cells. A meta-analysis of a large number of patients and clinical trials estimates the risk at ~10% higher than nontreated cancer patients. This finding is being evaluated by the FDA and warrants serious attention.

Surgery and Autologous Blood Donation. Epoetin alfa has been used perioperatively to treat anemia (hematocrit 30-36%) and reduce the need for erythrocyte transfusion. Patients undergoing elective orthopedic and cardiac procedures have been treated with 150-300 units/kg of epoetin alfa once daily for the 10 days preceding surgery, on the day of surgery, and for 4 days after surgery. As an alternative, 600 units/kg can be given on days 21, 14, and 7 before surgery, with an additional dose on the day of surgery. Epoetin alfa also has been used to improve autologous blood donation.

Other Uses. Epoetin alfa has received orphan drug status from the FDA for the treatment of the anemia of prematurity, HIV infection, and myelodysplasia. In the latter case, even very high doses >1000 units/kg 2 to 3 times a week have had limited success. Highly competitive athletes have used epoetin alfa to increase their hemoglobin levels ("blood doping") and improve performance. Unfortunately, this misuse of the drug has been implicated in the deaths of several athletes and is strongly discouraged.

MYELOID GROWTH FACTORS

The myeloid growth factors are glycoproteins that stimulate the proliferation and differentiation of one or more myeloid cell lines. Recombinant forms of several growth factors have been produced, including granulocyte-macrophage colony-stimulating factor (GM-CSF), G-CSF, IL-3, M-CSF or CSF-1, and stem cell factor (SCF) (*see* Table 37–1).

Myeloid growth factors are produced naturally by a number of different cells, including fibroblasts, endothelial cells, macrophages, and T cells (Figure 37–2). These factors are active at extremely low concentrations and act via membrane receptors of the cytokine receptor superfamily to activate the JAK/STAT signal transduction pathway. GM-CSF can stimulate proliferation, differentiation, and function of a number of the myeloid cell lineages (*see* Figure 37–1). It acts synergistically with other growth factors, including erythropoietin, at the level of the BFU. GM-CSF stimulates CFU-granulocyte(G)/erythrocyte(E)/monocyte(M)/megakaryocyte(Meg) [CFU-GEMM], CFU-GM, CFU-M, CFU-E, and CFU-Meg to increase cell production. GM-CSF also enhances the migration, phagocytosis, superoxide production, and antibody-dependent cell-mediated toxicity of neutrophils, monocytes, and eosinophils.

The G-CSF activity is restricted to neutrophils and their progenitors, stimulating their proliferation, differentiation, and function. It acts primarily on the CFU-G, although it also can play a synergistic role with IL-3 and GM-CSF in stimulating other cell lines. G-CSF enhances phagocytic and cytotoxic activities of neutrophils. G-CSF reduces inflammation by inhibiting IL-1, tumor necrosis factor, and interferon gamma. G-CSF also mobilizes primitive hematopoietic cells, including hematopoietic stem cells, from the marrow into the peripheral blood. This observation has virtually transformed the practice of stem cell transplantation, such that >90% of all such procedures today use G-CSF–mobilized peripheral blood stem cells as the donor product.

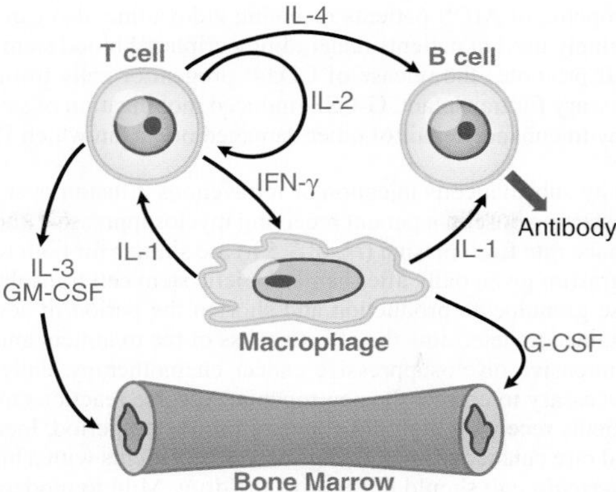

Figure 37–2 *Cytokine-cell interactions.* Macrophages, T cells, B cells, and marrow stem cells interact *via* several cytokines (IL-1, IL-2, IL-3, IL-4, IFN [interferon]-γ, GM-CSF, and G-CSF) in response to a bacterial or a foreign antigen challenge. *See* Table 37–1 for the functional activities of these various cytokines.

GRANULOCYTE-MACROPHAGE COLONY-STIMULATING FACTOR. Recombinant human GM-CSF (*sargramostim*) is a 127–amino acid glycoprotein. The primary therapeutic effect of sargramostim is to stimulate myelopoiesis.

The initial clinical application of sargramostim was in patients undergoing autologous bone marrow transplantation. By shortening the duration of neutropenia, transplant morbidity was significantly reduced without a change in long-term survival or risk of inducing an early relapse of the malignant process. The role of GM-CSF therapy in allogeneic transplantation is less clear. Its effect on neutrophil recovery is less pronounced in patients receiving prophylactic treatment for graft-versus-host disease (GVHD). However, it may improve survival in transplant patients who exhibit early graft failure. It also has been used to mobilize CD34-positive progenitor cells for peripheral blood stem cell collection for transplantation after myeloablative chemotherapy. Sargramostim has been used to shorten the period of neutropenia and reduce morbidity in patients receiving intensive cancer chemotherapy. It also stimulates myelopoiesis in some patients with cyclic neutropenia, myelodysplasia, aplastic anemia, or AIDS-associated neutropenia.

Sargramostim (LEUKINE) is administered by subcutaneous injection or slow intravenous infusion at doses of 125-500 μg/m²/day. Plasma levels of GM-CSF rise rapidly after subcutaneous injection and then decline with a $t_{1/2}$ of 2-3 h. When given intravenously, infusions should be maintained over 3-6 h. With the initiation of therapy, there is a transient decrease in the absolute leukocyte count secondary to margination and sequestration in the lungs. This is followed by a dose-dependent, biphasic increase in leukocyte counts over the next 7-10 days. Once the drug is discontinued, the leukocyte count returns to baseline within 2-10 days. When GM-CSF is given in lower doses, the response is primarily neutrophilic, whereas monocytosis and eosinophilia are observed at larger doses. After hematopoietic stem cell transplantation or intensive chemotherapy, sargramostim is given daily during the period of maximum neutropenia until a sustained rise in the granulocyte count is observed. Frequent blood counts are essential to avoid an excessive rise in the granulocyte count. Higher doses are associated with more pronounced side effects, including bone pain, malaise, flu-like symptoms, fever, diarrhea, dyspnea, and rash. An acute reaction to the first dose, characterized by flushing, hypotension, nausea, vomiting, and dyspnea, with a fall in arterial oxygen saturation due to granulocyte sequestration in the pulmonary circulation occurs in sensitive patients. With prolonged administration, a few patients may develop a capillary leak syndrome, with peripheral edema and pleural and pericardial effusions. Other serious side effects include transient supraventricular arrhythmia, dyspnea, and elevation of serum creatinine, bilirubin, and hepatic enzymes.

GRANULOCYTE COLONY-STIMULATING FACTOR. Recombinant human G-CSF, *filgrastim* (NEUPOGEN), is a 175–amino acid glycoprotein. The principal action of filgrastim is the stimulation of CFU-G to increase neutrophil production (*see* Figure 37–1).

Filgrastim is effective in the treatment of severe neutropenia after autologous hematopoietic stem cell transplantation and high-dose cancer chemotherapy. Like GM-CSF, filgrastim shortens the period of severe neutropenia and reduces morbidity secondary to bacterial and fungal infections. G-CSF also is effective in the treatment of severe congenital neutropenias. Filgrastim therapy can improve neutrophil counts in some patients with myelodysplasia or marrow damage (moderately severe aplastic anemia or tumor infiltration of the marrow). The neutropenia of AIDS patients receiving zidovudine also can be partially or completely reversed. Filgrastim is routinely used in patients undergoing peripheral blood stem cell (PBSC) collection for stem cell transplantation. It promotes the release of $CD34^+$ progenitor cells from the marrow, reducing the number of collections necessary for transplant. G-CSF–induced mobilization of stem cells into the circulation has been promoted as a way to enhance repair of other damaged organs in which PBSC might play a role.

Filgrastim is administered by subcutaneous injection or intravenous infusion over at least 30 min at doses of 1-20 μg/kg/day. The usual starting dose in a patient receiving myelosuppressive chemotherapy is 5 μg/kg/day. The distribution and clearance rate from plasma ($t_{1/2}$ of 3.5 h) are similar for both routes of administration. As with GM-CSF therapy, filgrastim given daily after hematopoietic stem cell transplantation or intensive cancer chemotherapy will increase granulocyte production and shorten the period of severe neutropenia. Frequent blood counts should be obtained to determine the effectiveness of the treatment and guide dosage adjustment. In patients who received intensive myelosuppressive cancer chemotherapy, daily administration of G-CSF for ≥14-21 days may be necessary to correct the neutropenia. Adverse reactions to filgrastim include mild to moderate bone pain in patients receiving high doses over a protracted period, local skin reactions following subcutaneous injection, and rare cutaneous necrotizing vasculitis. Patients with a history of hypersensitivity to proteins produced by *Escherichia coli* should not receive the drug. Mild to moderate splenomegaly has been observed in patients on long-term therapy.

Pegylated recombinant human G-CSF *pegfilgrastim* (NEULASTA) is available. The clearance of pegfilgrastim by glomerular filtration is minimized, thus making neutrophil-mediated clearance the primary route of elimination. Consequently the circulating $t_{1/2}$ of pegfilgrastim is longer than that of filgrastim, allowing for more sustained duration of action and less frequent dosing. The recommended dose for pegfilgrastim is fixed at 6 mg administered subcutaneously.

THROMBOPOIETIC GROWTH FACTORS

INTERLEUKIN-11. Interleukin-11 is a cytokine that stimulates hematopoiesis, intestinal epithelial cell growth, and osteoclasto-genesis and inhibits adipogenesis. Interleukin-11 also enhances megakaryocyte maturation in vitro. Recombinant human IL-11 *oprelvekin* (NEUMEGA) leads to a thrombopoietic response in 5-9 days when administered daily to normal subjects.

The drug is administered to patients at 25-50 μg/kg per day subcutaneously with a $t_{1/2}$ ~7 h. Oprelvekin is approved for use in patients undergoing chemotherapy for nonmyeloid malignancies with severe thrombocytopenia (platelet count <20,000/μL), and it is administered until the platelet count returns to >100,000/μL. The major complications of therapy are fluid retention and associated cardiac symptoms, such as tachycardia, palpitation, edema, and shortness of breath; this is a significant concern in elderly patients and often requires concomitant therapy with diuretics. Also reported are blurred vision, injection-site rash or erythema, and paresthesias.

THROMBOPOIETIN. Thrombopoietin, a glycoprotein produced by the liver, marrow stromal cells, and other organs, is the primary regulator of platelet production. Two forms of recombinant thrombopoietin have been developed for clinical use. One is a truncated version of the native protein, termed *recombinant human megakaryocyte growth and development factor* (rHuMGDF) that is covalently modified with polyethylene glycol to increase the circulatory $t_{1/2}$. The second is the full-length polypeptide termed *recombinant human thrombopoietin* (rHuTPO).

In clinical trials, both drugs are safe but data on efficacy are mixed. Due to several concerns including the immunogenicity of these agents, efforts are under way to develop small molecular mimics of recombinant thrombopoietin. Two of these agents are FDA-approved for use in patients with immune thrombocytopenic purpura (ITP) who have failed to respond to more conventional treatments. *Romiplostim* (NPLATE) contains 4 copies of a small peptide that binds with high affinity to the thrombopoietin receptor, grafted onto an immunoglobulin scaffold. Romiplostim is safe and efficacious in patients with ITP. The drug is administered weekly by subcutaneous injection, starting with a dose of 1 μg/kg, titrated to a maximum of 10 μg/kg, until platelet count increases above 50,000/μL. *Eltrombopag* (PROMACTA) is a small molecule that is a thrombopoietin receptor agonist. Eltrombopag is administered orally; the recommended starting dose is 50 mg/day, titrated to 75 mg depending on platelet response.

Drugs Effective in Iron Deficiency and Other Hypochromic Anemias

IRON AND IRON SALTS

Iron deficiency is the most common nutritional cause of anemia in humans. It can result from inadequate iron intake, malabsorption, blood loss, or an increased requirement, as with pregnancy. When severe, it results in a characteristic microcytic, hypochromic anemia. In addition to its role in

Table 37–2

The Body Content of Iron

	MG/KG OF BODY WEIGHT	
	MALE	FEMALE
Essential iron		
Hemoglobin	31	28
Myoglobin and enzymes	6	5
Storage iron	13	4
Total	50	37

hemoglobin, iron also is an essential component of myoglobin, heme enzymes (e.g., cytochromes, catalase, and peroxidase), and the metalloflavoprotein enzymes (e.g., xanthine oxidase and the α-glycerophosphate oxidase). Iron deficiency can affect metabolism in muscle independently of the effect of anemia on O_2 delivery. This may reflect a reduction in the activity of iron-dependent mitochondrial enzymes. Iron deficiency also has been associated with behavioral and learning problems in children, abnormalities in catecholamine metabolism, and possibly, impaired heat production.

METABOLISM OF IRON. The body store of iron is divided between essential iron-containing compounds and excess iron, which is held in storage (Table 37–2).

Hemoglobin (Hb) dominates the essential fraction. Each Hb molecule contains 4 atoms of iron, amounting to 1.1 mg (20 μmol) of iron/mL of red blood cells. Other forms of essential iron include *myoglobin* and a variety of heme and nonheme iron-dependent enzymes. *Ferritin* is a protein-iron storage complex that exists as individual molecules or as aggregates. *Apoferritin* (MW ~450 kDa) is composed of 24 polypeptide subunits that form an outer shell around a storage cavity for polynuclear hydrous ferric oxide phosphate. More than 30% of the weight of ferritin may be iron (4000 atoms of iron per ferritin molecule). Ferritin aggregates, referred to as *hemosiderin* and visible by light microscopy, constitute about one-third of normal stores. The 2 predominant sites of iron storage are the reticuloendothelial system and the hepatocytes.

Internal exchange of iron is accomplished by the plasma protein *transferrin*, a 76-kDa glycoprotein that has 2 binding sites for ferric iron. Iron is delivered from transferrin to intracellular sites by means of specific transferrin receptors in the plasma membrane. The iron-transferrin complex binds to the receptor, and the ternary complex is internalized through clathrin-coated pits by receptor-mediated endocytosis. A proton-pumping ATPase lowers the pH of the intracellular vesicular compartment (the endosomes) to ~5.5. Iron subsequently dissociates and the receptor returns the apotransferrin to the cell surface, where it is released into the extracellular environment. Cells regulate their expression of transferrin receptors and intracellular ferritin in response to the iron supply. The synthesis of apoferritin and transferrin receptors is regulated post-transcriptionally by 2 iron-regulating proteins 1 and 2 (IRP1 and IRP2). These IRPs are cytosolic RNA-binding proteins that bind to iron-regulating elements (IREs) present in the 5′ or 3′ untranslated regions of mRNA encoding apoferritin or the transferrin receptors, respectively. Binding of these IRPs to the 5′ IRE of apoferritin mRNA represses translation, whereas binding to the 3′ IRE of mRNA encoding the transferrin receptors enhances transcript stability, thereby increasing protein production.

The flow of iron through the plasma amounts to a total of 30-40 mg/day in the adult (~0.46 mg/kg of body weight). The major internal circulation of iron involves the erythron and reticuloendothelial cells (Figure 37–3). About 80% of the iron in plasma goes to the erythroid marrow to be packaged into new erythrocytes; these normally circulate for ~120 days before being catabolized by the reticuloendothelial system. At that time, a portion of the iron is immediately returned to the plasma bound to transferrin, while another portion is incorporated into the ferritin stores of reticuloendothelial cells and returned to the circulation more gradually. With abnormalities in erythrocyte maturation, the predominant portion of iron assimilated by the erythroid marrow may be rapidly localized in the reticuloendothelial cells as defective red-cell precursors are broken down; this is termed *ineffective erythropoiesis.* The rate of iron turnover in plasma may be reduced by half or more with red-cell aplasia, with all the iron directed to the hepatocytes for storage.

The human body conserves its iron stores to a remarkable degree. Only 10% of the total is lost per year by normal men (i.e., ~1 mg/day). Two-thirds of this iron is excreted from the GI tract as extravasated red cells, iron in bile, and iron in exfoliated mucosal cells. The other third is accounted for by small amounts of iron in

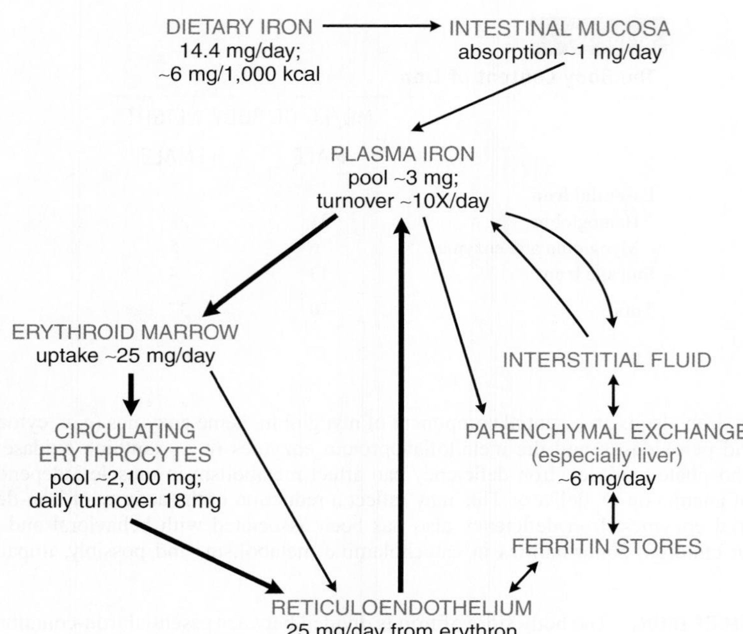

Figure 37–3 *Iron metabolism in humans (excretion omitted).*

desquamated skin and in the urine. Additional losses of iron occur in women due to menstruation. Although the average loss in menstruating women is ~0.5 mg per day, 10% of menstruating women lose >2 mg per day. Pregnancy and lactation impose an even greater requirement for iron (Table 37–3). Other causes of iron loss include blood donation, the use of anti-inflammatory drugs that cause bleeding from the gastric mucosa, and GI disease with associated bleeding.

The limited physiological losses of iron point to the primary importance of absorption in determining the body's iron content. After acidification and partial digestion of food in the stomach, iron is presented to the intestinal mucosa as either inorganic iron or heme iron. A ferrireductase, duodenal cytochrome B (Dcytb), located on luminal surface of absorptive cells of the duodenum and upper small intestine, reduces the iron to the ferrous state, which is the substrate for the *divalent metal (ion) transporter 1* (DMT1). DMT1 transports the iron to basolateral membrane, where it is taken up by another transporter, *ferroportin* (Fpn; SLC40A1), and subsequently reoxidized to Fe^{3+}, primarily by *hephaestin* (Hp; HEPH), a transmembrane copper-dependent ferroxidase. Apo-transferrin (Tf) binds the resultant oxidized Fe^{3+}.

Table 37–3

Iron Requirements for Pregnancy

	AVERAGE (mg)	RANGE (mg)
External iron loss	170	150-200
Expansion of red cell mass	450	200-600
Fetal iron	270	200-370
Iron in placenta and cord	90	30-170
Blood loss at delivery	150	90-310
Total requirement[a]	980	580-1340
Cost of pregnancy[b]	680	440-1050

[a]*Blood loss at delivery not included.*

[b]*Iron lost by the mother; expansion of red-cell mass not included.*

Source: Council on Foods and Nutrition. Iron deficiency in the United States. JAMA 1968; 203:407–412. Used with permission.

Table 37–4

Daily Iron Absorption Requirement

SUBJECT	IRON REQUIREMENT (μg/kg)	AVAILABLE IRON Poor diet–Good diet (μg/kg)	SAFETY FACTOR: AVAILABLE/ REQUIREMENT
Infant	67	33-66	0.5-1
Child	22	48-96	2-4
Adolescent (male)	21	30-60	1.5-3
Adolescent (female)	20	30-60	1.5-3
Adult (male)	13	26-52	2-4
Adult (female)	21	18-36	1-2
Mid-to-late pregnancy	80	18-36	0.22-0.45

The numbers in columns 2 and 3 refer to iron absorption via the GI tract in μg/kg body weight. As noted in Figure 37–3, of 14.4 mg of dietary iron presented to the GI tract each day, only ~1 mg is absorbed. See text concerning factors influencing iron absorption and differential absorption of heme versus nonheme iron.

IRON REQUIREMENTS AND THE AVAILABILITY OF DIETARY IRON. Adult men must absorb only 13 μg of iron/kg of body weight/day (~1 mg/day), whereas menstruating women require ~21 μg/kg (~1.4 mg) per day. In the last 2 trimesters of pregnancy, requirements increase to ~80 μg/kg (5-6 mg) per day; infants have similar requirements due to their rapid growth (Table 37–4).

The difference between dietary supply and requirements is reflected in the size of iron stores, which are low or absent when iron balance is precarious and high when iron balance is favorable. In infants after the third month of life and in pregnant women after the first trimester, stores of iron are negligible. Menstruating women have approximately one-third the stored iron found in adult men (*see* Table 37–2).

Although the iron content of the diet obviously is important, of greater nutritional significance is the bioavailability of iron in food. Heme iron, which constitutes only 6% of dietary iron, is far more available and is absorbed independent of the diet composition; it therefore represents 30% of iron absorbed. The nonheme fraction represents the larger amount of dietary iron ingested by the economically underprivileged. In a vegetarian diet, nonheme iron is absorbed very poorly because of the inhibitory action of a variety of dietary components, particularly phosphates. Ascorbic acid and meat facilitate the absorption of nonheme iron. In developed countries, the normal adult diet contains ~6 mg of iron per 1000 calories, providing an average daily intake for adult men of between 12 and 20 mg and for adult women of between 8 and 15 mg. Foods high in iron (>5 mg/100 g) include organ meats such as liver and heart, brewer's yeast, wheat germ, egg yolks, oysters, and certain dried beans and fruits; foods low in iron (<1 mg/100 g) include milk and milk products and most nongreen vegetables. Iron also may be added from cooking in iron pots. In assessing dietary iron intake, it is important to consider not just the amount of iron ingested but its bioavailability.

IRON DEFICIENCY. The prevalence of iron-deficiency anemia in the U.S. is on the order of 1-4% and depends on the economic status of the population. In developing countries, up to 20-40% of infants and pregnant women may be affected. Better iron balance has resulted from the practice of fortifying flour, the use of iron-fortified formulas for infants, and the prescription of medicinal iron supplements during pregnancy.

Iron-deficiency anemia results from dietary intake of iron that is inadequate to meet normal requirements (nutritional iron deficiency), blood loss, or interference with iron absorption. More severe iron deficiency is usually the result of blood loss, either from the GI tract, or in women, from the uterus. Finally, treatment of patients with erythropoietin can result in a functional iron deficiency. Iron deficiency in infants and young children can lead to behavioral disturbances and can impair development, which may not be fully reversible. Iron deficiency in children also can lead to an increased risk of lead toxicity secondary to pica and an increased absorption of heavy metals. Premature and low-birthweight infants are at greatest risk for developing iron deficiency, especially if they are not breast-fed and/or do not receive iron-fortified formula. After the age of 2-3 years, the requirement for iron declines until adolescence when rapid growth combined with irregular dietary habits again increases the risk of iron deficiency. Adolescent girls are at greatest risk; the dietary iron intake of most girls ages 11-18 is insufficient to meet their requirements.

TREATMENT OF IRON DEFICIENCY

GENERAL THERAPEUTIC PRINCIPLES. The response of iron-deficiency anemia to iron therapy is influenced by several factors, including the severity of anemia, the ability of the patient to tolerate and absorb medicinal iron, and the presence of other complicating illnesses. Therapeutic effectiveness is best measured by the resulting increase in the rate of production of red cells. The magnitude of the marrow response to iron therapy is proportional to the severity of the anemia (level of erythropoietin stimulation) and the amount of iron delivered to marrow precursors.

THERAPY WITH ORAL IRON. Orally administered ferrous sulfate is the treatment of choice for iron deficiency. Ferrous salts are absorbed about 3 times as well as ferric salts. Variations in the particular ferrous salt have relatively little effect on bioavailability; the sulfate (FEOSOL, others), fumarate (HEMOCYTE, FEOSTAT, others), succinate, gluconate (FERGON, others), aspartate, other ferrous salts, and polysaccharide-ferrihydrite complex (NIFEREX, others) are absorbed to approximately the same extent.

Other iron compounds have utility in fortification of foods. Reduced iron (metallic iron, elemental iron) is as effective as ferrous sulfate, provided that the material employed has a small particle size. Large-particle ferrum reductum and iron phosphate salts have a much lower bioavailability. Ferric edetate has been shown to have good bioavailability and to have advantages for maintenance of the normal appearance and taste of food. The amount of iron in iron tablets is important. It also is essential that the coating of the tablet dissolve rapidly in the stomach. Delayed-release preparations are available, but absorption from such preparations varies. Ascorbic acid (≥200 mg) increases the absorption of medicinal iron by at least 30%. However, the increased uptake is associated with an increase in the incidence of side effects. Preparations that contain other compounds with therapeutic action, such as vitamin B_{12}, folate, or cobalt, are not recommended because the patient's response to the combination cannot easily be interpreted.

The average dose for the treatment of iron-deficiency anemia is ~200 mg of iron per day (2-3 mg/kg), given in 3 equal doses of 65 mg. Children weighing 15-30 kg can take half the average adult dose; small children and infants can tolerate relatively large doses of iron, e.g., 5 mg/kg. When the object is the prevention of iron deficiency in pregnant women, e.g., doses of 15 to 30 mg of iron per day are adequate. Bioavailability of iron is reduced with food and by concurrent antacids. For a rapid response or to counteract continued bleeding, as much as 120 mg of iron may be administered 4 times a day. The duration of treatment is governed by the rate of recovery of hemoglobin (Table 37–5) and the desire to create iron stores.

UNTOWARD EFFECTS OF ORAL PREPARATIONS OF IRON. Side effects include heartburn, nausea, upper gastric discomfort, and diarrhea or constipation. A good policy is to initiate therapy at a small dosage, and then gradually to increase the dosage to that desired. Only individuals with underlying disorders that augment the absorption of iron run the hazard of developing iron overload (hemochromatosis).

IRON POISONING. Large amounts of ferrous salts are toxic, but fatalities are rare in adults. Most deaths occur in children, particularly between the ages of 12 and 24 months. As little as 1-2 g of iron may cause death, but 2-10 g usually is ingested in fatal cases. All iron preparations should be kept in childproof bottles. Signs and symptoms of severe poisoning may occur within 30 min after ingestion or may be delayed for several hours. They include abdominal pain, diarrhea, or vomiting of brown or bloody stomach contents containing pills. Of particular concern are pallor or cyanosis, lassitude, drowsiness, hyperventilation due to acidosis, and cardiovascular collapse. If death does not occur within 6 h, there may be a transient period of apparent recovery, followed by death in 12-24 h. The corrosive injury to the stomach may result in pyloric stenosis or gastric scarring. In the evaluation of a child thought to have ingested iron, a color test for iron in the gastric contents and determination of the concentration of iron in plasma can be performed. If the latter is <63 μmol (3.5 mg/L), the child is not in immediate danger. However, vomiting should be induced when there is iron

Table 37–5

Average Response to Oral Iron

TOTAL DOSE OF IRON (mg/day)	ESTIMATED ABSORPTION		INCREASE IN BLOOD Hb (g/L/day)
	%	mg	
35	40	14	0.7
105	24	25	1.4
195	18	35	1.9
390	12	45	2.2

in the stomach, and an X-ray should be taken to evaluate the number of pills remaining in the small bowel (iron tablets are radiopaque). When the plasma concentration of iron is greater than the total iron-binding capacity (63 μmol; 3.5 mg/L), *deferoxamine* should be administered (*see* Chapter 67). The speed of diagnosis and therapy is very important. With early treatment, the mortality from iron poisoning can be reduced from 45% to ~1%. *Deferiprone* is an oral iron chelator approved to treat iron overload due to blood transfusions in patients with thalassemia.

THERAPY WITH PARENTERAL IRON. When oral iron therapy fails, parenteral iron administration may be an effective alternative. Common indications are iron malabsorption (e.g., sprue, short bowel syndrome), severe oral iron intolerance, as a routine supplement to total parenteral nutrition, and in patients who are receiving erythropoietin. Parenteral iron can be given to iron-deficient patients and pregnant women to create iron stores, something that would take months to achieve by the oral route.

The rate of hemoglobin response is determined by the balance between the severity of the anemia (the level of erythropoietin stimulus) and the delivery of iron to the marrow from iron absorption and iron stores. When a large intravenous dose of iron dextran is given to a severely anemic patient, the hematologic response can exceed that seen with oral iron for 1-3 weeks. Subsequently, however, the response is no better than that seen with oral iron.

Parenteral iron therapy should be used only when clearly indicated because acute hypersensitivity, including anaphylactic and anaphylactoid reactions, can occur. Other reactions to intravenous iron include headache, malaise, fever, generalized lymphadenopathy, arthralgias, urticaria, and in some patients with rheumatoid arthritis, exacerbation of the disease. Four iron formulations are available in the U.S. These are iron dextran (DEXFERRUM or INFED), sodium ferric gluconate (FERRLECIT), ferumoxytol (FERAHEME), and iron sucrose (VENOFER). Ferumoxytol is a semisynthetic carbohydrate-coated superparamagnetic iron oxide nanoparticle that is approved for treatment of iron-deficiency anemia in patients with chronic kidney disease. The indications for the iron dextran preparations include treatment of any patient with documented iron deficiency and intolerance or irresponsiveness to oral iron. Indications for the ferric gluconate and iron sucrose are limited to patients with chronic kidney disease.

Iron Dextran. Iron dextran injection (INFED or DEXFERRUM) is a colloidal solution of ferric oxyhydroxide complexed with polymerized dextran (molecular weight, ~180,000 Da) that contains 50 mg/mL of elemental iron. The use of low-molecular-weight iron dextran has reduced the incidence of toxicity relative to that observed with high-molecular-weight preparations (IMFERON). Iron dextran can be administered by either intravenous (preferred) or intramuscular injection. Given intravenously in a dose <500 mg, the iron dextran complex is cleared exponentially with a plasma $t_{1/2}$ of 6 h. When ≥1 g is administered intravenously as total dose therapy, reticuloendothelial cell clearance is constant at 10-20 mg/h.

Intramuscular injection of iron dextran should be initiated only after a test dose of 0.5 mL (25 mg of iron). If no adverse reactions are observed, the injections can proceed. The daily dose ordinarily should not exceed 0.5 mL (25 mg of iron) for infants weighing <4.5 kg (10 lb), 1 mL (50 mg of iron) for children weighing <9 kg (20 lb), and 2 mL (100 mg of iron) for other patients. However, local reactions and the concern about malignant change at the site of injection make intramuscular administration inappropriate except when the intravenous route is inaccessible. The patient should be observed for signs of immediate anaphylaxis and for an hour after injection for any signs of vascular instability or hypersensitivity, including respiratory distress, hypotension, tachycardia, or back or chest pain. Delayed hypersensitivity reactions also are observed, especially in patients with rheumatoid arthritis or a history of allergies. Fever, malaise, lymphadenopathy, arthralgias, and urticaria can develop days or weeks following injection and last for prolonged periods of time. Use iron dextran with extreme caution in patients with rheumatoid arthritis or other connective tissue diseases, and during the acute phase of an inflammatory illness. Once hypersensitivity is documented, iron dextran therapy must be abandoned. With multiple total-dose infusions such as those sometimes used in the treatment of chronic GI blood loss—accumulations of slowly metabolized iron dextran stores in reticuloendothelial cells can be impressive. The plasma ferritin level also can rise to levels associated with iron overload. It seems prudent, however, to withhold the drug whenever the plasma ferritin rises above 800 μg/L.

Sodium Ferric Gluconate. Sodium ferric gluconate is an intravenous iron preparation with a molecular size of ~295 kDa and an osmolality of 990 mOsm/kg^{-1}. Administration of ferric gluconate at doses ranging from 62.5-125 mg during hemodialysis is associated with transferrin saturation exceeding 100%. Unlike iron dextran, which requires processing by macrophages that may require several weeks, ~80% of sodium ferric gluconate is delivered to transferrin with in 24 h. Sodium ferric gluconate also has a lower risk of inducing serious anaphylactic reactions than iron dextran.

Iron Sucrose. Iron sucrose is complex of polynuclear iron (III)-hydroxide in sucrose. Following intravenous injection, the complex is taken up by the reticuloendothelial system, where it dissociates into iron and sucrose. Iron sucrose is generally administered in daily amounts of 100-200 mg within a 14-day period to a total cumulative dose of 1000 mg. Like sodium ferric gluconate, iron sucrose appears to be better tolerated and to cause fewer adverse events than iron dextran. This agent is FDA-approved for the treatment of iron deficiency in patients with chronic kidney disease.

COPPER

Copper has redox properties similar to that of iron and is simultaneously essential and potentially toxic to the cell. Cells have virtually no free copper; rather, copper is stored by metallothioneins and distributed by specialized chaperones to sites that make use of copper's redox properties.

Copper deficiency is extremely rare. Even in clinical states associated with hypocupremia (sprue, celiac disease, and nephrotic syndrome), effects of copper deficiency usually are not demonstrable. Anemia due to copper deficiency has been described in individuals who have undergone intestinal bypass surgery, in those who are receiving parenteral nutrition, in malnourished infants, and in patients ingesting excessive amounts of zinc. Copper deficiency interferes with the absorption of iron and its release from reticuloendothelial cells. In humans, the prominent findings have been leukopenia, particularly granulocytopenia, and anemia. Concentrations of iron in plasma are variable, and the anemia is not always microcytic. When a low plasma copper concentration is determined in the presence of leukopenia and anemia, a therapeutic trial with copper is appropriate. Daily doses up to 0.1 mg/kg of cupric sulfate have been given by mouth, or 1-2 mg per day may be added to the solution of nutrients for parenteral administration.

PYRIDOXINE. Patients with either hereditary or acquired sideroblastic anemia characteristically have impaired hemoglobin synthesis and accumulate iron in the perinuclear mitochondria of erythroid precursor cells, so-called ringed sideroblasts. Oral therapy with pyridoxine is of proven benefit in correcting the sideroblastic anemias associated with the antituberculosis drugs isoniazid and pyrazinamide, which act as vitamin B_6 antagonists. A daily dose of 50 mg of pyridoxine completely corrects the defect without interfering with treatment, and routine supplementation of pyridoxine often is recommended (*see* Chapter 56). In contrast, if pyridoxine is given to counteract the sideroblastic abnormality associated with administration of levodopa, the effectiveness of levodopa in controlling Parkinson disease is decreased. Pyridoxine therapy does not correct the sideroblastic abnormalities produced by chloramphenicol or lead. Patients with idiopathic acquired sideroblastic anemia generally fail to respond to oral pyridoxine, and those individuals who appear to have a pyridoxine-responsive anemia require prolonged therapy with large doses of the vitamin, 50-500 mg/day.

RIBOFLAVIN. The spontaneous appearance in humans of red-cell aplasia due to riboflavin deficiency undoubtedly is rare, if it occurs at all. However, it seems reasonable to include riboflavin in the nutritional management of patients with gross, generalized malnutrition.

B_{12}, Folic Acid, and the Treatment of Megaloblastic Anemias

Vitamin B_{12} and folic acid are dietary essentials. A deficiency of either vitamin impairs DNA synthesis in any cell in which chromosomal replication and division are taking place. Because tissues with the greatest rate of cell turnover show the most dramatic changes, the hematopoietic system is especially sensitive to deficiencies of these vitamins.

METABOLIC ROLES OF VITAMIN B_{12} AND FOLIC ACID. The major roles of vitamin B_{12} and folic acid in intracellular metabolism are summarized in Figure 37–4. Intracellular vitamin B_{12} is maintained as 2 active coenzymes: *methylcobalamin* and *deoxyadenosylcobalamin*.

Methylcobalamin (CH_3B_{12}) supports the *methionine synthetase* reaction, which is essential for normal metabolism of folate. Methyl groups contributed by methyltetrahydrofolate ($CH_3H_4PteGlu_1$) are used to form methylcobalamin, which then acts as a methyl group donor for the conversion of homocysteine to methionine. This folate–cobalamin interaction is pivotal for normal synthesis of purines and pyrimidines, and therefore of DNA. The methionine synthetase reaction is largely responsible for the control of the recycling of folate cofactors; the maintenance of intracellular concentrations of folylpolyglutamates; and, through the synthesis of methionine and its product, *S-adenosylmethionine* (SAM), the maintenance of a number of methylation reactions.

Deoxyadenosylcobalamin (deoxyadenosyl B_{12}) is a cofactor for the *mitochondrial mutase* enzyme that catalyzes the isomerization of l-methylmalonyl CoA to succinyl CoA, an important reaction in carbohydrate and lipid metabolism. This reaction has no direct relationship to the metabolic pathways that involve folate.

Because methyltetrahydrofolate is the principal folate congener supplied to cells, the transfer of the methyl group to cobalamin is essential for the adequate supply of tetrahydrofolate ($H_4PteGlu_1$). Tetrahydrofolate is a precursor for the formation of intracellular folylpolyglutamates; it also acts as the acceptor of a 1-carbon unit in the conversion of serine to glycine, with the resultant formation of 5,10-methylenetetrahydrofolate (5,10-CH_2H_4PteGlu). The latter derivative donates the methylene group to deoxyuridylate (dUMP) for the

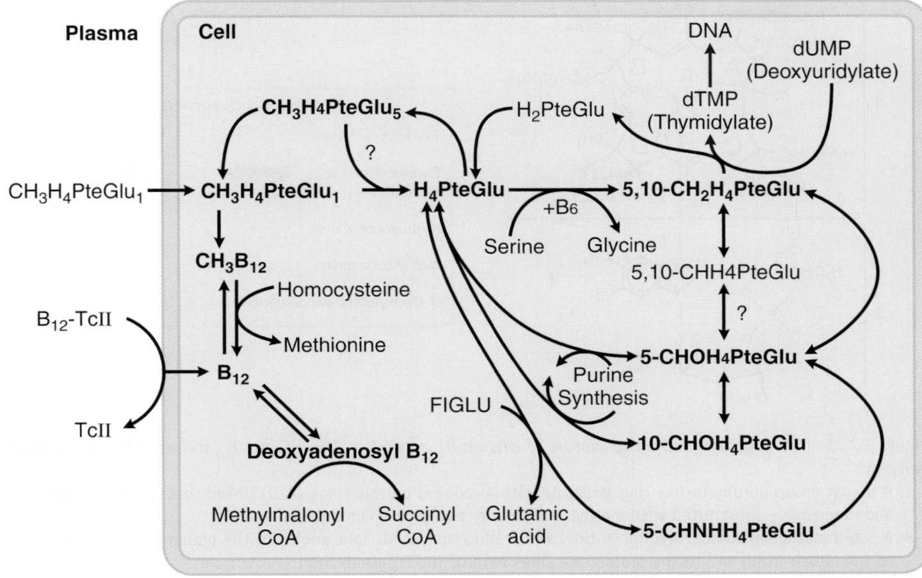

Figure 37–4 *Interrelationships and metabolic roles of vitamin B_{12} and folic acid. See* text for explanation and Figure 37–5 for structures of the various folate coenzymes. FIGLU, formiminoglutamic acid, which arises from the catabolism of histidine; TcII, transcobalamin II; $CH_3H_4PteGlu_1$, methyltetrahydrofolate.

synthesis of thymidylate (dTMP)—an extremely important reaction in DNA synthesis. In the process, the 5,10-CH_2H_4PteGlu is converted to dihydrofolate (H_2PteGlu). The cycle then is completed by the reduction of the H_2PteGlu to H_4PteGlu by dihydrofolate reductase, the step that is blocked by folate antagonists such as methotrexate (*see* Chapter 61). As shown in Figure 37–4, other pathways also lead to the synthesis of 5,10-methylenetetrahydrofolate. These pathways are important in the metabolism of formiminoglutamic acid (FIGLU) and purines and pyrimidines.

Deficiency of either vitamin B_{12} or folate decreases the synthesis of methionine and SAM, which interferes with protein biosynthesis, a number of methylation reactions, and the synthesis of polyamines. In addition, the cell responds to the deficiency by redirecting folate metabolic pathways to supply increasing amounts of methyltetrahydrofolate; this tends to preserve essential methylation reactions at the expense of nucleic acid synthesis. With vitamin B_{12} deficiency, methylenetetrahydrofolate reductase activity increases, directing available intracellular folates into the methyltetrahydrofolate pool (not shown in Figure 37–4). The methyltetrahydrofolate then is trapped by the lack of sufficient vitamin B_{12} to accept and transfer methyl groups, and subsequent steps in folate metabolism that require tetrahydrofolate are deprived of substrate. This process provides a common basis for the development of megaloblastic anemia with deficiency of either vitamin B_{12} or folic acid.

The mechanisms responsible for the neurological lesions of vitamin B_{12} deficiency are less well understood. Damage to the myelin sheath is the most obvious lesion in this neuropathy. This observation led to the early suggestion that the deoxyadenosyl B_{12}–dependent methylmalonyl CoA mutase reaction, a step in propionate metabolism, is related to the abnormality. However, other evidence suggests that the deficiency of methionine synthetase and the block of the conversion of methionine to SAM are more likely to be responsible.

VITAMIN B_{12}

Humans depend on exogenous sources of vitamin B_{12} (*see* structure in Figure 37–5). In nature, the primary sources are certain microorganisms that grow in soil, or the intestinal lumen of animals that synthesize the vitamin. The daily nutritional requirement of 3-5 μg must generally be obtained from animal by-products in the diet. However, some vitamin B_{12} is available from legumes, which are contaminated with bacteria that can synthesize vitamin B_{12}, and vegetarians often fortify their diets with a wide range of vitamins and minerals; thus, strict vegetarians rarely develop vitamin B_{12} deficiency. The terms *vitamin B_{12}* and *cyanocobalamin* are used interchangeably as generic terms for all of the cobamides active in humans. Preparations of vitamin B_{12} for therapeutic use contain either cyanocobalamin or hydroxocobalamin because only these derivatives remain active after storage.

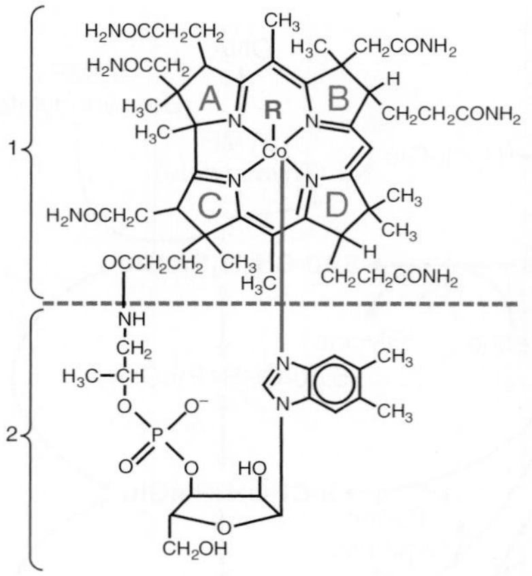

Vitamin B_{12} Congeners

Permissive Name	*R Group*
Cyanocobalamin (Vitamin B_{12})	–CN
Hydroxocobalamin	–OH
Methylcobalamin	$-CH_3$
5'-Deoxyadenosylcobalamin	–5'-Deoxyadenosyl

Figure 37–5 *The structures and nomenclature of vitamin B_{12} congeners.* The vitamin B_{12} molecule has the 3 major portions:

1. A planar group porphyrin-like ring structure with 4 reduced pyrrole rings (A-D) linked to a central cobalt atom and extensively substituted with methyl, acetamide, and propionamide residues.
2. A 5,6-dimethylbenzimidazolyl nucleotide, which links almost at right angles to the planar nucleus with bonds to the cobalt atom and to the propionate side chain of the C pyrrole ring.
3. A variable R group—the most important of which are found in the stable compounds cyanocobalamin and hydroxocobalamin and the active coenzymes methylcobalamin and 5-deoxyadenosylcobalamin.

METABOLIC FUNCTIONS. The active coenzymes methylcobalamin and 5-deoxyadenosylcobalamin are essential for cell growth and replication. Methylcobalamin is required for the conversion of homocysteine to methionine and its derivative S-adenosylmethionine. In addition, when concentrations of vitamin B_{12} are inadequate, folate becomes "trapped" as methyltetrahydrofolate to cause a functional deficiency of other required intracellular forms of folic acid (*see* Figure 37–4). The hematologic abnormalities in vitamin B_{12}–deficient patients result from this process. Deoxyadenosylcobalamin is required for the rearrangement of methylmalonyl CoA to succinyl CoA (*see* Figure 37–4).

ABSORPTION, DISTRIBUTION, ELIMINATION, AND DAILY REQUIREMENTS. In the presence of gastric acid and pancreatic proteases, dietary vitamin B_{12} is released from food and salivary binding protein and bound to gastric intrinsic factor. When the vitamin B_{12}–intrinsic factor complex reaches the ileum, it interacts with a receptor on the mucosal cell surface and is actively transported into circulation. Vitamin B_{12} deficiency in adults is rarely the result of a deficient diet per se; rather, it usually reflects a defect in one or another aspect of this complex sequence of absorption (Figure 37–6). Antibodies to parietal cells or intrinsic factor complex also can play a prominent role in producing a deficiency. Several intestinal conditions can interfere with absorption, including pancreatic disorders (loss of pancreatic protease secretion), bacterial overgrowth, intestinal parasites, sprue, and localized damage to ileal mucosal cells by disease or as a result of surgery.

Absorbed vitamin B_{12} binds to transcobalamin II, a plasma β-globulin, for transport to tissues. The supply of vitamin B_{12} available for tissues is directly related to the size of the hepatic storage pool and the amount of vitamin B_{12} bound to transcobalamin II (*see* Figure 37–6). Vitamin B_{12} bound to transcobalamin II is rapidly cleared from plasma and preferentially distributed to hepatic parenchymal cells. As much as 90% of the body's stores of vitamin B_{12}, from 1-10 mg, is in the liver. Vitamin B_{12} is stored as the active coenzyme with a turnover rate of 0.5-8 μg per day. The recommended daily intake of the vitamin in adults is 2.4 μg. Approximately 3 μg of cobalamins are secreted into bile each day, 50-60% of which is not destined for reabsorption. Interference with reabsorption by intestinal disease can progressively deplete hepatic stores of the vitamin.

VITAMIN B_{12} DEFICIENCY. Vitamin B_{12} deficiency is recognized clinically by its impact on the hematopoietic and nervous systems. The sensitivity of the hematopoietic system relates to its high rate of cell turnover. Other tissues with high rates of cell turnover (e.g., mucosa and cervical epithelium) also have high requirements for the vitamin. As a result of an inadequate supply of vitamin B_{12}, DNA replication becomes highly abnormal. Once a hematopoietic stem cell is committed to enter a programmed series of cell divisions, the defect in chromosomal replication results in an inability of maturing cells to complete nuclear divisions while cytoplasmic maturation continues at a relatively normal rate. This results in the production of morphologically abnormal cells and death of cells during maturation, a phenomenon referred to as *ineffective hematopoiesis*. Severe deficiency affects all cell lines, and a pronounced pancytopenia results.

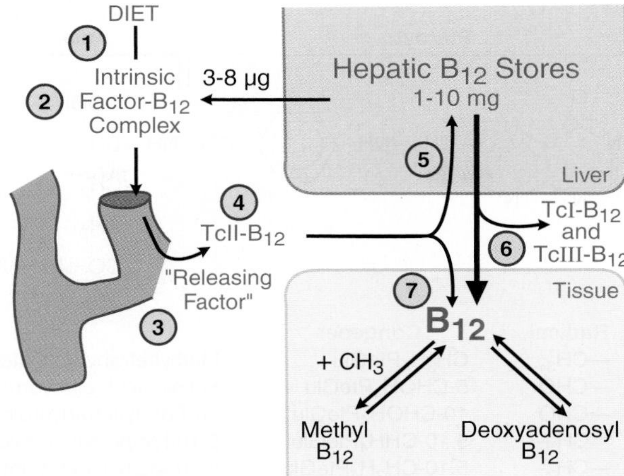

Figure 37–6 *Absorption and distribution of vitamin B_{12}.* Deficiency of vitamin B_{12} can result from a congenital or acquired defect in: (1) inadequate dietary supply; (2) inadequate secretion of intrinsic factor (classical pernicious anemia); (3) ileal disease; (4) congenital absence of transcobalamin II (TcII); or (5) rapid depletion of hepatic stores by interference with reabsorption of vitamin B_{12} excreted in bile. The utility of measurements of the concentration of vitamin B_{12} in plasma to estimate supply available to tissues can be compromised by liver disease and (6) the appearance of abnormal amounts of transcobalamins I and III (TcI and III) in plasma. The formation of methylcobalamin requires (7) normal transport into cells and an adequate supply of folic acid as $CH_3H_4PteGlu_1$.

The diagnosis of a vitamin B_{12} deficiency usually can be made using measurements of the serum vitamin B_{12} and/or serum methylmalonate (which is somewhat more sensitive and useful in identifying metabolic deficiency in patients with normal serum vitamin B_{12} levels). In managing a patient with severe megaloblastic anemia, a therapeutic trial using very small doses of the vitamin can be used to confirm the diagnosis. Serial measurements of the reticulocyte count, serum iron, and hematocrit are performed to define the characteristic recovery of normal red-cell production. The *Schilling test* can be used to measure the absorption of the vitamin and delineate the mechanism of the disease. By performing the Schilling test with and without added intrinsic factor, it is possible to discriminate between intrinsic factor deficiency by itself and primary ileal cell disease. *Vitamin B_{12} deficiency can irreversibly damage the nervous system.* Because the neurological damage can be dissociated from the changes in the hematopoietic system, vitamin B_{12} deficiency must be considered in elderly patients with dementia or psychiatric disorders, even if they are not anemic.

VITAMIN B_{12} THERAPY. Vitamin B_{12} is available for injection or oral administration; combinations with other vitamins and minerals also can be given orally or parenterally. The choice of a preparation always depends on the cause of the deficiency. Oral administration cannot be relied on for effective therapy in the patient with a marked deficiency of vitamin B_{12} and abnormal hematopoiesis or neurological deficits. The treatment of choice for vitamin B_{12} deficiency is cyanocobalamin administered by intramuscular or subcutaneous injection. Effective use of the vitamin B_{12} depends on accurate diagnosis and an understanding of the following general principles of therapy:

- Vitamin B_{12} should be given prophylactically only when there is a reasonable probability that a deficiency exists or will exist (i.e., dietary deficiency in the strict vegetarian, the predictable malabsorption of vitamin B_{12} in patients who have had a gastrectomy, and certain diseases of the small intestine). When GI function is normal, an oral prophylactic supplement of vitamins and minerals, including vitamin B_{12}, may be indicated. Otherwise, the patient should receive monthly injections of cyanocobalamin.
- The relative ease of treatment with vitamin B_{12} should not prevent a full investigation of the etiology of the deficiency. The initial diagnosis usually is suggested by a macrocytic anemia or an unexplained neuropsychiatric disorder.
- Therapy always should be as specific as possible. Although a large number of multivitamin preparations are available, the use of shotgun vitamin therapy in the treatment of vitamin B_{12} deficiency can be dangerous: sufficient folic acid may be given to result in a hematologic recovery that can mask continued vitamin B_{12} deficiency and permit neurological damage to develop or progress.
- Although a classical therapeutic trial with small amounts of vitamin B_{12} can help confirm the diagnosis, acutely ill elderly patients may not be able to tolerate the delay in the correction of a severe

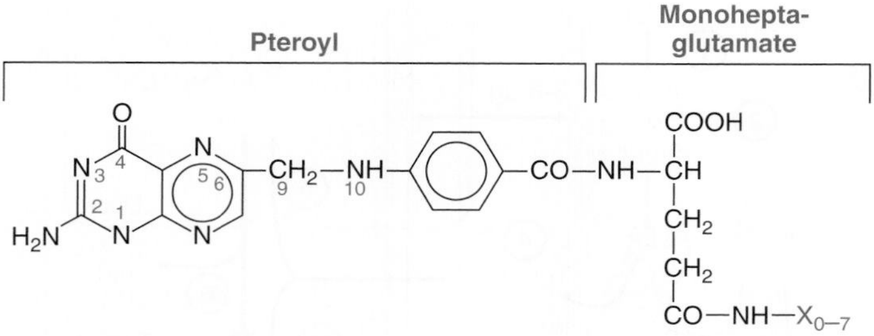

Pteroyl

Monohepta-glutamate

Position	Radical	Congener	
N^5	$—CH_3$	$CH_3H_4PteGlu$	Methyltetrahydrofolate
N^5	—CHO	$5\text{-}CHOH_4PteGlu$	Folinic acid (citrovorum factor)
N^{10}	—CHO	$10\text{-}CHOH_4PteGlu$	10-Formyltetrahydrofolate
$N^{5,10}$	=CH—	$5,10\text{-}CHH_4PteGlu$	5,10-Methenyltetrahydrofolate
$N^{5,10}$	$—CH_2—$	$5,10\text{-}CH_2H_4PteGlu$	5,10-Methylenetetrahydrofolate
N^5	—CHNH	$CHNHH_4PteGlu$	Formiminotetrahydrofolate
N^{10}	$—CH_2OH$	$CH_2OHH_4PteGlu$	Hydroxymethyltetrahydrofolate

Figure 37–7 *The structures and nomenclature of pteroylglutamic acid (folic acid) and its congeners.* X represents additional residues of glutamate; polyglutamates are the storage and active forms of the vitamin. The number of residues of glutamate is variable.

anemia. Such patients require supplemental blood transfusions and immediate therapy with folic acid and vitamin B_{12} to guarantee rapid recovery.

- Long-term therapy with vitamin B_{12} must be evaluated at intervals of 6-12 months in patients who are otherwise well. If there is an additional illness or a condition that may increase the requirement for the vitamin (e.g., pregnancy), reassessment should be performed more frequently.

FOLIC ACID

Pteroylglutamic acid (PteGlu) (Figure 37–7) is the common pharmaceutical form of folic acid. It is not the principal folate congener in food or the active coenzyme for intracellular metabolism. After absorption, PteGlu is rapidly reduced at the 5, 6, 7, and 8 positions to *tetrahydrofolic acid* (H_4PteGlu), which then acts as an acceptor of a number of one-carbon units. These are attached at either the 5 or the 10 position of the pteridine ring or may bridge these atoms to form a new five-membered ring. The most important forms of the coenzyme that are synthesized by these reactions are listed in Figure 37–4, and each plays a specific role in intracellular metabolism:

- *Conversion of Homocysteine to Methionine.* This reaction requires CH_3H_4PteGlu as a methyl donor and uses vitamin B_{12} as a cofactor.
- *Conversion of Serine to Glycine.* This reaction requires tetrahydrofolate as an acceptor of a methylene group from serine and uses pyridoxal phosphate as a cofactor. It results in the formation of 5,10-CH_2H_4PteGlu, an essential coenzyme for the synthesis of thymidylate.
- *Synthesis of Thymidylate.* 5,10-CH_2H_4PteGlu donates a methylene group and reducing equivalents to deoxyuridylate for the synthesis of thymidylate—a rate-limiting step in DNA synthesis.
- *Histidine Metabolism.* H_4PteGlu also acts as an acceptor of a formimino group in the conversion of formiminoglutamic acid to glutamic acid.
- *Synthesis of Purines.* Two steps in the synthesis of purine nucleotides require the participation of 10-$CHOH_4$PteGlu as a formyl donor in reactions catalyzed by ribotide transformylases: the formylation of glycinamide ribonucleotide and the formylation of 5-aminoimidazole-4-carboxamide ribonucleotide. By these reactions, carbon atoms at positions 8 and 2, respectively, are incorporated into the growing purine ring.
- *Utilization or Generation of Formate.* This reversible reaction uses H_4PteGlu and 10-$CHOH_4$PteGlu.

DAILY REQUIREMENTS. Many food sources are rich in folates, especially fresh green vegetables, liver, yeast, and some fruits. However, lengthy cooking can destroy up to 90% of the folate content of such food. Generally, a standard U.S. diet provides 50-500 μg of absorbable folate per day, although individuals with high intakes of fresh vegetables and meats will ingest as much as 2 mg per day. In the normal adult, the recommended daily intake is 400 μg; pregnant or lactating women and patients with high rates of cell turnover (such as patients

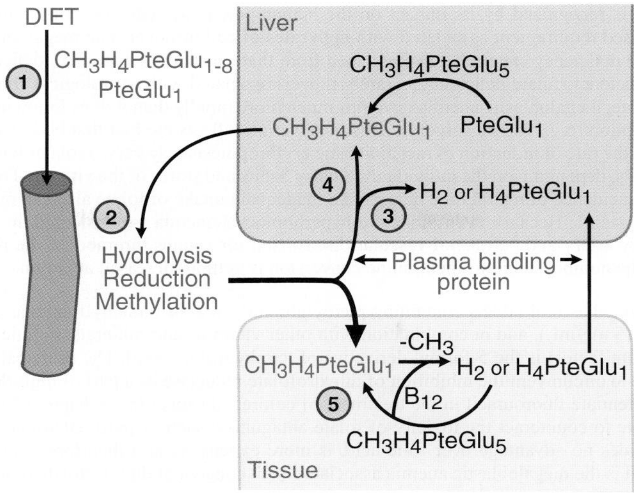

Figure 37–8 *Absorption and distribution of folate derivatives.* Dietary sources of folate polyglutamates are hydrolyzed to the monoglutamate, reduced, and methylated to $CH_3H_4PteGlu_1$ during gastrointestinal transport. Folate deficiency commonly results from (1) inadequate dietary supply and (2) small intestinal disease. In patients with uremia, alcoholism, or hepatic disease there may be defects in (3) the concentration of folate-binding proteins in plasma and (4) the flow of $CH_3H_4PteGlu_1$ into bile for reabsorption and transport to tissue (the folate enterohepatic cycle). Finally, vitamin B_{12} deficiency will (5) "trap" folate as $CH_3H_4PteGlu$, thereby reducing the availability of $H_4PteGlu_1$ for its essential roles in purine and pyrimidine synthesis.

with a hemolytic anemia) may require 500-600 μg or more per day. For the prevention of neural tube defects, a daily intake of at least 400 μg of folate in food or in supplements beginning a month before pregnancy and continued for at least the first trimester is recommended. Folate supplementation also is being considered in patients with elevated levels of plasma homocysteine.

ADME. As with vitamin B_{12}, the diagnosis and management of deficiencies of folic acid depend on an understanding of the transport pathways and intracellular metabolism of the vitamin (Figure 37–8). Folates present in food are largely in the form of reduced polyglutamates, and absorption requires transport and the action of a *pteroylglutamyl carboxypeptidase* associated with mucosal cell membranes. The mucosae of the duodenum and upper part of the jejunum are rich in *dihydrofolate reductase* and can methylate most or all of the reduced folate that is absorbed. Because most absorption occurs in the proximal portion of the small intestine, it is not unusual for folate deficiency to occur when the jejunum is diseased. Both nontropical and tropical sprues are common causes of folate deficiency and megaloblastic anemia.

Once absorbed, folate is transported rapidly to tissues as $CH_3H_4PteGlu$. Although certain plasma proteins do bind folate derivatives, they have a greater affinity for nonmethylated analogs. The role of such binding proteins in folate homeostasis is not well understood. An increase in binding capacity is detectable in folate deficiency and in certain disease states, such as uremia, cancer, and alcoholism. A constant supply of $CH_3H_4PteGlu$ is maintained by food and by an enterohepatic cycle of the vitamin. The liver actively reduces and methylates PteGlu (and H_2 or $H_4PteGlu$) and then transports the $CH_3H_4PteGlu$ into bile for reabsorption by the gut and subsequent delivery to tissues. This pathway may provide ≥200 μg of folate each day for recirculation to tissues. The importance of the enterohepatic cycle is suggested by animal studies that show a rapid reduction of the plasma folate concentration after either drainage of bile or ingestion of alcohol, which apparently blocks the release of $CH_3H_4PteGlu$ from hepatic parenchymal cells.

FOLATE DEFICIENCY. Folate deficiency is a common complication of diseases of the small intestine that interferes with the absorption of folate from food and the recirculation of folate through the enterohepatic cycle. In acute or chronic alcoholism, daily intake of folate in food may be severely restricted, and the enterohepatic cycle of the vitamin may be impaired by toxic effects of alcohol on hepatic parenchymal cells; this is the most common cause of folate-deficient megaloblastic erythropoiesis and the most amenable to therapy, via reinstitution of a normal diet. Disease states characterized by a high rate of cell turnover, such as hemolytic anemias, also may be complicated by folate deficiency. Additionally, drugs that inhibit dihydrofolate reductase (e.g., methotrexate and trimethoprim) or that interfere with the absorption and storage of folate in tissues (e.g., certain anticonvulsants and oral contraceptives) can lower the concentration of folate in plasma and may cause a megaloblastic anemia.

Folate deficiency is recognized by its impact on the hematopoietic system. As with vitamin B_{12}, this fact reflects the increased requirement associated with high rates of cell turnover. The megaloblastic anemia that results from folate deficiency cannot be distinguished from that caused by vitamin B_{12} deficiency. In contrast to vitamin B_{12} deficiency, folate deficiency is rarely if ever associated with neurological abnormalities. After deprivation of folate, megaloblastic anemia develops much more rapidly than it does following interruption of vitamin B_{12} absorption (e.g., gastric surgery). This observation reflects the fact that body stores of folate are limited. Although the rate of induction of megaloblastic erythropoiesis may vary, a folate-deficiency state may appear in 1-4 weeks, depending on the individual's dietary habits and stores of the vitamin. Folate deficiency is implicated in the incidence of neural tube defects. An inadequate intake of folate also can result in elevations in plasma homocysteine. Because even moderate hyperhomocysteinemia is considered an independent risk factor for coronary artery and peripheral vascular disease and for venous thrombosis, the role of folate as a methyl donor in the homocysteine-to-methionine conversion is getting increased attention.

Folic acid is marketed as oral tablets containing pteroylglutamic acid or L-methylfolate, as an aqueous solution for injection (5 mg/mL), and in combination with other vitamins and minerals. Folinic acid (leucovorin calcium, citrovorum factor) is the 5-formyl derivative of tetrahydrofolic acid. The principal therapeutic uses of folinic acid are to circumvent the inhibition of dihydrofolate reductase as a part of high-dose methotrexate therapy and to potentiate fluorouracil in the treatment of colorectal cancer (*see* Chapter 61). It also has been used as an antidote to counteract the toxicity of folate antagonists such as pyrimethamine or trimethoprim. Folinic acid provides no advantage over folic acid, is more expensive, and therefore is not recommended. A single exception is the megaloblastic anemia associated with congenital dihydrofolate reductase deficiency.

UNTOWARD EFFECTS. There have been rare reports of reactions to parenteral injections of folic acid and leucovorin. Oral folic acid usually is not toxic. Folic acid in large amounts may counteract the antiepileptic effect of phenobarbital, phenytoin, and primidone, and increase the frequency of seizures in susceptible children. The FDA recommends that oral tablets of folic acid be limited to strengths of ≤1 mg.

GENERAL PRINCIPLES OF THERAPY. The therapeutic use of folic acid is limited to the prevention and treatment of deficiencies of the vitamin. As with vitamin B_{12} therapy, effective use of the vitamin depends on accurate diagnosis and an understanding of the mechanisms that are operative in a specific disease state. The following general principles of therapy should be respected:

- Dietary supplementation is necessary when there is a requirement that may not be met by a "normal" diet. The daily ingestion of a multivitamin preparation containing 400-500 μg of folic acid has become standard practice before and during pregnancy to reduce the incidence of neural tube defects and for as long as a woman is breast-feeding. In women with a history of a pregnancy complicated by a neural tube defect, an even larger dose of 4 mg/day has been recommended. Patients on total parenteral nutrition should receive folic acid supplements as part of their fluid regimen because liver folate stores are limited. Adult patients with a disease state characterized by high cell turnover (e.g., hemolytic anemia) generally require 1 mg of folic acid given once or twice a day. The 1-mg dose also has been used in the treatment of patients with elevated levels of homocysteine.
- As with vitamin B_{12} deficiency, any patient with folate deficiency and a megaloblastic anemia should be evaluated carefully to determine the underlying cause of the deficiency state. This should include evaluation of the effects of medications, the amount of alcohol intake, the patient's history of travel, and the function of the GI tract.
- Therapy always should be as specific as possible. Multivitamin preparations should be avoided unless there is good reason to suspect deficiency of several vitamins.
- The potential danger of mistreating a patient who has vitamin B_{12} deficiency with folic acid must be kept in mind. The administration of large doses of folic acid can result in an apparent improvement of the megaloblastic anemia, inasmuch as PteGlu is converted by dihydrofolate reductase to H_4PteGlu; this circumvents the methylfolate "trap." However, folate therapy does not prevent or alleviate the neurological defects of vitamin B_{12} deficiency, and these may progress and become irreversible.

See the 12th edition of the parent text for details on treating the patient who is acutely ill with megaloblastic anemia.

For a complete Bibliographical Listing see Goodman & Gilman's ***The Pharmacological Basis of Therapeutics***, 12th ed., or Goodman & Gilman Online at www.AccessMedicine.com.

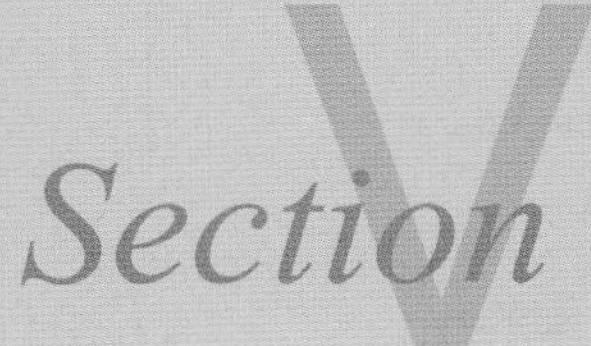

Section V Hormones and Hormone Antagonists

Chapter 38 Introduction to Endocrinology: The Hypothalamic-Pituitary Axis

ENDOCRINOLOGY AND HORMONES: GENERAL CONCEPTS

Endocrinology analyzes the biosynthesis of hormones, their sites of production, and the sites and mechanisms of their action and interaction. The major functions of hormones include the regulation of energy storage, production, and utilization; the adaptation to new environments or conditions of stress; the facilitation of growth and development; and the maturation and function of the reproductive system. Although hormones were originally defined as products of ductless glands, we now appreciate that many organs not classically considered as "endocrine" (e.g., the heart, kidneys, GI tract, adipocytes, and brain) synthesize and secrete hormones that play key physiological roles. In addition, the field of endocrinology has expanded to include the actions of growth factors acting by means of autocrine and paracrine mechanisms, the influence of neurons—particularly those in the hypothalamus—that regulate endocrine function, and the reciprocal interactions of cytokines and other components of the immune system with the endocrine system.

Conceptually, hormones may be divided into 2 classes:

- Hormones that act predominantly via *nuclear receptors* to modulate transcription in target cells (e.g., steroid hormones, thyroid hormone, and vitamin D)
- Hormones that typically act via *membrane receptors* to exert rapid effects on signal transduction pathways (e.g., peptide and amino acid hormones)

The receptors for both classes of hormones provide tractable targets for a diverse group of compounds that are among the most widely used drugs in clinical medicine.

THE HYPOTHALAMIC-PITUITARY-ENDOCRINE AXIS

Many of the classic endocrine hormones (e.g., cortisol, thyroid hormone, sex steroids, growth hormone) are regulated by complex reciprocal interactions among the hypothalamus, anterior pituitary, and endocrine glands (Table 38–1). The basic organization of the hypothalamic-pituitary-endocrine axis is summarized in Figure 38–1.

Discrete sets of hypothalamic neurons produce different releasing hormones, which are axonally transported to the median eminence. Upon stimulation, these neurons secrete their respective hypothalamic-releasing hormones into the hypothalamic-adenohypophyseal plexus, which flows to the anterior pituitary gland. The *hypothalamic-releasing hormones* bind to membrane receptors on specific subsets of pituitary cells and stimulate the secretion of the corresponding *pituitary hormones*. The pituitary hormones, which can be thought of as the *master signals*, then circulate to the target endocrine glands where they activate specific receptors to stimulate the synthesis and secretion of the target *endocrine hormones*. These interactions are *feed-forward regulation* in which the master (signal) hormones stimulate the production of target hormones by the endocrine organs.

Superimposed on this positive feed-forward regulation is *negative feedback* regulation, which permits precise control of hormone levels (Figure 38–2; *see* Figure 38–6). Typically, the endocrine target hormone circulates to both the hypothalamus and pituitary, where it acts via specific receptors

Table 38–1

Hormones that Integrate the Hypothalamic-Pituitary-Endocrine Axis

HYPOTHALAMIC-RELEASING HORMONE	PITUITARY TROPHIC (SIGNAL) HORMONE	TARGET HORMONE(S)
Growth hormone-releasing hormone (GHRH)	Growth hormone (GH)	IGF-1
Somatostatin (SST)[a]	Growth hormone	
Dopamine (DA)[b]	Prolactin	—
Corticotropin-releasing hormone (CRH)	Corticotropin	Cortisol/DHEA
Thyrotropin-releasing hormone (TRH)	Thyroid-stimulating hormone (TSH)	Thyroid hormone
Gonadotropin-releasing hormone (GnRH)	Follicle-stimulating hormone (FSH)	Estrogen Progesterone/Estrogen (f)
	Luteinizing hormone (LH)	Testosterone (m)

IGF-1, insulin-like growth factor-1; DHEA, dehydroepiandrosterone; f, female; m, male.
[a]Somatostatin inhibits growth hormone release.
[b]Dopamine inhibits prolactin release.

to inhibit the production and secretion of both its hypothalamic-releasing hormone and the regulatory pituitary hormone. In addition, other brain regions have inputs to the hypothalamic-releasing neurons, further integrating the regulation of hormone levels in response to diverse stimuli.

PITUITARY HORMONES AND THEIR HYPOTHALAMIC-RELEASING FACTORS

The anterior pituitary hormones can be classified into 3 different groups based on their structural features (Table 38–2):

- Pro-opiomelanocortin (POMC)-derived hormones include *corticotropin* (adrenocorticotrophic hormone [ACTH]) and *α-melanocyte-stimulating hormone* (α-MSH). These are derived from POMC by proteolytic processing (*see* Chapters 18 and 42).

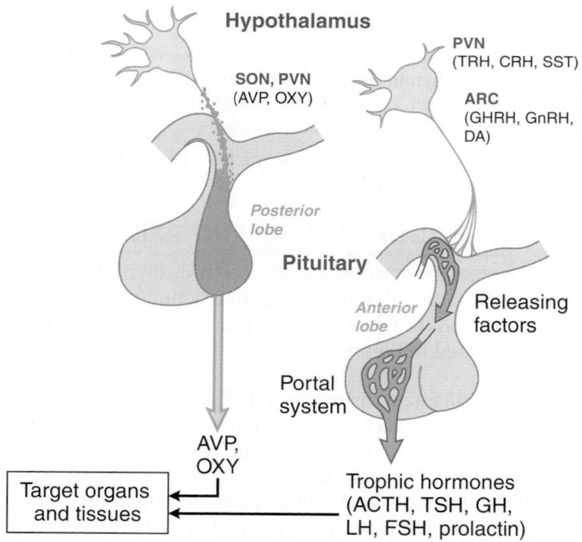

Figure 38–1 *Organization of the anterior and posterior pituitary gland.* Hypothalamic neurons in the supraoptic (SON) and paraventricular (PVN) nuclei synthesize arginine vasopressin (AVP) or oxytocin (OXY). Most of their axons project directly to the posterior pituitary, from which AVP and OXY are secreted into the systemic circulation to regulate their target tissues. Neurons that regulate the anterior lobe cluster in the mediobasal hypothalamus, including the PVN and the arcuate (ARC) nuclei. They secrete hypothalamic releasing hormones, which reach the anterior pituitary via the hypothalamic-adenohypophyseal portal system and stimulate distinct populations of pituitary cells. These cells, in turn, secrete the trophic (signal) hormones that regulate endocrine organs and other tissues. *See* Table 38–1 for abbreviations.

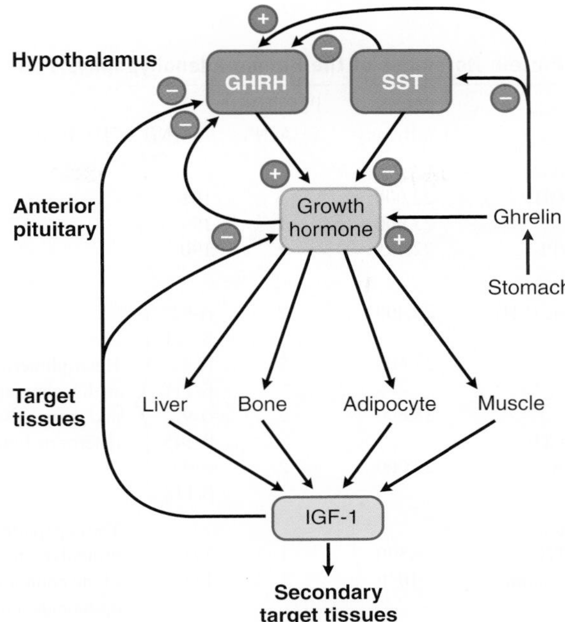

Figure 38–2 *Growth hormone secretion and actions.* Two hypothalamic factors, growth hormone-releasing hormone (GHRH) and somatostatin (SST) stimulate or inhibit the release of growth hormone (GH) from the pituitary, respectively. Insulin-like growth factor-1 (IGF-1), a product of GH action on peripheral tissues, causes negative feedback inhibition of GH release by acting at the hypothalamus and the pituitary. The actions of GH can be direct or indirect (mediated by IGF-1). See text for discussion of the other agents that modulate GH secretion and of the effects of locally produced IGF-1. Inhibition, –; stimulation, +.

- Somatotropic hormones *include growth hormone* (GH) and *prolactin*. In humans the somatotropic family also includes placental lactogen.
- The glycoprotein hormones—*thyroid-stimulating hormone* (TSH; also called thyrotropin), *luteinizing hormone* (LH; also called lutropin), and *follicle-stimulating hormone* (FSH; also called follitropin). In humans, the glycoprotein hormone family also includes *human chorionic gonadotropin* (hCG).

The synthesis and release of anterior pituitary hormones are influenced by the central nervous system (CNS). Their secretion is positively regulated by a group of peptides referred to as *hypothalamic-releasing hormones* (*see* Figure 38–1). These include *corticotropin-releasing hormone* (CRH), *growth hormone-releasing hormone* (GHRH), *gonadotropin-releasing hormone* (GnRH), and *thyrotropin-releasing hormone* (TRH). *Somatostatin* (SST), another hypothalamic peptide, negatively regulates secretion of pituitary GH and TSH. The neurotransmitter dopamine inhibits the secretion of prolactin by lactotropes.

The *posterior pituitary gland*, also known as the neurohypophysis, contains the endings of nerve axons arising from the hypothalamus that synthesize either *arginine vasopressin* or *oxytocin* (*see* Figure 38–1). Arginine vasopressin plays an important role in water homeostasis (*see* Chapter 25); oxytocin plays important roles in labor and parturition and in milk letdown, as discussed in the following sections and in Chapter 66.

SOMATOTROPIC HORMONES: GROWTH HORMONE AND PROLACTIN

GH and prolactin are structurally related members of the somatotropic hormone family and share many biological features. The somatotropes and lactotropes, the pituitary cells that produce and secrete GH and prolactin, respectively, are subject to strong inhibitory input from hypothalamic neurons; for prolactin, this negative dopaminergic input is the dominant regulator of secretion. GH and prolactin act via membrane receptors that belong to the cytokine receptor family and modulate target cell function via very similar signal transduction pathways (*see* Chapter 3). Several drugs that are used to treat excessive secretion of these hormones are effective to varying degrees for both GH and prolactin.

Table 38–2

Properties of the Protein Hormones of the Human Adenohypophysis and Placenta

HORMONE	MASS (daltons)	PEPTIDE CHAINS	AMINO ACID RESIDUES	
Somatotropic hormones				
Growth hormone (GH)	22,000	1	191	
Prolactin (PRL)	23,000	1	199	
Placental lactogen (PL)	22,125	1	190	
Glycoprotein hormones				
Luteinizing hormone (LH)	29,400	2	α-92 β-121	Heterodimeric glycoproteins with a common α-subunit and unique β-subunits that determine biological specificity
Follicle-stimulating hormone (FSH)	32,600	2	α-92 β-111	
Human chorionic gonadotropin (hCG)	38,600	2	α-92 β-145	
Thyroid-stimulating hormone (TSH)	28,000	2	α-92 β-118	
POMC-derived hormones[a]				These peptides are derived by proteolytic hormone processing of the common precursor, pro-opiomelanocortin (POMC)
Corticotropin (ACTH)	4500	1	39	
α-Melanocyte-stimulating (α-MSH)	1650	1	13	

[a]*See Chapter 42 for further discussion of POMC-derived peptides, including ACTH and α-MSH.*

PHYSIOLOGY

Table 38–2 presents some features of the somatotrophic hormones.

GH is secreted by somatotropes as a heterogeneous mixture of peptides; the principal form is a single polypeptide chain of 22 kDa that has 2 disulfide bonds and is not glycosylated. Alternative splicing produces a smaller form (~20 kDa) with equal bioactivity that makes up 5-10% of circulating GH. Recombinant human GH consists entirely of the 22 kDa form, which provides a way to detect GH abuse. In the circulation, a 55 kDa protein binds approximately 45% of the 22 kDa and 25% of the 20 kDa forms. A second protein unrelated to the GH receptor also binds approximately 5-10% of circulating GH with lower affinity. Bound GH is cleared more slowly and has a biological $t_{1/2}$ ~10 times that of unbound GH, suggesting that the bound hormone may provide a GH reservoir that dampens acute fluctuations in GH levels associated with its pulsatile secretion.

REGULATION OF SECRETION

GH secretion is high in children, peaks during puberty, and then decreases in an age-related manner in adulthood. GH is secreted in discrete but irregular pulses. The amplitude of secretory pulses is greatest at night. GHRH, produced by hypothalamic neurons, stimulates GH secretion (*see* Figure 38–2) by binding to a specific GPCR on somatotropes. The stimulated GHRH receptor couples to G_s to raise intracellular levels of cyclic AMP and Ca^{2+}, thereby stimulating GH synthesis and secretion. Loss-of-function mutations of the GHRH receptor cause a rare form of short stature in humans. GH and its major peripheral effector, *insulin-like growth factor 1* (IGF-1), act in negative feedback loops to suppress GH secretion. The negative effect of IGF-1 is predominantly through direct effects on the anterior pituitary gland, while the negative feedback action of GH is mediated in part by SST, synthesized in more widely distributed neurons.

SST is synthesized as a 92–amino acid precursor and processed by proteolytic cleavage to generate 2 peptides: SST-28 and SST-14 (Figure 38–3). SST exerts its effects by binding to and activating a family of 5 related GPCRs that signal through G_i to inhibit cyclic AMP formation and to activate K^+ channels and protein phosphotyrosine phosphatases.

Ghrelin, a 28-amino acid peptide, stimulates GH secretion. Ghrelin is synthesized predominantly in endocrine cells in the fundus of the stomach but also is produced at lower levels at a number of other sites. Both fasting and hypoglycemia stimulate circulating ghrelin levels. Ghrelin acts primarily through a GPCR called the GH secretagogue receptor. Ghrelin also stimulates appetite and increases food intake, apparently by central actions on NPY and agouti-related peptide neurons in the hypothalamus. Thus, ghrelin and its

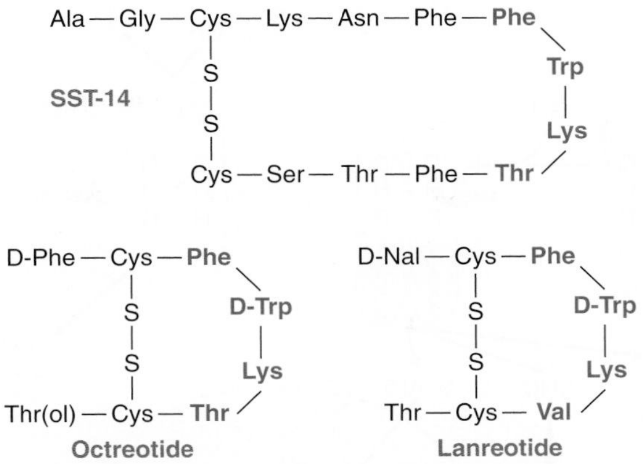

Ala — Gly — Cys — Lys — Asn — Phe — Phe — Trp — Lys — Thr — Phe — Thr — Ser — Cys (Cys–S–S–Cys)

SST-14

D-Phe — Cys — Phe — D-Trp — Lys — Thr — Cys — Thr(ol) (Cys–S–S–Cys)

Octreotide

D-Nal — Cys — Phe — D-Trp — Lys — Val — Cys — Thr (Cys–S–S–Cys)

Lanreotide

Figure 38–3 *Structures of somatostatin-14 and selected synthetic analogs.* Residues that play key roles in binding to SST receptors are shown in *red*. Octreotide and lanreotide are clinically available synthetic analogs of somatostatin. D-Nal, 3-(2-napthyl)-D-alanyl.

receptor act in a complex manner to integrate the functions of the GI tract, the hypothalamus, and the anterior pituitary.

Several neurotransmitters, drugs, metabolites, and other stimuli modulate the release of GHRH and/or SST and thereby affect GH secretion. DA, 5HT, and α_2 adrenergic receptor agonists stimulate GH release, as do hypoglycemia, exercise, stress, emotional excitement, and ingestion of protein-rich meals. In contrast, β adrenergic receptor agonists, free fatty acids, glucose, IGF-1, and GH itself inhibit release. Many of the physiological factors that influence *prolactin* secretion also affect GH secretion. Thus, sleep, stress, hypoglycemia, exercise, and estrogen increase the secretion of both hormones.

Prolactin is unique among the anterior pituitary hormones in that hypothalamic regulation of its secretion is predominantly inhibitory. The major regulator of prolactin secretion is DA, which interacts with the D_2 receptor, a GPCR on lactotropes, to inhibit prolactin secretion (Figure 38–4). Prolactin acts predominantly in women, both during pregnancy and in the postpartum period in women who breast-feed. During pregnancy, the maternal serum prolactin level starts to increase at 8 weeks of gestation, peaks to 250 ng/mL at term, and declines thereafter to prepregnancy levels unless the mother breast-feeds the infant. Suckling or breast manipulation in nursing mothers cause elevation of circulating prolactin levels. Prolactin levels can rise 10- to 100-fold within 30 min of stimulation. This response is distinct from milk letdown, which is mediated by oxytocin release from the posterior pituitary gland. The suckling response becomes less pronounced after several months of breast-feeding, and prolactin concentrations eventually decline to prepregnancy levels. Prolactin also is synthesized in lactotropes near the end of the luteal phase of the menstrual cycle and by decidual cells early in pregnancy (accounting for the high levels of prolactin in amniotic fluid during the first trimester of human pregnancy).

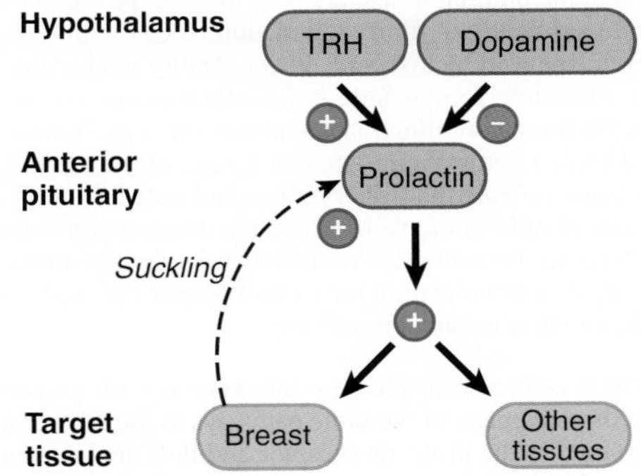

Figure 38–4 *Prolactin secretion and actions.* Prolactin is the only anterior pituitary hormone for which a unique stimulatory releasing factor has not been identified. Thyrotropin-releasing hormone (TRH), however, can stimulate prolactin release; dopamine inhibits it. Suckling induces prolactin secretion, and prolactin affects lactation and reproductive functions but also has effects on many other tissues. Prolactin is not under feedback control by peripheral hormones.

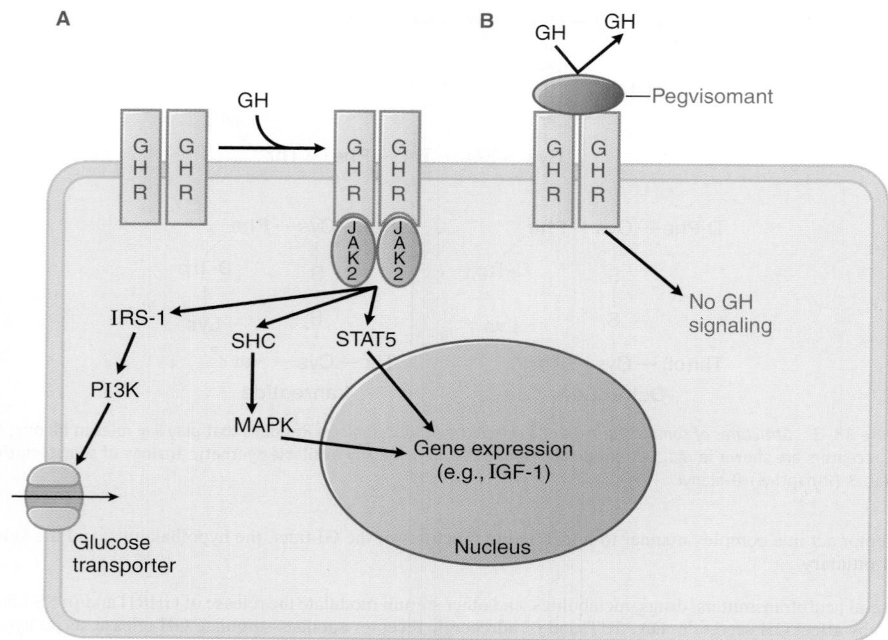

Figure 38–5 *Mechanisms of growth hormone and prolactin action and of GH receptor antagonism.* **A.** Binding of GH to a growth hormone receptor (GHR) homodimer induces autophosphorylation of JAK2. JAK2 then phosphorylates cytoplasmic proteins that activate downstream signaling pathways, including STAT5 and mediators upstream of MAPK, which ultimately modulate gene expression. The structurally related prolactin receptor also is a ligand activated homodimer that recruits the JAK-STAT signaling pathway. GHR also activates IRS-1, which may mediate the increased expression of glucose transporters on the plasma membrane. **B.** Pegvisomant, a recombinant pegylated variant of human GH, is a high affinity GH antagonist that interferes with GH signaling. JAK2, Janus kinase 2; IRS-1, insulin receptor substrate-1; PI3K, phosphatidyl inositol-3 kinase; STAT, signal transducer and activator of transcription; MAPK, mitogen-activated protein kinase; SHC, Src homology-containing proteins.

MOLECULAR AND CELLULAR BASES OF SOMATOTROPIC HORMONE ACTION

Receptors for GH and prolactin belong to the cytokine receptor superfamily; they contain an extracellular hormone-binding domain, a single membrane-spanning region, and an intracellular domain that mediates signal transduction.

GH receptor activation results in the binding of a single GH to 2 receptor monomers and to form a GH-GH receptor ternary complex (initiated by high-affinity interaction of GH with 1 monomer of the GH receptor dimer [mediated by GH site 1], followed by a second, lower affinity interaction of GH with the GH receptor [mediated by GH site 2]); these interactions induce a conformational change that activates downstream signaling. The ligand-occupied GH receptor dimer lacks inherent tyrosine kinase activity but provides docking sites for 2 molecules of JAK2, a cytoplasmic tyrosine kinase of the Janus kinase family. The juxtaposition of 2 JAK2 molecules leads to *trans*-phosphorylation and autoactivation of JAK2, with consequent tyrosine phosphorylation of cytoplasmic proteins that mediate downstream signaling events (Figure 38–5). *Pegvisomant* is a GH analog with amino acid substitutions that disrupt the interaction at site 2; pegvisomant binds to the receptor and causes its internalization but cannot trigger the conformational change that stimulates downstream events in the signal transduction pathway.

The effects of prolactin on target cells also result from interactions with a cytokine family receptor that is widely distributed and signals through many of the same pathways as the GH receptor. Unlike human GH and placental lactogen, which also bind to the prolactin receptor and thus are lactogenic, prolactin binds specifically to the prolactin receptor and has no somatotropic (GH-like) activity.

PHYSIOLOGICAL EFFECTS OF THE SOMATOTROPIC HORMONES

The most striking physiological effect of GH is the stimulation of the longitudinal growth of bones. GH also increases bone mineral density after the epiphyses have closed. GH also increases muscle mass (in human subjects with GH deficiency), increases glomerular filtration rate, and stimulates of preadipocyte differentiation into adipocytes. Growth hormone acts directly on adipocytes to increase lipolysis and on hepatocytes to stimulate gluconeogenesis, but its anabolic and growth-promoting effects are mediated indirectly through the induction of IGF-1. IGF-1 interacts with receptors on the cell surface that mediate its biological activities.

Prolactin effects are limited to tissues that express the prolactin receptor, particularly the mammary gland. Prolactin plays an important role in inducing growth and differentiation of the ductal and lobuloalveolar epithelia and is essential for lactation. Prolactin receptors are present in many other sites, including the hypothalamus, liver, adrenal, testes, ovaries, prostate, and immune system, suggesting that prolactin may play multiple roles outside of the breast. The physiological effects of prolactin at these sites remain poorly characterized.

PATHOPHYSIOLOGY OF THE SOMATOTROPIC HORMONES

EXCESS PRODUCTION OF SOMATOTROPIC HORMONES. Syndromes of excess secretion of GH and prolactin typically are caused by somatotrope or lactotrope adenomas that oversecrete the respective hormones.

Clinical Manifestations of Excess GH. GH excess causes distinct clinical syndromes depending on the age of the patient. If the epiphyses are unfused, GH excess causes increased longitudinal growth, resulting in gigantism. In adults, GH excess causes acromegaly. The symptoms and signs of acromegaly (e.g., arthropathy, carpal tunnel syndrome, generalized visceromegaly, macroglossia, hypertension, glucose intolerance, headache, lethargy, excess perspiration, and sleep apnea) progress slowly, and diagnosis often is delayed. Mortality is increased at least 2-fold relative to age-matched controls, predominantly due to increased death from cardiovascular disease.

Clinical Manifestations of Excess Prolactin. Hyperprolactinemia is a relatively common endocrine abnormality that can result from hypothalamic or pituitary diseases that interfere with the delivery of inhibitory dopaminergic signals, from renal failure, from primary hypothyroidism associated with increased TRH levels, or from treatment with dopamine receptor antagonists. Most often, hyperprolactinemia is caused by prolactin-secreting pituitary adenomas. Manifestations of prolactin excess in women include galactorrhea, amenorrhea, and infertility. In men, hyperprolactinemia causes loss of libido, erectile dysfunction, and infertility.

IMPAIRED PRODUCTION OF THE SOMATOTROPIC HORMONES

Clinical Manifestations of Growth Hormone Deficiency. Children with GH deficiency present with short stature, delayed bone age, and a low age-adjusted growth velocity. GH deficiency in adults is associated with decreased muscle mass and exercise capacity, decreased bone density, impaired psychosocial function, and increased mortality from cardiovascular causes. The diagnosis of GH deficiency should be entertained in children with height >2 to 2.5 standard deviations below normal, delayed bone age, a decreased growth velocity, and a predicted adult height substantially below the mean parental height. In adults, overt GH deficiency usually results from pituitary lesions caused by a functioning or nonfunctioning pituitary adenoma, secondary to trauma, or related to surgery or radiotherapy for a pituitary or suprasellar mass. Almost all patients with multiple deficits in other pituitary hormones also have deficient GH secretion.

Prolactin Deficiency. Prolactin deficiency may result from conditions that damage the pituitary gland, but prolactin is not given as part of endocrine replacement therapy.

PHARMACOTHERAPY OF SOMATOTROPIN HORMONE DISORDERS

GROWTH HORMONE EXCESS

Treatment options in gigantism/acromegaly include transsphenoidal surgery, radiation, and drugs that inhibit GH secretion or action.

SOMATOSTATIN ANALOGS. The development of synthetic analogs of SST has revolutionized the medical treatment of acromegaly. The goal of treatment is to decrease GH levels to <2.5 ng/mL after an oral glucose-tolerance test and to bring IGF-1 levels to within the normal range for age and sex. The 2 SST analogs used widely are *octreotide* and *lanreotide*, synthetic derivatives that have longer half-lives and bind preferentially to SST_2 and SST_5 receptors (*see* Figure 38–3). Octreotide (100 μg) administered subcutaneously 3 times daily is 100% bioactive; peak effects are seen within 30 min, serum $t_{1/2}$ is ~90 min, and duration of action is ~12 h. A long-acting, slow-release form (SANDOSTATIN-LAR DEPOT) greatly reduces the injection frequency. Administered intramuscularly in a dose of 20 or 30 mg once every 4 weeks, octreotide LAR is at least as effective as the regular formulation and as well tolerated. A lower dose of 10 mg per injection should be used in patients requiring hemodialysis or with hepatic cirrhosis. In addition to its effect on GH secretion, octreotide can decrease tumor size, although tumor growth generally resumes after octreotide treatment is stopped.

Lanreotide is a long-acting octapeptide SST analog that causes prolonged suppression of GH secretion when administered in a 30-mg dose intramuscularly. Its efficacy appears comparable to that of the long-acting formulation of octreotide; its duration of action is shorter; thus, it is administered at 10- or 14-day intervals. A supersaturated aqueous formulation of lanreotide, *lanreotide autogel* (SOMATULINE DEPOT), has been approved for use in the U.S. It is supplied in prefilled syringes containing 60, 90, or 120 mg lanreotide and administered by deep subcutaneous injection once every 4 weeks.

Pasireotide (SIGNIFOR) is a cyclohexapeptide SST analog that is approved for the treatment of Cushing disease in patients who are ineligible for pituitary surgery or in whom surgery has failed. Pasireotide binds to multiple SST receptors (1, 2, 3, and 5) but has the highest affinity for SST_5 receptor. The recommended dose range is 0.3 to 0.9 mg administered by subcutaneous injection twice daily.

Adverse Effects. GI side effects—including diarrhea, nausea, and abdominal pain—occur in up to 50% of patients receiving octreotide. These symptoms usually diminish over time and do not require cessation of therapy. Approximately 25% of patients receiving octreotide develop gallstones, presumably due to decreased gallbladder contraction and bile secretion. Compared with SST, octreotide reduces insulin secretion to a lesser extent and only infrequently affects glycemic control. Bradycardia and QT prolongation may occur in patients with underlying cardiac disease. Inhibitory effects on TSH secretion may lead to hypothyroidism, and thyroid function tests should be evaluated periodically. The incidence and severity of side effects associated with lanreotide and pasireotide are similar to those of octreotide. Pasireotide suppresses of ACTH secretion in Cushing disease and may lead to a decrease in cortisol secretion and to hypocortisolism.

Other Therapeutic Uses. SST blocks not only GH secretion but also the secretion of other hormones, growth factors, and cytokines. Thus, octreotide and the slow-release formulations of SST analogs have been used to treat symptoms associated with metastatic carcinoid tumors (e.g., flushing and diarrhea) and adenomas secreting vasoactive intestinal peptide (e.g., watery diarrhea). Octreotide also is the treatment of choice for patients who have thyrotrope adenomas that oversecrete TSH.

GROWTH HORMONE ANTAGONISTS. Pegvisomant (SOMAVERT) is a GH receptor antagonist approved for the treatment of acromegaly. Pegvisomant binds to the GH receptor but does not activate JAK-STAT signaling or stimulate IGF-1 secretion (*see* Figure 38–5). Pegvisomant is administered subcutaneously as a 40-mg loading dose followed by administration of 10 mg/day. Based on serum IGF-1 levels, the dose is titrated at 4- to 6-week intervals to a maximum of 40 mg/day. Pegvisomant should not be used in patients with an unexplained elevation of hepatic transaminases, and liver function tests should be monitored in all patients. In addition, lipohypertrophy has occurred at injection sites, sometimes requiring cessation of therapy; this is believed to reflect the inhibition of direct actions of GH on adipocytes. Because of concerns that loss of negative feedback by GH and IGF-1 may increase the growth of GH-secreting adenomas, careful follow-up by pituitary MRI is strongly recommended.

PROLACTIN EXCESS

The therapeutic options for patients with prolactinomas include transsphenoidal surgery, radiation, and treatment with DA receptor agonists that suppress prolactin production via activation of D_2 receptors.

DOPAMINE RECEPTOR AGONISTS. *Bromocriptine*, *cabergoline*, and *quinagolide* relieve the inhibitory effect of prolactin on ovulation and permit most patients with prolactinomas to become pregnant. Bromocriptine generally is recommended for fertility induction in patients with hyperprolactinemia. Quinagolide should not be used when pregnancy is intended. These agents generally decrease both prolactin secretion and the size of the adenoma. Over time, especially with cabergoline, the prolactinoma may decrease in size to the extent that the drug can be discontinued without recurrence of the hyperprolactinemia.

BROMOCRIPTINE. Bromocriptine (PARLODEL) is the dopamine receptor agonist against which newer agents are compared. Bromocriptine is a semisynthetic ergot alkaloid that interacts with D_2 receptors to inhibit spontaneous and TRH-induced release of prolactin; to a lesser extent, it also activates D_1 receptors. The oral dose of bromocriptine is well absorbed; however, only 7% of the dose reaches the systemic circulation because of extensive first-pass metabolism in the liver. Bromocriptine has a short elimination $t_{1/2}$ (between 2 and 8 h). A slow-release oral form is available outside of the U.S. Bromocriptine may be administered vaginally (2.5 mg once daily), with fewer GI side effects. Bromocriptine normalizes serum prolactin levels patients with prolactinomas and decreases tumor size in >50% of patients. The underlying adenoma, and hyperprolactinemia and tumor growth recur upon cessation of therapy. At higher concentrations, bromocriptine is used in the management of acromegaly, and at still higher concentrations is used in the management of Parkinson disease (*see* Chapter 22).

Adverse Effects. Frequent side effects include nausea and vomiting, headache, and postural hypotension. Less frequently, nasal congestion, digital vasospasm, and CNS effects such as psychosis, hallucinations, nightmares, or insomnia are observed. These adverse effects can be diminished by starting at a low dose (1.25 mg) administered at bedtime with a snack. Patients often develop tolerance to the adverse effects.

CABERGOLINE. Cabergoline (DOSTINEX) is an ergot derivative with a longer $t_{1/2}$ (~65 h), higher affinity, and greater selectivity for the D_2 receptor than bromocriptine. It undergoes significant first-pass metabolism in the liver. Cabergoline is the preferred drug for the treatment of hyperprolactinemia. Therapy is initiated at a dose of 0.25 mg twice a week or 0.5 mg once a week. The dose can be increased to a maximum of 1.5-2 mg 2 or 3 times a week as tolerated; the dose should only be increased once every 4 weeks. Cabergoline induces remission in a significant number of patients with prolactinomas. At higher doses, cabergoline is used in some patients with acromegaly.

Adverse Effects. Compared to bromocriptine, cabergoline has a much lower tendency to induce nausea, although it still may cause hypotension and dizziness. Cabergoline has been linked to valvular heart disease, an effect proposed to reflect agonist activity at the serotonin $5HT_{2B}$ receptor.

QUINAGOLIDE. Quinagolide (NORPROLAC) is a non-ergot D_2 agonist with a $t_{1/2}$ (22 h). Quinagolide is administered once daily at doses of 0.1-0.5 mg/day. It is not approved for use in the U.S. but has been used in the E.U.

GROWTH HORMONE DEFICIENCY

SOMATROPIN. Replacement therapy is well established in GH-deficient children and is gaining wider acceptance for GH-deficient adults. Currently, human GH is produced by recombinant DNA technology. *Somatropin* refers to the many GH preparations whose sequences match that of native GH (ACCRETROPIN, GENOTROPIN, HUMATROPE, NORDITROPIN, NUTROPIN, OMNITROPE, SAIZEN, SEROSTIM, TEV-TROPIN, VALTROPIN, and ZORBTIVE); *somatrem* refers to a derivative of GH with an additional methionine at the amino terminus that is no longer available in the U.S.

Pharmacokinetics. As a peptide hormone, GH is administered subcutaneously, with a bioavailability of 70%. Although the circulating $t_{1/2}$ of GH is only 20 min, its biological $t_{1/2}$ is considerably longer, and once-daily administration is sufficient.

Indications for Growth Hormone Treatment. GH deficiency in children is a well-accepted cause of short stature. With the advent of essentially unlimited supplies of recombinant GH, therapy has been extended to children with other conditions associated with short stature despite adequate GH production, including Turner syndrome, Noonan syndrome, Prader-Willi syndrome, chronic renal insufficiency, children born small for gestational age, and children with idiopathic short stature (i.e., >2.25 standard deviations below mean height for age and sex but with normal laboratory indices of GH levels). Severely affected GH-deficient adults may benefit from GH replacement therapy. The FDA also has approved GH therapy for AIDS-associated wasting and for malabsorption associated with the short bowel syndrome (based on the finding that GH stimulates the adaptation of GI epithelial cells).

Contraindications. GH should not be used in patients with acute critical illness due to complications after open heart or abdominal surgery, multiple accidental trauma, or acute respiratory failure. GH also should not be used in patients who have any evidence of neoplasia, and antitumor therapy should be completed before GH therapy is initiated. Other contraindications include proliferative retinopathy or severe nonproliferative diabetic retinopathy. In Prader-Willi syndrome, sudden death has been observed when GH was given to children who were severely obese or who had severe respiratory impairment.

Therapeutic Uses. In GH-deficient children, somatropin typically is administered in a dose of 25-50 μg/kg/day subcutaneously in the evening; higher daily doses (e.g., 50-67 μg/kg) are employed for patients with Noonan syndrome or Turner syndrome, who have partial GH resistance. In children with overt GH deficiency, measurement of serum IGF-1 levels sometimes is used to monitor initial response and compliance; long-term response is monitored by close evaluation of height, sometimes in conjunction with measurements of serum IGF-1 levels. GH is continued until the epiphyses are fused and also may be extended into the transition period from childhood to adulthood. For adults, a typical starting dose is 150-300 μg/day, with higher doses used in younger patients transitioning from pediatric therapy. Either an elevated serum IGF-1 level or persistent side effects mandates a decrease in dose; conversely, the dose can be increased (typically by 100-200 μg/day) if serum IGF-1 has not reached the normal range after 2 months of GH therapy. Because estrogen inhibits GH action, women taking oral—but not transdermal—estrogen may require larger GH doses to achieve the target IGF-1 level.

Adverse Effects of Growth Hormone Therapy. In children, GH therapy is associated with remarkably few side effects. Rarely, patients develop intracranial hypertension, with papilledema, visual changes, headache, nausea, and/or vomiting. Because of this, funduscopic examination is recommended at the initiation of therapy and at periodic intervals thereafter. The consensus is that GH should not be administered in the first year after treatment of pediatric tumors, including leukemia, or during the first 2 years after therapy for medulloblastomas or ependymomas. Because an increased incidence of type 2 diabetes mellitus has been reported, fasting glucose levels should be followed periodically during therapy. Finally, too-rapid growth may be associated with slipped epiphyses or scoliosis. Side effects associated with the initiation of GH therapy in adults include peripheral edema, carpal tunnel syndrome, arthralgias, and myalgias, which occur most frequently in patients who are older or obese and generally respond to a decrease in dose. Estrogens (e.g., birth control medications and estrogen supplements) inhibit GH action. GH therapy can increase the metabolic inactivation of glucocorticoids in the liver.

INSULIN-LIKE GROWTH FACTOR 1. Based on the hypothesis that GH predominantly acts via increases in IGF-1 (*see* Figure 38–2), IGF-1 has been developed for therapeutic use. Recombinant human IGF-1 (mecasermin [INCRELEX]) and a combination of recombinant human IGF-1 with its binding protein, IGFBP-3 (mecasermin rinfabate [IPLEX]), are FDA-approved. The latter formulation was subsequently discontinued for use in short stature due to patent issues, although it remains available for other conditions such as severe insulin resistance, muscular dystrophy, and HIV-related adipose redistribution syndrome.

ADME. Mecasermin is administered by subcutaneous injection and absorption is virtually complete. IGF-1 in circulation is bound by 6 proteins; a ternary complex that includes IGFBP-3 and the acid labile subunit accounts for >80% of the circulating IGF-1. This protein binding prolongs the $t_{1/2}$ of IGF-1 to ~6 h. Both the liver and kidney have been shown to metabolize IGF-1.

Therapeutic Uses. Mecasermin is FDA-approved for patients with impaired growth secondary to mutations in the GH receptor or postreceptor signaling pathway, patients who develop antibodies against GH that interfere with its action, and patients with IGF-1 gene defects that lead to primary IGF-1 deficiency. Typically the starting dose is 40-80 μg/kg per dose twice daily by subcutaneous injection, with a maximum of 120 μg/kg per dose twice daily. In patients with impaired growth secondary to GH deficiency or with idiopathic short stature, mecasermin stimulates linear growth but is less effective than conventional therapy using recombinant GH.

Adverse Effects. Side effects of mecasermin include hypoglycemia and lipohypertrophy. To diminish the frequency of hypoglycemia, mecasermin should be administered shortly before or after a meal or snack. Lymphoid tissue hypertrophy, including enlarged tonsils, also is seen and may require surgical intervention. Other adverse effects are similar to those associated with GH therapy.

Contraindications. Mecasermin should not be used for growth promotion in patients with closed epiphyses. It should not be given to patients with active or suspected neoplasia and should be stopped if evidence of neoplasia develops.

GROWTH HORMONE-RELEASING HORMONE

Sermorelin (GEREF) is a synthetic form of human GHRH that corresponds in sequence to the first 29 amino acids of human GHRH (a 44–amino acid peptide) and has full biological activity. Although sermorelin is FDA-approved for treatment of GH deficiency and as a diagnostic agent to differentiate between hypothalamic and pituitary disease, the drug was withdrawn from the U.S. market in late 2008.

THE GLYCOPROTEIN HORMONES: TSH AND THE GONADOTROPINS

The gonadotropins include *LH*, *FSH*, and *hCG*. They are referred to as the gonadotropins because of their actions on the gonads. Together with TSH, they constitute the glycoprotein family of pituitary hormones (*see* Table 38–2). Each hormone is a glycosylated heterodimer containing a common α subunit and a distinct β subunit that confers specificity of action.

LH and FSH are synthesized and secreted by gonadotropes, which make up ~10% of the hormone-secreting cells in the anterior pituitary. hCG is produced by the placenta only in primates and horses. GnRH stimulates pituitary gonadotropin production, which is further regulated by feedback effects of the gonadal hormones (Figure 38–6; *see* Figure 40–2 and Chapters 40 and 41). TSH is measured in the diagnosis of thyroid disorders, and recombinant TSH is used in the evaluation and treatment of well-differentiated thyroid cancer (*see* Chapter 39).

PHYSIOLOGY OF THE GONADOTROPINS

STRUCTURE-FUNCTION ASPECTS OF THE GONADOTROPINS. The carbohydrate residues on the gonadotropins influence their rates of clearance from the circulation, and also play a role in activating the gonadotropin receptors. Among the gonadotropin β subunits, that of hCG is most divergent because it contains a carboxy-terminal extension of 30 amino acids and extra carbohydrate residues that prolong its $t_{1/2}$. The longer $t_{1/2}$ of hCG has some clinical relevance for its use in assisted reproduction technologies (*see* Chapter 66).

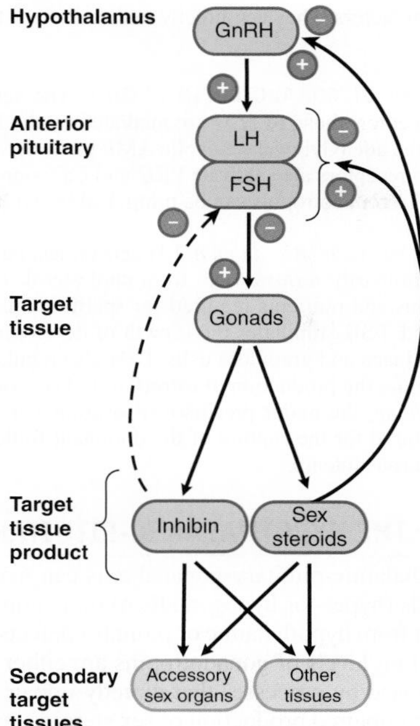

Figure 38–6 *The hypothalamic-pituitary-gonadal axis.* A single hypothalamic-releasing factor, gonadotropin-releasing hormone (GnRH), controls the synthesis and release of both gonadotropins (LH and FSH) in males and females. Gonadal steroid hormones (androgens, estrogens, and progesterone) exert feedback inhibition at the level of the pituitary and the hypothalamus. The preovulatory surge of estrogen also can exert a stimulatory effect at the level of the pituitary and the hypothalamus. Inhibins, a family of polypeptide hormones produced by the gonads, specifically inhibit FSH secretion by the pituitary.

REGULATION OF GONADOTROPIN SYNTHESIS AND SECRETION. The predominant regulator of gonadotropin synthesis and secretion is the hypothalamic peptide GnRH. It is a decapeptide with blocked amino and carboxyl termini derived by proteolytic cleavage of a 92–amino acid precursor peptide.

GnRH release is pulsatile and is governed by a hypothalamic neural pulse generator (primarily in the arcuate nucleus) that controls the frequency and amplitude of GnRH release. The GnRH pulse generator is active late in fetal life and for ~1 year after birth but decreases considerably thereafter. Shortly before puberty, CNS inhibition decreases and the amplitude and frequency of GnRH pulses increase, particularly during sleep. As puberty progresses, the GnRH pulses increase further in amplitude and frequency until the normal adult pattern is established. The intermittent release of GnRH is crucial for the proper synthesis and release of the gonadotropins; the continuous administration of GnRH leads to desensitization and downregulation of GnRH receptors on pituitary gonadotropes.

Molecular and Cellular Bases of GnRH Action. GnRH signals through a specific GPCR on gonadotropes that activates $G_{q/11}$ and stimulates the PLC-IP_3-Ca^{2+} pathway (*see* Chapter 3), resulting in increased synthesis and secretion of LH and FSH. Although cyclic AMP is not the major mediator of GnRH action, binding of GnRH to its receptor also increases adenylyl cyclase activity. GnRH receptors also are present in the ovary, testis, and other sites, where their physiological significance remains to be determined.

Other Regulators of Gonadotropin Production. Gonadal steroids regulate gonadotropin production at the level of the pituitary and the hypothalamus, but effects on the hypothalamus predominate (*see* Figure 38–6). The feedback effects of gonadal steroids are dependent on sex, concentration, and time. In women, low levels of estradiol and progesterone inhibit gonadotropin production, largely through opioid action on the neural pulse generator. Higher and more sustained levels of estradiol have positive feedback effects that ultimately result in the gonadotropin surge that triggers ovulation. In men, testosterone inhibits gonadotropin production, in part through direct actions and in part via its conversion by aromatase to estradiol. Gonadotropin production also is regulated by the *inhibins*, which are members of the bone morphogenetic protein family of secreted signaling proteins. Inhibin A and B are made by granulosa cells in the ovary and Sertoli cells in the testis in response to the gonadotropins and local growth factors. They act directly in the pituitary to inhibit FSH secretion without affecting that of LH.

MOLECULAR AND CELLULAR BASES OF GONADOTROPIN ACTION. The actions of LH and hCG on target tissues are mediated by the LH receptor; those of FSH are mediated by the FSH receptor. The FSH and LH receptors couple to G_s to activate the adenylyl cyclase-cyclic AMP pathway. At higher ligand concentrations, the agonist-occupied gonadotropin receptors also activate PKC and Ca^{2+} signaling pathways via G_q-mediated effects on PLC_{β}. Most actions of the gonadotropins can be mimicked by cyclic AMP analogs.

PHYSIOLOGICAL EFFECTS OF GONADOTROPINS. *In men*, LH acts on testicular Leydig cells to stimulate the de novo synthesis of androgens, primarily *testosterone*, from cholesterol. FSH acts on the Sertoli cells to stimulate the production of proteins and nutrients required for sperm maturation. *In women*, the actions of FSH and LH are more complicated. FSH stimulates the growth of developing ovarian follicles and induces the expression of LH receptors on theca and granulosa cells. FSH also regulates the expression of aromatase in granulosa cells, thereby stimulating the production of *estradiol*. LH acts on the theca cells to stimulate the de novo synthesis of *androstenedione*, the major precursor of ovarian estrogens in premenopausal women (*see* Figure 40–1). LH also is required for the rupture of the dominant follicle during ovulation and for the synthesis of progesterone by the corpus luteum.

CLINICAL DISORDERS OF THE HYPOTHALAMIC-PITUITARY-GONADAL AXIS

Clinical disorders of the hypothalamic-pituitary-gonadal axis can manifest either as alterations in levels and effects of sex steroids (hyper- or hypogonadism) or as impaired reproduction. Deficient sex steroid production resulting from hypothalamic or pituitary defects is termed *hypogonadotropic hypogonadism* because circulating levels of gonadotropins are either low or undetectable. In contrast, reproductive disorders caused by processes that directly impair gonadal function are termed *hypergonadotropic* because the impaired production of sex steroids leads to a loss of negative feedback inhibition, thereby increasing the synthesis and secretion of gonadotropins.

GnRH AND ITS SYNTHETIC AGONIST ANALOGS

A synthetic peptide comprising the native sequence of GnRH has been used both diagnostically and therapeutically in human reproductive disorders. In addition, a number of GnRH analogs with structural modifications have been synthesized and brought to market.

SYNTHETIC GnRH. Synthetic GnRH (gonadorelin [FACTREL, LUTREPULSE]) is FDA-approved; problems with availability have limited its clinical use in the U.S. As a peptide, gonadorelin is administered either subcutaneously or intravenously. It is well absorbed following subcutaneous injection and has a circulating $t_{1/2}$ of ~2-4 min. For therapeutic uses, it must be administered in a pulsatile manner to avoid downregulation of the GnRH receptor.

GnRH CONGENERS. Synthetic agonist congeners of GnRH have longer half-lives than native GnRH. After a transient stimulation of gonadotropin secretion, they downregulate the GnRH receptor and inhibit gonadotropin secretion. The available GnRH agonists contain substitutions of the native sequence at position 6 that protect against proteolysis and substitutions at the carboxyl terminus that improve receptor-binding affinity. Compared to GnRH, these analogs exhibit enhanced potency and prolonged duration of action (*see* Table 38–3 in the 12th edition of the parent text).

Pharmacokinetics. The myriad formulations of GnRH agonists provide for diverse applications, including relatively short-term effects (e.g., assisted reproduction technology) and more prolonged action (e.g., depot forms that inhibit gonadotropin secretion in GnRH-dependent precocious puberty). The rates and extents of absorption thus vary considerably. The intranasal formulations have bioavailability (~4%) that is considerably lower than those of the parenteral formulations.

Clinical Uses. The depot form of the GnRH agonist leuprolide (LUPRON) has been used diagnostically to differentiate between GnRH-dependent and GnRH-independent precocious puberty. Leuprolide depot (3.75 mg) is injected subcutaneously, and serum LH is measured 2 h later. A plasma LH level of >6.6 mIU/mL is diagnostic of GnRH-dependent (central) disease. Clinically, the various GnRH agonists are used to achieve pharmacological castration in disorders that respond to reduction in gonadal steroids. A clear indication is in children with GnRH-dependent precocious puberty, whose premature sexual maturation can be arrested with minimal side effects by chronic administration of a depot form of a GnRH agonist. Long-acting GnRH agonists are used for palliative therapy of hormone responsive tumors (e.g., prostate or breast cancer), generally in conjunction with agents that block steroid biosynthesis or action to avoid transient increases in hormone levels (*see* Chapters 40-42). The GnRH agonists also are used to suppress steroid-responsive conditions such as endometriosis, uterine fibroids, acute intermittent porphyria, and priapism. Depot preparations can be administered subcutaneously or intramuscularly monthly or every 3 months. The long-lasting GnRH agonists have been used to avoid a premature LH surge, and thus ovulation, in various ovarian stimulation protocols for in vitro fertilization.

Adverse Effects. The long-acting agonists generally are well tolerated, and side effects are those that would be predicted to occur when gonadal steroidogenesis is inhibited (e.g., hot flashes and decreased bone density in both sexes, vaginal dryness and atrophy in women, and erectile dysfunction in men). Because of these effects, therapy in non-life-threatening diseases such as endometriosis or uterine fibroids generally is limited to 6 months. Postmarketing surveillance noted an increase in the incidence of pituitary apoplexy, a syndrome of headache, neurological manifestations, and impaired pituitary function that usually results from infarction of a pituitary adenoma. GnRH agonists are contraindicated in pregnant women (FDA Category X).

Formulations and Indications. **Leuprolide** (LUPRON, ELIGARD) is formulated in multiple doses for injection: subcutaneous (500 mg/day), subcutaneous depot (7.5 mg/month; 22.5 mg/3 months; 30 mg/4 months; 45 mg/6 months), and intramuscular depot (3.75 mg/month; 11.25 mg/3 months). It is approved for endometriosis, uterine fibroids, advanced prostate cancer, and central precocious puberty. **Goserelin** (ZOLADEX) is formulated as a subcutaneous implant (3.6 mg/month; 10.8 mg/12 weeks). It is approved for endometriosis and advanced prostate and breast cancer. **Histrelin** (VANTAS, SUPPRELIN LA) is formulated as a subcutaneous implant (50 mg/12 months). It is approved for central precocious puberty and advanced prostate cancer. **Nafarelin** (SYNAREL) is formulated as a nasal spray (200 μg/spray). It is approved for endometriosis (400 μg/day) and central precocious puberty (1600 μg/day). **Triptorelin** (TRELSTAR DEPOT, TRELSTAR LA) is formulated for depot intramuscular injection (3.75 mg/month; 11.25 mg/12 weeks) and approved for advanced prostate cancer. *Buserelin* and *Deslorelin* are not available in the U.S.

GnRH ANTAGONIST ANALOGS

Two GnRH antagonists, *ganirelix* (ANTAGON) and *cetrorelix* (CETROTIDE), are FDA-approved to suppress the LH surge and thus prevent premature ovulation in ovarian-stimulation protocols (*see* Chapter 66).

Both GnRH antagonists are formulated for subcutaneous administration. Bioavailability exceeds 90% within 1-2 h, and the $t_{1/2}$ varies depending on the dose. Once-daily administration suffices for therapeutic effect. Hypersensitivity reactions, including anaphylaxis, have been noted in postmarketing surveillance, some with the initial dose. When used in conjunction with gonadotropin injections for assisted reproduction, the effects of estrogen withdrawal (e.g., hot flashes) are not seen. GnRH antagonists are contraindicated in pregnant women (FDA Category X).

Cetrorelix is also used off label for endometriosis and uterine fibroids, both of which are estrogen dependent. As antagonists rather than agonists, these drugs do not transiently increase gonadotropin secretion and sex steroid biosynthesis.

NATURAL AND RECOMBINANT GONADOTROPINS

The gonadotropins are used for both diagnosis and therapy in reproductive endocrinology. For further discussion of the uses of gonadotropins in female reproduction, *see* Chapter 66.

The original gonadotropin preparations for clinical therapy were prepared from human urine and included *chorionic gonadotropin*, obtained from the urine of pregnant women, and *menotropins*, obtained from the urine of postmenopausal women. Highly purified preparations of human gonadotropins now are prepared using recombinant DNA technology and exhibit less batch-to-batch variation. This technology is being used to produce forms of gonadotropins with increased half-lives or higher clinical efficacy. One such "designer" gonadotropin, FSH-CTP, contains the β subunit of FSH fused to the carboxy-terminal extension of hCG, thereby increasing considerably the $t_{1/2}$ of the recombinant protein.

PREPARATIONS

FOLLICLE-STIMULATING HORMONE

FSH has long been a mainstay of regimens for either ovarian stimulation or in vitro fertilization. The original *menotropin* formulations (REPRONEX) contained roughly equal amounts of FSH and LH, as well as a number of other urinary proteins, and were administered intramuscularly to diminish local reactions. *Urofollitropin* (uFSH; BRAVELLE, MENOPUR), prepared by immunoconcentration of FSH with monoclonal antibodies, is pure enough to be administered subcutaneously. The amount of LH contained in such preparations is diminished considerably. Recombinant FSH (rFSH) is prepared by expressing cDNAs encoding the α and β subunits of human FSH in mammalian cell lines, yielding products whose glycosylation pattern mimics that of FSH produced by gonadotropes. The 2 available rFSH preparations (*follitropin* α [GONAL-F] and *follitropin* β [FOLLISTIM, PUREGON]) differ slightly in their carbohydrate structures; both can be administered subcutaneously because they are considerably purer. The relative advantages of recombinant FSH versus urine-derived gonadotropins have not been definitively established.

HUMAN CHORIONIC GONADOTROPIN

The hCG used clinically originally came from the urine of pregnant women. Several urine-derived preparations are available (NOVAREL, PREGNYL, PROFASI); all of them are administered intramuscularly due to local reactions. Recombinant hCG (choriogonadotropin alfa [OVIDREL]) also has reached clinical use.

RECOMBINANT HUMAN LH

Human LH produced using recombinant DNA technology and designated lutropin alfa (LUVERIS, LHADI) now is available (*see* Chapter 66).

DIAGNOSTIC USES

Pregnancy Testing. During pregnancy, the placenta produces significant amounts of hCG, which can be detected in maternal urine. Over-the-counter pregnancy kits containing antibodies specific for the unique β subunit of hCG qualitatively assay for the presence of hCG and can detect pregnancy within a few days after a woman's first missed menstrual period.

Timing of Ovulation. Ovulation occurs ~36 h after the onset of the LH surge. Therefore, urinary concentrations of LH, as measured with an over-the-counter radioimmunoassay kit, can be used to predict the time of ovulation.

Localization of Endocrine Disease. Measurements of plasma LH and FSH levels with β subunit–specific radioimmunoassays are useful in the diagnosis of several reproductive disorders. Low or undetectable levels of LH and FSH are indicative of hypogonadotropic hypogonadism and suggest hypothalamic or pituitary disease, whereas high levels of gonadotropins suggest primary gonadal diseases. A plasma FSH level of ≥ 10-12 mIU/mL on day 3 of the menstrual cycle, is associated with reduced fertility.

The administration of hCG can be used to stimulate testosterone production and thus to assess Leydig cell function in males suspected of having primary hypogonadism (e.g., in delayed puberty). Serum testosterone levels are assayed after multiple injections of hCG. A diminished testosterone response to hCG indicates Leydig cell failure; a normal testosterone response suggests a hypothalamic-pituitary disorder and normal Leydig cells.

THERAPEUTIC USES

Male Infertility. In men with impaired fertility secondary to gonadotropin deficiency (hypogonadotropic hypogonadism), gonadotropins can establish or restore fertility. Treatment typically is initiated with hCG (1500-2000 IUs intramuscularly or subcutaneously) 3 times per week until the plasma testosterone level indicate full induction of steroidogenesis. Thereafter, the dose of hCG is reduced to 2000 IU twice a week or 1000 IU 3 times a week, and menotropins (FSH + LH) or recombinant FSH is injected 3 times a week (typical dose of 150 IU) to fully induce spermatogenesis.

The most common side effect of gonadotropin therapy in males is gynecomastia, which presumably reflects increased production of estrogens due to the induction of aromatase. Maturation of the prepubertal testes typically requires treatment for >6 months. Once spermatogenesis has been initiated, ongoing treatment with hCG alone usually is sufficient to support sperm production.

Cryptorchidism. Cryptorchidism, the failure of 1 or both testes to descend into the scrotum, affects up to 3% of full-term male infants and becomes less prevalent with advancing postnatal age. Cryptorchid testes have defective spermatogenesis and are at increased risk for developing germ cell tumors. Hence, the current approach is to reposition the testes as early as possible, typically at 1 year of age but definitely before 2 years of age. The local actions of androgens stimulate descent of the testes; thus, hCG has been used by some to induce testicular descent if the cryptorchidism is not secondary to anatomical blockage. Therapy usually consists of injections of hCG (3000 IU/m^2 body surface area) intramuscularly every other day for 6 doses.

POSTERIOR PITUITARY HORMONES: OXYTOCIN AND VASOPRESSIN

The structures of the neurohypophyseal hormones oxytocin and arginine vasopressin (also called antidiuretic hormone, or ADH) and the physiology and pharmacology of vasopressin are presented in Chapter 25. The following discussion emphasizes the physiology of oxytocin. Therapeutic uses of synthetic oxytocin as a uterine-stimulating agent to induce or augment labor in selected pregnant women and to decrease postpartum hemorrhage are described in Chapter 66.

PHYSIOLOGY OF OXYTOCIN

Oxytocin is a cyclic nonapeptide that differs from vasopressin by only 2 amino acids (*see* Chapter 25). It is synthesized as a larger precursor in neurons whose cell bodies reside in the paraventricular nucleus and, to a lesser extent, the supraoptic nucleus in the hypothalamus. The precursor peptide is rapidly cleaved to the active hormone and its neurophysin, packaged into secretory granules as an oxytocin-neurophysin complex, and secreted from nerve endings that terminate primarily in the posterior pituitary gland (neurohypophysis). In addition, oxytocinergic neurons that regulate the autonomic nervous system project to regions of the hypothalamus, brainstem, and spinal cord. Other sites of oxytocin synthesis include the luteal cells of the ovary, the endometrium, and the placenta. Oxytocin acts via a specific GPCR (OXT) closely related to the V_{1a} and V_2 vasopressin receptors. In the human myometrium, OXT couples to G_q/G_{11}, activating the PLC_β-IP_3-Ca^{2+} pathway and enhancing activation of voltage-sensitive Ca^{2+} channels.

Stimuli for oxytocin secretion include sensory stimuli arising from dilation of the cervix and vagina and from suckling at the breast. *Estradiol* stimulates oxytocin secretion, whereas the ovarian polypeptide *relaxin* inhibits its release. Other factors that primarily affect vasopressin secretion also have some impact on oxytocin release: ethanol inhibits release; pain, dehydration, hemorrhage, and hypovolemia stimulate release. Based on the behavior of intravenously administered oxytocin during labor induction, the plasma $t_{1/2}$ of oxytocin is ~13 min.

PHYSIOLOGICAL EFFECTS OF OXYTOCIN

Uterus. Oxytocin stimulates the frequency and force of uterine contractions. Uterine responsiveness to oxytocin roughly parallels this increase in spontaneous activity and is highly dependent on estrogen, which increases the expression of the oxytocin receptors. Because of difficulties associated with the measurement of oxytocin levels and because loss of pituitary oxytocin apparently does not compromise labor and delivery, the physiological role of oxytocin in pregnancy is debated. Exogenous oxytocin can enhance rhythmic contractions at any time, but an 8-fold increase in uterine sensitivity to oxytocin occurs in the last half of pregnancy, and is accompanied by a 30-fold increase in oxytocin receptor numbers. The oxytocin antagonist *atosiban* is effective in suppressing preterm labor. Progesterone antagonizes the stimulatory effect of oxytocin in vitro, and refractoriness to progesterone in late pregnancy may contribute to the normal initiation of human parturition.

Breast. Oxytocin plays an important physiological role in milk ejection. Stimulation of the breast through suckling or mechanical manipulation induces oxytocin secretion, causing contraction of the myoepithelium that surrounds alveolar channels in the mammary gland. This action forces milk from the alveolar channels into large collecting sinuses, where it is available to the suckling infant.

Brain. Studies in rodents and humans have implicated oxytocin as an important CNS regulator of trust and of autonomic systems linked to anxiety and fear.

CLINICAL USE OF OXYTOCIN

Oxytocin is used therapeutically only to induce or augment labor and to treat or prevent postpartum hemorrhage (*see* Chapter 66). Deficiencies of oxytocin associated with disorders of the posterior pituitary impair milk letdown after delivery and may be one of the earliest signs of pituitary insufficiency secondary to postpartum hemorrhage (Sheehan syndrome); oxytocin is not used clinically in this setting.

For a complete Bibliographical Listing see Goodman & Gilman's ***The Pharmacological Basis of Therapeutics***, 12th ed., or Goodman & Gilman Online at www.AccessMedicine.com.

Thyroid and Anti-Thyroid Drugs

Thyroid hormone is essential for normal development, especially of the central nervous system (CNS). In the adult, thyroid hormone maintains metabolic homeostasis and influences the function of virtually all organ systems. Thyroid hormone contains iodine that must be supplied by nutritional intake. The thyroid gland contains large stores of thyroid hormone in the form of *thyroglobulin*. These stores maintain systemic concentrations of thyroid hormone despite variations in iodine availability and nutritional intake. The thyroidal secretion is predominantly the prohormone *thyroxine*, which is converted in the liver and other tissues to the active form, *triiodothyronine*. Local activation of thyroxine also occurs in target tissues (e.g., brain and pituitary) and is increasingly recognized as an important regulatory step in thyroid hormone action. Serum concentrations of thyroid hormones are precisely regulated by the pituitary hormone, *thyrotropin* (TSH), in a negative-feedback system. The predominant actions of thyroid hormone are mediated via nuclear *thyroid hormone receptors* (TRs) and modulating transcription of specific genes.

Overt *hyperthyroidism* and *hypothyroidism*, thyroid hormone excess or deficiency, are usually associated with dramatic clinical manifestations. Milder disease often has a more subtle clinical presentation and is identified based on abnormal biochemical tests of thyroid function. Maternal and neonatal hypothyroidism, due to iodine deficiency, remains the major preventable cause of mental retardation worldwide. Treatment of the hypothyroid patient consists of thyroid hormone replacement. Treatments for hyperthyroidism include anti-thyroid drugs to decrease hormone synthesis and secretion, destruction of the gland by the administration of radioactive iodine, or surgical removal. In most patients, disorders of thyroid function can be either cured or have their diseases controlled. Likewise, thyroid malignancies are most often localized and resectable. Metastatic disease often responds to radioiodide treatment but may become highly aggressive and unresponsive to conventional treatment.

THYROID

The thyroid gland produces 2 fundamentally different types of hormones. The thyroid follicle produces the iodothyronine hormones *thyroxine* (T_4) and *3,5,3′-triiodothyronine* (T_3). The thyroid's parafollicular cells (C cells) produce calcitonin (*see* Chapter 44).

BIOSYNTHESIS OF THYROID HORMONES. The thyroid hormones are synthesized and stored as amino acid residues of *thyroglobulin*, a complex glycoprotein made up of 2 apparently identical subunits (330 kDa each) and constituting the vast majority of the thyroid follicular colloid. The thyroid gland is unique in storing great quantities of potential hormone in this way, and extracellular thyroglobulin can represent a large portion of the thyroid mass. The major steps in the synthesis, storage, release, and interconversion of thyroid hormones are summarized in Figure 39–1 and described as follows:

A. Uptake of Iodide. Iodine ingested in the diet reaches the circulation in the form of iodide ion (I^-). Under normal circumstances, the I^- concentration in the blood is very low (0.2-0.4 μg/dL; ~15-30 nM), but the thyroid actively transports the ion via a specific membrane-bound protein, termed the *sodium-iodide symporter* (NIS). As a result, the ratio of thyroid to plasma iodide concentration is usually between 20 and 50 and can exceed 100 when the gland is stimulated. Iodide transport is inhibited by a number of ions such as thiocyanate and perchlorate. Thyrotropin (thyroid-stimulating hormone [TSH]) stimulates NIS gene expression and promotes insertion of NIS protein into the membrane in a functional configuration. Thus, decreased stores of thyroid iodine enhance iodide uptake, and the administration of iodide can reverse this situation by decreasing NIS protein expression. Iodine accumulation throughout the body is mediated by a single NIS gene. Individuals with congenital NIS gene mutations have absent or defective iodine concentration in all tissues known to concentrate iodine.

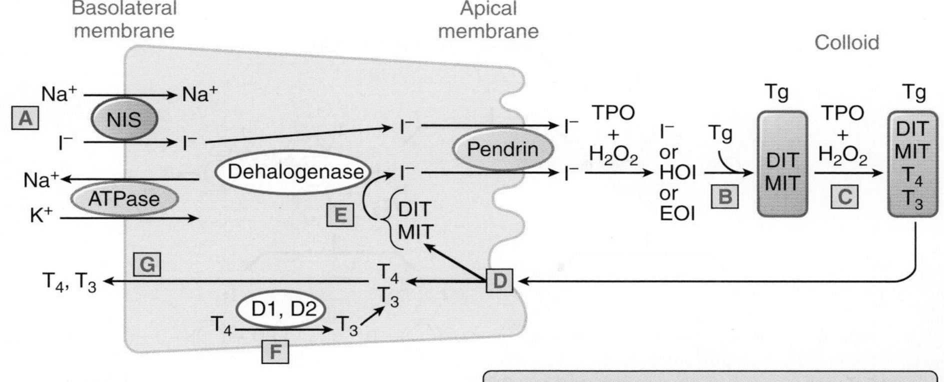

	METABOLIC STEP	INHIBITOR
A	Iodine transport	ClO_4^-, SCN
B	Iodination	PTU, MMI
C	Coupling	PTU, MMI
D	Colloid Resorption	Colchicine, Li^+, I^-
E	Deiodination of DIT + MIT	Dinitrotyrosine
F	Deodination of T_4	PTU
G	Secretion	D1

Figure 39–1 *Major pathways of thyroid hormone biosynthesis and release. Abbreviations:* Tg, thyroglobulin; DIT, diiodotyrosine; MIT, monoiodotyrosine; TPO, thyroid peroxidase; HOI, hypoiodous acid; EOI, enzyme-linked species; D1 and D2, deiodinases; PTU, propylthiouracil; MMI, methimazole.

B. Oxidation and Iodination. The oxidation of iodide to its active form is accomplished by *thyroid peroxidase*. The reaction results in the formation of monoiodotyrosyl (MIT) and diiodotyrosyl (DIT) residues in thyroglobulin just prior to its extracellular storage in the lumen of the thyroid follicle.

C. Formation of Thyroxine and Triiodothyronine from Iodotyrosines. The remaining synthetic step is the coupling of 2 diiodotyrosyl residues to form thyroxine (T_4) or of a monoiodotyrosyl and a diiodotyrosyl residue to form triiodothyronine (T_3). These oxidative reactions also are catalyzed by *thyroid peroxidase*. Intrathyroidal and secreted T_3 are also generated by the 5′-deiodination of thyroxine.

D. Resorption; and Proteolysis of Colloid; E. Deiodination of DIT/MIT; F. deiodination of T_4; G. Secretion of Thyroid Hormones. Because T_4 and T_3 are synthesized and stored within thyroglobulin, proteolysis is an important part of the secretory process. This process is initiated by endocytosis of colloid from the follicular lumen at the apical surface of the cell, with the participation of a thyroglobulin receptor, *megalin*. This "ingested" thyroglobulin appears as intracellular colloid droplets, which apparently fuse with lysosomes containing the requisite proteolytic enzymes. TSH enhances the degradation of thyroglobulin by increasing the activity of *thiol endopeptidases* of the lysosomes, which selectively cleave thyroglobulin, yielding hormone-containing intermediates that subsequently are processed by exopeptidases. The liberated hormones then exit the cell mostly as T_4, some as T_3, via a process of deiodination (Figure 39–2) that also occurs peripherally (Figure 39–3).

CONVERSION OF T_4 TO T_3 IN PERIPHERAL TISSUES. The normal daily production of T_4 is estimated to range between 80 and 100 μg; that of T_3 is between 30 and 40 μg. Although T_3 is secreted by the thyroid, metabolism of T_4 by 5′, or outer ring, deiodination in the peripheral tissues accounts for ~80% of circulating T_3. In contrast, removal of the iodine on position 5 of the inner ring produces the metabolically inactive 3,3′,5′-triiodothyronine (reverse T_3 or rT_3; Figure 39–2). Under normal conditions, ~40% of T_4 is converted to each of T_3 and rT_3, and ~20% is metabolized *via* other pathways, such as glucuronidation in the liver and excretion in the bile. Normal circulating concentrations of T_4 in plasma range from 4.5-11 μg/dL; those of T_3 are ~1/100 of that (60-180 ng/dL). Triiodothyronine has a much higher affinity for the nuclear thyroid hormone receptor compared with thyroxine and is much more potent biologically on a molar basis.

There are 3 *iodothyronine deiodinases*. Forms 1 and 2 (D1, D2) convert T_4 to T_3. D1 is expressed primarily in the liver and kidney, and also in the thyroid and pituitary (Figure 39–3). It is upregulated in hyperthyroidism; downregulated in hypothyroidism, and inhibited by the anti-thyroid drug *propylthiouracil*. D2 is expressed

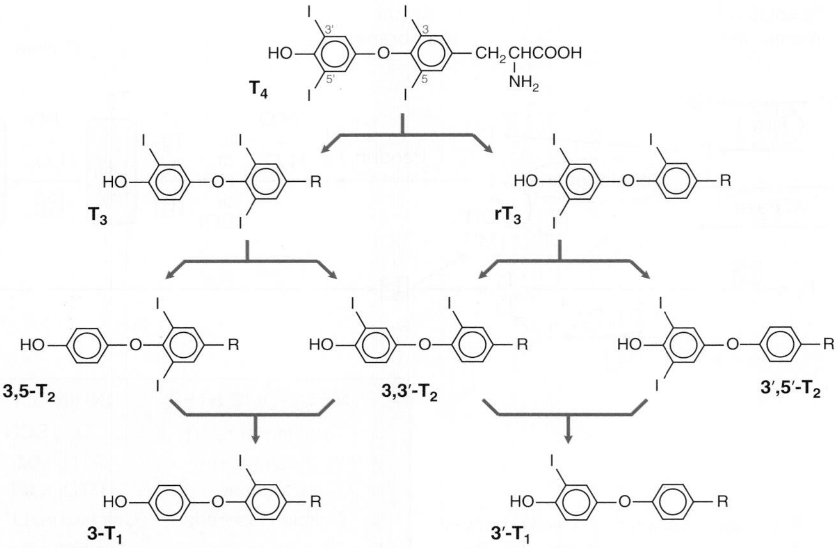

Figure 39–2 *Pathways of iodothyronine deiodination.*

primarily in the CNS (including the pituitary and hypothalamus) and brown adipose tissue, also in the thyroid, and at very low levels in skeletal muscle. The activity of D2 is unaffected by propylthiouracil. D2 localizes to the endoplasmic reticulum, which facilitates access of D2-generated T_3 to the nucleus. Hence organs that express D2 tend to use the locally generated T_3. D2 is regulated by T_4 such that elevated levels of the enzyme are found in hypothyroidism and suppressed levels are found in hyperthyroidism. Type 3 deiodinase (D3) catalyzes inner ring- or 5-deiodination, the main inactivating pathway of T_3 metabolism; D1 performs this function to some extent. D3 is found at highest levels in the CNS and placenta, and is also expressed in skin and uterus. The 3 deiodinases contain the rare amino acid selenocysteine in their active sites. Mutations in 1 such protein, SECIS binding protein 2, are associated with abnormal circulating thyroid hormone levels.

TRANSPORT OF THYROID HORMONES IN THE BLOOD. The thyroid hormones are transported in the blood in strong but noncovalent association with certain plasma proteins.

Thyroxine-binding globulin (TBG) is the major carrier of thyroid hormones. It is a glycoprotein that binds 1 molecule of T_4 per molecule of protein with a very high affinity (K_d, is ~10^{-10} M). T_3 is bound less avidly. T_4, but not T_3, also is bound by *transthyretin* (thyroxine-binding prealbumin), a retinol-binding protein. This protein is present in higher concentration than is TBG and primarily binds T_4 with a K_d ~10^{-7} M. Albumin also can bind T_4 when the more avid carriers are saturated, but its physiological importance is unclear. Binding of thyroid hormones to plasma proteins protects the hormones from metabolism and excretion, resulting

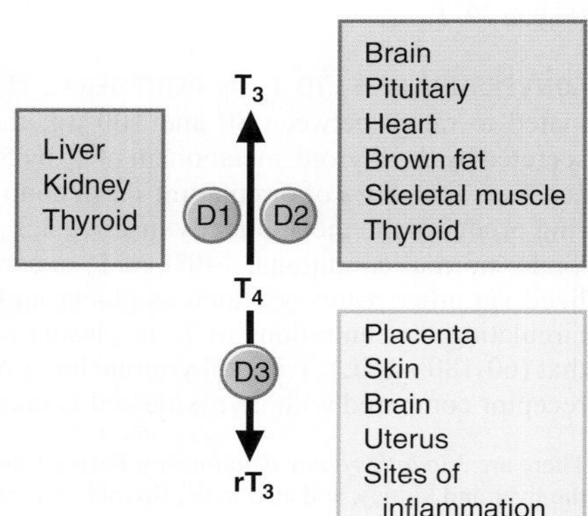

Figure 39–3 *Deiodinase isozymes.* D1, type I iodothyronine 5′-deiodinase; D2, type II iodothyronine 5′-deiodinase; D3, type III iodothyronine 5-deiodinase; BAT, brown adipose tissue.

Table 39–1

Factors that Alter Binding of Thyroxine to Thyroxine-Binding Globulin

INCREASE BINDING	DECREASE BINDING
Drugs	
Estrogens, tamoxifen	Corticosteroids, androgens
Selective estrogen receptor modulators	L-Asparaginase, furosemide
Methadone, heroin	Salicylates, mefenamic acid
Clofibrate, 5-fluorouracil	Antiseizure medications (phenytoin, carbamazepine)
Systemic Factors	
Liver disease, porphyria	Acute and chronic illness
HIV infection	Inheritance
Inheritance	

in their long half-lives in the circulation. The free (unbound) hormone is a small percentage (~0.03% of T_4 and ~0.3% of T_3) of the total hormone in plasma. The differential binding affinities for serum proteins also contribute to establishing the 10- to 100-fold differences in circulating hormone concentrations and half-lives of T_4 and T_3.

Only the unbound hormone has metabolic activity. Because of the high degree of binding of thyroid hormones to plasma proteins, changes in either the concentrations of these proteins or the binding affinity of the hormones for the proteins has major effects on the total serum hormone levels. Certain drugs and a variety of pathological and physiological conditions can alter both the binding of thyroid hormones to plasma proteins and the amounts of these proteins (Table 39–1).

DEGRADATION AND EXCRETION. T_3 and T_4 can deiodinated but can also be metabolized by ether cleavage, conjugation, and oxidative decarboxylation.

T_4 is eliminated slowly from the body, with a $t_{1/2}$ of 6-8 days. In hyperthyroidism, the $t_{1/2}$ is shortened to 3-4 days, whereas in hypothyroidism it may be 9-10 days. In conditions associated with increased binding to TBG, such as pregnancy, clearance is retarded. The opposite effect is observed when binding to protein is inhibited by certain drugs (*see* Table 39–1). T_3, which is less avidly bound to protein, has a $t_{1/2}$ of ~1 day.

The liver is the major site of non-deiodinative degradation of thyroid hormones; T_4 and T_3 are conjugated with glucuronic and sulfuric acids and excreted in the bile. Some thyroid hormone is liberated by hydrolysis of the conjugates in the intestine and reabsorbed. A portion of the conjugated material reaches the colon unchanged, where it is hydrolyzed and eliminated in feces as the free compounds.

FACTORS REGULATING OF THYROID HORMONE SECRETION. Thyrotropin or TSH is a glycoprotein hormone with α and β subunits analogous to those of the gonadotropins (*see* Table 38–2). TSH is secreted in a pulsatile manner and circadian pattern (levels are highest during sleep at night). TSH secretion is controlled by the hypothalamic peptide *thyrotropin-releasing hormone* (TRH) and by the concentration of free thyroid hormones in the circulation. Extra thyroid hormone inhibits transcription of both the TRH gene and the genes encoding the α and β subunits of TSH, which suppresses the secretion of TSH and causes the thyroid to become inactive and regress. Any decrease in the normal rate of thyroid hormone secretion by the thyroid evokes an enhanced secretion of TSH. Additional mechanisms mediating the effect of thyroid hormone on TSH secretion appear to be a reduction in TRH secretion by the hypothalamus and a reduction in the number of TRH receptors on pituitary cells (Figure 39–4).

THYROTROPIN-RELEASING HORMONE. TRH is a tripeptide (L-pyroglutamyl-L-histidyl-L-proline amide) synthesized by the hypothalamus and released into the hypophyseal-portal circulation where it interacts with TRH receptors on thyrotropes in the anterior pituitary. The binding of TRH to its receptor, a GPCR, stimulates the G_q-PLC-IP_3-Ca^{2+} pathway and activates PKC, ultimately stimulating the synthesis and release of TSH. Two TRH receptors have now been identified, TRH-R1 and TRH-R2, as well as selective analogs for these receptors. Somatostatin, dopamine, and glucocorticoids inhibit TRH-stimulated TSH secretion.

ACTIONS OF TSH ON THE THYROID. TSH increases the synthesis and secretion of thyroid hormone. These effects follow the binding of TSH to its receptor (a GPCR) on the plasma membrane of thyroid cells. Binding

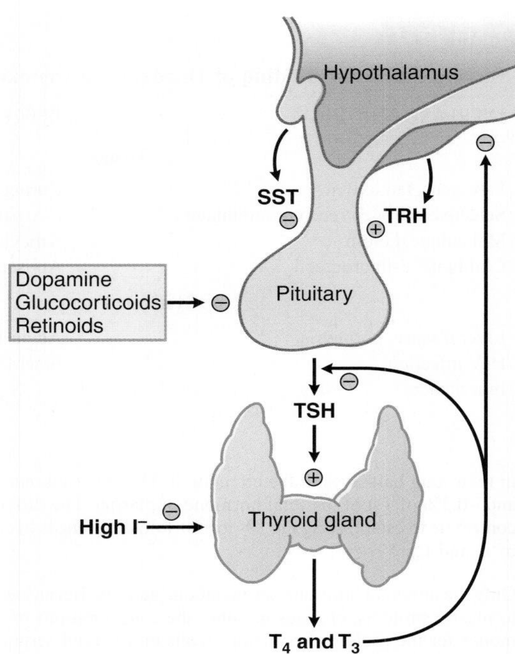

Figure 39–4 *Regulation of thyroid hormone secretion.* Myriad neural inputs influence hypothalamic secretion of thyrotropin-releasing hormone (TRH). TRH stimulates release of thyrotropin (TSH, thyroid-stimulating hormone) from the anterior pituitary; TSH stimulates the synthesis and release of the thyroid hormones T_3 and T_4. T_3 and T_4 feed back to inhibit the synthesis and release of TRH and TSH. Somatostatin (SST) can inhibit TRH action, as can dopamine and high concentrations of glucocorticoids. Low levels of I^- are required for thyroxine synthesis, but high levels inhibit thyroxin synthesis and release.

of TSH to its receptor stimulates the G_s-adenylyl cyclase–cyclic AMP pathway. Higher concentrations of TSH activate the G_q-PLC pathway. Multiple mutations of the TSH receptor result in clinical thyroid dysfunction.

IODINE AND THYROID FUNCTION. Normal thyroid function requires an adequate intake of iodine; without it, normal amounts of hormone cannot be made, TSH is secreted in excess, and the thyroid becomes hyperplastic and hypertrophic. The enlarged and stimulated thyroid becomes remarkably efficient at extracting the residual traces of iodide from the blood, developing an iodine gradient that may be 10 times normal; in mild-to-moderate iodine deficiency, the thyroid usually succeeds in producing sufficient hormone and preferentially secreting T_3. In more severe iodine deficiency, adult hypothyroidism and cretinism may occur. High levels of iodine inhibit thyroxine synthesis and release. In some areas of the world, simple or nontoxic goiter is prevalent because of insufficient dietary iodine. The addition of iodate to table salt (NaCl) provides a convenient iodine supplement. In the U.S., iodized salt provides 100 μg of iodine per gram. The recommended daily allowances for iodine range from 90-120 μg for children, 150 μg for adults, 220 μg for pregnancy, and 290 μg for lactation. Vegetables, meat, and poultry contain minimal amounts of iodine, whereas dairy products and fish are relatively high in iodine.

THYROID HORMONE TRANSPORT. Transmembrane passage of thyroid hormones appears to be mediated by monocarboxylic acid transporter 8 (MCT8, SLC16A2; *see* Table 5–2). MCT8 is widely expressed, including in liver, heart, and brain. MCT10 also transports T_4 and T_3 and is widely expressed, but its physiological importance for thyroid hormone transport in vivo is unknown. The organic anion transporter OATP1C1 preferentially transports T_4 rather than T_3, is highly expressed in brain capillaries, and has been hypothesized to be responsible for the transport of T_4 across the blood-brain barrier (*see* Chapter 5).

MEDIATION OF EFFECTS BY NUCLEAR RECEPTORS. Thyroid hormone action is mediated largely by the binding of T_3 to TRs, which are members of the nuclear receptor superfamily of transcription factors.

T_3 binds to TRs with ~10-fold greater affinity than does T_4, and T_4 is not thought to be biologically active in normal physiology. TRs bind to specific DNA sequences (thyroid hormone response elements [TREs]) in the promoter/regulatory regions of target genes. The transcription of most target genes is repressed by unliganded TRs and induced following the binding of T_3. In the unliganded state, the TR ligand-binding domain interacts with a corepressor complex that includes *histone deacetylases* and other proteins. The binding of T_3 causes replacement of the corepressor complex by a coactivator complex that includes *histone acetyltransferases*, *methyltransferases*, and other proteins. Other thyroid hormone target genes, such as those encoding TRH and the TSH subunits, are negatively regulated by T_3. The mechanism is not well defined, but these genes tend to be induced by the unliganded TR in addition to being repressed by T_3.

Two genes encode TRs: *THRA* and *THRB*. *THRA* encodes the receptor TRα1. TRα1 is expressed in most cell types, but its major activities are in the regulation of heart rate, body temperature, skeletal muscle function, and the development of bone and small intestine. Alternative splicing of the TRα primary transcript results in the production of TRα2, which lacks part of the ligand-binding domain (LBD), does not bind T_3, and has not known function. A cryptic promoter within intron 7 of *THRA* drives the production of small proteins that contain only a portion of the TRα LBD and appear to play a role, along with TRα1, in GI development. The *THRB* gene has 2 promoters that lead to the production of TRβ1 and TRβ2. These receptors have unique amino terminal domains but otherwise are identical. TRβ1 is ubiquitous; TRβ2 has a highly restricted pattern of expression. Mutations in *THRB* cause the syndrome of resistance to thyroid hormone. TRβ1 mediates specific effects in liver metabolism (including the hypocholesterolemic effect of T_3); TRβ2 has roles in the negative feedback by T_3 on hypothalamic TRH and pituitary TSH and in the development of retinal cones and the inner ear.

NONGENOMIC EFFECTS OF THYROID HORMONE. TRs are found outside the nucleus where they can exert biological effects via rapid nongenomic mechanisms.

TRs associate in a T_3-dependent manner with the p85α subunit PI3 kinase, resulting in the activation of PKB/Akt. The PI3K/Akt pathway has myriad effects. For example, it stimulates NO production by endothelial cells, which leads to vasodilation; hence, T_3 administration causes rapid vasodilation. There also is evidence for nongenomic actions of thyroid hormone via a plasma membrane receptor within integrin αVβ3. This putative receptor binds extracellular T_4 in preference to T_3, resulting in activation of MAP kinase. The importance of nongenomic actions in thyroid hormone physiology and pathophysiology remains uncertain.

Effects of Thyroid Hormone Metabolites. 3-Iodothyronamine and thyronamine, naturally occurring metabolites of T_4, are ligands for the GPCR trace amine-associated receptor 1 (TAAR1), an interaction of unknown relevance in humans.

MAJOR CLINICAL EFFECTS OF THYROID HORMONES

GROWTH AND DEVELOPMENT. Thyroid hormone plays a critical role in brain development by mechanisms that are incompletely understood. The absence of thyroid hormone during the period of active neurogenesis (up to 6 months postpartum) leads to irreversible mental retardation (cretinism) and is accompanied by multiple morphological alterations in the brain. These severe morphological alterations result from disturbed neuronal migration, deranged axonal projections, and decreased synaptogenesis. Thyroid hormone supplementation during the first 2 weeks of postnatal life prevents the development of these disturbed morphological changes. The actions of thyroid hormones on protein synthesis and enzymatic activity are not limited to the brain; most tissues are affected by the administration of thyroid hormone or by its deficiency. The extensive defects in growth and development in cretins vividly illustrate the pervasive effects of thyroid hormones in normal individuals.

Cretinism is usually classified as *endemic* (caused by extreme iodine deficiency) or *sporadic* (a consequence abnormal thyroid development or a defect in the synthesis of thyroid hormone). The affected child is dwarfed, with short extremities, mentally retarded, inactive, uncomplaining, and listless. Other manifestations include puffy face, enlarged tongue, dry and doughy skin, slow heart rate, and decreased body. For treatment to be fully effective, the diagnosis must be made long before these changes are obvious. In regions of endemic iodine deficiency, iodine replacement is best instituted before pregnancy. Screening of newborn infants for deficient thyroid function is carried out in the U.S. and in most industrialized countries.

THERMOGENIC EFFECTS. Thyroid hormone is necessary for both obligatory thermogenesis (the heat resulting from vital processes) as well as for facultative or adaptive thermogenesis.

Only a few organs, including the brain, gonads, and spleen, are unresponsive to the thermogenic effects of T_3. Obligatory thermogenesis is the result of T_3 making most biological processes thermodynamically less efficient for the sake of producing heat, but the pathways involved and their quantitative contributions have yet to be fully defined. The capacity of T_3 to induce the skeletal muscle Ca^{++}-dependent ATPase (SERCA1) contributes to thermogenesis by stimulating the cycling of calcium between cytosol and sarcoplasmic reticulum. Other than in brown adipose tissue, there is no evidence that uncoupling of phosphorylation is a major thermogenic mechanism. Regardless of the mechanism, thermogenesis is highly sensitive to thyroid hormone around the physiological range: small changes in L-thyroxine replacement doses may significantly alter resting energy expenditure in the hypothyroid patient. The ability of T_3 to stimulate thermogenesis has evolved along with ancillary effects to support this action, such as the stimulation of appetite and lipogenesis.

CARDIOVASCULAR EFFECTS. Hyperthyroid patients have tachycardia, increased stroke volume, increased cardiac index, cardiac hypertrophy, decreased peripheral vascular resistance, and increased pulse pressure. Hyperthyroidism is a relatively common cause of atrial fibrillation. Hypothyroid patients have bradycardia, decreased cardiac index, pericardial effusion, increased peripheral vascular resistance, decreased pulse pressure, and elevation of mean arterial pressure.

T_3 regulates myocardial gene expression primarily through TRα1, which is expressed at a higher level in cardiomyocytes than TRβ. T_3 shortens diastolic relaxation (lusitropic effect) by inducing expression of the sarcoplasmic reticulum ATPase SERCA2 and decreasing phospholamban, a SERCA2 inhibitor. T_3 increases the force of myocardial contraction (inotropic effect) in part by inducing expression of the ryanodine channel, the calcium channel of the sarcoplasmic reticulum. T_3 induces the gene encoding the myosin heavy chain (MHC) α isoform and decreases expression of the MHC β gene. Because MHCα endows the myosin holoenzyme with greater ATPase activity, this is one mechanism by which T_3 enhances the velocity of contraction. The chronotropic effect of T_3 is mediated by increases in the pacemaker ion current I_f in the sinoatrial node. Several proteins that comprise the I_f channel are induced by T_3, including HCN2 and HCN4. T_3 also appears to have a direct nongenomic vasodilating effect on vascular smooth muscle, which may contribute to the decreased systemic vascular resistance and increased cardiac output of hyperthyroidism.

METABOLIC EFFECTS. Thyroid hormone stimulates the expression of hepatic low-density lipoprotein (LDL) receptors and the metabolism of cholesterol to bile acids, such that hypercholesterolemia is a characteristic feature of hypothyroidism.

Thyroid hormone has complex effects on carbohydrate metabolism. Thyrotoxicosis is an insulin-resistant state. Post-receptor defects are manifested by depleted glycogen stores, enhanced gluconeogenesis, and increased rate of glucose absorption from the gut. Compensatory increases in insulin secretion result in hyperinsulinemia. There may be impaired glucose tolerance or even clinical diabetes, but most hyperthyroid patients are euglycemic. Conversely, hypothyroidism results in decreased absorption of glucose from the gut, decreased insulin secretion, and a reduced rate of peripheral glucose uptake. Glucose metabolism generally is not affected in a clinically significant manner in nondiabetic patients, although insulin requirements decrease in the hypothyroid patient with diabetes.

DISORDERS OF THYROID FUNCTION

THYROID HYPOFUNCTION. Hypothyroidism, known as *myxedema* when severe, is the most common disorder of thyroid function.

Worldwide, hypothyroidism resulting from iodine deficiency remains a common problem. In nonendemic areas where iodine is sufficient, chronic autoimmune thyroiditis (Hashimoto thyroiditis) accounts for most cases; this disorder is characterized by high levels of circulating antibodies directed against thyroid peroxidase and, sometimes, against thyroglobulin; antibodies directed at the TSH receptor may be present. The conditions are examples of *primary hypothyroidism,* failure of the thyroid gland itself. *Central hypothyroidism* occurs much less often and results from diminished stimulation of the thyroid by TSH because of pituitary failure (*secondary hypothyroidism*) or hypothalamic failure (*tertiary hypothyroidism*). Hypothyroidism present at birth (*congenital hypothyroidism*) is the most common preventable cause of mental retardation in the world.

Common symptoms of hypothyroidism include fatigue, lethargy, cold intolerance, mental slowness, depression, dry skin, constipation, mild weight gain, fluid retention, muscle aches and stiffness, irregular menses, and infertility. Common signs include goiter (primary hypothyroidism only), bradycardia, delayed relaxation phase of the deep tendon reflexes, cool and dry skin, hypertension, nonpitting edema, and facial puffiness. Deficiency of thyroid hormone during the first few months of life causes feeding problems, failure to thrive, constipation, and sleepiness. Retardation of mental development is irreversible if not treated promptly. Childhood hypothyroidism impairs linear growth and bone maturation. Diagnosis requires the finding of an elevated serum TSH or, in cases of central hypothyroidism, a decreased serum free T_4.

THYROID HYPERFUNCTION. Thyrotoxicosis is a condition caused by elevated concentrations of circulating free thyroid hormones. Increased thyroid hormone production is the most common cause, with the common link of TSH receptor stimulation and increased iodine uptake by the thyroid gland as shown by the measurement of the percentage uptake of ^{123}I or ^{131}I in a 24-h radioactive iodine uptake (RAIU) test.

TSH receptor stimulation is either the result of TSH receptor stimulating antibody in Graves disease or somatic activating TSH receptor mutations in autonomously functioning nodules or a toxic goiter. In contrast, thyroid inflammation or destruction resulting in excess "leak" of thyroid hormones or excess exogenous thyroid hormone intake results in a low 24-h RAIU. The term *subclinical hyperthyroidism* is defined as those with a subnormal serum TSH and normal concentrations of T_4 and T_3. Atrial arrhythmias, excess cardiac mortality, and excessive bone loss have been associated with this profile of thyroid function tests.

Graves disease is the most common cause of high RAIU thyrotoxicosis. Graves disease is an autoimmune disorder characterized by increased thyroid hormone production, diffuse goiter, and IgG antibodies that bind to and activate the TSH receptor. As with most types of thyroid dysfunction, women are affected more than men, with a ratio ranging from 5:1-7:1. Graves disease is more common between the ages of 20 and 50, but it may occur at any age. Graves disease is commonly associated with other autoimmune diseases. The characteristic exophthalmos associated with Graves disease is an infiltrative ophthalmopathy and is considered an autoimmune-mediated inflammation of the periorbital connective tissue and extraocular muscles. Toxic uninodular/multinodular goiter accounts for 10-40% of cases of hyperthyroidism and is more common in older patients. A low RAIU is seen in the destructive thyroiditides and in thyrotoxicosis in patients taking excessive doses of thyroid hormone.

Most of the signs and symptoms of thyrotoxicosis stem from the excessive production of heat, increased motor activity, and increased sensitivity to catecholamines produced by the sympathetic nervous system. The skin is flushed, warm, and moist; the muscles are weak and tremulous; the heart rate is rapid, the heartbeat is forceful, and the arterial pulses are prominent and bounding. Increased expenditure of energy gives rise to increased appetite and, if intake is insufficient, to loss of weight. There also may be insomnia, difficulty in remaining still, anxiety and apprehension, intolerance to heat, and increased frequency of bowel movements. Angina, arrhythmias, and heart failure may be present in older patients. Older patients may experience less manifestations of sympathetic nervous system stimulation. Some individuals may show extensive muscular wasting as a result of thyroid myopathy. The most severe form of hyperthyroidism is thyroid storm (see section below on therapeutic uses of anti-thyroid drugs).

THYROID FUNCTION TESTS. Measurement of the total hormone concentration in plasma may not give an accurate picture of the activity of the thyroid gland; total hormone concentration changes with alterations in amount and affinity of TBG in plasma.

Although equilibrium dialysis of undiluted serum and radioimmunoassay for free thyroxine (FT_4) in the dialysate represent the gold standard for determining FT_4 concentrations, this assay is typically not available in routine clinical laboratories. The most common assays used for estimating the free T_4 and free T_3 concentrations employ labeled analogs of these iodothyronines in chemiluminescence and enzyme-linked immunoassays. These assays are subject to influences of altered serum binding proteins, nonthyroid disease, and other drugs. In individuals with normal pituitary function, serum measurement of TSH is the thyroid function test of choice because pituitary secretion of TSH is sensitively regulated in response to circulating concentrations of thyroid hormones. The TSH assay can differentiate between normal and thyrotoxic patients, who should exhibit suppressed TSH values. Recombinant human TSH (*thyrotropin alfa* [THYROGEN]) is available as an injectable preparation to test the ability of thyroid tissue, both normal and malignant, to take up radioactive iodine and release thyroglobulin.

THERAPEUTIC USES OF THYROID HORMONE

The major indications for the therapeutic use of thyroid hormone are for hormone replacement therapy in patients with hypothyroidism and for TSH suppression therapy in patients with thyroid cancer.

THYROID HORMONE PREPARATIONS. Synthetic preparations of the sodium salts of the natural isomers of the thyroid hormones are available and widely used for thyroid hormone therapy.

Levothyroxine. Levothyroxine sodium (L-T_4, LEVOTHROID, LEVOXYL, SYNTHROID, UNITHROID, others) is available in tablets and as a lyophilized powder for injection. Table 39–2 lists drugs and other factors that may influence levothyroxine dosage requirements. Absorption of thyroxine occurs in the stomach and small intestine and is incomplete (~80% of the dose is absorbed). Absorption is slightly increased when the hormone is taken on an empty stomach, and it is associated with less variability in the TSH when taken this way regularly. The serum T_4 peaks 2-4 h after oral ingestion, with plasma $t_{1/2}$ ~7-days. For any given serum TSH, the serum T_4/T_3 ratio is higher in patients taking levothyroxine than in patients with endogenous thyroid function, due to the fact that ~20% of circulating T_3 normally is supplied by direct thyroidal secretion. Follow-up blood tests typically are done ~6 weeks after any dosage change due to the 1-week plasma $t_{1/2}$ of T_4. In situations where patients cannot take oral medications or where intestinal absorption is in question, levothyroxine may be given intravenously once daily at a dose ~80% of the patient's daily oral requirement.

Liothyronine. Liothyronine sodium (L-T_3) is the salt of triiodothyronine and is available in tablets (CYTOMEL) and in an injectable form (TRIOSTAT, others). Liothyronine absorption is nearly 100% with peak serum levels 2-4 h following oral ingestion. Liothyronine may be used occasionally when a more rapid onset of action is desired such as in the rare presentation of myxedema coma or if rapid termination of action is desired such as when preparing a thyroid cancer patient for ^{131}I therapy. Liothyronine is less desirable for chronic replacement therapy due to the requirement for more frequent dosing (plasma $t_{1/2}$ = 0.75 days), higher cost, and transient

Table 39–2

Factors Influencing Oral Levothyroxine Therapy

Drugs and other factors that may increase levothyroxine dosage requirements
Impaired levothyroxine absorption
Aluminum-containing antacids, proton pump inhibitors, sucralfate
Bile acid sequestrants (cholestyramine, colestipol, colesevelam)
Calcium carbonate (effect generally small), phosphate binders (lanthanum carbonate, sevelamer)
Chromium picolinate, raloxifene, iron salts
Food, soy products (effect generally very small), lactose intolerance (single case report)
Increased thyroxine metabolism, CYP3A4 induction
Bexarotene, rifampin, carbamazepine, phenytoin, sertraline
Impaired $T_4 \rightarrow T_3$ conversion
Amiodarone
Mechanisms uncertain or multifactorial
Estrogen, pregnancy, lovastatin, simvastatin, ethionamide, tyr kinase inhibitors (imatinib, sunitinib)
Drugs and other factors that may decrease levothyroxine dosage requirements
Advancing age (>65 years), androgen therapy in women
Drugs that may decrease TSH without changing free T_4 in levothyroxine-treated patients
Metformin

elevations of serum T_3 concentrations above the normal range. In addition, organs that express the type 2 deiodinase use the locally generated T_3 in addition to plasma T_3, and hence, there is theoretical concern that these organs will not maintain physiological intracellular T_3 levels in the absence of plasma T_4. Ten to 15 μg of liothyronine sodium 3 times per day typically yields a normal serum free T_3 in an athyreotic individual.

Other Preparations. A mixture of thyroxine and triiodothyronine 4:1 by weight is marketed as liotrix (THYROLAR). Desiccated thyroid preparations such as (ARMOUR THYROID, others), with a similar T_4:T_3 ratio, also are available. A 60-mg (1 grain) desiccated thyroid tablet is approximately equivalent in activity to 80 μg of thyroxine.

THYROID HORMONE REPLACEMENT THERAPY IN HYPOTHYROIDISM. Thyroxine (L-T_4, levothyroxine sodium) is the hormone of choice for thyroid hormone replacement therapy due to its consistent potency and prolonged duration of action. With this therapy, one relies on the types 1 and 2 deiodinases to convert T_4 to T_3 to maintain a steady serum level of free T_3.

The average daily adult replacement dose of levothyroxine sodium is 1.7 μg/kg body weight (0.8 μg/lb). Dosing should generally be based on lean body mass. The goal of therapy is to normalize the serum TSH (in primary hypothyroidism) or free T_4 (in secondary or tertiary hypothyroidism) and to relieve symptoms of hypothyroidism. In primary hypothyroidism, generally it is sufficient to follow TSH without free T_4. In individuals >60 years of age and those with known or suspected cardiac disease or with areas of autonomous thyroid function, institution of therapy at a lower daily dose of levothyroxine sodium (12.5-50 μg per day) is appropriate. The dose can be increased at a rate of 25 μg per day every 6-8 weeks until the TSH is normalized. Controlled trials give no evidence that combination therapy with $T_4 + T_3$ provides a better therapeutic response than does T_4 alone. Monotherapy with levothyroxine most closely mimics normal physiology and generally is preferred.

Hypothyroidism During Pregnancy. Due to the increased serum concentration of TBG induced by estrogen, the expression of type 3 deiodinase by the placenta, and the small amount of transplacental passage of L-T_4 from mother to fetus, a higher dose of L-T_4 is often required in pregnant patients. Overt hypothyroidism during pregnancy is associated with fetal distress, impaired psychoneural development in the progeny, and mildly impaired psychomotor development in the children and preterm delivery. Women should increase their levothyroxine dosage by ~30% as soon as pregnancy is confirmed. Most measure a serum TSH in the first trimester and then adjust the thyroxine dose based on this result. Subsequent dosage adjustments based on serum TSH, measured 4-6 weeks after each adjustment, should be made to bring the TSH into the lower portion of the reference range.

MYXEDEMA COMA. Myxedema coma is a rare syndrome that represents the extreme expression of severe, long-standing hypothyroidism. Myxedema coma occurs most often in elderly patients during the winter months. Cardinal features of myxedema coma are: *hypothermia*, *respiratory depression*, and *decreased consciousness*.

Intravenous administration of thyroid hormone is advised. Therapy with levothyroxine is begun with a loading dose of 250-500 μg followed by a daily full replacement dose.

CONGENITAL HYPOTHYROIDISM. Success in the treatment of congenital hypothyroidism depends on the age at which therapy is started. If therapy is instituted within the first 2 weeks of life, normal physical and mental development can be achieved.

To rapidly normalize the serum thyroxine concentration in the congenitally hypothyroid infant, an initial daily dose of levothyroxine of 10-15 μg/kg is recommended. Laboratory evaluations of TSH and FT_4 are performed 2 and 4 weeks after treatment is initiated, every 1-2 months in the first 6 months, every 3-4 months between 6 months and 3 years of age, and every 6-12 months from age 3 years until the end of growth.

THYROID CANCER. The mainstays of therapy for well-differentiated thyroid cancer (papillary, follicular) are surgical thyroidectomy, radioiodine, and levothyroxine to suppress TSH. For most low-risk patients with stage 1 or 2 disease, maintaining the TSH just below the reference range for not more than 5 years is one reasonable approach.

Thyroid Nodules. Thyroid nodules usually are asymptomatic, although they can cause neck discomfort, dysphagia, and a choking sensation. The use of levothyroxine to suppress TSH in euthyroid individuals with thyroid nodules cannot be recommended as a general practice. However, if the TSH is elevated, it is appropriate to administer levothyroxine to bring the TSH into the lower portion of the reference range.

ADVERSE EFFECTS OF THYROID HORMONE. Adverse effects of thyroid hormone generally occur only upon overtreatment and are similar to the consequences of hyperthyroidism.

ANTI-THYROID DRUGS AND OTHER THYROID INHIBITORS

Myriad compounds are capable of interfering, directly or indirectly, with the synthesis, release, or action of thyroid hormones (Tables 39-2 and 39–3). Several types are clinically useful:

- Anti-thyroid drugs, which interfere directly with the synthesis of thyroid hormones
- Ionic inhibitors, which block the iodide transport mechanism
- High concentrations of iodine, which decrease release of thyroid hormones from the gland and also may decrease hormone synthesis
- Radioactive iodine, which damages the thyroid gland with ionizing radiation

Adjuvant therapy with drugs that have no specific effects on thyroid hormone synthesis is useful in controlling the peripheral manifestations of thyrotoxicosis, including inhibitors of the peripheral deiodination of T_4 to T_3, β adrenergic receptor antagonists, and Ca^{2+} channel blockers.

Table 39–3

Anti-thyroid Compounds

PROCESS AFFECTED	EXAMPLES OF INHIBITORS
Active transport of iodide	Complex anions: perchlorate, fluoborate, pertechnetate, thiocyanate
Iodination of thyroglobulin	Thionamides: propylthiouracil, methimazole, carbimazole Thiocyanate, anilines, sulfonamides, iodide
Coupling reaction	Thionamides, sulfonamides ?All other inhibitors of iodination
Hormone release	Lithium salts, iodide
Iodotyrosine deiodination	Nitrotyrosines
Peripheral iodothyronine deiodination	Thiouracil derivatives, amiodarone Oral cholecystographic agents
Hormone excretion/inactivation	Inducers of hepatic drug-metabolizing enzymes: phenobarbital, rifampin, carbamazepine, phenytoin
Hormone action	Thyroxine analogs, amiodarone Cholestyramine (binding in gut), ?phenytoin

Source: Data adapted from Meier CA. Effects of drugs and other substances on thyroid hormone synthesis and metabolism. In: Braverman LE, Utiger RD, eds, Werner and Ingbar's The Thyroid, *9th ed. Philadelphia: Lippincott Williams & Wilkins; 2005.*

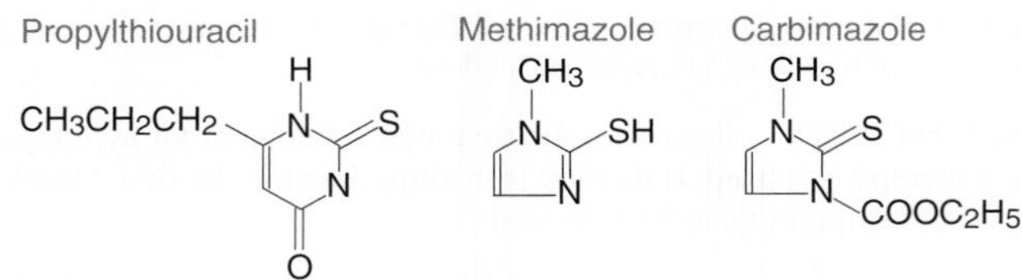

Figure 39–5 *Anti-thyroid drugs of the thiamide type.*

ANTI-THYROID DRUGS

The anti-thyroid drugs with clinical utility are the *thioureylenes*, which belong to the family of thioamides. Propylthiouracil is the prototype (Figure 39–5).

Mechanism of Action. Anti-thyroid drugs inhibit the formation of thyroid hormones by interfering with the incorporation of iodine into tyrosyl residues of thyroglobulin; they also inhibit the coupling of these iodotyrosyl residues to form iodothyronines. The drugs are thought to inhibit the peroxidase enzyme. Inhibition of hormone synthesis results in the depletion of stores of iodinated thyroglobulin as the protein is hydrolyzed and the hormones are released into the circulation. In addition to blocking hormone synthesis, propylthiouracil partially inhibits the peripheral deiodination of T_4 to T_3. *Methimazole* does not have this effect; this provides a rationale for the choice of propylthiouracil over other anti-thyroid drugs in the treatment of severe hyperthyroid states or of thyroid storm.

ADME. The anti-thyroid compounds currently used in the U.S. are propylthiouracil (6-*n*-propylthiouracil) and methimazole (1-methyl-2-mercaptoimidazole; TAPAZOLE, others). In Europe, carbimazole (NEOMERCAZOLE), a carbethoxy derivative of methimazole, is available, and its anti-thyroid action is due to its conversion to methimazole after absorption. Pharmacological properties of propylthiouracil and methimazole are shown in Table 39–4.

Untoward Reactions. The incidence of side effects from propylthiouracil and methimazole as currently used is relatively low. Agranulocytosis is the most serious reaction, usually occurring in the first few weeks or months of therapy but sometimes later. Patients should be instructed to immediately report the development of sore throat or fever, and should discontinue their anti-thyroid drug and obtain a granulocyte count. Agranulocytosis is reversible upon discontinuation of the offending drug, and the administration of recombinant human granulocyte colony-stimulating factor may hasten recovery. Mild granulocytopenia, if noted, may be due to thyrotoxicosis or may be the first sign of this dangerous drug reaction; frequent leukocyte counts are then required.

The most common reaction is a mild urticarial papular rash that often subsides spontaneously without interrupting treatment, but it sometimes calls for the administration of an antihistamine, corticosteroids, and changing to another. Other less frequent complications are pain and stiffness in the joints, paresthesias, headache, nausea, skin pigmentation, and loss of hair. Drug fever, hepatitis, and nephritis are rare, although abnormal liver function tests are not infrequent with higher doses of propylthiouracil. Although vasculitis was previously thought to be a rare complication, antineutrophilic cytoplasmic antibodies (ANCAs) have been reported to occur in ~50% of patients receiving propylthiouracil and rarely with methimazole.

Table 39–4

Pharmacokinetic Features of Anti-thyroid Drugs

	PROPYLTHIOURACIL	METHIMAZOLE
Plasma protein binding	~75%	Nil
Plasma $t_{1/2}$	75 minutes	~4-6 hours
Volume of distribution	~20 liters	~40 liters
Concentrated in thyroid	Yes	Yes
Metabolism of drug during illness		
Severe liver disease	Normal	Decreased
Severe kidney disease	Normal	Normal
Dosing frequency	1-4 times daily	Once or twice daily
Transplacental passage	Low	Low
Levels in breast milk	Low	Low

THERAPEUTIC USES. The anti-thyroid drugs are used in the treatment of hyperthyroidism:

- As definitive treatment, to control the disorder in anticipation of a spontaneous remission in Graves disease
- In conjunction with radioactive iodine, to hasten recovery while awaiting the effects of radiation
- To control the disorder in preparation for surgical treatment

Methimazole is the drug of choice for Graves disease; it is effective when given as a single daily dose, has improved adherence, and is less toxic than propylthiouracil. Methimazole has a relatively long plasma and intrathyroidal $t_{1/2}$, as well as a long duration of action. The usual starting dose for methimazole is 15–40 mg per day. The usual starting dose of propylthiouracil is 100 mg every 8 h. When doses >300 mg daily are needed, further subdivision of the time of administration to every 4-6 h is occasionally helpful. Once euthyroidism is achieved, usually within 12 weeks, the dose of anti-thyroid drug can be reduced, but not stopped, lest an exacerbation of Graves disease occur.

Response to Treatment. The thyrotoxic state usually improves within 3-6 weeks after the initiation of anti-thyroid drugs. The clinical response is related to the dose of anti-thyroid drug, the size of the goiter, and pretreatment serum T_3 concentrations. The rate of response is determined by the quantity of stored hormone, the rate of turnover of hormone in the thyroid, the $t_{1/2}$ of the hormone in the periphery, and the completeness of the block in synthesis imposed by the dosage given. Hypothyroidism may develop as a result of overtreatment. After treatment is initiated, patients should be examined and thyroid function tests (serum FT_4 and total or free triiodothyronine concentrations) measured every 2-4 months. Once euthyroidism is established, follow-up every 4-6 months is reasonable. Control of the hyperthyroidism usually is associated with a decrease in goiter size. When this occurs, the dose of the anti-thyroid drug should be significantly decreased and/or levothyroxine can be added once hypothyroidism is confirmed by laboratory testing.

Thyrotoxicosis in Pregnancy. Thyrotoxicosis occurs in ~0.2% of pregnancies and is caused most frequently by Graves disease. Anti-thyroid drugs are the treatment of choice; radioactive iodine is clearly contraindicated. Both propylthiouracil and methimazole cross the placenta equally, and either may be used safely in the pregnant patient, although the concern for propylthiouracil-associated liver failure in pregnancy may favor the use of methimazole. Carbimazole is used in the EU during pregnancy and is rarely associated with congenital gut abnormalities. The anti-thyroid drug dosage should be minimized to keep the serum FT_4 index in the upper half of the normal range or slightly elevated. As pregnancy progresses, Graves disease often improves. Relapse or worsening of Graves disease is common after delivery, and patients should be monitored closely. Methimazole up to 20 mg daily in nursing mothers reportedly has no effect on thyroid function in the infant, and propylthiouracil is thought to cross into breast milk even less than methimazole.

Adjuvant Therapy. Several drugs that have no intrinsic anti-thyroid activity are useful in the symptomatic treatment of thyrotoxicosis. *β Adrenergic receptor antagonists* (*see* Chapter 12) are effective in antagonizing the sympathetic/adrenergic effects of thyrotoxicosis, thereby reducing the tachycardia, tremor, and stare, and relieving palpitations, anxiety, and tension. Either propranolol, 20-40 mg 4 times daily, or atenolol, 50-100 mg daily, is usually given initially. *Ca^{2+} channel blockers* (diltiazem, 60-120 mg 4 times daily) can be used to control tachycardia and decrease the incidence of supraventricular tachyarrhythmias. Usually only short-term treatment with β adrenergic receptor antagonists or Ca^{2+} channel blockers is required, 2-6 weeks, and it should be discontinued once the patient is euthyroid. *Immunotherapy* has been used for Graves hyperthyroidism and ophthalmopathy. The B-lymphocyte depleting agent rituximab, when used with methimazole, prolongs remission of Graves disease.

IONIC INHIBITORS

The *ionic inhibitors* are substances that interfere with the concentration of iodide by the thyroid gland. These agents are anions that resemble iodide: *thiocyanate*, *perchlorate*, and *fluoroborate*, all monovalent hydrated anions of a size similar to that of iodide.

Thiocyanate differs from the rest qualitatively; it is not concentrated by the thyroid gland but in large amounts may inhibit the organification of iodine. Perchlorate is 10 times as active as thiocyanate. Perchlorate blocks the entrance of iodide into the thyroid by competitively inhibiting the NIS. Perchlorate can be used to control hyperthyroidism; however, when given in excessive amounts (2-3 g daily), it has caused fatal aplastic anemia. Perchlorate in doses of 750 mg daily has been used in the treatment of Graves disease. The various NIS inhibitors (perchlorate, thiocyanate, and nitrate) are additive in inhibiting iodine uptake. Lithium decreases secretion of T_4 and T_3, which can cause overt hypothyroidism in some patients taking Li^+ for the treatment of mania (*see* Chapter 16).

IODIDE

Iodide is the oldest remedy for disorders of the thyroid gland. In high concentration, iodide can influence several of the important functions of the thyroid gland. Iodide limits its own transport and acutely and transiently inhibits the synthesis of iodotyrosines and iodothyronines (the *Wolff-Chaikoff effect*). An important clinical effect of high $[I^-]_{plasma}$ is inhibition of the release of thyroid hormone.

RESPONSE TO IODIDE IN HYPERTHYROIDISM. The response to iodides in patients with hyperthyroidism is often striking and rapid: Release of thyroid hormone into the circulation is rapidly blocked, and its synthesis also is mildly decreased. In the thyroid gland, vascularity is reduced, the gland becomes much firmer, the cells become smaller, colloid reaccumulates in the follicles, and the quantity of bound iodine increases. The maximal effect occurs after 10-15 days of continuous therapy. Iodide therapy usually does not completely control the manifestations of hyperthyroidism, and the beneficial effect disappears. The uses of iodide in the treatment of hyperthyroidism are in the preoperative period in preparation for thyroidectomy, and in conjunction with anti-thyroid drugs and propranolol, in the treatment of thyrotoxic crisis.

Another use of iodide is to protect the thyroid from radioactive iodine fallout following a nuclear accident or military exposure. Because the uptake of radioactive iodine is inversely proportional to the serum concentration of stable iodine, the administration of 30-100 mg of iodide daily will markedly decrease the thyroid uptake of radioisotopes. Strong iodine solution (Lugol solution) consists of 5% iodine and 10% potassium iodide, which yield a dose of 8 mg of iodine per drop. *Potassium iodide–saturated solution* (KISS) also is available, containing 50 mg per drop. Typical doses include 16-36 mg (2-6 drops) of Lugol solution or 50-100 mg (1-2 drops) of KISS 3 times a day. A potassium iodide product (THYROSHIELD) is available over the counter to take in the event of a radiation emergency and block the uptake of radioiodide into the thyroid gland. The adult dose is 2 mL (130 mg) every 24 h, as directed by public health officials. Euthyroid patients with a history of a wide variety of underlying thyroid disorders may develop iodine-induced hypothyroidism when exposed to large amounts of iodine present in many commonly prescribed drugs (Table 39–5), and these patients do not escape from the acute Wolff-Chaikoff effect.

UNTOWARD REACTIONS. Occasional individuals show a marked sensitivity to iodide. Angioedema is the prominent symptom, and laryngeal edema may lead to suffocation. Multiple cutaneous hemorrhages may be present; manifestations of the serum-sickness type of hypersensitivity (e.g., fever, arthralgia, lymph node enlargement, and eosinophilia) may appear. Thrombotic thrombocytopenic purpura and fatal periarteritis nodosa attributed to hypersensitivity to iodide also have been described.

The severity of symptoms of chronic intoxication with iodide (*iodism*) is related to the dose. The symptoms start with an unpleasant brassy taste and burning in the mouth and throat as well as soreness of the teeth and gums. Increased salivation, coryza, sneezing, and irritation of the eyes with swelling of the eyelids commonly occur. Mild iodism simulates a "head cold." Excess transudation into the bronchial tree may lead to pulmonary edema. In addition, the parotid and submaxillary glands may become enlarged and tender, and the syndrome may be mistaken for mumps parotitis. Skin lesions are common and vary in type and intensity. Rarely, severe and sometimes fatal eruptions (ioderma) may occur after the prolonged use of iodides. The lesions are bizarre; they resemble those caused by bromism, a rare problem, and generally involute quickly when iodide is withdrawn. Symptoms of gastric irritation are common, and diarrhea, which is sometimes bloody, may occur. Fever, anorexia, and depression may be present. The symptoms of iodism disappear within a few days after stopping the administration of iodide. Renal excretion of I^- can be increased by procedures that promote Cl^- excretion (e.g., osmotic diuresis, chloruretic diuretics, and salt loading). These procedures may be useful when the symptoms of iodism are severe.

RADIOACTIVE IODINE

The primary isotopes used for the diagnosis and treatment of thyroid disease are ^{123}I and ^{131}I. ^{123}I is primarily a short-lived γ-emitter with a $t_{1/2}$ of 13 h and is used in diagnostic studies. ^{131}I has a $t_{1/2}$ of 8 days and emits both γ rays and β particles. More than 99% of its radiation is expended within 56 days. ^{131}I is used therapeutically for thyroid destruction of an overactive or enlarged thyroid and in thyroid cancer for thyroid ablation and treatment of metastatic disease.

The chemical behavior of the radioactive isotopes of iodine is identical to that of the stable isotope, ^{127}I. ^{131}I is rapidly and efficiently trapped by the thyroid, incorporated into the iodoamino acids, and deposited in the colloid of the follicles, from which it is slowly liberated. Thus, the destructive β particles originate within the follicle and act almost exclusively on the parenchymal cells of the thyroid, with little or no damage to surrounding tissue. The γ radiation passes through the tissue and can be quantified by external detection. The effects of the radiation depend on the dosage. With properly selected doses of ^{131}I, it is possible to destroy the thyroid gland completely without detectable injury to adjacent tissues.

THERAPEUTIC USES. Radioactive iodine finds its widest use in the treatment of hyperthyroidism and in the diagnosis of disorders of thyroid function. The clearest indication for radioactive iodine treatment is

Table 39–5

Commonly Used Iodine-Containing Drugs

DRUGS	IODINE CONTENT
Oral or local	
Amiodarone	75 mg/tablet
Calcium iodide syrup	26 mg/mL
Iodoquinol (diiodohydroxyquin)	134-416 mg/ tablet
Echothiophate iodide ophthalmic solution	5-41 μg/drop
Hydriodic acid syrup	13-15 mg/mL
Iodochlorhydroxyquin	104 mg/tablet
Iodine-containing vitamins	0.15 mg/tablet
Idoxuridine ophthalmic solution	18 μg/drop
Kelp/seaweed	0.15 mg/tablet
Lugol's solution	6.3 mg/drop
PONARIS nasal emollient	5 mg/0.8 mL
KI, saturated solution (KISS)	38 mg/drop
Topical antiseptics	
Iodoquinol cream (diiodohydroxyquin)	6 mg/g
Iodine tincture	40 mg/mL
Iodochlorhydroxyquin cream	12 mg/g
Iodoform gauze	4.8 mg/100 mg gauze
Povidone–iodine	10 mg/mL
Radiology contrast agents	
Diatrizoate meglumine sodium	370 mg/mL
Propyliodone	340 mg/mL
Iopanoic acid	333 mg/tablet
Ipodate	308 mg/capsule
Iothalamate	480 mg/mL
Metrizamide (undiluted)	483 mg/mL
Iohexol	463 mg/mL

Source: Braverman LE et al, eds. Werner & Ingbar's The Thyroid, 10th ed., p 244.

hyperthyroidism in older patients and in those with heart disease. Radioactive iodine also is the best form of treatment when Graves disease has persisted or recurred after subtotal thyroidectomy and when prolonged treatment with anti-thyroid drugs has not led to remission. Finally, radioactive iodine is indicated in patients with toxic nodular goiter. Sodium iodide ^{131}I (HICON, others) is available as a solution or in capsules containing carrier-free ^{131}I suitable for oral administration. Sodium iodide ^{123}I is available for scanning procedures.

HYPERTHYROIDISM. Radioactive iodine is a valuable alternative or adjunctive treatment of hyperthyroidism. Stable iodide (nonradioactive) may preclude treatment and imaging with radioactive iodine for weeks after the stable iodide has been discontinued. In those patients exposed to stable iodide, a 24-h radioiodine measurement of a tracer dose of ^{123}I should be performed before ^{131}I administration to ensure there is sufficient uptake to accomplish the desired ablation. The optimal dose of ^{131}I, expressed in terms of microcuries taken up per gram of thyroid tissue, varies in different laboratories from 80-150 μCi. The usual total dose is 4-15 mCi.

Beginning a few weeks after treatment, the symptoms of hyperthyroidism gradually abate over a period of 2-3 months. If therapy has been inadequate, the necessity for further treatment is apparent within 6-12 months. It is not uncommon, however, for the serum TSH to remain low for several months after ^{131}I therapy. Thus, assessing radioactive iodine failure based on TSH concentrations alone may be misleading and should always be accompanied by determination of free T_4 and usually serum T_3 concentrations. Depending to some extent on the dosage schedule adopted, 80% of patients are cured by a single dose, ~20% require 2 doses, and a very small fraction require 3 or more doses before the disorder is controlled. β Adrenergic antagonists, anti-thyroid drugs, or both, or stable iodide, can be used to hasten the control of hyperthyroidism.

Advantages. With radioactive iodine treatment, the patient is spared the risks and discomfort of surgery. The cost is low, hospitalization is not required in the U.S., and patients can participate in their customary activities during the entire procedure, although there are recommendations to limit exposure in young children.

Disadvantages. The chief consequence of the use of radioactive iodine is the high incidence of delayed hypothyroidism. Although cancer death rate is not increased after radioiodine therapy, there is a small but significant increase shown in specific types of cancer, including stomach, kidney, and breast. This finding is especially significant because these tissues all express the iodine transporter NIS and may be especially susceptible to radiation effects. Radioactive iodine treatment can induce a radiation thyroiditis, with release of preformed thyroxine and triiodothyronine into the circulation. In most patients, this is asymptomatic, but in some there can be worsening of symptoms of hyperthyroidism and rarely cardiac manifestations, such as atrial fibrillation or ischemic heart disease and very rarely thyroid storm. Pretreatment with anti-thyroid drugs should reduce or eliminate this complication.

The main contraindication for the use of ^{131}I therapy is pregnancy. After the first trimester, the fetal thyroid will concentrate the isotope and thus suffer damage; even during the first trimester, radioactive iodine is best avoided because there may be adverse effects of radiation on fetal tissues. The risk of causing neoplastic changes in the thyroid gland has been an ongoing; only small numbers of children have been treated in this way. Many clinics decline to treat younger patients and reserve radioactive iodine for patients older than 25-30 years.

Thyroid Carcinoma. Because most well-differentiated thyroid carcinomas accumulate very little iodine, stimulation of iodine uptake with TSH is required to treat metastases effectively. Currently, endogenous TSH stimulation is evoked by withdrawal of thyroid hormone replacement therapy in patients previously treated with near-total thyroidectomy with or without radioactive ablation of residual thyroid tissue. An ablative dose of ^{131}I ranging from 30 mCi to >150 mCi is administered, and a repeat total body scan is obtained 1 week later. Thyrogen (recombinant human TSH) is now available to test the capacity of thyroid tissue, both normal and malignant, to take up radioactive iodine and to secrete thyroglobulin. Thyrogen allows assessment of the presence of metastatic disease, without the necessity for patients to stop their suppressive levothyroxine therapy and become clinically hypothyroid. TSH-suppressive therapy with levothyroxine is indicated in all patients after treatment for thyroid cancer. The goal of therapy usually is to keep serum TSH levels in the subnormal range. A rise in serum thyroglobulin concentration is often the first indication of recurrent disease.

For a complete Bibliographical Listing see Goodman & Gilman's ***The Pharmacological Basis of Therapeutics***, 12th ed., or Goodman & Gilman Online at www.AccessMedicine.com.

Estrogens and Progestins

Estrogens and *progestins* are hormones that produce myriad physiological actions. In women, these include developmental effects, neuroendocrine actions involved in the control of ovulation, the cyclical preparation of the reproductive tract for fertilization and implantation, and major actions on mineral, carbohydrate, protein, and lipid metabolism. Estrogens also have important actions in males, including effects on bone, spermatogenesis, and behavior. The most common uses of these agents are menopausal hormone therapy and contraception in women, but the specific compounds and dosages used in these 2 settings differ substantially. Anti-estrogens are used in the treatment of hormone-responsive breast cancer and infertility. Selective estrogen receptor modulators (SERMs) that display tissue-selective agonist or antagonist activities are useful to prevent breast cancer and osteoporosis. The main use of antiprogestins has been for medical abortion.

ESTROGENS

Estrogens interact with 2 receptors of the nuclear receptor superfamily, termed estrogen receptors α (Erα) and β (ERβ). The most potent naturally occurring estrogen in humans, for both ERα- and ERβ-mediated actions, is *17β-estradiol*, followed by *estrone* and *estriol*. Steroidal *estrogens* arise from *androstenedione* or *testosterone* (Figure 40–1) by a reaction catalyzed by *aromatase* (CYP19).

The ovaries are the principal source of circulating estrogen in premenopausal women, with estradiol the main secretory product. Gonadotropins, acting via receptors that couple to the G_s-adenylyl cyclase–cyclic AMP pathway, increase the activities of aromatase and facilitate the transport of cholesterol (the precursor of all steroids) into the mitochondria of cells that synthesize steroids. In the ovary, type I *17β-hydroxysteroid dehydrogenase* favors the production of *testosterone* and *estradiol* from *androstenedione* and *estrone*, respectively. In the liver, the type II enzyme favors oxidation of circulating estradiol to *estrone*, and both of these steroids are then converted to *estriol* (*see* Figure 40–1). All 3 of these estrogens are excreted in the urine along with their glucuronide and sulfate conjugates.

In postmenopausal women, the principal source of circulating estrogen is adipose tissue stroma, where estrone is synthesized from *dehydroepiandrosterone* secreted by the adrenals. In men, estrogens are produced by the testes, but extragonadal production by aromatization of circulating C19 steroids (e.g., androstenedione and dehydroepiandrosterone) accounts for most circulating estrogens. Local production of estrogens by aromatization of androgens may play a causal or promotional role in the development of certain diseases such as breast cancer. Estrogens also may be produced from androgens via aromatase in the central nervous system (CNS) and other tissues and exert local effects near their production site (e.g., in bone they affect bone mineral density).

Human urine during pregnancy is an abundant source of natural estrogens. Pregnant mare's urine is the source of *conjugated equine estrogens*, which have been widely used therapeutically for many years.

PHYSIOLOGICAL AND PHARMACOLOGICAL ACTIONS

DEVELOPMENTAL ACTIONS. Estrogens are largely responsible for pubertal changes in girls and secondary sexual characteristics.

Estrogens cause growth and development of the vagina, uterus, and fallopian tubes, and contribute to breast enlargement. They also contribute to molding the body contours, shaping the skeleton, and causing the pubertal growth spurt of the long bones and epiphyseal closure. Growth of axillary and pubic hair, pigmentation of the genital region, and the regional pigmentation of the nipples and areolae that occur after the first trimester of pregnancy are also estrogenic actions. Androgens may also play a secondary role in female sexual development (*see* Chapter 41). Estrogens also play important developmental roles in males. In boys, estrogen deficiency diminishes the pubertal growth spurt and delays skeletal maturation and epiphyseal closure so that linear growth continues into adulthood. Estrogen deficiency in men leads to elevated gonadotropins, macroorchidism, and increased testosterone levels and also may affect carbohydrate and lipid metabolism and fertility in some individuals.

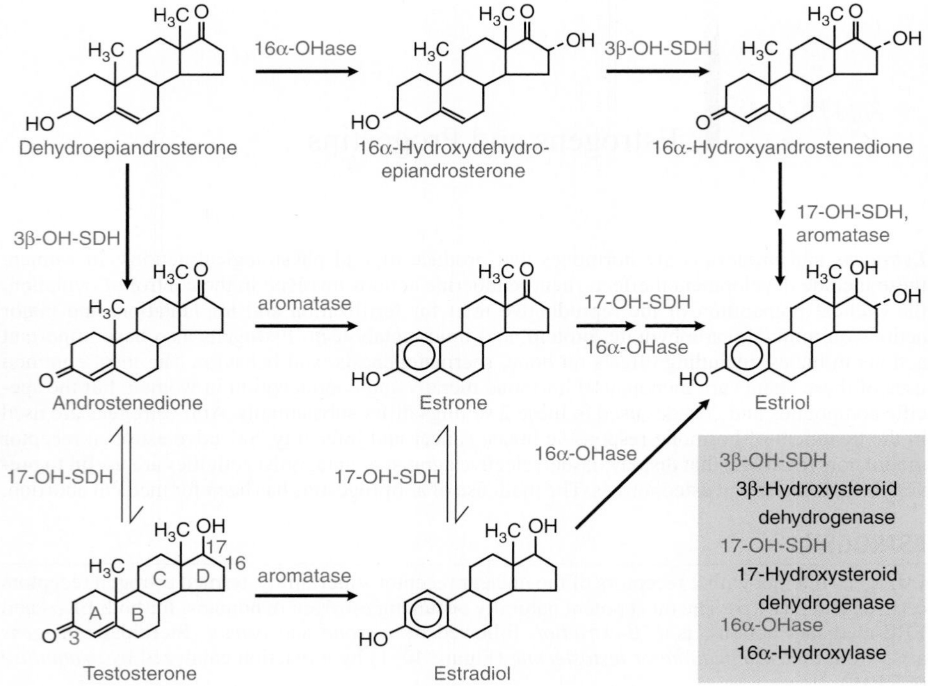

H₃C O

Dehydroepiandrosterone → 16α-OHase → 16α-Hydroxydehydro-epiandrosterone → 3β-OH-SDH → 16α-Hydroxyandrostenedione

Dehydroepiandrosterone → 3β-OH-SDH → Androstenedione

16α-Hydroxyandrostenedione → 17-OH-SDH, aromatase → Estriol

Androstenedione → aromatase → Estrone → 17-OH-SDH, 16α-OHase → Estriol

Androstenedione ⇌ 17-OH-SDH ⇌ Testosterone

Estrone ⇌ 17-OH-SDH ⇌ Estradiol

Testosterone → aromatase → Estradiol → 16α-OHase → Estriol

3β-OH-SDH 3β-Hydroxysteroid dehydrogenase
17-OH-SDH 17-Hydroxysteroid dehydrogenase
16α-OHase 16α-Hydroxylase

Figure 40–1 *The biosynthetic pathway for estrogens.*

NEUROENDOCRINE CONTROL OF THE MENSTRUAL CYCLE. A neuroendocrine cascade involving the *hypothalamus*, *pituitary*, and *ovaries* controls the menstrual cycle (Figure 40–2). A neuronal oscillator, or "clock," in the hypothalamus fires at intervals that coincide with the release of *gonadotropin-releasing hormone* (GnRH) into the hypothalamic-pituitary portal vasculature (*see* Chapter 38). GnRH interacts with its receptor on *pituitary gonadotropes* to cause release of *luteinizing hormone* (LH) and *follicle-stimulating hormone* (FSH). The frequency of the GnRH pulses, which varies in the different phases of the menstrual cycle, controls the relative synthesis of FSH and LH.

The gonadotropins (LH and FSH) regulate the growth and maturation of follicles in the ovary and the ovarian production of estrogen and progesterone, which exert feedback regulation on the pituitary and hypothalamus. Because the release of GnRH is intermittent, secretion of LH and FSH is pulsatile. The pulse *frequency* is determined by the neural "clock" (*see* Figure 40–2), termed the *hypothalamic GnRH pulse generator*, but the amount of gonadotropin released in each pulse (i.e., the pulse *amplitude*) is largely controlled by the actions of estrogens and progesterone on the pituitary. The intermittent, *pulsatile* nature of hormone release is essential for the maintenance of normal ovulatory menstrual cycles because constant infusion of GnRH results in a cessation of gonadotropin release and ovarian steroid production (*see* Chapter 38). Although the precise mechanism that regulates the timing of GnRH release (i.e., pulse frequency) is unclear, hypothalamic cells appear to have an intrinsic ability to release GnRH episodically. Ovarian steroids, primarily progesterone, regulate the frequency of GnRH release. At puberty the pulse generator is activated and establishes cyclic profiles of pituitary and ovarian hormones. Although the mechanism of activation is not entirely established, it may involve increases in circulating insulin-like growth factor 1 (IGF)-1 and leptin levels, the latter acting to inhibit neuropeptide Y (NPY) in the arcuate nucleus to relieve an inhibitory effect on GnRH neurons.

Figure 40–3 provides a schematic diagram of the profiles of gonadotropin and gonadal steroid levels in the menstrual cycle. In the early follicular phase of the cycle: (1) the pulse generator produces bursts of neuronal activity with a frequency of about 1/h that correspond with pulses of GnRH secretion, (2) these cause a corresponding pulsatile release of LH and FSH from pituitary gonadotropes, and (3) FSH in particular causes the graafian follicle to mature and secrete estrogen. The effects of estrogens on the pituitary are inhibitory at this time and cause the amount of LH and FSH released from the pituitary to decline, so gonadotropin levels

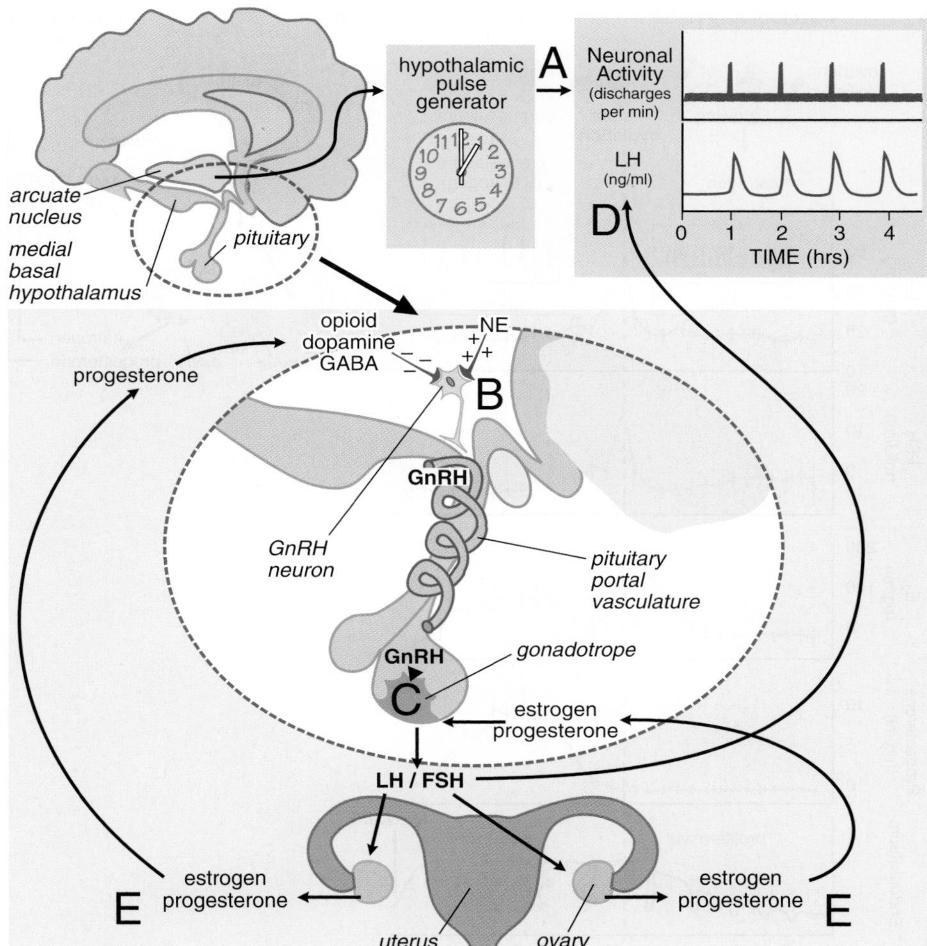

Figure 40–2 *Neuroendocrine control of gonadotropin secretion in females.* The hypothalamic pulse generator located in the arcuate nucleus of the hypothalamus functions as a neuronal "clock" that fires at regular hourly intervals (**A**). This results in the periodic release of gonadotropin-releasing hormone (GnRH) from GnRH-containing neurons into the hypothalamic-pituitary portal vasculature (**B**). GnRH neurons (**B**) receive inhibitory input from opioid, dopamine, and GABA neurons and stimulatory input from noradrenergic neurons (NE, norepinephrine). The pulses of GnRH trigger the intermittent release of luteinizing hormone (LH) and follicle-stimulating hormone (FSH) from pituitary gonadotropes (**C**), resulting in the pulsatile plasma profile (**D**). FSH and LH regulate ovarian production of estrogen and progesterone, which exert feedback controls (**E**). (*See* text and Figure 40–3 for additional details.)

gradually fall. Estrogens act primarily on the pituitary to control the amplitude of gonadotropin pulses and may also contribute to the amplitude of GnRH pulses secreted by the hypothalamus. *Inhibin*, produced by the ovary, exerts negative feedback to selectively decrease serum FSH.

At mid-cycle, serum estradiol rises above a threshold level of 150-200 pg/mL for ~36 h, exerting a brief positive feedback effect on the pituitary to trigger the preovulatory surge of LH and FSH. This effect primarily involves a change in pituitary responsiveness to GnRH. Progesterone may contribute to the mid-cycle LH surge. The mid-cycle surge in gonadotropins stimulates follicular rupture and ovulation within 1-2 days. The ruptured follicle then develops into the *corpus luteum*, which produces large amounts of progesterone and lesser amounts of estrogen under the influence of LH during the second half of the cycle. In the absence of pregnancy, the corpus luteum ceases to function, steroid levels drop, and menstruation occurs. When steroid

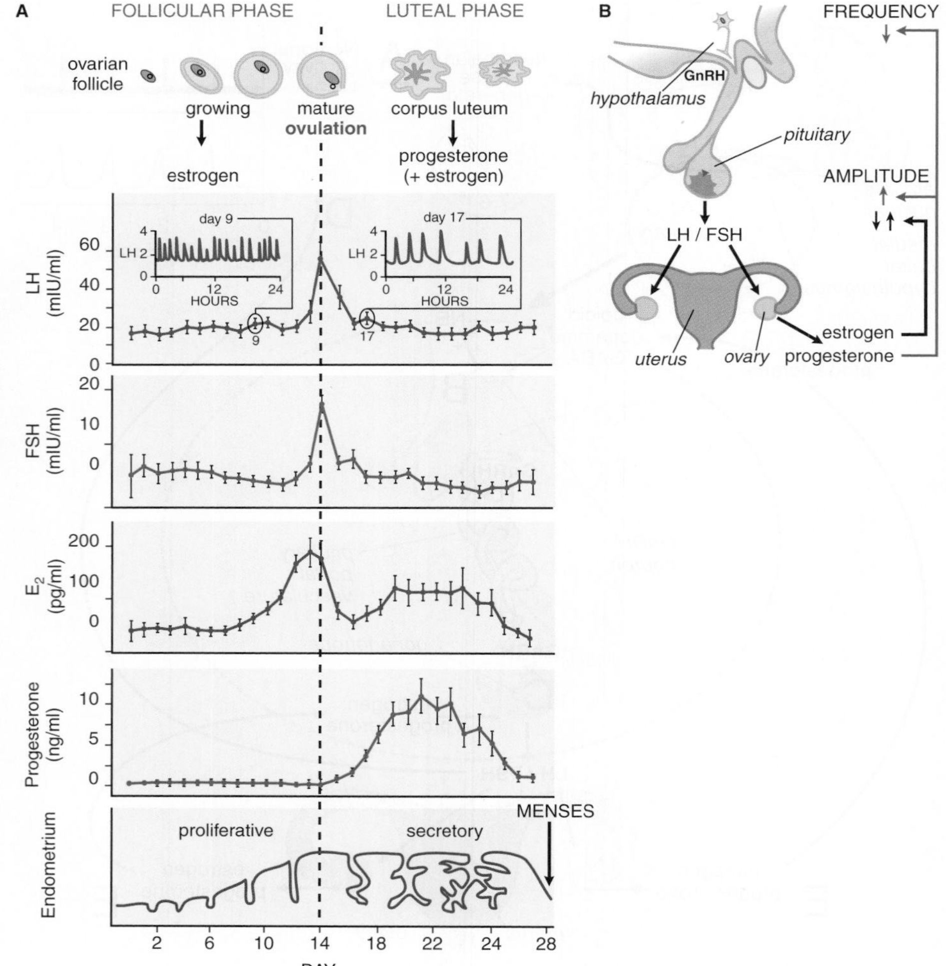

Figure 40–3 *Hormonal relationships of the human menstrual cycle.* **A.** Average daily values of LH, FSH, estradiol (E_2), and progesterone in plasma samples from women exhibiting normal 28-day menstrual cycles. Changes in the ovarian follicle (*top*) and endometrium (*bottom*) also are illustrated schematically. Frequent plasma sampling reveals pulsatile patterns of gonadotropin release. Characteristic profiles are illustrated schematically for the follicular phase (day 9, *inset on left*) and luteal phase (day 17, *inset on right*). Both the frequency (number of pulses per hour) and amplitude (extent of change of hormone release) of pulses vary throughout the cycle. (Redrawn with permission from Thorneycroft et al., 1971. © Elsevier). **B.** Major regulatory effects of ovarian steroids on hypothalamic-pituitary function. Estrogen decreases the amount of follicle-stimulating hormone (FSH) and luteinizing hormone (LH) released (i.e., gonadotropin pulse amplitude) during most of the cycle and triggers a surge of LH release only at mid-cycle. Progesterone decreases the frequency of GnRH release from the hypothalamus and thus decreases the frequency of plasma gonadotropin pulses. Progesterone also increases the amount of LH released (i.e., the pulse amplitude) during the luteal phase of the cycle.

levels drop, the pulse generator reverts to a firing pattern, the entire system then resets, and a new ovarian cycle occurs.

In the follicular phase of the cycle, estrogens inhibit gonadotropin release but then have a brief mid-cycle stimulatory action that increases the amount released and causes the LH surge. Progesterone, acting on the hypothalamus, exerts the predominant control of the frequency of LH release. It decreases the firing rate of the hypothalamic pulse generator, an action thought to be mediated largely via inhibitory opioid neurons (containing progesterone receptors) that synapse with GnRH neurons. Progesterone also exerts a direct effect on the pituitary to oppose the inhibitory actions of estrogens and thus enhance the amount of LH released (i.e., to increase the amplitude of the LH pulses). These steroid feedback effects, coupled with the intrinsic activity of the hypothalamic GnRH pulse generator, lead to relatively frequent LH pulses of small amplitude in the follicular phase of the cycle, and less frequent pulses of larger amplitude in the luteal phase.

In males, testosterone regulates the hypothalamic-pituitary-gonadal axis at both the hypothalamic and pituitary levels, and its negative feedback effect is mediated to a substantial degree by estrogen formed via aromatization.

EFFECTS OF CYCLICAL GONADAL STEROIDS ON THE REPRODUCTIVE TRACT

The cyclical changes in estrogen and progesterone production by the ovaries regulate corresponding events in the fallopian tubes, uterus, cervix, and vagina. Physiologically, these changes prepare the uterus for implantation, and the proper timing of events in these tissues is essential for pregnancy. If pregnancy does not occur, the endometrium is shed as the menstrual discharge (*see* Figure 40–3).

Menstruation marks the start of the menstrual cycle. During the follicular (or proliferative) phase of the cycle, estrogen begins the rebuilding of the endometrium by stimulating proliferation and differentiation. An important response to estrogen in the endometrium and other tissues is induction of the progesterone receptor (PR), which enables cells to respond to this hormone during the second half of the cycle. In the luteal (or secretory) phase of the cycle, elevated progesterone limits the proliferative effect of estrogens on the endometrium by stimulating differentiation. Major effects include stimulation of epithelial secretions important for implantation of the blastocyst and the characteristic growth of the endometrial blood vessels seen at this time. These effects are mediated by PR-A in animal models. Progesterone is thus important in preparation for implantation and for the changes that take place in the uterus at the implantation site (i.e., the decidual response). There is a narrow "window of implantation," spanning days 19-24 of the endometrial cycle, when the epithelial cells of the endometrium are receptive to blastocyst implantation. If implantation occurs, human chorionic gonadotropin (hCG), produced initially by the trophoblast and later by the placenta, interacts with the LH receptor of the corpus luteum to maintain steroid hormone synthesis during the early stages of pregnancy. Later the placenta becomes the major site of estrogen and progesterone synthesis.

METABOLIC EFFECTS. Estrogens affect myriad tissues. Many nonreproductive tissues, including bone, vascular endothelium, liver, CNS, immune system, the GI tract, and heart, express low levels of both estrogen receptors (ERs), and the ratio of ERα to ERβ varies in a cell-specific manner. The effects of estrogens on selected aspects of mineral, lipid, carbohydrate, and protein metabolism are particularly important for understanding their pharmacological actions.

Long-term administration of estrogen is associated with decreased plasma renin, angiotensin-converting enzyme, and endothelin-1; expression of the AT_1 receptor for AngII is also decreased. Estrogen actions on the vascular wall include increased production of NO and prostacyclin. All of these changes promote vasodilation and retard atherogenesis. Estrogens alter a number of metabolic pathways that affect the clotting cascade. Systemic effects include changes in hepatic production of plasma proteins. Estrogens cause a small increase in coagulation factors II, VII, IX, X, and XII, and they decrease the anticoagulation factors protein C, protein S, and antithrombin III (*see* Chapter 30). Fibrinolytic pathways also are affected, and several studies of women treated with estrogen alone or estrogen with a progestin have demonstrated decreased levels of plasminogen-activator inhibitor 1 (PAI-1) protein with a concomitant increase in fibrinolysis. Thus, estrogens increase both coagulation and fibrinolytic pathways, and imbalance in these 2 opposing activities may cause adverse effects.

Estrogens increase bone mass. Bone is continuously remodeled by the resorptive action of *osteoclasts* and the bone-forming action of *osteoblasts*. Estrogens directly regulate osteoblasts and increase osteocyte survival by inhibiting apoptosis. The major effect of estrogens is to decrease the number and activity of osteoclasts.

Estrogens slightly elevate serum triglycerides and slightly reduce total serum cholesterol levels. They increase high-density lipoprotein (HDL) levels and decrease the levels of low-density lipoprotein (LDL) and lipoprotein A (LPA) (*see* Chapter 31). The presence of ERs in the liver suggests that the beneficial effects of estrogen on lipoprotein metabolism may be due partly to direct hepatic actions. Estrogens also alter bile composition by increasing cholesterol secretion and decreasing bile acid secretion. This leads to increased saturation of bile with cholesterol and appears to be the basis for increased gallstone formation in some women receiving estrogens. In general, estrogens increase plasma levels of cortisol-binding globulin, thyroxine-binding globulin, and sex hormone-binding globulin (SHBG), which binds both androgens and estrogens.

ESTROGEN RECEPTORS

Estrogens exert their effects by interaction with receptors that are members of the superfamily of nuclear receptors. The 2 estrogen receptor genes are located on separate chromosomes: ESR1 encodes ERα, and ESR2 encodes ERβ. Both ERs are estrogen-dependent nuclear transcription factors that have different tissue distributions and transcriptional regulatory effects on a wide number of target genes. Both ERα and ERβ exist as multiple mRNA isoforms due to differential promoter use and alternative splicing. There are significant differences between the 2 receptor isoforms in the ligand-binding domains and in both transactivation domains. Human ERβ does not appear to contain a functional AF-1 domain. The receptors appear to have different biological functions and respond differently to various estrogenic compounds. However, their high homology in the DNA-binding domains suggests that both receptors recognize similar DNA sequences and hence regulate many of the same target genes.

ERα is expressed most abundantly in the female reproductive tract—especially the uterus, vagina, and ovaries—as well as in the mammary gland, the hypothalamus, endothelial cells, and vascular smooth muscle. ERβ is expressed most highly in the prostate and ovaries, with lower expression in lung, brain, bone, and vasculature. Both forms of ER are expressed on breast cancers, although ERα is believed to be the predominant form responsible for growth regulation (*see* Chapter 63). Polymorphic variants of ER have been identified, but attempts to correlate specific polymorphisms with the frequency of breast cancer, bone mass, endometrial cancer, or cardiovascular disease have led to contradictory results.

A cloned G protein-coupled receptor, GPR30, also appears to interact with estrogens in some cell systems, and its participation in the rapid effects of estrogen is an attractive idea. There may be interaction/cross-talk between membrane-associated ERα and membrane-localized GPR30 in some cancer cells, but in vivo confirmation is lacking.

MECHANISM OF ACTION

Both ERs are ligand-activated transcription factors that increase or decrease the transcription of target genes (Figure 40–4). After entering the cell by passive diffusion through the plasma membrane, the hormone binds to an ER in the nucleus. In the nucleus, the ER is present as an inactive monomer bound to heat-shock protein 90 (HSP90), and upon binding estrogen, a change in ER conformation dissociates the heat-shock proteins and causes receptor dimerization, which increases the affinity and the rate of receptor binding to DNA. Homodimers of ERα or ERβ and ERα/ERβ heterodimers can be produced depending on the receptor complement in a given cell. The ER dimer binds to estrogen response elements (EREs), typically located in the promoter region of target genes. The ER/DNA complex recruits a cascade of coactivator and other proteins to the promoter region of target genes (Figure 40–4B and legend) and allows the proteins that make up the general transcription apparatus to assemble and initiate transcription.

Some ERs are located on the plasma membrane of cells. These ERs are encoded by the same genes that encode ERα and ERβ but are transported to the plasma membrane and reside mainly in caveolae. Translocation to the membrane by all sex steroid receptors is mediated by palmitoylation of a 9–amino acid motif common to these receptors. Membrane-localized ERs mediate the rapid activation of some proteins such as MAPK (phosphorylated in several cell types) and the rapid increase in cyclic AMP caused by the hormone. These membrane interactions and sequelae provide additional levels of cross-talk and complexity in estrogen signaling.

ADME. Various estrogens are available for oral, parenteral, transdermal, or topical administration. Given the lipophilic nature of estrogens, absorption generally is good with the appropriate preparation. Aqueous or oil-based esters of estradiol are available for intramuscular injection, ranging in frequency from every week to once per month. Conjugated estrogens are available for IV or IM administration. Transdermal patches that are changed once or twice weekly deliver estradiol continuously through the skin. Preparations are available for topical use in the vagina or for application to the skin. Estrogen preparations also are available in combination with a progestin. All estrogens are labeled with precautionary statements urging the prescribing of the lowest effective dose and for the shortest duration consistent with the treatment goals and risks for each individual patient.

Oral administration is common and may use estradiol, conjugated estrogens, esters of estrone and other estrogens, and *ethinyl estradiol (in combination with a progestin)*. Estradiol is available in nonmicronized (FEMTRACE) and micronized preparations (ESTRACE, others). The micronized formulations yield a large surface for rapid absorption to partially overcome low absolute oral bioavailability due to first-pass metabolism. Addition of the ethinyl substituent at C17 (ethinyl estradiol) inhibits first-pass hepatic metabolism. Other common oral preparations contain conjugated equine estrogens (PREMARIN), which are primarily the sulfate esters of

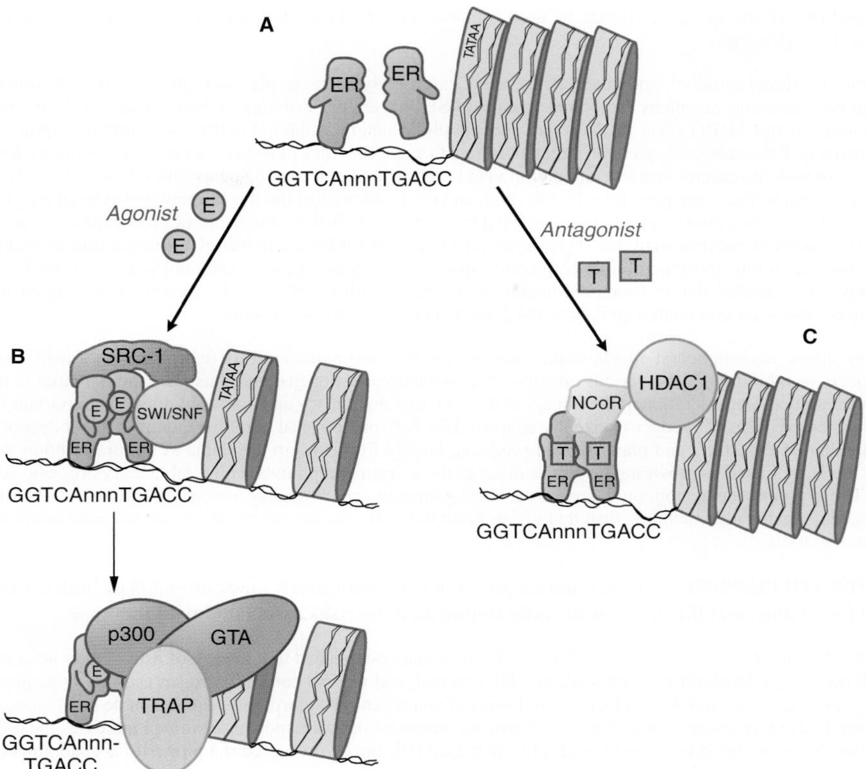

Figure 40–4 *Molecular mechanism of action of nuclear estrogen receptor.* **A.** Unliganded estrogen receptor (ER) exists as a monomer within the nucleus. **B.** Agonists such as 17β-estradiol (E) bind to the ER and cause a ligand-directed change in conformation that facilitates dimerization and interaction with specific estrogen response elements in DNA. The ER-DNA complex recruits coactivators such as SWI/SNF that modify chromatin structure, and coactivators such as steroid-receptor coactivator-1 (SRC-1) that has histone acetyltransferase (HAT) activity that further alters chromatin structure. This remodeling facilitates the exchange of the recruited proteins such that other coactivators (e.g., p300 and the TRAP complex) associate on the target gene promoter and proteins that comprise the general transcription apparatus (GTA) are recruited, with subsequent synthesis of mRNA. **C.** Antagonists such as tamoxifen (T) also bind to the ER but produce a different receptor conformation. The antagonist-induced conformation also facilitates dimerization and interaction with DNA, but a different set of proteins called corepressors, such as nuclear-hormone receptor corepressor (NcoR), are recruited to the complex. NcoR further recruits proteins such as histone deacetylase I (HDAC1) that act on histones to stabilize nucleosome structure and prevent interaction with the GTA.

estrone, equilin, and other naturally occurring compounds; *esterified esters* (MENEST); or mixtures of synthetic conjugated estrogens prepared from plant-derived sources (CENESTIN; ENJUVIA). These are hydrolyzed by enzymes present in the lower gut that remove the charged sulfate groups and allow absorption of estrogen across the intestinal epithelium. In another oral preparation, *estropipate* (ORTHO-EST, OGEN, others), estrone is solubilized as the sulfate and stabilized with piperazine. Due largely to differences in metabolism, the potencies of various oral preparations differ widely; e.g., ethinyl estradiol is much more potent than conjugated estrogens.

Administration of estradiol via transdermal patches (ALORA, CLIMARA, ESTRADERM, VIVELLE, others) provides slow, sustained release of the hormone, systemic distribution, and more constant blood levels than oral dosing. Estradiol is also available as a topical emulsion (ESTRASORB) or as a gel (ESTROGEL). The transdermal route does not lead to the high level of the drug in the portal circulation after oral administration, and thus should minimize hepatic effects of estrogens. Preparations available for intramuscular injection include compounds such as *estradiol valerate* (DELESTROGEN, others) or *estradiol cypionate* (DEPO-ESTRADIOL, others), which may be absorbed over several weeks following a single intramuscular injection. Preparations of estradiol (ESTRACE) and conjugated estrogen (PREMARIN) creams are available for topical administration to the vagina. A 3-month vaginal ring (ESTRING, FEMRING) may be used for slow release of estradiol, and tablets are also available for vaginal use (VAGIFEM).

Estradiol, ethinyl estradiol, and other estrogens are extensively bound to plasma proteins. Estradiol and other naturally occurring estrogens are bound mainly to SHBG; ethinyl estradiol is bound extensively to serum albumin but not SHBG. Due to their size and lipophilic nature, unbound estrogens distribute rapidly and extensively. Estrogens undergo rapid hepatic biotransformation, with a plasma $t_{1/2}$ measured in minutes. Estrogens also undergo enterohepatic recirculation via (1) sulfate and glucuronide conjugation in the liver, (2) biliary secretion of the conjugates into the intestine, and (3) hydrolysis in the gut (largely by bacterial enzymes) followed by reabsorption. Estradiol is converted primarily by 17β-hydroxysteroid dehydrogenase to estrone, which undergoes conversion by 16α-hydroxylation and 17-keto reduction to estriol, the major urinary metabolite; myriad sulfate and glucuronide conjugates appear in the urine. Ethinyl estradiol is cleared much more slowly than estradiol due to decreased hepatic metabolism with $t_{1/2}$ of 13-27 h. *Mestranol*, a component of some combination oral contraceptives, is the 3-methyl ether of ethinyl estradiol.

Many drugs, environmental agents (e.g., cigarette smoke), and nutraceuticals (e.g., St. John's wort) act as inducers or inhibitors of the various enzymes that metabolize estrogens, and thus have the potential to alter their clearance. Consideration of the impact of these factors on efficacy and untoward effects is important with the decreased doses of estrogens currently employed for both menopausal hormone therapy and contraception. A number of foodstuffs and plant-derived products, largely from soy, are available as nonprescription items and often are touted as providing benefits similar to those from compounds with established estrogenic activity. These products may contain flavonoids such as genistein, which display estrogenic activity in laboratory tests, albeit generally much less than that of estradiol; their efficacy at relevant doses has not been established in human trials.

UNTOWARD RESPONSES. Oral contraceptives now contain much lower amounts of both estrogen and progestins, and this has significantly diminished the risks associated with their use.

CONCERN ABOUT CARCINOGENIC ACTIONS. Early studies established that the use of estrogens is associated with the risk of developing breast, endometrial, cervical, and vaginal cancer. Estrogen use during pregnancy also can increase the incidence of cancer and nonmalignant genital abnormalities in both male and female offspring. The use of unopposed estrogen for hormone treatment in postmenopausal women increases the risk of endometrial carcinoma by 5- to 15-fold. This increased risk can be prevented if a progestin is coadministered with the estrogen, and this is now standard practice.

The association between estrogen and/or estrogen-progestin use and breast cancer is of great concern. The results of 2 large randomized clinical studies (the Women's Health Initiative study [WHI], and the Million Women Study [MWS]) of estrogen/progestin and estrogen-only in postmenopausal women clearly established a small but significant increase in the risk of breast cancer, apparently due to the medroxyprogesterone. In the WHI study, an estrogen-progestin combination increased the total risk of breast cancer by 25%; the absolute increase in attributable cases of disease was 6 per 1000 women and required 3 or more years of treatment. In women without a uterus who received estrogen alone, the relative risk of breast cancer was actually decreased. Thus, the data suggest that the progestin component in combined hormone-replacement therapy plays a major role in this increased risk of breast cancer. Importantly, the excess risk of breast cancer associated with menopausal hormone use appears to abate 5 years after discontinuing therapy. Thus, hormone replacement therapy for ≤5 years is often prescribed to mitigate hot flashes and likely has a minimal effect on the risk of breast cancer.

METABOLIC AND CARDIOVASCULAR EFFECTS. Although they may slightly elevate plasma triglycerides, estrogens themselves generally have favorable overall effects on plasma lipoprotein profiles. However, addition of progestins may reduce the favorable actions of estrogens. Estrogens do increase cholesterol levels in bile and cause a relative 2- to 3-fold increase in gallbladder disease. Many studies and clinical trials suggest that estrogen therapy in postmenopausal women would reduce the risk of cardiovascular disease. However, 2 recent randomized clinical trials have not found such protection. In women with established coronary heart disease (CHD), estrogen plus a progestin increased the relative risk of nonfatal myocardial infarction or CHD death within 1 year of treatment, but there was no overall change in 5 years. In women *without* existing CHD, treated with an estrogen plus progestin, protective effects were seen but only when hormone replacement was initiated within 10 years of menopause. It is clear, however, that oral estrogens increase the risk of thromboembolic disease in healthy women and in women with preexisting cardiovascular disease.

EFFECTS ON COGNITION. Several retrospective studies had suggested that estrogens had beneficial effects on cognition and delayed the onset of Alzheimer disease. However, in more recent studies, estrogen-progestin therapy was associated with increased incidence of dementia, and no benefit of hormone treatment on global cognitive function was observed.

OTHER POTENTIAL UNTOWARD EFFECTS. Nausea and vomiting are an initial reaction to estrogen therapy in some women, but these effects may disappear with time and may be minimized by taking estrogens with food or just before sleep. Fullness and tenderness of the breasts and edema may occur but sometimes can be diminished by lowering the dose. A more serious concern is that estrogens may cause severe migraine in some women. Estrogens also may reactivate or exacerbate endometriosis.

THERAPEUTIC USES. The 2 major uses of estrogens are for menopausal hormone therapy (MHT) and as components of combination oral contraceptives, The "effective" dose of estrogen used for MHT is less than that in oral contraceptives when one considers potency. The doses of estrogens employed in both settings have decreased substantially, thereby reducing the incidence of untoward effects.

MENOPAUSAL HORMONE THERAPY. The established benefits of estrogen therapy in postmenopausal women include amelioration of vasomotor symptoms and the prevention of bone fractures and urogenital atrophy.

Vasomotor Symptoms. The decline in ovarian function at menopause is associated with vasomotor symptoms in most women. The characteristic hot flashes may alternate with chilly sensations, inappropriate sweating, and (less commonly) paresthesias. Treatment with estrogen is specific and is the most efficacious pharmacotherapy. Medroxyprogesterone acetate (discussed in the section on progestins) may provide some relief of vasomotor symptoms; the α_2 adrenergic agonist clonidine diminishes vasomotor symptoms in some women, presumably by blocking the CNS outflow that regulates blood flow to cutaneous vessels. In many women, hot flashes diminish within several years; the dose and duration of estrogen use should thus be the minimum necessary to provide relief.

Osteoporosis. Osteoporosis is a disorder of the skeleton associated with the loss of bone mass (*see* Chapter 44). The result is thinning and weakening of the bones and an increased incidence of fractures. Osteoporosis is an indication for estrogen therapy. Most fractures in the postmenopausal period occur in women without a prior history of osteoporosis, and estrogens are the most efficacious agents available for prevention of fractures at all sites in such women. Estrogens act primarily to decrease bone resorption; consequently, estrogens are more effective at preventing rather than restoring bone loss and are most effective if treatment is initiated before significant bone loss occurs. Maximal benefit requires continuous use; bone loss resumes when treatment is discontinued. An appropriate diet with adequate intake of Ca^{2+} and vitamin D and weight-bearing exercise enhance the effects of estrogen treatment. The bisphosphonates (*see* Chapter 44) can also be considered.

Vaginal Dryness and Urogenital Atrophy. Loss of tissue lining the vagina or bladder leads to a variety of symptoms in many postmenopausal women, including vaginal dryness and itching, painful intercourse, swelling of tissues in the genital region, pain during urination, a need to urinate urgently or often, and sudden or unexpected urinary incontinence. For relief of vulvar and vaginal atrophy, local administration as a vaginal cream, ring device, or tablets may be considered.

Cardiovascular Disease. The incidence of cardiovascular disease is low in premenopausal women, rising rapidly after menopause; epidemiological studies show an association between estrogen use and reduced cardiovascular disease in postmenopausal women. Estrogens produce a favorable lipoprotein profile, promote vasodilation, inhibit the response to vascular injury, and reduce atherosclerosis. However, estrogens also promote coagulation and thromboembolic events. Randomized prospective studies unexpectedly indicated that the incidence of heart disease and stroke in older postmenopausal women, treated with conjugated estrogens and a progestin, was initially increased, although the trend reversed with time. Combined estrogen-progestin therapy is associated with a decrease in heart attacks in younger women.

MENOPAUSAL HORMONE REGIMENS. The use of *hormone-replacement therapy*, or HRT, that includes a progestin in addition to estrogen, limits estrogen-related endometrial hyperplasia. Postmenopausal HRT, when indicated, should include both an estrogen and progestin for women with a uterus. For women who have undergone a hysterectomy, endometrial carcinoma is not a concern, and estrogen alone avoids the possible deleterious effects of progestins. Menopausal hormone therapy with estrogens should use the lowest dose and shortest duration necessary to achieve an appropriate therapeutic goal.

Conjugated estrogens and *medroxyprogesterone acetate* (MPA) have been used most commonly in menopausal hormone regimens, although estradiol, estrone, and estriol have been used as estrogens, and *norethindrone*, *norgestimate*, *levonorgestrel*, *norethisterone*, and *progesterone* also have been widely used (especially in Europe). Various "continuous" or "cyclic" regimens have been used; the latter regimens include drug-free days. An example of a cyclic regimen is as follows: (1) administration of an estrogen for 25 days; (2) the addition of MPA for the last 12-14 days of estrogen treatment; and (3) 5-6 days with no hormone treatment, during which withdrawal bleeding normally occurs due to breakdown and shedding of the endometrium. Continuous administration of combined estrogen plus progestin does not lead to regular, recurrent endometrial shedding but may cause intermittent spotting or bleeding, especially in the first year of use. Other regimens include a progestin intermittently (e.g., every third month), but the long-term endometrial safety of these regimens remains to be firmly established. PREMPRO (conjugated estrogens plus MPA given as a fixed dose daily) and PREMPHASE (conjugated estrogens given for 28 days plus MPA given for 14 of 28 days) are widely used combination formulations. Other combination products available in the U.S. are FEMHRT (ethinyl estradiol plus norethindrone acetate), ACTIVELLA (estradiol plus norethindrone), PREFEST (estradiol and norgestimate), and ANGELIQ (estradiol and drospirenone). Doses and regimens are usually adjusted empirically based on control of symptoms, patient acceptance of bleeding patterns, and/or other untoward effects.

Another pharmacological consideration is the route of estrogen administration. Oral administration exposes the liver to higher concentrations of estrogens than does transdermal administration and may increase SHBG, other binding globulins, angiotensinogen; and possibly the cholesterol content of the bile. Transdermal estrogen appears to cause smaller beneficial changes in LDL and HDL profiles (~50% of those seen with the oral route).

Tibolone (LIVIAL) is widely used in the E.U. for treatment of vasomotor symptoms and prevention of osteoporosis but is not currently approved in the U.S. The parent compound itself is devoid of activity, but it is metabolized in a tissue-selective manner to 3 metabolites that have predominantly estrogenic, progestogenic, and androgenic activities.

ESTROGEN TREATMENT IN THE FAILURE OF OVARIAN DEVELOPMENT. In several conditions (e.g., Turner syndrome), the ovaries do not develop and puberty does not occur. Therapy with estrogen at the appropriate time replicates the events of puberty, and androgens (*see* Chapter 41) and/or growth hormone (*see* Chapter 38) may be used concomitantly to promote normal growth. Although estrogens and androgens promote bone growth, they also accelerate epiphyseal fusion, and their premature use can thus result in a shorter ultimate height.

SELECTIVE ESTROGEN RECEPTOR MODULATORS AND ANTI-ESTROGENS

SELECTIVE ESTROGEN RECEPTOR MODULATORS: TAMOXIFEN, RALOXIFENE, AND TOREMIFENE. Selective estrogen receptor modulators, or SERMs, are compounds with tissue-selective actions. The pharmacological goal of these drugs is to produce beneficial estrogenic actions in certain tissues (e.g., bone, brain, and liver) but antagonist activity in tissues such as breast and endometrium. Currently approved drugs in the U.S. in this class are tamoxifen citrate, raloxifene hydrochloride (EVISTA), and toremifene (FARESTON).

ANTI-ESTROGENS: CLOMIPHENE AND FULVESTRANT. These compounds are distinguished from the SERMs in that they are pure antagonists in all tissues studied. Clomiphene (CLOMID, SEROPHENE, others) is approved for the treatment of infertility in anovulatory women, and fulvestrant (FASLODEX) is used for the treatment of breast cancer in women with disease progression after tamoxifen.

PHARMACOLOGICAL EFFECTS. All of these agents bind to the ligand-binding pocket of both ERα and ERβ and competitively block estradiol binding. However, the conformation of ligand-bound ERs is different with different ligands, and this has 2 important mechanistic consequences. The distinct ER-ligand conformations recruit different coactivators and corepressors onto the promoter of a target gene. The tissue-specific actions of SERMs thus can be explained in part by the distinct conformation of the ER when occupied by different ligands, in combination with different coactivator and corepressor levels in different cell types.

Tamoxifen exhibits anti-estrogenic, estrogenic, or mixed activity depending on the species and target gene measured. In clinical tests or laboratory studies with human cells, the drug's activity depends on the tissue and end point measured. For example, tamoxifen inhibits the proliferation of cultured human breast cancer cells and reduces tumor size and number in women, and yet it stimulates proliferation of endometrial cells and causes endometrial thickening. The drug has an antiresorptive effect on bone, and in humans it decreases total cholesterol, LDL, and LPA but does not increase HDL and triglycerides. Tamoxifen treatment increases the relative risk of deep vein thrombosis, pulmonary embolism, and endometrial carcinoma. Tamoxifen produces hot flashes and other adverse effects, including cataracts and nausea. Due to its agonist activity in bone, it does not increase the incidence of fractures when used in this setting. Whereas 17α estradiol induces a conformation that recruits coactivators to the receptor, tamoxifen induces a conformation that permits the recruitment of the corepressor to both ERα and ERβ. The agonist activity of tamoxifen seen in tissues such as the endometrium is mediated by the ligand-independent AF-1 transactivation domain of ER α; because ERβ does not contain a functional AF-1 domain, tamoxifen does not activate ERβ.

Raloxifene is an estrogen agonist in bone, where it exerts an antiresorptive effect. The drug also acts as an estrogen agonist in reducing total cholesterol and LDL, but it does not increase HDL. Raloxifene does not cause proliferation or thickening of the endometrium. Studies indicate that raloxifene significantly reduces the risk of ER-positive but not ER-negative breast cancer. Raloxifene does not alleviate the vasomotor symptoms associated with menopause. Adverse effects include hot flashes, leg cramps, and a 3-fold increase in deep vein thrombosis and pulmonary embolism.

Clomiphene increases gonadotropin secretion and stimulates ovulation. Clomiphene's major pharmacological use is to induce ovulation in women with amenorrhea, polycystic ovarian syndrome, or dysfunctional bleeding with anovulatory cycles, but who have a functional hypothalamic-hypophyseal-ovarian system and adequate endogenous estrogen production.

Fulvestrant is anti-estrogenic. In clinical trials it is efficacious in treating tamoxifen-resistant breast cancers. Fulvestrant binds to ERα and ERβ with a high affinity comparable to estradiol but represses transactivation. It also increases dramatically the intracellular proteolytic degradation of ERα while apparently protecting ERβ from degradation. This effect on ERα protein levels may explain fulvestrant's efficacy in tamoxifen-resistant breast cancer.

ADME. Tamoxifen is given orally, and peak plasma levels are reached within 4-7 h. It has 2 elimination phases with half-lives of 7-14 h and 4-11 days; thus, 3-4 weeks of treatment are required to reach steady-state plasma levels. Tamoxifen is metabolized in humans by multiple hepatic CYPs, some of which it also induces. In humans, the more potent anti-estrogen metabolite 4-hydroxytamoxifen is produced in the liver. The major route of elimination from the body involves *N*-demethylation and deamination. The drug undergoes enterohepatic circulation, and excretion is primarily in the feces as conjugates of the deaminated metabolite.

Oral *Raloxifene* is absorbed rapidly with a bioavailability of ~2%. The drug has a $t_{1/2}$ of ~28 h and is eliminated primarily in the feces after hepatic glucuronidation. *Clomiphene* is well absorbed following oral administration, and the drug and its metabolites are eliminated primarily in the feces. The long plasma $t_{1/2}$ (5-7 days) is due largely to plasma-protein binding, enterohepatic circulation, and accumulation in fatty tissues. *Fulvestrant* is administered monthly by intramuscular depot injections. Plasma concentrations reach maximal levels in 7 days and are maintained for a month. The drug is eliminated primarily (90%) via the feces in humans.

THERAPEUTIC USES

BREAST CANCER. Tamoxifen is highly efficacious in the palliation of advanced breast cancer in women with ER-positive tumors, and it is now indicated as the hormonal treatment of choice for both early and advanced breast cancer in women of all ages. Response rates are ~50% in women with ER-positive tumors. Tamoxifen increases disease-free survival and overall survival; treatment for 5 years is more efficacious than shorter 1- to 2-year treatment periods in reducing cancer recurrence and death. Prophylactic treatment should be limited to 5 years because effectiveness decreases thereafter. The most frequent side effect is hot flashes. Tamoxifen has estrogenic activity in the uterus, increases the risk of endometrial cancer by 2- to 3-fold, and also causes a comparable increase in the risk of thromboembolic disease that leads to serious risks for women receiving anticoagulant therapy and women with a history of deep vein thrombosis or stroke. Toremifene has therapeutic actions similar to tamoxifen, and fulvestrant may be efficacious in women who become resistant to tamoxifen. Untoward effects of fulvestrant include hot flashes, GI symptoms, headache, back pain, and pharyngitis.

OSTEOPOROSIS. Raloxifene reduces the rate of bone loss and may increase bone mass at certain sites. Raloxifene does not appear to increase the risk of developing endometrial cancer. The drug has beneficial actions on lipoprotein metabolism, reducing both total cholesterol and LDL; HDL is not increased. Adverse effects include hot flashes, deep vein thrombosis, and leg cramps.

INFERTILITY. Clomiphene is used primarily for treatment of female infertility due to anovulation. By increasing gonadotropin levels, primarily FSH, it enhances follicular recruitment. It is relatively inexpensive, orally active, and requires less extensive monitoring than other treatment protocols. Untoward effects include ovarian hyperstimulation, increased incidence of multiple births, ovarian cysts, hot flashes, and blurred vision. Prolonged use (e.g., ≥12 cycles) may increase the risk of ovarian cancer. The drug should not be administered to pregnant women due to reports of teratogenicity in animals, but there is no evidence of this when used to induce ovulation.

ESTROGEN SYNTHESIS INHIBITORS

Continual administration of GnRH agonists prevents ovarian synthesis of estrogens but not their peripheral synthesis from adrenal androgens (*see* Chapter 38). The recognition that locally produced as well as circulating estrogens may play a significant role in breast cancer has greatly stimulated interest in the use of aromatase inhibitors to selectively block production of estrogens (*see* Chapter 63). Both steroidal (e.g., **formestane** and **exemestane** [AROMASIN]) and nonsteroidal agents (e.g., **anastrozole** [ARIMIDEX], **letrozole** [FEMARA], and **vorozole**) are available. Steroidal, or type I, agents are substrate analogs that act as suicide inhibitors to irreversibly inactivate aromatase, whereas the nonsteroidal, or type II, agents interact reversibly with the heme groups of CYPs. Exemestane, letrozole, and anastrozole are currently approved in the U.S. for the treatment of breast cancer. These agents may be used as first-line treatment of breast cancer or as second-line drugs after tamoxifen (*see* Chapter 62). They are highly efficacious and actually superior to tamoxifen in adjuvant use for postmenopausal women, and are indicated either following tamoxifen for 2-5 years or as initial agents. They have the added advantage of not increasing the risk of uterine cancer or venous thromboembolism. Because they dramatically reduce circulating as well as local levels of estrogens, they produce hot flashes. They lack the beneficial effect of tamoxifen to maintain bone density.

PROGESTINS

Progesterone is secreted by the ovary, mainly from the corpus luteum, during the second half of the menstrual cycle (*see* Figure 40–3). LH, acting via its G protein-coupled receptor, stimulates progesterone secretion during the normal cycle.

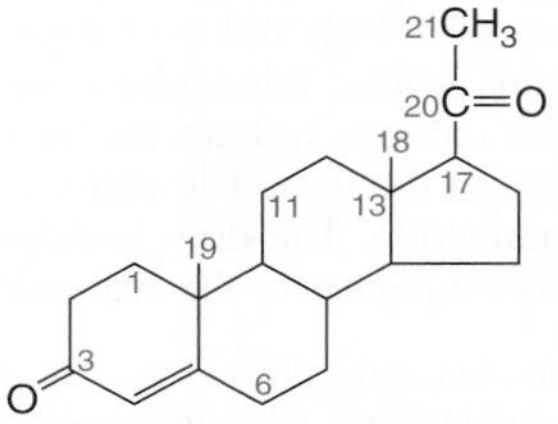

PROGESTERONE

After fertilization, the trophoblast secretes hCG into the maternal circulation, which then stimulates the LH receptor to sustain the corpus luteum and maintain progesterone production. During the second or third month of pregnancy, the developing placenta begins to secrete estrogen and progesterone in collaboration with the fetal adrenal glands, and thereafter the corpus luteum is not essential to continued gestation. Estrogen and progesterone continue to be secreted in large amounts by the placenta up to the time of delivery.

The progestins are widely used with estrogens for MHT. Depot MPA is used as a long-acting injectable contraceptive. The 19-nortestosterone derivatives (*estranes*) were developed for use as progestins in oral contraceptives, but they also exhibit androgenic and other activities. The gonanes are the "19-nor" compounds that have diminished androgenic activity relative to the estranes. These 2 classes of 19-nortestosterone derivatives are the progestational components of most oral and some long-acting injectable contraceptives. The remaining oral contraceptives contain a class of progestins derived from spironolactone (e.g., drospirenone) that have anti-mineralocorticoid and anti-androgenic properties. Other steroidal progestins include the gonane dienogest; 19-nor-progestin derivatives (e.g., *nomegestrol*, *Nestorone*, and *trimegestone*), which have increased selectivity for the progesterone receptor and less androgenic activity than estranes; and the spironolactone derivative *drospirenone*, which is used in combination with oral contraceptives. Like spironolactone, drospirenone is also a mineralocorticoid and androgen receptor antagonist.

PHYSIOLOGICAL AND PHARMACOLOGICAL ACTIONS

NEUROENDOCRINE ACTIONS. Progesterone produced in the luteal phase of the cycle decreases the frequency of GnRH pulses. This progesterone-mediated decrease in GnRH pulse frequency is critical for suppressing gonadotropin release and resetting the hypothalamic-pituitary-gonadal axis to transition from the luteal back to the follicular phase. Furthermore, GnRH suppression is the major mechanism of action of progestin-containing contraceptives.

Reproductive Tract. Progesterone decreases estrogen-driven endometrial proliferation and leads to the development of a secretory endometrium (*see* Figure 40–3); the abrupt decline in progesterone at the end of the cycle is the main determinant of the onset of menstruation. If the duration of the luteal phase is artificially lengthened, either by sustaining luteal function or by treatment with progesterone, decidual changes in the endometrial stroma similar to those seen in early pregnancy can be induced. Under normal circumstances, estrogen antecedes and accompanies progesterone in its action on the endometrium and is essential to the development of the normal menstrual pattern. Progesterone also influences the endocervical glands, and the abundant watery secretion of the estrogen-stimulated structures is changed to a scant viscid material. These and other effects of progestins decrease penetration of the cervix by sperm. The estrogen-induced maturation of the human vaginal epithelium is modified toward the condition of pregnancy by the action of progesterone. Progesterone is very important for the maintenance of pregnancy. Progesterone suppresses menstruation and uterine contractility.

Mammary Gland. Development of the mammary gland requires both estrogen and progesterone. During pregnancy and to a minor degree during the luteal phase of the cycle, progesterone, acting with estrogen, brings about a proliferation of the acini of the mammary gland. Toward the end of pregnancy, the acini fill with secretions and the vasculature of the gland notably increases; however, only after the levels of estrogen and progesterone decrease at parturition does lactation begin. During the luteal phase of the menstrual cycle, progesterone triggers a *single* round of mitotic activity in the mammary epithelium. This effect is transient; continued exposure to the hormone is rapidly followed by arrest of growth of the epithelial cells.

CNS. During a normal menstrual cycle, an increase in basal body temperature of ~0.6°C (1°F) may be noted at mid-cycle; this correlates with ovulation. This increase is due to progesterone, but the exact mechanism of this effect is unknown. Progesterone also increases the ventilatory response of the respiratory centers to carbon dioxide and leads to reduced arterial and alveolar P_{CO_2} in the luteal phase of the menstrual cycle and during pregnancy. Progesterone also may have depressant and hypnotic actions in the CNS, possibly accounting for reports of drowsiness after hormone administration. This potential untoward effect may be abrogated by giving progesterone preparations at bedtime, which may help some patients sleep.

Metabolic Effects. Progesterone itself increases basal insulin levels and the rise in insulin after carbohydrate ingestion but does not normally alter glucose tolerance. However, long-term administration of more potent progestins, such as norgestrel, may decrease glucose tolerance. Progesterone stimulates lipoprotein lipase activity and seems to enhance fat deposition. Progesterone and analogs such as MPA have been reported to increase LDL and cause either no effects or modest reductions in serum HDL levels. MPA decreases the favorable HDL increase caused by conjugated estrogens during postmenopausal hormone replacement, but not the beneficial effect of estrogens to lower LDL. In contrast, micronized progesterone does not significantly alter beneficial estrogen effects on either HDL or LDL profiles; the spironolactone derivative drospirenone may actually have advantageous effects on the cardiovascular system due to its anti-androgenic and anti-mineralocorticoid activities. Progesterone also may diminish the effects of aldosterone in the renal tubule and cause a decrease in sodium reabsorption that may increase mineralocorticoid secretion from the adrenal cortex.

CELLULAR MECHANISM OF ACTION. A single gene encodes 2 isoforms of the progesterone receptor, PR-A and PR-B. The first 164 N-terminal amino acids of PR-B are missing from PR-A. Because the ligand-binding domains of the 2 PR isoforms are identical, their ligand-binding properties are also the same. However, the structural differences outside the ligand-binding region contribute to different interactions with coactivators and corepressors and thus differential activities of PR-A and PR-B. The biological activities of PR-A and PR-B are distinct and depend on the target gene. In most cells, PR-B mediates the stimulatory activities of progesterone; PR-A strongly inhibits this action of PR-B and is also a transcriptional inhibitor of other steroid receptors. Several uterine genes appear to be regulated exclusively by PR-A, including calcitonin and amphiregulin, and the antiproliferative effect of progesterone on the estrogen-stimulated endometrium. In contrast, PR-B may be responsible for mediating progesterone's effects in the mammary gland.

In the absence of ligand, PR is present primarily in the nucleus in an inactive monomeric state bound to heat-shock proteins. When receptors bind progesterone, the heat-shock proteins dissociate and the receptors are phosphorylated and form dimers (homo- and hetero-) that bind to PREs (progesterone response elements) located on target genes. Transcriptional activation by PR occurs primarily via recruitment of coactivators. The receptor/coactivator complex then favors further interactions that mediate processes such as histone acetylase activity. Histone acetylation causes a remodeling of chromatin that increases the accessibility of general transcriptional proteins, including PolII, to the target promoter. Progesterone antagonists also facilitate receptor dimerization and DNA binding, but, as with ER, the conformation of antagonist-bound PR is different from that of agonist-bound PR. This different conformation favors PR interaction with corepressors that recruit histone deacetylases, reducing accessibility of a target promoter to the transcriptional apparatus. In general mechanistic terms, the PR functions similarly to the ER (*see* Figure 40–4).

Certain effects of progesterone, such as increased Ca^{2+} mobilization in sperm, can be seen in as little as 3 min and are therefore considered transcription-independent. Similarly, progesterone can promote oocyte maturation (meiotic resumption) independently of transcription.

ADME. The $t_{1/2}$ of progesterone is ~5 min, and the hormone is metabolized primarily in the liver to hydroxylated metabolites and their sulfate and glucuronide conjugates, which are eliminated in the urine. A major metabolite specific for progesterone is pregnane-3α, 20 α-diol; its measurement in urine and plasma is used as an index of endogenous progesterone secretion. The synthetic progestins have much longer half-lives (e.g., ~7 h for norethindrone, 16 h for norgestrel, 12 h for gestodene, and 24 h for MPA). The metabolism of synthetic progestins is primarily hepatic, and elimination is generally via the urine as conjugates and various polar metabolites.

Even though progesterone undergoes rapid first-pass metabolism, high-dose (e.g., 100-200 mg) preparations of micronized progesterone (PROMETRIUM) are available for oral use. The absolute bioavailability of these preparations is low but efficacious plasma levels can be obtained. Progesterone also is available in oil solution for injection, as a vaginal gel (CRINONE, PROCHIEVE), as a slow-release intrauterine device (PROGESTASERT) for contraception, and as a vaginal insert (ENDOMETRIN) for assisted reproductive technology. Esters such as MPA (DEPO-PROVERA) are available for intramuscular administration, and MPA (PROVERA, others) and megestrol acetate (MEGACE, others) may be used orally. The 19-nor steroids have good oral activity because the ethinyl substituent at C17 significantly slows hepatic metabolism. Implants and depot preparations of synthetic progestins are available in many countries for release over very long periods of time.

THERAPEUTIC USES. Progestins are mainly used for contraception, either alone or with an estrogen, and in combination with estrogen for hormone therapy of postmenopausal women. Progestins also are used diagnostically for secondary amenorrhea. Combinations of estrogens and progestins can also be given to test for endometrial responsiveness in patients with amenorrhea. Progestins are highly efficacious in decreasing the occurrence of endometrial hyperplasia and carcinoma caused by unopposed estrogens. Local intrauterine application via a hormone-releasing intrauterine device (IUD) containing levonorgestrel can be used to decrease estrogen-induced endometrial hyperplasia while reducing untoward effects of systemically administered progestins. Finally, levonorgestrel is used as so-called emergency contraception after known or suspected unprotected intercourse. The medication is given orally within 72 h after intercourse as either a single 1.5-mg dose (PLAN B ONE-STEP) or as 2 0.75-mg doses (PLAN B) separated by 12 h. The mechanism of action may involve several factors, including the prevention of ovulation, fertilization, and implantation.

ANTIPROGESTINS AND PROGESTERONE-RECEPTOR MODULATORS

The antiprogestin, RU 38486 (often referred to as RU-486) or *mifepristone* is available for the termination of pregnancy. *Ulipristal* acetate [ELLA (U.S.), ELLA ONE (E.U.)], a partial agonist at the progesterone receptor, is used for emergency contraception.

MIFEPRISTONE

Mifepristone is a derivative of the 19-norprogestin norethindrone containing a dimethyl-aminophenol substituent at the 11β-position. It effectively competes with both progesterone and glucocorticoids for binding to their respective receptors. Mifepristone is considered a progesterone-receptor modulator (PRM) due to its context-dependent activity. *Onapristone* (or ZK 98299) is a pure progesterone antagonist, similar in structure to mifepristone but with a methyl substituent in the 13α rather than 13β orientation.

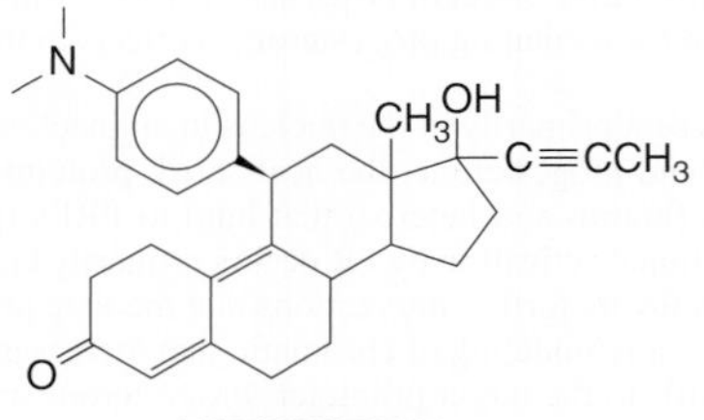

MIFEPRISTONE

PHARMACOLOGICAL ACTIONS. Mifepristone acts primarily as a competitive receptor antagonist for both progesterone receptors, although it may have some agonist activity in certain contexts. When administered in the early stages of pregnancy, mifepristone causes decidual breakdown by blockade of uterine progesterone receptors. This leads to detachment of the blastocyst, which decreases hCG production. This in turn causes a decrease in progesterone secretion from the corpus luteum, which further accentuates decidual breakdown. Decreased endogenous progesterone coupled with blockade of progesterone receptors in the uterus increases uterine prostaglandin levels and sensitizes the myometrium to their contractile actions. Mifepristone also causes cervical softening, which facilitates expulsion of the detached blastocyst. Mifepristone can delay or prevent ovulation depending on the timing and manner of administration. If administered for 1 or several days in the mid- to late luteal phase, mifepristone impairs the development of a secretory endometrium and produces menses. Mifepristone also binds glucocorticoid and androgen receptors and exerts anti-glucocorticoid and anti-androgenic actions. Thus, mifepristone blocks the feedback inhibition by cortisol of ACTH secretion from the pituitary, thereby increasing plasma levels of corticotropin and adrenal steroids.

ADME. Mifepristone is orally active with good bioavailability. Peak plasma levels occur within several hours. In plasma, it is bound by α_1 acid glycoprotein, which contributes to the drug's long $t_{1/2}$ (20-40 h). Metabolites are primarily the mono- and di-demethylated products (thought to have pharmacological activity) formed via CYP3A4. The drug undergoes hepatic metabolism and enterohepatic circulation; metabolic products are found predominantly in the feces.

THERAPEUTIC USES. Mifepristone (MIFEPREX), in combination with misoprostol or other prostaglandins, is available for the termination of early pregnancy. When mifepristone is used to produce a medical abortion, a prostaglandin is given 48 h after the antiprogestin to further increase myometrial contractions and ensure expulsion of the detached blastocyst. Intramuscular *sulprostone*, intravaginal *gemeprost*, and oral misoprostol have been used. The most severe untoward effect is vaginal bleeding, which most often lasts 8-17 days but is only rarely (0.1% of patients) severe enough to require blood transfusions. High percentages of women also have experienced abdominal pain and uterine cramps, nausea, vomiting, and diarrhea due to the prostaglandin. Women receiving chronic glucocorticoid therapy should not be given mifepristone because of its antiglucocorticoid activity. In fact, due to its high affinity for the glucocorticoid receptor, high doses of mifepristone can result in adrenal insufficiency.

ULIPRISTAL

Ulipristal, a derivative of 19-norprogesterone, functions as a selective progesterone receptor modulator (SPRM), acting as a partial agonist at progesterone receptors. Unlike mifepristone, ulipristal appears to be a relatively weak glucocorticoid antagonist.

PHARMACOLOGICAL ACTIONS. In high doses, ulipristal has antiproliferative effects in the uterus; however, its most relevant actions to date involve its capacity to inhibit ovulation. Ulipristal's anti-ovulatory actions likely occur due to progesterone regulation at many levels, including inhibition of LH release through the hypothalamus and pituitary, and inhibition of LH-induced follicular rupture within the ovary. A 30-mg dose of ulipristal can inhibit ovulation when taken up to 5 days after intercourse. Ulipristal can block ovarian rupture at or even just after the time of the LH surge. Ulipristal may also block endometrial implantation of the fertilized egg, although whether this contributes to its effects as an emergency contraceptive is not clear.

THERAPEUTIC USES. Ulipristal acetate [ELLA, ELLA ONE] has recently been licensed in the E.U. and the U.S. as an emergency contraceptive. Studies comparing ulipristal to levonorgestrel (progesterone-only emergency contraception, or POEC) demonstrate that ulipristal is at least as effective when taken up to 72 h after unprotected sexual intercourse. In addition, ulipristal remains effective up to 120 h (5 days) after intercourse, making ulipristal a more versatile emergency contraceptive than levonorgestrel, which does not work well beyond 72 h after unprotected intercourse. The most severe side effect in clinical trials has been a headache and abdominal pain.

HORMONAL CONTRACEPTIVES

The incredible growth of the earth's human population stands out as one of the fundamental events of the last 2 centuries. The Old Testament dictum "Be fruitful and multiply" (Genesis 9:1) has been followed too religiously by readers and nonreaders of the Bible alike. In 1798, Malthus started a great controversy by opposing the prevailing view of unlimited progress for humankind by making 2 postulates and a conclusion. Malthus postulated "that food is necessary for the existence of man" and that sexual attraction between female and male is necessary and likely to persist, since "toward the extinction of the passion between the sexes, no progress whatever has hitherto been made," barring "individual exceptions." Malthus concluded that "the power of populations is infinitely greater than the power of the earth to produce subsistence for man," producing a "natural inequality" that would someday loom "insurmountable in the way to perfectibility of society."

Malthus was right: passion between the sexes persists and the power of populations is very great indeed, so much so that our sheer numbers have increased to the point that they are straining the earth's capacity to supply food, energy, and raw materials, and to absorb the detritus of its human burden. Marine fisheries are being depleted, forests and aquifers are disappearing, and the atmosphere is accumulating greenhouse gases from combustion of the fossil fuels that provide the energy needs of 7 billion people, up from 1 billion in Malthus' day. Perhaps some of the blame can be laid at the feet of medical science: advances in public health and medicine have led to a significant decline in mortality and an increased life expectancy. However, medical science has also begun to assume a portion of the responsibility for overpopulation and its adverse effects. To this end, drugs in the form of hormones and their analogs have been developed to control human fertility.

COMBINATION ORAL CONTRACEPTIVES. The most frequently used agents in the U.S. are combination oral contraceptives containing both an estrogen and a progestin. Their theoretical efficacy is 99.9%. Combination oral contraceptives are available in many formulations. Monophasic, biphasic, or triphasic pills are generally provided in 21-day packs. (Virtually all preparations come as 28-day packs, with the pills for the last 7 days containing only inert ingredients.) For the monophasic agents, fixed amounts of the estrogen and progestin are present in each pill, which is taken daily for 21 days, followed by a 7-day "pill-free" period. The biphasic and triphasic preparations provide 2 or 3 different pills containing varying amounts of active ingredients, to be taken at different times during the 21-day cycle. This reduces the total amount of steroids administered and more closely approximates the estrogen-to-progestin ratios that occur during the menstrual cycle. With these preparations, predictable menstrual bleeding generally occurs during the 7-day "off" period each month. However, several oral contraceptions are now available whereby progestin withdrawal is only induced every 3 months.

The estrogen content of current preparations ranges from 20-50 μg; most contain 30-35 μg. Preparations containing ≤35 μg of an estrogen are generally referred to as "low-dose" or "modern" pills. The dose of progestin is more variable because of differences in potency of the compounds used. A transdermal preparation of norelgestromin and ethinyl estradiol (ORTHO EVRA) is marketed for weekly application to the buttock, abdomen, upper arm, or torso for the first 3 consecutive weeks followed by a patch-free week for each 28-day cycle. A similar 3-week on/1-week off cycle is employed for the intravaginal ring containing ethinyl estradiol and etonogestrel (NUVARING).

PROGESTIN-ONLY CONTRACEPTIVES. Several agents are available with theoretical efficacies of 99%. Specific preparations include the "minipill"; low doses of progestins (e.g., 350 μg of norethindrone [NOR-QD, ORTHO MICRONOR, others]) taken daily without interruption; subdermal implants of 216 mg of norgestrel (NORPLANT II, JADELLE) for long-term contraceptive action (e.g., up to 5 years) or 68 mg of etonogestrel (IMPLANON) for contraception lasting 3 years; and crystalline suspensions of medroxyprogesterone acetate for intramuscular injection of 104 mg (DEPO-SUBQ PROVERA 104) or 150 mg (DEPO-PROVERA, others) of drug; each provides effective contraception for 3 months. An IUD (PROGESTASERT) that releases low amounts of progesterone locally is available for insertion on a yearly basis. Its effectiveness is considered to be 97-98%, and contraceptive action probably is due to local effects on the endometrium. An IUD (MIRENA) releases levonorgestrel for up to 5 years.

MECHANISM OF ACTION

COMBINATION ORAL CONTRACEPTIVES. Combination oral contraceptives act by preventing ovulation. Direct measurements of plasma hormone levels indicate that LH and FSH levels are suppressed, a mid-cycle surge of LH is absent, endogenous steroid levels are diminished, and ovulation does not occur. Hypothalamic actions of steroids play a major role in the mechanism of oral contraceptive action. Progesterone diminishes the frequency of GnRH pulses. Because the proper frequency of LH pulses is essential for ovulation, this effect of progesterone likely plays a major role in the contraceptive action of these agents.

Multiple pituitary effects of both estrogen and progestin components are likely to contribute to oral contraceptive action. Oral contraceptives seem likely to decrease pituitary responsiveness to GnRH. Estrogens also suppress FSH release from the pituitary during the follicular phase of the menstrual cycle, and this effect seems likely to contribute to the lack of follicular development in oral contraceptive users. The progestin component may also inhibit the estrogen-induced LH surge at mid-cycle. Other effects may contribute to a minor extent to the extraordinary efficacy of oral contraceptives. Transit of sperm, the egg, and fertilized ovum are important to establish pregnancy, and steroids are likely to affect transport in the fallopian tube. In the cervix, progestin effects also are likely to produce a thick viscous mucus to reduce sperm penetration and in the endometrium to produce a state that is not receptive to implantation.

PROGESTIN-ONLY CONTRACEPTIVES. Progestin-only pills and levonorgestrel implants are highly efficacious but block ovulation in only 60-80% of cycles. Their effectiveness is thought to be due largely to a thickening of cervical mucus, which decreases sperm penetration, and to endometrial alterations that impair implantation; such local effects account for the efficacy of IUDs that release progestins. Depot injections of MPA are thought to exert similar effects, but they also yield plasma levels of drug high enough to prevent ovulation, presumably by decreasing the frequency of GnRH pulses.

UNTOWARD EFFECTS

COMBINATION ORAL CONTRACEPTIVES. Untoward effects of early hormonal contraceptives fell into several major categories: adverse cardiovascular effects; breast, hepatocellular, and cervical cancers; and a number of endocrine and metabolic effects. The current consensus is that low-dose preparations pose minimal health risks in women who have no predisposing risk factors.

Cardiovascular Effects. For nonsmokers without other risk factors such as hypertension or diabetes, there is no significant increase in the risk of myocardial infarction or stroke. There is a 28% increase in relative risk for venous thromboembolism, but the estimated absolute increase is very small because the incidence of these events in women without other predisposing factors is low (e.g., roughly half that associated with the risk of venous thromboembolism in pregnancy). The risk is significantly increased in women who smoke or have other factors that predispose to thrombosis or thromboembolism. Postmarketing studies indicate that women using transdermal contraceptives have a higher than expected exposure to estrogen and are at increased risk for the development of venous thromboembolism.

Early high-dose combination oral contraceptives caused hypertension in 4-5% of normotensive women and increased blood pressure in 10-15% of those with preexisting hypertension. This incidence is much lower with newer low-dose preparations, and most reported changes in blood pressure are not significant. The cardiovascular risk associated with oral contraceptive use does not appear to persist after use is discontinued. Estrogens increase serum HDL and decrease LDL levels; progestins tend to have the opposite effect. Recent studies of several low-dose preparations have not found significant changes in total serum cholesterol or lipoprotein profiles, although slight increases in triglycerides have been reported.

Cancer. Given the growth-promoting effects of estrogens, there has been a long-standing concern that oral contraceptives might increase the incidence of endometrial, cervical, ovarian, breast, and other cancers. There is *not* a widespread association between oral contraceptive use and cancer. Epidemiological evidence suggests that combined oral contraceptive use may increase the risk of cervical cancer by about 2-fold but only in long-term users (>5 years) with persistent human papilloma virus infection. There have been reports of increases in the incidence of hepatic adenoma and hepatocellular carcinoma. Current estimates indicate there is about a doubling in the risk of liver cancer after 4-8 years of use; these are rare cancers, and the absolute increases are small.

The effects of oral contraceptives on breast cancer are a concern. The risk of breast cancer in women of childbearing age is very low, and current oral contraceptive users in this group have only a very small increase in relative risk of 1.1-1.2, depending on other variables. This small increase is not substantially affected by duration of use, dose, or type of component, age at first use, or parity. Importantly, 10 years after discontinuation of oral contraceptive use, there is no difference in breast cancer incidence between past users and never users. Combination oral contraceptives decrease the incidence of endometrial cancer by 50%, an effect that lasts 15 years after the pills are stopped. This is thought to be due to the inclusion of a progestin throughout the entire 21-day cycle of administration. These agents also decrease the incidence of ovarian cancer. There are accumulating data that oral contraceptive use decreases the risk of colorectal cancer.

Metabolic and Endocrine Effects. The effects of sex steroids on glucose metabolism and insulin sensitivity are complex and may differ among agents in the same class. Early studies with high-dose oral contraceptives generally reported impaired glucose tolerance; these effects have decreased as steroid dosages have been lowered; current low-dose combination contraceptives may even improve insulin sensitivity. Similarly, the high-dose progestins in early oral contraceptives raised LDL and reduced HDL levels, but modern low-dose preparations do not produce unfavorable lipid profiles. There also have been periodic reports that oral contraceptives increase the incidence of gallbladder disease, but any such effect appears to be weak and associated with very long-term use.

The estrogenic component of oral contraceptives may increase hepatic synthesis of a number of serum proteins, including those that bind thyroid hormones, glucocorticoids, and sex steroids. Although physiological feedback mechanisms generally adjust hormone synthesis to maintain normal "free" hormone levels, these changes can affect the interpretation of endocrine function tests that measure *total* plasma hormone levels, and may necessitate dose adjustment in patients receiving thyroid-hormone replacement. The ethinyl estradiol present in oral contraceptives appears to cause a dose-dependent increase in several serum factors known to increase coagulation. However, in healthy women who do not smoke, there also is an increase in fibrinolytic activity that exerts a counter effect so that overall there is a minimal effect on hemostatic balance. This compensatory effect is diminished in smokers.

Miscellaneous Effects. Nausea, edema, and mild headache occur in some individuals; migraine headaches may be precipitated in a smaller fraction of women. Breakthrough bleeding may occur during the 21-day cycle when the active pills are being taken. Withdrawal bleeding may fail to occur in a small fraction of women during the 7-day "off" period, thus causing confusion about a possible pregnancy. Acne and hirsutism may be due to the androgenic activity of the 19-nor progestins.

PROGESTIN-ONLY CONTRACEPTIVES. Episodes of irregular, unpredictable spotting and breakthrough bleeding are the most frequently encountered untoward effect and the major reason women discontinue use of progestin-only contraceptives. With time, the incidence of these bleeding episodes decreases. No evidence indicates that the progestin-only minipill preparations increase thromboembolic events. Acne may be a problem because of the androgenic activity of norethindrone-containing preparations. These preparations may be attractive for nursing mothers because they do not decrease lactation.

Headache is a commonly reported untoward effect of depot MPA. Mood changes and weight gain also have been reported. Many studies have found decreases in HDL levels and increases in LDL levels, and there have been reports of decreased bone density. These effects may be due to reduced endogenous estrogens because depot MPA lowers gonadotropin levels. Because of the time required to completely eliminate the drug, the contraceptive effect of this agent may remain for 6-12 months after the last injection. Implants of norethindrone may be associated with infection, local irritation, pain at the insertion site, and, rarely, expulsion of the inserts. Headache, weight gain, and mood changes have been reported. Acne is seen in some patients. Ovulation occurs fairly soon after implant removal, reaching 50% in 3 months and almost 90% within 1 year.

CONTRAINDICATIONS. Modern oral contraceptives are considered generally safe in most healthy women; however, *these agents can contribute to the incidence and severity of cardiovascular, thromboembolic, or malignant disease, particularly if other risk factors are present.* Contraindications for combination oral contraceptive use include: the presence or history of thromboembolic disease, cerebrovascular disease, myocardial infarction, coronary artery disease, or congenital hyperlipidemia; known or suspected carcinoma of the breast, carcinoma of the female reproductive tract; abnormal undiagnosed vaginal bleeding; known or suspected pregnancy; and past or present liver tumors or impaired liver function. *The risk of serious cardiovascular side effects is particularly marked in women >35 years of age who smoke heavily* (e.g., >15 cigarettes per day); even low-dose oral contraceptives are contraindicated in such patients.

Other relative contraindications include migraine headaches, hypertension, diabetes mellitus, obstructive jaundice of pregnancy or prior oral contraceptive use, and gallbladder disease. If elective surgery is planned, discontinuation of oral contraceptives for several weeks to a month is recommended to minimize the possibility of thromboembolism after surgery. These agents should be used with care in women with prior gestational diabetes or uterine fibroids, and low-dose forms should generally be used in such cases. Progestin-only contraceptives are contraindicated in the presence of undiagnosed vaginal bleeding, benign or malignant liver disease, and known or suspected breast cancer. Depot MPA and levonorgestrel inserts are contraindicated in women with a history or predisposition to thrombophlebitis or thromboembolic disorders.

CHOICE OF CONTRACEPTIVE PREPARATIONS

Treatment should generally begin with preparations containing the minimum dose of steroids that provides effective contraceptive coverage. This is typically a pill with 30-35 μg of estrogen, but preparations with 20 μg may be adequate for lighter women or >40 years of age with perimenopausal symptoms; a preparation containing 50 μg of estrogen may be required for heavier women. In women for whom estrogens are contraindicated or undesirable, progestin-only contraceptives may be an option. The progestin-only minipill may have enhanced effectiveness in several such types of women (e.g., nursing mothers and women >40 years of age, in whom fertility may be decreased). The choice of a preparation also may be influenced by the specific 19-nor progestin component because this component may have varying degrees of androgenic and other activities. The androgenic activity of this component may contribute to untoward effects such as weight gain, acne due to increased sebaceous gland secretions, and unfavorable lipoprotein profiles. These side effects are greatly reduced in newer low-dose contraceptives that contain progestins with little to no androgenic activity.

NONCONTRACEPTIVE HEALTH BENEFITS

Combination oral contraceptives have substantial health benefits unrelated to their contraceptive use. Oral contraceptives significantly reduce the incidence of ovarian and endometrial cancer within 6 months of use. Depot MPA injections reduce substantially the incidence of uterine cancer. These agents also decrease the incidence of ovarian cysts and benign fibrocystic breast disease. Oral contraceptives have major benefits related to menstruation in many women, including more regular menstruation, reduced menstrual blood loss, less iron-deficiency anemia, and decreased frequency of dysmenorrhea. There also is a decreased incidence of pelvic inflammatory disease and ectopic pregnancies, and endometriosis may be ameliorated.

For a complete Bibliographical Listing see Goodman & Gilman's ***The Pharmacological Basis of Therapeutics***, 12th ed., or Goodman & Gilman Online at www.AccessMedicine.com.

Androgens

TESTOSTERONE AND OTHER ANDROGENS

In men, *testosterone* is the principal secreted androgen. *Leydig cells* synthesize the majority of testosterone by the pathways shown in Figure 41–1. In women, testosterone also is the principal androgen and is synthesized in the corpus luteum and the adrenal cortex by similar pathways. The testosterone precursors *androstenedione* and *dehydroepiandrosterone* are weak androgens that can be converted peripherally to testosterone.

SECRETION AND TRANSPORT OF TESTOSTERONE. Testosterone secretion is greater in men than in women at almost all stages of life, a difference that explains many of the other differences between men and women. In the first trimester in utero, the fetal testes begin to secrete testosterone, the principal factor in male sexual differentiation, probably stimulated by human chorionic gonadotropin (hCG) from the placenta. By the beginning of the second trimester, the serum testosterone concentration is close to that of mid-puberty, ~250 ng/dL (Figure 41–2). Testosterone production then falls by the end of the second trimester, but by birth the value is again ~250 ng/dL, possibly due to stimulation of the fetal Leydig cells by *luteinizing hormone* (LH) from the fetal pituitary gland. The testosterone value falls again in the first few days after birth, but it rises and peaks again at ~250 ng/dL at 2-3 months after birth and falls to <50 ng/dL by 6 months, where it remains until puberty. During puberty, from ~12 to 17 years of age, the serum testosterone concentration in males increases so that by early adulthood the serum testosterone concentration is 500 ng/dL to 700 ng/dL in men, compared to 30 ng/dL to 50 ng/dL in women. The magnitude of the testosterone concentration in the male is responsible for the pubertal changes that further differentiate men from women. As men age, their serum testosterone concentrations gradually decrease, which may contribute to other effects of aging in men.

LH, secreted by the pituitary gonadotropes (*see* Chapter 38), is the principal stimulus of testosterone secretion in men, perhaps potentiated by *follicle-stimulating hormone* (FSH), also secreted by gonadotropes. The secretion of LH by gonadotropes is positively regulated by hypothalamic *gonadotropin-releasing hormone* (GnRH); testosterone directly inhibits LH secretion in a negative feedback loop. LH is secreted in pulses, which occur approximately every 2 h and are greater in magnitude in the morning. The pulsatility appears to result from pulsatile secretion of GnRH from the hypothalamus. Testosterone secretion is likewise pulsatile and diurnal, the highest plasma concentrations occurring at ~8 A.M. and the lowest at ~8 P.M. The morning peaks diminish as men age. *Sex hormone-binding globulin* (SHBG) binds ~40% of circulating testosterone with high affinity, rendering the bound hormone unavailable for biological effects. Albumin binds almost 60% of circulating testosterone with low affinity, leaving ~2% unbound or free. In women, LH stimulates the *corpus luteum* (formed from the follicle after release of the ovum) to secrete testosterone. Under normal circumstances, however, *estradiol* and *progesterone*, not testosterone, are the principal inhibitors of LH secretion in women.

METABOLISM OF TESTOSTERONE TO ACTIVE AND INACTIVE COMPOUNDS. Testosterone has many different effects in tissues, both directly and through its metabolism to *dihydrotestosterone* and *estradiol* (Figure 41–3). The enzyme 5α-reductase catalyzes the conversion of testosterone to dihydrotestosterone. Dihydrotestosterone binds the *androgen receptor* (AR) with higher affinity than testosterone and activates gene expression more efficiently. Two forms of 5α-reductase have been identified: type I, which is found predominantly in nongenital skin, liver, and bone; and type II, which is found predominantly in urogenital tissue in men and genital skin in men and women. The enzyme complex aromatase, present in many tissues, catalyzes the conversion of testosterone to estradiol. This conversion accounts for ~85% of circulating estradiol in men; the remainder is secreted directly by the testes. Hepatic metabolism converts testosterone to the biologically inactive compounds androsterone and etiocholanolone (*see* Figure 41–3). Dihydrotestosterone is metabolized to androsterone, androstanedione, and androstanediol.

PHYSIOLOGICAL AND PHARMACOLOGICAL EFFECTS OF ANDROGENS

Testosterone is the principal circulating androgen in men. The varied effects of testosterone are due to its ability to act by at least 3 mechanisms: by binding to the AR; by conversion in certain tissues to dihydrotestosterone, which also binds to the AR; and by conversion to estradiol, which binds to the estrogen receptor (Figure 41–4).

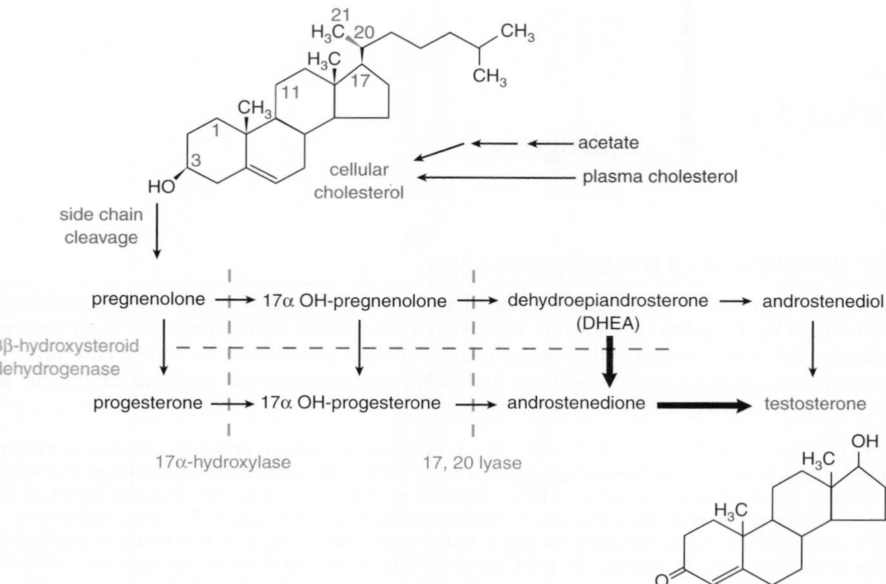

Figure 41–1 *Pathway of synthesis of testosterone in the Leydig cells of the testes.* In Leydig cells, the 11 and 21 hydroxylases (present in adrenal cortex) are absent but CYP17 (17 α-hydroxylase) is present. Thus, androgens and estrogens are synthesized; corticosterone and cortisol are not formed. Bold arrows indicate favored pathways.

EFFECTS THAT OCCUR VIA THE ANDROGEN RECEPTOR. Testosterone and dihydrotestosterone act as androgens via a single AR, a member of the nuclear receptor superfamily and is designated as NR3A.

In the absence of a ligand, the AR is located in the cytoplasm associated with a heat-shock protein complex. When testosterone or dihydrotestosterone binds to the ligand-binding domain, the AR dissociates from the heat-shock protein complex, dimerizes, and translocates to the nucleus. The dimer then binds via the DNA-binding domains to androgen response elements on certain responsive genes. The ligand-receptor complex recruits coactivators and acts as a transcription factor complex, stimulating or repressing expression of those genes.

Mutations in the hormone or DNA-binding regions of AR result in resistance to the action of testosterone, beginning in utero. Male sexual differentiation therefore is incomplete, as is pubertal development. Other

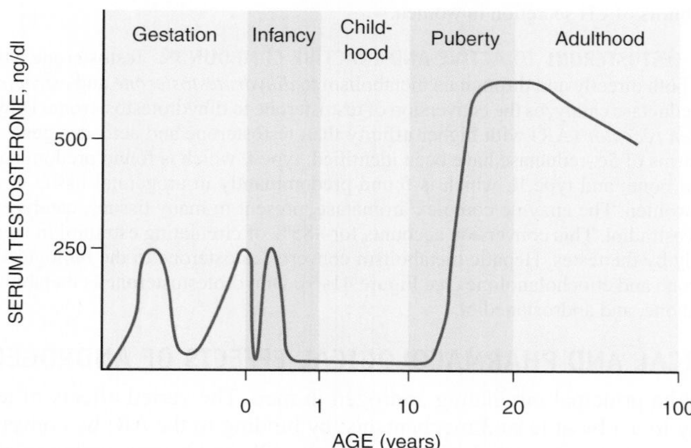

Figure 41–2 *Schematic representation of the serum testosterone concentration from early gestation to old age.*

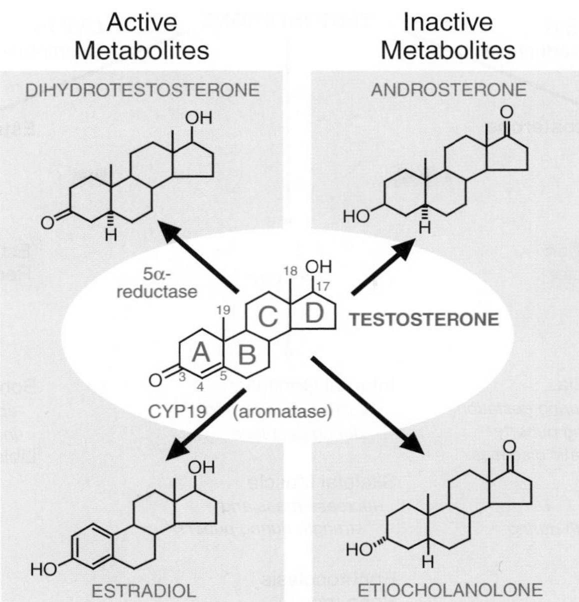

Figure 41–3 *Metabolism of testosterone to its major active and inactive metabolites.*

AR mutations occur in patients with spinal and bulbar muscular atrophy, known as Kennedy disease. These patients have an expansion of the CAG repeat, which codes for glutamine, at the amino terminus of the molecule. The result is very mild androgen resistance, manifest principally by gynecomastia, and progressively severe motor neuron atrophy. The mechanism by which the neuronal atrophy occurs is unknown. Other mutations in AR may explain why metastatic prostate cancer often regresses initially in response to androgen deprivation treatment, but then becomes unresponsive to continued deprivation. AR continues to be expressed in androgen-independent prostate cancer, and its signaling remains active. The ligand-independent signaling may result from mutations in the AR gene or changes in AR coregulatory proteins. In some patients resistant to standard androgen deprivation therapy, the tumor responds to further depletion of androgens by inhibitors of adrenal androgen synthesis, such as abiraterone.

EFFECTS THAT OCCUR VIA THE ESTROGEN RECEPTOR. Certain effects of testosterone are mediated by its conversion to estradiol, catalyzed by CYP19.

In the rare males deficient in CYP19 or the estrogen receptor, the epiphyses do not fuse and long-bone growth continues indefinitely; moreover, such patients are osteoporotic. Estradiol corrects the bone abnormalities in patients with aromatase deficiency but not in those with an estrogen-receptor defect. Because men have larger bones than women, and bone expresses the AR, testosterone also may have an effect on bone via the AR. Administration of estradiol to a male with CYP19 deficiency can increase libido, suggesting that the effect of testosterone on male libido may be mediated by conversion to estradiol.

EFFECTS OF ANDROGENS AT DIFFERENT STAGES OF LIFE

In Utero. When the fetal testes, stimulated by hCG, begin to secrete testosterone at about the eighth week of gestation, the high local concentration of testosterone around the testes stimulates the nearby Wolffian ducts to differentiate into the male internal genitalia. In the anlage of the external genitalia, testosterone is converted to dihydrotestosterone, which causes the development of the male external genitalia. The increase in testosterone at the end of gestation may result in further phallic growth.

Infancy. The consequences of the increase in testosterone secretion by the testes during the first few months of life are not yet known.

Puberty. Puberty in the male begins at a mean age of 12 years with an increase in the secretion of FSH and LH from the gonadotropes, stimulated by increased secretion of GnRH from the hypothalamus. The

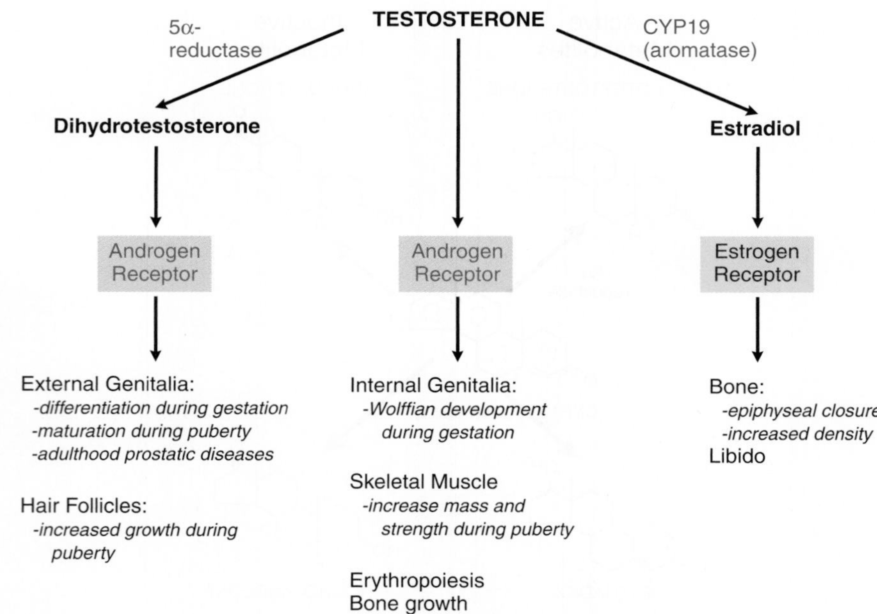

Figure 41–4 *Direct effects of testosterone and effects mediated indirectly via dihydrotestosterone or estradiol.*

increased secretion of FSH and LH stimulates the testes. The increase in testosterone production by Leydig cells and the effect of FSH on the Sertoli cells stimulate the development of the seminiferous tubules, which eventually produce mature sperm. Increased secretion of testosterone into the systemic circulation affects many tissues simultaneously, and the changes in most of them occur gradually during the course of several years. The phallus enlarges in length and width, the scrotum becomes rugated, and the prostate begins secreting the fluid it contributes to the semen. The skin becomes coarser and oilier due to increased sebum production, which contributes to the development of acne. Sexual hair begins to grow, initially pubic and axillary hair, then hair on the lower legs, and finally other body hair and facial hair. Muscle mass and strength, especially of the shoulder girdle, increase, and subcutaneous fat decreases. Epiphyseal bone growth accelerates, resulting in the pubertal growth spurt, but epiphyseal maturation leads eventually to a slowing and then cessation of growth. Bone also becomes thicker. Erythropoiesis increases, resulting in higher hematocrit and hemoglobin concentrations in men than boys or women. The larynx thickens, resulting in a lower voice. Libido develops. Other changes may result from the increase in testosterone during puberty. Men tend to have a better sense of spatial relations than do women and to exhibit behavior that differs in some ways from that of women, including being more aggressive.

Adulthood. The serum testosterone concentration and the characteristics of the adult man are maintained largely during early adulthood and midlife. One change during this time is the gradual development of male pattern baldness, beginning with recession of hair at the temples and/or at the vertex. Two other conditions are of great medical significance. One is benign *prostatic hyperplasia*, which occurs to a variable degree in almost all men, sometimes obstructing urine outflow by compressing the urethra as it passes through the prostate. This development is mediated by the conversion of testosterone to dihydrotestosterone by 5α-reductase II within prostatic cells. The other change is the development of *prostate cancer*. Although no direct evidence suggests that testosterone causes the disease, prostate cancer depends on androgen stimulation. This dependency is the basis of treating metastatic prostate cancer by lowering the serum testosterone concentration or by blocking its action at the receptor.

Senescence. As men age, the serum testosterone concentration gradually declines (*see* Figure 41–2), and the SHBG concentration gradually increases, so that by age 80, the total testosterone concentration is ~80% and the free testosterone is ~40% of those at age 20. This fall in serum testosterone could contribute to several other changes that occur with increasing age in men, including decreases in energy, libido, muscle mass and strength, and bone mineral density. Androgen deprivation also leads to insulin resistance, truncal obesity, and abnormal serum lipids, as observed in patients with metastatic prostate cancer receiving this treatment (*see* also Chapter 63).

CONSEQUENCES OF ANDROGEN DEFICIENCY

The consequences of androgen deficiency depend on the stage of life during which the deficiency first occurs and on the degree of the deficiency.

DURING FETAL DEVELOPMENT. Testosterone deficiency in a male fetus during the first trimester in utero causes incomplete sexual differentiation. Complete deficiency of testosterone secretion results in entirely female external genitalia. Testosterone deficiency at this stage of development also leads to failure of the Wolffian ducts to differentiate into the male internal genitalia, but the Müllerian ducts do not differentiate into the female internal genitalia as long as testes are present and secrete Müllerian inhibitory substance. Similar changes occur if testosterone is secreted normally but its action is diminished because of an abnormality of the AR or of the 5α-reductase. Abnormalities of the AR can have quite varied effects. The most severe form results in complete absence of androgen action and a female phenotype; moderately severe forms result in partial virilization of the external genitalia; and the mildest forms permit normal virilization in utero and result only in impaired spermatogenesis in adulthood. Abnormal 5α-reductase results in incomplete virilization of the external genitalia in utero but normal development of the male internal genitalia, which requires only testosterone. Testosterone deficiency during the third trimester impairs phallus growth. The result, microphallus, is a common occurrence in boys later discovered to be unable to secrete LH due to abnormalities of GnRH synthesis. In addition, with testosterone deficiency, the testes fail to descend into the scrotum; this condition, cryptorchidism, occurs commonly in boys whose LH secretion is subnormal (*see* Chapter 38).

BEFORE COMPLETION OF PUBERTY. When a boy can secrete testosterone normally in utero but loses the ability to do so before the anticipated age of puberty, the result is failure to complete puberty. All of the pubertal changes previously described, including those of the external genitalia, sexual hair, muscle mass, voice, and behavior, are impaired to a degree proportionate to the abnormality of testosterone secretion. In addition, if growth hormone secretion is normal when testosterone secretion is subnormal during the years of expected puberty, the long bones continue to lengthen because the epiphyses do not close. The result is longer arms and legs relative to the trunk. Another consequence of subnormal testosterone secretion during the age of expected puberty is enlargement of glandular breast tissue, called *gynecomastia*.

AFTER COMPLETION OF PUBERTY. When testosterone secretion becomes impaired after puberty (e.g., castration or anti-androgen treatment), regression of the pubertal effects of testosterone depends on both the degree and the duration of testosterone deficiency. When the degree of testosterone deficiency is substantial, libido and energy decrease within a week or 2, but other testosterone-dependent characteristics decline more slowly. A clinically detectable decrease in muscle mass in an individual does not occur for several years. A pronounced decrease in hematocrit and hemoglobin will occur within several months. A decrease in bone mineral density probably can be detected by dual energy absorptiometry within 2 years. A loss of sexual hair takes many years.

IN WOMEN. Loss of androgen secretion in women results in a decrease in sexual hair, but not for many years. The loss of androgens (especially with the severe loss of ovarian and adrenal androgens that occurs in panhypopituitarism) may result in the loss of effects associated with libido, energy, muscle mass and strength, and bone mineral density.

THERAPEUTIC ANDROGEN PREPARATIONS

Ingestion of testosterone is not an effective means of replacing testosterone deficiency due to the rapid hepatic catabolism. Most pharmaceutical preparations of androgens, therefore, are designed to bypass hepatic catabolism of testosterone.

TESTOSTERONE ESTERS. Esterifying a fatty acid to the 17α-hydroxyl group of testosterone creates a compound that is even more lipophilic than testosterone itself. When an ester, such as testosterone enanthate (heptanoate) or cypionate (cyclopentylpropionate) (Table 41–1), is dissolved in oil and administered intramuscularly every 2-4 weeks to hypogonadal men, the ester hydrolyzes in vivo and results in serum testosterone concentrations that range from higher than normal in the first few days after the injection to low normal just before the next injection (Figure 41–5). Attempts to decrease the frequency of injections by increasing the amount of each injection result in wider fluctuations and poorer therapeutic outcomes. The undecanoate ester of testosterone, when dissolved in oil and ingested orally, is absorbed into the lymphatic circulation, thus bypassing initial hepatic catabolism. *Testosterone undecanoate* in oil also can be injected and produces stable serum testosterone concentrations for 2 months. The undecanoate ester of testosterone is not currently marketed in the U.S.

ALKYLATED ANDROGENS. Several decades ago, chemists found that adding an alkyl group to the 17α position of testosterone retards its hepatic catabolism. Consequently, 17α-alkylated androgens are androgenic when administered orally; however, they are less androgenic than testosterone and cause hepatotoxicity, whereas native testosterone does not. Some 17α-alkylated androgens show greater anabolic effects than androgenic effects compared to native testosterone in laboratory tests in rats; however, these "anabolic"

Table 41–1

Androgens Available for Therapeutic Use

TESTOSTERONE
Testosterone Esters
Testosterone enanthate/undecanoate/cypionate
17α-Alkylated Androgens
Methyltestosterone, oxandrolone, stanozolol
Fluoxymesterone, danazol
Other
7α-Methyl-19-nortestosterone, tetrahydrogestrinone

steroids, so favored by athletes to illicitly improve performance, have not been convincingly demonstrated to have such a differential effect in human beings. Citing potentially serious health risks, the FDA has recommended against the use of body-building products that are marketed as containing steroids or steroid-like substances.

TRANSDERMAL DELIVERY SYSTEMS. Chemicals called excipients are used to facilitate the absorption of native testosterone across the skin in a controlled fashion. These transdermal preparations provide more stable serum testosterone concentrations than do injections of testosterone esters. The first such preparations were patches, 1 of which (ANDRODERM) is still available. Newer preparations include gels (ANDROGEL, TESTIM, Bio-T-Gel) and a buccal tablet (STRIANT) (*see* Figure 41–5).

SELECTIVE ANDROGEN RECEPTOR MODULATORS. Selective estrogen receptor modulators (SERMs) have been developed (*see* Chapter 40). Are selective AR modulators possible that exhibit desirable effects of testosterone in some tissues, such as muscle and bone, without the undesirable effects in other tissues, such as prostate? Nonsteroidal molecules with these properties have been developed and are being tested in humans.

THERAPEUTIC USES OF ANDROGENS

MALE HYPOGONADISM. The best established indication for administration of androgens is testosterone deficiency in men. Any of the testosterone preparations or testosterone esters described can be used to treat testosterone deficiency.

Monitoring for Efficacy. The goal of administering testosterone to a hypogonadal man is to mimic as closely as possible the normal serum concentration (*see* Figure 41–5). Therefore, measuring the serum testosterone concentration during treatment is the most important aspect of monitoring testosterone treatment for efficacy. When the enanthate or cypionate ester of testosterone is administered once every 2 weeks, the serum testosterone concentration measured midway between doses should be normal; if not, the dosage schedule should be adjusted accordingly. If testosterone deficiency results from testicular disease, as indicated by an elevated serum LH concentration, adequacy of testosterone treatment also can be judged indirectly by the normalization of LH within 2 months of treatment initiation. Normalization of the serum testosterone concentration induces normal virilization in prepubertal boys and restores virilization in adult men who became hypogonadal as adults. Within a few months, and often sooner, libido, energy, and hematocrit return to normal. Within 6 months, muscle mass increases and fat mass decreases. Bone density, however, continues to increase for 2 years.

Monitoring for Deleterious Effects. Testosterone administered by itself as a the transdermal preparation has no "side effects" (i.e., no effects that endogenously secreted testosterone does not have), as long as the dose is not excessive. Modified testosterone compounds, such as the 17α-alkylated androgens, do have undesirable effects even when dosages are targeted at physiological replacement. Some of these undesirable effects occur shortly after testosterone administration is initiated, whereas others usually do not occur until administration has been continued for many years. Raising the serum testosterone concentration can result in undesirable effects similar to those that occur during puberty, including acne, gynecomastia, and more aggressive sexual behavior. Physiological amounts of testosterone do not appear to affect serum lipids or apolipoproteins. Replacement of physiological levels of testosterone occasionally may have undesirable effects in the presence of concomitant illnesses. If the testosterone dose is excessive, erythrocytosis and, uncommonly, salt and water retention and peripheral edema occur even in men who have no predisposition to these conditions. When a man is >40 years of age, he is subject to certain testosterone-dependent diseases, including benign prostatic hyperplasia and prostate cancer. The principal adverse effects of the 17α-alkylated androgens are hepatic, including cholestasis and, uncommonly, peliosis hepatis, blood-filled hepatic cysts. Hepatocellular cancer

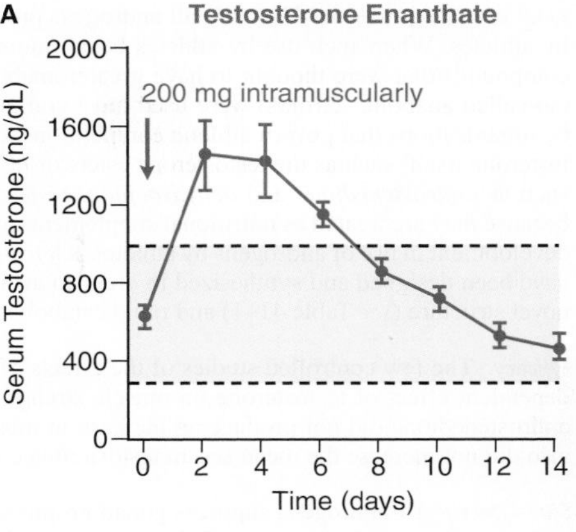

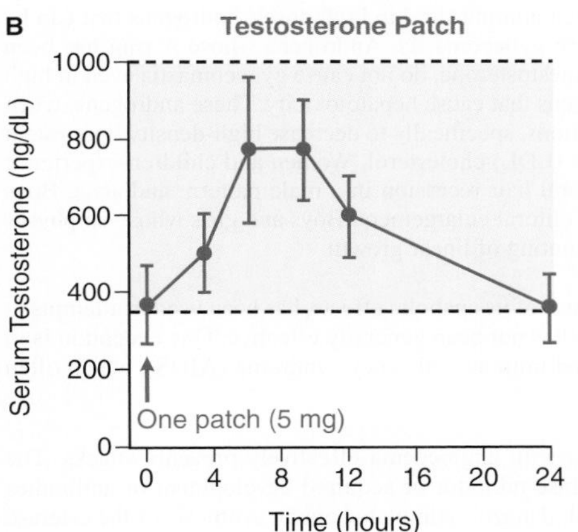

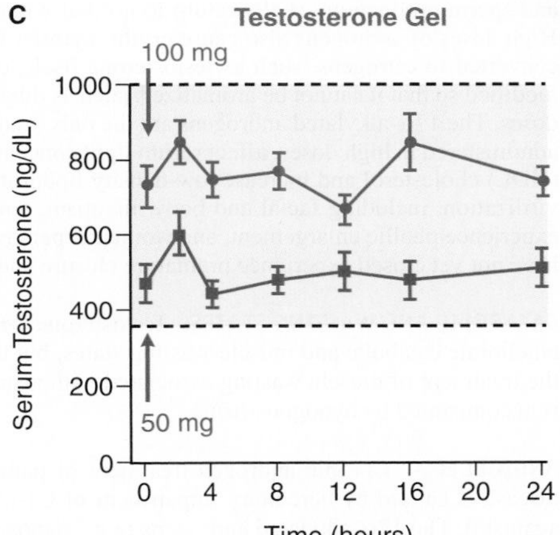

Figure 41–5 *Pharmacokinetic profiles of testosterone preparations during chronic administration to hypogonadal men.* Doses of each were given at time 0. *Shaded areas* indicate range of normal levels. **A.** Data adapted from Snyder PJ, et al. *J Clin Endocrinol Metab*, 1980;51:1535-1539. **B.** Data adapted from Dobs AS, et al. *J Clin Endocrinol Metab*, 1999;84:3469-3478. **C.** Data adapted from Swerdloff RS, et al. *J Clin Endocrinol Metab*, 2000;85:4500-4510.

has been reported rarely. The 17α-alkylated androgens, especially in large amounts, may lower serum high-density lipoprotein cholesterol.

Monitoring at the Anticipated Time of Puberty. Testosterone accelerates epiphyseal maturation, leading initially to a growth spurt but then to epiphyseal closure and permanent cessation of linear growth. Consequently, the height and growth-hormone status of the boy being treated, must be considered. Boys who are short because of growth-hormone deficiency should be treated with growth hormone before their hypogonadism is treated with testosterone.

MALE SENESCENCE. Preliminary evidence suggests that increasing the serum testosterone concentration of men whose serum levels are subnormal for no reason other than their age will increase their bone mineral density and lean mass and decrease their fat mass. It is uncertain, however, if such treatment will worsen benign prostatic hyperplasia or increase the incidence of prostate cancer.

FEMALE HYPOGONADISM. In a study of women with low serum testosterone concentrations due to panhypopituitarism, increasing the testosterone concentration to normal was associated with small increases in bone mineral density, fat-free mass, and sexual function compared to placebo.

ENHANCEMENT OF ATHLETIC PERFORMANCE. Some athletes take drugs, including androgens, to attempt to improve their performance. Citing potentially serious health risks, the FDA has recommended against the use of body-building products that are marketed as containing steroids or steroid-like substances.

Kinds of Androgens Used. Virtually all androgens produced for human or veterinary purposes have been taken by athletes. When such use by athletes began more than 25 years ago, 17α-alkylated androgens and other compounds that were thought to have greater anabolic effects than androgen effects relative to testosterone (so-called anabolic steroids) were used most commonly. Because these compounds can be detected readily by organizations that govern athletic competitions, other agents that increase the serum concentration of testosterone itself, such as the testosterone esters or hCG, have increased in popularity. Testosterone precursors, such as *androstenedione* and *dehydroepiandrosterone* (DHEA), also have increased in popularity recently because they are treated as nutritional supplements and thus are not regulated by athletic organizations. A new development in use of androgens by athletes is *tetrahydrogestrinone* (THG), a potent androgen that appears to have been designed and synthesized in order to avoid detection by antidoping laboratories on the basis of its novel structure (*see* Table 41–1) and rapid catabolism.

Efficacy. The few controlled studies of the effects of pharmacological doses of androgens do suggest a dose-dependent effect of testosterone on muscle strength that acts synergistically with exercise. In another trial, androstenedione did not produce an increase in muscle strength in men compared to placebo; the treatment also did not increase the mean serum testosterone concentration.

Side Effects. All androgens suppress gonadotropin secretion when taken in high doses and thereby suppress endogenous testicular function. This decreases endogenous testosterone and sperm production, resulting in diminished fertility. If administration continues for many years, testicular size may diminish. Testosterone and sperm production usually return to normal within a few months of discontinuation but may take longer. High doses of androgens also cause erythrocytosis. When administered in high doses, androgens that can be converted to estrogens, such as testosterone itself, cause gynecomastia. Androgens whose A ring has been modified so that it cannot be aromatized, such as dihydrotestosterone, do not cause gynecomastia even in high doses. The 17α-alkylated androgens are the only androgens that cause hepatotoxicity. These androgens, when administered in high doses, affect serum lipid concentrations, specifically to decrease high-density lipoprotein (HDL) cholesterol and increase low-density lipoprotein (LDL) cholesterol. Women and children experience virilization, including facial and body hirsutism, temporal hair recession in a male pattern, and acne. Boys experience phallic enlargement, and women experience clitoral enlargement. Boys and girls whose epiphyses have not yet closed experience premature closure and stunting of linear growth.

CATABOLIC AND WASTING STATES. Testosterone, because of its anabolic effects, has been used in attempts to ameliorate catabolic and muscle-wasting states, but this has not been generally effective. One exception is in the treatment of muscle wasting associated with acquired immunodeficiency syndrome (AIDS), which often is accompanied by hypogonadism.

ANGIOEDEMA. Chronic androgen treatment of patients with angioedema effectively prevents attacks. The disease is caused by hereditary impairment of C1-esterase inhibitor or acquired development of antibodies against it. The 17α-alkylated androgens (e.g., stanozolol, danazol) stimulate hepatic synthesis of the esterase inhibitor. Alternatively, concentrated C1-esterase inhibitor derived from human plasma (CINRYZE) may be used for protection in patients with hereditary angioedema.

BLOOD DYSCRASIAS. Androgens, such as danazol, still are used occasionally as adjunctive treatment for hemolytic anemia and idiopathic thrombocytopenic purpura that are refractory to first-line agents.

ANTI-ANDROGENS

INHIBITORS OF TESTOSTERONE SECRETION. Analogs of GnRH effectively inhibit testosterone secretion by inhibiting LH secretion. GnRH analogs, given repeatedly, downregulate the GnRH receptor and are available for treatment of prostate cancer.

Some antifungal drugs of the imidazole family, such as *ketoconazole* (*see* Chapter 57), inhibit CYPs and thereby block the synthesis of steroid hormones, including testosterone and cortisol. Because they may induce adrenal insufficiency and are associated with hepatotoxicity, these drugs generally are not used to inhibit androgen synthesis but sometimes are employed in cases of glucocorticoid excess (*see* Chapter 42).

INHIBITORS OF ANDROGEN ACTION. These drugs inhibit the binding of androgens to the AR or inhibit 5α-reductase.

ANDROGEN RECEPTOR ANTAGONISTS.

Flutamide, Bicalutamide, Nilutamide, and Enzalutamide. These relatively potent AR antagonists have limited efficacy when used alone because the increased LH secretion stimulates higher serum testosterone concentrations. They are used primarily in conjunction with a GnRH analog in the treatment of metastatic prostate cancer (*see* Chapter 63). Flutamide also has been used to treat hirsutism in women; however, its association with hepatotoxicity warrants caution against its use for this cosmetic purpose.

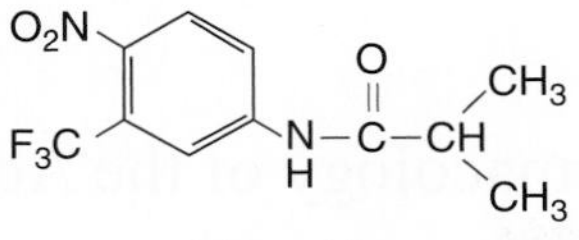

Flutamide

Spironolactone (ALDACTONE; *see* Chapter 25) is an inhibitor of aldosterone that also is a weak inhibitor of the AR and a weak inhibitor of testosterone synthesis. When the agent is used to treat fluid retention or hypertension in men, gynecomastia is a common side effect. In part because of this adverse effect, the selective mineralocorticoid receptor antagonist eplerenone (INSPRA) was developed. Spironolactone can be used in women to treat hirsutism. ***Cyproterone acetate*** is a progestin and a weak anti-androgen by virtue of binding to the AR. It is effective in reducing hirsutism but is not approved for use in the U.S.

5α-REDUCTASE INHIBITORS. Finasteride (PROSCAR) and dutasteride (AVODART) are antagonists of 5α-reductase. They block the conversion of testosterone to dihydrotestosterone, especially in the male external genitalia. These drugs are approved to treat benign prostatic hyperplasia.

Impotence is a documented, albeit infrequent, side effect of this use. Gynecomastia is a rare side effect. Finasteride also is approved for use in the treatment of male pattern baldness under the trade name PROPECIA, and is effective in the treatment of hirsutism.

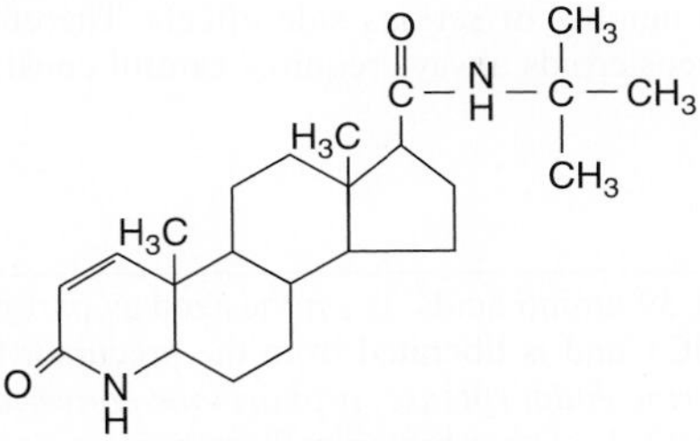

Finasteride

For a complete Bibliographical Listing see Goodman & Gilman's ***The Pharmacological Basis of Therapeutics***, 12th ed., or Goodman & Gilman Online at www.AccessMedicine.com.

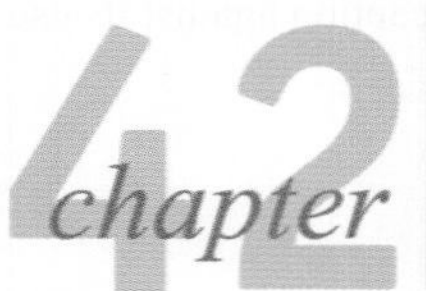

Pharmacology of the Adrenal Cortex

The major physiological and pharmacological effects of *adrenocorticotropic hormone* (ACTH, corticotropin) result from its action to increase the circulating levels of *adrenocortical steroids*. Synthetic derivatives of ACTH are used principally in the diagnostic assessment of adrenocortical function. Because corticosteroids mimic the therapeutic effects of ACTH, synthetic steroids generally are used therapeutically instead of ACTH.

Corticosteroids and their biologically active synthetic derivatives differ in their metabolic (glucocorticoid) and electrolyte-regulating (mineralocorticoid) activities. These agents are employed at physiological doses for replacement therapy when endogenous production is impaired. Glucocorticoids potently suppress inflammation, and their use in inflammatory and autoimmune diseases makes them among the most frequently prescribed classes of drugs. Because glucocorticoids exert effects on almost every organ system, the clinical use of and withdrawal from corticosteroids are complicated by a number of serious side effects. Therefore, the decision to institute therapy with systemic corticosteroids always requires careful consideration of the relative risks and benefits in each patient.

ACTH

Human ACTH, a peptide of 39 amino acids, is synthesized as part of a larger precursor protein, proopiomelanocortin (POMC), and is liberated from the precursor through proteolytic cleavage at dibasic residues by the *serine endoprotease*, *prohormone convertase 1* (also known as prohormone convertase 3) (Figure 42–1). Other biologically important peptides, including *endorphins, lipotropins, and the melanocyte-stimulating hormones* (MSHs), also are produced by proteolytic processing of the same POMC precursor (*see* Chapter 18).

The actions of ACTH and the other melanocortins liberated from POMC are mediated by their specific interactions with 5 *melanocortin receptor* (MCR) subtypes (MC1R-MC5R) comprising a subfamily of G protein-coupled receptors (GPCRs). The well-known effects of MSH on pigmentation result from interactions with the MC1R on melanocytes. ACTH, which is identical to α-MSH in its first 13 amino acids, exerts its effects on the adrenal cortex through the MC2R. The affinity of ACTH for the MC1R is much lower than for the MC2R; however, under pathological conditions in which ACTH levels are persistently elevated, such as primary adrenal insufficiency, ACTH also can signal through the MC1R and cause hyperpigmentation. β-MSH and possibly other melanocortins, acting via the MC4R and MC3R in the hypothalamus, play a role in regulating appetite and body weight. The role of MC5R is less well defined.

ACTIONS ON THE ADRENAL CORTEX. Acting via MC2R, ACTH stimulates the adrenal cortex to secrete *glucocorticoids*, *mineralocorticoids*, and the androgen precursor *dehydroepiandrosterone* (DHEA). The adrenal cortex histologically and functionally can be separated into 3 zones (Figure 42–2) that produce different steroid products under different regulatory influences:

- The *outer zona glomerulosa* secretes the mineralocorticoid aldosterone.
- The *middle zona fasciculata* secretes the glucocorticoid cortisol.
- The *inner zona reticularis* secretes DHEA and its sulfated derivative DHEAS (plasma concentration 1000× that of DHEA). DHEA sulfatase converts DHEAS to DHEA in the periphery.

Cells of the outer zone have receptors for angiotensin II (AngII) and express *aldosterone synthase* (CYP11B2), an enzyme that catalyzes the terminal reactions in mineralocorticoid biosynthesis. Although ACTH acutely stimulates mineralocorticoid production by the zona glomerulosa, this zone is regulated predominantly by AngII and *extracellular* K^+ (*see* Chapter 25) and does not undergo atrophy in the absence of ongoing stimulation by the pituitary gland. With persistently elevated ACTH, mineralocorticoid levels initially increase and then return to normal (a phenomenon termed *ACTH escape*). Cells of the zona fasciculata have fewer receptors for AngII and express *steroid 17α-hydroxylase* (CYP17) and *11β-hydroxylase* (CYP11B1) enzymes that

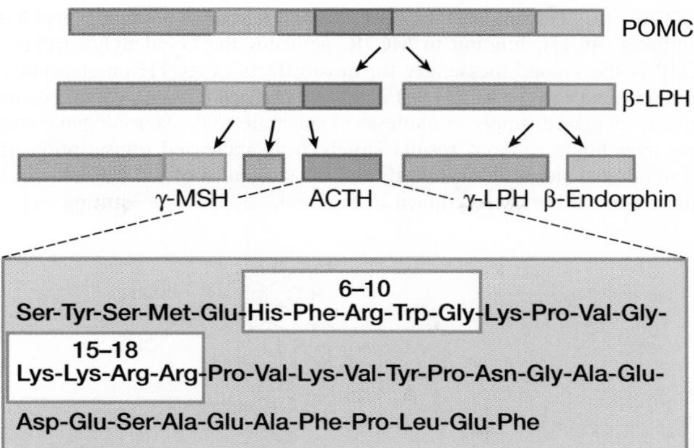

Figure 42–1 *Processing of proopiomelanocortin POMC to ACTH.* Proopiomelanocortin (POMC) is converted to adrenocorticotropic hormone (ACTH) and other peptides in the anterior pituitary. The boxes within the ACTH structure indicate regions important for steroidogenic activity (residues 6-10) and binding to the ACTH receptor (15-18). α-Melanocyte-stimulating hormone also derives from the POMC precursor and contains the first 13 residues of ACTH. LPH, lipotropin; MSH, melanocyte-stimulating hormone.

catalyze the production of glucocorticoids. In the zona reticularis, CYP17 carries out an additional C17-20 lyase reaction that converts C21 corticosteroids to C19 androgen precursors.

In the absence of the anterior pituitary and ACTH stimulation, the inner zones of the cortex atrophy, and the production of glucocorticoids and adrenal androgens is markedly impaired. Persistently elevated levels of ACTH, due either to repeated administration of large doses of ACTH or to excessive endogenous production, induce hypertrophy and hyperplasia of the inner zones of the adrenal cortex, with overproduction of cortisol and adrenal androgens. Adrenal hyperplasia is most marked in congenital disorders of steroidogenesis, in which ACTH levels are continuously elevated as a secondary response to impaired cortisol biosynthesis.

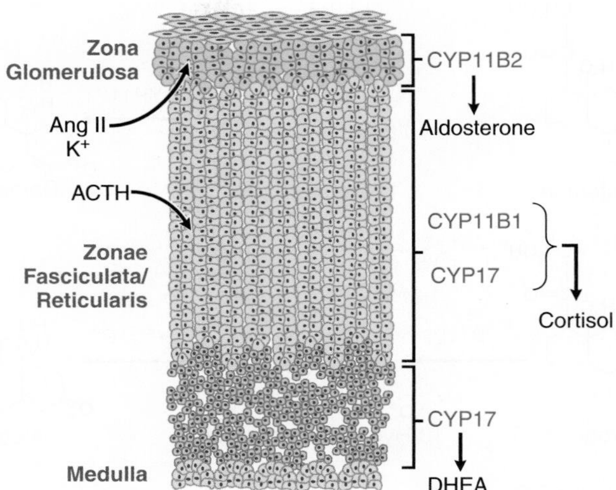

Figure 42–2 *The three anatomically and functionally distinct compartments of the adrenal cortex.* The major functional compartments of the adrenal cortex are shown, along with the steroidogenic enzymes that determine the unique profiles of corticosteroid products. Also shown are the predominant physiological regulators of steroid production: angiotensin II (AngII) and K^+ for the zona glomerulosa and ACTH for the zona fasciculata. The physiological regulator(s) of dehydroepiandrosterone (DHEA) production by the zona reticularis are not known, although ACTH acutely increases DHEA biosynthesis.

MECHANISM OF ACTION. ACTH stimulates the synthesis and release of adrenocortical hormones by increasing de novo biosynthesis. ACTH, binding to MC2R, activates the G_s-adenylyl cyclase-cyclic AMP-PKA pathway. Cyclic AMP is the second messenger for most effects of ACTH on steroidogenesis. Temporally, the response of adrenocortical cells to ACTH has 2 phases. *The acute phase*, which occurs within seconds to minutes, largely reflects increased supply of cholesterol substrate to the steroidogenic enzymes. *The chronic phase*, which occurs over hours to days, results largely from increased transcription of the steroidogenic enzymes. Pathways of adrenal steroid biosynthesis and the structures of the major steroid intermediates and products of the human adrenal cortex are shown in Figure 42–3. The rate-limiting step in steroid hormone

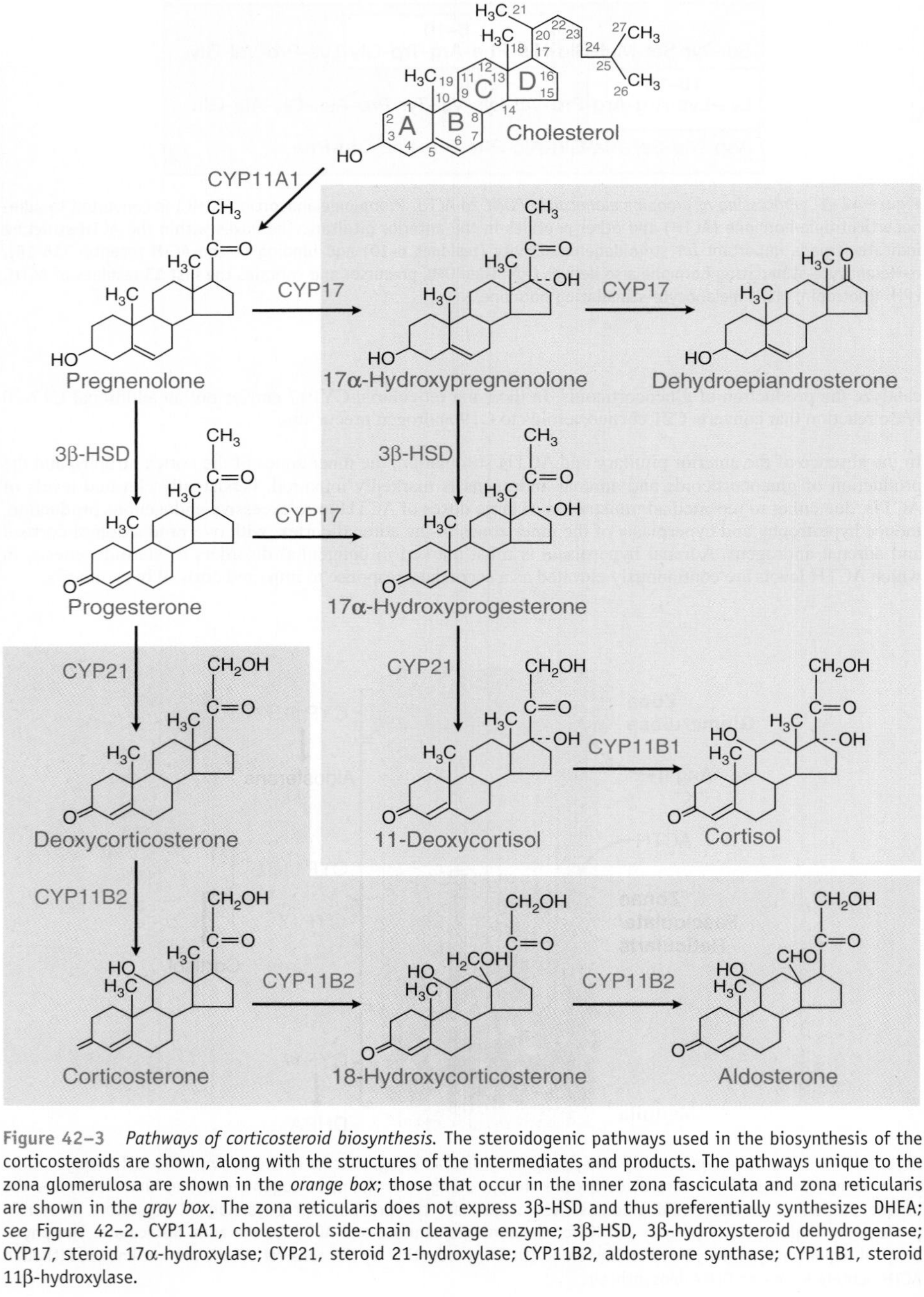

Figure 42–3 *Pathways of corticosteroid biosynthesis.* The steroidogenic pathways used in the biosynthesis of the corticosteroids are shown, along with the structures of the intermediates and products. The pathways unique to the zona glomerulosa are shown in the *orange box*; those that occur in the inner zona fasciculata and zona reticularis are shown in the *gray box*. The zona reticularis does not express 3β-HSD and thus preferentially synthesizes DHEA; *see* Figure 42-2. CYP11A1, cholesterol side-chain cleavage enzyme; 3β-HSD, 3β-hydroxysteroid dehydrogenase; CYP17, steroid 17α-hydroxylase; CYP21, steroid 21-hydroxylase; CYP11B2, aldosterone synthase; CYP11B1, steroid 11β-hydroxylase.

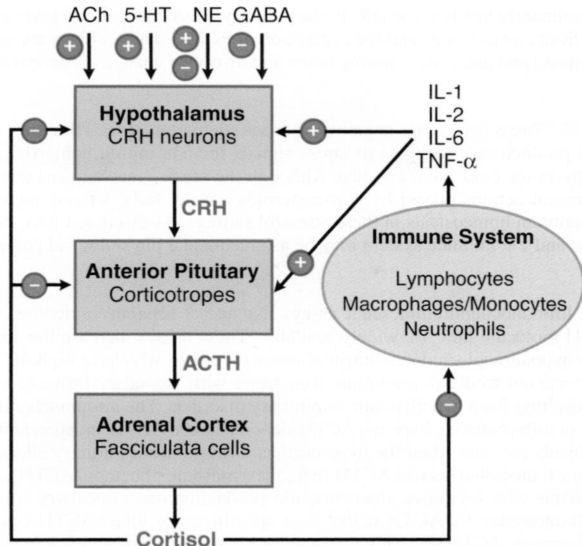

Figure 42–4 *The hypothalamic-pituitary-adrenal (HPA) axis and the immune inflammatory network.* Also shown are inputs from higher neuronal centers that regulate CRH secretion. + indicates a positive regulator, – indicates a negative regulator, + and – indicates a mixed effect, as for NE (norepinephrine). In addition, arginine vasopressin stimulates release of ACTH from corticotropes.

production is the conversion of cholesterol to pregnenolone, a reaction catalyzed by CYP11A1, the cholesterol side-chain cleavage enzyme. Most of the enzymes required for steroid hormone biosynthesis, including CYP11A1, are members of the cytochrome P450 superfamily (*see* Chapter 6).

REGULATION OF ACTH SECRETION

HYPOTHALAMIC-PITUITARY-ADRENAL AXIS. The rate of glucocorticoid secretion is determined by fluctuations in the release of ACTH by the pituitary corticotropes. These corticotropes are regulated by *corticotropin-releasing hormone* (CRH) and *arginine vasopressin* (AVP), peptide hormones released by specialized neurons of the endocrine hypothalamus. This hypothalamic-pituitary-adrenal (HPA) axis forms an integrated system that maintains appropriate levels of glucocorticoids (Figure 42–4). The 3 characteristic modes of regulation of the HPA axis are *diurnal rhythm* in basal steroidogenesis, *negative feedback regulation* by adrenal corticosteroids, and marked *increases in steroidogenesis in response to stress.*

The diurnal rhythm is entrained by higher neuronal centers in response to sleep-wake cycles, such that levels of ACTH peak in the early morning hours, causing the circulating glucocorticoid levels to peak at ~8 A.M. Negative feedback regulation occurs at multiple levels of the HPA axis and is the major mechanism that maintains circulating glucocorticoid levels in the appropriate range. Stress can override the normal negative feedback control mechanisms, leading to marked increases in plasma concentrations of glucocorticoids.

ARGININE VASOPRESSIN. AVP also acts as a secretagogue for corticotropes, significantly potentiating the effects of CRH. AVP is produced in the paraventricular nucleus and secreted into the pituitary plexus from the median eminence. AVP binds to V_{1b} receptor and activates the G_q-PLC-IP_3-Ca^{2+} pathway to enhance the release of ACTH. In contrast to CRH, AVP does not increase ACTH synthesis.

NEGATIVE FEEDBACK OF GLUCOCORTICOIDS. Glucocorticoids inhibit ACTH secretion via direct and indirect actions on CRH neurons to decrease CRH mRNA levels and CRH release and via direct effects on corticotropes. The indirect inhibitory effects on CRH neurons appear to be mediated by specific corticosteroid receptors in the hippocampus. At lower cortisol levels, the mineralocorticoid receptor (MR), which has a higher affinity for glucocorticoids than classical glucocorticoid receptors (GRs), is the major receptor species occupied. As glucocorticoid concentrations rise and saturate the MR, the GR becomes increasingly occupied. Both the MR and GR apparently control the basal activity of the HPA axis, whereas feedback inhibition by glucocorticoids predominantly involves the GR. In the pituitary, glucocorticoids act through the GR to inhibit the release of ACTH from corticotropes and the expression of POMC. These effects are both rapid (occurring within seconds to minutes) and delayed (requiring hours and involving changes in gene transcription mediated through the GR).

THE STRESS RESPONSE. Stress overcomes negative feedback regulation of the HPA axis, leading to a marked rise in corticosteroid production. Examples of stress signals include injury, hemorrhage, severe infection, major surgery, hypoglycemia, cold, pain, and fear. Although the precise mechanisms that underlie this stress response and the essential actions played by corticosteroids are not fully defined, increased corticosteroid secretion is vital to maintain homeostasis in these stressful settings. As discussed later, complex interactions between the HPA axis and the immune system may be a fundamental physiological component of this stress response.

ASSAYS FOR ACTH. Immunochemiluminescent assays that use 2 separate antibodies directed at distinct epitopes on the ACTH molecule now are widely available. These assays increase the ability to differentiate patients with primary hypoadrenalism due to intrinsic adrenal disease, who have high ACTH levels due to the loss of normal glucocorticoid feedback inhibition, from those with secondary forms of hypoadrenalism, due to low ACTH levels resulting from hypothalamic or pituitary disorders. The immunochemiluminescent ACTH assays also are useful in differentiating between ACTH-dependent and ACTH-independent forms of hypercorticism: High ACTH levels are seen when the hypercorticism results from pituitary adenomas (e.g., Cushing disease) or nonpituitary tumors that secrete ACTH (e.g., the syndrome of ectopic ACTH), whereas low ACTH levels are seen in patients with excessive glucocorticoid production due to primary adrenal disorders. One problem with the immunoassays for ACTH is that their specificity for intact ACTH can lead to falsely low values in patients with ectopic ACTH secretion; these tumors can secrete aberrantly processed forms of ACTH that have biological activity but do not react in the antibody assays.

THERAPEUTIC USES AND DIAGNOSTIC APPLICATIONS OF ACTH. ACTH has limited utility therapeutically. All proven therapeutic effects of ACTH can be achieved with appropriate doses of corticosteroids with a lower risk of side effects. Moreover, therapy with ACTH is less predictable and less convenient than therapy with corticosteroids. ACTH stimulates mineralocorticoid and adrenal androgen secretion and may therefore cause acute retention of salt and water, as well as virilization. Cosyntropin (CORTROSYN, SYNACTHEN), a synthetic peptide that corresponds to residues 1-24 of human ACTH, is used testing the integrity of the HPA axis. At the considerably supraphysiological dose of 250 μg, cosyntropin maximally stimulates adrenocortical steroidogenesis. An increase in the circulating cortisol to a level greater than 18-20 μg/dL indicates a normal response.

CRH Stimulation Test. Ovine CRH (corticorelin [ACTHREL]) and human CRH are available for diagnostic testing of the HPA axis, with the former used in the U.S. and the latter preferred in Europe. In patients with documented ACTH-dependent hypercorticism, CRH testing may help differentiate between a pituitary source (i.e., Cushing disease) and an ectopic source of ACTH.

ABSORPTION AND FATE TOXICITY. ACTH is readily absorbed from parenteral sites. The hormone rapidly disappears from the circulation after intravenous administration; in humans, the $t_{1/2}$ in plasma is ~15 min, primarily due to rapid enzymatic hydrolysis. Aside from rare hypersensitivity reactions, the toxicity of ACTH is primarily attributable to the increased secretion of corticosteroids. Cosyntropin generally is less antigenic than native ACTH.

ADRENOCORTICAL STEROIDS

The adrenal cortex synthesizes 2 classes of steroids: the *corticosteroids* (glucocorticoids and mineralocorticoids; *see* Figure 42–3), which have 21 carbon atoms, and the *androgens*, which have 19 carbons (*see* Figures 41–1 and 41–3). The actions of corticosteroids historically were described as *glucocorticoid* (reflecting their carbohydrate metabolism–regulating activity) and *mineralocorticoid* (reflecting their electrolyte balance–regulating activity). In humans, *cortisol* (*hydrocortisone*) is the main glucocorticoid and aldosterone is the main mineralocorticoid (Table 42–1).

Although the adrenal cortex is an important source of androgen precursors in women, patients with adrenal insufficiency can be restored to normal life expectancy by replacement therapy with glucocorticoids and mineralocorticoids. Adrenal androgens are not essential for survival. The levels of DHEA and DHEA-S peak in the third decade of life and decline progressively thereafter. Moreover, patients with a number of chronic diseases have very low DHEA levels, leading some to propose that DHEA treatment might at least partly alleviate the loss of libido, the decline in cognitive function, the decreased sense of well-being, and other adverse physiological consequences of aging. However, studies on the benefits of addition of DHEA to the standard replacement regimen in women with adrenal insufficiency have been inconclusive.

Table 42–1

Normal Daily Production Rates and Circulating Levels of the Predominant Corticosteroids

	CORTISOL	ALDOSTERONE
Rate of secretion under optimal conditions	10 mg/day	0.125 mg/day
Concentration in peripheral plasma:		
8 A.M.	16 μg/100 mL	0.01 μg /100 mL
4 A.M.	4 μg/100 mL	0.01 μg/100 mL

PHYSIOLOGICAL FUNCTIONS AND PHARMACOLOGICAL EFFECTS

PHYSIOLOGICAL ACTIONS. Corticosteroids have numerous effects, which include alterations in carbohydrate, protein, and lipid metabolism; maintenance of fluid and electrolyte balance; and preservation of normal function of the cardiovascular system, the immune system, the kidney, skeletal muscle, the endocrine system, and the nervous system. In addition, corticosteroids endow the organism with the capacity to resist stressful and noxious stimuli and environmental changes. In the absence of the adrenal cortex, survival is made possible only by maintaining an optimal environment, including adequate and regular feeding, ingestion of relatively large amounts of NaCl, and maintenance of an appropriate environmental temperature; stresses such as infection, trauma, and extremes in temperature in this setting can be life threatening.

The actions of corticosteroids are related to those of other hormones. For example, in the absence of lipolytic hormones, cortisol has virtually no effect on the rate of lipolysis by adipocytes. Conversely, in the absence of glucocorticoids, EPI and NE have only minor effects on lipolysis. Administration of a small dose of glucocorticoid, however, markedly potentiates the lipolytic action of these catecholamines. Those effects of corticosteroids that involve concerted actions with other hormonal regulators are termed *permissive* and most likely reflect steroid-induced changes in protein synthesis that, in turn, modify tissue responsiveness to other hormones.

Corticosteroids are termed *mineralocorticoids* and *glucocorticoids*, according to their relative potencies in Na^+ retention, effects on carbohydrate metabolism (i.e., hepatic deposition of glycogen and gluconeogenesis), and anti-inflammatory effects. In general, potencies of steroids as judged by their ability to sustain life in adrenalectomized animals closely parallel those determined for Na^+ retention, whereas potencies based on effects on glucose metabolism closely parallel those for anti-inflammatory effects. The effects on Na^+ retention and the carbohydrate/anti-inflammatory actions are not closely related and reflect selective actions at distinct receptors. As noted below (see structure-activity relationships and Table 42–3), some steroid derivatives provide relative selectivity for effects on Na^+ retention or anti-inflammatory effects.

GENERAL MECHANISMS FOR CORTICOSTEROID EFFECTS. Corticosteroids bind to specific receptor proteins in target tissues to regulate the expression of corticosteroid-responsive genes, thereby changing the levels and array of proteins synthesized by the various target tissues (Figure 38–5). Most effects of corticosteroids are not immediate but become apparent after several hours; clinically, one generally sees a delay before beneficial effects of corticosteroid therapy become manifest. Although corticosteroids predominantly act by increasing gene transcription, there are examples in which glucocorticoids decrease gene transcription. In addition, corticosteroids may exert some of their immediate effects by nongenomic mechanisms.

Glucocorticoid Receptors (GRs). The receptors for corticosteroids are members of the nuclear receptor family of transcription factors. The GR resides predominantly in the cytoplasm in an inactive form complexed with other proteins. Steroid binding results in receptor activation and translocation to the nucleus (*see* Figure 38–5). Several GR isoforms result from alternative RNA splicing. Of these, GRα is the prototypical glucocorticoid-responsive isoform. A second major GR isoform, GRβ, is a truncated dominant negative variant that lacks 35 amino acids at the C-terminus and is unable to bind glucocorticoids or activate gene expression. Polymorphisms have been identified in the human GR that are associated with differences in GR function and have been linked to glucocorticoid insensitivity.

Regulation of Gene Expression by Glucocorticoids. After ligand binding, the GR dissociates from its associated proteins and translocates to the nucleus. There, it interacts with specific DNA sequences called *glucocorticoid responsive elements* (GREs), which provide specificity to the induction of gene transcription by glucocorticoids. Genes can be activated or inhibited by GR-GRE interactions. The mechanisms by which GR activates transcription are complex and not completely understood, but they involve the interaction of the GR with transcriptional coactivators and with proteins that make up the basal transcription apparatus. In a case of transcriptional inhibition by GR, GR inhibits transcription of POMC by a direct interaction with a GRE in the *POMC* promoter, thereby contributing to the negative feedback regulation of the HPA axis. Other genes negatively regulated by glucocorticoids include genes for cyclooxygenase-2 (COX-2), inducible NO synthase (NOS2), and inflammatory cytokines. Some inhibitory effects of glucocorticoids such as downregulation of expression of genes encoding a number of cytokines, collagenase, and stromelysin, have been linked to protein–protein interactions between the GR and other transcription factors (e.g., NF-κB and AP-1) rather than to negative effects of the GR at specific GREs. Such protein–protein interactions and their consequent negative effects on gene expression appear to contribute significantly to the anti-inflammatory and immunosuppressive effects of the glucocorticoids.

Regulation of Gene Expression by Mineralocorticoids. Like the GR, the *mineralocorticoid receptor* (MR) also is a ligand-activated transcription factor and binds to a very similar hormone-responsive element. The MR also associates with HSP90 and activates the transcription of discrete sets of genes within target tissues. The selective actions of GR and MR result from differences in their ability to inhibit AP-1–mediated gene activation and differential interactions with other transcription factors. In addition, the MR has restricted expression: It is expressed in epithelial tissues involved in electrolyte transport (i.e., the kidney, colon, salivary glands, and sweat glands) and in nonepithelial tissues (e.g., hippocampus, heart, vasculature and adipose tissue).

Aldosterone exerts its effects on Na^+ and K^+ homeostasis primarily via its actions on the principal cells of the distal renal tubules and collecting ducts, whereas the effects on H^+ secretion largely are exerted in the intercalated cells. The binding of aldosterone to the MR in the kidney initiates a sequence of events that includes the rapid induction of *serum-* and *glucocorticoid-regulated kinase*, which in turn phosphorylates and activates amiloride-sensitive epithelial Na^+ channels in the apical membrane. Thereafter, increased Na^+ influx stimulates the Na^+, K^+-ATPase in the basolateral membrane. In addition to these rapid genomic actions, aldosterone also increases the synthesis of the individual components of these membrane proteins as part of a more delayed effect.

Receptor-Independent Mechanism for Corticosteroid Specificity. Aldosterone (a classic mineralocorticoid) and cortisol (generally viewed as predominantly glucocorticoid) bind the MR with equal affinity. The apparent specificity of the MR for aldosterone is maintained in the face of much higher circulating levels of glucocorticoids by the type 2 isozyme of *11β-hydroxysteroid dehydrogenase* (11βHSD2). This enzyme metabolizes glucocorticoids such as cortisol to receptor-inactive 11-keto derivatives such as cortisone (Figure 42–5). Because its predominant physiological form is the hemiacetal derivative that is resistant to 11βHSD action, aldosterone escapes this inactivation and maintains mineralocorticoid activity.

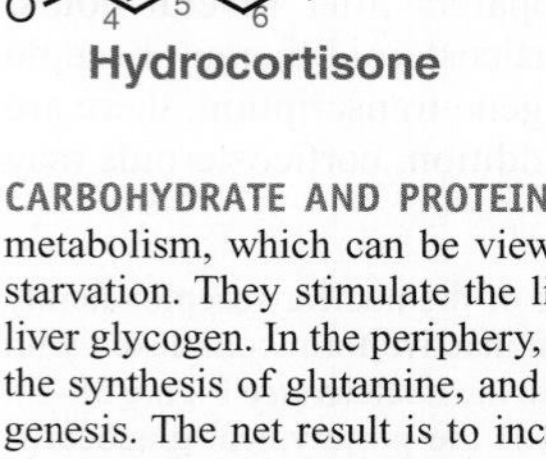

Hydrocortisone

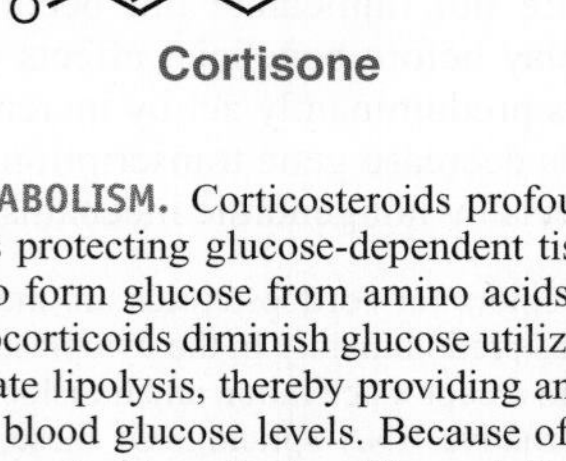

Cortisone

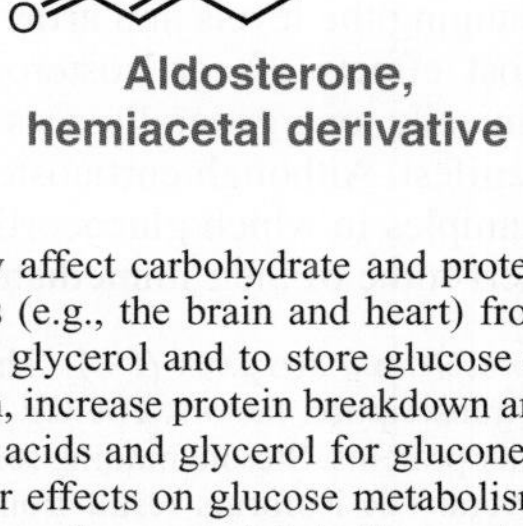

Aldosterone, hemiacetal derivative

CARBOHYDRATE AND PROTEIN METABOLISM. Corticosteroids profoundly affect carbohydrate and protein metabolism, which can be viewed as protecting glucose-dependent tissues (e.g., the brain and heart) from starvation. They stimulate the liver to form glucose from amino acids and glycerol and to store glucose as liver glycogen. In the periphery, glucocorticoids diminish glucose utilization, increase protein breakdown and the synthesis of glutamine, and activate lipolysis, thereby providing amino acids and glycerol for gluconeogenesis. The net result is to increase blood glucose levels. Because of their effects on glucose metabolism, glucocorticoids can worsen glycemic control in patients with overt diabetes and can precipitate the onset of hyperglycemia in susceptible patients.

LIPID METABOLISM. Two effects of corticosteroids on lipid metabolism are firmly established. The first is the dramatic redistribution of body fat that occurs in hypercorticism, such as Cushing syndrome. In this setting, there is increased fat in the back of the neck ("buffalo hump"), face ("moon facies"), and supraclavicular area, coupled with a loss of fat in the extremities. The other is the permissive facilitation of the lipolytic effect of other agents, such as growth hormone and β adrenergic receptor agonists, resulting in an increase in free fatty acids after glucocorticoid administration.

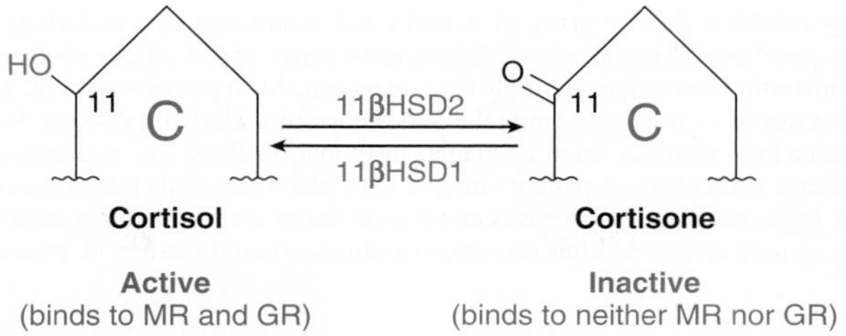

Figure 42–5 *11β-hydroxysteroid dehydrogenase confers specificity of corticosteroid action.* Type 2 11β-hydroxysteroid dehydrogenase (11βHSD2) converts cortisol, which binds to both the mineralocorticoid receptor (MR) and the glucocorticoid receptor (GR), to cortisone, which binds to neither MR nor GR, thereby protecting the MR from the high circulating concentrations of cortisol. This inactivation allows specific responses to aldosterone in sites such as the distal nephron. Aldosterone hemiacetal is resistant to 11βHSD. The type 1 isozyme of 11βHSD (11βHSD1) catalyzes the reverse reaction, which converts inactive cortisone to active cortisol in such tissues as liver and fat. Only ring C of the corticosteroid is depicted; *see* text figures for structures of cortisone and aldosterone hemiacetal.

ELECTROLYTE AND WATER BALANCE. Aldosterone is by far the most potent endogenous corticosteroid with respect to fluid and electrolyte balance. Mineralocorticoids act on the distal tubules and collecting ducts of the kidney to enhance reabsorption of Na^+ from the tubular fluid; they also increase the urinary excretion of K^+ and H^+. These actions on electrolyte transport, in the kidney and in other tissues (e.g., colon, salivary glands, and sweat glands), appear to account for the physiological and pharmacological activities that are characteristic of mineralocorticoids. Thus, the primary features of hyperaldosteronism are positive Na^+ balance with consequent expansion of extracellular fluid volume, normal or slight increases in plasma Na^+ concentration, normal or low plasma K^+, and alkalosis. Mineralocorticoid deficiency, in contrast, leads to Na^+ wasting and contraction of the extracellular fluid volume, hyponatremia, hyperkalemia, and acidosis. Chronically, hyperaldosteronism causes hypertension, whereas aldosterone deficiency can lead to hypotension and vascular collapse.

Glucocorticoids also exert effects on fluid and electrolyte balance, largely due to permissive effects on tubular function and actions that maintain glomerular filtration rate. Glucocorticoids play a permissive role in the renal excretion of free water. In part, the inability of patients with glucocorticoid deficiency to excrete free water results from the increased secretion of AVP, which stimulates water reabsorption in the kidney. In addition to their effects on monovalent cations and water, glucocorticoids also exert multiple effects on Ca^{2+} metabolism. Steroids lower Ca^{2+} uptake from the gut and increase Ca^{2+} excretion by the kidney. These effects collectively lead to decreased total body Ca^{2+} stores.

CARDIOVASCULAR SYSTEM. The most striking effects of corticosteroids on the cardiovascular system result from mineralocorticoid-induced changes in renal Na^+, as is evident in primary aldosteronism. MR activation has direct effects on the heart and vessel walls; aldosterone induces hypertension and interstitial cardiac fibrosis in animal models. The increased cardiac fibrosis appears to result from direct mineralocorticoid actions in the heart rather than from the effect of hypertension because treatment with spironolactone, an MR antagonist, blocks the development of fibrosis without altering blood pressure. The second major action of corticosteroids on the cardiovascular system is to enhance vascular reactivity to other vasoactive substances. Hypoadrenalism is associated with reduced responsiveness to vasoconstrictors such as NE and AngII, perhaps due to decreased expression of adrenergic receptors in the vascular wall. Conversely, hypertension is seen in patients with excessive glucocorticoid secretion, occurring in most patients with Cushing syndrome and in a subset of patients treated with synthetic glucocorticoids (even those lacking any significant mineralocorticoid action).

SKELETAL MUSCLE. Permissive concentrations of corticosteroids are required for the normal function of skeletal muscle, and diminished work capacity is a prominent sign of adrenocortical insufficiency. In patients with Addison disease, weakness and fatigue are frequent symptoms. Excessive amounts of either glucocorticoids or mineralocorticoids also impair muscle function. In primary aldosteronism, muscle weakness results primarily from hypokalemia rather than from direct effects of mineralocorticoids on skeletal muscle. In contrast, glucocorticoid excess over prolonged periods, either secondary to glucocorticoid therapy or endogenous hypercorticism, causes skeletal muscle wasting. This effect, *steroid myopathy*, accounts in part for weakness and fatigue in patients with glucocorticoid excess.

CNS. Corticosteroids exert a number of indirect effects on the CNS, through maintenance of blood pressure, plasma glucose concentrations, and electrolyte concentrations. Increasingly, direct effects of corticosteroids on the CNS have been recognized, including effects on mood, behavior, and brain excitability. Patients with adrenal insufficiency exhibit a diverse array of neurological manifestations, including apathy, depression, and irritability, even psychosis. Appropriate replacement therapy corrects these abnormalities. Conversely, glucocorticoid administration can induce multiple CNS reactions. Most patients respond with mood elevation, which may impart a sense of well-being despite the persistence of underlying disease. Some patients exhibit more pronounced behavioral changes, such as mania, insomnia, restlessness, and increased motor activity. A smaller but significant percentage of patients treated with glucocorticoids become anxious, depressed, or overtly psychotic. A high incidence of neuroses and psychoses is seen in patients with Cushing syndrome. These abnormalities usually disappear after cessation of glucocorticoid therapy or treatment of the Cushing syndrome.

FORMED ELEMENTS OF BLOOD. Glucocorticoids exert minor effects on hemoglobin and erythrocyte content of blood, as evidenced by the frequent occurrence of polycythemia in Cushing syndrome and of normochromic, normocytic anemia in adrenal insufficiency. More profound effects are seen in the setting of autoimmune hemolytic anemia, in which the immunosuppressive effects of glucocorticoids can diminish erythrocytes destruction. Corticosteroids also affect circulating white blood cells. Addison disease is associated with an increased mass of lymphoid tissue and lymphocytosis. In contrast, Cushing syndrome is characterized by lymphocytopenia and decreased mass of lymphoid tissue. The administration of glucocorticoids leads to a decreased number of circulating lymphocytes, eosinophils, monocytes, and basophils. A single dose of hydrocortisone leads to a decline of these circulating cells within 4-6 h; this effect persists for 24 h and results from the redistribution of cells away from the periphery rather than from increased destruction. In contrast, glucocorticoids increase circulating polymorphonuclear leukocytes as a result of increased release from the marrow, diminished rate of removal from the circulation, and decreased adherence to vascular walls. Finally, certain lymphoid malignancies are destroyed by glucocorticoid treatment, an effect that may relate to the capacity of glucocorticoids to activate apoptosis.

ANTI-INFLAMMATORY AND IMMUNOSUPPRESSIVE ACTIONS. In addition to their effects on lymphocyte number, corticosteroids profoundly alter the immune responses of lymphocytes. These effects are an important facet of the anti-inflammatory and immunosuppressive actions of the glucocorticoids. Although the use of glucocorticoids as anti-inflammatory agents does not address the underlying cause of the disease, the suppression of inflammation is of enormous clinical utility and has made these drugs among the most frequently prescribed agents. Similarly, glucocorticoids are of immense valuable in treating diseases that result from undesirable immune reactions. These diseases range from conditions that predominantly result from humoral immunity, such as urticaria (*see* Chapter 65), to those that are mediated by cellular immune mechanisms, such as transplantation rejection (*see* Chapter 35). The immunosuppressive and anti-inflammatory actions of glucocorticoids are inextricably linked, perhaps because they both involve inhibition of leukocyte functions.

Multiple mechanisms are involved in the suppression of inflammation by glucocorticoids. Glucocorticoids inhibit the production by multiple cells of factors that are critical in generating the inflammatory response. As a result, there is decreased release of vasoactive and chemoattractive factors, diminished secretion of lipolytic and proteolytic enzymes, decreased extravasation of leukocytes to areas of injury, and ultimately, decreased fibrosis. Glucocorticoids can also reduce expression of pro-inflammatory cytokines, as well as COX-2 and NOS2. Some of the cell types and mediators that are inhibited by glucocorticoids are summarized in Table 42–2.

ADME

ABSORPTION. Hydrocortisone and numerous congeners, including the synthetic analogs, are orally effective. Certain water-soluble esters of hydrocortisone and its synthetic congeners are administered intravenously to achieve high concentrations of drug rapidly in body fluids. More prolonged effects are obtained by intramuscular injection of suspensions of hydrocortisone, its esters, and congeners. Minor changes in chemical structure may markedly alter the rate of absorption, time of onset of effect, and duration of action. Glucocorticoids also are absorbed systemically from sites of local administration, such as synovial spaces, the conjunctival sac, skin, and respiratory tract. When administration is prolonged, when the site of application is covered with an occlusive dressing, or when large areas of skin are involved, absorption may be sufficient to cause systemic effects, including suppression of the HPA axis.

TRANSPORT, METABOLISM, AND EXCRETION. After absorption, ≥90% of cortisol in plasma is reversibly bound to protein under normal circumstances. Only the fraction of corticosteroid that is unbound is active and can enter cells. Two plasma proteins account for almost all of the steroid-binding capacity: *corticosteroid-binding globulin* (CBG; also called *transcortin*), and *albumin*. CBG is an α-globulin secreted by the liver that has high affinity for steroids (estimated dissociation constant of ~1.3×10^{-9} M) but relatively low total

Table 42–2

Inhibitory Effects of Glucocorticoids on Inflammatory/Immune Responses

CELL TYPE	FACTOR INHIBITED	COMMENTS
Macrophages and monocytes	Arachidonic acid, PGs, and LTs	Mediated by glucocorticoid inhibition of COX-2 and PLA_2.
	Cytokines: IL-l, IL-6, and tumor necrosis factor-α (TNF-α)	Production and release are blocked; cytokines exert multiple effects on inflammation (e.g., ↑ T cells, ↑ fibroblast proliferation).
	Acute phase reactants	Including the 3rd component of complement.
Endothelial cells	ELAM-1 and ICAM-1	Critical for leukocyte localization.
	Acute phase reactants Cytokines (e.g., IL-1) Arachidonic acid derivatives	*Ibid.* for macrophages/monocytes.
Basophils	Histamine, LTC_4	IgE-dependent release ↓ by glucocorticoids.
Fibroblasts	Arachidonic acid metabolites	Same as above for macrophages and monocytes. Glucocorticoids ↓ growth factor-induced DNA synthesis and fibroblast proliferation.
Lymphocytes	Cytokines (IL-1, IL-2, IL-3, IL-6, TNF-α, GM-CSF, interferon-γ)	Same as above for macrophages and monocytes.

ELAM-1, endothelial-leukocyte adhesion molecule-1; ICAM-1, intercellular adhesion molecule-1; LT, leukotriene; PG, prostaglandin.

binding capacity, whereas albumin, also produced by the liver, has a relatively large binding capacity but low affinity (estimated dissociation constant of 1×10^{-3} M). At normal or low concentrations of corticosteroids, most of the hormone is protein bound. At higher steroid concentrations, the capacity of protein binding is exceeded, and a greater fraction of the steroid exists in the free state. CBG has relatively high affinity for cortisol and some of its synthetic congeners and low affinity for aldosterone and glucuronide-conjugated steroid metabolites; thus, greater percentages of these latter steroids are found in the free form. A special state of physiological hypercorticism occurs during pregnancy. The elevated circulating estrogen levels induce CBG production, and CBG and total plasma cortisol increase severalfold. The physiological significance of these changes remains to be established.

Synthetic steroids with an 11-keto group, such as cortisone and prednisone, must be enzymatically reduced to the corresponding 11β-hydroxy derivative before they are biologically active. The type 1 isozyme of 11β-hydroxysteroid dehydrogenase (11βHSD1) catalyzes this reduction, predominantly in the liver, but also in specialized sites such as adipocytes, bone, eye, and skin. In settings in which this enzymatic activity is impaired, it is prudent to use steroids that do not require enzymatic activation (e.g., hydrocortisone or prednisolone rather than cortisone or prednisone). Such settings include severe hepatic failure and patients with the rare condition of cortisone reductase deficiency.

STRUCTURE–ACTIVITY RELATIONSHIPS. Chemical modifications to the cortisol molecule have generated derivatives with greater separations of glucocorticoid and mineralocorticoid activity (Table 42–3); for a number of synthetic glucocorticoids, the effects on electrolytes are minimal even at the highest doses used. In addition, these modifications have led to derivatives with greater potencies and with longer durations of action. A vast array of steroid preparations is available for oral, parenteral, and topical use. None of these currently available derivatives effectively separates anti-inflammatory effects from effects on carbohydrate, protein, and fat metabolism, or from suppressive effects on the HPA axis.

Estimates of Na^+-retaining and anti-inflammatory potencies of representative steroids are listed in Table 42–3. Some steroids that are classified predominantly as glucocorticoids (e.g., cortisol), also possess modest but significant mineralocorticoid activity and thus may affect fluid and electrolyte handling in the clinical setting. At doses used for replacement therapy in patients with primary adrenal insufficiency, the mineralocorticoid effects of these "glucocorticoids" are insufficient to replace that of aldosterone, and concurrent therapy with a more potent mineralocorticoid generally is needed. In contrast, aldosterone is exceedingly potent with respect to Na^+ retention but has only modest potency for effects on carbohydrate metabolism. At normal rates of

Table 42–3

Relative Potencies and Equivalent Doses of Representative Corticosteroids

COMPOUND	ANTI-INFLAMMATORY POTENCY	Na^+-RETAINING POTENCY	DURATION OF ACTION[a]	EQUIVALENT DOSE (mg)[b]
Cortisol	1	1	S	20
Cortisone	0.8	0.8	S	25
Fludrocortisone	10	125	I	[c]
Prednisone	4	0.8	I	5
Prednisolone	4	0.8	I	5
6α-Methylprednisolone	5	0.5	I	4
Triamcinolone	5	0	I	4
Betamethasone	25	0	L	0.75
Dexamethasone	25	0	L	0.75

[a]*Biological $t_{1/2}$: S, short (8-12 h); I, intermediate (12-36 h); L, long (36-72 h).*
[b]*Dose relationships apply only to oral or IV administration; potencies may differ greatly following IM or intra-articular administration.*
[c]*This agent is not used for glucocorticoid effects.*

secretion by the adrenal cortex or in doses that maximally affect electrolyte balance, aldosterone has no significant glucocorticoid activity and thus acts as a pure mineralocorticoid.

TOXICITY OF ADRENOCORTICAL STEROIDS

Two categories of toxic effects result from the therapeutic use of corticosteroids: those resulting from withdrawal of steroid therapy and those resulting from continued use at supraphysiological doses. The side effects from both categories are potentially life threatening and require a careful assessment of the risks and benefits in each patient.

WITHDRAWAL OF THERAPY. The most frequent problem in steroid withdrawal is flare-up of the underlying disease for which steroids were prescribed. Several other complications are associated with steroid withdrawal. The most severe complication of steroid cessation, acute adrenal insufficiency, results from overly rapid withdrawal of corticosteroids after prolonged therapy has suppressed the HPA axis. Many patients recover from glucocorticoid-induced HPA suppression within several weeks to months; however, in some individuals the time to recovery can be a year or longer. Protocols for discontinuing corticosteroid therapy in patients receiving long-term treatment with corticosteroids have been proposed. Patients who have received supraphysiological doses of glucocorticoids for a period of 2-4 weeks within the preceding year should be considered to have some degree of HPA impairment. A characteristic glucocorticoid withdrawal syndrome consists of fever, myalgia, arthralgia, and malaise, which may be difficult to differentiate from some of the underlying diseases for which steroid therapy was instituted. Finally, *pseudotumor cerebri*, a clinical syndrome that includes increased intracranial pressure with papilledema, is a rare condition that sometimes is associated with reduction or withdrawal of corticosteroid therapy.

CONTINUED USE OF SUPRAPHYSIOLOGICAL GLUCOCORTICOID DOSES. Besides the consequences that result from the suppression of the HPA axis, a number of other complications result from prolonged therapy with corticosteroids. These include fluid and electrolyte abnormalities, hypertension, hyperglycemia, increased susceptibility to infection, possible peptic ulcers, osteoporosis, myopathy, behavioral disturbances, cataracts, growth arrest, and the characteristic habitus of steroid overdose, including fat redistribution, striae, and ecchymoses.

THERAPEUTIC USES

With the exception of replacement therapy in deficiency states, the use of glucocorticoids largely is empirical. Given the number and severity of potential side effects, the decision to institute therapy with glucocorticoids always requires a careful consideration of the relative risks and benefits in each patient. For any disease and in any patient, the appropriate dose to achieve a given therapeutic effect must be determined by trial and error and must be reevaluated periodically as the activity of the underlying disease changes or as complications of therapy arise. *A single dose of glucocorticoid, even a large one, is virtually without harmful effects, and a short course of therapy (up to 1 week), in the absence of specific contraindications, is unlikely to be harmful. As the duration of glucocorticoid therapy is increased beyond 1 week, there are time- and dose-related increases in the incidence of disabling and potentially lethal effects*. Except in patients receiving replacement therapy, glucocorticoids are neither specific nor curative; rather, they are palliative by virtue of their anti-inflammatory and immunosuppressive actions. Finally, *abrupt cessation of glucocorticoids after prolonged therapy is associated with the risk of adrenal insufficiency, which may be fatal*.

When glucocorticoids are to be given over long periods, the dose must be determined by trial and error and must be the lowest that will achieve the desired effect. When the therapeutic goal is relief of painful or distressing symptoms not associated with an immediately life-threatening disease, complete relief is not sought, and the steroid dose is reduced gradually until worsening symptoms indicate that the minimal acceptable dose has been found. Where possible, the substitution of other medications, such as nonsteroidal anti-inflammatory drugs, may facilitate tapering the glucocorticoid dose once the initial benefit of therapy has been achieved. When therapy is directed at a life-threatening disease (e.g., pemphigus or lupus cerebritis), the initial dose should be a large one aimed at achieving rapid control of the crisis. If some benefit is not observed quickly, then the dose should be doubled or tripled. After initial control in a potentially lethal disease, dose reduction should be carried out under conditions that permit frequent accurate observations of the patient.

The lack of demonstrated deleterious effects of a single dose of glucocorticoids within the conventional therapeutic range justifies their administration to critically ill patients who may have adrenal insufficiency. If the underlying condition does result from deficiency of glucocorticoids, then a single intravenous injection of a soluble glucocorticoid may prevent immediate death and allow time for a definitive diagnosis to be made. If the underlying disease is not adrenal insufficiency, the single dose will not harm the patient. Long courses of therapy at high doses should be reserved for life-threatening disease. To diminish HPA axis suppression, the intermediate-acting steroid preparations (e.g., prednisone or prednisolone) should be given in the morning as a single dose. Alternate-day therapy with the same glucocorticoids also has been employed because certain patients obtain adequate therapeutic responses on this regimen. Alternatively, pulse therapy with higher glucocorticoid doses (e.g., doses as high as 1-1.5 g/day of methylprednisolone for 3 days) frequently is used to initiate therapy in patients with fulminant, immunologically related disorders such as acute transplantation rejection, necrotizing glomerulonephritis, and lupus nephritis.

REPLACEMENT THERAPY FOR ADRENAL INSUFFICIENCY. Adrenal insufficiency can result from structural or functional lesions of the adrenal cortex (primary adrenal insufficiency or Addison disease) or from structural or functional lesions of the anterior pituitary or hypothalamus (secondary adrenal insufficiency). In developed countries, primary adrenal insufficiency most frequently is secondary to autoimmune adrenal disease, whereas tuberculous adrenalitis is the most frequent etiology in developing countries. Other causes include adrenalectomy, bilateral adrenal hemorrhage, neoplastic infiltration of the adrenal glands, acquired immunodeficiency syndrome, inherited disorders of the steroidogenic enzymes, and X-linked adrenoleukodystrophy. Secondary adrenal insufficiency resulting from pituitary or hypothalamic dysfunction generally presents in a more insidious manner than does the primary disorder, probably because mineralocorticoid biosynthesis is preserved.

ACUTE ADRENAL INSUFFICIENCY. This life-threatening disease is characterized by GI symptoms (nausea, vomiting, and abdominal pain), dehydration, hyponatremia, hyperkalemia, weakness, lethargy, and hypotension. It usually is associated with disorders of the adrenal rather than the pituitary or hypothalamus and sometimes follows abrupt withdrawal of glucocorticoids used at high doses or for prolonged periods.

The immediate management of patients with acute adrenal insufficiency includes intravenous therapy with isotonic sodium chloride solution supplemented with 5% glucose and corticosteroids and appropriate therapy for precipitating causes such as infection, trauma, or hemorrhage. Because cardiac function often is reduced in the setting of adrenocortical insufficiency, the patient should be monitored for evidence of volume overload such as rising central venous pressure or pulmonary edema. After an initial intravenous bolus of 100 mg, hydrocortisone (cortisol) should be given by continuous infusion at a rate of 50-100 mg every 8 h, a dose that confers sufficient mineralocorticoid activity to meet all requirements. As the patient stabilizes, the hydrocortisone dose may be decreased to 25 mg every 6-8 h. Thereafter, patients are treated in the same fashion as those with chronic adrenal insufficiency. For the treatment of unconfirmed acute adrenal insufficiency, 4 mg of dexamethasone sodium phosphate can be substituted for hydrocortisone because dexamethasone does not cross-react in the cortisol assay and will not interfere with the measurement of cortisol (either basally or in response to the cosyntropin stimulation test). A failure to respond to cosyntropin in this setting is diagnostic of adrenal insufficiency.

CHRONIC ADRENAL INSUFFICIENCY. Patients with chronic adrenal insufficiency present with many of the same manifestations seen in adrenal crisis but with lesser severity. These patients require daily treatment with corticosteroids.

Traditional replacement regimens have used hydrocortisone in doses of 20-30 mg/day. *Cortisone acetate*, which is inactive until converted to cortisol by 11βHSD1, also has been used in doses ranging from 25-37.5 mg/day. In an effort to mimic the normal diurnal rhythm of cortisol secretion, these glucocorticoids generally have been given in divided doses, with two-thirds of the dose given in the morning and one-third given in the afternoon. Although some patients with primary adrenal insufficiency can be maintained on hydrocortisone and liberal salt intake, most of these patients also require mineralocorticoid replacement; fludrocortisone acetate generally is used in doses of 0.05-0.2 mg/day. For patients with secondary adrenal insufficiency, the administration of a glucocorticoid alone is generally adequate because the zona glomerulosa, which makes mineralocorticoids, is intact. When initiating treatment in patients with panhypopituitarism, it is important to administer glucocorticoids before initiating treatment with thyroid hormone because the administration of thyroid hormone may precipitate acute adrenal insufficiency by increasing the metabolism of cortisol.

The adequacy of corticosteroid replacement therapy is judged by clinical criteria and biochemical measurements. The subjective well-being of the patient is an important clinical parameter in primary and secondary disease. In primary adrenal insufficiency the disappearance of hyperpigmentation and the resolution of electrolyte abnormalities are valuable indicators of adequate replacement. Overtreatment may cause manifestations of Cushing syndrome in adults and decreased linear growth in children. Plasma ACTH levels may be used to monitor therapy in patients with primary adrenal insufficiency; the early-morning ACTH level should not be suppressed but should be <100 pg/mL (22 pmol/L).

Standard doses of glucocorticoids often must be adjusted upward in patients who also are taking drugs that increase their metabolic clearance (e.g., phenytoin, barbiturates, or rifampin) or who suffer the stress of intercurrent illness. *All patients with adrenal insufficiency should wear a medical alert bracelet or tag that lists their diagnosis and carries information about their steroid regimen.* During minor illness, the glucocorticoid dose should be doubled. The patient and family members should also be trained to administer parenteral dexamethasone (4 mg subcutaneously or intramuscularly) in the event that severe nausea or vomiting precludes the oral administration of medications; they then should seek medical attention immediately. Glucocorticoid doses also are adjusted when patients with adrenal insufficiency undergo surgery. In this setting, the doses are designed to approximate or exceed the maximal cortisol secretory rate of 200 mg/day; a standard regimen is hydrocortisone, 100 mg parenterally every 8 h. Following surgery, the dose is halved each day until it is reduced to routine maintenance levels.

CONGENITAL ADRENAL HYPERPLASIA (CAH). This is a group of genetic disorders in which the activity of 1 of the several enzymes required for the biosynthesis of glucocorticoids is deficient. The impaired production of cortisol and the consequent lack of negative feedback inhibition lead to increased release of ACTH. As a result, other hormonally active steroids that are proximal to the enzymatic block in the steroidogenic pathway are produced in excess. CAH includes a spectrum of disorders for which precise clinical presentation, laboratory findings, and treatment depend on which of the steroidogenic enzymes is deficient. In ~90% of patients, CAH results from mutations in CYP21, the enzyme that carries out the 21-hydroxylation reaction (*see* Figure 42–3).

Clinically, patients are divided into those with classic CAH, who have severe defects in enzymatic activity and first present during childhood, and those with nonclassic CAH, who present after puberty with signs and symptoms of mild androgen excess such as hirsutism, amenorrhea, infertility, and acne. Female patients with classic CAH, if not treated in utero with glucocorticoids, frequently are born with virilized external genitalia (female pseudohermaphroditism) that results from elevated production of adrenal androgen precursors at critical stages of sexual differentiation in utero. Males appear normal at birth and later may have precocious development of secondary sexual characteristics (isosexual precocious puberty). In both sexes, linear growth is accelerated in childhood, but the adult height is reduced by premature closure of the epiphyses. Some patients with classical CAH are unable to conserve Na^+ normally and thus are called "salt wasters." All patients with classical CAH require replacement therapy with hydrocortisone or a suitable congener, and those with salt wasting also require mineralocorticoid replacement. The goals of therapy are to restore levels of physiological steroid hormones to the normal range and to suppress ACTH and thereby abrogate the effects of overproduction of adrenal androgens. The typical oral dose of hydrocortisone is ~0.6 mg/kg daily in 2 or 3 divided doses. The mineralocorticoid used is fludrocortisone acetate (0.05-0.2 mg/day). Many experts also administer table salt to infants (one-fifth of a teaspoon dissolved in formula daily) until the child is eating solid food. Therapy is guided by gain in weight and height, by plasma levels of 17-hydroxyprogesterone, and by blood pressure. Elevated plasma renin activity suggests that the patient is receiving an inadequate dose of mineralocorticoid. Sudden spurts in linear growth often indicate inadequate pituitary suppression and excessive androgen secretion, whereas growth failure suggests overtreatment with glucocorticoid.

THERAPEUTIC USES IN NONENDOCRINE DISEASES. There are important uses of glucocorticoids in diseases that do not directly involve the HPA axis. The disorders discussed below illustrate the principles governing glucocorticoid use in selected diseases for which glucocorticoids are more frequently employed. The dosage of glucocorticoids varies considerably depending on the nature and severity of the underlying disorder. Approximate doses of a representative glucocorticoid (e.g., prednisone) are provided.

Rheumatic Disorders. Glucocorticoids are used widely in the treatment of rheumatic disorders and are a mainstay in the treatment of the more serious inflammatory rheumatic diseases, such as systemic lupus erythematosus, and a variety of vasculitic disorders, such as polyarteritis nodosa, Wegener granulomatosis, Churg-Strauss syndrome, and giant cell arteritis. For these more serious disorders, the starting dose of glucocorticoids should be sufficient to suppress the disease rapidly and minimize resultant tissue damage. Initially, prednisone (1 mg/kg/day in divided doses) often is used, generally followed by consolidation to a single daily dose, with subsequent tapering to a minimal effective dose as determined by the clinical picture.

Glucocorticoids are often used in conjunction with other immunosuppressive agents such as cyclophosphamide and methotrexate, which offer better long-term control than steroids alone. The exception is giant cell arteritis, for which glucocorticoids remain superior to other agents. Caution should be exercised in the use of glucocorticoids in some forms of vasculitis (e.g., polyarteritis nodosa), for which underlying infections with hepatitis viruses may play a pathogenetic role. Intermediate-acting glucocorticoids such as prednisone and methylprednisolone are generally preferred over longer-acting steroids such as dexamethasone.

In rheumatoid arthritis, because of the serious and debilitating side effects associated with chronic use, glucocorticoids are used as stabilizing agents for progressive disease that fails to respond to first-line treatments such as physiotherapy and nonsteroidal anti-inflammatory agents. In this case, glucocorticoids provide relief until other, slower-acting antirheumatic drugs (e.g., methotrexate or agents targeted at tumor necrosis factor) take effect. A typical starting dose is 5-10 mg of prednisone per day. In the setting of an acute exacerbation, higher doses of glucocorticoids may be employed (typically 20-40 mg/day of prednisone or equivalent), with rapid taper thereafter. Alternatively, patients with major symptomatology confined to 1 or a few joints may be treated with intra-articular steroid injections. Depending on joint size, typical doses are 5-20 mg of triamcinolone acetonide or its equivalent.

In noninflammatory degenerative joint diseases (e.g., osteoarthritis) or in a variety of regional pain syndromes (e.g., tendinitis or bursitis), glucocorticoids may be administered by local injection for the treatment of episodic disease flare-up. It is important to use a glucocorticoid that does not require bioactivation (e.g., prednisolone rather than prednisone) and to minimize the frequency of local steroid administration whenever possible. In the case of repeated intra-articular injection of steroids, there is a significant incidence of painless joint destruction, resembling Charcot arthropathy. It is recommended that intra-articular injections be performed with intervals of at least 3 months to minimize complications.

Renal Diseases. Patients with nephrotic syndrome secondary to minimal change disease generally respond well to steroid therapy, and glucocorticoids are the first-line treatment in both adults and children. Initial daily doses of prednisone are 1-2 mg/kg for 6 weeks, followed by a gradual tapering of the dose over 6-8 weeks, although some nephrologists advocate alternate-day therapy. Objective evidence of response, such as diminished proteinuria, is seen within 2-3 weeks in 85% of patients, and >95% of patients have remission within 3 months. Patients with renal disease secondary to systemic lupus erythematosus also are generally given a therapeutic trial of glucocorticoids. In the case of membranous glomerulonephritis, many nephrologists recommend a trial of alternate-day glucocorticoids for 8-10 weeks (e.g., prednisone, 120 mg every other day), followed by a 1- to 2-month period of tapering.

Allergic Disease. The onset of action of glucocorticoids in allergic diseases is delayed, and patients with severe allergic reactions such as anaphylaxis require immediate therapy with epinephrine. The manifestations of allergic diseases of limited duration—such as hay fever, serum sickness, urticaria, contact dermatitis, drug reactions, bee stings, and angioneurotic edema—can be suppressed by adequate doses of glucocorticoids given as supplements to the primary therapy. In severe disease, intravenous glucocorticoids (methylprednisolone, 125 mg intravenously every 6 h, or equivalent) are appropriate. In allergic rhinitis, intranasal steroids are viewed as the drug of choice by many experts.

Pulmonary Diseases. The use of glucocorticoids in bronchial asthma and other pulmonary diseases is discussed in Chapter 36. Antenatal glucocorticoids are used frequently in the setting of premature labor, decreasing the incidence of respiratory distress syndrome, intraventricular hemorrhage, and death in infants delivered prematurely. Betamethasone (12 mg intramuscularly every 24 h for 2 doses) or dexamethasone (6 mg intramuscularly every 12 h for 4 doses) is administered to women with definitive signs of premature labor between 26 and 34 weeks of gestation.

Infectious Diseases. Although the use of immunosuppressive glucocorticoids in infectious diseases may seem paradoxical, there are a limited number of settings in which they are indicated in the therapy of specific infectious pathogens. One example of beneficial effects is seen in AIDS patients with *Pneumocystis carinii* pneumonia and moderate to severe hypoxia; addition of glucocorticoids to the antibiotic regimen increases oxygenation and lowers the incidence of respiratory failure and mortality. Similarly, glucocorticoids clearly decrease the incidence of long-term neurological impairment associated with *Haemophilus influenzae* type b meningitis in infants and children ≥2 months of age.

Ocular Diseases. Glucocorticoids frequently are used to suppress inflammation in the eye and can preserve sight when used properly. They are administered topically for diseases of the outer eye and anterior segment and attain therapeutic concentrations in the aqueous humor after instillation into the conjunctival sac. For diseases of the posterior segment, intraocular injection or systemic administration is required. These uses of glucocorticoids are discussed in Chapter 64.

Skin Diseases. Glucocorticoids are remarkably efficacious in the treatment of a wide variety of inflammatory dermatoses. A typical regimen for an eczematous eruption is 1% hydrocortisone ointment applied locally twice daily. Effectiveness is enhanced by application of the topical steroid under an occlusive film, such as plastic wrap; unfortunately, the risk of systemic absorption also is increased by occlusive dressings, and this can be a significant problem when the more potent glucocorticoids are applied to inflamed skin. Glucocorticoids are administered systemically for severe episodes of acute dermatological disorders and for exacerbations of chronic disorders. The dose in these settings is usually 40 mg/day of prednisone. Systemic steroid administration can be lifesaving in pemphigus, which may require daily doses of up to 120 mg of prednisone. Chapter 65 presents the dermatologic uses of glucocorticoids.

GI Diseases. Patients with inflammatory bowel disease (chronic ulcerative colitis and Crohn disease) who fail to respond to more conservative management (i.e., rest, diet, and sulfasalazine) may benefit from glucocorticoids; steroids are most useful for acute exacerbations (*see* Chapter 47).

Hepatic Diseases. The use of corticosteroids in hepatic disease has been highly controversial. Glucocorticoids clearly are of benefit in autoimmune hepatitis; as many as 80% of patients show histological remission when treated with prednisone (40-60 mg daily initially, with tapering to a maintenance dose of 7.5-10 mg daily after serum transaminase levels fall). The role of corticosteroids in alcoholic liver disease is not fully defined; the most recent meta-analyses do not support a beneficial role of corticosteroids. In the setting of severe hepatic disease, prednisolone should be used instead of prednisone, which requires hepatic conversion to be active.

Malignancies. Glucocorticoids are used in the chemotherapy of acute lymphocytic leukemia and lymphomas because of their antilymphocytic effects, most commonly as a component of combination therapy (*see* Chapters 46 and 63).

Cerebral Edema. Corticosteroids are of value in the reduction or prevention of cerebral edema associated with parasites and neoplasms, especially those that are metastatic.

MISCELLANEOUS USES

Sarcoidosis. Corticosteroids are indicated therapy for patients with debilitating symptoms or life-threatening forms of sarcoidosis. Patients with severe pulmonary involvement are treated with 10-20 mg/day of prednisone, or an equivalent dose of alternative steroids, to induce remission. Higher doses may be required for other forms of this disease. Maintenance doses may be as low as 5 mg/day of prednisone. All patients who require chronic glucocorticoid therapy at doses exceeding the normal daily production rate are at increased risk of secondary tuberculosis; therefore, patients with a positive tuberculin reaction or other evidence of tuberculosis should receive prophylactic antituberculosis therapy.

Thrombocytopenia. In thrombocytopenia, prednisone (0.5 mg/kg) is used to decrease the bleeding tendency. In more severe cases, and for initiation of treatment of idiopathic thrombocytopenia, daily doses of prednisone (1-1.5 mg/kg) are employed. Patients with refractory idiopathic thrombocytopenia may respond to pulsed high-dose glucocorticoid therapy.

Autoimmune Destruction of Erythrocytes. Patients with autoimmune destruction of erythrocytes (i.e., hemolytic anemia with a positive Coombs test) are treated with prednisone (1 mg/kg/day). In the setting of severe hemolysis, higher doses may be used, with tapering as the anemia improves. Small maintenance doses may be required for several months in patients who respond.

Organ Transplantation. In organ transplantation, high doses of prednisone (50-100 mg) are given at the time of transplant surgery, in conjunction with other immunosuppressive agents, and most patients are kept on a maintenance regimen that includes lower doses of glucocorticoids (*see* Chapter 35). For some solid organ transplants (e.g., pancreas), protocols that either withdraw corticosteroids early after transplantation or that avoid them completely are becoming more common.

Spinal Cord Injury. Multicenter-controlled trials have demonstrated significant decreases in neurological defects in patients with acute spinal cord injury treated within 8 h of injury with large doses of methylprednisolone sodium succinate (30 mg/kg initially followed by an infusion of 5.4 mg/kg/h for 23 h).

DIAGNOSTIC APPLICATIONS OF DEXAMETHASONE. In addition to its therapeutic uses, dexamethasone is used as a first-line agent to diagnose hypercortisolism and to differentiate among the different causes of Cushing syndrome. The rationale and procedure are described in detail on page 1233 of the 12th edition of the parent text.

INHIBITORS OF THE BIOSYNTHESIS AND ACTION OF ADRENOCORTICAL STEROIDS

Hypercortisolism with its attendant morbidity and mortality is most frequently caused by corticotroph adenomas that overproduce ACTH (Cushing disease) or by adrenocortical tumors or bilateral hyperplasias that overproduce cortisol (Cushing syndrome). Less frequently, hypercortisolism may result from adrenocortical carcinomas or ectopic ACTH- or CRH-producing tumors. Although surgery is the treatment of choice, it is not always effective, and adjuvant therapy with inhibitors of steroidogenesis becomes necessary. In these settings, ketoconazole, metyrapone, etomidate, and mitotane are clinically useful. Ketoconazole, etomidate, and mitotane are discussed in more detail in other chapters. All of these agents pose the common risk of precipitating acute adrenal insufficiency; thus, they must be used in appropriate doses, and the status of the patient's HPA axis must be carefully monitored. Agents that act as glucocorticoid receptor antagonists (antiglucocorticoids) are discussed later in this chapter; mineralocorticoid antagonists are discussed in Chapter 25.

Ketoconazole. Ketoconazole (NIZORAL) is an antifungal agent (*see* Chapter 57). In doses higher than those employed in antifungal therapy, it is an effective inhibitor of adrenal and gonadal steroidogenesis, primarily because of its inhibition of the activity of CYP17 (17α-hydroxylase). At even higher doses, ketoconazole also inhibits CYP11A1, effectively blocking steroidogenesis in all primary steroidogenic tissues. Ketoconazole is the best tolerated and most effective inhibitor of steroid hormone biosynthesis in patients with hypercortisolism (although the FDA has not approved this indication for ketoconazole). In most cases, a dosage regimen of 600-800 mg/day (in 2 divided doses) is required, and some patients may require up to 1200 mg/day (in 2-3 doses). Side effects include hepatic dysfunction. The potential of ketoconazole to interact with CYP isoforms can lead to serious drug interactions (*see* Chapter 6).

Metyrapone. Metyrapone (METOPIRONE) is a relatively selective inhibitor of CYP11B1 (11β-hydroxylase), which converts 11-deoxycortisol to cortisol, thereby reducing cortisol production and elevating precursor levels (e.g., 11-deoxycortisol). Although the biosynthesis of aldosterone also is impaired, the elevated levels of 11-deoxycortisol sustain mineralocorticoid-dependent functions. In a diagnostic test of the entire HPA axis, metyrapone (30 mg/kg, maximum dose of 3 g) is administered orally with a snack at midnight, and plasma cortisol and 11-deoxycortisol are measured at 8 A.M. the next morning. A plasma cortisol <8 μg/dL validates adequate inhibition of CYP11B1; in this setting, an 11-deoxycortisol level <7 μg/dL is highly suggestive of impaired hypothalamic-pituitary-adrenal function.

Metyrapone has been used to treat the hypercorticism resulting from either adrenal neoplasms or tumors producing ACTH ectopically. Maximal suppression of steroidogenesis requires doses of 4 g/day. More frequently, metyrapone is used as adjunctive therapy in patients who have received pituitary irradiation or in combination with other agents that inhibit steroidogenesis. In this setting, a dose of 500-750 mg 3 or 4 times daily is employed. The use of metyrapone in the treatment of Cushing syndrome secondary to pituitary hypersecretion of ACTH is more controversial. Chronic administration of metyrapone can cause hirsutism, which results from increased synthesis of adrenal androgens upstream from the enzymatic block, and hypertension, which results from elevated levels of 11-deoxycortisol. Other side effects include nausea, headache, sedation, and rash.

Etomidate. Etomidate (AMIDATE), a substituted imidazole used primarily as an anesthetic agent and sedative, inhibits cortisol secretion at subhypnotic doses primarily by inhibiting CYP11B1 activity. Etomidate has been used off-label to treat hypercortisolism when rapid control is required in a patient who cannot take medication by the oral route. Etomidate is administered as a bolus of 0.03 mg/kg intravenously, followed by an infusion of 0.1 mg/kg/h to a maximum of 0.3 mg/kg/h.

Mitotane. Mitotane (LYSODREN) is an adrenocorticolytic agent used to treat inoperable adrenocortical carcinoma. Its cytolytic action is due to its metabolic conversion to a reactive acyl chloride by adrenal mitochondrial CYPs and subsequent reactivity with cellular proteins. Doses range from 0.5-3 g administered 3 times daily. Its onset of action takes weeks to months, and GI disturbances and ataxia are its major toxicities.

Aminoglutethimide. Aminoglutethimide (CYTADREN) primarily inhibits CYP11A1 (the initial and rate-limiting step in the biosynthesis of all physiological steroids) and also inhibits CYP11B1 and CYP19 (aromatase). Aminoglutethimide recently has been withdrawn from the market by the manufacturer and is no longer available.

ANTIGLUCOCORTICOIDS

The progesterone receptor antagonist *mifepristone* (MIFEPREX; RU-486) has received considerable attention because of its use as an antiprogestogen that can terminate early pregnancy (*see* Chapter 66). At higher doses, mifepristone also inhibits the GR, blocking feedback regulation of the HPA axis and secondarily increasing endogenous ACTH and cortisol levels. Because of its capacity to inhibit glucocorticoid action, mifepristone also has been studied as a potential therapeutic agent in a small number of patients with hypercortisolism. Currently, its use for this purpose is restricted to patients with inoperable causes of cortisol excess that have not responded to other agents.

For a complete Bibliographical Listing see Goodman & Gilman's ***The Pharmacological Basis of Therapeutics***, 12th ed., or Goodman & Gilman Online at www.AccessMedicine.com.

Endocrine Pancreas and Pharmacotherapy of Diabetes Mellitus and Hypoglycemia

Diabetes mellitus is a spectrum of metabolic disorders arising from myriad pathogenic mechanisms, all resulting in hyperglycemia. Both genetic and environmental factors contribute to its pathogenesis, which involves insufficient insulin secretion, reduced responsiveness to endogenous or exogenous insulin, increased glucose production, and/or abnormalities in fat and protein metabolism. The resulting hyperglycemia may lead to both acute symptoms and metabolic abnormalities. Major sources of the morbidity of diabetes are the chronic complications that arise from prolonged hyperglycemia, including retinopathy, neuropathy, nephropathy, and cardiovascular disease. These chronic complications can be mitigated in many patients by sustained control of the blood glucose. There are now a wide variety of treatment options for hyperglycemia that target different processes involved in glucose regulation or dysregulation.

PHYSIOLOGY OF GLUCOSE HOMEOSTASIS

REGULATION OF BLOOD GLUCOSE. The maintenance of glucose homeostasis, termed *glucose tolerance*, is a highly developed systemic process involving the integration of several major organs (Figure 43–1). Although the actions of insulin are of central importance, webs of inter-organ communication via other hormones, nerves, local factors and substrates, also play a vital role. The pancreatic β cell is central in this homeostatic process, adjusting the amount of insulin secreted very precisely to promote glucose uptake after meals and to regulate glucose output from the liver during fasting.

In the *fasting state* (Figure 43–1A), the fuel demands of the body are met by the oxidation of fatty acids. The brain does not effectively use fatty acids to meet energy needs and in the fasting state requires glucose for normal function; glucose requirements are ~2 mg/kg/min in adult humans, largely to supply the central nervous system (CNS) with an energy source. Fasting glucose requirements are primarily provided by the liver. Liver glycogen stores provide some of this glucose; conversion of lactate, alanine, and glycerol into glucose accounts for the remainder. The dominant regulation of hepatic *glycogenolysis* and *gluconeogenesis* are the pancreatic islet hormones *insulin* and *glucagon*. Insulin inhibits hepatic glucose production, and the decline of circulating insulin concentrations in the post-absorptive state (fasting) is permissive for higher rates of glucose output. Glucagon maintains blood glucose concentrations at physiological levels in the absence of exogenous carbohydrate (overnight and in between meals) by stimulating gluconeogenesis and glycogenolysis by the liver. Insulin secretion is stimulated by *food ingestion*, nutrient absorption, and elevated blood glucose, and insulin promotes glucose, lipid, and protein anabolism (Figure 43–1B). The centrality of insulin in glucose metabolism is emphasized by the fact that all the forms of human diabetes have as a root cause some abnormality of insulin secretion or action.

Pancreatic β *cell* function is primarily controlled by plasma glucose concentrations. Elevations of blood glucose are necessary for insulin release above basal levels, and other stimuli are relatively ineffective when plasma glucose is in the fasting range (4.4-5.5 mM or 80-100 mg %). These other stimuli include nutrient substrates, *insulinotropic hormones* released from the GI tract, and autonomic neural pathways. Neural stimuli cause some increase of insulin secretion prior to food consumption. Neural stimulation of insulin secretion occurs throughout the meal and contributes significantly to glucose tolerance. Arrival of nutrient chyme to the intestine leads to the release of insulinotropic peptides from specialized endocrine cells in the intestinal mucosa. *Glucose-dependent insulinotropic polypeptide* (GIP) and *glucagon-like peptide 1* (GLP-1), together termed *incretins,* are the essential gut hormones contributing to *glucose tolerance*. They are secreted in proportion to the nutrient load ingested and relay this information to the islet as part of a feed-forward mechanism that allows an insulin response appropriate to meal size. Insulin secretion rates in healthy humans are highest in the early digestive phase of meals, preceding and limiting the peak in blood glucose. This pattern of premonitory insulin secretion is an essential feature of normal glucose tolerance. How to mimic this pattern is one of the key challenges for successful insulin therapy in diabetic patients.

Elevated circulating insulin concentrations lower glucose in blood by inhibiting hepatic glucose production and stimulating the uptake and metabolism of glucose by muscle and adipose tissue. Production of glucose is

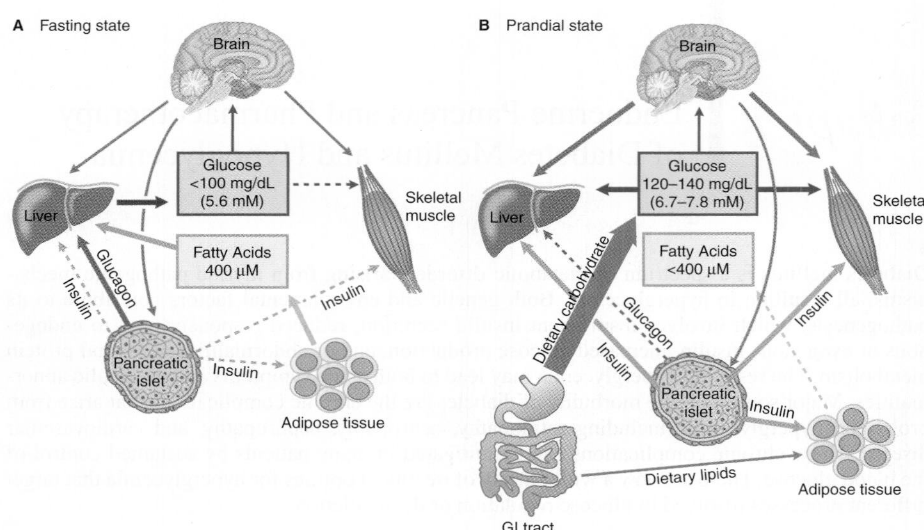

Figure 43–1 *Insulin, glucagon, and glucose homeostasis.* **A. Fasting State**—In healthy humans plasma glucose is maintained in a range from 4.4-5 mM, and fatty acids near 400 μM. In the absence of nutrient absorption from the GI tract, glucose is supplied primarily from the liver and fatty acids from adipose tissue. With fasting, plasma insulin levels are low, and plasma glucagon is elevated, contributing to increased hepatic glycogenolysis and gluconeogenesis; low insulin also releases adipocytes from inhibition, permitting increased lipogenesis. Most tissues oxidize primarily fatty acids during fasting, sparing glucose for use by the CNS. **B. Prandial State**—During feeding, nutrient absorption causes an increase in plasma glucose, resulting in release of incretins from the gut and neural stimuli that promote insulin secretion. Under the control of insulin, the liver, skeletal muscle, and adipose tissue actively take up glucose. Hepatic glucose production and lipolysis are inhibited, and total body glucose oxidation increases. The brain senses plasma glucose concentrations and provides regulatory inputs contributing to fuel homeostasis. The *boldness of the arrows* reflects relative intensity of action; a *dashed line* indicates little or no activity.

inhibited half-maximally by an insulin concentration of ~120 pmol/L, whereas glucose utilization is stimulated half-maximally at ~300 pmol/L. Some of the effects of insulin on the liver occur rapidly, within the first 20 min of meal ingestion, whereas stimulation of peripheral glucose uptake may require up to an hour to reach significant rates. Insulin has potent effects to reduce lipolysis from adipocytes, primarily through the inhibition of hormone-sensitive lipase, and increases lipid storage by promoting lipoprotein–lipase synthesis and adipocyte glucose uptake. Insulin also stimulates amino acid uptake and protein synthesis and inhibits protein degradation in muscle and other tissues.

The limited glycogen stores in skeletal muscle are mobilized at the onset of activity but most of the glucose support for exercise comes from hepatic gluconeogenesis. The dominant regulation of hepatic glucose production during exercise comes from EPI and NE. The catecholamines stimulate glycogenolysis and gluconeogenesis, inhibit insulin secretion, and enhance release of glucagon, all contributing to increased hepatic glucose output. In addition, catecholamines promote lipolysis, freeing fatty acids for oxidation in exercising muscle and glycerol for hepatic gluconeogenesis.

PANCREATIC ISLET PHYSIOLOGY AND INSULIN SECRETION. The pancreatic islets comprise 1-2% of the pancreatic volume. The pancreatic islet is a highly vascularized, highly innervated mini-organ containing 5 endocrine cell types: α *cells* that secrete *glucagon,* β *cells* that secrete *insulin*, δ cells that secrete somatostatin, cells that secrete pancreatic polypeptide, and ε *cells* that secrete *ghrelin*.

Insulin is initially synthesized as a single polypeptide chain, *preproinsulin* (110 amino acid), which is processed first to *proinsulin* and then to *insulin* and *C-peptide* (Figure 43–2). This complex and highly regulated process involves the Golgi complex, the endoplasmic reticulum, and the secretory granules of the β cell. Secretory granules are critical in bringing insulin to the cell surface for exocytosis, and in the cleavage and processing of the prohormone to the final secretion products, insulin and C-peptide. Equimolar quantities of insulin and C-peptide (31 amino acids) are co-secreted. Insulin has a $t_{1/2}$ of 5-6 min due to extensive hepatic clearance. C-peptide, in contrast, with no known physiological function or receptor, has a $t_{1/2}$ of ~30 min. The C-peptide is useful in assessment of β cell secretion, and to distinguish endogenous and exogenous

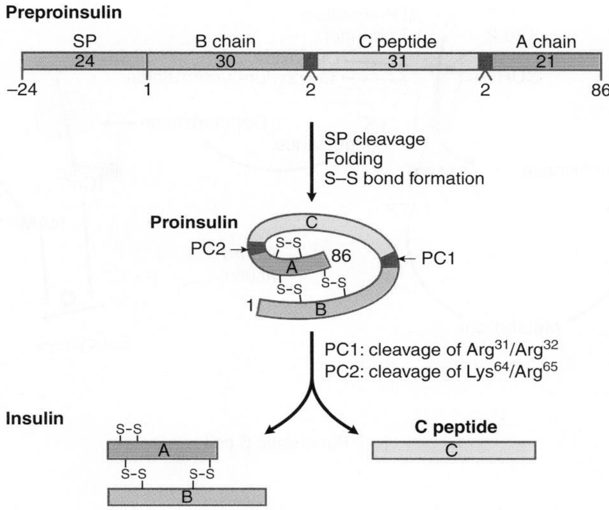

Figure 43–2 *Synthesis and processing of insulin.* The initial peptide, preproinsulin (110 amino acids) consists of a signal peptide (SP), B chain, C peptide, and A chain. The SP is cleaved and S-S bonds form as the proinsulin folds. Two prohormone convertases, PC1 and PC2, cleave proinsulin into insulin, C peptide, and 2 dipeptides. Insulin and C peptide are stored in granules and co-secreted in equimolar quantities.

hyperinsulinemia (for example in the evaluation of insulin-induced hypoglycemia). The β cell also synthesizes and secretes *islet amyloid polypeptide* (IAPP) or *amylin*, a 37–amino acid peptide. IAPP influences GI motility and the speed of glucose absorption. Pramlintide is an agent used in the treatment of diabetes that mimics the action of IAPP.

Insulin secretion is tightly regulated to provide stable concentrations of glucose in blood during both fasting and feeding. This regulation is achieved by the coordinated interplay of various nutrients, GI hormones, pancreatic hormones, and autonomic neurotransmitters. Glucose, amino acids (arginine, etc.), fatty acids, and ketone bodies promote the secretion of insulin. Glucose is the primary insulin secretagogue, and insulin secretion is tightly coupled to the extracellular glucose concentration. Insulin secretion is much greater when the same amount of glucose is delivered orally compared to intravenously (incretin effect). Islets are richly innervated by both adrenergic and cholinergic nerves. Stimulation of α_2 adrenergic receptors inhibits insulin secretion, whereas β_2 adrenergic receptor agonists and vagal nerve stimulation enhance release. In general, any condition that activates the sympathetic branch of the autonomic nervous system (such as hypoxia, hypoglycemia, exercise, hypothermia, surgery, or severe burns) suppresses the secretion of insulin by stimulation of α_2 adrenergic receptors. Glucagon and somatostatin inhibit insulin secretion.

The molecular events controlling glucose-stimulated insulin secretion begin with the transport of glucose into the β cell via GLUT, a facilitative glucose transporter, primarily GLUT1 in human β cells (Figure 43–3). Upon entry into the β cell, glucose is quickly phosphorylated by glucokinase (GK; hexokinase IV); this phosphorylation is the rate-limiting step in glucose metabolism in the β cell. GK's distinctive affinity for glucose leads to a marked increase in glucose metabolism over the range of 5-10 mM glucose, where glucose-stimulated insulin secretion is most pronounced. The glucose-6-phosphate produced by GK activity enters the glycolytic pathway, producing changes in NADPH and the ratio of ADP/ATP. Elevated ATP inhibits an ATP-sensitive K^+ channel (K_{ATP} channel), leading to cell membrane depolarization. This heteromeric K_{ATP} channel consists of an inward rectifying K^+ channel (Kir6.2) and a closely associated protein known as the sulfonylurea receptor (SUR). Mutations in the K_{ATP} channel are responsible for some types of neonatal diabetes or hypoglycemia. Membrane depolarization then leads to opening of a voltage-dependent Ca^{2+} channel and increased intracellular Ca^{2+}, resulting in exocytotic release of insulin from storage vesicles. These intracellular events are modulated by changes in cAMP production, amino acid metabolism, and the level of transcription factors. GPCRs for glucagon, GIP, and GLP-1 couple to G_s to stimulate adenylyl cyclase and insulin secretion; receptors for somatostatin and α_2 adrenergic agonists couple to G_i to reduce cellular cAMP production and secretion.

The pancreatic α cell secretes glucagon, primarily in response to hypoglycemia. Glucagon biosynthesis begins with *preproglucagon*, which is processed in a cell-specific fashion to several biologically active peptides such

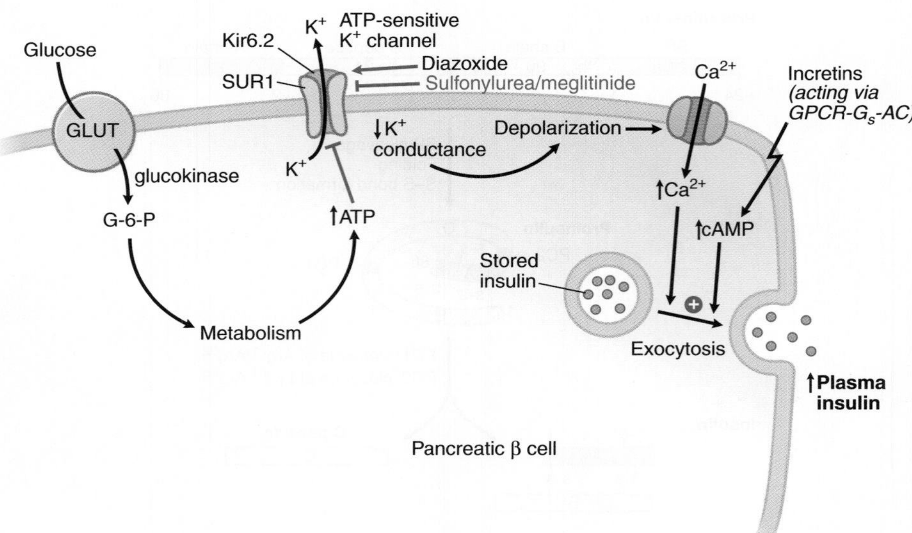

Figure 43–3 *Regulation of insulin secretion from a pancreatic β cell.* The pancreatic β cell in a resting state (fasting blood glucose) is hyperpolarized. Glucose, entering via GLUT transporters (primarily GLUT1 in humans, GLUT2 in rodents), is metabolized and elevates cellular ATP, which reduces K^+ conductance through the K_{ATP} channel; the decreased K^+ conductance results in depolarization, leading to Ca^{2+}-dependent exocytosis of stored insulin. The K_{ATP} channel, with SUR1 and Kir 6.2 subunits, is the site of action of several classes of drugs: ATP binds to and inhibits Kir 6.2; sulfonylureas and meglitinides bind to and inhibit SUR1; all 3 agents thereby promote insulin secretion. Diazoxide and ADP-Mg^{2+} (low ATP) bind to and activate SUR1, thereby inhibiting insulin secretion. Incretins enhance insulin secretion.

as glucagon, GLP-1, and glucagon-like peptide 2 (GLP-2) (*see* Figure 43–9). *In general, glucagon and insulin secretion are regulated in a reciprocal fashion; that is, the agents or processes that stimulate insulin secretion inhibit glucagon secretion. Notable exceptions are arginine and somatostatin: arginine stimulates and somatostatin inhibits the secretion of both hormones.*

INSULIN ACTION. The insulin receptor is expressed on virtually all mammalian cell types. Tissues that are critical for regulation of blood glucose are liver, skeletal muscle, fat (*see* Figure 43–1), and specific regions of the brain and the pancreatic islet. The actions of insulin are anabolic, and insulin signaling is critical for promoting the uptake, use, and storage of the major nutrients: glucose, lipids, and amino acids. Insulin stimulates glycogenesis, lipogenesis, and protein synthesis; it also inhibits the catabolism of these compounds. On a cellular level, insulin stimulates transport of substrates and ions into cells, promotes translocation of proteins between cellular compartments, regulates the action of specific enzymes, and controls gene transcription and mRNA translation. Some effects of insulin (e.g., activation of glucose and ion transport systems, phosphorylation or dephosphorylation of specific enzymes) occur within seconds or minutes; other effects (e.g., those promoting protein synthesis and regulating gene transcription and cell proliferation) manifest over minutes to hours to days. The effects of insulin on cell proliferation and differentiation occur over days.

THE INSULIN RECEPTOR. Insulin action is transmitted through a receptor tyrosine kinase that bears functional similarity to the *insulin-like growth factor 1 (IGF-1) receptor*. The insulin receptor is composed of linked α/β subunit dimers that are products of a single gene; dimers linked by disulfide bonds form a transmembrane heterotetramer glycoprotein composed of 2 extracellular α-subunits and 2 membrane-spanning β-subunits (Figure 43–4). The number of receptors varies from 40/cell on erythrocytes to 300,000/cell on adipocytes and hepatocytes.

The α-subunits inhibit the inherent tyrosine kinase activity of the β-subunits. Insulin binding to the α-subunits releases this inhibition and allows transphosphorylation of 1 β-subunit by the other, and autophosphorylation at specific sites from the juxtamembrane region to the intracellular tail of the receptor. Activation of the insulin receptor initiates signaling by phosphorylating a set of intracellular proteins such as the insulin receptor substrates (IRS) and Src-homology-2-containing protein (Shc). These IRS interact with effectors that amplify and extend the signaling cascade.

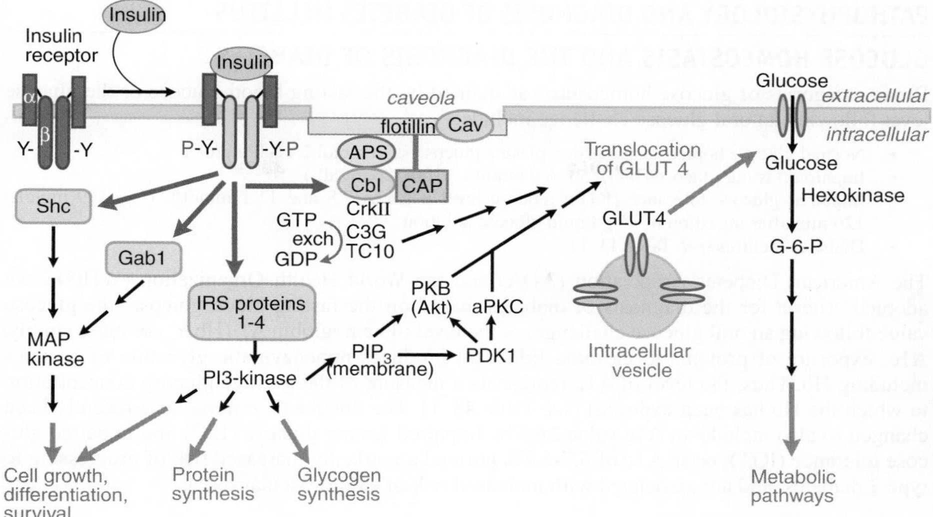

Figure 43–4 *Pathways of insulin signaling.* The binding of insulin to its plasma membrane receptor activates a cascade of downstream signaling events. Insulin binding activates the intrinsic tyrosine kinase activity of the receptor dimer, resulting in the tyrosine phosphorylation (Y-P) of the receptor's β subunits and a small number of specific substrates (*yellow shapes*): the insulin receptor substrate (IRS) proteins, Gab-1 and SHC; within the membrane, a caveolar pool of insulin receptor phosphorylates caveolin (Cav), APS, and Cbl. These tyrosine-phosphorylated proteins interact with signaling cascades via SH2 and SH3 domains to mediate the effects of insulin, with specific effects resulting from each pathway. In target tissues such as skeletal muscle and adipocytes, a key event is the translocation of the Glut4 glucose transporter from intracellular vesicles to the plasma membrane; this translocation is stimulated by both the caveolar and noncaveolar pathways. In the noncaveolar pathway, the activation of PI3K is crucial, and PKB/Akt (anchored at the membrane by PIP3) and/or an atypical form of PKC is involved. In the caveolar pathway, caveolar protein flotillin localizes the signaling complex to the caveola; the signaling pathway involves series of SH2 domain interactions that add the adaptor protein CrkII, the guanine nucleotide exchange protein C3G, and small GTP-binding protein, TC10. The pathways are inactivated by specific phosphoprotein phosphatases (e.g., PTB1B). In addition to the actions shown, insulin also stimulates the plasma membrane Na^+,K^+-ATPase by a mechanism that is still being elucidated; the result is an increase in pump activity and a net accumulation of K^+ in the cell. Abbreviations: APS, adaptor protein with PH and SH2 domains; CAP, Cbl associated protein; CrkII, chicken tumor virus regulator of kinase II; GLUT4, glucose transporter 4; Gab-1, Grb-2 associated binder; MAP kinase, mitogen-activated protein kinase; PDK, phosphoinositide-dependent kinase; PI3 kinase, phosphatidylinositol-3-kinase; PIP3, phosphatidylinositol trisphosphate; PKB, protein kinase B (also called Akt); aPKC, atypical isoform of protein kinase C; Y, tyrosine residue; Y-P, phosphorylated tyrosine residue.

Insulin action on glucose transport depends on the activation of phosphatidylinositol-3-kinase (PI3K). PI3K is activated by interaction with IRS proteins and generates phosphatidylinositol 3,4,5-trisphosphate (PIP3), which regulates the localization and activity of several downstream kinases, including Akt, atypical isoforms of protein kinase C (PKC ζ and λ/τ), and mammalian target of rapamycin (mTOR). The isoform Akt2 appears to control the downstream steps that are important for glucose uptake in skeletal muscle and adipose tissue, and to regulate glucose production in the liver. Substrates of Akt2 coordinate the translocation of the glucose transporter 4 (GLUT4) to the plasma membrane through processes involving actin remodeling and other membrane trafficking systems. Actions of small G-proteins, such as Rac and TC10, have also been implicated in the actin remodeling necessary for GLUT4 translocation. GLUT4 is expressed in insulin-responsive tissues such as skeletal muscle and adipose tissue. In the basal state, most GLUT4 resides in the intracellular space; following activation of insulin receptors, GLUT4 is shifted rapidly and in abundance to the plasma membrane, where it facilitates inward transport of glucose from the circulation. Insulin signaling also reduces GLUT4 endocytosis, increasing the residence time of the protein in the plasma membrane. Following the facilitated diffusion into cells along a concentration gradient, glucose is phosphorylated to glucose-6-phosphate (G-6-P) by hexokinases. Hexokinase II is found in association with GLUT4 in skeletal and cardiac muscle and in adipose tissue. Like GLUT4, hexokinase II is regulated transcriptionally by insulin. G-6-P can be isomerized to G-1-P and stored as glycogen (insulin enhances the activity of glycogen synthase); G-6-P can enter the glycolytic pathway (for ATP production) and the pentose phosphate pathway.

GLUCOSE HOMEOSTASIS AND THE DIAGNOSIS OF DIABETES

Broad categories of glucose homeostasis as defined by the fasting blood glucose or the glucose level following an oral glucose challenge include:

- Normal glucose homeostasis: fasting plasma glucose <5.6 mmol/L (100 mg/dL)
- Impaired fasting glucose (IFG): 5.6-6.9 mmol/L (100-125 mg/dL)
- Impaired glucose tolerance (IGT): glucose level between 7.8 and 11.1 mmol/L (140-199 mg/dL) 120 min after ingestion of 75 g liquid glucose solution
- Diabetes mellitus (*see* Table 43–1)

The American Diabetes Association (ADA) and the World Health Organization (WHO) have adopted criteria for the diagnosis of diabetes, based on the fasting blood glucose, the glucose value following an oral glucose challenge, or the level of hemoglobin A_{1c} (HbA_{1c}, or more simply, A1c; exposure of proteins to elevated [glucose] produces nonenzymatic glycation of proteins including Hb. Thus, the level of A1c represents a measure of the average glucose concentration to which the Hb has been exposed) (*see* Table 43–1). The diagnostic criteria have recently been changed to also include an A1c value ≥6.5%. Impaired fasting glucose (IFG) and impaired glucose tolerance (IGT), or an A1c of 5.7-6.4% portend a markedly increased risk of progressing to type 2 diabetes, and are associated with increased risk of cardiovascular disease.

The 4 categories of diabetes include type 1 diabetes, type 2 diabetes, other forms of diabetes, and gestational diabetes (Table 43–2). Although hyperglycemia is common to all forms of diabetes, the pathogenic mechanisms leading to diabetes are quite distinct.

SCREENING FOR DIABETES AND CATEGORIES OF INCREASED RISK OF DIABETES. Many individuals with type 2 diabetes are asymptomatic at the time of diagnosis, and diabetes is often found on routine blood testing for nonglucose-related reasons. The ADA recommends widespread screening for type 2 diabetes of these individuals with the following features:

- >45 years of age, or
- Body mass index >25 kg/m^2 with 1 of these additional risk factors: hypertension, low high-density lipoprotein, family history of type 2 diabetes, high-risk ethnic group (African American, Latino, Native American, Asian American, and Pacific Islander), abnormal glucose testing (IFG, IGT, A1c of 5.7-6.4%), cardiovascular disease, and women with polycystic ovary syndrome or who have previously delivered a large infant

Earlier diagnosis and treatment of type 2 diabetes should delay diabetes-related complications and reduce the burden of the disease. A number of interventions including pharmacological agents and lifestyle modification are effective. Screening for type 1 diabetes is not currently recommended.

PATHOGENESIS OF TYPE 1 DIABETES. Type 1 diabetes accounts for 5-10% of diabetes and results from autoimmune-mediated destruction of the β cells of the islet leading to total or near total insulin deficiency. Prior terminology included juvenile-onset diabetes mellitus or insulin-dependent diabetes mellitus. Type 1 diabetes resulting from autoimmune β cell destruction can occur at any age. Individuals with type 1 diabetes and their families have an increased prevalence of autoimmune diseases such as Addison disease, Graves and

Table 43–1

Criteria for the Diagnosis of Diabetes

- Symptoms of diabetes plus random blood glucose concentration ≥11.1 mM (200 mg/dL)[a] or
- Fasting plasma glucose ≥7.0 mM (126 mg/dL)[b] or
- Two-hour plasma glucose ≥11.1 mM (200 mg/dL) during an oral glucose tolerance test[c]
- HbA_{1c} ≥6.5%

[a]*Random is defined as without regard to time since the last meal.*
[b]*Fasting is defined as no caloric intake for at least 8 h.*
[c]*The test should be performed using a glucose load containing the equivalent of 75 g anhydrous glucose dissolved in water; this test is not recommended for routine clinical use.*
Note: *In the absence of unequivocal hyperglycemia and acute metabolic decompensation, these criteria should be confirmed by repeat testing on a different day.*
Source: Adapted from Diabetes Care, *2010;33:S62–S69.*

Table 43–2

Different Forms of Diabetes Mellitus

I. Type 1 diabetes β cell destruction, usually leading to absolute insulin deficiency)
   A. Immune-mediated
   B. Idiopathic

II. Type 2 diabetes (may range from predominantly insulin resistance with relative insulin deficiency to a predominantly insulin secretory defect with insulin resistance)

III. Other specific types of diabetes
   A. Genetic defects of β cell function characterized by mutations in:
      1. Hepatocyte nuclear transcription factor (HNF) 4α (MODY 1)
      2. Glucokinase (MODY 2)
      3. HNF-1α (MODY 3)
      4. Insulin promoter factor-1 (IPF-1; MODY 4)
      5. HNF-1β (MODY 5)
      6. NeuroD1 (MODY 6)
      7. Mitochondrial DNA
      8. Subunits of ATP-sensitive K^+ channel
      9. Proinsulin or insulin sequence conversion
   B. Genetic defects in insulin action
      1. Type A insulin resistance
      2. Leprechaunism
      3. Rabson-Mendenhall syndrome
      4. Lipodystrophy syndromes
   C. Diseases of the exocrine pancreas—pancreatitis, pancreatectomy, neoplasia, cystic fibrosis, hemochromatosis, fibrocalculous pancreatopathy, mutations in carboxyl ester lipase
   D. Endocrinopathies—acromegaly, Cushing syndrome, glucagonoma, pheochromocytoma, hyperthyroidism, somatostatinoma, aldosteronoma
   E. Drug- or chemical-induced—Vacor (a rodenticide); *see* Table 43–3
   F. Infections—congenital rubella, cytomegalovirus
   G. Uncommon forms of immune-mediated diabetes—"stiff-person" syndrome, anti-insulin receptor antibodies
   H. Other genetic syndromes sometimes associated with diabetes—Wolfram syndrome, Down syndrome, Klinefelter syndrome, Turner syndrome, Friedreich ataxia, Huntington disease, Laurence-Moon-Biedl syndrome, myotonic dystrophy, porphyria, Prader-Willi syndrome

IV. Gestational diabetes mellitus (GDM)

MODY, maturity onset of diabetes of the young.

Source: Copyright 2010 American Diabetes Association. From Diabetes Care, 2010;33(suppl 1):S62. Reprinted with permission from the American Diabetes Association.

Hashimoto disease, pernicious anemia, vitiligo, and celiac sprue. The concordance of type 1 diabetes in genetically identical twins is 40-60%, indicating a significant genetic component. The major genetic risk (40-50%) is conferred by HLA class II genes encoding HLA-DR and HLA-DQ (and possibly other genes with the HLA locus). However, there clearly is a critical interaction of genetics and an environmental or infectious agent. Most individuals with type 1 diabetes (~75%) do not have a family member with type 1 diabetes, and the genes conferring genetic susceptibility are found in a significant fraction of the nondiabetic population.

Genetically susceptible individuals are thought to have a normal β cell number or mass until β cell–directed autoimmunity develops and β cell loss begins. The initiating or triggering stimulus for the autoimmune process is not known, but most favor exposure to viruses (enterovirus, etc.) or other ubiquitous environmental agents. The β cell destruction is cell mediated, and there is also evidence that infiltrating cells produce local inflammatory agents such as TNF-α, IFN-γ, and IL-1, all of which can lead to β cell death. The β cell destruction occurs over a period of months to years and when >80% of the β cells are destroyed, hyperglycemia ensues and the clinical diagnosis of type 1 diabetes is made. Most patients report several weeks of polyuria and polydipsia, fatigue, and often abrupt and significant weight loss. Some adults with the phenotypic appearance of type 2 diabetes (obese, not insulin-requiring initially) have islet cell autoantibodies suggesting autoimmune-mediated β cell destruction and are diagnosed as expressing latent-autoimmune diabetes of adults (LADA).

PATHOGENESIS OF TYPE 2 DIABETES. The condition is best thought of as a heterogeneous syndrome of dysregulated glucose homeostasis associated with impaired insulin secretion and action. Overweight or obesity is a common correlate of type 2 diabetes that occurs in ~80% of affected individuals. For the vast majority of persons developing type 2 diabetes, there is no clear inciting incident; rather, the condition is thought to develop gradually over years with progression through identifiable prediabetic stages. Type 2 diabetes results when there is insufficient insulin action to maintain plasma glucose levels in the normal range. Insulin action is the composite effect of plasma insulin concentrations (determined by islet β cell function) and insulin sensitivity of key target tissues (liver, skeletal muscle, and adipose tissue). These sites of regulation are all impaired to variable extents in patients with type 2 diabetes (Figure 43–5). The etiology of type 2 diabetes has a strong genetic component. It is a heritable condition with a relative 4-fold increased risk of disease for persons having a diabetic parent or sibling, increasing to 6-fold if both parents have type 2 diabetes. Although more than 20 genetic loci with clear associations to type 2 diabetes have been identified through recent genome-wide association studies, the contribution of each is relatively small.

Impaired β Cell Function. In persons with type 2 diabetes, the sensitivity of the β cell to glucose is impaired, and there is also a loss of responsiveness to other stimuli such as insulinotropic GI hormones and neural signaling. This results in delayed secretion of insufficient amounts of insulin, allowing the blood glucose to rise dramatically after meals, and failure to restrain liver glucose release during fasting. The absolute mass of β cells also is greatly reduced in type 2 diabetes patients. Progressive reduction of β cell mass and function explains the natural history of type 2 diabetes in most patients who require steadily increasing therapy to maintain glucose control.

Type 2 diabetic patients frequently have elevated levels of fasting insulin, a result of their higher fasting glucose levels and insulin resistance. Another factor contributing to apparently high insulin levels early in the course of the disease is the presence of increased amounts of proinsulin. Proinsulin, the precursor to insulin, is inefficiently processed in the diabetic islet. Whereas healthy subjects have only 2-4% of total circulating insulin as proinsulin, type 2 diabetic patients can have 10-20% of the measurable plasma insulin in this form. Proinsulin has a considerably attenuated effect for lowering blood glucose compared to insulin.

Insulin Resistance. *Insulin sensitivity* is measured as the amount of glucose cleared from the blood in response to a dose of insulin. The failure of normal amounts of insulin to elicit the expected response is referred to as *insulin resistance.* There is inherent variability of insulin sensitivity among cells, tissues, and individuals. Insulin sensitivity is affected by many factors including age, body weight, physical activity levels, illness, and medications. Nonetheless, persons with type 2 diabetes or glucose intolerance have reduced responses to insulin and can easily be distinguished from groups with normal glucose tolerance.

The major insulin-responsive tissues are skeletal muscle, adipose tissue, and liver. Insulin resistance in muscle and fat is generally marked by a decrease in transport of glucose from the circulation. Hepatic insulin resistance generally refers to a blunted ability of insulin to suppress glucose production. Insulin resistance in

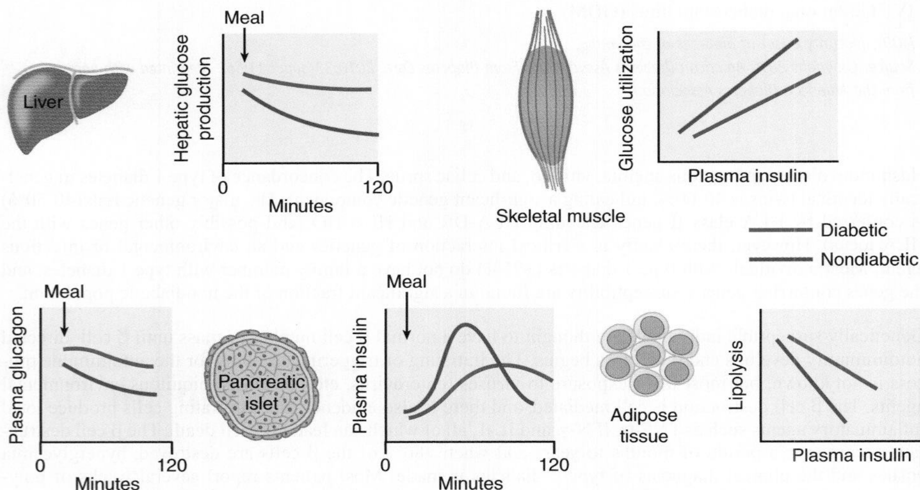

Figure 43–5 *Pathophysiology of type 2 diabetes mellitus.* Graphs show data from diabetic (——) and nondiabetic (——) patients, comparing postprandial insulin and glucagon secretion and hepatic glucose production, and the sensitivities of muscle glucose use and adipocyte lipolysis to insulin.

adipocytes causes increased rates of lipolysis and release of fatty acids into the circulation, which can contribute to insulin resistance in liver and muscle, hepatic steatosis, and dyslipidemia. The sensitivity of humans to the effects of insulin administration is inversely related to the amount of fat stored in the abdominal cavity; more visceral adiposity leads to more insulin resistance. Intracellular lipid or its by-products may have direct effects to impede insulin signaling. Enlarged collections of adipose tissue, visceral or otherwise, are often infiltrated with macrophages and can become sites of chronic inflammation. Adipocytokines, secreted from adipocytes and immune cells, including TNF-α, IL-6, resistin, and retinol-binding protein 4, can also cause systemic insulin resistance.

Sedentary persons are more insulin resistant than active ones, and physical training can improve insulin sensitivity. Physical activity can decrease the risk of developing diabetes and improve glycemic control in persons who have diabetes. Insulin resistance is more common in the elderly; within populations, insulin sensitivity decreases linearly with age. At the cellular level, insulin resistance involves blunted steps in the cascade from the insulin receptor tyrosine kinase to translocation of GLUT4 transporters, but the molecular mechanisms are incompletely defined. There have been >75 different mutations in the insulin receptor discovered, most of which cause significant impairment of insulin action. These mutations affect insulin receptor number, movement to and from the plasma membrane, binding, and phosphorylation. Mutations involving the insulin binding domains of the extracellular α-chain cause the most severe syndromes. Insulin sensitivity is under genetic control but it is unclear whether insulin-resistant individuals have mutations in specific components of the insulin signaling cascade or whether they have a complement of signaling effectors that operate at the lower range of normal. Regardless, it is apparent that insulin resistance clusters in families and is a major risk factor for the development of diabetes.

Dysregulated Hepatic Glucose Metabolism. In type 2 diabetes, hepatic glucose output is excessive in the fasting state and inadequately suppressed after meals. Abnormal secretion of the islet hormones, both insufficient insulin and excessive glucagon, accounts for a significant portion of dysregulated hepatic glucose metabolism in type 2 diabetes. Increased concentrations of glucagon, especially in conjunction with hepatic insulin resistance, can lead to excessive hepatic gluconeogenesis and glycogenolysis and abnormally high fasting glucose concentrations. The liver is resistant to insulin action in type 2 diabetes. This contributes to the reduced potency of insulin to suppress hepatic glucose production and promote hepatic glucose uptake and glycogen synthesis after meals. Despite ineffective insulin effects on hepatic glucose metabolism, the lipogenic effects of insulin in the liver are maintained and even accentuated by fasting hyperinsulinemia. This contributes to hepatic steatosis and further worsening of insulin resistance.

PATHOGENESIS OF OTHER FORMS OF DIABETES. Mutations in key genes involved in glucose homeostasis cause monogenic diabetes, which is inherited in an autosomal dominant fashion. These fall in 2 broad categories: diabetes onset in the immediate neonatal period (<6 months of age) and diabetes in children or adults. Some forms of neonatal diabetes are caused by mutations in the SUR or its accompanying inward rectifying K^+ channel and mutations in the insulin gene. Monogenic diabetes beyond the first year of life may appear clinically similar to type 1 or type 2 diabetes. In other instances, young individuals (adolescence to young adulthood) may have monogenic forms of diabetes known as maturity onset diabetes of the young (MODY). Phenotypically, these individuals are not obese and are not insulin resistant, or they may initially have modest hyperglycemia. The most common causes are mutations in key islet-enriched transcription factors or glucokinase. Most individuals with MODY are treated similarly to those with type 2 diabetes.

Diabetes may also be the result of other pathological processes such as acromegaly and Cushing disease (*see* Table 43–2). A number of medications promote hyperglycemia or lead to diabetes by either impairing insulin secretion or insulin action (Table 43–3).

DIABETES-RELATED COMPLICATIONS. Diabetes can cause metabolic derangements or acute complications, such as the life-threatening metabolic disorders of diabetic ketoacidosis and hyperglycemic hyperosmolar state. These require hospitalization for insulin administration, rehydration with intravenous fluids, and careful monitoring of electrolytes and metabolic parameters. Chronic complications of diabetes are commonly divided into microvascular and macrovascular complications. Microvascular complications occur only in individuals with diabetes and include retinopathy, nephropathy, and neuropathy. Macrovascular complications occur more frequently in individuals with diabetes but are not diabetes specific (e.g., increased atherosclerosis-related events such as myocardial infarction and stroke). In the U.S., diabetes is the leading cause of blindness in adults, the leading reason for renal failure requiring dialysis or renal transplantation, and the leading cause of nontraumatic lower extremity amputations. Fortunately, most of these diabetes-related complications can be prevented, delayed, or reduced by near normalization of the blood glucose on a consistent basis. How chronic hyperglycemia causes these complications is unclear. For microvascular complications, current hypothesis are that hyperglycemia leads to advanced glycosylation end products (AGEs), increased glucose metabolism via the sorbitol pathway, increased formation of diacylglycerol leading to PKC activation, and increased flux through the hexosamine pathway. Growth factors such as vascular endothelial growth factor α may be involved in diabetic retinopathy and TGF-β in diabetic nephropathy.

Table 43–3

Some Drugs That May Promote Hyperglycemia or Hypoglycemia

HYPERGLYCEMIA	HYPOGLYCEMIA
Glucocorticoids, T_3, T_4	β Adrenergic antagonists, ACE inhibitors
Antipsychotics (atypical, others)	Ethanol, LiCl, theophylline
Protease inhibitors, pentamidine	Salicylates, nonsteroidal anti-inflamatory drugs
β Adrenergic agonists, epinephrine	Pentamidine, bromocriptine, mebendazole
Diuretics (thiazide, loop)	
Hydantoins (phenytoin, others)	
Opioids (fentanyl, morphine, others)	
Diazoxide, nicotinic acid	
Interferons, amphotericin B	
Acamprosate, basiliximab, asparaginase	

For additional details, see Murad MH, Coto-Yglesias F, Wang AT, et al. Clinical review: Drug-induced hypoglycemia; a systematic review. J Clin Endocrinol Metab, 2009, 94:741–745.

THERAPY OF DIABETES

GOALS OF THERAPY. The goals of therapy for diabetes are to alleviate the symptoms related to hyperglycemia (fatigue, polyuria, etc.) and to prevent or reduce the acute and chronic complications of diabetes.

Glycemic control is assessed using both short-term (blood glucose self-monitoring) and long-term metrics (A1c, fructosamine). Using capillary blood glucose measurements, the patient assesses capillary blood glucose on a regular basis (fasting, before meals, or postprandially) and reports these values to the diabetes management team. A1c reflects glycemic control over the prior 3 months; glycosylated albumin (fructosamine) is a measure of glycemic control over the preceding 2 weeks. The term *comprehensive diabetes care* describes optimal therapy, which involves more than glucose management and includes aggressive treatment of abnormalities in blood pressure and lipids and detection and management of diabetes-related complications (Figure 43–6). Table 43–4 shows the ADA-recommended treatment goals for comprehensive diabetes care, for glucose, blood pressure, and lipids. A summary of available pharmacologic agents for the treatment of diabetes is at the end of this chapter (*see* Table 43–8).

NONPHARMACOLOGIC ASPECTS OF DIABETES THERAPY. The patient with diabetes should be educated about nutrition, exercise, and medications aimed at lowering the plasma glucose. In type 1 diabetes, matching caloric intake and insulin dosing is very important. In type 2 diabetes, the diet is directed at weight loss and reducing blood pressure and atherosclerotic risk. Remarkably, bariatric surgery also rapidly improves glucose tolerance and can prevent or reverse type 2 diabetes.

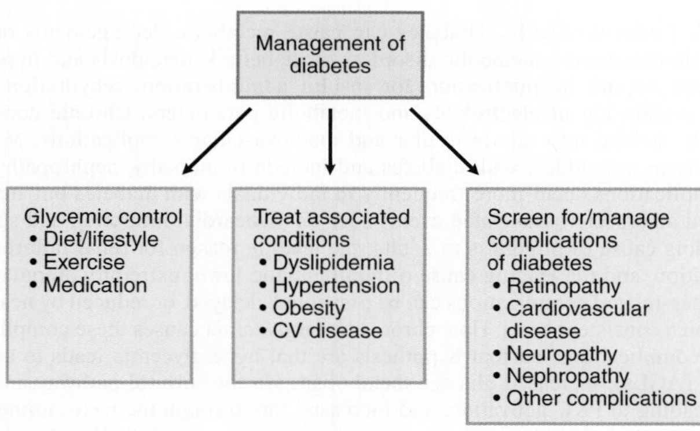

Figure 43–6 *Components of comprehensive diabetes care.*

Table 43–4

Goals of Therapy in Diabetes

INDEX	GOAL[a]
Glycemic control[b]	
A1C	<7.0%[c]
Preprandial capillary plasma glucose	3.9-7.2 mmol/L (70-130 mg/dL)
Peak postprandial capillary plasma glucose	10.0 mmol/L (<180 mg/dL)[d]
Blood pressure	<130/80
Lipids[e]	
Low-density lipoprotein	<2.6 mmol/L (<100 mg/dL)[f]
High-density lipoprotein	>1.1 mmol/L (>40 mg/dL)[g]
Triglycerides	<1.7 mmol/L (<150 mg/dL)

[a]*Goals should be individualized for each patient and may be different for certain patient populations.*
[b]*A1C is primary goal.*
[c]*While the ADA recommends an A1C <7.0% in general, it recommends an appropriate goal for the individual patient based on age, duration of diabetes, life expectancy, other medical conditions, cardiovascular disease).*
[d]*One to two hours after beginning of a meal.*
[e]*In decreasing order of priority*
[f]*In individuals with coronary artery disease, an LDL <1.8 mmol (70 mg/dL) is the goal.*
[g]*For women, some suggest a goal that is 0.25 mmol/L (10 mg/dL) higher.*
Source: Adapted from Diabetes Care, *2010;33:S11.*

INSULIN THERAPY

Insulin is the mainstay for treatment of virtually all type 1 and many type 2 diabetes patients. Insulin may be administered intravenously, intramuscularly, or subcutaneously. Long-term treatment relies predominantly on subcutaneous injection. Subcutaneous administration of insulin delivered into the peripheral circulation can lead to near-normal glycemia but differs from physiological secretion of insulin in 2 major ways:

- The absorption kinetics do not reproduce the rapid rise and decline of endogenous insulin in response to glucose following intravenous or oral administration.
- Injected insulin is delivered into the peripheral circulation instead of being released into the portal circulation. Thus, the portal/peripheral insulin concentration is not physiological, and this may alter the influence of insulin on hepatic metabolic processes.

INSULIN PREPARATION AND CHEMISTRY. Human insulin, produced by recombinant DNA technology, is soluble in aqueous solution. Doses and concentration of clinically used insulin preparations are expressed in international units. One unit of insulin is defined as the amount required to reduce the blood glucose concentration in a fasting rabbit to 45 mg/dL (2.5 mM). Commercial preparations of insulin are supplied in solution or suspension at a concentration of 100 units/mL, which is ~3.6 mg insulin per milliliter (0.6 mM) and termed U-100. Insulin also is available in a more concentrated solution (500 units/mL or U-500) for patients who are resistant to the hormone.

INSULIN FORMULATIONS. Preparations of insulin are classified according to their duration of action into *short-acting* and *long-acting* (Table 43–5).

Within the short-acting acting category, some distinguish the very rapid-acting insulins (aspart, glulisine, lispro) from regular insulin. Likewise, some distinguish formulations with a longer duration of action (detemir, glargine) from NPH insulin. Two approaches are used to modify the absorption and pharmacokinetic profile of insulin. The first approach is based on formulations that slow the absorption following subcutaneous injection. The other approach is to alter the amino acid sequence or protein structure of human insulin so that it retains its ability to bind the insulin receptor, but its behavior in solution or following injection is either accelerated or prolonged in comparison to native or regular insulin (Figure 43–7). There is wide variability in the kinetics of insulin action between and even within individuals. The time to peak hypoglycemic effect and insulin levels can vary by 50%, due in part, by large variations in the rate of subcutaneous absorption.

Short-Acting Regular Insulin. Native or regular insulin molecules associate as hexamers in aqueous solution at a neutral pH and this aggregation slows absorption following subcutaneous injection. Regular insulin should be injected 30-45 min before a meal. Regular insulin also may be given intravenously or intramuscularly.

Table 43–5

Properties of Insulin Preparations

PREPARATION		TIME OF ACTION		
		ONSET (h)	PEAK (h)	EFFECTIVE DURATION, (h)
Short-acting				
	Aspart	<0.25	0.5-1.5	3-4
	Glulisine	<0.25	0.5-1.5	3-4
	Lispro	<0.25	0.5-1.5	3-4
	Regular	0.5-1.0	2-3	4-6
Long-acting				
	Detemir	1-4	—[a]	20-24
	Glargine	1-4	—[a]	20-24
	NPH	1-4	6-10	10-16
Insulin combinations				
	75/25-75% protamine lispro, 25% lispro	<0.25	1.5 h	Up to 10-16
	70/30-70% protamine aspart, 30% aspart	<0.25	1.5 h	Up to 10-16
	50/50-50% protamine lispro, 50% lispro	<0.25	1.5 h	Up to 10-16
	70/30-70% NPH, 30% regular	0.5-1	Dual[b]	10-16

[a]Glargine and detemir have minimal peak activity.

[b]Dual: two peaks - one at 2-3 h; the second one several hours later.

Source: Copyright 2004 American Diabetes Association. Adapted with permission from Skyler JS. Insulin treatment. In: Lebovitz HE, ed. Therapy for Diabetes Mellitus. Alexandria, VA: American Diabetes Association; 2004.

Short-Acting Insulin Analogs. These analogs are absorbed more rapidly from subcutaneous sites than regular insulin (*see* Figures 43–7 and 43–8; *see* Table 43–5). Insulin analogs should be injected ≤15 min before a meal.

Insulin lispro (HUMALOG) is identical to human insulin except at positions B28 and B29. Unlike regular insulin, lispro dissociates into monomers almost instantaneously following injection. This property results in the characteristic rapid absorption and shorter duration of action compared with regular insulin. The prevalence of hypoglycemia is reduced with lispro; and glucose control, as assessed by A1c, is modestly but significantly improved (0.3-0.5%).

Insulin aspart (NOVOLOG) is formed by the replacement of proline at B28 with aspartic acid, reducing self-association. Like lispro, insulin aspart dissociates rapidly into monomers following injection. Insulin aspart and insulin lispro have similar effects on glucose control and hypoglycemia frequency, with lower rates of nocturnal hypoglycemia as compared with regular insulin.

Insulin glulisine (APIDRA) is formed when glutamic acid replaces lysine at B29, and lysine replaces asparagine at B3; these substitutions result in a reduction in self-association and rapid dissociation into active monomers. The time–action profile of insulin glulisine is similar to that of insulin aspart and insulin lispro.

Long-Acting Insulins. *Neutral protamine hagedorn* (NPH; insulin isophane) is a suspension of native insulin complexed with zinc and protamine in a phosphate buffer. This produces a cloudy or whitish solution in contrast to the clear appearance of other insulin solutions. This formulation dissolves more gradually when injected subcutaneously and thus its duration of action is prolonged. NPH insulin is usually given either once a day (at bedtime) or twice a day in combination with short-acting insulin.

Insulin glargine (LANTUS) is a long-acting analog of human insulin. Two arginine residues are added to the C terminus of the B chain, and an asparagine molecule in position 21 on the A chain is replaced with glycine. Insulin glargine is a clear solution with a pH of 4.0, which stabilizes the insulin hexamer. When injected into the neutral pH of the subcutaneous space, aggregation occurs, resulting in prolonged, but predictable, absorption from the injection site. Owing to insulin glargine's acidic pH, it cannot be mixed with short-acting insulin preparations that are formulated at a neutral pH. Glargine has a sustained peakless absorption profile, and

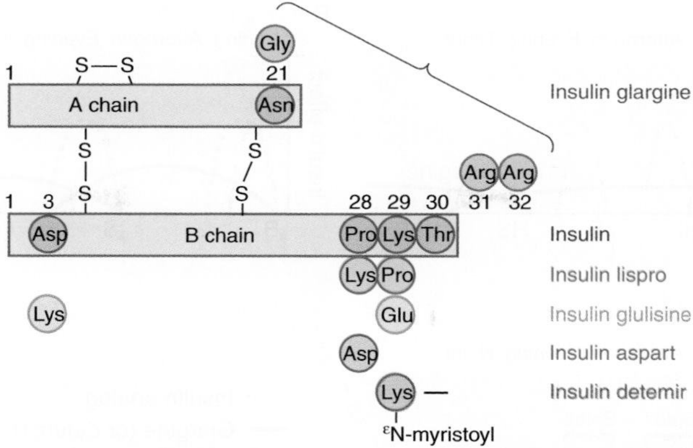

Figure 43–7 *Insulin analogs.* Modifications of native insulin can alter its pharmacokinetic profile. Reversing amino acids 28 and 29 in the B chain (lispro) or substituting Asp for Pro^{28B} (aspart) gives analogs with reduced tendencies for molecular self-association that are faster acting. Altering Asp^{3B} to Lys and Lys^{29B} to Glu produces an insulin (glulisine) with a more rapid onset and a shorter duration of action. Substituting Gly for Asn^{21A} and lengthening the B chain by adding Arg^{31} and Arg^{32} produces a derivative (glargine) with reduced solubility at pH 7.4 that is, consequently, absorbed more slowly and acts over a longer period of time. Deleting Thr^{30B} and adding a myristoyl group to the ε-amino group of Lys^{29B} (detemir) enhances reversible binding to albumin, thereby slowing transport across vascular endothelium to tissues and providing prolonged action.

provides a better once-daily 24-h insulin coverage than NPH insulin. Clinical trial data suggest that glargine has a lower risk of hypoglycemia, particularly overnight compared to NPH insulin. Glargine may be administered at any time during the day with equivalent efficacy and does not accumulate after several injections. The site of administration does not influence the time–action profile of glargine.

Insulin detemir (LEVEMIR) is an insulin analog modified by the addition of a saturated fatty acid to the ε amino group of LysB29, yielding a myristoylated insulin. When insulin detemir is injected subcutaneously, it binds to albumin via its fatty acid chain. Clinical studies in patients with type 1 diabetes have demonstrated that when insulin detemir is administered twice a day, it has a smoother time–action profile and produces a reduced prevalence of hypoglycemia than NPH insulin. The absorption profiles of glargine and detemir insulin are similar, but detemir often requires twice-daily administration.

Other Insulin Formulations. Stable combinations of NPH and regular insulin in proportions of 70:30 combinations are available, as are combinations of lispro protamine/lispro (50/50 and 75/25) and aspart protamine/aspart (70/30) (*see* Table 43–5).

INSULIN DELIVERY. Most insulin is injected subcutaneously. Pen devices containing prefilled regular, lispro, NPH, glargine, premixed lispro protamine-lispro, or premixed aspart protamine-aspart have proven to be popular with many diabetic patients. Jet injector systems that enable patients to receive subcutaneous insulin injections without a needle are available. Intravenous infusions of insulin are useful in patients with ketoacidosis or when requirements for insulin may change rapidly, such as during the perioperative period, during labor and delivery, and in intensive care situations.

Continuous Subcutaneous Insulin Infusion (CSII). Short-acting insulins are the only form of the hormone used in subcutaneous infusion pumps. A number of pumps are available for CSII therapy. Insulin pumps provide a constant basal infusion of insulin and have the option of different infusion rates during the day and night to help avoid the dawn phenomenon (rise in blood glucose that occurs just prior to awakening from sleep) and bolus injections that are programmed according to the size and nature of a meal. Selection of the most appropriate patients is extremely important for success with CSII. Pump therapy is capable of producing a more physiological profile of insulin replacement during exercise (where insulin production is decreased) and therefore less hypoglycemia than do traditional subcutaneous insulin injections.

FACTORS THAT AFFECT INSULIN ABSORPTION. Factors that determine the rate of absorption of insulin after subcutaneous administration include the site of injection, the type of insulin, subcutaneous blood flow, smoking, regional muscular activity at the site of the injection, the volume and concentration of the injected insulin, and depth of injection (insulin has a more rapid onset of action if delivered intramuscularly rather

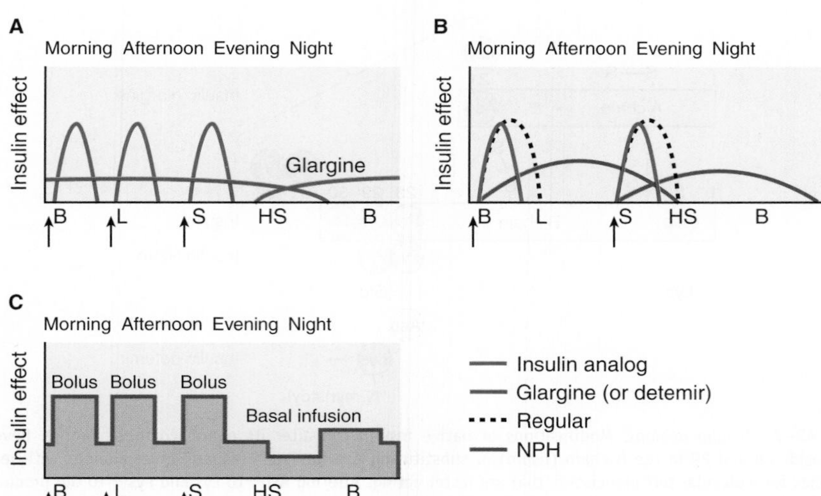

Figure 43–8 Commonly used insulin regimens. Panel A shows administration of a long-acting insulin like glargine (detemir could also be used but often requires twice-daily administration) to provide basal insulin and a pre-meal short-acting insulin analog (*see* Table 43–5). Panel B shows a less intensive insulin regimen with BID injection of NPH insulin providing basal insulin and regular insulin or an insulin analog providing meal-time insulin coverage. Only 1 type of shorting-acting insulin would be used. Panel C shows the insulin level attained following subcutaneous insulin (short-acting insulin analog) by an insulin pump programmed to deliver different basal rates. At each meal, an insulin bolus is delivered. B, breakfast; L, lunch; S, supper; HS, bedtime. *Upward arrow* shows insulin administration at mealtime. (Copyright 2008 American Diabetes Association. From Kaufman FR, ed. *Medical Management of Type 1 Diabetes*, 5th ed. Modified with permission from the American Diabetes Association.)

than subcutaneously). Increased subcutaneous blood flow (brought about by massage, hot baths, or exercise) increases the rate of absorption. The abdomen currently is the preferred site of injection in the morning because insulin is absorbed 20-30% faster from that site than from the arm. Rotation of insulin injection sites traditionally has been advocated to avoid lipohypertrophy or lipoatrophy. In a small group of patients, subcutaneous degradation of insulin has been observed, and this has necessitated the injection of large amounts of insulin for adequate metabolic control.

INSULIN DOSING AND REGIMENS. A number of commonly used dosage regimens that include mixtures of insulin given in 2 or more daily injections are depicted in Figure 43–8.

In most patients, insulin-replacement therapy includes long-acting insulin (basal) and a short-acting insulin to provide postprandial needs. In a mixed population of type 1 diabetes patients, the average dose of insulin is usually 0.6-0.7 units/kg body weight per day, with a range of 0.2-1 units/kg/day. Obese patients generally and pubertal adolescents require more (~1-2 units/kg/day) because of resistance of peripheral tissues to insulin. Patients who require less insulin than 0.5 units/kg/day may have some endogenous production of insulin or may be more sensitive to the hormone because of good physical conditioning. The basal dose is usually 40-50% of the total daily dose with the remainder as prandial or pre-meal insulin. The insulin dose at mealtime should reflect the anticipated carbohydrate intake. A supplemental scale of short-acting insulin is added to the prandial insulin dose to allow correction of the BG. *Insulin administered as a single daily dose of long-acting insulin, alone or in combination with short-acting insulin, is rarely sufficient to achieve euglycemia. More complex regimens that include multiple injections of long-acting or short-acting insulin are needed to reach this goal. In all patients, careful monitoring of therapeutic end points directs the insulin dose used. This approach is facilitated by self-monitoring of glucose and measurements of A1c.* In patients who have gastroparesis or loss of appetite, injection of a short-acting analog postprandially, based on the amount of food actually consumed, may provide smoother glycemic control.

ADVERSE EVENTS. Hypoglycemia is the major risk that must be weighed against benefits of efforts to normalize glucose control. Insulin treatment of both type 1 and type 2 diabetes is associated with modest weight gain. Although uncommon, allergic reactions to recombinant human insulin may still occur as a result of reaction to the small amounts of aggregated or denatured insulin in preparations, to minor contaminants, or because of sensitivity to a component added to insulin in its formulation (protamine, Zn^{2+}, etc.). Atrophy of subcutaneous fat at the site of insulin injection (lipoatrophy) was a rare side effect of older insulin preparations. Lipohypertrophy (enlargement of subcutaneous fat depots) has been ascribed to the lipogenic action of high local concentrations of insulin.

INSULIN TREATMENT OF KETOACIDOSIS AND OTHER SPECIAL SITUATIONS. Intravenous administration of insulin is most appropriate in patients with ketoacidosis or severe hyperglycemia with a hyperosmolar state. Insulin infusion inhibits lipolysis and gluconeogenesis completely and produces near-maximal stimulation of glucose uptake. In most patients with diabetic ketoacidosis, blood glucose concentrations will fall by ~10% per hour; the acidosis is corrected more slowly. As treatment proceeds, it often is necessary to administer glucose along with the insulin to prevent hypoglycemia but to allow clearance of all ketones. Patients with nonketotic hyperglycemic hyperosmolar state may be more sensitive to insulin than are those with ketoacidosis. Appropriate replacement of fluid and electrolytes is an integral part of the therapy in both situations because there is always a major deficit. A long-acting insulin should be administered subcutaneously before the insulin infusion is discontinued.

TREATMENT OF DIABETES IN CHILDREN OR ADOLESCENTS. Diabetes is one of the most common chronic diseases of childhood, and rates of type 1 diabetes in American youth are estimated at 1 in 300. An unfortunate corollary of the growing rates of obesity over the past 3 decades is an increase in the numbers of children and adolescents with non-autoimmune, or type 2, diabetes. Current estimates are that 15-20% of new cases of pediatric diabetes may be type 2 diabetes; rates vary by ethnicity, with disproportionately high rates in Native Americans, African Americans, and Latinos. Current practice is for more intensive, physiologically based insulin replacement with a goal of tight glucose control achieved with combinations of basal and prandial insulin replacement. The primary limiting factor of more aggressive insulin therapy is hypoglycemia. Diabetic patients <5 years old have increased rates of severe hypoglycemia with seizures and coma, and may suffer permanent cognitive dysfunction as a result of repeated episodes of low blood glucose. Older children and adolescents do not seem to have demonstrable cognitive impairment related to hypoglycemia; good glycemic control is associated with better mental function. The standard for insulin treatment now includes multiple dose regimens with 3-5 injections per day or CSII. Split/mixed regimens using NPH and regular insulin have been increasingly supplanted by regimens using insulin analogs because they offer more flexibility in dosing and meal patterns. Similarly, CSII is used with increasing frequency in the pediatric diabetic population and in older children and adolescents.

Because of the association of type 2 diabetes with obesity in the pediatric age group, lifestyle management is the recommended first step in therapy. Goals of reducing body weight and increasing physical activity are broadly recommended. The only medication currently approved by the FDA specifically for medical treatment of type 2 diabetes is *metformin*. Metformin is approved for children as young as 10 years of age and is available in a liquid formulation (100 mg/mL). Insulin is the typical second line of therapy after metformin; basal insulin can be added to oral agent therapy or multiple daily injections can be used when simpler regimens are not successful. Weight gain is a more significant problem than hypoglycemia with insulin treatment in pediatric type 2 diabetes.

MANAGEMENT OF DIABETES IN HOSPITALIZED PATIENTS. Hyperglycemia is common in hospitalized patients. Prevalence estimates of elevated blood glucose among inpatients with and without a prior diagnosis of diabetes range between 20% and 100% for patients treated in intensive care units (ICUs) and 30% and 83% outside the ICU. Stress of illness has been associated with insulin resistance, possibly the result of counter-regulatory hormone secretion, cytokines, and other inflammatory mediators. Food intake is often variable due to concurrent illness or preparation for diagnostic testing. Medications used in the hospital, such as glucocorticoids or dextrose-containing intravenous solutions, can exacerbate tendencies toward hyperglycemia. Finally fluid balance and tissue perfusion can affect the absorbance of subcutaneous insulin and the clearance of glucose. Therapy of hyperglycemia in hospitalized patients needs to be adjusted for these variables.

Emerging data indicate that hyperglycemia portends poor outcomes in hospitalized patients. The ADA currently suggests these blood glucose targets: 140-180 m/dL (7.8-10.0 mM) in critically ill patients and random glucose of 180 mg/dL (10 mM) or pre-meal glucose of 140 mg/dL (7.8 mM) in noncritically ill patients. Insulin is the cornerstone of treatment of hyperglycemia in hospitalized patients. For critically ill patients and those with variable blood pressure, edema, and tissue perfusion, intravenous insulin is the treatment of choice. Oral agents have a limited place in treatment of hyperglycemic patients in the hospital because of slow onset of action, insufficient potency, need for intact GI function, and side effects. Intravenous administration of insulin also is well suited to the treatment of diabetic patients during the perioperative period and during childbirth.

INSULIN SECRETAGOGUES AND ORAL HYPOGLYCEMIC AGENTS

A variety of sulfonylureas, meglitinides, GLP-1 agonists, and inhibitors of dipeptidyl peptidase-4 (DPP-4) are used as secretagogues to stimulate insulin release (Table 43–6).

Table 43–6

Properties of Insulin Secretagogues

CLASS/GENERIC NAME	DAILY DOSAGE[a], mg	DURATION OF ACTION, h
Sulfonylureas - 1st generation		
Chlorpropamide	100-500	>48
Tolazamide	100-1000	12-24
Tolbutamide	1000-3000	6-12
Sulfonylureas - 2nd generation		
Glimepiride	1-8	24
Glipizide	5-40	12-18
Glipizide (extended release)	5-20	24
Glyburide	1.25-20	12-24
Glyburide (micronized)	0.75-12	12-24
Nonsulfonylureas (Meglitinides)		
Repaglinide	0.5-16	2-6
Nateglinide	180-360	2-4
GLP-1 agonist		
Exenatide	0.01-0.02	4-6
Dipeptidyl Peptidase-4 Inhibitors		
Saxagliptin	2.5-5	
Sitagliptin	100	12-16
Vildagliptin	50-100	12-24

[a]Dose may be lower in some patients

K_{ATP} CHANNEL MODULATORS: SULFONYLUREAS

First-generation sulfonylureas (tolbutamide, tolazamide, and chlorpropamide) are rarely used now in the treatment of type 2 diabetes. The second, more potent generation of hypoglycemic sulfonylureas includes glyburide (glibenclamide; DIABETA, others), glipizide (GLUCOTROL, others), and glimepiride (AMARYL, others). Some are available in an extended-release (glipizide) or a micronized (glyburide) formulation.

MECHANISM OF ACTION. Sulfonylureas stimulate insulin release by binding to a specific site on the β cell K_{ATP} channel complex (SUR) and inhibiting its activity. K_{ATP} channel inhibition causes cell membrane depolarization and the cascade of events leading to insulin secretion (*see* Figure 43–3). The acute administration of sulfonylureas to type 2 diabetes patients increases insulin release from the pancreas. With chronic administration, circulating insulin levels decline to those that existed before treatment, but despite this reduction in insulin levels, reduced plasma glucose levels are maintained. The absence of acute stimulatory effects of sulfonylureas on insulin secretion during chronic treatment is attributed to downregulation of cell surface receptors for sulfonylureas on the pancreatic β cell.

ADME. Sulfonylureas are effectively absorbed from the GI tract. Food and hyperglycemia can reduce absorption. Sulfonylureas in plasma are largely (90-99%) bound to protein, especially albumin. The volumes of distribution of most of the sulfonylureas are ~0.2 L/kg. Although their half-lives are short (3-5 h), their hypoglycemic effects are evident for 12-24 h, and they often can be administered once daily. The liver metabolizes all sulfonylureas, and the metabolites are excreted in the urine. Thus, sulfonylureas should be administered with caution to patients with either renal or hepatic insufficiency.

ADVERSE EFFECTS AND DRUG INTERACTIONS. Sulfonylureas may cause hypoglycemic reactions, including coma. Weight gain of 1-3 kg is a common side effect of improving glycemic control with sulfonylurea treatment. Less frequent side effects include nausea and vomiting, cholestatic jaundice, agranulocytosis, aplastic and hemolytic anemias, generalized hypersensitivity reactions, and dermatological reactions. Rarely, patients treated with these drugs develop an alcohol-induced flush similar to that caused by disulfiram or hyponatremia.

The hypoglycemic effect of sulfonylureas may be enhanced by various mechanisms (decreased hepatic metabolism or renal excretion, displacement from protein-binding sites). Some drugs (sulfonamides, clofibrate, and salicylates) displace the sulfonylureas from binding proteins, thereby transiently increasing the concentration of free drug. Ethanol may enhance the action of sulfonylureas and cause hypoglycemia. Hypoglycemia may be more frequent in patients taking a sulfonylurea and 1 of these agents: androgens, anticoagulants, azole antifungals, chloramphenicol, fenfluramine, fluconazole, gemfibrozil, H_2 antagonists, magnesium salts, methyldopa, MAO inhibitors, probenecid, sulfinpyrazone, sulfonamides, tricyclic antidepressants, and urinary acidifiers. Other drugs may decrease the glucose-lowering effect of sulfonylureas by increased hepatic metabolism, increased renal excretion, or inhibiting insulin secretion (β blockers, Ca^{2+} channel blockers, cholestyramine, diazoxide, estrogens, hydantoins, isoniazid, nicotinic acid, phenothiazines, rifampin, sympathomimetics, thiazide diuretics, and urinary alkalinizers).

DOSAGE FORMS AVAILABLE. Treatment is initiated at lower end of the dose range and titrated upward based on the patient's glycemic response. Some have a longer duration of action and can be prescribed in a single daily dose (glimepiride), whereas others are formulated as extended-release or micronized formulations to extend their duration of action (*see* Table 43–6). Sulfonylureas such as glipizide or glimepiride appear safer in elderly individuals with type 2 diabetes.

THERAPEUTIC USES. Sulfonylureas are used to treat hyperglycemia in type 2 diabetes. Of properly selected patients, 50-80% respond to this class of agents. All members of the class appear be equally efficacious. A significant number of patients who respond initially later cease to respond to the sulfonylurea and develop unacceptable hyperglycemia (secondary failure). This may occur as a result of a change in drug metabolism or more likely from a progression of β cell failure. Some individuals with neonatal diabetes or MODY-3 respond to these agents. Contraindications to the use of these drugs include type 1 diabetes, pregnancy, lactation, and, for the older preparations, significant hepatic or renal insufficiency.

K_{ATP} CHANNEL MODULATORS: NONSULFONYLUREAS

REPAGLINIDE. Repaglinide (PRANDIN) is an oral insulin secretagogue of the meglitinide class (*see* Table 43–6). Like sulfonylureas, it stimulates insulin release by closing K_{ATP} channels in pancreatic β cells.

The drug is absorbed rapidly from the GI tract, and peak blood levels are obtained within 1 h. The $t_{1/2}$ is ~1 h. These features allow for multiple preprandial use. Repaglinide is metabolized primarily by the liver (CYP3A4) to inactive derivatives. Because a small proportion (~10%) is metabolized by the kidney, dosing of the drug in patients with renal insufficiency also should be performed cautiously. The major side effect of repaglinide is hypoglycemia. Repaglinide also is associated with a decline in efficacy (secondary failure) after initially improving glycemic control. Certain drugs may potentiate the action of repaglinide by displacing it from plasma protein binding sites (β blockers, chloramphenicol, coumarins, MAOIs, NSAIDs, probenecid, salicylates, and sulfonamide) or altering its metabolism (gemfibrozil, itraconazole, trimethoprim, cyclosporine, simvastatin, clarithromycin).

NATEGLINIDE. Nateglinide (STARLIX) is an orally effective insulin secretagogue. Nateglinide stimulates insulin secretion by blocking K_{ATP} channels in pancreatic β cells. Nateglinide promotes a more rapid but less sustained secretion of insulin than other available oral antidiabetic agents. The drug's major therapeutic effect is reducing postprandial glycemic elevations in type 2 diabetes patients.

Nateglinide is most effective when administered in a dose of 120 mg, 1-10 min before a meal. It is metabolized primarily by hepatic CYPs (2C9, 70%; 3A4, 30%) and should be used cautiously in patients with hepatic insufficiency. About 16% of an administered dose is excreted by the kidney as unchanged drug. Some drugs reduce the glucose-lowering effect of nateglinide (corticosteroids, rifamycins, sympathomimetics, thiazide diuretics, thyroid products); others (alcohol, NSAIDs, salicylates, MAOIs, and nonselective β blockers) may increase the risk of hypoglycemia with nateglinide. Nateglinide therapy may produce fewer episodes of hypoglycemia than other currently available oral insulin secretagogues including repaglinide. As with sulfonylureas and repaglinide, secondary failure occurs.

AMPK AND PPARγ ACTIVATORS

METFORMIN. Metformin (GLUCOPHAGE, others) is the only member of the biguanide class of oral hypoglycemic drugs available for use today.

Mechanism of Action. Metformin increases the activity of the AMP-dependent protein kinase (AMPK). AMPK is activated by phosphorylation when cellular energy stores are reduced. Activated AMPK stimulates fatty acid oxidation, glucose uptake, and nonoxidative metabolism, and it reduces lipogenesis and gluconeogenesis. The net result of these actions is increased glycogen storage in skeletal muscle, lower rates of hepatic glucose production, increased insulin sensitivity, and lower blood glucose levels.

Table 43–7

Comparison of Metformin and Thiazolidinediones

PARAMETER	METFORMIN	THIAZOLIDINEDIONES
Molecular target	AMPK	PPARγ
Pharmacologic action	Suppression of HGP	Enhanced insulin sensitivity
Reduction of HbA_{1c}[a]	1.0-1.25%	0.5-1.4%
Reduction of FFA	Minimal	Moderate
Stimulation of adiponectin	Minimal	Significant
Effect on body weight	Minimal	Increased
Peripheral edema	Minimal	Moderate
Fracture risk	None	Increased
Lactic acidosis	Rare[b]	None

HGP, hepatic glucose production.
[a]*Magnitude of absolute reduction dependent on starting A1C value*
[b]*In renal insufficiency*

The molecular mechanism by which metformin activates AMPK is not known; it may be indirect, possibly via reduction of intracellular energy stores. Metformin has little effect on blood glucose in normoglycemic states, does not affect the release of insulin or other islet hormones, and rarely causes hypoglycemia. However, even in persons with only mild hyperglycemia, metformin lowers blood glucose by reducing hepatic glucose production and increasing peripheral glucose uptake. This effect is at least partially mediated by reducing insulin resistance at key target tissues. Table 43–7 compares metformin and thiazolidinediones (glitazones).

ADME

Metformin is absorbed primarily from the small intestine. The drug does not bind to plasma proteins, and is excreted unchanged in the urine. It has a $t_{1/2}$ in the circulation of ~2 h. The transport of metformin into cells is mediated in part by organic cation transporters OCT 1 and OCT 2.

THERAPEUTIC USES AND DOSAGE. Metformin, currently the most commonly used oral agent for type 2 diabetes, is generally accepted as the first-line treatment for this condition. Metformin is effective as monotherapy and in combination therapy. Fixed-dose combinations of metformin in conjunction with glipizide, glyburide, pioglitazone, repaglinide, rosiglitazone, and sitagliptin are available. Metformin is available as an immediate-release form. The currently recommended dosing is 0.5-1.0 g twice daily, with a maximum dose of 2550 mg. A sustained-release preparation is available for once-daily dosing; the maximum dose is 2 g.

Metformin has superior or equivalent efficacy of glucose lowering compared to other oral agents used to treat diabetes, and reduces diabetes-related complications in patients with type 2 diabetes. Metformin does not typically cause weight gain and in some cases causes weight reduction. Metformin is not effective in the treatment of type 1 diabetes. In persons with IGT, treatment with metformin delays the progression to diabetes. Metformin has been used as a treatment for infertility in women with the polycystic ovarian syndrome. Although not formally approved for this purpose, metformin has demonstrable effects to improve ovulation and menstrual cyclicity and reduce circulating androgens and hirsutism.

ADVERSE EFFECTS; INTERACTIONS. The most common side effects (10-25%) of metformin are GI: nausea, indigestion, abdominal cramps or bloating, diarrhea, or some combination of these. Metformin has direct effects on GI function including glucose and bile salt absorption. Use of metformin is associated with 20-30% lower blood levels of vitamin B_{12}. Most GI adverse effects of metformin abate over time with continued use, and can be minimized by starting at low doses and gradually titrating to a target dose over several weeks, and by having patients take it with meals.

Metformin has been associated with lactic acidosis, mostly reported in patients with concurrent conditions that can cause poor tissue perfusion such as sepsis, myocardial infarction, and congestive heart failure; recent analyses of this association have raised doubts as to whether the association of lactic acidosis with metformin is causal. Renal failure is a comorbidity reported in patients having lactic acidosis associated with metformin use, and decreased glomerular filtration rates are thought to increase plasma metformin levels by reducing clearance of drug from the circulation (e.g., when creatinine clearance drops below 50 mL/min). It is important to assess renal function before starting metformin and to monitor function at least annually. Metformin should be discontinued preemptively in situations where renal function could decline precipitously, such as before radiographic procedures that use contrast dyes and during admission to hospital for severe illness. Metformin should not be used in severe pulmonary disease, decompensated heart failure, severe liver disease, or chronic alcohol abuse. Cationic drugs that are eliminated by renal tubular secretion have the potential for interaction with metformin by competing for common renal tubular transport systems. Adjustment of metformin is recommended in patients who are taking cationic medications such as cimetidine, furosemide, and nifedipine.

THIAZOLIDINEDIONES

Thiazolidinediones are ligands for the PPARγ receptor, a pair of nuclear hormone receptors that are involved in the regulation of genes related to glucose and lipid metabolism. Two thiazolidinediones are currently available to treat patients with type 2 diabetes, rosiglitazone (AVANDIA) and pioglitazone (ACTOS). Table 43–7 compares thiazolidinediones and metformin.

Mechanism of Action; Pharmacological Effects. Thiazolidinediones activate PPARγ receptors. PPARγ is expressed primarily in adipose tissue with lesser expression in cardiac, skeletal, and smooth muscle cells, islet β cells, macrophages, and vascular endothelial cells. The endogenous ligands for PPARγ include small lipophilic molecules such as oxidized linoleic acid, arachidonic acid, and the prostaglandin metabolite 15d-PGJ2; rosiglitazone and pioglitazone are synthetic ligands for PPARγ. Ligand binding to PPARγ causes heterodimer formation with the retinoid X receptor and interaction with PPAR response elements on specific genes. The principal response to PPARγ activation is adipocyte differentiation. PPARγ activity also promotes uptake of circulating fatty acids into fat cells and shifts of lipid stores from extra-adipose to adipose tissue. One consequence of the cellular responses to PPARγ activation is increased tissue sensitivity to insulin.

Pioglitazone and rosiglitazone are insulin sensitizers and increase insulin-mediated glucose uptake by 30-50% in patients with type 2 diabetes. Although adipose tissue seems to be the primary target for PPARγ agonists, both clinical and preclinical models support a role for skeletal muscle, the major site for insulin-mediated glucose disposal, in the response to thiazolidinediones. In addition to promoting glucose uptake into muscle and adipose tissue, the thiazolidinediones reduce hepatic glucose production and increase hepatic glucose uptake. It is not clear whether thiazolidinedione-induced improvement of insulin resistance is due to direct effects on key target tissues (skeletal muscle and liver), indirect effects mediated by secreted products of adipocytes (e.g., adiponectin), or some combination of these.

Thiazolidinediones also affect lipid metabolism. Treatment with rosiglitazone or pioglitazone reduces plasma levels of fatty acids by increasing clearance and reducing lipolysis. These drugs also cause a shift of triglyceride stores from nonadipose to adipose tissues, and from visceral to subcutaneous fat depots. In clinical trials, pioglitazone reduces plasma triglycerides by 10-15%, and raises HDL cholesterol levels. However, randomized clinical trials demonstrated a questionable benefit of pioglitazone, and no effect of rosiglitazone on major events related to atherosclerosis.

ADME. Both agents are absorbed within 2-3 h, and bioavailability is unaffected by food. The thiazolidinediones are metabolized by the liver and may be administered to patients with renal insufficiency, but should not be used if there is active hepatic disease. Rifampin induces hepatic CYPs and causes a significant decrease in plasma concentrations of rosiglitazone and pioglitazone; gemfibrozil impedes metabolism of the thiazolidinediones and can increase plasma levels by ~2-fold. Prudence suggests reducing the doses of the thiazolidinediones when they are used in conjunction with gemfibrozil.

Therapeutic Uses and Dosage. Rosiglitazone and pioglitazone are dosed once daily. The starting dose of rosiglitazone is 4 mg and should not exceed 8 mg daily. The starting dose of pioglitazone is 15-30 mg, up to a maximum of 45 mg daily. Thiazolidinediones enhance insulin action on liver, adipose tissue, and skeletal muscle, confer improvements in glycemic control in persons with type 2 diabetes, and cause average reductions in A1c of 0.5-1.4%. Thiazolidinediones require the presence of insulin for pharmacological activity and are not indicated to treat type 1 diabetes. Both pioglitazone and rosiglitazone are effective as monotherapy and as additive therapy to metformin, sulfonylureas, or insulin. The onset of action of thiazolidinediones is relatively slow; maximal effects on glucose homeostasis develop gradually over the course of 1-3 months.

ADVERSE EFFECTS AND DRUG INTERACTIONS. The most common adverse effects of the thiazolidinediones are weight gain and edema. Thiazolidinediones cause an increase in body adiposity and an average weight gain of 2-4 kg over the first year of treatment. The use of insulin with thiazolidinedione treatment roughly doubles the incidence of edema and amount of weight gain, compared with either drug alone. Macular edema has been reported in patients using both rosiglitazone and pioglitazone, usually in association with more general fluid retention. Beyond regular retinal exams, diabetic patients taking thiazolidinediones should be observed for visual changes.

Exposure to these drugs over several years in clinical trials has been associated with an increased incidence of heart failure (up to 2-fold). This has generally been attributed to the effect of the drugs to cause plasma volume expansion in type 2 diabetic patients who have significantly increased risk for heart failure. There does not appear to be an acute effect of pioglitazone or rosiglitazone to reduce myocardial contractility or ejection fraction. The use of thiazolidinediones in diabetic patients without a history of heart failure, or with compensated heart failure, can be initiated, but monitoring for signs and symptoms of congestive heart failure is important, especially when insulin is also used. Thiazolidinediones should not be used in patients with moderate to severe heart failure. Recent evidence suggests that rosiglitazone, but not pioglitazone, increases the risk of cardiovascular events (myocardial infarction, stroke). The FDA requires that new prescriptions for rosiglitazone be issued under a risk evaluation and mitigation strategy and be limited to patients whose diabetes could not be adequately controlled by other medications (including pioglitazone).

Treatment with thiazolidinediones has been associated with increased risk of bone fracture in women and with a small but consistent reduction in the hematocrit. Pioglitazone and rosiglitazone are associated with a lowering of transaminases, probably reflective of reductions in hepatic steatosis; thus, thiazolidinediones should be withheld from patients with clinically apparent liver disease and liver function be monitored intermittently during treatment.

GLP-1-BASED AGENTS

Incretins are GI hormones that are released after meals and stimulate insulin secretion. The best known incretins are GLP-1 and GIP. GIP is not effective for stimulating insulin release and lowering blood glucose in persons with type 2 diabetes, whereas GLP-1 is effective. Consequently, the GLP-1 signaling system has been a successful drug target.

Both GLP-1 and glucagon are products derived from preproglucagon, a 180–amino acid precursor with 5 separately processed domains (Figure 43–9). Given intravenously to diabetic subjects in supraphysiologic amounts, GLP-1 stimulates insulin secretion, inhibits glucagon release, delays gastric emptying, reduces food intake, and normalizes fasting and postprandial insulin secretion. The insulinotropic effect of GLP-1 is glucose-dependent in that insulin secretion at fasting glucose concentrations, even with high levels of circulating GLP-1, is minimal. GLP-1 is rapidly inactivated by the enzyme dipeptidyl peptidase IV (DPP-4), with a plasma $t_{1/2}$ of 1-2 min; thus, the natural peptide, itself, is not a useful therapeutic agent. Two broad strategies have been taken to applying GLP-1 to therapeutics, the development of injectable, DPP-4 resistant peptide agonists of the GLP-1 receptor, and the creation of small molecule inhibitors of DPP-4 (Figure 43–10; *see* Table 43–6).

GLP-1 RECEPTOR AGONISTS. Two GLP-1 receptor agonists that have been approved for treatment diabetic patients in the U.S. Exendin-4, a naturally occurring 39-amino acid reptilian peptide and GLP-1 homolog, is a potent GLP-1 receptor agonist that shares many of the physiological and pharmacological effects of GLP-1. It is not metabolized by DPP-4 and so has a plasma $t_{1/2}$ of 2-3 h following subcutaneous injection. Exendin-4 causes glucose-dependent insulin secretion, delayed gastric emptying, lower glucagon levels, and reduced food intake.

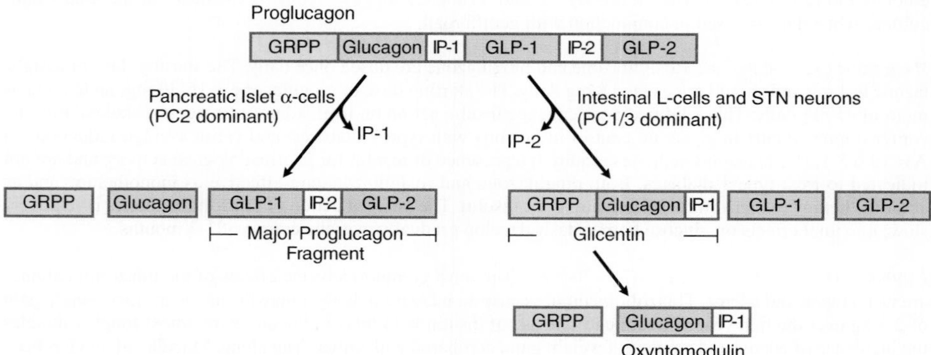

Figure 43–9 *Processing of proglucagon to glucagon, GLP-1, GLP-2, and GRPP.* Proglucagon is synthesized in islet α cells, intestinal enteroendocrine cells (L cells), and a subset of neurons in the hindbrain. In α cells, prohormone processing is primarily by proconvertase 2, releasing glucagon, glicentin-related pancreatic polypeptide (GRPP), and a major proglucagon fragment, containing the 2 glucagon-like peptides (GLPs). In L cells and neurons, proglucagon cleavage is mostly through proconvertase 1/3, giving glicentin, oxyntomodulin, GLP-1, and GLP-2. STN, solitary tract nucleus.

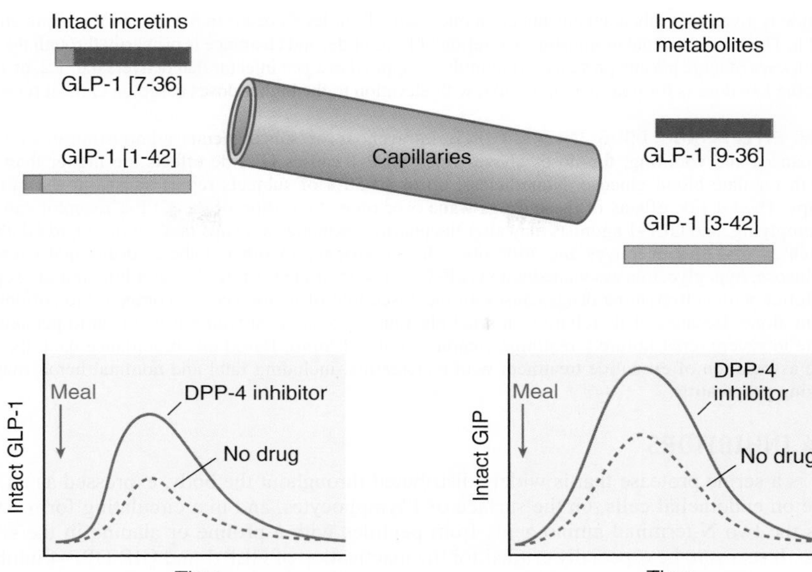

Figure 43–10 *Pharmacological effects of DDP-4 inhibition.* DPP-4, an ectoenzyme located on the luminal side of capillary endothelial cells metabolizes the incretins, glucagon-like peptide 1 (GLP-1), and glucose-dependent insulinotropic polypeptide (GIP), by removing the 2 N-terminal amino acids. The target for DPP-4 cleavage is a proline or alanine residue in the second position of the primary peptide sequence. The truncated metabolites GLP-1[9-36] and GIP[3-42] are the major forms of the incretins in plasma and are inactive as insulin secretagogues. Treatment with a DPP-4 inhibitor increases the concentrations of intact GLP-1 and GIP.

Exenatide (BYETTA), synthetic exendin-4, is approved for use as monotherapy and as adjunctive therapy for type 2 diabetes patients not achieving glycemic targets with other drugs.

In clinical trials, exenatide, alone or in combination with metformin, sulfonylurea, or thiazolidinedione, was associated with improved glycemic control, as reflected in an ~1% decrease in A1c, and weight loss that averaged 2.5-4 kg.

Liraglutide is also a GLP-1 receptor agonist. Structurally, liraglutide is nearly identical to native GLP-1, with Lys^{34} to Arg substitution and addition of a α-glutamic acid spacer coupled to a C16 fatty acyl group.

The fatty acid side chain permits binding to albumin and other plasma proteins and accounts for an extended $t_{1/2}$ permitting once-daily administration. The pharmacodynamic profile of liraglutide mimics GLP-1 and exenatide, and in clinical trials liraglutide caused both improvement in glycemic control and weight loss. In a single comparative trial, liraglutide reduced A1c ~30% more than exenatide. Liraglutide is indicated for adjunctive therapy in patients not achieving glycemic control with metformin, sulfonylurea, their combination, or metformin/thiazolidinedione.

MECHANISM OF ACTION. All GLP-1 receptor agonists share a common mechanism, activation of the GLP-1 receptor. GLP-1 receptors are expressed by β cells, cells in the peripheral and central nervous systems, the heart and vasculature, kidney, lung, and GI mucosa. Binding of agonists to the GLP-1 receptor activates the cyclic AMP-PKA pathway and several GEFs (guanine nucleotide exchange factors). GLP-1 receptor activation also initiates signaling via PKC and PI3K and alters the activity of several ion channels. In β cells, the end result of these actions is increased insulin biosynthesis and exocytosis in a glucose-dependent manner (*see* Figure 43–3).

ABSORPTION, DISTRIBUTION, METABOLISM, EXCRETION, AND DOSING. Exenatide is given as a subcutaneous injection twice daily, typically before meals. Exenatide is rapidly absorbed, reaches peak concentrations in ~2 h, undergoes little metabolism in the circulation, and has a volume of distribution of nearly 30 L. Clearance of the drug occurs primarily by glomerular filtration, with tubular proteolysis and minimal reabsorption. Exenatide is marketed as a pen that delivers 5 or 10 μg; dosing is typically started at the lower amount and increased as needed.

Liraglutide is given as a subcutaneous injection once daily. Peak levels occur in 8-12 h and the elimination $t_{1/2}$ is 12-14 h. There is little renal or intestinal excretion of liraglutide, and clearance is primarily through the metabolic pathways of large plasma proteins. Liraglutide is supplied in a pen injector that delivers 0.6, 1.2, or 1.8 mg of drug; the low dose is for treatment initiation, with elevation to the higher doses based on clinical response.

ADVERSE EFFECTS AND DRUG INTERACTIONS. Intravenous or subcutaneous administration of GLP-1 causes nausea and vomiting; the doses above which GLP-1 causes GI side effects are higher than those needed to regulate blood glucose. Nonetheless, up to 40-50% of subjects report nausea at the initiation of therapy. The GI side effects of these drugs wane over time. Activation of the GLP-1 receptor can delay gastric emptying, and GLP-1 agonists may alter the pharmacokinetics of drugs that require rapid GI absorption, such as oral contraceptives and antibiotics. In the absence of other diabetes drugs that cause low blood glucose, hypoglycemia associated with GLP-1 agonist treatment is rare. The combination of exenatide or liraglutide with sulfonylurea drugs causes an increased rate of hypoglycemia compared to sulfonylurea treatment alone. Because of its reliance on renal clearance, exenatide should not be given to persons with moderate to severe renal failure (creatinine clearance <30 mL/min). Based on surveillance data, there is a possible association of exenatide treatment with pancreatitis, including fatal and nonfatal hemorrhagic or necrotizing pancreatitis.

DPP-4 INHIBITORS

DPP-4 is a serine protease that is widely distributed throughout the body, expressed as an ecto-enzyme on endothelial cells, on the surface of T-lymphocytes, and in a circulating form. DPP-4 cleaves the two N-terminal amino acids from peptides with a proline or alanine in the second position. It seems to be especially critical for the inactivation of GLP-1 and GIP. DPP-4 inhibitors increase the AUC of GLP-1 and GIP when their secretion is by a meal (*see* Figure 43–10). Several agents provide nearly complete and long-lasting inhibition of DPP-4, thereby increasing the proportion of active GLP-1 from 10-20% of total circulating GLP-1 immunoreactivity to nearly 100%. **Sitagliptin** (JANUVIA), **saxagliptin** (ONGLYZA), **linagliptin** (TRADJENTA), and **alogliptin** (NESINA) are available in the U.S.; **vildagliptin**, is available in the E.U.

MECHANISMS OF ACTION; EFFECTS. Sitagliptin and alogliptin are competitive inhibitors of DPP-4; vildagliptin and saxagliptin bind the enzyme covalently. All 4 drugs can be given in doses that lower measurable activity of DPP-4 by >95% for 12 h. This causes a greater than 2-fold elevation of plasma concentrations of active GIP and GLP-1 and is associated with increased insulin secretion, reduced glucagon levels, and improvements in both fasting and postprandial hyperglycemia. Inhibition of DPP-4 does not appear to have direct effects on insulin sensitivity, gastric motility, or satiety, nor does chronic treatment with DPP-4 inhibitors affect body weight. DPP-4 inhibitors, used as monotherapy in type 2 diabetic patients, reduced A1c levels by an average ~0.8%. These compounds are also effective for chronic glucose control when added to the treatment of diabetic patients receiving metformin, thiazolidinediones, sulfonylureas, and insulin. The effects of DPP-4 inhibitors in combination regimens appear to be additive. The recommended dose of sitagliptin is 100 mg once daily. The recommended dose of saxagliptin is 5 mg once daily.

ADME. DPP-4 inhibitors are absorbed effectively from the small intestine. They circulate in primarily in unbound form and are excreted largely unchanged in the urine. Both sitagliptin and saxagliptin are excreted renally, and lower doses should be used in patients with reduced renal function. Sitagliptin has minimal metabolism by hepatic microsomal enzymes. Saxagliptin is metabolized by CYP3A4/5 to an active metabolite. The dose saxagliptin should be lowered to 2.5 mg daily when coadministered with strong CYP3A4 inhibitors (e.g., ketoconazole, atazanavir, clarithromycin, indinavir, itraconazole, nefazodone, nelfinavir, ritonavir, saquinavir, and telithromycin).

ADVERSE EFFECTS; DRUG INTERACTIONS. There are no consistent adverse effects that have been noted in clinical trials with any of the DPP-4 inhibitors. DPP-4 is expressed on lymphocytes; in the immunology literature, the enzyme is referred to as CD26. This area bears scrutiny as more patients are treated with these compounds.

OTHER HYPOGLYCEMIC AGENTS

ALPHA GLUCOSIDASE INHIBITORS

α-Glucosidase inhibitors reduce intestinal absorption of starch, dextrin, and disaccharides by inhibiting the action of α-glucosidase in the intestinal brush border. These drugs also increase the release of the glucoregulatory hormone GLP-1 into the circulation, which may contribute to their glucose-lowering effects. The drugs in this class are **acarbose** (PRECOSE, others), **miglitol** (GLYSET), and **voglibose**.

DOSING; ADME. Dosing of acarbose and miglitol are similar. Both are provided as 25, 50, or 100 mg tablets that are taken before meals. Treatment should start with lower doses and be titrated as indicated by balancing postprandial glucose, A1c, and GI symptoms. Acarbose is minimally absorbed; the small amount of drug reaching the systemic circulation is cleared by the kidney. Miglitol absorption is saturable, with 50-100% of any dose entering the circulation. Miglitol is cleared almost entirely by the kidney, and dose reductions are recommended for patients with creatinine clearance <30 mL/min.

ADVERSE EFFECTS AND DRUG INTERACTIONS. The most prominent adverse effects are malabsorption, flatulence, diarrhea, and abdominal bloating. Mild to moderate elevations of hepatic transaminases have been reported with acarbose, but symptomatic liver disease is very rare. Cutaneous hypersensitivity has been described but is also rare. Hypoglycemia has been described when α-glucosidase inhibitors are added to insulin or an insulin secretagogue. Acarbose can decrease the absorption of digoxin and miglitol can decrease the absorption of propranolol and ranitidine. Alpha glucosidase inhibitors are contraindicated in patients with stage 4 renal failure.

THERAPEUTIC USES. α-Glucosidase inhibitors are indicated as adjuncts to diet and exercise in type 2 diabetic patients not reaching glycemic targets. They can also be used in combination with other oral antidiabetic agents and/or insulin. In clinical studies α-glucosidase inhibitors reduce A1c by 0.5-0.8%, fasting glucose by ~1 mM and postprandial glucose by 2.0-2.5 mM. These agents do not cause weight gain or have significant effects on plasma lipids.

PRAMLINTIDE

Islet amyloid polypeptide (IAPP, amylin), is a 37–amino acid peptide produced in the pancreatic β cell and secreted with insulin. A synthetic form of amylin with several amino acid modifications to improve bioavailability, pramlintide (SYMLIN), has been developed as a drug for the treatment of diabetes; pramlintide may affect its actions via the amylin receptor in specific regions of the hindbrain. Activation of the amylin receptor causes reductions in glucagon release, delayed gastric emptying, and satiety.

ADME; DOSING. Pramlintide is administered as a subcutaneous injection prior to meals. Pramlintide is not extensively bound by plasma proteins and has a $t_{1/2}$ of 50 min. Metabolism and clearance is primarily by the kidney. The doses in patients with type 1 diabetes start at 15 μg and are titrated upward to a maximum of 60 μg; in type 2 diabetes the starting dose is 60 μg and the maximum is 120 μg. Because of differences in the pH of the solutions, pramlintide should not be administered in the same syringe as insulin.

ADVERSE EFFECTS; DRUG INTERACTIONS. The most common adverse effects are nausea and hypoglycemia. Although pramlintide alone does not lower blood glucose, addition to insulin at mealtimes has been noted to cause increased rates of hypoglycemia, occasionally severe. It is currently recommended that prandial insulin doses be reduced 30-50% at the time of pramlintide initiation and then retitrated. Because of its effects on GI motility, pramlintide is contraindicated in patients with gastroparesis or other disorders of motility. Pramlintide is a pregnancy Category C drug. Pramlintide can be used in persons with moderate renal disease (creatinine clearance >20 mL/min).

THERAPEUTIC USES. Pramlintide is approved for treatment of types 1 and 2 diabetes as an adjunct in patients who take insulin with meals. Pramlintide is now being evaluated as a drug for weight loss in nondiabetic persons.

BILE ACID BINDING RESINS

The only bile acid sequestrant specifically approved for the treatment of type 2 diabetes is *colesevelam* (WELCHOL).

MECHANISM OF ACTION. The mechanism by which bile acid binding and removal from enterohepatic circulation lowers blood glucose has not been established. Bile acid sequestrants could reduce intestinal glucose absorption, although there is no direct evidence of this. Bile acids also act as signaling molecules through nuclear receptors, some of which may act as glucose sensors.

ADME. Colesevelam is provided as a powder for oral solution and as 625-mg tablets; typical usage is 3 tablets twice daily before lunch and dinner or 6 tablets prior to the patient's largest meal. The drug's distribution is limited to the GI tract.

ADVERSE EFFECTS AND DRUG INTERACTIONS. Common side effects of colesevelam are gastrointestinal, with constipation, dyspepsia, abdominal pain, and nausea affecting up to 10% of treated patients. Like other bile acid binding resins, colesevelam can increase plasma triglycerides in persons with an inherent tendency to hypertriglyceridemia and should be used cautiously in patients with plasma triglycerides >200 mg/dL. Colesevelam can interfere with the absorption of commonly used agents (e.g., phenytoin, warfarin, verapamil, glyburide, L-thyroxine, and ethinyl estradiol, and fat-soluble vitamins). Colesevelam is a pregnancy Category B drug that has no contraindications in patients with renal or liver disease.

THERAPEUTIC USES. The bile acid binding resin colesevelam, approved for treatment of hypercholesterolemia, may be used for treatment of type 2 diabetes as an adjunct to diet and exercise. In clinical trials, colesevelam reduced A1c by 0.5% when added to metformin, sulfonylurea, or insulin treatment in type 2 diabetic patients.

BROMOCRIPTINE

A formulation of bromocriptine (CYCLOSET), a dopamine receptor agonist, is approved for the treatment of type 2 diabetes but is not yet available in the U.S. Bromocriptine is an established treatment for Parkinson disease and hyperprolactinemia (*see* Chapters 13, 22, and 38). Effects of bromocriptine on blood glucose are modest and may reflect an action in the CNS.

COMBINED PHARMACOLOGICAL APPROACHES TO TYPE 2 DIABETES

PROGRESSIVE MANAGEMENT OF TYPE 2 DIABETES

There are several useful algorithms or flow charts for the treatment of type 2 diabetes (Figure 43–11). There are a number of pathways or combination of drugs that are used for treatment of type 2 diabetes if the glucose control does not reach the therapeutic target. Table 43–8 summarizes available pharmacological agents for the treatment of diabetes.

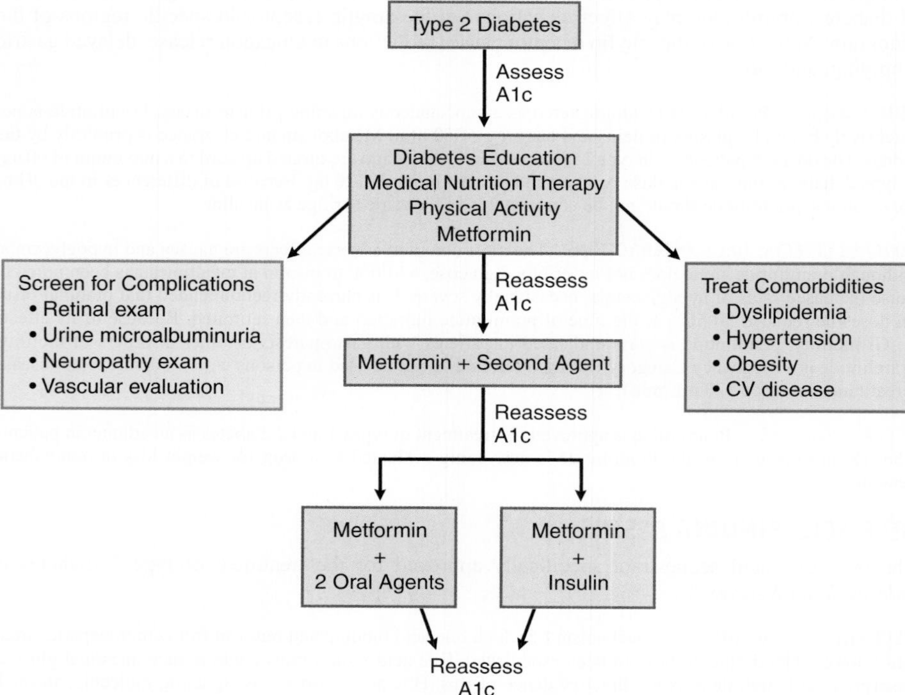

Figure 43–11 *Treatment algorithm for management of type 2 diabetes mellitus.* Patients diagnosed with type 2 diabetes, either by fasting glucose, oral glucose tolerance testing, or A1c measurement, should have diabetes education that includes instruction on medical nutrition therapy and physical activity. Most patients newly diagnosed with type 2 diabetes have had subclinical or undiagnosed diabetes for many years previously and should be evaluated for diabetic complications (retinal exam, test for excess protein or albumin excretion in the urine, and clinical evaluation for peripheral neuropathy and vascular insufficiency); common comorbidities (hypertension and dyslipidemia) should be treated. Metformin is the consensus first line of therapy and should be started at the time of diagnosis. Failure to reach the glycemic target, generally A1c ≤7% within 3-4 months, should prompt the addition of a second oral agent. Reinforce lifestyle interventions at every visit and check A1c every 3 months. Treatment may escalate to metformin plus 2 oral agents or metformin plus insulin, if necessary.

Table 43–8

Comparison of Agents Used for Treatment of Diabetes

	MECHANISM OF ACTION	EXAMPLES	HbA_{1C} REDUCTION (%)[a]	AGENT-SPECIFIC ADVANTAGES	AGENT-SPECIFIC DISADVANTAGES	CONTRAINDICATIONS
Oral						
Biguanides [c]	↓ Hepatic glucose production	Metformin	1-2	Weight neutral, Do not cause hypoglycemia, inexpensive	Diarrhea, nausea, lactic acidosis	GFR<50 mL/min, CHF, radiographic contrast studies, seriously ill patients, acidosis
α-Glucosidase inhibitors[c]	↓ GI glucose absorption	Acarbose, miglitol	0.5-0.8	Reduce postprandial glycemia	GI flatulence, liver function tests	Renal/liver disease
Dipeptidyl peptidase-4 inhibitors[c]	Prolong endogenous GLP-1 action	Saxagliptin, sitagliptin, vildagliptin	0.5-1.0	Do not cause hypoglycemia		Reduce dose with renal disease
Insulin secretagogues – Sulfonylureas[c]	↑ Insulin secretion	See text and Table 43–7	1-2	Inexpensive	Hypoglycemia, weight gain	Renal/liver disease
Insulin secretagogues – Non-sulfonylureas[c]	↑ Insulin secretion	See text and Table 43–7	1-2	Short onset of action, lower postprandial glucose	Hypoglycemia	Renal/liver disease
Thiazolidinediones[c]	↓ Insulin resistance, ↑ glucose utilization	Rosiglitazone, pioglitazone	0.5-1.4	Lower insulin requirements	Peripheral edema, CHF, weight gain, fractures, macular edema. Rosiglitazone may increase risk of CV disease	CHF, liver disease
Bile Acid sequestrants[c]	Bind bile acids; mechanism of glucose-lowering not known	Colesevelam	0.5		Constipation, dyspepsia, abdominal pain, nausea, ↑ triglycerides, interfere with absorption of other drugs, intestinal obstruction	

(continued)

Table 43–8

Comparison of Agents Used for Treatment of Diabetes (*Continued*)

	MECHANISM OF ACTION	EXAMPLES	HbA_{1C} REDUCTION (%)[a]	AGENT-SPECIFIC ADVANTAGES	AGENT-SPECIFIC DISADVANTAGES	CONTRAINDICATIONS
Parenteral						
Insulin	↑ Glucose utilization, ↓ Hepatic glucose production, and other anabolic actions	See text and Table 43–5	Not limited	Known safety profile	Injection, weight gain, hypoglycemia	
GLP-1 agonists[c]	↑ Insulin, ↓ Glucagon, slow gastric emptying, satiety	Exenatide, liraglutide	0.5-1.0	Weight loss	Injection, nausea, ↑ risk of hypoglycemia with insulin secretagogues, pancreatitis	Renal disease, agents that also slow GI motility, pancreatitis
Amylin agonists[b,c]	Slow gastric emptying, ↓ Glucagon	Pramlintide	0.25-0.5	Reduce postprandial glycemia; weight loss	Injection, nausea, ↑ risk of hypoglycemia with insulin	Agents that also slow GI motility
Medical nutrition therapy and physical activity[c]	↓ Insulin, resistance, ↑ insulin secretion	Low-calorie, low-fat diet, exercise	1-3	Other health benefits	Compliance difficult, long-term success low	

[a]*A1C reduction (absolute) depends partly on starting A1C value.*
[b]*Used in conjunction with insulin for treatment of type 1 diabetes*
[c]*Used for treatment of type 2 diabetes*
Source: Adapted with permission from Fauci AS, Braunwald E, Kasper DL, Hauser SL, Longo DL, Jameson JL, Loscalzo J, eds. Harrison's Principles of Internal Medicine, 17th ed. New York: McGraw-Hill; 2008.

In the absence of prolonged fasting, healthy humans almost never have blood glucose levels <3.5 mM. This is due to a highly adapted neuroendocrine counterregulatory system that prevents acute hypoglycemia, a hazardous and potentially lethal situation. The 2 major clinical scenarios for hypoglycemia are:

- Treatment of diabetes
- Inappropriate production of endogenous insulin or an insulin-like substance by a pancreatic islet tumor (insulinoma) or a non-islet tumor

Hypoglycemia in the first scenario can occur either in the fasting or fed state, whereas in the second scenario, hypoglycemia occurs almost exclusively in the fasting or postabsorptive state. Some drugs not used for the treatment of diabetes promote hypoglycemia (*see* Table 43–3).

The most common and serious adverse event related to diabetes therapy is hypoglycemia. Although an adverse reaction to a number of oral therapies, it is most pronounced and serious with insulin therapy. Hypoglycemia may result from an inappropriately large dose, from a mismatch between the time of peak delivery of insulin and food intake, or from superimposition of additional factors that increase sensitivity to insulin (e.g., adrenal or pituitary insufficiency) or that increase insulin-independent glucose uptake (e.g., exercise). Hypoglycemia is the major risk that always must be weighed against benefits of efforts to normalize glucose control.

The first physiological response to hypoglycemia is a reduction of endogenous insulin secretion, which occurs at a plasma glucose level of ~70 mg/dL (3.9 mM); thereafter, the counterregulatory hormones (EPI, glucagon, growth hormone, cortisol, and NE) are released. Symptoms of hypoglycemia are first discerned at a plasma glucose level of 60-80 mg/dL (3.3-4.4 mM). Sweating, hunger, paresthesias, palpitations, tremor, and anxiety, principally of autonomic origin, usually are seen first. Difficulty in concentrating, confusion, weakness, drowsiness, a feeling of warmth, dizziness, blurred vision, and loss of consciousness (i.e., most important neuroglycopenic symptoms) usually occur at lower plasma glucose levels than do autonomic symptoms.

In patients with type 1 and type 2 diabetes of longer duration, the glucagon secretory response to hypoglycemia becomes deficient. Diabetic patients thus become dependent on EPI for counterregulation, and if this mechanism becomes deficient, the incidence of severe hypoglycemia increases. Severe hypoglycemia can lead to convulsions and coma. With the ready availability of home glucose monitoring, hypoglycemia can be documented in most patients who experience suggestive symptoms. Hypoglycemia that occurs during sleep may be difficult to detect but should be suspected from a history of morning headaches, night sweats, or symptoms of hypothermia. Mild-to-moderate hypoglycemia may be treated simply by ingestion of glucose (15 g of carbohydrate). When hypoglycemia is severe, it should be treated with intravenous glucose or an injection of glucagon.

AGENTS USED TO TREAT HYPOGLYCEMIA

Glucagon is a single-chain polypeptide of 29 amino acids now produced by recombinant DNA technology. Glucagon interacts with a GPCR on the plasma membrane of target cells that signals through G_s. The primary effects of glucagon on the liver are mediated by cAMP. Glucagon is used to treat severe hypoglycemia, particularly in diabetic patients when the patient cannot safely consume oral glucose and intravenous glucose is not available.

For hypoglycemic reactions, 1 mg is administered intravenously, intramuscularly, or subcutaneously. After the initial response to glucagon, patients should be given glucose or urged to eat to prevent recurrent hypoglycemia. Nausea and vomiting are the most frequent adverse effects.

Diazoxide (PROGLYCEM) is an antihypertensive, antidiuretic benzothiadiazine derivative with potent hyperglycemic actions when given orally. Hyperglycemia results primarily from inhibition of insulin secretion. Diazoxide interacts with the K_{ATP} channel on the β cell membrane and either prevents its closing or prolongs the open time; this effect is opposite to that of the sulfonylureas (*see* Figure 43–3).

The usual oral dose is 3-8 mg/kg per day in adults and children and 8 to 15 mg/kg per day in infants and neonates. The drug can cause nausea and vomiting and thus usually is given in divided doses with meals. Diazoxide circulates largely bound to plasma proteins and has a $t_{1/2}$ of ~48 h. Diazoxide has a number of adverse effects, including retention of Na^+ and fluid, hyperuricemia, hypertrichosis, thrombocytopenia, and leucopenia, which sometimes limit its use. Despite these side effects, the drug may be useful in patients with inoperable insulinomas and in children with neonatal hyperinsulinism.

SOMATOSTATIN. Somatostatin (SST) is produced by δ cells of the pancreatic islet, cells of the GI tract, and in the CNS. Somatostatin, a 14–amino acid or a 28–amino acid peptide molecule, acts through a family of 5 GPCRs, $SSTR_{1-5}$. SST inhibits a wide variety of endocrine and exocrine secretions, including TSH and GH from the pituitary, gastrin, motilin, VIP, glicentin, and insulin, glucagon, and pancreatic polypeptide from the pancreatic islet. The physiological role of somatostatin has not been defined precisely, but its short $t_{1/2}$ (3-6 min) prevents its use therapeutically. Longer-acting analogs such as octreotide (SANDOSTATIN) and lanreotide (SOMATULINE) are useful for treatment of carcinoid tumors, glucagonomas, VIPomas, and acromegaly (*see* Chapter 38). Gallbladder abnormalities (stones and biliary sludge) occur frequently with chronic use of the somatostatin analogs, as do GI symptoms.

For a complete Bibliographical Listing see Goodman & Gilman's ***The Pharmacological Basis of Therapeutics***, 12th ed., or Goodman & Gilman Online at www.AccessMedicine.com.

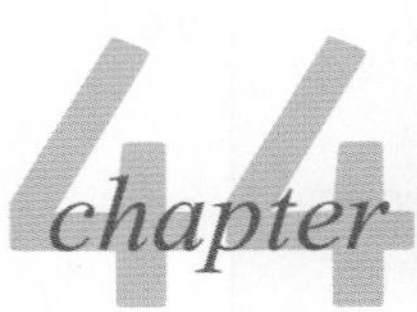

Agents Affecting Mineral Ion Homeostasis and Bone Turnover

PHYSIOLOGY OF MINERAL ION HOMEOSTASIS

CALCIUM

Elemental calcium is essential for a variety of biological functions. Its ionized form, Ca^{2+}, is an important component of current flow across excitable membranes. Ca^{2+} is vital for muscle contraction, fusion, and release of storage vesicles. In the submicromolar range, intracellular Ca^{2+} acts as a critical second messenger (*see* Chapter 3). In extracellular fluid, millimolar concentrations of Ca^{2+} promote blood coagulation and support the formation and continuous remodeling of the skeleton.

In the face of millimolar extracellular Ca^{2+}, intracellular free Ca^{2+} is maintained at a low level, ~100 nM in cells in their basal state, by active extrusion by Ca^{2+}–ATPases, by Na^+/Ca^{2+} exchange, and by accumulation into cellular storage networks such as the sarcoplasmic reticulum. Changes in cytosolic Ca^{2+} (whether released from intracellular stores or entering via membrane Ca^{2+} channels) can modulate effector targets, often by interacting with the Ca^{2+}-binding protein *calmodulin*. The rapid association–dissociation kinetics of Ca^{2+} and the relatively high affinity and selectivity of Ca^{2+}-binding domains permit effective regulation of Ca^{2+} over the 100 nM to 1 μM range.

The body content of calcium in healthy adult men and women, respectively, is ~1300 and 1000 g, of which >99% is in bone and teeth. Ca^{2+} in extracellular fluids is stringently regulated within narrow limits. In adult humans, the normal serum Ca^{2+} concentration ranges from 8.5-10.4 mg/dL (4.25-5.2 mEq/L, 2.1-2.6 mM) and includes 3 distinct chemical forms of Ca^{2+}: *ionized* (50%), *protein-bound* (40%), and *complexed* (10%). Thus, whereas total plasma Ca^{2+} concentration is ~2.5 mM, the concentration of ionized Ca^{2+} in plasma is ~1.2 mM. The various pools of Ca^{2+} are illustrated schematically in Figure 44–1. Only diffusible Ca^{2+} (i.e., ionized plus complexed) can cross cell membranes. Albumin accounts for some 90% of the serum Ca^{2+} bound to plasma proteins; a change of plasma albumin concentration of 1.0 g/dL from the normal value of 4.0 g/dL can be expected to alter total Ca^{2+} concentration by ~0.8 mg/dL. The remaining 10% of the serum Ca^{2+} is complexed with small polyvalent anions, primarily phosphate and citrate. The degree of complex formation depends on the ambient pH and the concentrations of ionized Ca^{2+} and complexing anions. Ionized Ca^{2+} is the physiologically relevant component, mediates calcium's biological effects, and, when perturbed, produces the characteristic signs and symptoms of hypo- or hypercalcemia. The extracellular Ca^{2+} concentration is tightly controlled by hormones that affect calcium entry at the intestine and its exit at the kidney; when needed, these same hormones regulate withdrawal from the large skeletal reservoir.

Calcium Stores. The skeleton contains 99% of total body calcium in a crystalline form resembling the mineral hydroxyapatite; other ions, including Na^+, K^+, Mg^{2+}, and F^-, also are present in the crystal lattice. The steady-state content of Ca^{2+} in bone reflects the net effect of bone resorption and bone formation.

Calcium Absorption and Excretion. In the U.S., ~75% of dietary Ca^{2+} is obtained from milk and dairy products. The adequate intake value for Ca^{2+} is 1300 mg/day in adolescents and 1000 mg/day in adults. After age 50, the adequate intake is 1200 mg/day. Figure 44–2 illustrates the components of whole-body daily Ca^{2+} turnover. Ca^{2+} enters the body only through the intestine. *Active vitamin D–dependent Ca^{2+} transport* occurs in the proximal duodenum, whereas *facilitated diffusion* throughout the small intestine accounts for most total Ca^{2+} uptake. This uptake is counterbalanced by an obligatory daily intestinal Ca^{2+} loss of ~150 mg/day that reflects the Ca^{2+} content of mucosal and biliary secretions and in sloughed intestinal cells. The efficiency of intestinal Ca^{2+} absorption is inversely related to calcium intake. Thus, a diet low in calcium leads to a compensatory increase in fractional absorption owing partly to activation of vitamin D. Disease states associated with steatorrhea, chronic diarrhea, or malabsorption promote fecal loss of Ca^{2+}. Drugs such as glucocorticoids and phenytoin depress intestinal Ca^{2+} transport.

Urinary Ca^{2+} excretion is the net difference between the quantity filtered at the glomerulus and the amount reabsorbed. About 9 g of Ca^{2+} are filtered each day, of which >98% is reabsorbed in the tubules. The efficiency of reabsorption is highly regulated by parathyroid hormone (PTH) and is influenced by filtered Na^+, the presence of nonreabsorbed anions, and diuretic agents (*see* Chapter 25).

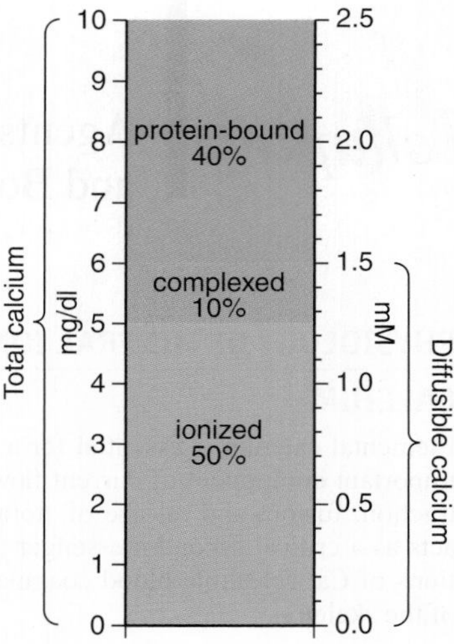

Figure 44–1 *Pools of calcium in serum.* Concentrations are expressed as mg/dL on the left-hand axis and as mM on the right. The total serum calcium concentration is 10 mg/dL or 2.5 mM, divided into 3 pools: protein-bound (40%), complexed with small anions (10%), and ionized calcium (50%). The complexed and ionized pools represent the diffusable forms of calcium.

PHOSPHATE

Phosphate is present in plasma, extracellular fluid, cell membrane phospholipids, intracellular fluid, collagen, and bone tissue. More than 80% of total body phosphorus is found in bone; ~15% is in soft tissue. Additionally, phosphate is a dynamic constituent of intermediary and energy metabolism and as a key regulator of enzyme activity when transferred by protein kinases from ATP to phosphorylatable serine, threonine, and tyrosine residues. Biologically, phosphorus (P) exists in both organic and inorganic (P_i) forms. Organic forms include phospholipids and various organic esters. In extracellular fluid, the bulk of phosphorus is present as inorganic phosphate in the form of NaH_2PO_4 and Na_2HPO_4. The aggregate level of inorganic phosphate (P_i) modifies tissue concentrations of Ca^{2+} and plays a major role in renal H^+ excretion. Within bone, phosphate is complexed with Ca^{2+} as hydroxyapatites and as calcium phosphate.

Absorption, Distribution, and Excretion. Phosphate is absorbed from and, to a limited extent, secreted into the GI tract. Phosphate is a ubiquitous component of ordinary foods; even an inadequate diet rarely causes phosphate depletion. Transport of phosphate from the intestinal lumen is an active, energy-dependent process that is regulated by several factors, primarily vitamin D, which stimulates absorption. In adults, about two-thirds of ingested phosphate is absorbed and is excreted almost entirely into the urine. In growing children, phosphate balance is positive, and plasma concentrations of phosphate are higher than in adults.

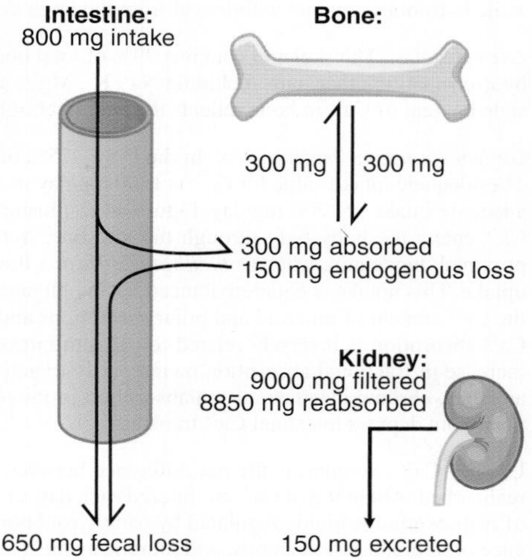

Figure 44–2 *Whole body daily turnover of calcium.* (Adapted with permission from Yanagawa N, Lee DBN. Renal handling of calcium and phosphorus. In: Coe FL, Favus MJ, eds. *Disorders of Bone and Mineral Metabolism*, New York: Raven Press; 1992, pp 3–40.)

Phosphate excretion in the urine represents the difference between the amount filtered and that reabsorbed. More than 90% of plasma phosphate is freely filtered at the glomerulus, and 80% is actively reabsorbed, predominantly in the proximal convoluted tubule. Renal phosphate absorption is regulated by a variety of hormones and other factors; the most important are PTH and dietary phosphate, with extracellular volume and acid–base status playing lesser roles. Dietary phosphate deficiency upregulates renal phosphate transporters and decreases excretion, whereas a high-phosphate diet increases phosphate excretion; these changes are independent of any effect on plasma P_i, Ca^{2+}, or PTH. PTH increases urinary phosphate excretion by blocking phosphate absorption. Expansion of plasma volume increases urinary phosphate excretion.

ROLE OF PHOSPHATE IN URINE ACIDIFICATION. Phosphate is concentrated progressively in the renal tubule and becomes the most abundant buffer system in the distal tubule and terminal nephron. The exchange of H^+ and Na^+ in the tubular urine converts Na_2HPO_4 to NaH_2PO_4, permitting the excretion of large amounts of acid without lowering the urine pH to a degree that would block H^+ transport.

PHARMACOLOGICAL ACTIONS OF PHOSPHATE. Phosphate salts are employed as mild laxatives (*see* Chapter 46).

HORMONAL REGULATION OF CALCIUM AND PHOSPHATE HOMEOSTASIS

A number of hormones interact to regulate extracellular Ca^{2+} and phosphate balance. The most important are PTH and *1,25-dihydroxyvitamin D_3* (*calcitriol*), which regulate mineral homeostasis by effects on the kidney, intestine, and bone (Figure 44–3).

PARATHYROID HORMONE

PTH is a polypeptide that helps to regulate plasma Ca^{2+} by affecting bone resorption/formation, renal Ca^{2+} excretion/reabsorption, and calcitriol synthesis (thus, GI Ca^{2+} absorption).

PTH is single polypeptide chain of 84 amino acids with molecular mass of ~9500 Da. Biological activity is associated with the N-terminal portion of the peptide; residues 1–27 are required for optimal binding to the PTH receptor and hormone activity. Derivatives lacking the first and second residue bind to PTH receptors but

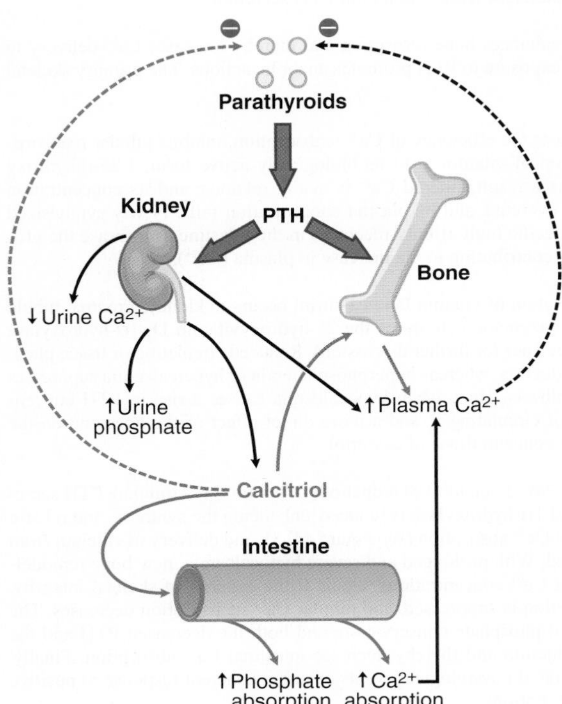

Figure 44–3 *Calcium homeostasis and its regulation by parathyroid hormone (PTH) and 1,25-dihydroxyvitamin D.* PTH has stimulatory effects on bone and kidney, including the stimulation of 1α-hydroxylase activity in kidney mitochondria leading to the increased production of 1,25-dihydroxyvitamin D (calcitriol) from 25-hydroxycholecalciferol, the monohydroxylated vitamin D metabolite (Figure 44–5). Calcitriol is the biologically active metabolite of vitamin D.

do not activate the cyclic AMP or IP_3–Ca^{2+} signaling pathways. The PTH fragment lacking the first 6 amino acids inhibits PTH action.

SYNTHESIS AND SECRETION. PTH is synthesized as a 115–amino acid peptide called *preproparathyroid hormone*, which is converted to *proparathyroid hormone* by cleavage of 25 amino-terminal residues in the endoplasmic reticulum. Proparathyroid hormone is converted in the Golgi complex to PTH by cleavage of 6 amino acids. PTH(1-84) resides within secretory granules until it is discharged into the circulation. PTH(1-84) has a $t_{1/2}$ in plasma of ~4 min; removal by the liver and kidney accounts for ~90% of its clearance. Proteolysis of PTH generates smaller fragments (e.g., a 33–36 amino acid N-terminal fragment that is fully active, a larger C-terminal peptide, and PTH[7-84]). PTH(7-84) and other amino-truncated PTH fragments are normally cleared from the circulation predominantly by the kidneys, whereas intact PTH is also removed by extrarenal mechanisms.

Physiological Functions. The primary function of PTH is to maintain a constant concentration of Ca^{2+} and P_i in the extracellular fluid. The principal processes regulated are renal Ca^{2+} and P_i absorption, and mobilization of bone Ca^{2+} (*see* Figure 44–3). The actions of PTH are mediated by at least 2 receptors: the PTH_1 and the PTH_2 receptor. Both of these are GPCRs that can couple with G_s and G_q in cell-type specific manners. PTH also can activate phospholipase D through a $G_{12/13}$–RhoA pathway. A third receptor, the CPTH receptor, interacts with forms of PTH that are truncated in the amino-terminal region, contain most of the carboxy terminus, and are inactive at the PTH_1 receptor; these CPTH receptors reportedly are expressed on osteocytes.

Regulation of Secretion. Plasma Ca^{2+} is the major factor regulating PTH secretion. As the concentration of Ca^{2+} diminishes, PTH secretion increases; hypocalcemia induces parathyroid hypertrophy and hyperplasia. Conversely, if the concentration of Ca^{2+} is high, PTH secretion decreases. Changes in plasma Ca^{2+} regulate PTH secretion by the plasma membrane–associated *calcium-sensing receptor* (CaSR) on parathyroid cells. The CaSR is a GPCR that couples with G_q and G_i. Occupancy of the CaSR by Ca^{2+} stimulates the G_q-PLC-IP_3-Ca^{2+} pathway leading to activation of PKC; this results in inhibition of PTH secretion, an unusual case in which elevation of cellular Ca^{2+} inhibits secretion (another being the granular cells in the juxtaglomerular complex of the kidney, where elevation of cellular Ca^{2+} inhibits renin secretion). Simultaneous activation of the G_i pathway by Ca^{2+} reduces cyclic AMP synthesis and lowers the activity of PKA, also a negative signal for PTH secretion. Conversely, reduced occupancy of CaSR by Ca^{2+} reduces signaling through G_i and G_q, thereby promoting PTH secretion. Other agents that increase parathyroid cell cyclic AMP levels, such as β adrenergic receptor agonists and dopamine, also increase PTH secretion, but much less than does hypocalcemia. The active vitamin D metabolite, 1,25-dihydroxyvitamin D (*calcitriol*), directly suppresses PTH gene expression. Severe hypermagnesemia or hypomagnesemia can inhibit PTH secretion.

Effects on Bone. Chronically elevated PTH enhances bone resorption and thereby increases Ca^{2+} delivery to the extracellular fluid, whereas intermittent exposure to PTH promotes anabolic actions. The primary skeletal target cell for PTH is the osteoblast.

Effects on Kidney. In the kidney, PTH enhances the efficiency of Ca^{2+} reabsorption, inhibits tubular reabsorption of phosphate, and stimulates conversion of vitamin D to its biologically active form, 1,25-dihydroxy vitamin D_3 (calcitriol; *see* Figure 44–3). As a result, filtered Ca^{2+} is avidly retained, and its concentration increases in plasma, whereas phosphate is excreted, and its plasma concentration falls. Newly synthesized 1,25-dihydroxy vitamin D_3 interacts with specific high-affinity receptors in the intestine to increase the efficiency of intestinal Ca^{2+} absorption, thereby contributing to the increase in plasma (Ca^{2+}).

Calcitriol Synthesis. The final step in the activation of vitamin D to calcitriol occurs in kidney proximal tubule cells. Three primary regulators govern the enzymatic activity of the 25-hydroxyvitamin D_3-1α-hydroxylase that catalyzes this step: P_i, PTH, and Ca^{2+} (see later for further discussion). Reduced circulating or tissue phosphate content rapidly increases calcitriol production, whereas hyperphosphatemia or hypercalcemia suppresses it. PTH powerfully stimulates calcitriol synthesis. Thus, when hypocalcemia causes a rise in PTH concentration, both the PTH-dependent lowering of circulating P_i and a more direct effect of the hormone on the 1α-hydroxylase lead to increased circulating concentrations of calcitriol.

Integrated Regulation of Extracellular [Ca^{2+}] by PTH. Even modest reductions of serum Ca^{2+} stimulate PTH secretion. With prolonged hypocalcemia, the renal 1α-hydroxylase is induced, enhancing the synthesis and release of calcitriol that directly stimulates intestinal Ca^{2+} absorption (*see* Figure 44–3), and delivery of calcium from bone into the extracellular fluid is augmented. With prolonged and severe hypocalcemia, new bone remodeling units are activated to restore circulating Ca^{2+} concentrations, albeit at the expense of skeletal integrity. When plasma Ca^{2+} activity rises, PTH secretion is suppressed, and tubular Ca^{2+} reabsorption decreases. The reduction in circulating PTH promotes renal phosphate conservation, and both the decreased PTH and the increased phosphate depress calcitriol production and thereby decrease intestinal Ca^{2+} absorption. Finally, bone remodeling is suppressed. These integrated physiological events ensure a coherent response to positive or negative excursions of plasma Ca^{2+} concentrations.

VITAMIN D

Vitamin D is a hormone rather than a vitamin, and it plays an active role in Ca^{2+} homeostasis. The biological actions of vitamin D are mediated by the vitamin D receptor (VDR), a nuclear receptor. Vitamin D is the name applied to 2 related fat-soluble substances, vitamin D_3 (*cholecalciferol)* and vitamin D_2 (*ergocalciferol*) (Figure 44–4), that share the capacity to prevent or cure rickets. In humans there is no practical difference between the antirachitic potencies of vitamin D_2 and vitamin D_3. Therefore, "vitamin D" is used here as a collective term for vitamins D_2 and D_3.

The principal provitamin found in animal tissues is 7-dehydrocholesterol, which is synthesized in the skin. Exposure of the skin to sunlight converts 7-dehydrocholesterol to cholecalciferol (vitamin D_3). Ergosterol,

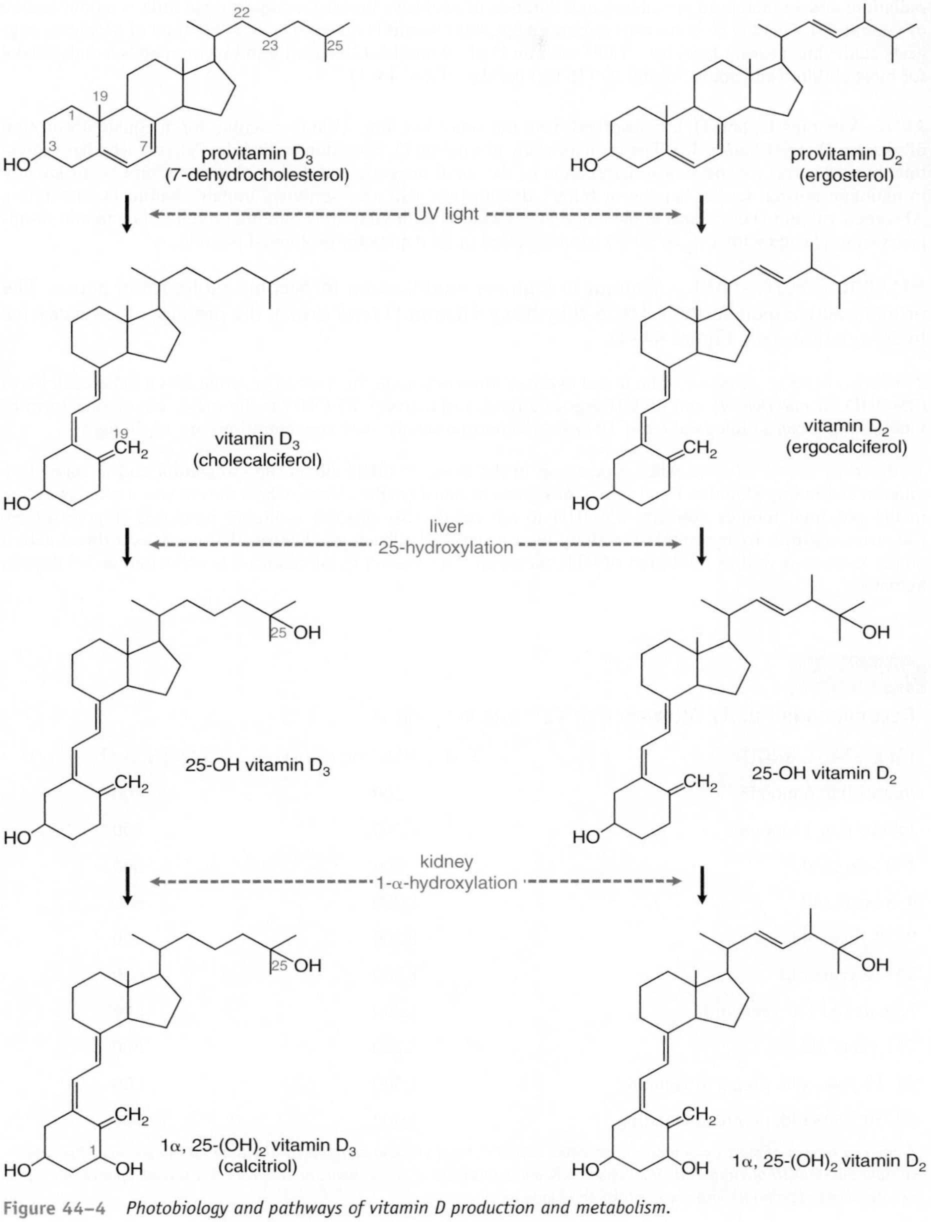

Figure 44–4 *Photobiology and pathways of vitamin D production and metabolism.*

present only in plants and fungi, is the provitamin for vitamin D_2 (ergocalciferol). Vitamin D_2 is the active constituent of a number of commercial vitamin preparations and is in irradiated bread and irradiated milk.

HUMAN REQUIREMENTS AND UNITS. Although sunlight provides adequate vitamin D supplies in the equatorial belt, in temperate climates insufficient cutaneous solar radiation, especially in winter, may necessitate dietary vitamin D supplementation. Serum levels of vitamin D vary widely, likely reflecting genetic background, diet, latitude, time spent out of doors, body size, developmental stage, and state of health, as well as plasma levels of *vitamin D binding protein*, a specific α-globulin. The actions of vitamin D may vary with the expression of components of the synthetic and action pathways of vitamin D. Other factors contributing to the rise of vitamin D deficiency may include diminished consumption of vitamin D–fortified foods owing to concerns about fat intake; reduced intake of dairy products; increased use of sunscreens and decreased exposure to sunlight to reduce the risk of skin cancer and prevent premature aging from exposure to ultraviolet radiation; and an increased prevalence and duration of exclusive breast-feeding (human milk is a poor source of vitamin D). There is no consensus regarding optimal vitamin D intake. The U.S. Institute of Medicine suggests achieving a serum level for 25-OH vitamin D of 50 nmol/L (20 ng/mL) and recommends a daily intake for most children and adults of 600 IU (15 μg) per day (Table 44–1).

ADME. Vitamins D_2 and D_3 are absorbed from the small intestine. Bile is essential for adequate absorption of vitamin D (*see* Chapter 46). The primary route of vitamin D_3 excretion is the bile. Patients who have intestinal bypass surgery or have or inflammation of the small intestine may fail to absorb vitamin D sufficiently to maintain normal levels; hepatic or biliary dysfunction also may seriously impair vitamin D absorption. Absorbed vitamin D circulates in the blood in association with vitamin D binding protein. The vitamin disappears from plasma with a $t_{1/2}$ of 20-30 h but is stored in fat depots for prolonged periods.

METABOLIC ACTIVATION. Vitamin D requires modification to become biologically active. The primary active metabolite is 1α,25-dihydroxy vitamin D (*calcitriol*), the product of 2 successive hydroxylations (*see* Figure 44–4).

25-Hydroxylation of Vitamin D. The initial hydroxylation occurs in the *liver* to generate 25-OH-cholecalciferol (25-OHD, or *calcifediol*) and 25-OH-ergocalciferol, respectively. 25-OHD is the major circulating form of vitamin D_3; it has a biological $t_{1/2}$ of 19 days, and normal steady-state concentrations are 15-50 ng/mL.

1α-Hydroxylation of 25-OHD. After production in the liver, 25-OHD enters the circulation and is carried by vitamin D–binding globulin. Final activation occurs primarily in the *kidney,* where the enzyme 1α-hydroxylase in the proximal tubules converts 25-OHD to *calcitriol.* This process is highly regulated (Figure 44–5). Calcitriol controls 1α-hydroxylase activity by a negative-feedback mechanism that involves a direct action on the kidney, as well as inhibition of PTH secretion. The plasma $t_{1/2}$ of calcitriol is estimated at 3-5 days in humans.

Table 44–1

Recommended Daily Allowance of Ca^{2+} and Vitamin D

LIFE STAGE GROUP	CALCIUM (mg/day)	VITAMIN D (IU/day)
Infants 0 to 6 months	200	400
Infants 6 to 12 months	260	400
1–3 years old	700	600
4–8 years old	1,000	600
9–18 years old	1,300	600
19–70 years old	1,000	600
Females 51–70 years old	1,200	600
71+ years old	1,200	800
14–18 years old, pregnant/lactating	1,300	600
19–50 years old, pregnant/lactating	1,000	600

A one-cup serving of most dairy products contains 200-300 mg of calcium and 100 IU of vitamin D. A serving of fish may contain 200-500 IU of vitamin D. The Goodman & Gilman website at AccessMedicine.com contains several updates on the debate about appropriate vitamin D intake and blood levels.

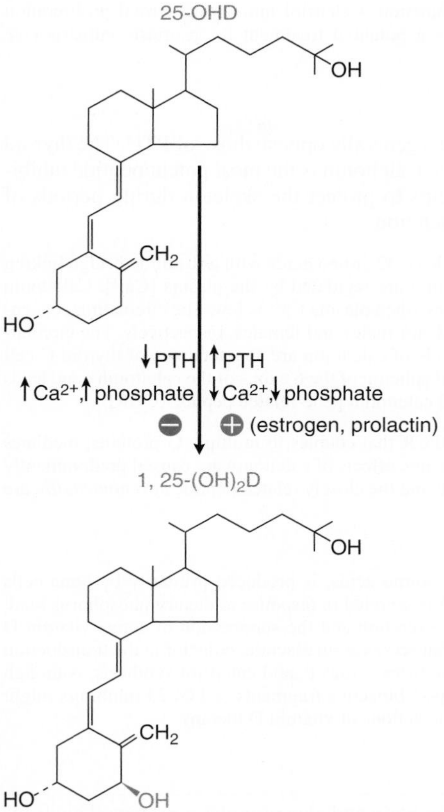

Figure 44–5 *Regulation of 1α-hydroxylase activity.* Changes in the plasma levels of PTH, Ca^{2+}, and phospate modulate the hydroxylation of 25-OH vitamin D to the active form, 1,25-dihydroxyvitamin D. 25-OHD, 25-hydroxycholecalciferol; 1,25-$(OH)_2$-D, calcitriol; PTH, parathyroid hormone.

PHYSIOLOGICAL FUNCTIONS AND MECHANISM OF ACTION. Calcitriol augments absorption and retention of Ca^{2+} and phosphate. Calcitriol acts to maintain normal concentrations of Ca^{2+} and phosphate in plasma by facilitating their absorption in the small intestine, by interacting with PTH to enhance their mobilization from bone, and by decreasing their renal excretion. The actions of calcitriol are mediated by binding to cytosolic VDRs within target cells, and the receptor–hormone complex translocates to the nucleus and interacts with DNA to modify gene transcription. The VDR belongs to the steroid and thyroid hormone receptor superfamily. Calcitriol also exerts nongenomic effects.

Calcium is absorbed predominantly in the duodenum. In the absence of calcitriol, GI calcium absorption is inefficient and involves passive diffusion via a paracellular pathway. Ca^{2+} absorption is potently augmented by calcitriol. It is likely that calcitriol enhances all 3 steps involved in intestinal Ca^{2+} absorption: entry across mucosal membranes (possibly involving TRPV6 Ca^{2+} channels), diffusion through the enterocytes, and active extrusion across serosal plasma membranes. Calcitriol upregulates the synthesis of calbindin-D_{9K}, calbindin-D_{28K}, and the serosal plasma membrane Ca^{2+}–ATPase. Calbindin-D_{9K} enhances the extrusion of Ca^{2+} by the Ca^{2+}–ATPase; the precise function of calbindin-D_{28K} is unsettled.

The primary role of calcitriol is to stimulate intestinal absorption of Ca^{2+}, which, in turn, indirectly promotes bone mineralization. Thus, PTH and calcitriol act independently to enhance bone resorption. Osteoblasts, the cells responsible for bone formation, express the VDR, and calcitriol induces their production of several proteins, including osteocalcin, a vitamin K–dependent protein that contains γ-carboxyglutamic acid residues, and interleukin-1 (IL-1), a lymphokine that promotes bone resorption. Thus, the current view is that calcitriol is a bone-mobilizing hormone but not a bone-forming hormone. Osteoporosis is a disease in which osteoclast responsiveness to calcitriol or other bone-resorbing agents is profoundly impaired, leading to deficient bone resorption.

Other Effects of Calcitriol. Effects of calcitriol extend well beyond calcium homeostasis. Receptors for calcitriol are distributed widely throughout the body. Calcitriol affects maturation and differentiation of mononuclear cells and influences cytokine production and immune function. Calcitriol inhibits epidermal proliferation and promotes epidermal differentiation and therefore is a potential treatment for psoriasis vulgaris (*see* Chapter 65).

CALCITONIN

Calcitonin is a hypocalcemic hormone whose actions generally oppose those of PTH. The thyroid parafollicular C cells produce and secrete calcitonin. Calcitonin is the most potent peptide inhibitor of osteoclast-mediated bone resorption and helps to protect the skeleton during periods of "calcium stress," such as growth, pregnancy, and lactation.

Regulation of Secretion. Calcitonin is a single-chain peptide of 32 amino acids with a disulfide bridge linking cys1 and cys7. The biosynthesis and secretion of calcitonin are regulated by the plasma [Ca^{2+}]. Calcitonin secretion increases when plasma Ca^{2+} is high and decreases when plasma Ca^{2+} is low. The circulating concentrations of calcitonin are low, normally <15 and 10 pg/mL for males and females, respectively. The circulating $t_{1/2}$ of calcitonin is ~10 min. Abnormally elevated levels of calcitonin are characteristic of thyroid C cell hyperplasia and medullary thyroid carcinoma. Differential splicing of the 6 exons of the calcitonin gene leads to tissue-specific production of calcitonin, katacalcin, and calcitonin gene-related peptide (CGRP).

Mechanism of Action. The calcitonin receptor (CTR), a GPCR that couples to multiple G proteins, mediates calcitonin's actions. The hypocalcemic and hypophosphatemic effects of calcitonin are caused predominantly by direct inhibition of osteoclastic bone resorption. CGRP and the closely related peptide *adrenomedullin* are potent endogenous vasodilators.

FIBROBLAST GROWTH FACTOR 23 AND KLOTHO

Fibroblast growth factor 23 (*FGF23*), a protein of 251 amino acids, is produced primarily by bone cells including osteoblasts, osteocytes, and lining cells. FGF23 is secreted in response to dietary phosphorus load; its main function is the promotion of urinary phosphate excretion and the suppression of active vitamin D production by the kidney. Klotho is a membrane protein that serves as an essential cofactor in the transduction of FGF23 signaling. Exogenous FGF23 administration reduces serum P_i and calcitriol synthesis. Although no clinical agents based on FGF23 have yet been developed, bioactive fragments or FGF23 inhibitors might become useful in counterbalancing the hyperphosphatemic actions of vitamin D therapy.

BONE PHYSIOLOGY

The skeleton is the primary structural support for the body and also provides a protected environment for hematopoiesis. It contains both a large mineralized matrix and a highly active cellular compartment.

BONE MASS. Bone mineral density (BMD) and fracture risk in later years reflect the maximal bone mineral content at skeletal maturity (peak bone mass) and the subsequent rate of bone loss. Major increases in bone mass, accounting for ~60% of final adult levels, occur during adolescence, mainly during years of highest growth velocity. Inheritance accounts for much of the variance in bone acquisition; other factors include circulating estrogen and androgens, physical activity, and dietary calcium. Bone mass peaks during the third decade, remains stable until age 50, and then declines progressively. In women, loss of estrogen at menopause accelerates the rate of bone loss. *Primary regulators of adult bone mass include physical activity, reproductive endocrine status, and calcium intake. Optimal maintenance of BMD requires sufficiency in all 3 areas, and deficiency of one is not compensated by excessive attention to another.*

BONE REMODELING. Once new bone is laid down, it is subject to a continuous process of breakdown and renewal called *remodeling*, by which bone mass is adjusted throughout adult life. Remodeling is carried out by myriad independent "bone remodeling units" throughout the skeleton. In response to physical or biochemical signals, recruitment of marrow precursor cells to the bone surface results in their fusion into the characteristic multinucleated osteoclasts that resorb, or excavate, a cavity into the bone. Osteoclast production is regulated by osteoblast-derived cytokines (e.g., IL-1 and IL-6). One important mechanism is the receptor for activating NF-κB (RANK) and its natural ligand, RANK ligand (RANKL; previously called *osteoclast differentiation factor*). On binding to RANK, RANKL induces osteoclast formation (Figure 44–6). RANKL initiates the activation of mature osteoclasts, as well as the differentiation of osteoclast precursors. Osteoblasts produce osteoprotegerin (OPG), which acts as a decoy ligand that inhibits osteoclast production by competing effectively with RANKL for binding to RANK. Under conditions favoring increased bone resorption, such as estrogen deprivation, OPG is suppressed, RANKL binds to RANK, and osteoclast production increases. When estrogen sufficiency is reestablished, OPG increases and competes effectively with RANKL for binding to RANK.

The resorption phase is followed by invasion of preosteoblasts into the base of the resorption cavity. These cells become osteoblasts and elaborate new bone matrix constituents that help form osteoid. Once the newly formed osteoid reaches a thickness of ~20 μm, mineralization begins. A complete remodeling cycle normally

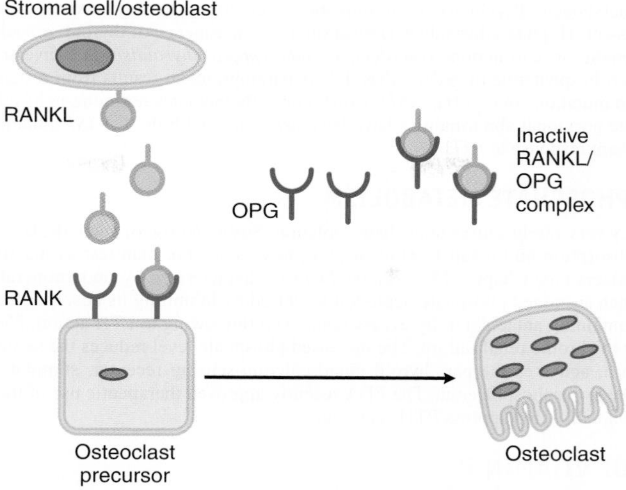

Figure 44–6 *Receptor for activating NF-κB ligand (RANKL) and osteoclast formation.* RANKL, acting on RANK, promotes osteoclast formation and subsequent resorption of bone matrix. Osteoprotegerin (OPG) binds to RANKL, reducing its binding to RANK and thereby inhibiting osteoclast differentiation.

requires ~6 months. Small bone deficits persist on completion of each cycle, reflecting inefficient remodeling dynamics. Consequently, lifelong accumulation of remodeling deficits underlies the well-documented phenomenon of age-related bone loss, a process that begins shortly after growth stops. *Alterations in remodeling activity represent the final pathway through which diverse stimuli, such as dietary sufficiency, exercise, hormones, and drugs, affect bone balance.*

DISORDERS OF MINERAL HOMEOSTASIS AND BONE

ABNORMAL CALCIUM METABOLISM

HYPERCALCEMIA. In an outpatient setting, the most common cause of hypercalcemia is primary hyperparathyroidism, which results from hypersecretion of PTH by 1 or more parathyroid glands. Symptoms and signs of primary hyperparathyroidism include fatigue, exhaustion, weakness, polydipsia, polyuria, joint pain, bone pain, constipation, depression, anorexia, nausea, heartburn, nephrolithiasis, and hematuria. This condition frequently is accompanied by significant hypophosphatemia owing to the effects of PTH in diminishing renal tubular phosphate reabsorption.

Vitamin D excess may cause hypercalcemia if sufficient 25-OHD is present to stimulate intestinal Ca^{2+} hyperabsorption, leading to hypercalcemia and suppressing PTH and 1,25-dihydroxyvitamin D levels. Measurement of 25-OHD is diagnostic. Serum assays for PTH, PTHrP, and 25-OH- and 1,25-$(OH)_2$D permit accurate diagnosis in the great majority of cases.

Hypercalcemia in hospitalized patients is caused most often by a systemic malignancy, either with or without bony metastasis. PTH-related protein (PTHrP) is a primitive, highly conserved protein that may be abnormally expressed in malignant tissue. The PTHrP interacts with the PTH-1 receptor in target tissues, thereby causing the hypercalcemia and hypophosphatemia seen in humoral hypercalcemia of malignancy. In some patients with lymphomas, hypercalcemia results from overproduction of 1,25-dihydroxyvitamin D by the tumor cells owing to expression of 1α-hydroxylase.

HYPOCALCEMIA. Combined deprivation of Ca^{2+} and vitamin D, as observed with malabsorption states, readily promotes hypocalcemia. When caused by malabsorption, hypocalcemia is accompanied by low concentrations of phosphate, total plasma proteins, and magnesium. Mild hypocalcemia (i.e., serum Ca^{2+} in the range of 8-8.5 mg/dL [2-2.1 mM]), is usually asymptomatic. Patients exhibit greater symptoms if the hypocalcemia develops acutely.

Symptoms of hypocalcemia include tetany and related phenomena such as paresthesias, increased neuromuscular excitability, laryngospasm, muscle cramps, and tonic-clonic convulsions. In chronic *hypoparathyroidism*, ectodermal changes (e.g., consisting of loss of hair, grooved and brittle fingernails, defects of dental enamel, and cataracts) occur. Psychiatric symptoms such as emotional lability, anxiety, depression, and delusions often are present. Hypoparathyroidis*m* is most often a consequence of thyroid or neck surgery but also may be due to genetic or autoimmune disorders. *Pseudohypoparathyroidism* is a diverse family of hypocalcemic and hyperphosphatemic disorders. Pseudohypoparathyroidism results from resistance to PTH; this resistance is due to mutations in $G_s\alpha$ (*GNAS1*), which normally mediates hormone-induced adenylyl cyclase activation. Multiple hormonal abnormalities have been associated with the *GNAS1* mutation, but none is as severe as the deficient response to PTH.

DISTURBED PHOSPHATE METABOLISM

Dietary inadequacy very rarely causes phosphate depletion. Sustained use of antacids, however, can severely limit phosphate absorption and result in clinical phosphate depletion, manifest as malaise, muscle weakness, and osteomalacia (*see* Chapter 45). *Osteomalacia* is characterized by undermineralized bone matrix and may occur when sustained phosphate depletion is caused by inhibiting its absorption in the GI tract (as with aluminum-containing antacids) or by excess renal excretion owing to PTH action. *Hyperphosphatemia* occurs commonly in chronic renal failure. The increased phosphate level reduces the serum Ca^{2+} concentration, which, in turn, activates the parathyroid gland calcium-sensing receptor, stimulates PTH secretion, and exacerbates the hyperphosphatemia. The FDA recently approved therapeutic use of the calcium-sensing receptor agonist *cinacalcet* to suppress PTH secretion.

DISORDERS OF VITAMIN D

HYPERVITAMINOSIS D. The acute or long-term administration of excessive amounts of vitamin D or enhanced responsiveness to normal amounts of the vitamin leads to derangements in calcium metabolism. In adults, hypervitaminosis D results from overtreatment of *hypo*parathyroidism and from faddist use of excessive doses. The amount of vitamin D necessary to cause hypervitaminosis varies widely. As a rough approximation, continued daily ingestion of ≥50,000 units may result in poisoning. The initial signs and symptoms of vitamin D toxicity are those associated with hypercalcemia.

Vitamin D Deficiency. Vitamin D deficiency results in inadequate absorption of Ca^{2+} and phosphate. The consequent decrease of plasma Ca^{2+} concentration stimulates PTH secretion, which acts to restore plasma Ca^{2+} at the expense of bone. Plasma concentrations of phosphate remain subnormal because of the phosphaturic effect of increased circulating PTH. In children, the result is a failure to mineralize newly formed bone and cartilage matrix, causing the defect in growth known as *rickets.* In adults, vitamin D deficiency results in osteomalacia, a disease characterized by generalized accumulation of undermineralized bone matrix. Muscle weakness, particularly of large proximal muscles, is typical and may reflect both hypophosphatemia and inadequate vitamin D action on muscle. Gross deformity of bone occurs only in advanced stages of the disease. Circulating 25-OHD concentrations <8 ng/mL are highly predictive of osteomalacia.

METABOLIC RICKETS AND OSTEOMALACIA. These disorders are characterized by abnormalities in calcitriol synthesis or response. Variants include *hypophosphatemic vitamin D–resistant rickets, vitamin D–dependent rickets, hereditary 1,25-dihydroxyvitamin D resistance, and renal osteodystrophy (renal rickets*). *See* Chapter 44 of the 12th edition of the parent text for details.

OSTEOPOROSIS

Osteoporosis is a condition of low bone mass and microarchitectural disruption that results in fractures with minimal trauma. Many women (30-50%) and men (15-30%) suffer a fracture related to osteoporosis. Characteristic sites of fracture include vertebral bodies, the distal radius, and the proximal femur, but osteoporotic individuals have generalized skeletal fragility, and fractures at sites such as ribs and long bones also are common. Fracture risk increases exponentially with age, and spine and hip fractures are associated with reduced survival.

Osteoporosis can be categorized as *primary* or *secondary.* Primary osteoporosis represents 2 different conditions: *type I osteoporosis*, characterized by loss of trabecular bone owing to estrogen lack at menopause, and *type II osteoporosis*, characterized by loss of cortical and trabecular bone in men and women due to long-term remodeling inefficiency, dietary inadequacy, and activation of the parathyroid axis with age. Secondary osteoporosis is due to systemic illness or medications such as glucocorticoids or phenytoin. The most successful approach to secondary osteoporosis is prompt resolution of the underlying cause or drug discontinuation. Whether primary or secondary, osteoporosis is associated with characteristic disordered bone remodeling, so the same therapies can be used.

PAGET DISEASE. Paget disease is characterized by single or multiple sites of disordered bone remodeling. It affects up to 2-3% of the population >60 years of age. The primary pathologic abnormality is increased bone resorption followed by exuberant bone formation. However, the newly formed bone is disorganized and of poor quality, resulting in characteristic bowing, stress fractures, and arthritis of joints adjoining the involved bone. The altered bone structure can produce secondary problems, such as deafness, spinal cord compression, high-output cardiac failure, and pain. Malignant degeneration to osteogenic sarcoma is a rare but lethal complication of Paget disease.

RENAL OSTEODYSTROPHY. Bone disease is a frequent consequence of chronic renal failure and dialysis. Pathologically, lesions are typical of hyperparathyroidism (osteitis fibrosa), vitamin D deficiency (osteomalacia), or a mixture of both. The underlying pathophysiology reflects increased serum phosphate and decreased calcium, leading to the loss of bone.

PHARMACOLOGICAL TREATMENT OF DISORDERS OF MINERAL ION HOMEOSTASIS AND BONE METABOLISM

HYPERCALCEMIA

Hypercalcemia can be life threatening. Such patients frequently are severely dehydrated because hypercalcemia compromises renal concentrating mechanisms. Thus, fluid resuscitation with large volumes of isotonic saline must be early and aggressive (6-8 L/day). Agents that augment Ca^{2+} excretion, such as loop diuretics (*see* Chapter 25), may help to counteract the effect of plasma volume expansion by saline but are contraindicated until volume is repleted.

Corticosteroids administered at high doses (e.g., 40-80 mg/day of prednisone) may be useful when hypercalcemia results from sarcoidosis, lymphoma, or hypervitaminosis D (*see* Chapter 42). The response to steroid therapy is slow; from 1-2 weeks may be required before plasma Ca^{2+} concentration falls. Calcitonin (CALCIMAR, MIACALCIN) may be useful in managing hypercalcemia. Reduction in Ca^{2+} can be rapid, although "escape" from the hormone commonly occurs within several days. The recommended starting dose is 4 units/kg of body weight administered subcutaneously every 12 h; if there is no response within 1-2 days, the dose may be increased to a maximum of 8 units/kg every 12 h. If the response after 2 more days still is unsatisfactory, the dose may be increased to a maximum of 8 units/kg every 6 h. Calcitonin can lower serum calcium by 1-2 mg/dL.

Intravenous *bisphosphonates* (*pamidronate, zoledronate*) have proven very effective in the management of hypercalcemia (see below for discussion of bisphosphonates). These agents potently inhibit osteoclastic bone resorption. Pamidronate (AREDIA) is given as an intravenous infusion of 60-90 mg over 4-24 h. With pamidronate, resolution of hypercalcemia occurs over several days, and the effect usually persists for several weeks. Zoledronate (ZOMETA) has superseded pamidronate because of its more rapid normalization of serum Ca^{2+} and longer duration of action.

Plicamycin (mithramycin, MITHRACIN) is a cytotoxic antibiotic that also decreases plasma Ca^{2+} concentrations by inhibiting bone resorption. Reduction in plasma Ca^{2+} concentrations occurs within 24-48 h when a relatively low dose of this agent is given (15-25 μg/kg of body weight) to minimize the high systemic toxicity of the drug; indeed, its toxicity generally precludes its use.

Once the hypercalcemic crisis has resolved or in patients with milder calcium elevations, long-term therapy is initiated. Parathyroidectomy remains the only definitive treatment for primary hyperparathyroidism. As described later, a calcium mimetic that stimulates the CaSR is a promising new therapy for hyperparathyroidism. Therapy of hypercalcemia of malignancy ideally is directed at the underlying cancer. When this is not possible, parenteral bisphosphonates often will maintain Ca^{2+} levels within an acceptable range.

HYPOCALCEMIA AND OTHER THERAPEUTIC USES OF CALCIUM

Hypoparathyroidism is treated primarily with vitamin D and dietary supplementation with Ca^{2+} as various calcium salts. *Calcium chloride* ($CaCl_2 \cdot 2H_2O$) contains 27% Ca^{2+}; it is valuable in the treatment of hypocalcemic tetany and laryngospasm. The salt is given intravenously and *must never be injected* into tissues. Injections of calcium chloride are accompanied by peripheral vasodilation and a cutaneous burning sensation. The salt usually is given intravenously in a concentration of 10% (equivalent to 1.36 mEq Ca^{2+}/mL). The rate of injection should be slow (not >1 mL/min) to prevent cardiac arrhythmias from a high concentration of Ca^{2+}. The injection may induce a moderate fall in blood pressure owing to vasodilation. *Calcium gluceptate* injection (a 22% solution; 18 mg or 0.9 mEq of Ca^{2+}/mL) is administered intravenously at a dose of 5-20 mL for the treatment of severe hypocalcemic tetany. *Calcium gluconate* injection (a 10% solution; 9.3 mg of Ca^{2+}/mL) given intravenously is the treatment of choice for severe hypocalcemic tetany. The intramuscular route should not be employed because abscess formation at the injection site may result.

Calcium carbonate and *calcium acetate* are used to restrict phosphate absorption in patients with chronic renal failure and oxalate absorption in patients with inflammatory bowel disease. Acute administration of Ca^{2+} may be lifesaving in patients with extreme hyperkalemia (serum K^+ > 7 mEq/L). Calcium gluconate (10-30 mL of a 10% solution) can reverse some of the cardiotoxic effects of hyperkalemia. Additional FDA-approved uses of Ca^{2+} include intravenous treatment for black widow spider envenomation and management of magnesium toxicity.

CLINICAL FORMS OF VITAMIN D. Calcitriol (1,25-dihydroxycholecalciferol; CALCIJEX, ROCALTROL) is available for oral administration or injection. Several derivatives of vitamin D are also used therapeutically.

Doxercalciferol (1α-hydroxyvitamin D_2, HECTOROL), a prodrug that first must be activated by hepatic 25-hydroxylation, is approved for use in treating secondary hyperparathyroidism. Dihydrotachysterol (DHT, ROXANE) is a reduced form of vitamin D_2. In the liver, DHT is converted to its active form, 25-OH dihydrotachysterol. DHT is effective in mobilizing bone mineral at high doses; it therefore can be used to maintain plasma Ca^{2+} in hypoparathyroidism. DHT is well absorbed from the GI tract and maximally increases serum Ca^{2+} concentration after 2 weeks of daily administration. The hypercalcemic effects typically persist for 2 weeks but can last for up to 1 month. DHT is available for oral administration in doses ranging from 0.2-1 mg/day (average 0.6 mg/day).

Ergocalciferol (calciferol, DRISDOL) is pure vitamin D_2. It is available for oral, intramuscular, or intravenous administration. Ergocalciferol is indicated for the prevention of vitamin D deficiency and the treatment of familial hypophosphatemia, hypoparathyroidism, and vitamin D–resistant rickets type II, typically in doses of 50,000-200,000 units/day in conjunction with calcium supplements. 1α-Hydroxycholecalciferol (1-OHD_3, alphacalcidol; ONE-ALPHA) is a synthetic vitamin D_3 derivative that is already hydroxylated in the 1α position and is rapidly hydroxylated by 25-hydroxylase to form 1,25-$(OH)_2D_3$. It is equal to calcitriol in assays for stimulation of intestinal absorption of Ca^{2+} and bone mineralization and does not require renal activation. It is available in the U.S. for experimental purposes.

ANALOGS OF CALCITRIOL. Several vitamin D analogs suppress PTH secretion by the parathyroid glands but have less or negligible hypercalcemic activity. They therefore offer a safer and more effective means of controlling secondary hyperparathyroidism.

Calcipotriol (calcipotriene) is a synthetic derivative of calcitriol with a modified side chain. Calcipotriol is <1% as active as calcitriol in regulating Ca^{2+} metabolism. Calcipotriol has been studied extensively as a treatment for psoriasis (*see* Chapter 65).

Paricalcitol (1,25-dihydroxy-19-norvitamin D_2, ZEMPLAR) is a synthetic calcitriol derivative that lacks the exocyclic C19 and has a vitamin D_2 rather than vitamin D_3 side chain (*see* Figure 44–4). It reduces serum PTH levels without producing hypercalcemia or altering serum phosphorus. Paricalcitol administered intravenously is FDA-approved for treating secondary hyperparathyroidism in patients with chronic renal failure.

22-Oxacalcitriol (1,25-dihydroxy-22-oxavitamin D_3, OCT, maxacalcitol, OXAROL) differs from calcitriol only in the substitution of C-22 with an O atom. Oxacalcitriol has a low affinity for vitamin D–binding protein; thus, more of the drug circulates in the free (unbound) form and is metabolized more rapidly than calcitriol with a consequent shorter $t_{1/2}$. Oxacalcitriol is a potent suppressor of PTH gene expression and shows very limited activity on intestine and bone. It is a useful compound in patients with overproduction of PTH in chronic renal failure.

THERAPEUTIC INDICATIONS FOR VITAMIN D

The major therapeutic uses of vitamin D are:

- Prophylaxis and cure of nutritional rickets
- Treatment of metabolic rickets and osteomalacia, particularly in the setting of chronic renal failure
- Treatment of hypoparathyroidism
- Prevention and treatment of osteoporosis
- Dietary supplementation

NUTRITIONAL RICKETS. Nutritional rickets results from inadequate exposure to sunlight or deficiency of dietary vitamin D. The incidence of this condition in the U.S. is now increasing. Infants and children receiving adequate amounts of vitamin D–fortified food do not require additional vitamin D; however, breast-fed infants or those fed unfortified formula should receive 400 units of vitamin D daily as a supplement (*see* Table 44–1), usually administered with vitamin A, for which purpose a number of balanced vitamin A and D preparations are available. *Because the fetus acquires >85% of its calcium stores during the third trimester, premature infants are especially susceptible to rickets and may require supplemental vitamin D.* Treatment of fully developed rickets requires a larger dose of vitamin D than that used prophylactically. One thousand units daily will normalize plasma Ca^{2+} and phosphate concentrations in ~10 days, with radiographic evidence of healing within ~3 weeks. However, a larger dose of 3000–4000 units daily often is prescribed for more rapid healing, particularly when respiration is compromised by severe thoracic rickets.

TREATMENT OF OSTEOMALACIA AND RENAL OSTEODYSTROPHY. Osteomalacia, distinguished by undermineralization of bone matrix, occurs commonly during sustained phosphate depletion. Patients with chronic renal disease are at risk for developing osteomalacia but also may develop a complex bone disease called *renal osteodystrophy*. In this setting, bone metabolism is stimulated by an increase in PTH and by a delay in bone mineralization that is due to decreased renal synthesis of calcitriol. In renal osteodystrophy, low bone mineral density may be accompanied by high-turnover bone lesions typically seen in patients with uncontrolled hyperparathyroidism or by low bone remodeling activity seen in patients with adynamic bone disease. The therapeutic approach to the patient with renal osteodystrophy depends on its specific type. In high-turnover (hyperparathyroid) or mixed high-turnover disease with deficient mineralization, dietary phosphate restriction, generally in combination with a phosphate binder, is recommended. Calcium-containing phosphate binders along with calcitriol administration may contribute to oversuppression of PTH secretion and likewise result in adynamic bone disease and an increased incidence of vascular calcification.

Highly effective non-calcium-containing phosphate binders have been developed. *Sevelamer hydrochloride* (RENAGEL), a nonabsorbable phosphate-binding polymer, effectively lowers serum phosphate concentration in hemodialysis patients. Sevelamer is modestly water soluble and only trace amounts are absorbed from the GI tract. Side effects of sevelamer include vomiting, nausea, diarrhea, and dyspepsia. Sevelamer does not affect the bioavailability of digoxin, warfarin, enalapril, or metoprolol. *Lanthanum carbonate* (FOSRENOL) is a poorly permeable trivalent cation that is useful in treating the hyperphosphatemia associated with renal osteodystrophy.

HYPOPARATHYROIDISM. Vitamin D and its analogs are a mainstay of the therapy of hypoparathyroidism. DHT has a faster onset, shorter duration of action, and a greater effect on bone mobilization than does vitamin D and traditionally has been a preferred agent. Calcitriol may be preferred for temporary treatment of hypocalcemia while awaiting effects of a slower-acting form of vitamin D.

PREVENTION AND TREATMENT OF OSTEOPOROSIS. This is described separately, earlier in the chapter.

DIETARY SUPPLEMENTATION. *See* Table 44–1.

ADVERSE EFFECTS OF VITAMIN D THERAPY

The primary toxicity associated with calcitriol reflects its potent effect to increase intestinal absorption of Ca^{2+} and phosphate, along with the potential to mobilize osseous Ca^{2+} and phosphate. Hypercalcemia, with or without hyperphosphatemia, commonly complicates calcitriol therapy and may limit its use at doses that effectively suppress PTH secretion. Noncalcemic vitamin D analogs provide alternative interventions, although they do not obviate the need to monitor serum Ca^{2+} and phosphorus concentrations. Hypervitaminosis D is treated by immediate withdrawal of the vitamin, a low-calcium diet, administration of glucocorticoids, and vigorous fluid support; forced saline diuresis with loop diuretics is also useful. With this regimen, the plasma Ca^{2+} concentration falls to normal, and Ca^{2+} in soft tissue tends to be mobilized. Conspicuous improvement in renal function occurs unless renal damage has been severe.

CALCITONIN

DIAGNOSTIC USE. Calcitonin is a sensitive and specific marker for the presence of medullary thyroid carcinoma (MTC), a neuroendocrine malignancy originating in thyroid parafollicular C cells.

THERAPEUTIC USE. Calcitonin lowers plasma Ca^{2+} and phosphate concentrations in patients with hypercalcemia. Although calcitonin is effective for up to 6 h in the initial treatment of hypercalcemia, patients become refractory after a few days. This is likely due to receptor downregulation. Use of calcitonin does not substitute for aggressive fluid resuscitation, and the bisphosphonates are the preferred agents. Calcitonin is effective in disorders of increased skeletal remodeling, such as Paget disease, and in some patients with osteoporosis. For Paget disease, calcitonin generally is administered by subcutaneous injection because intranasal delivery is relatively ineffective owing to limited bioavailability. After initial therapy at 100 units/day, the dose typically is reduced to 50 units 3 times a week. Side effects of calcitonin include nausea, hand swelling, urticaria, and, rarely, intestinal cramping.

BISPHOSPHONATES

Bisphosphonates are analogs of pyrophosphate that contain 2 phosphonate groups attached to a geminal (central) carbon that replaces the oxygen in pyrophosphate (Figure 44–7). These agents form a 3-dimensional structure capable of chelating divalent cations such as Ca^{2+} and have a strong affinity for bone, targeting especially bone surfaces undergoing remodeling.

Bisphosphonates are used extensively in conditions characterized by osteoclast-mediated bone resorption, including osteoporosis, steroid-induced osteoporosis, Paget disease, tumor-associated osteolysis, breast and prostate cancer, and hypercalcemia. Calcium supplements, antacids, food or medications containing divalent cations, such as iron, may interfere with intestinal absorption of bisphosphonates. Recent evidence suggests that second- and third-generation bisphosphonates also may be effective anticancer drugs.

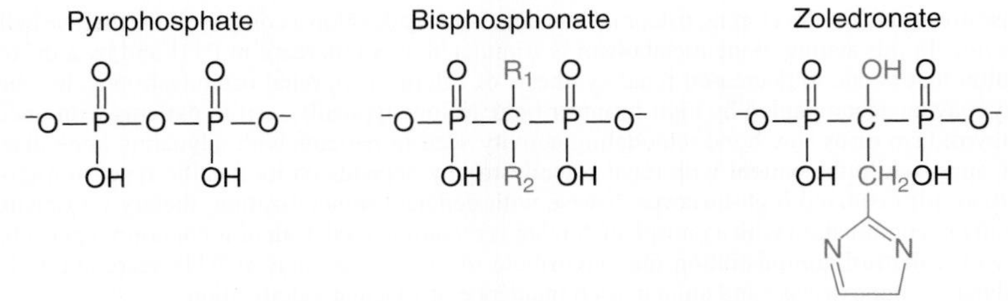

Pyrophosphate Bisphosphonate Zoledronate

Figure 44–7 *Pyrophosphate and bisphosphonates.* The substituents (R_1 and R_2) on the central carbon of the bisphosphonate parent structure are shown in *blue*.

Bisphosphonates act by direct inhibition of bone resorption. First-generation bisphosphonates contain minimally modified side chains (medronate, clodronate, and etidronate) or possess a chlorophenol group (tiludronate) and are the least potent agents. Second-generation aminobisphosphonates (e.g., alendronate and pamidronate) contain a nitrogen group in the side chain and are 10-100 times more potent than first-generation compounds. Third-generation bisphosphonates (e.g., risedronate and zoledronate) contain a nitrogen atom within a heterocyclic ring and are up to 10,000 times more potent than first-generation agents.

Bisphosphonates concentrate at sites of active remodeling, remain in the matrix until the bone is remodeled, and then are released in the acid environment of the resorption lacunae and induce apoptosis in osteoclasts. Although bisphosphonates prevent hydroxyapatite dissolution, their antiresorptive action is due to direct inhibitory effects on osteoclasts rather than strictly physiochemical effects. The antiresorptive activity apparently involves 2 primary mechanisms: osteoclast apoptosis and inhibition of components of the cholesterol biosynthetic pathway.

AVAILABLE BISPHOSPHONATES. *Etidronate sodium* (DIDRONEL) is used for treatment of Paget disease. Etidronate has been supplanted largely by pamidronate and zoledronate for treating hypercalcemia. *Pamidronate* (AREDIA; available in the U.S. only for parenteral administration) is approved for management of hypercalcemia and for prevention of bone loss in breast cancer and multiple myeloma, and also is effective in other skeletal disorders. For treatment of hypercalcemia, pamidronate may be given as an intravenous infusion of 60-90 mg over 4-24 h. Several newer bisphosphonates have been approved for treatment of Paget disease. These include *tiludronate* (SKELID), *alendronate* (FOSAMAX), and *risedronate* (ACTONEL). Tiludronate standard dosing is 400 mg/day orally for 3 months. Tiludronate in recommended doses does not interfere with bone mineralization, unlike etidronate. Zoledronate (ZOMETA) is approved for treating Paget disease; administered as a single 5-mg infusion, zoledronate decreases bone turnover markers for 6 months with no loss of therapeutic effect. Zoledronate is widely used for prevention of osteoporosis in prostate and breast cancer patients receiving hormonal therapy. It reduces both vertebral and nonvertebral fractures. A 4-mg formulation is available for intravenous treatment of hypercalcemia of malignancy, multiple myeloma, or bone metastasis resulting from solid tumors. The potent bisphosphonate *ibandronate* (BONIVA) is approved for the prevention and treatment of postmenopausal osteoporosis. The recommended oral dose is 2.5 mg daily or 150 mg once monthly.

For patients in whom oral bisphosphonates cause severe esophageal distress, *intravenous zoledronate* (RECLAST) or ibandronate offer skeletal protection without causing adverse GI effects. For treatment of osteoporosis, ibandronate (3 mg) is given intravenously every 3 months. Zoledronate is the first bisphosphonate to be approved from once-yearly intravenous treatment of osteoporosis (5 mg annually).

ADME. All oral bisphosphonates are very poorly absorbed from the intestine and have remarkably limited bioavailability (<1% [alendronate, risedronate] to 6% [etidronate, tiludronate]). Hence, these drugs should be administered with a full glass of water following an overnight fast and at least 30 min before breakfast. Oral bisphosphonates have not been used widely in children or adolescents because of uncertainty of long-term effects of bisphosphonates on the growing skeleton. Bisphosphonates are excreted primarily by the kidneys and are not recommended for patients with a creatinine clearance of <30 mL/min.

ADVERSE EFFECTS. Oral bisphosphonates can cause heartburn, esophageal irritation, or esophagitis. Other GI side effects include abdominal pain and diarrhea. Symptoms often abate when patients take the medication after an overnight fast, with tap or filtered water (not mineral water), and remain upright. Patients with active upper GI disease should not be given oral bisphosphonates. Serious osteonecrosis of the jaw is associated with use of bisphosphonates. Initial parenteral infusion of pamidronate may cause skin flushing, flu-like symptoms, muscle and joint aches and pains, nausea and vomiting, abdominal discomfort and diarrhea (or constipation) but mainly when given in higher concentrations or at faster rates than those recommended. These symptoms are short lived and generally do not recur with subsequent administration. Zoledronate can cause severe hypocalcemia and has been associated with renal toxicity, deterioration of renal function, and potential renal failure. Infusion of zoledronate should be given over at least 15 min, and the dose should be 4 mg; patients should have standard laboratory and clinical parameters of renal function assessed prior to treatment and periodically after treatment to monitor for deterioration in renal function.

OTHER THERAPEUTIC USES

Postmenopausal Osteoporosis. Much interest is focused on the role of bisphosphonates in the treatment of osteoporosis. Clinical trials show that treatment is associated with increased bone mineral density and protection against fracture.

Cancer. Bisphosphonates may also have direct antitumor action by inhibiting oncogene activation and through their anti-angiogenic effects. Randomized clinical trials of bisphosphonates in patients with breast cancer suggest that these agents delay or prevent development of metastases as a component of endocrine adjuvant therapy.

PARATHYROID HORMONE

Continuous administration of PTH or high-circulating PTH levels achieved in primary hyperparathyroidism causes bone demineralization and osteopenia. However, *intermittent* PTH administration promotes bone growth. Synthetic human 34-amino-acid amino-terminal PTH fragment [hPTH(1-34), *teriparatide* (FORTEO)] is approved for use in treating severe osteoporosis.

ADME. Pharmacokinetics and systemic actions of teriparatide on mineral metabolism are the same as for PTH. Teriparatide is administered by once-daily subcutaneous injection of 20 μg into the thigh or abdomen. Serum PTH concentrations peak at 30 min after the injection and are undetectable within 3 h, whereas the serum Ca^{2+} concentration peaks at 4-6 h after administration. Teriparatide bioavailability averages 95%; clearance averages 62 L/h in women and 94 L/h in men. The serum $t_{1/2}$ of teriparatide is ~1 h when administered subcutaneously versus 5 min when administered intravenously. The elimination of PTH(1-34) and full-length PTH proceeds by nonspecific enzymatic mechanisms in the liver, followed by renal excretion.

CLINICAL EFFECTS. In postmenopausal women with osteoporosis, teriparatide increases BMD and reduces the risk of vertebral and nonvertebral fractures. Candidates for teriparatide treatment include women who have a history of osteoporotic fracture, who have multiple risk factors for fracture, or who failed or are intolerant of previous osteoporosis therapy. Men with primary or hypogonadal osteoporosis are also candidates for treatment with teriparatide.

ADVERSE EFFECTS. Adverse effects include exacerbation of nephrolithiasis and elevation of serum uric acid levels. Teriparatide use should be limited to no more than 2 years and should not be used in patients who are at increased baseline risk for osteosarcoma (including those with Paget disease of bone, unexplained elevations of alkaline phosphatase, open epiphyses, or prior radiation therapy involving the skeleton). A tumor registry-based analysis of the occurrence of osteosarcoma in teriparatide-treated patients is ongoing; cases of osteosarcoma associated with the drug should be reported to the FDA.

CALCIUM SENSOR MIMETICS: CINACALCET

Calcimimetics are drugs that mimic the stimulatory effect of Ca^{2+} on the calcium-sensing receptor (CaSR) to inhibit PTH secretion by the parathyroid glands. By enhancing the sensitivity of the CaSR to extracellular Ca^{2+}, calcimimetics lower the concentration of Ca^{2+} at which PTH secretion is suppressed. Inorganic di- and trivalent cations, along with polycations such as spermine, aminoglycosides (e.g., streptomycin, gentamicin, and neomycin) and polybasic amino acids (e.g., polylysine) are full agonists and are referred to a *type I calcimimetics*. Phenylalkylamine derivatives that are allosteric CaSR modulators that require the presence of Ca^{2+} or other full agonists to enhance the sensitivity of activation without altering the maximal response are designated *type II calcimimetics*. Cinacalcet (SENSIPAR) is approved for the treatment of secondary hyperparathyroidism. Cinacalcet lowers serum PTH levels in patients with normal or reduced renal function.

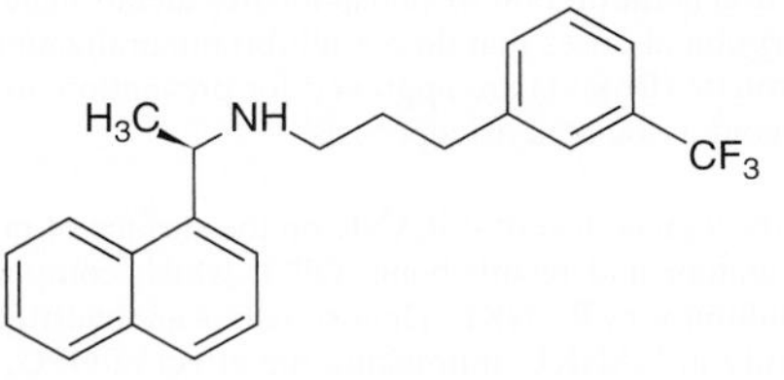

H_3C NH CF_3

Cinacalcet

ADME. Cinacalcet exhibits first-order absorption, with maximal serum concentrations achieved 2-6 h after oral administration. Maximal effects on serum PTH occur 2–4 h after administration. Cinacalcet has a $t_{1/2}$ of 30-40 h and is eliminated primarily by renal excretion (85%); the drug is also metabolized by multiple hepatic cytochromes, including CYPs 3A4, 2D6, and 1A2.

Cinacalcet is available in 30-, 60-, and 90-mg tablets. The recommended starting dose for treatment of secondary hyperparathyroidism in patients with chronic kidney disease on dialysis is 30 mg once daily, with a maximum of 180 mg/day. For treatment of parathyroid carcinoma, a starting dose of 30 mg twice daily is recommended, with a maximum of 90 mg 4 times daily. The starting dose is titrated upward every 2-4 weeks to maintain the PTH level between 150 and 300 pg/mL (secondary hyperparathyroidism) or to normalize serum calcium (parathyroid carcinoma).

ADVERSE REACTIONS. The principal adverse event with cinacalcet is hypocalcemia. Thus, the drug should not be used if the initial serum [Ca^{2+}] is <8.4 mg/dL; serum Ca^{2+} and phosphorus concentrations should be measured within 1 week, and PTH should be measured within 4 weeks after initiating therapy or after changing dosage. Seizure threshold is lowered by significant reductions in serum Ca^{2+}, so patients with a history of seizure disorders should be monitored especially closely. Finally, adynamic bone disease may develop if the PTH level is <100 pg/mL, and the drug should be discontinued or the dose decreased if the PTH level falls below 150 pg/mL.

DRUG INTERACTIONS. Potential drug interactions can be anticipated with drugs that interfere with Ca^{2+} homeostasis or that hinder cinacalcet absorption. Potentially interfering drugs may include vitamin D analogs, phosphate binders, bisphosphonates, calcitonin, glucocorticoids, gallium, and cisplatin. Caution is recommended when cinacalcet is coadministered with inhibitors of CYP3A4 (e.g., ketoconazole, erythromycin, or itraconazole), CYP2D6 (many β adrenergic receptor blockers, flecainide, vinblastine, and most tricyclic antidepressants), and many other drugs.

INTEGRATED APPROACH TO PREVENTION AND TREATMENT OF OSTEOPOROSIS

Osteoporosis is a major and growing public health problem in developed nations. Approximately 50% women and 25% of men >50 years of age will experience an osteoporosis-related fracture. However, important reductions in fracture risk can be achieved with appropriate lifelong attention to prevention (muscle strengthening exercise; avoiding smoking and excessive alcohol use). Attention to nutritional status (i.e., increased dietary calcium or calcium and/or vitamin D supplements) also may be required. Pharmacological agents used to manage osteoporosis act by decreasing the rate of bone resorption and thereby slowing the rate of bone loss (antiresorptive therapy) or by promoting bone formation (anabolic therapy). Because bone remodeling is a coupled process, antiresorptive drugs ultimately decrease the rate of bone formation and therefore do not promote substantial gains in BMD.

Pharmacological treatment of osteoporosis is aimed at restoring bone strength and preventing fractures. Antiresorptive drugs such as the bisphosphonates, estrogen, or the selective estrogen receptor modulator (SERM) raloxifene, and, to some extent, calcitonin inhibit osteoclast-mediated bone loss, thereby reducing bone turnover. Although the administration of estrogen to women at menopause is a powerful intervention to preserve bone and protect against fracture, the detrimental effects of hormone-replacement therapy (HRT) have mandated a major reexamination on treatment options (*see* later and Chapter 40). In addition to antiresorptive agents, the FDA has approved the biologically active PTH fragment PTH(1–34) (*teriparatide*, FORTEO) for use in treating postmenopausal women with osteoporosis and to increase bone mass in men with primary or hypogonadal osteoporosis.

ANTIRESORPTIVE AGENTS

Bisphosphonates. Bisphosphonates are the most frequently used drugs for the prevention and treatment of osteoporosis. Second- and third-generation oral bisphosphonates alendronate and risedronate have sufficient potency to suppress bone resorption at doses that do not inhibit mineralization. Alendronate (FOSAMAX), risedronate (ACTONEL), and ibandronate (BONIVA) are approved for prevention and treatment of osteoporosis and for the treatment of glucocorticoid-associated osteoporosis.

Denosumab. RANKL binds to its cognate receptor RANK on the surface of precursor and mature osteoclasts, and stimulates these cells to mature and resorb bone. OPG, which competes with RANK for binding to RANKL, is the physiological inhibitor of RANKL. Denosumab is an investigational human monoclonal antibody that binds with high affinity to RANKL, mimicking the effect of OPG, and thereby reducing the binding of RANKL to RANK. Denosumab blocks osteoclast formation and activation. It increases BMD and decreases bone turnover markers when given subcutaneously, 60 mg once every 6 months.

Selective Estradiol Receptor Modulators (SERMs). Raloxifene (EVISTA) acts as an estrogen agonist on bone and liver, is inactive on the uterus, and acts as an anti-estrogen on the breast (*see* Chapter 40). In postmenopausal women, raloxifene stabilizes and modestly increases BMD and has been shown to reduce the risk of vertebral compression fracture. Raloxifene is approved for both the prevention and treatment of osteoporosis. The major drawback of raloxifene is that it can worsen vasomotor symptoms.

Estrogen. Postmenopausal status or estrogen deficiency at any age significantly increases a patient's risk for osteoporosis and fractures. Likewise, overwhelming evidence supports the positive impact of estrogen replacement on the conservation of bone and protection against osteoporotic fracture after menopause (*see* Chapter 40). Since the outcome of the Women's Health Initiative (WHI) studies has indicated significantly increased risks of heart disease and breast cancer, the consensus now is to reserve HRT only for the short-term relief of vasomotor symptoms associated with menopause.

Calcium. The rationale for using supplemental calcium to protect bone varies with time of life. For preteens and adolescents, adequate substrate calcium is required for bone accretion. Higher calcium intake during the third decade of life is positively related to the final phase of bone acquisition. There is controversy about the role of calcium during the early years after menopause, when the primary basis for bone loss is estrogen withdrawal. In elderly subjects, supplemental calcium suppresses bone turnover and improves BMD.

Vitamin D and Its Analogs. Modest supplementation with vitamin D (400-800 IU/day) may improve intestinal Ca^{2+} absorption, suppress bone remodeling, and improve BMD in individuals with marginal or deficient vitamin D status. A prospective study found that neither dietary calcium nor vitamin D intake was of major importance for the primary prevention of osteoporotic fractures in women. However, supplemental vitamin D in combination with calcium reduced fracture incidence in multiple trials. The use of calcitriol to treat osteoporosis is distinct from ensuring vitamin D nutritional adequacy. Here, the rationale is to suppress parathyroid function directly and reduce bone turnover. Calcitriol and the polar vitamin D metabolite 1α-hydroxycholecalciferol are used frequently in Japan and other countries, but experience in the U.S. has been mixed.

Calcitonin. Calcitonin inhibits osteoclastic bone resorption and modestly increases bone mass in patients with osteoporosis, most prominently in patients with high intrinsic rates of bone turnover. Calcitonin nasal spray (200 units/day) reportedly reduces the incidence of vertebral compression fractures by ~40% in osteoporotic women.

Thiazide Diuretics. Although not strictly antiresorptive, thiazides reduce urinary Ca^{2+} excretion and constrain bone loss in patients with hypercalciuria. Hydrochlorothiazide, 25 mg once or twice daily, may reduce urinary Ca^{2+} excretion substantially. Effective doses of thiazides for reducing urinary Ca^{2+} excretion generally are lower than those necessary for blood pressure control (*see* Chapter 25).

Teriparatide. Teriparatide (FORTEO) is the only agent currently available that increases new bone formation. It is FDA-approved for treatment of osteoporosis for up to 2 years in both men and postmenopausal women at high risk for fractures. Teriparatide significantly decreased the incidence of vertebral (4-5% vs. 14%) and non-vertebral fractures (3% vs. 6%) compared to placebo in a prospective, randomized control study. Teriparatide increases predominantly trabecular bone at the lumbar spine and femoral neck; it has less significant effects at cortical sites. Teriparatide is approved at the 20 μg dose, administered once daily by subcutaneous injection in the thigh or abdominal wall. The most common adverse effects associated with teriparatide include injection-site pain, nausea, headaches, leg cramps, and dizziness.

COMBINATION THERAPIES

OSTEOPOROSIS. Because teriparatide stimulates bone formation, whereas bisphosphonates reduce bone resorption, it was predicted that therapy combining the 2 would enhance the effect on BMD more than treatment with either one alone. However, addition of alendronate to PTH treatment provided no additional benefit for BMD and reduced the anabolic effect of PTH in both women and men. Sequential treatment with PTH(1-84) followed by alendronate increased vertebral BMD to a greater degree than alendronate or estrogen alone.

PAGET DISEASE. Although most patients with Paget disease require no treatment, factors such as severe pain, neural compression, progressive deformity, hypercalcemia, high-output congestive heart failure, and repeated fracture risk are considered indications for treatment. Bisphosphonates and calcitonin decrease the elevated biochemical markers of bone turnover, such as plasma alkaline phosphatase activity and urinary excretion of hydroxyproline. An initial course of bisphosphonate typically is given once daily or once weekly for 6 months. With treatment, most patients experience a decrease in bone pain over several weeks. Such treatment may induce long-lasting remission. If symptoms recur, additional courses of therapy can be effective. Optimal therapy for Paget disease varies among patients. Bisphosphonates are the standard therapy. Intravenous pamidronate induces long-term remission following a single infusion. Zoledronate seems to exhibit greater response rates and a longer median duration of complete response. Compared with calcitonin, bisphosphonates have the advantage of oral administration, lower cost, lack of antigenicity, and generally fewer side effects.

FLUORIDE

Fluoride is discussed because of its effects on dentition and bone and its toxic properties.

ADME. Fluoride is obtained from the ingestion of plants and water, with most absorption taking place in the intestine. A second route of absorption is through the lungs, and inhalation of fluoride present in dusts and gases constitutes the major route of industrial exposure. Fluoride is distributed widely in organs and tissues but is concentrated in bone and teeth, and the skeletal burden is related to intake and age. Bone deposition reflects skeletal turnover; growing bone shows greater deposition than mature bone. The kidneys are the major site of fluoride excretion. Small amounts of fluoride also appear in sweat, milk, and intestinal secretions.

PHARMACOLOGICAL ACTIONS AND USES. Because it is concentrated in the bone, the radionuclide ^{18}F has been used in skeletal imaging. Sodium fluoride enhances osteoblast activity and increases bone volume. These effects may be bimodal, with low doses stimulating and higher doses suppressing osteoblasts. However, the apparent effects of fluoride in osteoporosis are slight compared with those achieved with PTH or others. Fluoride can inhibit several enzyme systems and diminish tissue respiration and anaerobic glycolysis.

Fluoride and Dental Caries. Supplementation of water fluoride content to 1.0 ppm is a safe and practical intervention that substantially reduces the incidence of caries in permanent teeth. There are partial benefits for children who begin drinking fluoridated water at any age; however, optimal benefits are obtained at ages before permanent teeth erupt. Topical application of fluoride solutions by dental personnel appears to be effective on newly erupted teeth and can reduce the incidence of caries by 30-40%. Dietary fluoride supplements should be considered for children <12 years of age whose drinking water contains <0.7 ppm fluoride. Adequate incorporation of fluoride into teeth hardens the outer layers of enamel and increases resistance to demineralization. The fluoride salts usually employed in dentifrices are sodium fluoride and stannous fluoride. Sodium fluoride also is available in a variety of preparations for oral and topical use.

Regulation of the fluoride concentration of community water supplies periodically encounters vocal opposition, including allegations of putative adverse health consequences of fluoridated water. Careful examination of these issues indicates that cancer and all-cause mortalities do not differ significantly between communities with fluoridated and nonfluoridated water.

ACUTE POISONING. Acute fluoride poisoning usually results from accidental ingestion of fluoride-containing insecticides or rodenticides. Initial symptoms (salivation, nausea, abdominal pain, vomiting, and diarrhea) are secondary to the local action of fluoride on the intestinal mucosa. Systemic symptoms are varied and severe: increased irritability of the central nervous system consistent with the Ca^{2+}-binding effect of fluoride and the resulting hypocalcemia; hypotension, presumably owing to central vasomotor depression as well as direct cardiotoxicity; and stimulation and then depression of respiration. Death can result from respiratory paralysis or cardiac failure. The lethal dose of sodium fluoride for humans is ~5 g, although there is considerable variation. Treatment includes the intravenous administration of glucose in saline and gastric lavage with lime water (0.15% calcium hydroxide solution) or other Ca^{2+} salts to precipitate the fluoride. Calcium gluconate is given intravenously for tetany; urine volume is kept high with vigorous fluid resuscitation.

CHRONIC POISONING. In humans, the major manifestations of chronic ingestion of excessive fluoride are osteosclerosis and mottled enamel. Osteosclerosis is characterized by increased bone density secondary both to elevated osteoblastic activity and to the replacement of hydroxyapatite by the denser fluoroapatite. The degree of skeletal involvement varies from changes that are barely detectable radiologically to marked cortical thickening of long bones, numerous exostoses scattered throughout the skeleton, and calcification of ligaments, tendons, and muscle attachments. In its severest form, it is a disabling and crippling disease.

Mottled enamel, or dental fluorosis, was first described >60 years ago. In very mild mottling, small, opaque, paper-white areas are scattered irregularly over the tooth surface. In severe cases, discrete or confluent, deep brown- to black-stained pits give the tooth a corroded appearance. Mottled enamel results from a partial failure of the enamel-forming ameloblasts to elaborate and lay down enamel. Mottling is one of the first visible signs of excess fluoride intake during childhood. Continuous use of water containing ~1 ppm of fluoride may result in very mild mottling in 10% of children; at 4-6 ppm the incidence approaches 100%, with a marked increase in severity. Severe dental fluorosis formerly occurred in regions where local water supplies had a very high fluoride content (e.g., Pompeii, Italy, and Pike's Peak, Colorado). Current regulations in the U.S. require lowering the fluoride content of the water supply or providing an alternative source of acceptable drinking water for affected communities. Sustained consumption of water with a fluoride content of 4 mg/L (4 ppm) is associated with deficits in cortical bone mass and increased rates of bone loss over time.

For a complete Bibliographical Listing see Goodman & Gilman's ***The Pharmacological Basis of Therapeutics***, 12th ed., or Goodman & Gilman Online at www.AccessMedicine.com.

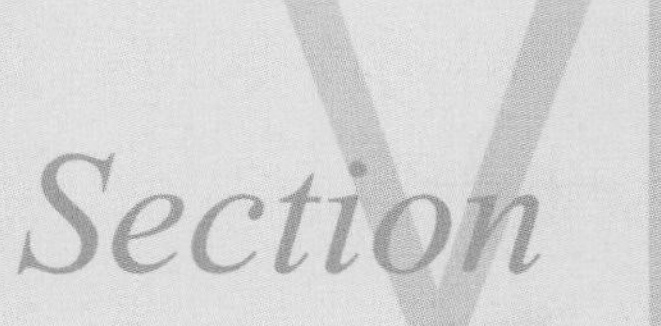

Section VI Drugs Affecting Gastrointestinal Function

chapter 45 Pharmacotherapy of Gastric Acidity, Peptic Ulcers, and Gastroesophageal Reflux Disease

The treatment and prevention of acid-related disorders are accomplished by decreasing gastric acidity and enhancing mucosal defense. The appreciation that an infectious agent, *Helicobacter pylori*, plays a key role in the pathogenesis of acid-peptic diseases has stimulated new approaches to prevention and therapy.

PHYSIOLOGY OF GASTRIC SECRETION

Gastric acid secretion is a complex and continuous process: neuronal (acetylcholine, ACh), paracrine (histamine), and endocrine (gastrin) factors all regulate the secretion of H^+ by parietal cells (Figure 45–1).

Specific receptors (M_3, H_2, and CCK_2, respectively) are on the basolateral membrane of parietal cells in the body and fundus of the stomach. Some of these receptors are also present on *enterochromaffin-like* (ECL) cells, where they regulate the release of histamine. The H_2 receptor is a GPCR that activates the G_s–adenylyl cyclase–cyclic AMP–PKA pathway. ACh and gastrin signal through GPCRs that couple to the G_q–PLC-IP_3–Ca^{2+} pathway in parietal cells. In parietal cells, the cyclic AMP and the Ca^{2+}-dependent pathways activate H^+, K^+-ATPase (the proton pump), which exchanges H^+ and K^+ across the parietal cell membrane. This pump generates the largest ion gradient known in vertebrates, with an intracellular pH of ~7.3 and an intracanalicular pH of ~0.8.

ACh release from postganglionic vagal fibers directly stimulates gastric acid secretion through muscarinic M_3 receptors on the basolateral membrane of parietal cells. The CNS predominantly modulates the activity of the enteric nervous system via ACh, stimulating gastric acid secretion in response to the sight, smell, taste, or anticipation of food (the "cephalic" phase of acid secretion). ACh also indirectly affects parietal cells by increasing the release of histamine from the ECL cells and of gastrin from G cells. ECL cells, the source of gastric histamine, usually are in close proximity to parietal cells. Histamine acts as a paracrine mediator, diffusing from its site of release to nearby parietal cells, where it activates H_2 receptors to stimulate gastric acid secretion.

Gastrin, produced by antral G cells, is the most potent inducer of acid secretion. Multiple pathways stimulate gastrin release, including CNS activation, local distention, and chemical components of the gastric contents. Gastrin stimulates acid secretion indirectly by inducing the release of histamine by ECL cells; a direct effect on parietal cells also plays a lesser role. *Somatostatin* (SST), which is produced by antral D cells, inhibits gastric acid secretion. Acidification of the gastric luminal pH to <3 stimulates SST release, which in turn suppresses gastrin release in a negative feedback loop. SST-producing cells are decreased in patients with *H. pylori* infection, and the consequent reduction of SST's inhibitory effect may contribute to excess gastrin production.

GASTRIC DEFENSES AGAINST ACID. The extremely high concentration of H^+ in the gastric lumen requires robust defense mechanisms to protect the esophagus and the stomach. The primary esophageal defense is the lower esophageal sphincter, which prevents reflux of acidic gastric contents into the esophagus. The stomach protects itself from acid damage by a number of mechanisms that require adequate mucosal blood flow. One key defense is the secretion of a mucus layer that helps to protect gastric epithelial cells by trapping secreted bicarbonate at the cell surface. Gastric mucus is soluble when secreted but quickly forms an insoluble gel that coats the mucosal surface of the stomach, slows ion diffusion, and prevents mucosal damage by macromolecules

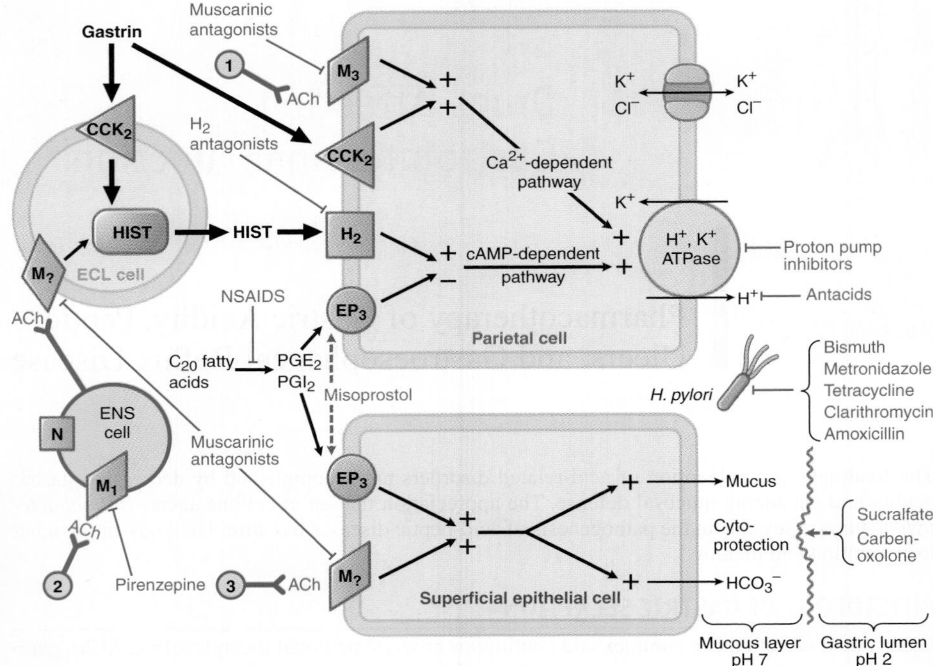

Figure 45–1 *Pharmacologist's view of gastric secretion and its regulation: the basis for therapy of acid-peptic disorders.* Shown are the interactions among an enterochromaffin-like (ECL) cell that secretes histamine, a ganglion cell of the enteric nervous system (ENS), a parietal cell that secretes acid, and a superficial epithelial cell that secretes mucus and bicarbonate. Physiological pathways, shown in solid black, may be stimulatory (+) or inhibitory (–). 1 and 3 indicate possible inputs from postganglionic cholinergic fibers; 2 shows neural input from the vagus nerve. Physiological agonists and their respective membrane receptors include acetylcholine (ACh), muscarinic (M), and nicotinic (N) receptors; gastrin, cholecystokinin receptor 2 (CCK_2); histamine (HIST), H_2 receptor; and prostaglandin E_2 (PGE_2), EP_3 receptor. A red indicates targets of pharmacological antagonism. A light blue dashed arrow indicates a drug action that mimics or enhances a physiological pathway. Shown in red are drugs used to treat acid-peptic disorders. NSAIDs are nonsteroidal anti-inflammatory drugs, which can induce ulcers via inhibition of cyclooxygenase.

such as pepsin. Mucus production is stimulated by prostaglandins E_2 and I_2, which also directly inhibit gastric acid secretion by parietal cells. Thus, drugs that inhibit prostaglandin formation (e.g., NSAIDs, ethanol) decrease mucus secretion and predispose to the development of acid-peptic disease. Figure 45–1 outlines the rationale and pharmacological basis for the therapy of acid-peptic diseases. The proton pump inhibitors are used most commonly, followed by the histamine H_2 receptor antagonists.

PROTON PUMP INHIBITORS

The most potent suppressors of gastric acid secretion are inhibitors of the gastric H^+, K^+-ATPase (proton pump) (Figure 45–2). These drugs diminish the daily production of acid (basal and stimulated) by 80-95%.

CHEMISTRY; MECHANISM OF ACTION; PHARMACOLOGY. Six proton pump inhibitors are available for clinical use: *omeprazole* (PRILOSEC, others) and its S-isomer, *esomeprazole* (NEXIUM), *lansoprazole* (PREVACID) and its R-enantiomer, *dexlansoprazole* (KAPIDEX), *rabeprazole* (ACIPHEX), and *pantoprazole* (PROTONIX, others). All proton pump inhibitors have equivalent efficacy at comparable doses.

Proton pump inhibitors (PPIs) are prodrugs that require activation in an acid environment. After absorption into the systemic circulation, the prodrug diffuses into the parietal cells of the stomach and accumulates in the acidic secretory canaliculi. Here, it is activated by proton-catalyzed formation of a tetracyclic sulfenamide (*see* Figure 45–2), trapping the drug so that it cannot diffuse back across the canalicular membrane. The activated form then binds covalently with sulfhydryl groups of cysteines in the H^+, K^+-ATPase, irreversibly inactivating the pump molecule. Acid secretion resumes only after new pump molecules are synthesized and

Figure 45–2 *Activation of prodrug proton pump inhibitor.* Omeprazole is converted to a sulfenamide in the acidic secretory canaliculi of the parietal cell. The sulfenamide interacts covalently with sulfhydryl groups in the proton pump, thereby irreversibly inhibiting its activity. Lansoprazole, rabeprazole, and pantoprazole undergo analogous conversions.

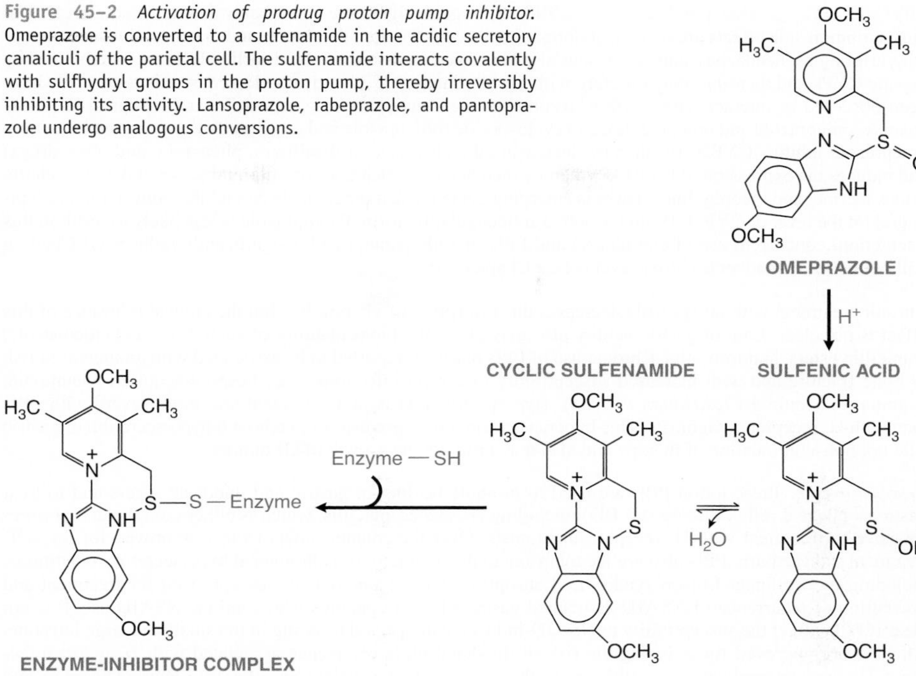

inserted into the luminal membrane, providing a prolonged (up to 24- to 48-h) suppression of acid secretion, despite the much shorter plasma $t_{1/2}$ ~ 0.5-2 h of the parent compounds.

To prevent degradation of PPIs by acid in the gastric lumen and improve oral bioavailability, oral dosage forms are supplied in different formulations:

- Enteric-coated drugs contained inside gelatin capsules (omeprazole, dexlansoprazole, esomeprazole, and lansoprazole)
- Enteric-coated granules supplied as a powder for suspension (lansoprazole)
- Enteric-coated tablets (pantoprazole, rabeprazole, and omeprazole)
- Powdered omeprazole combined with *sodium bicarbonate* (ZEGERID) contained in capsules and formulated for oral suspension

Patients for whom the oral route of administration is not available can be treated parenterally with esomeprazole, pantoprazole, or lansoprazole. The FDA-approved dose of intravenous pantoprazole for gastroesophageal reflux disease is 40 mg daily for up to 10 days. Higher doses (e.g., 160-240 mg in divided doses) are used to manage hypersecretory conditions such as the Zollinger-Ellison syndrome.

ADME. Because an acidic pH in the parietal cell acid canaliculi is required for drug activation and food stimulates acid production, these drugs ideally should be given ~30 min before meals. Concurrent administration of food may reduce somewhat the rate of absorption of PPIs. Once in the small bowel, PPIs are rapidly absorbed, highly protein bound, and extensively metabolized by hepatic CYPs, particularly CYP2C19 and CYP3A4. Asians are more likely than whites or African Americans to have the CYP2C19 genotype that correlates with slow metabolism of PPIs (23% vs. 3%, respectively), which may contribute to heightened efficacy and/or toxicity in this ethnic group.

Because not all pumps and all parietal cells are active simultaneously, maximal suppression of acid secretion requires several doses of the PPIs. For example, it may take 2-5 days of therapy with once-daily dosing to achieve the 70% inhibition of proton pumps that is seen at steady state. More frequent initial dosing (e.g., twice daily) will reduce the time to achieve full inhibition but is not proven to improve patient outcome. The resulting proton pump inhibition is irreversible; thus, acid secretion is suppressed for 24-48 h, or more, until new proton pumps are synthesized and incorporated into the luminal membrane of parietal cells. Chronic renal failure does not lead to drug accumulation with once-a-day dosing of the PPIs. Hepatic disease substantially reduces the clearance of esomeprazole and lansoprazole.

ADVERSE EFFECTS AND DRUG INTERACTIONS. PPIs generally cause remarkably few adverse effects. The most common side effects are nausea, abdominal pain, constipation, flatulence, and diarrhea. Subacute myopathy, arthralgias, headaches, and skin rashes also have been reported. As noted earlier, PPIs are metabolized by hepatic CYPs and therefore may interfere with the elimination of other drugs cleared by this route. PPIs have been observed to interact with warfarin (esomeprazole, lansoprazole, omeprazole, and rabeprazole), diazepam (esomeprazole and omeprazole), and cyclosporine (omeprazole and rabeprazole). Among the PPIs, only omeprazole inhibits CYP2C19 (thereby decreasing the clearance of disulfiram, phenytoin, and other drugs) and induces the expression of CYP1A2 (thereby increasing the clearance of imipramine, several antipsychotic drugs, tacrine, and theophylline). There is emerging evidence that omeprazole can inhibit conversion of clopidogrel (at the level of CYP2C19) to the active anticoagulating form. Pantoprazole is less likely to result in this interaction; concurrent use of clopidogrel and PPIs (mainly pantoprazole) significantly reduces GI bleeding without increasing adverse cardiac events (*see* Chapter 30).

Chronic treatment with omeprazole decreases the absorption of vitamin B_{12}, but the clinical relevance of this effect is not clear. Loss of gastric acidity also may affect the bioavailability of such drugs as ketoconazole, ampicillin esters, and iron salts. Chronic use of PPIs has been reported to be associated with an increased risk of bone fracture and with increased susceptibility to certain infections (e.g., hospital-acquired pneumonia, community-acquired *Clostridium difficile*). Hypergastrinemia is more frequent and more severe with PPIs than with H_2 receptor antagonists. This hypergastrinemia may predispose to rebound hypersecretion of gastric acid upon discontinuation of therapy and also may promote the growth of GI tumors.

Therapeutic Uses. Prescription PPIs are used to promote healing of gastric and duodenal ulcers and to treat gastroesophageal reflux disease (GERD), including erosive esophagitis, which is either complicated or unresponsive to treatment with H_2 receptor antagonists. Over-the-counter omeprazole is approved for the self-treatment of heartburn. PPIs also are the mainstay in the treatment of pathological hypersecretory conditions, including the Zollinger-Ellison syndrome. Lansoprazole and esomeprazole are approved for treatment and prevention of recurrence of NSAID-associated gastric ulcers in patients who continue NSAID use. It is not clear if PPIs affect the susceptibility to NSAID-induced damage and bleeding in the small and large intestine. All PPIs are approved for reducing the risk of duodenal ulcer recurrence associated with *H. pylori* infections. Therapeutic applications of PPIs are further discussed later under "Specific Acid-Peptic Disorders and Therapeutic Strategies."

H_2 RECEPTOR ANTAGONISTS

The H_2 receptor antagonists inhibit acid production by reversibly competing with histamine for binding to H_2 receptors on the basolateral membrane of parietal cells.

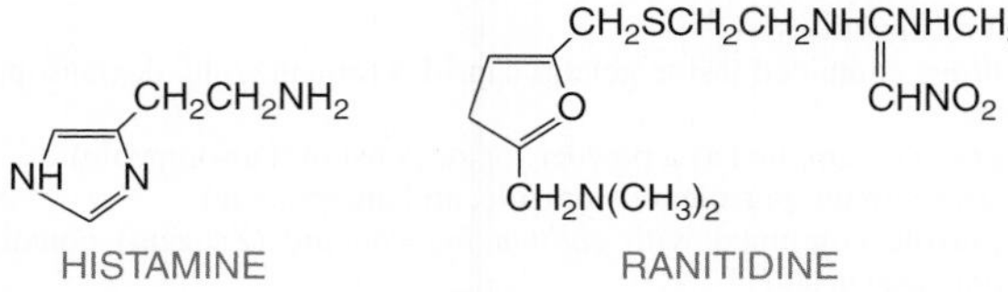

$CH_2CH_2NH_2$ NH N

HISTAMINE

$CH_2SCH_2CH_2NHCNHCH_3$ ‖ $CHNO_2$ O $CH_2N(CH_3)_2$

RANITIDINE

Four different H_2 receptor antagonists are available in the U.S.: *cimetidine* (TAGAMET, others), *ranitidine* (ZANTAC, others), *famotidine* (PEPCID, others), and *nizatidine* (AXID, others). These drugs are less potent than PPIs but still suppress 24-h gastric acid secretion by ~70%. Because the most important determinant of duodenal ulcer healing is the level of nocturnal acidity, evening dosing of H_2 receptor antagonists is adequate therapy in most instances. All 4 H_2 receptor antagonists are available as prescription and over-the-counter formulations for oral administration. Intravenous and intramuscular preparations of cimetidine, ranitidine, and famotidine also are available.

ADME. The H_2 receptor antagonists are rapidly absorbed after oral administration, with peak serum concentrations within 1-3 h. Absorption may be enhanced by food or decreased by antacids, but these effects probably are unimportant clinically. Therapeutic levels are achieved rapidly after intravenous dosing and are maintained for 4-5 h (cimetidine), 6-8 h (ranitidine), or 10-12 h (famotidine). Only a small percentage of H_2 receptor antagonists are protein bound. Small amounts (from <10% to ~35%) of these drugs undergo metabolism in the liver, but liver disease per se is not an indication for dose adjustment. The kidneys excrete these drugs and their metabolites by filtration and renal tubular secretion, and it is important to reduce drug doses in patients with decreased creatinine clearance. Neither hemodialysis nor peritoneal dialysis clears significant amounts of these drugs.

ADVERSE REACTIONS AND DRUG INTERACTIONS. H_2 receptor antagonists generally are well tolerated, with a low (<3%) incidence of adverse effects. Side effects are minor and include diarrhea, headache, drowsiness, fatigue, muscular pain, and constipation. Less common side effects include those affecting the CNS (confusion, delirium, hallucinations, slurred speech, and headaches), which occur primarily with intravenous administration of the drugs or in elderly subjects. Several reports have associated H_2 receptor antagonists with various blood dyscrasias, including thrombocytopenia. H_2 receptor antagonists cross the placenta and are excreted in breast milk. Although no major teratogenic risk has been associated with these agents, caution is warranted when they are used in pregnancy.

All agents that inhibit gastric acid secretion may alter the rate of absorption and subsequent bioavailability of the H_2 receptor antagonists (see "Antacids" section). Drug interactions with H_2 receptor antagonists occur mainly with cimetidine, and its use has decreased markedly. Cimetidine inhibits CYPs (e.g., CYP1A2, CYP2C9, and CYP2D6), and thereby can increase the levels of a variety of drugs that are substrates for these enzymes. Ranitidine also interacts with hepatic CYPs, but with an affinity of only 10% of that of cimetidine. Famotidine and nizatidine are even safer in this regard. Slight increases in blood-alcohol concentration may result from concomitant use of H_2 receptor antagonists.

Therapeutic Uses. The major therapeutic indications for H_2 receptor antagonists are to promote healing of gastric and duodenal ulcers, to treat uncomplicated GERD, and to prevent the occurrence of stress ulcers. For more information about the therapeutic applications of H_2 receptor antagonists, see below, "Specific Acid-Peptic Disorders and Therapeutic Strategies."

TOLERANCE AND REBOUND WITH ACID-SUPPRESSING MEDICATIONS

Tolerance to the acid-suppressing effects of H_2 receptor antagonists may develop within 3 days of starting treatment and may be resistant to increased doses of the medications. Diminished sensitivity to these drugs may result from the effect of the secondary hypergastrinemia to stimulate histamine release from ECL cells. PPIs do not cause this phenomenon; however, rebound increases in gastric acidity can occur when either of these drug classes is discontinued.

AGENTS THAT ENHANCE MUCOSAL DEFENSE

PROSTAGLANDIN ANALOGS: MISOPROSTOL

Prostaglandin E_2 (PGE_2) and prostacyclin (PGI_2) are the major prostaglandins synthesized by the gastric mucosa. Contrary to their cyclic AMP-elevating effects on many cells via EP_2 and EP_4 receptors, these prostanoids bind to the EP_3 receptor on parietal cells and stimulate the G_i pathway, thereby decreasing intracellular cyclic AMP and gastric acid secretion. PGE_2 also can prevent gastric injury by cytoprotective effects that include stimulation of mucin and bicarbonate secretion and increased mucosal blood flow. Acid suppression appears to be the most important effect clinically.

Because NSAIDs diminish prostaglandin formation by inhibiting cyclooxygenase, synthetic prostaglandin analogs offer a logical approach to counteract NSAID-induced damage. Misoprostol (15-deoxy-16-hydroxy-16-methyl-PGE_1; CYTOTEC, others) is a synthetic analog of PGE_1 that is FDA-approved to prevent NSAID-induced mucosal injury. The degree of inhibition of gastric acid secretion by misoprostol is directly related to dose; oral doses of 100-200 μg significantly inhibit basal acid secretion (up to 85-95% inhibition) or food-stimulated acid secretion (up to 75-85% inhibition). The usual recommended dose for ulcer prophylaxis is 200 μg 4 times a day.

ADME. Misoprostol is rarely used because of its side effects. The drug is rapidly absorbed after oral administration and is rapidly and extensively de-esterified to form misoprostol acid, the principal and active metabolite of the drug. A single dose inhibits acid production within 30 min; the therapeutic effect peaks at 60-90 min and lasts for up to 3 h. Food and antacids decrease the rate of misoprostol absorption. The free acid is excreted mainly in the urine, with an elimination $t_{1/2}$ of 20-40 min.

ADVERSE EFFECTS. Diarrhea, with or without abdominal pain and cramps, occurs in up to 30% of patients who take misoprostol. Apparently dose related, it typically begins within the first 2 weeks after therapy is initiated and often resolves spontaneously within a week; more severe cases may necessitate drug discontinuation. *Misoprostol can cause clinical exacerbations of inflammatory bowel disease* (*see* Chapter 47). *Misoprostol also is contraindicated during pregnancy* because it can increase uterine contractility.

SUCRALFATE

In the presence of acid-induced damage, pepsin-mediated hydrolysis of mucosal proteins contributes to mucosal erosion and ulcerations. This process can be inhibited by sulfated polysaccharides. Sucralfate (CARAFATE, others) consists of the octasulfate of sucrose to which $Al(OH)_3$ has been added. In an acid environment (pH <4), sucralfate undergoes extensive cross-linking to produce a viscous, sticky polymer that adheres to epithelial cells and ulcer craters for up to 6 h after a single dose. In addition to inhibiting hydrolysis of mucosal proteins by pepsin, sucralfate may have additional cytoprotective effects, including stimulation of local production of prostaglandins and EGF. Sucralfate also binds bile salts; thus, some clinicians use sucralfate to treat individuals with the syndromes of biliary esophagitis or gastritis (the existence of which is controversial).

Therapeutic Uses. The use of sucralfate to treat peptic acid disease has diminished in recent years. Nevertheless, because increased gastric pH may be a factor in the development of nosocomial pneumonia in critically ill patients, sucralfate may offer an advantage over PPIs and H_2 receptor antagonists for the prophylaxis of stress ulcers. Sucralfate also has been used in conditions associated with mucosal inflammation/ulceration that may not respond to acid suppression, including oral mucositis (radiation and aphthous ulcers) and bile reflux gastropathy. Administered by rectal enema, sucralfate also has been used for radiation proctitis and solitary rectal ulcers. Because it is activated by acid, sucralfate should be taken on an empty stomach 1 h before meals. The use of antacids within 30 min of a dose of sucralfate should be avoided. The dose of sucralfate is 1 g 4 times daily (for active duodenal ulcer) or 1 g twice daily (for maintenance therapy).

ADVERSE EFFECTS. The most common side effect of sucralfate is constipation (~2%). Sucralfate should be avoided in patients with renal failure who are at risk for aluminum overload. Likewise, aluminum-containing antacids should not be combined with sucralfate in these patients. Sucralfate forms a viscous layer in the stomach that may inhibit absorption of other drugs, including phenytoin, digoxin, cimetidine, ketoconazole, and fluoroquinolone antibiotics. Sucralfate therefore should be taken at least 2 h after the administration of other drugs. The "sticky" nature of the viscous gel produced by sucralfate in the stomach also may be responsible for the development of bezoars in some patients.

ANTACIDS

There are more effective and persistent agents than antacids, but their price, accessibility, and rapid action make them popular with consumers. Many factors, including palatability, determine the effectiveness and choice of antacid. Although sodium bicarbonate effectively neutralizes acid, it is very water soluble and rapidly absorbed from the stomach, and the alkali and sodium loads may pose a risk for patients with cardiac or renal failure. $CaCO_3$ rapidly and effectively neutralizes gastric H^+, but the release of CO_2 from bicarbonate- and carbonate-containing antacids can cause belching, nausea, abdominal distention, and flatulence. Calcium also may induce rebound acid secretion, necessitating more frequent administration. Combinations of Mg^{2+} (rapidly reacting) and Al^{3+} (slowly reacting) hydroxides provide a relatively balanced and sustained neutralizing capacity and are preferred by most experts. Magaldrate, a hydroxymagnesium aluminate complex, is converted rapidly in gastric acid to $Mg(OH)_2$ and $Al(OH)_3$, which are absorbed poorly and thus provide a sustained antacid effect. Although fixed combinations of magnesium and aluminum theoretically counteract the adverse effects of each other on the bowel (Al^{3+} can relax gastric smooth muscle, producing delayed gastric emptying and constipation; Mg^{2+} exerts the opposite effects), such balance is not always achieved in practice. Simethicone, a surfactant that may decrease foaming and hence esophageal reflux, is included in many antacid preparations. However, other fixed combinations, particularly those with aspirin, that are marketed for "acid indigestion" are potentially unsafe in patients predisposed to gastroduodenal ulcers, and should not be used.

For uncomplicated ulcers, antacids are given orally 1 and 3 h after meals and at bedtime. For severe symptoms or uncontrolled reflux, antacids can be given as often as every 30-60 min. In general, antacids should be administered in suspension form because this probably has a greater neutralizing capacity than powder or tablet dosage forms. Antacids are cleared from the empty stomach in ~30 min. However, the presence of food is sufficient to elevate gastric pH to ~5 for ~1 h and to prolong the neutralizing effects of antacids for ~2-3 h.

Antacids vary in the extent to which they are absorbed, and hence in their systemic effects. In general, most antacids can elevate urinary pH by ~1 pH unit. Antacids that contain Al^{3+}, Ca^{2+}, or Mg^{2+} are absorbed less completely than are those that contain $NaHCO_3$. With renal insufficiency, absorbed Al^{3+} can contribute to osteoporosis, encephalopathy, and proximal myopathy. About 15% of orally administered Ca^{2+} is absorbed, causing a transient hypercalcemia. The hypercalcemia from as little as 3-4 g of $CaCO_3$ per day can be problematic in patients with uremia. In the past, when large doses of $NaHCO_3$ and $CaCO_3$ were administered commonly with milk or cream for the management of peptic ulcer, the *milk-alkali syndrome* (alkalosis, hypercalcemia, and renal insufficiency) occurred frequently. Today, this syndrome is rare and generally results from the chronic ingestion of large quantities of Ca^{2+} (five to forty 500-mg tablets per day of calcium carbonate) taken with milk.

By altering gastric and urinary pH, antacids may affect a number of drugs (e.g., thyroid hormones, allopurinol, and imidazole antifungals, by altering rates of dissolution and absorption, bioavailability, and renal elimination). Al^{3+} and Mg^{2+} antacids also are notable for their propensity to chelate other drugs present in the GI tract and thereby decrease their absorption. Most interactions can be avoided by taking antacids 2 h before or after ingestion of other drugs.

OTHER ACID SUPPRESSANTS AND CYTOPROTECTANTS. The M_1 muscarinic receptor antagonists *pirenzepine* and *telenzepine* (*see* Chapter 9) can reduce basal acid production by 40-50%. The ACh receptor on the parietal cell itself is of the M_3 subtype, and these drugs are believed to suppress neural stimulation of acid production via actions on M_1 receptors of intramural ganglia (*see* Figure 45–1). Because of their relatively poor efficacy, significant and undesirable anticholinergic side effects, and risk of blood disorders (pirenzepine), they rarely are used today.

Rebamipide is used for ulcer therapy in parts of Asia. Its cytoprotective effects are exerted by increasing prostaglandin generation in gastric mucosa and by scavenging reactive oxygen species. *Ecabet* (GASTROM), which appears to increase the formation of PGE_2 and PGI_2, also is used for ulcer therapy, mostly in Japan. *Carbenoxolone*, a derivative of glycyrrhizic acid found in licorice root, has been used with modest success for ulcer therapy in Europe. Unfortunately, carbenoxolone inhibits the type I isozyme of 11β-hydroxysteroid dehydrogenase, which protects the mineralocorticoid receptor from activation by cortisol in the distal nephron; it therefore causes hypokalemia and hypertension due to excessive mineralocorticoid receptor activation (*see* Chapter 42). *Bismuth compounds* (*see* Chapter 46) are frequently prescribed in combination with antibiotics to eradicate *H. pylori* and prevent ulcer recurrence. Bismuth compounds bind to the base of the ulcer, promote mucin and bicarbonate production, and have significant antibacterial effects.

SPECIFIC ACID-PEPTIC DISORDERS AND THERAPEUTIC STRATEGIES

GASTROESOPHAGEAL REFLUX DISEASE

Although most cases of heartburn or gastroesophageal regurgitation follow a relatively benign course, these symptoms, often referred to as GERD, can be associated with severe erosive esophagitis; stricture formation and Barrett metaplasia (replacement of squamous by intestinal columnar epithelium), in turn, is associated with a small but significant risk of adenocarcinoma. The goals of GERD therapy are complete resolution of symptoms and healing of esophagitis. PPIs clearly are more effective than H_2 receptor antagonists in achieving these goals (*see* Figure 45–3).

In general, the optimal dose for each patient is determined based on symptom control. Strictures associated with GERD also respond better to PPIs than to H_2 receptor antagonists. One of the complications of GERD, Barrett esophagus, appears to be more refractory to therapy because neither acid suppression nor antireflux surgery has been shown convincingly to produce regression of metaplasia.

Regimens for the treatment of GERD with PPIs and histamine H_2 receptor antagonists are listed in Table 45–1. Although some patients with mild GERD symptoms may be managed by nocturnal doses of H_2 receptor antagonists, twice-daily dosing usually is required. Antacids are recommended only for the patient with mild, infrequent episodes of heartburn. In general, prokinetic agents (*see* Chapter 46) are not particularly useful for GERD, either alone or in combination with acid-suppressant medications.

SEVERE SYMPTOMS AND NOCTURNAL ACID BREAKTHROUGH. In patients with severe symptoms or extraintestinal manifestations of GERD, twice-daily dosing with a PPI may be needed. However, it is difficult if not impossible to render patients achlorhydric and two-thirds or more of subjects will continue to make acid, particularly at night. This phenomenon, called *nocturnal acid breakthrough*, has been invoked as a cause of

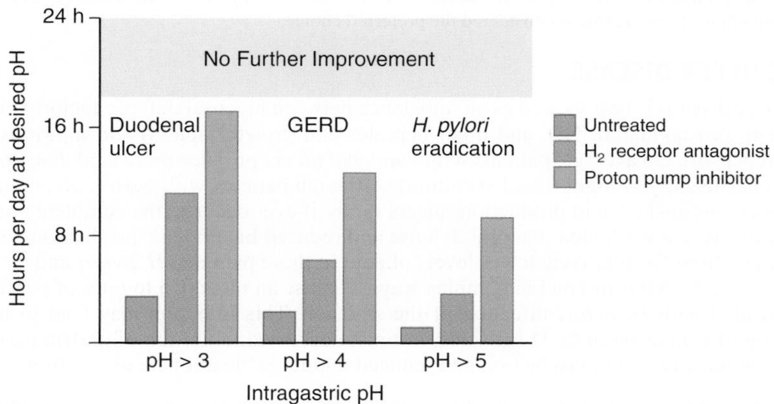

Figure 45–3 *Comparative success of therapy with proton pump inhibitors and H_2 receptor antagonists.* Data show the effects of a proton pump inhibitor (given once daily) and an H_2 receptor antagonist (given twice daily) in elevating gastric pH to the target ranges (i.e., pH 3 for duodenal ulcer, pH 4 for GERD, and pH 5 for antibiotic eradication of *H. pylori*).

Table 45–1

Antisecretory Drug Regimens for Treatment and Maintenance of GERD

DRUG	DOSAGE (twice daily)
H_2 Receptor Antagonists	
Cimetidine	400[a]/800[a] mg
Famotidine	20/40 mg
Nizatidine	150[a]/300[a] mg
Ranitidine	150/300 mg
Proton Pump Inhibitors	
Esomeprazole	20/40 mg daily/40[a] mg
Lansoprazole	30[a]/60[a] mg daily/30[a] mg
Omeprazole	20/40[a] mg daily/20[a] mg
Pantoprazole	40/80[a] mg daily/40[a] mg
Rabeprazole	20/40[a] mg daily/20[a] mg

[a]*Indicates unlabeled use.*

refractory symptoms in some patients with GERD. However, decreases in gastric pH at night while on therapy generally are not associated with acid reflux into the esophagus, and the rationale for suppressing nocturnal acid secretion remains to be established. Patients with continuing symptoms on twice-daily PPIs are often treated by adding an H_2 receptor antagonist at night. Although this can further suppress acid production, the effect is short lived, probably due to the development of tolerance.

THERAPY FOR EXTRAINTESTINAL MANIFESTATIONS OF GERD. Acid reflux has been implicated in a variety of atypical symptoms, including noncardiac chest pain, asthma, laryngitis, chronic cough, and other ear, nose, and throat conditions. PPIs (at higher doses) have been used with some success in certain patients with these disorders.

GERD AND PREGNANCY. Heartburn is estimated to occur in 30-50% of pregnancies, with an incidence approaching 80% in some populations. In the vast majority of cases, GERD ends soon after delivery and thus does not represent an exacerbation of a preexisting condition. Because of its high prevalence and the fact that it can contribute to the nausea of pregnancy, treatment often is required. Treatment choice in this setting is complicated by the paucity of data for the most commonly used drugs. In general, most drugs used to treat GERD fall in FDA Category B, with the exception of omeprazole (FDA Category C). Mild cases of GERD during pregnancy should be treated conservatively; antacids or sucralfate are considered the first-line drugs. If symptoms persist, H_2 receptor antagonists can be used, with ranitidine having the most established track record in this setting. PPIs are reserved for women with intractable symptoms or complicated reflux disease. In these situations, lansoprazole is considered the preferred choice.

PEPTIC ULCER DISEASE

Peptic ulcer disease is best viewed as an imbalance between mucosal defense factors (bicarbonate, mucin, prostaglandin, NO, and other peptides and growth factors) and injurious factors (acid and pepsin). On average, patients with *duodenal ulcers* produce more acid than do control subjects, particularly at night (basal secretion). Although patients with *gastric ulcers* have normal or even diminished acid production, ulcers rarely if ever occur in the complete absence of acid. Presumably, a weakened mucosal defense and reduced bicarbonate production contribute to the injury from the relatively lower levels of acid in these patients. *H. pylori* and exogenous agents such as NSAIDs interact in complex ways to cause an ulcer. Up to 60% of peptic ulcers are associated with *H. pylori* infection of the stomach. This infection may lead to impaired production of somatostatin by D cells and, in time, decreased inhibition of gastrin production, resulting in increased acid production and reduced duodenal bicarbonate production.

Table 45–2 summarizes current recommendations for drug therapy of gastroduodenal ulcers. PPIs relieve symptoms of duodenal ulcers and promote healing more rapidly than do H_2 receptor antagonists, although both classes of drugs are very effective in this setting (*see* Figure 45–3). Peptic ulcer represents a chronic disease, and recurrence within 1 year is expected in the majority of patients who do not receive prophylactic acid suppression. With the appreciation that *H. pylori* plays a major etiopathogenic role in the majority of

Table 45–2

Recommendations for Treatment of Gastroduodenal Ulcers

DRUG	ACTIVE ULCER	MAINTENANCE THERAPY
H_2 Receptor Antagonists		
Cimetidine	800 mg at bedtime/400 mg twice daily	400 mg at bedtime
Famotidine	40 mg at bedtime	20 mg at bedtime
Nizatidine/ranitidine	300 mg after evening meal or at bedtime/150 mg twice daily	150 mg at bedtime
Proton Pump Inhibitors		
Lansoprazole	15 mg (DU; NSAID risk reduction) daily 30 mg (GU including NSAID-associated) daily	
Omeprazole	20 mg daily	
Rabeprazole	20 mg daily	
Prostaglandin Analog		
Misoprostol	200 μg four times daily (NSAID-associated ulcer prevention)[a]	

DU, duodenal ulcer; GU, gastric ulcer.

[a]*Only misoprostol 800 μg/day has been directly shown to reduce the risk of ulcer complications such as perforation, hemorrhage, or obstruction (Rostom A, Moayyedi P, Hunt R. Canadian Association of Gastroenterology Consensus Group. Canadian consensus guidelines on long-term nonsteroidal anti-inflammatory drug therapy and the need for gastroprotection: Benefits versus risks. Aliment Pharmacol Ther, 2009, 29:481–496).*

peptic ulcers, prevention of relapse is focused on eliminating this organism from the stomach. Intravenous pantoprazole or lansoprazole is the preferred therapy in patients with acute bleeding ulcers. The theoretical benefit of maximal acid suppression in this setting is to accelerate healing of the underlying ulcer. In addition, a higher gastric pH enhances clot formation and retards clot dissolution.

NSAIDs also are very frequently associated with peptic ulcers and bleeding. The effects of these drugs are mediated systemically; in the stomach, NSAIDS suppress mucosal prostaglandin synthesis (particularly PGE_2 and PGI_2) and thereby reduce mucous production and cytoprotection (*see* Figure 45–1). Thus, minimizing NSAID use is an important adjunct to gastroduodenal ulcer therapy.

TREATMENT OF *HELICOBACTER PYLORI* INFECTION. *H. pylori*, a gram-negative rod, has been associated with gastritis and the subsequent development of gastric and duodenal ulcers, gastric adenocarcinoma, and gastric B-cell lymphoma. Because of the critical role of *H. pylori* in the pathogenesis of peptic ulcers, to eradicate this infection is standard care in patients with gastric or duodenal ulcers. Provided that patients are not taking NSAIDs, this strategy almost completely eliminates the risk of ulcer recurrence. Eradication of *H. pylori* also is indicated in the treatment of mucosa-associated lymphoid tissue lymphomas of the stomach, which can regress significantly after such treatment.

Five important considerations influence the selection of an eradication regimen (Table 45–3).

- Single-antibiotic regimens are ineffective in eradicating *H. pylori* infection and lead to microbial resistance. Combination therapy with 2 or 3 antibiotics (plus acid-suppressive therapy) is associated with the highest rate of *H. pylori* eradication.
- A PPI or H_2 receptor antagonist significantly enhances the effectiveness of *H. pylori* antibiotic regimens containing amoxicillin or clarithromycin (*see* Figure 45–3).
- A regimen of 10-14 days of treatment appears to be better than shorter treatment regimens.
- Poor patient compliance is linked to the medication-related side effects experienced by as many as half of patients taking triple-agent regimens, and to the inconvenience of 3 or 4 drug regimens administered several times per day. Packaging that combines the daily doses into 1 convenient unit is available and may improve patient compliance.
- The emergence of resistance to clarithromycin and metronidazole increasingly is recognized as an important factor in the failure to eradicate *H. pylori*. In the presence of in vitro evidence of resistance to metronidazole, amoxicillin should be used instead. In areas with a high frequency of resistance to clarithromycin and metronidazole, a 14-day quadruple-drug regimen (3 antibiotics combined with a PPI) generally is effective therapy.

Table 45–3

Therapy of *Helicobacter pylori* Infection

Triple therapy × 14 days: Proton pump inhibitor + clarithromycin 500 mg plus metronidazole 500 mg or amoxicillin 1 g twice a day (tetracycline 500 mg can be substituted for amoxicillin or metronidazole)	
Quadruple therapy × 14 days: Proton pump inhibitor twice a day + metronidazole 500 mg three times daily plus bismuth subsalicylate 525 mg + tetracycline 500 mg four times daily	
or	
H_2 receptor antagonist twice a day plus bismuth subsalicylate 525 mg + metronidazole 250 mg + tetracycline 500 mg four times daily	
Dosages:	
Proton pump inhibitors:	H_2 receptor antagonists:
Omeprazole: 20 mg	Cimetidine: 400 mg
Lansoprazole: 30 mg	Famotidine: 20 mg
Rabeprazole: 20 mg	Nizatidine: 150 mg
Pantoprazole: 40 mg	Ranitidine: 150 mg
Esomeprazole: 40 mg	

NSAID-RELATED ULCERS. Chronic NSAID users have a 2-4% risk of developing a symptomatic ulcer, GI bleeding, or perforation. Ideally, NSAIDs should be discontinued in patients with an ulcer if at all possible. Healing of ulcers despite continued NSAID use is possible with the use of acid-suppressant agents, usually at higher doses and for a considerably longer duration than standard regimens (e.g., ≥8 weeks). PPIs are superior to H_2 receptor antagonists and misoprostol in promoting the healing of active ulcers, and in preventing recurrence of gastric and duodenal ulcers in the setting of continued NSAID administration.

STRESS-RELATED ULCERS. Stress ulcers are ulcers of the stomach or duodenum that occur in the context of a profound illness or trauma requiring intensive care. The etiology of stress-related ulcers differs somewhat from that of other peptic ulcers, involving acid and mucosal ischemia. Because of limitations on the oral administration of drugs in many patients with stress-related ulcers, intravenous H_2 receptor antagonists have been used extensively to reduce the incidence of GI hemorrhage due to stress ulcers. Now that intravenous preparations of PPIs are available, it is likely that they will prove to be equally beneficial. *However, there is some concern over the risk of pneumonia secondary to gastric colonization by bacteria in an alkaline milieu.* In this setting, sucralfate appears to provide reasonable prophylaxis against bleeding without increasing the risk of aspiration pneumonia.

ZOLLINGER-ELLISON SYNDROME. Patients with this syndrome develop pancreatic or duodenal gastrinomas that stimulate the secretion of very large amounts of acid, sometimes in the setting of multiple endocrine neoplasia, type I. This can lead to severe gastroduodenal ulceration and other consequences of uncontrolled hyperchlorhydria. PPIs are the drugs of choice, usually given at twice the routine dosage for peptic ulcers with the therapeutic goal of reducing acid secretion to 1-10 mmol/h.

NONULCER DYSPEPSIA. This term refers to ulcer-like symptoms in patients who lack overt gastroduodenal ulceration. It may be associated with gastritis (with or without *H. pylori*) or with NSAID use, but the pathogenesis of this syndrome remains controversial.

For a complete Bibliographical Listing see Goodman & Gilman's ***The Pharmacological Basis of Therapeutics***, 12th ed., or Goodman & Gilman Online at www.AccessMedicine.com.

Gastrointestinal Motility and Water Flux; Emesis; Biliary and Pancreatic Disease

GASTROINTESTINAL MOTILITY

The gastrointestinal (GI) tract is in a continuous contractile, absorptive, and secretory state. The control of this state is complex, with contributions by the muscle and epithelium, local nerves of the enteric nervous system (ENS), the autonomic nervous system (ANS), and circulating hormones. Of these, perhaps the most important regulator of physiological gut function is the ENS (Figure 46–1).

The ENS is an extensive collection of nerves that constitutes the third division of the ANS. It is the only part of the ANS truly capable of autonomous function if separated from the central nervous system (CNS). The ENS lies within the wall of the GI tract organized into 2 connected networks of neurons and nerve fibers: the *myenteric (Auerbach) plexus*, found between the circular and longitudinal muscle layers, and the *submucosal (Meissner) plexus*, located in the submucosa. The former is largely responsible for motor control, whereas the latter regulates secretion, fluid transport, and blood flow. The ENS and the ANS are also involved in host defense and innervate organs and cells of the immune system.

GENERATION AND REGULATION OF GI ACTIVITY

The ENS is responsible for the largely autonomous nature of most GI activity. This activity is organized into relatively distinct programs that respond to input from the local environment of the gut, as well as the ANS-CNS. Each program consists of a series of complex, but coordinated, patterns of secretion and movement that show regional and temporal variation. The *fasting program* of the gut is called the MMC (*migrating myoelectric complex* when referring to electrical activity and *migrating motor complex* when referring to the accompanying contractions) and consists of a series of 4 phasic activities. The most characteristic, phase III, consists of clusters of rhythmic contractions that occupy short segments of the intestine for a period of 6-10 min before proceeding caudally (toward the anus). Phase II of the MMC is associated with the release of the peptide hormone *motilin*. Motilin agonists stimulate motility in the proximal gut. One whole MMC cycle (i.e., all 4 phases) takes ~80-110 min. The MMC occurs in the fasting state, helping to sweep debris caudad in the gut and limiting the overgrowth of luminal bacteria. The MMC is interrupted by the fed program in intermittently feeding animals such as humans. The *fed program* consists of high-frequency (12-15/min) contractions that are either propagated for short segments (*propulsive*) or are irregular and not propagated (*mixing*).

Peristalsis is a series of reflex responses to a bolus in the lumen of a given segment of the intestine; the ascending excitatory reflex results in contraction of the circular muscle on the oral side of the bolus, whereas the descending inhibitory reflex results in relaxation on the anal side. The net pressure gradient moves the bolus caudad. Motor neurons receive input from ascending and descending interneurons (which constitute the relay and programming systems) that are of 2 broad types, excitatory and inhibitory. The primary neurotransmitter of the excitatory motor neurons is acetylcholine (ACh). The principal neurotransmitter in the inhibitory motor neurons appears to be NO, although important contributions may also be made by ATP, vasoactive intestinal peptide (VIP), and pituitary adenylyl cyclase–activating peptide (PACAP). Enterochromaffin cells, scattered throughout the epithelium of the intestine, release serotonin (5HT) to initiate many gut reflexes by acting locally on enteric neurons. Excessive release of 5HT from the gut wall (e.g., by chemotherapeutic agents) leads to vomiting by actions of 5HT on vagal nerve endings in the proximal small intestine. Compounds targeting the 5HT system are important modulators of motility, secretion, and emesis.

Other cell types are important, including the interstitial cells of Cajal, distributed within the gut wall and responsible for setting the electrical rhythm and the pace of contractions in various regions of the gut. These cells also translate or modulate excitatory and inhibitory neuronal communication to the smooth muscle.

EXCITATION-CONTRACTION COUPLING IN GI SMOOTH MUSCLE

Control of tension in GI smooth muscle is dependent on the intracellular Ca^{2+} concentration. There are basically 2 types of excitation-contraction coupling in these cells. *Ionotropic receptors* can mediate changes in membrane potential, which in turn activate voltage-dependent Ca^{2+} channels to trigger an influx of Ca^{2+} (electromechanical coupling); *metabotropic receptors* activate various signal transduction pathways to release Ca^{2+} from intracellular stores (pharmaco-mechanical coupling). Inhibitory receptors act via PKA and PKG and lead to hyperpolarization, decreased cytosolic $[Ca^{2+}]$, and reduced interaction of actin and myosin. As an example, NO may induce relaxation via activation of guanylyl cyclase-cyclic GMP pathway and cause the opening of several types of K^+ channels.

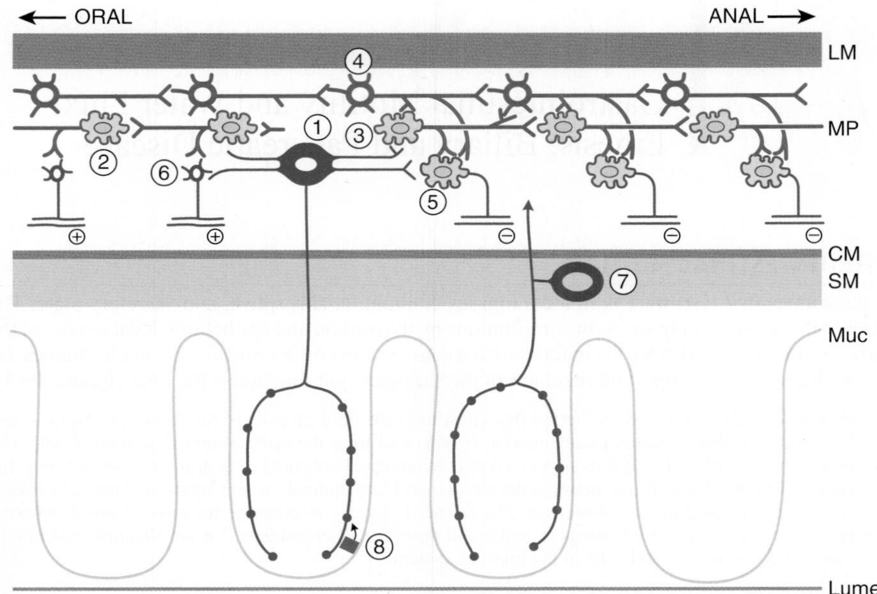

Figure 46–1 *The neuronal network that initiates and generates the peristaltic response.* Mucosal stimulation leads to release of serotonin by enterochromaffin cells (8), which excites the intrinsic primary afferent neurons (1), which then communicate with ascending (2) and descending (3) interneurons in the local reflex pathways. The reflex results in contraction at the oral end via the excitatory motor neuron (6) and aboral relaxation via the inhibitory motor neuron (5). The migratory myoelectric complex (see text) is shown here as being conducted by a different chain of interneurons (4). Another intrinsic primary afferent neuron with its cell body in the submucosa also is shown (7). MP, myenteric plexus; CM, circular muscle; LM, longitudinal muscle; SM, submucosa; Muc, mucosa. (Adapted with permission of Annual Reviews, from Kunze WA, Furness JB. The enteric nervous system and regulation of intestinal motility. *Annu Rev Physiol*, 1999;61:117–142. Permission conveyed through Copyright Clearance Center, Inc.)

FUNCTIONAL AND MOTILITY DISORDERS OF THE BOWEL

GI motility disorders are a heterogeneous group of syndromes. Typical motility disorders include achalasia of the esophagus (impaired relaxation of the lower esophageal sphincter associated with defective esophageal peristalsis that results in dysphagia and regurgitation), gastroparesis (delayed gastric emptying), myopathic and neuropathic forms of intestinal dysmotility, and others. These disorders can be congenital, idiopathic, or secondary to systemic diseases (e.g., diabetes mellitus or scleroderma). This term also has traditionally included disorders such as irritable bowel syndrome (IBS) and noncardiac chest pain. For most of these disorders, treatment remains empirical and symptom based, reflecting ignorance of the pathophysiology involved.

PROKINETIC AGENTS AND OTHER STIMULANTS OF GI CONTRACTILITY

Prokinetic agents are medications that enhance coordinated GI motility and transit of material in the GI tract. These agents appear to enhance the release of excitatory neurotransmitter at the nerve-muscle junction without interfering with the normal physiological pattern and rhythm of motility. By contrast, activation of muscarinic receptors with the older cholinomimetic agents (*see* Chapter 9) or AChE inhibitors (*see* Chapter 10) enhances contractions in a relatively uncoordinated fashion that produces little or no net propulsive activity.

DOPAMINE RECEPTOR ANTAGONISTS

Dopamine (DA) is present in significant amounts in the GI tract and has several inhibitory effects on motility, including reduction of lower esophageal sphincter and intragastric pressures. These effects, which result from suppression of ACh release from myenteric motor neurons, are mediated by D_2 dopaminergic receptors. DA receptor antagonists are effective as prokinetic agents; they have the additional advantage of relieving nausea and vomiting by antagonism of DA receptors in the chemoreceptor trigger zone. Examples are *metoclopramide* and *domperidone*.

METOCLOPRAMIDE. Metoclopramide (REGLAN, others) and other substituted benzamides are derivatives of *para*-aminobenzoic acid and are structurally related to procainamide.

The mechanisms of action of metoclopramide are complex and involve $5HT_4$ receptor agonism, vagal and central $5HT_3$ antagonism, and possible sensitization of muscarinic receptors on smooth muscle, in addition to DA receptor antagonism. Administration of metoclopramide results in coordinated contractions that enhance transit. Its effects are confined largely to the upper digestive tract, where it increases lower esophageal sphincter tone and stimulates antral and small intestinal contractions. Metoclopramide has no clinically significant effects on large-bowel motility.

ADME. Metoclopramide is absorbed rapidly after oral ingestion, undergoes sulfation and glucuronide conjugation by the liver, and is excreted principally in the urine, with a $t_{1/2}$ of 4-6 h. Peak concentrations occur within 1 h after a single oral dose; the duration of action is 1-2 h.

Therapeutic Use. Metoclopramide is indicated in symptomatic patients with gastroparesis, in whom it may cause modest improvements of gastric emptying. Metoclopramide injection is used as an adjunctive measure in medical or diagnostic procedures such as intestinal intubation or contrast radiography of the GI tract. Its greatest utility lies in its ability to ameliorate the nausea and vomiting that often accompany GI dysmotility syndromes. Metoclopramide is available in oral dosage forms (tablets and solution) and as a parenteral preparation for intravenous or intramuscular use. The initial regimen is 10 mg orally, 30 min before each meal and at bedtime. The onset of action is within 30-60 min. In patients with severe nausea, an initial dose of 10 mg can be given intramuscularly (onset of action 10-15 min) or intravenously (onset of action 1-3 min). For prevention of chemotherapy-induced emesis, metoclopramide can be given as an infusion of 1-2 mg/kg administered over at least 15 min, beginning 30 min before the chemotherapy is begun and repeated as needed every 2 h for 2 doses, then every 3 h for 3 doses.

Adverse Effects. The major side effects of metoclopramide include extrapyramidal effects. Dystonias, usually occurring acutely after intravenous administration, and parkinsonian-like symptoms that may occur several weeks after initiation of therapy generally respond to treatment with anticholinergic or antihistaminic drugs and reverse upon discontinuation of metoclopramide. Tardive dyskinesia also can occur with chronic treatment (months to years) and may be irreversible. Extrapyramidal effects appear to occur more commonly in children and young adults and at higher doses. Metoclopramide also can cause galactorrhea by blocking the inhibitory effect of dopamine on prolactin release (seen infrequently in clinical practice). Methemoglobinemia has been reported occasionally in premature and full-term neonates receiving metoclopramide.

DOMPERIDONE, A D_2 RECEPTOR ANTAGONIST. In contrast to metoclopramide, domperidone predominantly antagonizes the D_2 receptor without major involvement of other receptors.

Domperidone (MOTILIUM, others) is not available for use in the U.S. but is used elsewhere and has modest prokinetic activity in doses of 10-20 mg 3 times a day. Although it does not readily cross the blood-brain barrier to cause extrapyramidal side effects, domperidone exerts effects in the parts of the CNS that lack this barrier, such as those regulating emesis, temperature, and prolactin release. Domperidone does not appear to have any significant effects on lower GI motility.

SEROTONIN RECEPTOR AGONISTS

5HT plays an important role in the normal motor and secretory function of the gut (*see* Chapter 13). Indeed, >90% of the total 5HT in the body exists in the GI tract. The enterochromaffin cell produces most of this 5HT and rapidly releases 5HT in response to chemical and mechanical stimulation (e.g., food boluses; noxious agents such as cisplatin; certain microbial toxins; adrenergic, cholinergic, and purinergic receptor agonists). 5HT triggers the peristaltic reflex (*see* Figure 46–1) by stimulating intrinsic sensory neurons in the myenteric plexus (via $5HT_{1p}$ and $5HT_4$ receptors), as well as extrinsic vagal and spinal sensory neurons (via $5HT_3$ receptors). Additionally, stimulation of submucosal intrinsic afferent neurons activates secretomotor reflexes resulting in epithelial secretion.

5HT receptors also are found on other neurons in the ENS, where they can be either stimulatory ($5HT_3$ and $5HT_4$) or inhibitory ($5HT_{1a}$). In addition, serotonin also stimulates the release of other neurotransmitters. Thus, $5HT_1$ stimulation of the gastric fundus results in release of NO and reduces smooth muscle tone. $5HT_4$ stimulation of excitatory motor neurons enhances ACh release at the neuromuscular junction, and both $5HT_3$ and $5HT_4$ receptors facilitate interneuronal signaling. Developmentally, 5HT acts as a neurotrophic factor for enteric neurons via the $5HT_{2B}$ and $5HT_4$ receptors. Reuptake of serotonin by enteric neurons and epithelium is mediated by the same transporter (SERT; *see* Chapters 5 and 13) as 5HT reuptake by serotonergic neurons in the CNS. This reuptake also is blocked by selective serotonin reuptake inhibitors (SSRIs; *see* Figure 15–1 and Table 15–1), which explains the common side effect of diarrhea that accompanies the use of these agents. Modulation of the multiple, complex, and sometimes opposing effects of 5HT on gut motor function has become a major target for drug development. The availability of serotonergic prokinetic drugs has in

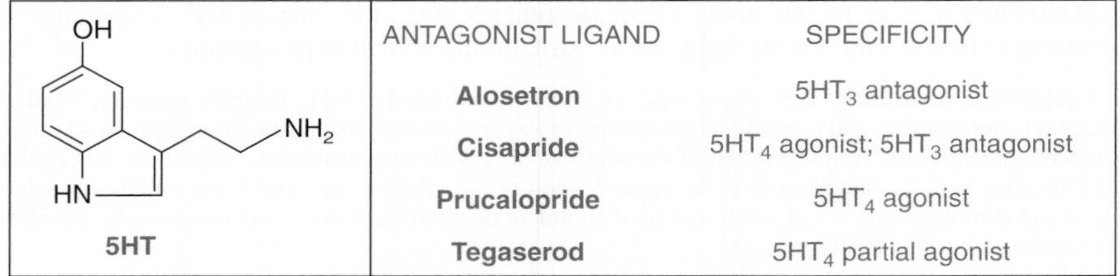

ANTAGONIST LIGAND	SPECIFICITY
Alosetron	$5HT_3$ antagonist
Cisapride	$5HT_4$ agonist; $5HT_3$ antagonist
Prucalopride	$5HT_4$ agonist
Tegaserod	$5HT_4$ partial agonist

Figure 46–2 *Serotonergic agents modulating GI motility.*

recent years been restricted because of serious adverse cardiac events. Tegaserod maleate (ZELNORM) has been discontinued; cisapride is available only via a restricted investigational drug protocol. A novel $5HT_4$ agonist, prucalopride (RESOLOR), is approved in Europe for symptomatic treatment of chronic constipation in women in whom laxatives fail to provide adequate relief.

CISAPRIDE. Cisapride (PROPULSID; Figure 46–2) is a $5HT_4$ agonist that stimulates adenylyl cyclase activity in neurons. It also has weak $5HT_3$ antagonistic properties and may directly stimulate smooth muscle. Cisapride was a commonly used prokinetic agent, however, it no longer is available in the U.S. because of its potential to induce serious and occasionally fatal cardiac arrhythmias that result from a prolonged QT interval. Cisapride is metabolized by CYP3A4 (*see* Chapter 6). Cisapride is contraindicated in patients with a history of prolonged QT interval, renal failure, ventricular arrhythmias, ischemic heart disease, congestive heart failure, respiratory failure, uncorrected electrolyte abnormalities, or concomitant medications known to prolong the QT interval. Cisapride is available only through an investigational, limited-access program for patients with GERD, gastroparesis, pseudo-obstruction, refractory severe chronic constipation, and neonatal enteral feeding intolerance who have failed all standard therapeutic modalities and who have undergone a thorough diagnostic evaluation, including an ECG.

PRUCALOPRIDE. Prucalopride (RESELOR; *see* Figure 46–2) is a specific $5HT_4$ receptor agonist that facilitates cholinergic neurotransmission. It acts throughout the length of the intestine, increasing oral-cecal transit and colonic transit without affecting gastric emptying in healthy volunteers. Given in doses of 2 and 4 mg orally, once daily, the drug improves bowel habits. Prucalopride is approved in Europe for use in women with chronic constipation in whom laxatives fail to provide adequate relief.

MOTILIDES

MACROLIDES AND ERYTHROMYCIN. Motilin, a 22–amino acid peptide hormone found in the M cells and in some enterochromaffin cells of the upper small bowel, is a potent contractile agent of the upper GI tract. Motilin levels fluctuate in association with the migrating motor complex and appear to be responsible for the amplification, if not the actual induction, of phase III activity. In addition, motilin receptors are found on smooth muscle cells and enteric neurons.

The effects of motilin can be mimicked by erythromycin, a property shared to varying extents by other macrolide antibiotics (e.g., oleandomycin, azithromycin, and clarithromycin; *see* Chapter 55). In addition to its motilin-like effects, which are most pronounced at higher doses (250-500 mg), erythromycin at lower doses (e.g., 40-80 mg) also may act by other poorly defined mechanisms that may involve cholinergic facilitation. Erythromycin has multiple effects on upper GI motility, increasing lower esophageal pressure and stimulating gastric and small-bowel contractility. By contrast, it has little or no effect on colonic motility. At doses higher than 3 mg/kg, it can produce a spastic type of contraction in the small bowel, resulting in cramps, impairment of transit, and vomiting.

THERAPEUTIC USE. Erythromycin is used as a prokinetic agent in patients with diabetic gastroparesis, where it can improve gastric emptying in the short term. Erythromycin-stimulated gastric contractions can be intense and result in "dumping" of relatively undigested food into the small bowel. This potential disadvantage can be exploited clinically to clear the stomach of undigestible residue such as plastic tubes or bezoars. Rapid development of tolerance to erythromycin, possibly by downregulation of the motilin receptor, and antibiotic effects (undesirable in this context) limit the use of this drug as a prokinetic agent. A standard dose of erythromycin for gastric stimulation is 3 mg/kg intravenously or 200-250 mg orally every 8 h. For small-bowel stimulation, a smaller dose (e.g., 40 mg intravenously) may be more useful; higher doses may actually retard the motility. Concerns about toxicity, pseudomembranous colitis, and the induction of resistant strains of bacteria, among other things, limit the use of erythromycin to acute situations or in circumstances where patients are resistant to other medications.

Mitemcinal (GM-611), a macrolide non-antibiotic, shows promise for the treatment of gastroparesis.

MISCELLANEOUS AGENTS FOR STIMULATING MOTILITY

The hormone *cholecystokinin* (CCK) is released from the intestine in response to meals and delays gastric emptying, causes contraction of the gallbladder, stimulates pancreatic enzyme secretion, increases intestinal motility, and promotes satiety. The C-terminal octapeptide of CCK, *sincalide* (KINEVAC), is useful for stimulating the gallbladder and/or pancreas and for accelerating barium transit through the small bowel for diagnostic testing of these organs. *Dexloxiglumide* is a CCK_1 (or CCK-A) receptor antagonist that can improve gastric emptying and has been investigated as a treatment for gastroparesis and for constipation-dominant IBS and may also have uses in feeding intolerance in critically ill individuals. Clonidine also has been reported to be of benefit in patients with gastroparesis. Octreotide acetate (SANDOSTATIN, others), a somatostatin analogue, also is used in some patients with intestinal dysmotility.

AGENTS THAT SUPPRESS MOTILITY

Smooth muscle relaxants such as organic nitrates and Ca^{2+} channel antagonists often produce temporary, if partial, relief of symptoms in motility disorders such as achalasia, in which the lower esophageal sphincter fails to relax, resulting in severe difficulty in swallowing. Preparations of botulinum toxin (BOTOX, DYSPORT, MYOBLOC), injected directly into the lower esophageal sphincter via an endoscope, in doses of 80-100 units, inhibit ACh release from nerve endings and can produce partial paralysis of the sphincter muscle, with significant improvements in symptoms and esophageal clearance.

LAXATIVES, CATHARTICS, AND THERAPY FOR CONSTIPATION

OVERVIEW OF GI WATER AND ELECTROLYTE FLUX. Water normally accounts for 70-85% of total stool weight. Net stool fluid content reflects a balance between luminal input (ingestion and secretion of water and electrolytes) and output (absorption) along the length of the GI tract. The daily challenge for the gut is to extract water, minerals, and nutrients from the luminal contents, leaving behind a manageable pool of fluid for proper expulsion of waste material via the process of defecation.

Normally ~8-9 L of fluid enter the small intestine daily from exogenous and endogenous sources (Figure 46–3). Net absorption of the water occurs in the small intestine in response to osmotic gradients that result from the uptake and secretion of ions and the absorption of nutrients (mainly sugars and amino acids), with only ~1-1.5 L crossing the ileocecal valve. The colon then extracts most of the remaining fluid, leaving ~100 mL of fecal water daily. Under normal circumstances, these quantities are within the range of the total absorptive capacity of the small bowel (~16 L) and colon (4-5 L). Neurohumoral mechanisms, pathogens, and drugs can alter secretion and absorption of fluid by the intestinal epithelium. Altered motility also contributes in a general way to this process. With decreased motility and excess fluid removal, feces can become inspissated and impacted, leading to constipation. When the capacity of the colon to absorb fluid is exceeded, diarrhea occurs.

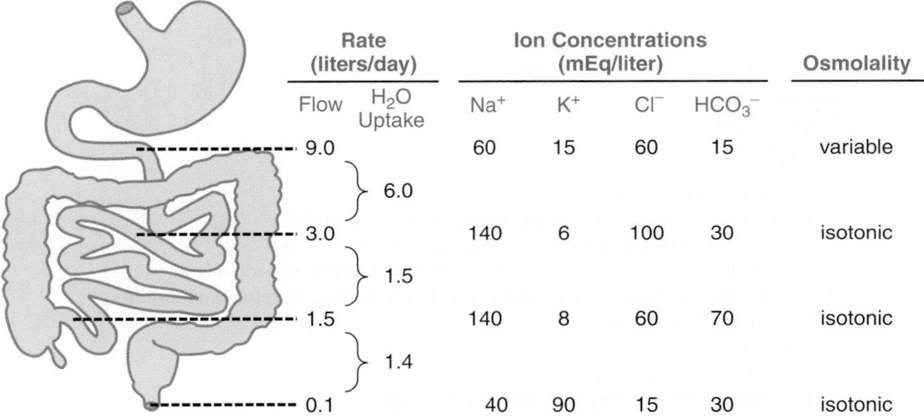

Figure 46–3 *The approximate volume and composition of fluid that traverses the small and large intestines daily.* Of the 9 L of fluid typically presented to the small intestine each day, 2 L are from the diet and 7 L are from secretions (salivary, gastric, pancreatic, and biliary). The absorptive capacity of the colon is 4-5 L per day.

CONSTIPATION: GENERAL PRINCIPLES OF PATHOPHYSIOLOGY AND TREATMENT. Patients use the term *constipation* not only for decreased frequency, but also for difficulty in initiation or passage, passage of firm or small-volume feces, or a feeling of incomplete evacuation.

Constipation has many reversible or secondary causes, including lack of dietary fiber, drugs, hormonal disturbances, neurogenic disorders, and systemic illnesses. In most cases of chronic constipation, no specific cause is found. Up to 60% of patients presenting with constipation have normal colonic transit. These patients either have IBS or define constipation in terms other than stool frequency. In the rest, attempts usually are made to categorize the underlying pathophysiology either as a disorder of delayed colonic transit because of an underlying defect in colonic motility or, less commonly, as an isolated disorder of defecation or evacuation (outlet disorder) due to dysfunction of the neuromuscular apparatus of the rectoanal region.

Colonic motility is responsible for mixing luminal contents to promote absorption of water and moving them from proximal to distal segments by means of propulsive contractions. Mixing in the colon is accomplished in a way similar to that in the small bowel: by short- or long-duration, stationary (nonpropulsive) contractions. In any given patient, the predominant factor often is not obvious. Consequently, the pharmacological approach to constipation remains empirical and is based, in most cases, on nonspecific principles.

Constipation generally may be corrected by adherence to a fiber-rich (20-35 g daily) diet, adequate fluid intake, appropriate bowel habits and training, and avoidance of constipating drugs. Constipation related to medications can be corrected by use of alternative drugs where possible, or adjustment of dosage. If nonpharmacological measures alone are inadequate, they may be supplemented with bulk-forming agents or osmotic laxatives.

When stimulant laxatives are used, they should be administered at the lowest effective dosage and for the shortest period of time to avoid abuse. In addition to perpetuating dependence on drugs, the laxative habit may lead to excessive loss of water and electrolytes; secondary aldosteronism may occur if volume depletion is prominent. Steatorrhea, protein-losing enteropathy with hypoalbuminemia, and osteomalacia due to excessive loss of calcium in the stool have been reported. Laxatives frequently are employed before surgical, radiological, and endoscopic procedures where an empty colon is desirable. The terms *laxatives*, *cathartics*, *purgatives*, *aperients*, and *evacuants* often are used interchangeably. There is a distinction, however, between *laxation* (the evacuation of formed fecal material from the rectum) and *catharsis* (the evacuation of unformed, usually watery fecal material from the entire colon). Most of the commonly used agents promote laxation, but some are actually cathartics that act as laxatives at low doses.

Laxatives relieve constipation and promote evacuation of the bowel via:

- Enhancing retention of intraluminal fluid by hydrophilic or osmotic mechanisms
- Decreasing net absorption of fluid by effects on small- and large-bowel fluid and electrolyte transport
- Altering motility by either inhibiting segmenting (nonpropulsive) contractions or stimulating propulsive contractions.

Laxatives can be classified based on their actions (Table 46–1) or by the pattern of effects produced by the usual clinical dosage (Table 46–2), with some overlap between classifications.

Table 46–1

Classification of Laxatives

1. **Luminally active agents**
   Hydrophilic colloids; bulk-forming agents (bran, psyllium, etc.)
   Osmotic agents (nonabsorbable inorganic salts or sugars)
   Stool-wetting agents (surfactants) and emollients (docusate, mineral oil)
2. **Nonspecific stimulants or irritants (with effects on fluid secretion and motility)**
   Diphenylmethanes (bisacodyl)
   Anthraquinones (senna and cascara)
   Castor oil
3. **Prokinetic agents (acting primarily on motility)**
   $5HT_4$ receptor agonists
   Dopamine receptor antagonists
   Motilides (erythromycin)

Table 46–2

Classification and Comparison of Representative Laxatives

LAXATIVE EFFECT AND LATENCY IN USUAL CLINICAL DOSAGE		
SOFTENING OF FECES, 1-3 DAYS	SOFT OR SEMIFLUID STOOL, 6-8 HOURS	WATERY EVACUATION, 1-3 HOURS
Bulk-forming laxatives	***Stimulant laxatives***	***Osmotic laxatives***[a]
Bran	Diphenylmethane derivatives	Sodium phosphates
Psyllium preparations	Bisacodyl	Magnesium sulfate
Methylcellulose		Milk of magnesia
Calcium polycarbophil		Magnesium citrate
Surfactant/osmotic laxatives	***Anthraquinone derivatives***	***Castor oil***
Docusates	Senna	
Poloxamers	Cascara sagrada	
Lactulose		

[a]*Employed in high dosage for rapid cathartic effect and in lower dosage for laxative effect.*

A variety of laxatives, both osmotic agents and stimulants, increase the activity of NO synthase and the biosynthesis of platelet-activating factor in the gut. Platelet-activating factor is a phospholipid proinflammatory mediator that stimulates colonic secretion and GI motility. NO also may stimulate intestinal secretion and inhibit segmenting contractions in the colon, thereby promoting laxation. Agents that reduce the expression of NO synthase or its activity can prevent the laxative effects of castor oil, cascara, and bisacodyl (but not senna), as well as magnesium sulfate.

DIETARY FIBER AND SUPPLEMENTS

Bulk, softness, and hydration of feces depend on the fiber content of the diet. Fiber is defined as that part of food that resists enzymatic digestion and reaches the colon largely unchanged. Colonic bacteria ferment fiber to varying degrees, depending on its chemical nature and water solubility. Fermentation of fiber has 2 important effects: (1) it produces short-chain fatty acids that are trophic for colonic epithelium; (2) it increases bacterial mass. Although fermentation of fiber generally decreases stool water, short-chain fatty acids may have a prokinetic effect, and increased bacterial mass may contribute to increased stool volume. However, fiber that is not fermented can attract water and increase stool bulk. The net effect on bowel movement therefore varies with different compositions of dietary fiber (Table 46–3). *In general, insoluble, poorly fermentable fibers, such as lignin, are most effective in increasing stool bulk and transit.*

Bran, the residue left when flour is made from cereal grains, contains >40% dietary fiber. Wheat bran, with its high lignin content, is most effective at increasing stool weight. Fruits and vegetables contain more *pectins* and *hemicelluloses*, which are more readily fermentable and produce less effect on stool transit. *Psyllium husk*, derived from the seed of the plantago herb, is a component of many commercial products for

Table 46–3

Properties of Different Dietary Fibers

TYPE OF FIBER	WATER SOLUBILITY	% FERMENTED
Nonpolysaccharides		
Lignin	Poor	0
Cellulose	Poor	15
Noncellulose polysaccharides		
Hemicellulose	Good	56-87
Mucilages and gums	Good	85-95
Pectins	Good	90-95

In general, insoluble, poorly fermentable fibers, such as lignin, are most effective in increasing stool bulk and transit.

constipation (METAMUCIL, others). Psyllium husk contains a hydrophilic mucilloid that undergoes significant fermentation in the colon, leading to an increase in colonic bacterial mass. The usual dose is 2.5-4 g (1-3 teaspoonfuls in 250 mL of fruit juice), titrated upward until the desired goal is reached. A variety of semisynthetic celluloses—e.g., methylcellulose (CITRUCEL, others) and the hydrophilic resin calcium polycarbophil (FIBERCON, FIBERALL, others), a polymer of acrylic acid resin—also are available. These poorly fermentable compounds absorb water and increase fecal bulk. Malt soup extract (MALTSUPEX, others), an extract of malt, is another orally administered bulk-forming agent. Bloating is the most common side effect of soluble fiber products (perhaps due to colonic fermentation), but it usually decreases with time.

OSMOTICALLY ACTIVE AGENTS

POLYETHYLENE GLYCOL–ELECTROLYTE SOLUTIONS. Long-chain polyethylene glycols (PEGs; MW ~3350 Da) are poorly absorbed and retain water via their high osmotic nature. When used in high volume, aqueous solutions of PEGs with electrolytes (COLYTE, GOLYTELY, others) produce an effective catharsis and have replaced oral sodium phosphates as the most widely used preparations for colonic cleansing prior to radiological, surgical, and endoscopic procedures.

Usually 240 mL of this solution is taken every 10 min until 4 L is consumed or the rectal effluent is clear. To avoid net transfer of ions across the intestinal wall, these preparations contain an isotonic mixture of sodium sulfate, sodium bicarbonate, sodium chloride, and potassium chloride. The osmotic activity of the PEG molecules retains the added water and the electrolyte concentration assures little or no net ionic shifts. A powder form of polyethylene glycol 3350 (MIRALAX, others) is now available for the short-term treatment (≤2 weeks) of occasional constipation. The usual dose is 17 g of powder per day in 8 ounces of water.

SALINE LAXATIVES. Laxatives containing magnesium cations or phosphate anions commonly are called *saline laxatives*: magnesium sulfate, magnesium hydroxide, magnesium citrate, sodium phosphate. Their cathartic action is believed to result from osmotic water retention, which then stimulates peristalsis. Other mechanisms may contribute, including the production of inflammatory mediators.

Magnesium-containing laxatives may stimulate the release of cholecystokinin, which leads to intraluminal fluid and electrolyte accumulation and to increased intestinal motility. For every additional mEq of Mg^{2+} in the intestinal lumen, fecal weight increases by ~7 g. The usual dose of magnesium salts contains 40-120 mEq of Mg^{2+} and produces 300-600 mL of stool within 6 h.

Phosphate salts are better absorbed than magnesium-based agents and therefore need to be given in larger doses to induce catharsis. The most frequently employed preparations of sodium phosphate are an oral solution (FLEET PHOSPHO-SODA) and tablets (VISICOL, OSMOPREP). The FDA has ruled that only prescription medications should be available for this purpose. To reduce the likelihood of acute phosphate nephropathy, oral phosphates should be avoided in patients at risk (the elderly, patients with known bowel pathology or renal dysfunction, and patients on angiotensin-converting enzyme [ACE] inhibitors, angiotensin receptor blockers [ARBs], and nonsteroidal anti-inflammatory drugs [NSAIDs]) and the 2-dose regimens should be split evenly with the first dose taken the evening before the exam and the second starting 3-5 h before the exam. Adequate fluid intake (1-3 L) is essential for any oral sodium phosphate regimen used for colonic preparation.

Magnesium- and phosphate-containing preparations must be used with caution or avoided in patients with renal insufficiency, cardiac disease, or preexisting electrolyte abnormalities, and in patients on diuretic therapy. Patients taking >45 mL of oral sodium phosphate as a prescribed bowel preparation may experience electrolyte shifts that pose a risk for the development of symptomatic dehydration, renal failure, metabolic acidosis, tetany from hypocalcemia, and even death in vulnerable populations.

NONDIGESTIBLE SUGARS AND ALCOHOLS. *Lactulose* (CEPHULAC, CHRONULAC, others) is a synthetic disaccharide of galactose and fructose that resists intestinal disaccharidase activity. This and other nonabsorbable sugars such as sorbitol and mannitol are hydrolyzed in the colon to short-chain fatty acids, which stimulate colonic propulsive motility by osmotically drawing water into the lumen. Sorbitol and lactulose are equally efficacious in the treatment of constipation caused by opioids and vincristine, of constipation in the elderly, and of idiopathic chronic constipation. They are available as 70% solutions, which are given in doses of 15-30 mL at night, with increases as needed up to 60 mL per day in divided doses. Effects may not be seen for 24-48 h after dosing is begun. Abdominal discomfort or distention and flatulence are relatively common but usually subside with continued administration.

Lactulose also is used to treat hepatic encephalopathy. Patients with severe liver disease have an impaired capacity to detoxify ammonia coming from the colon, where it is produced by bacterial metabolism of fecal urea. The drop in luminal pH that accompanies hydrolysis to short-chain fatty acids in the colon results in "trapping" of the ammonia by its conversion to the polar ammonium ion. Combined with the increases in colonic transit, this therapy significantly lowers circulating ammonia levels. The therapeutic goal in this condition is to give sufficient amounts of lactulose (usually 20-30 g, 3 to 4 times per day) to produce 2 to 3 soft stools a day with a pH of 5-5.5.

STOOL-WETTING AGENTS AND EMOLLIENTS

Docusate salts are anionic surfactants that lower the surface tension of the stool to allow mixing of aqueous and fatty substances, softening the stool and permitting easier defecation. These agents also stimulate intestinal fluid and electrolyte secretion (possibly by increasing mucosal cyclic AMP) and alter intestinal mucosal permeability. Docusate sodium (dioctyl sodium sulfosuccinate; COLACE, DOXINATE, others) and docusate calcium (dioctyl calcium sulfosuccinate; SURFAK, others) are available in several dosage forms. These agents have marginal efficacy in most cases of constipation.

Mineral oil is a mixture of aliphatic hydrocarbons obtained from petrolatum. The oil is indigestible and absorbed only to a limited extent. When mineral oil is taken orally for 2-3 days, it penetrates and softens the stool and may interfere with resorption of water. The side effects of mineral oil preclude its regular use and include interference with absorption of fat-soluble substances (such as vitamins), elicitation of foreign-body reactions in the intestinal mucosa and other tissues, and leakage of oil past the anal sphincter. Rare complications such as lipid pneumonitis due to aspiration also can occur, so "heavy" mineral oil should not be taken at bedtime and "light" (topical) mineral oil should never be administered orally.

STIMULANT (IRRITANT) LAXATIVES

Stimulant laxatives have direct effects on enterocytes, enteric neurons, and GI smooth muscle and probably induce a limited low-grade inflammation in the small and large bowel to promote accumulation of water and electrolytes and stimulate intestinal motility. This group incudes: *diphenylmethane derivatives*, *anthraquinones*, and *ricinoleic acid*.

DIPHENYLMETHANE DERIVATIVES. *Bisacodyl* (DULCOLAX, CORRECTOL, others) is marketed as enteric-coated and regular tablets and as a suppository for rectal administration. The usual oral daily dose of bisacodyl is 10-15 mg for adults and 5-10 mg for children ages 6-12 years old. The drug requires hydrolysis by endogenous esterases in the bowel for activation, and so the laxative effects after an oral dose usually are not produced in <6 h. Suppositories work within 30-60 min. Due to the possibility of developing an atonic non-functioning colon, bisacodyl should not be used for >10 consecutive days. Bisacodyl is mainly excreted in the stool; ~5% is absorbed and excreted in the urine as a glucuronide. Overdosage can lead to catharsis and fluid and electrolyte deficits. The diphenylmethanes can damage the mucosa and initiate an inflammatory response in the small bowel and colon.

Sodium *picosulfate* (LUBRILAX, SUR-LAX) is a diphenylmethane derivative widely available outside of the U.S. It is hydrolyzed by colonic bacteria to its active form and acts locally only in the colon. Effective doses of the diphenylmethane derivatives vary as much as 4- to 8-fold in individual patients. *Phenolphthalein*, once among the most popular components of laxatives, has been withdrawn from the market in the U.S. because of potential carcinogenicity. *Oxyphenisatin* was withdrawn due to hepatotoxicity.

ANTHRAQUINONE LAXATIVES. These derivatives of plants such as aloe, cascara, and senna share a tricyclic anthracene nucleus modified with hydroxyl, methyl, or carboxyl groups to form monoanthrones, such as rhein and frangula. For use, monoanthrones (oral mucosal irritants) are converted to more innocuous dimeric (dianthrones) or glycoside forms. This process is reversed by bacterial action in the colon to generate the active forms.

Senna (SENOKOT, EX-LAX, others) is obtained from the dried leaflets on pods of *Cassia acutifolia* or *Cassia angustifolia* and contains the rhein dianthrone glycosides sennoside A and B. *Cascara sagrada* is obtained from the bark of the buckthorn tree and contains the glycosides barbaloin and chrysaloin. The synthetic monoanthrone danthron was withdrawn from the U.S. market because of concerns over possible carcinogenicity. Aloe and cascara sagrada products sold as laxatives have been categorized by FDA as not generally recognized as safe and effective for over the counter use because of a lack of scientific information about potential carcinogenicity. These ingredients may still be sold over-the-counter in the U.S., but legally they cannot be labeled for use as laxatives. This judgment is medically prudent but may provoke a longing for times past amongst Joyceans, who recall that cascara sagrada, the *sacred bark*, worked well for Leopold Bloom, in Dublin, on the morning of June 16, 1904:

> *Midway, his last resistance yielding, he allowed his bowels to ease themselves quietly as he read, reading still patiently that slight constipation of yesterday quite gone. Hope its not too big to bring on piles again. No, just right. So. Ah! Costive one tabloid of cascara sagrada. Life might be so. (*Ulysses*, James Joyce, 1922)*

CASTOR OIL. A bane of childhood since the time of the ancient Egyptians, castor oil (PURGE, NEOLOID, others) is derived from the bean of the castor plant, *Ricinus communis*. The castor bean is the source of an extremely toxic protein, ricin, as well as the oil (chiefly of the triglyceride of ricinoleic acid). The triglyceride is hydrolyzed in the small bowel by the action of lipases into glycerol and the active agent, ricinoleic acid, which acts primarily in the small intestine to stimulate secretion of fluid and electrolytes and speed intestinal transit. When taken on an empty stomach, as little as 4 mL of castor oil may produce a laxative effect within 1-3 h; however, the usual dose for a cathartic effect is 15-60 mL for adults. Because of its unpleasant taste and its potential toxic effects on intestinal epithelium and enteric neurons, castor oil is seldom recommended now.

PROKINETIC AND OTHER AGENTS FOR CONSTIPATION

The term *prokinetic* generally is reserved for agents that enhance GI transit via interaction with specific receptors involved in the regulation of motility.

The potent $5HT_4$ receptor agonist *prucalopride* may be useful for the treatment of chronic constipation. *Misoprostol*, a synthetic prostaglandin analog, is primarily used for protection against gastric ulcers resulting from the use of NSAIDs (*see* Chapters 34 and 45). Prostaglandins can stimulate colonic contractions, particularly in the descending colon; this may account for the diarrhea that limits the usefulness of misoprostol as a gastroprotectant and find utility in patients with intractable constipation. *Colchicine*, a microtubule formation inhibitor used for gout (*see* Chapter 34), also has been shown to be effective in constipation, but its toxicity has limited widespread use. Neurotrophin-3 (NT-3) recently was shown to be effective in improving frequency and stool consistency by an unknown mechanism of action.

Lubiprostone (AMITIZA) is a prostanoid activator of Cl^- channels. The drug appears to bind to EP_4 receptors linked to activation of adenylyl cyclase, leading to enhanced apical Cl^- conductance. The drug promotes the secretion of a chloride-rich fluid, thereby improving stool consistency and promoting increased frequency by reflexly activating motility. A dose of 8 μg twice daily was found to be effective in IBS-C, though higher doses (24 μg twice daily) are given for chronic constipation. The drug is poorly bioavailable, acting only in the lumen of the bowel. Side effects of lubiprostone include nausea, headache, diarrhea, allergic reactions, and dyspnea.

Another class of secretory agent is represented by *linaclotide* (LINZESS), a 14–amino acid peptide agonist of guanylate cyclase C that stimulates secretion and motility. This compound is approved in the treatment of IBS-C and chronic constipation. Common side effects include gas, abdominal pain, and diarrhea.

OPIOID-INDUCED CONSTIPATION

Opioid analgesics can cause severe constipation. Laxatives and dietary strategies are frequently ineffective in the management of opioid-induced constipation. A promising strategy is the prevention of opioid-induced constipation with peripherally acting μ opioid receptor (MOR) antagonists that specifically target the underlying reason for this condition, without limiting centrally produced analgesia. *Methylnaltrexone* (RELISTOR), a peripherally restricted MOR antagonist, is approved for the treatment of opioid-induced constipation. In multicenter trials, when methylnaltrexone (0.15-0.3 mg/kg) was administered repeatedly every other day for 2 weeks, bowel movements occurred in 50% of the patients, compared with 8-15% of patients receiving placebo. Another MOR antagonist, *alvimopan* (ENTEREG, 0.5-1 mg twice daily for 6 weeks), increased spontaneous bowel movements and improved other symptoms of opioid-induced constipation without compromising analgesia.

POSTOPERATIVE ILEUS

Postoperative ileus refers to the intolerance to oral intake and nonmechanical obstruction of the bowel that occurs after abdominal and nonabdominal surgery. The pathogenesis is complex and is a combination of activation of neural inhibitory reflexes involving enteric MOR and the activation of local inflammatory mechanisms that reduce smooth muscle contractility. The condition is exacerbated by opioids, which are the mainstay of postoperative analgesia. Prokinetic agents typically do not have much effect in this condition, but recently, 2 new therapeutic agents have been introduced that have benefit in reducing GI recovery time after surgery.

Alvimopan (ENTEREG) is an orally active peripherally restricted μ opioid receptor antagonist that is approved for limited indications following surgery (12 mg prior to surgery and then once daily for up to 7 days or until discharge; not to exceed 15 doses total). Methylnaltrexone (see above) is FDA-approved for the treatment of opioid-induced constipation in patients receiving palliative care when laxative therapy is insufficient. *Dexpanthenol* (ILOPAN, others) is the alcohol of pantothenic acid (vitamin B_5). The drug is a congener of pantothenic acid, a precursor of coenzyme A, which serves as a cofactor in the synthesis of ACh by choline acetyl transferase. It is proposed to act by enhancing synthesis of ACh, major excitatory transmitter of the gut. Dexpanthenol is used as an injection immediately postoperatively after major abdominal surgery to minimize the occurrence of paralytic ileus. It is given by intramuscular injection (200-500 mg) immediately and then

2 h later and every 6 h after that until the situation has resolved. It may cause mild hypotension and shortness of breath as well as local irritation.

ENEMAS AND SUPPOSITORIES

Enemas are employed either by themselves or as adjuncts to bowel preparation regimens, to empty the distal colon or rectum of retained solid material. Bowel distention by any means will produce an evacuation reflex in most people, and almost any form of enema, including normal saline solution, can achieve this. Specialized enemas contain additional substances that are either osmotically active or irritant; however, their safety and efficacy have not been studied. Repeated enemas with hypotonic solutions can cause hyponatremia; repeated enemas with sodium phosphate–containing solution can cause hypocalcemia.

Glycerin is absorbed when given orally but acts as a hygroscopic agent and lubricant when given rectally. The resultant water retention stimulates peristalsis and usually produces a bowel movement in less than an hour. Glycerin is for rectal use only and is given in a single daily dose as a 2- or 3-g rectal suppository or as 5-15 mL of an 80% solution in enema form. Rectal glycerin may cause local discomfort, burning, or hyperemia and (minimal) bleeding. *CEO-TWO* suppositories contain sodium bicarbonate and potassium bitartrate and make use of rectal distension to initiate laxation. When administered rectally, the suppository produces CO_2, which initiates a bowel movement in 5-30 min.

ANTI-DIARRHEAL AGENTS

DIARRHEA: GENERAL PRINCIPLES AND APPROACH TO TREATMENT. An appreciation and knowledge of the underlying causative processes in diarrhea facilitates effective treatment. From a mechanistic perspective, diarrhea can be caused by an increased osmotic load within the intestine (resulting in retention of water within the lumen); excessive secretion of electrolytes and water into the intestinal lumen; exudation of protein and fluid from the mucosa; and altered intestinal motility resulting in rapid transit (and decreased fluid absorption). In most instances, multiple processes are affected simultaneously, leading to a net increase in stool volume and weight accompanied by increases in fractional water content.

Many patients with sudden onset of diarrhea have a benign, self-limited illness requiring no treatment or evaluation. In severe cases of diarrhea, dehydration and electrolyte imbalances are the principal risk. *Oral rehydration therapy* therefore is a cornerstone for patients with acute illnesses resulting in significant diarrhea. This therapy exploits the fact that nutrient-linked cotransport of water and electrolytes remains intact in the small bowel in most cases of acute diarrhea. Na^+ and Cl^- absorption links to glucose uptake by the enterocyte; this is followed by movement of water in the same direction. A balanced mixture of glucose and electrolytes in volumes matched to losses therefore can prevent dehydration. This can be provided by many commercial premixed formulas using glucose-electrolyte or rice-based physiological solutions.

Pharmacotherapy of diarrhea in adults should be reserved for patients with significant or persistent symptoms. Nonspecific anti-diarrheal agents typically do not address the underlying pathophysiology responsible for the diarrhea. Many of these agents act by decreasing intestinal motility and should be avoided in acute diarrheal illnesses caused by invasive organisms. In such cases, these agents may mask the clinical picture, delay clearance of organisms, and increase the risk of systemic invasion by the infectious organisms.

BULK-FORMING AND HYDROSCOPIC AGENTS. Hydrophilic and poorly fermentable colloids or polymers such as *carboxymethylcellulose* and calcium polycarbophil absorb water and increase stool bulk (calcium polycarbophil absorbs 60 times its weight in water). They usually are used for constipation but are sometimes useful in acute episodic diarrhea and in mild chronic diarrheas in patients suffering with IBS. Some of these agents also may bind bacterial toxins and bile salts. Clays such as kaolin (a hydrated aluminum silicate) and other silicates such as attapulgite (magnesium aluminum disilicate; DIASORB, others) bind water avidly and also may bind enterotoxins. However, binding is not selective and may involve other drugs and nutrients; hence these agents are best avoided within 2-3 h of taking other medications. A mixture of kaolin and pectin (a plant polysaccharide) is a popular over-the-counter remedy (KAOPECTOLIN, others) and may provide useful symptomatic relief of mild diarrhea.

BILE ACID SEQUESTRANTS. Cholestyramine, colestipol, and colesevelam effectively bind bile acids and some bacterial toxins. Cholestyramine is useful in the treatment of bile salt-induced diarrhea, as in patients with resection of the distal ileum. In these patients, excessive concentrations of bile salts reach the colon and stimulate water and electrolyte secretion. Patients with extensive ileal resection (usually >100 cm) eventually develop net bile salt depletion, which can produce steatorrhea because of inadequate micellar formation required for fat absorption. In such patients, the use of cholestyramine aggravates the diarrhea. In patients having bile salt-induced diarrhea, cholestyramine (QUESTRAN, QUESTRAN LIGHT, others) can be given at a dose of 4 g of the dried resin (4 times a day). If successful, the dose may be titrated down to achieve the desired stool frequency.

BISMUTH. Bismuth compounds are used to treat a variety of GI diseases, although their mechanism of action remains poorly understood. PEPTO-BISMOL is a popular over-the-counter preparation that consists of trivalent bismuth and salicylate suspended in a mixture of magnesium aluminum silicate clay. In the low pH of the stomach, the bismuth subsalicylate reacts with hydrochloric acid to form bismuth oxychloride and salicylic acid. Although 99% of the bismuth passes unaltered and unabsorbed into the feces, the salicylate is absorbed in the stomach and small intestine. Thus, the product carries the same warning regarding Reye syndrome as other salicylates.

Bismuth is thought to have anti-secretory, anti-inflammatory, and antimicrobial effects. Nausea and abdominal cramps also are relieved by bismuth. The clay in PEPTO-BISMOL and generic formulations also may have some additional benefits in diarrhea, but this is not clear. Bismuth subsalicylate is used for the prevention and treatment of traveler's diarrhea, but it also is effective in other forms of episodic diarrhea and in acute gastroenteritis. Today, the most common antibacterial use of this agent is in the treatment of *Helicobacter pylori* (*see* Chapter 45). A recommended dose of the bismuth subsalicylate (30 mL of regular strength liquid or 2 tablets) contains approximately equal amounts of bismuth and salicylate (262 mg each). For control of indigestion, nausea, or diarrhea, the dose is repeated every 30-60 min, as needed, up to 8 times a day. Dark stools (sometimes mistaken for melena) and black staining of the tongue in association with bismuth compounds are caused by bismuth sulfide formed in a reaction between the drug and bacterial sulfides in the GI tract.

PROBIOTICS. The GI tract contains a vast commensal microflora that is necessary for health. Alterations in the balance or composition of the microflora are responsible for antibiotic-associated diarrhea, and possibly other disease conditions. Probiotic preparations containing a variety of bacterial strains have shown some degree of benefit in acute diarrheal conditions, antibiotic-associated diarrhea, and infectious diarrhea, but most clinical studies have been small and conclusions are therefore limited.

ANTI-MOTILITY AND ANTI-SECRETORY AGENTS

OPIOIDS. Opioids continue to be widely used in the treatment of diarrhea. They act by several different mechanisms, mediated principally through either μ- or δ-opioid receptors on enteric nerves, epithelial cells, and muscle (*see* Chapter 18). These mechanisms include effects on intestinal motility (μ receptors), intestinal secretion (δ receptors), or absorption (μ and δ receptors). Commonly used anti-diarrheals such as diphenoxylate, difenoxin, and loperamide act principally via peripheral μ opioid receptors and are preferred over opioids that penetrate the CNS.

Loperamide. Loperamide (IMODIUM, IMODIUM A-D, others), a compound with MOR activity, is an orally active anti-diarrheal agent. The drug is 40-50 times more potent than morphine as an anti-diarrheal agent and penetrates the CNS poorly. It increases small intestinal and mouth-to-cecum transit times. Loperamide also increases anal sphincter tone. In addition, loperamide has anti-secretory activity against cholera toxin and some forms of *Escherichia coli* toxin, presumably by acting on G_i-linked receptors to counter the stimulation of adenylyl cyclase activity by the toxins.

Loperamide is available OTC in capsule, solution, and chewable tablet forms. It acts quickly after an oral dose, with peak plasma levels achieved within 3-5 h. It has a $t_{1/2}$ of ~11 h and undergoes extensive hepatic metabolism. The usual adult dose is 4 mg initially followed by 2 mg after each subsequent loose stool, up to 16 mg per day. If clinical improvement in acute diarrhea does not occur within 48 h, loperamide should be discontinued. Recommended maximum daily doses for children are 3 mg for ages 2-5 years, 4 mg for ages 6-8 years, and 6 mg for ages 8-12 years. Loperamide is not recommended for use in children <2 years of age. Loperamide is effective against traveler's diarrhea, used alone or in combination with antimicrobial agents (trimethoprim, trimethoprim-sulfamethoxazole, or a fluoroquinolone). Loperamide is used as adjunct treatment in most forms of chronic diarrheal disease, with few adverse effects. Loperamide lacks significant abuse potential and is more effective in treating diarrhea than diphenoxylate. Overdosage, however, can result in CNS depression (especially in children) and paralytic ileus. In patients with active inflammatory bowel disease involving the colon (*see* Chapter 47), loperamide should be used with great caution, if at all, to avoid development of toxic megacolon.

Diphenoxylate and Difenoxin. Diphenoxylate and its active metabolite difenoxin (diphenoxylic acid) are related structurally to meperidine. As anti-diarrheal agents, diphenoxylate and difenoxin are somewhat more potent than morphine. Both compounds are extensively absorbed after oral administration, with peak levels achieved within 1-2 h. Diphenoxylate is rapidly de-esterified to difenoxin, which is eliminated with a $t_{1/2}$ of ~12 h. Both drugs can produce CNS effects when used in higher doses (40-60 mg per day) and thus have a potential for abuse and/or addiction. They are available in preparations containing small doses of atropine (considered subtherapeutic) to discourage abuse and deliberate overdosage: 25 μg of atropine sulfate per tablet with either 2.5 mg diphenoxylate hydrochloride (LOMOTIL) or 1 mg of difenoxin hydrochloride (MOTOFEN). The usual dosage is 2 tablets initially, then 1 tablet every 3-4 h, not to exceed 8 tablets per day. With excessive use or overdose, constipation and (in inflammatory conditions of the colon) toxic megacolon may develop. In high doses, these drugs cause CNS effects as well as anticholinergic effects from the atropine (dry mouth, blurred vision, etc.) (*see* Chapter 9).

OTHER OPIOIDS. Opioids used for diarrhea include codeine (in doses of 30 mg given 3 or 4 times daily) and opium-containing compounds. *Paregoric* (camphorated opium tincture) contains the equivalent of 2 mg of morphine per 5 mL (0.4 mg/mL); *deodorized tincture of opium*, which is 25 times stronger, contains the equivalent of 50 mg of morphine per 5 mL (10 mg/mL). The 2 tinctures sometimes are confused in prescribing and dispensing, resulting in dangerous overdoses. The anti-diarrheal dose of opium tincture for adults is 0.6 mL (equivalent to 6 mg morphine) 4 times daily; the adult dose of paregoric is 5-10 mL (equivalent to 2-4 mg morphine) 1 to 4 times daily. Paregoric is used in children at a dose of 0.25-0.5 mL/kg (equivalent to 0.1-0.2 mg morphine/kg) 1 to 4 times daily.

Enkephalins are endogenous opioids that are important enteric neurotransmitters; they can inhibit intestinal secretion without affecting motility. *Racecadotril* (acetorphan), a dipeptide inhibitor of enkephalinase, potentiates the effects of endogenous enkephalins on the δ opioid receptor to produce an anti-diarrheal effect.

α_2 ADRENERGIC RECEPTOR AGONISTS. α_2 Adrenergic receptor agonists such as clonidine can interact with specific receptors on enteric neurons and enterocytes, thereby stimulating absorption and inhibiting secretion of fluid and electrolytes and increasing intestinal transit time. These agents may have a special role in diabetics with chronic diarrhea.

Oral clonidine (beginning at 0.1 mg twice a day) has been used in these patients; the use of a topical preparation (e.g., CATAPRES TTS, 2 patches a week) may result in more steady plasma levels of the drug. Clonidine also may be useful in patients with diarrhea caused by opiate withdrawal. Side effects such as hypotension, depression, and perceived fatigue may be dose limiting in susceptible patients.

OCTREOTIDE AND SOMATOSTATIN. Octreotide (SANDOSTATIN, others) (*see* Chapter 43) is an octapeptide analog of somatostatin (SST) that is effective in inhibiting the severe secretory diarrhea brought about by hormone-secreting tumors of the pancreas and the GI tract.

Octreotide inhibits secretion of 5HT and various GI peptides. Its greatest utility may be in the "dumping syndrome" seen in some patients after gastric surgery and pyloroplasty, in whom octreotide inhibits the release of hormones (triggered by rapid passage of food into the small intestine) that are responsible for distressing local and systemic effects. Octreotide has a $t_{1/2}$ of 1-2 h and is administered either subcutaneously or intravenously as a bolus dose. Standard initial therapy with octreotide is 50-100 μg, given subcutaneously 2 or 3 times a day, with titration to a maximum dose of 500 μg 3 times a day based on clinical and biochemical responses. A long-acting preparation of octreotide acetate enclosed in biodegradable microspheres (SANDOSTATIN LAR DEPOT) is available for use in the treatment of diarrheas associated with carcinoid tumors and VIP–secreting tumors, as well as in the treatment of acromegaly (*see* Chapter 38). This preparation is injected intramuscularly once per month in a dose of 20 or 30 mg. Side effects of octreotide depend on the duration of therapy; transient nausea, bloating, or pain at sites of injection in the short term, gallstone formation and hypo- or hyperglycemia in the long term. A long-acting SST analog, lanreotide (SOMATULIN, others), is available in Europe; another, vapreotide, is under development. SST (STILAMIN) also is available in Europe.

Variceal Bleeding. SST and octreotide are effective in reducing hepatic blood flow, hepatic venous wedge pressure, and azygos blood flow. These agents constrict the splanchnic arterioles by a direct action on vascular smooth muscle and by inhibiting the release of peptides contributing to the hyperdynamic circulatory syndrome of portal hypertension. Octreotide also may act through the ANS. Because of its short $t_{1/2}$ (1-2 min), SST can be given only by intravenous infusion (a 250 μg bolus dose followed by 250 μg hourly for 5 days). Higher doses (up to 500 μg/h) are more efficacious and can be used for patients who continue to bleed on the lower dose. For patients with variceal bleeding, therapy with octreotide usually is initiated while the patient is awaiting endoscopy.

Intestinal Dysmotility. Octreotide has complex and apparently conflicting effects on GI motility, including inhibition of antral motor activity and colonic tone. However, octreotide also can rapidly induce phase III activity of the migrating motor complex in the small bowel to produce longer and faster contractions than those occurring spontaneously. Its use has been shown to result in improvement in selected patients with scleroderma and small-bowel dysfunction.

Pancreatitis. Both SST and octreotide inhibit pancreatic secretion and have been used for the prophylaxis and treatment of acute pancreatitis. The rationale for their use is to rest the pancreas so as to not aggravate inflammation by the continuing production of proteolytic enzymes, to reduce intraductal pressures, and to ameliorate pain. Octreotide probably is less effective than SST in this regard because it may cause an increase in sphincter of Oddi pressure and perhaps also have a deleterious effect on pancreatic blood flow.

OTHER AGENTS

Berberine is a plant alkaloid that has complex pharmacological actions that include antimicrobial effects, stimulation of bile flow, inhibition of ventricular tachyarrhythmias, and possible antineoplastic activity. It is used most commonly in bacterial diarrhea and cholera, but is also apparently effective against intestinal parasites. The anti-diarrheal effects in part may be related to its antimicrobial activity, as well as its ability to inhibit smooth muscle contraction and delay intestinal transit by antagonizing the effects of ACh (by competitive and noncompetitive mechanisms) and blocking the entry of Ca^{2+} into cells. In addition, it inhibits intestinal secretion.

IRRITABLE BOWEL SYNDROME (IBS)

IBS affects up to 15% of the population in the U.S. Patients may complain of a variety of symptoms, the most characteristic of which is recurrent abdominal pain associated with altered bowel movements. IBS appears to result from a varying combination of disturbances in visceral motor and sensory function, often associated with significant affective disorders. The disturbances in bowel function can be either constipation or diarrhea or both at different times. Considerable evidence suggests a specific enhancement of visceral (as opposed to somatic) sensitivity to noxious, as well as physiological stimuli in this syndrome.

Many patients can be managed with dietary restrictions and fiber supplementation; many cannot. Treatment of bowel symptoms (either diarrhea or constipation) is predominantly symptomatic and nonspecific using agents discussed above. A possible role for serotonin in IBS has been suggested based on its known involvement in sensitization of nociceptor neurons in inflammatory conditions. This has led to the development of specific receptor modulators, such as the $5HT_3$ antagonist *alosetron* (*see* Figure 46–2).

An effective class of agents for IBS has been the tricyclic antidepressants (*see* Chapter 15), which can have neuromodulatory and analgesic properties independent of their antidepressant effect. Tricyclic antidepressants have a proven track record in the management of chronic "functional" visceral pain. Effective analgesic doses of these drugs (e.g., 25-75 mg per day of nortriptyline) are significantly lower than those required to treat depression. Although changes in mood usually do not occur at these doses, there may be some diminution of anxiety and restoration of sleep patterns. Selective serotonin reuptake inhibitors have fewer side effects and have been advocated particularly for patients with functional constipation because they can increase bowel movements and even cause diarrhea. However, they probably are not as effective as tricyclic antidepressants in the management of visceral pain.

α_2 Adrenergic agonists, such as clonidine (*see* Chapter 12), also can increase visceral compliance and reduce distention-induced pain. The SST analog octreotide has selective inhibitory effects on peripheral afferent nerves projecting from the gut to the spinal cord in healthy human beings and has been shown to blunt the perception of rectal distention in patients with IBS.

ALOSETRON, $5HT_3$ ANTAGONIST

The $5HT_3$ receptor participates in sensitization of spinal sensory neurons, vagal signaling of nausea, and peristaltic reflexes. The clinical effect of $5HT_3$ antagonism is a general reduction in GI contractility with decreased colonic transit, along with an increase in fluid absorption. Alosetron (LOTRONEX), a potent antagonist of the $5HT_3$ receptor, was initially withdrawn from the U.S. market because of an unusually high incidence of ischemic colitis (up to 3 per 1000 patients), leading to surgery and even death in a small number of cases. Nevertheless, the FDA has reapproved this drug for diarrhea-predominant IBS under a limited distribution system. The manufacturer requires a prescription program that includes physician certification and an elaborate patient education and consent protocol before dispensing. Alosetron is rapidly absorbed from the GI tract; its duration of action (~10 h) is longer than expected from its $t_{1/2}$ of 1.5 h. It is metabolized by hepatic CYPs. The drug should be started at 1 mg per day for the first 4 weeks and advanced to a maximum of 1 mg twice daily. Other $5HT_3$ antagonists currently available in the U.S. are approved for nausea and vomiting (*see* later in this chapter and Chapter 13).

ANTI-SPASMODICS AND OTHER AGENTS

Anticholinergic agents ("spasmolytics" or "anti-spasmodics") often are used in patients with IBS. The most common agents of this class available in the U.S. are nonspecific antagonists of the muscarinic receptor (*see* Chapter 9) and include the tertiary amines *dicyclomine* (BENTYL, others) and *hyoscyamine* (LEVSIN, others) and the quaternary ammonium compounds *glycopyrrolate* (ROBINUL, others) and *methscopolamine* (PAMINE, others). The advantage of the latter 2 compounds is that they have a limited propensity to cross the blood-brain barrier and hence a lower risk for neurological side effects such as lightheadedness, drowsiness, or nervousness. These agents typically are given either on an as-needed basis or before meals to prevent the pain and fecal urgency that occur in some patients with IBS.

Dicyclomine is given in doses of 20 mg orally every 6 h initially and increased to 40 mg every 6 h unless limited by side effects. Hyoscyamine is available as immediate-release oral capsules, tablets, elixir, drops, and a nonaerosol spray (all administered as 0.125-0.25 mg every 4 h as needed), and extended-release forms for oral use (0.25-0.375 mg every 12 h as needed). Glycopyrrolate is available as immediate-release tablets; the dose is 1-2 mg 2 or 3 times daily, not to exceed 8 mg/day. Methscopolamine is provided as 2.5-mg and 5-mg tablets; the dose is 2.5 mg a half hour before meals and 2.5-5 mg at bedtime.

OTHER DRUGS. *Cimetropium*, an antimuscarinic compound that is effective in patients with IBS, is not available in the U.S. *Otilonium* bromide is a quaternary ammonium salt with antimuscarinic effects that also appears to block Ca^{2+} channels and neurokinin NK_2 receptors; it is not available in the U.S. *Mebeverine* hydrochloride, a derivative of hydroxybenzamide, appears to have a direct effect on the smooth muscle cell, blocking K^+, Na^+, and Ca^{2+} channels, and is used outside of the U.S. as an anti-spasmodic agent.

ANTI-NAUSEANTS AND ANTI-EMETICS

NAUSEA AND VOMITING

Emesis and the sensation of nausea that accompanies it generally are viewed as protective reflexes that serve to rid the stomach and intestine of toxic substances and prevent their further ingestion. Vomiting is a complex process that appears to be coordinated by a central emesis center in the lateral reticular formation of the mid-brainstem adjacent to both the chemoreceptor trigger zone (CTZ) in the area postrema (AP) at the bottom of the fourth ventricle and the solitary tract nucleus (STN). The lack of a blood-brain barrier allows the CTZ to monitor blood and cerebrospinal fluid constantly for toxic substances and to relay information to the emesis center to trigger nausea and vomiting. The emesis center also receives information from the gut, principally by the vagus nerve (via the STN) but also by splanchnic afferents via the spinal cord. Two other important inputs to the emesis center come from the cerebral cortex (particularly in anticipatory nausea or vomiting) and the vestibular apparatus (in motion sickness). The CTZ has high concentrations of receptors for serotonin ($5HT_3$), dopamine (D_2), and opioids; the STN is rich in receptors for enkephalin, histamine, and ACh, and also contains $5HT_3$ receptors. A variety of these neurotransmitters are involved in nausea and vomiting (Figure 46–4). Anti-emetics generally are classified according to the predominant receptor on which they are proposed to act (Table 46–4). For treatment and prevention of the nausea and emesis associated with cancer chemotherapy, several anti-emetic agents from different pharmacological classes may be used in combination (Table 46–5).

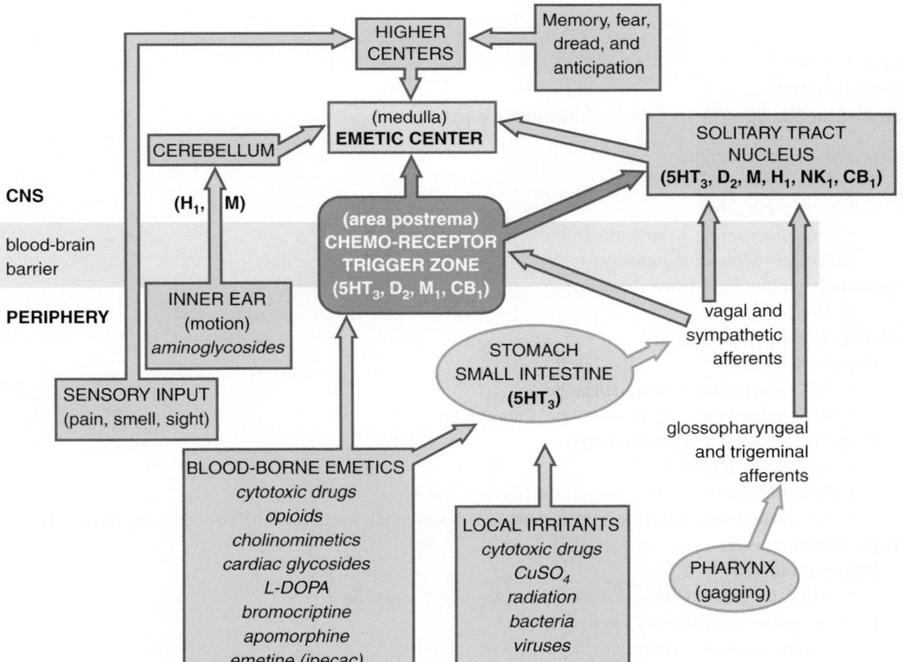

Figure 46–4 *Pharmacologist's view of emetic stimuli.* Myriad signaling pathways lead from the periphery to the emetic center. Stimulants of these pathways are noted in *italics*. These pathways involve specific neurotransmitters and their receptors (**bold** type). Receptors are shown for dopamine (D_2), acetylcholine (muscarinic, M), histamine (H_1), cannabinoids (CB_1), substance P (NK_1), and 5-hydroxytryptamine ($5HT_3$). Some of these receptors also may mediate signaling in the emetic center.

Table 46–4

General Classification of Anti-emetic Agents

ANTI-EMETIC CLASS	EXAMPLES	TYPE OF VOMITING MOST EFFECTIVE AGAINST
$5HT_3$ receptor antagonists[a]	Ondansetron	Cytotoxic drug-induced emesis
Centrally acting dopamine receptor antagonists	Metoclopramide[b] Promethazine[c]	Cytotoxic drug-induced emesis
Histamine H_1 receptor antagonists	Cyclizine	Vestibular (motion sickness)
Muscarinic receptor antagonists	Hyoscine (scopolamine)	Motion sickness
Neurokinin receptor antagonists	Aprepitant	Cytotoxic drug-induced emesis (delayed vomiting)
Cannabinoid receptor agonists	Dronabinol, nabilone	Cytotoxic drug-induced emesis

[a]*The most effective agents for chemotherapy-induced nausea and vomiting are the $5HT_3$ antagonists and metoclopramide. In addition to their use as single agents, they are often combined with other drugs to improve efficacy as well as reduce the incidence of side effects. See Table 46–5.*
[b]*Also has some peripheral activity at $5HT_3$ receptors.*
[c]*Also has some antihistaminic and anticholinergic activity.*

$5HT_3$ RECEPTOR ANTAGONISTS

Ondansetron (ZOFRAN, others) is the prototypical drug in this class. The $5HT_3$ receptor antagonists (Table 46–6) are the most widely used drugs for chemotherapy-induced emesis. Other agents in this class include granisetron (KYTRIL, others), dolasetron (ANZEMET), palonosetron (ALOXI), and tropisetron (not available in the U.S.).

Table 46–5

Anti-emetic Agents in Cancer Chemotherapy[a]

Low risk of emesis:
- Pre-chemotherapy
  - Dexamethasone
  - Metoclopramide ± diphenhydramine
  - Prochlorperazine ± lorazepam
- Post-chemotherapy (delayed emesis)
  - None

Moderate risk of emesis:
- Pre-chemotherapy
  - $5HT_3$ antagonist + dexamethasone
  - $5HT_3$ antagonist + dexamethasone + aprepitant
- Post-chemotherapy (delayed emesis)
  - Aprepitant (days 2 and 3)
  - Dexamethasone or $5HT_3$ antagonist (days 2-3 or 4)
  - Aprepitant (days 2-3, if used pre-chemo) ± dexamethasone (days 2-4) ± lorazepam (days 2-4)

High risk of emesis:
- Pre-chemotherapy
  - $5HT_3$ antagonist + dexamethasone + aprepitant ± lorazepam
- Post-chemotherapy (delayed emesis)
  - Dexamethasone + aprepitant
  - Dexamethasone (days 2-4) + aprepitant (days 2 and 3) ± lorazepam (days 2-4)

H, histamine; NK, neurokinin; 5HT, 5 hydroxytryptamine (serotonin).
[a]*Specific recommendations and doses are tailored to the patient and the chemotherapeutic regimen. For updated information, see the National Cancer Institute website (see Cancer Topics: Nausea and Vomiting).*
Some patients profit from cannabinoids (dronabinol, nabilone) ± a phenothiazine or dexamethasone. Ginger powder (Zingiber officinale) is being evaluated as an anti-emetic.

Table 46–6

$5HT_3$ Antagonists in Chemotherapy-Induced Nausea/Emesis

DRUG	CHEMICAL NATURE	RECEPTOR INTERACTIONS	$t_{1/2}$	DOSE (IV)
Ondansetron	Carbazole derivative	$5HT_3$ antagonist and weak $5HT_4$ antagonist	3.9 h	0.15 mg/kg
Granisetron	Indazole	$5HT_3$ antagonist	9-11.6 h	10 μg/kg
Dolasetron	Indole moiety	$5HT_3$ antagonist	7-9 h	1.8 mg/kg
Palonosetron	Isoquinoline	$5HT_3$ antagonist; highest affinity for $5HT_3$ receptor in this class	40 h	0.25 mg

IV, intravenous.

$5HT_3$ receptors are present in several critical sites involved in emesis, including vagal afferents, the STN (which receives signals from vagal afferents), and the AP itself (*see* Figure 46–4). Serotonin is released by the enterochromaffin cells of the small intestine in response to chemotherapeutic agents and may stimulate vagal afferents (via $5HT_3$ receptors) to initiate the vomiting reflex. The highest concentrations of $5HT_3$ receptors in the CNS are found in the STN and CTZ, and antagonists of $5HT_3$ receptors also may suppress nausea and vomiting by acting at these sites.

ADME. These agents are absorbed well from the GI tract. Ondansetron is extensively metabolized in the liver by CYP1A2, CYP2D6, and CYP3A4, followed by glucuronide or sulfate conjugation. Patients with hepatic dysfunction have reduced plasma clearance, and some adjustment in the dosage is advisable. Granisetron also is metabolized predominantly by the liver by the CYP3A family. Dolasetron is converted rapidly by plasma carbonyl reductase to its active metabolite, hydrodolasetron. A portion of this compound then undergoes subsequent biotransformation by CYP2D6 and CYP3A4 in the liver while about one-third of it is excreted unchanged in the urine. Palonosetron is metabolized principally by CYP2D6 and excreted in the urine as the metabolized and the unchanged forms in about equal proportions. The anti-emetic effects of these drugs persist long after they disappear from the circulation, suggesting their continuing interaction at the receptor level; these drugs can be administered effectively just once a day.

Therapeutic Use. These agents are most effective in treating chemotherapy-induced nausea and in treating nausea secondary to upper abdominal irradiation. They also are effective against hyperemesis of pregnancy, and to a lesser degree, postoperative nausea, but not against motion sickness. Unlike other agents in this class, palonosetron may be helpful in delayed emesis, perhaps reflecting its long $t_{1/2}$. These agents are available as tablets, oral solution, and intravenous preparations for injection. For patients on cancer chemotherapy, these drugs can be given in a single intravenous dose (*see* Table 46–6) infused over 15 min, beginning 30 min before chemotherapy, or in 2-3 divided doses, with the first usually given 30 min before and subsequent doses at various intervals after chemotherapy. The drugs also can be used intramuscularly (ondansetron only) or orally. Granisetron is available as a transdermal formulation that is applied 24-48 h before chemotherapy and worn for up to 7 days.

Adverse Effects. In general, these drugs are very well tolerated, with the most common adverse effects being constipation or diarrhea, headache, and lightheadedness.

DOPAMINE RECEPTOR ANTAGONISTS

Phenothiazines such as prochlorperazine, thiethylperazine (discontinued in the U.S.), and chlorpromazine (*see* Chapter 16) are among the most commonly used "general-purpose" anti-nauseants and anti-emetics. Their principal mechanism of action is D_2 receptor antagonism at the CTZ. These drugs are not uniformly effective in cancer chemotherapy-induced emesis but they possess antihistaminic and anticholinergic activities that are of value in other forms of nausea, such as motion sickness.

ANTIHISTAMINES

Histamine H_1 antagonists are primarily useful for motion sickness and postoperative emesis. They act on vestibular afferents and within the brainstem. *Cyclizine*, *hydroxyzine*, *promethazine*, and *diphenhydramine* are examples of this class of agents. Cyclizine has additional anticholinergic effects that may be useful for patients with abdominal cancer. For a detailed discussion of these drugs, *see* Chapter 32.

ANTICHOLINERGIC AGENTS

The most commonly used muscarinic receptor antagonist is *scopolamine* (hyoscine), which can be injected as the hydrobromide, but usually is administered as the free base in the form of a transdermal patch (TRANSDERM-SCOP).

Its principal utility is in the prevention and treatment of motion sickness, with some activity in postoperative nausea and vomiting. In general, however, anticholinergic agents have no role in chemotherapy-induced nausea.

SUBSTANCE P RECEPTOR ANTAGONISTS

The nausea and vomiting associated with cisplatin (*see* Chapter 61) have 2 components: an acute phase that universally is experienced (within 24 h after chemotherapy) and a delayed phase that affects only some patients (on days 2-5). $5HT_3$ receptor antagonists are not very effective against delayed emesis. Antagonists of the NK_1 receptors for substance P, such as *aprepitant* (and its parenteral formulation, fosaprepitant; EMEND), have anti-emetic effects in delayed nausea and improve the efficacy of standard anti-emetic regimens in patients receiving multiple cycles of chemotherapy.

After absorption, aprepitant is bound extensively to plasma proteins (>95%); it is metabolized primarily by hepatic CYP3A4, and is excreted in the stools; its $t_{1/2}$ is 9-13 h. Aprepitant has the potential to interact with other substrates of CYP3A4, requiring adjustment of other drugs, including dexamethasone, methylprednisolone (whose dose may need to be reduced by 50%), and warfarin. Aprepitant is contraindicated in patients on cisapride or pimozide, in whom life-threatening QT prolongation has been reported. Aprepitant is supplied in 40-, 80- and 125-mg capsules and is administered for 3 days in conjunction with highly emetogenic chemotherapy, along with a $5HT_3$ antagonist and a corticosteroid. The recommended adult dosage of aprepitant is 125 mg administered 1 h before chemotherapy on day 1, followed by 80 mg once daily in the morning on days 2 and 3 of the treatment regimen.

CANNABINOIDS

Dronabinol (Δ-9-tetrahydrocannabinol; MARINOL) is a naturally occurring cannabinoid that can be synthesized chemically or extracted from the marijuana plant, *Cannabis sativa*. The exact mechanism of the anti-emetic action of dronabinol is not known but probably relates to stimulation of the CB_1 subtype of cannabinoid receptors on neurons in and around the CTZ and emetic center (*see* Figure 46–4).

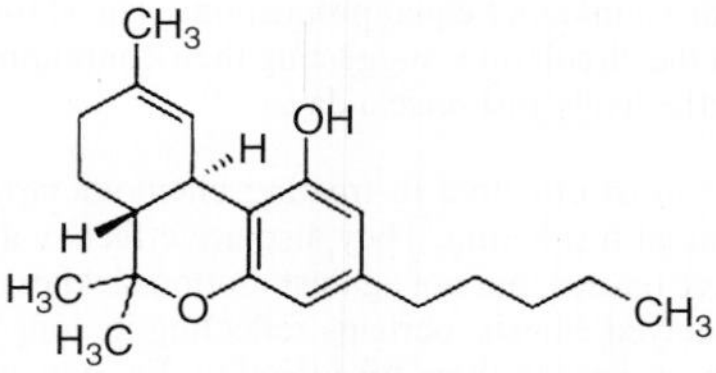

CH_3 OH H H H_3C H_3C O CH_3

DRONABINOL

ADME. Dronabinol is a highly lipid-soluble compound that is absorbed readily after oral administration; its onset of action occurs within an hour, and peak levels are achieved within 2-4 h. It undergoes extensive first-pass metabolism with limited systemic bioavailability after single doses (only 10-20%). The principal active metabolite is 11-OH-delta-9-tetrahydrocannabinol. These metabolites are excreted primarily via the biliary-fecal route, with only 10-15% excreted in the urine. Both dronabinol and its metabolites are highly bound (>95%) to plasma proteins. Because of its large volume of distribution, a single dose of dronabinol can result in detectable levels of metabolites for several weeks.

Therapeutic Use. Dronabinol is a useful prophylactic agent in patients receiving cancer chemotherapy when other anti-emetic medications are not effective. It also can stimulate appetite and has been used in patients with acquired immunodeficiency syndrome (AIDS) and anorexia. As an anti-emetic agent, it is administered at an initial dose of 5 mg/m^2 given 1-3 h before chemotherapy and then every 2-4 h afterward for a total of 4 to 6 doses. If this is inadequate, incremental increases can be made up to a maximum of 15 mg/m^2 per dose. For other indications, the usual starting dose is 2.5 mg twice a day; this can be titrated up to a maximum of 20 mg per day.

Adverse Effects. Dronabinol has complex effects on the CNS, including a prominent central sympathomimetic activity. This can lead to palpitations, tachycardia, vasodilation, hypotension, and conjunctival injection (bloodshot eyes). Patient supervision is necessary because marijuana-like "highs" (e.g., euphoria, somnolence, detachment, dizziness, anxiety, nervousness, panic, etc.) can occur, as can more disturbing effects such as paranoid reactions and thinking abnormalities. After abrupt withdrawal of dronabinol, an abstinence syndrome (irritability, insomnia, and restlessness) can occur. Because of its high affinity for plasma proteins, dronabinol can displace other plasma protein-bound drugs, whose doses may have to be adjusted as a consequence. Dronabinol should be prescribed with great caution to persons with a history of substance abuse (alcohol, drugs) because it, too, may be abused by these patients.

Nabilone (CESAMET) is a synthetic cannabinoid with a mode of action similar to that of dronabinol.

ADME. Nabilone is a highly lipid-soluble compound that is rapidly absorbed after oral administration; its onset of action occurs within an hour, and peak levels are achieved within 2 h. The $t_{1/2}$ is ~2 h for the parent compound and 35 h for metabolites. The metabolites are excreted primarily via the biliary-fecal route (60%), with only ~25% excreted in the urine.

Therapeutic Use. Nabilone is a useful prophylactic agent in patients receiving cancer chemotherapy when other anti-emetic medications are not effective. A dose (1-2 mg) can be given the night before chemotherapy; usual dosing starts 1-3 h before treatment and then every 8-12 h during the course of chemotherapy and for 2 days following its cessation.

Adverse Effects. The adverse effects are largely the same as for dronabinol, with significant CNS actions in >10% of patients. Cardiovascular, GI, and other side effects are also common and together with the CNS actions limit the usefulness of this agent.

GLUCOCORTICOIDS AND ANTI-INFLAMMATORY AGENTS

Glucocorticoids such as dexamethasone can be useful adjuncts (*see* Table 46–5) in the treatment of nausea in patients with widespread cancer, possibly by suppressing peritumoral inflammation and prostaglandin production. A similar mechanism has been invoked to explain beneficial effects of NSAIDs in the nausea and vomiting induced by systemic irradiation. For a detailed discussion of these drugs, *see* Chapters 34 and 42.

BENZODIAZEPINES

Benzodiazepines, such as lorazepam and alprazolam, by themselves are not very effective anti-emetics, but their sedative, amnesic, and antianxiety effects can be helpful in reducing the anticipatory component of nausea and vomiting in patients. For a detailed discussion of these drugs, *see* Chapter 17.

PHOSPHORATED CARBOHYDRATE SOLUTIONS

Aqueous solutions of glucose, fructose, and phosphoric acid (EMETROL, NAUSETROL) are available over the counter to relieve nausea. Their mechanisms of action are unclear.

MISCELLANEOUS GI DISORDERS

CHRONIC PANCREATITIS AND STEATORRHEA

PANCREATIC ENZYMES. Chronic pancreatitis is a debilitating syndrome that results in symptoms from loss of glandular function (exocrine and endocrine) and inflammation (pain). The goals of pharmacological therapy are prevention of malabsorption and palliation of pain.

Enzyme Formulations. Pancreatic enzymes are typically prescribed on the basis of the lipase content. Only pancrelipase (CREON, ZENPEP, PANCREAZE, PERTZYE) is licensed for sale in the U.S. Pancrelipase products contain various amounts of lipase, protease, and amylase and thus may not be interchangeable.

Replacement Therapy for Malabsorption. Fat malabsorption (steatorrhea) and protein maldigestion occur when the pancreas loses >90% of its ability to produce digestive enzymes. The resultant diarrhea and malabsorption can be managed well if 30,000 USP units of pancreatic lipase are delivered to the duodenum during a 4-h period with and after meals. Alternatively, one can titrate the dosage to the fat content of the diet, with ~8000 USP units of lipase activity required for each 17 g of dietary fat. Available preparations of pancreatic enzymes contain up to 20,000 units of lipase and 76,000 units of protease, and the typical dose of pancrelipase is 1-3 capsules with or just before meals. The loss of pancreatic amylase does not present a problem because of other sources of this enzyme (e.g., salivary glands).

Enzymes for Pain. Pain is the other cardinal symptom of chronic pancreatitis. The rationale for its treatment with pancreatic enzymes is based on the principle of negative feedback inhibition of the pancreas by the presence of duodenal proteases. The release of CCK, the principal secretagogue for pancreatic enzymes, is triggered by CCK-releasing monitor peptide in the duodenum, which normally is denatured by pancreatic trypsin. In chronic pancreatitis, trypsin insufficiency leads to persistent activation of this peptide and an increased release of CCK, which is thought to cause pancreatic pain because of continuous stimulation of pancreatic enzyme output and increased intraductal pressure. Delivery of active proteases to the duodenum (which can be done reliably only with uncoated preparations) therefore is important for the interruption of this loop. Although enzymatic therapy has become firmly entrenched for the treatment of painful pancreatitis, the evidence supporting this practice is equivocal at best.

Pancreatic enzyme preparations are tolerated extremely well by patients. Hyperuricosuria in patients with cystic fibrosis can occur, and malabsorption of folate and iron has been reported.

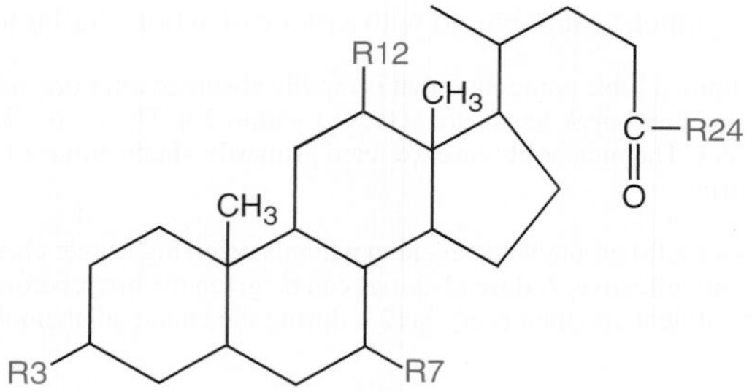

Bile Acid	R3	R7	R12	R24
Cholic acid	–OH	–OH	–OH	
Chenodeoxycholic acid	–OH	–OH	–H	glycine (75%)
Deoxycholic acid	–OH	–H	–OH	taurine (24%)
Lithocholic acid	$-SO_2^-$ / –OH	–H	–H	–OH (<1%)
Ursodeoxycholic acid	–OH	–OH	–H	

Figure 46–5 *Major bile acids in adults.*

BILE ACIDS

Bile acids and their conjugates are synthesized from cholesterol in the liver. Bile acids induce bile flow, feed-back-inhibit cholesterol synthesis, promote intestinal excretion of cholesterol, and facilitate the dispersion and absorption of lipids and fat-soluble vitamins. After secretion into the biliary tract, bile acids are largely (95%) reabsorbed in the intestine, returned to the liver, and then again secreted in bile (enterohepatic circulation). Cholic acid, chenodeoxycholic acid, and deoxycholic acid constitute 95% of bile acids; lithocholic acid and ursodeoxycholic acid are minor constituents. The bile acids exist largely as glycine and taurine conjugates, the salts of which are called *bile salts*. Ursodeoxycholic acid (UDCA; ursodiol, ACTIGALL, others) (Figure 46–5) is a hydrophilic, dehydroxylated bile acid that is formed by epimerization of the bile acid chenodeoxycholic acid (CDCA; chenodiol) in the gut by intestinal bacteria. When administered orally, litholytic bile acids such as chenodiol and ursodiol alter relative concentrations of bile acids, decrease biliary lipid secretion and reduce the cholesterol content of the bile so that it is less lithogenic. Ursodiol also may have cytoprotective effects on hepatocytes and effects on the immune system that account for some of its beneficial effects in cholestatic liver diseases.

FLATULENCE

"Gas" is a common but relatively vague GI complaint, used in reference not only to flatulence and eructation but also bloating or fullness. Over-the-counter and herbal preparations are popular. *Simethicone* (MYLICON, GAS-X, others), a mixture of siloxane polymers stabilized with silicon dioxide, is an inert non-toxic insoluble liquid. Because of its capacity to collapse bubbles by forming a thin layer on their surface, it is an effective anti-foaming agent; whether this accomplishes a therapeutic effect in the GI tract is not clear. Simethicone is available in chewable tablets, liquid-filled capsules, suspensions, and orally disintegrating strips, either by itself or in combination with other over-the-counter medications including antacids and other digestants. The usual dosage in adults is 40-25 mg 4 times daily. Activated charcoal may be used alone or in combination with simethicone, but has not been shown conclusively to have much benefit. An alpha-galactosidase preparation (BEANO) is available over the counter to reduce gas from baked beans.

SHORT BOWEL SYNDROME

GLP-2 RECEPTOR AGONIST

Teduglutide (GATTEX) is a 33-amino acid GLP-2 analog approved for the treatment of short-bowel syndrome. Teduglutide injection is administered by subcutaneously once daily to help improve intestinal absorption of nutrients to reduce the need of parenteral support. Common side effects include abdominal pain, nausea, headache, and flu-like symptoms. Teduglutide may cause serious side effects including cancer of the bowel, blockage of the bowel, and inflammation of the gallbladder or pancreas. Teduglutide has orphan drug status.

For a complete Bibliographical Listing see Goodman & Gilman's ***The Pharmacological Basis of Therapeutics***, 12th ed., or Goodman & Gilman Online at www.AccessMedicine.com.

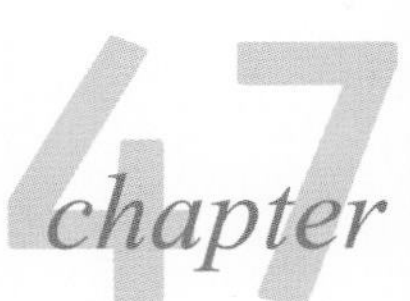

Pharmacotherapy of Inflammatory Bowel Disease

Inflammatory bowel disease (IBD) is a spectrum of chronic, idiopathic, inflammatory intestinal conditions. IBD causes significant gastrointestinal (GI) symptoms that include diarrhea, abdominal pain, bleeding, anemia, and weight loss. IBD conventionally is divided into 2 major subtypes: ulcerative colitis and Crohn disease. *Ulcerative colitis* is characterized by confluent mucosal inflammation of the colon starting at the anal verge and extending proximally for a variable extent (e.g., proctitis, left-sided colitis, or pancolitis). *Crohn disease*, by contrast, is characterized by transmural inflammation of any part of the GI tract but most commonly the area adjacent to the ileocecal valve. The inflammation in Crohn disease is not necessarily confluent, frequently leaving "skip areas" of relatively normal mucosa. The transmural nature of the inflammation may lead to fibrosis and strictures or fistula formation.

PATHOGENESIS OF IBD. Crohn disease and ulcerative colitis are chronic idiopathic inflammatory disorders of the GI tract; a summary of proposed pathogenic events and potential sites of therapeutic intervention is shown in Figure 47–1. Crohn disease and ulcerative colitis result from distinct pathogenetic mechanisms. Histologically, the transmural lesions in Crohn disease exhibit marked infiltration of lymphocytes and macrophages, granuloma formation, and submucosal fibrosis, whereas the superficial lesions in ulcerative colitis have lymphocytic and neutrophilic infiltrates. Within the diseased bowel in Crohn disease, the cytokine profile includes increased levels of interleukin (IL)-12, IL-23, interferon-γ, and tumor necrosis factor-α (TNFα), findings characteristic of T-helper 1 (T_H1)–mediated inflammatory processes. In contrast, the inflammatory response in ulcerative colitis resembles aspects of that mediated by the T_H2 pathway. Understanding of the inflammatory processes has evolved with the description of regulatory T cells and pro-inflammatory T_H17 cells, a novel T-cell population that expresses IL-23 receptor as a surface marker and produces, among others, the pro-inflammatory cytokines IL-17, IL-21, IL-22, and IL-26. T_H17 cells seem to play a prominent role in intestinal inflammation, particularly in Crohn disease.

PHARMACOTHERAPY FOR IBD. Medical therapy for IBD is problematic. Because no unique abnormality has been identified, therapy for IBD seeks to dampen the generalized inflammatory response. Regrettably, no agent can reliably accomplish this, and the response of an individual patient to a given medicine may be limited and unpredictable. Specific goals of pharmacotherapy in IBD include controlling acute exacerbations of the disease, maintaining remission, and treating specific complications such as fistulas. The major therapeutic options are considered below and summarized at chapter's end by Table 47–1.

MESALAMINE (5-ASA)-BASED THERAPY

First-line therapy for mild to moderate ulcerative colitis generally involves *mesalamine* (5-aminosalicylic acid, or 5-ASA). The archetype for this class of medications is sulfasalazine (AZULFIDINE), which consists of *5-ASA* linked to *sulfapyridine* by an azo bond (Figure 47–2).

MECHANISM OF ACTION AND PHARMACOLOGICAL PROPERTIES. Sulfasalazine is an oral prodrug that effectively delivers 5-ASA to the distal GI tract. The azo linkage in sulfasalazine prevents absorption in the stomach and small intestine, and the individual components are not liberated for absorption until colonic bacteria cleave the bond. 5-ASA is the therapeutic moiety, with little, if any, contribution by sulfapyridine. Although 5-ASA is a salicylate, its therapeutic effect does not appear to be related to cyclooxygenase inhibition; indeed, traditional nonsteroidal anti-inflammatory drugs may exacerbate IBD. Many potential sites of action (effects on immune function and inflammation) have been demonstrated in vitro for either sulfasalazine or mesalamine (inhibition of the production of IL-1 and TNFα, inhibition of the lipoxygenase pathway, scavenging of free radicals and oxidants, and inhibition of NF-κB, a transcription factor pivotal to production of inflammatory mediators), however, specific mechanisms of action have not been identified.

Although not active therapeutically, sulfapyridine causes many of the adverse effects observed in patients taking sulfasalazine. To preserve the therapeutic effect of 5-ASA without the adverse effects of sulfapyridine, several second-generation 5-ASA compounds have been developed (Figures 47–2, 47–3, and 47–4). They

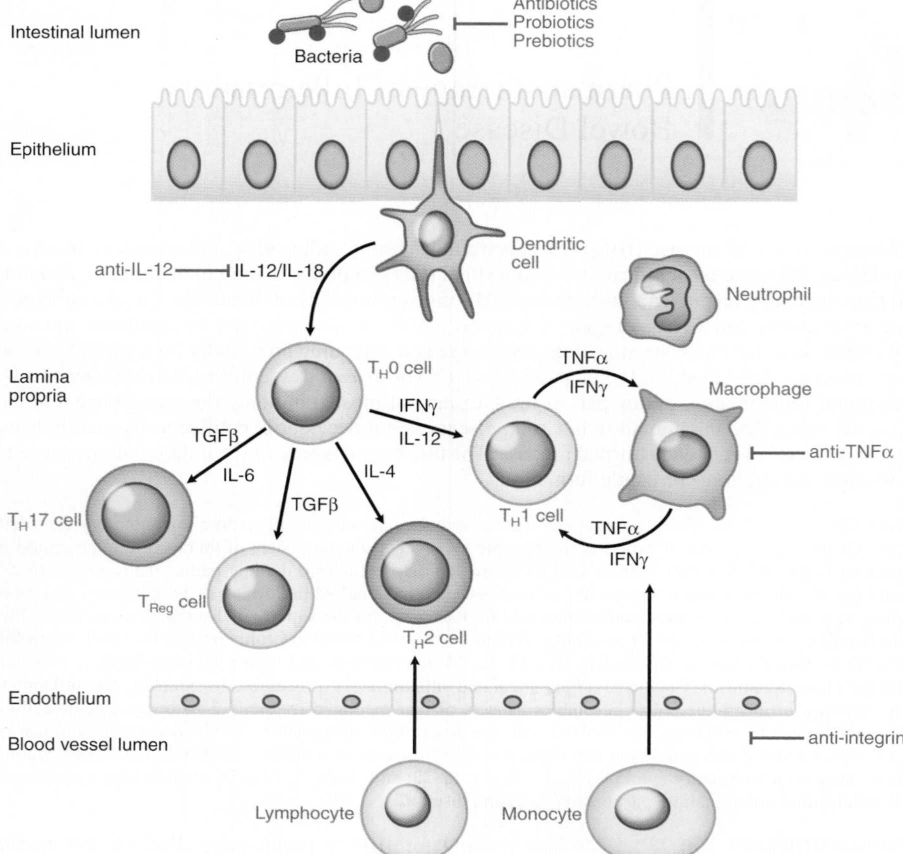

Figure 47–1 *Proposed pathogenesis of inflammatory bowel disease and target sites for pharmacological intervention.* Shown are the interactions among bacterial antigens in the intestinal lumen and immune cells in the intestinal wall. If the epithelial barrier is impaired, bacterial antigens can gain access to antigen-presenting cells (APC) such as dendritic cells in the lamina propria. These cells then present the antigen(s) to $CD4^+$ lymphocytes and also secrete cytokines such interleukin (IL)-12 and IL-18, thereby inducing the differentiation of T_H1 cells in Crohn's disease (or, under the control of IL-4, type 2 helper T cells [T_H2] in ulcerative colitis). The balance of pro-inflammatory and anti-inflammatory events is also governed by regulatory T_H17 and T_{Reg} cells, both of which serve to limit immune and inflammatory responses in the GI tract. Transforming growth factor (TGF)β and IL-6 are important cytokines that drive the expansion of the regulatory T cell subsets. The T_H1 cells produce a characteristic array of cytokines, including interferon (IFN)γ and TNFα, which in turn activate macrophages. Macrophages positively regulate T_H1 cells by secreting additional cytokines, including IFNγ and TNFα. Recruitment of a variety of leukocytes is mediated by activation of resident immune cells including neutrophils. Cell adhesion molecules such as integrins are important in the infiltration of leukocytes and novel biological therapeutic strategies aimed at blocking leukocyte recruitment are effective at reducing inflammation. General immunosuppressants (e.g., glucocorticoids, thioguanine derivatives, methotrexate, and cyclosporine) affect multiple sites of inflammation. More site-specific intervention involve intestinal bacteria (antibiotics, prebiotics, and probiotics) and therapy directed at TNFα or IL-12.

are divided into 2 groups: *prodrugs* and *coated drugs*. Prodrugs contain the same azo bond as sulfasalazine but replace the linked sulfapyridine with either another 5-ASA (*olsalazine*, DIPENTUM) or an inert compound (*balsalazide*, COLAZIDE). The alternative approaches employ either a delayed-release formulation (PENTASA) or a pH-sensitive coating (ASACOL; LIALDA/MEZAVANT). Delayed-release mesalamine is released throughout the small intestine and colon, whereas pH-sensitive mesalamine is released in the terminal ileum and colon. These different distributions of drug delivery have potential therapeutic implications.

Oral sulfasalazine is effective in patients with mild or moderately active ulcerative colitis, with response rates of 60-80%. The usual dose is 4 g/day in 4 divided doses with food; to avoid adverse effects, the dose

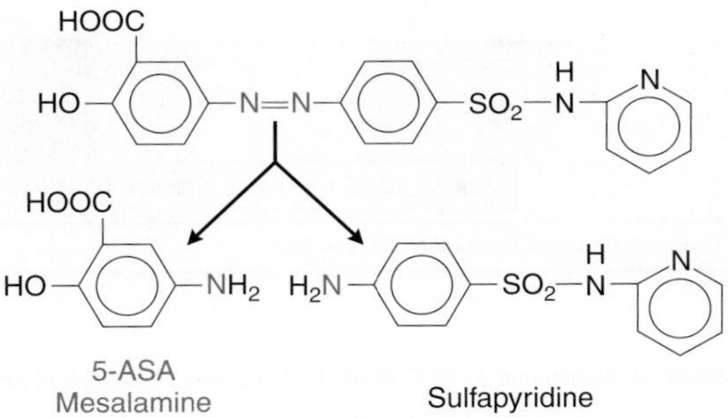

Sulfasalazine

5-ASA
Mesalamine

Sulfapyridine

Figure 47–2 *Generation of mesalamine from the prodrug sulfasalazine.* The *red* N atoms indicate the diazo linkage that is cleaved in the colon to generate the active moiety.

is increased gradually from an initial dose of 500 mg twice a day. Doses as high as 6 g/day can be used but cause an increased incidence of side effects. For patients with severe colitis, sulfasalazine is of less certain value, even though it is often added as an adjunct to systemic glucocorticoids. The drug plays a useful role in preventing relapses once remission has been achieved. Because they lack the dose-related side effects of sulfapyridine, the newer formulations can be used to provide higher doses of mesalamine with some improvement in disease control. The usual doses to treat active disease are 800 mg 3 times a day for ASACOL and 1 g 4 times a day for PENTASA. Lower doses are used for maintenance (e.g., ASACOL, 800 mg twice a day). The efficacy of 5-ASA preparations (e.g., sulfasalazine) in Crohn disease is less striking, with modest benefit at best in controlled trials. The second-generation 5-ASA prodrugs (e.g., olsalazine and balsalazide) do not have a significant effect in small-bowel Crohn disease.

Topical preparations of mesalamine suspended in a wax matrix suppository (ROWASA) or in a suspension enema (CANASA) are effective in active proctitis and distal ulcerative colitis, respectively. They appear to be superior to topical hydrocortisone in this setting, with response rates of 75-90%. Mesalamine enemas (4 g/60 mL) should be used at bedtime and retained for at least 8 h; the suppository (500 mg) should be used 2 to 3 times a day with the objective of retaining it for at least 3 h. Response to local therapy with mesalamine may occur within 3-21 days; however, the usual course of therapy is from 3-6 weeks. Once remission has occurred, lower doses are used for maintenance.

ADME. About 20-30% of orally administered sulfasalazine is absorbed in the small intestine. Much of this is taken up by the liver and excreted unmetabolized in the bile; the rest (~10%) is excreted unchanged in the urine. The remaining 70% reaches the colon, where, if cleaved completely by bacterial enzymes, it generates 400 mg mesalamine for every gram of the parent compound. Thereafter, the individual components of sulfasalazine follow different metabolic pathways. Sulfapyridine is absorbed rapidly from the colon. It undergoes extensive hepatic metabolism, including acetylation and hydroxylation, conjugation with glucuronic acid, and excretion in the urine. The acetylation phenotype of the patient determines plasma levels of sulfapyridine and the probability of side effects; rapid acetylators have lower systemic levels of the drug and fewer adverse effects. Only 25% of mesalamine is absorbed from the colon, and most of the drug is excreted in the stool. The small amount that is absorbed is acetylated in the intestinal mucosal wall and liver and then excreted in the urine. Intraluminal concentrations of mesalamine therefore are very high (~1500 μg/mL).

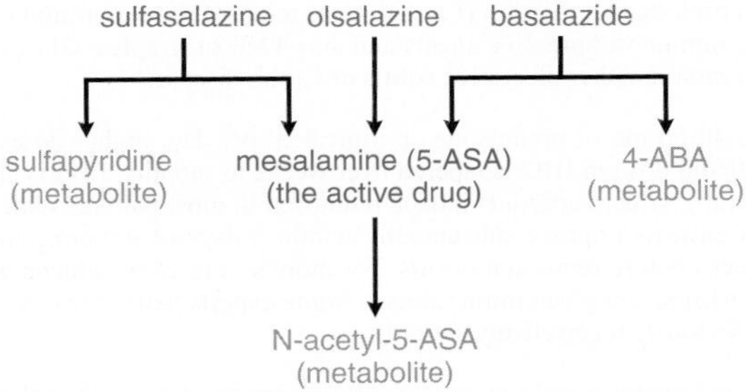

Figure 47–3 *Metabolic fates of the different oral formulations of mesalamine (5-ASA).*

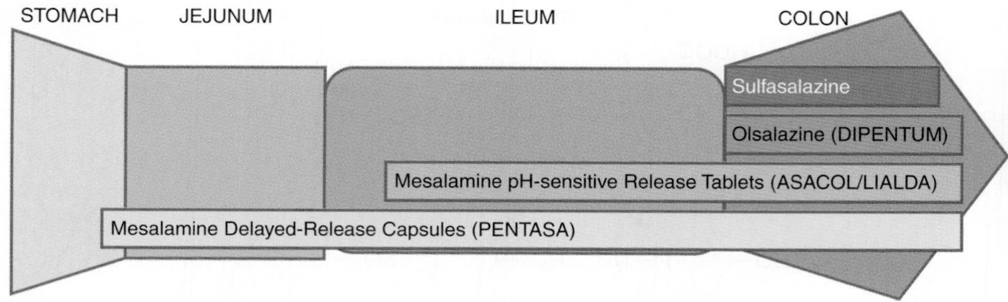

Figure 47–4 *Sites of release of mesalamine (5-ASA) in the GI tract from different oral formulations.*

The pH-sensitive coatings of ASACOL (EUDAGRIT) and LIALDA/MEZAVANT limit gastric and small intestinal absorption of 5-ASA. The pharmacokinetics of PENTASA differ somewhat. The ethylcellulose-coated microgranules are released in the upper GI tract as discrete prolonged-release units of mesalamine. Acetylated mesalamine can be detected in the circulation within an hour after ingestion, indicating some rapid absorption, but some intact microgranules also can be detected in the colon. Because it is released in the small bowel, a greater fraction of PENTASA is absorbed systemically compared with the other 5-ASA preparations.

ADVERSE EFFECTS. Side effects of sulfasalazine occur in 10-45% of patients with ulcerative colitis and are related primarily to the sulfa moiety. Some are dose related, including headache, nausea, and fatigue; these can be minimized by giving the medication with meals or by decreasing the dose. Allergic reactions include rash, fever, Stevens-Johnson syndrome, hepatitis, pneumonitis, hemolytic anemia, and bone marrow suppression. Sulfasalazine reversibly decreases the number and motility of sperm but does not impair female fertility. Sulfasalazine inhibits intestinal folate absorption and is usually administered with folate. The newer mesalamine formulations generally are well tolerated. Headache, dyspepsia, and skin rash are the most common. Diarrhea appears to be particularly common with olsalazine (occurring in 10-20% of patients). Nephrotoxicity, although rare, is a more serious concern. Mesalamine has been associated with interstitial nephritis; renal function should be monitored in all patients receiving these drugs. Both sulfasalazine and its metabolites cross the placenta but have not been shown to harm the fetus. The newer formulations also appear to be safe in pregnancy.

GLUCOCORTICOIDS

The effects of glucocorticoids on the inflammatory response are numerous (*see* Chapters 38 and 42). Glucocorticoids are indicated for moderate to severe IBD. Patients with IBD segregate into 3 general groups with respect to their response to glucocorticoids:

- *Glucocorticoid-responsive patients* improve clinically within 1-2 weeks and remain in remission as the steroids are tapered and then discontinued.
- *Glucocorticoid-dependent patients* respond to glucocorticoids but then experience a relapse of symptoms as the steroid dose is tapered.
- *Glucocorticoid-unresponsive patients* do not improve even with prolonged high-dose steroids.

Approximately 40% of patients are glucocorticoid responsive, 30-40% have only a partial response or become glucocorticoid dependent, and 15-20% of patients do not respond to therapy. Glucocorticoids sometimes are used for prolonged periods to control symptoms in corticosteroid-dependent patients. However, the failure to respond to steroids with prolonged remission (i.e., a disease relapse) should prompt consideration of alternative therapies, including immunosuppressive agents and anti-TNFα therapies. Glucocorticoids are not effective in maintaining remission in either ulcerative colitis or Crohn disease.

Initial doses in IBD are 40-60 mg of prednisone or equivalent per day; higher doses generally are no more effective. The glucocorticoid dose in IBD is tapered over weeks to months. Efforts should be made to minimize the duration of therapy. Glucocorticoids induce remission in most patients with either ulcerative colitis or Crohn disease. Most patients improve substantially within 5 days of initiating treatment; others require treatment for several weeks before remission occurs. For more severe cases, glucocorticoids such as *methylprednisolone* or *hydrocortisone* are given intravenously. Some experts believe that ACTH is more effective in patients who have not previously received any steroids.

Glucocorticoid enemas are useful mainly in patients whose disease is limited to the rectum and left colon. Hydrocortisone is available as a retention enema (100 mg/60 mL), and the usual dose is one 60-mL enema per night for 2 or 3 weeks. Patients with distal disease usually respond within 3-7 days. Absorption, although less than with oral preparations, is still substantial (up to 50-75%). Hydrocortisone also can be given once or twice daily as a 10% foam suspension (CORTIFOAM) that delivers 80 mg hydrocortisone per application; this formulation can be useful in patients with very short areas of distal proctitis and difficulty retaining fluid.

Budesonide (ENTOCORT ER) is an enteric-release form of a synthetic steroid that is used for ileocecal Crohn disease. It is proposed to deliver adequate steroid therapy to a specific portion of inflamed gut while minimizing systemic side effects owing to extensive first-pass hepatic metabolism to inactive derivatives. Topical therapy (e.g., enemas and suppositories) also is effective in treating colitis limited to the left side of the colon. Budesonide (9 mg/day for up to 8 weeks followed by 6 mg/day for maintenance of remission for up to 3 months) is effective in the acute management of mild-to-moderate exacerbations of Crohn disease.

IMMUNOSUPPRESSIVE AGENTS

Several drugs developed for cancer chemotherapy or as immunosuppressive agents in organ transplants have been adapted for treatment of IBD. Clinical experience has defined specific roles for each of these agents as mainstays in the pharmacotherapy of IBD. However, their potential for serious adverse effects mandates a careful assessment of risks and benefits in each patient.

THIOPURINE DERIVATIVES

The cytotoxic thiopurine derivatives *mercaptopurine* (6-MP, PURINETHOL) and *azathioprine* (IMURAN) (*see* Chapters 35 and 61) are used to treat patients with severe IBD or those who are steroid-resistant or steroid-dependent. These thiopurines impair purine biosynthesis and inhibit cell proliferation. Both are prodrugs: azathioprine is converted to mercaptopurine, which is subsequently metabolized to 6-thioguanine nucleotides, the putative active moieties (Figure 47–5).

These drugs generally are used interchangeably with appropriate dose adjustments, typically azathioprine (2-2.5 mg/kg) or mercaptopurine (1.5 mg/kg). Because of concerns about side effects, these drugs were used initially only in Crohn disease, which lacks a surgical curative option. They now are considered equally effective in Crohn disease and ulcerative colitis. These drugs effectively maintain remission in both diseases; they also may prevent or delay recurrence of Crohn disease after surgical resection. Finally, they are used successfully to treat fistulas in Crohn disease. The clinical response to azathioprine or mercaptopurine may take weeks to months, such that other drugs with a more rapid onset of action (e.g., mesalamine, glucocorticoids, or infliximab) are preferred in the acute setting.

In general, physicians who treat IBD believe that the long-term risks of azathioprine–mercaptopurine are lower than those of steroids. Thus, these purines are used in glucocorticoid-unresponsive or glucocorticoid-dependent disease and in patients who have had recurrent flares of disease requiring repeated courses of steroids. Additionally, patients who have not responded adequately to mesalamine but are not acutely ill may benefit by conversion from glucocorticoids to immunosuppressive drugs. Immunosuppressives therefore may be viewed as steroid-sparing agents.

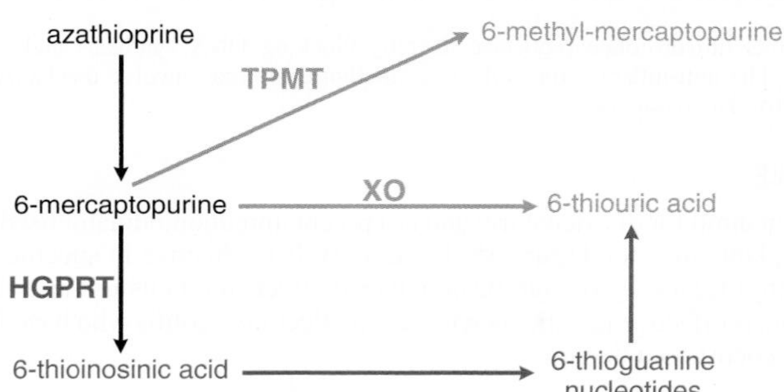

Figure 47–5 *Metabolism of azathioprine and 6-mercaptopurine.* HGPRT, hypoxanthine–guanine phosphoribosyl transferase; TPMT, thiopurine methyltransferase; XO, xanthine oxidase. The activities of these enzymes vary among humans due to differential expression of genetic polymorphisms, explaining responses and side effects when azathioprine–mercaptopurine therapy is employed (see text for details).

Adverse effects of azathioprine–mercaptopurine can be divided into 3 general categories: *idiosyncratic*, *dose related*, and *possible*. Adverse effects occur at any time after initiation of treatment and can affect up to 10% of patients. The most serious idiosyncratic reaction is pancreatitis, which affects ~5% of patients treated with these drugs. Fever, rash, and arthralgias are seen occasionally, whereas nausea and vomiting are somewhat more frequent. The major dose-related adverse effect is bone marrow suppression, and circulating blood counts should be monitored closely when therapy is initiated and at less frequent intervals during maintenance therapy. Elevations in liver function tests also may be dose related. The serious adverse effect of cholestatic hepatitis is relatively rare. Immunosuppressive regimens given in the setting of cancer chemotherapy or organ transplants have been associated with an increased incidence of malignancy, particularly non-Hodgkin's lymphoma.

METABOLISM AND PHARMACOGENETICS. Favorable responses to azathioprine–mercaptopurine are seen in up to two-thirds of patients. Mercaptopurine has 3 metabolic fates (*see* Figure 47–5):

- Conversion by xanthine oxidase to 6-thiouric acid
- Metabolism by thiopurine methyltransferase (TPMT) to 6-methyl-mercaptopurine (6-MMP)
- Conversion by hypoxanthine–guanine phosphoribosyl transferase (HGPRT) to 6-thioguanine nucleotides and other metabolites

The relative activities of these different pathways may explain, in part, individual variations in efficacy and adverse effects of these immunosuppressives.

The plasma $t_{1/2}$ of mercaptopurine is limited by its relatively rapid (i.e., within 1-2 h) uptake into erythrocytes and other tissues. Following this uptake, differences in TPMT activity determine the drug's fate. Approximately 80% of the U.S. population has what is considered "normal" metabolism, whereas 1 in 300 individuals has minimal TPMT activity. In the latter setting, mercaptopurine metabolism is shifted away from 6-methyl-mercaptopurine and driven toward 6-thioguanine nucleotides, which can severely suppress the bone marrow. About 10% of people have intermediate TPMT activity; given a similar dose, these individuals will tend to have higher 6-thioguanine levels than the normal metabolizers. Finally, ~10% of the population are rapid metabolizers. In these individuals, mercaptopurine is shunted away from 6-thioguanine nucleotides toward 6-MMP, which has been associated with abnormal liver function tests. In addition, relative to normal metabolizers, the 6-thioguanine levels of these rapid metabolizers are lower for an equivalent oral dose, possibly reducing therapeutic response. Pharmacogenetic typing can guide therapy (*see* Chapter 7).

Xanthine oxidase in the small intestine and liver converts mercaptopurine to thiouric acid, which is inactive as an immunosuppressant. Inhibition of xanthine oxidase by allopurinol diverts mercaptopurine to more active metabolites such as 6-thioguanine and increases both immunosuppressant and potential toxic effects. Thus, patients on mercaptopurine should be warned about potentially serious interactions with medications used to treat gout or hyperuricemia, and the dose should be decreased to 25% of the standard dose in subjects who are already taking allopurinol.

METHOTREXATE

Methotrexate is reserved for patients whose IBD is either steroid-resistant or steroid-dependent. In Crohn disease, it both induces and maintains remission. Therapy of IBD with methotrexate differs somewhat from its use in other autoimmune diseases. Most importantly, higher doses (e.g., 15-25 mg/week) are given parenterally. The increased efficacy with parenteral administration may reflect the unpredictable intestinal absorption at higher doses of methotrexate.

Methotrexate inhibits dihydrofolate reductase, thereby blocking DNA synthesis and causing cell death (*see* Figure 61–4). The anti-inflammatory effects of methotrexate may involve mechanisms in addition to inhibition of dihydrofolate reductase.

CYCLOSPORINE

Cyclosporine is an inhibitor of calcineurin and is a potent immunomodulator used most frequently after organ transplantation (*see* Figure 35–1 and text). It is effective in specific clinical settings in IBD, but the high frequency of significant adverse effects limits its use as a first-line medication. Cyclosporine is effective in patients with severe ulcerative colitis who have failed to respond adequately to glucocorticoid therapy.

Between 50% and 80% of these severely ill patients improve significantly (generally within 7 days) in response to intravenous cyclosporine (2-4 mg/kg per day), sometimes avoiding emergent colectomy. Careful monitoring of cyclosporine levels is necessary to maintain a therapeutic level in whole blood between 300 and 400 ng/mL. Oral cyclosporine is less effective as maintenance therapy in Crohn disease, perhaps because of its limited intestinal absorption. In this setting, long-term therapy with NEORAL or GENGRAF (formulations of cyclosporine with increased oral bioavailability) may be more effective. Cyclosporin can be used to treat fistulous complications of Crohn disease. A significant rapid response to intravenous cyclosporine has been observed; however, frequent relapses accompany oral cyclosporine therapy, and other medical strategies are required to maintain fistula closure. Thus, calcineurin inhibitors generally are used to treat specific problems over a short term while providing a bridge to longer-term therapy.

Other immunomodulators that are being evaluated in IBD include the calcineurin inhibitor tacrolimus (FK 506, PROGRAF), mycophenolate mofetil and mycophenolate (CELLCEPT, MYFORTIC), inhibitors of inosine monophosphate dehydrogenase to which lymphocytes are especially susceptible (*see* Chapter 35).

BIOLOGICAL THERAPIES

CROHN DISEASE

Infliximab (REMICADE, cA2) is a chimeric immunoglobulin (25% mouse, 75% human) that binds to and neutralizes TNFα, 1 of the principal cytokines mediating the T_H1 immune response characteristic of Crohn disease (*see* Figure 47–1).

Although infliximab was designed specifically to target TNFα, it may have more complex actions. Infliximab binds membrane-bound TNFα and may cause lysis of these cells by antibody-dependent or cell-mediated cytotoxicity. Thus, infliximab may deplete specific populations of subepithelial inflammatory cells. These effects, together with its mean terminal plasma $t_{1/2}$ of 8-10 days, may explain the prolonged clinical effects of infliximab. Infliximab (5 mg/kg infused intravenously at intervals of several weeks to months) decreases the frequency of acute flares in approximately two-thirds of patients with moderate to severe Crohn disease and also facilitates the closing of enterocutaneous fistulas associated with Crohn disease. Emerging evidence also supports its efficacy in maintaining remission and in preventing recurrence of fistulas. The combination of infliximab and azathioprine is more effective than infliximab alone in induction of remission and mucosal healing in steroid-resistant patients. Infliximab has also proven to be an effective treatment for refractory ulcerative colitis.

Both acute (fever, chills, urticaria, or even anaphylaxis) and subacute (serum sickness–like) reactions may develop after infliximab infusion. Antibodies to infliximab can decrease its clinical efficacy. Strategies to minimize the development of these antibodies (e.g., treatment with glucocorticoids or other immunosuppressives) may be critical to preserving infliximab efficacy. Infliximab therapy is associated with increased incidence of respiratory infections; of particular concern is potential reactivation of tuberculosis or other granulomatous infections with subsequent dissemination. The FDA recommends that candidates for infliximab therapy be tested for latent tuberculosis with purified protein derivative; patients testing positive should be treated prophylactically with isoniazid. Infliximab is contraindicated in patients with severe congestive heart failure. There is concern about a possible increased incidence of non-Hodgkin lymphoma, but a causal role has not been established. The significant cost of infliximab is an important consideration for some patients.

Adalimumab (HUMIRA) is a humanized recombinant human IgG_1 monoclonal antibody against TNFα. It is effective in inducing remission in mild to moderate, severe, and fistulizing Crohn disease.

Certolizumab pegol (CIMZIA) is a pegylated humanized fragment antigen binding (Fab) that binds TNFα. It is approved in the U.S. for the treatment of Crohn disease. With both adalimumab and certolizumab pegol, immunogenicity appears to be less of a problem than that associated with infliximab.

Natalizumab (TYSABRI) is a humanized monoclonal antibody against α4-integrin (also known as VLA-4). Binding of the antibody to this adhesion molecule will reduce extravasation of certain leukocytes (e.g., lymphocytes), preventing them from migrating to sites of inflammation where they may exacerbate tissue injury.

Natalizumab is approved in the U.S. for induction and maintenance of remission of moderate to severe Crohn disease. Natalizumab is contraindicated for use with other immunomodulators; patients taking natalizumab for the treatment of Crohn disease should have their doses of corticosteroids reduced before starting natalizumab treatment.

Etanercept (ENBREL), an anti-TNFα agent, is a fusion protein of the ligand-binding portion of the TNFα receptor and the Fc portion of human IgG_1. This construct binds to TNFα and blocks its biologic effects but is ineffective in Crohn disease.

Table 47–1

Medications Commonly Used to Treat Inflammatory Bowel Disease

	CROHN'S DISEASE					ULCERATIVE COLITIS			
	ACTIVE DISEASE			MAINTENANCE		ACTIVE DISEASE			MAINTENANCE
CLASS/DRUG	MILD-MODERATE	MODERATE-SEVERE	FISTULA	MEDICAL REMISSION	SURGICAL REMISSION	DISTAL COLITIS	MILD-MODERATE	MODERATE-SEVERE	
Mesalamine									
Enema	+[a]	–	–	–	–	+	+[a,b]	–	+
Oral	+	–	–	+/–	+[c]	+	+	–	+
Antibiotics									
(metronidazole ciprofloxacin, others)	+	+	+	?	+[c]	–	–	–	+[c]
Corticosteroids									
Enema, foam, suppository	+[a]	–	–	–	+	+[b]	–	–	–
Oral	+	+	–	–	–	+	+	+	–
Intravenous	–	+	–	–	–	+[d]	–	+	–
Immunomodulators									
6-MP/AZA	–	+	+	+	+[c]	+[d]	–	+[d]	+[d]
Methotrexate	–	?	?	?	?	–	–	–	–
Cyclosporine	–	+[d]	+[d]	–	–	+[d]	–	+[d]	–
Biological response modifiers									
Infliximab	+[d]	+	+	+[c]	?	+	–	+	?
Adalimumab	+	+	+	+	?	?	?	?	?
Certolizumab pegol	+	+	?	+	?	?	?	+	?
Natalizumab	–	+	?	+	?	?	?	?	?

6-MP, 6-mercaptopurine; AZA, azathioprine.

[a]*Distal colonic disease only.*

[b]*For adjunctive therapy.*

[c]*Some data to support use; remains controversial.*

[d]*Selected patients.*

Source: From Sands BE. Therapy of inflammatory bowel disease. Gastroenterology, *2000;118(2 suppl 1):S68-S82, table 1, p S71. With permission from Elsevier. Copyright © Elsevier.*

ULCERATIVE COLITIS

The role of anti-TNF therapies for steroid-refractory or steroid-dependent ulcerative colitis is less clear. Large controlled clinical trials have demonstrated that anti-TNF agents significantly reduce the severity of the inflammation. Unlike Crohn disease, ulcerative colitis is cured with surgery; thus, the cost and serious adverse events associated with anti-TNF therapy need to be balanced with the effectiveness of the drug at preventing the need for colectomy.

ANTIBIOTICS AND PROBIOTICS

A balance normally exists in the GI tract among the mucosal epithelium, the normal gut flora, and the immune response. Colonic bacteria may either initiate or perpetuate the inflammation of IBD, and recent studies have implicated specific bacterial antigens in the pathogenesis of Crohn disease. Thus, certain bacterial strains may be either pro- (e.g., *Bacteroides*) or anti-inflammatory (e.g., *Lactobacillus*), prompting attempts to manipulate the colonic flora in patients with IBD. Traditionally, antibiotics have been used most prominently in Crohn disease.

Antibiotics can be used as:

- Adjunctive treatment along with other medications for active IBD
- Treatment for a specific complication of Crohn disease
- Prophylaxis for recurrence in postoperative Crohn disease

Metronidazole, *ciprofloxacin*, and *clarithromycin* are the antibiotics used most frequently. Crohn disease-related complications that may benefit from antibiotic therapy include intra-abdominal abscess and inflammatory masses, perianal disease (including fistulas and perirectal abscesses), small-bowel bacterial overgrowth secondary to partial small-bowel obstruction, secondary infections with organisms such as *Clostridium difficile*, and postoperative complications. More recently, *probiotics* have been used to treat specific clinical situations in IBD. Probiotics are mixtures of putatively beneficial lyophilized bacteria given orally. Several studies have provided evidence for beneficial effects of probiotics in ulcerative colitis and pouchitis. However, the utility of probiotics as a primary therapy for IBD remains unclear.

SUPPORTIVE THERAPY IN IBD

Analgesic, anticholinergic, and antidiarrheal agents play supportive roles in reducing symptoms and improving quality of life. Oral iron, folate, and vitamin B_{12} should be administered as indicated. Loperamide or diphenoxylate (*see* Chapter 46) can be used to reduce the frequency of bowel movements and relieve rectal urgency in patients with mild disease; these agents are contraindicated in patients with severe disease because they may predispose to the development of toxic megacolon. Cholestyramine can be used to prevent bile salt–induced colonic secretion in patients who have undergone limited ileocolic resections. Anticholinergic agents (dicyclomine hydrochloride, etc.; Chapter 9) are used to reduce abdominal cramps, pain, and rectal urgency. As with the antidiarrheal agents, they are contraindicated in severe disease or when obstruction is suspected.

THERAPY OF IBD DURING PREGNANCY

IBD is a chronic disease that affects women in their reproductive years. In general, decreased disease activity increases fertility and improves pregnancy outcomes. At the same time, limiting medication during pregnancy is always desired but sometimes conflicts with the goal of controlling the disease. Mesalamine and glucocorticoids are FDA Category B drugs that are used frequently in pregnancy and generally are considered safe, whereas methotrexate is clearly contraindicated in pregnant patients. There does not appear to be an increase in adverse outcomes in pregnant patients maintained on thiopurine-based immunosuppressives.

SUMMARY OF AVAILABLE DRUG THERAPIES

Table 47–1 summarizes the medications routinely used to treat IBD.

For a complete Bibliographical Listing see Goodman & Gilman's ***The Pharmacological Basis of Therapeutics***, 12th ed., or Goodman & Gilman Online at www.AccessMedicine.com.

Section VII Chemotherapy of Microbial Diseases

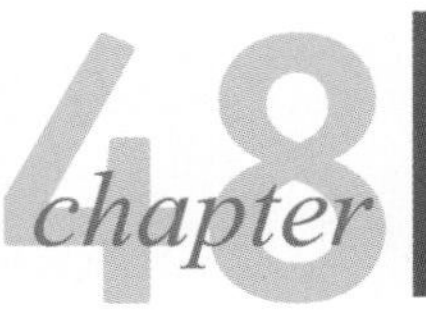

chapter 48 General Principles of Antimicrobial Therapy

ANTIMICROBIAL CHEMOTHERAPY

Microorganisms of medical importance fall into 4 categories: bacteria, viruses, fungi, and parasites. Likewise, antibiotics are broadly classified as (1) antibacterial, (2) antiviral, (3) antifungal, and (4) antiparasitic agents. Antimicrobial molecules should be viewed as ligands whose receptors are microbial proteins. The microbial proteins targeted by the antibiotic are essential components of biochemical reactions in the microbes, and interference with these physiological pathways kills the microorganisms. The biochemical processes commonly inhibited include cell wall synthesis in bacteria and fungi, cell membrane synthesis, synthesis of 30s and 50s ribosomal subunits, nucleic acid metabolism, function of topoisomerases, viral proteases, viral integrases, viral envelope fusion proteins, folate synthesis in parasites, and parasitic chemical detoxification processes.

Classification of an antibiotic is based on:

- The class and spectrum of microorganisms it kills
- The biochemical pathway it interferes with
- The chemical structure of its pharmacophore

The relationship between antimicrobial concentration and effect on a population of organisms is modeled using the standard Hill-type curve for receptor and agonist (*see* Chapters 2 and 3), characterized by 3 parameters: the inhibitory concentration 50, or IC_{50} (also termed EC_{50}), a measure of the antimicrobial agent's potency; the maximal effect, E_{max}; and H, the slope of the curve, or Hill factor. In antimicrobial therapy, the relationship is often expressed as an inhibitory sigmoid E_{max} model, to take into account the control bacterial population without treatment (E_{con}) as a fourth parameter (Equation 48–1 and Figure 48–1), where E is the effect as measured by microbial burden.

$$E = E_{con} - E_{max} \times [IC]^{H}/([IC]^{H} + [IC_{50}]^{H}) \quad \text{(Equation 48–1)}$$

THE PHARMACOKINETIC BASIS OF ANTIMICROBIAL THERAPY

PENETRATION OF ANTIMICROBIAL AGENTS INTO ANATOMIC COMPARTMENTS. In many infections, the pathogen causes disease not in the whole body, but in specific organs. Antibiotics are often administered far away from these sites of infection. Therefore, in choosing an antimicrobial agent for therapy, a crucial consideration is whether the drug can penetrate to the site of infection.

For example, the antibiotic levofloxacin achieves skin tissue/plasma peak concentration ratio of 1.4, epithelial lining fluid to plasma ratio of 2.8, and urine-to-plasma ratios of 67. In clinical trials with levofloxacin, the failure rate of therapy was 0% in patients with urinary tract infections, 3% in patients with pulmonary infections, and 16% in patients with skin and soft tissue infections. Clearly, the poorer the penetration into the anatomical compartment, the higher the likelihood of failure. Penetration of a drug into an anatomical compartment depends on the physical barriers that the molecule must traverse, the chemical properties of the drug, and the presence of multidrug transporters. The physical barriers are usually due to layers of epithelial and endothelial cells, and the type of junctions formed between these cells. Penetration across this physical barrier generally correlates with the octanol-water partition coefficient of the antimicrobial agent,

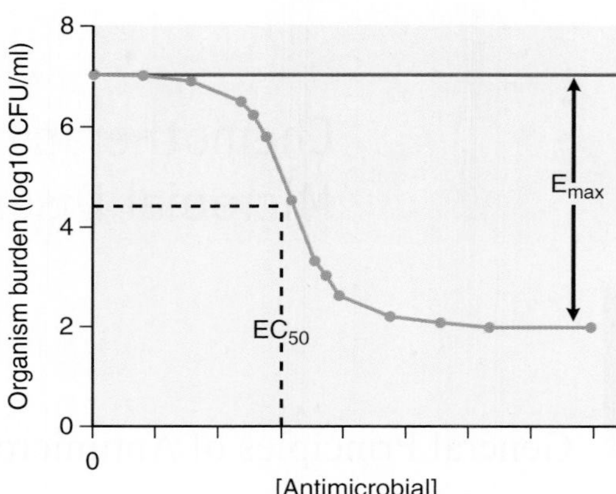

Figure 48–1 *Inhibitory sigmoid E_{max} curve.* CFU, colony-forming unit.

a measure of its hydrophobicity. Hydrophobic molecules get concentrated in the cell membrane bilayer, whereas hydrophilic molecules tend to concentrate in the blood, the cytosol, and other aqueous compartments (*see* Figure 2–3).

Membrane transporters comprise another barrier; they actively export drugs from the cellular or tissue compartment back into the blood (*see* Chapter 5). A well-known example is the *P-glycoprotein*. Although the octanol-water partition coefficient would favor lipophilic molecules to transverse across cell barriers, P-glycoprotein exports structurally unrelated amphiphilic and lipophilic molecules of 3-4 kDa, reducing their effective penetration. Antimicrobial agents that are P-glycoprotein substrates include HIV protease inhibitors, the antiparasitic agent ivermectin, the antibacterial agent telithromycin, and the antifungal agent itraconazole.

The CNS is guarded by the *blood-brain barrier*. The movement of antibiotics across the blood-brain barrier is restricted by tight junctions that connect endothelial cells of cerebral micro-vessels to one another in the brain parenchyma, as well as by protein transporters. Antimicrobial agents that are polar at physiological pH generally penetrate poorly; some, such as *penicillin G*, are actively transported out of the cerebrospinal fluid (CSF) and achieve CSF concentrations of only 0.5-5% of that achieved in plasma. However, the integrity of the blood-brain barrier is diminished during active bacterial infection; tight junctions in cerebral capillaries open, leading to a marked increase in the penetration of even polar drugs.

The eye, the epithelial lining fluid of the lung, and biofilms and vegetations on artificial heart valves and indwelling catheters pose special problems for drug penetration and effective therapy.

PHARMACOKINETIC COMPARTMENTS. Once an antibiotic has penetrated to the site of infection, it may be subjected to processes of elimination and distribution that differ from those in the blood. These sites where the concentration-time profiles differ from each other are considered separate pharmacokinetic compartments, thus, the human body is viewed as multicompartmental. The concentration of antibiotic within each compartment is assumed to be homogeneous. The model is also defined as *open* or *not open*; an open model is one in which the drug is eliminated out of the body from the compartment (e.g., kidneys). The order of the process must also be specified (*see* Chapter 2): a first-order process is directly correlated to concentration of drug D, or $[D]^1$, as opposed to zero order, which is independent of [D] and reflects a process that is saturated at ambient levels of D.

Suppose a patient has pneumonia with the pathogen in the lung epithelial lining fluid (ELF). The patient ingests an antibiotic that is absorbed via the GI tract (*g*) into blood or central compartment (compartment 1), as a first-order input. In this process, the transfer constant from the GI tract to central compartment is termed the *absorption constant* and is designated k_a. The antibiotic in the central compartment is then delivered to the lungs where it penetrates into the ELF (compartment 2). However, it also penetrates into other tissues of the body peripheral to the site of infection, termed the *peripheral compartment* (compartment 3). Thus, we have 4 compartments (including *g*, a specific compartment, the GI tract, from the set of initial absorption compartments labeled "p" in Figure 48–2), each with its own concentration-time profile, as shown in Figure 48–2. The penetration of drug from compartment 1 to 2 is based on the penetration factors discussed earlier and is defined by the transfer constant k_{12}. However, the drug also redistributes

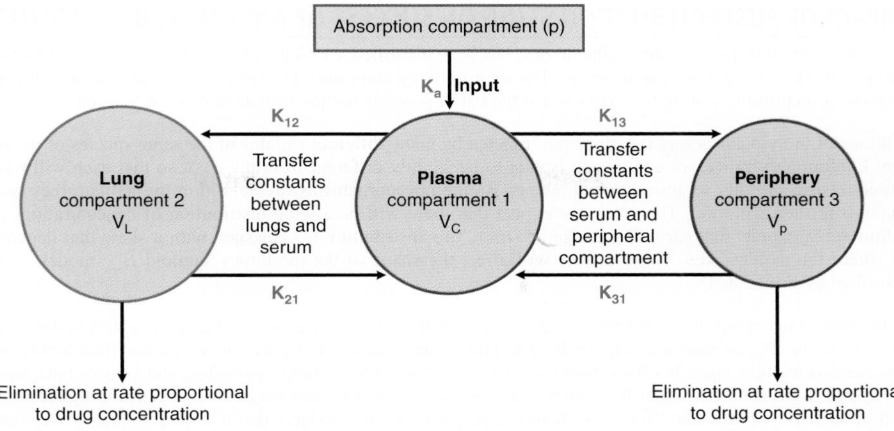

Figure 48–2 *Diagrammatic depiction of a multicompartment model.*

from compartment 2 back to 1, defined by transfer constant k_{21}. A similar process between the blood and peripheral tissues leads to transfer constants k_{13} and k_{31}. The drug may also be lost from the body (i.e., open system) via the lungs and other peripheral tissues (e.g., kidneys or liver) at a rate proportional to the concentration.

Antibiotic concentrations within each compartment change with time (the changes are described using standard differential equations). If X is the amount of antibiotic in a compartment, SCL the drug clearance, and V_c the volume of central compartment, then equations for absorption compartment (Equation 48–2), central compartment (Equation 48–3), site of infection or compartment 2 (Equation 48–4), and peripheral compartment (Equation 48–5) are as follows:

$$dX_g/dt = -K_a \cdot X_g \qquad \text{(Equation 48–2)}$$

$$dX_1/dt = K_a \cdot X_g - [(SCL/V_c) + K_{12} + K_{13}] \cdot X_1 + K_{21} \cdot X_2 + K_{31} \cdot X_3 \qquad \text{(Equation 48–3)}$$

$$dX_2/dt = K_{12} \cdot X_1 - K_{21} \cdot X_2 \qquad \text{(Equation 48–4)}$$

$$dX_3/dt = K_{13} \cdot X_3 - K_{31} \cdot X_3 \qquad \text{(Equation 48–5)}$$

Such models have been used in conjunction with population pharmacokinetics to describe and model a plethora of antimicrobials used to treat bacteria, fungi, viruses, and parasites. Recently, the models have been refined to include sub-populations of the pathogen (killed, inhibited, or resistant to the antibiotic) and other refinements described in Chapter 48 of the 12th edition of the parent text.

POPULATION PHARMACOKINETICS AND VARIABILITY IN DRUG RESPONSE. When multiple patients are treated with the same dose of a drug, each patient will achieve pharmacokinetic parameters that differ from others. This is termed *between-patient variability*. Even when the same dose is administered to the same patient on 2 separate occasions, the patient may achieve a different concentration-time profile of the drug between the 2 occasions. This is termed *inter-occasion* or *within-patient variability*. The variability is reflected at the level of the compartmental pharmacokinetic parameters such as k_a, k_{12}, k_{21}, SCL, V_c, and so on. Even when a recommended dose is administered, the drug may fail to reach a therapeutic concentration in some patients. In other patients, the drug may reach high and toxic concentrations. Such variability could be due to genetic variability. In addition, weight, height, and age also lead to variability. Furthermore, patients may have comorbid conditions such as renal and liver dysfunction, which may lead to variability. Drug interactions are an important source of variability with potentially dangerous consequences (*see* Chapters 5 and 6). Even when such factors are accounted for, there remains residual variability due to computational noise, assay variability, and unexplainable factors. The common practice of using an "average" value of data or "naive pooling" may prevent recognition of subgroups of patients at risk for therapeutic failure or increased toxicity of antibiotic. Knowledge of covariates associated with pharmacokinetic variability leads to better dose adjustments, or switching therapy from one antibiotic to another, or changing concomitant medications.

Once the microbial species causing the disease has been identified, a rational choice of the class of antibiotics likely to work in the patient can be made. The microbiology laboratory then plays a second role, which is to perform susceptibility testing to narrow down the list of possible antimicrobials that could be used.

Millions of individuals across the globe get infected by many different isolates of the same species of pathogen. Evolutionary processes cause each isolate to be slightly different from the next, so that each will have a unique susceptibility to antimicrobial agents. As the microorganisms divide within the patient, they may undergo further evolution. Therefore, we expect that there will be a wide distribution of concentrations of antimicrobial agents that can kill pathogens. Often, this distribution is Gaussian, with a skew that depends on where the patient lives. These factors will affect the shape of the inhibitory sigmoid E_{max} model curve described by Equation 48–1.

With changes in susceptibility, the sigmoid E_{max} curve shifts in 1 of 2 basic ways. The first is a shift to the right, an *increase in* IC_{50}, as shown in Figure 48–3A. This means that much higher concentrations than before are now needed to show specific effect. Susceptibility tests for bacteria, fungi, parasites, and viruses have been developed to determine whether these shifts have occurred at a sufficient magnitude to warrant higher doses of drug to achieve particular effect. The change in IC_{50} may become so large that it is not possible to overcome the concentration deficit by increasing the antimicrobial dose without causing toxicity to the patient. At that stage, the organism is now *"resistant"* to the particular antibiotic. A second possible change in the curve is a *decrease in* E_{max} (Figure 48–3B), such that increasing the dose of the antimicrobial agent beyond a certain point will achieve no further effect; i.e., changes in the microbe are such that eradication of the microbe by the particular drug can never be achieved. This occurs because the available target proteins have been reduced or the microbe has developed an alternative pathway to overcome the biochemical inhibition.

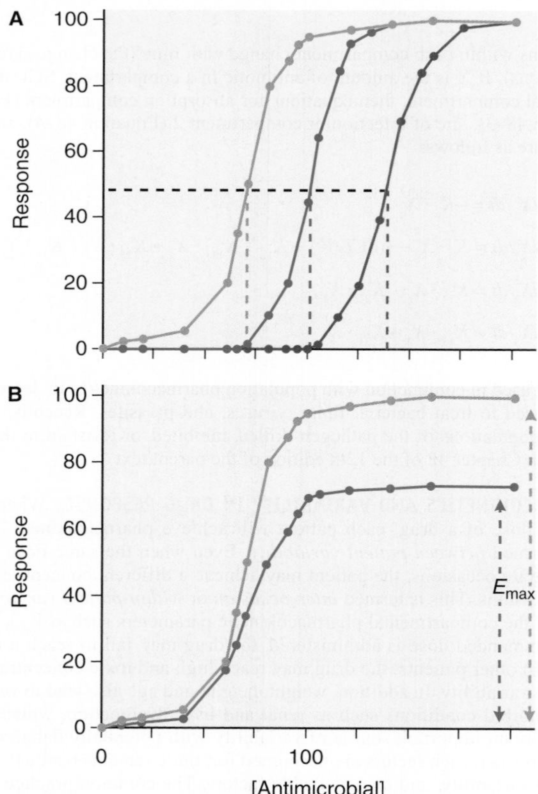

Figure 48–3 *Changes in sigmoid* E_{max} *model with increases in drug resistance.* Increase in resistance may show changes in IC_{50} (**panel A:** the IC_{50} increases from 70 [*orange line*] to 100 [*green line*], to 140 [*blue line*]) or decrease in E_{max} (**panel B:** efficacy decreases from full response [*orange line*] to 70% [*green line*]).

Bacteria. Dilution tests for bacterial drug susceptibility employ antibiotics in serially diluted drug concentrations on solid agar or in broth medium that contains a culture of the test microorganism. The lowest concentration of the agent that prevents visible growth after 18-24 h of incubation is known as the *minimum inhibitory concentration* (MIC).

Fungi. For fungi that are yeasts (i.e., *Candida*), susceptibility testing methods are similar to those used for bacteria. However, the definitions of MIC differ based on drug and the type of yeast, so there are cutoff points of 50% decreases in turbidity compared to controls at 24 h, or 80% at 48 h, or total clearance of the turbidity. Susceptibility tests and MICs for triazoles have been extensively shown to correlate with clinical outcomes.

Viruses. In HIV phenotypic assays, the patient's HIV-RNA is extracted from plasma, and genes for targets of antiretroviral drugs such as reverse transcriptase and protease are amplified. The genes are then inserted into a standard HIV vector that lacks analogous gene sequences to produce a recombinant virus, which is co-incubated with drug of interest in a mammalian cell viability assay. Growth is compared to a standardized wild-type control virus. For HIV reverse transcriptase, e.g., <4-fold increase in IC_{50} is defined as "sensitive," 4- to 10-fold increase in I IC_{50} is "intermediate," and >10-fold increase is "resistant." Further use has been made of the viral IC_{50} to establish the inhibitory quotient (IQ). The IQ is the ratio of plasma concentration of antiviral drug to the IC_{50}. The phenotypic IQ is the ratio of plasma trough concentration to the IC_{50}.

Parasites. Susceptibility testing for parasites, especially malaria, has been performed in the laboratory. The tests are similar to the broth tests for bacteria, fungi, and viruses. *Plasmodium* species in the patient's blood are cultured ex vivo in the presence of different dilutions of antimalarial drug. A sigmoid E_{max} curve for effect versus drug concentration is used to identify IC_{50} and E_{max}. These tests are primarily used in the research setting and not for individualization of therapy.

BASIS FOR SELECTION OF DOSE AND DOSING SCHEDULE

Although susceptibility testing is central to decision making, it does not completely predict patient response. Microorganisms in patients are exposed to dynamic concentrations of drug, and antibiotics are prescribed at a certain schedule (e.g., 3 times a day) so that there is a periodicity in the fluctuations of drug at the site of infection. Thus, the microbe is exposed to a particular shape of the concentration-time curve, an important determinant of the efficacy of the antibiotic for which we can write 3 corollaries:

1. In determining therapeutic outcomes, it is important to apply knowledge of susceptibility (MIC or EC_{90}) of the organism to the antimicrobial agent and index drug exposure to MIC.
2. The optimal dose of the antibiotic for a patient is the dose that achieves IC_{80} to IC_{90} exposures at the site of infection.
3. Optimal microbial kill by the antibiotic may be best achieved by maximizing certain shapes of the concentration-time curve, using the fact that certain dosing schedules maximize the antimicrobial effect (see below).

As an example, consider an antibiotic with a serum $t_{1/2}$ of 3 h that is being used to treat a bloodstream infection by a pathogen with an MIC of 0.5 mg/L, administered with a dosing interval of 24 h (that is, a once-daily schedule). Figure 48–4A depicts the concentration-time curve of the antibiotic, with definitions of peak concentration (C_{Pmax}), area under the curve (AUC), and the fraction of the dosing interval for which the drug concentration remains above the MIC (T > MIC), as shown. The AUC is a measure of the total concentration of drug and is calculated by taking an integral between 2 time points, 0-24 h (AUC_{0-24}) in this case. With a change in the dosing schedule of the same antibiotic amount by splitting it into 3 equal doses administered at 0, 8, and 16 h, the shape of the concentration-time curves changes to that shown in Figure 48–4B. Because the *same cumulative dose* has been given for the dosing interval of 24 h, the *AUC_{0-24} will be similar* whether it was given once a day or 3 times a day. However, *the C_{Pmax} will decrease* by one-third when the total dose is split into thirds and administered more frequently (*see* Figure 48–4B). Thus, when a dose is fractionated and administered more frequently, the C_{Pmax}/MIC ratio *decreases*. In contrast, the time that the drug concentration persists above MIC (T > MIC) *increases* with the more frequent dosing schedule.

Some classes of antimicrobial agents kill best when concentration persists above MIC for longer durations of the dosing interval. Indeed, increasing the drug concentration beyond 4 and 6 times the MIC does not increase microbial kill. Two good examples are β-lactam antibacterials (e.g., penicillin) and the antifungal agent 5-fluorocytosine (5-FC). In fact, there are usually good biochemical explanations for this pattern for the drugs. The clinical implication, however, is that a drug optimized by T > MIC should be dosed more frequently, or have its $t_{1/2}$ prolonged by other drugs, so that drug concentrations persist above MIC (or EC_{95}) as long as possible. Thus, the effectiveness of penicillin is enhanced when it is given as a continuous infusion. HIV protease inhibitors are often "boosted" with ritonavir; this "boosting" inhibits the metabolism of the protease inhibitors by CYPs 3A4 and 2D6, thereby prolonging time above EC_{95}.

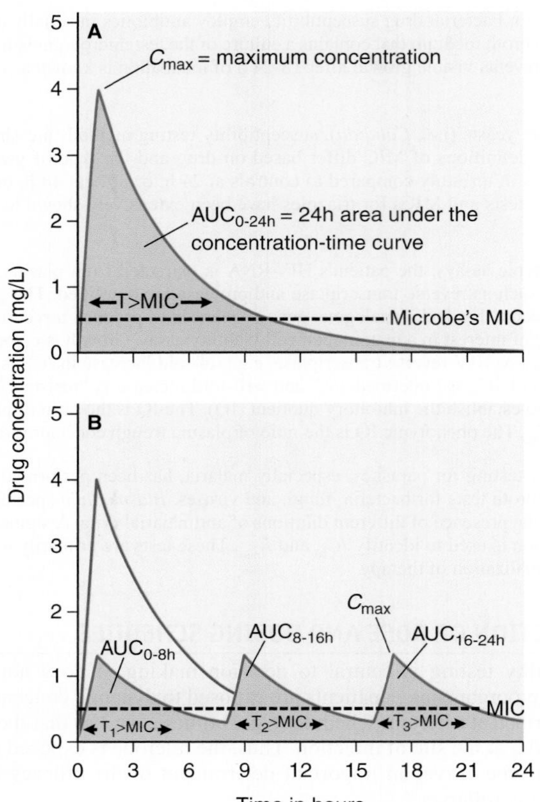

Figure 48–4 *Effect of different dose schedules on shape of concentration-time curve.* The total AUC for the fractionated dose in **curve B** is determined by adding $AUC_{0\text{-}8h}$, $AUC_{8\text{-}16h}$, and $AUC_{16\text{-}24h}$, which adds up to the same $AUC_{0\text{-}24h}$ in **curve A.** The time that the drug concentration exceeds MIC in **curve B** is also determined by adding up $T_1 > MIC$, $T_2 > MIC$, and $T_3 > MIC$, which results in a fraction greater than that for curve A.

Conversely, the peak concentration is paramount for some antimicrobial agents. Persistence of concentration above MIC has less relevance for these drugs, meaning that these drugs can be dosed more intermittently. Aminoglycosides are a prime example of this class: they used to be given 3 times a day but are highly effective when given once a day. These C_{Pmax}/MIC-linked drugs are administered less frequently due to their long duration of *post-antibiotic* effect (PAE). In other words, effect continues long after antibiotic concentrations decline below the MIC. Consider rifampin. The entry of rifampin into *Mycobacterium tuberculosis* increases with increased concentration in the bacillus microenvironment. Once inside the bacteria, the drug's macrocyclic ring binds the β subunit of DNA-dependent RNA polymerase (*rpoB)* to form a very stable drug-enzyme complex within 10 min, a process not enhanced by longer incubation of drug and enzyme. The PAE of the rifampin is long and concentration dependent.

There is a third group of drugs for which the dosing schedule has no effect on efficacy but the cumulative dose matters. Thus, it is the ratio of total concentration over time (AUC)-to-MIC that matters and not the time that concentration persists above a certain threshold. Antibacterial agents such as daptomycin fall into this class. These agents also have a good PAE. The AUC/IC_{50} explains why the nucleoside analogue reverse transcriptase inhibitors tenofovir and emtricitabine have been combined into 1 pill, administered once a day for the treatment of AIDS.

The shape of concentration-time curve that optimizes resistance suppression is often different from that which optimizes microbial kill. In many instances, the drug exposure associated with resistance suppression is much higher than for optimal kill. The optimal dose should be designed to achieve a high probability of exceeding the EC_{80} microbial PK/PD (pharmacokinetic/pharmacodynamic) index, or index associated with suppression of resistance, given the population pharmacokinetic variability and the MIC distribution of clinical microbe isolates. The population pharmacokinetic variability enables integration of pharmacogenetics, anthropometric measures, and residual variability into the decision to choose optimal dose. Once that has been achieved, the dose schedule is chosen according to whether efficacy is driven by AUC/MIC (or AUC/EC_{95}), C_{Pmax}/MIC, or T > MIC. Duration of therapy is then chosen, based on best available evidence.

TYPES AND GOALS OF ANTIMICROBIAL THERAPY

A useful way to organize the types and goals of antimicrobial therapy is to consider where along the disease progression timetable therapy is initiated (Figure 48–5); therapy can be *prophylactic, preemptive, empirical, definitive,* or *suppressive*.

PROPHYLACTIC THERAPY. Prophylaxis involves treating patients who are not yet infected or have not yet developed disease. The goal of prophylaxis is to prevent infection in some patients or to prevent development of a potentially dangerous disease in those who already have evidence of infection. The main principle behind prophylaxis is targeted therapy.

Prophylaxis is used in immunosuppressed patients such as those with HIV-AIDS or are post-transplantation and on anti-rejection medications. In these groups of patients, specific antiparasitic, antibacterial, antiviral, and antifungal therapy is administered based on the well-defined pattern of pathogens that are major causes of morbidity during immunosuppression. A risk-to-benefit analysis is used to determine choice and duration of prophylaxis. In AIDS patients, prophylaxis is discontinued when the CD4 count climbs above 200 cells/mm^3. Infections for which prophylaxis is given include *Pneumocystis jiroveci, Mycobacterium avium-intracellulare, Toxoplasma gondii, Candida* species, *Aspergillus* species, *Cytomegalovirus*, and other *Herpesviridae*.

Chemoprophylaxis is used to prevent wound infections after various surgical procedures. Several factors are important for the use of antibiotics for surgical prophylaxis. First, antimicrobial activity must be present at the wound site at the time of its closure. Thus, infusion of the first antimicrobial dose should begin within 60 min before surgical incision and should be discontinued within 24 h of the end of surgery. Second, the antibiotic must be active against the most likely contaminating microorganisms for that type of surgery. Chemoprophylaxis can be justified in dirty or contaminated surgical procedures (e.g., resection of the colon), where the incidence of wound infections is high. In clean surgical procedures, which account for ~75% of the total, the expected incidence of wound infection is <5%, and antibiotics should not be used routinely. When the surgery involves insertion of a prosthetic implant (e.g., prosthetic valve, vascular graft, prosthetic joint), cardiac surgery, or neurosurgical procedures, the complications of infection are so drastic that most authorities currently agree to chemoprophylaxis for these indications.

Prophylaxis may be used to protect healthy persons from acquisition of or invasion by specific microorganisms to which they are exposed. This is termed *postexposure prophylaxis.* Examples include rifampin administration to prevent meningococcal meningitis in people who are in close contact with a case, prevention of gonorrhea or syphilis after contact with an infected person, and macrolides after contact with confirmed cases of pertussis. Post-exposure prophylaxis is recommended in those patients inadvertently exposed to HIV infection.

Mother-to-child transmission of HIV and syphilis are important public health problems. Anti-retroviral therapy is administered for HIV prophylaxis during the pregnancy and peripartum periods. Prophylactic therapy for syphilis during pregnancy is effective in reducing neonatal death and infant neurological, auditory, and bone malformations.

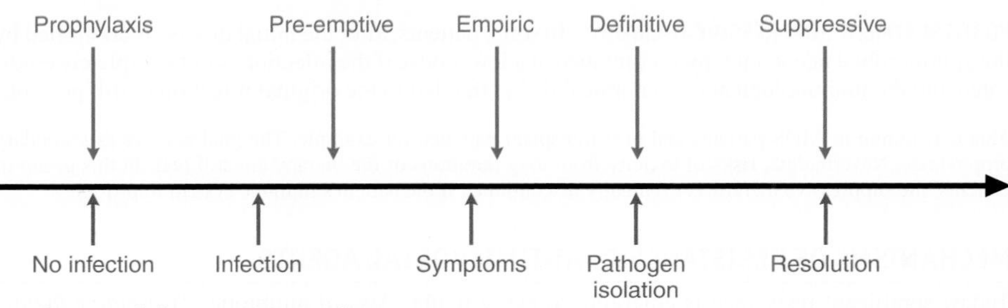

Figure 48–5 *Antimicrobial therapy-disease progression timeline.*

PRE-EMPTIVE THERAPY. Pre-emptive therapy is early, targeted therapy in high-risk patients who already have a laboratory or other test indicating that an asymptomatic patient has become infected. The principle is that delivery of therapy prior to development of symptoms (presymptomatic) aborts impending disease, and the therapy is for a short and defined duration.

This has been applied in the therapy for cytomegalovirus after both hematopoietic stem cell transplants and after solid organ transplantation.

EMPIRICAL THERAPY IN THE SYMPTOMATIC PATIENT. Once a patient is symptomatic, should the patient be treated immediately? The first consideration in selecting an antimicrobial is to determine if the drug is indicated. *The reflex action to associate fever with treatable infections and prescribe antimicrobial therapy without further evaluation is irrational and potentially dangerous.*

The diagnosis may be masked if therapy is started and appropriate cultures are not obtained. Antimicrobial agents are potentially toxic and may promote selection of resistant microorganisms. For some diseases, the cost of waiting a few days for microbiological evidence of infection is low. If the risks of waiting are high, based either on the patient's immune status or other known risk factors for poor outcome, initiation of optimal empirical antimicrobial therapy should rely on the clinical presentation and clinical experience. The most valuable and time-tested method for immediate identification of bacteria is examination of the infected secretion or body fluid with Gram stain. In malaria-endemic areas, or in travelers returning from such an area, a simple thick and thin blood smear may mean the difference between a patient's receiving appropriate lifesaving therapy or dying while on wrong therapy for presumed bacterial infection. Similarly, neutropenic patients with fever have high risks of mortality, and, when febrile, they are presumed to have either a bacterial or fungal infection; thus, a broad-spectrum combination of antibacterial and antifungal agents covering common infections encountered in granulocytopenic patients is recommended. Performance of cultures is still mandatory with a view to modify antimicrobial therapy with culture results.

DEFINITIVE THERAPY WITH KNOWN PATHOGEN. Once a pathogen has been isolated and susceptibilities results are available, therapy should be streamlined to a narrow targeted antibiotic. Monotherapy is preferred to decrease the risk of antimicrobial toxicity and selection of antimicrobial-resistant pathogens. Proper antimicrobial doses and dose schedules are crucial to maximizing efficacy and minimizing toxicity. In addition, the duration of therapy should be as short as is necessary.

Combination therapy is an exception, rather than a rule. Once a pathogen has been isolated, there should be no reason to use multiple antibiotics, except when evidence overwhelmingly suggests otherwise. Using 2 antimicrobial agents where one is required leads to increased toxicity and unnecessary damage to the patient's otherwise protective fungal and bacterial flora. Special circumstances where evidence is in favor of combination therapy include:

- Preventing resistance to monotherapy
- Accelerating the rapidity of microbial kill
- Enhancing therapeutic efficacy by use of synergistic interactions
- Reducing toxicity (i.e., when sufficient efficacy of 1 antibacterial agent can be achieved at doses that are toxic to the patient and a second drug is coadministered to permit lowering dose of first drug)

Clinical situations for which combination therapy is advised include antiretroviral therapy for AIDS, antiviral therapy for hepatitis B and C, the treatment of tuberculosis, *Mycobacterium avium-intracellulare* and leprosy, fixed-dose combinations of antimalarial drugs, the treatment of *Cryptococcus neoformans* with flucytosine and amphotericin B, during empirical therapy for patients with febrile neutropenia, and advanced AIDS with fever. The combination of a sulfonamide and an inhibitor of dihydrofolate reductase, such as trimethoprim, is synergistic owing to the blocking of sequential steps in microbial folate synthesis.

POST-TREATMENT SUPPRESSIVE THERAPY. In some patients, after the initial disease is controlled by the antimicrobial agent, therapy is continued at a lower dose if the infection is not completely eradicated and the immunological or anatomical defect that led to the original infection is still present.

This is common in AIDS patients and post-transplant patients, for example. The goal is more as secondary prophylaxis. Nevertheless, risks of toxicity from long durations of the therapy are still real. In this group of patients, the suppressive therapy is eventually discontinued if the patient's immune system improves.

MECHANISMS OF RESISTANCE TO ANTIMICROBIAL AGENTS

Today, significant resistance is emerging to every major class of antibiotic. *Two major factors are associated with emergence of antibiotic resistance: evolution and clinical/environmental practices*. Pathogens will evolve to develop resistance to the chemical warfare to which we subject them. This evolution is mostly aided by poor therapeutic practices by healthcare workers, as well as indiscriminant use of antibiotics for agricultural and animal husbandry purposes.

Antimicrobial resistance development may develop due to:

- Reduced entry of antibiotic into pathogen
- Enhanced export of antibiotic by efflux pumps
- Release of microbial enzymes that destroy the antibiotic
- Alteration of microbial proteins that transform prodrugs to the effective moieties
- Alteration of target proteins
- Development of alternative pathways to those inhibited by the antibiotic

Mechanisms by which such resistance develops can include acquisition of genetic elements that code for the resistant mechanism, mutations that develop under antibiotic pressure, or constitutive induction.

RESISTANCE DUE TO REDUCED ENTRY OF DRUG INTO PATHOGEN. The outer membrane of gram-negative bacteria is a permeable barrier that excludes large polar molecules from entering the cell. Small polar molecules, including many antibiotics, enter the cell through protein channels called *porins*. Absence of, mutation in, or loss of a favored porin channel can slow the rate of drug entry into a cell or prevent entry altogether, effectively reducing drug concentration at the target site. If the target is intracellular and the drug requires active transport across the cell membrane, a mutation or phenotypic change that slows or abolishes this transport mechanism can confer resistance.

For example, *Trypanosoma brucei* is treated with suramin and pentamidine during early stages, but with melarsoprol and eflornithine when CNS disease (sleeping sickness) is present. Melarsoprol is actively taken up by trypanosome P2 protein transporter. When the parasite either lacks the P2 transporter, or has a mutant form, resistance to melarsoprol and cross-resistance to pentamidine occur due to reduced uptake.

RESISTANCE DUE TO DRUG EFFLUX. Microorganisms can overexpress efflux pumps and then expel antibiotics to which the microbes would otherwise be susceptible. There are 5 major systems of efflux pumps that are relevant to antimicrobial agents:

- The multidrug and toxic compound extruder (MATE)
- The major facilitator superfamily (MFS) transporters
- The small multidrug resistance (SMR) system
- The resistance nodulation division (RND) exporters
- The ATP binding cassette (ABC) transporters

Efflux pumps are a prominent mechanism of resistance for parasites, bacteria, and fungi. One of the tragic consequences of resistance emergence has been the development of drug resistance by *Plasmodium falciparum*. Drug resistance to most antimalarial drugs is mediated by an ABC transporter encoded by *Plasmodium falciparum* multidrug resistance gene 1 (Pf*mdr1*). Point mutations in the Pf*mdr1* gene lead to drug resistance and failure of chemotherapy.

RESISTANCE DUE TO DESTRUCTION OF ANTIBIOTIC. Drug inactivation is a common mechanism of drug resistance. Bacterial resistance to aminoglycosides and to β-lactam antibiotics usually is due to production of an aminoglycoside-modifying enzyme or β-lactamase, respectively.

RESISTANCE DUE TO REDUCED AFFINITY OF DRUG TO ALTERED TARGET STRUCTURE. Common consequences of single point and multiple point mutations are alterations in amino acid composition and conformation of the target protein. This change leads to a reduced affinity of drug for its target, or of a prodrug for the enzyme that converts the prodrug to active drug.

Such alterations may be due to mutation of the natural target (e.g., fluoroquinolone resistance), target modification (e.g., ribosomal protection type of resistance to macrolides and tetracyclines), or acquisition of a resistant form of the native, susceptible target (e.g., staphylococcal methicillin resistance caused by production of a low-affinity penicillin-binding protein). In HIV, resistance mutations associated with reduced affinity are encountered in protease inhibitors, integrase inhibitors, fusion inhibitors, and nonnucleoside reverse transcriptase inhibitors. Similarly, point mutations in the β-tubulin gene of worms and protozoa lead to modification of the tubulin and resistance to benzimidazoles.

DRUG DEPENDENCE IN BACTERIA. An uncommon situation occurs when an organism not only becomes resistant to an antimicrobial agent but subsequently starts requiring it for growth.

Enterococcus, which easily develops vancomycin resistance, can, after prolonged exposure to the antibiotic, develop vancomycin-requiring strains.

RESISTANCE DUE TO ENHANCED EXCISION OF INCORPORATED DRUG. Nucleoside reverse transcriptase inhibitors such as zidovudine are 2′-deoxyribonucleoside analogs that are converted to their 5′-triphosphate form and compete with natural nucleotides. These drugs are incorporated into the viral DNA chain and cause chain termination. When resistance emerges via mutations at a variety of points in the reverse transcriptase gene, phosphorolytic excision of the incorporated chain-terminating nucleoside analog is enhanced.

HETERO-RESISTANCE AND VIRAL QUASI-SPECIES. Hetero-resistance is said to be present when a subset of the total microbial population is resistant, despite the total population being considered susceptible on testing. A subclone that has alterations in genes associated with drug resistance is expected to reflect the normal mutation rates and occur at between 10^{-6} and 10^{-5} colonies.

In bacteria, hetero-resistance has been described especially for vancomycin in *Staphylococcus aureus*, vancomycin in *Enterococcus faecium*, colistin in *Acinetobacter baumannii-calcoaceticus*, rifampin, isoniazid, and streptomycin in *M. tuberculosis*, and penicillin in *Streptococcus pneumoniae*. Increased therapeutic failures and mortality may occur in patients with hetero-resistant staphylococci and *M. tuberculosis*. In fungi, hetero-resistance leading to clinical failure has been described for fluconazole in *Cryptococcus neoformans* and *Candida albicans*.

In viruses, replication is more error prone than replication in bacteria and fungi. Viral evolution under drug and immune pressure occurs relatively easily, commonly resulting in variants or quasi-species that may contain drug-resistant subpopulations. This is not often termed hetero-resistance, but the principle is the same as described for bacteria and fungi. These minority quasi-species that are resistant to antiretroviral agents are associated with failure of antiretroviral therapy.

EVOLUTIONARY BASIS OF RESISTANCE EMERGENCE

DEVELOPMENT OF RESISTANCE VIA MUTATION SELECTION. Mutation and antibiotic selection of the resistant mutant are the molecular basis for resistance for many bacteria, viruses, and fungi. Mutations may occur in the gene encoding

- The target protein, altering its structure so that it no longer binds the drug
- A protein involved in drug transport
- A protein important for drug activation or inactivation
- In a regulatory gene or promoter affecting expression of the target, a transport protein, or an inactivating enzyme

Mutations are not caused by drug exposure. They are random events that confer a survival advantage when drug is present. Any large population of drug susceptible bacteria is likely to contain rare mutants that are only slightly less susceptible than the parent. However, suboptimal dosing strategies lead to selective kill of the more susceptible population, which leaves the resistant isolates to flourish.

In some instances, a single-step mutation results in a high degree of resistance. In other circumstances, however, sequential acquisition of more than 1 mutation leads to clinically significant resistance. As an example, the combination of pyrimethamine and sulfadoxine inhibits *Plasmodium falciparum*'s folate biosynthetic pathway via inhibition of dihydrofolate reductase (DHFR) by the pyrimethamine and inhibition of dihydropteroate synthetase (DHPS) by sulfadoxine. Clinically meaningful resistance occurs when there is a single point mutation in the *DHPS* gene accompanied by at least a double mutation in the *DHFR* gene.

HYPERMUTABLE PHENOTYPES. Protecting genetic information from disintegrating and also maintaining flexibility sufficient for genetic changes that lead to adaptation to the environment are essential to life. This is accomplished principally by the insertion of the correct base pair by DNA polymerase III, proofreading by the polymerase, and postreplicative repair. The development of a defect in any of these repair mechanisms leads to mutations in many genes; such isolates are termed *mutator (Mut) phenotypes* and may include mutations in genes causing antibiotic resistance.

This second-order selection of hypermutable (mutator) alleles based on alterations in DNA repair genes has been implicated in the emergence of multidrug resistant strains of *M. tuberculosis* Beijing genotype.

RESISTANCE BY EXTERNAL ACQUISITION OF GENETIC ELEMENTS. Drug resistance may be acquired by mutation and selection, with passage of the trait *vertically* to daughter cells. For mutation and selection to be successful in generating resistance, the mutation cannot be lethal and should not appreciably alter virulence. For the trait to be passed on, the original mutant or its progeny also must disseminate and replicate.

Drug resistance more commonly is acquired by *horizontal transfer* of resistance determinants from a donor cell, often of another bacterial species, by *transduction, transformation,* or *conjugation*. Resistance acquired by horizontal transfer can disseminate rapidly and widely either by clonal spread of the resistant strain or by subsequent transfers to other susceptible recipient strains. Horizontal transfer of resistance offers several advantages over mutation selection. Lethal mutation of an essential gene is avoided; the level of resistance often is higher; the gene, which still can be transmitted vertically, can be mobilized and rapidly amplified within a population by transfer to susceptible cells; and the resistance gene can be eliminated when it no longer offers a selective advantage.

HORIZONTAL GENE TRANSFER. Horizontal transfer of resistance genes is facilitated by mobile genetic elements that include plasmids and transducing phages. Other mobile elements—transposable elements, integrons, and gene cassettes—also participate in the process. *Transposable elements* are of 3 general types: insertion sequences, transposons, and transposable phages. Only insertion sequences and transposons are important for resistance.

Insertion sequences are short segments of DNA encoding enzymatic functions (e.g., transposase and resolvase) for site-specific recombination with inverted repeat sequences at either end. They can copy themselves and insert themselves into a chromosome or a plasmid. Insertion sequences do not encode resistance, but they function as sites for integration of other resistance-encoding elements (e.g., plasmids or transposons). *Transposons* are insertion sequences that also code for other functions, 1 of which can be drug resistance. Because transposons move between chromosome and plasmid, the resistance gene can "hitchhike" with a transferable element out of the host and into a recipient. Transposons are mobile elements that excise and integrate in the bacterial genomic or plasmid DNA. *Integrons* are not formally mobile and do not copy themselves, but they encode an integrase and provide a specific site into which mobile gene cassettes integrate. *Gene cassettes* encode resistance determinants, usually lacking a promoter, with a downstream repeat sequence. The integrase recognizes this repeat sequence and directs insertion of the cassette into position behind a strong promoter that is present on the integron. Integrons may be located within transposons or in plasmids, and therefore may be mobilizable, or located on the chromosome.

Transduction is acquisition of bacterial DNA from a *phage* (a virus that propagates in bacteria) that has incorporated DNA from a previous host bacterium within its outer protein coat. If the DNA includes a gene for drug resistance, the newly infected bacterial cell may acquire resistance. Transduction is particularly important in the transfer of antibiotic resistance among strains of *S. aureus. Transformation* is the uptake and incorporation into the host genome by homologous recombination of free DNA released into the environment by other bacterial cells. Transformation is the molecular basis of penicillin resistance in pneumococci and *Neisseria. Conjugation* is gene transfer by direct cell-to-cell contact through a sex pilus or bridge. This mechanism for the spread of antibiotic resistance is important because multiple resistance genes can be transferred in a single event. Conjugation with genetic exchange between nonpathogenic and pathogenic microorganisms probably occurs in the GI tracts of humans and animals. The efficiency of transfer is low; however, antibiotics can exert a powerful selective pressure to allow emergence of the resistant strain. Genetic transfer by conjugation is common among gram-negative bacilli, and resistance is conferred on a susceptible cell as a single event. Enterococci also contain a broad range of host-range conjugative plasmids that are involved in the transfer and spread of resistance genes among gram-positive organisms.

For a complete Bibliographical Listing see Goodman & Gilman's ***The Pharmacological Basis of Therapeutics***, 12th ed., or Goodman & Gilman Online at www.AccessMedicine.com.

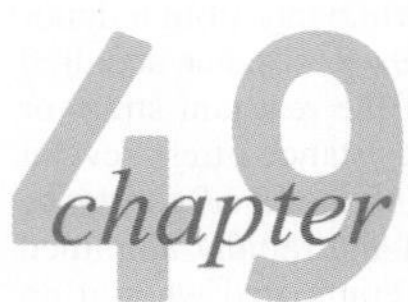

Chemotherapy of Malaria

Malaria affects about a quarter of a billion people and leads to almost 900,000 deaths annually. This disease is caused by infection with single-celled protozoan parasites of the genus *Plasmodium.* Five *Plasmodium* spp. are known to infect humans: *P. falciparum, P. vivax, P. ovale, P. malariae,* and *P. knowlesi. P. falciparum* and *P. vivax* cause most of the malarial infections worldwide. *P. falciparum* accounts for the majority of the burden of malaria in sub-Saharan Africa and is associated with the most severe disease. *P. vivax* accounts for half of the malaria burden in South and East Asia and >80% of the malarial infections in the America.

BIOLOGY OF MALARIAL INFECTION

Plasmodium sporozoites, which initiate infection in humans, are inoculated into the dermis and enter the bloodstream following the bite of a *Plasmodium*-infected female *anopheline* mosquito. Within minutes, sporozoites travel to the liver, where they infect hepatocytes via cell surface receptor-mediated events. This process initiates the *asymptomatic prepatent period*, or *exoerythrocytic stage* of infection, which typically lasts ~1 week.

During this period, the parasite undergoes asexual replication within hepatocytes, resulting in production of liver stage *schizonts*. When the infected hepatocytes rupture, tens of thousands of *merozoites* are released into the bloodstream and infect red blood cells. After the initial exoerythrocytic stage, *P. falciparum* and *P. malariae* are no longer found in the liver. *P. vivax* and *P. ovale*, however, can maintain a quiescent hepatocyte infection as a dormant form of the parasite known as the *hypnozoite* and can reinitiate symptomatic disease long after the initial symptoms of malaria are recognized and treated. Erythrocytic forms cannot reestablish infection of hepatocytes. Transmission of human-infecting malarial parasites is maintained in human populations by the persistence of hypnozoites (several months to few years for *P. vivax* and *P. ovale*), by antigenic variation in *P. falciparum* (probably months), and by the putative antigen variation in *P. malariae* (for as long as several decades).

The *asexual erythrocytic stages* of malarial parasites are responsible for the clinical manifestations of malaria. This part of the *Plasmodium* life cycle is initiated by merozoite recognition of red blood cells, mediated by cell surface receptors, followed by red blood cell invasion.

Once inside a red blood cell, the merozoite develops into a ring form, which becomes a trophozoite that matures into an asexually dividing blood stage schizont. Upon rupture of the infected erythrocyte, these schizonts release 8-32 merozoites that can establish new infections in nearby red blood cells. The erythrocytic replication cycle lasts for 24 h (for *P. knowlesi*), 48 h (for *P. falciparum, P. vivax,* and *P. ovale*), and 72 h (for *P. malariae*). Although most invading merozoites develop into schizonts, a small proportion become gametocytes, the form of the parasite that is infective to mosquitoes. Gametocytes are ingested into the mosquito midgut during an infectious blood meal and then transform into gametes that can fertilize to become zygotes. Zygotes mature into ookinetes, which penetrate the mosquito midgut wall and develop into oocysts. Numerous rounds of asexual replication occur in the oocyst to generate sporozoites over 10-14 days. Fully developed sporozoites rupture from oocysts and invade the mosquito salivary glands, from which they can initiate a new infection during subsequent mosquito blood meals (Figure 49–1).

P. falciparum has a family of binding proteins that can recognize a variety of host cell molecules; it invades all stages of erythrocytes and therefore can achieve high parasitemias. *P. vivax* selectively binds to the Duffy chemokine receptor protein as well as reticulocyte-specific proteins. *P. falciparum* assembles cytoadherence proteins (PfEMP1s, encoded by a highly variable family of *var* genes) into structures called knobs that are presented on the erythrocyte surface. Knobs allow the *P. falciparum*-parasitized erythrocyte to bind to post-capillary vascular endothelium, so as to avoid spleen-mediated clearance and allow the parasite to grow in a low O_2, high CO_2 microenvironment.

The cardinal signs and symptoms of malaria are high, spiking fevers, chills, headaches, myalgias, malaise, and GI symptoms. The clinical manifestations of malaria are detailed in Chapter 49 of the 12th edition of the parent text.

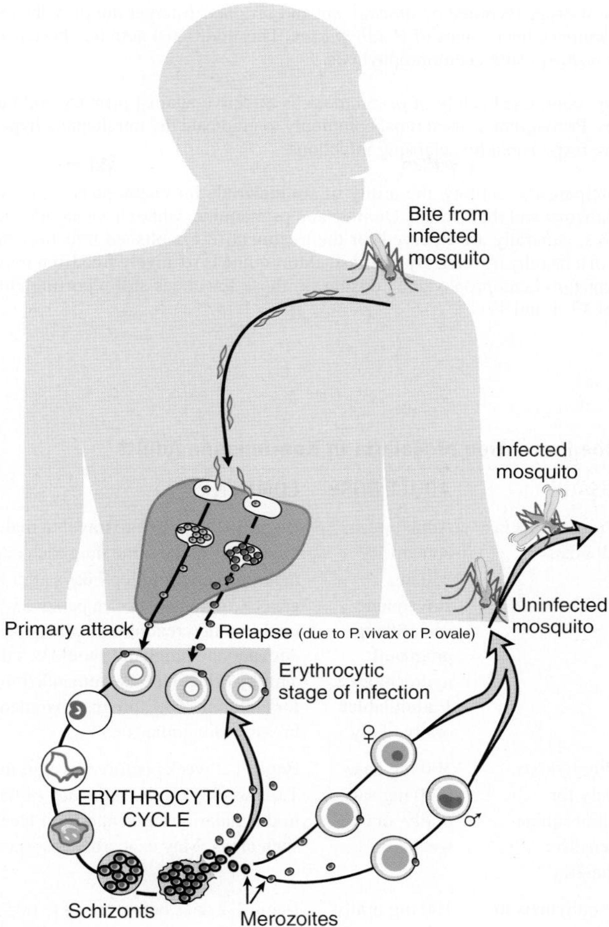

Figure 49–1 *Life cycle of malaria parasites.*

CLASSIFICATION OF ANTIMALARIAL AGENTS

The various stages of the malarial parasite life cycle in humans differ in their drug sensitivity. Thus, antimalarial drugs can be classified based on their activities during this life cycle as well as by their intended use for either chemoprophylaxis or treatment. The spectrum of antimalarial drug activity leads to several generalizations.

The first relates to chemoprophylaxis: *because no antimalarial drug kills sporozoites, it is not truly possible to prevent infection; drugs can only prevent the development of symptomatic malaria caused by the asexual erythrocytic forms*.

The second relates to the treatment of an established infection: *no single antimalarial is effective against all liver and intra-erythrocytic stages of the life cycle that may coexist in the same patient. Complete elimination of the parasite infection, therefore, may require more than 1 drug.*

The patterns of clinically useful activity fall into 3 general categories.

The first group of agents (*artemisinins, chloroquine, mefloquine, quinine* and *quinidine, pyrimethamine, sulfadoxine,* and *tetracycline*) are not reliably effective against primary or latent liver stages. Instead, their action is directed against the asexual blood stages responsible for disease. These drugs will treat, or prevent, clinically symptomatic malaria.

The second group of drugs (typified by *atovaquone* and *proguanil*) target not only the asexual erythrocytic forms but also the primary liver stages of *P. falciparum*. This additional activity shortens to several days the required period for postexposure chemoprophylaxis.

The third category, comprised solely of *primaquine*, is effective against primary and latent liver stages as well as gametocytes. Primaquine is used most commonly to eradicate the intrahepatic hypnozoites of *P. vivax* and *P. ovale* that are responsible for relapsing infections.

Aside from their antiparasitic activity, the utility of antimalarials for chemoprophylaxis or therapy depends on their pharmacokinetics and their safety. Quinine and primaquine, which have significant toxicity and relatively short half-lives, generally are reserved for the treatment of established infection and are not used for chemoprophylaxis in a healthy traveler. By contrast, chloroquine is relatively free from toxicity and has a long $t_{1/2}$ that is convenient for chemoprophylactic dosing (in those few areas still reporting chloroquine-sensitive malaria) (*see* Tables 49–1 and 49–2).

Table 49–1

Regimens for the Prevention of Malaria in Non-immune Adults

DRUG	USAGE	ADULT DOSE	COMMENTS
Atovaquone/ proguanil	Prophylaxis in all areas	Adult tablets contain 250 mg atovaquone and 100 mg proguanil hydrochloride. 1 adult tablet orally, daily	Begin 1-2 days before travel to malarious areas. Take daily at the same time each day while in the malarious area and for 7 days after leaving such areas. Contraindicated in persons with severe renal impairment (creatinine clearance <30 mL/minute). Atovaquone/proguanil should be taken with food or a milky drink. Not recommended for prophylaxis for children <5 kg, pregnant women, and women breastfeeding infants <5 kg.
Chloroquine phosphate	Prophylaxis only for chloroquine-sensitive malaria	300 mg base (500 mg salt) orally, once/ week	Begin 1-2 weeks before travel to malarious areas. Take weekly on the same day of the week while in the malarious area and for 4 weeks after leaving such areas. May exacerbate psoriasis.
Doxycycline	Prophylaxis in all areas	100 mg orally, daily	Begin 1-2 days before travel to malarious areas. Take daily at the same time each day while in the malarious area and for 4 weeks after leaving such areas. Contraindicated in children <8 years of age and pregnant women.
Hydroxy-chloroquine sulfate	An alternative to chloroquine for prophylaxis only in areas with chloroquine-sensitive malaria	310 mg base (400 mg salt) orally, once/ week	Begin 1-2 weeks before travel to malarious areas. Take weekly on the same day of the week while in the malarious area and for 4 weeks after leaving such areas.
Mefloquine	Prophylaxis in areas with mefloquine-sensitive malaria	228 mg base (250 mg salt) orally, once/ week	Begin 1-2 weeks before travel to malarious areas. Take weekly on same day of the week while in malarious area and for 4 weeks after leaving such areas. Contraindicated in persons allergic to mefloquine or related compounds (e.g., quinine, quinidine) and in persons with active depression, a history of depression, generalized anxiety disorder, psychosis, schizophrenia, other major psychiatric disorders, or seizures. Not recommended for persons with cardiac conduction abnormalities.

(*continued*)

Table 49–1

Regimens for the Prevention of Malaria in Non-immune Adults (*Continued*)

DRUG	USAGE	ADULT DOSE	COMMENTS
Primaquine	Prophylaxis for short-duration travel to areas with principally *P. vivax*	30 mg base (52.6 mg salt) orally, daily	Begin 1-2 days before travel to malarious areas. Take daily at same time each day while in malarious area and for 7 days after leaving such areas. Contraindicated in persons with G6PD[a] deficiency, and during pregnancy and lactation unless the infant being breastfed has documented normal G6PD level.
Primaquine	For presumptive anti-relapse therapy (terminal prophylaxis) to decrease the risk of relapses (*P. vivax*, *P. ovale*)	30 mg base (52.6 mg salt) orally, once/day for 14 days after departure from the malarious area	Indicated for persons who have had prolonged exposure to *P. vivax* and *P. ovale* or both. Contraindicated in persons with G6PD[a] deficiency, during pregnancy, and during lactation unless the breastfed infant has a documented normal G6PD level.

[a]Glucose-6-phosphate dehydrogenase. All persons who take primaquine should have a documented normal G6PD level before starting the medication. These regimens are based on recommendations of the U.S. Centers for Disease Control and Prevention (CDC). These recommendations may change over time. Recommendations and available treatment differ among countries in the industrialized world, developing world, and malaria-endemic regions; in the latter, some antimalarial treatments may be available without prescription, but the most effective drugs usually are controlled by governmental agencies. Consult the CDC Yellow Book for up-to-date information and for pediatric dosing.
Source: CDC Yellow Book 2014, http://www.cdc.gov/features/yellowbook/, accessed August 23, 2013.

For ease of reference, detailed information on the antimalarial drugs appears below in alphabetical order by drug name.

ARTEMISININ AND DERIVATIVES

Artemisinin and its 3 major semisynthetic derivatives in clinical use, dihydroartemisinin, artemether, and artesunate, are potent and fast-acting antimalarials. They are particularly well suited for the treatment of severe *P. falciparum* malaria and are also effective against the asexual erythrocytic stages of *P. vivax*. Increasingly, the standard treatment of malaria employs *artemisinin-based combination therapies* (ACTs) to increase treatment efficacy and reduce selection pressure for the emergence of drug resistance.

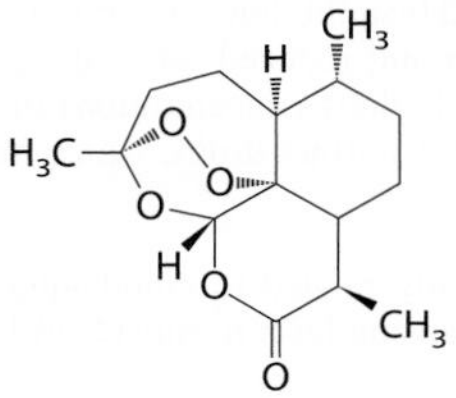

CH_3 H H_3C O O O H O CH_3 O

ARTEMISININ

Artemisinins cause a significant reduction of the parasite burden, with a 4-$\log_{10}$ reduction in the parasite population for each 48-h cycle of intraerythrocytic invasion, replication, and egress. Only 3 to 4 cycles (6-8 days) of treatment are required to remove all the parasites from the blood. Additionally, artemisinins possess some gametocytocidal activity, leading to a decrease in malarial parasite transmission.

Mechanism of Action. The activity of artemisinin and derivatives seems to result from cleavage of the drug's peroxide bridge by reduced heme-iron, produced inside the highly acidic digestive vacuole (DV) of the parasite as it digests hemoglobin. The site of action of the putatively toxic heme-adducts is unclear. Additionally, activated artemisinin might in turn generate free radicals that alkylate and oxidize macromolecules in the parasite.

ADME. The semisynthetic artemisinins have been formulated for oral (dihydroartemisinin, artesunate, and artemether), intramuscular (artesunate and artemether), intravenous (artesunate), and rectal (artesunate) routes. Bioavailability after oral dosing typically is ≤30%. Peak serum levels occur rapidly with artemisinins and in 2-6 h with intramuscular artemether. Both artesunate and artemether have modest levels of plasma protein binding, ranging from 43-82%. These derivatives are extensively metabolized and converted to dihydroartemisinin, which has a plasma $t_{1/2}$ of 1-2 h. Drug bioavailability via rectal administration is highly variable among individual patients. With repeated dosing, artemisinin and artesunate induce their own CYP-mediated metabolism, primarily via CYPs 2B6 and 3A4. This may enhance clearance by up to 5-fold.

Therapeutic Uses. Given their rapid and potent activity against even multidrug-resistant parasites, the artemisinins are valuable for the treatment of severe *P. falciparum* malaria. The artemisinins generally are not used alone because of their limited ability to eradicate infection completely. Artemisinins are highly effective, when combined with other antimalarials, for the first-line treatment of malaria. Artemisinins should not be used for chemoprophylaxis because of their short $t_{1/2}$.

Toxicity and Contraindications. In pregnant rats and rabbits, artemisinins can cause increased embryo lethality or malformations early postconception. Preclinical toxicity studies have identified the brain (and brainstem), liver, bone marrow, and fetus as the principal target organs. However, no systematic neurological changes were attributable to treatment in patients >5 years of age. Patients may develop dose-related and reversible decreases in reticulocyte and neutrophil counts and increases in transaminase levels. About 1 in 3000 patients develops an allergic reaction. Studies of artemisinin treatment during the first trimester have found no evidence of adverse effects on fetal development. Nonetheless, it is recommended that ACTs not be used for the treatment of children ≤5 kg or during the first trimester of pregnancy.

ACT PARTNER DRUGS. Current ACT regimens that are well tolerated in adults and children ≥5 kg include artemether/lumefantrine, artesunate-mefloquine, artesunate-amodiaquine, artesunate-sulfadoxine-pyrimethamine, and dihydroartemisinin-piperaquine.

Lumefantrine shares structural similarities with the arylamino alcohol drugs mefloquine and halofantrine and is formulated with artemether (COARTEM). This combination is highly effective for the treatment of uncomplicated malaria and is the most widely used first-line antimalarial across Africa. The pharmacokinetic properties of lumefantrine include a large apparent volume of distribution and a terminal elimination $t_{1/2}$ of 4-5 days. Administration with a high-fat meal is recommended because it significantly increases absorption. A sweetened dispersible formulation of artemether-lumefantrine (COARTEM *DISPERSIBLE*) has been approved for treatment of children.

Amodiaquine is a congener of chloroquine that is no longer recommended in the U.S. for chemoprophylaxis of *P. falciparum* malaria because of its toxicity (hepatic and agranulocytosis) that were generally associated with its prophylactic use. Amodiaquine is rapidly converted by hepatic CYPs into monodesethyl-amodiaquine. This metabolite, which retains substantial antimalarial activity, has a plasma $t_{1/2}$ of 9-18 days and reaches a peak concentration of ~500 nM 2 h after oral administration. By contrast, amodiaquine has a $t_{1/2}$ of ~3 h, attaining a peak concentration of ~25 nM within 30 min of oral administration. Clearance rates of amodiaquine ranges between individuals from 78-943 mL/min/kg.

Piperaquine is a potent and well-tolerated bisquinoline compound structurally related to chloroquine. Piperaquine has a large volume of distribution and reduced rates of excretion after multiple doses. It is rapidly absorbed, with a T_{max} (time to reach the highest concentration) of 2 h after a single dose. Piperaquine has the longest plasma $t_{1/2}$ (5 weeks) of all ACT partner drugs, which might also be effective in reducing rates of reinfection following treatment.

Pyronaridine is an antimalarial structurally related to amodiaquine. It is well tolerated and highly potent against both *P. falciparum* and *P. vivax*, causing fever to subside in 1-2 days and parasite clearance in 2-3 days.

ATOVAQUONE

A fixed combination of *atovaquone* with *proguanil hydrochloride* (MALARONE) is available in the U.S. for malaria chemoprophylaxis and for the treatment of uncomplicated *P. falciparum* malaria in adults and children.

Antimalarial Action and Resistance. Atovaquone is a lipophilic analog of ubiquinone, the electron acceptor for parasite dihydroorotate dehydrogenase, an enzyme essential for pyrimidine biosynthesis in the parasite. Atovaquone inhibits electron transport, collapses the mitochondrial membrane potential, and inhibits regeneration of ubiquinone. The drug is highly active against *P. falciparum* asexual blood stage parasites and the liver stages of *P. falciparum,* but not against *P. vivax* liver stage hypnozoites. Synergy between proguanil and atovaquone results from the ability of nonmetabolized proguanil to enhance the mitochondrial toxicity of atovaquone. Resistance to atovaquone alone in *P. falciparum* develops easily and is conferred by single nonsynonymous nucleotide polymorphisms in the cytochrome b gene located in the mitochondrial genome. Addition of proguanil markedly reduces the frequency of appearance of atovaquone resistance. However, once atovaquone resistance is present, the synergy of the partner drug proguanil diminishes.

ADME. Atovaquone absorption is slow and variable after an oral dose due to its lipophilicity. Absorption improves when the drug is taken with a fatty meal. More than 99% of the drug is bound to plasma protein; cerebrospinal fluid levels are <1% of those in plasma. Profiles of drug concentration versus time often show a double peak; the first at 1-8 h, the second 1-4 days after a single dose; this pattern suggests an enterohepatic circulation. In the absence of a CYP-inducing second medication, humans do not metabolize atovaquone significantly. The drug is excreted in bile, and >94% of the drug is recovered unchanged in feces. Atovaquone has a reported elimination $t_{1/2}$ from plasma of 2-3 days in adults and 1-2 days in children.

Therapeutic Uses. A tablet containing a fixed dose of 250 mg atovaquone and 100 mg proguanil hydrochloride, taken orally, is highly effective and safe in a 3-day regimen for treating mild-to-moderate attacks of chloroquine- or sulfadoxine-pyrimethamine-resistant *P. falciparum* malaria. The same regimen followed by a primaquine course is effective in treatment of *P. vivax* malaria. Atovaquone-proguanil is a standard agent for malaria chemoprophylaxis. Experience in prevention of non–*P. falciparum* malaria is limited. *P. vivax* infection may occur after drug discontinuation, indicating imperfect activity against exo-erythrocytic stages of this parasite.

Toxicity. Atovaquone may cause side effects (abdominal pain, nausea, vomiting, diarrhea, headache, rash) that require cessation of therapy. Vomiting and diarrhea may decrease drug absorption, resulting in therapeutic failure. However, readministration of this drug within an hour of vomiting may still be effective in patients with *P. falciparum* malaria. Atovaquone occasionally causes transient elevations of serum transaminase or amylase.

Precautions and Contraindications. Although atovaquone is generally considered to be safe, it needs further evaluation in children <11 kg, pregnant women, and lactating mothers. Atovaquone may compete with certain drugs for binding to plasma proteins, and therapy with rifampin, a potent inducer of CYP-mediated drug metabolism, can reduce plasma levels of atovaquone substantially, whereas atovaquone may raise plasma levels of rifampin. Coadministration with tetracycline is associated with a 40% reduction in plasma concentration of atovaquone.

DIAMINOPYRIMIDINES

Sulfadoxine-pyrimethamine (FANSIDAR) was a primary treatment for uncomplicated *P. falciparum* malaria, especially against chloroquine-resistant strains. Due to widespread resistance, it is no longer recommended for the treatment of uncomplicated malaria.

Antimalarial Action and Resistance. Pyrimethamine is a slow-acting blood *schizontocide* with antimalarial effects in vivo resulting from inhibition of *folate biosynthesis* in *Plasmodium,* similar to proguanil. The efficacy of pyrimethamine against hepatic forms of *P. falciparum* is less than that of proguanil, and at therapeutic doses pyrimethamine fails to eradicate *P. vivax* hypnozoites or gametocytes of any *Plasmodium* species. It increases the number of circulating *P. falciparum* mature infecting gametocytes, likely leading to increased transmission to mosquitoes during the period of treatment.

Synergy of pyrimethamine and the sulfonamides or sulfones results from inhibition of 2 metabolic steps in folate biosynthesis in the parasite:

- The utilization of *p*-aminobenzoic acid for the synthesis of dihydropteroic acid, which is catalyzed by dihydropteroate synthase and inhibited by sulfonamides
- The reduction of dihydrofolate to tetrahydrofolate, which is catalyzed by dihydrofolate reductase and inhibited by pyrimethamine (*see* Figure 52–2).

Dietary *p*-aminobenzoic acid or folate may affect the therapeutic response to antifolates. Resistance to pyrimethamine has developed in regions of prolonged or extensive drug use and can be attributed to mutations in dihydrofolate reductase that decrease the binding affinity of pyrimethamine.

ADME. Oral pyrimethamine is slowly but completely absorbed, reaching peak plasma levels in 2-6 h. The compound is significantly distributed in the tissues and is ~90% bound to plasma proteins. Pyrimethamine is slowly eliminated from plasma with a $t_{1/2}$ of 85-100 h. Concentrations that are suppressive for responsive *Plasmodium* strains remain in the blood for ~2 weeks. Pyrimethamine also enters the milk of nursing mothers.

Therapeutic Uses. Pyrimethamine-sulfadoxine is no longer recommended for the treatment of uncomplicated malaria or for chemoprophylaxis due to increasing drug resistance. However, for those living in malaria-endemic areas, some still recommend it for the intermittent preventive treatment of malaria in pregnancy.

Toxicity, Precautions, and Contraindications. Antimalarial doses of pyrimethamine alone cause minimal toxicity except for occasional skin rashes and reduced hematopoiesis. Excessive doses can produce a megaloblastic anemia, resembling that of folate deficiency, which responds readily to drug withdrawal or treatment with folinic acid. At high doses, pyrimethamine is teratogenic in animals, and in humans the related combination, trimethoprim-sulfamethoxazole, may cause birth defects.

Sulfonamides or sulfones, rather than pyrimethamine, usually account for the toxicity associated with coadministration of these antifolate drugs. The combination of pyrimethamine and sulfadoxine causes severe and even fatal cutaneous reactions, such as erythema multiforme, Stevens-Johnson syndrome, or toxic epidermal necrolysis. It has also been associated with serum sickness–type reactions, urticaria, exfoliative dermatitis, and hepatitis. Pyrimethamine-sulfadoxine is contraindicated for individuals with previous reactions to sulfonamides, for lactating mothers, and for infants <2 months of age. Administration of pyrimethamine with dapsone (MALOPRIM), a drug combination unavailable in the U.S., has occasionally been associated with agranulocytosis.

PROGUANIL

The antimalarial activity of proguanil (chloroguanide) is ascribed to cycloguanil, a cyclic triazine metabolite (structurally related to pyrimethamine) and selective inhibitor of the bifunctional plasmodial dihydrofolate reductase-thymidylate synthetase that is crucial for parasite de novo purine and pyrimidine synthesis.

Antimalarial Action and Resistance. In drug-sensitive *P. falciparum* malaria, proguanil exerts activity against both the primary liver stages and the asexual red blood cell stages, thus adequately controlling the acute attack and usually eradicating the infection. Proguanil is also active against acute *P. vivax* malaria, but because the latent tissue stages of *P. vivax* are unaffected, relapses may occur after the drug is withdrawn. Proguanil treatment does not destroy gametocytes, but oocytes in the gut of the mosquito can fail to develop normally.

Cycloguanil selectively inhibits the bifunctional dihydrofolate reductase–thymidylate synthetase of sensitive plasmodia, causing inhibition of DNA synthesis and depletion of folate cofactors. A series of amino acid changes near the dihydrofolate reductase–binding site have been identified that cause resistance to cycloguanil, pyrimethamine, or both. The presence of *Plasmodium* dihydrofolate reductase is not required for the intrinsic antimalarial activity of proguanil or chlorproguanil; however, the molecular basis for this alternative activity is unknown. Proguanil accentuates the mitochondrial membrane-potential-collapsing action of atovaquone against *P. falciparum* but displays no such activity by itself. In contrast to cycloguanil, resistance to the parent drug, proguanil, either alone or in combination with atovaquone, is not well documented.

ADME. Proguanil is slowly but adequately absorbed from the GI tract. After a single oral dose, peak plasma concentrations are attained within 5 h. The mean plasma elimination $t_{1/2}$ is ~180-200 h or longer. The drug's metabolism and activation involves the CYP2C subfamily; ~3% of whites are deficient in this oxidation phenotype, contrasted with ~20% of Asians and Kenyans. Proguanil is oxidized to 2 major metabolites, cycloguanil and an inactive 4-chlorophenyl biguanide. On a 200-mg-daily dosage regimen, plasma levels of cycloguanil in extensive metabolizers exceed the therapeutic range, whereas cycloguanil levels in poor metabolizers do not. Proguanil itself does not accumulate appreciably in tissues during long-term administration, except in red blood cells where its concentration is about 3 times that in plasma. In humans, 40-60% of the absorbed proguanil is excreted in urine, either as the parent drug or as the active metabolite.

Therapeutic Uses. Proguanil as a single agent is not available in the U.S. but has been prescribed as chemoprophylaxis in England and Europe for individuals traveling to malarious areas in Africa. Strains of *P. falciparum* resistant to proguanil emerge rapidly in areas where the drug is used exclusively, but breakthrough infections may also result from deficient conversion of proguanil to its active antimalarial metabolite. Proguanil is effective and tolerated well in combination with atovaquone, once daily for 3 days, to treat drug-resistant strains of *P. falciparum* or *P. vivax* (see section on atovaquone). *P. falciparum* readily develops clinical resistance to monotherapy with either proguanil or atovaquone; however, resistance to the combination is uncommon unless the strain is initially resistant to atovaquone.

Toxicity and Side Effects. In chemoprophylactic doses of 200-300 mg daily, proguanil causes relatively few adverse effects, except occasional nausea and diarrhea. Large doses (≥1 g daily) may cause vomiting, abdominal pain, diarrhea, hematuria, and the transient appearance of epithelial cells and casts in the urine. Doses as high as 700 mg twice daily have been taken for >2 weeks without serious toxicity. Proguanil is safe for use during pregnancy. It is remarkably safe when used in conjunction with other antimalarial drugs.

QUINOLINES AND RELATED COMPOUNDS

Quinine is the chief alkaloid of cinchona, the powdered bark of the South American cinchona tree. Quinine and its many derivatives have been the mainstay of malarial treatment for 4 centuries. Structure-activity analysis of the cinchona alkaloids provided the basis for the discovery of more recent antimalarials such as mefloquine.

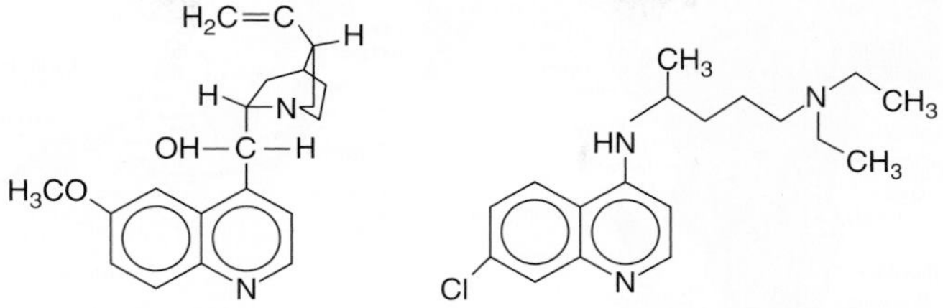

QUININE

CHLOROQUINE

ANTIMALARIAL ACTION. Asexual malarial parasites flourish in host erythrocytes by digesting hemoglobin; this generates free radicals and iron-bound heme as highly reactive by-products. Heme is sequestered as an insoluble, chemically inert malarial pigment termed *hemozoin*. Quinolines interfere with heme sequestration. Failure to inactivate heme and drug-heme complexes is thought to kill the parasites via oxidative damage to membranes, or other critical biomolecules.

CHLOROQUINE AND HYDROXYCHLOROQUINE

Chloroquine, a weak base, concentrates in the highly acidic digestive vacuoles of susceptible *Plasmodium*, where it binds to heme and disrupts its sequestration. Hydroxychloroquine, in which 1 of the *N*-ethyl substituents of chloroquine is β-hydroxylated, is essentially equivalent to chloroquine against *P. falciparum* malaria.

Resistance. Resistance of erythrocytic asexual forms of *P. falciparum* to antimalarial quinolines, especially chloroquine, now is common (Figure 49–2). Chloroquine resistance results from mutations in the polymorphic gene *pfcrt* gene (*pfcrt*, for *P. falciparum* chloroquine resistance transporter) that encodes a putative transporter that resides in the membrane of the acidic digestive vacuole, the site of hemoglobin degradation and chloroquine action. In addition to PfCRT, the P-glycoprotein transporter encoded by *pfmdr1,* and other transporters including PfMRP, may play a modulatory role in chloroquine resistance.

ADME. Chloroquine is well absorbed from the GI tract and rapidly from intramuscular and subcutaneous sites. This drug extensively sequesters in tissues, particularly liver, spleen, kidney, lung, and, to a lesser extent, brain and spinal cord. Chloroquine binds moderately (60%) to plasma proteins and is transformed via hepatic CYPs to 2 active metabolites, desethylchloroquine and bisdesethylchloroquine. The renal clearance of chloroquine is about half of its total systemic clearance. Unchanged chloroquine and desethylchloroquine account for >50% and 25% of the urinary drug products, respectively, and their renal excretion is increased by urine acidification. To avoid potentially lethal toxicity, parenteral chloroquine is given either slowly by constant intravenous infusion or in small divided doses by the subcutaneous or intramuscular route. Chloroquine is safer when given orally because the rates of absorption and distribution are more closely matched. Peak plasma levels are achieved in ~3-5 h. The $t_{1/2}$ of chloroquine increases from a few days to weeks as plasma levels decline. The terminal $t_{1/2}$ ranges from 30 to 60 days, and traces of the drug can be found in the urine for years after a therapeutic regimen.

Therapeutic Uses. Chloroquine is highly effective against the erythrocytic forms of *P. vivax, P. ovale, P. malariae, P. knowlesi,* and chloroquine-sensitive strains of *P. falciparum*. For infections caused by *P. ovale* and *P. malariae,* it remains the agent of choice for chemoprophylaxis and treatment. For *P. falciparum* this drug has been largely replaced by ACTs.

The utility of chloroquine has declined across most malaria-endemic regions of the world because of the spread of chloroquine-resistant *P. falciparum*. Except in areas where resistant strains of *P. vivax* are reported, chloroquine is very effective in chemoprophylaxis or treatment of acute attacks of malaria caused by *P. vivax, P. ovale*, and *P. malariae*. Chloroquine has no activity against primary or latent liver stages of the parasite. To prevent relapses in *P. vivax* and *P. ovale* infections, primaquine can be given either with chloroquine or used after a patient leaves an endemic area. Chloroquine rapidly controls the clinical symptoms and parasitemia of acute malarial attacks. Most patients become completely afebrile within 24-48 h after receiving therapeutic doses. If patients fail to respond during the second day of chloroquine therapy, resistant strains should be suspected and therapy instituted with quinine plus tetracycline or doxycycline, or

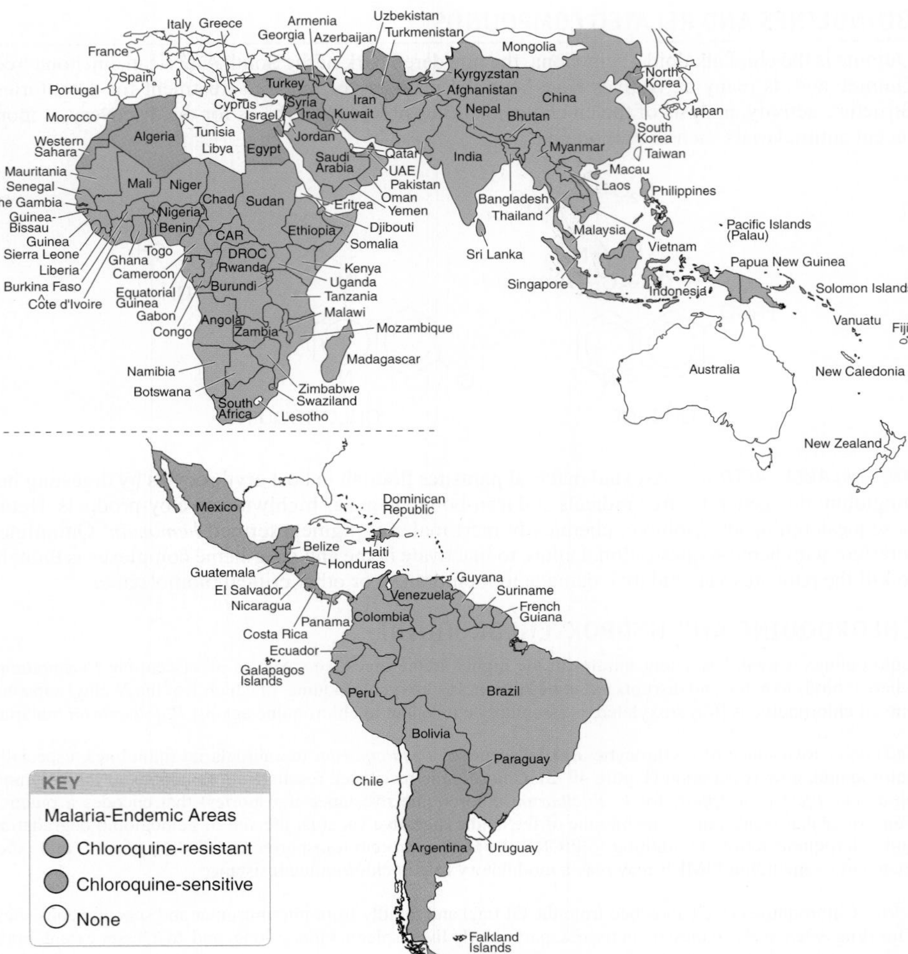

Figure 49–2 *Malaria-endemic countries in the Americas (bottom) and in Africa, the Middle East, Asia, and the South Pacific (top), 2007.* CAR, Central African Republic; DCOR, Democratic Republic of the Congo; UAE, United Arab Emirates. (Reproduced with permission from Fauci AS, Braunwald E, Kasper DL, Hauser SL, Longo DL, Jameson JL, Loscalzo J, eds. *Harrison's Principles of Internal Medicine,* 17th ed. New York: McGraw-Hill; 2008, Figure 203–2, p 1282. Copyright © 2008 by The McGraw-Hill Companies, Inc. All rights reserved.)

atovaquone-proguanil, or artemether-lumefantrine, or mefloquine if the others are not available. In comatose children, chloroquine is well absorbed and effective when given through a nasogastric tube. Tables 49–1 and 49–2 provide information about recommended chemoprophylactic and therapeutic dosage regimens involving chloroquine. Chloroquine and its analogs are also used to treat certain nonmalarial conditions, including hepatic amebiasis.

Toxicity and Side Effects. Taken in proper doses and for recommended total durations, chloroquine is very safe. However, its safety margin is narrow, and a single dose of 30 mg/kg may be fatal. Acute chloroquine toxicity is encountered most frequently when therapeutic or high doses are administered too rapidly by parenteral routes. Cardiovascular effects include hypotension, vasodilation, suppressed myocardial function, cardiac arrhythmias, and eventual cardiac arrest. Confusion, convulsions, and coma may also result from overdose. Chloroquine doses of >5 g given parenterally usually are fatal. Prompt treatment with mechanical ventilation, epinephrine, and diazepam may be lifesaving.

Doses of chloroquine used for oral therapy of the acute malarial attack may cause GI upset, headache, visual disturbances, and urticaria. Pruritus also occurs most commonly among dark-skinned persons. Prolonged treatment with suppressive doses occasionally causes side effects such as headache, blurring of vision, diplopia, confusion, convulsions, lichenoid skin eruptions, bleaching of hair, widening of the QRS interval, and T-wave abnormalities. These complications usually disappear soon after the drug is withheld. Rare instances of hemolysis and blood dyscrasias have been reported. Chloroquine may cause discoloration of nail beds and mucous membranes. This drug has also been reported to interfere with the immunogenicity of certain vaccines. Irreversible retinopathy and ototoxicity can result from high daily doses of chloroquine or hydroxychloroquine (>250 mg) leading to cumulative total doses of >1 g/kg. Retinopathy presumably is related to drug accumulation in melanin containing tissues and can be avoided if the daily dose is ≤250 mg. Prolonged therapy with high doses of chloroquine or hydroxychloroquine also can cause toxic myopathy, cardiopathy, and peripheral neuropathy. These reactions improve if the drug is withdrawn promptly. Rarely, neuropsychiatric disturbances, including suicide, may be related to overdose.

Precautions and Contraindications. Chloroquine is not recommended for treating individuals with epilepsy or myasthenia gravis, and should be used cautiously if at all in the presence of advanced liver disease or severe GI, neurological, or blood disorders. The dose should be adjusted in renal failure. In rare cases, chloroquine can cause hemolysis in patients with G6PD deficiency. Chloroquine should not be prescribed for patients with psoriasis or other exfoliative skin conditions. It should not be used to treat malaria in patients with porphyria cutanea tarda; however, it can be used in lower doses for treatment of manifestations of this form of porphyria. Chloroquine inhibits CYP2D6 and thus can interact with a variety of different drugs. It attenuates the efficacy of the yellow fever vaccine when administered at the same time. It should not be given with mefloquine because of increased risk of seizures. Chloroquine opposes the action of anticonvulsants and increases the risk of ventricular arrhythmias when coadministered with amiodarone or halofantrine. By increasing plasma levels of digoxin and cyclosporine, chloroquine can increase the risk of toxicity from these agents. Patients receiving long-term, high-dose therapy should undergo ophthalmological and neurological evaluations every 3-6 months.

QUININE AND QUINIDINE

Oral quinine is FDA-approved for the treatment of uncomplicated *P. falciparum* malaria. Quinidine, a stereoisomer of quinine, is more potent as an antimalarial and more toxic than quinine.

ANTIMALARIAL ACTION AND PARASITE RESISTANCE. Quinine acts against asexual erythrocytic forms and has no significant effect on hepatic forms of malarial parasites. This drug is more toxic and less effective than chloroquine against malarial parasites susceptible to both drugs. However, quinine, along with its stereoisomer quinidine, is especially valuable for the parenteral treatment of severe illness owing to drug-resistant strains of *P. falciparum*. Because of its toxicity and short $t_{1/2}$, quinine is generally not used for chemoprophylaxis. The antimalarial mechanism of quinine is presumably similar to that of chloroquine. The basis of *P. falciparum* resistance to quinine is complex. Patterns of *P. falciparum* resistance to quinine correlate in some strains with resistance to chloroquine yet in others correlate more closely with resistance to mefloquine and halofantrine. A number of transporter genes may confer resistance to quinine.

Action on Skeletal Muscle. Quinine increases the tension response to a single maximal stimulus delivered to muscle directly or through nerves, but it also increases the refractory period of muscle so that the response to tetanic stimulation is diminished. The excitability of the motor end-plate region decreases so that responses to repetitive nerve stimulation and to acetylcholine are reduced. Quinine can antagonize the actions of physostigmine on skeletal muscle. Quinine may also produce alarming respiratory distress and dysphagia in patients with myasthenia gravis.

ADME. Quinine is readily absorbed when given orally or intramuscularly. Oral absorption occurs mainly from the upper small intestine and is >80% complete, even in patients with marked diarrhea. After an oral dose, plasma levels reach a maximum in 3-8 h and, after distributing into an apparent volume of ~1.5 L/kg, decline with a $t_{1/2}$ of ~11 h. The pharmacokinetics of quinine may change according to the severity of malarial infection: the apparent volume of distribution and the systemic clearance of quinine decrease, such that the average elimination $t_{1/2}$ increases to 18 h. The high levels of plasma α_1-acid glycoprotein produced in severe malaria may prevent toxicity by binding quinine and thereby reducing the free fraction of drug. Concentrations of quinine are lower in erythrocytes (33-40%) and CSF (2-5%) than in plasma, and the drug readily reaches fetal tissues. The cinchona alkaloids are metabolized extensively, especially by hepatic CYP3A4; thus, only ~20% of an administered dose is excreted in an unaltered form in the urine. The major metabolite of quinine, 3-hydroxyquinine, retains some antimalarial activity and can accumulate and possibly cause toxicity in patients with renal failure. Renal excretion of quinine itself is more rapid when the urine is acidic.

THERAPEUTIC USES. Quinine and quinidine have long been treatments of choice for drug-resistant and severe *P. falciparum* malaria. However, the advent of oral and intravenous artemisinin therapy is changing this situation. In severe illness, the prompt use of loading doses of intravenous quinine (or quinidine, where intravenous quinine is not available) can be lifesaving. Oral medication to maintain therapeutic concentrations is then given as soon as tolerated and is continued for 5-7 days. Especially for treatment of infections with multidrug-resistant strains of *P. falciparum*, slower-acting blood schizonticides such as tetracyclines or clindamycin are given concurrently to enhance quinine efficacy. Formulations of quinine and quinidine and specific regimens for their use in the treatment of *P. falciparum* malaria are shown in Table 49–2. The therapeutic range for "free" quinine is 0.2 and 2.0 mg/L. Regimens needed to achieve this target vary based on patient age, severity of illness, and the responsiveness of *P. falciparum* to the drug. Dosage regimens for quinidine are similar to those for quinine, although quinidine binds less to plasma proteins and has a larger apparent volume of distribution, greater systemic clearance, and shorter terminal elimination $t_{1/2}$ than quinine. The CDC recommends a dose of quinidine of 10 mg salt/kg initially, followed by 0.02 mg salt/kg/min).

Nocturnal Leg Cramps. It is commonly believed that night cramps are relieved by quinine (200-300 mg) taken at bedtime. The FDA has required drug manufacturers to stop marketing over-the-counter quinine products for nocturnal leg cramps, stating that data supporting safety and efficacy of quinine for this indication were inadequate and that risks outweighed the potential benefits.

TOXICITY AND SIDE EFFECTS. The fatal oral dose of quinine for adults is ~2-8 g. Quinine is associated with a triad of dose-related toxicities when given at full therapeutic or excessive doses: cinchonism, hypoglycemia, and hypotension. Mild forms of cinchonism (consisting of tinnitus, high-tone deafness, visual disturbances, headache, dysphoria, nausea, vomiting, and postural hypotension) occur frequently and disappear soon after the drug is withdrawn. Hypoglycemia is also common and can be life threatening if not treated promptly with intravenous glucose. Hypotension is rare and most often is associated with excessively rapid intravenous infusions of quinine or quinidine. Prolonged medication or high single doses also may produce GI, cardiovascular, and skin manifestations. GI symptoms (nausea, vomiting, abdominal pain, and diarrhea) result from the local irritant action of quinine, but the nausea and emesis also have a central basis. Cutaneous manifestations may include flushing, sweating, rash, and angioedema, especially of the face. Quinine and quinidine, even at therapeutic doses, may cause hyperinsulinemia and severe hypoglycemia through their powerful stimulatory effect on pancreatic beta cells.

Quinine rarely causes cardiac complications unless therapeutic plasma concentrations are exceeded. QTc prolongation is mild and does not appear to be affected by concurrent mefloquine treatment. Acute overdosage also may cause serious and even fatal cardiac dysrhythmias such as sinus arrest, junctional rhythms, AV block, and ventricular tachycardia and fibrillation. Quinidine is even more cardiotoxic than quinine. Cardiac monitoring of patients on intravenous quinidine is advisable where possible.

Severe hemolysis can result from hypersensitivity to these cinchona alkaloids. Hemoglobinuria and asthma from quinine may occur more rarely. "Blackwater fever"—the triad of massive hemolysis, hemoglobinemia, and hemoglobinuria leading to anuria, renal failure, and in some instances death—is a rare hypersensitivity reaction to quinine therapy that can occur during treatment of malaria. Quinine occasionally may cause milder hemolysis, especially in people with G6PD deficiency. Thrombotic thrombocytopenic purpura also is rare but can occur even in response to ingestion of tonic water, which has ~4% the therapeutic oral dose per 12 oz ("cocktail purpura"). Other rare adverse effects include hypoprothrombinemia, leukopenia, and agranulocytosis.

PRECAUTIONS, CONTRAINDICATIONS, AND INTERACTIONS. Quinine must be used with considerable caution, if at all, in patients who manifest hypersensitivity. Quinine should be discontinued immediately if evidence of hemolysis appears. This drug should be avoided in patients with tinnitus or optic neuritis. In patients with cardiac dysrhythmias, the administration of quinine requires the same precautions as for quinidine. Quinine appears to be safe in pregnancy and is used commonly for the treatment of pregnancy-associated malaria. However, glucose levels must be monitored because of the increased risk of hypoglycemia.

The drugs are highly irritating and should not be given subcutaneously. Concentrated solutions may cause abscesses when injected intramuscularly, or thrombophlebitis when infused intravenously. Antacids that contain aluminum can delay absorption of quinine from the GI tract. Quinine and quinidine can delay the absorption and elevate plasma levels of cardiac glycosides and warfarin and related anticoagulants. The action of quinine at neuromuscular junctions enhances the effect of neuromuscular blocking agents and opposes the action of acetylcholinesterase inhibitors. Prochlorperazine can amplify quinine's cardiotoxicity, as can halofantrine. The renal clearance of quinine can be decreased by cimetidine and increased by urine acidification and by rifampin.

MEFLOQUINE

Mefloquine (LARIAM) emerged from the Walter Reed Malaria Research Program as safe and effective against drug-resistant strains of *P. falciparum*.

MECHANISMS OF ACTION AND PARASITE RESISTANCE. Mefloquine is a highly effective blood schizonticide. Mefloquine associates with intra-erythrocytic hemozoin, suggesting similarities to the mode of action of chloroquine. However, increased *pfmdr1* copy numbers are associated with both reduced parasite susceptibility to mefloquine and increased PfMDR1-mediated solute import into the digestive vacuole of intraerythrocytic parasites, suggesting that the drug's target resides outside of this vacuolar compartment. The (−)-enantiomer is associated with adverse CNS effects, whereas the (+)-enantiomer retains antimalarial activity with fewer side effects. Mefloquine can be paired with artesunate to reduce the selection pressure for resistance. This combination has proved efficacious for the treatment of *P. falciparum* malaria, even in regions with high prevalence of mefloquine-resistant parasites.

ADME. Mefloquine is taken orally because parenteral preparations cause severe local reactions. The drug is absorbed rapidly but with marked variability. Probably owing to extensive enterogastric and enterohepatic circulation, plasma levels of mefloquine rise in a biphasic manner to their peak in ~17 h. Mefloquine has a variable and long $t_{1/2}$, 13-24 days, reflecting its high lipophilicity, extensive tissue distribution, and extensive binding (~98%) to plasma proteins. The slow elimination of mefloquine fosters the emergence of drug-resistant parasites. Mefloquine is extensively metabolized in the liver by CYP3A4; this CYP can be inhibited by ketoconazole and induced by rifampicin. Excretion of mefloquine is mainly by the fecal route; only ~10% of mefloquine appears unchanged in the urine.

Therapeutic Uses. Mefloquine should be reserved for the prevention and treatment of malaria caused by drug-resistant *P. falciparum* and *P. vivax*; it is no longer considered first-line treatment of malaria. The drug is especially useful as a chemoprophylactic agent for travelers spending weeks to years in areas where these infections are endemic (*see* Table 49–1). In areas where malaria is due to multiply drug-resistant strains of *P. falciparum*, mefloquine is more effective when used in combination with an artemisinin compound.

Toxicity and Side Effects. At chemoprophylactic dosages, oral mefloquine is generally well tolerated. Vivid dreams are common; significant neuropsychiatric signs and symptoms can occur in ≥10% of people receiving treatment doses; serious adverse events (psychosis, seizures) are rare. Short-term adverse effects of treatment include nausea, vomiting, and dizziness. Dividing the dose improves tolerance. The full dose should be repeated if vomiting occurs within the first hour. After treatment of malaria with mefloquine, CNS toxicity can be as high as 0.5%; symptoms include seizures, confusion or decreased sensorium, acute psychosis, and disabling vertigo. Such symptoms are reversible upon drug discontinuation. Mild-to-moderate toxicities (e.g., disturbed sleep, dysphoria, headache, GI disturbances, and dizziness) occur even at prophylactic dosages. Adverse effects usually manifest after the first to third doses and often abate even with continued treatment. Cardiac abnormalities, hemolysis, and agranulocytosis are rare.

Contraindications and Interactions. At very high doses, mefloquine is teratogenic in rodents. Studies have suggested an increased rate of stillbirths with mefloquine use, especially during the first trimester. Pregnancy should be avoided for 3 months after mefloquine use because of the prolonged $t_{1/2}$ of this agent. This drug is contraindicated for patients with a history of seizures, depression, bipolar disorder and other severe neuropsychiatric conditions, or adverse reactions to quinoline antimalarials. Although this drug can be taken safely 12 h after a last dose of quinine, taking quinine shortly after mefloquine can be very hazardous because the latter is eliminated so slowly. Treatment with or after halofantrine or within 2 months of prior mefloquine administration is contraindicated. Controlled studies suggest that mefloquine does not impair performance in persons who tolerate the drug; nonetheless, some advise against the use of mefloquine for patients in occupations that require focused concentration, dexterity, and cognitive function.

PRIMAQUINE

Primaquine, in contrast to other antimalarials, acts on exo-erythrocytic tissue stages of plasmodia in the liver to prevent and cure relapsing malaria. Patients should be screened for G6PD deficiency prior to therapy with this drug.

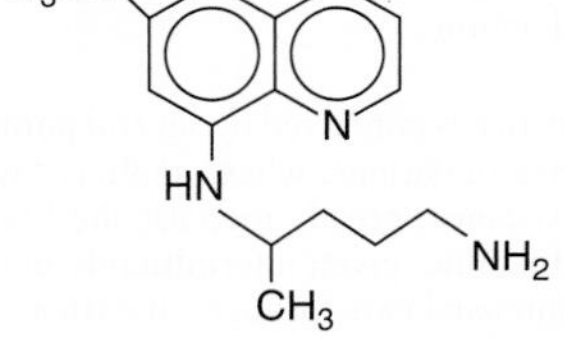

H_3CO N HN NH_2 CH_3

PRIMAQUINE

Antimalarial Action and Parasite Resistance. The mechanism of action of the 8-aminoquinolines has not been elucidated. Primaquine acts against primary and latent hepatic stages of *Plasmodium spp.* and prevents relapses in *P. vivax* and *P. ovale* infections. This drug and other 8-aminoquinolines also display gametocytocidal activity against *P. falciparum* and other *Plasmodium* species. However, primaquine is inactive against asexual blood stage parasites.

ADME. Absorption of primaquine from the GI tract approaches 100%. Peak plasma concentration occurs within 3 h and then falls with a variable $t_{1/2}$ averaging 7 h. Primaquine is metabolized rapidly; only a small fraction of a dose is excreted as the parent drug. Importantly, primaquine induces CYP1A2. The major metabolite, carboxyprimaquine, is inactive.

Therapeutic Uses. Primaquine is used primarily for terminal chemoprophylaxis and radical cure of *P. vivax* and *P. ovale* (relapsing) infections because of its high activity against the latent tissue forms (hypnozoites) of these *Plasmodium* species. The compound is given together with a blood schizonticide, usually chloroquine, to eradicate erythrocytic stages of these plasmodia and reduce the possibility of emerging drug resistance. For terminal chemoprophylaxis, primaquine regimens should be initiated shortly before or immediately after a subject leaves an endemic area (*see* Table 49–1). Radical cure of *P. vivax* or *P. ovale* malaria can be achieved if the drug is given either during an asymptomatic latent period of presumed infection or during an acute attack. Simultaneous administration of a schizonticidal drug plus primaquine is more effective than sequential treatment in promoting a radical cure. Limited studies have shown efficacy in prevention of *P. falciparum* and *P. vivax* malaria when primaquine is taken as chemoprophylaxis. Primaquine is generally well tolerated when taken for up to 1 year.

Toxicity and Side Effects. Primaquine has few side effects when given in the usual therapeutic doses. Primaquine can cause mild to moderate abdominal distress in some individuals. Taking the drug at mealtime often alleviates these symptoms. Mild anemia, cyanosis (methemoglobinemia), and leukocytosis are less common. High doses (60-240 mg daily) worsen the abdominal symptoms. Methemoglobinemia can occur even with usual doses of primaquine and can be severe in individuals with congenital deficiency of NADH methemoglobin reductase. Chloroquine and dapsone may synergize with primaquine to produce methemoglobinemia in these patients. Granulocytopenia and agranulocytosis are rare complications of therapy and usually are associated with overdosage. Other rare adverse reactions are hypertension, arrhythmias, and symptoms referable to the CNS.

Therapeutic or higher doses of primaquine may cause acute hemolysis and hemolytic anemia in humans with G6PD deficiency. Primaquine is the prototype of >50 drugs, including antimalarial sulfonamides, that cause hemolysis in G6PD-deficient individuals.

Precautions and Contraindications. G6PD deficiency should be ruled out prior to administration of primaquine. Primaquine has been used cautiously in subjects with the A form of G6PD deficiency, although benefits of treatment may not necessarily outweigh the risks but should not be used in patients with more severe deficiency. If a daily dose of >30 mg primaquine base (>15 mg in potentially sensitive patients) is given, then blood counts should be followed carefully. Patients should be counseled to look for dark or blood-colored urine, which would indicate hemolysis. Primaquine should not be given to pregnant women; in treating lactating mothers, primaquine should be prescribed only after ascertaining that the breast-feeding infant has a normal G6PD level. Primaquine is contraindicated for acutely ill patients suffering from systemic disease characterized by a tendency to granulocytopenia (e.g., active forms of rheumatoid arthritis and lupus erythematosus). Primaquine should not be given to patients receiving drugs capable of causing hemolysis or depressing the myeloid elements of the bone marrow.

SULFONAMIDES AND SULFONES

The sulfonamides and sulfones are slow-acting blood schizonticides and more active against *P. falciparum* than *P. vivax*.

MECHANISM OF ACTION. Sulfonamides are *p*-aminobenzoic acid analogs that competitively inhibit *Plasmodium* dihydropteroate synthase. These agents are combined with an inhibitor of parasite dihydrofolate reductase to enhance their antimalarial action.

DRUG RESISTANCE. Sulfadoxine resistance is conferred by several point mutations in the dihydropteroate synthase gene. These sulfadoxine-resistance mutations, when combined with mutations of dihydrofolate reductase and conferring pyrimethamine resistance, greatly increase the likelihood of sulfadoxine-pyrimethamine treatment failure. Sulfadoxine-pyrimethamine, given intermittently during the second and third trimesters of pregnancy, is a routine component of antenatal care throughout Africa. Intermittent preventive treatment strategies may also benefit infants. Generally, one can anticipate that, in the absence of novel antifolates effective against existing drug-resistant strains, the use of these antimalarials for either prevention or treatment will continue to decline.

TETRACYCLINES AND CLINDAMYCIN

Tetracycline and doxycycline are useful in malaria treatment, as is clindamycin. These agents are slow-acting blood schizonticides that can be used alone for short-term chemoprophylaxis in areas with chloroquine- and mefloquine-resistant malaria (only doxycycline is recommended for malaria chemoprophylaxis).

These antibiotics act via a delayed death mechanism resulting from their inhibition of protein translation in the parasite plastid. This effect on malarial parasites manifests as death of the progeny of drug-treated parasites, resulting in slow onset of antimalarial activity. Their relatively slow mode of action makes these drugs ineffective as single agents for malaria treatment. Dosage regimens for tetracyclines and clindamycin are listed in Tables 49–1 and 49–2. Because of their adverse effects on bones and teeth, tetracyclines should not be given to pregnant women or to children <8 years of age.

PRINCIPLES AND GUIDELINES FOR CHEMOPROPHYLAXIS AND CHEMOTHERAPY OF MALARIA

Pharmacological prevention of malaria poses a difficult challenge because *P. falciparum*, which causes nearly all the deaths from human malaria, has become progressively more resistant to available antimalarial drugs. Chloroquine remains effective against malaria caused by *P. ovale*, *P. malariae*, *P. knowlesi*, most strains of *P. vivax*, and chloroquine-sensitive strains of *P. falciparum* found in some geographic areas. However, chloroquine-resistant strains of *P. falciparum* are now the rule, not the exception, in most malaria-endemic regions (*see* Figure 49–2). Extensive geographic overlap also exists between chloroquine resistance and resistance to pyrimethamine-sulfadoxine. Multidrug-resistant *P. falciparum* malaria is especially prevalent and severe in Southeast Asia and Oceania. These infections may not respond adequately even to mefloquine or quinine. The following section presents an overview of the chemoprophylaxis and chemotherapy of malaria. Current CDC recommendations for drugs and dosing regimens for the chemoprophylaxis and treatment of malaria in nonimmune individuals are shown in Tables 49–1 and 49–2.

Drugs should not replace simple, inexpensive measures for malaria prevention. Individuals visiting malarious areas should take appropriate steps to prevent mosquito bites. One such measure is to avoid exposure to mosquitoes at dusk and dawn, usually the times of maximal feeding. Others include using insect repellents containing at least 30% *N,N′*-diethylmetatoluamide (DEET) and sleeping in well-screened rooms or under bed nets impregnated with a pyrethrin insecticide such as permethrin.

MALARIA CHEMOPROPHYLAXIS. Regimens for malaria chemoprophylaxis include primarily 3 drugs: *atovaquoneproguanil* and *doxycycline* that can both be used in all areas, and *mefloquine* that can be used in areas with mefloquine-sensitive malaria. Other available options are chloroquine or hydroxychloroquine (but their use is restricted to the few areas with chloroquine-sensitive malaria), and primaquine (for short duration travel to areas with principally *P. vivax*). In general, dosing should be started before exposure, ideally before the traveler leaves home (*see* Table 49–1).

In those few areas where chloroquine-sensitive strains of *P. falciparum* are found, chloroquine is still suitable for chemoprophylaxis. In areas where chloroquine-resistant malaria is endemic, mefloquine and atovaquone-proguanil are the regimens of choice for chemoprophylaxis. For chemoprophylaxis in long-term travelers, chloroquine is safe at the doses used, but some recommend yearly retinal examinations, and there is a finite dose limit for which chemoprophylaxis with chloroquine is recommended because of ocular toxicity. Mefloquine and doxycycline are well tolerated. Mefloquine is the best documented drug for long-term travelers and, if well tolerated, can be used for prolonged periods. Atovaquone-proguanil has been studied for up to 20 weeks but probably is acceptable for years based on experience with the individual components.

DIAGNOSIS AND TREATMENT OF MALARIA. The diagnosis of malaria must be considered for patients presenting with acute febrile illness after returning from a malaria-endemic region. An organized, rational approach to diagnosis, parasite identification, and appropriate treatment is

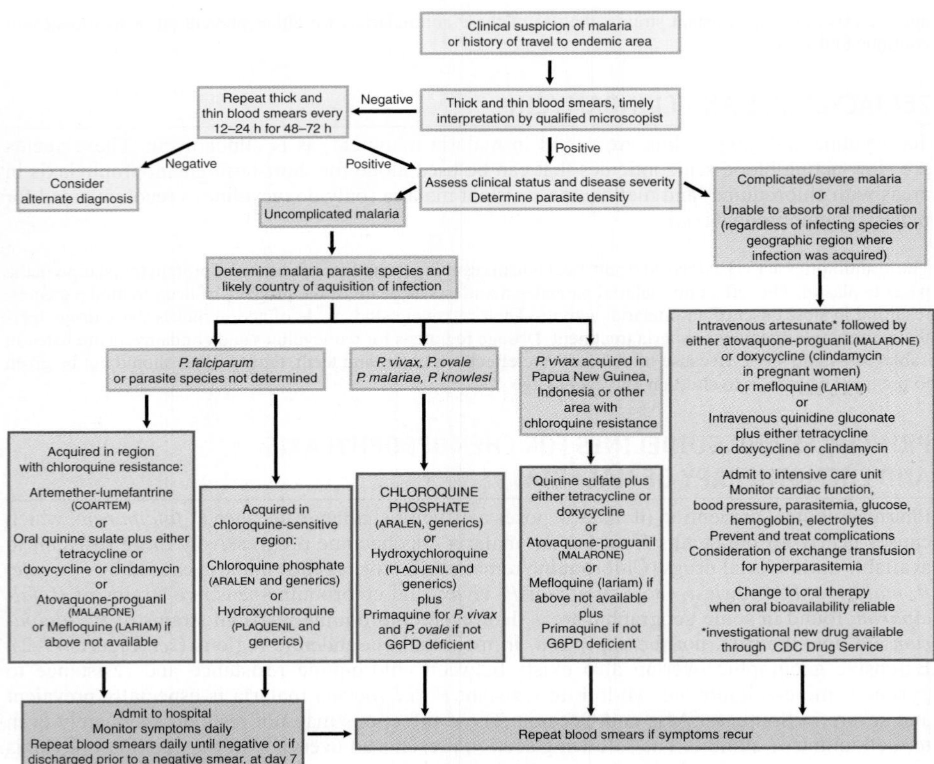

Figure 49–3 *Approach to the treatment of malaria.* Atovaquone-proguanil, mefloquine, artemether-lumefantrine, tetracycline, and doxycycline are not indicated during pregnancy. Tetracycline and doxycycline are not indicated in children <8 years of age. G6PD, glucose-6-phosphate dehydrogenase. (Modified from: Centers for Disease Control and Prevention. Malaria. http://www.cdc.gov/malaria/resources/pdf/algorithm.pdf. Accessed June 14, 2013.)

crucial. Guidelines for treatment of malaria in the U.S. are provided by the CDC and are shown in Table 49–2 and Figure 49–3.

Children and pregnant women are the most susceptible to severe malaria. The treatment of children generally is the same as for adults (pediatric dose should never exceed adult dose). However, tetracyclines should not be given to children <8 years of age except in an emergency, and atovaquone-proguanil as treatment has been approved only for children weighing >5 kg.

CHEMOPROPHYLAXIS AND TREATMENT DURING PREGNANCY. Chemoprophylaxis during pregnancy is complex, and women should evaluate with expert medical staff the benefits and risks of different strategies with regard to their particular situation. Severe malaria during pregnancy should be treated with intravenous antimalarial treatment according to the general guidelines for severe malaria, taking into account the drugs that should be avoided during pregnancy. In lactating mothers, treatment with most compounds is acceptable, although chloroquine and hydroxychloroquine are the preferred agents. The use of atovaquone-proguanil is not recommended unless breast-feeding infants weigh >5 kg. Also, the breast-feeding infant should be shown to have a normal G6PD level before receiving primaquine.

SELF-TREATMENT OF PRESUMPTIVE MALARIA FOR TRAVELERS. The CDC provides traveler's guidelines for self-treatment of presumptive malaria (atovaquone-proguanil, as described in Table 49–2) when professional care is not available within 24 h. In such cases, medical care should be sought immediately after treatment. These recommendations may change over time and with specific locations. Consult the CDC Yellow Book or www.cdc.gov/travel.

Table 49–2

Regimens for the Treatment of Malaria

DRUG	INDICATION	ADULT DOSAGE[a]	POTENTIAL ADVERSE EFFECTS AND COMMENTS
Artemether-lumefantrine (COARTEM)	*P. falciparum* from chloroquine resistant or unknown areas	Tablet: 20 mg artemether, lumefantrine. Dose: 4 tablets. Day 1: 2 doses separated by 8 hours; thereafter twice daily × 2 d	Headache anorexia, dizziness, asthenia, arthralgia myalgia. Take with food or whole milk. If patient vomits within 30 min, repeat dose. Contraindication: pregnancy.
Artesunate (IV; available from U.S. CDC)	Severe malaria (see CDC guidelines)	U.S. treatment IND: 4 equal doses of artesunate (2.4 mg/kg each) over a 3-day period followed by oral atovaquone-proguanil, doxycycline, clindamycin, or mefloquine (to avoid emergence of resistance)	See Artemether and CDC guidelines
Atovaquone-proguanil (oral)	*Plasmodium falciparum* from chloroquine-resistant areas; *P. vivax*	Tablet 250 mg atovaquone/100 mg, proguanil 4 tablets orally/day × 3 d	Abdominal pain, nausea, vomiting, diarrhea, headache, rash, mild reversible elevations in liver aminotransferase levels. Contraindications: pregnancy, hypersensitivity to atovaquone or proguanil, severe renal impairment (creatinine clearance <30 mL/min). Take with food to increase absorption of atovaquone.
Chloroquine phosphate	*P. falciparum* and *P. vivax* from chloroquine ensitive areas All *P. ovale* All *P. malariae* All *P. knowlesi*	600 mg base (1000 mg salt) orally immediately, followed by 300 mg base orally at 6, 24, and 48 h Total dose: 1500 mg base	Nausea, vomiting, rash, headache, dizziness, urticaria, abdominal pain, pruritus. Safe in children and pregnant women. Give for chemoprophylaxis (500 mg salt orally every week) in pregnant women with chloroquine-sensitive *P. vivax*. Contraindications: retinal or visual field change, hypersensitivity to 4-aminoquinolines. Use with caution in those with impaired liver function (drug is concentrated in liver)
Clindamycin (oral or IV)	*P. falciparum* from chloroquine-resistant areas *P. vivax* from chloroquine-esistant areas	Oral: 20 mg base/kg/d orally divided 3×/d × 7 d IV: 10 mg base/kg loading dose IV followed by 5 mg base/kg IV every 8 h; then oral clindamycin (as above) when patient can take oral meds; duration = 7 d	Diarrhea, nausea, rash. Always use in combination with quinine-quinidine. Safe in children and pregnant women.

(*continued*)

Table 49–2

Regimens for the Treatment of Malaria (*Continued*)

DRUG	INDICATION	ADULT DOSAGE[a]	POTENTIAL ADVERSE EFFECTS AND COMMENTS
Doxycycline (oral or IV)	*P. falciparum* and *P. vivax* from chloroquine-resistant areas	Oral: 100 mg orally twice daily × 7 d IV: 100 mg IV every 12 h and then oral doxycycline (as above) when patient can take oral meds; treatment course = 7 d	Nausea, vomiting, diarrhea, abdominal pain, dizziness, photosensitivity, headache, esophagitis, odynophagia; rarely hepatotoxicity, pancreatitis, and benign intracranial hypertension. Always use with quinine or quinidine. Contraindicated in children < 8 y, pregnant women, and persons with known hypersensitivity to tetracyclines. Food and milk decrease its absorption but will decrease GI disturbances. To prevent esophagitis, take with copious fluids, (patients should not lie down for 1 h after dosing). Barbiturates, carbamazepine, or phenytoin may reduce C_p.
Hydroxychloroquine (oral)	2nd-line alternative for *P. falciparum* and *P. vivax* from chloroquine-sensitive areas. All *P. ovale* All *P. malariae*	620-mg base (= 800 mg salt) orally immediately, followed by 310 mg base orally at 6, 24, and 48 h Total dose: 1550-mg base	Nausea, vomiting, rash, headache, dizziness, urticaria, abdominal pain, pruritus.[b] Safe in children and pregnant women. Contraindicated if retinal or visual field change, or if hypersensitive to 4-aminoquinolines. Use with caution if liver function is impaired.
Mefloquine[c]	*P. falciparum* from chloroquine-resistant areas (except Thailand-Burmese, Thailand-Cambodian border regions). *P. vivax* from chloroquine-resistant areas	684 mg base (= 750 mg salt) orally as initial dose, followed by 456 mg base orally given 6-12 h after initial dose Total dose = 1250 mg salt	GI complaints, mild CNS complaints, myalgia, mild skin rash, and fatigue; moderate to severe neuropsychiatric reactions, sinus arrhythmia, sinus bradycardia, 1° A-V block, QTc prolongation, abnormal T waves. Contraindications: hypersensitivity to drug, cardiac conduction abnormalities, psychiatric or seizure disorders. Do not administer if patient has received related drugs (chloroquine, quinine, quinidine) less than 12 h ago.

(*continued*)

Table 49–2

Regimens for the Treatment of Malaria (*Continued*)

DRUG	INDICATION	ADULT DOSAGE[a]	POTENTIAL ADVERSE EFFECTS AND COMMENTS
Primaquine phosphate	Radical cure of *P. vivax* and *P. ovale* (to eliminate hypnozoites)	30 mg base/d orally × 14 d	GI disturbances, methemoglobinemia (self-limited), hemolysis in G6PD deficiency (screen for G6PD deficiency prior to use). Contraindicated in persons with G6PD deficiency and in pregnant women. Should be taken with food to minimize GI adverse effects.
Quinine sulfate (oral)	*P. falciparum* and *P. vivax* from chloroquine-resistant areas	542 mg base (650 mg salt)[d] orally 3×/d × 3 d (infections acquired outside SE Asia) but to 7 d (infections acquired in SE Asia)	Cinchonism[e], sinus arrhythmia, junctional rhythms, AV block, prolonged QT interval, ventricular tachycardia, ventricular fibrillation (rare, more commonly seen with quinidine), hypoglycemia. Combine with tetracycline, doxycycline, or clindamycin, except for *P. vivax* infections in children <8 y or pregnant women. Contraindications: hypersensitivity, history of blackwater fever, thrombocytopenic purpura, thrombocytopenia associated with quinine/quinidine use, many cardiac conduction defects and arrhythmias[f], myasthenia gravis, optic neuritis.
Quinidine gluconate (IV)	Severe malaria (all species, independently of chloroquine resistance). Patient unable to take oral medication. Parasitemia >10%	6.25 mg base/kg (= 10 mg salt/kg) loading dose IV over 1-2 h, then 0.0125 mg base/kg/min continuous infusion for at least 24 h. Alternative regimen[g]	Cinchonism, tachycardia, prolongation of QRS and QTc intervals, flattening of T-wave (effects often transient). Ventricular arrhythmias, hypotension, hypoglycemia. Combine with tetracycline, doxycycline, or clindamycin. Contraindications: same as for quinine sulfate.[h]

(*continued*)

Table 49–2

Regimens for the Treatment of Malaria (*Continued*)

DRUG	INDICATION	ADULT DOSAGE[a]	POTENTIAL ADVERSE EFFECTS AND COMMENTS
Tetracycline (oral or IV)	*P. falciparum* (chloroquine-resistant areas) *P. vivax* from chloroquine-resistant areas (with quinine/ quinidine)	Oral: 250 mg 4 times daily × 7 d. IV: dosage same as for oral	See doxycycline

G6PD, glucose-6-phosphate dehydrogenase; IV, intravenous.

[a]See CDC Yellow Book 2012 online for pediatric dosing regimens and up-to-date information. Pediatric dosage should never exceed adult dosage.

[b]Extrapolated from chloroquine literature.

[c]Mefloquine should not be used to treat P. falciparum infections acquired in the following areas: borders of Thailand with Burma (Myanmar) and Cambodia, western provinces of Cambodia, eastern states of Burma (Myanmar), border between Burma and China, Laos along borders of Laos and Burma (and adjacent parts of Thailand-Cambodia border), and southern Vietnam due to resistant strains.

[d]Quinine sulfate capsule manufactured in the U.S. is in a 324-mg dose; therefore, two capsules should be sufficient for adult dosing.

[e]Nausea, vomiting, headache, tinnitus, deafness, dizziness, and visual disturbances.

[f]Refer to quinine sulfate, package insert (Mutual Pharmaceutical Inc, Philadelphia, PA, Rev 08, November 2009).

[g]Alternative dosing hypoglycemia optic neuritis regimen for quinidine gluconate (IV): 15 mg base/kg (24 mg salt/kg) loading dose IV infused over 4 h, followed by 7.5 mg base/kg (= 12 mg salt/kg) infused over 4 h every 8 h, starting 8 h after the loading dose (see package insert); once parasite density <1% and patient can take oral medication, complete treatment with oral quinine, dose as above Quinidine or quinine course = 7 d in SE Asia (3 d in Africa or South America)

[h]Refer to quinidine gluconate, package insert (Eli Lilly Co, Indianapolis, IN, February 2002).

These regimens are based on published recommendations of the U.S. Centers for Disease Control and Prevention (CDC). Although current at the time of writing, these recommendations may change over time. Up-to-date information should be obtained from the CDC website at www.cdc.gov/travel. Recommendations and available treatment differ among countries in the industrialized world, developing world, and malaria-endemic regions; in the latter, some anti-malarial treatments may be available without prescription, but the most effective drugs usually are controlled by governmental agencies.

From http://wwwnc.cdc.gov/travel/content/yellowbook/home-2010.aspx; accessed January 12, 2010.

For a complete Bibliographical Listing see Goodman & Gilman's ***The Pharmacological Basis of Therapeutics***, 12th ed., or Goodman & Gilman Online at www.AccessMedicine.com.

Chemotherapy of Protozoal Infections: Amebiasis, Giardiasis, Trichomoniasis, Trypanosomiasis, Leishmaniasis, and Other Protozoal Infections

Humans host a wide variety of protozoal parasites that can be transmitted by insect vectors, directly from other mammalian reservoirs or from one person to another. The immune system plays a crucial role in protecting against the pathological consequences of protozoal infections. Thus, opportunistic infections with protozoa are prominent in infants, individuals with cancer, transplant recipients, those receiving immunosuppressive drugs or extensive antibiotic therapy, and persons with advanced human immunodeficiency virus (HIV) infection. Because effective vaccines are unavailable, chemotherapy has been the only practical way to both treat infected individuals and reduce transmission. Many effective antiprotozoal drugs are toxic at therapeutic doses, a problem exacerbated by increasing drug resistance.

INTRODUCTION TO PROTOZOAL INFECTIONS OF HUMANS

AMEBIASIS. Amebiasis affects ~10% of the world's population, commonly individuals living in poverty, crowded conditions, and areas with poor sanitation. Three morphologically identical but genetically distinct species of *Entamoeba* (i.e., *E. histolytica, E. dispar,* and *E. moshkovskii*) have been isolated from infected persons, with *E. histolytica* responsible for ~10% of human infections. Only *E. histolytica* causes disease and requires treatment.

Humans are the only known hosts for these protozoa, which are transmitted almost exclusively by the fecal-oral route. Ingested *E. histolytica* cysts from contaminated food or water survive acid gastric contents and transform into *trophozoites* that reside in the large intestine. The outcome of *E. histolytica* infection is variable. Many individuals remain asymptomatic but excrete the infectious cyst form, making them a source for further infections. In other individuals, *E. histolytica* trophozoites invade into the colonic mucosa with resulting colitis and bloody diarrhea (amebic dysentery). In a smaller proportion of patients, *E. histolytica* trophozoites invade through the colonic mucosa, reach the portal circulation, and travel to the liver, where they establish an amebic liver abscess.

The cornerstone of therapy for amebiasis is metronidazole or its analogs tinidazole and ornidazole. Because metronidazole is so well absorbed in the gut, levels may not be therapeutic in the colonic lumen, and the drug is less effective against cysts. Hence patients with amebiasis (amebic colitis or amebic liver abscess) also should receive a luminal agent to eradicate any *E. histolytica* trophozoites residing within the gut lumen. Luminal agents are also used to treat asymptomatic individuals found to be infected with *E. histolytica*. The nonabsorbed aminoglycoside *paromomycin* and the 8-hydroxyquinoline compound *iodoquinol* are effective luminal agents. Diloxanide furoate, previously considered the luminal agent of choice for amebiasis, is no longer available in the U.S. *Nitazoxanide* (ALINIA), approved in the U.S. for treatment of cryptosporidiosis and giardiasis, is also active against *E. histolytica*.

GIARDIASIS. Giardiasis, caused by the flagellated protozoan *Giardia intestinalis*, is prevalent worldwide and is the most commonly reported intestinal protozoal infection in the U.S. Infection results from ingestion of the cyst form of the parasite, which is found in fecally contaminated water or food.

Infection with *Giardia* results in 1 of 3 syndromes: an asymptomatic carrier state, acute self-limited diarrhea, or chronic diarrhea. Chemotherapy with a 5-day course of *metronidazole* usually is successful, although therapy may have to be repeated or prolonged in some instances. A single dose of *tinidazole* (TINDAMAX, others) probably is superior to metronidazole for the treatment of giardiasis. *Paromomycin* (HUMATIN, others) has been used to treat pregnant women to avoid any possible mutagenic effects of the other drugs. *Nitazoxanide* (ALINIA), N-(nitrothiazolyl) salicylamide, and tinidazole are approved for the treatment of giardiasis in immune-competent children <12 years of age. Furazolidone has been discontinued in the U.S.

TRICHOMONIASIS. Trichomoniasis is caused by the flagellated protozoan *Trichomonas vaginalis*. This organism inhabits the genitourinary tract of the human host, where it causes vaginitis in women and, uncommonly, urethritis in men. Trichomoniasis is a sexually transmitted disease and has been associated with an increased risk of acquiring HIV infection. Only *trophozoite* forms of *T. vaginalis* have been identified in infected secretions.

Metronidazole remains the drug of choice for the treatment of trichomoniasis. Tinidazole, another nitroimidazole, appears to be better tolerated than metronidazole and has been used successfully at higher doses to treat metronidazole-resistant *T. vaginalis*.

TOXOPLASMOSIS. Toxoplasmosis is a zoonotic infection caused by *Toxoplasma gondii*. Although cats and other feline species are the natural hosts, tissue cysts (*bradyzoites*) have been recovered from all mammalian species examined. Common routes of infection in humans are:

- Ingestion of undercooked meat containing tissue cysts
- Ingestion of contaminated vegetable matter containing infective *oocysts*
- Direct oral contact with feces of cats shedding oocysts
- Transplacental fetal infection with *tachyzoites* from acutely infected mothers

The acute illness is usually self-limiting, and treatment rarely is required. Individuals who are immunocompromised, however, are at risk of developing toxoplasmic encephalitis from reactivation of tissue cysts deposited in the brain. The primary treatment for toxoplasmic encephalitis consists of the antifolates *pyrimethamine* (DARAPRIM) and *sulfadiazine* along with *folinic acid* (*leucovorin*). Therapy must be discontinued in ~40% of cases because of toxicity owing primarily to the sulfa compound; *clindamycin* can be substituted for sulfadiazine without loss of efficacy. Alternative regimens combining azithromycin, clarithromycin, atovaquone, or dapsone with either trimethoprim-sulfamethoxazole or pyrimethamine and folinic acid are less toxic but also less effective. *Spiramycin*, which concentrates in placental tissue, is used for the treatment of acute acquired toxoplasmosis in pregnancy to prevent transmission to the fetus. If fetal infection is detected, the combination of pyrimethamine, sulfadiazine, and folinic acid is administered to the mother (only after the first 12-14 weeks of pregnancy) and to the newborn in the postnatal period. Spiramycin is not available in the U.S.

CRYPTOSPORIDIOSIS. Cryptosporidia are coccidian protozoan parasites that can cause diarrhea. *Cryptosporidium parvum* and the newly named *C. hominis* appear to account for almost all infections in humans. Infectious *oocysts* in feces may be spread either by direct human-to-human contact or by contaminated water supplies.

After ingestion, the mature oocyte is digested, releasing *sporozoites* that invade host epithelial cells. In most individuals, infection is self-limited. However, in AIDS patients and other immunocompromised individuals, the severity of diarrhea may require hospitalization. The most effective therapy for cryptosporidiosis in AIDS patients is restoration of their immune function through highly active antiretroviral therapy (HAART) (*see* Chapter 59). *Nitazoxanide* has shown activity in treating cryptosporidiosis in immunocompetent children and is possibly effective in immunocompetent adults. Its efficacy in children and adults with HIV infection and AIDS is not clearly established.

TRYPANOSOMIASIS. African trypanosomiasis, or "sleeping sickness," is caused by subspecies of the hemoflagellate *Trypanosoma brucei* that are transmitted by bloodsucking tsetse flies of the genus *Glossina*. Largely restricted to sub-Saharan Africa, the infection causes serious human illness and also threatens livestock (*nagana*), leading to protein malnutrition. In humans, the infection is fatal unless treated. An estimated 500,000 Africans carry the infection, and >50 million people are at risk for the disease.

The parasite is entirely extracellular, and early human infection is characterized by the finding of replicating parasites in the bloodstream or lymph without CNS involvement (stage 1); stage 2 disease is characterized by CNS involvement. Symptoms of early-stage disease include febrile illness, lymphadenopathy, splenomegaly, and occasional myocarditis that result from systemic dissemination of the parasites. There are 2 types of African trypanosomiasis: the East African (Rhodesian; *T. brucei rhodesiense*) variety produces a progressive and rapidly fatal form of disease marked by early involvement of the CNS and frequent terminal cardiac failure; the West African type (Gambian; *T. brucei gambiense*) causes illness characterized by later involvement of the CNS and a more long-term course that progresses to the classical symptoms of sleeping sickness over months to years. Neurological symptoms include confusion, sensory deficits, psychiatric signs, disruption of the sleep cycle, and eventual progression into coma and death.

Standard therapy for early-stage disease is *pentamidine* for *T. brucei gambiense* and *suramin* for *T. brucei rhodesiense*. Both compounds must be given parenterally over long periods and are not effective against late-stage disease. The CNS phase has traditionally been treated with melarsoprol (available from the CDC), a highly toxic agent that causes a fatal reactive encephalopathy in 2-10% of treated patients. Moreover, lack of response to this agent is leading to increasing numbers of treatment failures. *Eflornithine*, an inhibitor of ornithine decarboxylase, a key enzyme in polyamine metabolism, offers the only alternative for the treatment of late-stage disease. It has efficacy against both early and late stages of human *T. brucei gambiense* infection; however, it is ineffective as monotherapy for infections of *T. brucei rhodesiense*. Notably, eflornithine has significantly fewer side effects than melarsoprol and is more effective than melarsoprol for treatment of late-stage Gambian trypanosomiasis, suggesting that eflornithine is the best available first-line treatment for this form of the disease. *Nifurtimox-eflornithine combination therapy* (NECT) allows a shorter exposure to eflornithine with good efficacy and a reduction in adverse events.

American trypanosomiasis, or *Chagas disease*, a zoonotic infection caused by *Trypanosoma cruzi*, affects ~15 million people from Mexico to Argentina and Chile. The chronic form of the disease in adults is a major cause of cardiomyopathy, megaesophagus, megacolon, and death. Blood-sucking triatomid bugs infesting poor rural dwellings most commonly transmit this infection to young children; transplacental transmission also may occur in endemic areas. Two nitroheterocyclic drugs, *nifurtimox* (available from the CDC) and *benznidazole* are used to treat this infection. Both agents suppress parasitemia and can cure the acute phase of Chagas disease in 60-80% of cases; both drugs are toxic and must be taken for long periods.

LEISHMANIASIS. Leishmaniasis is a complex vector-borne zoonosis caused by ~20 different species of intramacrophage protozoa of the genus *Leishmania*. Small mammals and canines generally serve as reservoirs for these pathogens, which can be transmitted to humans by the bites of female phlebotomine sandflies.

In increasing order of systemic involvement and potential clinical severity, major syndromes of human leishmaniasis have been classified into *cutaneous, mucocutaneous, diffuse cutaneous*, and *visceral* (*kala azar*) forms. Cutaneous forms of leishmaniasis generally are self-limiting, with cures occurring in 3-18 months after infection. However, this form of the disease can leave disfiguring scars. The mucocutaneous, diffuse cutaneous, and visceral forms of the disease do not resolve without therapy. Visceral leishmaniasis caused by *L. donovani* is fatal unless treated. The classic therapy for all species of *Leishmania* is *pentavalent antimony* (sodium antimony gluconate; sodium stibogluconate; PENTOSTAM); resistance to this compound is widespread in India, although it remains useful in other parts of the world. As an alternative, *liposomal amphotericin B* is a highly effective agent for visceral leishmaniasis, and it is currently the drug of choice for antimony-resistant disease. Treatment of leishmania has undergone major changes owing to the success of the first orally active agent, *miltefosine*. The drug also appears to have promise for the treatment of the cutaneous disease and for the treatment of dogs, an important animal reservoir of the disease. Paromomycin has been used with success as a parenteral agent for visceral disease, and topical formulations of paromomycin have efficacy against cutaneous disease.

OTHER PROTOZOAL INFECTIONS. Just a few of the many less common protozoal infections of humans are highlighted here.

Babesiosis, caused by either *Babesia microti* or *B. divergens*, is a tick-borne zoonosis that superficially resembles malaria in that the parasites invade erythrocytes, producing a febrile illness, hemolysis, and hemoglobinuria. This infection usually is mild and self-limiting but can be severe or even fatal in asplenic or severely immunocompromised individuals. Currently recommended therapy is with a combination of *clindamycin and quinine* for severe disease, and the combination of *azithromycin and atovaquone* for mild or moderate infections.

Balantidiasis, caused by the ciliated protozoan *Balantidium coli*, is an infection of the large intestine that may be confused with amebiasis. Unlike amebiasis, this infection usually responds to *tetracycline* therapy.

Isospora belli, a coccidian parasite, causes diarrhea in AIDS patients and responds to treatment with *trimethoprim-sulfamethoxazole*. *Cyclospora cayetanensis* causes self-limited diarrhea in normal hosts and can cause prolonged diarrhea in individuals with AIDS.

Microsporidia are spore-forming unicellular eukaryotic fungal parasites that can cause a number of disease syndromes, including diarrhea in immunocompromised individuals. Infections with microsporidia have been treated successfully with *albendazole*, an inhibitor of β-tubulin polymerization (*see* Chapter 51). Immunocompromised individuals with intestinal microsporidiosis due to *E. bieneusi* (which does not respond as well to albendazole) have been treated successfully with the antimicrobial *fumagillin*.

ANTIPROTOZOAL DRUGS

For ease of reference, the myriad agents used to treat nonmalarial protozoal diseases are presented alphabetically.

AMPHOTERICIN B

The pharmacology, formulation, and toxicology of amphotericin B are presented in Chapter 57.

Antiprotozoal Effects. Amphotericin B (AMBISOME) is a highly effective antileishmanial agent that cures >90% of the cases of visceral leishmaniasis and is the drug of choice for antimonial-resistant cases. It is a second-line drug for cutaneous or mucosal leishmaniasis, where it has been shown effective for the treatment of immunocompromised patients. The lipid preparations of the drug have reduced toxicity, but the cost of the drug and the difficulty of administration remain a problem in endemic regions.

Mechanism of Action. The basis of amphotericin B action against leishmania is similar to that for the drug's antifungal activities (*see* Chapter 57). Amphotericin complexes with ergosterol precursors in the cell membrane, forming pores that allow ions to enter the cell. Leishmania has similar sterol composition to fungal pathogens, and the drug binds to these sterols preferentially over the host cholesterol. No significant resistance to the drug has been encountered after nearly 30 years of use as an antifungal agent.

Therapeutic Uses. Typical regimens of 10-20 mg/kg total dose given in divided doses over 10-20 days by intravenous infusion have yielded >95% cure rates. In the U.S., the FDA recommends 3 mg/kg intravenously on days 1-5, 14, and 21 for a total dose of 21 mg/kg. Recent data suggest that a single dose of 5 mg/kg followed by 7-14 days treatment with oral miltefosine was effective at curing visceral leishmaniasis, and this dosing scheme warrants additional study.

CHLOROQUINE

The pharmacology and toxicology of chloroquine are presented in Chapter 49 (antimalarials). Chloroquine does have an FDA-approved use for *extra-intestinal amebiasis* at a dose of 1 g (600 mg base) daily for 2 days, followed by 500 mg daily for at least 2-3 weeks. Treatment is usually combined with an effective intestinal amebicide.

DILOXANIDE FUROATE

Diloxanide furoate (FURAMIDE, others) is a derivative of dichloroacetamide. Diloxanide furoate is a very effective luminal agent for the treatment of *E. histolytica* infection but is no longer available in the U.S.

EFLORNITHINE

Eflornithine (α-D,L difluoromethylornithine, DFMO, ORNIDYL) is an irreversible catalytic (suicide) inhibitor of ornithine decarboxylase, the enzyme that catalyzes the first and rate-limiting step in the biosynthesis of polyamines (putrescine, spermidine, and spermine) that are required for cell division and for normal cell differentiation. In trypanosomes, spermidine is required for the synthesis of trypanothione, a conjugate of spermidine and glutathione that replaces many of the functions of glutathione in the parasite.

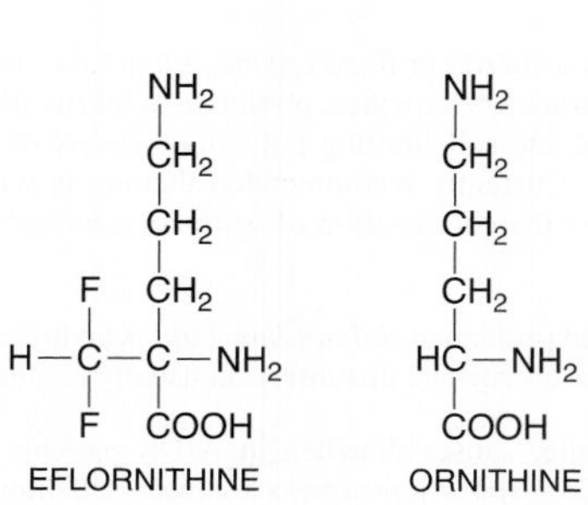

```
          NH2                 NH2
          |                   |
          CH2                 CH2
          |                   |
          CH2                 CH2
          |                   |
     F    CH2                 CH2
     |    |                   |
  H—C—C—NH2            HC—NH2
     |    |                   |
     F    COOH                COOH
   EFLORNITHINE          ORNITHINE
```

Eflornithine currently is used to treat West African (Gambian) trypanosomiasis caused by *T. brucei gambiense*; the drug is largely ineffective for East African trypanosomiasis. Eflornithine's difficult treatment regimen limits its use. Eflornithine is no longer available for systemic use in the U.S. but is available for treatment of Gambian trypanosomiasis by special request from the CDC. Eflornithine is safer and more efficacious than melarsoprol for late-stage gambiense sleeping sickness, and is the recommended first-line treatment for this disease when adequate care can be provided for its administration.

Antitrypanosomal Effects. Eflornithine is a cytostatic agent that has multiple biochemical effects on trypanosomes, all of which are a consequence of polyamine depletion. The parasite and human enzymes are equally susceptible to inhibition by eflornithine; however, the mammalian enzyme is turned over rapidly, whereas the parasite enzyme is stable, and this difference likely plays a role in the selective toxicity. *T. brucei rhodesiense* cells are less sensitive to eflornithine inhibition than *T. brucei gambiense* cells; studies *in vitro* suggest that the effective doses are increased by 10-20 times in the refractory cells. The molecular basis for the higher dose requirement in *T. brucei rhodesiense* is not understood.

ADME. Eflornithine is given by intravenous infusion. The drug does not bind to plasma proteins but is well distributed and penetrates into the CSF, where estimated concentrations of at least 50 μM must be reached to clear well distributed and penetrates into the CSF. Renal clearance after intravenous administration is rapid (2 mL/min/kg), with >80% of the drug cleared by the kidney largely in unchanged form. Some studies indicate that suramin enhances eflornithine uptake into the CNS and could lower the dose requirements for eflornithine.

Therapeutic Uses. Eflornithine is used for the treatment of late-stage West African trypanosomiasis caused by *T. brucei gambiense*. The preferred regimen for adult patients is 100 mg/kg given intravenously every 6 h as a 2-h infusion for 14 days. Response rates exceed 90% in the late-stage patients. Children (<12 years of age) receive higher doses of eflornithine (150 mg/kg given intravenously every 6 h for 14 days) based on prior findings that eflornithine trough concentrations in both the CSF and blood were significantly lower among children than in adults.The treatment course for eflornithine has been reduced to 7 days in combination with nifurtimox. This combination protocol, NECT, uses a shortened course of eflornithine with oral nifurtimox, with dosing as follows: 400 mg/kg/day given intravenously every 12 h by 2-h infusion for 7 days plus nifurtimox (orally at 15 mg/kg/day in 3 divided doses [every 8 h]) for 10 days. Eflornithine is less successful for treating AIDS patients with West African trypanosomiasis, presumably because host defenses play a critical role in clearing drug-treated *T. brucei gambiense* from the bloodstream.

Toxicity and Side Effects. Eflornithine causes adverse reactions that are generally reversible on withdrawal of the drug. Abdominal pain and headache are the predominant complaints, followed by reactions at the injection sites. Tissue infections and pneumonia are also observed. The most severe reactions reported include fever peaks (6%), seizures (4%), and diarrhea (2%). The case fatality rate for eflornithine (~1.2%) is significantly lower than for melarsoprol (4.9%), and overall eflornithine is superior to melarsoprol with respect to both safety and efficacy. Reversible hearing loss can occur after prolonged therapy with oral doses. Therapeutic doses of eflornithine are large and require coadministration of substantial volumes of intravenous fluid. This poses significant practical limitations in remote settings and can cause fluid overload in susceptible patients.

FUMAGILLIN

Fumagillin (FUMIDIL B, others) is an acyclic polyene macrolide. Fumagillin and its synthetic analog TNP-470 are toxic to microsporidia.

Fumagillin is used topically to treat keratoconjunctivitis caused by *E. hellem* at a dose of 3-10 mg/mL in a balanced salt suspension. For the treatment of intestinal microsporidiosis caused by *E. bieneusi*, fumagillin is used at a dose of 20 mg orally 3 times daily for 2 weeks. Adverse effects of fumagillin may include abdominal cramps, nausea, vomiting, and diarrhea. Reversible thrombocytopenia and neutropenia also have been reported. Fumagillin has not been approved for the systemic treatment of microsporidia infection in the U.S.

Fumagillin is used widely to treat the microsporidian *Nosema apis*, a pathogen of honey bees. Fumagillin and TNP-470 also inhibit angiogenesis and suppress tumor growth. TNP-470 is undergoing clinical trials as an anticancer agent (*see* Chapter 61). Human methionine-aminopeptidase-2 (MetAP2) is the target for the drugs' antitumor activity, and a gene encoding MetAP2 has been identified in the genome of the microsporidian parasite *E. cuniculi*.

8-HYDROXYQUINOLINES

The halogenated 8-hydroxyquinolines iodoquinol (diiodohydroxyquin) and clioquinol (iodochlorhydroxyquin) have been used as luminal agents to eliminate intestinal colonization with *E. histolytica*.

Iodoquinol (YODOXIN) is the safer and is the only one available for use as an oral agent in the U.S. When used at appropriate doses (never to exceed 2 g/day and duration of therapy not greater than 20 days in adults), adverse effects are unusual. However, the use of these drugs, especially at doses exceeding 2 g/day for long periods carries significant risk. The most important toxic reaction, ascribed primarily to clioquinol, is subacute myelo-optic neuropathy. Peripheral neuropathy is a less severe manifestation of neurotoxicity owing to these drugs. Administration of iodoquinol in high doses to children with chronic diarrhea has been associated with optic atrophy and permanent loss of vision.

Because of its superior adverse-event profile, paromomycin is preferred as the luminal agent for amebiasis; however, iodoquinol is a reasonable alternative. Iodoquinol is used in combination with metronidazole to treat individuals with amebic colitis or amebic liver abscess but may be used as a single agent for asymptomatic individuals found to be infected with *E. histolytica*. For adults, the recommended dose of iodoquinol is 650 mg orally 3 times daily for 20 days, whereas children receive 10 mg/kg of body weight orally 3 times a day (not to exceed 1.95 g/day) for 20 days.

MELARSOPROL

Despite the fact that it causes an often fatal encephalopathy in 2-10% of the patients, melarsoprol is the only drug for the treatment of late (CNS) stages of East African trypanosomiasis caused by *T. brucei rhodesiense*. Although melarsoprol is also effective against late-stage West African trypanosomiasis caused by *T. brucei gambiense*, eflornithine has become the first-line treatment for this disease. The continued use of melarsoprol in the field is indicative of the paucity of alternative therapies for late-stage sleeping sickness.

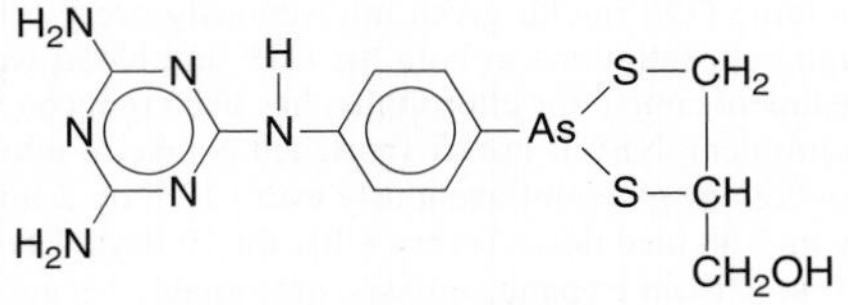

MELARSOPROL

Melarsoprol (MEL B; ARSOBAL) is supplied as a 3.6% (w/v) solution in propylene glycol for intravenous administration. It is available in the U.S. only from the CDC.

Mechanism of Action; Antiprotozoal Effects. Melarsoprol is metabolized to melarsen oxide, the active drug. Arsen-oxides react avidly and reversibly with vicinal sulfhydryl groups and thereby inactivate many enzymes. Melarsoprol reacts with trypanothione, the spermidine-glutathione adduct that substitutes for glutathione in these parasites. Binding of melarsoprol to trypanothione results in a melarsen oxide-trypanothione adduct that inhibits trypanothione reductase. Both the sequestering of trypanothione and the inhibition of trypanothione reductase would have lethal consequences to the cell; however, this mode of action remains unproven. Treatment failure owing to resistance of trypanosomes to melarsoprol has risen sharply and some of the resistant strains are an order of magnitude less sensitive to the drug. Resistance to melarsoprol likely involves transport defects. The adenine-adenosine transporter termed the *P2 transporter* is 1 example. It has activity on melarsoprol as well as pentamidine and berenil; point mutations in this transporter are found in melarsoprol-resistant isolates. Another transporter, HAPT1, has been identified, and the concomitant loss of both the P2 and HAPT transporters led to high-level cross-resistance to both melarsen and pentamidine.

ADME. Melarsoprol is always administered by slow intravenous injection, with care to avoid leakage into the surrounding tissues because the drug is intensely irritating. Melarsoprol is a prodrug and is metabolized rapidly ($t_{1/2}$ = 30 min) to melarsen oxide, the active form of the drug. A small but therapeutically significant amount of the drug enters the CSF and has a lethal effect on trypanosomes infecting the CNS. The compound is excreted rapidly, with 70-80% of the arsenic appearing in the feces.

Therapeutic Uses. Melarsoprol is the only effective drug available for treatment of the late meningoencephalitic stage of East African (Rhodesian) trypanosomiasis, which is 100% fatal if untreated. The drug is also effective in the early hemolymphatic stage of these infections, but because of its toxicity, it is reserved for therapy of late-stage infections. Patients infected with *T. brucei rhodesiense* who relapse after a course of melarsoprol usually respond to a second course of the drug. In contrast, patients infected with *T. brucei gambiense* who are not cured with melarsoprol rarely benefit from repeated treatment with this drug. Such patients often respond well to eflornithine.

For *T. brucei gambiense* a continuous 10-day course of 2.2 mg/kg/day is equivalent to the longer course treatment and is now recommended. For *T. brucei rhodesiense*, the CDC recommends 3 series of 3 daily doses with a 7-day rest period between series. The first series gives 1.8, 2.7, and 3.6 mg/kg on days 1, 2, and 3, respectively. The subsequent series are 3.6 mg/kg daily. Encephalopathy develops more frequently in patients with *T. brucei rhodesiense* compared to *T. brucei gambiense*. Concurrent administration of prednisolone is frequently employed throughout the treatment course.

Toxicity and Side Effects. Treatment with melarsoprol is associated with significant toxicity and morbidity. A febrile reaction often occurs soon after drug injection, especially if parasitemia is high. The most serious complications involve the nervous system. A reactive encephalopathy occurs 9-11 days after treatment starts in ~5-10% of patients, leading to death in about half of these. Peripheral neuropathy occurs in ~10% of patients receiving melarsoprol. Hypertension and myocardial damage are not uncommon, although shock is rare. Albuminuria occurs frequently, and evidence of renal or hepatic damage may necessitate modification of treatment. Vomiting and abdominal colic also are common, but their incidence can be reduced by injecting melarsoprol slowly into the supine, fasting patient.

Precautions and Contraindications. Melarsoprol should be given only to patients under hospital supervision. Initiation of therapy during a febrile episode has been associated with an increased incidence of reactive encephalopathy. Administration of melarsoprol to leprous patients may precipitate erythema nodosum. Use of the drug is contraindicated during epidemics of influenza. Severe hemolytic reactions have been reported in patients with deficiency of glucose-6-phosphate dehydrogenase. The drug may be used in pregnancy.

METRONIDAZOLE

Metronidazole and related nitroimidazoles are active in vitro against a wide variety of anaerobic protozoal parasites and anaerobic bacteria. Metronidazole is clinically effective in trichomoniasis, amebiasis, and giardiasis, as well as in a variety of infections caused by obligate anaerobic bacteria, including *Bacteroides, Clostridium*, and microaerophilic bacteria such as *Helicobacter* and *Campylobacter* spp. Metronidazole manifests antibacterial activity against all anaerobic cocci and both anaerobic gram-negative bacilli, including *Bacteroides* spp., and anaerobic spore-forming gram-positive bacilli. Nonsporulating gram-positive bacilli often are resistant, as are aerobic and facultatively anaerobic bacteria.

MECHANISM OF ACTION AND RESISTANCE. Metronidazole is a prodrug requiring reductive activation of the nitro group by susceptible organisms. Unlike their aerobic counterparts, anaerobic and microaerophilic pathogens (e.g., the amitochondriate protozoa *T. vaginalis, E. histolytica*, and *G. lamblia* and various anaerobic bacteria) contain electron transport components that have a sufficiently negative redox potential to donate electrons to metronidazole. The single electron transfer forms a highly reactive nitro radical anion that kills susceptible organisms by radical-mediated mechanisms that target DNA. Metronidazole is catalytically recycled; loss of the active metabolite's electron regenerates the parent compound. Increasing levels of O_2 inhibit metronidazole-induced cytotoxicity because O_2 competes with metronidazole for electrons generated by energy metabolism. Thus, O_2 can both decrease reductive activation of metronidazole and increase recycling of the activated drug. Anaerobic or microaerophilic organisms susceptible to metronidazole derive energy from the oxidative fermentation of ketoacids such as pyruvate. Pyruvate decarboxylation, catalyzed by pyruvate-ferredoxin oxidoreductase (PFOR), produces electrons that reduce ferredoxin, which, in turn, catalytically donates its electrons to biological electron acceptors or to metronidazole.

Clinical resistance to metronidazole is well documented for *T. vaginalis, G. lamblia*, and a variety of anaerobic and microaerophilic bacteria. Resistance correlates with impaired oxygen-scavenging capabilities, leading to higher local O_2 concentrations, decreased activation of metronidazole, and futile recycling of the activated drug. Other resistant strains have lowered levels of PFOR and ferredoxin, perhaps explaining why they may still respond to higher doses of metronidazole. In the case of *Bacteroides* spp., metronidazole resistance has been linked to a family of nitroimidazole (*nim*) resistance genes that can be encoded chromosomally or episomally. These *nim* genes appear to encode a nitroimidazole reductase capable of converting a 5-nitroimidazole to a 5-aminoimidazole, thus stopping the formation of the reactive nitroso group responsible for microbial killing.

ADME. Preparations of metronidazole are available for oral, intravenous, intravaginal, and topical administration. The drug usually is absorbed completely and promptly after oral intake and distributed to a volume approximating total body water; less than 20% of the drug is bound to plasma proteins. A linear relationship between dose and plasma concentration pertains for doses of 200-2000 mg. Repeated doses every 6-8 h result in some accumulation of the drug. The $t_{1/2}$ of metronidazole in plasma is ~8 h. With the exception of the placenta, metronidazole penetrates well into body tissues and fluids, including vaginal secretions, seminal fluid, saliva, breast milk, and CSF. After an oral dose, >75% of labeled metronidazole is eliminated in the urine, largely as metabolites formed by the liver from oxidation of the drug's side chains, a hydroxy derivative and an acid; ~10% is recovered as unchanged drug. Two principal metabolites result. The hydroxy metabolite has a longer $t_{1/2}$ (~12 h) and has ~50% of the antitrichomonal activity of metronidazole. Formation of glucuronides also is observed. Small quantities of reduced metabolites are formed by the gut flora. The urine of some patients may be reddish brown owing to the presence of unidentified pigments derived from the drug. Oxidative metabolism of metronidazole is induced by phenobarbital, prednisone, rifampin, and possibly ethanol and is inhibited by cimetidine.

THERAPEUTIC USES. Metronidazole cures genital infections with *T. vaginalis* in both in >90% of cases. The preferred treatment regimen is 2 g metronidazole as a single oral dose for both males and females. Tinidazole, which has a longer $t_{1/2}$ than metronidazole, is also used at a 2-g single dose and appears to provide equivalent or better responses. When repeated courses or higher doses of the drug are required for uncured or recurrent infections, it is recommended that intervals of 4-6 weeks elapse between courses. Leukocyte counts should be carried out before, during, and after each course of treatment. Treatment failures owing to the presence of metronidazole-resistant strains of *T. vaginalis* are becoming increasingly common. Most of these cases can be treated successfully by giving a second 2-g dose to both patient and sexual partner. In addition to oral therapy, the use of a topical gel containing 0.75% metronidazole or a 500- to 1000-mg vaginal suppository may be beneficial in refractory cases.

Metronidazole is the agent of choice for the treatment of all symptomatic forms of amebiasis, including amebic colitis and amebic liver abscess. The recommended dose is 500-750 mg metronidazole taken orally 3 times daily for 7-10 days, or for children, 35-50 mg/kg/day given in 3 divided doses for 7-10 days. Amebic liver abscess has been treated successfully by short courses (2.4 g daily as a single oral dose for 2 days) of metronidazole or tinidazole. *E. histolytica* persist in most patients who recover from acute amebiasis after metronidazole therapy, so it is recommended that all such individuals also be treated with a luminal amebicide. Although effective for the therapy of giardiasis, metronidazole has yet to be approved for treatment of this infection in the U.S. However, tinidazole is approved for the treatment of giardiasis as a single 2-g dose and is appropriate first-line therapy.

Metronidazole is a relatively inexpensive and versatile drug with efficacy against a broad spectrum of anaerobic and microaerophilic bacteria. It is used for the treatment of serious infections owing to susceptible anaerobic bacteria, including *Bacteroides*, *Clostridium*, *Fusobacterium*, *Peptococcus*, *Peptostreptococcus*, *Eubacterium*, and *Helicobacter*. The drug is also given in combination with other antimicrobial agents to treat polymicrobial infections with aerobic and anaerobic bacteria. Metronidazole achieves clinically effective levels in bones, joints, and the CNS. It can be given intravenously when oral administration is not possible. Metronidazole is used as a component of prophylaxis for colorectal surgery and is employed as a single agent to treat bacterial vaginosis. It is used in combination with other antibiotics and a proton pump inhibitor in regimens to treat infection with *H. pylori* (*see* Chapter 45). Metronidazole is used as primary therapy for *Clostridium difficile* infection, the major cause of pseudomembranous colitis. Metronidazole is also used in the treatment of patients with Crohn disease who have perianal fistulas and colonic disease.

Toxicity, Contraindications, and Drug Interactions. Common side effects are headache, nausea, dry mouth, and a metallic taste. Vomiting, diarrhea, and abdominal distress are experienced occasionally. Dizziness, vertigo, and very rarely, encephalopathy, convulsions, incoordination, and ataxia are neurotoxic effects that warrant discontinuation of metronidazole. The drug also should be withdrawn if numbness or paresthesias of the extremities occur. Reversal of serious sensory neuropathies may be slow or incomplete. Urticaria, flushing, and pruritus are indicative of drug sensitivity that can require withdrawal of metronidazole. Metronidazole is a rare cause of Stevens-Johnson syndrome, which may be more common among individuals receiving high doses of metronidazole and concurrent therapy with the antihelminthic mebendazole. Dysuria, cystitis, and a sense of pelvic pressure have been reported. Metronidazole has a disulfiram-like effect, and some patients experience abdominal distress, vomiting, flushing, or headache if they drink alcoholic beverages during or within 3 days of therapy with this drug. Metronidazole and disulfiram or any disulfiram-like drug should not be taken together because confusional and psychotic states may occur. Metronidazole should be used cautiously in patients with active disease of the CNS because of potential neurotoxicity. The drug also may precipitate CNS signs of lithium toxicity in patients receiving high doses of lithium. Metronidazole can prolong the prothrombin time of patients receiving therapy with warfarin (COUMADIN) anticoagulants. The dosage of metronidazole should be reduced in patients with severe hepatic disease. Metronidazole use during the first trimester generally is not advised.

MILTEFOSINE

Miltefosine (IMPAVIDO) is an alkylphosphocholine (APC) analog developed originally as an anticancer agent. It is highly curative against visceral leishmaniasis and also appears to be effective against the cutaneous forms of the disease. Its main drawback is its teratogenicity; it must not be used in pregnant women.

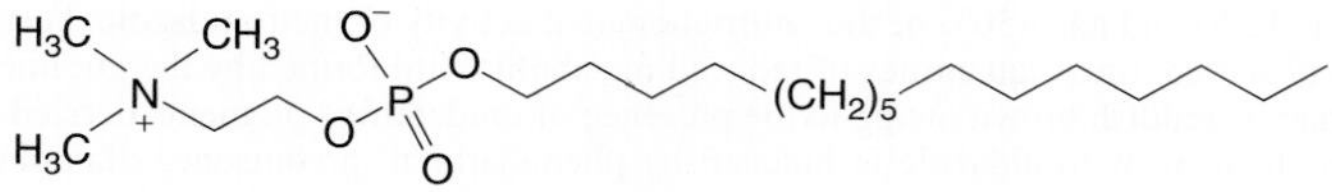

H_3C CH_3 O^- N+ O P O $(CH_2)_5$ H_3C O

MILTEFOSINE

Antiprotozoal Effects. Miltefosine is the first orally available therapy for leishmaniasis. It is a safe and effective treatment for visceral leishmaniasis and has shown >90% efficacy against some species of cutaneous leishmaniasis. The mechanism of action of miltefosine is not yet understood. Studies in *Leishmania* suggest that the drug may alter ether-lipid metabolism, cell signaling, or glycosylphosphatidylinositol anchor biosynthesis. Mutations in a P-type ATPase that belongs to the aminophospholipid translocase subfamily apparently decrease drug uptake and confer drug resistance.

ADME. Miltefosine is well absorbed orally and distributed throughout the human body. Detailed pharmacokinetic data are lacking, with the exception that miltefosine has a long $t_{1/2}$ (1-4 weeks). Plasma concentrations are proportional to the dose.

Therapeutic Uses. Oral miltefosine is registered for use in India for the treatment of visceral leishmaniasis: for adults >25 kg, 100 mg daily divided into 2 parts, and for adults <25 kg, 50 mg daily in 1 dose for 28 days; for children, 2.5 mg/kg/day in 2 divided doses. In the U.S., the recommended dose for both visceral and cutaneous disease is 2.5 mg/kg/day (maximum dose of 150 mg/day) for 28 days, given in 2 divided doses. The compound cannot be given intravenously because it has hemolytic activity.

Toxicity and Side Effects. Vomiting and diarrhea have been reported as frequent side effects in up to 60% of the patients. Elevations in hepatic transaminases and serum creatinine also have been reported. These effects are typically mild and reversible. Because of its teratogenic potential, miltefosine is contraindicated in pregnant women.

NIFURTIMOX AND BENZNIDAZOLE

Nifurtimox and benznidazole are used to treat American trypanosomiasis caused by *T. cruzi*. Nifurtimox (Bayer 2502, LAMPIT), a nitrofuran analog, and benznidazole (Roche 7-1051, ROCHAGAN), a nitroimidazole analog, can be obtained in the U.S. from the CDC.

Antiprotozoal Effects and Mechanisms of Action. Nifurtimox and benznidazole are trypanocidal against both the trypomastigote and amastigote forms of *T. cruzi*. Nifurtimox also has activity against *T. brucei* and can be curative against both early- and late-stage disease (see earlier discussion on nifurtimox-eflornithine combination therapy). The trypanocidal effects of nifurtimox and benznidazole derive from their activation by a NADH-dependent mitochondrial nitroreductase to nitro radical anions that are thought to account for the trypanocidal effects. The generated nitro anion radicals form covalent attachments to macromolecules leading to cellular damage that includes lipid peroxidation and membrane injury, enzyme inactivation, and damage to DNA.

ADME. Nifurtimox is well absorbed after oral administration, with peak plasma levels observed after ~3.5 h. Less than 0.5% of the dose is excreted in urine. The elimination $t_{1/2}$ is ~3 h. High concentrations of several unidentified metabolites are found, and nifurtimox undergoes rapid biotransformation, probably via a presystemic first-pass effect. Whether the metabolites have any trypanocidal activity is unknown.

Therapeutic Uses. Nifurtimox and benznidazole are employed in the treatment of American trypanosomiasis (Chagas disease) caused by *T. cruzi*. Because of toxicity, benznidazole is the preferred treatment. Both drugs markedly reduce the parasitemia, morbidity, and mortality of acute Chagas disease, with parasitological cures obtained in 80% of these cases. In the chronic form of the disease, parasitological cures are still possible in up to 50% of the patients, although the drug is less effective than in the acute stage. The clinical response of the acute illness to drug therapy varies with geographic region; parasite strains in Argentina, southern Brazil, Chile, and Venezuela appear to be more susceptible than those in central Brazil. The current recommendations are that patients <50 years of age with either acute- or recent chronic-phase disease, without advanced cardiomyopathy, should be treated. In patients >50 years of age, treatment is optional because of lowered drug tolerability. Therapy is strongly encouraged for patients who will receive immunosuppressive therapy or who are HIV positive. Therapy with nifurtimox or benznidazole should start promptly after exposure for persons at risk of *T. cruzi* infection from laboratory accidents or from blood transfusions.

Both drugs are given orally. For nifurtimox, adults (>17 years of age) with acute infection should receive 8-10 mg/kg/day in 3 to 4 divided doses for 90 days; children 1-10 years of age should receive 15-20 mg/kg/day in 3 to 4 divided doses for 90 days; for individuals 11-16 years old, the daily dose is 12.5-15 mg/kg given according to the same schedule. For benznidazole, the recommended treatment for adults (>13 years) is 5-7 mg/kg/day in 2 divided doses for 60 days, with children up to 12 years receiving 10 mg/kg/day. If gastric upset and weight loss occur during treatment, dosage should be reduced. The ingestion of alcohol should be avoided. Nifurtimox is used in combination with eflornithine in treating late stage *T.b. gambiense* sleeping sickness.

Toxicity and Side Effects. Side effects are common and range from hypersensitivity reactions (e.g., dermatitis, fever, icterus, pulmonary infiltrates, and anaphylaxis) to dose- and age-dependent complications primarily referable to the GI tract and both the peripheral and central nervous systems. Nausea and vomiting are common, as are myalgia and weakness. Peripheral neuropathy and GI symptoms are especially common after prolonged treatment; the latter complication may lead to weight loss and preclude further therapy. Because of the seriousness of Chagas disease and the lack of superior drugs, there are few absolute contraindications to the use of these drugs.

NITAZOXANIDE

Nitazoxanide (*N*-[nitrothiazolyl] salicylamide, ALINA) is an oral synthetic broad-spectrum antiparasitic agent (*see* Chapter 51). Nitazoxanide is FDA-approved for the treatment of cryptosporidiosis and giardiasis in children.

Antimicrobial Effects. Nitazoxanide and its active metabolite, tizoxanide (desacetyl-nitazoxanide), inhibit the growth of sporozoites and oocytes of *C. parvum* and inhibit the growth of the trophozoites of *G. intestinalis*, *E. histolytica*, and *T. vaginalis* in vitro. Nitazoxanide also demonstrated activity against intestinal helminths.

Mechanism of Action. Nitazoxanide interferes with the PFOR enzyme-dependent electron-transfer reaction, which is essential to anaerobic metabolism in protozoan and bacterial species.

ADME. Following oral administration, nitazoxanide is hydrolyzed rapidly to its active metabolite, tizoxanide, which undergoes conjugation to tizoxanide glucuronide. Bioavailability after an oral dose is excellent, and maximum plasma concentrations of the metabolites occur 1-4 h following administration. Tizoxanide is >99.9% bound to plasma proteins. Tizoxanide is excreted in the urine, bile, and feces; tizoxanide glucuronide is excreted in the urine and bile.

Therapeutic Uses. In the U.S., nitazoxanide is approved for the treatment of *G. intestinalis* infection (therapeutic efficacy of 85-90% for clinical response) and for the treatment of diarrhea caused by cryptosporidia (therapeutic efficacy, 56-88% for clinical response) in adults and children >1 year of age. The efficacy of nitazoxanide in children (or adults) with cryptosporidia infection and AIDS has not been clearly established. For children ages 12-47 months, the recommended dose is 100 mg nitazoxanide every 12 h for 3 days; for children ages 4-11 years, the dose is 200 mg nitazoxanide every 12 h for 3 days. A 500-mg tablet, suitable for adult dosing (every 12 h), is available. Nitazoxanide has been used as a single agent to treat mixed infections with intestinal parasites (protozoa and helminths). Effective parasite clearance after nitazoxanide treatment was shown for *G. intestinalis, E. histolytica/E. dispar, B. hominis, C. parvum, C. cayetanensis, I. belli, H. nana, T. trichiura, A. lumbricoides*, and *E. vermicularis*, although more than 1 course of therapy was required in some cases. Nitazoxanide has been used to treat infections with *G. intestinalis* that are resistant to metronidazole and albendazole.

Toxicity and Side Effects. Adverse effects appear are rare with nitazoxanide. A greenish tint to the urine is seen in most individuals taking nitazoxanide. Nitazoxanide is a pregnancy Category B agent, based on animal teratogenicity and fertility studies.

PAROMOMYCIN

Paromomycin (aminosidine, HUMATIN) is an aminoglycoside that is used as an oral agent to treat *E. histolytica* infection, cryptosporidiosis, and giardiasis. A topical formulation has been used to treat trichomoniasis; parenteral administration has been used for visceral leishmaniasis.

Mechanism of Action; ADME. Paromomycin shares the same mechanism of action as neomycin and kanamycin (binding to the 30S ribosomal subunit) and has the same spectrum of antibacterial activity. The drug is not absorbed from the GI tract and thus the actions of an oral dose are confined to the GI tract; 100% of the oral dose is recovered in the feces. Paromomycin is available only for oral use in the U.S.

Antimicrobial Effects; Therapeutics Uses. Paromomycin is the drug of choice for treating intestinal colonization with *E. histolytica* and is used in combination with metronidazole to treat amebic colitis and amebic liver abscess. Adverse effects are rare with oral usage but include abdominal pain and cramping, epigastric pain, nausea and vomiting, steatorrhea, and diarrhea. Rarely, rash and headache have been reported. Dosing in adults is 500 mg orally 3 times daily for 10 days, whereas children have been treated with 25-30 mg/kg/day in 3 divided oral doses. Paromomycin formulated as a 6.25% cream has been used to treat vaginal trichomoniasis in patients in whom metronidazole therapy has failed. Cures have been reported, but vulvovaginal ulcerations and pain can complicate treatment. Paromomycin is also efficacious as a topical formulation containing 15% paromomycin in combination with 12% methylbenzonium chloride for the treatment of cutaneous leishmaniasis. The drug has been administered parenterally alone or in combination with antimony to treat visceral leishmaniasis. Paromomycin has been advocated as a treatment for giardiasis in pregnant women, when metronidazole is contraindicated and as an alternative agent for metronidazole-resistant isolates of *G. intestinalis*.

PENTAMIDINE

Pentamidine is a positively charged aromatic diamine. It is a broad-spectrum agent with activity against several species of pathogenic protozoa and some fungi.

Pentamidine as the di-isethionate salt is marketed for injection (PENTAM 300, others) or for use as an aerosol (NEBUPENT). The di-isethionate salt is highly water soluble; however, solutions should be used promptly because pentamidine is unstable in solution.

Antiprotozoal and Antifungal Effects. Pentamidine is used for the treatment of early-stage *T. brucei gambiense* infection but is ineffective in the treatment of late-stage disease and has reduced efficacy against *T. brucei rhodesiense*. Pentamidine is an alternative agent for the treatment of cutaneous leishmaniasis. Pentamidine is an alternative agent for the treatment and prophylaxis of Pneumocystis pneumonia caused by *Pneumocystis jiroveci*. *Diminazene* (BERENIL) is a related diamidine that is used as an inexpensive alternative to pentamidine for the treatment of early African trypanosomiasis.

Mechanism of Action and Resistance. The mechanism of action of the diamidines is unknown. The compounds display multiple effects on any given parasite and act by disparate mechanisms in different parasites. Multiple transporters are responsible for pentamidine uptake, and this may account for the fact that little resistance to this drug is observed in field isolates despite its years of use as a prophylactic agent.

ADME. Pentamidine isethionate is fairly well absorbed from parenteral sites of administration. Following a single intravenous dose, the drug disappears from plasma with an apparent $t_{1/2}$ of several minutes to a few h and maximum plasma concentrations after intramuscular injection occurring at 1 h. The $t_{1/2}$ of elimination is long (weeks to months); the drug is 70% bound to plasma proteins. This highly charged compound is poorly absorbed orally and does not cross the blood-brain barrier, explaining its ineffectiveness against late-stage trypanosomiasis. Inhalation of pentamidine aerosols is used for prophylaxis of *Pneumocystis* pneumonia; delivery of drug by this route results in little systemic absorption and decreased toxicity compared with intravenous administration.

Therapeutic Uses. Pentamidine isethionate is used for the treatment of early-stage *T. brucei gambiense* and is given by intramuscular injection in single doses of 4 mg/kg/day for 7 days. Pentamidine has been used successfully in courses of 15-20 intramuscular doses of 4 mg/kg every other day to treat visceral leishmaniasis. This compound provides an alternative to antimonials, lipid formulations of amphotericin B, or miltefosine but it is overall the least well tolerated.

Pentamidine is one of several drugs or drug combinations used to treat or prevent *Pneumocystis* infection. *Pneumocystis* pneumonia (PCP) is a major cause of mortality in individuals with AIDS and can occur in patients who are immunosuppressed by other mechanisms. Trimethoprim-sulfamethoxazole is the drug of choice for the treatment and prevention of PCP (*see* Chapter 52). Pentamidine is reserved for 2 indications: (1) as a 4 mg/kg single daily intravenous dose for 21 days to treat severe PCP in individuals who cannot tolerate trimethoprim-sulfamethoxazole and are not candidates for alternative agents (e.g., atovaquone or the combination of clindamycin and primaquine); (2) as a "salvage" agent for individuals with PCP who fail to respond to initial therapy (usually trimethoprim-sulfamethoxazole; pentamidine may be less effective than the combination of clindamycin and primaquine or atovaquone for this indication).

Pentamidine administered as an aerosol preparation is used for the prevention of PCP in at-risk individuals who cannot tolerate trimethoprim-sulfamethoxazole and are not deemed candidates for either dapsone (alone or in combination with pyrimethamine) or atovaquone. Candidates for PCP prophylaxis are individuals with HIV infection and a CD4 count of <200/mm^3 and individuals with HIV infection and persistent unexplained fever or oropharyngeal candidiasis. For prophylaxis, pentamidine isethionate is given monthly as a 300-mg dose in a 5-10% nebulized solution over 30-45 min. Although convenient, aerosolized pentamidine has several disadvantages, including its failure to treat any extrapulmonary sites of *Pneumocystis*, the lack of efficacy against any other potential opportunistic pathogens, and a slightly increased risk for pneumothorax.

Toxicity and Side Effects. Approximately 50% of individuals receiving the drug at recommended doses show some adverse effect. Intravenous administration of pentamidine may be associated with hypotension, tachycardia, and headache. These effects are probably secondary to the binding of pentamidine to imidazoline receptors and can be ameliorated by slowing the infusion rate. Hypoglycemia, which can be life threatening, may occur at any time during pentamidine treatment. Careful monitoring of blood sugar is key. Paradoxically, pancreatitis, hyperglycemia, and the development of insulin-dependent diabetes have been seen in some patients. Pentamidine is nephrotoxic (~25% of treated patients show signs of renal dysfunction), and if the serum creatinine concentration rises >1.0-2.0 mg/dL, it may be necessary to withhold the drug temporarily or change to an alternative agent. Other adverse effects include skin rashes, thrombophlebitis, anemia, neutropenia, and elevation of hepatic enzymes. Intramuscular administration of pentamidine is associated with the development of sterile abscesses at the injection site, which can become infected secondarily; most authorities recommend intravenous administration. Aerosolized pentamidine is associated with few adverse events.

SODIUM STIBOGLUCONATE

Sodium stibogluconate (sodium antimony gluconate, PENTOSTAM) is a pentavalent antimonial compound that has been the mainstay of the treatment of leishmaniasis. Increasing resistance to antimonials has reduced their efficacy and they are no longer useful in India, where lipid-based amphotericin B and miltefosine are now recommended instead. In the U.S., sodium stibogluconate can be obtained from the CDC.

Mechanism of Action. The relatively nontoxic pentavalent antimonials act as prodrugs that are reduced to the more toxic Sb^{3+} species that kill amastigotes within the phagolysosomes of macrophages. Following reduction, the drugs seem to interfere with the trypanothione redox system, Sb^{3+} induces a rapid efflux of trypanothione and glutathione from the cells, and also inhibits trypanothione reductase, thereby causing a significant loss of thiol reduction potential in the cells.

ADME. The drug is given intravenously or intramuscularly; it is not active orally. The agent is absorbed rapidly, distributed in an apparent volume of ~0.22 L/kg, and eliminated in 2 phases. The first has a $t_{1/2}$ of ~2 h, and the second is much slower ($t_{1/2}$ = 33-76 h). The prolonged terminal elimination phase may reflect conversion of the Sb^{5+} to the more toxic Sb^{3+} that is concentrated and slowly released from tissues. The drug is eliminated in the urine.

Therapeutic Uses. Sodium stibogluconate is given parenterally. The standard course is 20 mg/kg/day for 21 days for cutaneous disease and for 28 days for visceral leishmaniasis. Increased resistance has greatly compromised the effectiveness of antimonials, and the stibogluconate is now obsolete in India. Liposomal amphotericin B is the recommended alternative for treatment of either visceral leishmaniasis (*kala azar*) in India or mucosal leishmaniasis in general; the orally effective compound miltefosine is likely to see much wider use. Intralesional treatment has also been advocated as a safer, alternative method for treating cutaneous disease. Children usually tolerate the drug well at the same dose per kilogram used for adults. Patients who respond favorably show clinical improvement within 1-2 weeks of initiation of therapy. The drug may be given on alternate days or for longer intervals if unfavorable reactions occur in especially debilitated individuals. Patients infected with HIV present a challenge because they usually relapse after successful initial therapy with either pentavalent antimonials or amphotericin B.

Toxicity and Side Effects. In general, high-dose regimens of sodium stibogluconate are fairly well tolerated; toxic reactions usually are reversible, and most subside despite continued therapy. Adverse effects noted most commonly include pain at the injection site; chemical pancreatitis in nearly all patients; elevation of serum hepatic transaminase levels; bone marrow suppression manifested by decreased red cell, white cell, and platelet counts in the blood; muscle and joint pain; weakness and malaise; headache; nausea and abdominal pain; and skin rashes. Reversible polyneuropathy has been reported. Hemolytic anemia and renal damage are rare manifestations of antimonial toxicity, as are shock and sudden death.

SURAMIN

Suramin sodium (BAYER 205, formerly GERMANIN, others) is a water-soluble trypanocide; solutions deteriorate quickly in air and only freshly prepared solutions should be used. In the U.S., suramin is available only from the CDC.

Antiparasitic Effects. Suramin is a relatively slow-acting trypanocide (>6 h in vitro) with high clinical activity against both *T. b. gambiense* and *T. b. rhodesiense*. Its mechanism of action is unknown. Selective toxicity is likely to result from the ability of the parasite to take up the drug by receptor-mediated endocytosis of the protein-bound drug, with low-density lipoproteins the most important interacting proteins for this event. Suramin inhibits many trypanosomal and mammalian enzymes and receptors unrelated to its antiparasitic effects. No consensus for the mechanism of action has emerged, and the lack of any significant field resistance points to multiple potential targets.

ADME. Because it is not absorbed after oral intake, suramin is given intravenously to avoid local inflammation and necrosis associated with subcutaneous or intramuscular injections. After its administration, the drug displays complex pharmacokinetics with marked interindividual variability. The drug is 99.7% serum protein bound and has a terminal elimination $t_{1/2}$ of 41-78 days. Suramin is not appreciably metabolized; renal clearance accounts for elimination of ~80% of the compound from the body. Very little suramin penetrates the CSF, consistent with its polar character and lack of efficacy once the CNS has been invaded by trypanosomes.

Therapeutic Uses. Suramin is the first-line therapy for early-stage *T. brucei rhodesiense* infection. Because only small amounts of the drug enter the brain, suramin is used only for the treatment of early-stage African trypanosomiasis (before CNS involvement). Treatment of active African trypanosomiasis should not be started until 24 h after diagnostic lumbar puncture to ensure no CNS involvement, and caution is required if the patient has onchocerciasis (river blindness) because of the potential for eliciting a Mazzotti reaction (i.e., pruritic rash, fever, malaise, lymph node swelling, eosinophilia, arthralgias, tachycardia, hypotension, and possibly permanent blindness). Suramin is given by slow intravenous injection as a 10% aqueous solution. The normal single dose for adults with *T. brucei rhodesiense* infection is 1 g. It is advisable to employ a test dose of 200 mg initially to detect sensitivity, after which the normal dose is given intravenously (e.g., on days 1, 3, 7, 14, and 21). The pediatric dose is 20 mg/kg, given according to the same schedule. Patients in poor condition should be treated with lower doses during the first week. Patients who relapse after suramin therapy should be treated with melarsoprol.

Toxicity and Side Effects. The most serious immediate reaction consisting of nausea, vomiting, shock, and loss of consciousness is rare (~1 in 2000 patients). Malaise, nausea, and fatigue are also common immediate reactions. The most common problem encountered after several doses of suramin is renal toxicity, manifested by albuminuria, and delayed neurological complications, including headache, metallic taste, paresthesias, and peripheral neuropathy. These complications usually disappear spontaneously despite continued therapy. Other, less prevalent reactions include vomiting, diarrhea, stomatitis, chills, abdominal pain, and edema. Patients receiving suramin should be followed closely. Therapy should not be continued in patients who show intolerance to initial doses, and the drug should be employed with great caution in individuals with renal insufficiency.

For a complete Bibliographical Listing see Goodman & Gilman's ***The Pharmacological Basis of Therapeutics***, 12th ed., or Goodman & Gilman Online at www.AccessMedicine.com.

51 chapter Chemotherapy of Helminth Infections

Infections with helminths, or parasitic worms, affect more than 2 billion people worldwide (Figure 51–1). In regions of rural poverty in the tropics, where prevalence is greatest, simultaneous infection with more than 1 type of helminth is common.

Worms pathogenic for humans are *Metazoa* and can be classified into *roundworms* (*nematodes*) and 2 types of *flatworms, flukes* (*trematodes*) and *tapeworms* (*cestodes*). These biologically diverse eukaryotes vary with respect to life cycle, bodily structure, development, physiology, localization within the host, and susceptibility to chemotherapy. Immature forms invade humans via the skin or GI tract and evolve into well-differentiated adult worms with characteristic tissue distributions. With few exceptions, such as *Strongyloides* and *Echinococcus*, these organisms cannot complete their life cycle and replicate within the human host to produce mature offspring. Therefore, the extent of exposure to these parasites dictates the number of parasites infecting the host. Second, any reduction in the number of adult organisms by chemotherapy is sustained unless reinfection occurs. The burden of parasitic helminths within an infected population is not uniformly distributed, and it typically displays a negative binomial distribution whereby relatively few persons carry the heaviest parasite burden, resulting in increased morbidity in these individuals who also contribute disproportionately to transmission.

Anthelmintics are drugs that act either locally within the gut lumen to cause expulsion of worms from the GI tract, or systemically against helminths residing outside the GI tract. Therapy for many tissue-dwelling helminths, such as filarial parasites, is not fully effective. There is increasing appreciation of the impact of helminth infections on the health and education of school-aged children. In a massive public health effort, international health organizations are promoting the periodic and frequent use of anthelmintic drugs in schools as a means to control morbidity caused by soil-transmitted helminths and schistosomes in developing countries. Control programs employing anthelmintics rank among the world's largest health efforts, and hundreds of millions of people receive treatment annually.

This chapter is divided into 2 main parts:

- Clinical presentation and recommended chemotherapy for common helminth infections
- Pharmacological properties of specific anthelmintics

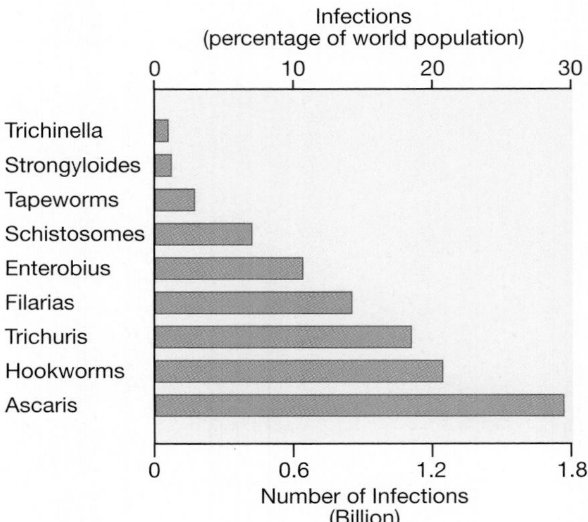

Figure 51–1 *Relative incidence of helminth infections worldwide.*

NEMATODES (ROUNDWORMS)

The major nematode parasites of humans include the *soil-transmitted helminths* (STHs; sometimes referred to as "geohelminths") and the *filarial nematodes*. The major STH infections (*ascariasis* [roundworm], *trichuriasis* [whipworm], and *hookworm infection*) are among the most prevalent infections in developing countries. The agents most widely employed for reducing morbidity are the benzimidazole (BZ) anthelmintics, either albendazole (ALBENZA and ZENTEL) or mebendazole (VERMOX, others) (Figure 51–2).

ROUNDWORM: *ASCARIS LUMBRICOIDES*. *Ascaris lumbricoides*, known as the "roundworm," may affect from 70-90% of persons in some tropical regions; it is also seen in temperate climates. People become infected by ingesting food or soil contaminated with embryonated *A. lumbricoides* eggs.

The preferred anthelmintics are the BZs, mebendazole and albendazole, and the broad-spectrum drug pyrantel pamoate. Cure with any of these drugs can be achieved in nearly 100% of cases. Mebendazole and albendazole are preferred for therapy of asymptomatic to moderate ascariasis but should be used with caution to treat heavy *Ascaris* infections, alone or with hookworms. Some clinicians recommend the use of pyrantel for heavy *Ascaris* infections because this agent paralyzes the worms prior to their expulsion.

TOXOCARIASIS: *TOXOCARA CANIS*. This zoonotic infection, caused by the canine ascarid *Toxocara canis*, is a common helminthiasis in North America and Europe.

Three major syndromes are caused by *T. canis* infection: visceral larva migrans (VLM), ocular larva migrans (OLM), and covert toxocariasis (CTox). CTox may represent an under-appreciated cause of asthma and seizures. Specific treatment of VLM is reserved for patients with severe, persistent, or progressive symptoms. Albendazole is the drug of choice. In contrast, anthelmintic therapies for OLM and CTox are controversial.

HOOKWORM: *NECATOR AMERICANUS, ANCYLOSTOMA DUODENALE*. These closely related hookworm species infect ~1 billion people in developing countries (*see* Figure 51–1).

N. americanus is the predominant hookworm worldwide, whereas *A. duodenale* is focally endemic in Egypt and in parts of northern India and China. Hookworm larvae live in the soils and penetrate exposed skin. After reaching the lungs, the larvae migrate to the oral cavity and are swallowed. After attaching to the small intestinal mucosa, the derived adult worms feed on host blood. There is a general relationship between the number of hookworms (hookworm burden) as determined by quantitative fecal egg counts and fecal blood loss. Unlike heavy *Ascaris* and *Trichuris* infections, which occur predominantly in children, heavy hookworm infections also occur in adults, including women of reproductive age. Although iron supplementation (and transfusion in severe cases) often is helpful in individuals with severe iron-deficiency anemia, the major goal of treatment is to remove blood-feeding adult hookworms from the intestines. Albendazole is the agent of first choice and is considered far superior to mebendazole at removing adult hookworms from the GI tract. Oral albendazole is the drug of choice for treating *cutaneous larva migrans,* or "creeping eruption," which is due most commonly to skin migration by larvae of the dog hookworm, *A. braziliense*. Oral ivermectin or topical *thiabendazole* also can be used.

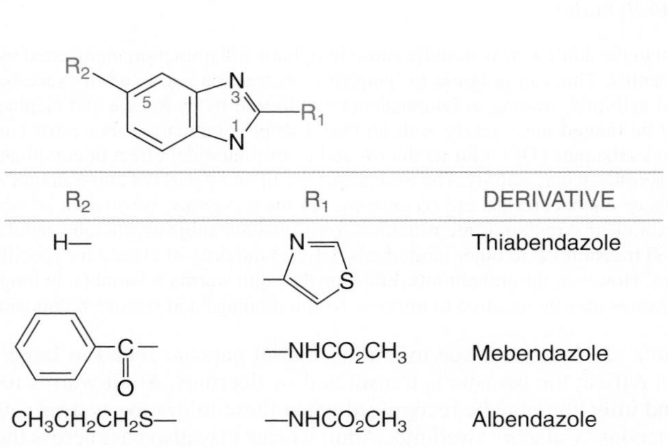

R_2	R_1	DERIVATIVE
H—	N, S	Thiabendazole
C—, O	$—NHCO_2CH_3$	Mebendazole
$CH_3CH_2CH_2S—$	$—NHCO_2CH_3$	Albendazole

Figure 51–2 *Structure of the Benzimidazoles.*

WHIPWORM: TRICHURIS TRICHIURA. *Trichuris* (whipworm) infection is acquired by ingestion of embryonated eggs. In children, heavy *Trichuris* worm burdens can lead to colitis, *Trichuris* dysentery syndrome, and rectal prolapse. Mebendazole and albendazole are the most effective agents for treatment of whipworm. Both drugs provide significant reductions in host worm burdens even when used in a single dose. However, a "cure" (i.e., total worm burden removal) typically requires a 3-day course of therapy.

THREADWORM: *STRONGYLOIDES STERCORALIS*. *S. stercoralis* is distinctive among helminths in being able to complete its life cycle within the human host, infecting 30-100 million people worldwide, most frequently in the tropics and other hot, humid locales. In the U.S., strongyloidiasis is still endemic in the Appalachian region and in parts of the American South.

Infective larvae in fecally contaminated soil penetrate the skin or mucous membranes, travel to the lungs, and ultimately mature into adult worms in the small intestine, where they reside. Many infected individuals are asymptomatic, but some experience skin rashes, nonspecific GI symptoms, and cough. Life-threatening disseminated disease, known as the *hyperinfection syndrome*, can occur in immunosuppressed persons, even decades after the initial infection when parasite replication in the small intestine is unchecked by a competent immune response. Ivermectin is the drug of choice for treatment of strongyloidiasis.

PINWORM: *ENTEROBIUS VERMICULARIS*. *Enterobius* is one of the most common helminth infections in temperate climates, including the U.S.

Although this parasite rarely causes serious complications, pruritus in the perianal and perineal region can be severe, and scratching may cause secondary infection. In female patients, worms may wander into the genital tract and penetrate into the peritoneal cavity. Salpingitis or even peritonitis may ensue. Because the infection easily spreads throughout members of a family, a school, or an institution, the physician must decide whether to treat all individuals in close contact with an infected person. Pyrantel pamoate, mebendazole, and albendazole are highly effective. Single oral doses of each should be repeated after 2 weeks. When their use is combined with rigid standards of personal hygiene, a very high proportion of cures can be obtained.

TRICHINOSIS: *TRICHINELLA SPIRALIS*. *T. spiralis* is an ubiquitous zoonotic nematode parasite. Trichinosis in the U.S. and the developing world is usually caused by eating the under- or uncooked meat of deer and wild pigs.

When released by acid stomach contents, encysted larvae mature into adult worms in the intestine. Adults then produce infectious larvae that invade tissues, especially skeletal muscle and heart. Severe infection can be fatal, but more typically causes marked muscle pain and cardiac complications. Infection is readily preventable by cooking all pork products thoroughly before eating. The encysted larvae are killed by exposure to heat of 60°C for 5 min. Albendazole and mebendazole are effective against the intestinal forms of *T. spiralis* that are present early in infection. The efficacy of these agents or any anthelmintic agent on larvae that have migrated to muscle is questionable.

LYMPHATIC FILARIASIS: *WUCHERERIA BANCROFTI, BRUGIA MALAYI, AND B. TIMORI*. Adult worms that cause human lymphatic filariasis (LF) dwell in the lymphatic vessels. Transmission occurs through the bite of infected mosquitoes; ~90% of cases are due to *W. bancrofti*; most of the rest are due to *B. malayi*.

In LF, host reaction to the adult worms initially cause lymphatic inflammation manifested by fevers, lymphangitis, and lymphadenitis. This can progress to lymphatic obstruction and is often exacerbated by secondary attacks of bacterial cellulitis, leading to lymphedema manifested by hydrocele and elephantiasis. All at-risk individuals should be treated once yearly with an oral 2-drug combination. For most countries, the WHO recommends diethylcarbamate (DEC) for its micro- and macrofilaricidal effect in combination with albendazole to enhance macrofilaricidal activity. The exceptions are in many parts of sub-Saharan Africa and Yemen, where either loiasis or onchocerciasis are co-endemic. In these regions, ivermectin is substituted for DEC. DEC and ivermectin clear circulating microfilariae from infected subjects, thereby reducing the likelihood that mosquitoes will transmit LF to other individuals. DEC is the drug of choice for specific therapy directed against adult worms. However, the anthelmintic effect on the adult worms is variable. In longstanding elephantiasis, surgical measures may be required to improve lymph drainage and remove redundant tissue.

LOIASIS: *LOA LOA*. *L. loa* is a tissue-migrating filarial parasite found in large river regions of Central and West Africa; the parasite is transmitted by deerflies. Adult worms reside in subcutaneous tissues, and infection may be recognized when these migrating worms cause episodic and transient subcutaneous "Calabar" swellings. Adult worms may also pass across the sclera, causing "eyeworm."

Rarely, encephalopathy, cardiopathy, or nephropathy occurs in association with heavy infection, particularly following chemotherapy. DEC currently is the best single drug for the treatment of loiasis. Glucocorticoids may be administered to ameliorate post-treatment acute reactions. In rare instances, life-threatening encephalopathy follows the treatment of loiasis, probably due to the inflammatory reaction to dead or dying microfilariae lodged in the cerebral microvasculature. Guidelines have been developed aimed at screening out populations with heavy infection so that they are not administered ivermectin, which has also been associated with fatal encephalopathy.

RIVER BLINDNESS (ONCHOCERCIASIS). *Onchocerca volvulus*, transmitted by blackflies near fast-flowing streams and rivers, infects 17-37 million people in 22 countries in sub-Saharan Africa and fewer people (<100,000) in 4 Latin American countries.

Inflammatory reactions, primarily to microfilariae rather than adult worms, affect the subcutaneous tissues, lymph nodes, and eyes. Onchocerciasis is a leading cause of infectious blindness. Ivermectin is the drug of choice for control and treatment of onchocerciasis. DEC is no longer recommended because ivermectin produces far milder systemic reactions and few if any ocular complications. Although suramin (*see* Chapter 50) kills adult *O. volvulus* worms, treatment with this relatively toxic agent is generally not advised.

GUINEA WORM: *DRACUNCULUS MEDINENSIS*. Known as the guinea, dragon, or Medina worm, this parasite causes dracunculiasis, an infection in decline (<5000 cases as of 2009, mostly in rural Sudan, Ghana, and Mali).

People become infected by drinking water containing copepods that carry infective larvae. After ~1 year, the adult female worms migrate and emerge through the skin, usually of the lower legs or feet. Strategies such as filtering drinking water and reducing contact of infected individuals with water have markedly reduced the transmission and prevalence of dracunculiasis in most endemic regions. There is no effective anthelmintic for treatment of *D. medinensis* infection. *Metronidazole*, 250 mg given 3 times a day for 10 days, may provide symptomatic and functional relief.

CESTODES (FLATWORMS)

BEEF TAPEWORM: *TAENIA SAGINATA*. Humans are the definitive hosts for *T. saginata*.

Preventable by cooking beef to 60°C for >5 min, this infection rarely produces serious clinical disease, but it must be distinguished from that produced by *Taenia solium*. Praziquantel (BILTRICIDE) is the drug of choice for treatment of infection by *T. saginata*, although niclosamide can also be used.

PORK TAPEWORM: *TAENIA SOLIUM*. *T. solium* causes 2 types of infection. The intestinal form with adult tapeworms is caused by eating undercooked meat containing cysticerci, or more commonly by fecal-oral transmission of infective *T. solium* eggs from another infected human host. *Cysticercosis*, the far more dangerous systemic form that usually coexists with the intestinal form, is caused by invasive larval forms of the parasite.

Systemic infection results either from ingestion of fecally contaminated infectious material, or from eggs liberated from a gravid segment passing upward into the duodenum, where the outer layers are digested. In either case, larvae gain access to the circulation and tissues, exactly as in their cycle in the intermediate host, usually the pig. Invasion of the brain (neurocysticercosis) is common and dangerous. Niclosamide is preferred for treatment of intestinal infections with *T. solium* because it will have no effect on occult neurocysticercosis. Albendazole is the drug of choice for treating cysticercosis. The advisability of chemotherapy for neurocysticercosis is controversial, being appropriate only when it is directed at live cysticerci and not against dead or dying cysticerci. Pretreatment with glucocorticoids is strongly advised in this situation to minimize inflammatory reactions to dying parasites. Some experts advocate use of albendazole therapy for patients with multiple cysts or viable cysts.

FISH TAPEWORM: *DIPHYLLOBOTHRIUM LATUM*. *D. latum* is found most commonly in rivers and lakes of the Northern Hemisphere. In North America, the pike is the most common second intermediate host. The eating of inadequately cooked infested fish introduces the larvae into the human intestine; the larvae can develop into adult worms up to 25 m long. Most infected individuals are asymptomatic. The most frequent manifestations include abdominal symptoms and weight loss; megaloblastic anemia develops due to a deficiency of vitamin B_{12}. Therapy with praziquantel readily eliminates the worm and ensures hematological remission.

DWARF TAPEWORM: *HYMENOLEPIS NANA*. *H. nana* is the smallest and most common tapeworm parasitizing humans. *H. nana* is the only cestode that can develop from ovum to mature adult in humans without an intermediate host. Cysticerci develop in the villi of the intestine and then regain access to the intestinal lumen where larvae mature into adults. Praziquantel is effective against *H. nana* infections, but higher doses than used for other tapeworm infections usually are required. Albendazole is partially efficacious against *H. nana*.

ECHINOCOCCUS SPECIES. Humans are one of several intermediate hosts for larval forms of *Echinococcus* species that cause "cystic" (*E. granulosus*) and "alveolar" (*E. multilocularis* and *E. vogeli*) hydatid disease. Dogs and related canids are definitive hosts for these tapeworms.

Parasite eggs from canine stools are a major worldwide cause of disease in associated livestock (e.g., sheep and goats). Removal of the cysts by surgery is the preferred treatment, but leakage from ruptured cysts may spread disease to other organs. Prolonged regimens of albendazole, either alone or as an adjunct to surgery, are reportedly of some benefit. However, some patients are not cured despite multiple courses of therapy, especially in alveolar echinococcosis where lifelong therapy with albendazole may be required. Benzimidazole treatment should be administered in the perioperative period.

TREMATODES (FLUKES)

SCHISTOSOMIASIS: *SCHISTOSOMA HAEMATOBIUM, S. MANSONI, S. JAPONICUM*. These are the main species of blood flukes that cause human schistosomiasis; less common species are *Schistosoma intercalatum* and *Schistosoma mekongi*. Infected freshwater snails act as intermediate hosts for transmission of the infection, which continues to spread as agriculture and water resources increase.

The clinical manifestations of schistosomiasis generally correlate with the intensity of infection, with pathology primarily involving the liver, spleen, and GI tract (for *S. mansoni* and *S. japonicum*) or the urinary and genital tracts (*S. haematobium*). Heavy infection with *S. haematobium* predisposes to squamous cell carcinoma of the bladder. Chronic infections can cause porto-systemic shunting due to hepatic granuloma formation and periportal fibrosis in the liver.

Praziquantel is the drug of choice for treatment of schistosomiasis. Oxamniquine is effective for treatment of *S. mansoni* infections, particularly in South America, where the sensitivity of most strains may permit single-dose therapy; higher doses of the drug are required to treat African strains than to treat Brazilian strains of *S. mansoni*. Metrifonate (trichlorfon) is effective in the treatment of *S. haematobium* infections but not against *S. mansoni* and *S. japonicum*. Artemether (*see* Chapter 49) shows promise as an anti-schistosomal agent, targeting the larval schistosomula stages of the parasite.

LUNG FLUKES: *PARAGONIMUS WESTERMANI, ET AL*. Lung flukes, including several *Paragonimus* species, infect humans and carnivores; *P. westermani* is the most common. Humans become infected by eating raw or undercooked crabs or crayfish. Disease is caused by reactions to adult worms in the lungs or ectopic sites. Praziquantel is effective, as is triclabendazole (EGATEN). Bithionol is a second-line agent.

***CLONORCHIS SINENSIS, OPISTHORCHIS VIVERRINI, OPISTHORCHIS FELINEUS*.** These closely related trematodes exist in the Far East (*C. sinensis*, "the Chinese liver fluke," and *O. viverrini*) and parts of Eastern Europe (*O. felineus*). Metacercariae released from poorly cooked infected cyprinoid fish (carp) mature into adult flukes that inhabit the human biliary system. Heavy infections can cause obstructive liver disease, inflammatory gallbladder pathology associated with cholangiocarcinoma, and obstructive pancreatitis. One-day therapy with praziquantel is highly effective against these parasites.

FASCIOLA HEPATICA. Humans are only accidentally infected with *F. hepatica*, the large liver fluke that exists worldwide and primarily affects herbivorous ruminants such as cattle and sheep. Triclabendazole, given as a single oral dose of 10 mg/kg, or in cases of severe infection 20 mg/kg divided into 2 doses, is the drug of choice for treatment of fascioliasis.

***FASCIOLOPSIS BUSKI, HETEROPHYES HETEROPHYES, METAGONIMUS YOKOGAWAI, NANOPHYETUS SALMINCOLA*.** Obtained by eating contaminated water chestnuts and other caltrops in Southeast Asia, *F. buski* is one of the largest parasites causing human infection. Undercooked fish transmit infection with the other, much smaller GI trematodes that are widely distributed geographically. Abdominal symptoms produced by reactions to these flukes usually are mild, but heavy infections with *F. buski* can cause intestinal obstruction and peritonitis. Infections with all the intestinal trematodes respond well to single-day therapy with praziquantel.

BENZIMIDAZOLES (BZs)

Thiabendazole, mebendazole, and albendazole have been used extensively for the treatment of human helminth infections. The chemical structures of these drugs are shown in Figure 51–2.

Thiabendazole is active against a wide range of nematodes that infect the GI tract. However, its clinical value has declined markedly because of thiabendazole's toxicity (CNS, liver, hypersensitivity, and visual side effects). Mebendazole, the prototype benzimidazole carbamate, was introduced for the treatment of intestinal roundworm infections. Albendazole is a benzimidazole carbamate that is used worldwide for treatment of intestinal nematodes and cestodes; it is notable for the systemic bioavailability and efficacy of its sulfoxide metabolite against tissue-dwelling nematodes and cestodes. Albendazole is the drug of choice for treating cysticercosis and cystic hydatid disease. When used in single dose in conjunction with either ivermectin or DEC, it has shown additive effect in the control of LF and related tissue filarial infections. Of note, albendazole lacks activity against the liver fluke *F. hepatica*.

ANTHELMINTIC ACTION. The primary mechanism of action of BZ is thought to be inhibition of microtubule polymerization by binding to β-tubulin. The selective toxicity of these agents against helminths results from their higher affinity for parasite β-tubulin than for β-tubulin in humans.

Appropriate doses of mebendazole and albendazole are highly effective in treating most of the major STH infections (ascariasis, enterobiasis, trichuriasis, and hookworm) as well as less common human nematode infections. These drugs are active against both larval and adult stages of nematodes that cause these infections, and they are ovicidal for *Ascaris* and *Trichuris*. Immobilization and death of susceptible GI parasites occur slowly, and their clearance from the GI tract may not be complete until several days after treatment. Evidence for the emergence of β-tubulin gene mutations associated with resistance among human nematodes is confined to *T. trichiura* and *W. bancrofti*. Drug treatment failures have been reported in hookworm infections, but there is little evidence of widespread dissemination of resistant forms.

Albendazole is superior to mebendazole in curing hookworm and trichuriasis infections in children, especially when used as a single dose. Moreover, albendazole is more effective than mebendazole against strongyloidiasis and is superior to mebendazole against all tissue-dwelling helminths due to its active metabolite albendazole sulfoxide. It is therefore the drug of choice against cystic and alveolar hydatid disease caused by *Echinococcus granulosus* and *E. multilocularis*, and neurocysticercosis caused by larval forms of *Taenia solium*. The BZs probably are active against the intestinal stages of *Trichinella spiralis* in humans but probably do not affect the larval stages in tissues. Albendazole is highly effective against the migrating forms of dog and cat hookworms that cause cutaneous larval migrans, although thiabendazole can be applied topically for this purpose. Microsporidial species that cause intestinal infections in HIV-infected individuals respond partially (*Enterocytozoon bieneusi*) or completely (*Encephalitozoon intestinalis* and related *Encephalitozoon* species) to albendazole. Albendazole also has efficacy against anaerobic protozoa such as *Trichomonas vaginalis* and *Giardia lamblia*. BZs exert antifungal activity in vitro but have no utility in human mycoses.

ADME. Thiabendazole is soluble in water; mebendazole and albendazole are poorly soluble in aqueous solution. The low systemic bioavailability (22%) of mebendazole results from a combination of poor absorption and rapid first-pass hepatic metabolism. Absorbed mebendazole is ~95% bound to plasma proteins and is extensively metabolized. Mebendazole, rather than its metabolites, appears to be the active drug form. Conjugates of mebendazole and its metabolites have been found in bile, but little unchanged mebendazole appears in the urine. Coadministration of *cimetidine* will increase plasma levels of mebendazole, possibly due to inhibition of first-pass CYP-mediated metabolism.

Albendazole is variably and erratically absorbed after oral administration; absorption is enhanced by the presence of fatty foods and possibly by bile salts. Albendazole is rapidly metabolized in the liver and possibly in the intestine, to albendazole sulfoxide, which has potent anthelmintic activity. Albendazole sulfoxide is ~70% bound to plasma proteins and has a highly variable plasma $t_{1/2}$ of 4-15 h. It is well distributed into various tissues including hydatid cysts, where it reaches a concentration of ~20% that in plasma. The bioavailability of the parent drug and activity of albendazole sulfoxide explain why albendazole is more effective than mebendazole for treatment of tissue-dwelling helminths. Oxidation of the sulfoxide derivatives to the nonchiral sulfone metabolite of albendazole, which is pharmacologically inactive, is probably rate limiting in determining the clearance and plasma $t_{1/2}$ of the bioactive (+) sulfoxide metabolite. Albendazole metabolites are excreted mainly in the urine.

Therapeutic Uses. Thiabendazole remains a useful drug when applied topically for treatment of cutaneous larva migrans (creeping eruption). For treatment of strongyloidiasis, thiabendazole has been replaced by ivermectin.

Mebendazole is an effective drug for treatment of GI nematode infections. For treatment of enterobiasis, a single 100-mg tablet is taken; a second dose should be given after 2 weeks. For control of ascariasis, trichuriasis, or hookworm infections, the recommended regimen is 100 mg of mebendazole taken in the morning and evening for 3 consecutive days (or a single 500-mg tablet administered once). If the patient is not cured 3 weeks after treatment, a second course should be given. A single dose of albendazole is superior to a single dose of mebendazole against hookworms and trichuriasis.

Albendazole is a safe and highly effective therapy for infections with GI nematodes, including *A. lumbricoides*, *T. trichiura*, and hookworms. For treatment of STH infections (enterobiasis, ascariasis, trichuriasis, and hookworm), albendazole is taken as a single oral 400-mg dose by adults and children >2 years of age. In children between the ages of 12 and 24 months, the WHO recommends a reduced dose of 200 mg. A 400-mg dose of albendazole appears to be superior to a 500-mg dose of mebendazole for curing hookworm infections and reducing egg counts.

Albendazole is the drug of choice for treating cystic hydatid disease due to *Echinococcus granulosus*. Although the drug provides only a modest cure rate when used alone, it is a useful adjunctive treatment in the perioperative period to reduce the risk of disseminated infection resulting from spillage of cyst contents at the time of surgery, or with nonoperative puncture, aspiration, injection, and re-aspiration (PAIR) procedures. A typical dosage regimen for adults is 400 mg given twice a day (for children, 15 mg/kg/day, maximum of 800 mg) for 1-6 months. Although it is the only drug available with useful activity against alveolar echinococcosis caused by *E. multilocularis*, it is parasiti-static rather than -cidal, and lifelong therapy with or without surgical intervention is usually required to control the infection. Albendazole, in the same regimen for 8-30 days, also is the preferred treatment of neurocysticercosis caused by larval forms of *Taenia solium*. For both adults and children, the course can be repeated as necessary, as long as liver and bone marrow toxicities are monitored. Glucocorticoid therapy is usually begun before initiating albendazole therapy and continued for several days after institution of therapy to reduce the incidence of side effects resulting from inflammatory reactions to dead and dying cysticerci. Glucocorticoids increase plasma levels of albendazole sulfoxide.

Albendazole, 400 mg/day, also has shown efficacy for therapy of microsporidial intestinal infections in patients with AIDS. Infection with *Capillaria philippinensis* can be treated with a 10-day treatment regimen with albendazole (400 mg/day). Albendazole is given with DEC to control LF in most parts of the world. The strategy is annual dosing with combination therapy for 4-6 years to maintain the microfilaremia at such low levels that transmission cannot occur. The period of therapy is estimated to correspond to the duration of fecundity of adult worms. To avoid serious reactions to dying microfilariae, the albendazole/ivermectin combination is recommended in locations where filariasis coexists with either onchocerciasis or loiasis.

Toxicity, Side Effects, Precautions, and Contraindications. Excluding thiabendazole, the BZs have excellent safety profiles. Overall, the incidence of side effects, primarily mild GI symptoms, occur in only 1% of treated children. Side effects frequently encountered with therapeutic doses include anorexia, nausea, vomiting, and dizziness. Mebendazole does not cause significant systemic toxicity in routine clinical use, due to its low systemic bioavailability. Transient symptoms of abdominal pain, distention, and diarrhea have occurred in cases of massive infestation and expulsion of GI worms. Albendazole produces few side effects when used for short-term therapy of GI helminth infections, even in patients with heavy worm burdens. Even in long-term therapy of cystic hydatid disease and neurocysticercosis, albendazole is well tolerated by most patients. The most common side effect is liver dysfunction, generally manifested by an increase in serum transaminase levels; rarely jaundice may be noted, but enzyme activities return to normal after therapy is completed. Liver function tests should be conducted during protracted albendazole therapy; the drug is not recommended for patients with cirrhosis. The safety of albendazole in children <2 years of age has not been established.

The BZs as a group display few clinically significant interactions with other drugs. Albendazole may induce its own metabolism; plasma levels of its sulfoxide metabolites can be increased by coadministration of glucocorticoids and possibly praziquantel. Caution is advised when using high doses of albendazole together with general inhibitors of hepatic CYPs. Coadministration of cimetidine can increase the bioavailability of mebendazole.

Use in Pregnancy. Neither albendazole nor mebendazole is recommended for use in human pregnancy. A review of the risk of congenital abnormalities from BZs concluded that their use during pregnancy was not associated with an increased risk of major congenital defects; nonetheless, it is recommended that treatment should be avoided during the first trimester of pregnancy. Hookworm occurs in many pregnant women in developing countries, including up to one-third of pregnant women in sub-Saharan Africa. Because some of these infected women may develop iron-deficiency anemia leading to adverse pregnancy outcomes, BZ treatment would be beneficial during the second and third trimesters of pregnancy. There is no evidence that maternal BZ therapy presents a risk to breast-fed infants.

Use in Young Children. The BZs have not been extensively studied in children <2 years of age. The WHO concluded that BZs may be used in children >1 year if the risks from adverse consequences caused by STHs are justified. The recommended dose is 200 mg of albendazole in children between the ages of 12 and 24 months.

DIETHYLCARBAMAZINE (DEC)

Diethylcarbamazine (DEC) (HETRAZAN) is a first-line agent for control and treatment of LF caused by *Wuchereria bancrofti* and *Brugia malayi* and for therapy of tropical pulmonary eosinophilia, an uncommon manifestation of lymphatic filarial infection. DEC is also the drug of choice for treatment of loiasis, caused by infection with the filarial parasite *L. loa*.

Caution must be used in treatment of high-grade *L. loa* infection because the rapid killing of large numbers of microfilariae can cause life-threatening post-treatment complications. Annual single-dose combination chemotherapy with both DEC and albendazole show considerable promise for the control of LF in geographic regions where onchocerciasis and loiasis are not endemic.

Anthelmintic Action. The mechanisms of action of DEC against filarial species are unknown. Microfilarial forms of susceptible filarial species are most affected by DEC. These developmental forms of *W. bancrofti, B. malayi*, and *L. loa* rapidly disappear from human blood after consumption of the drug. Microfilariae of *O. volvulus* rapidly disappear from skin after DEC administration, but the drug does not kill microfilariae in nodules that contain the adult (female) worms. The drug has some activity against the adult lifecycle stages of *W. bancrofti*, *B. malayi,* and *L. Loa* but negligible activity against adult *O. volvulus*.

ADME. DEC is absorbed rapidly from the GI tract. Peak plasma levels occur within 1-2 h; the plasma $t_{1/2}$ varies from 2-10 h, depending on the urinary pH. Alkalinizing the urine can elevate plasma levels, prolong the plasma $t_{1/2}$, and increase both the therapeutic effect and toxicity of DEC. Dosage reduction may be required for people with renal dysfunction. Metabolism is rapid and extensive; a major metabolite, DEC-*N*-oxide, is active.

Therapeutic Uses. Recommended regimens differ according to whether the drug is used for population-based chemotherapy, treatment of confirmed filarial infection, or prophylaxis against infection.

W. bancrofti, B. malayi, and B. timori. The standard regimen for the treatment of LF traditionally has been a 12-day, 6 mg/kg/day course of DEC. In the U.S., it is common practice to administer small test doses of 50-100 mg (1-2 mg/kg for children) over a 3-day period prior to beginning the 12-day regimen. However, a single dose of 6 mg/kg reportedly has comparable macrofilaricidal and microfilaricidal efficacy to the standard regimen. Single-dose therapy may be repeated every 6-12 months, as necessary. Although DEC does not usually reverse existing lymphatic damage, early treatment of asymptomatic individuals may prevent new lymphatic damage. For mass treatment to interrupt transmission, effective strategies have included the introduction of DEC into table salt (0.2-0.4% by weight of the base). DEC, given annually as a single oral dose of 6 mg/kg, is most effective in reducing microfilaremia when coadministered with either albendazole (400 mg) or ivermectin (0.2-0.4 mg/kg). Therapy is usually well tolerated.

O. volvulus and L. loa. DEC is contraindicated for the treatment of onchocerciasis because it causes severe reactions related to microfilarial destruction, including worsening ocular lesions. Ivermectin is the preferred drug for this infection. DEC remains the best available drug for therapy of loiasis. Treatment is initiated with test doses of 50 mg (1 mg/kg in children) daily for 2-3 days, escalating to maximally tolerated daily doses of 9 mg/kg in 3 doses for 2-3 weeks. In patients with high-grade microfilaremia, low test doses are used, often accompanied by pretreatment with glucocorticoids or antihistamines, to minimize reactions to dying microfilariae. Albendazole may be useful in patients who either fail therapy with DEC or who cannot tolerate the drug. DEC is clinically effective against microfilariae and adult worms of *D. streptocerca*. DEC is no longer recommended as a first-line drug for the treatment of toxocariasis.

Toxicity and Side Effects. Below a daily dose of 8-10 mg/kg, direct toxic reactions to DEC are rarely severe and usually disappear within a few days despite continuation of therapy. These reactions include anorexia, nausea, headache, and, at high doses, vomiting. Major adverse effects result directly or indirectly from the host response to destruction of parasites, primarily microfilariae. Delayed reactions to dying adult worms may result in lymphangitis, swelling, and lymphoid abscesses in bancroftian and brugian filariasis, and small skin wheals in loiasis. The drug occasionally causes severe side effects in heavy *L. loa* infections, including retinal hemorrhages and severe encephalopathy. In patients with onchocerciasis, the *Mazzotti reaction* typically occurs within a few hours after the first dose.

Precautions and Contraindications. Population-based therapy with DEC should be avoided where onchocerciasis or loiasis is endemic, although the drug can be used to protect foreign travelers from these infections. Pretreatment with glucocorticoids and antihistamines often is undertaken to minimize indirect reactions to DEC that result from release of antigen by dying microfilariae. Dosage reduction may be appropriate for patients with impaired renal function or persistent alkaline urine.

DOXYCYCLINE

Filarial parasites, including *W. bancrofti* and *O. volvulus,* harbor bacterial symbionts of the genus *Wolbachia*, against which long courses of doxycycline (*see* Chapter 55) (≥6 weeks) in bancroftian filariasis and onchocerciasis are effective. A 6-week regimen of doxycycline (100 mg daily), by killing the *Wolbachia,* leads to sterility of adult female *Onchocerca* worms.

IVERMECTIN

Ivermectin (MECTIZAN; STROMECTOL) is a semisynthetic analog of avermectin B_{1a} (abamectin), an insecticide developed for crop management. Ivermectin now is used extensively to control and treat a broad spectrum of infections caused by parasitic nematodes (roundworms) and arthropods (insects, ticks, and mites) that plague livestock and domestic animals.

MECHANISM OF ACTION. Ivermectin immobilizes affected organisms by inducing a tonic paralysis of the musculature. Avermectins induce paralysis by activating a family of ligand-gated Cl^- channels, particularly glutamate-gated Cl^- channels found only in invertebrates. Ivermectin probably binds to glutamate-activated Cl^- channels found in nematode nerve or muscle cells, and causes hyperpolarization by increasing intracellular chloride concentration, resulting in paralysis. Avermectins also bind with high affinity to γ-aminobutyric acid (GABA)-gated and other ligand-gated Cl^- channels in nematodes such as *Ascaris* and in insects, but the physiological consequences are less well defined.

ANTI-PARASITIC ACTIVITY. In humans infected with *O. volvulus*, ivermectin causes a rapid, marked decrease in microfilarial counts in the skin and ocular tissues that lasts for 6-12 months. The drug has little discernible effect on adult parasites, but affects developing larvae and blocks egress of microfilariae from the uterus of adult female worms. By reducing microfilariae in the skin, ivermectin decreases transmission to the *Simulium* black fly vector. Ivermectin also is effective against microfilaria but not against adult worms of *W. bancrofti, B. malayi, L. loa*, and *M. ozzardi*. The drug exhibits excellent efficacy in humans against *A. lumbricoides, S. stercoralis*, and cutaneous larva migrans.

ADME. Peak levels of ivermectin in plasma are achieved within 4-5 h after oral administration. The long $t_{1/2}$ (~57 h in adults) primarily reflects a low systemic clearance (~1-2 L/hour) and a large apparent volume of distribution. Ivermectin is ~93% bound to plasma proteins. The drug is extensively metabolized by hepatic CYP3A4. Virtually no ivermectin appears in human urine in either unchanged or conjugated form.

THERAPEUTIC USES

Onchocerciasis. Ivermectin, administered as a single oral dose (150-200 μg/kg) given every 6-12 months, is the drug of choice for onchocerciasis in adults and children ≥5 years of age. Marked reduction of microfilariae in the skin results in major relief of the intense pruritus that is a feature of onchocerciasis. Clearance of microfilariae from skin and ocular tissues occurs within a few days and lasts for 6-12 months; the dose then should be repeated. The drug is not curative, however, because ivermectin has little effect on adult *O. volvulus.* Annual doses of the drug are quite safe and substantially reduce transmission of this infection. Resistance to ivermectin and the related agent moxidectin have been reported in a variety of parasites of veterinary importance, suggesting the potential for development of similar resistance in human parasites, particularly in the setting of mass treatment campaigns.

Lymphatic Filariasis. Ivermectin is as effective as DEC for controlling LF, and unlike DEC, it can be used in regions where onchocerciasis, loiasis, or both are endemic. A single annual dose of ivermectin (200 μg/kg) and a single annual dose of albendazole (400 mg) are even more effective in controlling LF than either drug alone. The duration of treatment is at least 5 years, based on the estimated fecundity of the adult worms. This dual-drug regimen also reduces infections with intestinal nematodes.

Strongyloidiasis. Ivermectin administered as a single dose of 150 to 200 μg/kg is the drug of choice for human strongyloidiasis. It is generally recommended that a second dose be administered a week following the first dose. This regimen is more efficacious than a 3-day course of albendazole.

Infections with Other Intestinal Nematodes. Ivermectin is more effective in ascariasis and enterobiasis than in trichuriasis or hookworm infection. In the latter 2 infections, although it is not curative, it significantly reduces the intensity of infection.

Other Indications. Taken as a single 200-μg/kg oral dose, ivermectin is a first-line drug for treatment of cutaneous *larva migrans* caused by dog or cat hookworms, and for treatment of scabies. In uncomplicated scabies, 2 doses should be administered, 1-2 weeks apart. In severe (crusted) scabies, ivermectin should be used in repeated doses, with 1 recommended regimen entailing 7 doses of 200 μg/kg given with food, on days 1, 2, 8, 9, 15, 22, and 29. The drug appears to be effective against human head lice as well.

Toxicity, Side Effects, and Precautions. Ivermectin is well tolerated by uninfected humans. In filarial infection, ivermectin therapy frequently causes a Mazzotti-like reaction to dying microfilariae. The intensity and nature of these reactions relate to the microfilarial burden. After treatment of *O. volvulus* infections, these side effects usually are limited to mild itching and swollen, tender lymph nodes, which occur in 5-35% of people, last just a few days, and are relieved by aspirin and antihistamines. Rarely, more severe reactions occur that include high fever, tachycardia, hypotension, dizziness, headache, myalgia, arthralgia, diarrhea, and facial and peripheral edema; these may respond to glucocorticoid therapy. Ivermectin induces milder side effects than does DEC, and unlike DEC, ivermectin seldom exacerbates ocular lesions in onchocerciasis. The drug can cause rare but serious side effects including marked disability and encephalopathies in patients with heavy *L. loa* microfilaria. *Loa* encephalopathy is associated with ivermectin treatment of individuals with *Loa* microfilaremia levels ≥30,000 microfilariae per milliliter of blood. Because of its effects on GABA receptors in the CNS, ivermectin is contraindicated in conditions associated with an impaired blood-brain barrier (e.g., African trypanosomiasis and meningitis). Ivermectin is not approved for use in children <5 years of age or in pregnant or lactating women (low levels of the drug appear in the mother's milk).

PRAZIQUANTEL

Praziquantel (BILTRICIDE, DISTOCIDE) shows activity against most cestodes and trematodes that infect humans, whereas nematodes generally are unaffected. The drug is most commonly used for treatment of schistosomiasis.

Mechanism of Anthelmintic Action. Praziquantel has 2 major effects on adult schistosomes. At the lowest effective concentrations, it causes increased muscular activity, followed by contraction and spastic paralysis. Affected worms detach from blood vessel walls and migrate from the mesenteric veins to the liver. At slightly higher concentrations, praziquantel causes tegumental damage and exposes a number of tegumental antigens. The clinical efficacy of this drug correlates better with tegumental action. The drug is ineffective against juvenile schistosomes and therefore is relatively ineffective in early infection. An intact immune response is believed to be important for the clinical efficacy of the drug.

Absorption, Fate, and Excretion. Praziquantel is readily absorbed after oral administration, reaching maximal levels in human plasma in 1-2 h. Extensive first-pass metabolism to many inactive hydroxylated and conjugated products limits the bioavailability of this drug and results in plasma concentrations of metabolites at least 100-fold higher than that of praziquantel. The drug is ~80% bound to plasma proteins. Plasma $t_{1/2}$ is 0.8-3 h, depending on the dose, and 4-6 h for its metabolites; this may be prolonged in patients with severe liver disease, including those with hepatosplenic schistosomiasis. About 70% of an oral dose is recovered as metabolites in the urine within 24 h; most of the remainder is eliminated in the bile.

Therapeutic Uses. Praziquantel is the drug of choice for treating schistosomiasis caused by all *Schistosoma* species that infect humans. A single oral dose of 40 mg/kg or 3 doses of 20 mg/kg each, given 4-6 h apart, generally produce cure rates of 70-95% and consistently high reductions (>85%) in egg counts. Three doses of 25 mg/kg taken 4-8 h apart result in high rates of cure for infections with the liver flukes *C. sinensis* and *O. viverrini*, or the intestinal flukes *F. buski, H. heterophyes*, and *M. yokogawai*. The same 3-dose regimen, used over 2 days, is highly effective against infections with the lung fluke, *P. westermani*. The liver fluke *F. hepatica* is resistant to praziquantel and should be treated with the BZ drug triclabendazole. Low doses of praziquantel can be used to treat intestinal infections with adult cestodes (a single oral dose of 25 mg/kg for *H. nana* and 10 to 20 mg/kg for *D. latum, T. saginata*, or *T. solium*). Retreatment after 7-10 days is advisable for individuals heavily infected with *H. nana*. Although albendazole is preferred for therapy of human cysticercosis, praziquantel represents an alternative agent; its use for this indication is hampered by the important pharmacokinetic interaction with dexamethasone and other corticosteroids that should be coadministered in this condition.

Toxicity, Precautions, and Interactions. Abdominal discomfort and drowsiness may occur shortly after taking praziquantel; these direct effects are transient and dose related. Indirect effects such as fever, pruritus, urticaria, rashes, arthralgia, and myalgia are noted occasionally. Such side effects and increases in eosinophilia often relate to parasite burden and may be a consequence of parasite killing and antigen release. In neurocysticercosis, inflammatory reactions to praziquantel may produce meningismus, seizures, and cerebrospinal fluid pleocytosis. These effects usually are delayed in onset, last 2-3 days, and respond to analgesics and anticonvulsants. Praziquantel is considered safe in children >4 years of age. Low levels of the drug appear in the breast milk, but there is no evidence that this compound is mutagenic or carcinogenic. The bioavailability of praziquantel is reduced by inducers of hepatic CYPs. Dexamethasone reduces the bioavailability of praziquantel. Under certain conditions, praziquantel may increase the bioavailability of albendazole. Praziquantel is contraindicated in ocular cysticercosis because the host response can irreversibly damage the eye. Driving and other tasks requiring mental alertness should be avoided. Severe hepatic disease can prolong the $t_{1/2}$, requiring dosage adjustment.

METRIFONATE

Metrifonate (trichlorfon; BILARCIL) is an organophosphorus compound used first as an insecticide and later as an anthelmintic, especially for treatment of *S. haematobium*. Metrifonate is a prodrug; at physiological pH, it is converted nonenzymatically to *dichlorvos* (2,2-dichlorovinyl dimethyl phosphate [DDVP]), a potent cholinesterase inhibitor (*see* Chapter 10). However, inhibition of cholinesterase alone is unlikely to explain the antischistosomal properties of metrifonate.

OXAMNIQUINE. Oxamniquine is used as a second-line drug after praziquantel for the treatment of *S. mansoni* infection. *S. haematobium* and *S. japonicum* are refractory to this drug.

NICLOSAMIDE. Niclosamide, a halogenated salicylanilide derivative, was introduced for human use as a taeniacide. Niclosamide is no longer approved for use in the U.S.

PIPERAZINE. Piperazine has been superseded as a first-line anthelmintic by the better-tolerated BZ anthelmintics.

PYRANTEL PAMOATE

Pyrantel pamoate first was introduced into veterinary practice as a broad-spectrum anthelmintic against pinworm, roundworm, and hookworm infections. Its effectiveness and lack of toxicity led to its trial against related intestinal helminths in humans. *Oxantel pamoate*, an *m*-oxyphenol analog of pyrantel, is effective for single-dose treatment of trichuriasis.

Antihelmintic Action. Pyrantel and its analogs are depolarizing neuromuscular blocking agents. They open nonselective cation channels and induce persistent activation of nicotinic acetylcholine receptors and spastic paralysis of the worm. Pyrantel also inhibits cholinesterases. Pyrantel is effective against hookworm, pinworm, and roundworm but is ineffective against *T. trichiura,* which responds to the analog oxantel.

ADME. Pyrantel pamoate is poorly absorbed from the GI tract, a property that confines its action to intraluminal GI nematodes. Less than 15% is excreted in the urine as parent drug and metabolites. The major proportion of an administered dose is recovered in the feces.

Therapeutic Uses. Pyrantel pamoate is an alternative to mebendazole or albendazole in the treatment of ascariasis and enterobiasis. High cure rates are achieved after a single oral dose of 11 mg/kg, to a maximum of 1 g. Pyrantel also is effective against hookworm infections caused by *A. duodenale* and *N. americanus*, although repeated doses are needed to cure heavy infections by *N. americanus*. The drug should be used in combination with oxantel for mixed infections with *T. trichiura*. For pinworm, repeat the treatment after an interval of 2 weeks. In the U.S., pyrantel is sold as an over-the-counter pinworm treatment (PIN-X, others).

Precautions. Transient and mild GI symptoms occasionally occur, as do headache, dizziness, rash, and fever. Pyrantel pamoate has not been studied in pregnant women. Pyrantel pamoate and piperazine are mutually antagonistic with respect to their neuromuscular effects on parasites and should not be used together.

For a complete Bibliographical Listing see Goodman & Gilman's ***The Pharmacological Basis of Therapeutics***, 12th ed., or Goodman & Gilman Online at www.AccessMedicine.com.

Sulfonamides, Trimethoprim-Sulfamethoxazole, Quinolones, and Agents for Urinary Tract Infections

SULFONAMIDES

The sulfonamide drugs were the first effective chemotherapeutic agents to be employed systemically for the prevention and cure of bacterial infections in humans. The advent of penicillin and other antibiotics diminished the usefulness of the sulfonamides, but the introduction of the combination of trimethoprim and sulfamethoxazole has increased the use of sulfonamides for the prophylaxis and treatment of specific microbial infections. *Sulfonamides* are derivatives of *para*-aminobenzenesulfonamide (sulfanilamide; Figure 52–1) and are congeners of para-aminobenzoic acid. Most of them are relatively insoluble in water, but their sodium salts are readily soluble.

The minimal structural prerequisites for antibacterial action are all embodied in sulfanilamide itself. The sulfur must be linked directly to the benzene ring. The *para*-NH_2 group (the N of which has been designated as N4) is essential and can be replaced only by moieties that can be converted in vivo to a free amino group. Substitutions made in the amide NH_2 group (position N1) have variable effects on antibacterial activity of the molecule; substitution of heterocyclic aromatic nuclei at N1 yields highly potent compounds.

MECHANISM OF ACTION. Sulfonamides are competitive inhibitors of *dihydropteroate synthase*, the bacterial enzyme responsible for the incorporation of *para*-aminobenzoic acid (PABA) into *dihydropteroic acid*, the immediate precursor of *folic acid* (Figure 52–2). Sensitive microorganisms are those that must synthesize their own folic acid; bacteria that can use preformed folate are not affected. Toxicity is selective for bacteria because mammalian cells require preformed folic acid, cannot synthesize it, and are thus insensitive to drugs acting by this mechanism.

SYNERGISTS OF SULFONAMIDES. *Trimethoprim* exerts a synergistic effect with sulfonamides. It is a potent and selective competitive inhibitor of microbial *dihydrofolate reductase*, the enzyme that reduces *dihydrofolate* to *tetrahydrofolate*, which is required for 1-carbon transfer reactions. Coadministration of a sulfonamide and trimethoprim introduces sequential blocks in the biosynthetic pathway for tetrahydrofolate (*see* Figure 52–2); the combination is much more effective than either agent alone.

EFFECTS ON MICROBES

Sulfonamides have a wide range of antimicrobial activity against both gram-positive and gram-negative bacteria. Resistant strains have become common and the usefulness of these agents has diminished correspondingly. Sulfonamides are *bacteriostatic*; cellular and humoral defense mechanisms of the host are essential for final eradication of the infection.

ANTIBACTERIAL SPECTRUM. Resistance to sulfonamides is increasingly a problem. Microorganisms that may be susceptible in vitro to sulfonamides include *Streptococcus pyogenes*, *Streptococcus pneumoniae,*

SULFANILAMIDE | PARA-AMINOBENZOIC ACID | DAPSONE

Figure 52–1 *Sulfanilamide and para-aminobenzoic acid.* Sulfonamides are derivatives of sulfanilamide and act by virtue of being congeners of para-aminobenzoate (PABA). The antimicrobial and dermatological anti-inflammatory agent dapsone (4,4′-diaminodiphenyl sulfone; *see* Figure 56–5 and Chapter 65) also bears a resemblance to PABA and sulfanilamide.

Haemophilus influenzae, Haemophilus ducreyi, Nocardia, Actinomyces, Calymmatobacterium granulomatis, and *Chlamydia trachomatis*. Minimal inhibitory concentrations (MICs) range from 0.1 μg/mL for *C. trachomatis* to 4-64 μg/mL for *Escherichia coli*. Peak plasma drug concentrations achievable in vivo are ~100-200 μg/mL. Isolates of *Neisseria meningitidis* and *Shigella* are generally resistant, as are many strains of *E. coli* isolated from patients with urinary tract infections (community acquired).

ACQUIRED BACTERIAL RESISTANCE TO SULFONAMIDES. Bacterial resistance to sulfonamides can originate by random mutation and selection or by transfer of resistance by plasmids (*see* Chapter 48); it usually does not involve cross-resistance to other classes of antibiotics. Resistance to sulfonamide can result from: (1) a lower affinity of dihydropteroate synthase for sulfonamides, (2) decreased bacterial permeability or active efflux of the drug, (3) an alternative metabolic pathway for synthesis of an essential metabolite, or (4) an increased production of an essential metabolite or drug antagonist (e.g., PABA). Plasmid-mediated resistance is due to plasmid-encoded drug-resistant dihydropteroate synthetase.

ABSORPTION, DISTRIBUTION, METABOLISM, AND EXCRETION

Except for sulfonamides especially designed for their local effects in the bowel (*see* Chapter 47), this class of drugs is absorbed rapidly from the GI tract. Approximately 70-100% of an oral dose is absorbed, and sulfonamide can be found in the urine within 30 min of ingestion. Peak plasma levels are achieved in 2-6 h, depending on the drug. The small intestine is the major site of absorption, but some of the drug is absorbed from the stomach. Absorption from other sites, such as the vagina, respiratory tract, or abraded skin, is variable and unreliable, but a sufficient amount may enter the body to cause toxic reactions in susceptible persons or to produce sensitization.

All sulfonamides are bound in varying degree to plasma proteins, particularly to albumin. This is determined by the hydrophobicity of a particular drug and its pK_a; at physiological pH, drugs with a high pK_a exhibit a low degree of protein binding, and vice versa. Sulfonamides are distributed throughout all tissues of the body. The diffusible fraction of *sulfadiazine* is distributed uniformly throughout the total-body water, whereas *sulfisoxazole* is confined largely to the extracellular space. Because the protein content of such body fluids usually is low, the drug is present in the unbound active form. After systemic administration of adequate doses, sulfadiazine and sulfisoxazole attain concentrations in CSF that may be effective in meningitis. However, because of the emergence of sulfonamide-resistant microorganisms, these drugs are used rarely for the treatment of meningitis. Sulfonamides pass readily through the placenta and reach the fetal circulation. The concentrations attained in the fetal tissues may cause both antibacterial and toxic effects.

Sulfonamides are metabolized in the liver. The major metabolite is the N4-acetylated sulfonamide. Acetylation results in products that have no antibacterial activity but retain the toxic potential of the parent substance.

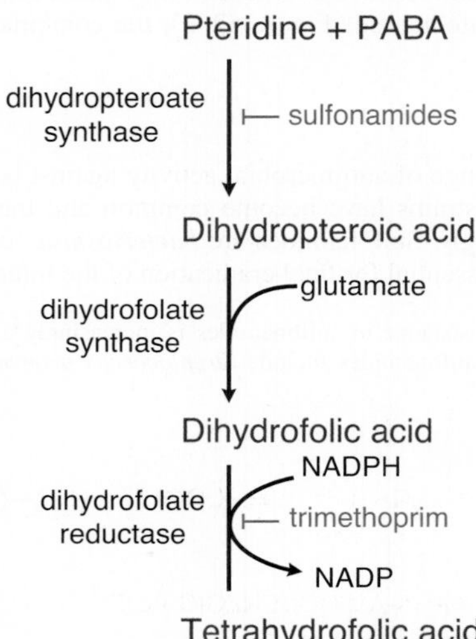

Figure 52–2 *Steps in folate metabolism blocked by sulfonamides and trimethoprim.* Coadministration of a sulfonamide and trimethoprim introduces sequential blocks in the biosynthetic pathway for tetrahydrofolate; the combination is much more effective than either agent alone.

Sulfonamides are eliminated from the body partly as the unchanged drug and partly as metabolic products. The largest fraction is excreted in the urine, and the $t_{1/2}$ depends on renal function. In acid urine, the older sulfonamides are insoluble and crystalline deposits may form. Small amounts are eliminated in the feces, bile, milk, and other secretions.

PHARMACOLOGICAL PROPERTIES OF INDIVIDUAL SULFONAMIDES

The sulfonamides may be classified on the basis of the rapidity with which they are absorbed and excreted (Table 52–1).

RAPIDLY ABSORBED AND ELIMINATED SULFONAMIDES

Sulfisoxazole. Sulfisoxazole is a rapidly absorbed and excreted sulfonamide with excellent antibacterial activity. Its high solubility eliminates much of the renal toxicity inherent in the use of older sulfonamides. Sulfisoxazole is bound extensively to plasma proteins. Following an oral dose of 2-4 g, peak concentrations in plasma of 110-250 μg/mL are found in 2-4 h. Approximately 30% of sulfisoxazole in the blood and ~30% in the urine is in the acetylated form. The kidney excretes ~95% of a single dose in 24 h. Concentrations of the drug in urine thus greatly exceed those in blood and may be bactericidal. The concentration in CSF is about a third of that in the blood. Sulfisoxazole acetyl is marketed in combination with erythromycin ethylsuccinate for use in children with otitis media.

The untoward effects of sulfisoxazole are similar to other sulfonamides. Because of its relatively high solubility in the urine as compared with sulfadiazine, sulfisoxazole rarely produces hematuria or crystalluria (0.2-0.3%). Nonetheless, patients should still ingest an adequate quantity of water. Sulfisoxazole must be used with caution in patients with impaired renal function. Like all sulfonamides, sulfisoxazole may produce hypersensitivity reactions, some of which are potentially lethal.

Sulfamethoxazole. Sulfamethoxazole is a close congener of sulfisoxazole, but its rates of enteric absorption and urinary excretion are slower. It is administered orally and employed for both systemic and urinary tract infections. Precautions must be observed to avoid sulfamethoxazole crystalluria because of the high percentage of the acetylated, relatively insoluble form of the drug in the urine. The clinical uses of sulfamethoxazole are the same as those for sulfisoxazole. In the U.S., it is marketed only in fixed-dose combinations with trimethoprim.

Sulfadiazine. Sulfadiazine given orally is absorbed rapidly from the GI tract. Peak blood concentrations are reached within 3-6 h. About 55% of the drug is bound to plasma protein. Therapeutic concentrations are attained in CSF within 4 h of a single oral dose of 60 mg/kg. Both free and acetylated forms of sulfadiazine are readily excreted by the kidney; 15-40% of the excreted drug is in acetylated form. Alkalinization of the urine accelerates the renal clearance of both forms by diminishing their tubular reabsorption. Every precaution must be taken to ensure fluid intake adequate to produce a daily urine output of at least 1200 mL in adults and a corresponding quantity in children. If this cannot be accomplished, sodium bicarbonate may be given to reduce the risk of crystalluria.

POORLY ABSORBED SULFONAMIDES

SULFASALAZINE. Sulfasalazine (AZULFIDINE, others) is very poorly absorbed from the GI tract. It is used in the therapy of ulcerative colitis and regional enteritis. Intestinal bacteria break sulfasalazine down to 5-aminosalicylate (5-ASA, mesalamine; *see* Figures 47–2 through 47–4), the active agent in inflammatory bowel disease, and sulfapyridine, a sulfonamide that is absorbed and eventually excreted in the urine.

Table 52–1

Classes of Sulfonamides

CLASS	SULFONAMIDE	SERUM $t_{1/2}$ (h)
Absorbed and excreted rapidly	Sulfisoxazole Sulfamethoxazole Sulfadiazine	5-6 11 10
Poorly absorbed orally but active in bowel lumen	Sulfasalazine	—
Topically used	Sulfacetamide Silver sulfadiazine	— —
Long-acting	Sulfadoxine	100-230

SULFONAMIDES FOR TOPICAL USE

Sulfacetamide. Sulfacetamide is the N1-acetyl-substituted derivative of sulfanilamide. Its aqueous solubility is ~90 times that of sulfadiazine. Solutions of the sodium salt of the drug are employed extensively in the management of ophthalmic infections. Very high aqueous concentrations are not irritating to the eye and are effective against susceptible microorganisms. The drug penetrates into ocular fluids and tissues in high concentration. Sensitivity reactions to sulfacetamide are rare, but the drug should not be used in patients with known hypersensitivity to sulfonamides. A 30% solution of the sodium salt has a pH of 7.4, whereas the solutions of sodium salts of other sulfonamides are highly alkaline. *See* Chapters 64 and 65 for ocular and dermatological uses.

Silver Sulfadiazine. Silver sulfadiazine (SILVADENE, others) is used topically to reduce microbial colonization and the incidence of infections from burns. Silver sulfadiazine should not be used to treat an established deep infection. Silver is released slowly from the preparation in concentrations that are selectively toxic to the microorganisms. However, bacteria may develop resistance to silver sulfadiazine. Although little silver is absorbed, the plasma concentration of sulfadiazine may approach therapeutic levels if a large surface area is involved. Adverse reactions—burning, rash, and itching—are infrequent. Silver sulfadiazine is considered an agent of choice for the prevention of burn infections.

Mafenide. This sulfonamide (α-amino-*p*-toluene-sulfonamide; SULFAMYLON) is applied topically to prevent colonization of burns by a large variety of gram-negative and gram-positive bacteria. It should not be used in treatment of an established deep infection. Adverse effects include intense pain at sites of application, allergic reactions, and loss of fluid by evaporation from the burn surface because occlusive dressings are not used. The drug and its primary metabolite inhibit *carbonic anhydrase*, and the urine becomes alkaline. Metabolic acidosis with compensatory tachypnea and hyperventilation may ensue; these effects limit the usefulness of mafenide. Mafenide is absorbed from the burn surface, reaching peak plasma concentrations in 2-4 h; the absorbed drug is converted to *para*-carboxybenzenesulfonamide.

LONG-ACTING SULFONAMIDES

Sulfadoxine. This agent has a particularly long plasma $t_{1/2}$ (7-9 days). It is used in combination with pyrimethamine (500 mg sulfadoxine plus 25 mg pyrimethamine as FANSIDAR) for the prophylaxis and treatment of malaria caused by mefloquine-resistant strains of *Plasmodium falciparum* (*see* Chapter 49). However, because of severe and sometimes fatal reactions, including the Stevens-Johnson syndrome, and the emergence of resistant strains, the drug has limited usefulness for the treatment of malaria.

SULFONAMIDE THERAPY

URINARY TRACT INFECTIONS (UTIs). Because a significant percentage of UTIs are caused by sulfonamide-resistant microorganisms, sulfonamides are no longer a therapy of first choice. Trimethoprim-sulfamethoxazole, a quinolone, trimethoprim, fosfomycin, or ampicillin are the preferred agents. *Sulfisoxazole* may be used effectively in areas where the prevalence of resistance is not high. The usual dosage is 2-4 g initially followed by 1-2 g, orally 4 times a day for 5-10 days. Patients with acute pyelonephritis with high fever are at risk of bacteremia and shock and should not be treated with a sulfonamide.

NOCARDIOSIS. Sulfonamides are of value in the treatment of infections due to *Nocardia* spp. Sulfisoxazole or sulfadiazine may be given in dosages of 6-8 g daily and this schedule should be continued for several months after all manifestations have been controlled. Combination of sulfonamide with a second antibiotic has been recommended, especially for advanced cases; ampicillin, erythromycin, and streptomycin have been suggested but there are no clinical data to show that combination therapy is better than therapy with a sulfonamide alone. Trimethoprim-sulfamethoxazole also is effective; some authorities consider this combination to be the treatment of choice.

TOXOPLASMOSIS. The combination of pyrimethamine and sulfadiazine is the treatment of choice for toxoplasmosis (*see* Chapter 50). Pyrimethamine is given as a loading dose of 75 mg followed by 25 mg orally per day, with sulfadiazine 1 g orally every 6 h, plus folinic acid (leucovorin) 10 mg orally each day for at least 3-6 weeks. Patients should receive at least 2 L of fluid intake daily to prevent crystalluria.

USE OF SULFONAMIDES FOR PROPHYLAXIS. The sulfonamides are as efficacious as oral penicillin in preventing streptococcal infections and recurrences of rheumatic fever among susceptible subjects. Their toxicity and the possibility of infection by drug-resistant streptococci make sulfonamides less desirable than penicillin for this purpose: however, sulfonamides should be used in patients who are hypersensitive to penicillin. Untoward responses usually occur during the first 8 weeks of therapy. White blood cell counts should be carried out once weekly during the first 8 weeks.

UNTOWARD REACTIONS TO SULFONAMIDES

The untoward effects that follow the administration of sulfonamides are numerous and varied; the overall incidence of reactions is ~5%.

DISTURBANCES OF THE URINARY TRACT. The risk of crystalluria is very low with the more soluble agents such as sulfisoxazole. Crystalluria has occurred in dehydrated patients with acquired immunodeficiency syndrome (AIDS) who were receiving sulfadiazine for *Toxoplasma* encephalitis. Fluid intake should be sufficient to ensure a daily urine volume of at least 1200 mL (in adults). Alkalinization of the urine may be desirable if urine volume or pH is unusually low because the solubility of sulfisoxazole increases greatly with slight elevations of pH.

DISORDERS OF THE HEMATOPOIETIC SYSTEM. Although rare, acute hemolytic anemia may occur. In some cases, it may be due to a sensitization phenomenon; in other instances, the hemolysis is related to an erythrocytic deficiency of glucose-6-phosphate dehydrogenase activity. Agranulocytosis occurs in ~0.1% of patients who receive sulfadiazine; it also can follow the use of other sulfonamides. Although return of granulocytes to normal levels may be delayed for weeks or months after sulfonamide is withdrawn, most patients recover spontaneously with supportive care. Aplastic anemia involving complete suppression of bone marrow activity with profound anemia, granulocytopenia, and thrombocytopenia is an extremely rare occurrence with sulfonamide therapy. It probably results from a direct myelotoxic effect and may be fatal. Reversible suppression of the bone marrow is quite common in patients with limited bone marrow reserve (e.g., patients with AIDS or those receiving myelosuppressive chemotherapy).

HYPERSENSITIVITY REACTIONS. Among the skin and mucous membrane manifestations attributed to sensitization to sulfonamide are morbilliform, scarlatinal, urticarial, erysipeloid, pemphigoid, purpuric, and petechial rashes, as well as erythema nodosum, erythema multiforme of the Stevens-Johnson type, Behçet syndrome, exfoliative dermatitis, and photosensitivity. These hypersensitivity reactions occur most often after the first week of therapy but may appear earlier in previously sensitized individuals. Fever, malaise, and pruritus frequently are present simultaneously. The incidence of untoward dermal effects is ~2% with sulfisoxazole; patients with AIDS manifest a higher frequency of rashes with sulfonamide treatment than do other individuals. A syndrome similar to serum sickness may appear after several days of sulfonamide therapy. Drug fever is a common untoward manifestation of sulfonamide treatment; the incidence approximates 3% with sulfisoxazole. Focal or diffuse necrosis of the liver owing to direct drug toxicity or sensitization occurs in <0.1% of patients. Headache, nausea, vomiting, fever, hepatomegaly, jaundice, and laboratory evidence of hepatocellular dysfunction usually appear 3-5 days after sulfonamide administration is started, and the syndrome may progress to acute yellow atrophy and death.

MISCELLANEOUS REACTIONS. Anorexia, nausea, and vomiting occur in 1-2% of persons receiving sulfonamides. The administration of sulfonamides to newborn infants, especially if premature, may lead to the displacement of bilirubin from plasma albumin, potentially causing an encephalopathy called *kernicterus*. Sulfonamides should not be given to pregnant women near term because these drugs cross the placenta and are secreted in milk.

DRUG INTERACTIONS. Drug interactions of the sulfonamides are seen with the oral anticoagulants, the sulfonylurea hypoglycemic agents, and the hydantoin anticonvulsants. In each case, sulfonamides can potentiate the effects of the other drug by inhibiting its metabolism or by displacing it from albumin. Dosage adjustment may be necessary when a sulfonamide is given concurrently.

TRIMETHOPRIM-SULFAMETHOXAZOLE

Trimethoprim inhibits bacterial dihydrofolate reductase, an enzyme downstream from the one that sulfonamides inhibit in the same biosynthetic sequence (*see* Figure 52–2). The combination of trimethoprim with sulfamethoxazole was an important advance in the development of clinically effective and synergistic antimicrobial agents. In much of the world, the combination of trimethoprim with sulfamethoxazole is known as *cotrimoxazole*. In addition to its combination with sulfamethoxazole (BACTRIM, SEPTRA, others), trimethoprim also is available as a single-entity preparation.

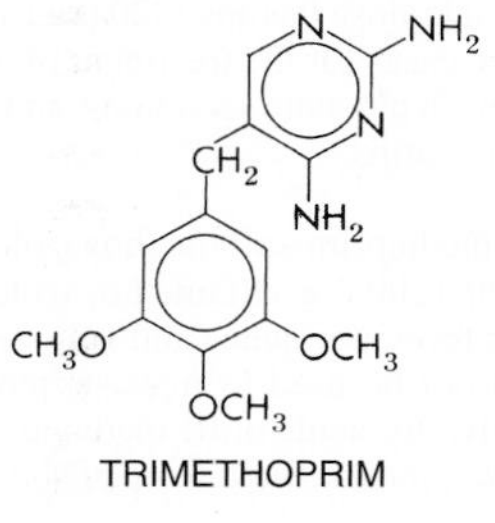

N NH2
N
CH2
NH2
CH3O OCH3
OCH3

TRIMETHOPRIM

ANTIBACTERIAL SPECTRUM. The antibacterial spectrum of trimethoprim is similar to that of sulfamethoxazole, although trimethoprim is 20-100 times more potent. Most gram-negative and gram-positive microorganisms are sensitive to trimethoprim, but resistance can develop when the drug is used alone. *Pseudomonas aeruginosa, Bacteroides fragilis*, and enterococci usually are resistant. There is significant variation in the susceptibility of *Enterobacteriaceae* to trimethoprim in different geographic locations because of the spread of resistance mediated by plasmids and transposons (*see* Chapter 48).

Efficacy of Trimethoprim-Sulfamethoxazole in Combination. *Chlamydia trachomatis* and *N. meningitidis* are susceptible to trimethoprim-sulfamethoxazole. Although most *S. pneumoniae* are susceptible, there has been a disturbing increase in resistance. From 50-95% of strains of *Staphylococcus aureus, Staphylococcus epidermidis, S. pyogenes*, the *viridans* group of streptococci, *E. coli, Proteus mirabilis, Proteus morganii, Proteus rettgeri, Enterobacter* spp., *Salmonella, Shigella, Pseudomonas pseudomallei, Serratia*, and *Alcaligenes* spp. are inhibited. Also sensitive are *Klebsiella* spp., *Brucella abortus, Pasteurella haemolytica, Yersinia pseudotuberculosis, Yersinia enterocolitica*, and *Nocardia asteroides*.

MECHANISM OF ACTION. The antimicrobial activity of the combination of trimethoprim and sulfamethoxazole results from actions on sequential steps of the enzymatic pathway for the synthesis of tetrahydrofolic acid (*see* Figure 52–2). Tetrahydrofolate is essential for one-carbon transfer reactions (e.g., the synthesis of thymidylate from deoxyuridylate). Selective toxicity for microorganisms is achieved in 2 ways. Mammalian cells use preformed folates from the diet and do not synthesize the compound. Furthermore, trimethoprim is a highly selective inhibitor of dihydrofolate reductase of lower organisms: ~100,000 times more drug is required to inhibit human reductase than the bacterial enzyme. The optimal ratio of the concentrations of the 2 agents equals the ratio of the minimal inhibitory concentrations of the drugs acting independently. Although this ratio varies for different bacteria, the most effective ratio for the greatest number of microorganisms is 20:1, sulfamethoxazole:trimethoprim. The combination is thus formulated to achieve a sulfamethoxazole concentration in vivo that is 20 times greater than that of trimethoprim; sulfamethoxazole has pharmacokinetic properties such that the concentrations of the 2 drugs will thus be relatively constant in the body over a long period.

BACTERIAL RESISTANCE. Bacterial resistance to trimethoprim-sulfamethoxazole is a rapidly increasing problem. Resistance often is due to the acquisition of a plasmid that codes for an altered dihydrofolate reductase. Resistance to trimethoprim-sulfamethoxazole is reportedly formed in almost 30% of urinary isolates of *E. coli*.

ADME. The pharmacokinetic profiles of sulfamethoxazole and trimethoprim are closely but not perfectly matched to achieve a constant ratio of 20:1 in their concentrations in blood and tissues. After a single oral dose of the combined preparation, trimethoprim is absorbed more rapidly than sulfamethoxazole. Peak blood concentrations of trimethoprim usually occur by 2 h in most patients, whereas peak concentrations of sulfamethoxazole occur by 4 h after a single oral dose. The half-lives of trimethoprim and sulfamethoxazole are ~11 and 10 h, respectively.

When 800 mg sulfamethoxazole is given with 160 mg trimethoprim (the conventional 5:1 ratio) twice daily, the peak concentrations of the drugs in plasma are ~40 and 2 μg/mL, the optimal ratio. Peak concentrations are similar (46 and 3.4 μg/mL) after intravenous infusion of 800 mg sulfamethoxazole and 160 mg trimethoprim over a period of 1 h.

Trimethoprim is distributed and concentrated rapidly in tissues; ~40% is bound to plasma protein in the presence of sulfamethoxazole. The volume of distribution of trimethoprim is almost 9 times that of sulfamethoxazole. The drug readily enters CSF and sputum. High concentrations of each component of the mixture also are found in bile. About 65% of sulfamethoxazole is bound to plasma protein. About 60% of administered trimethoprim and from 25-50% of administered sulfamethoxazole are excreted in the urine in 24 h. Two-thirds of the sulfonamide is unconjugated. Metabolites of trimethoprim also are excreted. The rates of excretion and the concentrations of both compounds in the urine are reduced significantly in patients with uremia.

THERAPEUTIC USES

Urinary Tract Infections. Treatment of uncomplicated lower UTI with trimethoprim-sulfamethoxazole often is highly effective for sensitive bacteria. Single-dose therapy (320 mg trimethoprim plus 1600 mg sulfamethoxazole in adults) has been effective in some cases for the treatment of acute uncomplicated UTI. Trimethoprim also is found in therapeutic concentrations in prostatic secretions, and trimethoprim-sulfamethoxazole is often effective for the treatment of bacterial prostatitis.

Bacterial Respiratory Tract Infections. Trimethoprim-sulfamethoxazole is effective for acute exacerbations of chronic bronchitis. Administration of 800-1200 mg sulfamethoxazole plus 160-240 mg trimethoprim twice a day appears to be effective in decreasing fever, purulence and volume of sputum, and sputum bacterial count. Trimethoprim-sulfamethoxazole should *not* be used to treat streptococcal pharyngitis because it does not eradicate the microorganism. It is effective for acute otitis media in children and acute maxillary sinusitis in adults caused by susceptible strains of *H. influenzae* and *S. pneumoniae*.

GI Infections. The combination is an alternative to a fluoroquinolone for treatment of shigellosis. Trimethoprim-sulfamethoxazole appears to be effective in the management of carriers of sensitive strains of *Salmonella typhi* and other *Salmonella* spp; however, failures have occurred. Acute diarrhea owing to sensitive strains of enteropathogenic *E. coli* can be treated or prevented with either trimethoprim or trimethoprim + sulfamethoxazole. However, antibiotic treatment of diarrheal illness owing to enterohemorrhagic *E. coli* O157:H7 may increase the risk of hemolytic-uremic syndrome, perhaps by increasing the release of Shiga toxin by the bacteria.

Infection by Pneumocystis jiroveci. High-dose therapy (trimethoprim 15-20 mg/kg/day plus sulfamethoxazole 75-100 mg/kg/day in 3 or 4 divided doses) is effective for this severe infection in patients with AIDS. Adjunctive corticosteroids should be given at the onset of anti-*Pneumocystis* therapy in patients with a PO_2 <70 mm Hg or an alveolar-arterial gradient >35 mm Hg. Prophylaxis with 800 mg sulfamethoxazole and 160 mg trimethoprim once daily or 3 times a week is effective in preventing pneumonia caused by this organism in patients with AIDS. Adverse reactions are less frequent with the lower prophylactic doses of trimethoprim-sulfamethoxazole. The most common problems are rash, fever, leukopenia, and hepatitis.

Prophylaxis in Neutropenic Patients. Low-dose therapy (150 mg/m^2 of body surface area of trimethoprim and 750 mg/m^2 of body surface area of sulfamethoxazole) is effective for the prophylaxis of infection by *P. jiroveci*. A regimen of 800 mg sulfamethoxazole and 160 mg trimethoprim twice daily to severely neutropenic patients provides significant protection against sepsis caused by gram-negative bacteria.

Miscellaneous Infections. Nocardia infections have been treated successfully with the combination, but failures also have been reported. Although a combination of doxycycline and streptomycin or gentamicin now is considered to be the treatment of choice for brucellosis, trimethoprim-sulfamethoxazole may be an effective substitute for the doxycycline combination. Trimethoprim-sulfamethoxazole also has been used successfully in the treatment of Whipple disease, infection by *Stenotrophomonas maltophilia*, and infection by the intestinal parasites *Cyclospora* and *Isospora*. Wegener granulomatosis may respond, depending on the stage of the disease.

UNTOWARD EFFECTS. The margin between toxicity for bacteria and that for humans may be relatively narrow when the patient is folate-deficient. In such cases, trimethoprim-sulfamethoxazole may cause or precipitate megaloblastosis, leukopenia, or thrombocytopenia. In routine use, the combination appears to exert little toxicity. About 75% of the untoward effects involve the skin. Trimethoprim-sulfamethoxazole reportedly causes up to 3 times as many dermatological reactions as does sulfisoxazole alone (5.9% vs. 1.7%). Exfoliative dermatitis, Stevens-Johnson syndrome, and toxic epidermal necrolysis are rare, occurring primarily in older individuals. Nausea and vomiting constitute the bulk of GI reactions; diarrhea is rare. Glossitis and stomatitis are relatively common. Mild and transient jaundice has been noted and appears to have the histological features of allergic cholestatic hepatitis. CNS reactions consist of headache, depression, and hallucinations, manifestations ascribed to sulfonamides. Hematological reactions include various anemias, coagulation disorders, granulocytopenia, agranulocytosis, purpura, Henoch-Schönlein purpura, and sulfhemoglobinemia. Permanent impairment of renal function may follow the use of trimethoprim-sulfamethoxazole in patients with renal disease, and a reversible decrease in creatinine clearance has been noted in patients with normal renal function. Patients with AIDS frequently have hypersensitivity reactions to trimethoprim-sulfamethoxazole (rash, neutropenia, Stevens-Johnson syndrome, Sweet syndrome, and pulmonary infiltrates). It may be possible to continue therapy in such patients following rapid oral desensitization.

THE QUINOLONES

Quinolones are derivatives of nalidixic acid. The fluorinated 4-quinolones, such as *ciprofloxacin* (CIPRO, others) and *moxifloxacin* (AVELOX), have broad antimicrobial activity and are effective after oral administration for the treatment of a wide variety of infectious diseases (Table 52–2).

Rare and potentially fatal side effects, however, have resulted in the withdrawal from the U.S. market of lomefloxacin, sparfloxacin (phototoxicity, QTc prolongation), gatifloxacin (hypoglycemia), temafloxacin (immune hemolytic anemia), trovafloxacin (hepatotoxicity), grepafloxacin (cardiotoxicity), and clinafloxacin (phototoxicity).

MECHANISM OF ACTION. The quinolone antibiotics target bacterial *DNA gyrase* and *topoisomerase IV*. For many gram-positive bacteria, topoisomerase IV is the primary target. In contrast, DNA gyrase is the primary quinolone target in many gram-negative microbes. The gyrase introduces negative supercoils into the DNA to combat excessive positive supercoiling that can occur during DNA replication (Figure 52–3). The quinolones inhibit gyrase-mediated DNA supercoiling at concentrations that correlate well with those required to inhibit bacterial growth (0.1-10 μg/mL). Mutations of the gene that encodes the A subunit of the gyrase can confer resistance to these drugs. Topoisomerase IV, which separates interlinked (catenated) daughter DNA molecules that are the product of DNA replication, also is target for quinolones.

Table 52–2

Structural Formulas of Selected Quinolones and Fluoroquinolones

CONGENER	R_1	R_6	R_7	X
Nalidixic acid	$-C_2H_5$	–H	$-CH_3$	–N–
Norfloxacin	$-C_2H_5$	–F	–N NH (piperazine ring)	–CH–
Ciprofloxacin	(cyclopropyl)	–F	–N NH (piperazine ring)	–CH–
Levofloxacin	O, CH_3, X, N_1 (ring)	–F	–N NH–CH_3 (piperazine ring)	O, CH_3, C, N_1 (ring)

Eukaryotic cells do not contain DNA gyrase. They do contain a conceptually and mechanistically similar type II DNA topoisomerase but quinolones inhibit it only at concentrations (100-1000 μg/mL) much higher than those needed to inhibit the bacterial enzymes.

ANTIBACTERIAL SPECTRUM. The fluoroquinolones are potent bactericidal agents against *E. coli* and various species of *Salmonella, Shigella, Enterobacter, Campylobacter*, and *Neisseria* (MIC_{90} usually are <0.2 μg/mL). Fluoroquinolones also have good activity against staphylococci, but not against methicillin-resistant strains (MIC_{90} = 0.1-2 μg/mL). Activity against streptococci is limited to a subset of the quinolones, including levofloxacin (LEVAQUIN), gatifloxacin, and moxifloxacin (AVELOX). Several intracellular bacteria are inhibited by fluoroquinolones at concentrations that can be achieved in plasma; these include species of *Chlamydia, Mycoplasma, Legionella, Brucella*, and *Mycobacterium* (including *Mycobacterium tuberculosis*). Ciprofloxacin (CIPRO, others), ofloxacin (FLOXIN), and pefloxacin have MIC_{90} values from 0.5-3 μg/mL for *M. fortuitum, M. kansasii*, and *M. tuberculosis*. Several fluoroquinolones, including garenoxacin (not available in U.S.) and gemifloxacin, have activity against anaerobic bacteria.

Resistance to quinolones may develop during therapy via mutations in the bacterial chromosomal genes encoding DNA gyrase or topoisomerase IV or by active transport of the drug out of the bacteria. Resistance has increased after the introduction of fluoroquinolones, especially in *Pseudomonas* and staphylococci. Increasing fluoroquinolone resistance also is being observed in *C. jejuni, Salmonella, N. gonorrhoeae*, and *S. pneumoniae*.

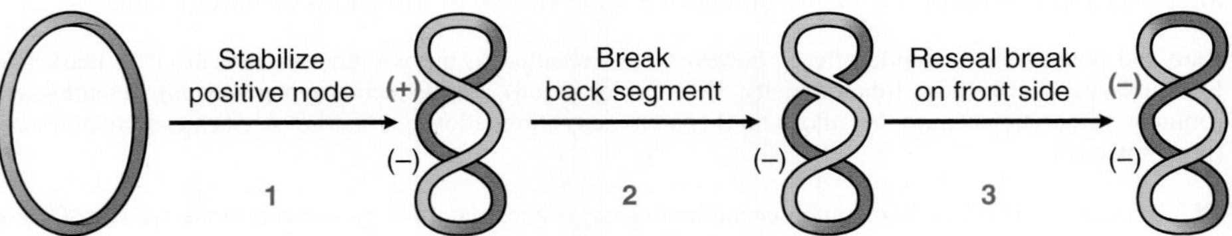

Figure 52–3 *Model of the formation of negative DNA supercoils by DNA gyrase.* DNA gyrase binds to 2 segments of DNA (1), creating a node of positive (+) superhelix. The enzyme then introduces a double-strand break in the DNA and passes the front segment through the break (2). The break is then resealed (3), creating a negative (–) supercoil. Quinolones inhibit the nicking and closing activity of the gyrase and, at higher concentrations, block the decatenating activity of topoisomerase IV. (From Cozzarelli NR. DNA gyrase and the supercoiling of DNA. *Science*, 1980;207:953-960. Reprinted with permission from AAAS.)

ADME. The quinolones are well absorbed after oral administration. Peak serum levels of the fluoroquinolones are obtained within 1-3 h of an oral dose of 400 mg. The volume of distribution of quinolones is high, with concentrations in urine, kidney, lung and prostate tissue, stool, bile, and macrophages and neutrophils higher than serum levels. Relatively low serum levels are reached with norfloxacin and limit its usefulness to the treatment of UTIs. Food may delay the time to peak serum concentrations. Oral doses in adults are 200-400 mg every 12 h for ofloxacin, 400 mg every 12 h for norfloxacin and pefloxacin, and 250 to 750 mg every 12 h for ciprofloxacin. Bioavailability of the fluoroquinolones is >50% for all agents and >95% for several. The serum $t_{1/2}$ is 3-5 h for norfloxacin and ciprofloxacin. Quinolone concentrations in CSF, bone, and prostatic fluid are lower than in serum. Pefloxacin and ofloxacin levels in ascites fluid are close to serum levels, and ciprofloxacin, ofloxacin, and pefloxacin have been detected in human breast milk. Most quinolones are cleared predominantly by the kidney, and dosages must be adjusted for renal failure. By contrast, pefloxacin and moxifloxacin are metabolized predominantly by the liver and should not be used in patients with hepatic failure. None of the agents is removed efficiently by peritoneal or hemodialysis.

Pharmacokinetic Aspects. The pharmacokinetic and pharmacodynamic parameters of antimicrobial agents are important in preventing the selection and spread of resistant strains and have led to description of the mutation-prevention concentration, which is the lowest concentration of antimicrobial that prevents selection of resistant bacteria from high bacterial inocula. β-Lactams are time-dependent agents without significant post-antibiotic effects, resulting in bacterial eradication when unbound serum concentrations exceed MICs of these agents against infecting pathogens for >40-50% of the dosing interval. By contrast, fluoroquinolones are concentration- and time-dependent agents, resulting in bacterial eradication when unbound serum area under the curve-to-MIC ratios exceed 25-30. An extended release formulation of ciprofloxacin (PROQUIN XR) exemplifies this principle (*see* Figure 48–4).

THERAPEUTIC USES

Urinary Tract Infections. Nalidixic acid is useful only for UTI caused by susceptible microorganisms. The fluoroquinolones are significantly more potent and have a much broader spectrum of antimicrobial activity. Norfloxacin and ciprofloxacin XR are approved for use in the U.S. only for UTIs. Fluoroquinolones are more efficacious than trimethoprim-sulfamethoxazole for the treatment of UTI.

Prostatitis. Norfloxacin, ciprofloxacin, and ofloxacin are effective in the treatment of prostatitis caused by sensitive bacteria. Fluoroquinolones administered for 4-6 weeks appear to be effective in patients not responding to trimethoprim-sulfamethoxazole.

Sexually Transmitted Diseases. The quinolones are contraindicated in pregnancy. Fluoroquinolones lack activity for *Treponema pallidum* but have activity in vitro against *C. trachomatis* and *H. ducreyi*. For chlamydial urethritis/cervicitis, a 7-day course of ofloxacin is an alternative to a 7-day treatment with doxycycline or a single dose of azithromycin; other available quinolones have not been reliably effective. A single oral dose of a fluoroquinolone such as ofloxacin or ciprofloxacin had been effective treatment for sensitive strains of *N. gonorrhoeae*, but increasing resistance to fluoroquinolones has led to ceftriaxone being the first-line agent for this infection. Chancroid (infection by *H. ducreyi*) can be treated with 3 days of ciprofloxacin.

GI and Abdominal Infections. For traveler's diarrhea (frequently caused by enterotoxigenic *E. coli*), the quinolones are equal to trimethoprim-sulfamethoxazole in effectiveness, reducing the duration of loose stools by 1-3 days. Norfloxacin, ciprofloxacin, and ofloxacin given for 5 days all have been effective in the treatment of patients with shigellosis. Ciprofloxacin and ofloxacin treatment cures most patients with enteric fever caused by *S. typhi*, as well as bacteremic nontyphoidal infections in AIDS patients, and clears chronic fecal carriage. The in vitro ability of the quinolones to induce the Shiga toxin *stx2* gene (the cause of the hemolytic-uremic syndrome) in *E. coli* suggests that the quinolones should not be used for Shiga toxin–producing *E. coli*. Ciprofloxacin and ofloxacin are less effective in treating episodes of peritonitis occurring in patients on chronic ambulatory peritoneal dialysis (likely cause: coagulase- negative staphylococci).

Respiratory Tract Infections. Many newer fluoroquinolones, including gatifloxacin (available only for ophthalmic use in U.S.) and moxifloxacin, have excellent activity against *S. pneumoniae*. The fluoroquinolones have in vitro activity against the rest of the commonly recognized respiratory pathogens. Either a fluoroquinolone (ciprofloxacin or levofloxacin) or azithromycin is the antibiotic of choice for *L. pneumophila*. Fluoroquinolones have been very effective at eradicating both *H. influenzae* and *M. catarrhalis* from sputum. Mild to moderate respiratory exacerbations owing to *P. aeruginosa* in patients with cystic fibrosis have responded to oral fluoroquinolone therapy.

Bone, Joint, and Soft Tissue Infections. The treatment of chronic osteomyelitis requires prolonged (weeks to months) antimicrobial therapy with agents active against *S. aureus* and gram-negative rods. The fluoroquinolones, with an appropriate antibacterial spectrum for these infections, may be used in some cases; recommended doses are 500 mg every 12 h or, if severe, 750 mg twice daily. Dosage should be reduced for patients with severely impaired renal function. Clinical cures are as high as 75% in chronic osteomyelitis in which gram-negative rods predominate. Failures are associated with the development of resistance in *S. aureus*, *P. aeruginosa*, and *Serratia marcescens*. In diabetic foot infections, the fluoroquinolones in combination with an agent with anti-anaerobic activity are a reasonable choice.

Other Infections. Ciprofloxacin is used for the prophylaxis of anthrax and is effective for the treatment of tularemia. The quinolones may be used as part of multiple-drug regimens for the treatment of multidrug-resistant tuberculosis and atypical mycobacterial infections as well as *Myobacterium avium* complex infections in AIDS (*see* Chapter 56). Quinolones, when used as prophylaxis in neutropenic patients, have decreased the incidence of gram-negative rod bacteremias. Levofloxacin is approved to treat and prevent anthrax as well as plague due to *Yersinia pestis*.

ADVERSE EFFECTS. Quinolones and fluoroquinolones generally are well tolerated. Common adverse reactions involve the GI tract, with 3-17% of patients reporting mild nausea, vomiting, and abdominal discomfort. Ciprofloxacin is the most common cause of *C. difficile* colitis. Gatifloxacin is associated with both hypo- and hyperglycemia in older adults. CNS side effects (1-11%) include mild headache and dizziness. Rarely, hallucinations, delirium, and seizures have occurred, predominantly in patients who were also receiving theophylline or NSAIDS. Ciprofloxacin and pefloxacin inhibit the metabolism of theophylline, and toxicity from elevated concentrations of the methylxanthine may occur. NSAIDS may augment displacement of γ-aminobutyric acid (GABA) from its receptors by the quinolones. Rashes, including photosensitivity reactions, also can occur. Achilles tendon rupture or tendinitis is a recognized adverse effect, especially in those >60 years old, inpatients taking corticosteroids, and in solid organ transplant recipients. Ciprofloxacin should not be given to pregnant women and are generally not used in children.

Leukopenia, eosinophilia, and mild elevations in serum transaminases occur rarely. QT interval prolongation has been observed with sparfloxacin and to a lesser extent with gatifloxacin and moxifloxacin. Quinolones should be used with caution in patients on class III (amiodarone) and class IA (quinidine, procainamide) anti-arrhythmics (*see* Chapter 29).

ANTISEPTIC AND ANALGESIC AGENTS FOR URINARY TRACT INFECTIONS

Urinary tract antiseptics are concentrated in the renal tubules where they inhibit the growth of many species of bacteria. These agents cannot be used to treat systemic infections because effective concentrations are not achieved in plasma with safe doses; however, they can be administered orally to treat UTIs. Furthermore, effective antibacterial concentrations reach the renal pelves and the bladder.

METHENAMINE. Methenamine (hexamethylenamine) is a urinary tract antiseptic and prodrug that acts by generating formaldehyde via the following reaction:

$$NH_4(CH_2)_6 + 6H_2O + 4H^+ \rightarrow 4NH_4^+ + 6HCHO$$

At pH 7.4, almost no decomposition occurs; the yield of formaldehyde is 6% of the theoretical amount at pH 6 and 20% at pH 5. Thus, acidification of the urine promotes formaldehyde formation and the formaldehyde-dependent antibacterial action. The decomposition reaction is fairly slow, and 3 h are required to reach 90% completion. Nearly all bacteria are sensitive to free formaldehyde at concentrations of ~20 μg/mL. Microorganisms do not develop resistance to formaldehyde. Urea-splitting microorganisms (e.g., *Proteus* spp.) tend to raise the pH of the urine and thus inhibit the release of formaldehyde.

Pharmacology, Toxicology, and Therapeutic Uses. Methenamine is absorbed orally, but 10-30% decomposes in the gastric juice unless the drug is protected by an enteric coating. Because of the ammonia produced, methenamine is contraindicated in hepatic insufficiency. Excretion in the urine is nearly quantitative. When the urine pH is 6 and the daily urine volume is 1000-1500 mL, a daily dose of 2 g will yield a urine concentration of 18-60 μg/mL of formaldehyde; this is more than the MIC for most urinary tract pathogens. Low pH alone is bacteriostatic, so acidification serves a double function. The acids commonly used are mandelic acid and hippuric acid (UREX, HIPREX). GI distress frequently is caused by doses >500 mg 4 times a day, even with enteric-coated tablets. Painful and frequent micturition, albuminuria, hematuria, and rashes may result from doses of 4 to 8 g/day given for longer than 3-4 weeks. Renal insufficiency is not a contraindication to the use of methenamine alone, but the acids given concurrently may be detrimental; methenamine mandelate is contraindicated in renal insufficiency. Methenamine combines with sulfamethizole and perhaps other sulfonamides in the urine, which results in mutual antagonism; therefore, these drugs should not be used in combination. Methenamine is not a primary drug for the treatment of acute UTIs but is of value for chronic suppressive treatment of UTIs. The agent is most useful when the causative organism is *E. coli*, but it usually can suppress the common gram-negative offenders and often *S. aureus* and *S. epidermidis* as well. *Enterobacter aerogenes* and *Proteus vulgaris* are usually resistant. The physician should strive to keep the pH <5.5.

NITROFURANTOIN. Nitrofurantoin (FURADANTIN, MACROBID, others) is a synthetic nitrofuran that is used for the prevention and treatment of UTIs.

Antimicrobial Activity. Nitrofurantoin is activated by enzymatic reduction, with the formation of highly reactive intermediates that seem to be responsible for the observed capacity of the drug to damage DNA. Bacteria reduce nitrofurantoin more rapidly than do mammalian cells, and this is thought to account for the selective antimicrobial activity of the compound. Nitrofurantoin is active against many strains of *E. coli* and enterococci. However, most species of *Proteus* and *Pseudomonas* and many species of *Enterobacter* and *Klebsiella* are resistant. Nitrofurantoin is bacteriostatic for most susceptible microorganisms at concentrations of ≤32 μg/mL or less and is bactericidal at concentrations of ≥100 μg/mL. The antibacterial activity is higher in acidic urine.

Pharmacology, Toxicity, and Therapy. Nitrofurantoin is absorbed rapidly and completely from the GI tract. Antibacterial concentrations are not achieved in plasma following ingestion of recommended doses because the drug is eliminated rapidly. The plasma $t_{1/2}$ is 0.3-1 h; ~40% is excreted unchanged into the urine. The average dose of nitrofurantoin yields a concentration in urine of ~200 μg/mL. This concentration is soluble at pH >5, but the urine should not be alkalinized because this reduces antimicrobial activity. The rate of excretion is linearly related to the creatinine clearance, so in patients with impaired glomerular function, the efficacy of the drug may be decreased and the systemic toxicity increased. Nitrofurantoin colors the urine brown.

The oral dosage of nitrofurantoin for adults is 50-100 mg 4 times a day with meals and at bedtime, less for the macrocrystalline formulation (100 mg every 12 h for 7 days). A single 50-100-mg dose at bedtime may be sufficient to prevent recurrences. The daily dose for children is 5-7 mg/kg but may be as low as 1 mg/kg for long-term therapy. A course of therapy should not exceed 14 days; repeated courses should be separated by rest periods. Pregnant women, individuals with impaired renal function (creatinine clearance <40 mL/min), and children <1 month of age should not receive nitrofurantoin. Nitrofurantoin is approved for the treatment of UTIs. It is not recommended for treatment of pyelonephritis or prostatitis.

The most common untoward effects are nausea, vomiting, and diarrhea; the macrocrystalline preparation is better tolerated than traditional formulations. Various hypersensitivity reactions occur occasionally, including chills, fever, leukopenia, granulocytopenia, hemolytic anemia (associated with G6PD deficiency), cholestatic jaundice, and hepatocellular damage. Chronic active hepatitis is an uncommon. Acute pneumonitis with fever, chills, cough, dyspnea, chest pain, pulmonary infiltration, and eosinophilia may occur within hours to days of the initiation of therapy; these symptoms usually resolve quickly after discontinuation of the drug. Interstitial pulmonary fibrosis can occur in patients (especially the elderly) taking the drug chronically. Megaloblastic anemia is rare. Headache, vertigo, drowsiness, muscular aches, and nystagmus occur occasionally but are readily reversible. Severe polyneuropathies with demyelination and degeneration of both sensory and motor nerves have been reported; neuropathies are most likely to occur in patients with impaired renal function and in persons on long-continued treatment.

PHENAZOPYRIDINE. Phenazopyridine hydrochloride (PYRIDIUM, others) is *not* a urinary antiseptic. However, it does have an analgesic action on the urinary tract and alleviates symptoms of dysuria, frequency, burning, and urgency. The usual dose is 200 mg 3 times daily. The compound is an azo dye, which colors urine orange or red. GI upset is seen in up to 10% of patients and can be reduced by administering the drug with food; overdosage may result in methemoglobinemia. OTC products containing phenazopyridine are under review by the FDA for safety and efficacy.

For a complete Bibliographical Listing see Goodman & Gilman's ***The Pharmacological Basis of Therapeutics***, 12th ed., or Goodman & Gilman Online at www.AccessMedicine.com.

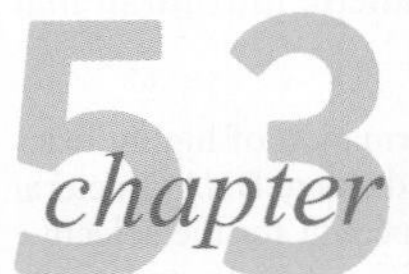

chapter 53 Penicillins, Cephalosporins, and Other β-Lactam Antibiotics

The β-lactam antibiotics—*penicillins*, *cephalosporins*, and *carbapenems*—share a common structure and mechanism of action, inhibition of the synthesis of the bacterial peptidoglycan cell wall. Bacterial resistance against the β-lactam antibiotics continues to increase at a dramatic rate. β-Lactamase inhibitors such as clavulanate can extend the utility of these drugs against β-lactamase-producing organisms. Unfortunately, resistance includes not only production of β-lactamases but also alterations in or acquisition of novel penicillin-binding proteins (PBPs) and decreased entry and/or active efflux of the antibiotic. To a dangerous degree, we are re-entering the pre-antibiotic era, with many nosocomial gram-negative bacterial infections resistant to all available antibiotics.

MECHANISM OF ACTION: INHIBITION OF PEPTIDOGLYCAN SYNTHESIS. Peptidoglycan is a heteropolymeric component of the cell wall that provides rigid mechanical stability. The β-lactam antibiotics inhibit the last step in peptidoglycan synthesis (Figure 53–1).

In gram-positive microorganisms, the cell wall is 50-100 molecules thick; in gram-negative bacteria, it is only 1 or 2 molecules thick (Figure 53–2A). The peptidoglycan is composed of glycan chains, which are linear strands of 2 alternating amino sugars (*N*-acetylglucosamine and *N*-acetylmuramic acid) that are cross-linked by peptide chains. Peptidoglycan precursor formation takes place in the cytoplasm. The synthesis of UDP–acetylmuramyl-pentapeptide is completed with the addition of a dipeptide, D-alanyl-D-alanine (formed by racemization and condensation of L-alanine). UDP-acetylmuramyl-pentapeptide and UDP-acetylglucosamine are linked (with the release of the uridine nucleotides) to form a long polymer. The cross-link is completed

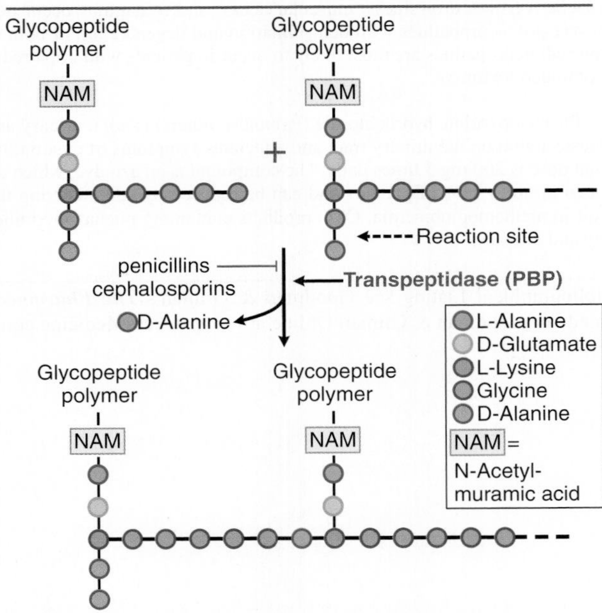

Figure 53–1 *Action of β-lactam antibiotics in Staphylococcus aureus.* The bacterial cell wall consists of glycopeptide polymers (a NAM-NAG amino-hexose backbone) linked via bridges between amino acid side chains. In *S. aureus*, the bridge is $(Gly)_5$-D-Ala between lysines. The cross-linking is catalyzed by a transpeptidase, the enzyme that penicillins and cephalosporins inhibit.

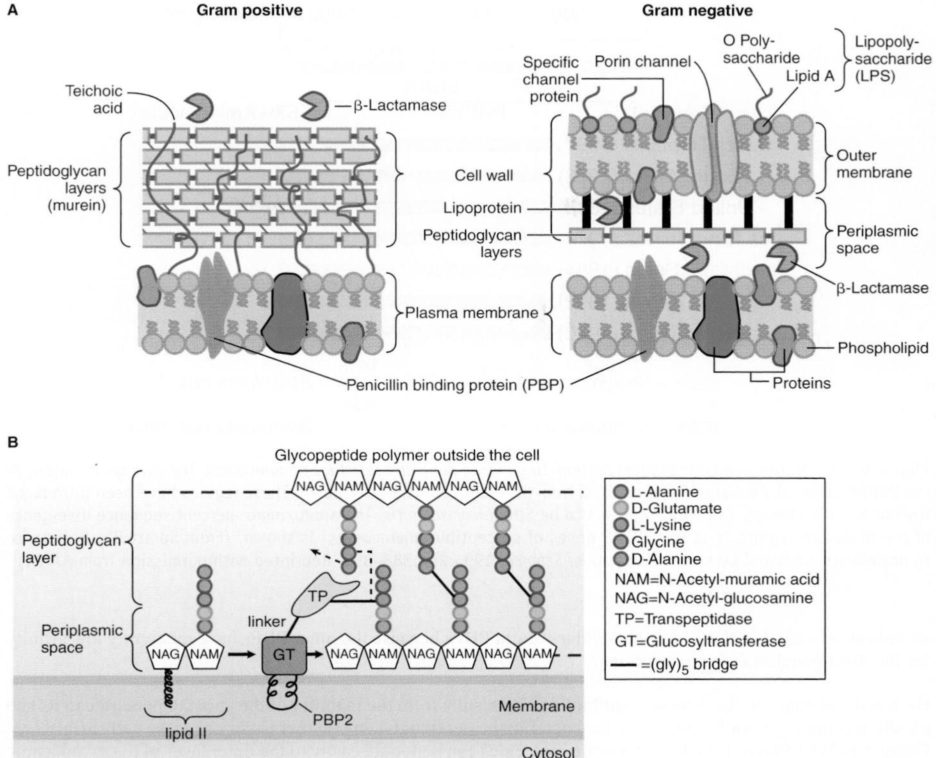

Figure 53–2 **A.** *Structure and composition of gram-positive and gram-negative cell walls.* (From Figure 4–11, p 83 of TORTORA, GERALD, MICROBIOLOGY: INTRODUCTION, 3rd Edition, © 1989. Reprinted by permission of Pearson Education, Inc., Upper Saddle River, NJ.) **B.** *Penicillin binding protein 2 (PBP2) from S. aureus.* PBP2 has 2 enzymatic activities that are crucial to synthesis of the peptidoglycan layers of bacterial cell walls: a transpeptidase (TP) that cross-links amino acid side chains, and a glycosyltransferase (GT) that links subunits of the glycopeptide polymer (*see* Figure 53–1). The transpeptidase and glycosyltransferase domains are separated by a linker region. The glycosyltransferase is thought to be partially embedded in the membrane.

by transpeptidation reaction that occurs outside the cell membrane (Figure 53–2B). The β-lactam antibiotics inhibit this last step in peptidoglycan synthesis (*see* Figure 53–1), presumably by acylating the transpeptidase via cleavage of the —CO—N— bond of the β-lactam ring. There are additional, related targets for the actions of penicillins and cephalosporins; these are collectively termed *PBPs*. The transpeptidase responsible for synthesis of the peptidoglycan is 1 of these PBPs. The lethality of penicillin for bacteria appears to involve both lytic and nonlytic mechanisms.

MECHANISMS OF BACTERIAL RESISTANCE TO PENICILLINS AND CEPHALOSPORINS. Bacteria can be resistant to β-lactam antibiotics by myriad mechanisms.

A sensitive strain may acquire resistance by mutations that decrease the affinity of PBPs for the antibiotic. Because the β-lactam antibiotics inhibit many different PBPs in a single bacterium, the affinity for β-lactam antibiotics of several PBPs must decrease for the organism to be resistant. Methicillin-resistant *Staphylococcus aureus* (*MRSA*) are resistant via acquisition of an additional high-molecular-weight PBP (via a transposon) with a very low affinity for all β-lactam antibiotics; this mechanism is responsible for methicillin resistance in the coagulase-negative staphylococci. Altered PBPs with decreased affinity for β-lactam antibiotics are acquired by homologous recombination between PBP genes of different bacterial species. Four of the 5 high-molecular-weight PBPs of the most highly penicillin-resistant *Streptococcus pneumoniae* isolates have decreased affinity for β-lactam antibiotics as a result of interspecies homologous recombination events (Figure 53–3). In contrast, isolates with high-level resistance to third-generation cephalosporins contain

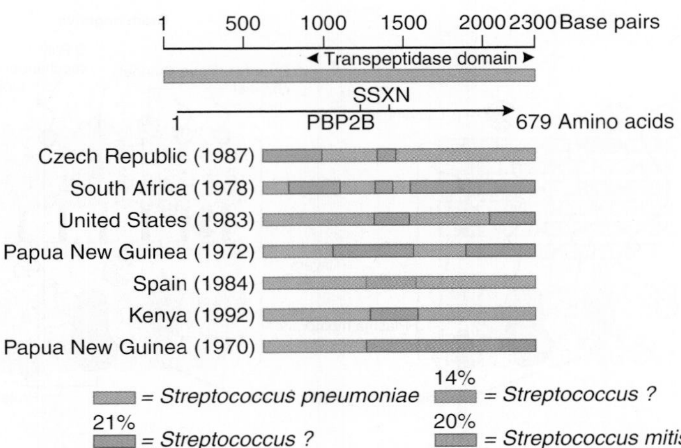

Figure 53–3 *Mosaic penicillin binding protein 2B genes in penicillin-resistant pneumococci.* The divergent regions in the PBP2B genes of 7 resistant pneumococci from different countries are shown. These regions have been introduced from at least 3 sources, 1 of which appears to be *Streptococcus mitis*. The approximate percent sequence divergence of the divergent regions from the PBP2B genes of susceptible pneumococci is shown. (From Spratt BG. Resistance to antibiotics mediated by target alterations. *Science*, 1994;264:388–393. Reprinted with permission from AAAS.)

alterations of only 2 of the 5 high-molecular-weight PBPs because the other PBPs have inherently low affinity for the third-generation cephalosporins.

Bacterial resistance to the β-lactam antibiotics also results from the inability of the agent to penetrate to its site of action (Figure 53–4). In gram-positive bacteria, the peptidoglycan polymer is very near the cell surface (*see* Figure 53–2) and small β-lactam antibiotic molecules can penetrate easily to the outer layer of the cytoplasmic membrane and the PBPs. In gram-negative bacteria, the inner membrane is covered by the outer membrane, lipopolysaccharide, and capsule (*see* Figure 53–2). The outer membrane functions as an impenetrable barrier for some antibiotics. Some small hydrophilic antibiotics, however, diffuse through aqueous channels in the outer membrane that are formed by proteins called *porins*. The number and size of pores in the outer membrane vary among different gram-negative bacteria, thereby providing greater or lesser access for antibiotics to the site of action. Active efflux pumps serve as another mechanism of resistance, removing the antibiotic from its site of action before it can act (*see* Figure 53–4).

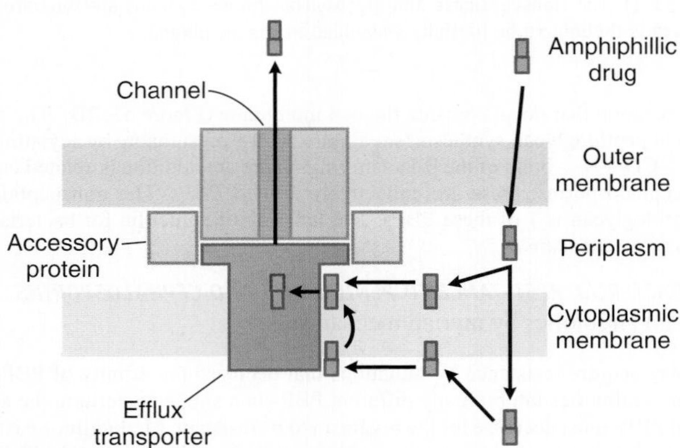

Figure 53–4 *Antibiotic efflux pumps of gram-negative bacteria.* Multidrug efflux pumps traverse both the inner and outer membranes of gram-negative bacteria. The pumps are composed of a minimum of 3 proteins and are energized by the proton motive force. Increased expression of these pumps is an important cause of antibiotic resistance. (Reprinted with permission from Oxford University Press. Nikaido H. Antibiotic resistance caused by gram-negative multidrug efflux pumps. *Clin Infect Dis*, 1998;27[suppl I]:S32–S41. © 1998 by the Infectious Diseases Society of America. All rights reserved.)

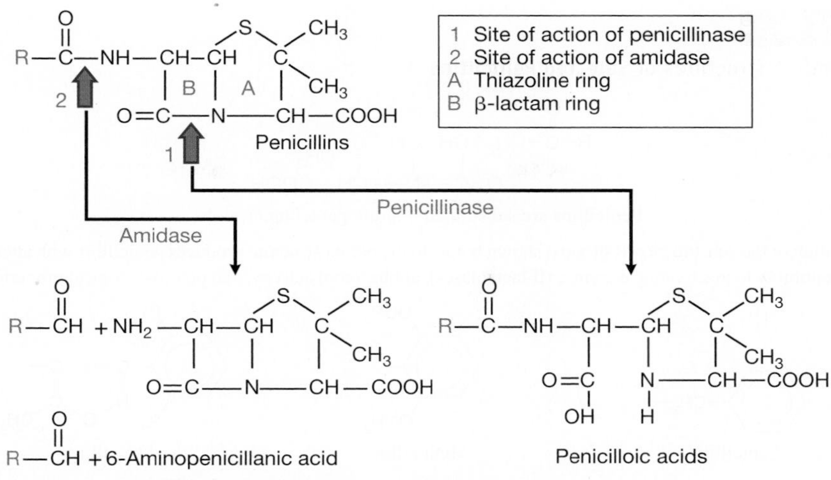

Figure 53–5 *Structure of penicillins and products of their enzymatic hydrolysis.*

Bacteria also can destroy β-lactam antibiotics enzymatically via the action of β-lactamases (Figures 53–2 and 53–5). β-Lactamases are grouped into four classes: A through D. The substrate specificities of some of these classes are relatively narrow; these often are described as either penicillinases or cephalosporinases. Other "extended-spectrum" enzymes are less discriminant and can hydrolyze a variety of β-lactam antibiotics. In general, gram-positive bacteria produce and secrete a large amount of β-lactamase (*see* Figure 53–2A). Most of these enzymes are penicillinases. The information for staphylococcal penicillinase is encoded in a plasmid; this may be transferred by bacteriophage to other bacteria and is inducible by substrates. In gram-negative bacteria, β-lactamases are found in relatively small amounts but are located in the periplasmic space between the inner and outer cell membranes (*see* Figure 53–2A) for maximal protection of the microbe. β-Lactamases of gram-negative bacteria are encoded either in chromosomes or in plasmids, and may be constitutive or inducible. The plasmids can be transferred between bacteria by conjugation. These enzymes can hydrolyze penicillins, cephalosporins, or both.

OTHER FACTORS THAT INFLUENCE THE ACTIVITY OF β-LACTAM ANTIBIOTICS. Microorganisms adhering to implanted prosthetic devices (e.g., catheters, artificial joints, prosthetic heart valves) produce biofilms. Bacteria in biofilms produce extracellular polysaccharides and, in part owing to decreased growth rates, are much less sensitive to antibiotic therapy. The β-lactam antibiotics are most active against bacteria in the logarithmic phase of growth and have little effect on microorganisms in the stationary phase. Similarly, bacteria that survive inside viable cells of the host generally are protected from the action of the β-lactam antibiotics.

THE PENICILLINS

Despite the emergence of microbial resistance, the penicillins are currently the drugs of choice for a large number of infectious diseases. Penicillins (Figure 53–5) consist of a thiazolidine ring (A) connected to a β-lactam ring (B) to which is attached a side chain (R). The penicillin nucleus itself is the chief structural requirement for biological activity. Side chains can be added that alter the susceptibility of the resulting compounds to inactivating enzymes (β-lactamases) and that change the antibacterial activity and the pharmacological properties of the drug (Table 53–1).

UNITAGE OF PENICILLIN. The international unit of penicillin is the specific penicillin activity contained in 0.6 μg of the crystalline sodium salt of penicillin G. One milligram of pure penicillin G sodium thus equals 1667 units; 1.0 mg of pure penicillin G potassium represents 1595 units. The dosage and the antibacterial potency of the semisynthetic penicillins are expressed in terms of weight.

CLASSIFICATION OF THE PENICILLINS AND SUMMARY OF THEIR PHARMACOLOGICAL PROPERTIES

Penicillins are classified according to their spectra of antimicrobial activity.

- ***Penicillin G*** and its close congener ***penicillin V*** are highly active against sensitive strains of gram-positive cocci, but they are readily hydrolyzed by penicillinase. Thus, they are *ineffective against most strains of S. aureus.*

Table 53–1

Chemical Structures of Selected Penicillins

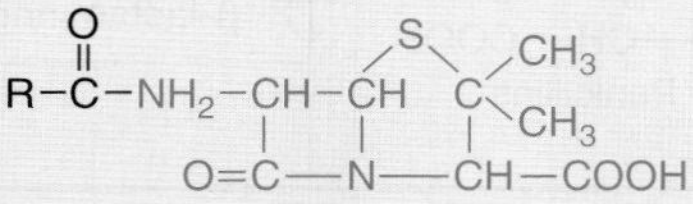

Penicillins are substituted 6-aminopenicillanic acids

Addition of the substituents (R groups) shown below to the parent structure produces penicillins with altered susceptibility to inactivating enzymes (β-lactamases), antibacterial activity, and pharmacological properties.

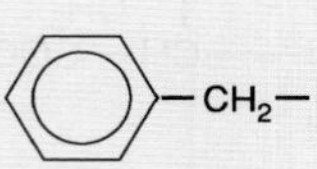

Penicillin G	Methicillin	Oxacillin
Amoxicillin	Ticarcillin	Piperacillin

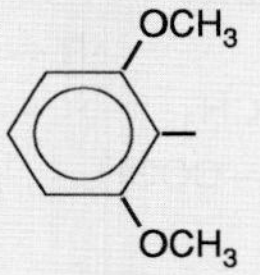

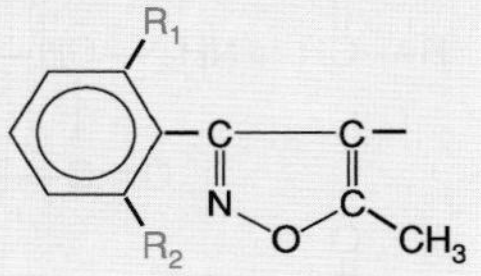

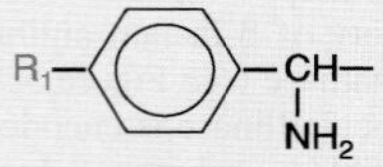

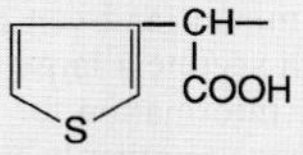

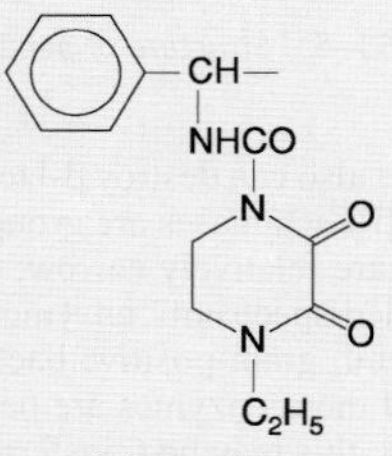

- **The penicillinase-resistant penicillins** (*methicillin*, discontinued in U.S.), *nafcillin*, *oxacillin*, *cloxacillin* (not currently marketed in the U.S.), and *dicloxacillin* have less potent antimicrobial activity against microorganisms that are sensitive to penicillin G, but they are the *agents of first choice for treatment of penicillinase-producing S. aureus and Staphylococcus epidermidis that are not methicillin-resistant.*
- Ampicillin, amoxicillin, and others make up a group **of penicillins whose antimicrobial activity is extended to include gram-negative microorganisms** (e.g., *Haemophilus influenzae*, *Escherichia coli*, and *Proteus mirabilis*). These drugs are **frequently administered with a β-lactamase inhibitor** such as clavulanate or sulbactam to prevent hydrolysis by class A β-lactamases.
- **Agents with extended antimicrobial activity** that includes *Pseudomonas*, *Enterobacter*, and *Proteus* spp. [carbenicillin (discontinued in U.S.), its indanyl ester (carbenicillin indanyl), and ticarcillin (marketed with clavulanate in U.S.)] These agents are inferior to ampicillin against gram-positive cocci and *Listeria monocytogenes* and are less active than piperacillin against *Pseudomonas*.
- ***Mezlocillin, azlocillin*** (both discontinued in U.S.), and ***piperacillin*** have excellent antimicrobial activity against many isolates of *Pseudomonas*, *Klebsiella*, and certain other gram-negative microorganisms. Piperacillin retains the activity of ampicillin against gram-positive cocci and *L. monocytogenes.*

General common properties: Following absorption of an oral dose, penicillins are distributed widely throughout the body. Therapeutic concentrations of penicillins are achieved readily in tissues and in secretions such as joint fluid, pleural fluid, pericardial fluid, and bile. Penicillins do not penetrate living phagocytic cells to a significant extent, and only low concentrations of these drugs are found in prostatic secretions, brain tissue, and intraocular fluid. Concentrations of penicillins in cerebrospinal fluid (CSF) are variable but are <1% of those in plasma when the meninges are normal. When there is inflammation, concentrations in CSF may increase to as much as 5% of the plasma value. Penicillins are eliminated rapidly, particularly by glomerular filtration and renal tubular secretion, such that their half-lives in the body are short, typically 30-90 min. As a consequence, concentrations of these drugs in urine are high.

PENICILLIN G AND PENICILLIN V

ANTIMICROBIAL ACTIVITY. The antimicrobial spectra of penicillin G (benzylpenicillin) and penicillin V (the phenoxymethyl derivative) are very similar for aerobic gram-positive microorganisms. However, penicillin G is 5-10 times more active than penicillin V against *Neisseria* spp. and certain anaerobes. Most streptococci (but not enterococci) are very susceptible. However, penicillin-resistant *viridans* streptococci and *S. pneumoniae* are becoming more common. Penicillin-resistant pneumococci are especially common in pediatric populations. Many penicillin-resistant pneumococci also are resistant to third-generation cephalosporins. More than 90% of strains of staphylococci isolates are now resistant to penicillin G, (and nearly half are methicillin-resistant). Most strains of *S. epidermidis* and many strains of gonococci are also resistant. With rare exceptions, meningococci are quite sensitive to penicillin G.

Most anaerobic microorganisms, including *Clostridium* spp., are highly sensitive. *Bacteroides fragilis* is an exception, displaying resistance to penicillins and cephalosporins by virtue of expressing a broad-spectrum cephalosporinase. Some strains of *Prevotella melaninogenicus* also have acquired this trait. *Actinomyces israelii*, *Streptobacillus moniliformis*, *Pasteurella multocida*, and *L. monocytogenes* are inhibited by penicillin G. Most species of *Leptospira* are moderately susceptible to the drug. One of the most sensitive microorganisms is *Treponema pallidum*. *Borrelia burgdorferi*, the organism responsible for Lyme disease, also is susceptible. None of the penicillins is effective against amebae, plasmodia, rickettsiae, fungi, or viruses.

ADME

Oral Administration of Penicillin G. About one-third of an orally administered dose of penicillin G is absorbed from the GI tract. Gastric juice at pH 2 rapidly destroys the antibiotic. Absorption is rapid, and maximal concentrations in blood are attained in 30-60 min. Ingestion of food may interfere with enteric absorption of all penicillins. Thus, oral penicillin G should be administered at least 30 min before a meal or 2 h after. Despite the convenience of oral administration of penicillin G, this route should be used only in infections in which clinical experience has proven its efficacy.

Oral Administration of Penicillin V. The virtue of penicillin V in comparison with penicillin G is that it is more stable in an acidic medium and therefore is better absorbed from the GI tract, yielding plasma concentrations 2-5 times those provided by penicillin G.

Parenteral Administration of Penicillin G. After intramuscular injection, peak concentrations in plasma are reached within 15-30 min, declining rapidly thereafter ($t_{1/2}$ ~ 30 min). Repository preparations of penicillin G increase the duration of the effect. The compound currently favored is penicillin G benzathine (BICILLIN L-A, PERMAPEN), which releases penicillin G slowly from the area in which it is injected and produces relatively low but persistent concentrations in the blood. The average duration of demonstrable antimicrobial activity in the plasma is ~26 days. It is administered once monthly for rheumatic fever prophylaxis and can be given in a single injection to treat streptococcal pharyngitis. The persistence of penicillin in the blood after a suitable intramuscular dose of penicillin G benzathine reduces cost, need for repeated injections, and local trauma. The local anesthetic effect of penicillin G benzathine is comparable with that of penicillin G procaine.

Distribution. Penicillin G is distributed widely throughout the body, but the concentrations in various fluids and tissues differ widely. Its apparent volume of distribution is ~0.35 L/kg. Approximately 60% of the penicillin G in plasma is reversibly bound to albumin. Significant amounts appear in liver, bile, kidney, semen, joint fluid, lymph, and intestine. Probenecid markedly decreases the tubular secretion of the penicillins and also produces a significant decrease in the apparent volume of distribution of the penicillins.

Penetration into Cerebrospinal Fluid. Penicillin does not readily enter the CSF but penetrates more easily when the meninges are inflamed. The concentrations are usually in the range of 5% of the value in plasma and are therapeutically effective against susceptible microorganisms. Penicillin and other organic acids are secreted rapidly from the CSF into the bloodstream by an active transport process. Probenecid competitively inhibits this transport and thus elevates the concentration of penicillin in CSF. In uremia, other organic acids accumulate in the CSF and compete with penicillin for secretion; the drug occasionally reaches toxic concentrations in the brain and can produce convulsions.

Excretion. Approximately 60-90% of an intramuscular dose of penicillin G in aqueous solution is eliminated in the urine, largely within the first hour after injection. The remainder is metabolized to penicilloic acid (*see* Figure 53–5). The $t_{1/2}$ for elimination of penicillin G is ~30 min in normal adults. Approximately 10% of the drug is eliminated by glomerular filtration and 90% by tubular secretion. Renal clearance approximates the total renal plasma flow. Clearance values are considerably lower in neonates and infants; as a result penicillin persists in the blood several times longer in premature infants than in children and adults. The $t_{1/2}$ of the antibiotic in children <1 week of age is 3 h; by 14 days of age it is 1.4 h. After renal function is fully established in young children, the rate of renal excretion of penicillin G is considerably more rapid than in adults. Anuria increases the $t_{1/2}$ of penicillin G from 0.5 h to ~10 h. When renal function is impaired, 7-10% of the antibiotic may be inactivated each hour by the liver. The dose of the drug must be readjusted during dialysis and the period of progressive recovery of renal function. If hepatic insufficiency also is present, the $t_{1/2}$ will be prolonged even further.

THERAPEUTIC USES

Pneumococcal Infections. Penicillin G remains the agent of choice for the management of infections caused by sensitive strains of *S. pneumoniae*, but resistance is an increasing problem.

Pneumococcal Pneumonia. Pneumococcal pneumonia should be treated with a third-generation cephalosporin or with 20-24 million units of penicillin G daily by constant intravenous infusion. If the organism is sensitive to penicillin, then the dose can be reduced. For parenteral therapy of sensitive isolates of pneumococci, penicillin G is favored. Therapy should be continued for 7-10 days, including 3-5 days after the patient's temperature has returned to normal.

Pneumococcal Meningitis. Pneumococcal meningitis should be treated with a combination of vancomycin and a third-generation cephalosporin until it is established that the infecting pneumococcus is penicillin-sensitive. Dexamethasone given at the same time as antibiotics is associated with an improved outcome. The recommended therapy is 20-24 million units of penicillin G daily by constant intravenous infusion or divided into boluses given every 2-3 h for 14 days.

Streptococcal Infections. Streptococcal pharyngitis (including scarlet fever) is the most common disease produced by *Streptococcus pyogenes* (group A β-hemolytic streptococcus). Penicillin-resistant isolates have yet to be observed. The preferred oral therapy is with penicillin V, 500 mg every 6 h for 10 days. Penicillin therapy of streptococcal pharyngitis reduces the risk of subsequent acute rheumatic fever; however, current evidence suggests that the incidence of glomerulonephritis that follows streptococcal infections is not reduced to a significant degree by treatment with penicillin.

Streptococcal Toxic Shock and Necrotizing Fascitis. These are life-threatening infections associated with toxin production and are treated optimally with penicillin plus clindamycin (to decrease toxin synthesis).

Streptococcal Pneumonia, Arthritis, Meningitis, and Endocarditis. These uncommon conditions should be treated with penicillin G when they are caused by *S. pyogenes*; daily doses of 12-20 million units are administered intravenously for 2-4 weeks (4 weeks for endocarditis).

Infections Caused by Other Streptococci. The *viridans* group of streptococci is the most common cause of infectious endocarditis. These are nongroupable α-hemolytic microorganisms that are increasingly resistant to penicillin G. It is important to determine quantitative microbial sensitivities to penicillin G in patients with endocarditis. Patients with penicillin-sensitive viridans group streptococcal endocarditis can be treated successfully with daily doses of 12-20 million units of intravenous penicillin G for 2 weeks in combination with gentamicin 1 mg/kg every 8 h. The recommended therapy for penicillin- and aminoglycoside-sensitive enterococcal endocarditis is 20 million units of penicillin G or 12 g ampicillin daily administered intravenously in combination with a low dose of gentamicin. Therapy usually should be continued for 6 weeks.

Infections with Anaerobes. Many anaerobic infections are caused by mixtures of microorganisms. Most are sensitive to penicillin G. An exception is the *B. fragilis* group, in which up to 75% of strains may be resistant. Pulmonary and periodontal infections usually respond well to penicillin G; clindamycin may be more effective than penicillin for therapy of lung abscess. Mild-to-moderate infections at these sites may be treated with oral medication (either penicillin G or penicillin V 400,000 units [250 mg] 4 times daily). More severe infections should be treated with 12-20 million units of penicillin G intravenously. Brain abscesses also frequently contain several species of anaerobes, and most authorities recommend high doses of penicillin G (20 million units per day) plus metronidazole or chloramphenicol.

Staphylococcal Infections. Most staphylococcal infections are caused by microorganisms that produce penicillinase. Hospital-acquired methicillin-resistant staphylococci are resistant to penicillin G, all the penicillinase-resistant penicillins, and the cephalosporins. Isolates occasionally may appear to be sensitive to various cephalosporins in vitro, but resistant populations arise during therapy and lead to failure. Vancomycin, linezolid, quinupristin-dalfopristin, and daptomycin are active for infections caused by these bacteria, although reduced susceptibility to vancomycin has been observed. Community-acquired MRSA in many cases retains susceptibility to trimethoprim-sulfamethoxazole, doxycycline, and clindamycin.

Meningococcal Infections. Penicillin G remains the drug of choice for meningococcal disease. Patients should be treated with high doses of penicillin given intravenously (see above). The occurrence of penicillin-resistant strains should be considered in patients who are slow to respond to treatment. Penicillin G does not eliminate the meningococcal carrier state, and its administration thus is ineffective as a prophylactic measure.

Gonococcal Infections. Gonococci gradually have become more resistant to penicillin G, and penicillins are no longer the therapy of choice. For uncomplicated gonococcal urethritis, a single intramuscular injection of 250 mg ceftriaxone is the recommended treatment. Gonococcal arthritis, disseminated gonococcal infections with skin lesions, and gonococcemia should be treated with ceftriaxone 1 g daily given either intramuscularly or intravenously for 7-10 days. Ophthalmia neonatorum also should be treated with ceftriaxone for 7-10 days (25-50 mg/kg/day intramuscularly or intravenously).

Syphilis. Therapy of syphilis with penicillin G is highly effective. Primary, secondary, and latent syphilis of <1-year duration may be treated with penicillin G procaine (2.4 million units per day intramuscularly) plus probenecid (1.0 g/day orally) for 10 days or with 1-3 weekly intramuscular doses of 2.4 million units of penicillin G benzathine (3 doses in patients with HIV infection). Patients with neurosyphilis, or cardiovascular syphilis typically receive intensive therapy with 20 million units of penicillin G daily for 10 days. There are no proven alternatives for treating syphilis in pregnant women, so penicillin-allergic individuals must be acutely desensitized to prevent anaphylaxis. Infants with congenital syphilis discovered at birth or during the postnatal period should be treated for at least 10 days with 50,000 units/kg daily of aqueous penicillin G in 2 divided doses or 50,000 units/kg of procaine penicillin G in a single daily dose.

Most patients with secondary syphilis develop the Jarisch-Herxheimer reaction, including chills, fever, headache, myalgias, and arthralgias occurring several hours after the first dose of penicillin. This reaction is thought to be due to release of spirochetal antigens with subsequent host reactions to the products. Aspirin gives symptomatic relief, and therapy with penicillin should not be discontinued.

Actinomycosis. Penicillin G is the agent of choice for the treatment of all forms of actinomycosis (10-20 million units of penicillin G intravenously per day for 6 weeks). Surgical drainage or excision of the lesion may be necessary before cure is accomplished.

Diphtheria. Penicillin and other antibiotics do not alter the incidence of complications or the outcome of diphtheria; specific antitoxin is the only effective treatment. However, penicillin G eliminates the carrier state. The parenteral administration of 2-3 million units per day in divided doses for 10-12 days eliminates the diphtheria bacilli from the pharynx and other sites in practically 100% of patients. A single daily injection of penicillin G procaine for the same period produces comparable results.

Anthrax. Strains of *Bacillus anthracis* resistant to penicillin have been recovered from human infections. When penicillin G is used, the dose should be 12-20 million units per day.

Clostridial Infections. Penicillin G is the agent of choice for gas gangrene (12-20 million units per day given parenterally). Adequate debridement of the infected areas is essential. Antibiotics probably have no effect on the outcome of tetanus. Debridement and administration of human tetanus immune globulin may be indicated.

Fusospirochetal Infections. Gingivostomatitis, produced by the synergistic action of *Leptotrichia buccalis* and spirochetes that are present in the mouth, is readily treatable with penicillin. For simple "trench mouth," 500 mg penicillin V given every 6 h for several days usually suffices.

Rat-Bite Fever. The 2 microorganisms responsible for this infection, *Spirillum minor* in the Far East and *Streptobacillus moniliformis* in the U.S. and Europe, are sensitive to penicillin G, the drug of choice. Because most cases due to *Streptobacillus* are complicated by bacteremia and, in many instances, by metastatic infections, especially of the synovia and endocardium, a daily dose of 12-15 million units given parenterally for 3-4 weeks is recommended.

Listeria Infections. Ampicillin (with gentamicin for immunosuppressed patients with meningitis) and penicillin G are the drugs of choice in the management of infections owing to *L. monocytogenes*. The recommended dose of penicillin G is 15-20 million units parenterally per day for at least 2 weeks. For endocarditis, the dose is the same, but the duration of treatment should be no less than 4 weeks.

Lyme Disease. Although a tetracycline is the usual drug of choice for early disease, amoxicillin is effective; the dose is 500 mg 3 times daily for 21 days. Severe disease is treated with a third-generation cephalosporin or up to 20 million units of intravenous penicillin G daily for 10-14 days.

Erysipeloid. The causative agent of this disease, *Erysipelothrix rhusiopathiae*, is sensitive to penicillin. The infection responds well to a single injection of 1.2 million units of penicillin G benzathine. When endocarditis is present, penicillin G, 12-20 million units per day, for 4-6 weeks is required.

Pasteurella multocida. *Pasteurella multocida* is the cause of wound infections after a cat or dog bite. It is susceptible to penicillin G and ampicillin and resistant to penicillinase-resistant penicillins and first-generation cephalosporins. When the infection causes meningitis, a third-generation cephalosporin is preferred.

Prophylactic Uses of the Penicillins. As prophylaxis has been investigated under controlled conditions, it has become clear that penicillin is highly effective in some situations, useless and potentially dangerous in others, and of questionable value in still others (*see* Chapter 48).

Streptococcal Infections. The administration of penicillin to individuals exposed to *S. pyogenes* protects against infection. The oral ingestion of 200,000 units of penicillin G or penicillin V twice a day or a single injection of 1.2 million units of penicillin G benzathine is effective. Indications for this type of prophylaxis include outbreaks of streptococcal disease in closed populations (e.g., boarding schools or military bases).

Recurrences of Rheumatic Fever. The oral administration of 200,000 units of penicillin G or penicillin V every 12 h decreases the incidence of recurrences of rheumatic fever in susceptible individuals. The intramuscular injection of 1.2 million units of penicillin G benzathine once a month also yields excellent results. Prophylaxis must be continued throughout the year. Some suggest that prophylaxis should be continued for life because instances of acute rheumatic fever have been observed in the fifth and sixth decades, but the necessity of prolonged prophylaxis has not been established.

Syphilis. Prophylaxis for a contact with syphilis consists of a course of therapy as described for primary syphilis. A serological test for syphilis should be performed monthly for at least 4 months thereafter.

Surgical Procedures in Patients with Valvular Heart Disease. About 25% of cases of subacute bacterial endocarditis follow dental extractions. Since transient bacterial invasion of the bloodstream occurs occasionally after surgical procedures (e.g., tonsillectomy and genitourinary and GI procedures) and during childbirth, these, too, are indications for prophylaxis in patients with valvular heart disease. Whether the incidence of bacterial endocarditis actually is altered by this type of chemoprophylaxis remains to be determined.

THE PENICILLINASE-RESISTANT PENICILLINS

These penicillins are resistant to hydrolysis by staphylococcal penicillinase. Their appropriate use should be restricted to the treatment of infections that are known or suspected to be caused by staphylococci that elaborate the enzyme, including the vast majority of strains that are encountered clinically. These drugs are much less active than penicillin G against other penicillin-sensitive microorganisms.

The role of the penicillinase-resistant penicillins for most staphylococcal disease is changing with the increasing incidence of isolates of so-called ***methicillin-resistant microorganisms***. This term denotes resistance of these bacteria to all the penicillinase-resistant penicillins and cephalosporins. Vancomycin is considered the drug of choice for such infections. Vancomycin also is the drug of choice for serious infection caused by methicillin-resistant *S. epidermidis*; rifampin is given concurrently when a foreign body is involved.

THE ISOXAZOLYL PENICILLINS: OXACILLIN, CLOXACILLIN, AND DICLOXACILLIN. These semisynthetic congeners are relatively stable in an acidic medium and absorbed adequately after oral administration. All are markedly resistant to cleavage by penicillinase. These drugs are not substitutes for penicillin G in the treatment of diseases amenable to it and are not active against enterococci or *Listeria.* Oral administration is not a substitute for the parenteral route in the treatment of serious staphylococcal infections.

Pharmacological Properties. The isoxazolyl penicillins are potent inhibitors of the growth of most penicillinase-producing staphylococci. Dicloxacillin is the most active and many strains of *S. aureus* are inhibited by concentrations of 0.05-0.8 μg/mL. These agents are, in general, less effective against microorganisms susceptible to penicillin G, and they are not useful against gram-negative bacteria. These agents are absorbed rapidly but incompletely (30-80%) from the GI tract. These drugs are absorbed more efficiently when administered 1 h before or 2 h after meals. Peak concentrations in plasma are attained by 1 h. All these congeners are bound to plasma albumin to a great extent (~90-95%); none is removed from the circulation to a significant degree by hemodialysis. The isoxazolyl penicillins are excreted by the kidney; there is also significant hepatic degradation and elimination in the bile. The half-lives for all are between 30 and 60 min. Intervals between doses do not have to be altered for patients with renal failure.

NAFCILLIN. This semisynthetic penicillin is highly resistant to penicillinase and has proven effective against infections caused by penicillinase-producing strains of *S. aureus.*

Pharmacological Properties. Nafcillin is slightly more active than oxacillin against penicillin G–resistant *S. aureus* (most strains are inhibited by 0.06-2 μg/mL). Although it is the most active of the penicillinase-resistant penicillins against other microorganisms, it is not as potent as penicillin G. The peak plasma concentration is ~8 μg/mL 60 min after a 1-g intramuscular dose. Nafcillin is ~90% bound to plasma protein. Peak concentrations of nafcillin in bile are well above those found in plasma. Concentrations of the drug in CSF appear to be adequate for therapy of staphylococcal meningitis.

THE AMINOPENICILLINS: AMPICILLIN, AMOXICILLIN, AND CONGENERS

These agents have similar antibacterial activity and a spectrum that is broader than the antibiotics already discussed. They all are destroyed by β-lactamase (from both gram-positive and gram-negative bacteria).

ANTIMICROBIAL ACTIVITY. Ampicillin and the related aminopenicillins are bactericidal for both gram-positive and gram-negative bacteria. The meningococci and *L. monocytogenes* are sensitive to this class of drugs. Many pneumococcal isolates have varying levels of resistance to ampicillin. Penicillin-resistant strains should be considered ampicillin/amoxicillin-resistant. *H. influenzae* and the *viridans* group of streptococci exhibit varying degrees of resistance. Enterococci are about twice as sensitive to ampicillin as they are to penicillin G. From 30-50% of *E. coli*, a significant number of *P. mirabilis*, and practically all species of *Enterobacter* presently are insensitive. Resistant strains of *Salmonella* are recovered with increasing frequency. Most strains of *Shigella*, *Pseudomonas*, *Klebsiella*, *Serratia*, *Acinetobacter*, and indole-positive *Proteus* also are resistant to this group of penicillins; these antibiotics are less active against *B. fragilis* than penicillin G. Concurrent administration of a β-lactamase inhibitor such as clavulanate or *sulbactam* markedly expands their spectrum of activity.

ADME

Ampicillin. Ampicillin (PRINCIPEN, others) is stable in acid and is well absorbed after oral administration. An oral dose of 0.5 g produces peak concentrations in plasma of ~3 μg/mL at 2 h. Intake of food prior to ingestion of ampicillin diminishes absorption. Intramuscular injection of 0.5-1 g sodium ampicillin yields peak plasma concentrations of ~7-10 μg/mL, respectively, at 1 h. Plasma levels decline with a $t_{1/2}$ of ~80 min. Severe renal impairment markedly prolongs the $t_{1/2}$. Peritoneal dialysis is ineffective in removing the drug from the blood, but hemodialysis removes ~40% of the body store in ~7 h. Adjustment of the dose of ampicillin is required in the presence of renal dysfunction. Ampicillin appears in the bile, undergoes enterohepatic circulation, and is excreted in the feces.

Amoxicillin. This drug, a penicillinase-susceptible semi-synthetic penicillin (*see* Table 53–1), is a close chemical and pharmacological relative of ampicillin. Amoxicillin is stable in acid, designed for oral use, and absorbed more rapidly and completely from the GI tract than ampicillin. The antimicrobial spectrum of amoxicillin is essentially identical to that of ampicillin, except that amoxicillin is less effective than ampicillin for shigellosis. Peak plasma concentrations of amoxicillin (AMOXIL, others) are 2-2.5 times greater for amoxicillin than for ampicillin after oral administration of the same dose. Food does not interfere with absorption. Perhaps because of more complete absorption of this congener, the incidence of diarrhea with amoxicillin is less than that following administration of ampicillin. The incidence of other adverse effects appears to be similar. Although the $t_{1/2}$ of amoxicillin is similar to that for ampicillin, effective concentrations of orally administered amoxicillin are detectable in the plasma for twice as long as with ampicillin because of the more complete absorption. About 20% of amoxicillin is protein bound in plasma, a value similar to that for ampicillin. Most of a dose of the antibiotic is excreted in an active form in the urine. Probenecid delays excretion of the drug.

THERAPEUTIC INDICATIONS

Upper Respiratory Infections. Ampicillin and amoxicillin are active against *S. pyogenes* and many strains of *S. pneumoniae* and *H. influenzae*. The drugs constitute effective therapy for sinusitis, otitis media, acute exacerbations of chronic bronchitis, and epiglottitis caused by sensitive strains of these organisms. Amoxicillin is the most active of all the oral β-lactam antibiotics against both penicillin-sensitive and penicillin-resistant *S. pneumoniae*. Based on the increasing prevalence of pneumococcal resistance to penicillin, an increase in dose of oral amoxicillin (from 40-45 up to 80-90 mg/kg/day) for empirical treatment of acute otitis media in children is recommended. Ampicillin-resistant *H. influenzae* is a problem in many areas. The addition of a β-lactamase inhibitor (amoxicillin-clavulanate or ampicillin-sulbactam) extends the spectrum to β-lactamase-producing *H. influenzae* and Enterobacteriaceae. Bacterial pharyngitis should be treated with penicillin G or penicillin V because *S. pyogenes* is the major pathogen.

Urinary Tract Infections. Most uncomplicated urinary tract infections are caused by Enterobacteriaceae, and *E. coli* is the most common species; ampicillin often is an effective agent, although resistance is increasingly common. Enterococcal urinary tract infections are treated effectively with ampicillin alone.

Meningitis. Acute bacterial meningitis in children is frequently due to *S. pneumoniae* or *Neisseria meningitidis*. Because 20-30% of strains of *S. pneumoniae* now may be resistant to ampicillin, it is not indicated for single-agent treatment of meningitis. Ampicillin has excellent activity against *L. monocytogenes*, a cause of meningitis in immunocompromised persons. The combination of ampicillin and vancomycin plus a third-generation cephalosporin is a rational regimen for empirical treatment of suspected bacterial meningitis.

Salmonella Infections. Disease associated with bacteremia, disease with metastatic foci, and the enteric fever syndrome (including typhoid fever) respond favorably to antibiotics. A fluoroquinolone or ceftriaxone is considered by some to be the drug of choice, but the administration of trimethoprim-sulfamethoxazole or high doses of ampicillin (12 g/day for adults) also is effective. The typhoid carrier state has been eliminated successfully in patients without gallbladder disease with ampicillin, trimethoprim-sulfamethoxazole, or ciprofloxacin.

ANTI-PSEUDOMONAL PENICILLINS: THE CARBOXYPENICILLINS AND THE UREIDOPENICILLINS

ANTIMICROBIAL ACTIVITY. The carboxypenicillins, carbenicillin (discontinued in the U.S.) and ticarcillin (marketed in combination with clavulanate in the U.S.) and their close relatives, are active against some isolates of *P. aeruginosa* and certain indole-positive *Proteus* spp. that are resistant to ampicillin and its congeners. They are ineffective against most strains of *S. aureus*, *Enterococcus faecalis*, *Klebsiella*, and

L. monocytogenes. B. fragilis is susceptible to high concentrations of these drugs, but penicillin G is actually more active. The ureidopenicillins, mezlocillin (discontinued in the U.S.) and piperacillin, have superior activity against *P. aeruginosa* compared with carbenicillin and ticarcillin. Mezlocillin and piperacillin are useful for treatment of infections with *Klebsiella.* The carboxypenicillins and the ureidopenicillins are sensitive to destruction by β-lactamases.

PHARMACOLOGICAL PROPERTIES

Carbenicillin. Carbenicillin was the first penicillin with activity against *P. aeruginosa* and some *Proteus* strains that are resistant to ampicillin. Preparations of carbenicillin may cause adverse effects in addition to those that follow the use of other penicillins. Congestive heart failure may result from the administration of excessive Na^+. Hypokalemia may occur because of obligatory excretion of cation with the large amount of nonreabsorbable anion (carbenicillin) presented to the distal renal tubule. The drug interferes with platelet function, and bleeding may occur because of abnormal aggregation of platelets.

Carbenicillin Indanyl Sodium. This indanyl ester of carbenicillin is acid stable and is suitable for oral administration. After absorption, the ester is converted rapidly to carbenicillin by hydrolysis of the ester linkage. The antimicrobial spectrum of the drug is therefore that of carbenicillin. The active moiety is excreted rapidly in the urine, where it achieves effective concentrations. Thus, the only use of this drug is for the management of urinary tract infections caused by *Proteus* spp. other than *P. mirabilis* and by *P. aeruginosa.*

Piperacillin. Piperacillin extends the spectrum of ampicillin to include most strains of *P. aeruginosa,* Enterobacteriaceae (non-β-lactamase-producing), many *Bacteroides* spp., and *E. faecalis*. Combined with a β-lactamase inhibitor (piperacillin-tazobactam, ZOSYN) it has the broadest antibacterial spectrum of the penicillins. Pharmacokinetic properties are reminiscent of the other ureidopenicillins. High biliary concentrations are achieved.

THERAPEUTIC INDICATIONS. Piperacillin and related agents are important agents for the treatment of patients with serious infections caused by gram-negative bacteria, including infections often acquired in the hospital. Therefore, these penicillins find their greatest use in treating bacteremias, pneumonias, infections following burns, and urinary tract infections owing to microorganisms resistant to penicillin G and ampicillin; the bacteria especially responsible include *P. aeruginosa*, indole-positive strains of *Proteus*, and *Enterobacter* spp. Because *Pseudomonas* infections are common in neutropenic patients, therapy for severe bacterial infections in such individuals should include a β-lactam antibiotic such as piperacillin with good activity against these microorganisms.

RELATED AGENTS

Ticarcillin. This semisynthetic penicillin is very similar to carbenicillin, but it is 2 to 4 times more active against *P. aeruginosa*. Ticarcillin is inferior to piperacillin for the treatment of serious infections caused by *Pseudomonas*. Ticarcillin is only marketed in combination with clavulanate (TIMENTIN) in the U.S.

Mezlocillin. This ureidopenicillin is more active against *Klebsiella* than is carbenicillin; its activity against *Pseudomonas* in vitro is similar to that of ticarcillin. It is more active than ticarcillin against *E. faecalis.* Mezlocillin sodium has been discontinued in the U.S.

UNTOWARD REACTIONS TO PENICILLINS

HYPERSENSITIVITY REACTIONS. Hypersensitivity reactions are by far the most common adverse effects noted with the penicillins, and these agents probably are the most common cause of drug allergy.

Allergic reactions (overall incidence, 0.7-10%) can complicate treatment courses. Manifestations of allergy to penicillins include maculopapular rash, urticarial rash, fever, bronchospasm, vasculitis, serum sickness, exfoliative dermatitis, Stevens-Johnson syndrome, and anaphylaxis. Hypersensitivity to penicillins generally extends to the other β-lactams (e.g., cephalosporins, some carbapenems). Hypersensitivity reactions may occur with any dosage form of penicillin; allergy to 1 penicillin exposes the patient to a greater risk of reaction if another is given but does not necessarily imply repetition on subsequent exposures. Hypersensitivity reactions may appear in the absence of a previous known exposure to the drug. This may be caused by unrecognized prior exposure to penicillin in the environment (e.g., in foods of animal origin or from the fungus-producing penicillin). Although elimination of the antibiotic usually results in rapid clearing of the allergic manifestations, they may persist for 1-2 weeks or longer after therapy has been stopped. In some cases, the reaction is mild and disappears even when the penicillin is continued; in others, immediate cessation of penicillin treatment is required. In a few instances, it is necessary to interdict the future use of penicillin because of the risk of death, and the patient should be so warned.

Penicillins and their breakdown products act as haptens after covalent reaction with proteins. The most abundant breakdown product is the penicilloyl moiety (major determinant moiety [MDM]), which is formed when the β-lactam ring is opened (*see* Figure 53–5). A large percentage of immunoglobulin (Ig)E-mediated reactions are to the MDM, but at least 25% of reactions are to other breakdown products. The terms *major* and *minor determinants* refer to the frequency with which antibodies to these haptens appear to be formed. They do not describe the severity of the reaction that may result. In fact, anaphylactic reactions to penicillin usually are mediated by IgE antibodies against the minor determinants. Anti-penicillin antibodies are detectable in virtually all patients who have received the drug and in many who have never knowingly been exposed to it. Immediate allergic reactions are mediated by skin-sensitizing or IgE antibodies, usually of minor-determinant specificities. Accelerated and late urticarial reactions usually are mediated by major-determinant–specific skin-sensitizing antibodies. Some reactions may be due to toxic antigen-antibody complexes of major-determinant-specific IgM antibodies. Skin rashes of all types may be caused by allergy to penicillin. The incidence of skin rashes appears to be highest following the use of ampicillin, at ~9%; rashes follow the administration of ampicillin in nearly all patients with infectious mononucleosis.

The most serious hypersensitivity reactions produced by the penicillins are angioedema and anaphylaxis. Acute anaphylactic or anaphylactoid reactions induced by various preparations of penicillin constitute the most important immediate danger connected with their use. Anaphylactoid reactions may occur at any age. Their incidence is thought to be 0.004-0.04%. About 0.001% of patients treated with these agents die from anaphylaxis. Anaphylaxis most often has followed the injection of penicillin, although it also has been observed after oral or intradermal administration. The most dramatic reaction is sudden, severe hypotension and rapid death. In other instances, bronchoconstriction with severe asthma; abdominal pain, nausea, and vomiting; extreme weakness; or diarrhea and purpuric skin eruptions have characterized the anaphylactic episodes. Serum sickness of variable intensity and severity, mediated by IgG antibodies, is rare; when it occurs, it appears after penicillin treatment has been continued for 1 week or more; it may be delayed until 1 or 2 weeks after the drug has been stopped and may persist for a week or longer. Vasculitis may be related to penicillin hypersensitivity. The Coombs reaction frequently becomes positive during prolonged therapy, but hemolytic anemia is rare. Reversible neutropenia has been noted, occurring in up to 30% of patients treated with 8-12 g nafcillin for >21 days. The bone marrow shows an arrest of maturation. Eosinophilia is an occasional accompaniment of other allergic reactions to penicillin. Penicillins rarely cause interstitial nephritis; methicillin has been implicated most frequently. Fever may be the only evidence of a hypersensitivity reaction to the penicillins. The febrile reaction usually disappears within 24-36 h after administration of the drug is stopped but may persist for days.

Management of the Patient Potentially Allergic to Penicillin. Evaluation of the patient's history is the most practical way to avoid the use of penicillin in patients who are at the greatest risk of adverse reaction. Occasionally, *desensitization* is recommended for penicillin-allergic patients who must receive the drug. This procedure consists of administering gradually increasing doses of penicillin in the hope of avoiding a severe reaction and should be performed only in an intensive care setting. When full doses are reached, penicillin should not be discontinued and then restarted because immediate reactions may recur. The efficacy of this procedure is unproven. Patients with life-threatening infections (e.g., endocarditis or meningitis) may be continued on penicillin despite the development of a maculopapular rash, although alternative antimicrobial agents should be used whenever possible. The rash often resolves as therapy is continued, perhaps owing to the development of blocking antibodies of the IgG class. Rarely, exfoliative dermatitis with or without vasculitis develops in these patients if therapy with penicillin is continued.

OTHER ADVERSE REACTIONS. The penicillins have minimal direct toxicity. Apparent toxic effects include bone marrow depression, granulocytopenia, and hepatitis; the latter effect is rare but is seen most commonly following the administration of oxacillin and nafcillin. The administration of penicillin G, carbenicillin, piperacillin, or ticarcillin has been associated with impaired hemostasis due to defective platelet aggregation. Most common among the irritative responses to penicillin are pain and sterile inflammatory reactions at the sites of intramuscular injections. In some individuals who receive penicillin intravenously, phlebitis or thrombophlebitis develops. Adverse responses to oral penicillin preparations may include nausea, vomiting, and mild to severe diarrhea.

When penicillin is injected accidentally into the sciatic nerve, severe pain occurs and dysfunction in the area of distribution of this nerve develops and persists for weeks. Intrathecal injection of penicillin G may produce arachnoiditis or severe and fatal encephalopathy. Because of this, intrathecal or intraventricular administration of penicillins should be avoided. When the concentration of penicillin G in CSF exceeds 10 μg/mL, significant dysfunction of the CNS is frequent. The rapid intravenous administration of 20 million units of penicillin G potassium, which contains 34 mEq of K^+, may lead to severe or even fatal hyperkalemia in persons with renal dysfunction. Injection of penicillin G procaine may result in an immediate reaction, characterized by dizziness, tinnitus, headache, hallucinations, and sometimes seizures. This is due to the rapid liberation of toxic concentrations of procaine.

REACTIONS UNRELATED TO HYPERSENSITIVITY OR TOXICITY. Penicillin changes the composition of the microflora in the GI tract by eliminating sensitive microorganisms. Normal microflora are typically reestablished shortly after therapy is stopped; however, in some patients, superinfection results. Pseudomembranous colitis, related to overgrowth and production of a toxin by *Clostridium difficile*, has followed oral and, less commonly, parenteral administration of penicillins.

Cephalosporin antibiotics are produced from 7-aminocephalosporanic acid by the addition of different side chains (Table 53–2).

Compounds containing 7-aminocephalosporanic acid are relatively stable in dilute acid and relatively resistant to penicillinase regardless of the nature of their side chains and their affinity for the enzyme. Modifications at position 7 of the β-lactam ring are associated with alteration in antibacterial activity; substitutions at position 3 of the dihydrothiazine ring alter the metabolism and pharmacokinetic properties of the drugs. The cephamycins are similar to the cephalosporins but have a methoxy group at position 7 of the β-lactam ring of the 7-aminocephalosporanic acid nucleus.

MECHANISM OF ACTION. Cephalosporins and cephamycins inhibit bacterial cell wall synthesis in a manner similar to that of penicillin.

CLASSIFICATION. *Classification is by generations*, based on general features of antimicrobial activity (Table 53–3).

The ***first-generation*** cephalosporins (e.g., cephalothin and cefazolin) have good activity against gram-positive bacteria and relatively modest activity against gram-negative microorganisms. Most gram-positive cocci (with

Table 53–2

Structural Formulas and Dosage Data for Selected Cephalosporins

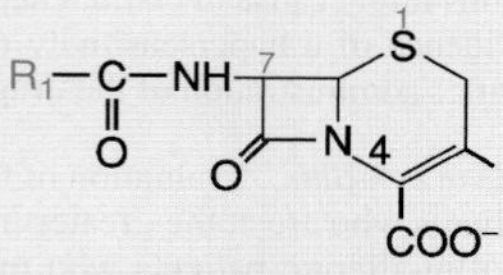

R_1–C(=O)–NH– (7) ... S (1) ... N (4) ... R_2 ... COO^-

Cephem nucleus

COMPOUND	R_1	R_2	DOSAGE FORMS,[a] ADULT DOSAGE FOR SEVERE INFECTION, AND $t_{1/2}$
First generation Cephalexin	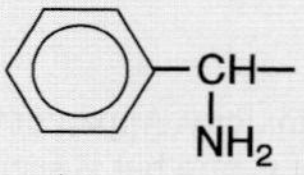 C_6H_5–CH(NH$_2$)–	$-CH_3$	O: 1 g every 6 hours $t_{1/2}$ = 0.9 hour
Second generation Cefaclor	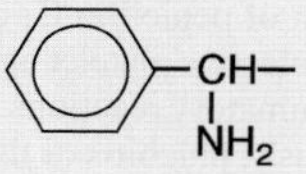 C_6H_5–CH(NH$_2$)–	–Cl	O: 1 g every 8 hours $t_{1/2}$ = 0.7 hours
Third generation Cefdinir	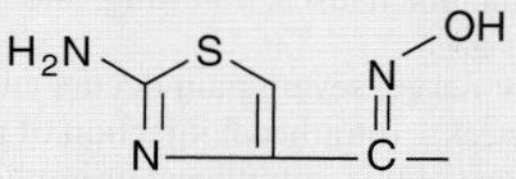 H_2N-thiazolyl–C(=N–OH)–	$-CH=CH_2$	O: 300 mg every 12 hours or 600 mg every 24 hours $t_{1/2}$ = 1.7 hours
Ceftazidime	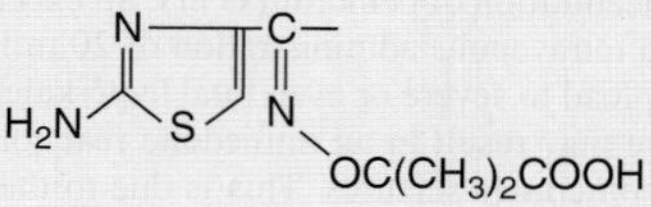 H_2N-thiazolyl–C(=N–OC(CH$_3$)$_2$COOH)–	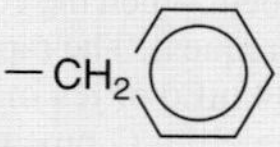 $-CH_2$–pyridinium	I: 2 g every 8 hours $t_{1/2}$ = 1.8 hours
Fourth generation Cefepime	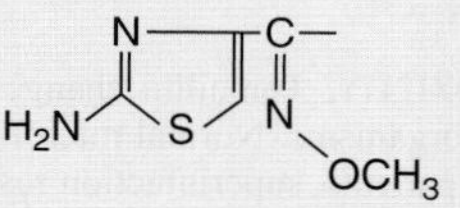 H_2N-thiazolyl–C(=N–OCH$_3$)–	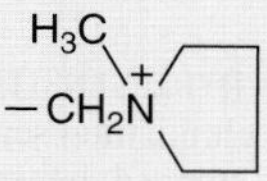 $-CH_2N^+$(H$_3$C)-pyrrolidinium	I: 2 g every 8 hours $t_{1/2}$ = 2 hours

[a]T, tablet; C, capsule; O, oral suspension; I, injection.

Table 53–3

Cephalosporin Generations

EXAMPLES	USEFUL SPECTRUM[a]
First Generation	
Cefazolin	Streptococci[b]; *Staphylococcus aureus*[c]
Cephalexin monohydrate	
Cefadroxil	
Cephradine	
Second Generation	
Cefuroxime	*Escherichia coli*, *Klebsiella*, *Proteus*, *Haemophilus influenzae*, *Moraxella catarrhalis*. Not as active against gram-positive organisms as first-generation agents.
Cefuroxime axetil	
Cefprozil	
Cefmetazole	Inferior activity against *S. aureus* compared to cefuroxime but with added activity against *Bacteroides fragilis* and other *Bacteroides* spp.
Loracarbef	
Third Generation	
Cefotaxime	Enterobacteriaceae[d]; *Pseudomonas aeruginosa*[e]; *Serratia*; *Neisseria gonorrhoeae*; activity for *S. aureus*, *Streptococcus pneumoniae*, and *Streptococcus pyogenes*[f] comparable to first-generation agents. Activity against *Bacteroides* spp. inferior to that of cefoxitin and cefotetan
Ceftriaxone	
Cefdinir	
Cefditoren pivoxil	
Ceftibuten	
Cefpodoxime proxetil	
Ceftizoxime	
Cefoperazone	Active against *Pseudomonas*
Ceftazidime	
Fourth Generation	
Cefepime	Comparable to third generation but more resistant to some β-lactamases

[a]*All cephalosporins lack activity against enterococci,* Listeria monocytogenes, Legionella *spp., methicillin-resistant* S. aureus, Xanthomonas maltophilia, *and* Acinetobacter *species.* [b]*Except for penicillin-resistant strains.* [c]*Except for methicillin-resistant strains.* [d]*Resistance to cephalosporins may be induced rapidly during therapy by de-repression of bacterial chromosomal β-lactamases, which destroy the cephalosporins.* [e]*Ceftazidime only.* [f]*Ceftazidime lacks significant gram-positive activity. Cefotaxime is most active in class against* S. aureus *and* S. pyogenes.

the exception of enterococci, MRSA, and *S. epidermidis*) are susceptible. Most oral cavity anaerobes are sensitive, but the *B. fragilis* group is resistant. Activity against *Moraxella catarrhalis*, *E. coli*, *K. pneumoniae*, and *P. mirabilis* is good.

The ***second-generation*** cephalosporins have somewhat increased activity against gram-negative microorganisms but are much less active than the third-generation agents. A subset of second-generation agents (cefoxitin, cefotetan, and cefmetazole, which have been discontinued in the U.S.) also is active against *B. fragilis*.

Third-generation cephalosporins generally are less active than first-generation agents against gram-positive cocci; these agents are much more active against the Enterobacteriaceae, although resistance is dramatically increasing due to β-lactamase-producing strains. A subset of third-generation agents (ceftazidime and cefoperazone) also is active against *P. aeruginosa* but less active than other third-generation agents against gram-positive cocci.

Fourth-generation cephalosporins, such as cefepime, have an extended spectrum of activity compared with the third generation and have increased stability from hydrolysis by plasmid and chromosomally mediated β-lactamases (but not the KPC class A β-lactamases). Fourth-generation agents are useful in the empirical treatment of serious infections in hospitalized patients when gram-positive microorganisms, Enterobacteriaceae, and *Pseudomonas* all are potential etiologies.

None of the cephalosporins has reliable activity against the following bacteria: penicillin-resistant *S. pneumoniae*, MRSA, methicillin-resistant *S. epidermidis* and other coagulase-negative staphylococci, *Enterococcus*, *L. monocytogenes*, *Legionella pneumophila*, *L. micdadei*, *C. difficile*, *Xanthomonas maltophilia*, *Campylobacter jejuni*, KPC-producing *Enterobacteriaceae*, and *Acinetobacter* spp.

MECHANISMS OF BACTERIAL RESISTANCE. Resistance to the cephalosporins may be related to the inability of the antibiotic to reach its sites of action or to alterations in the PBPs that are targets of the cephalosporins. Alterations in 2 PBPs (1A and 2X) that decrease their affinity for cephalosporins render pneumococci resistant to third-generation cephalosporins because the other 3 PBPs have inherently low affinity.

The most prevalent mechanism of resistance to cephalosporins is destruction of the cephalosporins by hydrolysis of the β-lactam ring. The cephalosporins have variable susceptibility to β-lactamase. Of the first-generation agents, cefazolin is more susceptible to hydrolysis by β-lactamase from *S. aureus* than is cephalothin (no longer marketed). Cefoxitin, cefuroxime, and the third-generation cephalosporins are more resistant to hydrolysis by the β-lactamases produced by gram-negative bacteria than first-generation cephalosporins. Third-generation cephalosporins are susceptible to hydrolysis by inducible, chromosomally encoded (type I) β-lactamases. Induction of type I β-lactamases by treatment of infections owing to aerobic gram-negative bacilli with second- or third-generation cephalosporins or imipenem may result in resistance to all third-generation cephalosporins. The fourth-generation cephalosporins, such as cefepime, are poor inducers of type I β-lactamases and are less susceptible to hydrolysis by type I β-lactamases than are the third-generation agents. They are, however, susceptible to degradation by KPC and metallo-β-lactamases.

GENERAL PHARMACOLOGY

Many cephalosporins (cephalexin, cephradine, cefaclor, cefadroxil, loracarbef, cefprozil, cefpodoxime proxetil, ceftibuten, cefuroxime axetil, cefdinir, and cefditoren) are absorbed readily after oral administration; others can be administered intramuscularly or intravenously. Cephalosporins are excreted primarily by the kidney; thus the dosage should be reduced in patients with renal insufficiency. Probenecid slows the tubular secretion of most cephalosporins. Exceptions are cefpiramide and cefoperazone, which are excreted predominantly in the bile. Cefotaxime is deacetylated to a metabolite with less antimicrobial activity than the parent compound that is excreted by the kidneys. The other cephalosporins do not undergo appreciable metabolism. Several cephalosporins penetrate into the CSF in sufficient concentration to be useful for the treatment of meningitis. Cephalosporins also cross the placenta, and they are found in high concentrations in synovial and pericardial fluids. Penetration into the aqueous humor of the eye is relatively good after systemic administration of third-generation agents, but penetration into the vitreous humor is poor. Concentrations in bile usually are high, especially with cefoperazone and cefpiramide.

SPECIFIC AGENTS

FIRST-GENERATION CEPHALOSPORINS

Cefazolin has an antibacterial spectrum that is typical of other first-generation cephalosporins except that it also has activity against some *Enterobacter* spp. Cefazolin is relatively well tolerated after either intramuscular or intravenous administration; it is excreted by glomerular filtration and is ~85% bound to plasma proteins. Cefazolin usually is preferred among the first-generation cephalosporins because it can be administered less frequently owing to its longer $t_{1/2}$.

Cephalexin has the same antibacterial spectrum as the other first-generation cephalosporins. It is somewhat less active against penicillinase-producing staphylococci. Oral therapy with cephalexin (usually 0.5 g) results in peak concentrations in plasma adequate for the inhibition of many gram-positive and gram-negative pathogens. The drug is not metabolized, and 70-100% is excreted in the urine.

Cephradine is similar in structure to cephalexin, and its activity in vitro is almost identical. Cephradine is not metabolized and, after rapid absorption from the GI tract, is excreted unchanged in the urine. Because cephradine is so well absorbed, the concentrations in plasma are nearly equivalent after oral or intramuscular administration.

Cefadroxil is the *para*-hydroxy analog of cephalexin. Concentrations of cefadroxil in plasma and urine are at somewhat higher levels than are those of cephalexin. The drug is given orally once or twice a day for the treatment of urinary tract infections. Its activity in vitro is similar to that of cephalexin.

SECOND-GENERATION CEPHALOSPORINS. Second-generation cephalosporins have a broader spectrum than do the first-generation agents and are active against sensitive strains of *Enterobacter* spp., indole-positive *Proteus* spp., and *Klebsiella* spp.

Cefoxitin is resistant to some β-lactamases produced by gram-negative rods. This antibiotic is less active than the first-generation cephalosporins against gram-positive bacteria, but is more active against anaerobes, especially *B. fragilis*. Cefoxitin's special role seems to be for treatment of certain anaerobic and mixed aerobic-anaerobic infections, such as pelvic inflammatory disease and lung abscess.

Cefaclor's concentration in plasma after oral administration is ~50% of that achieved after an equivalent oral dose of cephalexin. However, cefaclor is more active against *H. influenzae* and *M. catarrhalis*, although some β-lactamase-producing strains of these organisms may be resistant.

Loracarbef is similar in activity to cefaclor and more stable against some β-lactamases.

Cefuroxime is similar to loracarbef with broader gram-negative activity against some *Citrobacter* and *Enterobacter* spp. Unlike cefoxitin, cefmetazole, and cefotetan, cefuroxime lacks activity against *B. fragilis*. The drug can be given every 8 h. Concentrations in CSF are ~10% of those in plasma, and the drug is effective (but inferior to ceftriaxone) for treatment of meningitis owing to *H. influenzae* (including strains resistant to ampicillin), *N. meningitidis*, and *S. pneumoniae*.

Cefuroxime axetil is the 1-acetyloxyethyl ester of cefuroxime. Between 30% and 50% of an oral dose is absorbed, and the drug then is hydrolyzed to cefuroxime; resulting concentrations in plasma are variable.

Cefprozil is an orally administered agent that is more active than first-generation cephalosporins against penicillin-sensitive streptococci, *E. coli*, *P. mirabilis*, *Klebsiella* spp., and *Citrobacter* spp; serum $t_{1/2}$ is ~1.3 h.

THIRD-GENERATION CEPHALOSPORINS

Cefotaxime is highly resistant to many β-lactamases and has good activity against many gram-positive and gram-negative aerobic bacteria. However, activity against *B. fragilis* is poor compared with agents such as clindamycin and metronidazole. Cefotaxime has a $t_{1/2}$ in plasma of ~1 h and should be administered every 4–8 h for serious infections. The drug is metabolized in vivo to desacetylcefotaxime, which is less active than is the parent compound. Cefotaxime has been used effectively for meningitis caused by *H. influenzae*, penicillin-sensitive *S. pneumoniae*, and *Neisseria meningitides*.

Ceftizoxime has a spectrum of activity in vitro that is very similar to that of cefotaxime, except that it is less active against *S. pneumoniae* and more active against *B. fragilis*. The $t_{1/2}$ is 1.8 h, and the drug thus can be administered every 8-12 h for serious infections. Ceftizoxime is not metabolized; 90% is recovered in urine.

Ceftriaxone has activity very similar to that of ceftizoxime and cefotaxime but a longer $t_{1/2}$ (~8 h). Administration of the drug once or twice daily has been effective for patients with meningitis. About half the drug can be recovered from the urine; the remainder is eliminated by biliary secretion. A single dose of ceftriaxone (125-250 mg) is effective in the treatment of urethral, cervical, rectal, or pharyngeal gonorrhea, including disease caused by penicillinase-producing microorganisms.

Cefpodoxime proxetil is an orally administered third-generation agent that is very similar in activity to the fourth-generation agent cefepime except that it is not more active against *Enterobacter* or *Pseudomonas* spp.

Cefditoren pivoxil is a prodrug that is hydrolyzed by esterases during absorption to the active drug, cefditoren. Cefditoren is eliminated unchanged in the urine. The drug is active against methicillin-susceptible strains *of S. aureus*, penicillin-susceptible strains *of S. pneumoniae*, *S. pyogenes*, *H. influenzae*, *H. parainfluenzae*, and *M. catarrhalis*. Cefditoren pivoxil is only indicated for the treatment of mild-to-moderate pharyngitis, tonsillitis, uncomplicated skin and skin structure infections, and acute exacerbations of chronic bronchitis.

Cefixime is orally effective against urinary tract infections caused by *E. coli* and *P. mirabilis*, otitis media caused by *H. influenza* and *S. pyogenes*, pharyngitis due to *S. pyogenes*, and uncomplicated gonorrhea. It is available as an oral suspension (SUPRAX, others). Cefixime has a plasma $t_{1/2}$ of 3-4 h and is both excreted in the urine and eliminated in the bile. The standard dose for adults is 400 mg/day for 5-7 days, and for a longer interval in patients with *S. pyogenes*. Doses must be reduced in patients with renal impairment. Pediatric dosing varies with patient weight.

Ceftibuten is an orally effective cephalosporin that is less active against gram-positive and gram-negative organisms than cefixime, with activity limited to *S. pneumonia* and *S. pyogenes*, *H. influenzae*, and *M. catarrhalis*. Ceftibuten is only indicated for acute bacterial exacerbations of chronic bronchitis, acute bacterial otitis media, pharyngitis, and tonsillitis.

Cefdinir is effective orally; it is eliminated primarily unchanged in the urine. Cefdinir has activity against facultative gram-negative bacteria but lacks anaerobic activity. It is also inactive against *Pseudomonas* and *Enterobacter* spp.

Third-Generation Cephalosporins with Good Anti-Pseudomonal Activity. **Ceftazidime** is one-quarter to one-half as active against gram-positive microorganisms as is cefotaxime. Its activity against the Enterobacteriaceae is very similar, but its major distinguishing feature is excellent activity against *Pseudomonas* and other gram-negative bacteria. Ceftazidime has poor activity against *B. fragilis*. Its $t_{1/2}$ in plasma is ~1.5 h; the drug is not metabolized.

FOURTH-GENERATION CEPHALOSPORINS: CEFEPIME AND CEFPIROME

Only cefepime is available for use in the U.S. Cefepime resists hydrolysis by many of the plasmid-encoded β-lactamases. It is a poor inducer of, and is relatively resistant to, the type I chromosomally encoded and some extended-spectrum β-lactamases. Thus, it is active against many Enterobacteriaceae that are resistant to other cephalosporins via induction of type I β-lactamases. Cefepime is susceptible hydrolysis by many bacteria expressing extended-spectrum plasmid-mediated β-lactamases. Cefepime is excreted renally; doses should be adjusted for renal failure. Cefepime has excellent penetration into the CSF in animal models of meningitis. The recommended dosage for adults is 2 g intravenously every 12 h. The serum $t_{1/2}$ is 2 h.

Against the fastidious gram-negative bacteria (*H. influenzae*, *Neisseria gonorrhoeae*, and *N. meningitidis*), cefepime has comparable or greater in vitro activity than cefotaxime. For *P. aeruginosa*, cefepime has comparable activity to ceftazidime, although it is less active than ceftazidime for other *Pseudomonas* spp. and *X. maltophilia*. Cefepime has higher activity than ceftazidime and comparable activity to cefotaxime for streptococci and methicillin-sensitive *S. aureus*. It is not active against MRSA, penicillin-resistant pneumococci, enterococci, *B. fragilis*, *L. monocytogenes*, *Mycobacterium avium* complex, or *Mycobacterium tuberculosis*.

ADVERSE REACTIONS

Hypersensitivity reactions to the cephalosporins are the most common side effects; they are identical to those caused by the penicillins. Patients who are allergic to 1 class of β-lactam antibiotics may manifest cross-reactivity to a member of the other class.

Immediate reactions such as anaphylaxis, bronchospasm, and urticaria are observed. More commonly, maculopapular rash develops, usually after several days of therapy; this may or may not be accompanied by fever and eosinophilia. Patients with a history of a mild or a temporally distant reaction to penicillin appear to be at low risk of allergic reaction following the administration of a cephalosporin. However, patients who have had a recent severe, immediate reaction to a penicillin should be given a cephalosporin with great caution, if at all. A positive Coombs reaction appears frequently in patients who receive large doses of a cephalosporin, but hemolysis is rare. Cephalosporins have produced rare instances of bone marrow depression, characterized by granulocytopenia.

The cephalosporins are potentially nephrotoxic. Renal tubular necrosis has followed the administration of cephaloridine in doses >4 g/day; this agent is no longer available in the U.S. Other cephalosporins when used by themselves in recommended doses rarely produce significant renal toxicity. High doses of cephalothin (no longer available in the U.S.) have produced acute tubular necrosis in certain instances, and usual doses (8-12 g/day) have caused nephrotoxicity in patients with preexisting renal disease. Diarrhea can result from the administration of cephalosporins and may be more frequent with cefoperazone, perhaps because of its greater biliary excretion. Intolerance to alcohol has been noted with cephalosporins that contain the methylthiotetrazole (MTT) group. Serious bleeding related either to hypoprothrombinemia owing to the MTT group, thrombocytopenia, and/or platelet dysfunction has been reported.

THERAPEUTIC USES

The **first-generation cephalosporins** are excellent agents for skin and soft tissue infections owing to *S. pyogenes* and methicillin-susceptible *S. aureus*. A single dose of cefazolin just before surgery is the preferred prophylaxis for procedures in which skin flora are the likely pathogens. For colorectal surgery, where prophylaxis for intestinal anaerobes is desired, the second-generation agent cefoxitin is preferred.

Second-generation cephalosporins generally have been displaced by third-generation agents. The oral second-generation cephalosporins can be used to treat respiratory tract infections, although they are suboptimal (compared with oral amoxicillin) for treatment of penicillin-resistant *S. pneumoniae* pneumonia and otitis media. In situations where facultative gram-negative bacteria and anaerobes are involved, such as intra-abdominal infections, pelvic inflammatory disease, and diabetic foot infection, cefoxitin and cefotetan both are effective.

The **third-generation cephalosporins** are the drugs of choice for serious infections caused by *Klebsiella*, *Enterobacter*, *Proteus*, *Providencia*, *Serratia*, and *Haemophilus* spp. Ceftriaxone is the therapy of choice for all forms of gonorrhea and for severe forms of Lyme disease. Third-generation cephalosporins cefotaxime or ceftriaxone are used for the initial treatment of meningitis in nonimmunocompromised adults and children >3 months of age (in combination with vancomycin and ampicillin pending identification of the causative agent). They are the drugs of choice for the treatment of meningitis caused by *H. influenzae*, sensitive *S. pneumoniae*, *N. meningitidis*, and gram-negative enteric bacteria. Cefotaxime has failed in the treatment of meningitis owing to resistant *S. pneumoniae*; thus vancomycin should be added. Ceftazidime plus an aminoglycoside is the treatment of choice for *Pseudomonas* meningitis. Third-generation cephalosporins lack activity against *L. monocytogenes* and penicillin-resistant pneumococci, which may cause meningitis. The antimicrobial spectra of cefotaxime and ceftriaxone are excellent for the treatment of community-acquired pneumonia.

The **fourth-generation cephalosporins** are indicated for the empirical treatment of nosocomial infections where antibiotic resistance owing to extended-spectrum β-lactamases or chromosomally induced β-lactamases are anticipated. For example, cefepime has superior activity against nosocomial isolates of *Enterobacter*, *Citrobacter*, and *Serratia* spp. compared with ceftazidime and piperacillin. KPC- or metallo-β-lactamase expressing strains are resistant to cefepime.

OTHER β-LACTAM ANTIBIOTICS

CARBAPENEMS

Carbapenems are β-lactams that contain a fused β-lactam ring and a 5-member ring system that differs from the penicillins because it is unsaturated and contains a carbon atom instead of the sulfur atom. This class of antibiotics has a broader spectrum of activity than most other β-lactam antibiotics.

IMIPENEM. Imipenem is marketed in combination with cilastatin, a drug that inhibits the degradation of imipenem by a renal tubular dipeptidase.

Antimicrobial Activity. Imipenem, like other β-lactam antibiotics, binds to PBPs, disrupts bacterial cell wall synthesis, and causes death of susceptible microorganisms. It is very resistant to hydrolysis by most β-lactamases. The activity of imipenem is excellent in vitro for a wide variety of aerobic and anaerobic microorganisms. Streptococci (including penicillin-resistant *S. pneumoniae*), enterococci (excluding *E. faecium* and non-β-lactamase-producing penicillin-resistant strains), staphylococci (including penicillinase-producing strains), and *Listeria* all are susceptible. Some strains of methicillin-resistant staphylococci are susceptible: many strains are not. Activity was excellent against the Enterobacteriaceae until the emergence of KPC carbapenemase-producing strains. Most strains of *Pseudomonas* and *Acinetobacter* are inhibited. Anaerobes, including *B. fragilis*, are highly susceptible.

Pharmacokinetics and Adverse Reactions. Imipenem is not absorbed orally. The drug is hydrolyzed rapidly by a dipeptidase found in the brush border of the proximal tubule. To prolong drug activity, imipenem is combined with cilastatin, an inhibitor of the dehydropeptidase; the combined preparation is available as PRIMAXIN. Both imipenem and cilastatin have a $t_{1/2}$ of ~1 h. When administered concurrently with cilastatin, ~70% of administered imipenem is recovered in the urine as the active drug. Dosage should be modified for patients with renal insufficiency. Nausea and vomiting are the most common adverse reactions (1-20%). Seizures have been noted in up to 1.5% of patients, especially when high doses are given to patients with CNS lesions and to those with renal insufficiency. Patients who are allergic to other β-lactam antibiotics may have hypersensitivity reactions when given imipenem.

Therapeutic Uses. Imipenem–cilastatin is effective for a wide variety of infections, including urinary tract and lower respiratory infections; intra-abdominal and gynecological infections; and skin, soft tissue, bone, and joint infections. The drug combination appears to be especially useful for the treatment of infections caused by cephalosporin-resistant nosocomial bacteria. It is prudent to use imipenem for empirical treatment of serious infections in hospitalized patients who have recently received other β-lactam antibiotics. Imipenem should not be used as monotherapy for infections owing to *P. aeruginosa* because of the risk of resistance developing during therapy.

MEROPENEM. Meropenem (MERREM IV) is a derivative of thienamycin. It does not require coadministration with cilastatin because it is not sensitive to renal dipeptidase. Its toxicity is similar to that of imipenem except that it may be less likely to cause seizures.

DORIPENEM. Doripenem (DORIBAX) has a spectrum of activity that is similar to that of imipenem and meropenem, with greater activity against some resistant isolates of Pseudomonas.

ERTAPENEM. Ertapenem (INVANZ) differs from imipenem and meropenem by having a longer $t_{1/2}$ that allows once-daily dosing and by having inferior activity against *P. aeruginosa* and *Acinetobacter* spp. Its activity against gram-positive organisms, Enterobacteriaceae, and anaerobes makes it useful in intra-abdominal and pelvic infections.

AZTREONAM. Aztreonam (AZACTAM) is resistant to many of the β-lactamases elaborated by most gram-negative bacteria, including the metallo-β-lactamases but not the KPC β-lactamases.

The antimicrobial activity of aztreonam differs from those of other β-lactam antibiotics and more closely resembles that of an aminoglycoside. Aztreonam has activity only against gram-negative bacteria; it has no activity against gram-positive bacteria and anaerobic organisms. Activity against Enterobacteriaceae is excellent, as is that against *P. aeruginosa.* It is also highly active in vitro against *H. influenzae* and gonococci. Aztreonam is administered either intramuscularly or intravenously. The $t_{1/2}$ for elimination is 1.7 h; most of the drug is recovered unaltered in the urine. The $t_{1/2}$ is prolonged to ~6 h in anephric patients. The usual dose of aztreonam for severe infections is 2 g every 6-8 h (reduced in patients with renal insufficiency). A notable feature is little allergic cross-reactivity with β-lactam antibiotics, with the possible exception of ceftazidime with which it has considerable structural similarity. Aztreonam is therefore useful for treating gram-negative infections that normally would be treated with a β-lactam antibiotic were it not for a prior allergic reaction. Aztreonam generally is well tolerated.

β-LACTAMASE INHIBITORS

Certain molecules can inactivate β-lactamases and prevent the destruction of β-lactam antibiotic substrates. β-Lactamase inhibitors are most active against plasmid-encoded β-lactamases (including those that hydrolyze ceftazidime and cefotaxime), but they are inactive at clinically achievable concentrations against the type I chromosomal β-lactamases induced in gram-negative bacilli (e.g., *Enterobacter*, *Acinetobacter*, and *Citrobacter*) by 2nd and 3rd generation cephalosporins.

Clavulanic acid has poor intrinsic antimicrobial activity but is a "suicide" inhibitor that irreversibly binds β-lactamases produced by a wide range of gram-positive and gram-negative microorganisms. Clavulanic acid is well absorbed by mouth and also can be given parenterally. It is combined with amoxicillin as an oral preparation (AUGMENTIN, others) and with ticarcillin as a parenteral preparation (TIMENTIN).

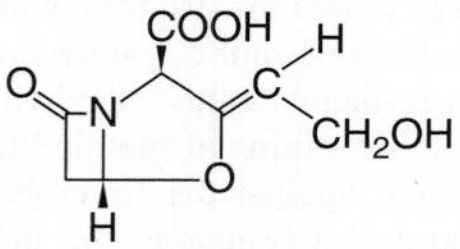

COOH H O N C CH_2OH O H

CLAVULANIC ACID

Amoxicillin plus clavulanate is effective for β-lactamase-producing strains of staphylococci, *H. influenzae*, gonococci, and *E. coli*. It is effective in the treatment of acute otitis media in children, sinusitis, animal or human bite wounds, cellulitis, and diabetic foot infections. Addition of clavulanate to ticarcillin extends its spectrum to aerobic gram-negative bacilli, *S. aureus*, and *Bacteroides* spp. There is no increased activity against *Pseudomonas* spp. The combination is especially useful for mixed nosocomial infections, often with an aminoglycoside. Dosage should be adjusted in renal insufficiency.

Sulbactam is a β-lactamase inhibitor similar in structure to clavulanic acid. It is available for intravenous or intramuscular use combined with ampicillin (UNASYN, others). Dosage must be adjusted for patients with impaired renal function. The combination has good activity against gram-positive cocci, including β-lactamase-producing strains of *S. aureus*, gram-negative aerobes (but not resistant strains of *E. coli* or *Pseudomonas*), and anaerobes; it also has been used effectively for the treatment of mixed intra-abdominal and pelvic infections.

Tazobactam is a β-lactamase inhibitor with good activity against many of the plasmid β-lactamases, including some of the extended-spectrum class. It is combined with piperacillin as a parenteral preparation (ZOSYN) that should be equivalent in antimicrobial spectrum to ticarcillin plus clavulanate.

For a complete Bibliographical Listing see Goodman & Gilman's ***The Pharmacological Basis of Therapeutics***, 12th ed., or Goodman & Gilman Online at www.AccessMedicine.com.

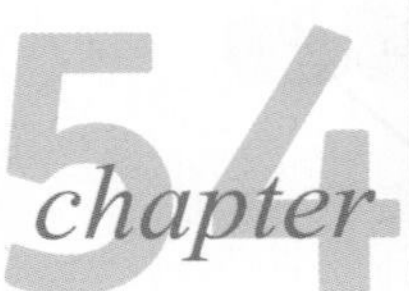

Aminoglycosides

Aminoglycosides (*gentamicin, tobramycin, amikacin, netilmicin, kanamycin, streptomycin, paromomycin, and neomycin*) are used primarily to treat infections caused by aerobic gram-negative bacteria. Streptomycin is an important agent for the treatment of tuberculosis, and paromomycin is used orally for intestinal amebiasis and in the management of hepatic coma. Aminoglycosides are *bactericidal inhibitors* of protein synthesis. Mutations affecting proteins in the bacterial ribosome can confer marked resistance to their action. Most commonly resistance is due to acquisition of plasmids or transposon-encoding genes for aminoglycoside-metabolizing enzymes or from impaired transport of drug into the cell. Thus, there can be cross-resistance between members of the class.

Aminoglycosides are natural products or semisynthetic derivatives of compounds produced by a variety of soil actinomycetes. Amikacin, a derivative of kanamycin, and netilmicin, a derivative of sisomicin, are semisynthetic products. These agents contain amino sugars linked to an aminocyclitol ring by glycosidic bonds (Figure 54–1). They are polycations, and their polarity is responsible in part for pharmacokinetic properties shared by all members of the group. For example, none is absorbed adequately after oral administration, inadequate concentrations are found in cerebrospinal fluid (CSF), and all are excreted relatively rapidly by the normal kidney. All members of the group share the same spectrum of toxicity, most notably nephrotoxicity and ototoxicity, which can involve the auditory and vestibular functions of the eighth cranial nerve.

GENERAL PROPERTIES

MECHANISM OF ACTION. The aminoglycoside antibiotics are rapidly bactericidal. Bacterial killing is concentration dependent: the higher the concentration, the greater the rate of bacterial killing. The bactericidal activity persists after the serum concentration has fallen below the *minimum inhibitory concentration* (MIC). These properties probably account for the efficacy of high-dose, extended-interval dosing regimens.

Aminoglycosides diffuse through aqueous channels formed by *porin* proteins in the outer membrane of gram-negative bacteria to enter the periplasmic space. Transport of aminoglycosides across the cytoplasmic (inner) membrane depends on a transmembrane electrical gradient coupled to electron transport to drive permeation of these antibiotics. This energy-dependent phase is rate-limiting and can be blocked or inhibited by divalent cations (e.g., Ca^{2+} and Mg^{2+}), hyperosmolarity, a reduction in pH, and anaerobic conditions. Thus, the antimicrobial activity of aminoglycosides is reduced markedly in the anaerobic environment of an abscess and in hyperosmolar acidic urine.

Once inside the cell, aminoglycosides bind to polysomes and interfere with protein synthesis by causing misreading and premature termination of mRNA translation (Figure 54–2). The primary intracellular site of action of the aminoglycosides is the 30S ribosomal subunit. At least 3 of these ribosomal proteins, and perhaps the 16S ribosomal RNA as well, contribute to the streptomycin-binding site. Aminoglycosides interfere with the initiation of protein synthesis, leading to the accumulation of abnormal initiation complexes; the drugs also can cause misreading of the mRNA template and incorporation of incorrect amino acids into the growing polypeptide chains. The resulting aberrant proteins may be inserted into the cell membrane, leading to altered permeability and further stimulation of aminoglycoside transport.

MICROBIAL RESISTANCE TO THE AMINOGLYCOSIDES. Bacteria may be resistant to aminoglycosides because of:

- Inactivation of the drug by microbial enzymes
- Failure of the antibiotic to penetrate intracellularly
- Low affinity of the drug for the bacterial ribosome

Clinically, drug inactivation is the most common mechanism for acquired microbial resistance. The genes encoding aminoglycoside-modifying enzymes are acquired primarily by conjugation and transfer of resistance plasmids (*see* Chapter 48). These enzymes phosphorylate, adenylate, or acetylate specific hydroxyl or

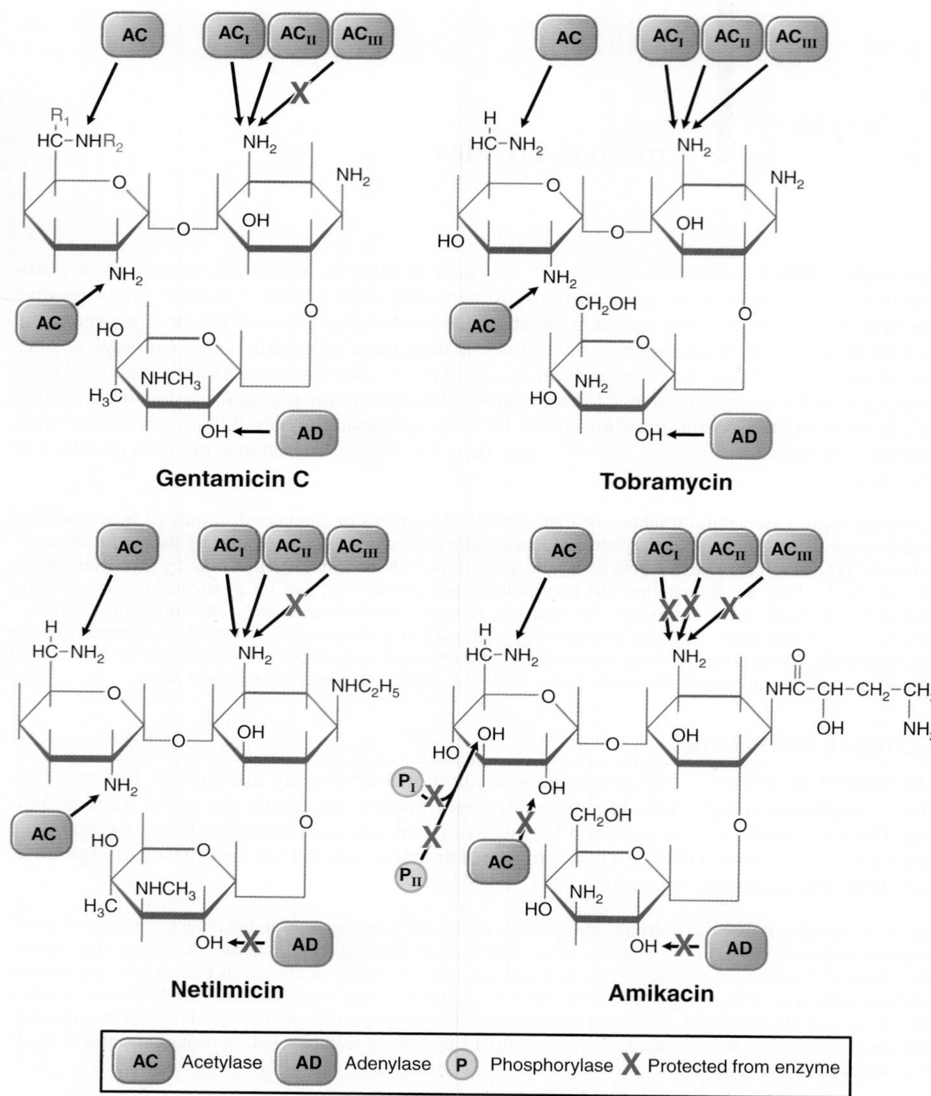

Figure 54–1 *Sites of activity of various plasmid-mediated enzymes capable of inactivating aminoglycosides.* The *red* **X** indicates regions of the molecules that are protected from the designated enzyme. In gentamicin C_1, $R_1=R_2=CH_3$; in gentamicin C_2, $R_1=CH_3$, $R_2=H$; in gentamicin C_{1a}, $R_1=R_2=H$. (Reproduced with permission from Moellering RC Jr. Microbiological considerations in the use of tobramycin and related aninoglycosidic aminocyclitol antibiotics. *Med J Aust,* 1977;2S:4–8. Copyright 1977. *The Medical Journal of Australia*.)

amino groups (*see* Figure 54–1). Amikacin is a suitable substrate for only a few of these inactivating enzymes (*see* Figure 54–1); thus, strains that are resistant to multiple other aminoglycosides tend to be susceptible to amikacin. However, a significant percentage of clinical isolates of *Enterococcus faecalis* and *E. faecium* are highly resistant to all aminoglycosides. Resistance to gentamicin indicates cross-resistance to tobramycin, amikacin, kanamycin, and netilmicin because the inactivating enzyme is bifunctional and can modify all these aminoglycosides. Owing to differences in the chemical structures of streptomycin and other aminoglycosides, this enzyme does not modify streptomycin, which is inactivated by another enzyme; consequently, gentamicin-resistant strains of enterococci may be susceptible to streptomycin. Intrinsic resistance to aminoglycosides may be caused by failure of the drug to penetrate the cytoplasmic (inner) membrane. Transport of aminoglycosides across the cytoplasmic membrane is an active process that depends on oxidative metabolism. Strictly anaerobic bacteria thus are resistant to these drugs because they lack the necessary transport system.

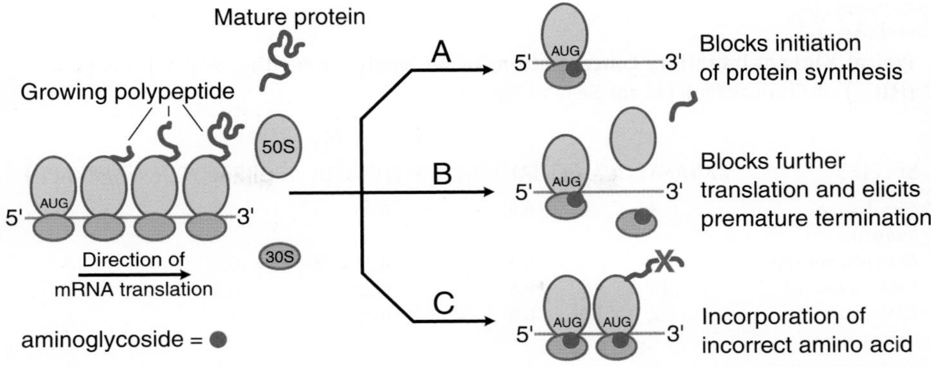

Figure 54–2 *Effects of aminoglycosides on protein synthesis.* **A.** Aminoglycoside (represented by *red circles*) binds to the 30S ribosomal subunit and interferes with initiation of protein synthesis by fixing the 30S-50S ribosomal complex at the start codon (AUG) of mRNA. As 30S-50S complexes downstream complete translation of mRNA and detach, the abnormal initiation complexes, so-called streptomycin monosomes, accumulate, blocking further translation of the message. Aminoglycoside binding to the 30S subunit also causes misreading of mRNA, leading to **B,** premature termination of translation with detachment of the ribosomal complex and incompletely synthesized protein or **C,** incorporation of incorrect amino acids (indicated by the *red X*), resulting in the production of abnormal or nonfunctional proteins.

Missense mutations in *Escherichia coli* that substitute a single amino acid in a crucial ribosomal protein may prevent binding of streptomycin. Although highly resistant to streptomycin, these strains are not widespread in nature. Similarly, 5% of strains of *Pseudomonas aeruginosa* exhibit such ribosomal resistance to streptomycin. Because ribosomal resistance usually is specific for streptomycin, these strains of enterococci remain sensitive to a combination of penicillin and gentamicin in vitro.

ANTIBACTERIAL SPECTRUM OF THE AMINOGLYCOSIDES. The antibacterial activity of gentamicin, tobramycin, kanamycin, netilmicin, and amikacin is directed primarily against aerobic gram-negative bacilli. Kanamycin, like streptomycin, has a more limited spectrum. The aerobic gram-negative bacilli vary in their susceptibility to the aminoglycosides (*see* Table 54–1).

Aminoglycosides have little activity against anaerobic microorganisms or facultative bacteria under anaerobic conditions. Their action against most gram-positive bacteria is limited, and they should not be used as single agents to treat infections caused by gram-positive bacteria. In combination with a cell wall–active agent, such as a penicillin or vancomycin, an aminoglycoside produces a synergistic bactericidal effect in vitro. Clinically, the superiority of aminoglycoside combination regimens over β-lactams alone is not proven except in relatively few infections (discussed later).

ADME AND DOSING

ABSORPTION. The aminoglycosides are polar cations and therefore are poorly absorbed from the GI tract. Less than 1% of a dose is absorbed after either oral or rectal administration. The drugs are eliminated quantitatively in the feces. Nonetheless, long-term oral or rectal administration of aminoglycosides may result in accumulation to toxic concentrations in patients with renal impairment. Absorption of gentamicin from the GI tract may be increased by GI disease (e.g., ulcers or inflammatory bowel disease). Instillation of these drugs into body cavities with serosal surfaces also may result in rapid absorption and unexpected toxicity (i.e., neuromuscular blockade). Intoxication may occur when aminoglycosides are applied topically for long periods to large wounds, burns, or cutaneous ulcers, particularly if there is renal insufficiency.

All the aminoglycosides are absorbed rapidly from intramuscular sites of injection. Peak concentrations in plasma occur after 30-90 min. These concentrations range from 4-12 μg/mL following a 1.5-2 mg/kg dose of gentamicin, tobramycin, or netilmicin and from 20-35 μg/mL following a 7.5 mg/kg dose of amikacin or kanamycin. There is increasing use of aminoglycosides administered via inhalation, primarily for the management of patients with cystic fibrosis who have chronic *P. aeruginosa* pulmonary infections. Amikacin and tobramycin solutions for injection have been used, as well as a commercial formulation of tobramycin designed for inhalation (TOBI, others).

DISTRIBUTION. Because of their polar nature, the aminoglycosides do not penetrate into most cells, the CNS, or the eye. Except for streptomycin, there is negligible binding of aminoglycosides to plasma albumin. The apparent volume of distribution of these drugs is 25% of lean body weight and approximates the volume of

Table 54–1

Typical Minimal Inhibitory Concentrations of Aminoglycosides That Will Inhibit 90% (MIC_{90}) of Clinical Isolates for Several Species

	MIC_{90} µg/mL				
SPECIES	KANAMYCIN	GENTAMICIN	NETILMICIN	TOBRAMYCIN	AMIKACIN
Citrobacter freundii	8	0.5	0.25	0.5	1
Enterobacter spp.	4	0.5	0.25	0.5	1
Escherichia coli	16	0.5	0.25	0.5	1
Klebsiella pneumoniae	32	0.5	0.25	1	1
Proteus mirabilis	8	4	4	0.5	2
Providencia stuartii	128	8	16	4	2
Pseudomonas aeruginosa	>128	8	32	4	2
Serratia spp.	>64	4	16	16	8
Enterococcus faecalis	—	32	2	32	≥64
Staphylococcus aureus	2	0.5	0.25	0.25	16

Source: Adapted from Wiedemann B, Atkinson BA. Susceptibility to antibiotics: Species incidence and trends. In: Lorian V, ed. Antibiotics in Laboratory Medicine, 3rd ed. Baltimore: Lippincott Williams & Wilkins; 1991:962–1208.

extracellular fluid. The aminoglycosides distribute poorly into adipose tissue, which must be considered when using weight-based dosing regimens in obese patients.

Concentrations of aminoglycosides in secretions and tissues are low. High concentrations are found only in the renal cortex and the endolymph and perilymph of the inner ear; the high concentration in these sites likely contribute to the nephrotoxicity and ototoxicity caused by these drugs. As a result of active hepatic secretion, concentrations in bile approach 30% of those found in plasma, but this represents a very minor excretory route for the aminoglycosides. Inflammation increases the penetration of aminoglycosides into peritoneal and pericardial cavities. Concentrations of aminoglycosides achieved in CSF with parenteral administration usually are subtherapeutic. Treatment of meningitis with intravenous administration is generally suboptimal. Intrathecal or intraventricular administration of aminoglycosides has been used to achieve therapeutic levels, but the availability of third- and fourth-generation cephalosporins has generally made this unnecessary.

Administration of aminoglycosides to women late in pregnancy may result in accumulation of drug in fetal plasma and amniotic fluid. Streptomycin and tobramycin can cause hearing loss in children born to women who receive the drug during pregnancy. Insufficient data are available regarding the other aminoglycosides; therefore, these agents should be used with caution during pregnancy and only for strong clinical indications in the absence of suitable alternatives.

ELIMINATION. The aminoglycosides are excreted almost entirely by glomerular filtration, achieving urine concentrations of 50-200 µg/mL. The half-lives of the aminoglycosides in plasma are 2-3 h in patients with normal renal function. Because the elimination of aminoglycosides depends almost entirely on the kidney, a linear relationship exists between the concentration of creatinine in plasma and the $t_{1/2}$ of all aminoglycosides in patients with moderately compromised renal function. *Because the incidence of nephrotoxicity and ototoxicity is likely related to the overall drug exposure to aminoglycosides, it is critical to reduce the maintenance dosage of these drugs in patients with impaired renal function.*

Although excretion of aminoglycosides is similar in adults and children >6 months of age, half-lives of aminoglycosides may be prolonged significantly in the newborn: 8-11 h in the first week of life in newborns weighing <2 kg and ~5 h in those weighing >2 kg. Thus, it is critically important to monitor plasma concentrations of aminoglycosides during treatment of neonates. Aminoglycoside clearances are increased and half-lives are reduced in patients with cystic fibrosis. Larger doses of aminoglycosides may likewise be required in burn patients because of more rapid drug clearance, possibly because of drug loss through burn tissue. Aminoglycosides can be removed from the body by either hemodialysis or peritoneal dialysis.

Aminoglycosides can be inactivated by various penicillins in vitro and thus should not be admixed in solution. Some reports indicate that this inactivation may occur in vivo in patients with end-stage renal failure, making monitoring of aminoglycoside plasma concentrations even more necessary in such patients. Amikacin appears to be the aminoglycoside least affected by this interaction; penicillins with more nonrenal elimination (such as piperacillin) may be less prone to cause this interaction.

DOSING. High-dose, extended-interval administration of aminoglycosides is the preferred means of administering aminoglycosides for most indications and patient populations. Administering once daily higher doses at extended intervals is likely to be at least equally efficacious and potentially less toxic than administration of divided doses. Because of the post-antibiotic effect of aminoglycosides, good therapeutic response can be attained even when concentrations of amino-glycosides fall below inhibitory concentrations for a substantial fraction of the dosing interval. High-dose, extended-interval dosing schemes for aminoglycosides may also reduce the characteristic oto- and nephro-toxicity of these drugs. This diminished toxicity is probably due to a threshold effect from accumulation of drug in the inner ear or in the kidney. High-dose, extended-interval regimens, despite the higher peak concentration, provide a longer period when concentrations fall below the threshold for toxicity than does a multiple-dose regimen (compare the 2 dosage regimens shown in Figure 54–3).

Exceptions to the high-dose/extended-interval dosing include pregnancy, neonates, and in pediatric infections, and combination therapy for endocarditis. In these infections, multiple daily doses (with a lower total daily dose) are preferred because data documenting equivalent safety and efficacy of extended-interval dosing are inadequate. Extended-interval dosing should also be avoided in patients with significant renal dysfunction (i.e., creatinine clearance <25 mL/min). Aminoglycoside doses must be adjusted for patients with creatinine clearances of <80 mL/min (Table 54–2), and plasma concentrations must be monitored. Concentrations of aminoglycosides achieved in plasma after a given dose vary widely among patients.

For twice- or thrice-daily dosing regimens, both peak and trough plasma concentrations are determined. The peak concentration documents that the dose produces therapeutic concentrations, while the trough concentration is used to avoid toxicity. Trough concentrations should be <1-2 μg/mL for gentamicin, netilmicin, and tobramycin and <10 μg/mL for amikacin and streptomycin. Monitoring of aminoglycoside plasma concentrations also is important when using an extended-interval dosing regimen. The most accurate method for

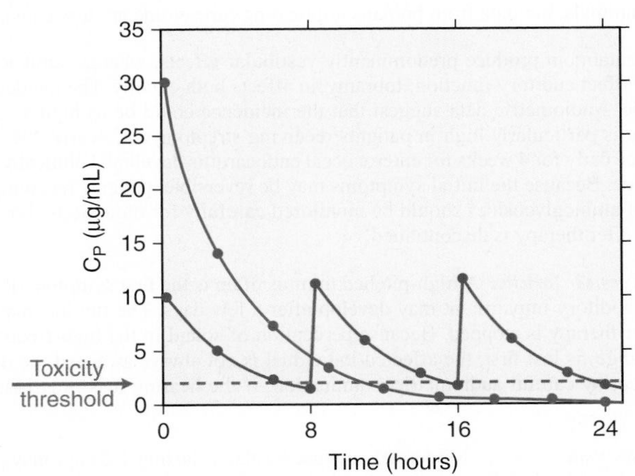

Figure 54–3 *Comparison of single dose and divided dose regimens for gentamicin.* In a hypothetical patient, a dose of gentamicin (5.1 mg/kg) is administered intravenously as a single bolus (*red line*) or in 3 portions, a third of the dose every 8 h (*purple line*), such that the total drug administered is the same in the 2 cases. The threshold for toxicity (*green dashed line*) is the plasma concentration of 2 μg/mL, the maximum recommended for prolonged exposure. The single-dose regimen produces a higher plasma concentration than the every-8-h regimen; this higher peak provides efficacy that otherwise might be compromised due to prolonged sub-threshold concentrations later in the dosing interval or that is provided by the lower peak levels achieved with the every-8-h regimen. The once-daily regimen also provides a 13-h period during which plasma concentrations are below the threshold for toxicity. The every-8-h regimen, by contrast, provides only 3 short (~1 h) periods in 24 h during which plasma concentrations are below the threshold for toxicity. The single high-dose, extended interval is generally preferred for aminoglycosides, with a few exceptions (during pregnancy, in neonates, etc.), as noted in the text. On the other hand, a divided-dose regimen can be useful for maximizing the time above a threshold (e.g., MIC) for some antibiotics (*see* Figure 48–4).

Table 54–2

Dose Reduction of Aminoglycosides Based on Calculated Creatinine Clearance

CREATININE CLEARANCE (mL/min)	% OF MAXIMUM DAILY DOSE*	FREQUENCY OF DOSING
100	100	Every 24 hours
75	75	
50	50	
25	25	
20	80	Every 48 hours
10	60	
<10	40	

**The maximum adult daily dose for amikacin, kanamycin, and streptomycin is 15 mg/kg; for gentamicin and tobramycin, 5.5 mg/kg; and for netilmicin, 6.5 mg/kg.*

monitoring plasma levels for dose adjustment is to measure the concentration in 2 plasma samples drawn several hours apart (e.g., at 2 and 12 h after a dose). The clearance then can be calculated and the dose adjusted to achieve the desired target range.

UNTOWARD EFFECTS. All aminoglycosides have the potential to produce reversible and irreversible vestibular, cochlear, and renal toxicity.

OTOTOXICITY. Vestibular and auditory dysfunction can follow the administration of any of the aminoglycosides, and ototoxicity may become a dose-limiting adverse effect. Aminoglycoside-induced ototoxicity results in irreversible, bilateral high-frequency hearing loss and temporary vestibular hypofunction. Degeneration of hair cells and neurons in the cochlea correlates with the loss of hearing. Accumulation within the perilymph and endolymph occurs predominantly when aminoglycoside concentrations in plasma are high. Diffusion back into the bloodstream is slow; the half-lives of the aminoglycosides are 5 to 6 times longer in the otic fluids than in plasma. Drugs such as *ethacrynic acid* and *furosemide* potentiate the ototoxic effects of the aminoglycosides in animals, but data from humans implicating furosemide are less convincing.

Streptomycin and gentamicin produce predominantly vestibular effects, whereas amikacin, kanamycin, and neomycin primarily affect auditory function; tobramycin affects both equally. The incidence of ototoxicity is difficult to determine. Audiometric data suggest that the incidence could be as high as 25%. The incidence of vestibular toxicity is particularly high in patients receiving streptomycin; nearly 20% of individuals who received 500 mg twice daily for 4 weeks for enterococcal endocarditis developed clinically detectable irreversible vestibular damage. Because the initial symptoms may be reversible, patients receiving high doses and/or prolonged courses of aminoglycosides should be monitored carefully for ototoxicity; however, deafness may occur several weeks after therapy is discontinued.

Clinical Symptoms of Cochlear Toxicity. A high-pitched tinnitus often is the first symptom of toxicity. If the drug is not discontinued, auditory impairment may develop after a few days. The tinnitus may persist for several days to 2 weeks after therapy is stopped. Because perception of sound in the high-frequency range (outside the conversational range) is lost first, the affected individual is not always aware of the difficulty, and it will not be detected except by careful audiometric examination. If the hearing loss progresses, the lower sound ranges are affected.

Clinical Symptoms of Vestibular Toxicity. Moderately intense headache lasting 1-2 days may precede the onset of labyrinthine dysfunction. This is followed immediately by an acute stage in which nausea, vomiting, and difficulty with equilibrium develop and persist for 1-2 weeks. Prominent symptoms include vertigo in the upright position, inability to perceive termination of movement ("mental past-pointing"), and difficulty in sitting or standing without visual cues. The acute stage ends suddenly and is followed by chronic labyrinthitis, in which, the patient has difficulty when attempting to walk or make sudden movements; ataxia is the most prominent feature. The chronic phase persists for ~2 months. Recovery from this phase may require 12-18 months, and most patients have some permanent residual damage. Early discontinuation of the drug may permit recovery before irreversible damage of the hair cells.

NEPHROTOXICITY. Approximately 8-26% of patients who receive an aminoglycoside for several days develop mild renal impairment that is almost always reversible. The toxicity results from accumulation and retention of aminoglycoside in the proximal tubular cells. The initial manifestation of damage at this site is excretion of enzymes of the renal tubular brush border followed by mild proteinuria, and the appearance of hyaline and granular casts. The glomerular filtration rate is reduced after several additional days. The non-oliguric phase of renal insufficiency is thought to be due to the effects of aminoglycosides on the distal portion of the nephron with a reduced sensitivity of the collecting-duct epithelium to vasopressin. Although severe acute tubular necrosis may occur rarely, the most common significant finding is a mild rise in plasma creatinine. The impairment in renal function is almost always reversible because the proximal tubular cells have the capacity to regenerate. Toxicity correlates with the total amount of drug administered and with longer courses of therapy. High-dose, extended-interval dosing approaches lead to less nephrotoxicity at the same level of total drug exposure (as measured by area under the curve) than divided-dose approaches (*see* Figure 54–3). Neomycin, which concentrates to the greatest degree, is highly nephrotoxic in human beings and should not be administered systemically. Streptomycin does not concentrate in the renal cortex and is the least nephrotoxic. Drugs such as amphotericin B, vancomycin, angiotensin-converting enzyme inhibitors, cisplatin, and cyclosporine may potentiate aminoglycoside-induced nephrotoxicity.

NEUROMUSCULAR BLOCKADE. Acute neuromuscular blockade and apnea have been attributed to the aminoglycosides; patients with myasthenia gravis are particularly susceptible. In humans, neuromuscular blockade generally has occurred after intrapleural or intraperitoneal instillation of large doses of an aminoglycoside; however, the reaction can follow intravenous, intramuscular, and even oral administration of these agents. Neuromuscular blockade may be reversed by intravenous administration of a Ca^{++} salt.

OTHER UNTOWARD EFFECTS. In general, the aminoglycosides have little allergenic potential. Rare hypersensitivity reactions—including skin rashes, eosinophilia, fever, blood dyscrasias, angioedema, exfoliative dermatitis, stomatitis, and anaphylactic shock—have been reported as cross-hypersensitivity among drugs in this class.

THERAPEUTIC USES OF AMINOGLYCOSIDES

Gentamicin is an important agent for the treatment of many serious gram-negative bacillary infections. It is the aminoglycoside of first choice because of its lower cost and reliable activity against all but the most resistant gram-negative aerobes. Gentamicin preparations are available for parenteral, ophthalmic, and topical administration. Gentamicin, tobramycin, amikacin, and netilmicin can be used interchangeably for the treatment of most of the following infections. For most indications, gentamicin is preferred because of long experience with its use and its lower cost. Many different types of infections can be treated successfully with these aminoglycosides; however, owing to their toxicities, prolonged use should be restricted to the therapy of life-threatening infections and those for which a less toxic agent is contraindicated or less effective.

Aminoglycosides frequently are used in combination with a cell wall–active agent (*β-lactam or glycopeptide*) for the therapy of serious proven or suspected bacterial infections. The 3 rationales for this approach are: to expand the empiric spectrum of activity of the antimicrobial regimen; to provide synergistic bacterial killing; and to prevent the emergence of resistance to the individual agents. Combination therapy is used in infections such as healthcare-associated pneumonia or sepsis, where multidrug-resistant gram-negative organisms such as *P. aeruginosa*, *Enterobacter*, *Klebsiella*, and *Serratia* may be causative and the consequences of failing to provide initially active therapy are dire. The use of aminoglycosides to achieve synergistic bacterial killing and improve clinical response is most well established for the treatment of endocarditis due to gram-positive organisms, most importantly *Enterococcus*. Clinical data do not support the use of combination therapy for synergistic killing of gram-negative organisms, with the possible exceptions of serious *P. aeruginosa* infections.

GENTAMICIN

DOSING. The typical recommended intramuscular or intravenous dose of gentamicin sulfate when used for the treatment of known or suspected gram-negative organisms as a single agent or in combination therapy for adults with normal renal function is 5-7 mg/kg daily given over 30-60 min. For patients with renal dysfunction, the interval may be extended. For patients who are not candidates for extended-interval dosing, a loading dose of 2 mg/kg and then 3-5 mg/kg per day, one-third given every 8 h is recommended. Dosages at the upper end of this range may be required to achieve therapeutic levels for trauma or burn patients, those with septic shock, patients with cystic fibrosis, and others in whom drug clearance is more rapid or volume of distribution is larger than normal. Several dosage schedules have been suggested for newborns and infants: 3 mg/kg once daily for preterm newborns <35 weeks of gestation; 4 mg/kg once daily for newborns >35 weeks of gestation; 5 mg/kg daily in 2 divided doses for neonates with severe infections; and 2-2.5 mg/kg every 8 h for children up to 2 years of age. Peak plasma concentrations range from 4-10 μg/mL (dosing: 1.7 mg/kg every 8 h) and 16-24 μg/mL (dosing: 5.1 mg/kg once daily). It should be emphasized that the recommended doses of gentamicin do not always yield desired concentrations. Periodic determinations of the plasma concentration of aminoglycosides are recommended strongly.

THERAPEUTIC USES

Urinary Tract Infections. Aminoglycosides usually are not indicated for the treatment of uncomplicated urinary tract infections, although a single intramuscular dose of gentamicin (5 mg/kg) has been effective in uncomplicated infections of the lower urinary tract. However, as strains of *E. coli* have acquired resistance to β-lactams, trimethoprim-sulfamethoxazole, and fluoroquinolones, use of aminoglycosides may increase. Once the microorganism is isolated and its sensitivities to antibiotics are determined, the aminoglycoside should be discontinued if the infecting microorganism is sensitive to less toxic antibiotics.

Pneumonia. The organisms that cause community-acquired pneumonia are susceptible to broad-spectrum β-lactam antibiotics, macrolides, or a fluoroquinolone, and usually it is not necessary to add an aminoglycoside. Aminoglycosides are ineffective for the treatment of pneumonia due to anaerobes or *S. pneumoniae*, which are common causes of community-acquired pneumonia. They should not be considered as effective single-drug therapy for any aerobic gram-positive cocci (including *Staphylococcus aureus* or streptococci), the microorganisms commonly responsible for suppurative pneumonia or lung abscess. An amino-glycoside in combination with a β-lactam antibiotic is recommended as standard therapy for hospital-acquired pneumonia in which a multiple-drug-resistant gram-negative aerobe is a likely causative agent. Once it is established that the β-lactam is active against the causative agent, there is generally no benefit from continuing the aminoglycoside.

Meningitis. Availability of third-generation cephalosporins, especially cefotaxime and ceftriaxone, has reduced the need for treatment with aminoglycosides in most cases of meningitis, except for infections caused by gram-negative organisms resistant to β-lactam antibiotics (e.g., species of *Pseudomonas* and *Acinetobacter*). If an aminoglycoside is necessary, in adults, 5 mg of a preservative-free formulation of gentamicin (or equivalent dose of another aminoglycoside) is administered directly intrathecally or intraventricularly once daily.

Peritonitis Associated with Peritoneal Dialysis. Patients who develop peritonitis as a result of peritoneal dialysis may be treated with aminoglycoside diluted into the dialysis fluid to a concentration of 4-8 mg/L for gentamicin, netilmicin, or tobramycin or 6-12 mg/L for amikacin. Intravenous or intramuscular administration of drug is unnecessary because serum and peritoneal fluid will equilibrate rapidly.

Bacterial Endocarditis. "Synergistic" or low-dose gentamicin (3 mg/kg/day in 3 divided doses) in combination with a penicillin or vancomycin has been recommended in certain circumstances for treatment of infections due to gram-positive organisms, primarily bacterial endocarditis. Penicillin and gentamicin in combination are effective as a short-course (i.e., 2-week) regimen for uncomplicated native-valve streptococcal endocarditis. In cases of enterococcal endocarditis, concomitant administration of penicillin and gentamicin for 4-6 weeks is recommended. A 2-week regimen of gentamicin or tobramycin in combination with nafcillin is effective for the treatment of selected cases of staphylococcal tricuspid native-valve endocarditis. For patients with native mitral or aortic valve staphylococcal endocarditis, the risks of aminoglycoside administration likely outweigh the benefits.

Sepsis. Inclusion of an aminoglycoside in an empirical regimen is commonly recommended for the febrile patient with granulocytopenia and for sepsis when *P. aeruginosa* is a potential pathogen. More recent studies using potent broad-spectrum β-lactams (e.g., carbapenems and anti-pseudomonal cephalosporins) have demonstrated no benefit from adding an aminoglycoside to the regimen unless there is concern that an infection may be caused by a multiple-drug-resistant organism.

Topical Applications. Gentamicin is absorbed slowly when it is applied topically in an ointment and somewhat more rapidly when it is applied as a cream. When the antibiotic is applied to large areas of denuded body surface, as may be the case in burn patients, plasma concentrations can reach 4 μg/mL, and 2-5% of the drug may appear in the urine.

UNTOWARD EFFECTS. The most important and serious side effects of the use of gentamicin are nephrotoxicity and irreversible ototoxicity. Intrathecal or intraventricular administration is used rarely because it may cause local inflammation.

TOBRAMYCIN

The antimicrobial activity, pharmacokinetic properties, and toxicity profile of tobramycin are similar to those of gentamicin. Tobramycin may be given either intramuscularly, intravenously, or by inhalation. Tobramycin (TOBREX, others) also is available in ophthalmic ointments and solutions. Indications for the use of tobramycin are the same as those for gentamicin. The superior activity of tobramycin against *P. aeruginosa* makes it the preferred aminoglycoside for treatment of serious infections known or suspected to be caused by this organism. Tobramycin usually is used with an anti-pseudomonal β-lactam antibiotic. In contrast to gentamicin, tobramycin shows poor activity in combination with penicillin against many strains of enterococci. Most strains of *E. faecium* are highly resistant. Tobramycin is ineffective against mycobacteria. Dosages and serum concentrations are identical to those for gentamicin.

AMIKACIN

The spectrum of antimicrobial activity of amikacin is the broadest of the group. Because of its resistance to many of the aminoglycoside-inactivating enzymes, amikacin has a special role for the initial treatment of serious nosocomial gram-negative bacillary infections in hospitals where resistance to gentamicin and tobramycin has become a significant problem. Amikacin is active against most strains of *Serratia*, *Proteus*, and *P. aeruginosa* as well as most strains of *Klebsiella*, *Enterobacter*, and *E. coli* that are resistant to gentamicin and tobramycin. Most resistance to amikacin is found among strains of *Acinetobacter*, *Providencia*, and *Flavobacterium* and strains of *Pseudomonas* other than *P. aeruginosa*; these all are unusual pathogens. Amikacin is less active than gentamicin against enterococci and should not be used for this organism. Amikacin is not active against the majority of gram-positive anaerobic bacteria. It is active against *Mycobacterium tuberculosis*, including streptomycin-resistant strains and atypical mycobacteria.

The recommended dose of amikacin is 15 mg/kg/day as a single daily dose or divided into 2 or 3 equal portions, which must be reduced for patients with renal failure. The drug is absorbed rapidly after intramuscular injection, and peak concentrations in plasma approximate 20 μg/mL after injection of 7.5 mg/kg, The concentration 12 h after a 7.5 mg/kg dose is 5-10 μg/mL. A 15 mg/kg once-daily dose produces peak concentrations 50-60 μg/mL and a trough of <1 μg/mL. For treatment of mycobacterial infections, thrice-weekly dosing schedules are used, with doses up to 25 mg/kg. As with the other aminoglycosides, amikacin causes ototoxicity, hearing loss, and nephrotoxicity.

NETILMICIN

Netilmicin is similar to gentamicin and tobramycin in its pharmacokinetic properties and dosage. Its antibacterial activity is broad against aerobic gram-negative bacilli. Like amikacin, it is not metabolized by most of the aminoglycoside-inactivating enzymes; thus, it may be active against certain bacteria that are resistant to gentamicin (with the exception of resistant enterococci). Netilmicin is useful for the treatment of serious infections owing to susceptible Enterobacteriaceae and other aerobic gram-negative bacilli. The recommended dose of netilmicin for complicated urinary tract infections in adults is 1.5-2 mg/kg every 12 h. For other serious systemic infections, a total daily dose of 4-7 mg/kg is administered as a single dose or 2 to 3 divided doses. Children should receive 3-7 mg/kg/day in 2 to 3 divided doses; neonates receive 3.5-5 mg/kg/day as a single daily dose. The $t_{1/2}$ for elimination is usually 2–2.5 h in adults and increases with renal insufficiency. Netilmicin may produce ototoxicity and nephrotoxicity.

STREPTOMYCIN

Streptomycin is used for the treatment of certain unusual infections generally in combination with other antimicrobial agents. It generally is less active than other members of the class against aerobic gram-negative rods.

THERAPEUTIC USES

Bacterial Endocarditis. The combination of penicillin G (bacteriostatic against enterococci) and streptomycin is effective as bactericidal therapy for enterococcal endocarditis. Gentamicin is generally preferred for its lesser toxicity; also, gentamicin should be used when the strain of enterococcus is resistant to streptomycin (MIC >2 mg/mL). Streptomycin should be used instead of gentamicin when the strain is resistant to the latter and has demonstrable susceptibility to streptomycin, which may occur because the enzymes that inactivate these 2 aminoglycosides are different.

Streptomycin may be administered by deep intramuscular injection or intravenously. Intramuscular injection may be painful, with a hot tender mass developing at the site of injection. The dose of streptomycin is 15 mg/kg/day for patients with creatinine clearances >80 mL/min. It typically is administered as a 1000-mg single daily dose for tuberculosis or 500 mg twice daily, resulting in peak serum concentrations of ~50-60 and 15-30 μg/mL and trough concentrations of <1 and 5-10 μg/mL, respectively. The total daily dose should be reduced in direct proportion to the reduction in creatinine clearance for creatinine clearances >30 mL/min (*see* Table 54–2).

Tularemia. Streptomycin (or gentamicin) is the drug of choice for the treatment of tularemia. Most cases respond to the administration of 1-2 g (15-25 mg/kg) streptomycin per day (in divided doses) for 10-14 days.

Plague. Streptomycin is effective agent for the treatment of all forms of plague. The recommended dose is 2 g/day in 2 divided doses for 10 days. Gentamicin is probably as efficacious.

Tuberculosis. Streptomycin is a second-line agent for the treatment of active tuberculosis, and streptomycin always should be used in combination with at least 1 or 2 other drugs to which the causative strain is susceptible. The dose for patients with normal renal function is 15 mg/kg/day as a single intramuscular injection for 2-3 months and then 2 or 3 times a week thereafter.

UNTOWARD EFFECTS. Streptomycin has been replaced by gentamicin for most indications because the toxicity of gentamicin is primarily renal and reversible, whereas that of streptomycin is vestibular and irreversible. The administration of streptomycin may produce dysfunction of the optic nerve, including scotomas, presenting as enlargement of the blind spot. Among the less common toxic reactions to streptomycin is peripheral neuritis.

NEOMYCIN

Neomycin is a broad-spectrum antibiotic. Susceptible microorganisms usually are inhibited by concentrations of ≤10 μg/mL. Gram-negative species that are highly sensitive are *E. coli*, *Enterobacter aerogenes*, *Klebsiella pneumoniae*, and *Proteus vulgaris*. Gram-positive microorganisms that are inhibited include *S. aureus* and *E. faecalis*. *M. tuberculosis* also is sensitive to neomycin. Strains of *P. aeruginosa* are resistant to neomycin. Neomycin sulfate is available for topical and oral administration. Neomycin currently is available in many brands of creams, ointments, and other products alone and in combination with polymyxin, bacitracin, other antibiotics, and a variety of corticosteroids. There is no evidence that these topical preparations shorten the time required for wound healing or that those containing a steroid are more effective.

THERAPEUTIC USES. Neomycin is used widely for topical application in a variety of infections of the skin and mucous. The oral administration of neomycin (usually in combination with erythromycin base) has been employed primarily for "preparation" of the bowel for surgery. Neomycin and polymyxin B have been used for irrigation of the bladder to prevent bacteriuria and bacteremia associated with indwelling catheters. For this purpose, 1 mL of a preparation (NEOSPORIN G.U. IRRIGANT) containing 40 mg neomycin and 200,000 units polymyxin B per milliliter is diluted in 1 L of 0.9% sodium chloride solution and is used for continuous irrigation of the urinary bladder through appropriate catheter systems. The bladder is irrigated at the rate of 1 L every 24 h.

ABSORPTION AND EXCRETION. Neomycin is poorly absorbed from the GI tract and is excreted by the kidney. A total daily intake of 10 g for 3 days yields a blood concentration below that associated with systemic toxicity if renal function is normal. About 97% of an oral dose of neomycin is not absorbed and is eliminated unchanged in the feces.

UNTOWARD EFFECTS. Hypersensitivity reactions, primarily skin rashes, occur in 6-8% of patients when neomycin is applied topically. The most important toxic effects of neomycin are ototoxicity and nephrotoxicity; as a consequence, the drug is no longer available for parenteral administration. Neuromuscular blockade with respiratory paralysis also has occurred after irrigation of wounds or serosal cavities. Individuals treated with 4-6 g/day of the drug by mouth sometimes develop a sprue-like syndrome with diarrhea, steatorrhea, and azotorrhea. Overgrowth of yeasts in the intestine also may occur.

KANAMYCIN

Kanamycin is among the most toxic aminoglycosides and there are few indications for its use. It has no therapeutic advantage over streptomycin or amikacin and probably is more toxic; either should be used instead, depending on susceptibility of the isolate.

For a complete Bibliographical Listing see Goodman & Gilman's *The* ***Pharmacological Basis of Therapeutics***, 12th ed., or Goodman & Gilman Online at www.AccessMedicine.com.

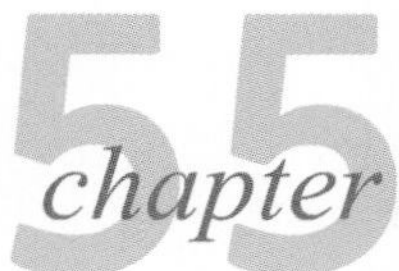

Protein Synthesis Inhibitors and Miscellaneous Antibacterial Agents

The antimicrobial agents discussed in this chapter may be grouped as:

- *Bacteriostatic protein-synthesis inhibitors that target the ribosome*, such as tetracyclines and glycylcyclines, chloramphenicol, macrolides and ketolides, lincosamides (clindamycin), streptogramins (quinupristin/dalfopristin), oxazolidinones (linezolid), and aminocyclitols (spectinomycin).
- *Agents acting on the cell wall or cell membrane* such as polymyxins, glycopeptides (vancomycin and teicoplanin), and lipopeptides (daptomycin).
- *Miscellaneous compounds* acting by diverse mechanisms with limited indications: bacitracin and mupirocin.

TETRACYCLINES AND GLYCYLCYCLINES

The tetracyclines are a series of derivatives of a basic 4-ring structure shown below for doxycycline. Glycylcyclines are tetracycline congers with substituents that confer broad-spectrum activity and activity against bacteria that are resistant to other antibiotics; the available glycylcycline is tigecycline (TYGACIL).

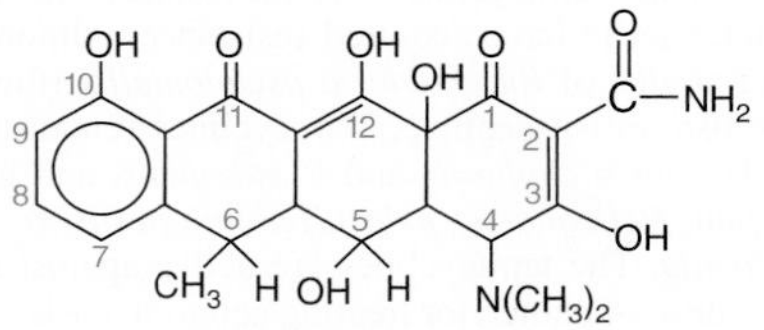

DOXYCYCLINE

MECHANISM OF ACTION. Tetracyclines and glycylcyclines inhibit bacterial protein synthesis by binding to the 30S bacterial ribosome and preventing access of aminoacyl tRNA to the acceptor (A) site on the mRNA-ribosome complex (Figure 55–1). These drugs enter gram-negative bacteria by passive diffusion through channels formed by porins in the outer cell membrane and by active transport that pumps tetracyclines across the cytoplasmic membrane.

ANTIMICROBIAL ACTIVITY. Tetracyclines are bacteriostatic antibiotics with activity against a wide range of aerobic and anaerobic gram-positive and gram-negative bacteria.

Doxycycline, the most important member of the tetracyclines, is a drug of choice for sexually transmitted diseases, rickettsial infections, plague, brucellosis, tularemia, and spirochetal infections, and is also used for treatment of respiratory tract infections including atypical pneumonia pathogens, and for skin and soft-tissue infections caused by community strains of methicillin-resistant *Staphylococcus aureus* (MRSA), for which minocycline also is effective. Glycylcyclines have activity against bacteria that resistant to the first- and second-generation tetracyclines.

These agents are effective against some microorganisms, such as *Rickettsia*, *Coxiella burnetii*, *Mycoplasma pneumoniae*, *Chlamydia* spp., *Legionella* spp., *Ureaplasma*, some atypical mycobacteria, and *Plasmodium* spp., that are resistant to cell-wall-active antimicrobial agents. The tetracyclines are active against many spirochetes, including *Borrelia recurrentis*, *Borrelia burgdorferi* (Lyme disease), *Treponema pallidum* (syphilis), and *Treponema pertenue.* Demeclocycline, tetracycline, minocycline, and doxycycline are available in the U.S. for systemic use. Resistance of a bacterial strain to any 1 member of the class may or may not result in cross-resistance to other tetracyclines. Tigecycline is generally active against organisms that are susceptible to tetracyclines as well as those with acquired resistance to tetracyclines.

Tetracyclines intrinsically are more active against gram-positive than gram-negative microorganisms, but acquired resistance is common. Recent data from the U.S. on the activity of tetracycline and other agents are displayed in Table 55–1. *Bacillus anthracis* and *Listeria monocytogenes* are susceptible. Doxycycline and

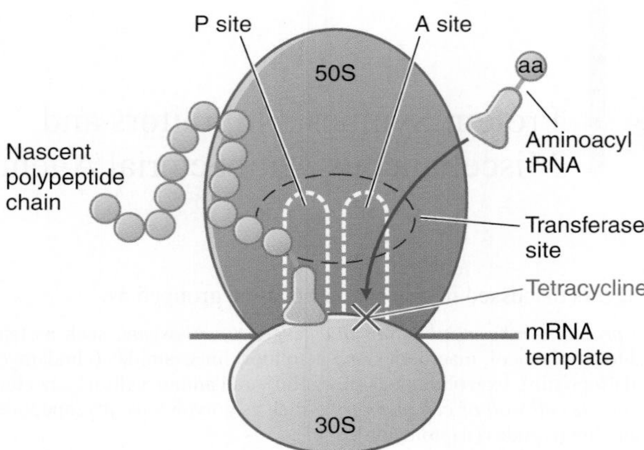

Figure 55–1 *Inhibition of bacterial protein synthesis by tetracyclines.* mRNA attaches to the 30S subunit of bacterial ribosomal RNA. The P (peptidyl) site of the 50S ribosomal RNA subunit contains the nascent polypeptide chain; normally, the aminoacyl tRNA charged with the next amino acid (aa) to be added moves into the A (acceptor) site, with complementary base pairing between the anticodon sequence of tRNA and the codon sequence of mRNA. *Tetracyclines* bind to the 30S subunit, block tRNA binding to the A site, and thereby inhibit protein synthesis.

minocycline can be active against some tetracycline-resistant isolates. *Haemophilus influenzae* is generally susceptible, but many Enterobacteriaceae have acquired resistance. Although all strains of *Pseudomonas aeruginosa* are resistant, 90% of strains of *Burkholderia pseudomallei* (the cause of melioidosis) are sensitive. Most strains of *Brucella* also are susceptible. Tetracyclines remain useful for infections caused by *Haemophilus ducreyi* (chancroid), *Vibrio cholerae*, and *V. vulnificus*, and inhibit the growth of *Legionella pneumophila*, *Campylobacter jejuni*, *Helicobacter pylori*, *Yersinia pestis*, *Yersinia enterocolitica*, *Francisella tularensis*, and *Pasteurella multocida*. The tetracyclines are active against many anaerobic and facultative microorganisms. Tetracycline is a drug of choice for treating actinomycosis.

In general, tigecycline is equally or more active in vitro against bacteria than the tetracyclines, including against tetracycline-resistant organisms, especially gram-negative organisms. There are a few exceptions where other tetracyclines may be more active against certain organisms, such as *Stenotrophomonas* and *Ureaplasma*.

RESISTANCE TO TETRACYCLINES AND GLYCYLCYCLINES. Resistance is primarily plasmid mediated and often inducible. The 3 main resistance mechanisms are:

- Decreased accumulation of tetracycline as a result of either decreased antibiotic influx or acquisition of an energy-dependent efflux pathway
- Production of a ribosomal protection protein that displaces tetracycline from its target
- Enzymatic inactivation of tetracyclines

Cross-resistance, or lack thereof, among tetracyclines depends on which mechanism is operative. Tetracycline resistance due to a ribosomal protection mechanism (*tetM*) produces cross-resistance to doxycycline and minocycline because the target site protected is the same for all tetracyclines. The glycylamido moiety characteristic of tigecycline reduces its affinity for most efflux pumps, restoring activity against many organisms displaying tetracycline resistance due to this mechanism. Binding of glycylcyclines to ribosomes is also enhanced, improving activity against organisms that harbor ribosomal protection proteins that confer resistance to other tetracyclines.

ADME

Oral absorption of most tetracyclines is incomplete. The percentage of unabsorbed drug rises as the dose increases. Tigecycline is available only for parenteral administration. Concurrent ingestion of divalent and trivalent cations (e.g., Ca^{2+}, Mg^{2+}, Al^{3+}, $Fe^{2+/3+}$, and Zn^{2+}) impairs absorption. Thus, dairy products, antacids, aluminum hydroxide gels; Ca, Mg, and Fe or Zn salts; bismuth subsalicylate (e.g., PEPTO-BISMOL) and dietary Fe and Zn supplements can interfere with absorption of tetracyclines. After a single oral dose, the peak plasma concentration is attained in 2-4 h. These drugs have half-lives in the range of 6-12 h and frequently are administered 2 to 4 times daily. Demeclocycline also is incompletely absorbed but can be administered in lower daily dosages because its $t_{1/2}$ of 16 h provides effective plasma concentrations for 24-48 h.

Table 55–1

Activity of Selected Antimicrobials Against Key Gram-Positive Pathogens

	CONCENTRATION OF ANTIMICROBIAL AGENT REQUIRED TO INHIBIT GROWTH OF 90% OF ISOLATES, µg/mL (% SUSCEPTIBLE AT CLINICALLY ACHIEVABLE CONCENTRATIONS OF DRUG)						
	Strep. pyogenes	*Streptococcus pneumoniae*		*Staphylococcus aureus*		*Enterococcus faecalis*	*Enterococcus faecium*
		PCNS	PCNR	MSSA	MRSA		
Tetracycline	4 (89.7)	≤2 (94.6)	>8 (36.7)	≤2 (95.7)	≤2 (93.4)	>8 (24.6)	>8 (58.7)
Tigecycline	≤0.03 (100)	≤0.03 (NR)	≤0.03 (NR)	0.25 (100)	0.25 (99.9)	0.25 (99.9)	0.12 (NR)
Erythromycin	1 (89.7)	>2 (87.3)	>2 (17.2)	>2 (70.8)	>2 (6.1)	>2 (9.1)	>2 (3.0)
Clindamycin	≤0.25 (97.7)	≤0.25 (97.1)	>2 (44.4)	≤0.25 (94.6)	>2 (57.9)	NA	NA
Quinupristin/dalfopristin	≤0.12 (100)	0.5 (99)	0.5 (100)	0.25 (100)	0.5 (100)	8 (3.9)	2 (92.6)
Linezolid	1 (100)	1 (100)	1 (100)	2 (99.9)	2 (99.9)	2 (99.9)	2 (98.0)
Vancomycin	0.25 (100)	≤1 (100)	≤1 (100)	1 (99.9)	1 (99.9)	2 (94.5)	>16 (26.6)
Daptomycin	0.06 (100)	0.12 (NA)	0.12 (NA)	0.25 (100)	0.5 (100)	2 (100)	4 (100)

PCNS, penicillin-susceptible; PCNR, penicillin-resistant; MSSA, methicillin-susceptible Staphylococcus aureus; *MRSA, methicillin-resistant* Staphylococcus aureus; *NR, not reported; NA, not applicable.*

Entries are drug concentrations, in µg/mL, required to inhibit growth of 90% of isolates of that organism. In parentheses below each drug concentration is the percentage of isolates inhibited at clinically useful drug concentrations.

Sources: Gales AC, Sader HS, Fritsche TR. Diagn Microbiol Infect Dis, 2008;60:421–427 and Critchley IA, Blosser-Middleton RS, Jones ME, et al. Antimicrob Agents Chemother, 2003;47:1689–1693.

Oral doses of doxycycline and minocycline are well absorbed (90-100%) and have half-lives of 16-18 h; they can be administered less frequently and at lower doses than tetracycline or demeclocycline. Plasma concentrations are equivalent whether doxycycline is given orally or parenterally. Food, including dairy products, does not interfere with absorption of doxycycline and minocycline.

Tetracyclines distribute widely throughout the body, including urine and prostate. They accumulate in reticuloendothelial cells of the liver, spleen, and bone marrow, and in bone, dentine, and enamel of unerupted teeth. Tigecycline distributes rapidly and extensively into tissues, with an estimated apparent volume of 7-10 L/kg. Inflammation of the meninges is not required for the passage of tetracyclines into the cerebrospinal fluid. Tetracyclines cross the placenta and enter the fetal circulation and amniotic fluid. Relatively high concentrations are found in breast milk.

Except for doxycycline, most tetracyclines are eliminated primarily by the kidney, although they also are concentrated in the liver, excreted in bile, and partially reabsorbed via enterohepatic recirculation. Comparable amounts of tetracycline (i.e., 20-60%) are excreted in the urine within 24 h following oral or intravenous administration. Doxycycline is largely excreted unchanged both in the bile and urine, tigecycline is mostly excreted unchanged along with a small amount of glucuronidated metabolites, and minocycline is extensively metabolized by the liver before excretion. Doses of these agents do not require adjustment in patients with renal dysfunction. Specific dosage adjustment recommendations in hepatic disease are available only for tigecycline. There is some evidence for drug interactions between doxycycline and hepatic enzyme-inducing agents such as phenytoin and rifampin, but not for minocycline or tigecycline.

THERAPEUTIC USES AND DOSAGE

The tetracyclines have been used extensively to treat infectious diseases and as an additive to animal feeds to facilitate growth (a use that likely contributes to the development of bacterial resistance). The drugs remain useful as first-line therapy for infections caused by rickettsiae, mycoplasmas, and chlamydiae. The glycylcyclines have restored much of the antibacterial activity lost to the tetracyclines due to resistance and can be used for a number of infections due to gram-positive and gram-negative organisms.

The oral dose of tetracycline ranges from 1-2 g/day in adults. Children >8 years of age should receive 25-50 mg/kg daily in 4 divided doses. The low pH of tetracycline, but not doxycycline or minocycline, invariably causes phlebitis if infused into a peripheral vein. The oral or intravenous dose of doxycycline for adults is 100 mg every 12 h on the first day and then 50 mg every 12 h, 100 mg once a day, or 100 mg twice daily when severe infection is present; for children >8 years of age, the dose is 4-5 mg/kg/day in 2 divided doses the first day, then 2-2.5 mg/kg given once or twice daily. The dose of minocycline for adults is 200 mg orally or intravenously initially, followed by 100 mg every 12 h; for children, it is 4 mg/kg initially followed by 2 mg/kg every 12 h. Tigecycline is administered intravenously to adults as a 100-mg loading dose, followed by 50 mg every 12 h. For patients with severe hepatic impairment, the loading dose should be followed by a reduced maintenance dose of 25 mg every 12 h. Dosage data are not available for tigecycline in pediatrics.

Tetracyclines should not be administered intramuscularly because of local irritation and poor absorption. GI distress, nausea, and vomiting can be minimized by administration of tetracyclines with food. Generally, oral administration of tetracyclines should occur 2 h before or 2 h after coadministration with any of the agents listed. Cholestyramine and colestipol also bind orally administered tetracyclines and interfere with the absorption of the antibiotic.

Respiratory Tract Infections. Doxycycline has good activity against *Streptococcus pneumoniae* and *H. influenzae* and excellent activity against atypical pathogens such as *Mycoplasma* and *Chlamydophilia pneumoniae.* Tigecycline has been demonstrated to be effective for use as a single agent for adults hospitalized with community-acquired bacterial pneumonia.

Skin and Soft-Tissue Infections. Tigecycline is approved for the treatment of complicated skin and soft-tissue infections. Low doses of tetracycline have been used to treat acne (250 mg orally twice a day).

Intra-abdominal Infections. Resistance among Enterobacteriaceae and gram-negative anaerobes limit the utility of the tetracyclines for intra-abdominal infections. However, tigecycline possesses excellent activity against these pathogens as well as *Enterococcus*.

GI Infections. Therapy with the tetracyclines is often ineffective in infections caused by *Shigella*, *Salmonella*, or other Enterobacteriaceae because of drug-resistant strains. Resistance limits the usefulness of tetracyclines for travelers' diarrhea. Doxycycline (300 mg as a single dose) is effective in reducing stool volume and eradicating *V. cholerae* from the stool within 48 h. Some strains of *V. cholerae* are resistant to tetracyclines.

Sexually Transmitted Diseases. Doxycycline no longer is recommended for gonococcal infections. *Chlamydia trachomatis* often is a coexistent pathogen in acute pelvic inflammatory disease. Doxycycline, 100 mg intravenously twice daily, is recommended for at least 48 h after substantial clinical improvement, followed by oral therapy at the same dosage to complete a 14-day course. Acute epididymitis is caused by infection with *C. trachomatis* or *Neisseria gonorrhoeae* in men <35 years of age. Effective regimens include a single injection of ceftriaxone (250 mg) plus doxycycline, 100 mg orally twice daily for 10 days. Sexual partners also should be treated. Doxycycline (100 mg twice daily for 21 days) is first-line therapy for treatment of lymphogranuloma venereum. Non-pregnant penicillin-allergic patients who have primary, secondary, or latent syphilis can be treated with a tetracycline regimen such as doxycycline, 100 mg orally twice daily for 2 weeks. Tetracyclines should not be used for treatment of neurosyphilis.

Rickettsial Infections. Tetracyclines are life-saving in rickettsial infections, including Rocky Mountain spotted fever, recrudescent epidemic typhus (Brill disease), murine typhus, scrub typhus, rickettsialpox, and Q fever. Clinical improvement often is evident within 24 h after initiation of therapy. Doxycycline is the drug of choice for treatment of Rocky Mountain spotted fever in adults and in children, including those <9 years of age, in whom the risk of staining of permanent teeth is outweighed by the seriousness of this potentially fatal infection.

Anthrax. Doxycycline, 100 mg every 12 h (2.2 mg/kg every 12 h for children weighing <45 kg), is indicated for prevention or treatment of anthrax. It should be used in combination with another agent when treating inhalational or GI infection. The recommended duration of therapy is 60 days for bioterrorism exposures.

Local Application. Except for local use in the eye, topical use of the tetracyclines is not recommended. Minocycline sustained-release microspheres for subgingival administration are used in dentistry.

Other Infections. Tetracyclines in combination with rifampin or streptomycin are effective for acute and chronic infections caused by *Brucella melitensis*, *Brucella suis*, and *Brucella abortus*. Although streptomycin is preferable, tetracyclines also are effective in tularemia. Actinomycosis, although most responsive to penicillin G, may be successfully treated with a tetracycline. Minocycline is an alternative for the treatment of nocardiosis, but a sulfonamide should be used concurrently. Yaws and relapsing fever respond favorably to the tetracyclines. Tetracyclines are useful in the acute treatment and for prophylaxis of leptospirosis (*Leptospira* spp.). *Borrelia* spp., including *B. recurrentis* (relapsing fever) and *B. burgdorferi* (Lyme disease), respond to therapy with a tetracycline. The tetracyclines have been used to treat susceptible atypical mycobacterial pathogens, including *Mycobacterium marinum*.

UNTOWARD EFFECTS

GI. All tetracyclines can produce GI irritation, most commonly after oral administration. Tolerability can be improved by administering these drugs with food, but tetracyclines should not be taken with dairy products or antacids. Tetracycline has been associated with esophagitis, esophageal ulcers, and pancreatitis. *Pseudomembranous colitis caused by overgrowth of* Clostridium difficile *is a potentially life-threatening complication.*

Photosensitivity. Demeclocycline, doxycycline, and other tetracyclines and glycylcyclines to a lesser extent may produce photosensitivity reactions in treated individuals exposed to sunlight.

Hepatic Toxicity. Hepatic toxicity has developed in patients with renal failure receiving ≥2 g of drug per day parenterally, but this effect also may occur when large quantities are administered orally. Pregnant women are particularly susceptible.

Renal Toxicity. Tetracyclines may aggravate azotemia in patients with renal disease because of their catabolic effects. Doxycycline, minocycline, and tigecycline have fewer renal side effects than other tetracyclines. Nephrogenic diabetes insipidus has been observed in some patients receiving demeclocycline, and this phenomenon has been exploited for the treatment of the syndrome of inappropriate secretion of antidiuretic hormone (*see* Chapter 25). Fanconi syndrome has been observed in patients ingesting outdated tetracycline, presumably due to toxic effects on the proximal renal tubules.

Effects on Teeth. Children treated with a tetracycline or glycylcycline may develop permanent brown discoloration of the teeth. The duration of therapy appears to be less important than the total quantity of antibiotic administered. The risk is highest when a tetracycline is given to infants before the first dentition but may develop if the drug is given between the ages of 2 months and 5 years when these teeth are being calcified. Treatment of pregnant patients with tetracyclines may produce discoloration of the teeth in their children.

Other Toxic and Irritative Effects. Tetracyclines are deposited in the skeleton during gestation and throughout childhood and may depress bone growth in premature infants. This is readily reversible if the period of exposure to the drug is short. Thrombophlebitis frequently follows intravenous administration. This irritative effect of tetracyclines has been used therapeutically in patients with malignant pleural effusions. Long-term tetracycline therapy may produce leukocytosis, atypical lymphocytes, toxic granulation of granulocytes, and thrombocytopenic purpura. Tetracyclines may cause increased intracranial pressure (pseudotumor cerebri) in young infants, even when given in the usual therapeutic doses. Patients receiving minocycline may experience vestibular toxicity, manifested by dizziness, ataxia, nausea, and vomiting. The symptoms occur soon after the initial dose and generally disappear within 24-48 h after drug cessation. Various skin reactions rarely may follow the use of any of the tetracyclines. Among the more severe allergic responses are angioedema and anaphylaxis; anaphylactoid reactions can occur even after the oral use. Other hypersensitivity reactions are burning of the eyes, cheilosis, atrophic or hypertrophic glossitis, pruritus ani or vulvae, and vaginitis. Fever of varying degrees and eosinophilia may occur when these agents are administered. Asthma also has been observed. Cross-sensitization among the various tetracyclines is common.

CHLORAMPHENICOL

Chloramphenicol can cause serious and fatal blood dyscrasias; consequently, the drug is now reserved for treatment of life-threatening infections in patients who cannot take safer alternatives because of resistance or allergies.

MECHANISM OF ACTION. Chloramphenicol inhibits protein synthesis in bacteria, and to a lesser extent, in eukaryotic cells. Chloramphenicol acts primarily by binding reversibly to the 50S ribosomal subunit (near the binding site for the macrolide antibiotics and clindamycin). The drug prevents the binding of the amino acid–containing end of the aminoacyl tRNA to the acceptor site on the 50S ribosomal subunit. The interaction between peptidyltransferase and its amino acid substrate cannot occur, and peptide bond formation is inhibited (Figure 55–2).

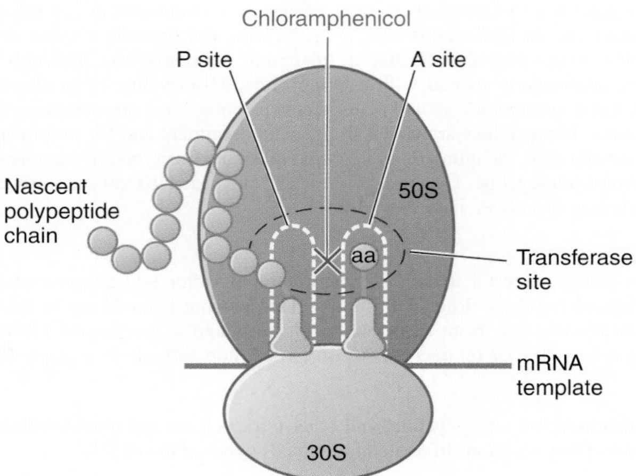

Figure 55–2 *Inhibition of bacterial protein synthesis by chloramphenicol.* Chloramphenicol binds to the 50S ribosomal subunit at the peptidyltransferase site, inhibiting transpeptidation. Chloramphenicol binds near the site of action of clindamycin and the macrolide antibiotics. These agents interfere with the binding of chloramphenicol and thus may interfere with each other's actions if given concurrently. *See* Figure 55–1 for additional information.

Chloramphenicol also can inhibit mitochondrial protein synthesis in mammalian cells, perhaps because mitochondrial ribosomes resemble bacterial ribosomes (both are 70S); erythropoietic cells are particularly sensitive.

ANTIMICROBIAL ACTIVITY. Chloramphenicol is bacteriostatic against most species, although it may be bactericidal against *H. influenzae*, *Neisseria meningitidis*, and *S. pneumoniae.* Many gram-negative bacteria and most anaerobic bacteria are inhibited in vitro. Strains of *S. aureus* tend to be less susceptible. Chloramphenicol is active against *Mycoplasma*, *Chlamydia*, and *Rickettsia.* Enterobacteriaceae are variably sensitive to chloramphenicol. *P. aeruginosa* is resistant to even very high concentrations of chloramphenicol. Strains of *V. cholerae* have remained largely susceptible to chloramphenicol. Prevalent strains of *Shigella* and *Salmonella* are resistant to multiple drugs, including chloramphenicol.

RESISTANCE TO CHLORAMPHENICOL. Resistance to chloramphenicol usually is caused by a plasmid-encoded acetyltransferase that inactivates the drug. Resistance also can result from decreased permeability and from ribosomal mutation.

ADME. Chloramphenicol is absorbed rapidly from the GI tract. For parenteral use, chloramphenicol succinate is a prodrug that is hydrolyzed by esterases to chloramphenicol in vivo. Chloramphenicol succinate is rapidly cleared from plasma by the kidneys; this may reduce overall bioavailability of the drug because as much as 30% of the dose may be excreted before hydrolysis. Poor renal function in the neonate and other states of renal insufficiency result in increased plasma concentrations of chloramphenicol succinate. Decreased esterase activity has been observed in the plasma of neonates and infants, prolonging time to peak concentrations of active chloramphenicol (up to 4 h) and extending the period over which renal clearance of chloramphenicol succinate can occur.

Chloramphenicol is widely distributed in body fluids and readily reaches therapeutic concentrations in CSF. The drug actually may accumulate in the brain. Chloramphenicol is present in bile, milk, and placental fluid. It also is found in the aqueous humor after subconjunctival injection. Hepatic metabolism to the inactive glucuronide is the major route of elimination. This metabolite and chloramphenicol are excreted in the urine. Patients with impaired hepatic function have decreased metabolic clearance, and dosage should be adjusted. About 50% of chloramphenicol is bound to plasma proteins; such binding is reduced in cirrhotic patients and in neonates. Half-life is not altered significantly by renal insufficiency or hemodialysis, and dosage adjustment usually is not required. However, if the dose of chloramphenicol has been reduced because of cirrhosis, clearance by hemodialysis may be significant. This effect can be minimized by administering the drug at the end of hemodialysis. Variability in the metabolism and pharmacokinetics of chloramphenicol in neonates, infants, and children necessitates monitoring of drug concentrations in plasma.

THERAPEUTIC USES AND DOSAGE. *Therapy with chloramphenicol must be limited to infections for which the benefits of the drug outweigh the risks of the potential toxicities. When other antimicrobial drugs that are equally effective and less toxic are available, they should be used instead of chloramphenicol.*

Typhoid Fever. Third-generation cephalosporins and quinolones are drugs of choice for the treatment of typhoid fever. The adult dose of chloramphenicol for typhoid fever is 1 g every 6 h for 4 weeks.

Bacterial Meningitis. Chloramphenicol remains an alternative drug for the treatment of meningitis caused by *H. influenzae*, *N. meningitidis*, and *S. pneumoniae* in patients who have severe allergy to β-lactams and in developing countries. The total daily dose for children should be 50 mg/kg of body weight, divided into 4 equal doses given intravenously every 6 h.

Rickettsial Diseases. The tetracyclines usually are the preferred agents for the treatment of rickettsial diseases. However, in patients allergic to these drugs, in those with reduced renal function, in pregnant women, and in children <8 years of age who require prolonged or repeated courses of therapy, chloramphenicol may be the drug of choice. Rocky Mountain spotted fever, epidemic, murine, scrub, and recrudescent typhus, and Q fever respond well to chloramphenicol. For adults and children with these diseases, a dosage of 50 mg/kg/day divided into 6-h intervals is recommended. Therapy should be continued until the general condition has improved and is afebrile for 24-48 h.

UNTOWARD EFFECTS. Chloramphenicol inhibits the synthesis of proteins of the inner mitochondrial membrane, probably by inhibiting the ribosomal peptidyltransferase. Much of the toxicity observed with this drug can be attributed to these effects.

Hypersensitivity Reactions. Skin rashes may result from hypersensitivity to chloramphenicol. Fever may appear simultaneously or be the sole manifestation. Angioedema is a rare complication. Jarisch-Herxheimer reactions may occur after institution of chloramphenicol therapy for syphilis, brucellosis, and typhoid fever.

Hematological Toxicity. Chloramphenicol affects the hematopoietic system in 2 ways: a dose-related toxicity that presents as anemia, leukopenia, or thrombocytopenia, and an idiosyncratic response manifested by aplastic anemia, leading in many cases to fatal pancytopenia. Pancytopenia occurs more commonly in individuals who undergo prolonged therapy and especially in those who are exposed to the drug on more than 1 occasion. Although the incidence of the reaction is low, ~1 in ≥30,000 courses of therapy, the fatality rate is high when bone marrow aplasia is complete, and there is an increased incidence of acute leukemia in those who recover. Aplastic anemia accounts for ~70% of cases of blood dyscrasias due to chloramphenicol; hypoplastic anemia, agranulocytosis, and thrombocytopenia make up the remainder. The proposed mechanism involves conversion of the nitro group to a toxic intermediate by intestinal bacteria.

The risk of aplastic anemia does not contraindicate the use of chloramphenicol in situations in which it may be lifesaving. The drug should never be used, however, in undefined situations or in diseases readily, safely, and effectively treatable with other antimicrobial agents.

Dose-related, reversible erythroid suppression probably reflects an inhibitory action of chloramphenicol on mitochondrial protein synthesis in erythroid precursors, which in turn impairs iron incorporation into heme. Bone marrow suppression occurs regularly when plasma concentrations are ≥25 μg/mL and is observed with the use of large doses of chloramphenicol, prolonged treatment, or both. Dose-related suppression of the bone marrow may progress to fatal aplasia if treatment is continued, but most cases of bone marrow aplasia develop without prior dose-related marrow suppression.

Other Toxic and Irritative Effects. Nausea and vomiting, unpleasant taste, diarrhea, and perineal irritation may follow the oral administration of chloramphenicol. Blurring of vision and digital paresthesias may rarely occur. Tissues that have a high rate of oxygen consumption (e.g., heart, brain) may be particularly susceptible to chloramphenicol's effects on mitochondrial enzymes.

Neonates, especially if premature, may develop a serious illness termed *gray baby syndrome* if exposed to excessive doses of chloramphenicol. This syndrome usually begins 2-9 days after treatment is started. Within the first 24 h, vomiting, refusal to suck, irregular and rapid respiration, abdominal distention, periods of cyanosis, and passage of loose green stools occur. Over the next 24 h, neonates turn an ashen-gray color and become flaccid and hypothermic. A similar "gray syndrome" has been reported in adults who were accidentally overdosed with the drug. Death occurs in ~40% of patients within 2 days of initial symptoms. Those who recover usually exhibit no sequelae. Two mechanisms apparently are responsible for chloramphenicol toxicity in neonates: (1) a developmental deficiency of glucuronyl transferase, the hepatic enzyme that metabolizes chloramphenicol; and (2) inadequate renal excretion of unconjugated drug. At the onset of the clinical syndrome, chloramphenicol concentrations in plasma usually exceed 100 μg/mL, and may be as low as 75 μg/mL. Children ≤2 weeks of age should receive chloramphenicol in a daily dose no larger than 25 mg/kg of body weight; after this age, full-term infants may be given daily quantities up to 50 mg/kg.

Drug Interactions. Chloramphenicol inhibits hepatic CYPs and thereby prolongs the half-lives of drugs that are metabolized by this system. Severe toxicity and death have occurred because of failure to recognize such effects. Concurrent administration of phenobarbital or rifampin, which potently induce CYPs, shortens the $t_{1/2}$ of the antibiotic and may result in subtherapeutic drug concentrations.

MACROLIDES AND KETOLIDES

Macrolides and ketolides are effective for treatment of respiratory tract infections caused by the common pathogens of community-acquired pneumonia. All except azithromycin have important drug interactions because they inhibit hepatic CYPs.

Chapter 55 of the parent text includes a fuller presentation of the structure-activity data of these compounds. *Macrolide antibiotics* contain a multi-membered lactone ring to which are attached 1 or more deoxy sugars. Modest structural modifications (e.g., in *clarithromycin* and *azithromycin*) improve acid stability and tissue penetration and broaden the spectrum of activity. *Ketolides* are structurally similar multi-membered ring systems but with different substituents. *Telithromycin* (KETEK) is the only ketolide currently approved in the U.S. Telithromycin differs from erythromycin in that a 3-keto group replaces the α-L-cladinose of the 14-member macrolide ring, and there is a substituted carbamate at C11-C12. These modifications render ketolides less susceptible to methylase-mediated (*erm*) and efflux-mediated (*mef* or *msr*) mechanisms of resistance. Ketolides therefore are active against many macrolide-resistant gram-positive strains.

MECHANISM OF ACTION. Macrolide antibiotics are bacteriostatic agents that inhibit protein synthesis by binding reversibly to 50S ribosomal subunits of sensitive microorganisms (Figure 55–3), at or very near the site that binds chloramphenicol (*see* Figure 55–2). Erythromycin does not inhibit peptide bond formation per se but rather inhibits the translocation step wherein a newly synthesized peptidyl tRNA molecule moves from the acceptor site on the ribosome to the peptidyl donor site. Gram-positive bacteria accumulate ~100 times more erythromycin than do gram-negative bacteria. Ketolides and macrolides have the same ribosomal target site.

ANTIMICROBIAL ACTIVITY. Erythromycin usually is bacteriostatic but may be bactericidal in high concentrations against susceptible organisms. The antibiotic is most active in vitro against aerobic gram-positive cocci and bacilli (*see* Table 55–1). Macrolide resistance among *S. pneumoniae* often co-exists with penicillin resistance. Staphylococci are not reliably sensitive to erythromycin. Macrolide-resistant strains of *S. aureus* are potentially cross-resistant to clindamycin and streptogramin B (quinupristin). Gram-positive bacilli also are sensitive to erythromycin, including *Clostridium perfringens*, *Corynebacterium diphtheriae*, and *L. monocytogenes*.

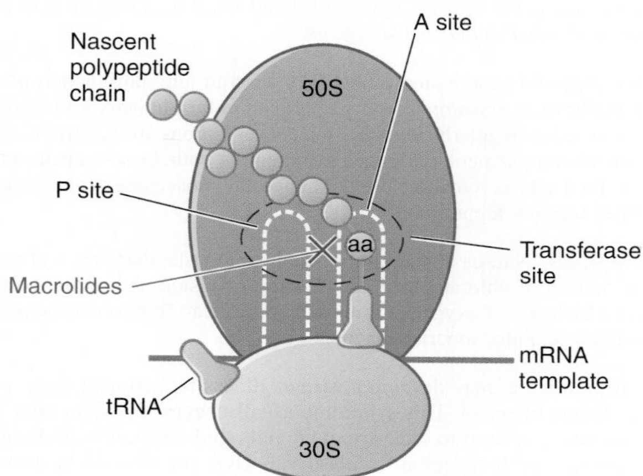

Figure 55–3 *Inhibition of bacterial protein synthesis by the erythromycin, clarithromycin, and azithromycin.* Macrolide antibiotics are bacteriostatic agents that inhibit protein synthesis by binding reversibly to the 50S ribosomal subunits of sensitive organisms. Erythromycin appears to inhibit the translocation step such that the nascent peptide chain temporarily residing at the A site fails to move to the P, or donor, site. Alternatively, macrolides may bind and cause a conformational change that terminates protein synthesis by indirectly interfering with transpeptidation and translocation. *See* Figure 55–1 for additional information.

Erythromycin is inactive against most aerobic enteric gram-negative bacilli. It has modest activity in vitro against *H. influenzae* and *N. meningitidis*, and good activity against most strains of *N. gonorrhoeae*. Useful antibacterial activity also is observed against *P. multocida*, *Borrelia* spp., and *Bordetella pertussis*. Resistance is common for *B. fragilis*. Macrolides are usually active against *C. jejuni*. Erythromycin is active against *M. pneumoniae* and *L. pneumophila*. Most strains of *C. trachomatis* are inhibited by erythromycin. Some of the atypical mycobacteria are sensitive to erythromycin in vitro.

Clarithromycin is slightly more potent than erythromycin against sensitive strains of streptococci and staphylococci, and has modest activity against *H. influenzae* and *N. gonorrhoeae*. Clarithromycin and azithromycin have good activity against *Moraxella catarrhalis*, *Chlamydia* spp., *L. pneumophila*, *B. burgdorferi*, *M. pneumoniae*, and *H. pylori*. Azithromycin and clarithromycin have enhanced activity against *Mycobacterium avium-intracellulare*, as well as against some protozoa (e.g., *Toxoplasma gondii*, *Cryptosporidium*, and *Plasmodium* spp.). Clarithromycin has good activity against *Mycobacterium leprae*. Telithromycin's spectrum of activity is similar to those of clarithromycin and azithromycin. Telithromycin's capacity to withstand many macrolide resistance mechanisms increases its activity against macrolide-resistant *S. pneumoniae* and *S. aureus*.

RESISTANCE TO MACROLIDES AND KETOLIDES. Resistance to macrolides usually results from 1 of 4 mechanisms:

- Drug efflux by an active pump mechanism
- Ribosomal protection by inducible or constitutive production of methylase enzymes, that modify the ribosomal target and decrease drug binding
- Macrolide hydrolysis by esterases produced by Enterobacteriaceae
- Chromosomal mutations that alter a 50S ribosomal protein (in *Bacillus subtilis, Campylobacter* spp., mycobacteria, and gram-positive cocci)

ADME

Absorption. Erythromycin base is incompletely but adequately absorbed from the upper small intestine. Because it is inactivated by gastric acid, it is administered as enteric-coated tablets, as capsules containing enteric-coated pellets that dissolve in the duodenum, or as an ester. Food may delay absorption. Esters of erythromycin base (e.g., stearate, estolate, and ethylsuccinate) have improved acid stability, and their absorption is less altered by food. A single oral 250-mg dose of erythromycin estolate produces peak serum concentrations of ~1.5 μg/mL after 2 h.

Clarithromycin is absorbed rapidly from the GI tract after oral administration, but hepatic first-pass metabolism reduces its bioavailability to 50-55%. Peak concentrations occur ~2 h after drug administration. Clarithromycin may be given with or without food, but the extended-release form, typically given once daily as a 1-g dose, should be administered with food to improve bioavailability. Azithromycin administered orally is absorbed rapidly and distributes widely throughout the body, except to the brain and CSF. Azithromycin should not be administered with food. Azithromycin also can be administered intravenously, producing plasma concentrations of 3-4 μg/mL after a 1-h infusion of 500 mg. Telithromycin is formulated as a 400-mg tablet for oral administration. There is no parenteral form. It is well absorbed with ~60% bioavailability. Peak serum concentrations are achieved within 30 min to 4 h.

Distribution. Erythromycin diffuses readily into intracellular fluids, achieving antibacterial activity in essentially all sites except the brain and CSF. Concentrations in middle ear exudate may be inadequate for the treatment of otitis media caused by *H. influenzae.* Protein binding is ~70-80% for erythromycin base and even higher for the estolate. Erythromycin traverses the placenta, and drug concentrations in fetal plasma are ~5-20% of those in the maternal circulation. Concentrations in breast milk are 50% of those in serum.

Clarithromycin and its active metabolite, 14-hydroxyclarithromycin, achieve high intracellular concentrations throughout the body, including the middle ear. Azithromycin's unique pharmacokinetic properties include extensive tissue distribution and high drug concentrations within cells (including phagocytes), resulting in much greater concentrations of drugs in tissue or secretions compared to simultaneous serum concentrations. Telithromycin penetrates well into most tissues, exceeding plasma concentrations by ~2-fold to ≥10-fold. Telithromycin is concentrated into macrophages and white blood cells, where concentrations of 40 μg/mL (500 times the plasma concentration) are maintained 24 h after dosing.

Elimination. Only 2-5% of orally administered erythromycin is excreted in active form in the urine; this value is from 12-15% after intravenous infusion. The antibiotic is concentrated in the liver and excreted in the bile. The serum $t_{1/2}$ of erythromycin is ~1.6 h. Although the $t_{1/2}$ may be prolonged in patients with anuria, dosage reduction is not routinely recommended in renal failure patients. The drug is not removed significantly by either peritoneal dialysis or hemodialysis.

Clarithromycin is metabolized in the liver to several metabolites; the active 14-hydroxy metabolite is the most significant. Primary metabolic pathways are oxidative *N*-demethylation and hydroxylation at the 14 position.

The elimination half-lives are 3-7 h for clarithromycin and 5-9 h for 14-hydroxyclarithromycin. Metabolism is saturable, resulting in nonlinear pharmacokinetics, and longer half-lives with higher dosages. The amount of clarithromycin excreted unchanged in the urine ranges from 20-40%, depending on the dose administered and the formulation (tablet versus oral suspension). An additional 10-15% of a dose is excreted in the urine as 14-hydroxyclarithromycin. Dose adjustment is not necessary unless the creatinine clearance is <30 mL/min.

Azithromycin undergoes some hepatic metabolism to inactive metabolites, but biliary excretion is the major route of elimination. Only 12% of drug is excreted unchanged in the urine. The elimination $t_{1/2}$, 40-68 h, is prolonged because of extensive tissue sequestration and binding. With a $t_{1/2}$ of 9.8 h, telithromycin can be given once daily. The drug is cleared primarily by hepatic metabolism, 50% by CYP3A4 and 50% by CYP-independent metabolism. No adjustment of the dose is required for hepatic failure or mild-to-moderate renal failure.

THERAPEUTIC USES AND DOSAGE. The usual oral dose of erythromycin (erythromycin base) for adults ranges from 1-2 g/day, in divided doses, usually given every 6 h. Daily doses of erythromycin as large as 8 g orally, given for 3 months, have been well tolerated. Food should not be taken concurrently, if possible, with erythromycin base or the stearate formulations, but this is not necessary with erythromycin estolate. The oral dose of erythromycin for children is 30-50 mg/kg/day, divided into 4 portions; this dose may be doubled for severe infections. Intramuscular administration of erythromycin is not recommended because of pain upon injection. Intravenous administration is generally reserved for the therapy of severe infections, such as legionellosis. The usual dose is 0.5-1 g every 6 h; 1 g of erythromycin gluceptate (not available in the U.S.) has been given intravenously every 6 h for as long as 4 weeks with no adverse effects except for local thrombophlebitis. Erythromycin lactobionate is available for intravenous injection. The combination of erythromycin and sulfisoxazole appears to have synergistic antibacterial activity; it is available as a suspension used primarily for treatment of otitis media in children.

Clarithromycin (BIAXIN, others) usually is given twice daily at a dose of 250 mg for children >12 years and adults with mild to moderate infection. Larger doses (e.g., 500 mg twice daily) are indicated for more severe infection such as pneumonia or infections caused by more resistant organisms such as *H. influenzae*. The 500-mg extended-release formulation is given as 2 tablets once daily. Clarithromycin (500 mg) is also packaged with lansoprazole (30 mg) and amoxicillin (1 g) as a combination regimen (PREVPAC) that is administered twice daily for 10 or 14 days to eradicate *H. pylori*.

Azithromycin (ZITHROMAX, other) should be given 1 h before or 2 h after meals when administered orally. For outpatient therapy of community-acquired pneumonia, pharyngitis, or skin and skin-structure infections, a loading dose of 500 mg is given on the first day, and then 250 mg per day is given for days 2 through 5. Treatment or prophylaxis of *M. avium-intracellulare* infection in AIDS patients requires higher doses: 600 mg daily in combination with 1 or more other agents for treatment, or 1200 mg once weekly for primary prevention. Azithromycin is useful in treatment of sexually transmitted diseases, especially during pregnancy when tetracyclines are contraindicated. The treatment of uncomplicated nongonococcal urethritis presumed to be caused by *C. trachomatis* consists of a single 1-g dose of azithromycin. This dose also is effective for chancroid. Azithromycin (1 g per week for 3 weeks) is an alternative regimen for treatment of granuloma inguinale or lymphogranuloma venereum. In children, the recommended dose of azithromycin oral suspension for acute otitis media and pneumonia is 10 mg/kg on the first day (maximum: 500 mg) and 5 mg/kg (maximum: 250 mg/day) on days 2 through 5. A single 30 mg/kg dose is approved as an alternative for otitis media. The dose for tonsillitis or pharyngitis is 12 mg/kg/day, up to 500 mg total, for 5 days.

Respiratory Tract Infections. Macrolides and ketolides are suitable drugs for the treatment of a number of respiratory tract infections. Azithromycin and clarithromycin are suitable choices for treatment of mild to moderate community-acquired pneumonia among ambulatory patients. In hospitalized patients, a macrolide is commonly added to a cephalosporin for coverage of atypical respiratory pathogens. Macrolides, fluoroquinolones, and tetracyclines are drugs of choice for treatment of pneumonia caused by *C. pneumoniae* or *M. pneumoniae*. Erythromycin has been considered as the drug of choice for treatment of pneumonia caused by *L. pneumophila*, *Legionella micdadei*, or other *Legionella* spp. Because of excellent in vitro activity, superior tissue concentration, the ease of administration as a single daily dose, and better tolerability compared to erythromycin, azithromycin (or a fluoroquinolone) has supplanted erythromycin as the first-line agent for treatment of legionellosis. The recommended dose is 500 mg daily, intravenously or orally, for a total of 10-14 days. Macrolides are also appropriate alternative agents for the treatment of acute exacerbations of chronic bronchitis, acute otitis media, acute streptococcal pharyngitis, and acute bacterial sinusitis. Azithromycin or clarithromycin are generally preferred to erythromycin for these indications due to their broader spectrum and superior tolerability.

Telithromycin is effective in the treatment of community-acquired pneumonia, acute exacerbations of chronic bronchitis, and acute bacterial sinusitis, and has a potential advantage where macrolide-resistant strains are common. Due to a number of cases of severe hepatotoxicity, the drug's FDA approval is limited to community-acquired pneumonia; *telithromycin should be used only in circumstances where it provides a substantial advantage over less toxic therapies.*

Skin and Soft-Tissue Infections. Macrolides are alternatives for treatment of erysipelas and cellulitis among patients who have a serious allergy to penicillin. Erythromycin has been an alternative agent for the treatment of relatively minor skin and soft-tissue infections caused by either penicillin-sensitive or penicillin-resistant *S. aureus*. However, many strains of *S. aureus* are resistant to macrolides.

Chlamydial Infections. Chlamydial infections can be treated effectively with any of the macrolides. A single 1-g dose of azithromycin is recommended for patients with uncomplicated urethral, endocervical, rectal, or epididymal infections because of the ease of compliance. During pregnancy, erythromycin base, 500 mg 4 times daily for 7 days, is recommended as first-line therapy for chlamydial urogenital infections. Azithromycin, 1 g orally as a single dose, is a suitable alternative. Erythromycin base is preferred for chlamydial pneumonia of infancy and ophthalmia neonatorum (50 mg/kg/day in 4 divided doses for 10-14 days). Azithromycin, 1 g/week for 3 weeks, may be effective for lymphogranuloma venereum.

Diphtheria. Erythromycin, 250 mg 4 times daily for 7 days, is very effective for acute infections or for eradicating the carrier state. Other macrolides are not FDA-approved for this indication. Antibiotics do not alter the course of an acute infection with diphtheria or decrease the risk of complications. Antitoxin is indicated in the treatment of acute infection.

Pertussis. Erythromycin is the drug of choice for treating persons with *B. pertussis* disease and for postexposure prophylaxis of household members and close contacts. A 7-day regimen of erythromycin estolate (40 mg/kg/day; maximum: 1 g/day; not available in U.S.) is effective. Clarithromycin and azithromycin also are effective. If administered early in the course of whooping cough, erythromycin may shorten the duration of illness; it has little influence on the disease once the paroxysmal stage is reached. Nasopharyngeal cultures should be obtained from people with pertussis who do not improve with erythromycin therapy because resistance has been reported.

Campylobacter Infections. Fluoroquinolones have largely has replaced erythromycin for this disease in adults. Erythromycin remains useful for treatment of *Campylobacter* gastroenteritis in children.

Helicobacter pylori Infection. Clarithromycin, 500 mg, in combination with omeprazole, 20 mg, and amoxicillin, 1 g (PREVPAC), each administered twice daily for 10-14 days, is effective for treatment of peptic ulcer disease caused by *H. pylori*.

Mycobacterial Infections. Clarithromycin or azithromycin is recommended as first-line therapy for prophylaxis and treatment of disseminated infection caused by *M. avium-intracellulare* in AIDS patients and for treatment of pulmonary disease in patients not infected with HIV. Azithromycin (1.2 g once weekly) or clarithromycin (500 mg twice daily) is recommended for primary prevention for AIDS patients with <50 CD4 cells/mm^3. Single-agent therapy should not be used for treatment of active disease or for secondary prevention in AIDS patients. Clarithromycin (500 mg twice daily) plus ethambutol (15 mg/kg once daily) with or without rifabutin is an effective combination regimen. Clarithromycin also has been used with minocycline for the treatment of *M. leprae* in lepromatous leprosy.

Prophylactic Uses. Erythromycin is an effective alternative for the prophylaxis of recurrences of rheumatic fever in individuals who are allergic to penicillin. Clarithromycin or azithromycin (or clindamycin) are recommended alternatives for the prevention of bacterial endocarditis in patients undergoing dental procedures.

UNTOWARD EFFECTS

Hepatotoxicity. Cholestatic hepatitis is the most striking side effect. It is caused primarily by erythromycin estolate and rarely by the ethylsuccinate or the stearate. The illness starts after 10-20 days of treatment and is characterized initially by nausea, vomiting, and abdominal cramps. These symptoms are followed shortly thereafter by jaundice, which may be accompanied by fever, leukocytosis, eosinophilia, and elevated transaminases in plasma. Findings usually resolve within a few days after cessation of drug therapy. Hepatotoxicity has also been observed with clarithromycin and azithromycin, although at a lower rate than with erythromycin. Telithromycin may induce severe hepatotoxicity and should only be used in circumstances where it represents a clear advantage over alternative agents.

GI Toxicity. Oral administration of erythromycin, frequently is accompanied by epigastric distress, which may be quite severe. Intravenous administration of erythromycin may cause similar symptoms. Erythromycin stimulates GI motility by acting on motilin receptors (*see* Chapter 46). The GI symptoms are dose related and occur more commonly in children and young adults; they may be reduced by prolonging the infusion time to 1 h or by pretreatment with glycopyrrolate. Intravenous infusion of 1-g doses, even when dissolved in a large volume, often is followed by thrombophlebitis. This can be minimized by slow rates of infusion. Clarithromycin, azithromycin, and telithromycin also may cause GI distress, but to a lesser degree than erythromycin.

Cardiac Toxicity. Erythromycin, clarithromycin, and telithromycin have been reported to cause cardiac arrhythmias, including QT prolongation with ventricular tachycardia. Most patients have had underlying risk factors or were receiving anti-arrhythmics or other agents that prolong QTc.

Other Toxic and Irritative Effects. Allergic reactions observed are fever, eosinophilia, and skin eruptions, which disappear shortly after therapy is stopped. Transient auditory impairment with erythromycin has been observed. Visual disturbances due to slowed accommodation have been reported following telithromycin. Telithromycin is contraindicated in patients with myasthenia gravis due to exacerbation of neurological symptoms. Loss of consciousness has been associated with telithromycin.

Drug Interactions. Erythromycin, clarithromycin, and telithromycin inhibit CYP3A4 and cause significant drug interactions. Erythromycin and clarithromycin potentiate the effects of carbamazepine, corticosteroids, cyclosporine, digoxin, ergot alkaloids, theophylline, triazolam, valproate, and warfarin, probably by interfering with CYP-mediated metabolism of these drugs (*see* Chapter 6). Telithromycin is both a substrate and a strong inhibitor of CYP3A4. Coadministration of rifampin, a potent inducer of CYP, decreases the serum concentrations of telithromycin by 80%. CYP3A4 inhibitors (e.g., itraconazole) increase peak serum concentrations of telithromycin. Azithromycin and dirithromycin appear to be free of these drug interactions; however, caution is advised.

LINCOSAMIDES (CLINDAMYCIN)

Clindamycin is a congener of lincomycin. Clindamycin principally is used to treat anaerobic infections.

ANTIMICROBIAL ACTIVITY. Clindamycin generally is similar to erythromycin in its in vitro activity against susceptible strains of pneumococci, *Streptococcus pyogenes*, and viridans streptococci (*see* Table 55–1). Methicillin-susceptible strains of *S. aureus* usually are susceptible to clindamycin, but MRSA and coagulase-negative staphylococci frequently are resistant. Clindamycin is more active than erythromycin or clarithromycin against anaerobic bacteria, especially *B. fragilis*. From 10-20% of clostridial species other than *C. perfringens* are resistant. Resistance to clindamycin in *Bacteroides* spp. increasingly is encountered. Strains of *Actinomyces israelii* and *Nocardia asteroides* are sensitive. Essentially all aerobic gram-negative bacilli are resistant. Clindamycin plus primaquine and clindamycin plus pyrimethamine are second-line regimens for *Pneumocystis jiroveci* pneumonia and *T. gondii* encephalitis, respectively.

MECHANISM OF ACTION; RESISTANCE. Clindamycin binds exclusively to the 50S subunit of bacterial ribosomes and suppresses protein synthesis. Although clindamycin, erythromycin, and chloramphenicol are not structurally related, they act at sites in close proximity (*see* Figures 55–2 and 55–3), and binding by one of these antibiotics to the ribosome may inhibit the interaction of the others. Macrolide resistance due to ribosomal methylation also may produce resistance to clindamycin. Because clindamycin does not induce the methylase, there is cross-resistance only if the enzyme is produced constitutively. Clindamycin is not a substrate for macrolide efflux pumps; thus strains that are resistant to macrolides by this mechanism are susceptible to clindamycin.

ADME. Clindamycin is nearly completely absorbed following oral administration. Peak C_p of 2-3 μg/mL are attained within 1 h after the ingestion of 150 mg. Food in the stomach does not reduce absorption significantly. The $t_{1/2}$ of the antibiotic is ~3 h. Clindamycin palmitate, an oral preparation for pediatric use, is an inactive prodrug that is hydrolyzed rapidly in vivo. The phosphate ester of clindamycin, which is given parenterally, also is rapidly hydrolyzed in vivo to the active parent compound.

Clindamycin is widely distributed in many fluids and tissues, including bone but not to CSF, even when the meninges are inflamed. Concentrations sufficient to treat cerebral toxoplasmosis are achievable. The drug readily crosses the placental barrier. Ninety percent or more of clindamycin is bound to plasma proteins. Clindamycin accumulates in polymorphonuclear leukocytes, alveolar macrophages, and in abscesses.

Clindamycin is inactivated by metabolism to *N*-demethylclindamycin and clindamycin sulfoxide, which are excreted in the urine and bile. Dosage adjustments may be required in patients with severe hepatic failure. Only ~10% of the clindamycin administered is excreted unaltered in the urine, and small quantities are found in the feces. However, antimicrobial activity persists in feces for ≥5 days after parenteral therapy with clindamycin is stopped and growth of clindamycin-sensitive microorganisms may be suppressed for up to 2 weeks.

THERAPEUTIC USES AND DOSAGE. The oral dose of clindamycin (clindamycin hydrochloride [CLEOCIN]) for adults is 150-300 mg every 6 h; for severe infections, it is 300-600 mg every 6 h. Children should receive 8-12 mg/kg/day of clindamycin palmitate hydrochloride (CLEOCIN PEDIATRIC) in 3 or 4 divided doses or for severe infections, 13-25 mg/kg/day. However, children weighing ≤10 kg should receive ½ teaspoonful of clindamycin palmitate hydrochloride (37.5 mg) every 8 h as a minimal dose. For serious infections, intravenous or intramuscular administration is recommended in dosages of 1200-2400 mg/day, divided into 3 or 4 equal doses for adults. Children should receive 15-40 mg/kg/day in 3 or 4 divided doses; in severe infections, a minimal daily dose of 300 mg is recommended, regardless of body weight.

Clindamycin is the drug of choice for treatment of lung abscess and anaerobic lung and pleural space infections. Clindamycin (600 mg intravenously every 8 h, or 300-450 mg orally every 6 h for less severe disease) in combination with primaquine (15 mg of base once daily) is useful for the treatment of mild to moderate cases of *P. jiroveci* pneumonia in AIDS patients. Clindamycin is an alternative agent for the treatment of skin and soft-tissue infections, especially in patients with β-lactam allergies. However, *the high incidence of diarrhea and the occurrence of pseudomembranous colitis should limit its use to infections where it represents a clear therapeutic advantage.*

Clindamycin (600-1200 mg given intravenously every 6 h) in combination with pyrimethamine (a 200-mg loading dose followed by 75 mg orally each day) and *leucovorin* (folinic acid, 10 mg/day) is effective for acute treatment of encephalitis caused by *T. gondii* in patients with AIDS. Clindamycin also is available as a topical solution, gel, or lotion (CLEOCIN T, others) and as a vaginal cream (CLEOCIN, others). It is effective topically (or orally) for acne vulgaris and bacterial vaginosis.

UNTOWARD EFFECTS

GI Effects. The reported incidence of diarrhea associated with the administration of clindamycin ranges from 2-20%. A number of patients have developed pseudomembranous colitis caused by the toxin from the organism *C. difficile*. This colitis is characterized by watery diarrhea, fever, and elevated peripheral white blood cell counts. *This syndrome may be lethal.* Discontinuation of the drug, combined with administration of metronidazole or oral vancomycin usually is curative, but relapses occur. Agents that inhibit peristalsis (e.g., opioids) may prolong and worsen the condition.

Other Toxic and Irritative Effects. Skin rashes occur in ~10% of patients treated with clindamycin and may be more common in patients with HIV infection. Other uncommon reactions include exudative erythema multiforme (Stevens-Johnson syndrome), reversible elevation of aspartate aminotransferase and alanine aminotransferase, granulocytopenia, thrombocytopenia, and anaphylactic reactions. Local thrombophlebitis may follow intravenous administration of the drug. Clindamycin may potentiate the effect of a neuromuscular blocking agent administered concurrently.

STREPTOGRAMINS (QUINUPRISTIN/DALFOPRISTIN)

Quinupristin/dalfopristin (SYNERCID) is a combination of quinupristin (a streptogramin B), with dalfopristin (a streptogramin A), in a 30:70 ratio. These compounds are semisynthetic derivatives of naturally occurring agents produced by *Streptomyces pristinaespiralis*. Quinupristin and dalfopristin are more soluble derivatives of the congeners, pristinamycin IA and IIA, and therefore are suitable for intravenous administration.

ANTIMICROBIAL ACTIVITY. Quinupristin/dalfopristin is active against gram-positive cocci and organisms responsible for atypical pneumonia (e.g., *M. pneumoniae*, *Legionella* spp., and *C. pneumoniae*), but is inactive against gram-negative organisms. The combination is bactericidal against streptococci and many strains of staphylococci but bacteriostatic against *Enterococcus faecium*.

MECHANISM OF ACTION. Quinupristin and dalfopristin are protein synthesis inhibitors that bind the 50S ribosomal subunit. Quinupristin binds at the same site as macrolides and has a similar effect, with inhibition of polypeptide elongation and early termination of protein synthesis. Dalfopristin binds at a site nearby, resulting in a conformational change in the 50S ribosome, synergistically enhancing the binding of quinupristin at its target site. Dalfopristin directly interferes with polypeptide-chain formation. The net result of the cooperative and synergistic binding of these 2 molecules to the ribosome is bactericidal activity.

RESISTANCE TO STREPTOGRAMINS. Resistance to quinupristin is mediated by genes encoding a ribosomal methylase that prevents binding of drug to its target, or genes encoding lactonases that inactivate type B streptogramins. Resistance to dalfopristin is mediated by genes that encode acetyltransferases that inactivate type A streptogramins, or staphylococcal genes that encode ATP-binding efflux proteins that pump type A streptogramins out of the cell. These resistance determinants are located on plasmids. Resistance to quinupristin/dalfopristin always is associated with a resistance gene for type A streptogramins. Methylase-encoding genes can render the combination bacteriostatic instead of bactericidal, making it ineffective in certain infections in which bactericidal activity is necessary (e.g., endocarditis).

ADME. Quinupristin/dalfopristin is administered by intravenous infusion over at least 1 h. It is incompatible with saline and heparin and should be dissolved in 5% dextrose in water. The $t_{1/2}$ is 0.85 h for quinupristin and 0.7 h for dalfopristin. The volume of distribution is 0.87 L/kg for quinupristin and 0.71 L/kg for dalfopristin. Hepatic metabolism by conjugation is the principal means of clearance for both compounds, with 80% of an administered dose eliminated by biliary excretion. Renal elimination of active compound accounts for most of the remainder. No dosage adjustment is necessary for renal insufficiency. Pharmacokinetics are not significantly altered by peritoneal dialysis or hemodialysis. Hepatic insufficiency increases the plasma AUC of active component and metabolites by 180% for quinupristin and 50% for dalfopristin.

THERAPEUTIC USES AND DOSAGE. Quinupristin/dalfopristin is approved in the U.S. for treatment of infections caused by vancomycin-resistant strains of *E. faecium* (dose of 7.5 mg/kg every 8-12 h) and complicated skin and skin-structure infections caused by methicillin-susceptible strains of *S. aureus* or *S. pyogenes*. In Europe it also is approved for treatment of nosocomial pneumonia and infections caused by MRSA. Quinupristin/dalfopristin should be reserved for treatment of serious infections caused by multiple-drug-resistant gram-positive organisms such as vancomycin-resistant *E. faecium.*

UNTOWARD EFFECTS. The most common side effects are infusion-related events, such as pain and phlebitis at the infusion site and arthralgias and myalgias. Phlebitis and pain can be minimized by infusion of drug through a central venous catheter. Arthralgias and myalgias, more likely to be problematic in patients with hepatic insufficiency are managed by reducing the infusion frequency to every 12 h.

DRUG INTERACTIONS. Quinupristin/dalfopristin inhibits CYP3A4. The concomitant administration of other CYP3A4 substrates with quinupristin/dalfopristin may result in significant toxicity. Caution and monitoring are recommended for drugs in which the toxic therapeutic window is narrow or for drugs that prolong the QTc interval.

OXAZOLIDINONES (LINEZOLID)

Linezolid (ZYVOX) is a synthetic antimicrobial agent of the oxazolidinone class.

ANTIMICROBIAL ACTIVITY. Linezolid is active against gram-positive organisms including staphylococci, streptococci, enterococci, gram-positive anaerobic cocci, and gram-positive rods such as *Corynebacterium* spp. and *L. monocytogenes* (*see* Table 55–1). It has poor activity against most gram-negative aerobic or anaerobic bacteria. It is bacteriostatic against enterococci and staphylococci and bactericidal against streptococci. *Mycobacterium tuberculosis* is moderately susceptible.

MECHANISM OF ACTION AND RESISTANCE TO OXAZOLIDINONES. Linezolid inhibits protein synthesis by binding to the P site of the 50S ribosomal subunit and preventing formation of the larger ribosomal-fMet-tRNA complex that initiates protein synthesis. Because of its unique mechanism of action, linezolid is active against strains that are resistant to multiple other agents, including penicillin-resistant strains of *S. pneumoniae*; methicillin-resistant, vancomycin-intermediate, and vancomycin-resistant strains of staphylococci; and vancomycin-resistant strains of enterococci. Resistance in enterococci and staphylococci is due to point mutations of the 23S rRNA. Since bacteria have multiple copies of 23S rRNA genes, resistance generally requires mutations in 2 or more copies.

ADME. Linezolid is well absorbed after oral administration and may be administered without regard to food. Dosing for oral and intravenous preparations is the same. The $t_{1/2}$ is ~4-6 h. Linezolid is 30% protein-bound and distributes widely to well-perfused tissues. Linezolid is nonenzymatically oxidized to aminoethoxyacetic acid and hydroxyethyl glycine derivatives. Approximately 80% of a dose of linezolid appears in the urine, 30% as active compound and 50% as the 2 primary oxidation products. Ten percent of the administered dose appears as oxidation products in feces. No dose adjustment in renal insufficiency is recommended. Linezolid and its breakdown products are eliminated by dialysis; therefore the drug should be administered after hemodialysis.

THERAPEUTIC USES AND DOSAGE. Linezolid (600 mg twice daily) has had clinical and microbiological cure rates in the range of 85-90% in treatment of a variety of infections caused by vancomycin-resistant *E. faecium.* Linezolid is FDA-approved for treatment of skin and skin structure infections (complicated and uncomplicated) caused by streptococci and *S. aureus* (methicillin-susceptible and MRSA). A 400-mg twice-daily dosage regimen is recommended only for treatment of uncomplicated skin and skin-structure infections. For nosocomial pneumonia caused by MRSA or methicillin-susceptible *S. aureus*, cure rates with linezolid (~60%) were similar to those with vancomycin. Linezolid also may be an effective alternative for patients with MRSA infections who have reduced susceptibility to vancomycin. Linezolid also is approved for treatment of community-acquired pneumonia caused by penicillin-susceptible strains of *S. pneumoniae.*

Linezolid should be reserved as an alternative agent for treatment of infections caused by multiple-drug-resistant strains. It should not be used when other agents are likely to be effective. Indiscriminant use and overuse will hasten selection of resistant strains and the eventual loss of this valuable newer agent.

UNTOWARD EFFECTS. Myelosuppression, including anemia, leukopenia, pancytopenia, and thrombocytopenia, has been reported in patients receiving linezolid. Platelet counts should be monitored in patients with risk of bleeding, preexisting thrombocytopenia, or intrinsic or acquired disorders of platelet function and in patients receiving courses of therapy lasting beyond 2 weeks. The drug is well tolerated, with generally minor side effects (e.g., GI complaints, headache, rash). Patients receiving long-term (e.g., >8 weeks) treatment with linezolid have developed peripheral neuropathy, optic neuritis, and lactic acidosis. Linezolid should generally not be used for long-term therapy if there are alternative agents.

Drug Interactions. Linezolid is a weak nonspecific inhibitor of monoamine oxidase. Patients receiving concomitant therapy with an adrenergic or serotonergic agent (including selective serotonin reuptake inhibitors [SSRIs]) or consuming >100 mg of tyramine a day may experience serotonin syndrome (palpitations, headache, or hypertensive crisis). Coadministration of these agents is best avoided if possible. However, in patients receiving SSRIs who acutely require linezolid therapy for short-term (10-14 days) treatment, coadministration with careful monitoring is reasonable. Linezolid is neither a substrate nor an inhibitor of CYPs.

AMINOCYCLITOLS (SPECTINOMYCIN)

Spectinomycin is indicated only for the treatment of gonococcal infection when a β-lactam or fluoroquinolone cannot be given.

ANTIMICROBIAL ACTIVITY, MECHANISM OF ACTION, AND RESISTANCE TO SPECTINOMYCIN. Spectinomycin selectively inhibits protein synthesis in gram-negative bacteria by binding to the 30S ribosomal subunit. Its action is similar to that of the aminoglycosides, but spectinomycin is not bactericidal and does not cause misreading of messenger RNA. Bacterial resistance may be mediated by mutations in the 16S ribosomal RNA or by drug modification by adenylyltransferase.

ADME. Spectinomycin is rapidly absorbed after intramuscular injection. The drug is not significantly bound to plasma protein, and all of an administered dose is recovered in the urine within 48 h.

THERAPEUTIC USES AND DOSAGE. Spectinomycin is active against a number of gram-negative bacterial species, but *it is inferior to other drugs to which such microorganisms are susceptible. Its only therapeutic use is in the treatment of gonorrhea caused by strains resistant to first-line drugs (ceftriaxone, cefixime) or if there are contraindications to these drugs.* Spectinomycin is recommended in patients who are intolerant or allergic to β-lactams. The drug is not available in the U.S. The recommended dose for men and women is a single deep intramuscular injection of 2 g. Spectinomycin has no effect on incubating or established syphilis, and is not active against *Chlamydia* spp. It also is less effective for pharyngeal infections.

UNTOWARD EFFECTS. Local pain, urticaria, chills, fever, dizziness, nausea, and insomnia have been noted. The injection may be painful.

POLYMYXINS

The polymyxins are a group of closely related antibiotics elaborated by strains of *Bacillus polymyxa*. Colistin (polymyxin E) is produced by *Bacillus colistinus*. Polymyxin B is a mixture of polymyxins B_1 and B_2. These drugs, which are cationic detergents, are simple basic peptides with molecular masses of ~1000 Da.

ANTIMICROBIAL ACTIVITY, MECHANISM OF ACTION, AND RESISTANCE TO POLYMYXINS. The antimicrobial activities of polymyxin B and colistin are similar and restricted to gram-negative bacteria. Polymyxins are surface-active amphipathic agents. They interact strongly with phospholipids and disrupt the structure of cell membranes. Sensitivity to polymyxin B apparently is related to the phospholipid content of the cell wall–membrane complex. Polymyxin B binds to the lipid A portion of endotoxin (the lipopolysaccharide of the outer membrane of gram-negative bacteria) and inactivates this molecule. The cell walls of certain resistant bacteria may prevent access of the drug to the cell membrane. Although resistance to polymyxins is rare, emergence of resistance while on treatment has been documented.

ADME. Polymyxin B and colistin are not absorbed when given orally and are poorly absorbed from mucous membranes and the surfaces of large burns. They are cleared renally, and modification of the dose is required in patients with impaired renal function.

THERAPEUTIC USES

Topical Uses. Polymyxin B sulfate is available for ophthalmic, otic, and topical use in combination with a variety of other compounds. Colistin is available as otic drops. Infections of the skin, mucous membranes, eye, and ear due to polymyxin B–sensitive microorganisms respond to local application of the antibiotic in solution or ointment. External otitis, frequently due to *Pseudomonas*, may be cured by the topical use of the drug. *P. aeruginosa* is a common cause of infection of corneal ulcers; local application or subconjunctival injection of polymyxin B often is curative.

Systemic Uses. Colistin is available as colistin sulfate for oral use and as colistimethate sodium for parenteral administration. Due to the emergence of multidrug-resistant gram-negative organisms (especially

Stenotrophomonas maltophilia, *Acinetobacter* spp., *P. aeruginosa*, and *Klebsiella* spp.), there has been a resurgence in the systemic use of polymyxins, despite their toxicity when administered via this route. Because dosing of these agents varies by drug (polymyxin B or colistin), by the particular commercial preparation, and by the patient's degree of renal dysfunction, expert consultation is recommended.

Untoward Effects. Because polymyxins are nephrotoxic when administered via systemically, these drugs are rarely used except topically. Polymyxin B applied to intact or denuded skin or mucous membranes produces no systemic reactions because of its almost complete lack of absorption from these sites. Hypersensitization is uncommon with topical application. Neurological reactions include muscle weakness, apnea, paresthesias, vertigo, and slurred speech.

GLYCOPEPTIDES (VANCOMYCIN AND TEICOPLANIN)

Vancomycin is a tricyclic glycopeptide antibiotic produced by *Streptococcus orientalis*. Teicoplanin is a mixture of related glycopeptides available as an antibiotic in Europe. It is similar to vancomycin in chemical structure, mechanism of action, spectrum of activity, and route of elimination (i.e., primarily renal).

ANTIMICROBIAL ACTIVITY. Vancomycin possesses activity against a broad spectrum of gram-positive bacteria (*see* Table 55–1). Essentially all species of gram-negative bacilli and mycobacteria are resistant to vancomycin. Teicoplanin is active against methicillin-susceptible and MRSA. Some strains of staphylococci, coagulase positive and coagulase negative, as well as enterococci and other organisms that are intrinsically resistant to vancomycin (i.e., *Lactobacillus* spp. and *Leuconostoc* spp.), are resistant to teicoplanin.

MECHANISM OF ACTION. Vancomycin and teicoplanin inhibit the synthesis of the cell wall in sensitive bacteria by binding with high affinity to the D-alanyl-D-alanine terminus of cell wall precursor units (Figure 55–4). Because of their large molecular size, they are unable to penetrate the outer membrane of gram-negative bacteria.

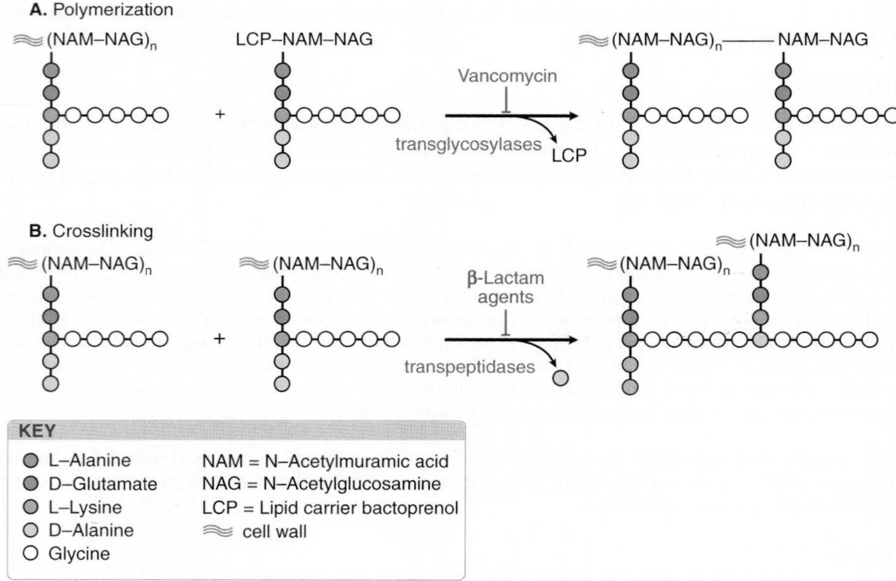

Figure 55–4 *Inhibition of bacterial cell wall synthesis: vancomycin and β-lactam agents.* Vancomycin inhibits the polymerization or transglycosylase reaction (**A**) by binding to the D-alanyl-D-alanine terminus of the cell wall precursor unit attached to its lipid carrier and blocks linkage to the glycopeptide polymer (indicated by the subscript n). These $(NAM–NAG)_n$ peptidoglycan polymers are located within the cell wall. Van A-type resistance is due to expression of enzymes that modify cell wall precursor by substituting a terminal D-lactate for D-alanine, reducing affinity for vancomycin by 1000-fold. β-Lactam antibiotics inhibit the cross-linking or transpeptidase reaction (**B**) that links glycopeptide polymer chains by formation of a cross-bridge with the stem peptide (the 5 glycines in this example) of one chain, displacing the terminal D-alanine of an adjacent chain. *See* also Figure 53–2.

RESISTANCE TO GLYCOPEPTIDES. Glycopeptide-resistant strains of enterococci, primarily *E. faecium*, have emerged as major nosocomial pathogens in hospitals in the U.S. Determinants of vancomycin resistance are located on a transposon that is readily transferable among enterococci, and, potentially, other gram-positive bacteria. These strains are typically resistant to multiple antibiotics, including streptomycin, gentamicin, and ampicillin. Resistance to streptomycin and gentamicin is of special concern because the combination of an aminoglycoside with a cell-wall-synthesis inhibitor is the only reliably bactericidal regimen for treatment of enterococcal endocarditis.

Enterococcal resistance to glycopeptides is the result of alteration of the D-alanyl-D-alanine target to D-alanyl-D-lactate or D-alanyl D-serine, which bind glycopeptides poorly. Several enzymes within the *van* gene cluster are required for this target alteration to occur. The *Van A* phenotype confers inducible resistance to teicoplanin and vancomycin in *E. faecium* and *Enterococcus faecalis*. The *Van B* phenotype, which tends to be a lower level of resistance, also has been identified in *E. faecium* and *E. faecalis*. The trait is inducible by vancomycin but not teicoplanin, and consequently, many strains remain susceptible to teicoplanin. The *Van C* phenotype, the least important clinically and least well characterized, confers resistance only to vancomycin.

S. aureus and coagulase-negative staphylococci may express reduced or "intermediate" susceptibility to vancomycin (MIC, 4-8 μg/mL) or high-level resistance (MIC ≥16 μg/mL). Intermediate resistance is associated with a heterogeneous phenotype in which a small proportion of cells within the population (1 in 10^5 to 1 in 10^6) will grow in the presence of vancomycin concentrations >4 μg/mL. Prior treatment courses and low vancomycin levels may predispose patients to infection and treatment failure with vancomycin-intermediate strains. These strains typically are resistant to methicillin and multiple other antibiotics; their emergence is a major concern because until recently vancomycin has been the only antibiotic to which staphylococci were reliably susceptible. High-level vancomycin-resistant *S. aureus* strains (MIC ≥32 μg/mL) harbor a conjugative plasmid into which the *Van A* transposon is integrated by an interspecies horizontal gene transfer from *E. faecalis* to a MRSA. These isolates have been variably susceptible to teicoplanin and the investigational lipoglycopeptides.

ADME. Vancomycin is poorly absorbed after oral administration. The drug should be administered intravenously, never intramuscularly. Approximately 30% of vancomycin is bound to plasma protein. Vancomycin appears in various body fluids, including the CSF when the meninges are inflamed (7-30%); bile; and pleural, pericardial, synovial, and ascitic fluids. About 90% of an injected dose of vancomycin is excreted by glomerular filtration; elimination $t_{1/2}$ is ~6 h. The drug accumulates if renal function is impaired, and dosage adjustments must be made. The drug can be cleared from plasma with hemodialysis. Teicoplanin can be administered by intramuscular injection as well as intravenous administration. An intravenous dose of 1 g in adults produces plasma concentrations of 15-30 μg/mL 1 h after a 1- to 2-h infusion. Teicoplanin is highly bound by plasma proteins (90-95%) and has an extremely long serum elimination $t_{1/2}$ (up to 100 h).

THERAPEUTIC USES AND DOSAGE. Vancomycin and teicoplanin have been used to treat a variety of infections, including osteomyelitis and endocarditis caused by methicillin-resistant and methicillin-susceptible staphylococci, streptococci, and enterococci. Teicoplanin is not licensed for use in the U.S.

Vancomycin hydrochloride (VANCOCIN, others) is marketed for *intravenous* use as a sterile powder for solution. It should be diluted and infused over at least a 60-min period to avoid infusion-related adverse reactions; the recommended dose for adults is 30-45 mg/kg/day in 2-3 divided doses. Current recommendations call for monitoring serum trough concentrations (within 30 min prior to a dose) at steady state, typically before the fourth dose of a given dosage regimen. A trough serum concentration of 10 μg/mL is recommended. For patients with more serious infections (including endocarditis, osteomyelitis, meningitis, and MRSA pneumonia), trough levels of 15-20 μg/mL are recommended. Pediatric doses are: for newborns during the first week of life, 15 mg/kg initially, followed by 10 mg/kg every 12 h; for infants 8-30 days old, 15 mg/kg followed by 10 mg/kg every 8 h; for older infants (>30 days) and children, 10-15 mg/kg every 6 h. Alteration of dosage is required for patients with impaired renal function. In functionally anephric patients and patients receiving dialysis with non-high-flux membranes, administration of 1 g (~15 mg/kg) every 5-7 days typically achieves adequate serum levels. In patients receiving intermittent high-efficiency or high-flux dialysis, maintenance doses administered after each dialysis session are typically required. Blood levels should be monitored to decide on dose adjustments.

Skin/Soft-Tissue and Bone/Joint Infections. Vancomycin is used in the treatment of skin/soft-tissue and bone/joint infections, where gram-positive organisms including MRSA are the leading pathogens.

Respiratory Tract Infections. Vancomycin is employed for the treatment of pneumonia when MRSA is suspected. Because vancomycin penetration into lung tissue is relatively low, aggressive dosing is generally recommended.

CNS Infections. Vancomycin is a key component in the initial empirical treatment of community-acquired bacterial meningitis in locations where penicillin-resistant *S. pneumoniae* is common. Penetration of vancomycin across inflamed meningitis is poor; thus, aggressive dosing is typically warranted. Vancomycin is also used to treat nosocomial meningitis often caused by staphylococci.

Endocarditis and Vascular Catheter Infections. Vancomycin is standard therapy for staphylococcal endocarditis when the isolate is methicillin resistant or patients have a severe penicillin allergy. Vancomycin is an effective alternative for the treatment of endocarditis caused by viridans streptococci in patients who are allergic to penicillin. In combination with an aminoglycoside, it may be used for enterococcal endocarditis in patients with serious penicillin allergy or for penicillin-resistant isolates. Vancomycin is used for the treatment of vascular catheter infections due to gram-positive organisms.

Other Infections. Vancomycin can be administered orally to patients with pseudomembranous colitis due to *C. difficile*. The dose for adults is 125-250 mg every 6 h; the total daily dose for children is 40 mg/kg, given in 3 to 4 divided doses. The standard dose of teicoplanin in adults is 3-6 mg/kg/day, with higher dosages possible for treatment of serious staphylococcal infections. Once-daily dosing is possible due to the prolonged serum $t_{1/2}$. Teicoplanin doses must be adjusted in patients with renal insufficiency. For functionally anephric patients, administration once weekly is appropriate, but serum drug concentrations should be monitored to determine that the therapeutic range has been maintained.

UNTOWARD EFFECTS. Hypersensitivity reactions produced by vancomycin and teicoplanin include macular skin rashes and anaphylaxis. Phlebitis and pain at the site of intravenous injection are relatively uncommon. Chills, rash, and fever may occur. Rapid intravenous infusion of vancomycin may cause erythematous or urticarial reactions, flushing, tachycardia, and hypotension. The extreme flushing that can occur is not an allergic reaction but a direct effect of vancomycin on mast cells, causing them to release histamine. This reaction is generally not observed with teicoplanin. Auditory impairment, sometimes permanent, is associated with excessive concentrations of these drugs in plasma (60-100 μg/mL of vancomycin). Nephrotoxicity has become less common with modern formulations at standard dosages. Careful dosing and monitoring of vancomycin is necessary to balance the risks and benefits. Caution should be exercised when ototoxic or nephrotoxic drugs, such as aminoglycosides, are administered concurrently with vancomycin.

LIPOPEPTIDES (DAPTOMYCIN)

Daptomycin (CUBICIN), a cyclic lipopeptide antibiotic derived from *Streptomyces roseosporus*, has been resurrected in response to increasing need for bactericidal antibiotics effective against vancomycin-resistant gram-positive bacteria.

Antimicrobial Activity. Daptomycin is a bactericidal antibiotic selectively active against aerobic, facultative, and anaerobic gram-positive bacteria (*see* Table 55–1). Daptomycin may be active against vancomycin-resistant strains, although MICs tend to be higher for these organisms than for their vancomycin-susceptible counterparts.

Mechanisms of Action and Resistance to Daptomycin. Daptomycin binds to bacterial membranes resulting in depolarization, loss of membrane potential, and cell death. It has concentration-dependent bactericidal activity. Daptomycin resistance has been reported to emerge while on therapy. The mechanisms of resistance to daptomycin have not been fully characterized.

ADME. Daptomycin is poorly absorbed orally and should be administered only intravenously. Direct toxicity to muscle precludes intramuscular injection. The serum $t_{1/2}$ is 8-9 h, permitting once-daily dosing. Approximately 80% of the administered dose is recovered in urine; a small amount is excreted in feces. Although the drug penetrates adequately into the lung, the drug is inactivated by pulmonary surfactant. If the creatinine clearance is <30 mL/min; the dose is administered only every 48 h. For hemodialysis patients the dose should be given immediately after dialysis. Daptomycin does not affect CYPs and has no important drug–drug interactions. Caution is recommended when daptomycin is coadministered with aminoglycosides or statins because of potential risks of nephrotoxicity and myopathy, respectively.

Therapeutic Uses and Dosage. Daptomycin is indicated for treatment of complicated skin and soft tissue infections (at 4 mg/kg/day) and complicated bacteremia and right-sided endocarditis (at 6 mg/kg/day). Its efficacy is comparable to that of vancomycin.

Untoward Effects. Elevations of creatine kinase may occur; this does not require discontinuation unless findings suggest an otherwise unexplained myopathy. Rhabdomyolysis has been reported to occur rarely.

BACITRACIN

Bacitracin is an antibiotic produced by the Tracy-I strain of *B. subtilis*. The bacitracins are a group of polypeptide antibiotics. The commercial products have multiple components; the major constituent is bacitracin A.

Antimicrobial Activity. Bacitracin inhibits the synthesis of the bacterial cell wall; a variety of gram-positive cocci and bacilli, *Neisseria*, *H. influenzae*, and *T. pallidum*, are sensitive to the drug at ≤0.1 unit/mL.

Actinomyces and *Fusobacterium* are inhibited by concentrations of 0.5-5 units/mL. Enterobacteriaceae, *Pseudomonas*, *Candida* spp., and *Nocardia* are resistant to the drug. A unit of the antibiotic is equivalent to 26 μg of the USP standard.

Therapeutic Uses and Dosage. Current use is restricted to topical application. Bacitracin is available in ophthalmic and dermatologic ointments; the antibiotic also is available as a powder (BACI-RX) for the extemporaneous compounding of topical solutions. A number of topical preparations of bacitracin, to which neomycin or polymyxin or both have been added, are available. For open infections, such as infected eczema and infected dermal ulcers, the local application of the antibiotic may be of some help in eradicating sensitive bacteria. Bacitracin rarely produces hypersensitivity. Suppurative conjunctivitis and infected corneal ulcer, when caused by susceptible bacteria, respond well to the topical use of bacitracin. Bacitracin has been used with limited success for eradication of nasal carriage of staphylococci. Oral bacitracin has been used with some success for the treatment of antibiotic-associated diarrhea caused by *C. difficile*.

Untoward Effects. Nephrotoxicity results from the parenteral use of bacitracin.

MUPIROCIN

Antimicrobial Activity, Mechanism of Action, and Resistance. Mupirocin (BACTROBAN) is for topical use only. The drug is bactericidal against many gram-positive and selected gram-negative bacteria. It has good activity against *S. pyogenes* and methicillin-susceptible and MRSA. Mupirocin inhibits bacterial protein synthesis by reversible binding and inhibition of isoleucyl transfer-RNA synthase. There is no cross-resistance with other classes of antibiotics. High-level resistance is mediated by a plasmid, which encodes a "bypass" Ile tRNA synthase that binds mupirocin poorly.

ADME. Systemic absorption through intact skin or skin lesions is minimal. Any absorbed drug is rapidly metabolized to inactive monic acid.

Therapeutic Uses and Dosage. Mupirocin is available as a 2% cream and a 2% ointment for dermatologic use and as a 2% ointment for intranasal use. The dermatologic preparations are indicated for treatment of traumatic skin lesions and impetigo secondarily infected with *S. aureus* or *S. pyogenes*. The nasal ointment is approved for eradication of *S. aureus* nasal carriage. The consensus is that patients who stand to benefit from mupirocin prophylaxis are those with proven *S. aureus* nasal colonization plus risk factors for distant infection or a history of skin or soft-tissue infections.

Untoward Effects. Mupirocin may cause irritation and sensitization at the site of application. Contact with the eyes causes irritation that may take several days to resolve. Polyethylene glycol present in the ointment can be absorbed from damaged skin. Application of the ointment to large surface areas should be avoided in patients with moderate to severe renal failure to avoid accumulation of polyethylene glycol.

For a complete Bibliographical Listing see Goodman & Gilman's ***The Pharmacological Basis of Therapeutics***, 12th ed., or Goodman & Gilman Online at www.AccessMedicine.com.

Chemotherapy of Tuberculosis, *Mycobacterium Avium Complex* Disease, and Leprosy

Mycobacteria cause tuberculosis (TB) and leprosy. Although the burden of leprosy has decreased, TB is still the most important infectious killer of humans. *Mycobacterium avium-intracellulare* (or *Mycobacterium avium* complex [MAC]) infection continues to be difficult to treat, mainly due to 3 natural barriers:

- **Cell wall**—More than 60% of the cell wall is lipid, mainly mycolic acids composed of 2-branched, 73-hydroxy fatty acids with chains made of 76-90 carbon atoms. This shield prevents many pharmacological compounds from getting to the bacterial cell membrane or inside the cytosol.
- **Efflux pumps**—These transport proteins export potentially harmful chemicals from the bacterial cytoplasm into the extracellular space, preventing accumulation of effective drug concentrations in the cell. These exporters are responsible for the native resistance of mycobacteria to many standard antibiotics. As an example, ATP-binding cassette (ABC) permeases comprise a full 2.5% of the genome of *Mycobacterium tuberculosis*.
- **Location in host**—Some of the bacilli hide inside the patient's cells, adding an extra physicochemical barrier that antimicrobial agents must cross to be effective.

Mycobacteria are defined by their rate of growth on agar as *rapid* and *slow* growers (Table 56–1). Slow growers tend to be susceptible to antibiotics developed specifically for Mycobacteria; rapid growers tend to be also susceptible to antibiotics used against many other bacteria.

The mechanisms of action of the anti-mycobacterial drugs are summarized in Figure 56–1. Figure 56–2 depicts the mechanisms of resistance to these drugs. Tables 56–2 and 56–3 summarize the pharmacokinetic parameters of the antimycobacterial agents.

ANTI-MYCOBACTERIAL DRUGS

RIFAMYCINS: RIFAMPIN, RIFAPENTINE, AND RIFABUTIN

Rifampin or *rifampicin* (RIFADIN; RIMACTANE, others), *rifapentine* (PRIFTIN), and *rifabutin* (MYCOBUTIN) are important in treatment of mycobacterial diseases.

MECHANISM OF ACTION. Rifampin's action against *M. tuberculosis* typifies the mechanism by which rifamycins act. Rifampin enters bacilli in a concentration-dependent manner, achieving steady-state concentrations

Table 56–1

Pathogenic Mycobacterial Rapid and Slow Growers (Runyon Classification)

SLOW GROWERS
Runyon I: Photochromogens *Mycobacterium kansasii, Mycobacterium marinum*
Runyon II: Scotochromogens *Mycobacterium scrofulaceum, Mycobacterium szulgai, Mycobacterium gordonae*
Runyon III: Non-chromogens *Mycobacterium avium complex, Mycobacterium haemophilum, Mycobacterium xenopi*
RAPID GROWERS
Runyon IV: *Mycobacterium fortuitum* complex, *Mycobacterium smegmatis* group

Slow growers tend to be susceptible to antibiotics specifically developed for Mycobacteria; rapid growers tend to be susceptible to antibiotics also used against many other bacteria.

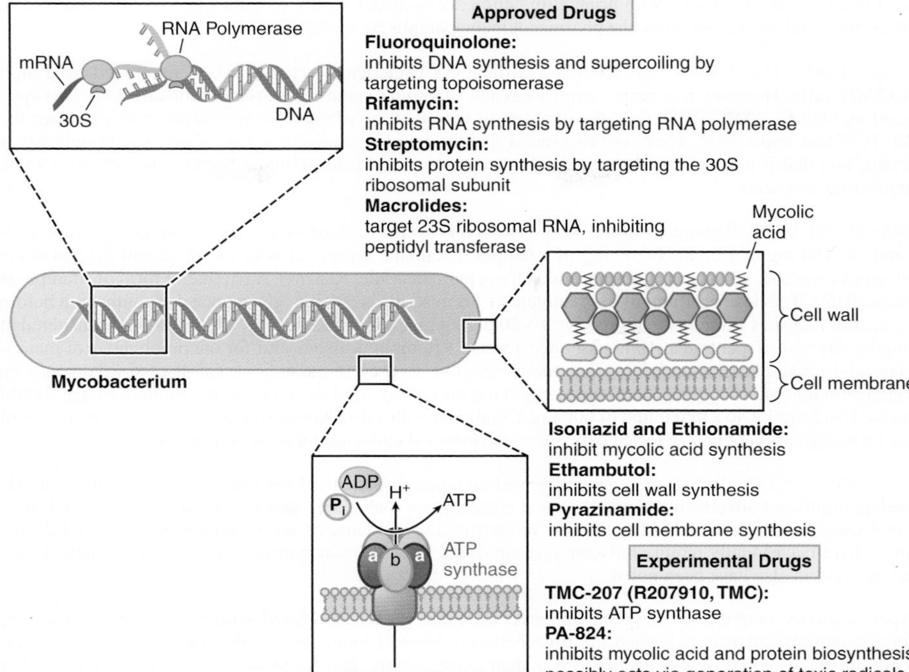

RNA Polymerase
mRNA
30S
DNA
Approved Drugs
Fluoroquinolone:
inhibits DNA synthesis and supercoiling by targeting topoisomerase
Rifamycin:
inhibits RNA synthesis by targeting RNA polymerase
Streptomycin:
inhibits protein synthesis by targeting the 30S ribosomal subunit
Macrolides:
target 23S ribosomal RNA, inhibiting peptidyl transferase
Mycolic acid
Cell wall
Cell membrane
Mycobacterium
Isoniazid and Ethionamide:
inhibit mycolic acid synthesis
Ethambutol:
inhibits cell wall synthesis
Pyrazinamide:
inhibits cell membrane synthesis
ADP
H+
ATP
Pi
ATP synthase
a
b
a
Experimental Drugs
TMC-207 (R207910, TMC):
inhibits ATP synthase
PA-824:
inhibits mycolic acid and protein biosynthesis; possibly acts via generation of toxic radicals

Figure 56–1 *Mechanisms of action of established and experimental drugs used for the chemotherapy of mycobacterial infections.* Shown at the top are the sites of action of approved drugs for the chemotherapy of mycobacterial diseases. Rifamycin is a generic term for several drugs, of which rifampin is used most frequently. Also included are 2 experimental drugs now under investigation: TMC-207 and PA-824. Clofazimine, whose mode of action is not understood, is omitted.

within 15 min. The drug binds to the β subunit of DNA-dependent RNA polymerase (*rpoB*) to form a stable drug–enzyme complex, suppressing chain formation in RNA synthesis.

ANTIBACTERIAL ACTIVITY. Rifampin inhibits the growth of most gram-positive bacteria as well as many gram-negative microorganisms. Rifampin inhibits the growth of many *M. tuberculosis* clinical isolates in vitro at concentrations of 0.06-0.25 mg/L. Rifampin is also bactericidal against *Mycobacterium leprae*. *Mycobacterium kansasii* is inhibited by 0.25-1 mg/L. Most strains of *Mycobacterium scrofulaceum*, *Mycobacterium intracellulare*, and *M. avium* are suppressed by concentrations of 4 mg/L. *Mycobacterium fortuitum* is highly resistant to the drug. Rifabutin inhibits the growth of most MAC isolates at concentrations ranging from 0.25-1 mg/L and of many strains of *M. tuberculosis* at concentrations of ≤0.125 mg/L.

BACTERIAL RESISTANCE. The prevalence of rifampin-resistant isolates (1 in every 10^7 to 10^8 bacilli) is due to altered *rpoB*. Mutations in genes involved in DNA repair mechanisms will impair the repair of multiple genes, which may lead to hyper-mutable strains (*see* Chapter 48). *M. tuberculosis* Beijing genotype clinical isolates have been associated with higher rates of simultaneous rifampin and isoniazid resistance associated with mutations in the repair genes *mut* and *ogt*. Inducible or environment-dependent mutators may be more common than these stable mutator phenotypes. Antibiotics, endogenous oxidative and metabolic stressors lead to DNA damage, which induces *dnaE2*. The induction is associated with error-prone DNA repair and leads to higher rates of rifampin resistance.

ADME. After oral administration, the rifamycins are absorbed to variable extents (Table 56–2). Food decreases the rifampin C_{Pmax} by one-third; a high-fat meal increases the area under the curve (AUC) of rifapentine by 50%. Food has no effect on rifabutin absorption. Rifapentine should be taken with food, if possible. Rifamycins are metabolized by microsomal B-esterases and cholinesterases. A major pathway for rifabutin elimination is CYP3A. Due to autoinduction, all 3 rifamycins reduce their own AUCs with repeated administration (Table 56–3). They have good penetration into many tissues, but levels in the CNS reach only ~5% of those in plasma, likely due to the activity of P-glycoprotein. The drugs and metabolites are excreted by bile and eliminated via feces, with urine elimination accounting for only one-third and less of metabolites. Tables 56–2 and 56–3 summarize the pharmacokinetic parameters of the rifamycins.

PHARMACOKINETICS-PHARMACODYNAMICS. Rifampin's bactericidal activity is best optimized by a high AUC/MIC ratio. However, resistance suppression and rifampin's enduring post-antibiotic effect are best optimized by high C_{max}/MIC. Therefore, the duration of time that the rifampin concentration persists above the MIC is of less importance. These results predict that the $t_{1/2}$ of a rifamycin is less of an issue in optimizing therapy, and that if patients could tolerate it, higher doses would lead to higher bactericidal activities while suppressing resistance.

THERAPEUTIC USES. Rifampin for oral administration is available alone or as a fixed-dose combination with isoniazid (150 mg of isoniazid, 300 mg of rifampin; Rifamate, others) or with isoniazid and pyrazinamide (50 mg of isoniazid, 120 mg of rifampin, and 300 mg pyrazinamide; RIFATER). A parenteral form of rifampin is also available. The dose of rifampin for treatment of TB in adults is 600 mg, given once daily, either 1 h before or 2 h after a meal. Children should receive 10-20 mg/kg given in the same way. Rifabutin is administered at 5 mg/kg/day and rifapentine at 10 mg/kg once a week. Rifampin is also useful for the prophylaxis of meningococcal disease and *Haemophilus influenzae* meningitis. To prevent meningococcal disease, adults may be treated with 600 mg twice daily for 2 days or 600 mg once daily for 4 days; children >1 month of age should receive 10-15 mg/kg, to a maximum of 600 mg. Combined with a β-lactam antibiotic or vancomycin, rifampin may be useful for therapy in selected cases of staphylococcal endocarditis or osteomyelitis.

UNTOWARD EFFECTS. Rifampin is generally well tolerated in patients. Fewer than 4% of patients with TB develop significant adverse reactions; the most common are rash, fever, and nausea and vomiting. Chronic liver disease, alcoholism, and old age appear to increase the incidence of severe hepatic problems. GI disturbances have occasionally required discontinuation of the drug. Various nonspecific symptoms related to the nervous system also have been noted.

Hypersensitivity reactions may be encountered. Adverse events associated with high rifampin dose are more commonly encountered when the time between doses is long; thus, high-dose rifampin should not be administered on a dosing schedule of less than twice weekly; less frequent administration is associated with a flu-like syndrome of fever, chills, and myalgias in 20% of patients; adverse effects may also include eosinophilia, interstitial nephritis, acute tubular necrosis, thrombocytopenia, hemolytic anemia, and shock. Light chain proteinuria, thrombocytopenia, transient leukopenia, and anemia have occurred during rifampin therapy. Rifampin crosses the placenta and its teratogenic potential; thus, its use is best avoided during pregnancy.

Table 56–2

Population Pharmacokinetic Parameter Estimates for Antimycobacterial Drugs in Adult Patients

	PARAMETER ESTIMATE[c]		
	k_a (h^{-1})	SCL (L/h)	V_d (L)
First-line Drugs			
Rifampin	1.15	19	53
Rifapentine	0.6	2.03	37.8
Rifabutin	0.2	61	231/1,050[a]
Pyrazinamide	3.56	3.4	29.2
Isoniazid	2.3	22.1	35.2
Ethambutol	0.7	1.3[b]	6.0[b]
Clofazimine	0.7	0.6/76.7	1470
Dapsone	1.04	1.83	69.6
Second-line Agents			
Ethionamide	0.25	1.9[b]	3.2[b]
Para-aminosalicylic acid	0.4	0.3[b]	0.9[b]
Cycloserine	1.9	0.04[b]	0.5[b]

k_a, absorption constant (see Chapter 48); SCL, systemic clearance; V_d, volume of distribution.
[a]Volume of central compartment/volume of peripheral compartment.
[b]Expressed per kilogram of body weight.
[c]Pharmacokinetic parameters are presented in terms of Figure 48–1 and Equation 48–1.

Table 56–3

Pharmacokinetic Parameters of Rifampin, Rifabutin, and Rifapentine

	RIFABUTIN	RIFAMPIN	RIFAPENTINE
Protein binding (%)	71	85	97
Oral bioavailability (%)	20	68	—
t_{max} (hours)	2.5-4.0	1.5-2.0	5.0-6.0
C_{max} total (μg/mL)	0.2-0.6	8-20	8-30
C_{max} free drug (μg/mL)	0.1	1.5	0.5
Half-life (hours)	32-67	2-5	14-18
Intracellular/extracellular penetration	9	5	24-60
Autoinduction (AUC decrease)	40%	38%	20%
CYP3A induction	Weak	Pronounced	Moderate
CYP3A substrate	Yes	No	No

AUC, area under the curve.
Pharmacokinetic parameters are presented in terms of Figure 48–1 and Equation 48–1.

Rifabutin is generally well tolerated; primary reasons for discontinuation of therapy include rash (4%), GI intolerance (3%), and neutropenia (2%; 25% in patients with severe HIV infection). Uveitis and arthralgias have occurred in patients receiving rifabutin doses >450 mg daily in combination with clarithromycin or fluconazole. Patients should be cautioned to discontinue the drug if visual symptoms (pain or blurred vision) occur. Rifabutin causes an orange-tan discoloration of skin, urine, feces, saliva, tears, and contact lenses, like rifampin. Rarely, thrombocytopenia, a flu-like syndrome, chest pain, and hepatitis develop in patients treated with rifabutin. Unique side effects include polymyalgia, pseudojaundice, and anterior uveitis.

RIFAMYCIN OVERDOSE. Rifampin overdose is uncommon. The most prominent symptoms are the orange discoloration of skin, fluids, and mucosal surfaces, leading to the term *red-man syndrome.* Overdose can be life-threatening; treatment consists of supportive measures; there is no antidote.

DRUG INTERACTIONS. Because rifampin potently induces CYPs, its administration results in a decreased $t_{1/2}$ for a number of compounds that are metabolized by these CYPs. Rifabutin is a less potent inducer of CYPs than rifampin; however, rifabutin does induce hepatic microsomal enzymes and decreases the $t_{1/2}$ of zidovudine, prednisone, digitoxin, quinidine, ketoconazole, propranolol, phenytoin, sulfonylureas, and warfarin. It has less effect than rifampin on serum levels of indinavir and nelfinavir. Compared to rifabutin and rifampin, the CYP-inducing effects of rifapentine are intermediate.

PYRAZINAMIDE

Pyrazinamide is the synthetic pyrazine analog of nicotinamide.

MECHANISM OF ACTION. Pyrazinamide is activated to pyrazinoic acid under acidic conditions that likely prevail at the edges of necrotic TB cavities where inflammatory cells produce lactic acid. Some of the parent drug diffuses into *M. tuberculosis* where a nicotinamidase (pyrazinaminidase) deaminates pyrazinamide to pyrazinoic acid (POA^-), which is exported by an efflux pump. In an acidic extracellular milieu, a fraction of POA^- is protonated to POAH and enters the bacillus. As the pH of the extracellular medium declines toward the pK_a of pyrazinoic acid, 2.9, the Henderson-Hasselbalch equilibrium (*see* Figure 2–3) progressively favors the formation of POAH, its equilibration across bacillar membrane, and its accumulation within the bacillus; acidic conditions also enhance microbial killing. Although the actual mechanism of microbial kill is still unclear, 4 mechanisms have been proposed:

- Inhibition of fatty acid synthase type I leading to interference with mycolic acid synthesis
- Binding to ribosomal protein S1 (RpsA) and inhibition of trans-translation
- Reduction of intracellular pH disruption of membrane transport by HPOA

ANTIBACTERIAL ACTIVITY. Pyrazinamide exhibits antimicrobial activity in vitro only at acidic pH. At pH of 5.8-5.95, 80-90% of clinical isolates have an MIC of ≤100 mg/L.

MECHANISMS OF RESISTANCE. Pyrazinamide-resistant *M. tuberculosis* express nicotinamidase with reduced affinity for pyrazinamide. This reduced affinity decreases the conversion of pyrazinamide to POA. Single point mutations in the *pncA* gene are encountered in up to 70% of resistant clinical isolates.

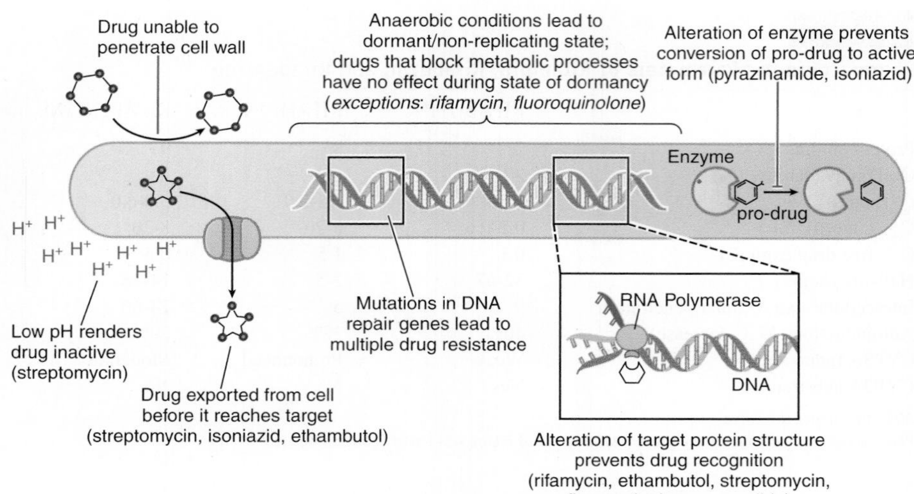

Figure 56–2 *Mechanisms of drug resistance in Mycobacteria.*

ADME. Oral bioavailability of pyrazinamide is >90%. GI absorption segregates patients into 2 groups: fast absorbers (56%) with an absorption rate constant of 3.56/h and slow absorbers (44%) with an absorption rate of 1.25/h. The drug is concentrated 20-fold in lung epithelial lining fluid. Pyrazinamide is metabolized by microsomal deamidase to POA and subsequently hydroxylated to 5-hydroxy-POA, which is excreted by the kidneys. CL (clearance) and V_d (volume of distribution) increase with patient mass (0.5 L/h and 4.3 L for every 10 kg above 50 kg), and V_d is larger in males (by 4.5 L) (*see* Table 56–2). This has several implications: the $t_{1/2}$ of pyrazinamide will vary considerably based on weight and gender, and the AUC_{0-24} will decrease with increase in weight for the same dose (same mg drug/kg body weight). Pyrazinamide clearance is reduced in renal failure; therefore, the dosing frequency must be reduced to 3 times a week at low glomerular filtration rates. Hemodialysis removes pyrazinamide; therefore, the drug needs to be re-dosed after each session of hemodialysis.

MICROBIAL PHARMACOKINETICS-PHARMACODYNAMICS. Pyrazinamide's sterilizing effect is closely linked to AUC_{0-24}/MIC. However, resistance suppression is linked to the fraction of time that C_p persists above MIC (T > MIC). Because patient weight impacts both SCL and volume, both AUC and $t_{1/2}$ will be impacted by high weight. Simulations indicate that optimal AUC_{0-24}/MIC and T > MIC are likely to be achieved only by doses much higher than the currently recommended 15-30 mg/kg/day; the safety of such higher doses in patients is unclear.

THERAPEUTIC USES. The coadministration of pyrazinamide with isoniazid or rifampin has led to a one-third reduction in the duration of anti-TB therapy, and a two-thirds reduction in TB relapse. The combination has reduced the length of therapy to 6 months, producing the current "short course" regimen. Pyrazinamide is administered at an oral dose of 15-30 mg/kg/day.

UNTOWARD EFFECTS. Injury to the liver is the most serious side effect of pyrazinamide. With an oral dose of 40-50 mg/kg, signs and symptoms of hepatic disease appear in ~15% of patients, with jaundice in 2-3% and death due to hepatic necrosis in rare instances. Current regimens (15-30 mg/kg/day) are much safer. Prior to pyrazinamide administration, all patients should undergo studies of hepatic function, and these studies should be repeated at frequent intervals during the entire period of treatment. If there is evidence of significant hepatic damage, therapy must be stopped. Pyrazinamide should not be given to patients with hepatic dysfunction unless its use is unavoidable.

In nearly all patients, pyrazinamide inhibits excretion of urate, and causes a hyperuricemia that may result in acute episodes of gout. Other untoward effects observed with pyrazinamide include arthralgias, anorexia, nausea and vomiting, dysuria, malaise, and fever. Pyrazinamide is not approved in the U.S. during pregnancy because of inadequate data on teratogenicity.

ISONIAZID

Isoniazid (isonicotinic acid hydrazide, INH; NYDRAZID, others) is a primary agent for TB. All patients infected with isoniazid-sensitive strains should receive the drug if they can tolerate it.

The combination of isoniazid + pyrazinamide + rifampin provides a "short-course" therapy with improved remission rates.

MECHANISM OF ACTION. Isoniazid enters bacilli by passive diffusion. The drug is not directly toxic to the bacillus but must be activated to its toxic form within the bacillus by KatG, a multifunctional catalase-peroxidase. The activated drug forms adducts with bacillar NAD^+ and $NADP^+$ that inhibit essential steps in mycolic acid synthesis (cell wall) and nucleic acid synthesis (Figure 56–3). Other products of KatG activation of INH include superoxide, H_2O_2, alkyl hydroperoxides, and the NO radical, which may also contribute to the mycobactericidal effects of INH.

MECHANISMS OF RESISTANCE. Resistance to INH is associated with mutation or deletion of katG, overexpression of the genes for inhA (confers low-level resistance to INH and some cross-resistance to ethionamide) and ahpC, and mutations in the *kasA* gene. The prevalence of drug-resistant mutants is ~1 in 10^6 bacilli. Because TB cavities may contain as many as 10^7-10^9 microorganisms, preexistent resistance can be expected in pulmonary TB cavities of untreated patients. These spontaneous mutants will be selected and amplified by monotherapy. Thus, 2 or more agents are usually used. Because the mutations resulting in drug resistance are independent events, the probability of resistance to 2 antimycobacterial agents is small, ~1 in 10^{12} ($1 \times 10^6 \times 10^6$), a low probability considering the number of bacilli involved.

ADME. The bioavailability of orally administered isoniazid is ~100% for the 300 mg dose. The pharmacokinetics of isoniazid are best described by a one-compartment model, with the pharmacokinetic parameters in Table 56–2. Isoniazid is metabolized by hepatic arylamine *N*-acetyltransferase type 2 (NAT2), encoded by a variety of NAT2* alleles (*see* Figure 56–3). Isoniazid clearance in patients has been traditionally classified as 1 of 2 phenotypic groups: "slow" and "fast" acetylators (Figure 56–4), and more recently as 3 groups, including "intermediate" metabolizers; this variability largely reflects expression of various NAT2 alleles. Most (75-95%) of a dose of isoniazid is excreted in the urine within 24 h, predominantly as acetylisoniazid and isonicotinic acid.

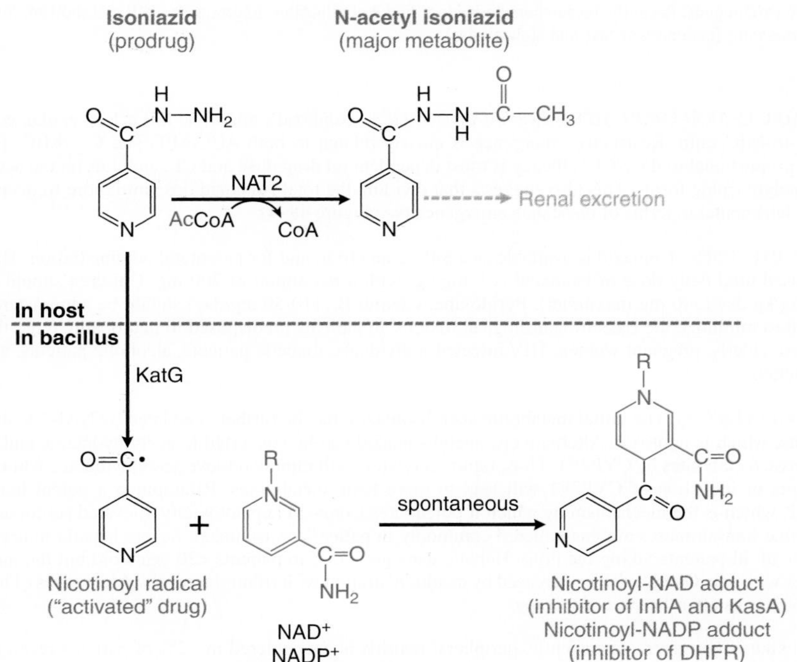

Figure 56–3 *Metabolism and activation of isoniazid.* The prodrug isoniazid is metabolized in humans by NAT2 isoforms to its principal metabolite, N-acetyl isoniazid, which is excreted by the kidney. Isoniazid diffuses into mycoplasma where it is "activated" by KatG (oxidase/peroxidase) to the nicotinoyl radical. The nicotinoyl radical reacts spontaneously with NAD^+ to produce adducts that inhibit essential enzymes in synthesis of the cell-wall component mycolic acid, and with $NADP^+$ to produce an inhibitor of nucleic acid synthesis. InhA, enoyl acyl carrier protein; KasA, enoyl acyl carrier protein synthase; DHFR, dihydrofolate reductase.

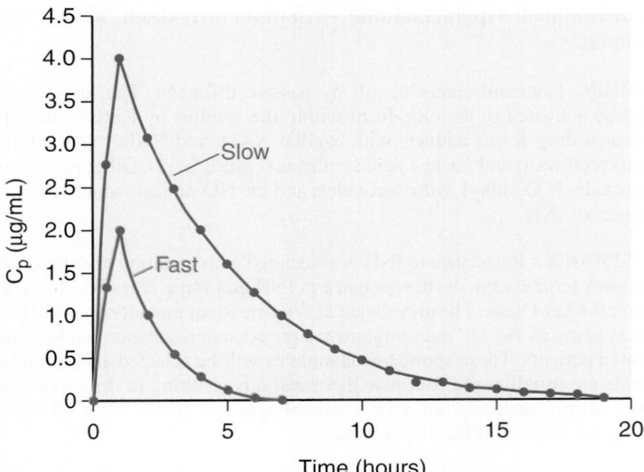

Figure 56–4 *Multi-modal distribution of INH clearance due to NAT2 polymorphisms.* A group of matched male volunteers received INH (250 mg orally) and the time courses of plasma drug levels (C_p) were assessed. One-third of the subjects had INH elimination $t_{1/2}$ values <1.5 h; these are the *fast acetylators*. Two-thirds had $t_{1/2}$ values ranging from 2.1 to 4.0 h, with a suggestion of multiple groups; these are the *slow acetylators*. Plots of the mean data (C_p vs. time after administration) demonstrate the pharmacokinetic effects of acetylation rate. Both groups reached C_{Pmax} at 1 h. The slow acetylators (*red line*) achieved a higher C_p (4 μg/mL) with a mean elimination $t_{1/2}$ = 3.0 h; the fast acetylators (*green line*) reached a lower maximal C_p (2 μg/mL) with a mean elimination $t_{1/2}$ = 1.0 h. The acetylation rate reflects variable expression of active and defective polymorphic forms of NAT2. Slow acetylators may be a greater risk for adverse effects from INH, sulfonamides, and procainamide; fast acetylators may have diminished responses to standard doses of these agents but greater risk from bioactivation by NAT2 of arylamine/hydrazine carcinogens. Recently, researchers have identified 3 elimination subgroups for INH metabolism: *fast, slow,* and *intermediate* (codominant fast and slow alleles).

MICROBIAL PHARMACOKINETICS-PHARMACODYNAMICS. Isoniazid's microbial kill is best explained by the AUC_{0-24}-to-MIC ratio. Resistance emergence is closely related to both AUC/MIC and C_{max}/MIC. Because AUC is proportional to dose/CL, efficacy is most dependent on drug dose and CL, and thus on the activity of *NAT-2* polymorphic forms. This also suggests that dividing the total isoniazid dose into more frequent doses may be detrimental in terms of resistance emergence (*see* Figure 48–4).

THERAPEUTIC USES. Isoniazid is available as a pill, as an elixir, and for parenteral administration. The commonly used total daily dose of isoniazid is 5 mg/kg, with a maximum of 300 mg. Children should receive 10-15 mg/kg/day (300 mg maximum). Pyridoxine, vitamin B_6, (10-50 mg/day) should be administered with isoniazid to minimize the risks of neurological toxicity in patients predisposed to neuropathy (e.g., the malnourished, elderly, pregnant women, HIV-infected individuals, diabetic patients, alcoholic patients, and uremic patients).

UNTOWARD EFFECTS. The initial metabolite acetylisoniazid may be further acetylated by NAT-2 to diacetylhydrazine, which is nontoxic. Alternatively, acetylisoniazid can be converted to acetylhydrazine and then to hepatotoxic metabolites by CYP2E1. Thus, rapid acetylators will rapidly remove acetylhydrazine while slower acetylators or induction of CYP2E1 will lead to more toxic metabolites. Rifampin is a potent inducer of CYP2E1, which is the mechanism by which it potentiates isoniazid hepatotoxicity. Elevated serum aspartate and alanine transaminases are encountered commonly in patients on isoniazid. Severe hepatic injury occurs in ~0.1% of all patients taking the drug. Hepatic damage is rare in patients <20 years old but the incidence increases with age. Overall risk is increased by coadministration with rifampin to ~3%. Most cases of hepatitis occur 4-8 weeks after the start of therapy.

If pyridoxine is not given concurrently, peripheral neuritis is encountered in ~2% of patients receiving isoniazid 5 mg/kg of the drug daily. Neuropathy is more frequent in "slow" acetylators and in individuals with diabetes mellitus, poor nutrition, or anemia. Other neurological toxicities include convulsions in patients with seizure disorders, optic neuritis and atrophy, muscle twitching, dizziness, ataxia, paresthesias, stupor, and toxic encephalopathy. Mental abnormalities may appear during the use of this drug.

Patients may develop hypersensitivity to isoniazid. Hematological reactions also may occur. Arthritic symptoms also have been attributed to this agent. Miscellaneous reactions associated with isoniazid therapy include dryness of the mouth, epigastric distress, methemoglobinemia, tinnitus, and urinary retention. A drug-induced syndrome resembling systemic lupus erythematosus has also been reported.

ISONIAZID OVERDOSE. Isoniazid overdose has been associated with the clinical triad of:

- Seizures refractory to treatment with phenytoin and barbiturates
- Metabolic acidosis with an anion gap that is resistant to treatment with sodium bicarbonate
- Coma

Treatment involves cessation of isoniazid dosing and administration of intravenous pyridoxine over 5-15 min on a gram-to-gram basis with the ingested isoniazid. If the dose of ingested isoniazid is unknown, then a pyridoxine dose of 70 mg/kg should be used. In patients with seizures, benzodiazepines are used.

DRUG INTERACTIONS. Isoniazid is a potent inhibitor of CYP2C19, CYP3A, and a weak inhibitor of CYP2D6. However, isoniazid induces CYP2E1. Drugs that are metabolized by these enzymes will potentially be affected (Table 56–4).

ETHAMBUTOL

Ethambutol hydrochloride (MYAMBUTOL) is a water-soluble and heat-stable compound.

MECHANISM OF ACTION. Ethambutol inhibits arabinosyl transferase III (catalyzes the transfer of arabinose in arabinogalactan biosynthesis), thereby disrupting the assembly of mycobacterial cell wall.

ANTIBACTERIAL ACTIVITY. Ethambutol has activity against a wide range of mycobacteria. Ethambutol MICs are 0.5-2 mg/L in clinical isolates of *M. tuberculosis*, ~0.8 mg/L for *M. kansasii*, and 2-7.5 mg/L for *M. avium*. The following species are also susceptible: *Mycobacterium gordonae, M. marinum, M. scrofulaceum, M. szulgai*. However, the majority of *M. xenopi, M. fortuitum*, and *M. chelonae* are resistant.

MECHANISMS OF RESISTANCE. In vitro, mycobacterial resistance to the drug develops via mutations in the *embB* gene, which encodes arabinosyl transferases. Enhanced efflux pump activity induces resistance to both isoniazid and ethambutol in vitro.

ADME. The oral bioavailability of ethambutol is ~80%. The decline in ethambutol is biexponential, with a $t_{1/2}$ of 3 h in the first 12 h, and a $t_{1/2}$ of 9 h between 12 and 24 h, due to redistribution of drug. Clearance and V_d are greater in children than in adults on a per kilogram basis. Slow and incomplete absorption is common in children, so that good peak concentrations of drug are often not achieved with standard dosing. *See* Table 56–2 for PK data on this drug. About 80% of the drug is not metabolized and is renally excreted. Therefore, in renal failure ethambutol should be dosed at 15-25 mg/kg, 3 times a week instead of daily. The remainder of ethambutol (~20%) is excreted as aldehyde and dicarboxylic acid derivatives (produced by alcohol and aldehyde dehydrogenases).

MICROBIAL PHARMACOKINETICS-PHARMACODYNAMICS. Ethambutol's microbial kill of *M. tuberculosis* is optimized by AUC/MIC, while that against disseminated MAC is optimized by C_{max}/MIC. Thus, to optimize microbial kill, high intermittent doses such as 25 mg/kg every other day to 50 mg/kg twice a week may be superior to daily doses of 15 mg/kg.

THERAPEUTIC USES. Ethambutol is available for oral administration in tablets containing the D-isomer. It is used for the treatment of TB, disseminated MAC, and in *M. kansasii* infection.

Table 56–4

Isoniazid-Drug Interactions via Inhibition and Induction of CYPs

CO-ADMINISTERED DRUG	CYP ISOFORM	ADVERSE EFFECTS
Acetaminophen	CYP2E1 inhibition-induction	Hepatotoxicity
Carbamazepine	CYP3A inhibition	Neurological toxicity
Diazepam	CYP3A and CYP2C19 inhibition	Sedation and respiratory depression
Ethosuximide	CYP3A inhibition	Psychotic behavior
Isoflurane and enflurane	CYP2E1 induction	Decreased effectiveness
Phenytoin	CYP2C19 inhibition	Neurological toxicity
Theophylline	CYP3A inhibition	Seizures, palpitation, nausea
Vincristine	CYP3A inhibition	Limb weakness and tingling
Warfarin	CYP2C9 inhibition	Possibility of increased bleeding (single case reported)

UNTOWARD EFFECTS. Ethambutol produces very few serious untoward reactions: ~1% experience diminished visual acuity resulting from a reversible optic neuritis, 0.5% a rash, and 0.3% drug fever. Other side effects that have been observed are pruritus, joint pain, GI upset, abdominal pain, malaise, headache, dizziness, mental confusion, disorientation, and possible hallucinations. Therapy with ethambutol results in an increased concentration of urate in the blood in ~50% of patients, owing to decreased renal excretion of uric acid.

AMINOGLYCOSIDES: STREPTOMYCIN, AMIKACIN, AND KANAMYCIN

Streptomycin, amikacin, and kanamycin are used for the treatment of mycobacterial diseases. These aminoglycosides inhibit protein synthesis by binding to the 30S ribosomal subunit (*see* Figure 54–2). The pharmacological properties and therapeutic uses of aminoglycosides are discussed in full in Chapter 54.

The MICs for *M. tuberculosis* in Middlebrook broth are 0.25-3.0 mg/L for all 3 aminoglycosides. For *M. avium* streptomycin and amikacin, MICs are 1-8 mg/L; those of kanamycin are 3-12 mg/L. *M. kansasii* is frequently susceptible to these agents but other nontuberculous mycobacteria are only occasionally susceptible.

BACTERIAL RESISTANCE. Primary resistance to streptomycin is found in 2-3% of *M. tuberculosis* clinical isolates. Resistance results from mutations in 2 components of the 30S ribosomal subunit, *rpsL* and *rrs*; in the rRNA methyltransferase gene *gidB*, and in efflux pumps.

CLOFAZIMINE

Clofazimine (LAMPRENE), a fat-soluble riminophenazine dye, was discontinued in 2005 but remains licensed as an orphan drug.

MECHANISM OF ACTION. Clofazimine has both antibacterial activity as well as anti-inflammatory effects via inhibition of macrophages, T cells, neutrophils, and complement. Clofazimine is recommended as a component of multiple drug therapy for leprosy. The compound also is useful for treatment of chronic skin ulcers (Buruli ulcer) produced by *Mycobacterium ulcerans*. Possible mechanisms of action include:

- Membrane disruption
- Inhibition of mycobacterial phospholipase A_2
- Inhibition of microbial K^+ transport
- Generation of hydrogen peroxide
- Interference with the bacterial electron transport chain

ANTIBACTERIAL ACTIVITY. The MICs for *M. avium* are 1-5 mg/L. The MICs for *M. tuberculosis* are ~1.0 mg/L. It also has activity against many gram-positive bacteria.

ADME. Clofazimine is administered orally at doses up to 300 mg/day. Bioavailability is variable (45-60%) and is increased 2-fold by high-fat meals and decreased 30% by antacids. After a single dose of 200 mg of clofazimine, the t_{max} is 5.3-7.8 h. After prolonged repeated dosing, the $t_{1/2}$ is ~70 days. For PK data, *see* Table 56–2. Clofazimine is metabolized by the liver.

UNTOWARD EFFECTS. GI problems are encountered in 40-50% of patients. In patients who have died following the abdominal pain, crystal deposition in intestinal mucosa, liver, spleen, and abdominal lymph nodes has been demonstrated. Body secretion discoloration, eye discoloration, and skin discoloration occur in most patients.

DRUG INTERACTIONS. Anti-inflammatory effects may be inhibited by dapsone.

FLUOROQUINOLONES

Fluoroquinolones are DNA gyrase inhibitors (*see* Chapter 52). Drugs such as ofloxacin and ciprofloxacin have been second-line anti-TB agents for many years, but they are limited by the rapid development of resistance.

Adding C8 halogen and C8 methoxy groups markedly reduces the propensity for drug resistance. Of the C8 methoxy quinolones, *moxifloxacin* (FDA-approved for nontubercular infections) is furthest along in clinical testing as an anti-TB agent. Moxifloxacin is being studied to replace either isoniazid or ethambutol.

THERAPEUTIC USES IN TREATMENT OF TB. In TB patients, moxifloxacin (400 mg/day) has bactericidal effects similar to that of standard doses of isoniazid. When replacing ethambutol in the standard multidrug regimen, 400 mg/day of moxifloxacin produces faster sputum conversion at 4 weeks than ethambutol. Moxifloxacin is currently being studied in a phase 3 trial that may eventually lead to 4-month duration of anti-TB therapy compared to the current 6 months.

TMC-207 (R207910)

MECHANISM OF ACTION. TMC-207 is a experimental diarylquinone for treatment of multidrug-resistant TB. The compound targets bacillar energy metabolism, acting on subunit c of the ATP synthase of *M. tuberculosis* and leading to inhibition of the proton pump activity of the ATP synthase. The TMC-207 MIC for *M. tuberculosis* is 0.03-0.12 mg/L. It has good activity against *MAC, M. leprae, M. bovis, M. marinum, M. kansasii, M. ulcerans, M. fortuitum, M. szulgai*, and *M. abscessus*.

PHARMACOKINETICS, EFFICACY, AND THERAPEUTIC USE. A regimen of TMC207 400 mg daily for 2 weeks followed by 200 mg 3 times day thereafter was added to a background second-line regimen of either kanamycin or amikacin, ofloxacin with or without ethambutol in patients with TB resistant to both isoniazid and rifampin (MDRTB), and led to an 8-week sputum conversion of ~50% with TMC207 compared to 9% without.

UNTOWARD EFFECTS. The adverse events encountered in the limited number of patients exposed to this experimental agent are mild and include nausea in 26% of patients and diarrhea in 13% of patients, with others (e.g., arthralgia, pain in extremities, and hyperuricemia) in a small proportion of patients.

PA-824

PA-824, an experimental agent, is a nitroimidazopyran prodrug that requires activation by the bacteria via a nitro-reduction step, similar to the structurally related agent, metronidazole. Activation requires a specific glucose-6-phosphate dehydrogenase, FGD1.

MECHANISM OF ACTION. PA-824 inhibits *M. tuberculosis* mycolic acid and protein synthesis. Another mechanism involves generation of reactive nitrogen species such as NO by PA-824's des-nitro metabolite, which then augment the kill of intracellular nonreplicating persistent bacilli by the innate immune system.

ANTIBACTERIAL ACTIVITY. In vitro, the drug kills both nonreplicating *M. tuberculosis* that are under anaerobic conditions as well as replicating bacteria in ambient air. The MICs of PA-824 against *M. tuberculosis* range from 0.015–0.25 mg/L, but the drug lacks activity against other mycobacteria.

BACTERIAL RESISTANCE. The proportion of mutants resistant to 5 mg/L of PA-824 is 10^{-6}. Resistance can arise due to changes in structure of FGD, resulting from point mutations in *fgd* gene. However, resistant isolates have also been identified that lack *fgd* mutations, so that resistance may also be due to other mechanisms.

ETHIONAMIDE

Ethionamide (TRECATOR) is a congener of thioisonicotinamide.

MECHANISM OF ACTION. Ethionamide is a prodrug that is activated to a sulfoxide by a mycobacterial NADPH-specific monooxygenase (EthaA), and then to 2-ethyl-4-aminopyridine. Although these products are not toxic to mycobacteria, it is believed that a closely related and transient intermediate is the active antibiotic. Like isoniazid, ethionamide inhibits mycobacterial growth by inhibiting the activity of the *inhA* gene product, the enoyl-ACP reductase of fatty acid synthase II. Both drugs inhibit mycolic acid biosynthesis with consequent impairment of cell-wall synthesis.

ANTIBACTERIAL ACTIVITY. The multiplication of *M. tuberculosis* is suppressed by concentrations of ethionamide ranging from 0.6-2.5 mg/L. A concentration of ≤10 mg/L will inhibit ~75% of photochromogenic mycobacteria; the scotochromogens are more resistant.

BACTERIAL RESISTANCE. Resistance occurs mainly via changes in the enzyme that activates ethionamide. Mutations in *inhA* gene lead to resistance to both ethionamide and isoniazid.

ADME. The oral bioavailability of ethionamide approaches 100%. The pharmacokinetics are adequately explained by a one-compartment model with first-order absorption and elimination; see PK values in Table 56–2. The $t_{1/2}$ is ~2 h. Ethionamide is cleared by hepatic metabolism. Metabolites are eliminated in the urine. Ethionamide is administered only orally. The initial dosage for adults is 250 mg twice daily; it is increased by 125 mg/day every 5 days until a dose of 15-20 mg/kg/day is achieved. The maximal dose is 1 g daily. The drug is best taken with meals in divided doses to minimize gastric irritation. Children should receive 10-20 mg/kg/day in 2 divided doses, not to exceed 1 g/day.

UNTOWARD EFFECTS. Approximately 50% of patients are unable to tolerate a single dose larger than 500 mg because of GI upset. The most common reactions are anorexia, nausea and vomiting, gastric irritation, and a variety of neurologic symptoms. Severe postural hypotension, mental depression, drowsiness, and asthenia are common. Convulsions and peripheral neuropathy are rare. Other reactions referable to the nervous system include olfactory disturbances, blurred vision, diplopia, dizziness, paresthesias, headache, restlessness, and tremors. Pyridoxine (vitamin B_6) relieves the neurologic symptoms, and its concomitant administration is recommended. Severe allergic skin rashes, purpura, stomatitis, gynecomastia, impotence, menorrhagia, acne, and alopecia have also been observed. A metallic taste also may be noted. Hepatitis has been associated with the use of the ethionamide in ~5% of cases. Hepatic function should be assessed at regular intervals in patients receiving the drug.

PARA-AMINOSALICYLIC ACID

Para-aminosalicylic acid (PAS) was the first effective treatment for TB.

MECHANISM OF ACTION. PAS is a congener of *para*-aminobenzoic acid, the substrate of dihydropteroate synthase (*fol*P1/P2); this structural similarity accounted for PAS's postulated action as a competitive inhibitor of the enzyme (Figure 56–5). PAS is a poor inhibitor of dihydropteroate synthase in vitro; moreover, only 37% of the PAS-resistant clinical isolates or spontaneous mutants encode a mutation in any genes for enzymes in the folate pathway or biosynthesis of thymine nucleotides. Furthermore, mutations in *thyA* (the gene for thymidylate synthase) lead to drug resistance in only a minority of drug-resistant isolates. Unidentified actions of PAS likely play important roles in its anti-TB effects.

ANTIBACTERIAL ACTIVITY. PAS is bacteriostatic. In vitro, most strains of *M. tuberculosis* are sensitive to a concentration of 1 mg/L. It has no activity against other bacteria.

ADME. PAS is administered orally in a daily dose of 12 g, with the daily dose divided into 3 equal portions. Children should receive 150-300 mg/kg/day in 3-4 divided doses. PAS oral bioavailability is >90%. PK data are shown in Table 56–2. The C_{Pmax} increases 1.5-fold and AUC 1.7-fold with food; indeed, PAS should be administered with food, which also reduces gastric irritation. PAS is *N*-acetylated in the liver to *N*-acetyl PAS, a potential hepatotoxin. Over 80% of the drug is excreted in the urine; >50% is in the form of the acetylated compound. Excretion of PAS is reduced by renal dysfunction, requiring a reduction in dosage.

UNTOWARD EFFECTS. The incidence of untoward effects associated with the use of PAS is ~10-30%. GI problems predominate and often limit patient adherence. Hypersensitivity reactions to PAS are seen in 5-10% of patients and manifest as skin eruptions, fever, eosinophilia, and other hematological abnormalities.

CYCLOSERINE

Cycloserine (SEROMYCIN) is a broad-spectrum antibiotic produced by *Streptococcus orchidaceous* that is used in the multi-agent treatment of TB when primary agents have failed.

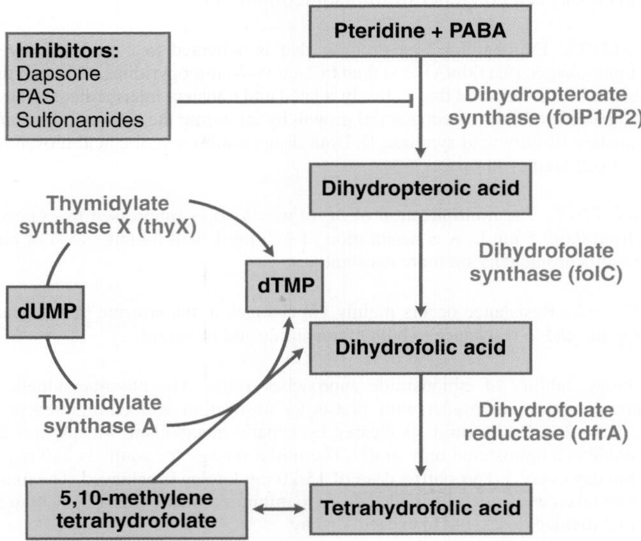

Figure 56–5 *Effects of antimicrobials on folate metabolism and deoxynucleotide synthesis.* Two forms of thymidylate synthase are relevant here: the human form, thyA (EC 2.1.1.45) and the bacterial form, thyX (EC 2.1.1.148); molecular differences may permit development of form-specific inhibitors.

MECHANISM OF ACTION. Cycloserine is a congener of D-alanine. D-alanyl-D-alanine is an essential component of the peptidoglycan of the bacterial cell wall (*see* Figure 55–4). Cycloserine inhibits 2 enzymes that are necessary for incorporation of alanine into the cell wall: a racemase that converts L-alanine to D-alanine, and a ligase that joins 2 D-alanines to make D-alanyl-D-alanine.

ANTIBACTERIAL ACTIVITY; RESISTANCE. Cycloserine inhibits *M. tuberculosis* at concentrations of 5-20 mg/L. It has good activity against MAC, enterococci, *Escherichia coli, Staphylococcus aureus, Nocardia* species, and *Chlamydia*. Resistance of *M. tuberculosis* occurs in 10-82% of clinical isolates. Mutations involved in cycloserine resistance of pathogenic *Mycobacteria* are currently unknown.

ADME. The usual dose for adults is 250-500 mg orally, twice daily. Oral cycloserine is almost completely absorbed. C_{max} in plasma is reached in 45 min in fasting subjects, but is delayed for up to 3.5 h with a high-fat meal. *See* Table 56–2 for PK values. Cycloserine is well distributed throughout body. About 50% of cycloserine is excreted unchanged in the urine in the first 12 h; a total of 70% is recoverable in the active form over a period of 24 h. The drug may accumulate to toxic concentrations in patients with renal failure. About 60% of it is removed by hemodialysis.

UNTOWARD EFFECTS. Neuropsychiatric symptoms are common and occur in 50% of patients on 1 g/day, so much so that the drug has earned the nickname "psych-serine." Symptoms range from headache and somnolence to severe psychosis, seizures, and suicidal ideas. Large doses of cycloserine or the concomitant ingestion of alcohol increases the risk of seizures. Cycloserine is contraindicated in individuals with a history of epilepsy and should be used with caution in individuals with a history of depression.

CAPREOMYCIN

Capreomycin (CAPASTAT) is an antimycobacterial cyclic peptide. Antimycobacterial activity is similar to that of aminoglycosides as are adverse effects, and capreomycin should not be administered with other drugs that damage cranial nerve VIII. Bacterial resistance to capreomycin develops when it is given alone; such microorganisms show cross-resistance with kanamycin and neomycin. The adverse reactions associated with the use of capreomycin are hearing loss, tinnitus, transient proteinuria, cylindruria, and nitrogen retention. Eosinophilia is common. Leukocytosis, leukopenia, rashes, and fever have also been observed. Capreomycin is a second-line antituberculosis agent. The recommended daily dose is 1 g (no more than 20 mg/kg) per day for 60-120 days, followed by 1 g 2 to 3 times a week.

MACROLIDES

The pharmacology, bacterial activity, resistance mechanisms of macrolides are discussed in Chapter 55. Azithromycin and clarithromycin are used for the treatment of MAC.

DAPSONE

Dapsone is a broad-spectrum agent with antibacterial, anti-protozoal, and antifungal effects.

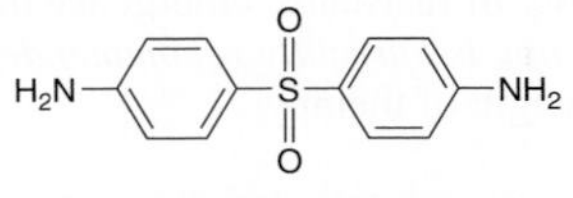

H_2N—C$_6$H$_4$—S(=O)(=O)—C$_6$H$_4$—NH_2

DAPSONE

MECHANISM OF ACTION. Dapsone (DDS, diamino-diphenylsulfone) is a structural analog of *para*-aminobenzoic acid (PABA) and a competitive inhibitor of dihydropteroate synthase (*fol*P1/P2) in the folate pathway, shown in Figure 56–5 (*see* also Figures 52–1 and 52–1). The anti-inflammatory effects of dapsone occur via inhibition of tissue damage by neutrophils. Dapsone is extensively used for acne, but this therapy is not recommended.

ANTIMICROBIAL EFFECTS

Antibacterial. Dapsone is bacteriostatic against *M. leprae* at concentrations of 1-10 mg/L. More than 90% of clinical isolates of MAC and *M. kansasii* have an MIC of ≤8 mg/L, but the MICs for *M. tuberculosis* isolates are high. It has little activity against other bacteria.

Anti-parasitic. Dapsone is highly effective against *Plasmodium falciparum* with IC_{50} of 0.006-0.013 mg/mL (0.6-1.3 mg/L) even in sulfadoxine-pyrimethamine–resistant strains. Dapsone has an IC_{50} of 0.55 mg/L against *Toxoplasma gondii* tachyzoites.

Antifungal. Dapsone is effective at concentrations of 0.1/mg/L against the fungus *Pneumocystic jiroveci*.

DRUG RESISTANCE. Resistance to dapsone results primarily from mutations in genes encoding dihydropteroate synthase (*see* Figure 56–5).

ADME. After oral administration, absorption is complete; the elimination $t_{1/2}$ is 20-30 h. The population pharmacokinetics of dapsone are shown in Table 56–2. Dapsone undergoes *N*-acetylation by NAT2 and *N*-oxidation to dapsone hydroxylamine via CYP2E1 and CYP2C. Dapsone hydroxylamine enters red blood cells, leading to methemoglobin formation. Sulfones (e.g., dapsone) tend to be retained for up to 3 weeks in skin and muscle and especially in liver and kidney. Intestinal reabsorption of sulfones excreted in the bile contributes to long-term retention in the bloodstream; periodic interruption of treatment is advisable for this reason. Approximately 70-80% of a dose of dapsone is excreted in the urine as an acid-labile mono-*N*-glucuronide and mono-*N*-sulfamate.

THERAPEUTIC USES. Dapsone is administered as an oral agent. Therapeutic uses of dapsone in the treatment of leprosy are described later. Dapsone is combined with chlorproguanil for the treatment of malaria. The anti-inflammatory effects are the basis for therapy for pemphigoid, dermatitis herpetiformis, linear IgA bullous disease, relapsing chondritis, and ulcers caused by the brown recluse spider.

DAPSONE AND G6PD DEFICIENCY. Glucose-6-phosphate dehydrogenase (G6PD) protects red cells against oxidative damage. However, G6PD deficiency is encountered in nearly half a billion people worldwide. Dapsone, an oxidant, causes severe hemolysis in patients with G6PD deficiency. Thus, G6PD deficiency testing should be performed prior to use of dapsone wherever possible.

OTHER UNTOWARD EFFECTS. Doses of ≤100 mg in healthy persons and ≤50 mg in healthy individuals with a G6PD deficiency do not cause hemolysis. Hemolysis develops in almost every individual treated with 200-300 mg of dapsone per day; methemoglobinemia also is common. A genetic deficiency in the NADH-dependent methemoglobin reductase can result in severe methemoglobinemia after administration of dapsone. Isolated instances of headache, nervousness, insomnia, blurred vision, paresthesias, reversible peripheral neuropathy, drug fever, hematuria, pruritus, psychosis, and a variety of skin rashes have been reported. An infectious mononucleosis-like syndrome, which may be fatal, occurs occasionally.

PRINCIPLES OF ANTITUBERCULOSIS CHEMOTHERAPY

Tuberculosis is not caused by a single species, but by a mixture of species with 99.9% similarity at the nucleotide level. The complex includes *M. tuberculosis (typus humanus), M. canettii, M. africanum, M. bovis*, and *M. microti*. They all cause TB, with *M. microti* responsible for only a handful of human cases.

ANTITUBERCULOSIS THERAPY. With anti-TB drug monotherapy, emergence of resistance renders the drugs ineffective. The mutation rates to first-line anti-TB drugs are between 10^{-7} and 10^{-10}, so that the likelihood of resistance is high to any single anti-TB drugs in patients with cavitary TB who have ~10^9 CFU of bacilli in a 3-cm pulmonary lesion. However, the likelihood that bacilli would develop mutations to 2 or more different drugs is the product of 2 mutation rates (between 1 in 10^{14} and 1 in 10^{20}), a probability of resistance emergence that is acceptably small. *Thus, only combination therapy anti-TB therapy is currently recommended for treatment of TB.* Multidrug therapy has led to a reduction in length of therapy.

Isoniazid, pyrazinamide, rifampin, ethambutol, and streptomycin are currently considered first-line anti-TB agents. Moxifloxacin is being studied as a first-line agent. First-line agents are more efficacious and better tolerated, relative to second-line agents. Second-line drugs include ethionamide, PAS, cycloserine, amikacin, kanamycin, and capreomycin.

TYPES OF ANTITUBERCULOSIS THERAPY

PROPHYLAXIS. After infection with *M. tuberculosis*, ~10% of people will develop active disease over a lifetime. The highest risk of reactivation TB is in patients with Mantoux tuberculin skin test reaction ≥5 mm who also fall into 1 of the following categories: recently exposed to TB, have HIV co-infection, or are immunosuppressed. If the tuberculin skin test is ≥10 mm, high risk of TB is encountered in recent (≤5 years) immigrants from areas of high TB prevalence, children <4 years of age, intravenous drug users, as well as residents and employees of high-risk congregate settings. Any person with a skin test >15 mm is also at high risk. In these patients at high risk of active TB, prophylaxis is recommended to prevent active disease. Prophylaxis consists of oral isoniazid, 300 mg daily or twice weekly, for 6 months in adults. Those who cannot take isoniazid should be given rifampin, 10 mg/kg daily, for 4 months. In children, isoniazid 10-15 mg/kg daily (maximum 300 mg) is administered, or 20-30 mg/kg 2 times a week directly observed, for 9 months. In children who cannot tolerate isoniazid, rifampin 10-20 mg/kg daily for 6 months is recommended.

DEFINITIVE THERAPY. The current standard regimen for drug-susceptible TB consists of isoniazid (5 mg/kg, maximum 300 mg/day), rifampin (10 mg/kg, maximum 600 mg/day), and pyrazinamide (15-30 mg/kg, maximum of 2 g/day) for 2 months, followed by intermittent 10 mg/kg rifampin and 15 mg/kg isoniazid 2 or 3 times a week for 4 months. Children should receive 10-20 mg/kg isoniazid per day (300 mg maximum). Rifabutin 5 mg/kg/day can be used for the entire 6 months of therapy in adult HIV-infected patients because rifampin can adversely interact with some antiretroviral agents to reduce their effectiveness. In case there is resistance to isoniazid, initial therapy also may include ethambutol (15-20 mg/kg/day) or streptomycin (1 g/day) until isoniazid susceptibility is documented. Ethambutol doses in children are 15-20 mg/kg/day (maximum 1 g) or 50 mg/kg twice weekly (2.5 g). Because monitoring of visual acuity is difficult in children <5 years old, caution should be exercised in using ethambutol in these children.

The first 2 months of the 4-drug regimen is termed the initial phase of therapy, and the last 4 months the continuation phase of therapy. Rifapentine (10 mg/kg once a week) may be substituted for rifampin in the continuation phase in patients with no evidence of HIV infection or cavitary TB. Pyridoxine, vitamin B_6, (10-50 mg/day) should be administered with isoniazid to minimize the risks of neurological toxicity in patients predisposed to neuropathy. The duration of therapy for drug-susceptible pulmonary TB is 6 months. A 9-month duration should be used for patients with cavitary disease who are still sputum culture positive at 2 months. Most cases of extrapulmonary TB are treated for 6 months. TB meningitis is an exception that requires a 9- to 12-month duration. In addition, corticosteroids are recommended for TB pericarditis, and results of a meta-analysis suggest they should also be used in TB meningitis.

DRUG-RESISTANT TB. In documented drug resistance, therapy should be based on evidence of susceptibility and should include:

- At least 3 drugs to which the pathogen is susceptible, with at least 1 injectable anti-TB agent
- In the case of multidrug resistant-TB, use of 4 to 6 medications for better outcomes
- At least 18 months of therapy

The addition to the regimen of a fluoroquinolone and surgical resection of the main lesions have been associated with improved outcome. There are currently no data to support intermittent therapy.

PRINCIPLES OF THERAPY AGAINST *MYCOBACTERIUM AVIUM* COMPLEX (*MAC*)

The *MAC* is made up of at least 2 species: *M. intracellulare* and *M. avium*. *M. intracellulare* causes pulmonary disease often in immunocompetent individuals. *M. avium* is further divided into a number of subspecies: *M. avium* subsp. *hominissuis* causes disseminated disease in immunocompromised patients, *M. avium* subsp. *paratuberculosis* has been implicated in the etiology of Crohn disease, and *M. avium* subsp. *avium* causes TB of birds. These bacteria are ubiquitous in the environment and can be encountered in water, food, and soil.

THERAPY OF *MAC* PULMONARY INFECTION

M. intracellulare often infects immunocompetent patients. In newly diagnosed patients with *MAC* pneumonia, triple drug therapy is recommended: a rifamycin, ethambutol, and a macrolide. For the macrolides, either oral clarithromycin or azithromycin may be used. Rifampin is often the rifamycin of choice. Clarithromycin, 1000 mg, or azithromycin, 500 mg, are combined with ethambutol, 25 mg/kg, and rifampin, 600 mg, and administered 3 times a week for nodular and bronchiectatic disease. Therapy is continued for 12 months after the last negative culture. The same drugs are administered for patients with cavitary disease, but the dosing regimens are azithromycin 250 mg, ethambutol 15 mg/kg, and rifampin 600 mg. Parenteral streptomycin or amikacin at 15 mg/kg is recommended as a fourth drug. Duration of therapy is as for nodular disease. In advanced pulmonary disease or during re-treatment, rifabutin 300 mg daily may replace rifampin. Because clarithromycin susceptibility correlates with outcome, risk of failure is high when high clarithromycin MICs are documented. Patients at risk for failure also include those with cavitary disease, presumably due to higher bacillary load. Even with these therapies, long-term success is still fairly limited (~50%).

THERAPY FOR DISSEMINATED *M. AVIUM* COMPLEX

Disseminated *MAC* disease is caused by *M. avium* in 95% of patients. This is a disease of the immunocompromised patient. Patients at risk for infection are those who have had other opportunistic infections, are colonized with *MAC*, or have an HIV RNA burden >5 $\log_{10}$ copies/mm^3.

The symptoms of disseminated disease are nonspecific and include fever, night sweats, weight loss, elevated serum alkaline phosphates, and anemia at the time of diagnosis. However, when disease occurs in patients already on anti-retroviral therapy, it may manifest as a focal disease of the lymph nodes, osteomyelitis, pneumonitis, pericarditis, skin or soft-tissue abscesses, genital ulcers, or CNS infection.

PROPHYLACTIC THERAPY. Monotherapy with either oral azithromycin 1200 mg once a week or clarithromycin 500 mg twice a day is started when patients present with a CD4 count $<50/mm^3$. For patients intolerant of macrolides, rifabutin 300 mg/day is administered. Once the CD4 count is >100 per mm^3 for ≥ 3 months, *MAC* prophylaxis should be discontinued.

DEFINITIVE AND SUPPRESSIVE THERAPY. In patients with disease due to *MAC*, the goals of therapy include suppression of symptoms and conversion to negative blood cultures. The infection itself is not completely eradicated until immune reconstitution. Recommended therapy consists of a combination of clarithromycin 500 mg twice a day with ethambutol 15 mg/kg daily, administered orally. Azithromycin 500-600 mg daily is an acceptable alternative to clarithromycin. The addition of rifabutin 300 mg/day may improve outcomes. Mortality in disseminated *MAC* is high in patients with either a CD4 cell count $<50/mm^3$ or a *MAC* burden of $>2 \log_{10}$ CFU/mm^3 of blood, or in the absence of effective antiretroviral therapy. In these patients, a fourth drug may be added, based on susceptibility testing. Potential fourth agents include amikacin, 10-15 mg/kg intravenously daily; streptomycin, 1 g intravenously or intramuscularly daily; ciprofloxacin, 500-750 mg orally twice daily; levofloxacin, 500 mg orally daily; or moxifloxacin, 400 g orally daily. Patients should be continued on suppressive therapy until all of these criteria are met:

- Therapy duration of at least 12 months
- CD4 count $>100/mm^3$ for at least 6 months
- Asymptomatic for *MAC* infection

PRINCIPLES OF ANTI-LEPROSY THERAPY

The global prevalence of leprosy has declined by 90% since 1985, largely due to the global initiative of the WHO to eliminate leprosy (Hansen disease) as a public health problem by providing multidrug therapy (rifampin, clofazimine, and dapsone) free of charge.

TYPES OF ANTI-LEPROSY THERAPY

Therapy for leprosy is based on multidrug regimens using rifampin, clofazimine, and dapsone. The reasons for using combinations of agents include reduction in the development of resistance, the need for adequate therapy when primary resistance already exists, and reduction in the duration of therapy. The most bactericidal drug in current regimens is rifampin. Because of high kill rates and massive release of bacterial antigens, rifampin is not often given during a "reversal" reaction (see below) or in patients with erythema nodosum leprosum. Clofazimine is only bacteriostatic against *M. leprae*. However, it also has anti-inflammatory effects and can treat reversal reactions and erythema nodosum leprosum. The third major agent in the regimen is dapsone. The objective of administering these drugs is total cure.

PAUCI-BACILLARY LEPROSY. The WHO regimen consists of a single dose of oral rifampin, 600 mg, combined with dapsone, 100 mg, administered under direct supervision once every month for 6 months, and dapsone, 100 mg a day, in between for 6 months. In the U.S., the regimen consists of dapsone, 100 mg, and rifampin, 600 mg, daily for 6 months, followed by dapsone monotherapy for 3-5 years.

MULTIBACILLARY THERAPY. The WHO recommends the same regimen as for paucibacillary leprosy, with 2 major changes. First, clofazimine, 300 mg a day, is added for the entirety of therapy. Second, the regimen lasts 1 year instead of 6 months. In the U.S., the regimen is also the same as for paucibacillary, but dual therapy continues for 3 years, followed by dapsone monotherapy for 10 years. Clofazimine is added when there is dapsone resistance or chronically reactional patients. Viable bacilli are killed within 3 months of therapy, suggesting that the length of current therapy for multibacillary leprosy may be unnecessarily long. Recently, the WHO proposed that all forms of leprosy be treated with the same dose as for paucibacillary leprosy. This new shorter regimen promises to reduce duration of therapy radically.

TREATMENT OF REACTIONS IN LEPROSY. Patients with tuberculoid leprosy may develop "reversal reactions," manifestations of delayed hypersensitivity to antigens of *M. leprae*. Early therapy with corticosteroids or clofazimine is effective. Reactions in the lepromatous form of the disease (erythema nodosum leprosum) are characterized by the appearance of raised, tender, intracutaneous nodules, severe constitutional symptoms, and high fever. Treatment with clofazimine or thalidomide is effective.

Table 56–5

Drugs Used in the Treatment of Mycobacteria Other Than for Tuberculosis, Leprosy, or MAC

MYCOBACTERIAL SPECIES	FIRST-LINE THERAPY	ALTERNATIVE AGENTS
M. kansasii	Isoniazid + rifampin[a] + ethambutol	Trimethoprim-sulfamethoxazole; ethionamide; cycloserine; clarithromycin; amikacin; streptomycin; moxifloxacin or gatifloxacin
M. fortuitum complex	Amikacin + doxycycline	Cefoxitin; rifampin; a sulfonamide; moxifloxacin or gatifloxacin; clarithromycin; trimethoprim-sulfamethoxazole; imipenem
M. marinum	Rifampin + ethambutol	Trimethoprim-sulfamethoxazole; clarithromycin; minocycline; doxycycline
Mycobacterium ulcerans	Rifampin + streptomycin[c]	Clarithromycin[b]; rifapentine[b]
M. malmoense	Rifampin + ethambutol ± clarithromycin	Fluoroquinolone
M. haemophilum	Clarithromycin + rifampin + quinolone	—

[a]*In HIV-infected patients, the substitution of rifabutin for rifampin minimizes drug interactions with the HIV protease inhibitors and non-nucleoside reverse transcriptase inhibitors.*
[b]*Based on animal models.*
[c]*For* Mycobacterium ulcerans, *surgery is the primary therapy.*

THERAPY FOR OTHER NONTUBERCULOUS MYCOBACTERIA

Mycobacteria other than those already discussed can be recovered from a variety of lesions in humans. Therapy for infections from these organisms is summarized in Table 56–5.

For a complete Bibliographical Listing see Goodman & Gilman's ***The Pharmacological Basis of Therapeutics***, 12th ed., or Goodman & Gilman Online at www.AccessMedicine.com.

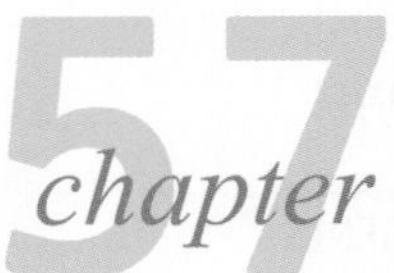

Antifungal Agents

There are 200,000 known species of fungi, and estimates of the total size of Kingdom Fungi range to well over a million. Residents of the kingdom are quite diverse and include yeasts, molds, mushrooms, smuts, the pathogens *Aspergillus fumigatus* and *Candida albicans*, and the source of penicillin, *Penicillium chrysogenum*. Fortunately, only ~400 fungi cause disease in animals, and even fewer cause significant human disease. However, fungal infections are becoming more common in patients with compromised immune systems. Fungi are eukaryotes with unique cell walls containing glucans and chitin, and their eradication requires different strategies than those for treatment of bacterial infections. Available agents have effects on the synthesis of membrane and cell-wall components, on membrane permeability, on the synthesis of nucleic acids, and on microtubule/mitotic spindle function (Figure 57–1). Antifungal agents described in this chapter are discussed under two major headings, systemic and topical, although this distinction is somewhat arbitrary. The imidazole, triazole, and polyene antifungal agents may be used either systemically or topically, and many superficial mycoses can be treated either systemically or topically. Table 57–1 summarizes common mycoses and their pharmacotherapy.

SYSTEMIC ANTIFUNGAL AGENTS

DRUGS FOR DEEPLY INVASIVE FUNGAL INFECTIONS

AMPHOTERICIN B. Amphotericin B is an amphoteric polyene macrolide with broad spectrum antifungal activity.

MECHANISM OF ACTION. Amphotericin B has useful clinical activity against a broad range of pathogenic fungi and limited activity against the protozoa *Leishmania* spp. and *Naegleria fowleri*. The antifungal activity of amphotericin B depends principally on its binding to a sterol moiety, primarily ergosterol in the membrane of sensitive fungi. By virtue of their interaction with these sterols, polyenes appear to form pores or channels that increase the permeability of the membrane, allowing leakage of a variety of small molecules (*see* Figure 57–1).

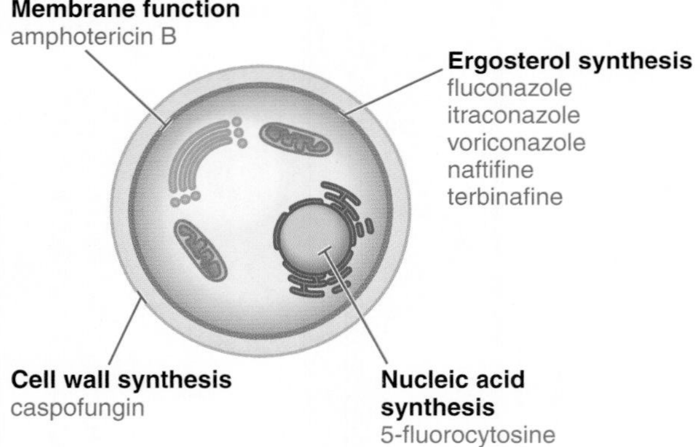

Figure 57–1 *Sites of action of antifungal drugs*. Amphotericin B and other polyenes (e.g., nystatin) bind to ergosterol in fungal cell membranes and increase membrane permeability. The imidazoles and triazoles (itraconazole, et al.) inhibit 14-α-sterol demethylase, prevent ergosterol synthesis, and lead to the accumulation of 14-α-methylsterols. The allylamines (e.g., naftifine and terbinafine) inhibit squalene epoxidase and prevent ergosterol synthesis. The echinocandins, such as caspofungin, inhibit the formation of glucans in the fungal cell wall.

Table 57–1

Pharmacotherapy of Mycoses

DEEP MYCOSES	DRUGS	SUPERFICIAL MYCOSES	DRUGS
Invasive aspergillosis		***Candidiasis***	
Immunosuppressed	Voriconazole, amphotericin B	Vulvovaginal	*Topical* Butoconazole, clotrimazole, miconazole, nystatin, terconazole, tioconazole
Non-immunosuppressed	Voriconazole, amphotericin B, itraconazole		*Oral* Fluconazole
Blastomycosis			
Rapidly progressive or CNS	Amphotericin B		
Indolent and non-CNS	Itraconazole	Oropharyngeal	*Topical* Clotrimazole, nystatin
Candidiasis			*Oral (systemic)* Fluconazole, itraconazole Posaconazole
Deeply invasive	Amphotericin B, fluconazole, voriconazole, caspofungin, micafungin, anidulafungin	Cutaneous	*Topical* Amphotericin B, clotrimazole, ciclopirox, econazole, ketoconazole, miconazole, nystatin
Coccidioidomycosis			
Rapidly progressing	Amphotericin B		
Indolent	Itraconazole, fluconazole	***Ringworm***	*Topical* Butenafine, ciclopirox, clotrimazole, econazole, haloprogin, ketoconazole, miconazole, naftifine, oxiconazole, sertaconazole, sulconazole, terbinafine, tolnaftate, undecylenate
Meningeal	Fluconazole, intrathecal amphotericin B		
Cryptococcosis			
Non-AIDS and initial AIDS	Amphotericin B, flucytosine		
Maintenance AIDS	Fluconazole		
Histoplasmosis			
Chronic pulmonary	Itraconazole		*Systemic* Griseofulvin, itraconazole, terbinafine
Disseminated			
Rapidly progressing or CNS	Amphotericin B		
Indolent non-CNS	Itraconazole		
Maintenance AIDS	Itraconazole		
Mucormycosis	Amphotericin B		
Pseudallescheriasis	Voriconazole, itraconazole		
Sporotrichosis			
Cutaneous	Itraconazole		
Extracutaneous	Amphotericin B, itraconazole		
Prophylaxis in the immunocompromised host	Fluconazole Posaconazole Micafungin		
***Empirical therapy in the immunocompromised host** (category not recognized by FDA)*	Amphotericin B Caspofungin Fluconazole		

FORMULATIONS. Table 57–2 summarizes the pharmacokinetic properties of the 4 available preparations.

C-AMB (conventional amphotericin B, FUNGIZONE). Amphotericin B is insoluble in water but is formulated for intravenous infusion by complexing it with the bile salt deoxycholate. The complex is marketed as a lyophilized powder for injection. C-AMB forms a colloid in water, with particles largely <0.4 μm in diameter. Filters

Table 57–2

Pharmocokinetic Parameters for Amphotericin B Formulations after Multiple Administrations in Humans

PRODUCT	DOSE (mg/kg)	C_{max} (μg/mL)	$AUC_{(0-24h)}$ (μg·h/mL)	V (L/kg)	CL (mL/h/kg)
AmBisome (L-AMB)	5	83 ± 35.2	555 ± 311	0.11 ± 0.08	11 ± 6
Amphotec (ABCD)	5	3.1	43	4.3	117
Ablecet (ABLC)	5	1.7 ± 0.8	14 ± 7	131 ± 7.7	426 ± 188.5
Fungizone (C-AMB)	0.6	1.1 ± 0.2	17.1 ± 5	5 ± 2.8	38 ± 15

For details, see Boswell GW, Buell D, Bekersky I. AmBisome (liposomal amphotericin B): A comparative review. J Clin Pharmacol, 1998;38:583–592. © 1998 The American College of Clinical Pharmacology. Reprinted by permission of SAGE Publications.

in intravenous infusion lines that trap particles >0.22 μm in diameter will remove significant amounts of drug. Addition of electrolytes to infusion solutions causes the colloid to aggregate.

ABCD. Amphotericin B colloidal dispersion (AMPHOTEC, AMPHOCIL) contains roughly equimolar amounts of amphotericin B and cholesteryl sulfate formulated for injection. Like C-AMB, ABCD forms a colloidal solution when dispersed in aqueous solution.

L-AMB. Liposomal amphotericin B is a small, unilamellar vesicle formulation of amphotericin B (AMBISOME). The drug is supplied as a lyophilized powder, which is reconstituted with sterile water for injection.

ABLC (ABELCET). Amphotericin B lipid complex is a complex of amphotericin B with lipids (dimyristoylphosphatidylcholine and dimyristoylphosphatidylglycerol).

The 3 lipid formulations collectively appear to reduce the risk of the patient's serum creatinine doubling during therapy by 58%. However, the cost of the lipid formulations greatly exceeds that of C-AMB, making them unavailable in many countries.

ADME. GI absorption of all amphotericin B formulations is negligible and IV delivery is indicated for systemic use. Amphotericin B in plasma is more than 90% bound to proteins. Pharmacokinetic parameters vary with the formulation. Azotemia, liver failure, or hemodialysis does not have a measurable impact on plasma concentrations. Concentrations of amphotericin B (via C-AMB) in fluids from inflamed pleura, peritoneum, synovium, and aqueous humor are approximately two-thirds of trough concentrations in plasma. Little amphotericin B from any formulation penetrates into cerebrospinal fluid (CSF), vitreous humor, or normal amniotic fluid.

ANTIFUNGAL ACTIVITY; FUNGAL RESISTANCE. Amphotericin B has useful clinical activity against *Candida* spp., *Cryptococcus neoformans, Blastomyces dermatitidis, Histoplasma capsulatum, Sporothrix schenckii, Coccidioides* spp., *Paracoccidioides braziliensis, Aspergillus* spp., *Penicillium marneffei*, and the agents of mucormycosis. Amphotericin B has limited activity against the protozoa *Leishmania* spp. and *N. fowleri.* The drug has no antibacterial activity. Some isolates of *Candida lusitaniae* have been relatively resistant to amphotericin B. *Aspergillus terreus* and perhaps *Aspergillus nidulans* may be more resistant to amphotericin B than other *Aspergillus* species.

THERAPEUTIC USES. The recommended doses for each formulation are summarized in Table 57–2. Candida esophagitis responds to much lower doses than deeply invasive mycoses. Intrathecal infusion of C-AMB is useful in patients with meningitis caused by *Coccidioides.* Too little is known about intrathecal administration of lipid formulations to recommend them. C-AMB can be injected into the CSF of the lumbar spine, cisterna magna, or lateral cerebral ventricle. Fever and headache are common reactions that may be decreased by intrathecal administration of 10-15 mg of hydrocortisone. Local injections of amphotericin B into a joint or peritoneal dialysate fluid commonly produce irritation and pain. Intraocular injection following pars plana vitrectomy has been used successfully for fungal endophthalmitis. Intravenous administration of amphotericin B is the treatment of choice for mucormycosis and is used for initial treatment of cryptococcal meningitis, severe or rapidly progressing histoplasmosis, blastomycosis, coccidioidomycosis, and penicilliosis marneffei, as well as in patients not responding to azole therapy of invasive aspergillosis, extracutaneous sporotrichosis, fusariosis, alternariosis, and trichosporonosis. Amphotericin B (C-AMB or L-AMB) is often given to selected patients with profound neutropenia who have fever that does not respond to broad-spectrum antibacterial agents over 5-7 days.

UNTOWARD EFFECTS. The major acute reactions to *intravenous amphotericin B formulations* are fever and chills. Infusion-related reactions are worst with ABCD and least with L-AMB. Tachypnea and respiratory stridor or modest hypotension also may occur, but true bronchospasm or anaphylaxis is rare. Patients with pre-existing cardiac or pulmonary disease may tolerate the metabolic demands of the reaction poorly and develop hypoxia or hypotension. The reaction ends spontaneously in 30-45 min; meperidine may shorten it. Pretreatment with oral acetaminophen or use of intravenous glucocorticoids at the start of the infusion decreases reactions.

Azotemia occurs in 80% of patients who receive C-AMB for deep mycoses. Lipid formulations are less nephrotoxic, being much less with ABLC, even less with L-AMB, and minimal with ABCD. Toxicity is dose-dependent and usually transient and increased by concurrent therapy with other nephrotoxic agents, such as aminoglycosides or cyclosporine. Permanent functional impairment is uncommon in adults with normal renal function prior to treatment unless the cumulative dose exceeds 3-4 g. Renal tubular acidosis and renal wasting of K^+ and Mg^{2+} also may be seen during and for several weeks after therapy, often requiring repletion. Administration of 1 L of normal saline intravenously on the day that C-AMB is to be given has been recommended for adults who are able to tolerate the Na^+ load.

Hypochromic, normocytic anemia commonly occurs during treatment with C-AMB. Anemia is less with lipid formulations and usually not seen over the first 2 weeks. The anemia is most likely due to decreased production of erythropoietin and often responds to administration of recombinant erythropoietin. Headache, nausea, vomiting, malaise, weight loss, and phlebitis at peripheral infusion sites are common. Arachnoiditis has been observed as a complication of injecting C-AMB into the CSF.

FLUCYTOSINE

Flucytosine (5-fluorocytosine) has a spectrum of antifungal activity that is considerably more restricted than that of amphotericin B.

MECHANISM OF ACTION. All susceptible fungi are capable of deaminating flucytosine to 5-fluorouracil (5-FU) (Figure 57–2), a potent antimetabolite that is used in cancer chemotherapy (*see* Chapter 61). Fluorouracil is metabolized first to 5-fluorouracil-ribose monophosphate (5-FUMP) by the enzyme uracil phosphoribosyl transferase (UPRTase). 5-FUMP then is either incorporated into RNA (via synthesis of 5-fluorouridine triphosphate) or metabolized to 5-fluoro-2′-deoxyuridine-5′-monophosphate (5-FdUMP), a potent inhibitor of thymidylate synthetase and thus of DNA synthesis. The selective action of flucytosine is due to the lack of *cytosine deaminase* in mammalian cells, which prevents metabolism to fluorouracil.

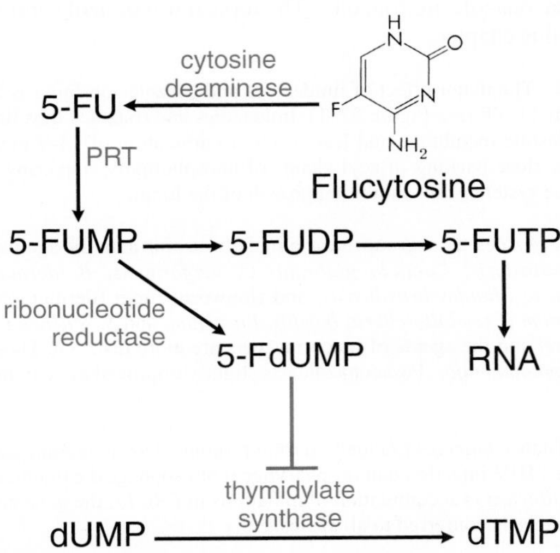

Figure 57–2 *Action of flucytosine in fungi.* Flucytosine (5-fluorocytosine) is transported by cytosine permease into the fungal cell, where it is deaminated to 5-fluorouracil (5-FU). The 5-FU is converted to 5-fluorouracil-ribose monophosphate (5-FUMP) and then is either converted to 5-fluorouridine triphosphate (5-FUTP) and incorporated into RNA or converted to 5-fluoro-2′-deoxyuridine-5′-monophosphate (5-FdUMP), a potent inhibitor of thymidylate synthase. 5-FUDP, 5-fluorouridine-5′-diphosphate; dUMP, deoxyuridine-5′-monophosphate; dTMP, deoxythymidine-5′-monophosphate; PRT, phosphoribosyltransferase.

ANTIFUNGAL ACTIVITY. Flucytosine has clinically useful activity against *C. neoformans, Candida* spp., and the agents of chromoblastomycosis.

FUNGAL RESISTANCE. Drug resistance arising during therapy (secondary resistance) is an important cause of therapeutic failure when flucytosine is used alone for cryptococcosis and candidiasis. The mechanism for this resistance can be loss of the permease necessary for cytosine transport or decreased activity of either UPRTase or cytosine deaminase (*see* Figure 57–2).

ADME. Flucytosine is absorbed rapidly and well from the GI tract and widely distributed in the body. Approximately 80% of a given dose is excreted unchanged in the urine. The $t_{1/2}$ of the drug is 3-6 h but may reach 200 h in renal failure. The clearance of flucytosine is approximately equivalent to that of creatinine. Reduction of dosage is necessary in patients with decreased renal function, and concentrations of drug in plasma should be measured periodically (desirable range of peak concentrations, 50 and 100 μg/mL). Flucytosine is cleared by hemodialysis, and patients undergoing such treatment should receive a single dose of 37.5 mg/kg after dialysis; the drug also is removed by peritoneal dialysis.

THERAPEUTIC USES. Flucytosine (ANCOBON) is given orally at 50-150 mg/kg/day, in 4 divided doses at 6-h intervals. Flucytosine is used predominantly in combination with amphotericin B. An all-oral regimen of flucytosine plus fluconazole also has been advocated for therapy of AIDS patients with cryptococcosis, but the combination has substantial GI toxicity with no evidence that flucytosine adds benefit. The addition of flucytosine to ≥6 weeks of therapy with C-AMB runs the risk of substantial bone marrow suppression or colitis if the flucytosine dose is not promptly adjusted downward as amphotericin B–induced azotemia occurs. The guidelines for the treatment of cryptococcal meningoencephalitis recommend addition of flucytosine (100 mg/kg orally in 4 divided doses) for the first 2 weeks of treatment with amphotericin B in AIDS patients.

Untoward Effects. Flucytosine may depress the bone marrow and lead to leukopenia. Other untoward effects include rash, nausea, vomiting, diarrhea, and severe enterocolitis. In ~5% of patients, plasma levels of hepatic enzymes are elevated, but this effect reverses when therapy is stopped. Toxicity is more frequent in patients with AIDS or azotemia and when plasma drug concentrations exceed 100 μg/mL.

IMIDAZOLES AND TRIAZOLES

The azole antifungals include two broad classes, imidazoles and triazoles. Of the drugs now on the market in the U.S., clotrimazole, miconazole, ketoconazole, econazole, butoconazole, oxiconazole, sertaconazole, and sulconazole are imidazoles; terconazole, itraconazole, fluconazole, voriconazole, and posaconazole are triazoles. The topical use of azole antifungals is described in the second section of this chapter.

MECHANISM OF ACTION. The major effect of imidazoles and triazoles on fungi is inhibition of 14-α-sterol demethylase, a microsomal CYP (*see* Figure 57–1). Imidazoles and triazoles thus impair the biosynthesis of ergosterol for the cytoplasmic membrane and lead to the accumulation of 14-α-methylsterols. These methylsterols may disrupt the close packing of acyl chains of phospholipids, impairing the functions of certain membrane-bound enzyme systems, thus inhibiting growth of the fungi.

ANTIFUNGAL ACTIVITY. Azoles as a group have clinically useful activity against *C. albicans, Candida tropicalis, Candida parapsilosis, Candida glabrata, C. neoformans, B. dermatitidis, H. capsulatum, Coccidioides* spp., *Paracoccidioides brasiliensis,* and ringworm fungi (dermatophytes). *Aspergillus* spp., *Scedosporium apiospermum (Pseudallescheria boydii), Fusarium*, and *S. schenckii* are intermediate in susceptibility. *Candida krusei* and the agents of mucormycosis are more resistant. These drugs have antiprotozoal effects against *Leishmania major*. Posaconazole has slightly improved activity in vitro against the agents of mucormycosis.

RESISTANCE. Azole resistance emerges gradually during prolonged azole therapy, causing clinical failure in patients with far-advanced HIV infection and oropharyngeal or esophageal candidiasis. The primary mechanism of resistance in *C. albicans* is accumulation of mutations in *ERG11*, the gene coding for the 14-α-sterol demethylase; cross-resistance is conferred to all azoles.

INTERACTION OF AZOLE ANTI-FUNGALS WITH OTHER DRUGS. The azoles interact with hepatic CYPs as substrates and inhibitors (Table 57–3), providing myriad possibilities for the interaction of azoles with many other medications. Thus, azoles can elevate plasma levels of some coadministered drugs (Table 57–4). Other coadministered drugs can decrease plasma concentrations of azole antifungal agents (Table 57–5). As a consequence of myriad interactions, combinations of certain drugs with azole antifungal medications may be contraindicated (Table 57–6).

Table 57–3

Interaction of Azole Antifungal Agents with Hepatic CYPs

FLUCONAZOLE	VORICONAZOLE	ITRACONAZOLE	POSACONAZOLE
CYP3A4 inhibitor CYP2C9 inhibitor CYP2C19 inhibitor	CYP2C9 inhibitor and substrate CYP3A4 inhibitor CYP2C19 inhibitor	CYP3A4 inhibitor	CYP3A4 inhibitor

Table 57–4

Drugs Exhibiting Elevated Plasma Concentrations When Co-Administered with Azole Anti-Fungal Agents

Alfentanil	Eplerenone	Losartan	Saquinavir
Alprazolam	Ergot alkaloids	Lovastatin	Sildenafil
Astemizole	Erlotinib	Methadone	Sirolimus
Buspirone	Eszopiclone	Methylprednisolone	Solifenacin
Busulfan	Felodipine	Midazolam	Sunitinib
Carbamazepine	Fexofenadine	Nevirapine	Tacrolimus
Cisapride	Gefitinib	Omeprazole	Triazolam
Cyclosporine	Glimepiride	Phenytoin	Vardenafil
Digoxin	Glipizide	Pimozide	Vinca alkaloids
Docetaxel	Halofantrine	Quinidine	Warfarin
Dofetilide	Haloperidol	Ramelteon	Zidovudine
Efavirenz	Imatinib	Ranolazine	Zolpidem
Eletriptan	Irinotecan	Risperidone	

Mechanism of interaction presumably occurs largely at the level of hepatic CYPs, especially CYPs 3A4, 2C9, and 2D6, but can also involve P-glycoprotein and other mechanisms. Not all drugs listed interact equally with all azoles. For details, see Chapter 6 and reference to Table 57–5.

Table 57–5

Some Agents that Decrease Triazole Concentration

Coadministered Agent	Fluconazole	Voriconazole	Itraconazole	Posaconazole
Antacids (concurrent)	–		+	–
Carbamazepine	+	×	+	+
Didanosine			+	
Efavirenz		×	+	
H_2 antagonists	–	–	+	+
Nevirapine		+	+	
Phenobarbital		×	+	
Phenytoin	–	+	+	+
Proton pump inhibitors	–	–[a]	+	+
Rifampin	+	×	+	+
Rifabutin		×	+	+
Ritonavir		×		
St. John's wort		+	+	

+, causes decrease; –, causes no decrease, possible increase; ×, combination contraindicated.

[a]Omeprazole and voriconazole increase each other's C_p; reduce omeprazole dose by 50% when initiating voriconazole therapy.

Source: Reproduced with permission from Zonios DI, Bennett JE. Update on azole antifungals. Sem Respir Crit Care Med, 2008;29:192–210, which contains additional information and references.

Table 57–6

Some Additional Contraindicated Azole Drug Combinations

DRUG	FLUCONAZOLE	VORICONAZOLE	ITRACONAZOLE	POSACONAZOLE
Alfuzosin		x	x	x
Artemether	x	x		
Bepridil	x			
Clopidogrel	x			
Conivaptan	x	x	x	x
Dabigatran			x	
Darunavir		x		
Dronedarone	x	x	x	x
Everolimus	x	x	x	x
Lopinavir		x		
Lumefantrine	x	x		
Mesoridazine	x			
Nilotinib	x	x	x	x
Nisoldipine	use with caution	x	x	x
Quinine	x	x		
Rifapentine		x	use with caution	use with caution
Ritonavir		x	use with caution	
Rivaroxaban		x	x	
Salmeterol		x	x	x
Silodosin		x	x	x
Simvastatin	use with caution		x	
St. John's wort		x		
Tetrabenazine	x	x		
Thioridazine	x	x		
Tolvaptan	x	x	x	x
Topotecan			x	
Ziprasidone	x	x		

KETOCONAZOLE

Ketoconazole, administered orally, has been replaced by itraconazole for the treatment of all mycoses except when the lower cost of ketoconazole outweighs the advantage of itraconazole. Ketoconazole sometimes is used to inhibit excessive production of glucocorticoids in patients with Cushing syndrome (*see* Chapter 42) and is available for topical use.

ITRACONAZOLE

Itraconazole lacks ketoconazole's corticosteroid suppression while retaining most of ketoconazole's pharmacological properties and expanding the antifungal spectrum. This synthetic triazole is an equimolar racemic mixture of 4 diastereoisomers.

ADME. Itraconazole (SPORANOX, others) is available as a capsule and a solution in hydroxypropyl-β-cyclodextrin for oral use. The capsule form of the drug is best absorbed in the fed state, but the oral solution is better absorbed in the fasting state, providing peak plasma concentrations >150% of those obtained with the capsule. Itraconazole is metabolized in the liver; it is both a substrate for and a potent inhibitor of CYP3A4. Itraconazole is present in plasma with an approximately equal concentration of a biologically active metabolite, hydroxy-itraconazole. The native drug and metabolite are >99% bound to plasma proteins. Neither appears in urine or CSF. The $t_{1/2}$ of itraconazole at steady state is ~30-40 h. Steady-state levels of itraconazole are not reached for 4 days and those of hydroxy-itraconazole for 7 days; thus, loading doses are recommended when treating deep mycoses. Severe liver disease will increase itraconazole plasma concentrations, but azotemia and hemodialysis have no effect.

DRUG INTERACTIONS. Tables 57–4, 57–5, and 57–6 list select interactions of azoles with other drugs.

THERAPEUTIC USES. Itraconazole is the drug of choice for patients with indolent, nonmeningeal infections due to *B. dermatitidis, H. capsulatum, P. brasiliensis*, and *Coccidioides immitis.* The drug also is useful in the therapy of indolent invasive aspergillosis outside the CNS, particularly after the infection has been stabilized with amphotericin B. Although not an approved use, itraconazole is a reasonable choice for the treatment of pseudallescheriasis, an infection not responding to amphotericin B therapy, as well as cutaneous and extracutaneous sporotrichosis, tinea corporis, and extensive tinea versicolor. HIV-infected patients with disseminated histoplasmosis or *P. marneffei* infections have a decreased incidence of relapse if given prolonged itraconazole "maintenance" therapy (*see* Chapter 59). Itraconazole is not recommended for maintenance therapy of cryptococcal meningitis in HIV-infected patients because of a high incidence of relapse. Long-term therapy has been used in non-HIV–infected patients with allergic bronchopulmonary aspergillosis to decrease the dose of glucocorticoids and reduce attacks of acute bronchospasm. Itraconazole solution is effective and approved for use in oropharyngeal and esophageal candidiasis. Because the solution has more GI side effects than fluconazole tablets, itraconazole solution usually is reserved for patients not responding to fluconazole.

Dosage. In treating deep mycoses, a loading dose of 200 mg of itraconazole is administered 3 times daily for the first 3 days. After the loading doses, two 100-mg capsules are given twice daily with food. Divided doses may increase the AUC. For maintenance therapy of HIV-infected patients with disseminated histoplasmosis, 200 mg once daily is used. Onychomycosis can be treated with either 200 mg once daily for 12 weeks or for infections isolated to fingernails, 2 monthly cycles consisting of 200 mg twice daily for 1 week followed by a 3-week period of no therapy—so-called pulse therapy. Once-daily terbinafine (250 mg) is superior to pulse therapy with itraconazole. For oropharyngeal candidiasis, itraconazole oral solution should be taken fasting in a dose of 100 mg (10 mL) once daily and swished vigorously in the mouth before swallowing to optimize any topical effect. Patients with esophageal thrush unresponsive or refractory to treatment with fluconazole tablets are given 100 mg of the solution twice a day for 2-4 weeks.

UNTOWARD EFFECTS; PRECAUTIONS. Adverse effects of itraconazole therapy can occur as a result of interactions with many other drugs (*see* Tables 57–3 and 57–4). Serious hepatotoxicity has rarely led to hepatic failure and death. Intravenous itraconazole causes a dose-dependent inotropic effect that can lead to congestive heart failure in patients with impaired ventricular function. In the absence of interacting drugs, itraconazole capsules and suspension are well tolerated at 200 mg daily. Diarrhea, abdominal cramps, anorexia, and nausea are more common with the suspension than with the capsules. In patients receiving 50-400 mg of the capsules per day, nausea and vomiting, hypertriglyceridemia, hypokalemia, increased serum aminotransferase, and rash occurred in 2-10% of patients. Occasionally, rash necessitates drug discontinuation, but most adverse effects can be handled with dose reduction. Profound hypokalemia has been seen in patients receiving ≥600 mg daily and in those who recently have received prolonged amphotericin B therapy. Doses of 300 mg twice daily have led to other side effects, including adrenal insufficiency, lower limb edema, hypertension, and in at least 1 case, rhabdomyolysis. Doses >400 mg/day are not recommended for long-term use. Anaphylaxis has been observed rarely, as well as severe rash, including Stevens-Johnson syndrome. Itraconazole is pregnancy Category C and is contraindicated for the treatment of onychomycosis during pregnancy or for women contemplating pregnancy.

FLUCONAZOLE

ADME. Fluconazole is almost completely absorbed from the GI tract. Plasma concentrations are essentially the same whether the drug is given orally or intravenously; its bioavailability is unaltered by food or gastric acidity. Renal excretion accounts for >90% of elimination; the elimination $t_{1/2}$ ~25-30 h. Fluconazole diffuses readily into body fluids, including breast milk, sputum, and saliva; concentrations in CSF can reach 50-90% of the values in plasma. The dosage interval should be increased in renal insufficiency. A dose of 100-200 mg should be given after each hemodialysis.

DRUG INTERACTIONS. Fluconazole is an inhibitor of CYP3A4 and CYP2C9 (*see* Tables 57–3 and 57–4). Patients who receive >400 mg daily or azotemic patients who have elevated fluconazole blood levels may experience drug interactions not otherwise seen.

THERAPEUTIC USES

Candidiasis. Fluconazole, 200 mg on day 1 and then 100 mg daily for at least 2 weeks, is effective in oropharyngeal candidiasis. Doses of 100-200 mg daily have been used to decrease candiduria in high-risk patients. A single dose of 150 mg is effective in uncomplicated vaginal candidiasis. A dose of 400 mg daily decreases the incidence of deep candidiasis in allogeneic bone marrow transplant recipients and is useful in treating candidemia of non-immunosuppressed patients. The drug has been used successfully as empirical treatment of febrile neutropenia in patients not responding to antibacterial agents and who are not at high risk of mold infections. *C. glabrata* becomes resistant upon prolonged exposure to fluconazole. Empirical use of fluconazole for suspected candidemia may not be advisable in patients who have been receiving long-term fluconazole prophylaxis and may be colonized with azole-resistant *C. glabrata, Candida krusei* would not be expected to respond to fluconazole or other azoles.

Cryptococcosis. Fluconazole, 400 mg daily, is used for the initial 8 weeks in the treatment of cryptococcal meningitis in patients with AIDS after the patient's clinical condition has been stabilized with at least 2 weeks of intravenous amphotericin B. After 8 weeks in patients no longer symptomatic, the dose is decreased to 200 mg daily and continued indefinitely. If the patient has completed 12 months of treatment for cryptococcosis, responds to HAART, has a CD4 count maintained >200/mm^3 for at least 6 months, and is asymptomatic from cryptococcal meningitis, it is reasonable to discontinue maintenance fluconazole as long as the CD4 response is maintained. Fluconazole, 400 mg daily, has been recommended as continuation therapy in non-AIDS patients with cryptococcal meningitis who have responded to an initial course of C-AMB or L-AMB and for patients with pulmonary cryptococcosis.

Other Mycoses. Fluconazole is the drug of choice for treatment of coccidioidal meningitis because of good penetration into the CSF and much less morbidity than intrathecal amphotericin B. In other forms of coccidioidomycosis, fluconazole is comparable to itraconazole. Fluconazole has no useful activity against histoplasmosis, blastomycosis, or sporotrichosis and is not effective in the prevention or treatment of aspergillosis. Fluconazole has no activity in mucormycosis.

UNTOWARD EFFECTS. Side effects in patients receiving >7 days of drug, regardless of dose, include nausea, headache, skin rash, vomiting, abdominal pain, and diarrhea (all in the range of 2-4%). Reversible alopecia may occur with prolonged therapy at 400 mg daily. Rare cases of deaths due to hepatic failure or Stevens-Johnson syndrome have been reported. Fluconazole has been associated with skeletal and cardiac deformities in several infants born to women taking high doses during pregnancy. Fluconazole is a Category C agent that should be avoided during pregnancy.

DOSAGE. Fluconazole (DIFLUCAN, others) is marketed in the U.S. as tablets of 50, 100, 150, and 200 mg for oral administration, powder for oral suspension providing 10 and 40 mg/mL, and intravenous solutions containing 2 mg/mL in saline and in dextrose solution. Generally recommended dosages are 50-400 mg once daily for either oral or intravenous administration. A loading dose of twice the daily maintenance dose is generally administered on the first day of therapy. Prolonged maintenance therapy may be required to prevent relapse. Children are treated with 3-12 mg/kg once daily (maximum: 600 mg/day).

VORICONAZOLE

Voriconazole (VFEND) is a triazole with a structure similar to fluconazole but with an expanded spectrum and poor aqueous solubility.

ADME. Oral bioavailability is 96% . Volume of distribution is high (4.6 L/kg), with extensive drug distribution in tissues. Metabolism occurs through CYPs 2C19 and 2C9; CYP3A4 plays a limited role. Plasma elimination $t_{1/2}$ is 6 h. Voriconazole exhibits nonlinear metabolism so that higher doses cause greater-than-linear increases in systemic drug exposure. Genetic polymorphisms in CYP2C19 can cause up to 4-fold differences in drug exposure: ~20% of Asians are homozygous poor metabolizers, compared with 2% of whites and African Americans. Less than 2% of parent drug is recovered from urine; 80% of the inactive metabolites are excreted in the urine. The oral dose does not have to be adjusted for azotemia or hemodialysis. Patients with mild-to-moderate cirrhosis should receive the same loading dose of voriconazole but half the maintenance dose. The intravenous formulation of voriconazole contains sulfobutyl ether β-cyclodextrin (SBECD), which is excreted by the kidney. Significant accumulation of SBECD occurs with a creatinine clearance <50 mL/min; in that setting, oral voriconazole is preferred.

DRUG INTERACTIONS. Voriconazole is metabolized by, and inhibits, CYPs 2C19, 2C9, and CYP3A4 (in that order of decreasing potency). The major metabolite of voriconazole, the voriconazole N-oxide, also inhibits these CYPs. Inhibitors or inducers of these CYPs may increase or decrease voriconazole plasma concentrations, respectively. Voriconazole and its major metabolite can increase the plasma concentrations of other drugs metabolized by these enzymes (*see* Tables 57–3, 57–4, and 57–5). Because the sirolimus AUC increases 11-fold when voriconazole is given, coadministration is contraindicated. *When starting voriconazole in a patient receiving ≥40 mg/day of omeprazole, reduce the dose of omeprazole by half.*

THERAPEUTIC USES. Voriconazole provided superior efficiency to C-AMB in the primary therapy of invasive aspergillosis. Although not approved, voriconazole has been used in the empirical therapy of neutropenic patients whose fever did not respond to >96 h of antibacterial therapy. Voriconazole is approved for use in esophageal candidiasis. Voriconazole is approved for initial treatment of candidemia and invasive aspergillosis, as well as for salvage therapy in patients with *P. boydii* (*S. apiospermum*) and *Fusarium* infections. Positive response of patients with cerebral fungal suggest that the drug penetrates infected brain.

UNTOWARD EFFECTS. Voriconazole is teratogenic in animals and is contraindicated in pregnancy (Category D). Although voriconazole is generally well-tolerated, occasional cases of hepatotoxicity have been reported; liver function should be monitored. Voriconazole can prolong the QTc interval, which can become significant in patients with other risk factors for torsade de pointes. Transient visual or auditory hallucinations are frequent after the first dose, usually at night and particularly with intravenous administration; symptoms diminish with time. Patients receiving their first intravenous infusion have had anaphylactoid reactions requiring drug discontinuation. Rash occurs in 6% of patients.

DOSAGE. Treatment is usually initiated with an intravenous infusion of 6 mg/kg every 12 h for two doses, followed by 3-4 mg/kg every 12 h, administered no faster than 3 mg/kg/h. As the patient improves, oral administration is continued as 200 mg every 12 h. Patients failing to respond may be given 300 mg every 12 h. Because high-fat meals reduce voriconazole bioavailability, oral drug should be given either 1 h before or 1 h after meals.

POSACONAZOLE

Posaconazole (NOXAFIL) is a synthetic structural analog of itraconazole with the same broad antifungal spectrum but with up to 4-fold greater activity in vitro against yeasts and filamentous fungi, including the agents of mucormycosis. As for other imidazoles, the mechanism of action is inhibition of sterol 14-α demethylase.

ADME. Bioavailability is variable and significantly enhanced by the presence of food. The drug has a long $t_{1/2}$ (25-31 h), a large volume of distribution (331-1341 L), and extensive binding (>98%) to protein. Systemic exposure is 4 times higher in homozygous CYP2C19 slow metabolizers than in homozygous wild-type metabolizers. Steady-state concentrations are reached in 7-10 days when dosed 4 times daily. Hepatic impairment causes a modest increase in plasma concentrations. Almost 80% of the drug and its metabolites are excreted in the stool, with 66% as unchanged drug. The major metabolic pathway is hepatic UDP glucuronidation. Hemodialysis does not remove drug from the circulation. Gastric acid improves absorption. Drugs that reduce gastric acid (e.g., cimetidine and esomeprazole) decrease posaconazole exposure by 32-50%. Diarrhea reduces the average plasma concentration by 37%.

THERAPEUTIC USE. Posaconazole is used for treatment of oropharyngeal candidiasis, although fluconazole is preferred because of safety and cost. Posaconazole is approved for prophylaxis against candidiasis and aspergillosis in patients >13 years of age who have prolonged neutropenia or severe graft-versus-host disease (GVHD). It is approved in the E.U. as salvage therapy for aspergillosis and several other infections, as are itraconazole and voriconazole. Posaconazole is available as a flavored suspension containing 40 mg/mL. Dosage for adults and children >8 years of age is 200 mg (5 mL suspension) 3 times daily for prophylaxis. Treatment of active infection is begun at 200 mg 4 times daily and changed to 400 mg twice daily once infection has improved. All doses should be taken with a full meal.

DRUG INTERACTIONS. Posaconazole inhibits CYP3A4. Coadministration with rifabutin or phenytoin increases the plasma concentration of these drugs and decreases posaconazole exposure by 2-fold. Posaconazole is not known to prolong cardiac repolarization but should not be coadministered with drugs that are CYP3A4 substrates and prolong the QTc interval (*see* Tables 57–4 and 57–6).

UNTOWARD EFFECTS. Common adverse effects include nausea, vomiting, diarrhea, abdominal pain, and headache. Although adverse effects occur in at least a third of patients, discontinuation due to adverse effects in long-term studies has been only 8%. Posaconazole is pregnancy Category C.

DOSAGE. Dosage for adults and children >8 years of age is 200 mg (5 mL suspension) 3 times daily for prophylaxis. Treatment of active infection is begun at 200 mg 4 times daily and changed to 400 mg twice daily once infection has improved. All doses should be taken with a full meal.

ISAVUCONAZOLE

Isavuconazole (BAL8557) is an investigational water-soluble prodrug of the synthetic triazole, BAL4815. The prodrug is readily cleaved by esterases in the human body to release the active triazole. In vitro activity is comparable to voriconazole. Following oral administration, the drug has a long half-life, ~100 h, and is well tolerated. Phase III trials are enrolling patients with deeply invasive candidiasis and aspergillosis.

ECHINOCANDINS

Echinocandins inhibit formation of 1,3-β-D-glucans in the fungal cell wall, reducing its structural integrity (Figure 57–3), resulting in osmotic instability and cell death. Three echinocandins are approved for clinical use: caspofungin, micafungin, and anidulafungin. All are cyclic lipopeptides with a hexapeptide nucleus. Susceptible fungi include *Candida* and *Aspergillus* species.

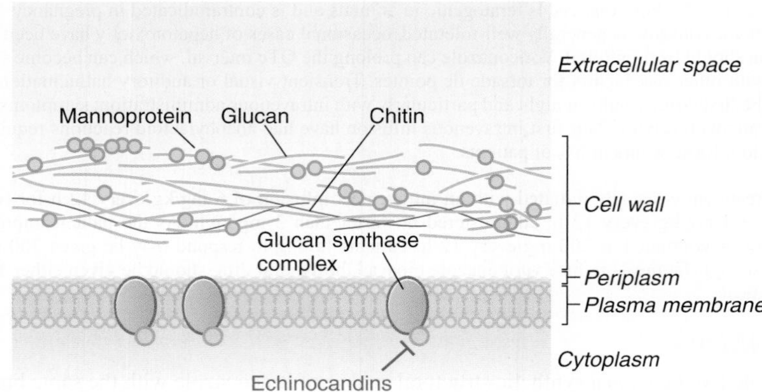

Figure 57–3 *The action of echinocandins*. The strength of the fungal cell wall is maintained by fibrillar polysaccharides, largely β-1,3-glucan and chitin, which bind covalently to each other and to proteins. A glucan synthase complex in the plasma membrane catalyzes the synthesis of β-1,3-glucan; the glucan is extruded into the periplasm and incorporated into the cell wall. Echinocandins inhibit the activity of the glucan synthase complex, resulting in loss of the structural integrity of the cell wall. A subunit of glucan synthase designated Fks1p is thought to be the target of the echinocandin. Mutations in Fks1p, coded by *FSK1*, cause resistance to echinocandins.

GENERAL PHARMACOLOGICAL CHARACTERISTICS. Echinocandins differ somewhat pharmacokinetically (Table 57–7) but all share lack of oral bioavailability, extensive protein binding (>97%), inability to penetrate into CSF, lack of renal clearance, and only a slight to modest effect of hepatic insufficiency on plasma drug concentration. Adverse effects are minimal. All 3 agents are pregnancy Category C.

CASPOFUNGIN

Caspofungin acetate (CANCIDAS) is a water-soluble, semisynthetic lipopeptide.

CLINICAL PHARMACOLOGY. Catabolism is largely by hydrolysis and *N*-acetylation, with excretion of the metabolites in the urine and feces. Mild and moderate hepatic insufficiency increase the AUC by 55% and 76%, respectively. Caspofungin increases tacrolimus levels by 16%, which should be managed by standard monitoring. Cyclosporine slightly increases caspofungin levels. Rifampin and other drugs activating CYP3A4 can cause reduction in caspofungin levels. Caspofungin is approved for initial therapy of deeply invasive candidiasis and as salvage therapy for patients with invasive aspergillosis who are failing approved drugs, such as amphotericin B formulations or voriconazole. Caspofungin is also approved for esophageal candidiasis and for the treatment of persistently febrile neutropenic patients with suspected fungal infections. Caspofungin is well tolerated, with the exception of phlebitis at the infusion site. Histamine-like effects have been reported with rapid infusions. Other symptoms have been equivalent to those observed in patients receiving fluconazole.

Caspofungin is administered intravenously once daily over 1 h. In candidemia and salvage therapy of aspergillosis, the initial dose is 70 mg, followed by 50 mg daily. The dose should be increased to 70 mg daily in

Table 57–7

Pharmacokinetics of Echinocandins in Humans

DRUG	DOSE (mg)	C_{max} (μg/mL)	AUC_{0-24h} (mg·h/L)	$t_{1/2}$ (h)	CL (mL/min/kg)
Caspofungin	70	12	93.5	10	0.15
Micafungin	75	7.1	59.9	13	0.16
Anidulafungin	200	7.5	104.5	25.6	0.16

For details, see Wagner C, Graninger W, Presterl E, Joukhadar C. The echinocandins: Comparison of their pharmacokinetics, pharmacodynamics and clinical applications. Pharmacology, 2006;78:161–177.

patients receiving rifampin as well as in those failing to respond to 50 mg. Esophageal candidiasis is treated with 50 mg daily. In moderate hepatic failure, the dose should be reduced to 35 mg daily.

MICAFUNGIN

Micafungin (MYCAMINE) is a water-soluble semisynthetic echinocandin. Micafungin has linear pharmacokinetics over a large range of doses (1-3 mg/kg) and ages. Small amounts of drug are metabolized in the liver by arylsulfatase and catechol *O*-methyltransferase. About 71% of both native drug and metabolites are excreted in the feces. Reduction of dose in moderate hepatic failure is not required. Clearance is more rapid in premature infants compared to older children and adults. Micafungin is a mild inhibitor of CYP3A4, increasing AUC of nifedipine by 18% and sirolimus by 21%. Micafungin has no effect on tacrolimus clearance.

The drug is approved for the treatment of deeply invasive candidiasis and esophageal candidiasis and for prophylaxis of deeply invasive candidiasis in hematopoietic stem cell transplant recipients. Micafungin is given intravenously as 100 mg daily over 1 h for adults, with 50 mg recommended for prophylaxis and 150 mg for esophageal candidiasis.

ANIDULAFUNGIN

Anidulafungin (ERAXIS) is a water-insoluble semisynthetic compound extracted from the fungus *A. nidulans*. The drug is cleared from the body by slow chemical degradation. No metabolism by the liver or renal excretion occurs. There are no known drug interactions. Anidulafungin appears noninferior to fluconazole in candidemia of non-neutropenic patients and is approved for the treatment of esophageal candidiasis. Drug dissolved in the supplied diluent is infused once daily in saline or 5% dextrose in water at a rate not exceeding 1.1 mg/min. For deeply invasive candidiasis, anidulafungin is given daily as a loading dose of 200 mg followed by 100 mg daily. For esophageal candidiasis, a loading dose of 100 mg is followed by 50 mg daily.

GRISEOFULVIN

MECHANISM OF ACTION. Griseofulvin is a practically insoluble fungistatic that inhibits microtubule function and thereby disrupts assembly of the mitotic spindle. Although the effects of the drug are similar to those of *colchicine* and the vinca alkaloids, griseofulvin's binding sites on the tubulin are distinct; griseofulvin also interacts with microtubule-associated protein.

ADME. Blood levels after oral administration are quite variable. Absorption is improved when the drug is taken with a fatty meal. Because the rates of dissolution and disaggregation limit the bioavailability of griseofulvin, micro-sized and ultra-micro-sized powders are now used in preparations (GRIFULVIN V and GRIS-PEG, respectively). Griseofulvin has a plasma $t_{1/2}$ of ~1 day, and ~50% of the oral dose can be detected in the urine within 5 days, mostly in the form of metabolites; the primary metabolite is 6-methylgriseofulvin. Barbiturates decrease griseofulvin absorption from the GI tract.

Griseofulvin is deposited in keratin precursor cells; when these cells differentiate, the drug remains tightly bound to keratin, providing prolonged resistance to fungal invasion. For this reason, the new growth of hair or nails is the first to become free of disease. As the fungus-containing keratin is shed, it is replaced by normal tissue. Griseofulvin is detectable in the stratum corneum of the skin within 4-8 h of oral administration. Only a very small fraction of a dose of the drug is present in body fluids and tissues.

ANTIFUNGAL ACTIVITY. Griseofulvin is fungistatic in vitro for various species of the dermatophytes *Microsporum, Epidermophyton*, and *Trichophyton*. The drug has no effect on bacteria or on other fungi.

THERAPEUTIC USES. Mycotic disease of the skin, hair, and nails responds to griseofulvin therapy. For tinea capitis in children, griseofulvin remains the drug of choice; efficacy is best for tinea capitis caused by *Microsporum canis, Microsporum audouinii, Trichophyton schoenleinii*, and *Trichophyton verrucosum*. Griseofulvin is also effective for ringworm of the glabrous skin; tinea cruris and tinea corporis caused by *M. canis, Trichophyton rubrum, T. verrucosum*, and *Epidermophyton floccosum*; and tinea of the hands (*T. rubrum* and *Trichophyton mentagrophytes*) and beard (*Trichophyton* species). *T. rubrum* and *T. mentagrophytes* infections may require higher-than-conventional doses of griseofulvin.

DOSAGE. The recommended daily dose of griseofulvin is 2.3 mg/kg (up to 500 mg) for children and 500 mg to 1 g for adults. Doses of 1.5-2 g daily may be used for short periods in severe or extensive infections. Best results are obtained when the daily dose is divided and given at 6-h intervals. Treatment must be continued until infected tissue is replaced by normal hair, skin, or nails, which requires 1 month for scalp and hair ringworm, 6-9 months for fingernails, and at least a year for toenails. Itraconazole or terbinafine is much more effective for onychomycosis.

UNTOWARD EFFECTS. The incidence of serious reactions due to griseofulvin is very low. Headache occurs in 15% of patients. Other side effects include GI and nervous system manifestations, and augmentation of the effects of alcohol. Hepatotoxicity also has been observed. Hematological effects include leukopenia, neutropenia, punctate basophilia, and monocytosis; these often disappear despite continued therapy. Blood studies should be carried out at least once a week during the first month of treatment or longer. Common renal effects include albuminuria and cylindruria without evidence of renal insufficiency. Reactions involving the skin are cold and warm urticaria, photosensitivity, lichen planus, erythema, erythema multiforme–like rashes, and vesicular and morbilliform eruptions. Serum sickness syndromes and severe angioedema develop rarely. Estrogen-like effects have been observed in children. A moderate but inconsistent increase of fecal protoporphyrins has been noted with chronic use.

Griseofulvin induces hepatic CYPs, thereby increasing the rate of metabolism of warfarin; adjustment of the dosage of the latter agent may be necessary in some patients. The drug may reduce the efficacy of low-estrogen oral contraceptive agents, probably by a similar mechanism.

TERBINAFINE

Terbinafine is a synthetic allylamine, structurally similar to the topical agent naftifine (see below). It acts by inhibiting fungal squalene epoxidase, thereby reducing ergosterol biosynthesis (*see* Figure 57–1).

Terbinafine is well absorbed, but bioavailability is ~40% due to first-pass metabolism in the liver. The drug accumulates in skin, nails, and fat. The initial $t_{1/2}$ is ~12 h but extends to 200-400 h at steady state. Terbinafine is not recommended in patients with marked azotemia or hepatic failure. Rifampin decreases and cimetidine increases plasma terbinafine concentrations. The drug is well tolerated, with a low incidence of GI distress, headache, or rash. Very rarely, fatal hepatotoxicity, severe neutropenia, Stevens-Johnson syndrome, or toxic epidermal necrolysis may occur. The drug is pregnancy Category B and it is recommended that systemic terbinafine therapy for onychomycosis be postponed until after pregnancy is complete. Terbinafine (LAMISIL, others), given as one 250-mg tablet daily for adults, is somewhat more effective for nail onychomycosis than itraconazole. Duration of treatment varies with the site being treated but typically is 6-12 weeks. Efficacy in onychomycosis can be improved by the simultaneous use of amorolfine 5% nail lacquer. Terbinafine also is effective in tinea capitis and is used off-label for ringworm elsewhere on the body.

TOPICAL ANTIFUNGAL AGENTS

Topical treatment is useful in many superficial fungal infections, i.e., those confined to the stratum corneum, squamous mucosa, or cornea. Such diseases include dermatophytosis (ringworm), candidiasis, tinea versicolor, piedra, tinea nigra, and fungal keratitis.

The preferred formulation for cutaneous application usually is a cream or solution. Ointments are messy and are too occlusive. The use of powders is largely confined to the feet and moist lesions of the groin and other intertriginous areas. Topical administration of antifungal agents usually is not successful for mycoses of the nails (onychomycosis) and hair (tinea capitis) and has no place in the treatment of subcutaneous mycoses, such as sporotrichosis and chromoblastomycosis. Regardless of formulation, penetration of topical drugs into hyperkeratotic lesions often is poor. Removal of thick, infected keratin is sometimes a useful adjunct to therapy.

IMIDAZOLES AND TRIAZOLES FOR TOPICAL USE

These closely related classes of drugs are synthetic antifungal agents that are used both topically and systemically. Indications for their topical use include ringworm, tinea versicolor, and mucocutaneous candidiasis. Resistance to imidazoles or triazoles is very rare among the fungi that cause ringworm.

CUTANEOUS APPLICATION. The preparations for cutaneous use described below are effective for tinea corporis, tinea pedis, tinea cruris, tinea versicolor, and cutaneous candidiasis. They should be applied twice a day for 3-6 weeks. The cutaneous formulations are not suitable for oral, vaginal, or ocular use.

VAGINAL APPLICATION. Vaginal creams, suppositories, and tablets for vaginal candidiasis are all used once a day for 1-7 days, preferably at bedtime. None is useful in trichomoniasis. Most vaginal creams are administered in 5-g amounts. Three vaginal formulations—clotrimazole tablets, miconazole suppositories, and terconazole cream—come in both low- and high-dose preparations. A shorter duration of therapy is recommended for the higher doses. These preparations are administered for 3-7 days. Approximately 3-10% of the vaginal dose is absorbed. No adverse effects on the human fetus have been attributed to the vaginal use of imidazoles or triazoles.

ORAL USE. Use of the oral troche of clotrimazole is properly considered as topical therapy. The only indication for this 10-mg troche is oropharyngeal candidiasis.

CLOTRIMAZOLE. Absorption of clotrimazole is <0.5% after application to the intact skin; from the vagina, it is 3-10%. Fungicidal concentrations remain in the vagina for as long as 3 days after application of the drug. The small amount absorbed is metabolized in the liver and excreted in bile. Clotrimazole on the skin may cause stinging, erythema, edema, vesication, desquamation, pruritus, and urticaria. When it is applied to the vagina, ~1.6% of recipients complain of a mild burning sensation, and rarely of lower abdominal cramps, a slight increase in urinary frequency, or skin rash. The sexual partner may experience penile or urethral irritation. By the oral route, clotrimazole can cause GI irritation. In patients using troches, the incidence of this side effect is ~5%.

THERAPEUTIC USES. Clotrimazole is available as a 1% cream, lotion, powder, aerosol solution, and solution (LOTRIMIN AF, MYCELEX, others), 1% or 2% vaginal cream, or vaginal tablets of 100, 200, or 500 mg (GYNE-LOTRIMIN, others), and 10-mg troches (MYCELEX, others). For the vagina, the standard regimens are one 100-mg tablet once a day at bedtime for 7 days, one 200-mg tablet daily for 3 days, one 500-mg tablet inserted only once, or 5 g of cream once a day for 3 days (2% cream) or 7 days (1% cream). For oropharyngeal candidiasis, troches are to be dissolved slowly in the mouth 5 times a day for 14 days.

Topical clotrimazole cures dermatophyte infections in 60-100% of cases. The cure rates in cutaneous candidiasis are 80-100%. In vulvovaginal candidiasis, the cure rate is usually >80% with the 7-day regimen. A 3-day regimen of 200 mg once a day appears to be similarly effective, as does single-dose treatment (500 mg). Recurrences are common after all regimens. The cure rate with oral troches for oral and pharyngeal candidiasis may be as high as 100% in the immunocompetent host.

ECONAZOLE

Econazole is the deschloro derivative of miconazole. Econazole readily penetrates the stratum corneum and is found in effective concentrations down to the mid-dermis. Less than 1% of an applied dose appears to be absorbed into the blood. Approximately 3% of recipients have local erythema, burning, stinging, or itching. Econazole nitrate (SPECTAZOLE, ECOSTATIN, others) is available as a water-miscible cream (1%) to be applied twice a day.

MICONAZOLE

Miconazole readily penetrates the stratum corneum of the skin and persists there for >4 days after application. Less than 1% is absorbed into the blood. Absorption is no more than 1.3% from the vagina. Adverse effects from topical application to the vagina include burning, itching, or irritation in ~7% of recipients, and infrequently, pelvic cramps (0.2%), headache, hives, or skin rash. Irritation, burning, and maceration are rare after cutaneous application. Miconazole is considered safe for use during pregnancy, although some recommend avoiding its use during the first trimester.

THERAPEUTIC USES. Miconazole nitrate is available as a cream, ointment, lotion, powder, gel, aerosol powder, and aerosol solution (MICATIN, ZEASORB-AF, others). To avoid maceration, only the lotion should be applied to intertriginous areas. Miconazole is available as a 2% and 4% vaginal cream, and as 100-mg, 200-mg, or 1200-mg vaginal suppositories (MONISTAT 7, MONISTAT 3, MONISTAT 1, others), to be applied high in the vagina at bedtime for 7, 3, or 1 day(s), respectively. In the treatment of tinea pedis, tinea cruris, and tinea versicolor, the cure rate may be >90%. In the treatment of vulvovaginal candidiasis, the mycologic cure rate at the end of 1 month is ~80-95%. Pruritus sometimes is relieved after a single application. Some vaginal infections caused by *C. glabrata* also respond.

TERCONAZOLE AND BUTOCONAZOLE

Terconazole (TERAZOL, others) is a ketal triazole with a mechanism of action similar to that of the imidazoles. The 80-mg vaginal suppository is inserted at bedtime for 3 days; the 0.4% vaginal cream is used for 7 days and the 0.8% cream for 3 days. Clinical efficacy and patient acceptance of both preparations are at least as good as for clotrimazole in patients with vaginal candidiasis.

Butoconazole is an imidazole that is pharmacologically comparable to clotrimazole. Butoconazole nitrate (FEMSTAT 3, others) is available as a 2% vaginal cream. Because of the slower response during pregnancy, a 6-day course is recommended (during the second and third trimester).

TIOCONAZOLE

Tioconazole (VAGISTAT 1, others) is an imidazole marketed for treatment of *Candida* vulvovaginitis. A single 4.6-g dose of ointment (300 mg) is given at bedtime.

OXICONAZOLE, SULCONAZOLE, AND SERTACONAZOLE

These imidazole derivatives are used for the topical treatment of infections caused by the common pathogenic dermatophytes. Oxiconazole nitrate (OXISTAT) is available as a 1% cream and lotion; sulconazole nitrate (EXELDERM, SULCOSYN) is supplied as a 1% solution and/or cream. Sertaconazole (ERTACZO) is a 2% cream marketed for tinea pedis.

KETOCONAZOLE

This imidazole is available as a 0.5% cream, foam, gel, and shampoo (NIZORAL, others) for common skin dermatophytes infections, for tinea versicolor, and seborrheic dermatitis.

STRUCTURALLY DIVERSE ANTIFUNGAL AGENTS

CICLOPIROX OLAMINE

Ciclopirox olamine (LOPROX, others) has broad-spectrum antifungal activity. It is fungicidal to C. albicans, E. floccosum, M. canis, T. mentagrophytes, and T. rubrum. It also inhibits the growth of Malassezia furfur. After application to the skin, it penetrates through the epidermis into the dermis, but even under occlusion, <1.5% is absorbed into the systemic circulation. Because the $t_{1/2}$ is 1.7 h, no systemic accumulation occurs. The drug penetrates into hair follicles and sebaceous glands. It can sometimes cause hypersensitivity. It is available as a 0.77% cream, gel, suspension, and lotion for the treatment of cutaneous candidiasis and for tinea corporis, cruris, pedis, and versicolor. An 8% topical solution (PENLAC NAIL LACQUER, others) is available for onychomycosis. Ciclopirox gel and 1% shampoo are also used for the treatment of seborrheic dermatitis of the scalp. Cure rates in the dermatomycoses and candidal infections are 81-94%. No topical toxicity has been noted.

HALOPROGIN

Haloprogin is a halogenated phenolic ether. It is fungicidal to *Epidermophyton, Pityrosporum, Microsporum, Trichophyton*, and *Candida.* Irritation, pruritus, burning sensations, vesiculation, increased maceration, and "sensitization" (or exacerbation of the lesion) occasionally occur, especially on the foot if occlusive footgear is worn. Haloprogin is poorly absorbed through the skin; it is converted to trichlorophenol in the body; the systemic toxicity from topical application appears to be low. Haloprogin (HALOTEX) cream or solution is applied twice a day for 2-4 weeks. Its principal use is against tinea pedis. It also is used against tinea cruris, tinea corporis, tinea manuum, and tinea versicolor. Haloprogin is no longer available in the U.S.

TOLNAFTATE

Tolnaftate is a thiocarbamate. It is effective in the treatment of most cutaneous mycoses caused by *T. rubrum, T. mentagrophytes, Trichophyton tonsurans, E. floccosum, M. canis, M. audouinii, Microsporum gypseum*, and *M. furfur*, but it is ineffective against *Candida.* In tinea pedis, the cure rate is ~80%, compared with ~95% for miconazole. Tolnaftate (AFTATE, TINACTIN, others) is available in a 1% concentration as a cream, gel, powder, aerosol powder, and topical solution, or as a topical aerosol liquid. Pruritus is usually relieved in 24-72 h. Involution of interdigital lesions caused by susceptible fungi is very often complete in 7-21 days. Toxic or allergic reactions to tolnaftate have not been reported.

NAFTIFINE

Naftifine, a synthetic allylamine, inhibits squalene-2,3-epoxidase and thus inhibit fungal biosynthesis of ergosterol. The drug has broad-spectrum fungicidal activity in vitro. Naftifine hydrochloride (NAFTIN) is available as a 1% cream or gel. It is effective for the topical treatment of tinea cruris and tinea corporis; twice-daily application is recommended. The drug is well tolerated, although local irritation has been observed in 3% of treated patients. Although not approved for these uses, naftifine may be efficacious for cutaneous candidiasis and tinea versicolor.

TERBINAFINE

Terbinafine 1% cream or spray is applied twice daily and is effective in tinea corporis, tinea cruris, and tinea pedis. Terbinafine is less active against *Candida* species and *M. furfur*, but the cream also can be used in cutaneous candidiasis and tinea versicolor.

BUTENAFINE

Butenafine hydrochloride (MENTAX, LOTRIMIN ULTRA) is a benzylamine derivative with a mechanism of action and spectrum of activity similar to those of terbinafine, naftifine, and other allylamines.

POLYENE ANTIFUNGAL AGENTS

NYSTATIN

Nystatin, a tetraene macrolide produced by *Streptomyces noursei*, is structurally similar to amphotericin B and has the same mechanism of action. The drug is not absorbed from the GI tract, skin, or vagina. Nystatin (MYCOSTATIN, NILSTAT, others) is useful only for candidiasis and is supplied in preparations intended for cutaneous, vaginal, or oral administration for this purpose. Infections of the nails and hyperkeratinized or crusted skin lesions do not respond. Powders are preferred for moist lesions and are applied 2 to 3 times daily. Creams or ointments are used twice daily. Combinations of nystatin with antibacterial agents or corticosteroids also are available. Imidazoles or triazoles are more effective agents than nystatin for vaginal candidiasis. Nystatin suspension is usually effective for oral candidiasis of the immunocompetent host. Other than the bitter taste and occasional complaints of nausea, adverse effects are uncommon.

MISCELLANEOUS ANTIFUNGAL AGENTS

UNDECYLENIC ACID

Undecylenic acid is primarily fungistatic and against a variety of fungi, including those that cause ringworm. Undecylenic acid (DESENEX, others) is available in a cream, powder, spray powder, soap, and liquid. Zinc undecylenate is marketed in combination with other ingredients. The zinc provides an astringent action that aids in the suppression of inflammation. Compound undecylenic acid ointment contains both undecylenic acid (~5%) and zinc undecylenate (~20%). Calcium undecylenate (CALDESENE, CRUEX) is available as a powder. Undecylenic acid preparations are used in the treatment of various dermatomycoses, especially tinea pedis. Concentrations of the acid as high as 10%, as well as those of the acid and salt in the compound ointment, may be applied to the skin. The preparations usually are not irritating to tissue, and sensitization to them is uncommon. In tinea pedis, the infection frequently persists despite intensive treatment and the clinical "cure" rate is ~50%, which is much lower than that obtained with the imidazoles, haloprogin, or tolnaftate. Undecylenic acid preparations also are approved for use in the treatment of diaper rash, tinea cruris, and other minor dermatologic conditions.

Benzoic Acid and Salicylic Acid. An ointment containing benzoic and salicylic acids is known as Whitfield's ointment. It combines the fungistatic action of benzoate with the keratolytic action of salicylate (in a ratio of 2:1, usually 6-3%) and is used mainly in the treatment of tinea pedis. Because benzoic acid is only fungistatic, eradication of the infection occurs only after the infected stratum corneum is shed. Continuous medication is required for several weeks to months. The salicylic acid accelerates the desquamation. The ointment also is sometimes used to treat tinea capitis. Mild irritation may occur at the site of application.

For a complete Bibliographical Listing see Goodman & Gilman's ***The Pharmacological Basis of Therapeutics***, 12th ed., or Goodman & Gilman Online at www.AccessMedicine.com.

Antiviral Agents (Nonretroviral)

Viruses are simple microorganisms that consist of either double- or single-stranded DNA or RNA enclosed in a protein coat called a *capsid.* Some viruses also possess a lipid envelope derived from the infected host cell, which, like the capsid, may contain antigenic glycoproteins. Effective antiviral agents inhibit virus-specific replicative events or preferentially inhibit *virus-directed rather than host cell–directed* nucleic acid or protein synthesis (Table 58–1). Host cell molecules that are essential to viral replication also offer targets for intervention. Figure 58–1 gives a schematic diagram of the replicative cycle of typical DNA and RNA viruses.

DNA viruses include poxviruses (smallpox), herpesviruses (chickenpox, shingles, oral and genital herpes), adenoviruses (conjunctivitis, sore throat), hepadnaviruses (hepatitis B virus [HBV]), and papillomaviruses (warts). Most DNA viruses enter the host cell nucleus, where the viral DNA is transcribed into mRNA by host cell polymerase; mRNA is translated in the usual host cell fashion into virus-specific proteins. Poxviruses are an exception; they carry their own RNA polymerase and replicate in the host cell cytoplasm.

For RNA viruses, the replication strategy relies either on enzymes in the virion to synthesize mRNA or has the viral RNA serving as its own mRNA. The mRNA is translated into various viral proteins, including RNA polymerase, which directs the synthesis of more viral mRNA and genomic RNA. Most RNA viruses complete their replication in the host cell cytoplasm, but some, such as influenza, are transcribed in the host cell nucleus. Examples of RNA viruses include rubella virus (German measles), rhabdoviruses (rabies), picornaviruses (poliomyelitis, meningitis, colds, hepatitis A), arenaviruses (meningitis, Lassa fever), flaviviruses (West Nile meningoencephalitis, yellow fever, hepatitis C), orthomyxoviruses (influenza), paramyxoviruses (measles, mumps), and coronaviruses (colds, severe acute respiratory syndrome [SARS]). Retroviruses are RNA viruses that include human immunodeficiency virus (HIV); chemotherapy for retro-viruses is described in Chapter 59.

Table 58–2 summarizes currently approved drugs for nonretroviral infections. Their pharmacological properties are presented below, class by class, as listed in the table.

ANTI-HERPESVIRUS AGENTS

Herpes simplex virus type 1 (HSV-1) typically causes diseases of the mouth, face, skin, esophagus, or brain. Herpes simplex virus type 2 (HSV-2) usually causes infections of the genitals, rectum, skin, hands, or meninges. Both cause serious infections in neonates. Acyclovir is the prototype of a group of antiviral agents that are nucleoside congeners that are phosphorylated intracellularly by a viral kinase and subsequently by host cell enzymes to become inhibitors of viral DNA synthesis. Related agents include penciclovir and ganciclovir.

ACYCLOVIR AND VALACYCLOVIR. Acyclovir is an acyclic guanine nucleoside analog that lacks the 2′ and 3′ positions normally supplied by ribose. Valacyclovir is the L-valyl ester prodrug of acyclovir.

ACYCLOVIR

Table 58–1

Stages of Virus Replication and Possible Targets of Action of Antiviral Agents

STAGE OF REPLICATION	CLASSES OF SELECTIVE INHIBITORS
Cell entry	
Attachment	Soluble receptor decoys, antireceptor antibodies, fusion
Penetration	protein inhibitors
Uncoating	Ion channel blockers, capsid stabilizers
Release of viral genome	
Transcription of viral genome[a]	Inhibitors of viral DNA polymerase, RNA polymerase,
Transcription of viral messenger RNA	reverse transcriptase, helicase, primase, or integrase
Replication of viral genome	
Translation of viral proteins	Interferons, antisense oligonucleotides, ribozymes
Regulatory proteins (early)	Inhibitors of regulatory proteins
Structural proteins (late)	
Post-translational modifications	
Proteolytic cleavage	Protease inhibitors
Myristoylation, glycosylation	
Assembly of virion components	Interferons, assembly protein inhibitors
Release	Neuraminidase inhibitors, antiviral antibodies, cytotoxic
Budding, cell lysis	lymphocytes

[a]*Depends on specific replication strategy of virus, but virus-specified enzyme required for part of process.*

Acyclovir's clinical use is limited to herpesviruses. Acyclovir is most active against HSV-1 (0.02-0.9 μg/mL), approximately half as active against HSV-2 (0.03-2.2 μg/mL), a tenth as potent against varicella zoster virus (VZV; 0.8-4.0 μg/mL) and Epstein-Barr virus (EBV), and least active against cytomegalovirus (CMV) (generally >20 μg/mL) and human herpesvirus 6 (HHV-6). Uninfected mammalian cell growth generally is unaffected by high acyclovir concentrations (>50 μg/mL).

THERAPEUTIC USES. In immunocompetent persons, the clinical benefits of acyclovir and valacyclovir are greater in initial HSV infections than in recurrent ones. These drugs are particularly useful in immunocompromised patients because these individuals experience both more frequent and more severe HSV and VZV infections. Because VZV is less susceptible than HSV to acyclovir, higher doses must be used for treating VZV infections. Oral valacyclovir is as effective as oral acyclovir in HSV infections and more effective for treating herpes zoster. Acyclovir is ineffective therapeutically in established cytomegalovirus (CMV) infections but ganciclovir is effective for CMV prophylaxis in immunocompromised patients. EBV-related oral hairy leukoplakia may improve with acyclovir. Oral acyclovir in conjunction with systemic corticosteroids appears beneficial in treating Bell palsy; valacyclovir is ineffective in acute vestibular neuritis. See the 12th edition of the parent text for details of dosage regimens for specific indications in treating HSV, VZV, and CMV.

MECHANISMS OF ACTION AND RESISTANCE. Acyclovir inhibits viral DNA synthesis via a mechanism outlined in Figure 58–2. Its selectivity of action depends on interaction with HSV *thymidine kinase* and *DNA polymerase*. Cellular uptake and initial phosphorylation are facilitated by HSV thymidine kinase. The affinity of acyclovir for HSV thymidine kinase is ~200 times greater than for the mammalian enzyme. Cellular enzymes convert the monophosphate to acyclovir triphosphate, which competes for endogenous dGTP. The immunosuppressive agent mycophenolate mofetil (*see* Chapter 35) potentiates the anti-herpes activity of acyclovir and related agents by depleting intracellular dGTP pools. Acyclovir triphosphate competitively inhibits viral DNA polymerases and, to a much lesser extent, cellular DNA polymerases. Acyclovir triphosphate also is incorporated into viral DNA, where it acts as a chain terminator because of the lack of a 3′-hydroxyl group. By a mechanism termed *suicide inactivation*, the terminated DNA template containing acyclovir binds the viral DNA polymerase and leads to its irreversible inactivation.

Acyclovir resistance in HSV can result from impaired production of viral thymidine kinase, altered thymidine kinase substrate specificity (e.g., phosphorylation of thymidine but not acyclovir), or altered viral DNA polymerase. Alterations in viral enzymes are caused by point mutations and base insertions or deletions in the corresponding genes. Resistant variants are present in native virus populations and in isolates from treated patients. The most common resistance mechanism in clinical HSV isolates is absent or deficient viral thymidine kinase activity; viral DNA polymerase mutants are rare. Phenotypic resistance typically is defined by in vitro inhibitory concentrations of >2-3 μg/mL, which predict failure of therapy in immunocompromised

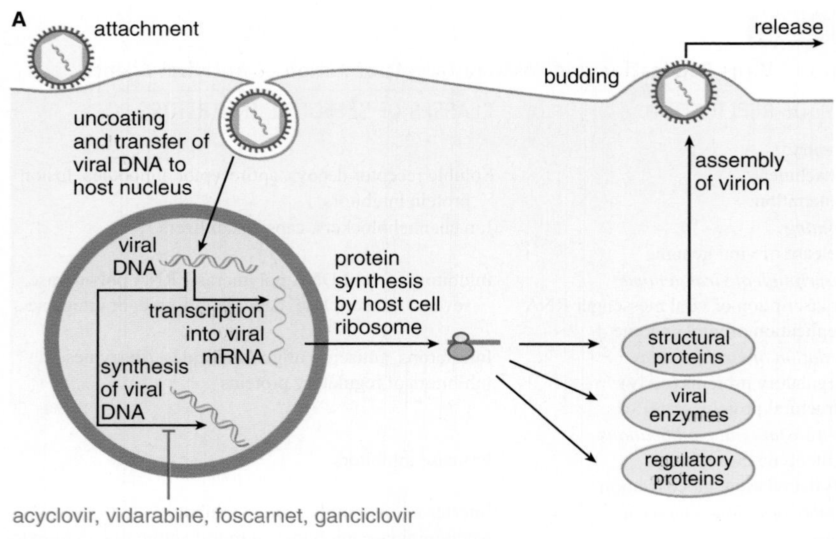

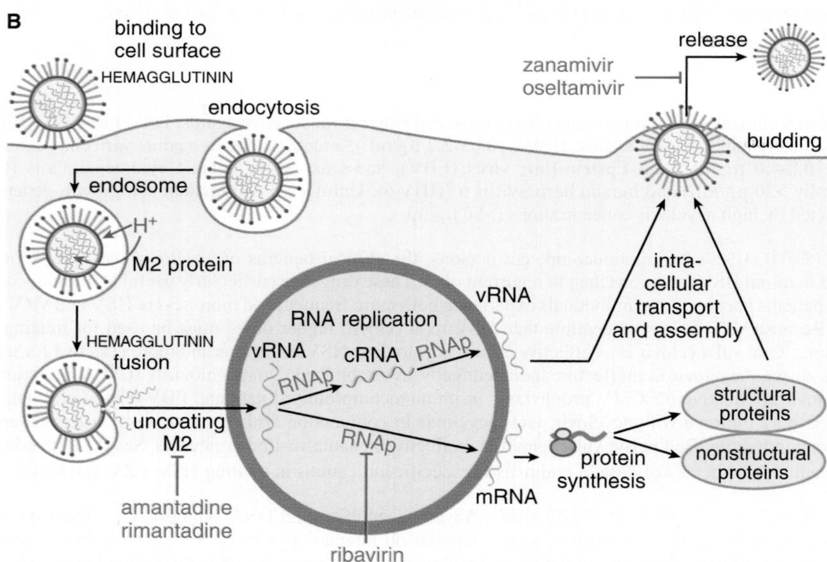

Figure 58–1 *Replicative cycles of DNA (A) and RNA (B) viruses.* The replicative cycles of herpesvirus (A) and influenza (B) are examples of DNA-encoded and RNA-encoded viruses, respectively. Sites of action of antiviral agents also are shown. cDNA, complementary DNA; cRNA, complementary RNA; DNAp, DNA polymerase; mRNA, messenger RNA; RNAp, RNA polymerase; vRNA, viral RNA. The symbol ——┤ indicates a block to virus growth. **A.** Replicative cycles of herpes simplex virus, a DNA virus, and the probable sites of action of antiviral agents. Herpesvirus replication is a regulated multistep process. After infection, a small number of immediate-early genes are transcribed; these genes encode proteins that regulate their own synthesis and are responsible for synthesis of early genes involved in genome replication, such as thymidine kinases, DNA polymerases, etc. After DNA replication, the bulk of the herpesvirus genes (called *late genes*) are expressed and encode proteins that either are incorporated into or aid in the assembly of progeny virions. **B.** Replicative cycles of influenza, an RNA virus, and the loci for effects of antiviral agents. The mammalian cell shown is an airway epithelial cell. The M2 protein of influenza virus allows an influx of hydrogen ions into the virion interior, which in turn promotes dissociation of the RNP (ribonuclear protein) segments and release into the cytoplasm (uncoating). Influenza virus mRNA synthesis requires a primer cleared from cellular mRNA and used by the viral RNAp complex. The neuraminidase inhibitors zanamivir and oseltamivir specifically inhibit release of progeny virus.

Table 58–2

Nomenclature of Antiviral Agents

GENERIC NAME	OTHER NAMES	DOSAGE FORMS AVAILABLE
Antiherpesvirus agents		
Acyclovir	ACV, acycloguanosine	IV, O, T, ophth[a]
Cidofovir	HPMPC, CDV	IV
Famciclovir	FCV	O
Foscarnet	PFA, phosphonoformate	IV, O[a]
Fomivirsena	ISIS 2922	Intravitreal
Ganciclovir	GCV, DHPG	IV, O, intravitreal
Idoxuridine	IDUR	Ophth
Penciclovir	PCV	T, IV[a]
Trifluridine	TFT, trifluorothymidine	Ophth
Valacyclovir		O
Valganciclovir		O
Anti-influenza agents		
Amantadine		O
Oseltamivir	GS4104	O
Rimantadine		O
Zanamivir	GC167	Inhalation
Antihepatitis agents		
Adefovir dipivoxil	Bis-pom-PMEA	O
Entecavir		O
Interferon alfa-N1		Injected
Interferon alfa-N3		Injected
Interferon alfacon-1		Injected
Interferon alfa-2B		Injected
Interferon alfa-2A		Injected
Lamivudine	3TC	O
Peginterferon alfa 2A		SC
Peginterferon alfa 2B		SC
Other antiviral agents		
Ribavirin		O, inhalation, IV
Telbivudine		O
Tenofovir disoproxil fumarate	TDF	O
Imiquimod		Topical

[a]Not currently approved for use in U.S. IV, intravenous; O, oral; T, topical; ophth, ophthalmic.

patients. Acyclovir resistance in VZV isolates is caused by mutations in VZV thymidine kinase and less often by mutations in viral DNA polymerase.

ADME. The oral bioavailability of acyclovir is ~10-30% and decreases with increasing dose. Valacyclovir is converted rapidly and virtually completely to acyclovir after oral administration. This conversion is thought to result from first-pass intestinal and hepatic metabolism through enzymatic hydrolysis. Unlike acyclovir, valacyclovir is a substrate for intestinal and renal peptide transporters. The oral bioavailability of acyclovir increases ~70% following valacyclovir administration. Peak plasma concentrations of valacyclovir are only 4% of acyclovir levels. Less than 1% of an administered dose of valacyclovir is recovered in the urine; most is eliminated as acyclovir. Acyclovir distributes widely in body fluids, including vesicular fluid, aqueous humor, and cerebrospinal fluid (CSF). Compared with plasma, salivary concentrations are low, and vaginal secretion concentrations vary widely. Acyclovir is concentrated in breast milk, amniotic fluid, and placenta. Newborn plasma levels are similar to maternal ones. Percutaneous absorption of acyclovir after topical administration is low. The elimination $t_{1/2}$ of acyclovir is ~2.5 h (range: 1.5-6 h) in adults with normal renal function.

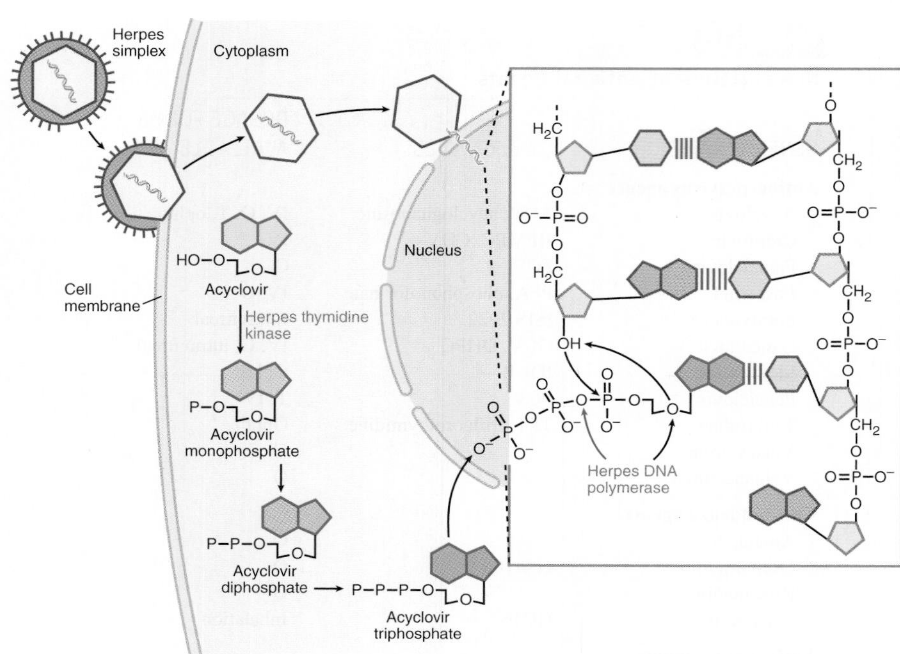

Figure 58–2 *Mechanism of action of acyclovir in cells infected by herpes simplex virus.* A herpes simplex virion is shown attaching to a susceptible host cell, fusing its envelope with the cell membrane, and releasing naked capsids that deliver viral DNA into the nucleus, where it initiates synthesis of viral DNA. Acyclovir molecules entering the cell are converted to acyclovir monophosphate by virus-induced thymidine kinase. Host-cell enzymes add 2 more phosphates to form acyclovir triphosphate, which is transported into the nucleus. After the herpes DNA polymerase cleaves pyrophosphate from acyclovir triphosphate (*indicated by the red arrow in the inset*), viral DNA polymerase inserts acyclovir monophosphate rather than 2′-deoxyguanosine monophosphate into the viral DNA (*indicated by black arrows in the inset*). Further elongation of the chain is impossible because acyclovir monophosphate lacks the 3′ hydroxyl group necessary for the insertion of an additional nucleotide, and the exonuclease associated with the viral DNA polymerase cannot remove the acyclovir moiety. In contrast, ganciclovir and penciclovir have a 3′ hydroxyl group; therefore, further synthesis of viral DNA is possible in the presence of these drugs. Foscarnet acts at the pyrophosphate-binding site of viral DNA polymerase and prevents cleavage of the pyrophosphate from nucleoside triphosphates, thus stalling further primer template extension. Red lines [III] indicate hydrogen bonding of the base pairs. (Adapted from Balfour HH. Antiviral drugs. *N Engl J Med,* 1999;340:1255–1268.)

The elimination $t_{1/2}$ of acyclovir is ~4 h in neonates and increases to 20 h in anuric patients. Renal excretion is the principal route of elimination.

UNTOWARD EFFECTS. Acyclovir generally is well tolerated. Topical acyclovir in a polyethylene glycol base may cause mucosal irritation and transient burning when applied to genital lesions. Oral acyclovir has been associated infrequently with nausea, diarrhea, rash, or headache and very rarely with renal insufficiency or neurotoxicity. Valacyclovir also may be associated with headache, nausea, diarrhea, nephrotoxicity, and CNS symptoms (confusion, hallucinations). Uncommon side effects include severe thrombocytopenic syndromes, sometimes fatal, in immunocompromised patients. Acyclovir has been associated with neutropenia in neonates. The principal dose-limiting toxicities of intravenous acyclovir are renal insufficiency and CNS side effects. Nephrotoxicity usually resolves with drug cessation and volume expansion. Hemodialysis may be useful in severe cases. Severe somnolence and lethargy may occur with combinations of zidovudine (*see* Chapter 59) and acyclovir. Concomitant cyclosporine and probably other nephrotoxic agents enhance the risk of nephrotoxicity. Probenecid decreases the acyclovir renal clearance and prolongs the elimination $t_{1/2}$. Acyclovir may decrease the renal clearance of other drugs eliminated by active renal secretion, such as methotrexate.

CIDOFOVIR. Cidofovir is a cytidine nucleotide analog with inhibitory activity against human herpes, papilloma, polyoma, pox, and adenoviruses.

Because cidofovir is a phosphonate that is phosphorylated by cellular but not viral enzymes, it inhibits acyclovir-resistant thymidine kinase (TK)–deficient or TK-altered HSV or VZV strains, ganciclovir-resistant CMV strains with UL97 mutations (but not those with DNA polymerase mutations), and some foscarnet-resistant CMV strains. Cidofovir synergistically inhibits CMV replication in combination with ganciclovir or foscarnet.

THERAPEUTIC USES. Intravenous cidofovir is approved for the treatment of CMV retinitis in HIV-infected patients. Intravenous cidofovir has been used for treating acyclovir-resistant mucocutaneous HSV infection, adenovirus disease in transplant recipients, and extensive molluscum contagiosum in HIV patients. Reduced doses without probenecid may be beneficial in BK virus nephropathy in renal transplant patients. Topical cidofovir gel eliminates virus shedding and lesions in some HIV-infected patients with acyclovir-resistant mucocutaneous HSV infections and has been used in treating anogenital warts and molluscum contagiosum in immunocompromised patients and cervical intraepithelial neoplasia in women. Intralesional cidofovir induces remissions in adults and children with respiratory papillomatosis. See the 12th edition of the parent text for details of dosage regimens for specific indications.

MECHANISMS OF ACTION AND RESISTANCE. Cidofovir inhibits viral DNA synthesis by slowing and eventually terminating chain elongation. Cidofovir is metabolized to its active diphosphate form by cellular enzymes; the levels of phosphorylated metabolites are similar in infected and uninfected cells. The diphosphate acts as both a competitive inhibitor with respect to dCTP and as an alternative substrate for viral DNA polymerase.

Cidofovir resistance in CMV is due to mutations in viral DNA polymerase. Low-level resistance to cidofovir develops in up to ~30% of retinitis patients by 3 months of therapy. Highly ganciclovir-resistant CMV isolates that possess DNA polymerase and UL97 kinase mutations are resistant to cidofovir, and prior ganciclovir therapy may select for cidofovir resistance. Some foscarnet-resistant CMV isolates show cross-resistance to cidofovir, and triple-drug-resistant variants with DNA polymerase mutations occur.

ADME. Cidofovir has very low oral bioavailability. Penetration into the CSF is low. Topical cidofovir gel may result in low plasma concentrations (<0.5 μg/mL) in patients with large mucocutaneous lesions. Plasma levels after intravenous dosing decline in a biphasic pattern with a terminal $t_{1/2}$ that averages 2.6 h. The active form, cidofovir diphosphate, has a prolonged intracellular $t_{1/2}$ and competitively inhibits CMV and HSV DNA polymerases at concentrations one-eighth to one six-hundredth of those required to inhibit human DNA polymerases. A phosphocholine metabolite also has a long intracellular $t_{1/2}$ (~87 h) and may serve as an intracellular reservoir of drug. The prolonged intracellular $t_{1/2}$ of cidofovir diphosphate allows infrequent dosing regimens. Cidofovir is cleared by the kidney via glomerular filtration and tubular secretion. Over 90% of the dose is recovered unchanged in the urine. Probenecid blocks tubular transport of cidofovir and reduces renal clearance and associated nephrotoxicity. Elimination relates linearly to creatinine clearance; the $t_{1/2}$ increases to 32.5 h in patients on chronic ambulatory peritoneal dialysis (CAPD). Hemodialysis removes >50% of the administered dose.

UNTOWARD EFFECTS. Nephrotoxicity is the principal dose-limiting side effect of intravenous cidofovir. Concomitant oral probenecid and saline prehydration reduce the risk of renal toxicity; however, probenecid alters renal clearance of many agents, albeit not of cidofidir. For example, probenecid alters zidovudine pharmacokinetics such that zidovudine doses should be reduced when probenecid is present, as should the doses of other drugs whose renal secretion probenecid inhibits (e.g., β-lactam antibiotics, nonsteroidal anti-inflammatory drugs [NSAIDs], acyclovir, lorazepam, furosemide, methotrexate, theophylline, and rifampin). On maintenance doses of 5 mg/kg every 2 weeks, up to 50% of patients develop proteinuria, 10-15% show an elevated serum creatinine concentration, and 15-20% develop neutropenia. Anterior uveitis that is responsive to topical corticosteroids and cycloplegia occurs commonly and low intraocular pressure occurs infrequently with intravenous cidofovir. Administration with food and pretreatment with antiemetics, antihistamines, and/or acetaminophen may improve tolerance. Concurrent nephrotoxic agents are contraindicated, and at least 7 days should elapse before initiation of cidofovir treatment is recommended after prior exposure to aminoglycosides, intravenous pentamidine, amphotericin B, foscarnet, NSAID, or contrast dye. Cidofovir and oral ganciclovir are poorly tolerated in combination at full doses.

Topical application of cidofovir is associated with dose-related application-site reactions (e.g., burning, pain, and pruritus) in up to one-third of patients and occasionally ulceration. Cidofovir is considered a potential human carcinogen. It may cause infertility and is classified as pregnancy Category C.

FAMCICLOVIR AND PENCICLOVIR. Famciclovir is the diacetyl ester prodrug of 6-deoxy penciclovir and lacks intrinsic antiviral activity. Penciclovir is an acyclic guanine nucleoside analog. Penciclovir is similar to acyclovir in its spectrum of activity and potency against HSV and VZV. It also is inhibitory for HBV.

THERAPEUTIC USES. Oral famciclovir, topical penciclovir, and intravenous penciclovir are approved for managing HSV and VZV infections. See the 12th edition of the parent text for details of dosage regimens for specific indications.

MECHANISMS OF ACTION AND RESISTANCE. Penciclovir is an inhibitor of viral DNA synthesis. In HSV- or VZV-infected cells, penciclovir is phosphorylated initially by viral TK. Penciclovir triphosphate is a competitive inhibitor of viral DNA polymerase (*see* Figure 58–2). Although penciclovir triphosphate is approximately one one-hundredth as potent as acyclovir triphosphate in inhibiting viral DNA polymerase, it is present in infected cells at much higher concentrations and for more prolonged periods. The prolonged intracellular $t_{1/2}$ of penciclovir triphosphate, 7-20 h, is associated with prolonged antiviral effects. Because penciclovir has a 3′-hydroxyl group, it is not an obligate chain terminator but does inhibit DNA elongation. Resistance during clinical use is low. TK–deficient, acyclovir-resistant herpes viruses are cross-resistant to penciclovir.

ADME. Oral penciclovir has low (<5%) bioavailability. In contrast, famciclovir is well absorbed orally (bioavailability ~75%) and is converted rapidly to penciclovir by deacetylation of the side chain and oxidation of the purine ring during and following absorption. Food slows absorption but does not reduce overall bioavailability. The plasma elimination $t_{1/2}$ of penciclovir averages ~2 h, and >90% is excreted unchanged in the urine. Following oral famciclovir administration, nonrenal clearance accounts for ~10% of each dose, primarily through fecal excretion, but penciclovir (60% of dose) and its 6-deoxy precursor (<10% of dose) are eliminated primarily in the urine. The plasma $t_{1/2}$ averages 9.9 h in renal insufficiency (Cl_{cr} <30 mL/min); hemodialysis efficiently removes penciclovir.

UNTOWARD EFFECTS. Oral famciclovir is associated with headache, diarrhea, and nausea. Urticaria, rash, and hallucinations or confusional states (predominantly in the elderly) have been reported. Topical penciclovir (~1%) rarely is associated with local reactions. The short-term tolerance of famciclovir is comparable with that of acyclovir. Penciclovir is mutagenic at high concentrations. Long-term administration (1 year) does not affect spermatogenesis in men. Safety during pregnancy has not been established.

FOMIVIRSEN. Fomivirsen, a 21-base phosphorothioate oligonucleotide, provides antisense therapy.

The drug is complementary to the messenger RNA sequence for the major immediate-early transcriptional region of CMV and inhibits CMV replication through sequence-specific and nonspecific mechanisms, including inhibition of virus binding to cells. Fomivirsen is active against CMV strains resistant to ganciclovir, foscarnet, and cidofovir. Fomivirsen is given by intravitreal injection in the treatment of CMV retinitis for patients intolerant of or unresponsive to other therapies. Following injection, it is cleared slowly from the vitreous ($t_{1/2}$ ~55 h) through distribution to the retina and probable exonuclease digestion. In HIV-infected patients with refractory, sight-threatening CMV retinitis, fomivirsen injections (330 μg weekly for 3 weeks and then every 2 weeks or on days 1 and 15 followed by monthly) significantly delay time to retinitis progression. Ocular side effects include iritis in up to one-quarter of patients, which can be managed with topical corticosteroids; vitritis; cataracts; and increases in intraocular pressure in 15-20% of patients. Recent cidofovir use may increase the risk of inflammatory reactions. The drug is no longer available in the U.S.

FOSCARNET. Foscarnet (trisodium phosphonoformate) is an inorganic pyrophosphate analog that is inhibitory for all herpesviruses and HIV.

THERAPEUTIC USES. Intravenous foscarnet is effective for treatment of CMV retinitis, including ganciclovir-resistant infections, other types of CMV infection, and acyclovir-resistant HSV and VZV infections. Foscarnet is poorly soluble in aqueous solutions and requires large volumes for administration. See the 12th edition of the parent text for details of dosage regimens for specific indications.

MECHANISMS OF ACTION AND RESISTANCE. Foscarnet inhibits viral nucleic acid synthesis by interacting directly with herpesvirus DNA polymerase or HIV reverse transcriptase (*see* Figures 58–1A and 58–2). Foscarnet has ~100-fold greater inhibitory effects against herpesvirus DNA polymerases than against cellular DNA polymerase-α. Herpesviruses resistant to foscarnet have point mutations in the viral DNA polymerase.

ADME. Oral bioavailability of foscarnet is low. Vitreous levels approximate those in plasma; CSF levels average 66% of those in plasma at steady state. Over 80% of foscarnet is excreted unchanged in the urine. Dose adjustments are indicated for small decreases in renal function. Plasma elimination has initial bimodal half-lives totaling 4-8 h and a prolonged terminal elimination $t_{1/2}$ averaging 3-4 days. Sequestration in bone with gradual release accounts for the fate of an estimated 10-20% of a given dose. Foscarnet is cleared efficiently by hemodialysis (~50% of a dose).

UNTOWARD EFFECTS. Major dose-limiting toxicities are nephrotoxicity and symptomatic hypocalcemia. Increases in serum creatinine occur in up to one-half of patients but are generally reversible after cessation.

High doses, rapid infusion, dehydration, prior renal insufficiency, and concurrent nephrotoxic drugs are risk factors. Saline loading may reduce the risk of nephrotoxicity. Foscarnet is highly ionized at physiological pH, and metabolic abnormalities are very common. These include increases or decreases in Ca^{2+} and phosphate, hypomagnesemia, and hypokalemia. Concomitant intravenous pentamidine administration increases the risk of symptomatic hypocalcemia. CNS side effects include headache (25%), tremor, irritability, seizures, and hallucinosis. Other reported side effects are generalized rash, fever, nausea or emesis, anemia, leukopenia, abnormal liver function tests, electrocardiographic changes, infusion-related thrombophlebitis, and painful genital ulcerations. Topical foscarnet may cause local irritation and ulceration, and oral foscarnet may cause GI disturbance. Preclinical studies indicate that high foscarnet concentrations are mutagenic. Safety in pregnancy or childhood is uncertain.

GANCICLOVIR AND VALGANCICLOVIR. Ganciclovir is an acyclic guanine nucleoside analog that is similar in structure to acyclovir. Valganciclovir is the L-valyl ester prodrug of ganciclovir. Ganciclovir has inhibitory activity against all herpesviruses and is especially active against CMV.

THERAPEUTIC USES. Ganciclovir is effective for treatment and chronic suppression of CMV retinitis in immunocompromised patients and for prevention of CMV disease in transplant patients. A ganciclovir ophthalmic gel formulation (ZIRGAN) is effective in treating HSV keratitis. See the 12th edition of the parent text for details of dosage regimens for specific indications.

MECHANISMS OF ACTION AND RESISTANCE. Ganciclovir inhibits viral DNA synthesis. It is monophosphorylated intracellularly by viral TK during HSV infection and by a viral phosphotransferase encoded by the UL97 gene during CMV infection. Ganciclovir diphosphate and ganciclovir triphosphate are formed by cellular enzymes. At least 10-fold higher concentrations of ganciclovir triphosphate are present in CMV-infected than in uninfected cells. The triphosphate is a competitive inhibitor of deoxyguanosine triphosphate incorporation into DNA and preferentially inhibits viral rather than host cellular DNA polymerases. Incorporation into viral DNA causes eventual cessation of DNA chain elongation (*see* Figures 58–1A and 58–2).

CMV can become resistant to ganciclovir by either of 2 mechanisms: reduced intracellular ganciclovir phosphorylation owing to mutations in the viral phosphotransferase and mutations in viral DNA polymerase. Highly resistant variants with both mutations are cross-resistant to cidofovir and variably to foscarnet. Ganciclovir also is much less active against acyclovir-resistant TK–deficient HSV strains.

ADME. The oral bioavailability of ganciclovir is 6-9% following ingestion with food. Oral valganciclovir is well absorbed and hydrolyzed rapidly to ganciclovir; the bioavailability of ganciclovir averages 61% following administration of valganciclovir. Food increases the bioavailability of valganciclovir by ~25%. Following intravenous administration of ganciclovir, vitreous fluid levels are similar to or higher than those in plasma and decline with a $t_{1/2}$ of 23-26 h. Intraocular sustained-release ganciclovir implants provide vitreous levels of ~4.1 μg/mL. The plasma elimination $t_{1/2}$ is ~2-4 h. Intracellular ganciclovir triphosphate concentrations are 10-fold higher than those of acyclovir triphosphate and decline much more slowly, with an intracellular elimination $t_{1/2}$ >24 h. Over 90% of ganciclovir is eliminated unchanged by renal excretion. Plasma $t_{1/2}$ increases in patients with severe renal insufficiency.

UNTOWARD EFFECTS. Myelosuppression is the principal dose-limiting toxicity of ganciclovir. Neutropenia occurs in ~15-40% of patients and is observed most commonly during the second week of treatment and usually is reversible within 1 week of drug cessation. Persistent fatal neutropenia has occurred. Recombinant granulocyte colony-stimulating factor (G-CSF; filgrastim, lenograstim) may be useful in treating ganciclovir-induced neutropenia (*see* Chapter 37). Thrombocytopenia occurs in 5-20% of patients. Zidovudine and probably other cytotoxic agents increase the risk of myelosuppression, as do nephrotoxic agents that impair ganciclovir excretion. Probenecid and possibly acyclovir reduce renal clearance of ganciclovir. Oral ganciclovir increases the absorption and peak plasma concentrations of didanosine by approximately 2-fold and that of zidovudine by ~20%. CNS side effects (5-15%) range in severity from headache to behavioral changes to convulsions and coma. About one-third of patients must interrupt or prematurely stop intravenous ganciclovir therapy because of bone marrow or CNS toxicity. Infusion-related phlebitis, azotemia, anemia, rash, fever, liver function test abnormalities, nausea or vomiting, and eosinophilia also have been described. Ganciclovir is classified as pregnancy Category C.

DOCOSANOL

Docosanol is a long-chain saturated alcohol that is approved as an over-the-counter 10% cream for the treatment of recurrent orolabial herpes. Docosanol inhibits the in vitro replication of many lipid-enveloped viruses, including HSV. It does not inactivate HSV directly but appears to block fusion between the cellular and viral envelope membranes and inhibits viral entry into the cell. Topical treatment beginning within 12 h of prodromal symptoms or lesion onset reduces healing time by ~1 day and is well tolerated. Treatment initiation at papular or later stages provides no benefit.

IDOXURIDINE

Idoxuridine is an iodinated thymidine analog that inhibits the in vitro replication of various DNA viruses, including herpesviruses and poxviruses. Idoxuridine lacks selectivity, in that low concentrations inhibit the growth of uninfected cells. The triphosphate inhibits viral DNA synthesis and is incorporated into both viral and cellular DNA. In the U.S., idoxuridine is approved only for topical (ophthalmic) treatment of HSV keratitis. Idoxuridine formulated in dimethylsulfoxide is available outside the U.S. for topical treatment of herpes labialis, genitalis, and zoster. Adverse reactions include pain, pruritus, inflammation, and edema of the eye or lids; allergic reactions are rare.

TRIFLURIDINE

Trifluridine is a fluorinated pyrimidine nucleoside that has in vitro inhibitory activity against HSV types 1 and 2, CMV, vaccinia, and to a lesser extent, certain adenoviruses. Trifluridine inhibits replication of herpesviruses, including acyclovir-resistant strains, and also inhibits cellular DNA synthesis at relatively low concentrations. Trifluridine monophosphate irreversibly inhibits thymidylate synthase, and trifluridine triphosphate is a competitive inhibitor of thymidine triphosphate incorporation into DNA; trifluridine is incorporated into viral and cellular DNA. Trifluridine-resistant HSV has been described.

Trifluridine currently is used for treatment of primary keratoconjunctivitis and recurrent epithelial keratitis owing to HSV types 1 and 2. Topical trifluridine is more active than idoxuridine and comparable with vidarabine in HSV ocular infections. Adverse reactions include discomfort on instillation and palpebral edema. Hypersensitivity reactions and irritation are uncommon. Topical trifluridine also appears to be effective in some patients with acyclovir-resistant HSV cutaneous infections.

ANTI-INFLUENZA AGENTS

Recently, there has been concern about the possibility of new influenza pandemics, stemming from small but severe outbreaks of H5N1 avian influenza and the novel 2009 influenza A H1N1, thought to be of swine origin. Four drugs are currently approved for the treatment and prevention of influenza virus infection: the adamantine antivirals, amantadine and rimantadine; oseltamivir; and zanamivir; peramivir, an investigational neuraminidase inhibitor, is available for intravenous use via emergency use authorization (EUA). Development of resistance to these drugs, and the spread of resistant viruses, are major challenges in the chemotherapy and chemoprophylaxis of influenza and are likely to drive future recommendations for use of these drugs in global populations.

AMANTADINE AND RIMANTADINE. Amantadine and its derivative rimantadine are uniquely configured tricyclic amines.

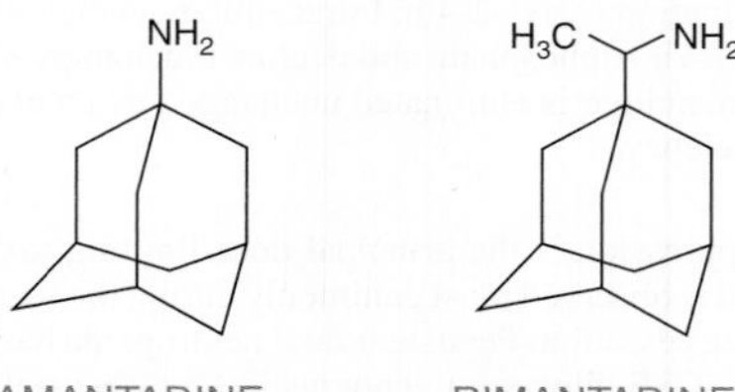

THERAPEUTIC USES. Although both drugs are useful for the prevention and treatment of infections caused by influenza A virus, vaccination against influenza is a more cost-effective means of reducing disease burden. Amantadine and rimantadine are active only against susceptible influenza A viruses (not influenza B); rimantadine is 4- to 10-fold more active than amantadine. Virtually all H3N2 strains of influenza circulating worldwide are resistant to these drugs.

Seasonal prophylaxis with either amantadine or rimantadine (a total of 200 mg/day in 1 or 2 divided doses in young adults) is ~70-90% protective against influenza A illness. These agents are efficacious in preventing nosocomial influenza and in curtailing nosocomial outbreaks during pandemic influenza. Doses of 100 mg/day are better tolerated and still appear to be protective against influenzal illness. Seasonal prophylaxis is an alternative in high-risk patients if the influenza vaccine cannot be administered or may be ineffective (i.e., in immunocompromised patients). Prophylaxis should be started as soon as influenza is identified in a community or region and should be continued throughout the period of risk (usually 4-8 weeks) because any protective effects are lost several days after cessation of therapy. Alternatively, the drugs can be started in conjunction with immunization and continued for 2 weeks until protective immune responses develop.

The amantadines are effective against influenza A H1N1 if treatment is initiated within 2 days of the onset of symptoms. In uncomplicated influenza A illness of adults, early amantadine or rimantadine treatment (200 mg/day for 5 days) reduces the duration of fever and systemic complaints by 1-2 days, speeds functional recovery, and sometimes decreases the duration of virus shedding. The usual regimen in children (≥1 year of age) is 5 mg/kg/day, up to 150 mg, administered once or twice daily. Resistant variants have been recovered from ~30% of treated children or outpatient adults by the fifth day of therapy.

MECHANISMS OF ACTION AND RESISTANCE. Amantadine and rimantadine inhibit an early step in viral replication, probably viral uncoating; for some strains, they also have an effect on a late step in viral assembly probably mediated through altering hemagglutinin processing. The primary locus of action is the influenza A virus M2 protein, an integral membrane protein that functions as an ion channel. By interfering with this function of the M2 protein, the drugs inhibit the acid-mediated dissociation of the ribonucleoprotein complex early in replication and potentiate acidic pH–induced conformational changes in hemagglutinin during its intracellular transport later in replication. Resistance to these drugs results from a mutation in the RNA sequence encoding for the M2 protein transmembrane domain; resistant isolates typically appear in the treated patient within 2-3 days of starting therapy.

ADME. Table 58–3 summarizes important pharmacokinetics properties of these anti-viral agents. The 2 adamantanes differ in several respects. Amantadine is excreted largely unmetabolized in the urine ($t_{1/2}$ of elimination is ~12-18 h in young adults, increasing up to 2-fold in the elderly and even more in those with renal impairment). By contrast, elimination of rimantadine depends on hepatic function; the drug is subject to phase 1 and phase 2 reactions prior to renal excretion of metabolites (elimination $t_{1/2}$ ~24-36 h; 60-90% is excreted in the urine as metabolites). The elderly require only one-half the weight-adjusted dose of amantadine needed for young adults. Amantadine is excreted in breast milk. Rimantadine concentrations in nasal mucus average 50% higher than those in plasma.

UNTOWARD EFFECTS. The most common side effects related to amantadine and rimantadine are minor dose-related CNS and GI effects: nervousness, light-headedness, difficulty concentrating, insomnia, and loss of appetite, and nausea. CNS side effects (5-33%) occur in patients treated with amantadine at doses of 200 mg/day but are significantly less frequent with rimantadine. The neurotoxic effects of amantadine appear to be increased by concomitant ingestion of antihistamines and psychotropic or anticholinergic drugs, especially in the elderly. At comparable doses of 100 mg/day, rimantadine is significantly better tolerated in nursing home residents than amantadine. High amantadine plasma concentrations (1.0-5.0 μg/mL) have been associated with serious neurotoxic reactions, including delirium, hallucinosis, seizures, and coma, and cardiac

Table 58–3

Pharmacological Characteristics of Antivirals for Influenza

	AMANTADINE	RIMANTADINE	ZANAMIVIR	OSELTAMIVIR
Spectrum (types of influenza)	A	A	A, B	A, B
Route/formulations	Oral (tablet/ capsule/syrup)	Oral (tablet/ syrup)	Inhaled (powder) Intravenous[a]	Oral (capsule/syrup) Intravenous[a]
Oral bioavailability	>90%	>90%	<5%[b]	80%[c]
Effect of meals on AUC	Negligible	Negligible	Not applicable	Negligible
Elimination $t_{1/2}$, h	12-18	24-36	2.5-5	6-10[c]
Protein binding, %	67%	40%	<10%	3%[c]
Metabolism, %	<10%	~75%	Negligible	Negligible
Renal excretion, % (parent drug)	>90%	~25%	100%	95%[c]
Dose adjustments	Cl_{cr} ≤50 Age ≥65 yrs	Cl_{cr} ≤10 Age ≥65 years	None[d]	Cl_{cr} ≤30

Cl_{cr}, creatinine clearance
A fifth agent, permavir, is investigational in the U.S. and approved in Japan at a dose of 600 mg intravenously once daily in adults. Its elimination is primarily renal, with dosage adjustment required for renal insufficiency.
[a]Investigational at present.
[b]Systemic absorption 4-17% after inhalation.
[c]For antivirally active oseltamivir carboxylate.
[d]Inhaled formulation only.

arrhythmias. Exacerbations of preexisting seizure disorders and psychiatric symptoms may occur with amantadine and possibly with rimantadine. Both drugs are considered pregnancy Category C.

OSELTAMIVIR

Oseltamivir carboxylate is a transition-state analog of sialic acid that is a potent selective inhibitor of the neuraminidases of influenza A and B virus. Oseltamivir phosphate is an ethyl ester prodrug that lacks antiviral activity. Oseltamivir carboxylate has an antiviral spectrum and potency similar to that of zanamivir: it inhibits amantadine and rimantadine-resistant influenza A viruses and some zanamivir-resistant variants.

THERAPEUTIC USES. Oral oseltamivir is effective in the treatment and prevention of influenza A and B virus infections. Treatment of previously healthy adults (75 mg twice daily for 5 days) or children 1-12 years of age (weight-adjusted dosing) with acute influenza reduces illness duration by ~1-2 days, speeds functional recovery, and reduces the risk of complications leading to antibiotic use by 40-50%. Treatment is associated with approximate halving of the risk of subsequent hospitalization in adults. When used for prophylaxis during the typical influenza season, oseltamivir (75 mg once daily) is effective (~70-90%) in reducing the likelihood of influenza illness in both unimmunized working adults and in immunized nursing home residents; short-term use protects against influenza in household contacts.

MECHANISMS OF ACTION AND RESISTANCE. Influenza neuraminidase cleaves terminal sialic acid residues and destroys the receptors recognized by viral hemagglutinin, which are present on the cell surface, in progeny virions, and in respiratory secretions. This enzymatic action is essential for release of virus from infected cells. Interaction of oseltamivir carboxylate with the neuraminidase causes a conformational change within the enzyme's active site and inhibits its activity. Inhibition of neuraminidase activity leads to viral aggregation at the cell surface and reduced virus spread within the respiratory tract. Influenza variants selected in vitro for resistance to oseltamivir carboxylate contain hemagglutinin and/or neuraminidase mutations. Seasonal influenza A (H1N1) has become virtually 100% resistant to oseltamivir worldwide. Importantly, novel H1N1 (nH1N1 or swine influenza) remains susceptible to oseltamivir.

ADME. Table 58–3 summarizes important pharmacokinetics properties of oseltamivir carboxylate. Oral oseltamivir phosphate is absorbed rapidly and cleaved by esterases in the GI tract and liver to the active carboxylate. Food does not decrease bioavailability but reduces the risk of GI intolerance. Bronchoalveolar lavage levels in animals and middle ear fluid and sinus concentrations in humans are comparable with plasma levels. Probenecid doubles the plasma $t_{1/2}$ of the carboxylate, which indicates tubular secretion by the anionic pathway. Children <2 years of age exhibit age-related changes in oseltamivir carboxylate clearance and total drug exposure.

UNTOWARD EFFECTS. Oral oseltamivir is associated with nausea, abdominal discomfort, and, less often, emesis. GI complaints typically resolve in 1-2 days despite continued dosing, and are preventable by administration with food. An increased frequency of headache was reported in one prophylaxis study in elderly adults. Neither the phosphate nor the carboxylate form interacts with CYPs in vitro. Oseltamivir does not appear to impair fertility, but safety in pregnancy is uncertain (pregnancy Category C).

ZANAMIVIR. Zanamivir is a sialic acid analog that potently and specifically inhibits the neuraminidases of influenza A and B viruses. Zanamivir inhibits in vitro replication of influenza A and B viruses, including amantadine- and rimantadine-resistant strains and several oseltamivir-resistant variants.

THERAPEUTIC USES. Inhaled zanamivir is effective for the prevention and treatment of influenza A and B virus infections. Early zanamivir treatment (10 mg [2 inhalations] twice daily for 5 days) of febrile influenza in ambulatory adults and children ≥5 years of age shortens the time to illness resolution by 1-3 days and in adults reduces by 40% the risk of lower respiratory tract complications leading to antibiotic use. Once-daily inhaled zanamivir is highly protective against community-acquired influenza illness, and when given for 10 days, it protects against household transmission. Intravenous zanamivir ($t_{1/2}$ ~1.7 h) is available in the U.S. as an emergency investigational new drug (EIND) and in the E.U. on a compassionate use basis for life-threatening resistant influenza.

MECHANISMS OF ACTION AND RESISTANCE. Zanamivir inhibits viral neuraminidase and thus causes viral aggregation at the cell surface and reduced spread of virus within the respiratory tract. In vitro selection of viruses resistant to zanamivir is associated with mutations in the viral hemagglutinin and/or neuraminidase. Hemagglutinin variants are cross-resistant to other neuraminidase inhibitors. Neuraminidase variants contain mutations in the enzyme active site that diminish binding of zanamivir, but the altered enzymes show reduced activity or stability. Zanamivir-resistant variants usually have decreased infectivity in animals.

ADME. Table 58–3 summarizes important pharmacokinetics properties of zanamivir. Oral bioavailability of zanamivir is <5%, and the commercial form is delivered by oral inhalation of dry powder in a lactose carrier. The proprietary inhaler device is breath-actuated and requires a cooperative patient. Following inhalation of the dry powder, ~15% is deposited in the lower respiratory tract and ~80% in the oropharynx. Overall bioavailability is 4-17%.

UNTOWARD EFFECTS. Orally inhaled zanamivir generally is well tolerated in ambulatory adults and children with influenza. Wheezing and bronchospasm have been reported in some influenza-infected patients without known airway disease, and acute deteriorations in lung function, including fatal outcomes, have occurred in those with underlying asthma or chronic obstructive airway disease. Zanamivir is not generally recommended for treatment of patients with underlying airway disease because of the risk of serious adverse events. Preclinical studies of zanamivir revealed no evidence of mutagenic, teratogenic, or oncogenic effects (pregnancy Category C). No clinically significant drug interactions have been recognized to date. Zanamivir does not diminish the immune response to injected influenza vaccine.

ANTI-HEPATITIS VIRUS AGENTS

A number of agents are available for treatment of HBV and HCV infections. Several agents (e.g., interferons, ribavirin, and the nucleoside/nucleotide analogs lamivudine, telbivudine, and tenofovir) have other uses as well (*see* Chapter 59). Therapeutic strategies for hepatitis B and C are very different and are described separately.

DRUGS USED MAINLY FOR HEPATITIS C VIRUS INFECTION

HCV infection is associated with significant morbidity and mortality. Untreated, this virus can cause progressive hepatocellular injury with fibrosis and eventual cirrhosis. Chronic HCV is also a major risk factor for hepatocellular carcinoma. Although the virus is quite prolific, producing several billion new particles every few days in an infected individual, this RNA virus does not integrate into chromosomal DNA, and it does not establish latency per se. Therefore, the infection is, in theory, curable in all affected individuals. The current standard of care for treatment is a combination of peginterferon alfa and ribavirin, which produces a high cure rate in selected virus genotypes only.

INTERFERONS. Interferons (IFNs) are potent cytokines that possess antiviral, immunomodulatory, and antiproliferative activities (*see* Chapter 35). Three major classes of human interferons with significant antiviral activity are: α, β, and γ. Clinically used recombinant α-IFNs (*see* Table 58–2) are non-glycosylated proteins of ~19,500 Da, the pegylated forms predominating in the U.S. market.

IFN-α and IFN-β may be produced by nearly all cells in response to viral infection and a variety of other stimuli, including double-stranded RNA and certain cytokines (e.g., interleukin 1, interleukin 2, and tumor necrosis factor). IFN-γ production is restricted to T lymphocytes and natural killer cells responding to antigenic stimuli, mitogens, and specific cytokines. IFN-α and IFN-β exhibit antiviral and antiproliferative actions; stimulate the cytotoxic activity of lymphocytes, natural killer cells, and macrophages; and upregulate class I major histocompatibility (MHC) antigens and other surface markers. IFN-γ has less antiviral activity but more potent immunoregulatory effects, particularly macrophage activation, expression of class II MHC antigens, and mediation of local inflammatory responses. Most animal viruses are inhibited by IFNs, although many DNA viruses are relatively insensitive. The biological activity of IFN usually is measured in terms of antiviral effects in cell culture and generally is expressed as international units (IUs) relative to reference standards.

MECHANISMS OF ACTION. Following binding to specific cellular receptors, IFNs activate the JAK-STAT signal-transduction pathway and lead to the nuclear translocation of a cellular protein complex that binds to genes containing an IFN-specific response element. This, in turn, leads to synthesis of over 2 dozen proteins that contribute to viral resistance mediated at different stages of viral penetration (Figure 58–3).

A given virus may be inhibited at several steps, and the principal inhibitory effect differs among virus families. Certain viruses are able to counter IFN effects by blocking production or activity of selected IFN-inducible proteins. For example, IFN resistance in HCV is attributable to inhibition of the IFN-induced protein kinase, among other mechanisms. Complex interactions exist between IFNs and other parts of the immune system, so IFNs may ameliorate viral infections by exerting direct antiviral effects and/or by modifying the immune response to infection. For example, IFN-induced expression of MHC antigens may contribute to the antiviral actions of IFN by enhancing the lytic effects of cytotoxic T-lymphocytes. Conversely, IFNs may mediate some

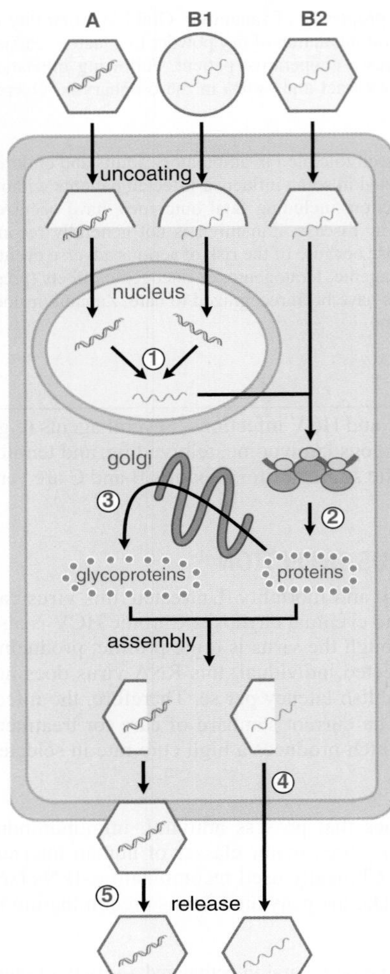
A
B1
B2
uncoating
nucleus
①
golgi
③
②
glycoproteins
proteins
assembly
④
⑤
release
Viruses
A. DNA
B. RNA
1. orthomyxoviruses and retroviruses
2. picornaviruses and most RNA viruses
IFN Effects
① inhibition of transcription
activates Mx protein
blocks mRNA synthesis
② inhibition of translation
activates methylase, thereby reducing
mRNA cap methylation
activates 2′5′ oligoadenylate synthetase
⟶ 2′5′A ⟶ inhibits mRNA splicing
and activates RNase L ⟶ cleaves
viral RNA
activates protein kinase P1 ⟶ blocks
eIF-2α function ⟶ inhibits initiation
of mRNA translation
activates phosphodiesterase ⟶ blocks
tRNA function
③ inhibition of post-translational processing
inhibits glycosyltransferase, thereby reducing
protein glycosylation
④ inhibition of virus maturation
inhibits glycosyltransferase, thereby reducing
glycoprotein maturation
⑤ inhibition of virus release
causes membrane changes ⟶ blocks
budding

Figure 58–3 *Interferon-mediated antiviral activity occurs via multiple mechanisms.* The binding of IFN to specific cell surface receptor molecules signals the cell to produce a series of antiviral proteins. The stages of viral replication that are inhibited by various IFN-induced antiviral proteins are shown. Most of these act to inhibit the translation of viral proteins (mechanism 2), but other steps in viral replication also are affected (mechanisms 1, 3, and 4). The roles of these mechanisms in the other actions of IFNs are under study. 2′5′A, 2′-5′-oligoadenylates; eIF-2α, protein synthesis initiation factor; IFN, interferon; mRNA, messenger RNA; Mx, IFN-induced cellular protein with anti-viral activity; RNase L, latent cellular endoribonuclease; tRNA, transfer RNA. (Modified from Baron S, Coppenhaver DH, Dianzani F, et al. Introduction to the interferon system. In: Baron S, Dianzani F, Stanton GJ, et al., eds. *Interferons: Principles and Medical Applications*, Galveston, TX: University of Texas Medical Branch Dept. of Microbiology; 1992:1–15. With permission.)

of the systemic symptoms associated with viral infections and contribute to immunologically mediated tissue damage in certain viral diseases.

ADME. After intramuscular or subcutaneous injection of IFN-α, absorption is >80%. Plasma levels are dose related, peaking at 4-8 h and returning to baseline by 18-36 h. Increased levels of 2′-5′-oligoadenylate synthase [2-5(A) synthase] in peripheral blood mononuclear cells are apparent at 6 h and last for 4 days after a single injection. An antiviral state in peripheral blood mononuclear cells peaks at 24 h and decreases slowly to baseline by 6 days after injection. After systemic administration, low levels of IFN are detected in respiratory secretions, CSF, eye, and brain. Because IFNs induce long-lasting cellular effects, their activities are not easily predictable from usual pharmacokinetic measures. After intravenous dosing, clearance of IFN from plasma occurs in a complex manner. With subcutaneous or intramuscular dosing, the plasma $t_{1/2}$ of IFN-α ranges from 3-8 h, due to distribution to the tissues, cellular uptake, and catabolism primarily in the kidney and liver. Negligible amounts are excreted in the urine. Clearance of IFN-α2B is reduced by ~80% in dialysis patients.

Attachment of IFN proteins to large inert polyethylene glycol (PEG) molecules (pegylation) slows absorption, decreases clearance, and provides higher and more prolonged serum concentrations that enable once-weekly dosing. Two pegylated IFNs are available commercially: peginterferon alfa-2a (PEGASYS) and peginterferon alfa-2B (PEG-INTRON). PegIFN alfa-2B has a 12 kDa PEG that increases the plasma $t_{1/2}$ to ~30-54 h. PegIFN alfa-2A contains a branched-chain 40 kDa PEG bonded to IFN-α2A and has a plasma $t_{1/2}$ averaging ~80-90 h. Increasing PEG size is associated with longer $t_{1/2}$ and less renal clearance. About 30% of pegIFN alfa-2B is cleared by the kidneys; pegIFN alfa-2A also is cleared primarily by the liver. Dose reductions in both pegylated IFNs are indicated in end-stage renal disease.

UNTOWARD EFFECTS. Injection of recombinant IFN doses of ≥1-2 million units (MU) usually is associated with an acute influenza-like syndrome beginning several hours after injection. Symptoms include fever, chills, headache, myalgia, arthralgia, nausea, vomiting, and diarrhea. Fever usually resolves within 12 h. Tolerance develops gradually in most patients. Febrile responses can be moderated by pretreatment with antipyretics. Up to one-half of patients receiving intralesional therapy for genital warts experience the influenzal illness initially, as well as discomfort at the injection site, and leukopenia.

Dose-limiting toxicities of systemic IFN are myelosuppression; neurotoxicity (e.g., somnolence, confusion, and depression); autoimmune disorders including thyroiditis and hypothyroidism; and uncommonly, cardiovascular effects with hypotension. Elevations in hepatic enzymes and triglycerides, alopecia, proteinuria and azotemia, interstitial nephritis, autoantibody formation, pneumonia, and hepatotoxicity may occur. Alopecia and personality change are common in IFN-treated children. The development of serum neutralizing antibodies to exogenous IFNs may be associated infrequently with loss of clinical responsiveness. IFN may impair fertility; safety during pregnancy is not established. IFNs can increase the hematological toxicity of drugs such as zidovudine and ribavirin and may increase the neurotoxicity and cardiotoxic effects of other drugs. Thyroid function and hepatic enzymes should be monitored during IFN therapy. Pegylated IFNs are better tolerated than standard IFNs, with discontinuation rates ranging from 2-11%, although the frequencies of fever, nausea, injection-site inflammation, and neutropenia may be somewhat higher. Severe neutropenia and the need for dose modifications are higher in HIV-coinfected persons.

THERAPEUTIC USES. Recombinant, natural, and pegylated IFNs currently are approved in the U.S. for treatment of condyloma acuminatum, chronic HCV infection, chronic HBV infection, Kaposi sarcoma in HIV-infected patients, other malignancies, and multiple sclerosis. In addition, interferons have been granted orphan drug status for a variety of rare disease states including idiopathic pulmonary fibrosis, laryngeal papillomatosis, juvenile rheumatoid arthritis, and infections associated with chronic granulomatous disease.

Hepatitis B Virus. In patients with chronic HBV infection, parenteral administration of various IFNs is associated with serological, biochemical, and histological improvement in ~25-50% of the patients. Lasting responses require moderately high IFN doses and prolonged administration (typically 5-10 MU/day in adults and 6 MU/m^2 in children 3 times per week of IFNα-2B for 4 to 6 months). Low pretherapy serum HBV DNA levels and high aminotransferase levels are predictors of response. PegIFN alfa-2A (180 μg once weekly for 24-48 weeks) appears superior to conventional IFN alfa-2A in HbeAg-positive patients. High-dose IFN can cause myelosuppression and clinical deterioration in those with decompensated liver disease.

Antiviral effects and improvements occur in about one-half of chronic hepatitis D virus (HDV) infections, but relapse is common unless HbsAg disappears. IFN does not appear to be beneficial in acute HBV or HDV infections.

Hepatitis C Virus. In chronic HCV infection, IFN alfa-2B monotherapy (3 MU 3 times weekly) is associated with ~50-70% rate of aminotransferase normalization and loss of plasma viral RNA, but sustained virologic remission is observed in only 10-25% of patients. Sustained viral responses are associated with long-term histological improvement and probably reduced risk of hepatocellular carcinoma and hepatic failure. Viral genotype and pretreatment RNA level influence response to treatment, but early viral clearance is the best predictor of sustained response. Nonresponders generally do not benefit from IFN monotherapy retreatment, but they and patients relapsing after monotherapy often respond to combined pegylated IFN and ribavirin treatment. IFN treatment may benefit HCV-associated cryoglobulinemia and glomerulonephritis. IFN administration during acute HCV infection appears to reduce the risk of chronicity.

Pegylated IFNs are superior to conventional thrice-weekly IFN monotherapy in inducing sustained remissions in treatment-naive patients. Monotherapy with pegIFN alfa-2A (180 μg subcutaneously weekly for 48 weeks) or pegIFN alfa-2B (1.5 μg/kg/week for 1 year) is associated with sustained response in 30-39%, including stable cirrhotic patients, and it is a treatment option in patients unable to take ribavirin. The efficacy of conventional and pegylated IFNs is enhanced by the addition of ribavirin to the treatment regimens, particularly for genotype 1 infections. Combined therapy with pegIFN alfa-2A (180 μg once weekly for 48 weeks) and ribavirin (1000-1200 mg/day in divided doses) gives higher sustained viral response rates than IFN-ribavirin combinations. The dose and duration of therapy depend on genotype of HCV infections. Approximately 15-20% of those failing to respond to combined IFN-ribavirin will have sustained responses to combined pegIFN-ribavirin.

Papillomavirus. In refractory condylomata acuminata (genital warts), intralesional injection of various natural and recombinant IFNs is associated with complete clearance of injected warts in 36-62% of patients, but other treatments are preferred. Relapse occurs in 20-30% of patients. Verruca vulgaris may respond to intralesional IFN-α. Intramuscular or subcutaneous administration is associated with some regression in wart size but greater toxicity. Systemic IFN may provide adjunctive benefit in recurrent juvenile laryngeal papillomatosis and in treating laryngeal disease in older patients.

Other Viruses. IFNs have been shown to have virological and clinical effects in various herpesvirus infections including genital HSV infections, localized herpes-zoster infection of cancer patients or of older adults, and CMV infections of renal transplant patients. However, IFN generally is associated with more side effects and inferior clinical benefits compared with conventional antiviral therapies. Topically applied IFN and trifluridine combinations appear active in acyclovir-resistant mucocutaneous HSV infections.

In HIV-infected persons, IFNs have been associated with antiretroviral effects. In advanced infection, however, the combination of zidovudine and IFN is associated with only transient benefit and excessive hematological toxicity. IFN-α (3 MU 3 times weekly) is effective for treatment of HIV-related thrombocytopenia resistant to zidovudine therapy.

Except for adenovirus, IFN has broad-spectrum antiviral activity against respiratory viruses. However, prophylactic intranasal IFN-α is protective only against rhinovirus colds, and chronic use is limited by the occurrence of nasal side effects. Intranasal IFN is therapeutically ineffective in established rhinovirus colds.

RIBAVIRIN. Ribavirin, a purine nucleoside analog with a modified base and D-ribose sugar, inhibits the replication of a wide range of RNA and DNA viruses, including orthomyxo-, paramyxo-, arena-, bunya-, and flavi-viruses in vitro. Therapeutic concentrations may reversibly inhibit macromolecular synthesis and proliferation of uninfected cells, suppress lymphocyte responses, and alter cytokine profiles in vitro.

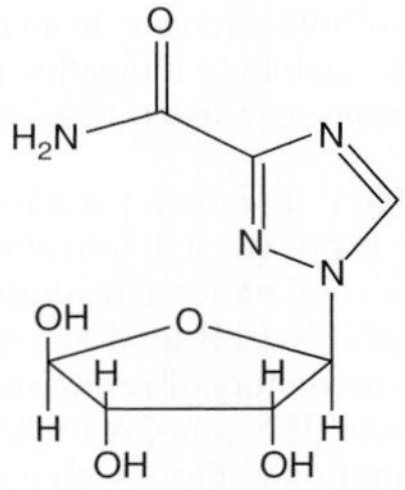

RIBAVIRIN

THERAPEUTIC USES. Oral ribavirin in combination with injected pegIFN alfa-2A or alfa-2B is standard treatment for chronic HCV infection. Ribavirin aerosol is approved in the U.S. for treatment of RSV bronchiolitis and pneumonia in hospitalized children. Aerosolized ribavirin (usual dose of 20 mg/mL as the starting solution in the drug reservoir of the small particle aerosol generator unit for an 18 h exposure/day for 3-7 days) may reduce some illness measures, but its use generally is not recommended. Aerosol ribavirin combined with intravenous immunoglobulin appears to reduce mortality of RSV infection in bone marrow transplant and other highly immunocompromised patients.

Intravenous and/or aerosol ribavirin has been used occasionally in treating severe influenza virus infection and in the treatment of immunosuppressed patients with adenovirus, vaccinia, parainfluenza, or measles virus infections. Aerosolized ribavirin is associated with reduced duration of fever but no other clinical or antiviral effects in influenza infections in hospitalized children. Intravenous ribavirin decreases mortality in Lassa fever and has been used in treating other arenavirus-related hemorrhagic fevers. Intravenous ribavirin is beneficial in hemorrhagic fever with renal syndrome owing to hantavirus infection but appears ineffective in hantavirus-associated cardiopulmonary syndrome or SARS. Intravenous ribavirin is investigational in the U.S.

MECHANISMS OF ACTION AND RESISTANCE. Ribavirin alters cellular nucleotide pools and inhibits viral mRNA synthesis. Host cell enzymes phosphorylate ribavirin to mono-, di-, and tri-phosphate derivatives. In both uninfected and RSV-infected cells, the predominant derivative (>80%) is the triphosphate, which has an intracellular $t_{1/2}$ <2 h. Ribavirin monophosphate competitively inhibits cellular IMP dehydrogenase and interferes with the synthesis of GTP and thus nucleic acid synthesis in general. Ribavirin triphosphate also competitively inhibits the GTP-dependent 5′ capping of viral messenger RNA and specifically influenza virus transcriptase activity. Ribavirin has multiple sites of action, and some of these (e.g., inhibition of GTP synthesis) may potentiate others (e.g., inhibition of GTP-dependent enzymes). Ribavirin also may enhance viral mutagenesis to an extent that some viruses may be inhibited from effective replication, so-called lethal mutagenesis. Emergence of viral resistance to ribavirin has been reported in Sindbis and HCV.

ADME. Ribavirin is actively taken up by nucleoside transporters in the proximal small bowel; oral bioavailability averages ~50%. Food increases plasma levels substantially. With aerosol administration, levels in respiratory secretions are very high but variable. The elimination of ribavirin is complex. The plasma $t_{1/2}$ increases to ~200-300 h at steady state. Erythrocytes concentrate ribavirin triphosphate; the drug exits red cells gradually, with a $t_{1/2}$ of ~40 days. Hepatic metabolism and renal excretion of ribavirin and its metabolites are the principal routes of elimination. Hepatic metabolism involves deribosylation and hydrolysis to yield a triazole carboxamide. Ribavirin should be used cautiously in patients with creatinine clearances of <50 mL/min.

UNTOWARD EFFECTS. Aerosolized ribavirin may cause conjunctival irritation, rash, transient wheezing, and occasional reversible deterioration in pulmonary function. When used in conjunction with mechanical ventilation, equipment modifications and frequent monitoring are required to prevent plugging of ventilator valves and tubing with ribavirin. Techniques to reduce environmental exposure of healthcare workers are recommended. Pregnant women should not directly care for patients receiving ribavirin aerosol (FDA pregnancy Category X).

Systemic ribavirin causes dose-related reversible anemia owing to extravascular hemolysis and suppression of bone marrow. Associated increases occur in reticulocyte counts and in serum bilirubin, iron, and uric acid concentrations. Bolus intravenous infusion may cause rigors. About 20% of chronic HCV infection patients receiving combination IFN-ribavirin therapy discontinue treatment early because of side effects. In addition to IFN toxicities, oral ribavirin increases the risk of fatigue, cough, rash, pruritus, nausea, insomnia, dyspnea, depression, and particularly, anemia. Preclinical studies indicate that ribavirin is teratogenic, embryotoxic, oncogenic, and possibly gonadotoxic. To prevent possible teratogenic effects, up to 6 months is required for washout following cessation of long-term treatment. Ribavirin inhibits the phosphorylation and antiviral activity of pyrimidine nucleoside HIV reverse-transcriptase inhibitors such as zidovudine and stavudine but increases the activity of purine nucleoside reverse-transcriptase inhibitors (e.g., didanosine) in vitro. It appears to increase the risk of mitochondrial toxicity from didanosine (*see* Chapter 59).

BOCEPREVIR. Boceprevir (VICTRELIS) inhibits hepatitis C virus non-structural protein 3 (NS3) serine protease.

Boceprevir is indicated for the treatment of chronic hepatitis gentotype 1 infection in adults >18 years old with compensated liver disease, including cirrhosis, who are previously untreated or who have failed previous interferon and ribavirin therapy. Boceprevir is administered in combination with peginterferon alfa and ribavirin. The recommended dose is 800 mg (four 200-mg capsules) three times daily (every 7-9 hours) with food. The $t_{1/2}$ is ~3.4 h. The drug is metabolized mostly by aldoketoreductase and partly by CYP3A4/5, which the drug strongly inhibits. Side effects of combination treatment include fatigue, anemia, nausea, headache, and dysgeusia. Boceprevir is contraindicated in pregnancy.

DRUGS FOR HEPATITIS B VIRUS INFECTION

Unlike HCV, HBV is transcribed into DNA that can be integrated into host chromosomal DNA and is capable of establishing lifelong chronic infection in ~10% of patients. Those with chronic HBV may develop active hepatitis that can lead to fibrosis and cirrhosis, and all such individuals have a greatly increased incidence of hepatocellular carcinoma.

Interferon, or a combination of interferon and ribavirin, can cure patients with chronic infection but is associated with a high rate of side effects, often leading to premature treatment discontinuation. Several antiretroviral nucleoside or nucleotide analog polymerase inhibitors, including lamivudine, telbivudine, and tenofovir, have potent anti-HBV activity and have provided a popular alternative therapy: chronic suppressive oral single agent or combination treatment. These regimens are much better tolerated than IFN-containing regimens but are not usually curative.

ADEFOVIR. Adefovir dipivoxil is a prodrug of adefovir, an acyclic phosphonate nucleotide analog of adenosine monophosphate.

THERAPEUTIC USES. Adefovir dipivoxil is approved for treatment of chronic HBV infections. In patients with HBV e-antigen (HbeAg)–positive chronic hepatitis B, adefovir dipivoxil (10 mg/day) reduces serum HBV DNA levels by 99% and, in about one-half of patients, improves hepatic histology and normalization of aminotransferase levels by 48 weeks. In patients with HbeAg-negative chronic HBV, adefovir is associated with similar biochemical and histological benefits. Regression of cirrhosis may occur in some patients. In patients with lamivudine-resistant HBV infections, adefovir dipivoxil monotherapy results in sustained reductions in serum HBV DNA levels. In patients with dual HIV and lamivudine-resistant HBV infections, adefovir dipivoxil (10 mg/day) causes significant HBV DNA level reductions.

MECHANISMS OF ACTION AND RESISTANCE. Adefovir dipivoxil enters cells and is de-esterified to adefovir, which cellular enzymes convert to the diphosphate, a competitive inhibitor of dATP at viral DNA polymerases and reverse transcriptases and also serves as a chain terminator of viral DNA synthesis. Its selectivity relates to a higher affinity for HBV DNA polymerase compared with cellular polymerases. Adefovir resistance has been detected in ~4% of chronically infected HBV patients during 3 years of treatment. Such variants have unique point mutations in the HBV polymerase but retain susceptibility to lamivudine.

ADME. The dipivoxil prodrug is absorbed rapidly and hydrolyzed in the intestine and blood to adefovir with liberation of pivalic acid, providing a bioavailability ~30-60%. Food does not affect bioavailability. Adefovir is eliminated unchanged by renal excretion. After oral administration of adefovir dipivoxil, ~30-45% of the dose is recovered within 24 h; the $t_{1/2}$ of elimination is 5-7.5 h. Dose reductions are recommended for Cl_{Cr} values <50 mL/min. Adefovir is removed by hemodialysis.

UNTOWARD EFFECTS. Adefovir dipivoxil causes dose-related nephrotoxicity and tubular dysfunction, manifested by azotemia and hypophosphatemia, acidosis, glycosuria, and proteinuria that usually are reversible months after discontinuation. The dose (10 mg/day) used in chronic HBV infection patients has been associated with fewer adverse events (e.g., headache, abdominal discomfort, diarrhea, and asthenia) and negligible renal toxicity than higher doses. Acute, sometimes severe exacerbations of hepatitis can occur in patients stopping adefovir or other anti-HBV therapies.

Adefovir is genotoxic, and high doses cause hepatotoxicity, lymphoid toxicity, and renal tubular nephropathy in animals. Adefovir dipivoxil is not associated with reproductive toxicity, although high intravenous doses of adefovir cause maternal and embryotoxicity with fetal malformations in rats (pregnancy Category C). Drugs that reduce renal function could decrease adefovir clearance. Ibuprofen increases adefovir exposure modestly. An increased risk of lactic acidosis and steatosis may exist when adefovir is used in conjunction with nucleoside analogs or other antiretroviral agents. Adefovir is transported efficiently into tubular epithelium by a probenecid-sensitive organic anion transporter (hOAT1).

ENTECAVIR.

Entecavir is a guanosine nucleoside analog with selective activity against HBV polymerase.

THERAPEUTIC USES. Entecavir is indicated for the treatment of chronic HBV infection in adults with active viral replication and either evidence of persistent elevations in serum aminotransferases or histologically active disease. The recommended dose for nucleoside-treatment-naive adults is 0.5 mg once daily. For patients with lamivudine or telbivudine resistance, the dose is 1 mg once daily. Entecavir is superior to lamivudine in the degree of suppression and associated with a more frequent fall of HBV DNA to undetectable levels. Entecavir had negligible resistance (≤1%) for up to 4 years and is active against adefovir-resistant HBV.

MECHANISMS OF ACTION AND RESISTANCE. Entecavir requires intracellular phosphorylation. Entecavir triphosphate competes with endogenous deoxyguanosine triphosphate and inhibits all 3 activities of the HBV polymerase (reverse transcriptase): base priming, reverse transcription of the negative strand from the pregenomic messenger RNA, and synthesis of the positive strand of HBV DNA. Entecavir triphosphate is a weak inhibitor of cellular DNA polymerases α, β, and δ and mitochondrial DNA polymerase γ. HIV reverse transcriptase variants containing the M184V substitution show loss of susceptibility to entecavir. Lamivudine and telbivudine resistance confers decreased susceptibility to entecavir.

ADME. Steady-state is reached after 6-10 days of once daily dosing. Administration with food decreases C_{max} by 44-46% and AUC by 18-20%; thus entecavir should be administered on an empty stomach. It is primarily eliminated unchanged in the kidney. Renal clearance is independent of dose, suggesting that entecavir undergoes both glomerular filtration and net tubular secretion. Entecavir exhibits biphasic elimination, with a terminal $t_{1/2}$ of 128-149 h; the active triphosphate has an elimination $t_{1/2}$ of 15 h. Dose reductions are needed for patients with Cl_{Cr} <50 mL/min, typically by extension of the dosing interval.

UNTOWARD EFFECTS. Severe acute exacerbations of hepatitis B have been reported in patients who have discontinued anti-HBV therapy, including entecavir. Hepatic function should be monitored closely with both clinical and laboratory follow-up for several months in patients who discontinue anti-HBV therapy. There is a potential for development of resistance to nucleoside reverse transcriptase inhibitors in HBV/HIV coinfection, especially if HIV is not being treated. Other common adverse reactions include headache, fatigue, dizziness, and nausea.

LAMIVUDINE. Lamivudine is a nucleoside analog that inhibits HIV reverse transcriptase and HBV DNA polymerase. It inhibits HBV replication with negligible cellular cytotoxicity. Its use as an antiretroviral agent is discussed in Chapter 59.

THERAPEUTIC USES. Lamivudine is approved for the treatment of chronic HBV hepatitis in adults and children. In adults, doses of 100 mg/day for 1 year cause suppression of HBV DNA levels, normalization of aminotransferase levels and reductions in hepatic inflammation in 40-50% of patients. Seroconversion with antibody to HbeAg occurs in <20% of recipients at 1 year. Prolonged therapy is associated with sustained suppression of HBV DNA and continued histological improvement. Prolonged therapy halves the risk of clinical progression and development of hepatocellular carcinoma in those with advanced fibrosis or cirrhosis. The frequency of lamivudine-resistant variants increases progressively with continued drug administration, reaching 67% after 4 years of treatment. The risk of resistance development is higher after transplantation and in HIV/HBV coinfected patients.

Combined use of IFN or pegIFN alfa-2A with lamivudine has not improved responses in HBeAg-positive patients consistently. In HIV and HBV coinfections, higher lamivudine doses are associated with antiviral effects and uncommonly anti-HBe seroconversion. Administration of lamivudine before and after liver transplantation may suppress recurrent HBV infection.

MECHANISMS OF ACTION AND RESISTANCE. Cellular enzymes convert lamivudine to the triphosphate. Lamivudine triphosphate is a potent competitive inhibitor of the DNA polymerase/reverse transcriptase of HBV and causes chain termination. Lamivudine shows enhanced antiviral activity in combination with adefovir or penciclovir against hepadnaviruses. Point mutations in the *YMDD* motif of HBV DNA polymerase markedly reduce susceptibility. Lamivudine resistance confers cross-resistance to related agents such as emtricitabine, and is often associated with an additional non-*YMDD* mutation that confers cross-resistance to famciclovir. Lamivudine-resistant HBV retains susceptibility to adefovir, tenofovir, and partially to entecavir. Viruses bearing *YMDD* mutations are less replication competent than wild-type HBV. However, lamivudine resistance is associated with elevated HBV DNA levels, decreased likelihood of HbeAg loss or seroconversion, hepatitis exacerbations, and progressive fibrosis and graft loss in transplant recipients.

ADME. The pharmacokinetic properties of lamivudine are described in Chapter 59. The intracellular $t_{1/2}$ of the triphosphate averages 17-19 h in HBV-infected cells, so once-daily dosing is possible. Dose reductions are indicated for moderate renal insufficiency. Trimethoprim decreases the renal clearance of lamivudine.

UNTOWARD EFFECTS. At the doses used for chronic HBV infection, lamivudine generally has been well tolerated. Post-treatment aminotransferase elevations occur in ~15% of patients after cessation.

TELBIVUDINE. Telbivudine is a synthetic thymidine nucleoside analog with activity against HBV DNA polymerase.

THERAPEUTIC USES. Telbivudine is indicated for the treatment of chronic HBV in adult patients with evidence of viral replication and either evidence of persistent elevations in serum aminotransferases (ALT or AST) or histologically active disease. The recommended dose is 600 mg orally once daily without regard to food. An oral solution is also available. Telbivudine resistance is 25% after 2 years of treatment and higher than observed with other oral anti-HBV agents. Cross-resistance and treatment-emergent resistance limit the use of telbivudine for patients with chronic HBV, compared to alternative agents.

MECHANISMS OF ACTION AND RESISTANCE. Telbivudine is phosphorylated by cellular kinases to the active triphosphate form, which has a $t_{1/2}$ of 14 h. Telbivudine 5′-triphosphate inhibits HBV DNA polymerase/reverse transcriptase by competing with the natural substrate, TTP. Incorporation of telbivudine 5′-triphosphate into viral DNA causes chain termination.

Lamivudine-resistant HBV strains expressing either the M204I substitution or the L180M/M204V double substitution have ≥1000-fold reduced susceptibility. HBV encoding the adefovir mutation A181V showed 3- to 5-fold reduced susceptibility. The A181T substitution is associated with decreased clinical response in patients with HBV treated with adefovir and entecavir.

ADME. At 600 mg once daily, steady state is achieved after ~5-7 days with ~1.5-fold accumulation. Telbivudine concentrations decline biexponentially with an elimination $t_{1/2}$ of 40-49 h. The drug is eliminated unchanged in the urine. Patients with moderate-to-severe renal dysfunction require dose adjustments.

UNTOWARD EFFECTS. Telbivudine is generally well tolerated and safe. The most common adverse events resulting in telbivudine discontinuation included increased creatine kinase, nausea, diarrhea, fatigue, myalgia, and myopathy.

TENOFOVIR. Tenofovir is a nucleotide analog with activity against both HIV-1 and HBV. It is administered orally as the disoproxil prodrug. For more detail, *see* Chapter 59.

THERAPEUTIC USES. Tenofovir is approved for treatment of HBV infection in adults at a dose of 300 mg once daily without regard to food. In HBeAg-negative patients, tenofovir suppresses HBV DNA to <400 copies/mL in 93% of subjects at 48 weeks, compared to 63% for adefovir. Tenofovir resistance is not evident over 48 weeks of treatment. Due to its safety, efficacy, and resistance profile, tenofovir will likely supersede adefovir for the treatment of chronic HBV infection. Overall, tenofovir has a favorable resistance profile and has been effective in treating lamivudine-resistant HBV. The tenofovir dose should be adjusted for impaired renal function and during hemodialysis.

CLEVUDINE

Clevudine is a nucleoside analog with potent activity against HBV. The oral drug is approved for use in South Korea and the Philippines. However, the drug caused myopathy in large phase 3 clinical trials, casting doubt on its future approval in the U.S.

OTHER AGENTS

IMIQUIMOD. *Imiquimod* is a novel immunomodulatory agent that is effective for topical treatment of condylomata acuminata, molluscum contagiosum, and certain other dermatologic conditions associated with DNA virus infections. It lacks direct antiviral or antiproliferative effects in vitro; rather, imiquimod induces cytokines and chemokines with antiviral and immunomodulating effects.

When applied topically as a 5% cream to genital warts in humans, imiquimod induces local IFN-α, IFN-β, and IFN-γ and TNFα responses and causes reductions in viral load and wart size. When applied topically (3 times weekly for up to 16 weeks), imiquimod cream results in complete clearance of treated genital and perianal warts in ~50% of patients in 8-10 weeks, with response rates higher in women than in men. Application is associated with local erythema, excoriation/flaking, itching, burning, and less often, erosions or ulcerations.

For a complete Bibliographical Listing see Goodman & Gilman's ***The Pharmacological Basis of Therapeutics***, 12th ed., or Goodman & Gilman Online at www.AccessMedicine.com.

Antiretroviral Agents and Treatment of HIV Infection

The pharmacotherapy of HIV infection is a rapidly moving field. Three-drug combinations are the minimum standard of care for this infection, so current agents constitute several thousand possible regimens. Knowing the essential features of the pathophysiology of this disease and how chemotherapeutic agents affect the virus and the host is critical in developing a rational approach to therapy. *Unique features of this drug class include the need for lifelong administration to control virus replication and the possibility of rapid emergence of permanent drug resistance if these agents are not used properly.*

PATHOGENESIS OF HIV-RELATED DISEASE

Human immunodeficiency viruses (HIVs) are lentiviruses, a family of retroviruses evolved to establish chronic persistent infection with gradual onset of clinical symptoms. Replication is constant following infection, and although some infected cells may harbor nonreplicating virus for years, in the absence of treatment there generally is no true period of viral latency following infection. Humans and nonhuman primates are the only natural hosts for these viruses.

There are 2 major families of HIV. Most of the epidemic involves HIV-1; HIV-2 is more closely related to simian immunodeficiency virus (SIV) and is concentrated in western Africa. HIV-1 is genetically diverse, with at least 5 distinct subfamilies or clades. HIV-1 and HIV-2 have similar sensitivity to most antiretroviral drugs, although the non-nucleoside reverse transcriptase inhibitors (NNRTIs) are HIV-1-specific and have no activity against HIV-2.

VIRUS STRUCTURE. HIV is a typical retrovirus with a small RNA genome of 9300 base pairs. Two copies of the genome are contained in a nucleocapsid core surrounded by a lipid bilayer, or envelope, that is derived from the host cell plasma membrane (Figure 59–1). The viral genome encodes 3 major open reading frames: *gag* encodes a polyprotein that is processed to release the major structural proteins of the virus; *pol* overlaps *gag* and encodes 3 important enzyme activities—an RNA-dependent DNA polymerase or reverse transcriptase with RNAase activity, protease, and the viral integrase; and *env* encodes the large transmembrane envelope protein responsible for cell binding and entry. Several small genes encode regulatory proteins that enhance virion production or combat host defenses. These include *tat, rev, nef,* and *vpr*.

VIRUS LIFE CYCLE (*see* Figure 59–1). HIV tropism is controlled by the envelope protein gp160 (env). The major target for env binding is the CD4 receptor present on lymphocytes and macrophages, although cell entry also requires binding to a coreceptor, generally the chemokine receptor CCR5 or CXCR4. CCR5 is present on macrophage lineage cells. Most infected individuals harbor predominantly the CCR5-tropic virus; HIV with this tropism is responsible for nearly all naturally acquired infections. A shift from CCR5 to CXCR4 utilization is associated with advancing disease, and the increased affinity of HIV-1 for CXCR4 allows infection of T-lymphocyte lines. A phenotypic switch from CCR5 to CXCR4 heralds accelerated loss of CD4+ helper T cells and increased risk of immunosuppression. Whether coreceptor switch is a cause or a consequence of advancing disease is still unknown, but it is possible to develop clinical AIDS without this switch.

The gp41 domain of env controls the fusion of the virus lipid bilayer with that of the host cell. Following fusion, full-length viral RNA enters the cytoplasm, where it undergoes replication to a short-lived RNADNA duplex; the original RNA is degraded by RNase H to allow creation of a full-length double-stranded DNA copy of the virus. Because the HIV reverse transcriptase is error prone and lacks a proofreading function, mutation is quite frequent and occurs at ~3 bases out of every full-length (9300-base-pair) replication. Virus DNA is transported into the nucleus, where it is integrated into a host chromosome by the viral integrase in a random or quasi-random location.

Following integration, the virus may remain quiescent, not producing RNA or protein but replicating as the cell divides. When a cell that harbors the virus is activated, viral RNA and proteins are produced. Structural

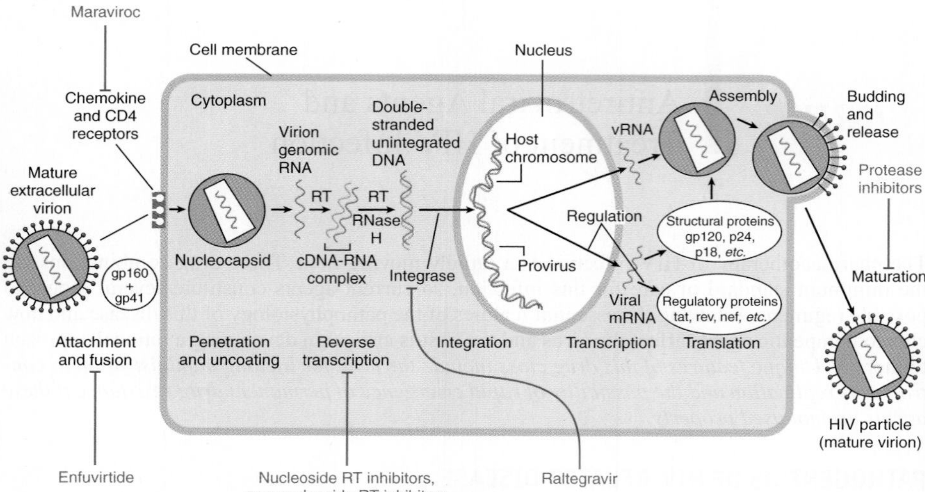

Figure 59–1 *Replicative cycle of HIV-1 and sites of action of available antiretroviral agents.* Available antiretroviral agents are shown in *blue*. cDNA, complementary DNA; gp120 + gp41, extracellular and intracellular domains, respectively, of envelope glycoprotein; mRNA, messenger RNA; RNase H, ribonuclease H; RT, reverse transcriptase. (Adapted from Hirsch MS, D'Aquila RT. Therapy for human immunodeficiency virus infection. *N Engl J Med*, 1993; 328:1686–1695.)

proteins assemble around full-length genomic RNA to form a nucleocapsid. The envelope and structural proteins assemble at the cell surface, concentrating in cholesterol-rich lipid rafts. The nucleocapsid cores are directed to these sites and bud through the cell membrane, creating new enveloped HIV particles containing 2 complete single-stranded RNA genomes. Reverse transcriptase is incorporated into virus particles so replication can begin immediately after the virus enters a new cell.

HOW THE VIRUS CAUSES DISEASE. Sexual acquisition of HIV infection is likely mediated by one or, at most, a handful of infectious virus particles. Soon after infection, there is a rapid burst of replication peaking at 2-4 weeks, with $\geq 10^9$ cells becoming infected. This peak is associated with a transient dip in the number of peripheral CD4+ (helper) T lymphocytes. As a result of new host immune responses and target cell depletion, the number of infectious virions as reflected by the plasma HIV RNA concentration (also known as *viral load*) declines to a quasi-steady state. This *set point* reflects the interplay between host immunity and the pathogenicity of the infecting virus. In the average infected individual, several billion infectious virus particles are produced every few days.

Eventually, the host CD4+ T lymphocyte count begins a steady decline, accompanied by a rise in the plasma HIV RNA concentration. Once the peripheral CD4 cell count falls below 200 cells/mm^3, there is an increasing risk of opportunistic diseases and ultimately death. Sexual acquisition of CCR5-tropic HIV-1 is associated with a median time to clinical AIDS of 8-10 years. Some patients, termed *long-term nonprogressors*, can harbor HIV for more than 2 decades without significant decline in peripheral CD4 cell count or clinical immunosuppression; this may reflect a combination of favorable host immunogenetics and immune responses.

An important question relevant to treatment is whether HIV disease is a consequence of CD4+ lymphocyte depletion alone. Most natural history data suggest that this is true. Regardless, successful therapy is based on inhibition of HIV replication; interventions designed specifically to boost the host immune response without exerting a direct antiviral effect have had no reliable clinical benefit.

PRINCIPLES OF HIV CHEMOTHERAPY

Current treatment assumes that all aspects of disease derive from the direct toxic effects of HIV on host cells, mainly CD4+ T lymphocytes. The goal of therapy is to suppress virus replication as much as possible for as long as possible. The current standard of care is to use at least 3 drugs simultaneously for the entire duration of treatment.

Current guidelines in the U.S. recommend starting therapy in all those with a CD4 count of ≤350 cells/mm^3. Treatment is also recommended for HIV-infected pregnant women, those with HIV nephropathy, and those with concurrent hepatitis B virus infection requiring treatment regardless of CD4 count. Increasing evidence supports the value of antiretroviral therapy in preventing transmission of the virus from person to person. In the foreseeable future, treatment may be recommended for all infected adults and children.

Drug resistance is a key problem. There is a high likelihood that all untreated infected individuals harbor viruses with single-amino-acid mutations conferring some degree of resistance to every known antiretroviral drug because of the high mutation rate of HIV and the tremendous number of infectious virions. Thus, a combination of active agents is required to prevent drug resistance, analogous to strategies employed in the treatment of tuberculosis (*see* Chapter 56). Intentional drug holidays, also known as *structured treatment interruptions*, allow the virus to replicate anew, increase the risk of drug resistance and disease progression, and are not recommended.

The expected outcome of initial therapy in a previously untreated patient is an undetectable *viral load* (plasma HIV RNA <50 copies/mL) within 24 weeks of starting treatment. Mathematical models of HIV replication suggested that 3 is the minimum number of agents required to guarantee effective long-term suppression of HIV replication without resistance. In treatment-naive patients, a regimen containing a non-nucleoside plus 2 nucleoside reverse transcriptase inhibitors is as effective as a regimen containing an additional nucleoside, indicating the equivalence of these 3-drug and 4-drug regimens. Four or more drugs may be used simultaneously in pretreated patients harboring drug-resistant virus, but the number of agents a patient can take is limited by toxicity and inconvenience.

Failure of an antiretroviral regimen is defined as a persistent increase in plasma HIV RNA concentrations in a patient with previously undetectable virus, despite continued treatment with that regimen. This indicates resistance to 1 or more drugs in the regimen and necessitates a change in treatment. The selection of new agents is therefore informed by the patient's treatment history and viral resistance testing. Treatment failure generally requires implementation of a completely new combination of drugs. Adding a single active agent to a failing regimen is functional monotherapy if the patient is resistant to all drugs in the regimen. The risk of failing a regimen depends on the percentage of prescribed doses taken during any given period of treatment.

As antiretroviral therapy becomes more effective and easier to take, long-term toxicity of these drugs is of greater concern. An important consequence of long-term therapy is the development of a metabolic syndrome (*HIV lipodystrophy syndrome*) characterized by insulin resistance, fat redistribution, and hyperlipidemia, that occurs in 10-40% of treated patients. Clinical features include peripheral fat wasting (lipoatrophy), central fat accumulation including enlarged breasts and buffalo hump, insulin resistance and hyperglycemia, and elevations in serum cholesterol and triglycerides. Lipodystrophy has been associated with an increased risk of myocardial infarction in virologically controlled patients. A potential concern that applies to all protease inhibitors and NNRTIs is clinically significant pharmacokinetic drug interactions. All agents in these 2 drug classes can act as inhibitors and/or inducers of hepatic CYPs and other drug metabolizing enzymes, as well as drug transport proteins.

An increasingly recognized complication of initiating antiretroviral therapy is accelerated inflammatory reaction to overt or subclinical opportunistic infections or malignancies. This *immune reconstitution inflammatory syndrome* (*IRIS*) is most commonly seen when initiating therapy in individuals with low CD4 counts and/or advanced HIV disease. Infections commonly associated with IRIS include tuberculosis and other mycobacterial diseases, cryptococcosis, hepatitis virus infections, and Pneumocystis pneumonia.

Drugs Used to Treat HIV Infection

NUCLEOSIDE AND NUCLEOTIDE REVERSE TRANSCRIPTASE INHIBITORS

The HIV-encoded, RNA-dependent DNA polymerase, also called *reverse transcriptase*, converts viral RNA into proviral DNA that is then incorporated into a host cell chromosome. Available inhibitors of this enzyme are either nucleoside/nucleotide analogs or non-nucleoside inhibitors (Table 59–1). Nucleoside/nucleotide reverse transcriptase inhibitors (NRTIs) prevent infection of susceptible cells but do not eradicate the virus from cells that already harbor integrated proviral DNA. Nearly all patients starting antiretroviral treatment do so with at least 1 agent from this class. Figure 59–2 shows the mechanism of action of NRTIs, which involves phosphorylation by host cells to the active inhibitory form.

All but 1 of the drugs in this class are nucleosides that must be triphosphorylated at the 5′-hydroxyl to exert activity. The sole exception, tenofovir, is a nucleotide monophosphate analog that requires 2 additional phosphates to acquire full activity. These compounds inhibit both HIV-1 and HIV-2, and several have

Table 59–1

Antiretroviral Agents Approved for Use in the U.S.

GENERIC NAME	ABBREVIATION; CHEMICAL NAMES
Nucleoside Reverse Transcriptase Inhibitors	
Zidovudine[a]	ZDV; azidothymidine (AZT)
Didanosine	ddI; dideoxyinosine
Stavudine	d4T; didehydrodeoxythymidine
Zalcitabine[c]	DDC; dideoxycytidine
Lamivudine[a]	3TC; dideoxythiacytidine
Abacavir[a]	ABC; cyclopropylami nopurinylcyclopentene
Tenofovir disoproxil[a]	TDF; phosphinyl methoxypropyladenine (PMPA)
Emtricitabine[a]	FTC; fluorooxathiolanyl cytosine
Non-nucleoside Reverse Transcriptase Inhibitors	
Nevirapine	NVP
Efavirenz[a]	EFV
Delavirdine	DLV
Etravirine	ETV
Protease Inhibitors	
Saquinavir	SQV
Indinavir	IDV
Ritonavir	RTV
Nelfinavir	NFV
Amprenavir[c]	APV
Lopinavir[b]	LPV/r
Atazanavir	ATV
Fosamprenavir	FPV
Tipranavir	TPV
Darunavir	DRV
Entry Inhibitors	
Enfuvirtide	T-20
Maraviroc	MVC
Integrase Inhibitor	
Raltegravir	RAL

[a]*A number of fixed-dose co-formulations are available: zidovudine + lamivudine (COMBIVIR); zidovidine + lamivudine + abacavir (TRIZIVIR); abacavir + lamivudine (EPZICOM); tenofovir + emtricitabine (TRUVADA); tenofivir + efavirenz + emtricitabine (ATRIPLA).*
[b]*Lopinavir is available only as part of a fixed-dose co-formulation with ritonavir (KALETRA/ALUVIA).*
[c]*No longer marketed worldwide.*

broad-spectrum activity against other human and animal retroviruses; emtricitabine, lamivudine, and tenofovir are active against hepatitis B virus (HBV), and tenofovir also has activity against herpesviruses (*see* Chapter 58).

The selective toxicity of these drugs depends on their ability to inhibit the HIV reverse transcriptase without inhibiting host cell DNA polymerases. Although the intracellular triphosphates for all these drugs have low affinity for human DNA polymerase-α and polymerase-β, some do inhibit human DNA polymerase-γ, which is the mitochondrial enzyme. As a result, the important toxicities common to this class of drugs result in part from the inhibition of mitochondrial DNA synthesis. These toxicities include anemia, granulocytopenia,

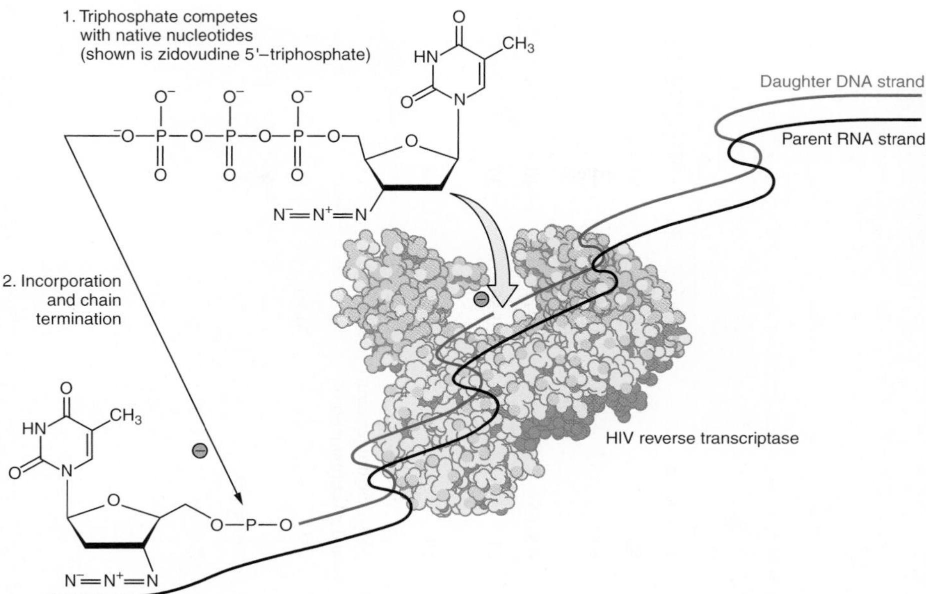

Figure 59–2 *Mechanism of nucleoside/nucleotide reverse transcriptase inhibitors (NRTIs).* Zidovudine is depicted; Table 59–1 lists other agents in the NRTI class. Nucleoside and nucleotide analogs must enter cells and be phosphorylated to generate synthetic substrates for reverse transcriptase. The fully phosphorylated analogs block replication of the viral genome both by competitively inhibiting incorporation of native nucleotides and by terminating elongation of nascent proviral DNA because they lack a 3′-hydroxyl group.

myopathy, peripheral neuropathy, and pancreatitis. Lactic acidosis with or without hepatomegaly and hepatic steatosis is a rare but potentially fatal complication seen with stavudine, zidovudine, and didanosine. Phosphorylated emtricitabine, lamivudine, and tenofovir have low affinity for DNA polymerase-γ and are largely devoid of mitochondrial toxicity.

Table 59–2 summarizes the pharmacokinetic properties of NRTIs approved for treating HIV infection. A notable pharmacological feature of these agents is the elimination of the intracellular nucleoside di- or tri-phosphate, which is the active form. In general, the phosphorylated anabolites are eliminated from cells much more gradually than the parent drug is eliminated from the plasma. As a result, available NRTIs are dosed once or twice daily.

These drugs are not major substrates for hepatic CYPs. Pharmacokinetic drug interactions involving tenofovir and protease inhibitors are likely to be explained by inhibition of OATP drug transporters (*see* Chapter 5). High-level resistance to NRTIs, especially thymidine analogs, occurs slowly by comparison to non-NRTIs and first-generation protease inhibitors. High-level resistance can occur rapidly with lamivudine and emtricitabine. Cross-resistance is common but often confined to drugs having similar chemical structures. Several nucleoside analogs have favorable safety and tolerability profiles and are useful in suppressing the emergence of HIV isolates resistant to the more potent drugs in combination regimens.

ZIDOVUDINE. Zidovudine (AZT) is a synthetic thymidine analog (*see* structure in Figure 59–2) with potent activity against a broad spectrum of retroviruses including HIV-1, HIV-2, and human T-cell lymphotrophic viruses (HTLVs) I and II. Zidovudine is active in lymphoblastic and monocytic cell lines but has no impact on cells already infected with HIV. Zidovudine appears to be more active in activated than in resting lymphocytes because the phosphorylating enzyme, thymidine kinase, is S-phase-specific. Zidovudine is FDA-approved for the treatment of adults and children with HIV infection and for preventing mother-to-child transmission; it also is recommended for post-exposure prophylaxis in HIV-exposed healthcare workers. Zidovudine (RETROVIR) is marketed in oral tablets, capsules, and solution as well as a solution for intravenous injection. Zidovudine is available in coformulated tablets with lamivudine (COMBIVIR) or with lamivudine and abacavir (TRIZIVIR).

Table 59–2

Pharmacokinetic Properties of Nucleoside Reverse Transcriptase Inhibitors[a]

PARAMETER	ZIDOVUDINE	LAMIVUDINE	STAVUDINE[b]	DIDANOSINE[c]	ABACAVIR	TENOFOVIR	EMTRICITABINE
Oral bioavailability, %	64	86-87	86	42	83	25	93
Effect of meals on AUC	↓24% (high fat)	↔	↔	↓55% (acidity)	↔	↑40% (high fat)	↔
Plasma $t_{1/2}$, elim, h	1.0	5-7	1.1-1.4	1.5	0.8-1.5	14-17	10
Intracellular $t_{1/2}$, elim of triphosphate, h	3-4	12-18	3.5	25-40	21	10-50	39
Plasma protein binding, %	20-38	<35	<5	<5	50	<8	<4
Metabolism, %	60-80 (glucuronidation)	<36	ND	50 (purine metabolism)	>80 (dehydrogenation and glucuronidation)	ND	13
Renal excretion of parent drug, %	14	71	39	18-36	<5	70-80	86

AUC, area under plasma concentration time curve; $t_{1/2}$, elim, half-life of elimination; ↑, increase; ↓, decrease; ↔, no effect; ND, not determined.

[a]Reported mean values in adults with normal renal and hepatic function.

[b]Parameters reported for the stavudine capsule formulation.

[c]Parameters reported for the didanosine chewable tablet formulation.

MECHANISMS OF ACTION AND RESISTANCE. Intracellular zidovudine is phosphorylated to zidovudine 5′-triphosphate. Zidovudine 5′-triphosphate terminates the elongation of proviral DNA because it is incorporated by reverse transcriptase into nascent DNA but lacks a 3′-hydroxyl group. The monophosphate competitively inhibits cellular thymidylate kinase, and this may reduce the amount of intracellular thymidine triphosphate. Zidovudine 5′-triphosphate only weakly inhibits cellular DNA polymerase-α but is a more potent inhibitor of mitochondrial polymerase-γ. Because the conversion of zidovudine 5′-monophosphate to diphosphate is very inefficient, high concentrations of the monophosphate accumulate inside cells and may serve as a precursor depot for formation of triphosphate. As a consequence, there is little correlation between extracellular concentrations of parent drug and intracellular concentrations of triphosphate, and higher plasma concentrations of zidovudine do not increase intracellular triphosphate concentrations proportionately.

Resistance to zidovudine is associated with mutations at reverse transcriptase codons 41, 44, 67, 70, 210, 215, and 219. These mutations are referred to as *thymidine analog mutations* (TAMs) because of their ability to confer cross-resistance to other thymidine analogs such as stavudine. The M184V substitution in the reverse transcriptase gene associated with the use of lamivudine or emtricitabine greatly restores sensitivity to zidovudine. The combination of zidovudine and lamivudine produces greater long-term suppression of plasma HIV RNA than does zidovudine alone.

ADME. Zidovudine is absorbed rapidly and reaches peak plasma concentrations within 1 h. Table 59–2 summarizes the drug's pharmacokinetic profile, which is not altered significantly during pregnancy; drug concentrations in the newborn approach those of the mother. Parent drug crosses the blood-brain barrier relatively well and also is detectable in breast milk, semen, and fetal tissue.

UNTOWARD EFFECTS. Patients initiating zidovudine treatment often complain of fatigue, malaise, myalgia, nausea, anorexia, headache, and insomnia; these symptoms usually resolve within a few weeks. Erythrocytic macrocytosis is seen in ~90% of patients but usually is not associated with anemia. Chronic zidovudine administration has been associated with nail hyperpigmentation. Skeletal muscle myopathy can occur and is associated with depletion of mitochondrial DNA, most likely as a consequence of inhibition of DNA polymerase-γ. Serious hepatic toxicity, with or without steatosis and lactic acidosis, is rare but can be fatal.

PRECAUTIONS AND INTERACTIONS. Zidovudine is not a substrate or inhibitor of CYPs. However, probenecid, fluconazole, atovaquone, and valproic acid may increase plasma concentrations of zidovudine, probably through inhibition of glucuronosyl transferases. Zidovudine can cause bone marrow suppression and should be used cautiously in patients with preexisting anemia or granulocytopenia and in those taking other marrow-suppressive drugs. Stavudine and zidovudine compete for intracellular phosphorylation and should not be used concomitantly.

STAVUDINE. Stavudine (d4T) is a synthetic thymidine analog that is active in vitro against HIV-1 and HIV-2. Stavudine (ZERIT) is approved for use in HIV-infected adults and children, including neonates.

MECHANISMS OF ACTION AND RESISTANCE. Intracellular stavudine is sequentially phosphorylated stavudine 5′-triphosphate. Like zidovudine, stavudine is most potent in activated cells, probably because thymidine kinase, which produces the monophosphate, is an S-phase-specific enzyme. Stavudine resistance is seen most frequently with mutations at reverse transcriptase codons 41, 44, 67, 70, 210, 215, and 219, which are mutations associated with zidovudine resistance. Resistance mutations for stavudine appear to accumulate slowly. Cross-resistance to multiple nucleoside analogs has been reported following prolonged therapy.

ADME. Table 59–2 summarizes the agent's PK data. Stavudine is well absorbed and reaches peak plasma concentrations within 1 h; bioavailability is not affected by food. The drug penetrates well into the CSF, achieving concentrations that are ~40% of those in plasma. Placental concentrations of stavudine are about half those of zidovudine. The drug undergoes active tubular secretion, and renal elimination accounts for ~40% of parent drug; thus, dose should be adjusted in patients with renal insufficiency.

UNTOWARD EFFECTS. The most common serious toxicity of stavudine is peripheral neuropathy. Although this may reflect mitochondrial toxicity, stavudine is a less potent inhibitor of DNA polymerase-γ than either didanosine or zalcitabine, suggesting that other mechanisms may be involved. Stavudine is also associated with a progressive motor neuropathy characterized by weakness and in some cases respiratory failure, similar to Guillain-Barré syndrome.

Lactic acidosis and hepatic steatosis are associated with stavudine use, and may be more common when stavudine and didanosine are combined. Acute pancreatitis is not highly associated with stavudine but is more common when stavudine is combined with didanosine than when didanosine is given alone. Of all nucleoside analogs, stavudine use is associated most strongly with fat wasting (*lipoatrophy*). Stavudine has fallen out of favor in the developed world largely because of this toxicity.

PRECAUTIONS AND INTERACTIONS. Stavudine is mainly renally cleared and is not subject to metabolic drug interactions. The incidence and severity of peripheral neuropathy may be increased when stavudine is combined with other neuropathic medications; thus, drugs such as ethambutol, isoniazid, phenytoin, and vincristine should be avoided. Combining stavudine with didanosine leads to increased risk and severity of peripheral neuropathy and potentially fatal pancreatitis; therefore, *these 2 drugs should not be used together*. Stavudine and zidovudine compete for intracellular phosphorylation and should not be used concomitantly.

LAMIVUDINE. Lamivudine is a cytidine analog reverse transcriptase inhibitor that is active against HIV-1, HIV-2, and HBV. Lamivudine (EPIVIR) is approved for HIV in adults and children ≥3 months of age. Lamivudine has been effective in combination with other antiretroviral drugs in both treatment-naive and experienced patients and is a common component of therapy, given its safety, convenience, and efficacy. Lamivudine (EPIVIR-HBV) is approved for treatment of chronic hepatitis B.

MECHANISMS OF ACTION AND RESISTANCE. Lamivudine enters cells by passive diffusion and is sequentially phosphorylated to lamivudine 5′-triphosphate, which is the active anabolite. Lamivudine has low affinity for human DNA polymerases, explaining its low toxicity to the host. High-level resistance to lamivudine occurs with single-amino-acid substitutions, M184V or M184I. These mutations can reduce in vitro sensitivity to lamivudine as much as 1000-fold. The M184V mutation restores zidovudine susceptibility in zidovudine-resistant HIV and also partially restores tenofovir susceptibility in tenofovir-resistant HIV harboring the K65R mutation. This effect may contribute to the sustained virologic benefits of zidovudine and lamivudine combination therapy.

ADME. Table 59–2 summarizes the PK parameters for this drug. Lamivudine is excreted primarily unchanged in the urine; dose adjustment is recommended for patients with a creatinine clearance <50 mL/min. Lamivudine freely crosses the placenta into the fetal circulation.

UNTOWARD EFFECTS. Lamivudine is one of the least toxic antiretroviral drugs. Neutropenia, headache, and nausea have been reported at higher than recommended doses. Pancreatitis has been reported in pediatric patients.

PRECAUTIONS AND INTERACTIONS. Because lamivudine also has activity against HBV, caution is warranted in using this drug in patients coinfected with HBV or in HBV-endemic areas: discontinuation of lamivudine may be associated with a rebound of HBV replication and exacerbation of hepatitis.

ABACAVIR. Abacavir (ZIAGEN), a synthetic purine analog, is approved for the treatment of HIV-1 infection, in combination with other antiretroviral agents. Abacavir is available in a co-formulation with zidovudine and lamivudine (TRIZIVIR) for twice-daily dosing and in a co-formulation with lamivudine (EPZICOM) for once-daily dosing. Abacavir is approved for use in adult and pediatric patients ≥3 months of age, with dosing in the latter based on body weight.

MECHANISMS OF ACTION AND RESISTANCE. Abacavir is the only approved antiretroviral that is active as a guanosine analog. It is sequentially phosphorylated in the host cell to carbovir 5′-triphosphate, which terminates the elongation of proviral DNA because it is incorporated by reverse transcriptase into nascent DNA but lacks a 3′-hydroxyl group. Clinical resistance to abacavir is associated with 4 specific substitutions: K65R, L74V, Y115F, and M184V. In combination, these substitutions can reduce susceptibility by up to 10-fold. K65R confers cross-resistance to all nucleosides except zidovudine. An alternate pathway for abacavir resistance involves mutations at codons 41, 210, and 215.

ADME. Table 59–2 summarizes the PK parameters for this agent. The presence of food does not affect the oral bioavailability of abacavir. Abacavir is neither a substrate nor an inhibitor of CYPs. Its CSF/plasma AUC ratio is ~0.3.

UNTOWARD EFFECTS. The most important adverse effect of abacavir is a unique and potentially fatal hypersensitivity syndrome characterized by fever, abdominal pain, and other GI complaints; a mild maculopapular rash; and malaise or fatigue. Respiratory complaints (cough, pharyngitis, dyspnea), musculoskeletal complaints, headache, and paresthesias are less common. The presence of concurrent fever, abdominal pain, and rash within 6 weeks of starting abacavir is diagnostic and necessitates immediate discontinuation of the drug. *Abacavir must never be restarted once discontinued for hypersensitivity*. The hypersensitivity syndrome (in 2-9% of patients) results from a genetically mediated immune response linked to both the *HLA-B*5701* locus and the M493T allele in the heat-shock locus *Hsp70-Hom*. The latter gene is implicated in antigen presentation, and this haplotype is associated with aberrant tumor necrosis factor-α release after exposure of human lymphocytes to abacavir ex vivo.

PRECAUTIONS AND INTERACTIONS. Abacavir is not associated with any clinically significant pharmacokinetic drug interactions. However, a large dose of ethanol (0.7 g/kg) increased the abacavir plasma AUC by 41% and prolonged the elimination $t_{1/2}$ by 26% possibly owing to competition for alcohol dehydrogenase, which produces the dehydro metabolite of the drug (*see* Table 59–2).

TENOFOVIR. Tenofovir disoproxil is a derivative of adenosine 5′-monophosphate that lacks a complete ribose ring; it is the only nucleotide analog currently marketed for the treatment of HIV infection. Tenofovir is available as the disoproxil prodrug, which substantially improves oral absorption. It is active against HIV-1, HIV-2, and HBV. Tenofovir (VIREAD) is FDA-approved for treating HIV infection in adults in combination with other antiretroviral agents and for the treatment of chronic hepatitis B in adults.

MECHANISMS OF ACTION AND RESISTANCE. Tenofovir disoproxil is hydrolyzed rapidly to tenofovir, which is phosphorylated by cellular kinases to its active metabolite, tenofovir diphosphate (which is actually a triphosphate: the parent drug is a monophosphate). Tenofovir diphosphate is a competitive inhibitor of viral reverse transcriptases and is incorporated into HIV DNA to cause chain termination because it has an incomplete ribose ring. Although tenofovir diphosphate has broad-spectrum activity against viral DNA polymerases, it has low affinity for human DNA polymerase-α, polymerase-β, and polymerase-γ, which is the basis for its selective toxicity.

Specific resistance occurs with a K65R substitution that has been associated with clinical failure of tenofovir-containing regimens. Tenofovir sensitivity and virologic efficacy also are reduced in patients harboring HIV isolates with high-level resistance to zidovudine or stavudine. The M184V mutation associated with lamivudine or emtricitabine resistance partially restores susceptibility in tenofovir-resistant HIV harboring the K65R mutation.

ADME. Table 59–2 shows PK data for tenofovir. Following an intravenous dose, 70-80% of the drug is recovered unchanged in the urine; thus, doses should be decreased in those with renal insufficiency. Tenofovir is not known to inhibit or induce CYPs.

UNTOWARD EFFECTS. Tenofovir generally is well tolerated, with few significant adverse effects reported except for flatulence. Rare episodes of acute renal failure and Fanconi syndrome have been reported, and this drug should be used with caution in patients with preexisting renal disease. Tenofovir use is associated with small declines in estimated creatinine clearance after months of treatment in some patients; because the dose needs to be reduced in renal insufficiency, renal function (creatinine and phosphorus) should be monitored regularly. Since tenofovir also has activity against HBV, caution is warranted in using this drug in patients coinfected with HBV: discontinuation of tenofovir may be associated with a rebound of HBV replication and exacerbation of hepatitis. Tenofovir can increase the AUC of didanosine and the 2 drugs probably should not be used together.

EMTRICITABINE. Emtricitabine (EMTRIVA) is a cytidine analog that is chemically related to lamivudine and shares many of its properties. Emtricitabine is active against HIV-1, HIV-2, and HBV. The drug is FDA-approved for treating HIV infection in adults in combination with other antiretroviral agents and is available co-formulated with tenofovir ± efavirenz.

MECHANISMS OF ACTION AND RESISTANCE. Emtricitabine enters cells by passive diffusion and is sequentially phosphorylated to its active metabolite, emtricitabine 5′-triphosphate. High-level resistance to emtricitabine occurs with the same mutations affecting lamivudine (mainly M184V), although these appear to occur less frequently with emtricitabine. The M184V mutation restores sensitivity to zidovudine and in zidovudine-resistant HIV partially restores sensitivity to tenofovir in tenofovir-resistant HIV harboring the K65R mutation. The same K65R mutation confers resistance to emtricitabine and the other cytidine analog lamivudine, as well as didanosine, stavudine, and abacavir.

ADME. Table 59–2 summarizes pharmacokinetic data for emtricitabine. Orally administered drug is absorbed rapidly and well; the drug can be taken without regard to meals. Emtricitabine is excreted primarily unchanged in the urine, thus, the dose should be reduced in patients with creatinine clearances of <50 mL/min.

UNTOWARD EFFECTS. Emtricitabine is one of the least toxic antiretroviral drugs and has few significant adverse effects. Prolonged exposure has been associated with hyperpigmentation of the skin, especially in sun-exposed areas. Because emtricitabine also has in vitro activity against HBV, caution is warranted in using this drug in patients co-infected with HBV and in regions with high HBV seroprevalence.

PRECAUTIONS AND INTERACTIONS. Emtricitabine is not metabolized to a significant extent by CYPs, and it is not susceptible to any known metabolic drug interactions.

DIDANOSINE. Didanosine (2′,3′-dideoxyinosine; ddI) is a purine nucleoside analog that is active against HIV-1, HIV-2, and other retroviruses including HTLV-1. The drug (VIDEX, VIDEX EC) is

FDA-approved for adults and children with HIV infection in combination with other antiretroviral agents. This drug is no longer widely prescribed in the developed world because of the availability of agents with less toxicity.

MECHANISMS OF ACTION AND RESISTANCE. Didanosine enters cells via a nucleoside transporter and is sequentially phosphorylated by cellular enzymes to the triphosphate, the active anabolite that functions as an antiviral adenosine analog. Resistance to didanosine is associated with mutations at reverse transcriptase codons 65 and 74. The L74V substitution, which reduces susceptibility 5- to 26-fold in vitro, is seen most commonly in patients failing to respond to didanosine. Other nucleoside analog mutations, including TAMs, can contribute to didanosine resistance even though the drug does not appear to select for these mutations de novo. The reverse transcriptase insertion mutations at codon 69 produce cross-resistance to all current nucleoside analogs, including didanosine.

ADME. Table 59–2 summarizes some major pharmacokinetic parameters for didanosine. The drug is acid labile, and thus is administered with an antacid buffer. Food decreases didanosine bioavailability. All formulations of didanosine must be administered at least 30 min before or 2 h after eating. This complicates dosing of didanosine in combination with antiretroviral drugs that must be given with food, as is the case for most HIV protease inhibitors. Didanosine is excreted both by glomerular filtration and by tubular secretion; doses therefore must be adjusted in patients with renal insufficiency.

UNTOWARD EFFECTS. The most serious toxicities associated with didanosine include peripheral neuropathy and pancreatitis, both of which are thought to be a consequence of mitochondrial toxicity. Didanosine should be avoided in patients with a history of pancreatitis or neuropathy. Patients complain of pain, numbness, and tingling in the affected extremities. If the drug is stopped as soon as symptoms appear, the neuropathy should improve or resolve. However, irreversible neuropathy can occur with continued use. Retinal changes and optic neuritis also have been reported. Coadministration of other drugs that cause pancreatitis or neuropathy (i.e., stavudine) also will increase the risk and severity of these symptoms. Ethambutol, isoniazid, vincristine, cisplatin, and pentamidine also should be avoided. Serious hepatic toxicity occurs very rarely but can be fatal. Other reported adverse effects include elevated hepatic transaminases, headache, and asymptomatic hyperuricemia and portal hypertension.

PRECAUTIONS AND INTERACTIONS. Buffering agents included in didanosine formulations can interfere with the bioavailability of some coadministered drugs because of altered pH or chelation with cations in the buffer. For example, didanosine greatly reduces the AUCs of ciprofloxacin and indinavir; concentrations of ketoconazole and itraconazole, whose absorption is pH dependent, also are diminished. These interactions generally can be avoided by separating administration of didanosine from that of other agents by at least 2 h after or 6 h before the interacting drug. The enteric-coated formulation of didanosine does not alter ciprofloxacin or indinavir absorption. Didanosine is excreted renally, and shared renal excretory mechanisms provide a basis for interactions with oral ganciclovir, allopurinol, and tenofovir. Methadone decreases the didanosine AUC by ~60%.

NON-NUCLEOSIDE REVERSE TRANSCRIPTASE INHIBITORS

NNRTIs include a variety of chemical substrates that bind to a hydrophobic pocket in the p66 subunit of the HIV-1 reverse transcriptase, in a site distant from the active site (Figure 59–3). These compounds induce a conformational change in the 3-dimensional structure of the enzyme that greatly reduces its activity, and thus they act as noncompetitive inhibitors. Because the binding site for NNRTIs is virus-strain-specific, the approved agents are active against HIV-1 but not HIV-2 or other retroviruses and should not be used to treat HIV-2 infection. These compounds also have no activity against host cell DNA polymerases. The 4 approved NNRTIs are nevirapine, efavirenz, etravirine, and delavirdine. Table 59–3 summarizes their pharmacokinetic properties.

Agents in this class share a number of properties. All approved NNRTIs are eliminated from the body by hepatic metabolism. Efavirenz, etravirine, and nevirapine are moderately potent inducers of hepatic drug-metabolizing enzymes including CYP3A4; delavirdine is mainly a CYP3A4 inhibitor. Pharmacokinetic drug interactions are thus an important consideration with this class of compounds. All NNRTIs except etravirine are susceptible to high-level drug resistance caused by single-amino-acid changes in the NNRTI-binding pocket (usually in codons 103 or 181). Exposure to even a single dose of nevirapine in the absence of other antiretroviral drugs is associated with resistance mutations in up to one-third of patients. *These agents are potent and highly effective but must be combined with at least 2 other active agents to avoid resistance.*

The use of efavirenz or nevirapine in combination with other antiretroviral drugs is associated with favorable long-term suppression of viremia and elevation of CD4+ lymphocyte counts. Efavirenz is a common component of first regimens for treatment-naive patients indue to its convenience, tolerability, and potency. Rashes occur frequently with all NNRTIs, usually during the first 4 weeks of therapy. Rare cases of potentially fatal

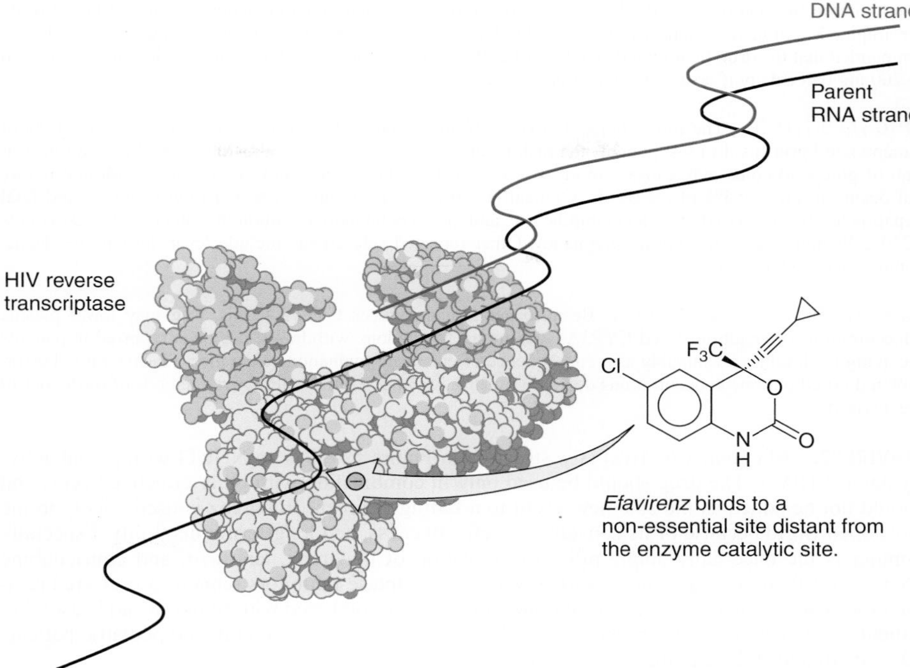

Figure 59–3 *Mechanism of non-nucleoside reverse transcriptase inhibitors (NNRTIs).*

Stevens-Johnson syndrome have been reported with nevirapine, efavirenz, and etravirine. Fat accumulation can be seen after long-term use of NNRTIs, and fatal hepatitis has been associated with nevirapine use.

NEVIRAPINE. Nevirapine (VIRAMUNE) is a dipyridodiazepinone NNRTI with potent activity against HIV-1. The drug is FDA-approved for the treatment of HIV-1 infection in adults and children in combination with other antiretroviral agents. *Nevirapine should never be used as a single agent or as the sole addition to a failing regimen.* Nevirapine is approved for use in infants and children ≥15 days old, with dosing based on body surface area. Single-dose nevirapine has been used commonly in pregnant HIV-infected women to prevent mother-to-child transmission.

Table 59–3

Pharmacokinetic Properties of Non-nucleoside Reverse Transcriptase Inhibitors[a]

PARAMETER	NEVIRAPINE[b]	EFAVIRENZ[b]	ETRAVIRINE
Oral bioavailability, %	90-93	50	NR
Effect of meals on *AUC*	↔	↑17-28%	↑33-102%
Plasma $t_{1/2}$, elim, h	25-30	40-55	41
Plasma protein binding, %	60	99	99.9
Metabolism by CYPs	3A4 > 2B6	2B6 > 3A4	3A4, 2C9, 2C19, UGT
Renal excretion of parent drug, %	<3	<3	1%
Autoinduction of metabolism	Yes	Yes	NR
Inhibition of CYP3A	No	Yes	No

AUC, area under plasma concentration–time curve; $t_{1/2}$, elim, half-life of elimination; ↑, increase; ↓, decrease; ↔, no effect; NR, not reported; CYP, cytochrome P450; UGT, UDP-glucuronosyltransferase.

[a]Reported mean values in adults with normal renal and hepatic function.

[b]Values at steady state after multiple oral doses.

ADME. Table 59–3 summarizes the PK data for this agent. Nevirapine is well absorbed and its bioavailability is not altered by food or antacids. The drug readily crosses the placenta and has been found in breast milk. Nevirapine is a moderate inducer of CYPs and induces its own metabolism. To compensate for this, it is recommended that the drug be initiated at a dose of 200 mg once daily for 14 days, with the dose then increased to 200 mg twice daily if no adverse reactions have occurred.

UNTOWARD EFFECTS. The most frequent adverse events associated with nevirapine are rash (in ~16% of patients) and pruritus. In most patients the rash resolves with continued administration of drug; administration of glucocorticoids may cause a more severe rash. Life-threatening Stevens-Johnson syndrome is rare but occurs in up to 0.3% of recipients. Clinical hepatitis occurs in up to 1% of patients. Severe and fatal hepatitis has been associated with nevirapine use, and this may be more common in women with CD4 counts >250 cells/mm^3, especially during pregnancy. Other reported side effects include fever, fatigue, headache, somnolence, and nausea.

PRECAUTIONS AND INTERACTIONS. Because nevirapine induces CYP3A4, this drug may lower plasma concentrations of coadministered CYP3A4 substrates. Methadone withdrawal has been reported in patients receiving nevirapine, presumably as a consequence of enhanced methadone clearance. Plasma ethinyl estradiol and norethindrone concentrations decrease by 20% with nevirapine; alternative methods of birth control are advised.

EFAVIRENZ. Efavirenz (SUSTIVA) (*see* structure in Figure 59–3) is an NNRTI with potent activity against HIV-1. The drug should be used only in combination with other effective agents and should not be added as the sole new agent to a failing regimen. Efavirenz is used widely in the developed world because of its convenience, effectiveness, and long-term tolerability. Especially popular is the once-daily single pill co-formulation of efavirenz, tenofovir, and emtricitabine (ATRIPLA). Efavirenz plus 2 nucleoside reverse transcriptase inhibitors remains a preferred regimen for treatment-naive patients. Efavirenz can be safely combined with rifampin and is useful in patients also being treated for tuberculosis. Efavirenz is approved for adult and pediatric patients ≥3 years of age and weighing at least 10 kg.

ADME. Table 59–3 summarizes the PK data for this agent. Efavirenz is well absorbed from the GI tract, but there is diminished absorption of the drug with increasing doses. Bioavailability (AUC) is increased by 22% with a high-fat meal. Efavirenz is >99% bound to plasma proteins and, as a consequence, has a low CSF-to-plasma ratio of 0.01. The drug should be taken initially on an empty stomach at bedtime to reduce side effects. Efavirenz is cleared mainly by CYP2B6 and to a lesser extent by CYP3A4. The parent drug is not excreted renally to a significant degree. The long elimination $t_{1/2}$ permits once-daily dosing.

UNTOWARD EFFECTS. The most important adverse effects of efavirenz involve the CNS. Up to 53% of patients report some CNS or psychiatric side effects, but <5% discontinue the drug for this reason. Patients commonly report dizziness, impaired concentration, dysphoria, vivid or disturbing dreams, and insomnia. CNS side effects generally become more tolerable and resolve within the first 4 weeks of therapy. Rash occurs frequently with efavirenz (27%), usually in the first few weeks of treatment, resolving spontaneously and rarely requiring drug discontinuation. Life-threatening skin eruptions such as Stevens-Johnson syndrome are rare. Other side effects reported with efavirenz include headache, increased hepatic transaminases, and elevated serum cholesterol. Efavirenz is the only antiretroviral drug that is unequivocally teratogenic in primates. *Women of childbearing potential therefore should use 2 methods of birth control and avoid pregnancy while taking efavirenz.*

PRECAUTIONS AND INTERACTIONS. Efavirenz is a moderate inducer of hepatic enzymes, especially CYP3A4, but also a weak to moderate CYP inhibitor. Efavirenz decreases concentrations of phenobarbital, phenytoin, and carbamazepine; the methadone AUC is reduced by 33-66% at steady state. Efavirenz reduces the rifabutin AUC by 38% on average. Efavirenz has a variable effect on HIV protease inhibitors: indinavir, saquinavir, and amprenavir concentrations are reduced; ritonavir and nelfinavir concentrations are increased. Drugs that induce CYPs 2B6 or 3A4 (e.g., phenobarbital, phenytoin, and carbamazepine) would be expected to increase the clearance of efavirenz and should be avoided.

ETRAVIRINE. Etravirine is a diarylpyrimidine NNRTI that is active against HIV-1. Etravirine is unique in its ability to inhibit reverse transcriptase that is resistant to other NNRTIs. The drug appears to have conformational and positional flexibility in the NNRTI binding pocket that allow it to inhibit the function of the HIV-1 reverse transcriptase in the presence of common NNRTI resistance mutations. Etravirine (INTELENCE) is approved for use only in treatment-experienced HIV-infected adults. NNRTI-experienced patients should not receive etravirine plus NRTIs alone. Etravirine has not yet been approved for pediatric use.

ADME. Table 59–3 summarizes the PK data for this agent. Food increases the etravirine AUC by 50%, and it is recommended that the drug be administered with food. Methyl- and dimethyl-hydroxylated metabolites are produced in the liver primarily by CYPs 3A4, 2C9, and 2C19, accounting for most of the elimination of this drug. No unchanged drug is detected in the urine.

UNTOWARD EFFECTS. The only notable side effect of etravirine is rash (17% vs. placebo value of 9%), usually occurring within a few weeks of starting therapy and resolving within 1-3 weeks. Severe rash including Stevens-Johnson syndrome and toxic epidermal necrolysis have been reported.

PRECAUTIONS AND INTERACTIONS. Etravirine is an inducer of CYP3A4 and glucuronosyl transferases, and an inhibitor of CYPs 2C9 and 2C19, and can therefore be involved in a number of clinically significant pharmacokinetic drug interactions. Etravirine can be combined with darunavir/ritonavir, lopinavir/ritonavir, and saquinavir/ritonavir without the need for dose adjustments. The dose of maraviroc should be doubled when these 2 drugs are combined. Etravirine should not be administered with tipranavir/ritonavir, fosamprenavir/ritonavir, or atazanavir/ritonavir in the absence of better data to guide dosing. Etravirine should not be combined with efavirenz, nevirapine, or delavirdine. Unlike other NNRTIs, etravirine does not appear to alter the clearance of methadone.

DELAVIRDINE

Delavirdine is a bisheteroarylpiperazine NNRTI that selectively inhibits HIV-1. This agent shares resistance mutations with efavirenz and nevirapine. Delavirdine is well absorbed, especially at pH <2. Antacids, histamine H_2-receptor antagonists, proton pump inhibitors, and achlorhydria may decrease its absorption. The drug can be administered irrespective of food. Delavirdine clearance is primarily through oxidative metabolism by CYP3A4, with <5% of a dose recovered unchanged in the urine. At the recommended dose of 400 mg 3 times daily, the elimination $t_{1/2}$ is 5.8 h.

The most common side effect of delavirdine is rash (18-36%), usually in the first few weeks of treatment and often resolving despite continued therapy. Severe dermatitis, including erythema multiforme and Stevens-Johnson syndrome, is rare. Elevated hepatic transaminases and hepatic failure also have been reported, as has neutropenia (rare). Delavirdine is both a substrate for and an inhibitor of CYP3A4 and can alter the metabolism of other CYP3A4 substrates. Delavirdine increases the plasma concentrations of most HIV protease inhibitors.

HIV PROTEASE INHIBITORS

HIV protease inhibitors (PIs) are peptide-like chemicals that competitively inhibit the action of the virus aspartyl protease (Figure 59–4). This protease is a homodimer consisting of two 99-amino acid monomers; each monomer contributes an aspartic acid residue that is essential for catalysis. The preferred cleavage site for this enzyme is the N-terminal side of proline residues, especially between phenylalanine and proline. Human aspartyl proteases (i.e., renin, pepsin, gastricsin, and cathepsins D and E) contain only 1 polypeptide chain and are not significantly inhibited by HIV PIs.

Table 59–4 summarizes pharmacokinetic data for these agents. Clearance is mainly through hepatic oxidative metabolism. All except nelfinavir are metabolized predominantly by CYP3A4 (and nelfinavir's major metabolite is cleared by CYP3A4). All approved HIV PIs have the potential for metabolic drug interactions. Most of these drugs inhibit CYP3A4 at clinically achieved concentrations, although the magnitude of inhibition varies greatly, with ritonavir by far the most potent. It is now a common practice to combine HIV PIs with a low dose of ritonavir to take advantage of that drug's remarkable capacity to inhibit CYP3A4 metabolism. Doses of 100 or 200 mg once or twice daily are sufficient to inhibit CYP3A4 and increase ("boost") the concentrations of most concurrently administered CYP3A4 substrates. The enhanced pharmacokinetic profile of HIV PIs administered with ritonavir reflects inhibition of both first-pass and systemic clearance, resulting in improved oral bioavailability and a longer elimination $t_{1/2}$ of the coadministered drug. This allows a reduction in both drug dose and dosing frequency while increasing systemic concentrations. Combinations of darunavir, lopinavir, fosamprenavir, and atazanavir with ritonavir are approved for once-daily administration.

Most HIV PIs are substrates for the P-glycoprotein efflux pump (P-gp) (*see* Chapter 5). These agents generally penetrate less well into semen than do NRTIs and NNRTIs. HIV PIs have a high interindividual variability that may reflect differential activity of intestinal and hepatic CYPs. The speed with which HIV develops resistance to unboosted PIs is intermediate between that of nucleoside analogs and NNRTIs. Initial (primary) resistance mutations in the enzymatic active site confer only a 3- to 5-fold drop in sensitivity to most drugs; these are followed by secondary mutations often distant from the active site that compensate for the reduction in proteolytic efficiency. Accumulation of secondary resistance mutations increases the likelihood of cross-resistance to other PIs.

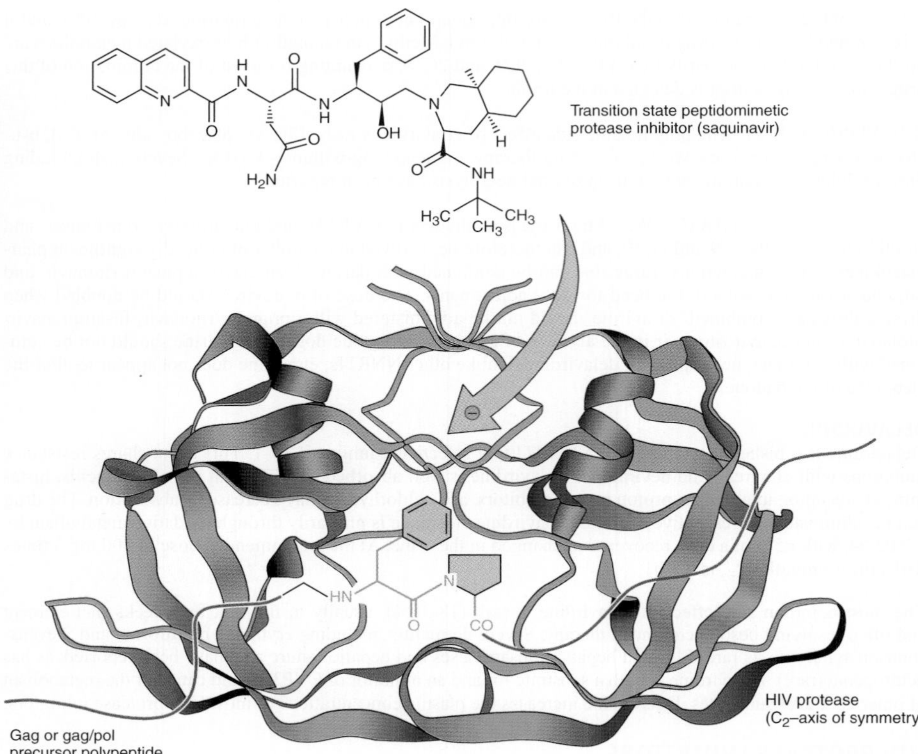

Figure 59–4 *Mechanism of action of the HIV protease inhibitor saquinavir.* Shown here is a phenylalanine-proline target peptide sequence (*in blue*) for the protease enzyme (*in golden brown*) with chemical structures of the native amino acids (*in lower box*) to emphasize homology of their structures to that of saquinavir (*at top*).

GI side effects including nausea, vomiting, and diarrhea are common, although symptoms resolve within 4 weeks of starting treatment. With potent activity and favorable resistance profiles, these drugs are a common component of regimens for treatment-experienced patients. However, the virologic benefits of these drugs must be balanced against short- and long-term toxicities, including the risk of insulin resistance and lipodystrophy.

SAQUINAVIR. Saquinavir is a peptidomimetic hydroxyethylamine that inhibits both HIV-1 and HIV-2 replication (Figure 59–4). Typical of HIV PIs, high-level resistance requires accumulation of multiple resistance mutations. The drug is available as a hard-gelatin capsule (INVIRASE). When combined with ritonavir and nucleoside analogs, saquinavir produces viral load reductions comparable with those of other HIV protease inhibitor regimens.

ADME. Table 59–4 summarizes the pharmacokinetic profile of this agent. Fractional oral bioavailability is low owing mainly to first-pass metabolism, and so this drug should always be given in combination with

Table 59–4

Pharmacokinetic Properties of HIV-1 Protease Inhibitors[a]

PARAMETER	SAQUINAVIR[b]	INDINAVIR	RITONAVIR	NELFINAVIR	FOSAMPRENAVIR	LOPINAVIR[c]	ATAZANAVIR	TIPRANAVIR	DARUNAVIR
Bioavailability (oral), %	13	60-65	>60	20-80 (formulation- and food-dependent)	ND	ND	ND	ND	82
Effect of meals on *AUC*	↑570% (high fat)	↓77% (high fat)	↑13% (capsule)	↑100-200%	↔	↑27% (moderate fat)	↑70% (light meal)	↔	↑30%
Plasma $t_{1/2}$, h	1-2	1.8	3-5	3.5-5	7.7	5-6	6.5-7.9	4.8-6.0	15
Plasma protein binding, %	98	60	98-99	>98	90	98-99	86	99.9	95
Metabolism by CYPs	3A4	3A4	3A4 < 2D6	2C19 < 3A4	3A4	3A4	3A4	3A4	3A4
Autoinduction of metabolism	No	No	Yes	Yes	No	Yes	No	Yes	ND
Renal excretion of parent drug, %	<3	9-12	3.5	1-2	1	<3	7	0.5	8
Inhibition of CYP3A4	+	++	+++	++	++	+++	++	+++	+++

AUC area under plasma concentration–time curve; $t_{1/2}$ half-life of elimination; ↑, increase; ↓, decrease; ↔, no effect; CYP, cytochrome P450; ND, not determined; +, weak; ++, moderate; +++, substantial.

[a]Reported mean values in adults with normal renal and hepatic function.

[b]Parameters reported for the saquinavir soft-gel capsule formulation.

[c]Values for lopinavir, tipranavir, and darunavir reflect coadministration with ritonavir.

ritonavir. Low doses of ritonavir increase the saquinavir steady-state AUC by 20- to 30-fold. Substances that inhibit intestinal but not hepatic CYP3A4 (e.g., grapefruit juice) can increase the saquinavir AUC by ~3-fold.

UNTOWARD EFFECTS. The most frequent side effects of saquinavir are GI: nausea, vomiting, diarrhea, and abdominal discomfort. Most side effects of saquinavir are mild and short lived, although long-term use is associated with lipodystrophy.

PRECAUTIONS AND INTERACTIONS. Saquinavir clearance is increased with CYP3A4 induction. Coadministration of inducers of CYP3A4 such as rifampin, phenytoin, or carbamazepine lowers saquinavir concentrations and should be avoided. The effect of nevirapine or efavirenz on saquinavir may be reversed with ritonavir.

RITONAVIR. Ritonavir (NORVIR) is a peptidomimetic HIV protease inhibitor designed to complement the C_2 axis of symmetry of the enzyme active site. Ritonavir is active against both HIV-1 and HIV-2 (perhaps slightly less active against HIV-2). Ritonavir is mostly used as a pharmacokinetic enhancer (CYP3A4 inhibitor); the low doses used for this purpose are not known to induce ritonavir resistance mutations. The drug is used infrequently as the sole protease inhibitor in combination regimens because of GI toxicity.

ADME. Table 59–4 summarizes the pharmacokinetic profile of this agent. Interindividual variability in pharmacokinetics is high, with variability exceeding 6-fold in trough concentrations among patients given 600 mg ritonavir every 12 h as capsules.

UNTOWARD EFFECTS. The major side effects of ritonavir are GI and include dose-dependent nausea, vomiting, diarrhea, anorexia, abdominal pain, and taste perversion. GI toxicity may be reduced if the drug is taken with meals. Peripheral and perioral paresthesias can occur at the therapeutic dose of 600 mg twice daily. These side effects generally abate within a few weeks of starting therapy. Ritonavir also causes dose-dependent elevations in serum total cholesterol and triglycerides, as well as other signs of lipodystrophy.

PRECAUTIONS AND INTERACTIONS. Ritonavir is one of the most potent known inhibitors of CYP3A4. Thus, ritonavir should be used with caution in combination with any CYP3A4 substrate and should not be combined with drugs that have a narrow therapeutic index such as midazolam, triazolam, fentanyl, and ergot derivatives. Ritonavir is a mixed competitive and irreversible inhibitor of CYP 3A4 and its effects can persist for 2-3 days after the drug is discontinued. Ritonavir is also a weak inhibitor of CYP2D6. Potent inducers of CYP3A4 activity such as rifampin may lower ritonavir concentrations and should be avoided or their dosage adjusted. Capsule and solution formulations of ritonavir contain alcohol and should not be administered with disulfiram or metronidazole. Ritonavir is also a moderate inducer of CYP3A4, glucuronosyl *S*-transferase, and possibly other hepatic enzymes and drug transport proteins. The concentrations of some drugs therefore will be decreased in the presence of ritonavir. Ritonavir reduces the ethinyl estradiol AUC by 40%, and alternative forms of contraception should be used.

Use of Ritonavir as a CYP3A4 Inhibitor. Ritonavir inhibits the metabolism of all current HIV PIs and is frequently used in combination with most of these drugs, with the exception of nelfinavir, to enhance their pharmacokinetic profile and allow a reduction in dose and dosing frequency of the coadministered drug. Ritonavir also overcomes the deleterious effect of food on indinavir bioavailability. Low doses of ritonavir (100 or 200 mg once or twice daily) are just as effective at inhibiting CYP3A4 and are much better tolerated than the 600 mg twice-daily.

FOSAMPRENAVIR. Fosamprenavir (LEXIVA) is a phosphonooxy prodrug of amprenavir that has increased water solubility and improved oral bioavailability. Fosamprenavir is as effective, and generally better tolerated than amprenavir, and as a result, amprenavir is no longer marketed. The drug is active against both HIV-1 and HIV-2. Fosamprenavir has long-term virologic benefit in treatment-naive and treatment-experienced patients, with or without ritonavir, in combination with nucleoside analogs. Twice-daily fosamprenavir/ritonavir produces virologic outcomes equivalent to lopinavir/ritonavir in both treatment-naive and treatment-experienced patients. Fosamprenavir is approved for use in treatment-naive pediatric patients ≥2 years of age and treatment-experienced patients ≥6 years of age, at a dose of 30 mg/kg twice daily or 18 mg/kg plus ritonavir 3 mg/kg twice daily.

Amprenavir's primary resistance mutation occurs at HIV protease codon 50. Primary resistance occurs less frequently at codon 84.

ADME. Table 59–4 summarizes the pharmacokinetic profile of this agent. The phosphorylated prodrug is ~2000 times more water soluble than amprenavir. Fosamprenavir is dephosphorylated rapidly to amprenavir in the intestinal mucosa. Meals have no significant effect on fosamprenavir pharmacokinetics.

UNTOWARD EFFECTS. The most common adverse effects associated are GI and include diarrhea, nausea, and vomiting. Hyperglycemia, fatigue, paresthesias, and headache also have been reported. Fosamprenavir can produce skin eruptions; moderate to severe rash (in up to 8% of recipients) may occur within 2 weeks of starting therapy. Fosamprenavir has fewer effects on plasma lipid profiles than lopinavir-based regimens.

PRECAUTIONS AND INTERACTIONS. Inducers of hepatic CYP3A4 activity (e.g., rifampin and efavirenz) may lower plasma amprenavir concentrations. Because amprenavir is both a CYP3A4 inhibitor and inducer, pharmacokinetic drug interactions can occur and may be unpredictable, especially if the drug is given without ritonavir.

LOPINAVIR. Lopinavir is structurally similar to ritonavir but is 3- to 10-fold more potent against HIV-1. This agent is active against both HIV-1 and HIV-2. Lopinavir is available only in co-formulation with low doses of ritonavir (KALETRA) as a CYP3A4 inhibitor. Lopinavir has antiretroviral activity comparable with that of other potent HIV PIs and better than that of nelfinavir. Lopinavir also has considerable and sustained antiretroviral activity in patients who failed previous HIV protease inhibitor–containing regimens.

Treatment-naive patients who fail a first regimen containing lopinavir generally do not have HIV protease mutations but may have genetic resistance to the other drugs in the regimen. For treatment-experienced patients, accumulation of 4 or more HIV protease inhibitor resistance mutations is associated with a reduced likelihood of virus suppression after starting lopinavir.

ADME. Table 59–4 summarizes the pharmacokinetic profile of this agent. The adult lopinavir/ritonavir dose is 400/100 mg (2 tablets) twice daily, or 800/200 mg (4 tablets) once daily. Lopinavir/ritonavir should not be dosed once daily in treatment-experienced patients. Lopinavir/ritonavir is approved for use in pediatric patients ≥14 days, with dosing based on either weight or body surface area. A pediatric tablet formulation is available for use in children >6 months of age. Lopinavir is absorbed rapidly after oral administration. Food has a minimal effect on bioavailability. Although the tablets contain lopinavir/ritonavir in a fixed 4:1 ratio, the observed plasma concentration ratio for these 2 drugs following oral administration is nearly 20:1, reflecting the sensitivity of lopinavir to the inhibitory effect of ritonavir on CYP3A4. Both lopinavir and ritonavir are highly bound to plasma proteins, mainly to α_1-acid glycoprotein, and have a low fractional penetration into CSF and semen.

UNTOWARD EFFECTS. The most common adverse events reported with the lopinavir/ritonavir co-formulation are GI: loose stools, diarrhea, nausea, and vomiting. Laboratory abnormalities include elevated total cholesterol and triglycerides. It is unclear whether these side effects are due to ritonavir, lopinavir, or both.

PRECAUTIONS AND INTERACTIONS. Concomitant administration of agents that induce CYP3A4, such as rifampin, may lower plasma lopinavir concentrations considerably. St. John's wort is a known inducer of CYP3A4, leading to lower concentrations of lopinavir and possible loss of antiviral effectiveness. Coadministration of other antiretrovirals that can induce CYP3A4, including amprenavir, nevirapine or efavirenz, may require increasing the dose of lopinavir. The liquid formulation of lopinavir contains 42% ethanol and should not be administered with disulfiram or metronidazole. Ritonavir is also a moderate CYP inducer at the dose employed in the co-formulation and can adversely decrease concentrations of some coadministered drugs (e.g., oral contraceptives). There is no direct proof that lopinavir is a CYP inducer in vivo; however, concentrations of some coadministered drugs (e.g., amprenavir and phenytoin) are lower with the lopinavir/ritonavir co-formulation than would have been expected with low-dose ritonavir alone.

ATAZANAVIR. Atazanavir is an azapeptide protease inhibitor that is active against both HIV-1 and HIV-2.

THERAPEUTIC USE. In treatment-experienced patients, atazanavir (REYATAZ) 400 mg once daily without ritonavir was inferior to the lopinavir/ritonavir co-formulation given twice daily. The combination of atazanavir and low-dose ritonavir had a similar viral-load effect as the lopinavir/ritonavir co-formulation in 1 study, suggesting that this drug should be combined with ritonavir in treatment-experienced patients and perhaps in treatment-naive patients with high baseline viral load. Atazanavir, in combination with ritonavir, is approved for treatment of pediatric patients >6 years of age, with dosing based on weight. The primary atazanavir resistance mutation occurs at HIV protease codon 50 and confers ~9-fold decreased susceptibility. High-level resistance is more likely if 5 or more additional mutations are present.

ADME. Table 59–4 summarizes the pharmacokinetic profile of this agent. Atazanavir is absorbed rapidly after oral administration. A light meal increases the AUC by 70%; a high-fat meal increases the AUC by 35%. It is therefore recommended that the drug be administered with food. Absorption is pH dependent, and proton pump inhibitors or other acid-reducing agents substantially reduce atazanavir concentrations after oral dosing. The mean elimination $t_{1/2}$ of atazanavir increases with dose, from 7 h at the standard 400-mg once-daily dose to nearly 10 h at a dose of 600 mg. The drug is present in CSF at <3% of plasma concentrations but has excellent penetration into seminal fluid.

UNTOWARD EFFECTS. Like indinavir, atazanavir frequently causes unconjugated hyperbilirubinemia, although this is not associated with hepatotoxicity. Postmarketing reports include hepatic adverse reactions of cholecystitis, cholelithiasis, cholestasis, and other hepatic function abnormalities. Other side effects reported with atazanavir include diarrhea and nausea, mainly during the first few weeks of therapy. Overall, 6% of patients discontinue atazanavir because of side effects during 48 weeks of treatment. Patients treated with atazanavir have significantly lower fasting triglyceride and cholesterol concentrations than patients treated with nelfinavir, lopinavir, or efavirenz. Atazanavir is not known to cause glucose intolerance or changes in insulin sensitivity.

PRECAUTIONS AND INTERACTIONS. Because atazanavir is metabolized by CYP3A4, concomitant administration of agents that induce CYP3A4 (e.g., rifampin) is contraindicated. Atazanavir is also a moderate inhibitor of CYP3A4 and may alter plasma concentrations of other CYP3A4 substrates. Atazanavir is a moderate UGT1A1 inhibitor and increases the raltegravir AUC by 41-72%. Ritonavir significantly increases the atazanavir AUC and reduces atazanavir systemic clearance. Proton pump inhibitors (PPIs) reduce atazanavir concentrations substantially with concomitant administration. PPIs and H_2 blockers should be avoided in patients receiving atazanavir without ritonavir.

DARUNAVIR. Darunavir is a nonpeptidic protease inhibitor that is active against both HIV-1 and HIV-2. Darunavir binds tightly but reversibly to the active site of HIV protease but has also been shown to prevent protease dimerization. At least 3 darunavir-associated resistance mutations are required to confer resistance. Darunavir (PREZISTA) in combination with ritonavir is approved for use in HIV-infected adults.

ADME. Table 59–4 summarizes the pharmacokinetic profile of this agent. Darunavir/ritonavir can be used as a once-daily (800/100 mg) or twice-daily (600/100 mg) regimen with nucleosides in treatment-naive adults and as a twice-daily regimen (with food) in treatment-experienced adults. Darunavir/ritonavir twice daily is approved for use in pediatric patients >6 years of age, with dosing based on weight. Darunavir is absorbed rapidly after oral administration with ritonavir, with peak concentrations occurring 2-4 h. Ritonavir increases darunavir bioavailability by up to 14-fold. When combined with ritonavir, the mean elimination $t_{1/2}$ of darunavir is ~15 h and the AUC is increased by an order of magnitude.

UNTOWARD EFFECTS. Because darunavir must be combined with a low dose of ritonavir, drug administration can be accompanied by all of the side effects caused by ritonavir, including GI complaints in up to 20% of patients. Darunavir, like fosamprenavir, contains a sulfa moiety, and rash has been reported in up to 10% of recipients. Darunavir/ritonavir is associated with increases in plasma triglycerides and cholesterol, although the magnitude of increase is lower than that seen with lopinavir/ritonavir. Darunavir has been associated with episodes of hepatotoxicity.

PRECAUTIONS AND INTERACTIONS. Because darunavir is metabolized by CYP3A4, concomitant administration of agents that induce CYP3A4 (e.g., rifampin) is contraindicated. The drug interaction profile of darunavir/ritonavir is dominated by those expected with ritonavir. Darunavir/ritonavir 600/100 twice daily increases the maraviroc AUC by 340%; the maraviroc dose should be reduced to 150 mg twice daily when combined with darunavir.

INDINAVIR. Indinavir is a peptidomimetic HIV protease inhibitor. Indinavir (CRIXIVAN) lacks significant advantages over other HIV PIs and is no longer widely prescribed because of problems with nephrolithiasis and other nephrotoxicities.

ADME. Table 59–4 summarizes the pharmacokinetic profile of this agent. Indinavir is absorbed rapidly after oral administration, with peak concentrations achieved in ~1 h. High-calorie, high-fat meals reduce plasma concentrations by 75%; thus, indinavir must be taken with ritonavir or while fasting or with a light low-fat meal. Indinavir has the lowest protein binding of the HIV PIs, with only 60% of drug bound to plasma proteins. As a consequence, indinavir has higher fractional CSF penetration than other drugs in this class. The short $t_{1/2}$ of indinavir makes thrice-daily (every 8 h) dosing necessary unless the drug is combined with ritonavir, which reduces indinavir clearance, allowing twice-daily dosing regardless of meals.

UNTOWARD EFFECTS. A unique and common adverse effect of indinavir is crystalluria and nephrolithiasis, stemming from the poor solubility of the drug (lower at pH 7.4 than at pH 3.5). Nephrolithiasis occurs in ~3% of patients. Patients must drink sufficient fluids to maintain dilute urine and prevent renal complications. Risk of nephrolithiasis is related to higher plasma drug concentrations. Indinavir frequently causes unconjugated hyperbilirubinemia. This is generally asymptomatic and not associated with serious long-term sequelae. Prolonged administration of indinavir is associated with the HIV lipodystrophy syndrome. Indinavir has been associated with hyperglycemia and can induce a state of relative insulin resistance. Dermatologic complications have been reported, including hair loss, dry skin, dry and cracked lips, and ingrown toenails.

PRECAUTIONS AND INTERACTIONS. Patients taking indinavir should drink at least 2 L of water daily to prevent renal complications. *This is especially problematic for those who live in warm climates.* Because indinavir solubility decreases at higher pH, antacids or other buffering agents *should not* be taken at the same time. Didanosine formulations containing an antacid buffer should not be taken within 2 h before or 1 h after indinavir. Indinavir is metabolized by CYP3A4 and is a moderately potent CYP3A4 inhibitor. Indinavir should not be coadministered with other CYP3A4 substrates that have a narrow therapeutic index.

NELFINAVIR. Nelfinavir is a nonpeptidic protease inhibitor that is active against both HIV-1 and HIV-2. Nelfinavir (VIRACEPT) is approved for the treatment of HIV infection in adults and children in combination with other antiretroviral drugs. Long-term virologic suppression with nelfinavir-based combination regimens is significantly inferior to lopinavir/ritonavir, atazanavir, or efavirenz-based regimens. Nelfinavir is well tolerated in pregnant HIV-infected women but detection of a potentially carcinogenic contaminant led to a recommendation that the drug not be used pregnant women.

The primary nelfinavir resistance mutation (D30N) is unique to this drug and results in a 7-fold decrease in susceptibility. Isolates with only this mutation retain full sensitivity to other HIV PIs. Less commonly, a primary resistance mutation occurs at position 90, which can confer cross-resistance. Secondary resistance mutations can accumulate and these are associated with further resistance to nelfinavir, as well as cross-resistance to other HIV PIs.

ADME. Table 59–4 summarizes the pharmacokinetic profile of this agent. A moderate-fat meal increases the AUC 2- to 3-fold; higher concentrations are achieved with high-fat meals. Intraindividual and interindividual variabilities in plasma nelfinavir concentrations are large as a consequence of variable absorption. Nelfinavir is the only HIV protease inhibitor whose pharmacokinetics are not substantially improved with ritonavir. Its major hydroxy-*t*-butylamide metabolite, M8, is formed by CYP2C19 and has antiretroviral activity similar to that of the parent drug. This is the only known active metabolite of any HIV protease inhibitor. Nelfinavir induces its own metabolism.

UNTOWARD EFFECTS. The most important side effect of nelfinavir is diarrhea and loose stools, which resolve in most patients within the first 4 weeks of therapy. Otherwise, nelfinavir is generally well tolerated. It has been associated with glucose intolerance, elevated cholesterol levels, and elevated triglycerides.

PRECAUTIONS AND INTERACTIONS. Because nelfinavir is metabolized by CYPs 2C19 and 3A4, concomitant administration of agents that induce these enzymes may be contraindicated (as with rifampin) or may necessitate an increased nelfinavir dose (as with rifabutin). Nelfinavir is a moderate inhibitor of CYP3A4 and may alter plasma concentrations of other CYP3A4 substrates. Nelfinavir also induces hepatic drug-metabolizing enzymes, reducing the AUC of ethinyl estradiol by 47% and norethindrone by 18%. Combination oral contraceptives therefore should not be used as the sole form of contraception in patients taking nelfinavir. Nelfinavir reduces the zidovudine AUC by 35%.

TIPRANAVIR. Tipranavir is a non-peptidic protease inhibitor that is active against both HIV-1 and HIV-2. Tipranavir (APTIVUS) is approved for use only in treatment-experienced adult and pediatric patients whose HIV is resistant to 1 or more PIs. Combining tipranavir/ritonavir with at least 1 other active antiretroviral drug, usually enfuvirtide, greatly improves virologic responses. Tipranavir/ritonavir is approved for use in adults and pediatric patients >2 years of age, with pediatric dosing based on weight or body surface area.

Because most HIV strains sensitive to tipranavir are also sensitive to darunavir, darunavir is preferred for most treatment-experienced patients because of its better tolerability and toxicity profile.

ADME. Table 59–4 summarizes the pharmacokinetic profile of this agent. Tipranavir must be administered with ritonavir because of poor oral bioavailability. The recommended regimen of tipranavir/ritonavir 500/200 mg twice daily includes a ritonavir dose higher than that of other boosted HIV PIs; lower doses of ritonavir should not be used. Food does not alter pharmacokinetics in the presence of ritonavir but may reduce GI side effects.

UNTOWARD EFFECTS. Tipranavir use has been associated rarely with fatal hepatotoxicity and also with intracranial hemorrhage (including fatalities) and bleeding episodes in patients with hemophilia. The drug has anticoagulant properties in vitro and in animal models that are potentiated by vitamin E. Tipranavir is more likely to cause elevation in lipids and triglycerides than other boosted PIs, possibly due to the higher dose of ritonavir. Tipranavir contains a sulfa moiety, and ~10% of treated patients report a transient rash. The current formulation contains a high amount of vitamin E; patients should not take supplements containing this vitamin.

PRECAUTIONS AND INTERACTIONS. Like ritonavir, tipranavir is a substrate, inhibitor, and inducer of CYP enzymes. Tipranavir/ritonavir reduces the concentrations (AUC) of all coadministered PIs by 44-76% and should not be administered with any of these agents. This reflects the combined effect of the increased ritonavir dose, as well as tipranavir's unique capacity among PIs to induce expression of the P-glycoprotein drug transporter.

ENTRY INHIBITORS

The 2 drugs available in this class, enfuvirtide and maraviroc, have different mechanisms of action (*see* Figure 59–1). Enfuvirtide inhibits fusion of the viral and cell membranes mediated by gp41 and CD4 interactions. Maraviroc is a chemokine receptor antagonist and binds to the host cell CCR5 receptor to block binding of viral gp120.

MARAVIROC. Maraviroc blocks the binding of the HIV outer envelope protein gp120 to the CCR5 chemokine receptor (Figure 59–5). Maraviroc (SELZENTRY) is approved for use in HIV-infected adults who have baseline evidence of predominantly CCR5-tropic virus. The drug has no activity against viruses that are CXCR4-tropic or dual-tropic. Maraviroc retains activity against viruses that have become resistant to antiretroviral agents of other classes because of its unique mechanism of action.

HIV can develop resistance to this drug through 2 distinct pathways. A patient starting maraviroc therapy with HIV that is predominantly CCR5-tropic may experience a shift in tropism to CXCR4- or dual/mixed-tropism predominance. This is especially likely in patients harboring low-level but undetected CXCR4- or dual/mixed-tropic virus prior to initiation of maraviroc. Alternatively, HIV can retain its CCR5-tropism but gain resistance to the drug through specific mutations in the V3 loop of gp 120 that allow virus binding in the presence of inhibitor.

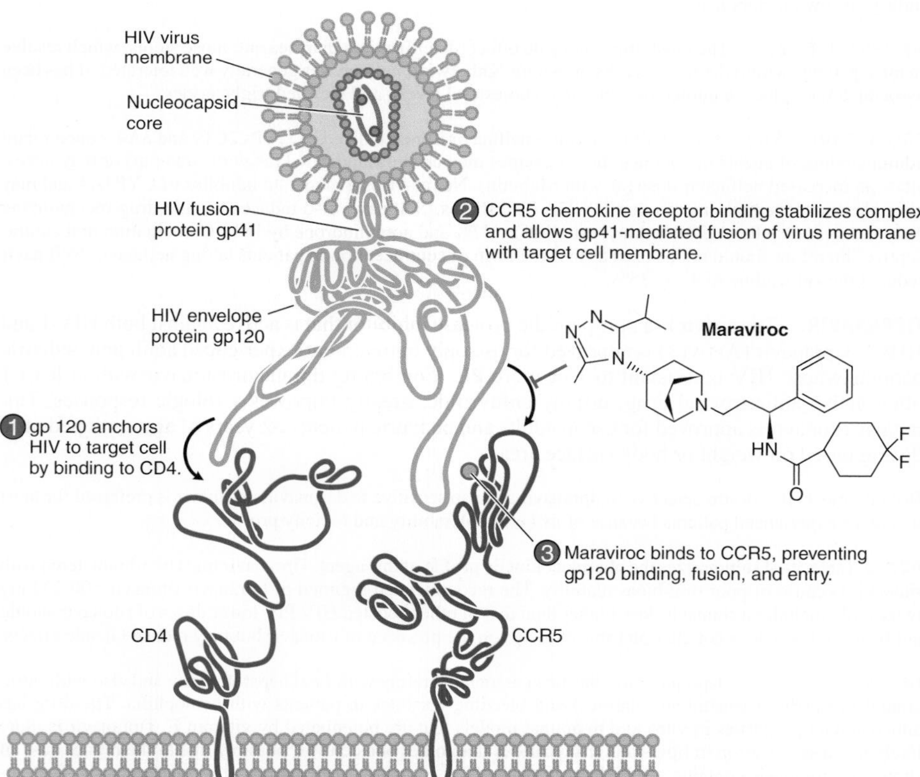

Figure 59–5 *Mechanism of action of the HIV entry inhibitor maraviroc.*

ADME. Maraviroc is the only antiretroviral drug approved at 3 different starting doses, depending on concomitant medications. When combined with most CYP3A inhibitors, the starting dose is 150 mg twice daily; when combined with most CYP3A inducers, the starting dose is 600 mg twice daily; for other concomitant medications, the starting dose is 300 mg twice daily. The oral bioavailability of maraviroc, 23-33%, is dose-dependent. Food decreases bioavailability, but there are no food requirements for drug administration. Elimination is mainly via CYP3A4 with an elimination $t_{1/2}$ of 10.6 h.

UNTOWARD EFFECTS. Maraviroc is generally well tolerated. One case of serious hepatotoxicity with allergic features has been reported, but in controlled trials significant (grade 3 or 4) hepatotoxicity was no more frequent with maraviroc than with placebo.

PRECAUTIONS AND INTERACTIONS. Maraviroc is a CYP3A4 substrate and susceptible to pharmacokinetic drug interactions involving CYP3A4 inhibitors or inducers. Maraviroc is not itself a CYP inhibitor or inducer in vivo, although high-dose maraviroc (600 mg daily) can increase concentrations of the CYP2D6 substrate debrisoquine.

ENFUVIRTIDE. Enfuvirtide is a 36-amino-acid synthetic peptide that is not active against HIV-2 but is broadly effective against laboratory and clinical isolates of HIV-1. Enfuvirtide (FUZEON) is FDA-approved for use only in treatment-experienced adults who have evidence of HIV replication despite ongoing antiretroviral therapy. The drug's cost and route of administration (subcutaneous injection twice daily) limit its use to those with no other treatment options.

MECHANISMS OF ACTION AND RESISTANCE. The amino acid sequence of enfuvirtide is derived from the transmembrane gp41 region of HIV-1 that is involved in fusion of the virus membrane lipid bilayer with that of the host cell membrane. The peptide blocks the interaction between the N36 and C34 sequences of the gp41 glycoprotein by binding to a hydrophobic groove in the N36 coil. This prevents formation of a 6-helix bundle critical for membrane fusion and viral entry into the host cell. Enfuvirtide inhibits infection of CD4+ cells by free virus particles. Enfuvirtide retains activity against viruses that have become resistant to antiretroviral agents of other classes. HIV can develop resistance to this drug through specific mutations in the enfuvirtide-binding domain of gp41.

ADME. Enfuvirtide is the only approved antiretroviral drug that must be administered parenterally. The bioavailability of subcutaneous enfuvirtide is 84% compared with an intravenous dose. Pharmacokinetics of the subcutaneous drug are not affected by site of injection. The major route of elimination for enfuvirtide has not been determined. The mean elimination $t_{1/2}$ of parenteral drug is 3.8 h, necessitating twice-daily administration.

UNTOWARD EFFECTS. The most prominent adverse effects of enfuvirtide are injection-site reactions. Most patients (98%) develop local side effects including pain, erythema, and induration at the site of injection; 80% of patients develop nodules or cysts. Use of enfuvirtide has been associated with a higher incidence of lymphadenopathy and pneumonia. Enfuvirtide is not known to alter the concentrations of any coadministered drugs.

INTEGRASE INHIBITORS

Chromosomal integration is a defining characteristic of retrovirus life cycles and allows viral DNA to remain in the host cell nucleus for a prolonged period of inactivity or latency (*see* Figure 59–1). Because human DNA is not known to undergo excision/reintegration, this process is an excellent target for antiviral intervention. The HIV integrase inhibitor, raltegravir, prevents the formation of covalent bonds between host and viral DNA—a process known as *strand transfer*—presumably by interfering with essential divalent cations in the enzyme's catalytic core.

RALTEGRAVIR. Raltegravir blocks the catalytic activity of the HIV-encoded integrase, thus preventing integration of viral DNA into the host chromosome (Figure 59–6). Raltegravir has potent activity against both HIV-1 and HIV-2. Raltegravir retains activity against viruses that have become resistant to antiretroviral agents of other classes because of its unique mechanism of action. Raltegravir (ISENTRESS) is approved for use in HIV-infected adults.

ADME. Peak concentrations of raltegravir occur ~1 h after oral dosing. Elimination is biphasic, with an α-phase $t_{1/2}$ of ~1 h and a terminal β-phase $t_{1/2}$ of ~12 h, with the α-phase predominating. The pharmacokinetics of raltegravir are highly variable. Moderate- and high-fat meals increase raltegravir apparent bioavailability (AUC) by as much as 2-fold; a low-fat meal decreases AUC modestly (46%); however, there are no food requirements for raltegravir administration. The drug is 83% protein bound in human plasma. Raltegravir is eliminated mainly via glucuronidation by UGT1A1.

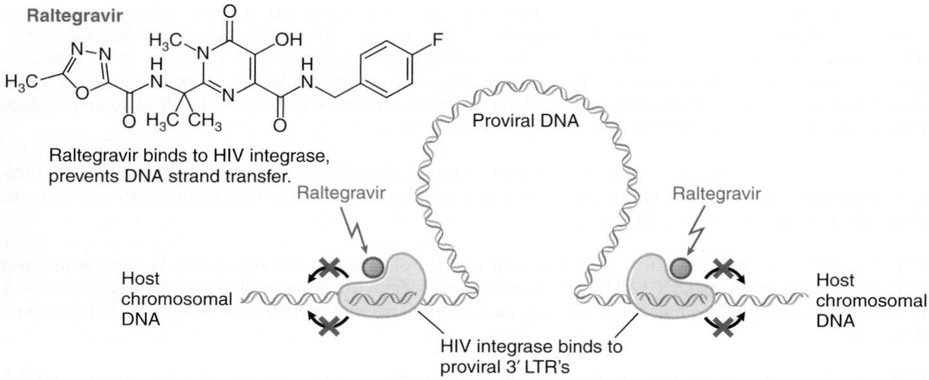

Figure 59–6 *Mechanism of action of the HIV integrase inhibitor raltegravir.*

UNTOWARD EFFECTS. Raltegravir is generally well tolerated, with little clinical toxicity. The most common complaints are headache, nausea, asthenia, and fatigue. Creatine kinase elevations, myopathy, and rhabdomyolysis have been reported, as has exacerbation of depression.

PRECAUTIONS AND INTERACTIONS. As a UGT1A1 substrate, raltegravir is susceptible to pharmacokinetic drug interactions involving inhibitors or inducers of this enzyme. Atazanavir, a moderate UGT1A1 inhibitor, increases the raltegravir AUC 41-72%. Tenofovir increases the raltegravir AUC by 49%, but the mechanism for this interaction is unknown. When raltegravir is combined with the CYP inducer rifampin, the raltegravir dose should be doubled to 800 mg twice daily. Raltegravir has little effect on the pharmacokinetics of the usual coadministered drugs.

Future Treatment Guidelines

Several expert panels issue periodic recommendations for use of antiretroviral drugs for treatment-naive and treatment-experienced adults and children. In the U.S., the Panel on Clinical Practices for Treatment of HIV Infection issues updated guidelines approximately every 6 months; their most recent guidelines can be accessed at http://www.aidsinfo.nih.gov/Guidelines (Department of Health and Human Services).

Current treatment recommendations center around making 2 important clinical decisions:

- **When to start therapy in treatment-naive individuals**
- **When to change therapy in individuals who are failing their current regimen**

The specific drugs recommended may change as new choices become available and clinical research data accumulate. Selection of drugs in the developed world will be driven by genotypic and phenotypic resistance testing. However, future treatment guidelines will likely continue to be driven by 3 principles:

- **Use of combination therapy to prevent the emergence of resistant virus**
- **Emphasis on regimen convenience, tolerability, and adherence to chronically suppress HIV replication**
- **Realization of the need for lifelong treatment under most circumstances**

Treatment guidelines are not sufficient to dictate all aspects of patient management. Prescribers of antiretroviral therapy must maintain a comprehensive and current fund of knowledge regarding this disease and its pharmacotherapy. Because the treatment of HIV infection is a long-lived and complex affair, and because mistakes can have dire and irreversible consequences for the patient, the prescribing of these drugs should be limited to those with specialized training.

For a complete Bibliographical Listing see Goodman & Gilman's ***The Pharmacological Basis of Therapeutics***, 12th ed., or Goodman & Gilman Online at www.AccessMedicine.com.

Section VIII Chemotherapy of Neoplastic Diseases

chapter 60 General Principles of Cancer Chemotherapy

INTRODUCTION. Cancer pharmacology has changed dramatically as curative treatments have been identified for many previously fatal malignancies such as testicular cancer, lymphomas, and leukemia. Adjuvant chemotherapy and hormonal therapy can extend life and prevent disease recurrence following surgical resection of localized breast, colorectal, and lung cancers. Chemotherapy is also employed as part of the multimodal treatment of locally advanced head and neck, breast, lung, and esophageal cancers, soft-tissue sarcomas, and pediatric solid tumors, thereby allowing for more limited surgery and even cure in these formerly incurable cases. Colony-stimulating factors restore bone marrow function and expand the utility of high-dose chemotherapy. Chemotherapeutic drugs are increasingly used in nonmalignant diseases: cytotoxic antitumor agents have become standard in treating autoimmune diseases, including rheumatoid arthritis (methotrexate and cyclophosphamide), Crohn disease (6-mercaptopurine), organ transplantation (methotrexate and azathioprine), sickle cell anemia (hydroxyurea), and psoriasis (methotrexate). Despite these therapeutic successes, few categories of medication have a narrower therapeutic index and greater potential for causing harmful effects than the cytotoxic antineoplastic drugs. A thorough understanding of their pharmacology, including drug interactions and clinical pharmacokinetics, is essential for their safe and effective use in humans.

The compounds used in the chemotherapy of neoplastic disease are quite varied in structure and mechanism of action, including alkylating agents; antimetabolite analogs of folic acid, pyrimidine, and purine; natural products; hormones and hormone antagonists; and a variety of agents directed at specific molecular targets. Tables 60–1 through 60–5 summarize of the main classes and examples of these drugs. Figure 60–1 depicts the cellular targets of chemotherapeutic agents.

The rapidly expanding knowledge of cancer biology has led to the discovery of entirely new and more cancer-specific targets (e.g., growth factor receptors, intracellular signaling pathways, epigenetic processes, tumor vascularity, DNA repair defects, and cell death pathways). For example, in many tumors, proliferation and survival depends on the constitutive activity of a single growth factor pathway, or so-called oncogene addiction (i.e., the "Achilles heel"), and inhibition of that pathway leads to cell death. Thus, imatinib (GLEEVEC) attacks the unique and specific *bcr-abl* translocation in chronic myelocytic leukemia. Imatinib also inhibits *c-kit* and produces extended control of GI stromal tumors that express a mutated and constitutively activated form of *c-kit*. Monoclonal antibodies effectively inhibit tumor-associated antigens such as the amplified *her-2/neu* receptor in breast cancer cells. These examples emphasize that entirely new strategies for drug discovery and development, and advances in patient care, will result from new knowledge of cancer biology.

New clinical trial designs, aimed at determining effects of new drugs at the molecular level, increasingly employ biomarkers derived from samples of biological fluids or tumors to assess the effects of these new agents on signaling pathways, tumor proliferation and cell death, and angiogenesis. Imaging of molecular, metabolic, and physiological effects of drugs will become increasingly important in establishing that drugs effectively engage their targets.

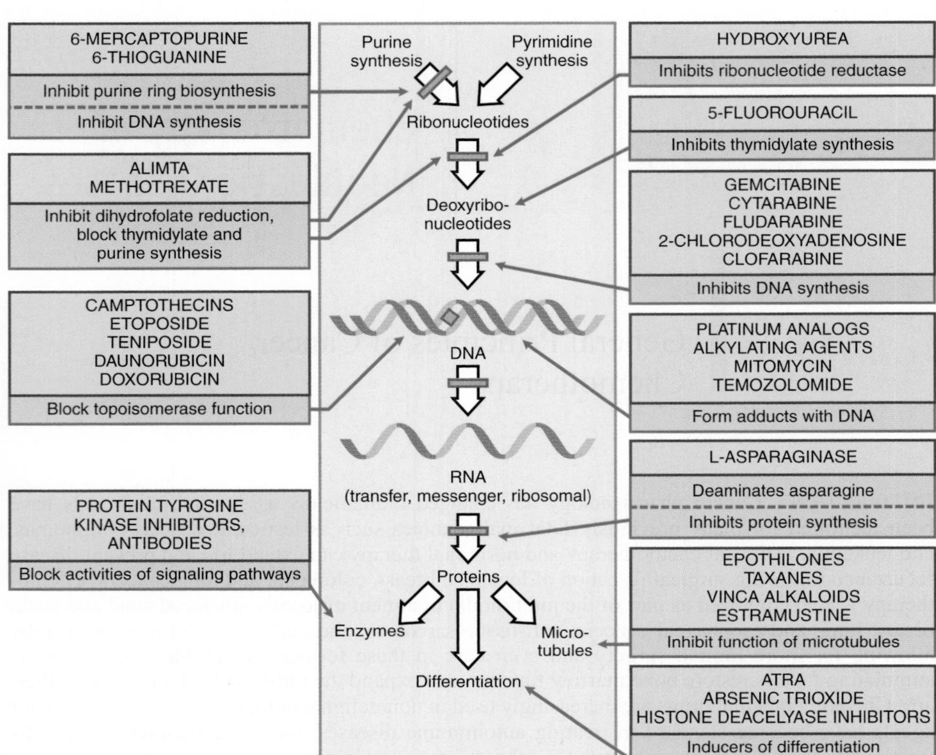

Figure 60–1 *Mechanisms and sites of action of some chemotherapeutic agents for neoplastic disease.*

New therapies are not likely to replace cytotoxics in the foreseeable future. Rather, the targeted drugs and cytotoxics will continue to be used in combination. For instance, monoclonal antibodies or small targeted molecules, used as single agents against solid tumors, produce low response rates and modest benefits; however, in combination with cytotoxics and in early stages of disease, monoclonal antibodies such as trastuzumab (HERCEPTIN) and bevacizumab (AVASTIN) are dramatically effective. At the same time, the toxicities of cytotoxic drugs have become more manageable with the development of better anti-nausea medications (*see* Chapters 13 and 46) and with granulocyte colony-stimulating factor and erythropoietin to restore bone marrow function (*see* Chapters 37 and 62). Finally, targeted drugs are helping to overcome resistance to chemotherapeutic agents by normalizing blood flow, promoting apoptosis, and inhibiting pro-survival signals from growth factor pathways. Tumor angiogenesis leads to increased interstitial pressure and diminishes delivery of drugs to tumor cells; inhibitors of angiogenesis (e.g., bevacizumab) normalize blood flow and interstitial pressure, improve drug delivery, and are thus synergistic with cytotoxic drugs in the treatment of lung, breast, and other cancers.

Drug resistance remains a major obstacle to successful cancer treatment.

Resistance results from a variety of pharmacokinetic and molecular changes that can defeat the best designed treatments, including poor drug absorption and delivery; genetically determined variability in drug transport, activation, and clearance; and mutations, amplifications, or deletions in drug targets. The resistance process is best understood for targeted agents. Tumors developing resistance to *bcr-abl* inhibitors and to inhibitors of the epidermal growth factor receptor (EGFR) express mutations in the target enzyme. Cells exhibiting drug-resistant mutations exist in the patient prior to drug treatment and are selected by drug exposure. Resistance to inhibitors of the EGFR may develop through expression of an alternative receptor, *c-met*, which bypasses EGFR blockade and stimulates proliferation. Defects in recognition of DNA breaks and overexpression of specific repair enzymes may also contribute to resistance to cytotoxic drugs, and a loss of apoptotic pathways can lead to resistance to both cytotoxic and targeted agents.

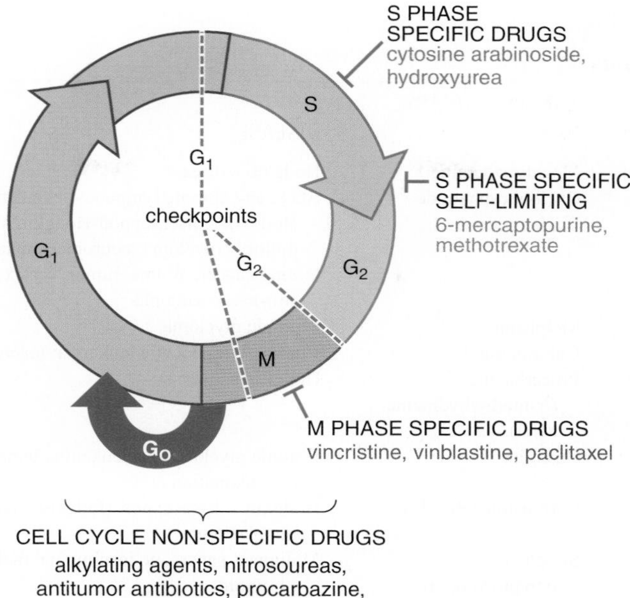

Figure 60–2 *Cell cycle specificity of antineoplastic agents.*

Drugs in combination can negate the effects of a resistance mechanism specific for a single agent, and they may be synergistic because of their biochemical interactions.

Ideally, drug combinations should not overlap in their major toxicities. In general, cytotoxic drugs are used as close as possible to their maximally tolerated individual doses and should be given as frequently as tolerated to discourage tumor regrowth. Because the tumor cell population in patients with clinically detectable disease exceeds 1 g, or 10^9 cells, and each cycle of therapy kills <99% of the cells, it is necessary to repeat treatments in multiple, carefully timed cycles to achieve cure.

THE CELL CYCLE. An understanding of the life cycle of tumors is essential for the rational use of antineoplastic agents (Figure 60–2).

Many cytotoxic agents act by damaging DNA. Their toxicity is greatest during the S, or DNA synthetic, phase of the cell cycle. Others, such as the vinca alkaloids and taxanes, block the formation of a functional mitotic spindle in the M phase. These agents are most effective on cells entering mitosis, the most vulnerable phase of the cell cycle. Accordingly, human neoplasms most susceptible to chemotherapeutic measures are those having a high percentage of proliferating cells. Normal tissues that proliferate rapidly (bone marrow, hair follicles, and intestinal epithelium) are thus highly susceptible to damage from cytotoxic drugs.

Slowly growing tumors with a small growth fraction (e.g., carcinomas of the colon or non–small cell lung cancer) are less responsive to cycle-specific drugs. More effective are agents that inflict high levels of DNA damage (e.g., alkylating agents) or those that remain at high concentrations inside the cell for extended periods of time (e.g., fluoropyrimidines).

The clinical benefit of cytotoxic drugs has primarily been measured by radiological assessment of drug effects on tumor size; newer "targeted" agents, however, may simply slow or halt tumor growth so their effects may best be measured in the assessment of time to disease progression. More recently, there is growing interest in designing drugs that selectively kill the stem cell component of tumors because these cells are believed to be responsible for the continuous proliferation and repopulation of tumors after a toxic exposure to chemotherapy or targeted therapy. For example, bone marrow and epithelial tissues contain a compartment of normal nondividing stem cells that display resistance to cytotoxic drugs and retain the capacity to regenerate the normal cell population. Tumor stem cells exhibit the same resistance to chemotherapy, radiotherapy, and oxidative insults, and thus they may represent a significant barrier to the cure of neoplasms.

Table 60–1

Alkylating Agents

TYPE OF AGENT	NONPROPRIETARY NAMES	DISEASE
Nitrogen mustards	Mechlorethamine	Hodgkin's disease
	Cyclophosphamide Ifosfamide	Acute and chronic lymphocytic leukemia; Hodgkin's disease; non-Hodgkin's lymphoma; multiple myeloma; neuroblastoma; breast, ovary, lung cancer; Wilms' tumor; cervix, testis cancer; soft-tissue sarcoma
	Melphalan	Multiple myeloma
	Chlorambucil	Chronic lymphocytic leukemia; macroglobulinemia
Methylhydrazine derivative	Procarbazine (*N*-methylhydrazine, MIH)	Hodgkin's disease
Alkyl sulfonate	Busulfan	Chronic myelogenous leukemia, bone marrow transplantation
Nitrosoureas	Carmustine (BCNU)	Hodgkin's disease; non-Hodgkin's lymphoma; glioblastoma
	Streptozocin (streptozotocin)	Malignant pancreatic insulinoma; malignant carcinoid
	Bendamustine	Non-Hodgkin's lymphoma
Triazenes	Dacarbazine (DTIC; dimethyltriazenoi-midazole carboxamide),	Malignant melanoma; Hodgkin's disease; soft-tissue sarcomas; melanoma
	Temozolomide	Malignant gliomas
Platinum coordination complexes	Cisplatin, carboplatin, oxaliplatin	Testicular, ovarian, bladder, esophageal, lung, head and neck, colon, breast cancer

Although cells from different tumors display differences in the duration of their transit through the cell cycle and in the fraction of cells in active proliferation, all cells display a similar pattern of cell cycle progression (*see* Figure 60–2):

- A phase that precedes DNA synthesis (G_1)
- A DNA synthetic phase (S)
- An interval following the termination of DNA synthesis (G_2)
- The mitotic phase (M) in which the cell, containing a double complement of DNA, divides into 2 daughter G_1 cells
- A probability of moving into a quiescent state (G_0) and failing to move forward for long periods of time

At each transition point in the cell cycle, specific proteins such as *p53* and *chk-1* and *2*, monitor the integrity of DNA and, upon detection of DNA damage, may initiate DNA repair processes or, in the presence of massive damage, direct cells down a cell death (apoptosis) pathway. Some cancer chemotherapeutic drugs act at specific phases, in the cell cycle, mainly at the S phase and M phase; other agents are cytoxic at any point in the cell cycle and are termed *cell cycle phase nonspecific agents*.

Each transition point in the cell cycle requires the activation of specific *cyclin-dependent kinases (CDKs)*, which, in their active forms, couple with corresponding regulatory proteins called *cyclins*. The proliferative impact of CDKs is, in turn, dampened by inhibitory proteins such as *p16*. Tumor cells often exhibit changes in cell-cycle regulation that lead to relentless proliferation (e.g., mutations or loss of p16 or other inhibitory components of the so-called retinoblastoma pathway, enhanced cyclin or CDK activity). Consequently, CDKs and their effector proteins have become attractive targets for discovery of anti-neoplastic agents.

Table 60–2

Antimetabolites

TYPE OF AGENT	NONPROPRIETARY NAMES	DISEASE
Folic acid analogs	Methotrexate (amethopterin)	Acute lymphocytic leukemia; choriocarcinoma; breast, head, neck, and lung cancers; osteogenic sarcoma; bladder cancer
	Pemetrexed	Mesothelioma, lung cancer
Pyrimidine analogs	Fluorouracil (5-fluorouracil; 5-FU), capecitabine	Breast, colon, esophageal, stomach, pancreas, head, and neck; premalignant skin lesion (topical)
	Cytarabine (cytosine arabinoside)	Acute myelogenous and acute lymphocytic leukemia; non-Hodgkin's lymphoma
	Gemcitabine	Pancreatic, ovarian, lung cancer
	5-aza-cytidine	Myelodysplasia
	Deoxy-5-aza-cytidine	Myelodysplasia
Purine analogs and related inhibitors	Mercaptopurine (6-mercaptopurine; 6-MP)	Acute lymphocytic and myelogenous leukemia; small cell non-Hodgkin's lymphoma
	Pentostatin (2′-deoxycoformycin)	Hairy cell leukemia; chronic lymphocytic leukemia; small cell non-Hodgkin's lymphoma
	Fludarabine	Chronic lymphocytic leukemia
	Clofarabine	Acute myelogenous leukemia
	Nelarabine	T-cell leukemia, lymphoma

Because of the central importance of DNA to the identity and functionality of a cell, elaborate mechanisms ("checkpoints") have evolved to monitor DNA integrity. If a cell possesses normal checkpoint function, drug-induced DNA damage will activate apoptosis when the cell reaches the G_1/S or G_2/M boundary. If the p53 gene product or other checkpoint proteins are mutated or absent and the checkpoint function fails, damaged cells will not divert to the apoptotic pathway but will proceed through the S phase and mitosis. The cell progeny will emerge as a mutated and potentially drug-resistant population. Thus, alterations in the regulation of cell-cycle kinetics and checkpoint controls are critical factors in determining sensitivity to cytotoxic drugs and understanding the success or failure of new agents.

ACHIEVING THERAPEUTIC INTEGRATION AND EFFICACY

The treatment of cancer patients requires a skillful interdigitation of pharmacotherapy with other modalities of treatment (e.g., surgery and irradiation). Each treatment modality carries its own risks and benefits, with the potential for both antagonistic and synergistic interactions between modalities, particularly between drugs and irradiation. Furthermore, individual patient characteristics determine the choice of modalities. Not all patients can tolerate drugs, and not all drug regimens are appropriate for a given patient. Renal and hepatic function, bone marrow reserve, general performance status, and concurrent medical problems all come into consideration in making a therapeutic plan. Other less quantifiable considerations, such as the natural history of the tumor, the patient's willingness to undergo difficult and potentially dangerous treatments, and the patient's physical and emotional tolerance for side effects, enter the equation, with the goal of balancing the likely long-term gains and risks in the individual patient.

One of the great challenges of therapeutics is to adjust drug regimens to achieve a therapeutic but nontoxic outcome. Orally administered drugs are now frequently prescribed using uniform dosing for all adult patients. Dose adjustment based on renal function, on hepatic function, or on pharmacokinetic monitoring does facilitate meeting specific targets such as desired drug concentration in plasma or area under the concentration-time curve (AUC). There are few good guidelines for adjusting dose on the basis of obesity or age. Elderly patients, particularly those >70 years of age, exhibit less tolerance for chemotherapy because of decreased renal and hepatic drug clearance, lower protein binding, and less bone marrow reserve. Drug clearance decreases in morbidly obese patients, and dosage should probably be capped for these patients at no more than 150% of the dosage for patients of average body surface area (1.73 m^2), with adjustment upward for tolerance after each subsequent dose.

Table 60–3

Natural Products

TYPE OF AGENT	NONPROPRIETARY NAMES	DISEASE
Vinca alkaloids	Vinblastine	Hodgkin's disease; non-Hodgkin's lymphoma; testis cancer
	Vinorelbine	Breast and lung cancer
	Vincristine	Acute lymphocytic leukemia; neuroblastoma; Wilms' tumor; rhabdomyosarcoma; Hodgkin's disease; non-Hodgkin's lymphoma
Taxanes	Paclitaxel, docetaxel	Ovarian, breast, lung, prostate, bladder, head, and neck cancer
Epipodophyllotoxins	Etoposide	Testis, small cell lung and other lung cancer; breast cancer; Hodgkin's disease; non-Hodgkin's lymphomas; acute myelogenous leukemia; Kaposi's sarcoma
	Teniposide	Acute lymphoblastic leukemia in children
Camptothecins	Topotecan	Ovarian cancer; small cell lung cancer
	irinotecan	Colon cancer
Antibiotics	Dactinomycin (actinomycin D)	Choriocarcinoma; Wilms' tumor; rhabdomyosarcoma; testis; Kaposi's sarcoma
	Daunorubicin (daunomycin, rubidomycin)	Acute myelogenous and acute lymphocytic leukemia
	Doxorubicin	Soft-tissue, osteogenic, and other sarcoma; Hodgkin's disease; non-Hodgkin's lymphoma; acute leukemia; breast, genitourinary, thyroid, lung, and stomach cancer; neuroblastoma and other childhood and adult sarcomas
Echinocandins	Yondelis	Soft-tissue sarcomas, ovarian cancer
Anthracenedione	Mitoxantrone	Acute myelogenous leukemia; breast and prostate cancer
	Bleomycin	Testis and cervical cancer; Hodgkin's disease; non-Hodgkin's lymphoma
	Mitomycin C	Stomach, anal, and lung cancer
Enzymes	L-Asparaginase	Acute lymphocytic leukemia

Even patients with normal renal and hepatic function exhibit significant variability in pharmacokinetics of anticancer drugs that can reduce efficacy or cause excess toxicity. The following examples illustrate the potential of using pharmacokinetic targeting to improve therapy:

- The thrombocytopenia caused by carboplatin is a direct function of AUC, which in turn is determined by renal clearance of the parent drug. One can target a desired AUC based on creatinine clearance.
- Monitoring of 5-fluorouracil levels in plasma allows dose adjustment to improve response rates in patients with rapid drug clearance, and to avoid toxicity in those with slow drug clearance.
- High-dose methotrexate therapy requires drug-level monitoring to detect patients at high risk for renal failure and severe myelosuppression. Patients with inappropriately high concentrations of methotrexate at specific time points can be rescued from toxicity by the administration of leucovorin, and in extreme cases, by dialysis or administration of a methotrexate-cleaving enzyme and orphan drug, glucarpidase (VORAXAZE; recombinant carboxypeptidase G2).

MOLECULAR TESTING TO SELECT PATIENTS FOR CHEMOTHERAPY. Molecular tests are increasingly employed to identify patients likely to benefit from treatment and those at highest risk of toxicity.

Table 60–4

Hormones and Antagonists

TYPE OF AGENT	NONPROPRIETARY NAMES	DISEASE
Adrenocortical suppressants	Mitotane (*o,p′*-DDD)	Adrenal cortex cancer
Adrenocortico-steroids	Prednisone (other equivalent preparations available)	Acute and chronic lymphocytic leukemia; non-Hodgkin's lymphoma; Hodgkin's disease; breast cancer, multiple myeloma
Progestins	Hydroxyprogesterone caproate, medroxyprogesterone acetate, megestrol acetate	Endometrial, breast cancer
Estrogens	Diethylstilbestrol, ethinyl estradiol (other preparations available)	Breast, prostate cancer
Anti-estrogens	Tamoxifen, toremifene	Breast cancer
Aromatase inhibitors	Anastrozole, letrozole, exemestane	Breast cancer
Androgens	Testosterone propionate, fluoxymesterone (other preparations available)	Breast cancer
Anti-androgen	Flutamide, casodex	Prostate cancer
GnRH analog	Leuprolide	Prostate cancer

Pretreatment testing has become standard practice to select patients for hormonal therapy of breast cancer and for treatment with antibodies such as trastuzumab (*her-2/neu receptor*) and rituximab (*CD20*). The presence of a mutated *k-ras* gene indicates that a colorectal cancer patient's tumor will not respond to anti-EGFR antibodies; mutations of EGFR signal a 70% likelihood of response to erlotinib (TARCEVA) and gefitinib (IRESSA), both inhibitors of this receptor. Although *not* yet routinely employed in traditional cytotoxic therapy, molecular testing of tumors could improve outcomes by pairing patients with drugs likely to be effective against mutations that drive tumor proliferation or survival. Mutations of the *b-Raf*, *HER 2/neu*, and *Alk*, which are found in subsets of solid tumors in human subjects, represent examples of promising targets for solid tumor chemotherapy.

Inherited differences in protein sequence polymorphisms or levels of RNA expression influence toxicity and anti-tumor response. For example, tandem repeats in the promoter region of the gene encoding thymidylate synthase, the target of 5-fluorouracil, determine the level of expression of the enzyme. Increased numbers of repeats are associated with increased gene expression, a lower incidence of toxicity, and a decreased rate of response in patients with colorectal cancer. Polymorphisms of the dihydropyrimidine dehydrogenase gene, the product of which is responsible for degradation of 5-fluorouracil, are associated with decreased enzyme activity and a significant risk of overwhelming drug toxicity, particularly in the rare individual homozygous for the polymorphic genes. Other polymorphisms appear to affect the clearance and therapeutic activity of cancer drugs, including tamoxifen, methotrexate, irinotecan, and 6-mercaptopurine.

Gene expression profiling, in which the levels of messenger RNA from thousands of genes are randomly surveyed using gene arrays, has revealed tumor profiles that are highly associated with metastasis. The expression of the transcription factor HOX B13 correlates with disease recurrence in patients receiving adjuvant hormonal therapy in breast cancer. Gene expression profiles also predict the benefit of adjuvant chemotherapy for breast cancer patients and the response of ovarian cancer patients to platinum-based therapy. New molecular tests and their more widespread use likely will shorten the time for drug development and approval, help to avoid the costs and toxicity of ineffective drugs, and improve patient outcome.

A CAUTIONARY NOTE. Although advances in drug discovery and molecular profiling of tumors offer great promise for improving the outcomes of cancer treatment, a final word of caution regarding all treatment regimen deserves emphasis. *The pharmacokinetics and toxicities of cancer drugs vary among individual patients.* It is imperative to *recognize toxicities early*, to *alter doses or discontinue offending medication* to relieve symptoms and reduce risk, and to *provide vigorous supportive care* (platelet transfusions, antibiotics, and hematopoietic growth factors). Toxicities

Table 60–5

Miscellaneous Agents

TYPE OF AGENT	NONPROPRIETARY NAMES	DISEASE
Substituted urea	Hydroxyurea	Chronic myelogenous leukemia; polycythemia vera; essential thrombocytosis
Differentiating agents	Tretinoin, arsenic trioxide	Acute promyelocytic leukemia
	Histone deacetylase inhibitor (vorinostat)	Cutaneous T-cell lymphoma
Protein tyrosine kinase inhibitors	Imatinib	Chronic myelogenous leukemia; GI stromal tumors (GIST); hypereosinophilia syndrome
	Dasatinib, nilotinib	Chronic myelogenous leukemia
	Gefitinib, erlotinib	EGFR inhibitors: Non–small cell lung cancer
	Sorafenib	Hepatocellular cancer, renal cancer
	Sunitinib	GIST, renal cancer
	Lapatinib	Breast cancer
Proteasome inhibitor	Bortezomib	Multiple myeloma
Biological response modifiers	Interferon-alfa, interleukin-2	Hairy cell leukemia; Kaposi's sarcoma; melanoma; carcinoid; renal cell; non-Hodgkin's lymphoma; mycosis fungoides; chronic myelogenous leukemia
Immunomodulators	Thalidomide	Multiple myeloma
	Lenalidomide	Myelodysplasia (5q^{-} syndrome); multiple myeloma
mTOR Inhibitors	Temsirolimus, everolimus	Renal cancer
Monoclonal antibodies		(*see* Tables 62–1 and 62–2)

affecting the heart, lungs, or kidneys may be irreversible if recognized late in their course, leading to permanent organ damage or death. Fortunately, such toxicities can be minimized by early recognition and by adherence to standardized protocols and to the guidelines for drug use.

For a complete Bibliographical Listing see Goodman & Gilman's ***The Pharmacological Basis of Therapeutics***, 12th ed., or Goodman & Gilman Online at www.AccessMedicine.com.

Cytotoxic Agents

I. Alkylating Agents and Platinum Coordination Complexes

In 1942, Louis Goodman and Alfred Gilman, the originators of this text, began clinical studies of intravenous nitrogen mustards in patients with lymphoma, launching the modern era of cancer chemotherapy. Six major types of alkylating agents are used in the chemotherapy of neoplastic diseases:

- Nitrogen mustards
- Ethyleneimines
- Alkyl sulfonates
- Nitrosoureas
- The triazenes
- DNA-methylating drugs, including procarbazine, temozolomide, and dacarbazine

In addition, because of similarities in their mechanisms of action and resistance, platinum complexes are discussed with classical alkylating agents, even though they do not alkylate DNA but instead form covalent metal adducts with DNA.

The chemotherapeutic alkylating agents have in common the property of forming highly reactive carbonium ion intermediates. These reactive intermediates covalently link to sites of high electron density, such as phosphates, amines, sulfhydryl, and hydroxyl groups. Their chemotherapeutic and cytotoxic effects are directly related to the alkylation of reactive amines, oxygens, or phosphates on DNA. The general mechanisms actions of alkylating agents on DNA are illustrated in Figure 61–1 with mechlorethamine (nitrogen mustard). The extreme cytotoxicity of bifunctional alkylators correlates very closely with interstrand cross-linkage of DNA.

A **Activation**

B **Nucleophilic attack of unstable aziridine ring by electron donor**

(–S̈H of protein, –N̈– of protein or DNA base, =Ö of DNA base or phosphate)

Figure 61–1 *Mechanism of action of alkylating agents.* **A.** Activation reaction. **B.** Alkylation of N^7 of guanine.

The ultimate cause of cell death related to DNA damage is not known. Specific cellular responses include cell-cycle arrest and attempts to repair DNA. The specific repair enzyme complex utilized will depend on 2 factors: the chemistry of the adduct formed and the repair capacity of the cell involved. The process of recognizing and repairing DNA generally requires an intact nucleotide excision repair (NER) complex, but may differ with each drug and with each tumor. Alternatively, recognition of extensively damaged DNA by p53 can trigger apoptosis. Mutations of p53 lead to alkylating agent resistance.

Structure-Activity Relationships. Although these alkylating agents share the capacity to alkylate biologically important molecules, modification of the basic chloroethylamino structure changes reactivity, lipophilicity, active transport across biological membranes, sites of macromolecular attack, and mechanisms of DNA repair, all of which determine drug activity in vivo. With several of the most valuable agents (e.g., cyclophosphamide, ifosfamide), the active alkylating moieties are generated in vivo through hepatic metabolism (Figure 61–2). Consult Chapter 61 of the 12th edition of the parent text for details on metabolic activation and structure-activity relationships among these compounds.

The newest approved alkylating agent, **bendamustine**, has the typical chloroethyl reactive groups attached to a benzimidazole backbone. The unique properties and activity of this drug may derive from this purine-like structure; the agent produces slowly repaired DNA cross-links, lacks cross-resistance with other classical alkylators, and has significant activity in chronic lymphocytic leukemia (CLL) and large-cell lymphomas refractory to standard alkylators. One class of alkylating agents transfers methyl rather than ethyl groups to DNA. The **triazene** derivative 5-(3,3-dimethyl-1-triazeno)-imidazole-4-carboxamide, usually called

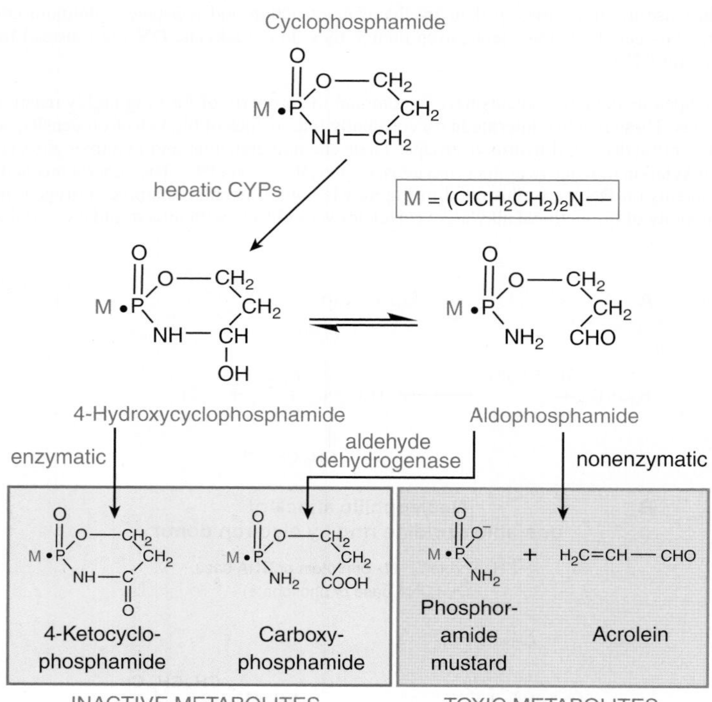

Figure 61–2 *Metabolic activation of cyclophosphamide.* Cyclophosphamide is activated (hydroxylated) by CYP2B, with subsequent transport of the activated intermediate to sites of action. The selectivity of cyclophosphamide against certain malignant tissues may result in part from the capacity of normal tissues to degrade the activated intermediates via aldehyde dehydrogenase, glutathione transferase, and other pathways. Ifosfamide is structurally similar to cyclophosphamide: whereas cyclophosphamide has 2 chloroethyl groups on the exocyclic nitrogen atom, 1 of the 2-chloroethyl groups of ifosfamide is on the cyclic phosphoramide nitrogen of the oxazaphosphorine ring. Ifosfamide is activated by hepatic CYP3A4. The activation of ifosfamide proceeds more slowly, with greater production of de-chlorinated metabolites and chloroacetaldehyde. These differences in metabolism likely account for the higher doses of ifosfamide required for equitoxic effects, the greater neurotoxicity of ifosfamide, and perhaps differences in the antitumor spectra of cyclophosphamide and ifosfamide.

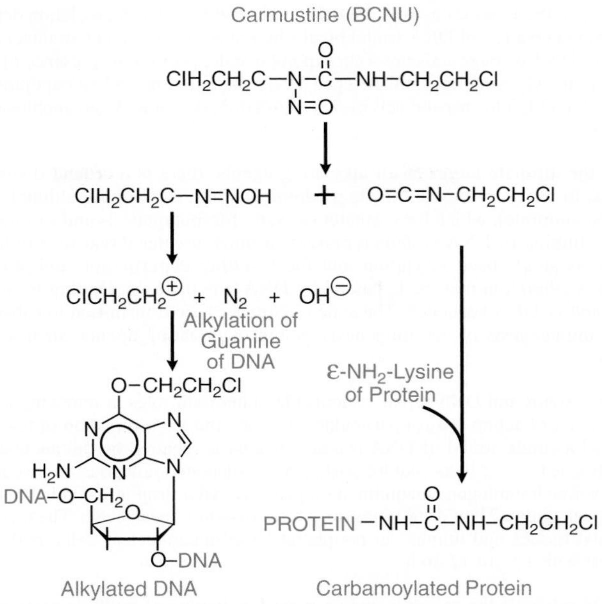

Carmustine (BCNU)

Alkylated DNA

Carbamoylated Protein

Figure 61–3 *Generation of alkylating and carbamylating intermediates from carmustine (BCNU).* The 2-chloroethyl diazonium ion, a strong electrophile, can alkylate guanine, cytidine, and adenine bases. Displacement of the halogen atom that can then lead to interstrand or intrastrand cross-linking of DNA. The formation of cross-links after the initial alkylation reaction proceeds slowly and can be reversed by the DNA repair enzyme O^6-alkyl, methyl guanine methyltransferase (MGMT), which displaces the chloroethyl adduct from its binding to guanine in a suicide reaction. The same enzyme, when expressed in human gliomas, produces resistance to nitrosoureas and to other methylating agents, including DTIC, temozolomide, and procarbazine.

dacarbazine or **DTIC**, is prototypical of methylating agents. Dacarbazine requires initial activation by hepatic CYPs through an *N*-demethylation reaction. In the target cell, spontaneous cleavage of the metabolite, methyl-triazeno-imidazole-carboxamide (MTIC), yields an alkylating moiety, a methyl diazonium ion. A related triazene, temozolomide, undergoes spontaneous, nonenzymatic activation to MTIC and has significant activity against gliomas.

The **nitrosoureas**, which include compounds such as 1,3-*bis*-(2-chloroethyl)-1-nitrosourea (carmustine [BCNU]), 1-(2-chloroethyl)-3-cyclohexyl-1-nitrosourea (lomustine [CCNU]), and its methyl derivative (semustine [methyl-CCNU]), as well as the antibiotic streptozocin (streptozotocin), exert their cytotoxicity through the spontaneous breakdown to an alkylating intermediate, the 2-chloroethyl diazonium ion. As with the nitrogen mustards, interstrand cross-linking appears to be the primary lesion responsible for the cytotoxicity of nitrosoureas. The reactions of the nitrosoureas with macromolecules are shown in Figure 61–3.

Stable ethyleneimine derivatives have antitumor activity; triethylenemelamine (**TEM**) and triethylenethiophosphoramide (**thiotepa**) have been used clinically. In standard doses, thiotepa produces little toxicity other than myelosuppression; it also is used for high-dose chemotherapy regimens, in which it causes both mucosal and CNS toxicity. Altretamine (hexamethylmelamine [**HMM**]) is chemically similar to TEM. The methylmelamines are *N*-demethylated by hepatic microsomes with the release of formaldehyde; there is a direct relationship between the degree of the demethylation and their antitumor activity in model systems.

Esters of alkane sulfonic acids alkylate DNA through the release of methyl radicals. Busulfan is of value in high-dose chemotherapy.

GENERAL PHARMACOLOGICAL ACTIONS

Cytotoxic Actions. The capacity of alkylating agents to interfere with DNA integrity and function and to induce cell death in rapidly proliferating tissues provides the basis for their therapeutic and toxic properties. Acute effects manifest primarily against rapidly proliferating tissues; however, certain alkylating agents may have damaging effects on tissues with normally low mitotic indices (e.g., liver, kidney, and mature lymphocytes); effects in these tissues usually are delayed. Lethality of DNA alkylation depends on the recognition of the adduct, the creation of DNA strand breaks by repair enzymes, and an intact apoptotic response. In non-dividing cells, DNA damage activates a checkpoint that depends on the presence of a normal p53 gene. Cells thus blocked in the G_1/S interface either repair DNA alkylation or undergo apoptosis. Malignant cells with mutant or absent p53 fail to suspend cell-cycle progression, do not undergo apoptosis, and exhibit resistance to these drugs.

Although DNA is the ultimate target of all alkylating agents, there is a crucial distinction between the bifunctional agents, in which cytotoxic effects predominate, and the monofunctional methylating agents (procarbazine, temozolomide), which have greater capacity for mutagenesis and carcinogenesis. This suggests that the cross-linking of DNA strands represents a much greater threat to cellular survival than do other effects, such as single-base alkylation and the resulting depurination and single-chain scission. Conversely, simple methylation may be bypassed by DNA polymerases, leading to mispairing reactions that permanently modify DNA sequence. These new sequences are transmitted to subsequent generations and may result in mutagenesis or carcinogenesis. Some methylating agents, such as procarbazine, are highly carcinogenic.

Adduct recognition systems and DNA repair systems play important roles in removing adducts, and thereby determine the selectivity of action against particular cell types and the acquisition of resistance to alkylating agents. Alkylation of a single strand of DNA (mono-adducts) is repaired by the nucleotide excision repair pathway; the less frequent cross-links require participation of nonhomologous end joining, an error-prone pathway, or the error-free homologous recombination pathway. After drug infusion in humans, mono-adducts appear rapidly and peak within 2 h of drug exposure, while cross-links peak at 8 h. The $t_{1/2}$ for repair of adducts varies among normal tissues and tumors; in peripheral blood mononuclear cells, both mono-adducts and cross-links disappear with a $t_{1/2}$ of 12-16 h.

The repair process depends on the presence and accurate functioning of multiple proteins. Their absence or mutation, as in Fanconi anemia or ataxia telangiectasia, leads to extreme sensitivity to DNA cross-linking agents such as mitomycin, cisplatin, or classical alkylators. Other repair enzymes are specific for removing methyl and ethyl adducts from the O-6 of guanine (MGMT) and for repair of alkylation of the N-3 of adenine and N-7 of guanine (3-methyladenine-DNA glycosylase). High expression of MGMT protects cells from cytotoxic effects of nitrosoureas and methylating agents and confers drug resistance, while methylation and silencing of the gene in brain tumors are associated with clinical response to BCNU and temozolomide. Bendamustine differs from classical chloroethyl alkylators in activating base excision repair, rather than the more complex double-strand break repair or MGMT. It impairs physiological arrest of adduct-containing cells at mitotic checkpoints and leads to mitotic catastrophe rather than apoptosis, and does not require an intact p53 to cause cytotoxicity.

Recognition of DNA adducts is an essential step in promoting attempts at repair and ultimately leading to apoptosis. The Fanconi pathway, consisting of 12 proteins, recognizes adducts and signals the need for repair of a broad array of DNA-damaging drugs and irradiation. Absence or inactivation of components of this pathway leads to increased sensitivity to DNA damage. Conversely, for the methylating drugs, nitrosoureas, cisplatin and carboplatin, and thiopurine analogs, the mismatch repair (MMR) pathway is essential for cytotoxicity, causing strand breaks at sites of adduct formation, creating mispairing of thymine residues, and triggering apoptosis.

Mechanisms of Resistance to Alkylating Agents. Resistance to an alkylating agent develops rapidly when it is used as a single agent. Specific biochemical changes implicated in the development of resistance include:

- Decreased permeation of actively transported drugs (mechlorethamine and melphalan).
- Increased intracellular concentrations of nucleophilic substances, principally thiols such as glutathione, which can conjugate with and detoxify electrophilic intermediates.
- Increased activity of DNA repair pathways, which may differ for the various alkylating agents.
- Increased rates of metabolic degradation of the activated forms of cyclophosphamide and ifosfamide to their inactive keto and carboxy metabolites by aldehyde dehydrogenase (*see* Figure 61–2), and detoxification of most alkylating intermediates by glutathione transferases.
- Loss of ability to recognize adducts formed by nitrosoureas and methylating agents, as the result of defective mismatch repair (MMR) proteins capability, confers resistance, as does defective checkpoint function, for virtually all alkylating drugs.
- Impaired apoptotic pathways, with overexpression of bcl-2 as an example, confer resistance.

TOXICITIES OF ALKYLATING AGENTS

BONE MARROW. Alkylating agents differ in their patterns of antitumor activity and in the sites and severity of their side effects. Most cause dose-limiting toxicity to bone marrow elements and, to a lesser extent, intestinal mucosa. Most alkylating agents (i.e., melphalan, chlorambucil, cyclophosphamide, and ifosfamide) cause acute myelosuppression, with a nadir of the peripheral blood granulocyte count at 6-10 days and recovery in

Table 61–1

Dose-Limiting Extramedullary Toxicities of Single Alkylating Agents

DRUG	MTD[a] (mg/m²)	FOLD INCREASE OVER STANDARD DOSE	MAJOR ORGAN TOXICITIES
Cyclophosphamide	7000	7	Cardiac, hepatic VOD
Ifosfamide	16,000	2.7	Renal, CNS, hepatic VOD
Thiotepa	1000	18	GI, CNS, hepatic VOD
Melphalan	180	5.6	GI, hepatic VOD
Busulfan	640	9	GI, hepatic VOD
Carmustine (BCNU)	1050	5.3	Lung, hepatic VOD
Cisplatin	200	2	PN, renal
Carboplatin	2000	5	Renal, PN, hepatic VOD

CNS, central nervous system; GI, gastrointestinal; PN, peripheral neuropathy; VOD, veno-occlusive disease.
[a]Maximum tolerated dose (MTD; cumulative) in treatment protocols.

14-21 days. Cyclophosphamide has lesser effects on peripheral blood platelet counts than do the other agents. Busulfan suppresses all blood elements, particularly stem cells, and may produce a prolonged and cumulative myelosuppression lasting months or even years. For this reason, it is used as a preparative regimen in allogenic bone marrow transplantation. Carmustine and other chloroethylnitrosoureas cause delayed and prolonged suppression of both platelets and granulocytes, reaching a nadir 4-6 weeks after drug administration and reversing slowly thereafter. Both cellular and humoral immunity are suppressed by alkylating agents, which have been used to treat various autoimmune diseases. Immunosuppression is reversible at usual doses, but opportunistic infections may occur with extended treatment.

MUCOSA. Alkylating agents are highly toxic to dividing mucosal cells and to hair follicles, leading to oral mucosal ulceration, intestinal denudation, and alopecia. Mucosal effects are particularly damaging in high-dose chemotherapy protocols associated with bone marrow reconstitution, as they predispose to bacterial sepsis arising from the GI tract. In these protocols, cyclophosphamide, melphalan, and thiotepa have the advantage of causing less mucosal damage than the other agents. In high-dose protocols, however, other toxicities become limiting (Table 61–1).

NERVOUS SYSTEM. Nausea and vomiting commonly follow agent administration of nitrogen mustard or BCNU. Ifosfamide is the most neurotoxic agent of this class and may produce altered mental status, coma, generalized seizures, and cerebellar ataxia. These side effects result from the release of chloroacetaldehyde from the phosphate-linked chloroethyl side chain of ifosfamide. High-dose busulfan can cause seizures; in addition, it accelerates the clearance of phenytoin, an antiseizure medication.

OTHER ORGANS. All alkylating agents, including temozolomide, have caused pulmonary fibrosis, usually several months after treatment. In high-dose regimens, particularly those employing busulfan or BCNU, vascular endothelial damage may precipitate veno-occlusive disease (VOD) of the liver, an often fatal side effect that is successfully reversed by the investigational drug defibrotide. The nitrosoureas and ifosfamide, after multiple cycles of therapy, may lead to renal failure. Cyclophosphamide and ifosfamide release a nephrotoxic and urotoxic metabolite, acrolein, which causes a severe hemorrhagic cystitis in high-dose regimens. This adverse effect can be prevented by coadministration of 2-mercaptoethanesulfonate (mesna [MESNEX]), which conjugates acrolein in urine. Ifosfamide in high doses for transplant causes a chronic, and often irreversible, renal toxicity. Nephrotoxicity correlates with the total dose of drug received and increases in frequency in children <5 years of age. The syndrome may be due to chloroacetaldehyde and/or acrolein excreted in the urine.

The more unstable alkylating agents (e.g., mechlorethamine and the nitrosoureas) have strong vesicant properties, damage veins with repeated use and, if extravasated, produce ulceration. All alkylating agents have toxic effects on the male and female reproductive systems, causing an often permanent amenorrhea, particularly in perimenopausal women, and an irreversible azoospermia in men.

Leukemogenesis. Alkylating agents are highly leukemogenic. Acute nonlymphocytic leukemia, often associated with partial or total deletions of chromosome 5 or 7, peaks in incidence ~4 years after therapy and may affect up to 5% of patients treated on regimens containing alkylating drugs. Leukemia often is preceded by a period of neutropenia or anemia and by bone marrow morphology consistent with myelodysplasia. Melphalan, the nitrosoureas, and the methylating agent procarbazine have the greatest propensity to cause leukemia, while it is less common after cyclophosphamide.

MECHLORETHAMINE

Mechlorethamine HCl (MUSTARGEN) was the first clinically used nitrogen mustard and is the most reactive of the drugs in this class. It is used topically for treatment of cutaneous T-cell lymphoma (CTCL) as a solution that is rapidly mixed and applied to affected areas. It has been largely replaced by cyclophosphamide, melphalan, and other, more stable alkylating agents.

Severe local reactions of exposed tissues necessitate rapid intravenous injection of mechlorethamine for most uses. Mechlorethamine, rapidly and within minutes, undergoes chemical degradation (affected markedly by pH) as it combines with either water or cellular nucleophiles. The major acute toxic manifestations of mechlorethamine are nausea and vomiting, lacrimation, and myelosuppression. Leukopenia and thrombocytopenia limit the amount of drug that can be given in a single course.

CYCLOPHOSPHAMIDE

ADME. Cyclophosphamide is well absorbed orally and is activated to the 4-hydroxy intermediate (*see* Figure 61–2). Its rate of metabolic activation exhibits significant interpatient variability and increases with successive doses in high-dose regimens but appears to be saturable at infusion rates of >4 g/90 min and concentrations of the parent compound >150 μM. 4-Hydroxycyclophosphamide may be oxidized further by aldehyde oxidase, either in liver or in tumor tissue, to inactive metabolites. The hydroxyl metabolite of ifosfamide similarly is inactivated by aldehyde dehydrogenase. 4-Hydroxycyclophosphamide and its tautomer, aldophosphamide, travel in the circulation to tumor cells where aldophosphamide cleaves spontaneously, generating stoichiometric amounts of phosphoramide mustard and acrolein. Phosphoramide mustard is responsible for antitumor effects, while acrolein causes hemorrhagic cystitis often seen during therapy with cyclophosphamide. Patients should receive vigorous intravenous hydration during high-dose treatment. Brisk hematuria in a patient receiving daily oral therapy should lead to immediate drug discontinuation. Refractory bladder hemorrhage can become life-threatening and may require cystectomy for control of bleeding. Inappropriate secretion of antidiuretic hormone has been observed, usually at doses >50 mg/kg (*see* Chapter 25). It is important to be aware of the possibility of water intoxication, because these patients usually are vigorously hydrated.

Pretreatment with CYP inducers such as phenobarbital enhances the rate of activation of the azoxyphosphorenes but does not alter total exposure to active metabolites over time and does not affect toxicity or efficacy. Cyclophosphamide can be used in full doses in patients with renal dysfunction, because it is eliminated by hepatic metabolism. Patients with significant hepatic dysfunction (bilirubin <3 mg/dL) should receive reduced doses. Maximal C_P is achieved 1 hour after oral administration; the $t_{1/2}$ of parent drug in plasma is ~7 h.

Therapeutic Uses. Cyclophosphamide (LYOPHILIZED CYTOXAN) is administered orally or intravenously. Recommended doses vary widely, and standard protocols for determining the schedule and dose of cyclophosphamide in combination with other chemotherapeutic agents should be consulted. As a single agent, a daily oral dose of 100 mg/m^2 for 14 days has been recommended for patients with lymphomas and CLL. Higher doses of 500 mg/m^2 intravenously every 2-4 weeks are used in combination with other drugs in the treatment of breast cancer and lymphomas. The neutrophil nadir of 500-1000 cells/mm^3 generally serves as a lower limit for dosage adjustments in prolonged therapy. In regimens associated with bone marrow or peripheral stem cell rescue, cyclophosphamide may be given in total doses of 5-7 g/m^2 over a 3-5-day period. GI ulceration, cystitis (counteracted by mesna and diuresis), and, less commonly, pulmonary, renal, hepatic, and cardiac toxicities (hemorrhagic myocardial necrosis) may occur after high-dose therapy with total doses >200 mg/kg.

The clinical spectrum of activity for cyclophosphamide is very broad. It is an essential component of many effective drug combinations for non-Hodgkin lymphomas, other lymphoid malignancies, breast and ovarian cancers, and solid tumors in children. Complete remissions and presumed cures have been reported when cyclophosphamide was given as a single agent for Burkitt lymphoma. It frequently is used in combination with doxorubicin and a taxane as adjuvant therapy after surgery for breast cancer. Because of its potent immunosuppressive properties, cyclophosphamide has been used to treat autoimmune disorders, including Wegener granulomatosis, rheumatoid arthritis, and the nephrotic syndrome. Caution is advised when the drug is considered for non-neoplastic conditions, not only because of its acute toxic effects but also because of its potential for inducing sterility, teratogenic effects, and leukemia.

IFOSFAMIDE

Ifosfamide (IFEX, others) is an analog of cyclophosphamide. Severe urinary tract and CNS toxicity initially limited the use of ifosfamide, but adequate hydration and coadministration of mesna have reduced its bladder toxicity.

Therapeutic Uses. Ifosfamide is approved for treatment of relapsed germ cell testicular cancer and is frequently used for first-time treatment of pediatric and adult sarcomas. It is a common component of high-dose chemotherapy regimens with bone marrow or stem cell rescue; in these regimens, in total doses of 12-14 g/m^2, it may cause severe neurological toxicity, including hallucinations, coma, and death, with symptoms appearing 12 h to 7 days after beginning the ifosfamide infusion. This toxicity may result from a metabolite, chloroacetaldehyde. Ifosfamide also causes nausea, vomiting, anorexia, leukopenia, nephrotoxicity, and VOD of the liver. In nonmyeloablative regimens, ifosfamide is infused intravenously over at least 30 min at a dose of ≤1.2 g/m^2/day for 5 days. Intravenous mesna is given as bolus injections in a dose equal to 20% of the ifosfamide dose concomitantly and an additional 20% again 4 and 8 h later, for a total mesna dose of 60% of the ifosfamide dose. Alternatively, mesna may be given concomitantly in a single dose equal to the ifosfamide dose. Patients also should receive at least 2 L of oral or intravenous fluid daily. Treatment cycles are repeated every 3-4 weeks.

Pharmacokinetics. Ifosfamide has a plasma elimination $t_{1/2}$ ~1.5 h after doses of 3.8-5 g/m^2 and a somewhat shorter $t_{1/2}$ at lower doses; its pharmacokinetics are highly variable due to variable rates of hepatic metabolism (*see* legend to Figure 61–2).

Toxicity. Ifosfamide has virtually the same toxicity profile as cyclophosphamide, although it causes greater platelet suppression, neurotoxicity, nephrotoxicity, and in the absence of mesna, urothelial damage.

MELPHALAN

This alkylating agent primarily is used to treat multiple myeloma and, less commonly, in high-dose chemotherapy with marrow transplantation. The general pharmacological and cytotoxic actions of melphalan are similar to those of other bifunctional alkylators. The drug is not a vesicant.

ADME. Oral melphalan is absorbed in an inconsistent manner and, for most indications, is given as an intravenous infusion. The drug has a plasma $t_{1/2}$ ~45-90 min; 10-15% of an administered dose is excreted unchanged in the urine. Patients with decreased renal function may develop unexpectedly severe myelosuppression.

Therapeutic Uses. Melphalan (ALKERAN) for multiple myeloma is given in doses of 4-10 mg orally for 4-7 days every 28 days, with dexamethasone or thalidomide. Treatment is repeated at 4-week intervals based on response and tolerance. Dosage adjustments should be based on blood cell counts. Melphalan also may be used in myeloablative regimens followed by bone marrow or peripheral blood stem cell reconstitution, at a dose of 180-200 mg/m^2. The toxicity of melphalan is mostly hematological and is similar to that of other alkylating agents. Nausea and vomiting are less frequent. The drug causes less alopecia and, rarely, renal or hepatic dysfunction.

CHLORAMBUCIL

The cytotoxic effects of chlorambucil on the bone marrow, lymphoid organs, and epithelial tissues are similar to those observed with other nitrogen mustards. As an orally administered agent, chlorambucil is well tolerated in small daily doses and provides flexible titration of blood counts. Nausea and vomiting may result from single oral doses of ≥20 mg.

ADME. Oral absorption of chlorambucil is adequate and reliable. The drug has a $t_{1/2}$ in plasma of ~1.5 h and is hydrolyzed to inactive products.

Therapeutic Uses. Chlorambucil is almost exclusively used in treating CLL, for which it has largely been replaced by fludarabine and cyclophosphamide. In treating CLL, the initial daily dose of chlorambucil (LEUKERAN) is 0.1-0.2 mg/kg, given once daily and continued for 3-6 weeks. With a fall in the peripheral total leukocyte count or clinical improvement, the dosage is titrated to maintain neutrophils and platelets at acceptable levels. Maintenance therapy (usually 2 mg daily) often is required to maintain clinical response. Chlorambucil treatment may continue for months or years, achieving its effects gradually and often without significant toxicity to a compromised bone marrow. Marked hypoplasia of the bone marrow may be induced with excessive doses, but the myelosuppressive effects are moderate, gradual, and rapidly reversible. GI discomfort, azoospermia, amenorrhea, pulmonary fibrosis, seizures, dermatitis, and hepatotoxicity rarely may be encountered. A marked increase in the incidence of acute myelocytic leukemia (AML) and other tumors was noted in the treatment of polycythemia vera and in patients with breast cancer receiving chlorambucil as adjuvant chemotherapy.

BENDAMUSTINE

This drug is approved for treatment of CLL and non-Hodgkin lymphoma. Bendamustine is given as a 30-min intravenous infusion in dosages of 100 mg/m^2/day on days 1 and 2 of a 28-day cycle. Lower doses may be indicated in heavily pretreated patients. Bendamustine is rapidly degraded through sulfhydryl interaction and adduct formation with macromolecules; <5% of the parent drug is excreted in the urine intact. *N*-demethylation and oxidation produces metabolites that have antitumor activity, but less than that of the parent molecule. The parent drug has a plasma $t_{1/2}$ ~30 min. The clinical toxicity pattern of bendamustine is typical of alkylators, with a rapidly reversible myelosuppression and mucositis, both generally tolerable.

Although nitrogen mustards containing chloroethyl groups constitute the most widely used class of alkylating agents, alternative alkylators with greater chemical stability and well-defined activity in specific types of cancer have value in clinical practice.

ETHYLENEIMINES AND METHYLMELAMINES

ALTRETAMINE

Altretamine (hexamethylmelamine [HEXALEN]) is structurally similar to TEM (tretamine). Its precise mechanism of cytotoxicity is unknown. It is a palliative treatment for persistent or recurrent ovarian cancer following cisplatin-based combination therapy. The usual dosage of altretamine as a single agent in ovarian cancer is 260 mg/m^2/day in 4 divided doses, for 14 or 21 consecutive days out of a 28-day cycle, for up to 12 cycles.

ADME. Altretamine is well absorbed from the GI tract; its elimination $t_{1/2}$ is 4-10 h. The drug undergoes rapid demethylation in the liver; the principal metabolites are pentamethylmelamine and tetramethyl melamine.

Clinical Toxicities. The main toxicities of altretamine are myelosuppression and neurotoxicity. Altretamine causes both peripheral and central neurotoxicity (ataxia, depression, confusion, drowsiness, hallucinations, dizziness, and vertigo). Neurological symptoms abate upon discontinuation of therapy. Peripheral blood counts and a neurological examination should be performed prior to the initiation of each course of therapy. Therapy should be interrupted for at least 14 days and subsequently restarted at a lower dosage of 200 mg/m^2/day if the white cell count falls to <2000 cells/mm^3 or the platelet count falls to <75,000 cells/mm^3 or if neurotoxic or intolerable GI symptoms occur. If neurological symptoms fail to stabilize on the reduced-dose schedule, altretamine should be discontinued. Nausea and vomiting also are common side effects and may be dose limiting. Renal dysfunction may necessitate discontinuing the drug. Other rare adverse effects include rashes, alopecia, and hepatic toxicity. Severe, life-threatening orthostatic hypotension may develop in patients who receive MAO-inhibitors, amitriptyline, imipramine, or phenelzine concurrently with altretamine.

THIOTEPA

Thiotepa (THIOPLEX, others) consists of 3 ethyleneimine groups stabilized by attachment to the nucleophilic thiophosphoryl base. Its current use is primarily for high-dose chemotherapy regimens. Both thiotepa and its desulfurated primary metabolite, triethylenephosphoramide (TEPA), to which it is rapidly converted by hepatic CYPs, form DNA cross-links.

ADME. TEPA becomes the predominant form of the drug present in plasma within hours of thiotepa administration. The parent compound has a plasma $t_{1/2}$ of 1.2-2 h, TEPA has a longer $t_{1/2}$, 3-24 h. Thiotepa pharmacokinetics essentially are the same in children as in adults at conventional doses (≤80 mg/m^2), and drug and metabolite $t_{1/2}$ are unchanged in children receiving high-dose therapy of 300 mg/m^2/day for 3 days. Less than 10% of the administered drug appears in urine as the parent drug or the primary metabolite.

Clinical Toxicities. Toxicities include myelosuppression and, to a lesser extent, mucositis. Myelosuppression tends to develop somewhat later than with cyclophosphamide, with leukopenic nadirs at 2 weeks and platelet nadirs at 3 weeks. In high-doses, thiotepa may cause neurotoxic symptoms, including coma and seizures.

ALKYL SULFONATES

BUSULFAN

Busulfan (MYLERAN, BUSULFEX) exerts few pharmacological actions other than myelosuppression at conventional doses and, prior to the advent of imatinib mesylate (GLEEVEC), was a standard agent for patients in the chronic phase of myelocytic leukemia and caused a severe and prolonged pancytopenia in some patients. Busulfan now is primarily used in high-dose regimens, in which pulmonary fibrosis, GI mucosal damage, and hepatic veno-occlusive disease (VOD) are important toxicities.

ADME. Busulfan is well absorbed after oral administration in dosages of 2-6 mg/day and has a plasma $t_{1/2}$ of 2-3 h. The drug is conjugated to GSH by GSTA1A and further metabolized by CYP-dependent pathways; its major urinary metabolite is methane sulfonic acid. In high doses, children <18 years of age clear the drug 2-4 times faster than adults and tolerate higher doses. Busulfan clearance varies considerably among patients. VOD is associated with high area under the curve (AUC) (AUC >1500 μM × min) peak drug levels and slow clearance, leading to recommendations for dose adjustment based on drug level monitoring. A target steady-state concentration of 600-900 ng/mL in plasma in adults or AUC <1000 μM × min in children achieves an appropriate balance between toxicity and therapeutic benefit.

Therapeutic Uses. In treating chronic myelogenous leukemia (CML), the initial oral dose of busulfan varies with the total leukocyte count and the severity of the disease; daily doses of 2-8 mg for adults (~60 μg/kg or

1.8 mg/m^2 for children) are used to initiate therapy and are adjusted appropriately to subsequent hematological and clinical responses, with the aim of reducing the total leukocyte count to ≤10,000 cells/mm^3. A decrease in the leukocyte count usually is not seen during the first 10-15 days of treatment, and the leukocyte count may actually increase during this period. Because the leukocyte count may fall for >1 month after discontinuing the drug, it is recommended that busulfan be withdrawn when the total leukocyte count has declined to ~15,000 cells/mm^3. A normal leukocyte count usually is achieved within 12-20 weeks. During remission, daily treatment resumes when the total leukocyte count reaches ~50,000 cells/mm^3. Daily maintenance doses are 1-3 mg.

In high-dose therapy, doses of 1 mg/kg are given every 6 h for 4 days, with adjustment based on pharmacokinetics. Anticonvulsants must be used concomitantly to protect against acute CNS toxicities, including tonic-clonic seizures that may occur several hours after each dose. Although phenytoin is a frequent choice, phenytoin induces the GSTs that metabolize busulfan, reducing its AUC by ~20%. In patients requiring concomitant anti-seizure medication, non-enzyme-inducing benzodiazepines such as lorazepam and clonazepam are recommended as an alternative to phenytoin. If phenytoin is used concurrently, plasma busulfan levels should be monitored and the busulfan dose adjusted accordingly.

Clinical Toxicity. The toxic effects of busulfan are related to its myelosuppressive properties; prolonged thrombocytopenia may occur. Occasionally, patients experience nausea, vomiting, and diarrhea. Long-term use leads to impotence, sterility, amenorrhea, and fetal malformation. Rarely, patients develop asthenia and hypotension. High-dose busulfan causes VOD of the liver in ≤10% of patients, as well as seizures, hemorrhagic cystitis, permanent alopecia, and cataracts. The coincidence of VOD and hepatotoxicity is increased by its coadministration with drugs that inhibit CYPs, including imidazoles and metronidazole, possibly through inhibition of the clearance of busulfan and/or its toxic metabolites.

NITROSOUREAS

The nitrosoureas have an important role in the treatment of brain tumors and find occasional use in treating lymphomas and in high-dose regimens with bone marrow reconstitution. They function as bifunctional alkylating agents but differ from conventional nitrogen mustards in both pharmacological and toxicological properties.

Carmustine (BCNU) and lomustine (CCNU) are highly lipophilic and thus readily cross the blood-brain barrier, an important property in the treatment of brain tumors. Unfortunately, with the exception of streptozocin, nitrosoureas cause profound and delayed myelosuppression with recovery 4-6 weeks after a single dose. Long-term treatment with the nitrosoureas, especially semustine (methyl-CCNU), has resulted in renal failure. As with other alkylating agents, the nitrosoureas are highly carcinogenic and mutagenic. They generate both alkylating and carbamylating moieties (*see* Figure 61–3).

CARMUSTINE (BCNU)

Carmustine's major action is its alkylation of DNA at the O^6-guanine position, an adduct repaired by MGMT. Methylation of the MGMT promoter inhibits its expression in ~30% of primary gliomas and is associated with sensitivity to nitrosoureas. In high doses with bone marrow rescue, carmustine produces hepatic VOD, pulmonary fibrosis, renal failure, and secondary leukemia.

ADME. Carmustine is unstable in aqueous solution and in body fluids. After intravenous infusion, it disappears from the plasma with a highly variable $t_{1/2}$ of ≥15-90 min. Approximately 30-80% of the drug appears in the urine within 24 h as degradation products. The alkylating metabolites enter rapidly into the cerebrospinal fluid (CSF), and their concentrations in the CSF reach 15-30% of the concurrent plasma values.

Therapeutic Uses. Carmustine (BiCNU) is administered intravenously at doses of 150-200 mg/m^2, given by infusion over 1-2 h and repeated every 6 weeks. Because of its ability to cross the blood-brain barrier, carmustine has been used in the treatment of malignant gliomas. An implantable carmustine wafer (GLIADEL) is available for use as an adjunct to surgery and radiation in newly diagnosed high-grade malignant glioma patients and as an adjunct to surgery for recurrent glioblastoma multiforme.

STREPTOZOCIN

Streptozocin (or streptozotocin) has a methylnitrosourea (MNU) moiety attached to the 2-carbon of glucose. It has a high affinity for cells of the islets of Langerhans and causes diabetes in experimental animals.

ADME. Streptozocin is rapidly degraded following intravenous administration. The $t_{1/2}$ of the drug is ~15 min. Only 10-20% of a dose is recovered intact in the urine.

Therapeutic Uses. Streptozocin (ZANOSAR) is used in the treatment of human pancreatic islet cell carcinoma and malignant carcinoid tumors. It is administered intravenously, 500 mg/m^2 once daily for 5 days; this course is repeated every 6 weeks. Alternatively, 1000 mg/m^2 can be given weekly for 2 weeks, and the weekly dose then can be increased to a maximum of 1500 mg/m² as tolerated. Nausea is frequent. Mild, reversible renal or hepatic toxicity occurs in approximately two-thirds of cases; in <10% of patients, renal toxicity may be cumulative with each dose and may lead to irreversible renal failure. Streptozocin should not be given with other nephrotoxic drugs. Hematological toxicities (anemia, leukopenia, thrombocytopenia) occur in 20% of patients.

TRIAZENES

DACARBAZINE (DTIC)

Dacarbazine functions as a methylating agent after metabolic activation to the monomethyl triazeno metabolite, MTIC. It kills cells in all phases of the cell cycle. Resistance has been ascribed to the removal of methyl groups from the O^6-guanine bases in DNA by MGMT.

ADME. Dacarbazine is administered intravenously. After an initial rapid phase ($t_{1/2}$ of ~20 min), dacarbazine is cleared from plasma with a terminal $t_{1/2}$ of ~5 h. The $t_{1/2}$ is prolonged in the presence of hepatic or renal disease. Almost 50% of the compound is excreted intact in the urine by tubular secretion.

Therapeutic Uses. The primary clinical indication for dacarbazine (DTIC-DOME) is in the chemotherapy of Hodgkin disease. In combination with other drugs for Hodgkin disease, dacarbazine is given in dosages of 150 mg/m²/day for 5 days, repeated every 4 weeks; it can be used alone as a single dose of 375 mg/m², repeated every 15 days. It is modestly effective against malignant melanoma and adult sarcomas. Dacarbazine (DTIC-DOME) for malignant melanoma is given in dosages of 2-4.5 mg/kg/day for a 10-day period, repeated every 28 days; alternatively, 250 mg/m² can be given daily for 5 days and repeated every 3 weeks. Extravasation of the drug may cause tissue damage and severe pain.

Toxicity. DTIC induces nausea and vomiting in >90% of patients; vomiting usually develops 1-3 h after treatment and may last up to 12 h. Myelosuppression, with both leukopenia and thrombocytopenia, is mild and readily reversible within 1-2 weeks. A flu-like syndrome may occur. Hepatotoxicity, alopecia, facial flushing, neurotoxicity, and dermatological reactions are less common adverse effects.

TEMOZOLOMIDE

Temozolomide (TEMODAR) is the standard agent in combination with radiation therapy for patients with malignant glioma and for astrocytoma. Temozolomide, like dacarbazine, forms the methylating metabolite MTIC and kills cells in all phases of the cell cycle.

ADME. Temozolomide is administered orally or intravenously in dosages of ~200 mg/day; it has a bioavailability approaching 100%. Plasma levels of the parent drug decline with a $t_{1/2}$ of 1-2 h. The primary active metabolite MTIC reaches a maximum plasma concentration (150 ng/mL) 90 min after a dose and declines with a $t_{1/2}$ of 2 h. Little intact drug is recovered in the urine, the primary urinary metabolite being the inactive imidazole carboxamide.

Toxicity. The toxicities of temozolomide mirror those of DTIC. Hematological monitoring is necessary to guide dosing adjustments.

METHYLHYDRAZINES

PROCARBAZINE

Procarbazine is employed for second-line therapy in malignant brain tumors.

Cytotoxic Action. The antineoplastic activity of procarbazine results from its conversion by CYP-mediated hepatic oxidative metabolism to highly reactive alkylating species that methylate DNA. Activated procarbazine can produce chromosomal damage, including chromatid breaks and translocations, consistent with its mutagenic and carcinogenic actions. Resistance to procarbazine develops rapidly when it is used as a single agent; one mechanism of resistance results from increased expression of MGMT, which repairs methylation of guanine.

Pharmacokinetics. The pharmacokinetic behavior of procarbazine has not yet been thoroughly defined. The drug is extensively metabolized by CYP isoenzymes to azo, methylazoxy, and benzylazoxy intermediates, which are found in the plasma and yield the alkylating metabolites in tumor cells. In brain cancer patients, the concurrent use of anti-seizure drugs that induce hepatic CYPs does not significantly alter the pharmacokinetics of the parent drug.

Therapeutic Uses. The recommended dosage of procarbazine (MATULANE) for adults is 100 mg/m²/day for 10-14 days in combination regimens such as MOPP (nitrogen mustard, Oncovin, procarbazine, and prednisone) for Hodgkin disease. The drug rarely is used in current practice.

Toxicity. The most common toxic effects include leukopenia and thrombocytopenia, which begin during the second week of therapy and reverse within 2 weeks off treatment. GI symptoms such as mild nausea and vomiting occur in most patients; diarrhea and rash are noted in 5-10% of cases. Behavioral disturbances also have been reported. Because procarbazine augments sedative effects, the concomitant use of CNS depressants should be avoided. The drug is a weak MAO inhibitor; it blocks the metabolism of catecholamines, sympathomimetics, and dietary tyramine and may provoke hypertension in patients concurrently exposed to these. Procarbazine has disulfiram-like actions, and therefore the ingestion of alcohol should be avoided. The drug is highly carcinogenic, mutagenic, and teratogenic and is associated with a 5-10% risk of acute leukemia in patients treated with MOPP. The highest risk is for patients who also receive radiation therapy. Procarbazine is a potent immunosuppressive agent. It causes infertility, particularly in males.

PLATINUM COORDINATION COMPLEXES

Platinum coordination complexes have broad antineoplastic activity and have become the foundation for treatment of ovarian, head and neck, bladder, esophagus, lung, and colon cancers. Although cisplatin and other platinum complexes do not form carbonium ion intermediates like other alkylating agents or formally alkylate DNA, they covalently bind to nucleophilic sites on DNA and share many pharmacological attributes with alkylators.

MECHANISM OF ACTION. Cisplatin, carboplatin, and oxaliplatin enter cells by an active Cu^{2+} transporter, CTR1, and in doing so rapidly degrade the transporter. The compounds are actively extruded from cells by ATP7A and ATP7B copper transporters and by multidrug resistance protein 1 (MRP1); variable expression of these transporters may contribute to clinical resistance. Inside the cell, the chloride, cyclohexane, or oxalate ligands of the analogs are displaced by water molecules, yielding a positively charged molecule that reacts with nucleophilic sites on DNA and proteins.

Aquation of cisplatin is favored at the low concentrations of Cl^- inside the cell and in the urine. High concentrations of Cl^- stabilize the drug, explaining the effectiveness of Cl^- diuresis in preventing nephrotoxicity. The activated platinum complexes can react with electron-rich regions, such as sulfhydryls, and with various sites on DNA, forming both intrastrand and interstrand cross-links. The DNA-platinum adducts inhibit replication and transcription, lead to single- and double-stranded breaks and miscoding, and if recognized by p53 and other checkpoint proteins, cause induction of apoptosis. Adduct formation is an important predictor of clinical response. The analogs differ in the conformation of their adducts and the effects of adduct on DNA structure and function. Oxaliplatin and carboplatin are slower to form adducts. The oxaliplatin adducts are bulkier and less readily repaired, create a different pattern of distortion of the DNA helix, and differ from cisplatin adducts in the pattern of hydrogen bonding to adjacent segments of DNA.

Unlike the other platinum analogs, oxaliplatin exhibits a cytotoxicity that does not depend on an active MMR system, which may explain its greater activity in colorectal cancer. It also seems less dependent on the presence of high mobility group (HMG) proteins that are required by the other platinum derivatives. Testicular cancers have a high concentration of HMG proteins and are quite sensitive to cisplatin. Basal-type breast cancers, such as those with *BRCA1* and *BRCA2* mutations, lack *Her 2* amplification and hormone-receptor expression and appear to be uniquely susceptible to cisplatin through their upregulation of apoptotic pathways governed by p63 and p73. The cell cycle specificity of cisplatin differs among cell types; the effects of cross-linking are most pronounced during the S phase. The platinum analogs are mutagenic, teratogenic, and carcinogenic. Cisplatin- or carboplatin-based chemotherapy for ovarian cancer is associated with a 4-fold increased risk of developing secondary leukemia.

Resistance to Platinum Analogs. Resistance to the platinum analogs likely is multifactorial; the compounds differ in their degree of cross-resistance. Carboplatin shares cross-resistance with cisplatin in most experimental tumors, while oxaliplatin does not. A number of factors influence sensitivity to platinum analogs in experimental cells, including intracellular drug accumulation and intracellular levels of glutathione and other sulfhydryls such as metallothionein that bind to and inactivate the drug and rates of repair of DNA adducts. Repair of platinum-DNA adducts requires participation of the NER pathway. Inhibition or loss of NER increases sensitivity to cisplatin in ovarian cancer patients, while overexpression of NER components is associated with poor response to cisplatin or oxaliplatin-based therapy in lung, colon, and gastric cancer.

Resistance to cisplatin, but not oxaliplatin, appears to be partly mediated through loss of function in the MMR proteins. In the absence of effective repair of DNA-platinum adducts, sensitive cells cannot replicate or transcribe affected portions of the DNA strand. Some DNA polymerases can bypass adducts, possibly contributing to resistance. Overexpression of copper efflux transporters, ATP7A and ATP7B, correlates with poor survival after cisplatin-based therapy for ovarian cancer.

CISPLATIN

ADME. After intravenous administration, cisplatin has an initial plasma elimination $t_{1/2}$ of 25-50 min; concentrations of total (bound and unbound) drug fall thereafter, with a $t_{1/2}$ of ≥24 h. More than 90% of the platinum in the blood is covalently bound to plasma proteins. High concentrations of cisplatin are found in the kidney, liver, intestine, and testes; cisplatin penetrates poorly into the CNS. Only a small portion of the drug is excreted by the kidney during the first 6 h; by 24 h, up to 25% is excreted, and by 5 days, up to 43% of the administered dose is recovered in the urine, mostly covalently bound to protein and peptides. Biliary or intestinal excretion of cisplatin is minimal.

Therapeutic Uses. Cisplatin (PLATINOL) is given only intravenously. The usual dosage is 20 mg/m^2/day for 5 days, 20-30 mg weekly for 3-4 weeks, or 100 mg/m^2 given once every 4 weeks. *To prevent renal toxicity, it is important to establish a chloride diuresis by the infusion of 1-2 L of normal saline prior to treatment.* The appropriate amount of cisplatin then is diluted in a solution containing dextrose, saline, and mannitol and administered intravenously over 4-6 h. Because aluminum inactivates cisplatin, the drug should not come in contact with needles or other infusion equipment that contain aluminum during its preparation or administration.

Cisplatin, in combination with bleomycin, etoposide, ifosfamide, or vinblastine, cures 90% of patients with testicular cancer. Used with paclitaxel, cisplatin or carboplatin induces complete response in the majority of patients with carcinoma of the ovary. Cisplatin produces responses in cancers of the bladder, head and neck, cervix, and endometrium; all forms of carcinoma of the lung; anal and rectal carcinomas; and neoplasms of childhood. The drug also sensitizes cells to radiation therapy and enhances control of locally advanced lung, esophageal, and head and neck tumors when given with irradiation.

TOXICITY. Cisplatin-induced nephrotoxicity has been largely abrogated by adequate pretreatment hydration and chloride diuresis. Amifostine (ETHYOL), a thiophosphate cytoprotective agent, reduces renal toxicity associated with repeated administration of cisplatin. Ototoxicity caused by cisplatin is unaffected by diuresis and is manifested by tinnitus and high-frequency hearing loss. Marked nausea and vomiting occur in almost all patients and usually can be controlled with $5HT_3$ antagonists, NK1-receptor antagonists, and high-dose corticosteroids (*see* Table 46–6).

At higher doses or after multiple cycles of treatment, cisplatin causes a progressive peripheral motor and sensory neuropathy that may worsen after discontinuation of the drug and may be aggravated by subsequent or simultaneous treatment with taxanes or other neurotoxic drugs. Cisplatin causes mild to moderate myelosuppression, with transient leukopenia and thrombocytopenia. Anemia may become prominent after multiple cycles of treatment. Electrolyte disturbances, including hypomagnesemia, hypocalcemia, hypokalemia, and hypophosphatemia, are common. Hypocalcemia and hypomagnesemia secondary to tubular damage and renal electrolyte wasting may produce tetany if untreated. Routine measurement of Mg^{2+} concentrations in plasma is recommended. Hyperuricemia, hemolytic anemia, and cardiac abnormalities are rare side effects. Anaphylactic-like reactions, characterized by facial edema, bronchoconstriction, tachycardia, and hypotension, may occur within minutes after administration and should be treated by intravenous injection of epinephrine and with corticosteroids or anti-histamines. Cisplatin has been associated with the development of AML, usually ≥4 years after treatment.

CARBOPLATIN

The mechanisms of action and resistance and the spectrum of clinical activity of carboplatin (PARAPLATIN; CBDCA, JIM-8) are similar to cisplatin. However, the 2 drugs differ significantly in their chemical, pharmacokinetic, and toxicological properties.

ADME. Because carboplatin is much less reactive than cisplatin, the majority of drug in plasma remains in its parent form, unbound to proteins. Most drug is eliminated via renal excretion, with a $t_{1/2}$ ~2 h. A small fraction of platinum binds irreversibly to plasma proteins and disappears slowly, with a $t_{1/2}$ ≥5 days.

Therapeutic Uses. Carboplatin and cisplatin are equally effective in the treatment of suboptimally debulked ovarian cancer, non–small cell lung cancer, and extensive-stage small cell lung cancer; however, carboplatin may be less effective than cisplatin in germ cell, head and neck, and esophageal cancers. Carboplatin is an effective alternative for responsive tumors in patients unable to tolerate cisplatin because of impaired renal function, refractory nausea, significant hearing impairment, or neuropathy, but doses must be adjusted for renal function. In addition, it may be used in high-dose therapy with bone marrow or peripheral stem cell rescue. Carboplatin is administered as an intravenous infusion over at least 15 min and is given once every 21-28 days; the dose of carboplatin should be adjusted in proportion to the reduction in creatinine clearance (CrCl) for patients with a CrCl <60 mL/min.

Toxicity. Carboplatin is relatively well tolerated clinically, causing less nausea, neurotoxicity, ototoxicity, and nephrotoxicity than cisplatin. The dose-limiting toxicity of carboplatin is myelosuppression, primarily thrombocytopenia. It may cause a hypersensitivity reaction; in patients with a mild reaction, premedication, graded doses of drug, and more prolonged infusion lead to desensitization.

OXALIPLATIN

ADME. Oxaliplatin has a short $t_{1/2}$ in plasma, probably as a result of its rapid uptake by tissues and its reactivity; the initial $t_{1/2}$ ~17 min. No dose adjustment is required for hepatic dysfunction or for patients with a CrCl ≥20 mL/min.

Therapeutic Uses. Oxaliplatin exhibits a range of antitumor activity (colorectal and gastric cancer) that differs from other platinum agents. Oxaliplatin's effectiveness in colorectal cancer is perhaps due to its MMR- and HMG-independent effects. It also suppresses expression of thymidylate synthase (TS), the target enzyme of 5-fluorouracil (5-FU) action, which may promote synergy of these 2 drugs. In combination with 5-FU, it is approved for treatment of patients with colorectal cancer.

Toxicity. The dose-limiting toxicities of oxaliplatin are peripheral neuropathies. An acute form, often triggered by exposure to cold liquids, manifests as paresthesias and/or dysesthesias in the upper and lower extremities, mouth, and throat. A second type relates to cumulative dose and has features similar to cisplatin neuropathy; 75% of patients receiving a cumulative dose of 1560 mg/m^2 experience some progressive sensory neurotoxicity, with dysesthesias, ataxia, and numbness of the extremities. Hematological toxicity is mild to moderate, except for rare immune-mediated cytopenias; nausea is well controlled with $5HT_3$-receptor antagonists. Oxaliplatin causes leukemia and pulmonary fibrosis months to years after administration. Oxaliplatin may cause an acute allergic response with urticaria, hypotension, and bronchoconstriction.

II. Antimetabolites

FOLIC ACID ANALOGS

Folic acid is an essential dietary factor that is converted by enzymatic reduction to a series of tetrahydrofolate (FH_4) cofactors that provide methyl groups for the synthesis of precursors of DNA (thymidylate and purines) and RNA (purines). Interference with FH_4 metabolism reduces the cellular capacity for one-carbon transfer and the necessary methylation reactions in the synthesis of purine ribonucleotides and thymidine monophosphate (TMP), thereby inhibiting DNA replication.

Antifolate chemotherapy produced the first striking, although temporary, remissions in leukemia and the first cure of a solid tumor, choriocarcinoma. Recognition that methotrexate (MTX), an inhibitor of dihydrofolate reductase (DHFR), also directly inhibits the folate-dependent enzymes of de novo purine and thymidylate synthesis led to development of antifolate analogs that specifically target these other folate-dependent enzymes (Figure 61–4). New congeners have greater capacity for transport into tumor cells (pralatrexate) and exert their primary inhibitory effect on TS (raltitrexed, TOMUDEX), early steps in purine biosynthesis (lometrexol), or both (the multitargeted antifolate, pemetrexed, ALIMTA).

Mechanism of Action. The primary target of MTX is the enzyme DHFR (*see* Figure 61–4). To function as a cofactor in 1-carbon transfer reactions, folate must be reduced by DHFR to FH_4. Inhibitors such as MTX, with a high affinity for DHFR (K_i ~0.01-0.2 nM), cause partial depletion of the FH_4 cofactors (5-10 methylene tetrahydrofolic acid and N-10 formyl tetrahydrofolic acid) required for the synthesis of thymidylate and purines. In addition, MTX, like cellular folates, undergoes conversion to a series of polyglutamates (MTX-PGs) in both normal and tumor cells. These MTX-PGs constitute an intracellular storage form of folates and folate analogs and dramatically increase inhibitory potency of the analog for additional sites, including TS and 2 early enzymes in the purine biosynthetic pathway. The dihydrofolic acid polyglutamates that accumulate in cells behind the blocked DHFR reaction also act as inhibitors of TS and other enzymes (*see* Figure 61–4).

Selective Toxicity; Rescue. As with most antimetabolites, MTX is only partially selective for tumor cells and kills rapidly dividing normal cells, such as those of the intestinal epithelium and bone marrow. Folate antagonists kill cells during the S phase of the cell cycle and are most effective when cells are proliferating rapidly. The toxic effects of MTX may be terminated by administering leucovorin, a fully reduced folate coenzyme that repletes the intracellular pool of FH_4 cofactors.

Cellular Entry and Retention. Because folic acid and many of its analogs are polar, they cross the blood-brain barrier poorly and require specific transport mechanisms to enter mammalian cells. Three inward folate transport systems are found on mammalian cells: (1) a folate receptor, which has high affinity for folic acid but much reduced ability to transport MTX and other analogs; (2) the reduced folate transporter, the major transit protein for MTX, raltitrexed, pemetrexed, and most analogs; and (3) a transporter that is active at low pH. The reduced folate transporter is highly expressed in the hyperdiploid subtype of acute lymphoblastic leukemia (ALL), which has extreme sensitivity to MTX. Once in the cell, additional glutamyl residues are added to the molecule by the enzyme folylpolyglutamate synthetase. Because these higher polyglutamates are strongly charged and cross cellular membranes poorly, polyglutamation serves as a mechanism of entrapment and may account for the prolonged retention of MTX in chorionic epithelium (where it is a potent abortifacient); in tumors derived from this tissue, such as choriocarcinoma cells; and in normal tissues subject to cumulative drug toxicity, such as liver. Polyglutamyl folates and analogs have substantially greater affinity than the monoglutamate form for folate-dependent enzymes that are required for purine and thymidylate synthesis and have at least equal affinity for DHFR.

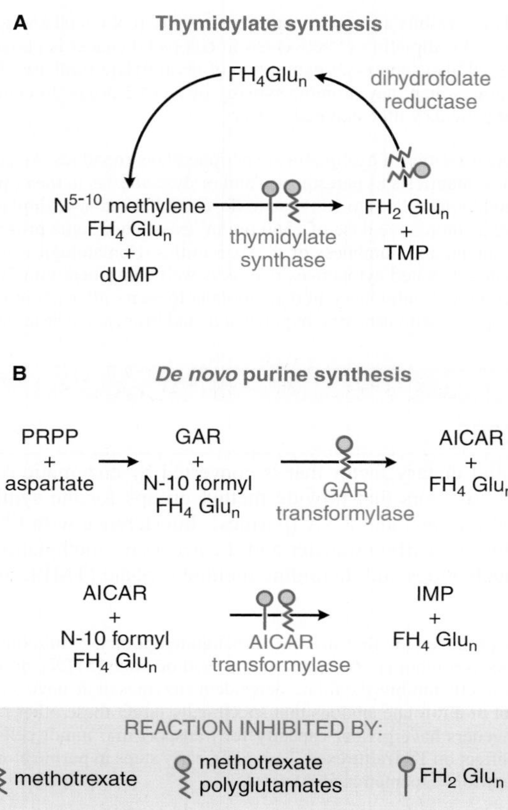

Figure 61–4 *Actions of methotrexate and its polyglutamates.* AICAR, aminoimidazole carboxamide; dUMP, deoxyuridine monophosphate; FH_2Glu_n/FH_4Glu_n, dihydro-/tetrahydro-folate polyglutamates; GAR, glycinamide ribonucleotide; IMP, inosine monophosphate; PRPP, 5-phosphoribosyl-1-pyrophosphate; TMP, thymidine monophosphate.

Newer Congeners. New folate antagonists that are better substrates for the reduced folate carrier have been identified. In efforts to bypass the obligatory membrane transport system and to facilitate penetration of the blood-brain barrier, lipid-soluble folate antagonists also have been synthesized. Trimetrexate (NEUTREXIN), a lipid-soluble analog that lacks a terminal glutamate, has modest antitumor activity, primarily in combination with leucovorin rescue. However, it is beneficial in the treatment of *Pneumocystis jiroveci* (*Pneumocystis carinii*) pneumonia where leucovorin provides differential rescue of the host but not the parasite. The most important new folate analog, MTA or pemetrexed (ALIMTA), is a pyrrole–pyrimidine structure. It is avidly transported into cells via the reduced folate carrier and is converted to polyglutamates that inhibit TS and glycine amide ribonucleotide transformylase, as well as DHFR. It has activity against ovarian cancer, mesothelioma, and non–small cell adenocarcinomas of the lung. Pemetrexed and its polyglutamates have a somewhat different spectrum of biochemical actions. Like MTX, pemetrexed inhibits DHFR, but as a polyglutamate, it even more potently inhibits glycinamide ribonucleotide formyltransferase (GART) and TS. Unlike MTX, it produces little change in the pool of reduced folates, indicating that the distal sites of inhibition (TS and GART) predominate. Its pattern of deoxynucleotide depletion also differs; it causes a greater fall in thymidine triphosphate (TTP) than in other triphosphates. Like MTX, it induces p53 and cell-cycle arrest, but this effect does not depend on induction of p21. A newer congener, pralatrexate, is more effectively taken up and polyglutamated than MTX and is approved for treatment of cutaneous T-cell lymphoma.

MECHANISMS OF RESISTANCE TO ANTIFOLATES. Resistance to MTX can involve alterations in each known step in MTX action, including:

- Impaired transport of MTX into cells
- Production of altered forms of DHFR that have decreased affinity for the inhibitor
- Increased concentrations of intracellular DHFR through gene amplification or altered gene regulation

- Decreased ability to synthesize MTX polyglutamates
- Increased expression of a drug efflux transporter of the MRP class (*see* Chapter 5)

DHFR levels in leukemic cells increase within 24 h after treatment of patients with MTX, probably as a result of induction of DHFR synthesis. Unbound DHFR protein may bind to its own message and reduce its own translation, while the DHFR-MTX complex is ineffective in blocking the DHFR translation. With longer periods of drug exposure, tumor cell populations that contain markedly increased levels of DHFR emerge. These cells contain multiple gene copies of DHFR either in mitotically unstable double-minute chromosomes (extrachromosomal elements) or in stably integrated, homogeneously staining chromosomal regions or amplicons. Similar gene amplification target proteins have been implicated in the resistance to many antitumor agents, including 5-FU and pentostatin (2′-deoxycoformycin).

High doses of MTX may permit entry of the drug into transport-defective cells and may permit the intracellular accumulation of MTX in concentrations that inactivate high levels of DHFR. The understanding of resistance to pemetrexed is incomplete. In various cell lines, resistance to this agent seems to arise from loss of influx transport, TS amplification, changes in purine biosynthetic pathways, or loss of polyglutamation.

ADME. MTX is readily absorbed from the GI tract at doses of <25 mg/m^2; larger doses are absorbed incompletely and are routinely administered intravenously. After intravenous administration, the drug disappears from plasma in a triphasic fashion. The rapid distribution phase is followed by a second phase, which reflects renal clearance ($t_{1/2}$ of ~2-3 h). A third phase has a $t_{1/2}$ of ~8-10 h. This terminal phase of disappearance, if unduly prolonged by renal failure, may be responsible for major toxic effects of the drug on the marrow, GI epithelium, and skin. Distribution of MTX into body spaces, such as the pleural or peritoneal cavity, occurs slowly. However, if such spaces are expanded (e.g., by ascites or pleural effusion), they may act as a site of storage and slow release of the drug, resulting in prolonged elevation of plasma concentrations and more severe bone marrow toxicity.

Approximately 50% of MTX binds to plasma proteins and may be displaced from plasma albumin by myriad agents (e.g., sulfonamides, salicylates, tetracycline, chloramphenicol, and phenytoin); caution should be used if these drugs are given concomitantly. Up to 90% of a given dose is excreted unchanged in the urine, mostly within the first 8-12 h. Metabolism of MTX usually is minimal. After high doses, however, metabolites are readily detectable; these include 7-hydroxy-MTX, which is potentially nephrotoxic. Renal excretion of MTX occurs through a combination of glomerular filtration and active tubular secretion. Therefore, the concurrent use of drugs that reduce renal blood flow (e.g., NSAIDs), that are nephrotoxic (e.g., cisplatin), or that are weak organic acids (e.g., aspirin, piperacillin) can delay drug excretion and lead to severe myelosuppression. In patients with renal insufficiency, the dose should be adjusted in proportion to decreases in renal function, and high-dose regimens should be avoided. Concentrations of MTX in CSF are only 3% of those in the systemic circulation at steady state; hence, neoplastic cells in the CNS probably are not killed by standard dosage regimens. When high doses of MTX are given, cytotoxic concentrations of MTX reach the CNS. MTX is retained in the form of polyglutamates for long periods (e.g., weeks in the kidneys, several months in the liver).

Pharmacogenetics may influence the response to antifolates and their toxicity. The C677T substitution in methylenetetrahydrofolate reductase reduces the activity of the enzyme that generates methylenetetrahydrofolate, the cofactor for TS, and thereby increases MTX toxicity. The presence of this polymorphism in leukemic cells confers increased sensitivity to MTX and might also modulate the toxicity and therapeutic effect of pemetrexed, a predominant TS inhibitor. Likewise, polymorphisms in the promoter region of TS affect its expression, and by altering the intracellular levels of TS, modulate the response and toxicity of both antifolates and fluoropyrimidines.

Therapeutic Uses. MTX is a critical drug in the management of childhood ALL. High-dose MTX is of great value in remission induction and consolidation and in the maintenance of remissions in this highly curable disease. A 6- to 24-h infusion of relatively large doses of MTX may be employed every 2-4 weeks (≥1-7.5 g/m^2) but only when leucovorin rescue follows within 24 h of the MTX infusion. For maintenance therapy, it is administered weekly, 20 mg/m^2 orally. Outcome of treatment in children correlates inversely with the rate of drug clearance. During MTX infusion, high steady-state levels are associated with a lower leukemia relapse rate. MTX is of limited value in adults with AML, except for treatment and prevention of leukemic meningitis. The intrathecal administration of MTX has been employed for treatment or prophylaxis of meningeal leukemia or lymphoma and for treatment of meningeal carcinomatosis. This route of administration achieves high concentrations of MTX in the CSF and also is effective in patients whose systemic disease has become resistant to MTX. The recommended intrathecal dose in all patients >3 years of age is 12 mg. The dose is repeated every 4 days until malignant cells no longer are evident in the CSF. Leucovorin may be administered to counteract the potential toxicity of MTX that escapes into the systemic circulation, although this generally is not necessary. Because MTX administered into the lumbar space distributes poorly over the cerebral convexities, the drug may be given via an intraventricular Ommaya reservoir in the treatment of active intrathecal disease. MTX is of established value in choriocarcinoma and related trophoblastic tumors of women;

cure is achieved in ~75% of advanced cases treated sequentially with MTX and dactinomycin and in >90% when early diagnosis is made. For choriocarcinoma, 1 mg/kg of MTX is administered intramuscularly every other day for 4 doses, alternating with leucovorin (0.1 mg/kg every other day). Courses are repeated at 3-week intervals, toxicity permitting, and urinary β-human chorionic gonadotropin titers are used as a guide for persistence of disease.

Beneficial effects also are observed in the combination therapy of Burkitt and other non-Hodgkin lymphomas. MTX is a component of regimens for carcinomas of the breast, head and neck, ovary, and bladder. High-dose MTX with leucovorin rescue (HDM-L) is a standard agent for adjuvant therapy of osteosarcoma and produces a high complete response rate in CNS lymphomas. The administration of HDM-L has the potential for renal toxicity, probably related to the precipitation of the drug, a weak acid, in the acidic tubular fluid. Thus, vigorous hydration and alkalinization of urine pH are required prior to drug administration. If MTX values measured 48 h after drug administration are 1 μM or higher, higher doses (100 mg/m^2) of leucovorin must be given until the plasma concentration of MTX falls to <50 nM. With appropriate hydration and urine alkalinization, and in patients with normal renal function, the incidence of nephrotoxicity following HDM-L is <2%. In patients who become oliguric, intermittent hemodialysis is ineffective in reducing MTX levels. Continuous-flow hemodialysis can eliminate MTX at ~50% of the clearance rate in patients with intact renal function. Alternatively, a MTX-cleaving enzyme, carboxypeptidase G2, can be obtained from the Cancer Therapy Evaluation Program at the National Cancer Institute. MTX concentrations in plasma fall by ≥99% within 5-15 min following enzyme administration, with insignificant rebound. Systemically administered carboxypeptidase G2 has little effect on MTX levels in the CSF.

MTX (amethopterin; RHEUMATREX, TREXALL, others) is used in the treatment of severe, disabling psoriasis (*see* Chapter 65) in doses of 2.5 mg orally for 5 days, followed by a rest period of at least 2 days, or 10-25 mg intravenously weekly. It also is used at low dosage to induce remission in refractory rheumatoid arthritis. MTX inhibits cell-mediated immune reactions and is employed to suppress graft-versus-host disease in allogenic bone marrow and organ transplantation and for the treatment of dermatomyositis, Wegener granulomatosis, and Crohn disease (*see* Chapters 35 and 47). MTX is also used as an abortifacient, generally in combination with a prostaglandin (*see* Chapter 66).

CLINICAL TOXICITIES. The primary toxicities of antifolates are on the bone marrow and the intestinal epithelium. Patients may be at risk for spontaneous hemorrhage or life-threatening infection, and may require prophylactic transfusion of platelets and broad-spectrum antibiotics if febrile. Side effects usually reverse completely within 2 weeks, but prolonged myelosuppression may occur in patients with compromised renal function who have delayed drug excretion. The dosage of MTX (and likely pemetrexed) must be reduced in proportion to any reduction in CrCL. Additional toxicities of MTX include alopecia, dermatitis, an allergic interstitial pneumonitis, nephrotoxicity (after high-dose therapy), defective oogenesis or spermatogenesis, abortion, and teratogenesis. Low-dose MTX may lead to cirrhosis after long-term continuous treatment, as in patients with psoriasis. Intrathecal administration of MTX often causes meningismus and an inflammatory response in the CSF. Seizures, coma, and death may occur rarely. Leucovorin does not reverse neurotoxicity.

Pemetrexed toxicity mirrors that of MTX, with the additional feature of a prominent erythematous and pruritic rash in 40% of patients. Dexamethasone, 4 mg twice daily on days –1, 0, and +1, markedly diminishes this toxicity. Unpredictably severe myelosuppression with pemetrexed, seen especially in patients with pre-existing homocystinemia, largely is eliminated by concurrent administration of low dosages of folic acid, 350-1000 mg/day, beginning 1-2 weeks prior to pemetrexed and continuing while the drug is administered. Patients should receive intramuscular vitamin B_{12} (1 mg) with the first dose of pemetrexed to correct possible B_{12} deficiency. These small doses of folate and B_{12} do not compromise the therapeutic effect.

PYRIMIDINE ANALOGS

The pyrimidine antimetabolites encompass a diverse group of drugs that inhibit RNA and DNA function. The fluoropyrimidines and certain purine analogs (6-mercaptopurine and 6-thioguanine) inhibit the synthesis of essential precursors of DNA. Others, such as the cytidine and adenosine nucleoside analogs, become incorporated into DNA and block its further elongation and function. Other inhibitory effects of these analogs may contribute to their cytotoxicity and their capacity to induce differentiation.

Cellular Actions of Pyrimidine Antimetabolites. Four bases (Figure 61–5) form DNA: 2 pyrimidines (thymine and cytosine) and 2 purines (guanine and adenine). RNA differs in that it incorporates uracil instead of thymine as one of its bases. Strategies for inhibiting DNA synthesis are based on the ability to create analogs of these precursors that readily enter tumor cells and become activated by intracellularly. As an example, the pyrimidine analog, 5-FU, is converted to a deoxynucleotide, fluorodeoxyuridine monophosphate (FdUMP), which in turn

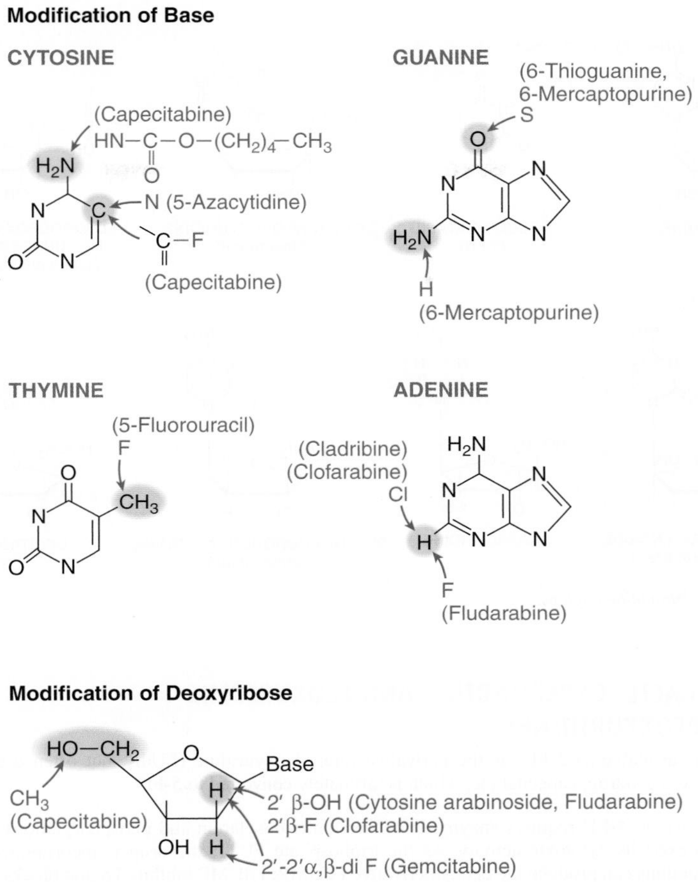

Modification of Base

Modification of Deoxyribose

Figure 61–5 *Structural modification of base and deoxyribonucleoside analogs. Yellow ellipses* indicate sites modified to create antimetabolites. Specific substitutions are noted in *red* for each drug. Modifications occur in the base ring systems, in their amino or hydroxyl side groups, and in the deoxyribose sugar found in deoxyribonucleosides. *See* structures in Figure 61–6.

blocks the enzyme, TS, required for the physiological conversion of dUMP to dTMP, a component of DNA. Other analogs incorporate into DNA itself and thereby block its function.

Cells can make the purine and pyrimidine bases de novo and convert them to their active triphosphates (dNTPs), providing substrates for DNA polymerase. Alternatively, cells can salvage free bases or their deoxynucleosides from the bloodstream. Thus, cells can take up uracil, guanine, and their analogs and convert them to (deoxy) nucleotides by the addition of deoxyribose and phosphate groups. Antitumor analogs of these bases (5-FU, 6-thioguanine) can be formulated as simple substituted bases. Other bases, including cytosine, thymine, and adenine, and their analogs can only be used as deoxynucleosides, which are readily transported into cells and activated to deoxynucleotides by intracellular kinase. Thus, cytarabine (cytosine arabinoside; Ara-C), gemcitabine, 5-azacytidine, and adenosine analogs (cladribine) (Figures 61–5 and 61–6) are nucleosides readily taken up by cells, converted to nucleotides, and incorporated into DNA.

Fludarabine phosphate, a nucleotide, is dephosphorylated rapidly in plasma, releasing the nucleoside that is readily taken up by cells. Analogs may differ from the physiological bases in a variety of ways: by altering in the purine or pyrimidine ring; by altering the sugar attached to the base, as in the arabinoside, Ara-C; or by altering both the base and sugar, as in fludarabine phosphate (*see* Figure 61–5). These alterations produce inhibitory effects on vital enzymatic pathways and prevent DNA synthesis.

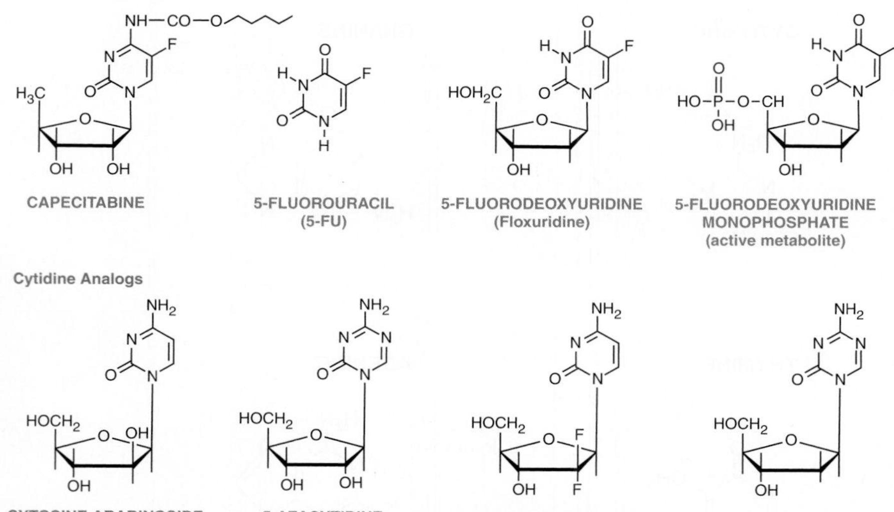

Figure 61–6 *Pyrimidine analogs.*

FLUOROURACIL, CAPECITABINE, AND FLOXURIDINE (FLUORODEOXYURIDINE)

Fluorouracil is available as 5-FU, as the derivative fluorodeoxyuridine (FUdR, not often used in clinical practice), and as a prodrug, capecitabine, which is ultimately converted to 5-FU.

Mechanisms of Action. 5-FU requires enzymatic conversion (ribosylation and phosphorylation) to the nucleotide form to exert its cytotoxic activity. As the triphosphate FUTP, the drug is incorporated into RNA. Alternative reactions can produce the deoxy derivative FdUMP; FdUMP inhibits TS and blocks the synthesis of TTP, a necessary constituent of DNA (Figure 61–7). The folate cofactor, 5,10-methylenetetrahydrofolate, and FdUMP form a covalently bound ternary complex with TS. The physiological complex of TS-folate-dUMP progresses to the synthesis of thymidylate by transfer of the methylene group and 2 hydrogen atoms from folate to dUMP, but this reaction is blocked in the inhibited complex of TS-FdUMP-folate by the stability of the fluorine carbon bond on FdUMP; sustained inhibition of the enzyme results.

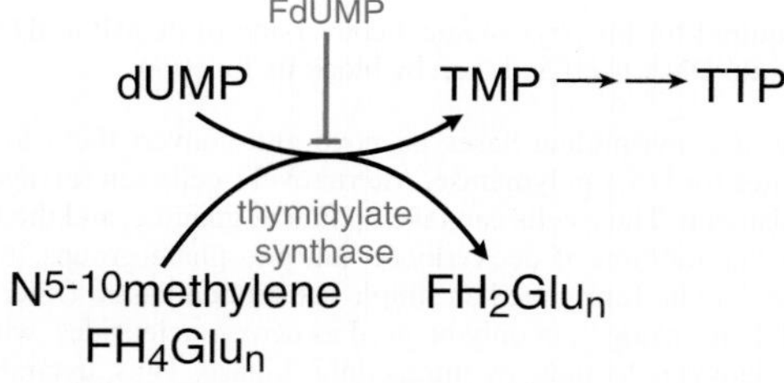

Figure 61–7 *Actions of 5-fluoro-2′-deoxyuridine-5′-phosphate (5-FdUMP) and 5-FU nucleotides.* 5-FU, 5-fluorouracil; dUMP FdUMP, deoxyuridine monophosphate/fluoro dUMP; FH_2Glu_n/FH_4Glu_n, dihydro-/tetrahydro-folate polyglutamates; TMP/TTP, thymidine monophosphate/triphosphate.

5-FU is incorporated into both RNA and DNA. In 5-FU-treated cells, both FdUTP and dUTP (that accumulates behind the blocked TS reaction) incorporate into DNA in place of the depleted physiological TTP. Presumably, such incorporation into DNA calls into action the excision-repair process, which can lead to DNA strand breakage because DNA repair requires TTP, which is lacking as a result of TS inhibition. 5-FU incorporation into RNA also causes toxicity as the result of major effects on both the processing and functions of RNA.

Mechanisms of Resistance. Resistance to the cytotoxic effects of 5-FU or FUdR has been ascribed to loss or decreased activity of the enzymes necessary for activation of 5-FU, amplification of TS, mutation of TS to a form that is not inhibited by FdUMP, and high levels of the degradative enzymes dihydrouracil dehydrogenase and thymidine phosphorylase. TS levels are finely controlled by an autoregulatory feedback mechanism wherein the unbound enzyme interacts with and inhibits the translational efficiency of its own mRNA, which provides for the rapid TS modulation needed for cellular division. When TS is bound to FdUMP, inhibition of translation is relieved, and levels of free TS rise, restoring thymidylate synthesis. Thus, TS autoregulation may be an important mechanism by which malignant cells become insensitive to the effects of 5-FU.

Some malignant cells appear to have insufficient concentrations of 5,10-methylenetetrahydrofolate, and thus cannot form maximal levels of the inhibited ternary complex with TS. Addition of exogenous folate in the form of leucovorin increases formation of the complex and enhances responses to 5-FU. A number of other agents have been combined with 5-FU in attempts to enhance the cytotoxic activity through biochemical modulation. MTX, by inhibiting purine synthesis and increasing cellular pools of 5-phosphoribosyl-1-pyrophosphate (PRPP), enhances the activation of 5-FU and increases antitumor activity of 5-FU when given prior to but not following 5-FU. The combination of cisplatin and 5-FU has yielded impressive responses in tumors of the upper aerodigestive tract, but the molecular basis of their interaction is unclear. Oxaliplatin, which downregulates TS expression, is commonly used with 5-FU and leucovorin for treating metastatic colorectal cancer. A most important interaction is the enhancement of irradiation by fluoropyrimidines, the basis for which is unclear. 5-FU with simultaneous irradiation cures anal cancer and enhances local tumor control in head, neck, cervical, rectal, gastroesophageal, and pancreatic cancer.

ADME. 5-FU is administered parenterally because absorption after oral ingestion of the drug is unpredictable and incomplete. 5-FU is inactivated by reduction of the pyrimidine ring in a reaction carried out by dihydropyrimidine dehydrogenase (DPD), which is found in liver, intestinal mucosa, tumor cells, and other tissues. Inherited deficiency of this enzyme leads to greatly increased sensitivity to the drug. DPD deficiency can be detected either by enzymatic or molecular assays using peripheral white blood cells or by determining the plasma ratio of 5-FU to its metabolite, 5-fluoro-5,6-dihydrouracil.

Plasma clearance is rapid ($t_{1/2}$ ~10-20 min). Only 5-10% of a single intravenous dose of 5-FU is excreted intact in the urine. The dose does not have to be modified in patients with hepatic dysfunction, presumably because of sufficient degradation of the drug at extrahepatic sites. 5-FU enters the CSF in minimal amounts.

THERAPEUTIC USES

5-FLUOROURACIL. 5-FU produces partial responses in 10-20% of patients with metastatic colon carcinomas, upper GI tract carcinomas, and breast carcinomas but rarely is used as a single agent. 5-FU in combination with leucovorin and oxaliplatin or irinotecan in the adjuvant setting is associated with a survival advantage for patients with colorectal cancers. For average-risk patients in good nutritional status with adequate hematopoietic function, the weekly dosage regimen employs 500-600 mg/m^2 with leucovorin once each week for 6 of 8 weeks. Other regimens use daily doses of 500 mg/m^2 for 5 days, repeated in monthly cycles. When used with leucovorin, doses of daily 5-FU for 5 days must be reduced to 375-425 mg/m^2 because of mucositis and diarrhea. 5-FU increasingly is used as a biweekly infusion, a schedule that has less overall toxicity as well as superior response rates and progression-free survival for patients with metastatic colon cancer.

FLOXURIDINE (FUdR). FUdR (fluorodeoxyuridine [FUDR]) is converted directly to FdUMP by thymidine kinase. The drug is administered primarily by continuous infusion into the hepatic artery for treatment of metastatic carcinoma of the colon or following resection of hepatic metastases; the response rate to such infusion is 40-50%, double that observed with intravenous administration. Intrahepatic arterial infusion for 14-21 days causes minimal systemic toxicity; however, there is a significant risk of biliary sclerosis if this route is used for multiple cycles of therapy. Treatment should be discontinued at the earliest manifestation of toxicity (usually stomatitis or diarrhea) because the maximal effects of bone marrow suppression and gut toxicity will not be evident until days 7-14.

CAPECITABINE (XELODA). Capecitabine, an orally administered prodrug of 5-FU, is approved for the treatment of (1) metastatic breast cancer in patients who have not responded to a regimen of paclitaxel and an anthracycline antibiotic; (2) metastatic breast cancer when used in combination with docetaxel in patients who have had a prior anthracycline-containing regimen; and (3) metastatic colorectal cancer. The recommended dosage is 2500 mg/m^2/day, given in 2 divided doses with food, for 2 weeks, followed by a rest period of 1 week. Capecitabine is well absorbed orally. It is rapidly de-esterified and deaminated, yielding high plasma concentrations of an inactive prodrug 5′-deoxyfluorodeoxyuridine (5′-dFdU), which disappears with a $t_{1/2}$ of ~1 h. The conversion of 5′-dFdU to 5-FU by thymidine phosphorylase occurs in liver tissues, peripheral tissues, and tumors. 5-FU levels are <10% of those of 5′-dFdU, reaching a maximum of 0.3 mg/L or 1 μM at 2 h. Liver dysfunction delays the conversion of the parent compound to 5′-dFdU and 5-FU, but there is no consistent effect on toxicity.

Combination Therapy. Higher response rates are seen when 5-FU or capecitabine is used in combination with other agents (e.g., with cisplatin in head and neck cancer, with oxaliplatin or irinotecan in colon cancer). The combination of 5-FU and oxaliplatin or irinotecan has become the standard first-line treatment for patients with metastatic colorectal cancer. The use of 5-FU in combination regimens has improved survival in the adjuvant treatment for breast cancer and, with oxaliplatin and leucovorin, for colorectal cancer. 5-FU also is a potent radiation sensitizer. Beneficial effects also have been reported when combined with irradiation as primary treatment for locally advanced cancers of the esophagus, stomach, pancreas, cervix, anus, and head and neck. 5-FU produces very favorable results for the topical treatment of premalignant keratoses of the skin and multiple superficial basal cell carcinomas.

Clinical Toxicities. The clinical manifestations of toxicity caused by 5-FU and floxuridine are similar. The earliest untoward symptoms during a course of therapy are anorexia and nausea, followed by stomatitis and diarrhea, reliable warning signs that a sufficient dose has been administered. Mucosal ulcerations occur throughout the GI tract and may lead to fulminant diarrhea, shock, and death, particularly in patients who are DPD deficient. The major toxic effects of bolus-dose regimens result from the myelosuppressive action of 5-FU. The nadir of leukopenia usually occurs 9-14 days after the first injection of drug. Thrombocytopenia and anemia also may occur, as may loss of hair (occasionally progressing to total alopecia), nail changes, dermatitis, and increased pigmentation and atrophy of the skin may. Hand-foot syndrome, a particularly prominent adverse effect of capecitabine, consists of erythema, desquamation, pain, and sensitivity to touch of the palms and soles. Acute chest pain with evidence of ischemia in the electrocardiogram may result from coronary artery vasospasms during or shortly after 5-FU infusion. In general, myelosuppression, mucositis, and diarrhea occur less often with infusional than with bolus regimens, while hand-foot syndrome occurs more often with infusional than with bolus regimens. The significant risk of toxicity with fluoropyrimidines emphasizes the need for very skillful supervision by physicians familiar with the action and possible hazards.

Capecitabine causes a similar spectrum of toxicities as 5-FU (diarrhea, myelosuppression), but the hand-foot syndrome occurs more frequently and may require dose reduction or cessation of therapy.

CYTIDINE ANALOGS

CYTARABINE (CYTOSINE ARABINOSIDE; Ara-C)

Cytarabine (1-β-D-arabinofuranosylcytosine; Ara-C [CYTOSAR-U, TARABINE PFS, others]) is the most important antimetabolite used in the therapy of AML; it is the single most effective agent for induction of remission in this disease.

MECHANISM OF ACTION. Ara-C is an analog of 2′-deoxycytidine; the 2′-hydroxyl in a position *trans* to the 3′-hydroxyl of the sugar (*see* Figures 61–5 and 61–6) hinders rotation of the pyrimidine base around the nucleoside bond and interferes with base pairing. The drug enters cells via nucleoside transporters; hENT1 appears to be the primary mediator of Ara-C influx. In the cell, Ara-C is converted to its active form, the 5′-monophosphate ribonucleotide, by deoxycytidine kinase (CdK), an enzyme that shows polymorphic expression among patients (see below). Ara-CMP then reacts with deoxynucleotide kinases to form diphosphate and triphosphates (Ara-CDP and Ara-CTP). Ara-CTP competes with deoxycytidine 5′-triphosphate (dCTP) for incorporation into DNA by DNA polymerases. The incorporated Ara-CMP residue is a potent inhibitor of DNA polymerase, both in replication and repair synthesis, and blocks the further elongation of the nascent DNA molecule. If DNA breaks are not repaired, apoptosis ensues. Ara-C cytotoxicity correlates with the total Ara-C incorporated into DNA; incorporation of ~5 molecules of Ara-C per 10^4 bases of DNA decreases cellular clonogenicity by ~50%.

In infants and adults with ALL and t(4;11) mixed-lineage leukemia (MLL) translocation, high-dose Ara-C is particularly effective; in these patients, the nucleoside transporter, hENT1, is highly expressed, and its expression correlates with sensitivity to Ara-C. At extracellular drug concentrations >10 μM (levels achievable with high-dose Ara-C), the nucleoside transporter no longer limits drug accumulation, and intracellular metabolism to a triphosphate becomes rate limiting. Particular subtypes of AML derive benefit from high-dose Ara-C treatment; these include t(8;21), inv(16), t(9;16), and del(16). Approximately 20% of AML patients have leukemic cells with a *k-RAS* mutation, and these patients seem to derive greater benefit from high dose Ara-C regimens than do patients with wild type *k-RAS*.

MECHANISMS OF RESISTANCE. Response to Ara-C is strongly influenced by the relative activities of anabolic and catabolic enzymes that determine the proportion of drug converted to Ara-CTP. The rate-limiting activating enzyme, CdK, produces Ara-CMP. It is opposed by the degradative enzyme, cytidine deaminase, which converts Ara-C to a nontoxic metabolite, ara-uridine (Ara-U). Cytidine deaminase activity is high in many normal tissues, including intestinal mucosa, liver, and neutrophils, but lower in AML cells and other human tumors. A second degradative enzyme, dCMP deaminase, converts Ara-CMP to the inactive metabolite, Ara-UMP. Increased synthesis and retention of Ara-CTP in leukemic cells lead to a longer duration of complete remission in patients with AML. The capacity of cells to transport Ara-C also may affect response. Clinical studies have implicated a loss of CdK as the primary mechanism of resistance to Ara-C in AML.

ADME. Due to the presence of high concentrations of cytidine deaminase in the GI mucosa and liver, only ~20% of the drug reaches the circulation after *oral* Ara-C administration; thus, the drug must be given intravenously. Peak concentrations of 2-50 μM are measurable in plasma after intravenous injection of 30-300 mg/m^2 but fall rapidly ($t_{1/2}$ ≈10 min). Less than 10% of the injected dose is excreted unchanged in the urine within 12-24 h; most appears as the inactive deaminated product, Ara-U. Higher concentrations of Ara-C are found in CSF after continuous infusion than after rapid intravenous injection, but are ≤10% of concentrations in plasma. After *intrathecal* administration of the drug at a dose of 50 mg/m^2, deamination proceeds slowly, with a $t_{1/2}$ of 3-4 h, and peak concentrations of 1-2 μM are achieved. CSF concentrations remain above the threshold for cytotoxicity (0.4 μM) for ≥24 h. A depot liposomal formulation of Ara-C (DepoCyt) provides sustained release into the CSF. After a standard 50-mg dose, liposomal Ara-C remains above cytotoxic levels for an average of 12 days, thus avoiding the need for frequent lumbar punctures.

Therapeutic Uses. Continuous inhibition of DNA synthesis for a duration equivalent to at least 1 cell cycle or 24 h is necessary to expose most tumor cells during the S, or DNA-synthetic, phase of the cycle. The optimal interval between bolus doses of Ara-C is ~8-12 h, a schedule that maintains intracellular concentrations of Ara-CTP at inhibitory levels during a multi-day cycle of treatment. Typical schedules for administration of Ara-C employ bolus doses every 12 h or continuous drug infusion for 5-7 days. Two dosage schedules are recommended: (1) rapid intravenous infusion of 100 mg/m^2 every 12 h for 5-7 days or (2) continuous intravenous infusion of 100-200 mg/m^2/day for 5-7 days. In general, children tolerate higher doses than adults. Intrathecal doses of 30 mg/m^2 every 4 days have been used to treat meningeal or lymphomatous leukemia. The intrathecal administration of liposomal cytarabine (DepoCyt), 50 mg for adults, 35 mg for children, every 2 weeks seems equally effective as the every-4-days regimen with the standard drug. Ara-C is indicated for induction and maintenance of remission in AML and is useful in the treatment of other leukemias, such as ALL, CML in the blast phase, acute promyelocytic leukemia, and high-grade lymphomas. Because drug concentration in plasma rapidly falls below the level needed to saturate transport and intercellular activation, clinicians have employed high-dose regimens (2-3 g/m^2 every 12 h for 6-8 doses) to achieve 20-50 times higher serum levels, with improved results in remission induction and consolidation for AML. Injection of the liposomal formulation is indicated for the intrathecal treatment of lymphomatous meningitis.

CLINICAL TOXICITIES. Cytarabine is a potent myelosuppressive agent capable of producing acute, severe leukopenia, thrombocytopenia, and anemia with striking megaloblastic changes. Other toxic manifestations include GI disturbances, stomatitis, conjunctivitis, reversible hepatic enzyme elevations, noncardiogenic pulmonary edema, and dermatitis. The onset of dyspnea, fever, and pulmonary infiltrates on chest computed tomography scans may follow 1-2 weeks after high-dose Ara-C and may be fatal in 10-20% of patients, especially in patients being treated for relapsed leukemia. No specific therapy, other than Ara-C discontinuation, is indicated. Intrathecal Ara-C, either the free drug or the liposomal preparation, may cause arachnoiditis, seizures, delirium, myelopathy, or coma, especially if given concomitantly with systemic high-dose MTX or systemic Ara-C. Cerebellar toxicity, manifesting as ataxia and slurred speech, and cerebral toxicity (seizures, dementia, and coma) may follow intrathecal administration or high-dose systemic administration, especially in patients >40 years of age and/or patients with poor renal function.

AZACITIDINE (5-AZACYTIDINE)

5-Azacytidine (*see* Figure 61–6) and decitabine (2′-deoxy-5-azacytidine) have antileukemic activity and induce differentiation by inhibiting DNA cytosine methyltransferase activity. Both drugs are approved for treatment of myelodysplasia, for which they induce normalization of bone marrow in 15-20% of patients and reduce transfusion requirement in one-third of patients. 5-Azacytidine improves survival.

Mechanism of Action. The aza-nucleosides enter cells by the human equilibrative transporter. The drugs incorporate into DNA, where they become covalently bound to the methyltransferase, depleting intracellular enzyme and leading to global demethylation of DNA, tumor cell differentiation, and apoptosis. Decitabine also induces double-strand DNA breaks, perhaps as a consequence of the effort to repair the protein-DNA adduct.

Pharmacokinetics. After subcutaneous administration of the standard dose of 75 mg/m^2, 5-azacytidine undergoes rapid deamination by cytidine deaminase (plasma $t_{1/2}$ ~20-40 min). Due to the formation of intracellular nucleotides, which become incorporated into DNA, the effects of the aza-nucleosides persist for many hours.

Therapeutic Use. The usual regimen for 5-azacytidine in myelodysplastic syndrome (MDS) is 75 mg/m^2/day for 7 days every 28 days, while decitabine is given in a dose of 20 mg intravenously every day for 5 days every 4 weeks. Best responses may become apparent only after 2-5 courses of treatment.

Toxicity. The major toxicities of the aza-nucleosides include myelosuppression and mild GI symptoms. 5-Azacytidine produces rather severe nausea and vomiting when given intravenously in large doses (150-200 mg/m^2/day for 5 days).

GEMCITABINE

Gemcitabine (2′,2′-difluorodeoxycytidine; dFdC) (*see* Figure 61–6), a difluoro analog of deoxycytidine, is used for patients with metastatic pancreatic; non-squamous, non–small cell lung; ovarian; and bladder cancer.

Mechanism of Action. Gemcitabine enters cells via 3 distinct nucleoside transporters: hENT (the major route), hCNT, and a nucleobase transporter found in malignant mesothelioma cells. Intracellularly, CdK phosphorylates gemcitabine to the monophosphate (dFdCMP), which is converted to di- and triphosphates (dFdCDP and dFdCTP). Although gemcitabine's anabolism and effects on DNA in general mimic those of cytarabine, there are distinct differences in kinetics of inhibition, additional enzymatic sites of action, different effects of incorporation into DNA, and a distinct spectrum of clinical activity. Unlike that of cytarabine, the cytotoxicity of gemcitabine is not confined to the S phase of the cell cycle. The cytotoxic activity may reflect several actions on DNA synthesis. dFdCTP competes with dCTP as a weak inhibitor of DNA polymerase. dFdCDP is a stoichiometric inhibitor of ribonucleotide reductase (RNR), resulting in depletion of deoxyribonucleotide pools necessary for DNA synthesis. Incorporation of dFdCTP into DNA causes DNA strand termination and appears resistant to repair. The capacity of cells to incorporate dFdCTP into DNA is critical for gemcitabine-induced apoptosis. Gemcitabine is inactivated by cytidine deaminase, which is found both in tumor cells and throughout the body.

ADME. Gemcitabine is administered as an intravenous infusion. The pharmacokinetics of the parent compound are largely determined by deamination in liver, plasma, and other organs, and the predominant urinary elimination product is dFdU. In patients with significant renal dysfunction, dFdU and its triphosphate accumulate to high and potentially toxic levels. Gemcitabine has a short plasma $t_{1/2}$ (~15 min); women and elderly patients clear the drug more slowly.

Therapeutic Uses. The standard dosing schedule for gemcitabine (GEMZAR) is a 30-min intravenous infusion of 1-1.25 g/m^2 on days 1, 8, and 15 of each 21- to 28-day cycle, depending on the indication. Conversion of gemcitabine to dFdCMP by CdK is saturated at infusion rates of ~10 mg/m^2/min. To increase dFdCTP formation, the duration of infusion at this maximum concentration has been extended to 100-150 min at a fixed rate of 10 mg/min. The 150-min infusion produces a higher level of dFdCTP within peripheral blood mononuclear cells and increases the degree of myelosuppression but does not improve antitumor activity. The inhibition of DNA repair by gemcitabine may increase cytotoxicity of other agents, particularly platinum compounds, and with radiation therapy.

Clinical Toxicities. The principal toxicity is myelosuppression. Longer-duration infusions lead to greater myelosuppression and hepatic toxicity. Nonhematological toxicities include a flu-like syndrome, asthenia, and rarely a posterior leukoencephalopathy syndrome. Mild, reversible elevation in liver transaminases may occur in ≥40% of patients. Interstitial pneumonitis, at times progressing to acute respiratory distress syndrome (ARDS), may occur within the first 2 cycles of treatment and usually responds to corticosteroids. Rarely, patients treated for many months may develop a slowly progressive hemolytic uremic syndrome, necessitating drug discontinuation. Gemcitabine is a very potent radiosensitizer and should not be used with radiotherapy.

PURINE ANALOGS

The pioneering studies of Hitchings and Elion identified analogs of naturally occurring purine bases with antileukemic and immunosuppressant properties. Figure 61–8 shows structural formulas of several of these, with adenosine for comparison.

Other purine analogs that have valuable roles in leukemia and lymphoid malignancies include cladribine (standard therapy for hairy cell leukemia), fludarabine phosphate (standard treatment for CLL), nelarabine (pediatric ALL), and clofarabine (T-cell leukemia/lymphoma). The apparent selectivity of these agents may relate to their effective uptake, activation, and apoptotic effects in lymphoid tissue.

6-THIOPURINE ANALOGS

6-Mercaptopurine (6-MP) and 6-thioguanine (6-TG) are approved agents for human leukemias and function as analogs of the natural purines, hypoxanthine and guanine. The substitution of sulfur for oxygen on C6 of the purine ring creates compounds that are readily transported into cells, including activated malignant cells. Nucleotides formed from 6-MP and 6-TG inhibit de novo purine synthesis and also become incorporated into nucleic acids.

Mechanism of Action. Hypoxanthine guanine phosphoribosyl transferase (HGPRT) converts 6-TG and 6-MP to the ribonucleotides 6-thioguanosine-5′-monophosphate (6-thioGMP) and 6-thioinosine-5′-monophosphate

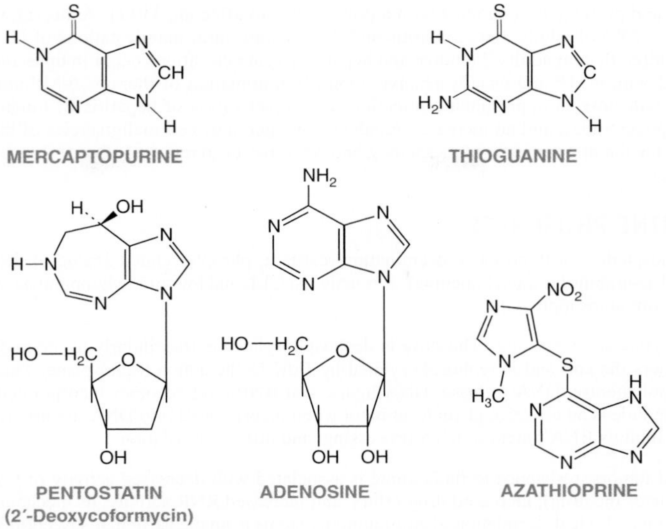

MERCAPTOPURINE THIOGUANINE

PENTOSTATIN (2′-Deoxycoformycin) ADENOSINE AZATHIOPRINE

Figure 61–8 *Adenosine and various purine analogs.*

(T-IMP), respectively. Because T-IMP is a poor substrate for guanylyl kinase (the enzyme that converts GMP to GDP), T-IMP accumulates intracellularly. T-IMP inhibits the new formation of ribosyl-5-phosphate, as well as conversion of IMP to adenine and guanine nucleotides. The most important point of attack seems to be the reaction of glutamine and PRPP to form ribosyl-5-phosphate, the first committed step in the de novo pathway. 6-Thioguanine nucleotide is incorporated into DNA, where it induces strand breaks and base mispairing.

Mechanisms of Resistance. The most common mechanism of 6-MP resistance observed in vitro is deficiency or complete lack of the activating enzyme, HGPRT, or increased alkaline phosphatase activity. Other mechanisms for resistance include (1) decreased drug uptake, or increased efflux due to active transporters; (2) alteration in allosteric inhibition of ribosylamine 5-phosphate synthase; and (3) impaired recognition of DNA breaks and mismatches due to loss of a component (MSH6) of MMR.

Pharmacokinetics and Toxicity. Absorption of oral mercaptopurine is incomplete (10-50%); the drug is subject to first-pass metabolism by xanthine oxidase in the liver. Food or oral antibiotics decrease absorption. Oral bioavailability is increased when mercaptopurine is combined with high-dose MTX. After an intravenous dose, the $t_{1/2}$ of the drug is ~50 min in adults, due to rapid metabolic degradation by xanthine oxidase and by thiopurine methyltransferase (TPMT). Restricted brain distribution of mercaptopurine results from an efficient efflux transport system in the blood-brain barrier. In addition to the HGPRT-catalyzed anabolism of mercaptopurine, there are 2 other pathways for its metabolism. The first involves methylation of the sulfhydryl group and subsequent oxidation of the methylated derivatives. Activity of the enzyme TPMT reflects the inheritance of polymorphic alleles; up to 15% of the Caucasian population has decreased enzyme activity. Low levels of erythrocyte TPMT activity are associated with increased drug toxicity in individual patients and a lower risk of relapse. In patients with autoimmune disease treated with mercaptopurine, those with polymorphic alleles may experience bone marrow aplasia and life-threatening toxicity. Testing for these polymorphisms prior to treatment is recommended in this patient population.

A relatively large percentage of the administered sulfur appears in the urine as inorganic sulfate. The second major pathway for 6-MP metabolism involves its oxidation by xanthine oxidase to 6-thiourate, an inactive metabolite. Oral doses of 6-MP should be reduced by 75% in patients receiving the xanthine oxidase inhibitor, allopurinol; no dose adjustment is required for intravenous dosing.

Therapeutic Uses. In the maintenance therapy of ALL, the initial daily oral dose of 6-MP (PURINETHOL) is 50-100 mg/m^2 and is thereafter adjusted according to white blood cell and platelet count. The combination of MTX and 6-MP appears to be synergistic. By inhibiting the earliest steps in purine synthesis, MTX elevates the intracellular concentration of PRPP, a cofactor required for 6-MP activation.

CLINICAL TOXICITIES. The principal toxicity of 6-MP is bone marrow depression; thrombocytopenia, granulocytopenia, or anemia may not become apparent for several weeks. When depression of normal bone marrow elements occurs, dose reduction usually results in prompt recovery, although myelosuppression may be severe and prolonged in patients with a polymorphism affecting TPMT. Anorexia, nausea, or vomiting is seen in ~25% of adults, but stomatitis and diarrhea are rare; manifestations of GI effects are less frequent in children than in adults. Jaundice and hepatic enzyme elevations occur in up to one-third of adult patients treated with 6-MP and usually resolve upon discontinuation of therapy. 6-MP and its derivative, azathioprine, predispose to opportunistic infection (e.g., reactivation of hepatitis B, fungal infection, and *Pneumocystis* pneumonia), and an increased incidence of squamous cell malignancies of the skin. 6-MP is teratogenic during the first trimester of pregnancy, and AML has been reported after prolonged 6-MP therapy for Crohn disease.

FLUDARABINE PHOSPHATE

Fludarabine phosphate is a fluorinated, deamination-resistant, phosphorylated analog of the antiviral agent vidarabine (9-β-D-arabinofuranosyl-adenine). It is active in CLL and low-grade lymphomas and is also effective as a potent immunosuppressant.

Mechanisms of Action and Resistance. The drug is dephosphorylated extracellularly to the nucleoside fludarabine, which enters the cell and is rephosphorylated by CdK to the active triphosphate. This antimetabolite inhibits DNA polymerase, DNA primase, DNA ligase, and RNR, and becomes incorporated into DNA and RNA. The nucleotide is an effective chain terminator when incorporated into DNA. Incorporation of fludarabine into RNA inhibits RNA function, RNA processing, and mRNA translation.

In experimental tumors, resistance to fludarabine is associated with decreased activity of CdK (the enzyme that phosphorylates the drug), increased drug efflux, and increased RNR activity. Its mechanism of immunosuppression and paradoxical stimulation of autoimmunity stems from the particular susceptibility of lymphoid cells to purine analogs and the specific effects on the $CD4^+$ subset of T cells, as well as its inhibition of regulatory T-cell responses.

ADME. Fludarabine phosphate is administered both intravenously and orally and is rapidly converted to fludarabine in the plasma. The median time to reach maximal concentrations of drug in plasma after oral administration is 1.5 h, and oral bioavailability averages 55-60%. The $t_{1/2}$ of fludarabine in plasma is ~10 h. The compound is eliminated primarily by renal excretion.

THERAPEUTIC USES. Fludarabine phosphate (FLUDARA, OFORTA) is approved for intravenous and oral use and is equally active by both routes. The recommended dose is 25 mg/m^2 daily for 5 days by intravenous infusion, or 40 mg/m^2 daily for 5 days by mouth. The drug is administered intravenously over 30-120 min. Dosage should be reduced in patients with renal impairment in proportion to the reduction in CrCl. Treatment may be repeated every 4 weeks, and gradual improvement in CLL usually occurs within 2-3 cycles. Fludarabine phosphate is highly active alone or with rituximab and cyclophosphamide for the treatment of patients with CLL; overall response rates in previously untreated patients approximate 80% and the duration of response averages 22 months. The synergy of fludarabine with alkylators may stem from the observation that it blocks the repair of double-strand DNA breaks and interstrand cross-links induced by alkylating agents. It also is effective in follicular B-cell lymphomas refractory to standard therapy. It is increasingly used as a potent immunosuppressive agent in nonmyeloablative allogeneic bone marrow transplantation.

CLINICAL TOXICITIES. Oral and intravenous therapy cause myelosuppression in ~50% of patients, nausea and vomiting in a minor fraction, and, uncommonly, chills and fever, malaise, anorexia, peripheral neuropathy, and weakness. Lymphopenia and thrombocytopenia and cumulative side effects are expected. Depletion of $CD4^+$ T cells with therapy predisposes to opportunistic infections. Tumor lysis syndrome, a rare complication, occurs primarily in previously untreated patients with CLL. Altered mental status, seizures, optic neuritis, and coma have been observed at higher doses and in older patients. Autoimmune events may occur after fludarabine treatment. CLL patients may develop an acute hemolytic anemia or pure red cell aplasia during or following fludarabine treatment. Prolonged cytopenias, probably mediated by autoimmunity, also complicate fludarabine treatment. Myelodysplasia and acute leukemias may arise as late complications. Pneumonitis is an occasional side effect and responds to corticosteroids. In patients with compromised renal function, the initial doses should be reduced in proportion to the reduction in CrCl.

CLADRIBINE

Cladribine (2-chlorodeoxyadenosine [2-CdA]) is an adenosine deaminase-resistant purine analog that has potent and probably curative activity in hairy cell leukemia, CLL, and low-grade lymphomas.

Mechanisms of Action and Resistance. Cladribine enters cells via active nucleoside transport. After phosphorylation by CdK and conversion to cladribine triphosphate, it is incorporated into DNA. It produces DNA strand breaks and depletion of NAD and ATP, leading to apoptosis. It is a potent inhibitor of RNR. The drug does not require cell division to be cytotoxic. Resistance is associated with loss of the activating enzyme, CdK; increased expression of RNR; or increased active efflux by ABCG2 or other members of the ABC cassette family of transporters.

ADME. Cladribine is moderately well absorbed orally (55%) but is routinely administered intravenously. It is excreted by the kidneys, with a terminal $t_{1/2}$ in plasma of 6.7 h. Cladribine crosses the blood-brain barrier and reaches CSF concentrations of ~25% of those seen in plasma. Doses should be adjusted for renal dysfunction.

Therapeutic Uses. Cladribine (LEUSTATIN, others) is administered as a single course of 0.09 mg/kg/day for 7 days by continuous intravenous infusion. It is the drug of choice in hairy cell leukemia. Eighty percent of patients achieve a complete response after a single course of therapy. The drug also is active in CLL; low-grade lymphomas; Langerhans cell histiocytosis; CTCLs, including mycosis fungoides and the Sézary syndrome; and Waldenström macroglobulinemia.

Clinical Toxicities. The major dose-limiting toxicity of cladribine is myelosuppression. Cumulative thrombocytopenia may occur with repeated courses. Opportunistic infections are common and correlate with decreased $CD4^+$ cell counts. Other toxic effects include nausea, infections, high fever, headache, fatigue, skin rashes, and tumor lysis syndrome.

CLOFARABINE (2-CHLORO-2′-FLUORO-ARABINOSYLADENINE)

This analog incorporates the 2-chloro, glycosylase-resistant substituent of cladribine and a 2′-fluoro-arabinosyl substitution, which adds stability and enhances uptake and phosphorylation. The resulting compound is approved for pediatric ALL after failure of 2 prior therapies. Clofarabine produces complete remissions in 20-30% of these patients. It has activity as well in pediatric and adult AML and in myelodysplasia. The uptake and metabolic activation of clofarabine in tumor cells follow the same path as cladribine and the other purine nucleosides, although clofarabine is more readily phosphorylated by dCK. Clofarabine triphosphate has a long intracellular $t_{1/2}$ (24 h). It incorporates into DNA, where it terminates DNA synthesis and leads to apoptosis; clofarabine also inhibits RNR.

Clinical Pharmacology. In children, it is administered in doses of 52 mg/m^2 given as a 2-h infusion daily for 5 days. The primary elimination $t_{1/2}$ in plasma is 6.5 h. Most of the drug is excreted unchanged in the urine. Doses should be adjusted according to reductions in CrCl. The primary toxicities are myelosuppression; a clinical syndrome of hypotension, tachyphemia, pulmonary edema, organ dysfunction, and fever, all suggestive of capillary leak syndrome and cytokine release that necessitate immediate discontinuation of the drug; elevated hepatic enzymes and increased bilirubin; nausea, vomiting, and diarrhea; and hypokalemia and hypophosphatemia.

NELARABINE (6-METHOXY-ARABINOSYL-GUANINE)

Nelarabine is the only guanine nucleoside in clinical use. It has selective activity against acute T-cell leukemia (20% complete responses) and the closely related T-cell lymphoblastic lymphoma and is approved for use in relapsed/refractory patients. Its basic mechanism of action closely resembles that of the other purine nucleosides, in that it is incorporated into DNA and terminates DNA synthesis.

ADME. Following infusion, the parent methoxy compound is rapidly activated in blood and tissues by adenosine deaminase–mediated cleavage of the methyl group, yielding the phosphorylase resistant Ara-G, which has a plasma $t_{1/2}$ of 3 h. The active metabolite is transported into tumor cells, where it is activated by CdK to Ara-G triphosphate (Ara-GTP) that incorporates into DNA and terminates DNA synthesis. The drug and its metabolite, Ara-G, are primarily eliminated by metabolism to guanine, and a smaller fraction is eliminated by renal excretion of Ara-G. The dose should be used with close clinical monitoring in patients with severe renal impairment (CrCL <50 mg/mL). Adults are given a dose of 1500 mg/m^2 intravenously as a 2-h infusion on days 1, 3, and 5 of a 21-day cycle, and children are given a lower dose of 650 mg/m^2/day intravenously for 5 days and repeated every 21 days.

Clinical Toxicity. Side effects include myelosuppression and liver function test abnormalities, as well as frequent, serious neurological sequelae, such as seizures, delirium, somnolence, peripheral neuropathy, or Guillain-Barré syndrome. Neurological side effects may not be reversible.

PENTOSTATIN (2′-DEOXYCOFORMYCIN)

Pentostatin (2′-deoxycoformycin; *see* Figure 61–8), a transition-state analog of the intermediate in the adenosine deaminase (ADA) reaction, potently inhibits ADA. Its effects mimic the phenotype of genetic ADA deficiency (severe immunodeficiency affecting both T- and B-cell functions).

Mechanism of Action. Inhibition of ADA by pentostatin leads to accumulation of intracellular adenosine and deoxyadenosine nucleotides, which can block DNA synthesis by inhibiting RNR. Deoxyadenosine also inactivates *S*-adenosyl homocysteine hydrolase. The resulting accumulation of *S*-adenosyl homocysteine is particularly toxic to lymphocytes. Pentostatin also can inhibit RNA synthesis, and its triphosphate derivative is incorporated into DNA, resulting in strand breakage. Although the precise mechanism of cytotoxicity is not known, it is probable that the imbalance in purine nucleotide pools accounts for its antineoplastic effect in hairy cell leukemia and T-cell lymphomas.

ADME. Pentostatin is administered intravenously and has a mean terminal $t_{1/2}$ of 5.7 h. The recommended dose is 4 mg/m^2 administered intravenously, every other week. After hydration with 500-1000 mL of 5% dextrose in half-normal (0.45%) saline, the drug is administered by rapid intravenous injection or by infusion over a period of ≤30 min, followed by an additional 500 mL of fluids. The drug is eliminated almost entirely by renal excretion. Proportional reduction of dosage is recommended in patients with renal impairment as measured by reduced CrCl.

Clinical Use. Pentostatin is effective in producing complete remissions (58%) and partial responses (28%) in hairy cell leukemia. It largely has been superseded by cladribine. Toxic manifestations include myelosuppression, GI symptoms, skin rashes, and abnormal liver function studies. Depletion of normal T cells occurs, and neutropenic fever and opportunistic infections may result. Immunosuppression may persist for several years after discontinuation. At high doses (10 mg/m^2), major renal and neurological complications are encountered. Pentostatin in combination with fludarabine phosphate may result in severe or even fatal pulmonary toxicity.

III. Natural Products

MICROTUBULE-DAMAGING AGENTS

VINCA ALKALOIDS

Purified alkaloids from the periwinkle plant, including *vinblastine* and *vincristine*, were among the earliest clinical agents for treatment of leukemias, lymphomas, and testicular cancer. A closely related derivative, vinorelbine, has important activity against lung and breast cancer.

Mechanism of Action. The vinca alkaloids are cell-cycle–specific agents and, in common with other drugs, such as colchicine, podophyllotoxin, the taxanes, and the epothilones, block cells in mitosis. The biological activities of the vincas can be explained by their ability to bind specifically to β tubulin and to block its polymerization with α tubulin into microtubules. The mitotic spindle cannot form, duplicated chromosomes cannot align along the division plate, and cell division arrests in metaphase. Cells blocked in mitosis undergo changes characteristic of apoptosis. Microtubules are found in high concentration in the brain and contribute to other cellular functions such as movement, phagocytosis, and axonal transport. Side effects of the vinca alkaloids, such as their neurotoxicity, may relate to disruption of these functions.

Resistance. Despite their structural similarity, the individual vinca alkaloids have unique patterns of clinical efficacy (see below). However, in most experimental systems, they share cross-resistance. Their antitumor effects are blocked by multidrug resistance mediated by the *mdr* gene/P-glycoprotein, which confers resistance to a broad range of agents (the vinca alkaloids, epipodophyllotoxins, anthracyclines, and taxanes). Chromosomal abnormalities consistent with gene amplification and markedly increased levels of P-glycoprotein (a membrane efflux transporter) have been observed in resistant cells in culture. Other membrane transporters, such as the MRP and the closely related breast cancer resistance protein, may contribute to resistance. Other forms of resistance to vinca alkaloids stem from mutations in β tubulin or in the relative expression of isoforms of β tubulin that prevent the inhibitors from effectively binding to their target.

Cytotoxic Actions. The very limited myelosuppressive action of vincristine makes it a valuable component of several combination therapy regimens for leukemia and lymphoma, while the lack of severe neurotoxicity of vinblastine is a decided advantage in lymphomas and in combination with cisplatin against testicular cancer. Vinorelbine, which causes a mild neurotoxicity as well as myelosuppression, has an intermediate toxicity profile.

Metabolism and Excretion. The liver cytochromes extensively metabolize all 3 agents, and the metabolites are excreted in the bile. Only a small fraction of a dose (<15%) is found in the urine unchanged. In patients with hepatic dysfunction (bilirubin >3 mg/dL), a 50-75% reduction in dose of any of the vinca alkaloids is advisable. The elimination $t_{1/2}$ is 20 h for vincristine, 23 h for vinblastine, and 24 h for vinorelbine.

VINBLASTINE

Therapeutic Uses. Vinblastine sulfate (VELBAN) is given intravenously; special precautions must be taken against subcutaneous extravasation, which may cause painful irritation and ulceration. The drug should not be injected into an extremity with impaired circulation. After a single dose of 0.3 mg/kg of body weight, myelosuppression reaches its maximum in 7-10 days. If a moderate level of leukopenia (~3000 cells/mm^3) is not attained, the weekly dose may be increased gradually by increments of 0.05 mg/kg of body weight. For testicular cancer, vinblastine is used in doses of 0.3 mg/kg every 3 weeks. Doses should be reduced by 50% for patients with plasma bilirubin >1.5 mg/dL. Vinblastine is used with bleomycin and cisplatin in the curative therapy of metastatic testicular tumors, although it has been supplanted by etoposide or ifosfamide. It is a component of the standard curative regimen for Hodgkin disease (doxorubicin [ADRIAMYCIN], bleomycin, vinblastine, and dacarbazine [ABVD]). It also is active in Kaposi sarcoma, neuroblastoma, Langerhans cell histiocytosis, bladder cancer, carcinoma of the breast, and choriocarcinoma.

Clinical Toxicities. Maximal leukopenia occurs within 7-10 days, after which recovery ensues within 7 days. Other toxic effects of vinblastine include mild neurological manifestations. GI disturbances including nausea, vomiting, anorexia, and diarrhea may be encountered. The syndrome of inappropriate secretion of antidiuretic hormone has been reported. Loss of hair, stomatitis, and dermatitis occur infrequently. Extravasation during injection may lead to cellulitis and phlebitis.

VINCRISTINE

Therapeutic Uses. Vincristine is a standard component of regimens for treating pediatric leukemias, lymphomas, and solid tumors, such as Wilms, tumor, neuroblastoma, and rhabdomyosarcoma. In large-cell non-Hodgkin lymphomas, vincristine remains an important agent, particularly when used in the CHOP regimen with cyclophosphamide, doxorubicin, and prednisone. Vincristine sulfate (VINCASAR PFS) used with glucocorticoids is the treatment of choice to induce remissions in childhood leukemia and in combination with alkylating agents and anthracycline for pediatric sarcomas. The common intravenous dosage for vincristine is 2 mg/m^2 of body surface area at weekly or longer intervals. Vincristine is tolerated better by children than by adults, who may experience severe, progressive neurological toxicity and require a lower dose of 1.4 mg/m^2. Administration of the drug more frequently than every 7 days or at higher doses increases the toxic manifestations without proportional improvement in the response rate. Precautions also should be used to avoid extravasation during intravenous administration. Doses should be reduced for patients with elevated plasma bilirubin.

Clinical Toxicities. The clinical toxicity of vincristine is mostly neurological. Severe neurological manifestations may be reversed by suspending therapy or reducing the dosage, upon first evidence of motor dysfunction. Severe constipation, sometimes resulting in colicky abdominal pain and obstruction, may be prevented by a prophylactic program of laxatives and hydrophilic (bulk-forming) agents, and usually is a problem only with doses >2 mg/m^2. Reversible alopecia occurs in ~20% of patients. Modest leukopenia may occur. Thrombocytopenia, anemia, and the syndrome of inappropriate secretion of ADH are less common. Inadvertent injection of vincristine into the CSF causes a devastating and often fatal irreversible coma and seizures.

VINORELBINE

Vinorelbine has activity against non–small cell lung cancer and breast cancer. Vinorelbine (NAVELBINE, others) is administered in normal saline as an intravenous infusion over 6-10 min. When used alone, it is given at doses of 30 mg/m^2 either weekly or for 2 out of every 3 weeks. When used with cisplatin for the treatment of non–small cell lung cancer, it is given at doses of 25 mg/m^2 either weekly or for 3 out of every 4 weeks. A lower dose (20-25 mg/m^2) may be required for patients who have received prior chemotherapy and for hematological toxicity. Its primary toxicity is granulocytopenia, with only modest thrombocytopenia and less neurotoxicity than other vinca alkaloids. Vinorelbine may cause allergic reactions and mild, reversible changes in liver enzymes. Doses should be reduced in patients with elevated plasma bilirubin.

TAXANES

Paclitaxel (TAXOL, others) was first isolated from the bark of the Western yew tree. Paclitaxel and its congener, the semisynthetic docetaxel (TAXOTERE), exhibit unique pharmacological properties as inhibitors of mitosis, differing from the vinca alkaloids and colchicine derivatives in that they bind to a different β-tubulin site and promote rather than inhibit microtubule formation. The taxanes have a central role in the therapy of ovarian, breast, lung, GI, genitourinary, and head and neck cancers.

Paclitaxel has very limited water solubility and is administered in a vehicle of 50% ethanol and 50% polyethoxylated castor oil (CREMOPHOR EL); this vehicle likely is responsible for a high rate of hypersensitivity reactions. Patients receiving this formulation are protected by pretreatment with an H_1 receptor antagonist such as diphenhydramine, an H_2 receptor antagonist such as cimetidine (*see* Chapter 32), and a glucocorticoid such as dexamethasone (*see* Chapter 42).

An albumin-bound nanoparticle solution for infusion (nab-paclitaxel, ABRAXANE) is soluble in aqueous solutions and can be administered safely without prophylactic antihistamines or steroids. This form of paclitaxel has increased cellular uptake via an albumin-specific mechanism. Docetaxel, somewhat more soluble than paclitaxel, is administered in polysorbate 80 and is associated with a lower incidence of hypersensitivity reactions than paclitaxel dissolved in CREMOPHOR. However, pretreatment with dexamethasone for 3 days starting 1 day prior to therapy is required to prevent progressive fluid retention and minimize the severity of hypersensitivity reactions.

Mechanism of Action; Drug Interactions; Resistance. Paclitaxel binds specifically to the β-tubulin subunit of microtubules and antagonizes their disassembly, with the result that bundles of microtubules and aberrant structures derived from microtubules appear in the mitotic phase of the cell cycle. Arrest in mitosis follows. Cell death occurs by apoptosis and depends on both drug concentration and duration of drug exposure. Drugs that block cell-cycle progression prior to mitosis antagonize the toxic effects of taxanes.

Drug interactions have been noted; the sequence of cisplatin preceding paclitaxel decreases paclitaxel clearance and produces greater toxicity than the opposite schedule. Paclitaxel decreases doxorubicin clearance and enhances cardiotoxicity, while docetaxel has no apparent effect on anthracycline pharmacokinetics.

The basis of clinical drug resistance is not known. Resistance to taxanes is associated in some cultured tumor cells with increased expression of the *mdr*-1 gene and its product, P-glycoprotein; other resistant cells have β-tubulin mutations and may display heightened sensitivity to vinca alkaloids. Other resistant cell lines display an increase in survivin, an anti-apoptotic factor, α *Aurora kinase,* that promotes completion of mitosis. The taxanes preferentially bind to the βII-tubulin subunit of microtubules; therefore, cells may become resistant by upregulating the βIII-isoform of tubulin.

ADME. Paclitaxel is administered as a 3-h infusion of 135-175 mg/m^2 every 3 weeks or as a weekly 1-h infusion of 80-100 mg/m^2. Prolonged infusions (96 h) also are active. Hepatic CYPs (primarily CYP2C8, secondarily CYP3A4) extensively metabolize the drug. The primary metabolite is 6-OH paclitaxel, which is inactive; multiple additional hydroxylation products are found in plasma; <10% of a dose is excreted in the urine intact. Dose reductions in patients with abnormal hepatic function have been suggested, and 50-75% doses of taxanes should be used in the presence of hepatic metastases >2 cm in size or in patients with abnormal serum bilirubin. Drugs that induce CYP2C8 or CYP3A4, such as phenytoin and phenobarbital, or those that inhibit these CYPs, such as antifungal imidazoles, significantly alter drug clearance and toxicity.

Paclitaxel clearance is nonlinear and decreases with increasing dose or dose rate; the plasma $t_{1/2}$ ~10-14 h and clearance is 15-18 L/hr/m^2. The critical plasma concentration for inhibiting bone marrow elements depends on duration of exposure but likely is 50-100 nM. Paclitaxel clearance is markedly delayed by cyclosporine A and other drugs that inhibit P-glycoprotein.

Nab-paclitaxel achieves a higher serum concentration of paclitaxel compared to CREMOPHOR-solubilized paclitaxel, but the increased clearance of nab-paclitaxel results in a similar drug exposure. Nab-paclitaxel is most often administered intravenously over 30 min at 260 mg/m^2 every 3 weeks. Like the other taxanes, nab-paclitaxel should not be given to patients with an absolute neutrophil count <1500 cells/mm^3.

Docetaxel pharmacokinetics are similar to those of paclitaxel, with an elimination $t_{1/2}$ of ~12 h. Clearance is primarily through CYP3A4- and CYP3A5-mediated hydroxylation, leading to inactive metabolites. In contrast to paclitaxel, the pharmacokinetics of docetaxel are linear for doses ≤115 mg/m^2.

Therapeutic Uses. The taxanes have become central components of regimens for treating metastatic ovarian, breast, lung, GI, genitourinary, and head and neck cancers. These drugs are administered once weekly or once every 3 weeks. The appropriate use of the steroid-sparing nab-paclitaxel still is being evaluated in clinical trials.

Clinical Toxicities. Paclitaxel exerts its primary toxic effects on the bone marrow. Neutropenia usually occurs 8-11 days after a dose and reverses rapidly by days 15-21. Used with filgrastim (granulocyte-colony stimulating factor [G-CSF]), doses as high as 250 mg/m^2 over 24 h are well tolerated, and peripheral neuropathy becomes dose limiting. Many patients experience myalgias after receiving paclitaxel. In high-dose schedules, or with prolonged use, a stocking-glove sensory neuropathy can be disabling, particularly in patients with underlying diabetic neuropathy or concurrent cisplatin therapy. Mucositis is prominent in 72- or 96-h infusions and in the weekly schedule. Hypersensitivity reactions can occur in patients receiving paclitaxel infusions of short duration (1-6 h) but are largely averted by pretreatment with dexamethasone, diphenhydramine, and histamine H_2 receptor antagonists, as noted above. Premedication is not necessary with 96-h infusions. Many patients experience asymptomatic bradycardia; occasional episodes of silent ventricular tachycardia also occur and resolve spontaneously during 3- or 24-h infusions. Nab-paclitaxel produces increased rates of peripheral neuropathy compared to CREMOPHOR-delivered paclitaxel but rarely causes hypersensitivity reactions.

Docetaxel causes greater degrees of neutropenia than paclitaxel but less peripheral neuropathy and asthenia and less frequent hypersensitivity. Fluid retention is a progressive problem with multiple cycles of docetaxel therapy, leading to peripheral edema, pleural and peritoneal fluid, and pulmonary edema in extreme cases. Oral dexamethasone, 8 mg/day, begun 1 day prior to drug infusion and continuing for 3 days, greatly ameliorates fluid retention. In rare cases, docetaxel may cause a progressive interstitial pneumonitis and respiratory failure if the drug is not discontinued.

ESTRAMUSTINE

Estramustine (EMCYT, estramustine phosphate) combines estradiol and normustine (nornitrogen mustard) through a carbamate link. Although the intent of the combination was to enhance the uptake of the alkylating agent into estradiol-sensitive prostate cancer cells, estramustine does not function in vivo as an alkylating agent; rather, it binds to β tubulin and microtubule-associated proteins, causing microtubule disassembly and antimitotic actions.

Therapeutic Use. Estramustine is used solely for the treatment of metastatic or locally advanced hormone refractory prostate cancer at an initial dosage of 14 mg/kg/day in 3 or 4 divided doses.

ADME. Following oral administration, at least 75% of a dose of estramustine phosphate is absorbed from the GI tract and rapidly dephosphorylated. The drug undergoes extensive first-pass metabolism by hepatic CYPs to an active 17-keto derivative, estromustine, and to multiple inactive products; the active drug forms accumulate in the prostate. Some hydrolysis of the carbamate linkage occurs in the liver, releasing estradiol, estrone, and the normustine group. Estramustine and estromustine have a plasma $t_{1/2}$ of 10 and 14 h, respectively, and are excreted as inactive metabolites, mainly in the feces.

Clinical Toxicities; Drug Interactions. In addition to myelosuppression, estramustine also possesses estrogenic side effects (gynecomastia, impotence, elevated risk of thrombosis, and fluid retention), hypercalcemia, acute attacks of porphyria, impaired glucose tolerance, and hypersensitivity reactions, including angioedema. Estramustine inhibits the clearance of taxanes.

EPOTHILONES

The epothilones are 16-membered polyketides discovered as cytotoxic metabolites from a strain of *Sorangium cellulosum*, a myxobacterium originally isolated from soil on the bank of the Zambezi River in southern Africa. These compounds overcome some of the problems of other microtubule disrupting and stabilizing agents, such as difficulties in formulation, drug delivery, and susceptibility to multidrug resistance. Ixabepilone (IXEMPRA) is approved for breast cancer treatment.

Others in development include the epothilone B analogs patupilone (EPO906) and 21-aminoepothilone B (BMS-310705), the epothilone D analog KOS-1584 (R1645), and the synthetic sagopilone.

Mechanism of Action; Resistance. They bind to β tubulin and trigger microtubule nucleation at multiple sites away from the centriole. This chaotic microtubule stabilization triggers cell-cycle arrest at the G2-M interface and apoptosis. Epothilones bind to a site distinct from that of taxanes. In colon cancer cell lines, p53 and Bax trigger apoptosis in ixabepilone-treated cells. In vitro studies suggest that ixabepilone is less susceptible to P-glycoprotein-mediated multidrug resistance than are taxanes. Other mechanisms implicated in epothilone resistance include mutation of the β-tubulin binding site and upregulation of isoforms of β tubulin.

ADME. Ixabepilone is administered intravenously. Because of its minimal aqueous solubility, it is delivered in the solubilizing agent, polyoxyethylated castor oil/ethanol (CREMOPHOR EL). CREMOPHOR has been implicated as the cause of infusion reactions; such reactions are infrequent when administration is preceded by premedication with H_1 and H_2 antagonists. The drug is cleared by hepatic CYPs and has a plasma $t_{1/2}$ of 52 h.

Therapeutic Uses. In patients with metastatic breast cancer resistant to or pretreated with anthracyclines and resistant to taxanes, ixabepilone plus capecitabine provides an improved progression-free survival of 1.6 months compared to capecitabine alone. Ixabepilone also is indicated as monotherapy for metastatic breast cancer in patients who have previously progressed through treatment with anthracyclines, taxanes, and capecitabine. The recommended dose of ixabepilone as monotherapy or in combination with capecitabine is 40 mg/m^2 administered over 3 h every 3 weeks. Because of additive myelosuppression, the phase III trial used an attenuated dose of capecitabine (2000 mg/m^2) administered with ixabepilone. Patients should be premedicated with both an H_1 and H_2 antagonist before receiving ixabepilone to minimize hypersensitivity reactions.

The combination of ixabepilone and capecitabine is contraindicated in patients with a baseline neutrophil count <1500 cells/mm^3, a platelet count <100,000 cells/mm^3, serum transaminases >2.5 × ULN or bilirubin above normal. In patients receiving ixabepilone monotherapy with mild to moderate hepatic dysfunction (bilirubin <1.5 × ULN or 1.5-3 × ULN, respectively), starting doses of 32 and 20 mg/m^2 are recommended due to delayed drug clearance.

Toxicities. Epothilones have toxicities similar to those of the taxanes: neutropenia, peripheral sensory neuropathy, fatigue, diarrhea, and asthenia.

CAMPTOTHECIN ANALOGS

The camptothecins are potent, cytotoxic antineoplastic agents that target the nuclear enzyme *topoisomerase I.* The lead compound in this class, camptothecin, was isolated from the tree *Camptotheca acuminata. Irinotecan* and *topotecan*, currently the only camptothecin analogs approved for clinical use, have activity in colorectal, ovarian, and small cell lung cancer.

Chemistry. All camptothecins have a fused 5-ring backbone that includes a labile lactone ring (*see* Figures 6–5 and 6–6 for examples). The hydroxyl group and S-conformation of the chiral center at C20 in the lactone ring are required for biological activity. Appropriate substitutions on the A and B rings of the quinoline subunit enhance water solubility and increase potency for inhibiting topoisomerase I. Topotecan is a semisynthetic molecule with a basic dimethylamino group that increases its water solubility. Irinotecan (CPT-11) differs from topotecan in that it is a prodrug. The carbamate bond between the camptothecin moiety and the dibasic bis-piperidine side chain at position C10 (which makes the molecule water soluble) is cleaved by a carboxylesterase to form the active metabolite, SN-38 (*see* Figure 6–5).

Mechanism of Action. The DNA topoisomerases are nuclear enzymes that reduce torsional stress in supercoiled DNA, allowing selected regions of DNA to become sufficiently untangled to permit replication, repair, and transcription. Two classes of topoisomerase (I and II) mediate DNA strand breakage and resealing. Camptothecin analogs inhibit the function of topoisomerase I; myriad other chemical entities (e.g., anthracyclines, epipodophyllotoxins, acridines) inhibit topoisomerase II. The camptothecins bind to and stabilize the normally transient DNA-topoisomerase I cleavable complex. Although the initial cleavage action of topoisomerase I is not affected, the re-ligation step is inhibited, leading to the accumulation of single-stranded breaks in DNA. These lesions are reversible and not by themselves toxic to the cell. However, the collision of a DNA replication fork with this cleaved strand of DNA causes an irreversible double-strand DNA break, ultimately leading to cell death. The precise sequence of events that leads from drug-induced DNA damage to cell death has not been fully elucidated; one does observe internucleosomal DNA fragmentation, a characteristic of programmed cell death.

Camptothecins are *S phase–specific drugs*, because ongoing DNA synthesis is necessary for cytotoxicity. This has important clinical implications. S phase–specific cytotoxic agents generally require prolonged exposures of tumor cells to drug concentrations above a minimum threshold for optimal therapeutic efficacy. In fact, low-dose, protracted administration of camptothecin analogs have less toxicity, and equal or greater antitumor activity, than shorter, more intense courses.

Mechanisms of Resistance. Decreased intracellular drug accumulation may underlie resistance in cell lines. Topotecan, but not SN-38 or irinotecan, is a substrate for P-glycoprotein; however, compared with other substrates, such as etoposide or doxorubicin, topotecan is a relatively poor substrate. Other reports have associated topotecan and irinotecan resistance with the MRP class of transporters. Cell lines that lack carboxylesterase activity demonstrate resistance to irinotecan, but the liver and red blood cells may have sufficient carboxylesterase activity to convert irinotecan to SN-38. Camptothecin resistance also may result from decreased expression or mutation of topoisomerase I. A transient downregulation of topoisomerase I has been demonstrated following prolonged exposure to camptothecins in vitro and in vivo. Mutations leading to reduced topoisomerase I enzyme catalytic activity or DNA-binding affinity have been associated with experimental camptothecin resistance. Finally, exposure of cells to topoisomerase I–targeted agents upregulates topoisomerase II, an alternative enzyme for DNA strand passage.

TOPOTECAN

ADME. Topotecan is approved for intravenous administration. An oral dosage form in development has a bioavailability of 30-40% in cancer patients. Topotecan exhibits linear pharmacokinetics, and it is rapidly eliminated from systemic circulation with a $t_{1/2}$ ~3.5-4.1 h. Only 20-35% of the total drug in plasma is found to be in the active lactone form. Within 24 h, 30-40% of the administered dose appears in the urine. Doses should be reduced in proportion to reductions in CrCl. Hepatic metabolism appears to be a relatively minor route of drug elimination. Plasma protein binding of topotecan is low (7-35%), which may explain its relatively greater CNS penetration.

Therapeutic Uses. Topotecan (HYCAMTIN) is indicated for previously treated patients with ovarian and small cell lung cancer. Significant hematological toxicity limits its use in combination with other active agents in these diseases (e.g., cisplatin). The recommended dosing regimen of topotecan for ovarian cancer and small cell lung cancer is a 30-min infusion of 1.5 mg/m^2/day for 5 consecutive days every 3 weeks. For cervical cancer in conjunction with cisplatin, the dose of topotecan is 0.75 mg/m^2 on days 1, 2, and 3, repeated every 21 days. The dose of topotecan should be reduced to 0.75 mg/m^2/day in patients with moderate renal dysfunction (CrCl of 20-40 mL/min); topotecan should not be administered to patients with severe renal impairment (CrCl <20 mL/min). Hepatic dysfunction does not alter topotecan clearance and toxicity. A baseline neutrophil count >1500 cells/mm^3 and a platelet count >100,000 is necessary prior to topotecan administration.

Clinical Toxicities. The dose-limiting toxicity with all dosing schedules is neutropenia, with or without thrombocytopenia. The incidence of severe neutropenia at 1.5 mg/m^2 daily for 5 days every 3 weeks may be as high as 81%, with a 26% incidence of febrile neutropenia. In patients with hematological malignancies, GI side effects such as mucositis and diarrhea become dose limiting. Other less common and generally mild topotecan-related toxicities include nausea and vomiting, elevated liver transaminases, fever, fatigue, and rash.

IRINOTECAN

ADME. The conversion of irinotecan to SN-38 is mediated predominantly by carboxylesterases in the liver (*see* Figure 6–5). Although SN-38 can be measured in plasma shortly after beginning an intravenous infusion of irinotecan, the AUC of SN-38 is only ~4% of the AUC of irinotecan, suggesting that only a relatively small fraction of the dose is ultimately converted to the active form of the drug. Irinotecan exhibits linear pharmacokinetics. In comparison to topotecan, a relatively large fraction of both irinotecan and SN-38 are present in plasma as the biologically active intact lactone form. The $t_{1/2}$ of SN-38 is 11.5 h, 3 times that of topotecan. CSF penetration of SN-38 in humans has not been characterized.

In contrast to topotecan, hepatic metabolism of irinotecan and SN-38 represents an important route of elimination for both. Oxidative metabolites have been identified in plasma, all of which result from CYP3A-mediated reactions directed at the bis-piperidine side chain. These metabolites are not significantly converted to SN-38. The total body clearance of irinotecan was found to be 2 times greater in brain cancer patients taking antiseizure drugs that induce hepatic CYPs.

UGT1A1 glucuronidates the hydroxyl group at position C10 (resulting from cleavage of the bispiperidine promoiety), producing the inactive metabolite SN-38G (*see* Figure 6–6). Biliary excretion appears to be the primary elimination route of irinotecan, SN-38, and metabolites, although urinary excretion also contributes (14-37%). The extent of SN-38 glucuronidation inversely correlates with the risk of severe diarrhea after irinotecan therapy. UGT1A1 polymorphisms associated with familial hyperbilirubinemia syndromes may have a major impact on the clinical use of irinotecan. A positive correlation has been found between baseline serum unconjugated bilirubin concentration and both severity of neutropenia and the AUC of irinotecan and SN-38 in patients treated with irinotecan. Severe irinotecan toxicity has been observed in cancer patients with Gilbert syndrome, presumably due to decreased glucuronidation of SN-38. The presence of bacterial glucuronidase in the intestinal lumen potentially can contribute to irinotecan's GI toxicity by releasing unconjugated SN-38 from the inactive glucuronide metabolite.

Therapeutic Uses. Approved single-agent dosage schedules of irinotecan (CAMPTOSAR, others) in the U.S. include 125 mg/m^2 as a 90-min infusion administered weekly (on days 1, 8, 15, and 22) for 4 out of 6 weeks, and 350 mg/m^2 given every 3 weeks. In patients with advanced colorectal cancer, irinotecan is used as first-line therapy in combination with fluoropyrimidines or as a single agent or in combination with cetuximab following failure of a 5-FU/oxaliplatin regimen.

Clinical Toxicities. The dose-limiting toxicity with all dosing schedules is delayed diarrhea (35%), with or without neutropenia. An intensive regimen of loperamide (4 mg of loperamide starting at the onset of any loose stool beginning more than a few hours after receiving therapy, followed by 2 mg every 2 h; *see* Chapter 47) reduces this incidence by more than half. However, once severe diarrhea occurs, standard doses of antidiarrheal agents tend to be ineffective. Diarrhea generally resolves within a week and, unless associated with fever and neutropenia, rarely is fatal.

The second most common irinotecan-associated toxicity is myelosuppression. Severe neutropenia occurs in 14-47% of the patients treated with the every-3-weeks schedule and is less frequently encountered among patients treated with the weekly schedule. Febrile neutropenia is observed in 3% of patients and may be fatal, particularly when associated with concomitant diarrhea. A cholinergic syndrome resulting from the inhibition of acetylcholinesterase activity by irinotecan may occur within the first 24 h after irinotecan administration. Symptoms include acute diarrhea, diaphoresis, hypersalivation, abdominal cramps, visual accommodation disturbances, lacrimation, rhinorrhea, and less often, asymptomatic bradycardia. These effects are short lasting and respond within minutes to atropine. Other common toxicities include nausea and vomiting, fatigue, vasodilation or skin flushing, mucositis, elevation in liver transaminases, and alopecia. There have been case reports of dyspnea and interstitial pneumonitis associated with irinotecan therapy.

ANTIBIOTICS

DACTINOMYCIN (ACTINOMYCIN D)

Actinomycin D has beneficial effects in the treatment of solid tumors in children and choriocarcinoma in adult women.

Actinomycins are chromopeptides. Most contain the same chromophore, the planar phenoxazone actinosin, which is responsible for their yellow-red color. The differences among naturally occurring actinomycins are confined to variations in the structure of the amino acids of the peptide side chains.

Mechanism of Action. The capacity of actinomycins to bind to double-helical DNA is responsible for their biological activity and cytotoxicity. The planar phenoxazone ring intercalates between adjacent guanine–cytosine base pairs of DNA, while the polypeptide chains extend along the minor groove of the helix, resulting in a dactinomycin-DNA complex with stability sufficient to block the transcription of DNA by RNA polymerase. The DNA-dependent RNA polymerases are much more sensitive to the effects of dactinomycin than are the DNA polymerases. In addition, dactinomycin causes single-strand breaks in DNA, possibly through a free-radical intermediate or as a result of the action of topoisomerase II. Dactinomycin inhibits rapidly proliferating cells of normal and neoplastic origin, and is among the most potent antitumor agents known.

ADME. Dactinomycin is administered by intravenous injection. Metabolism of the drug is minimal. The drug is excreted in both bile and urine and disappears from plasma with a terminal $t_{1/2}$ of 36 h. Dactinomycin does not cross the blood-brain barrier.

Therapeutic Uses. The usual daily dose of dactinomycin (actinomycin D; COSMEGEN) is 10-15 μg/kg; given intravenously for 5 days. If no manifestations of toxicity are encountered, additional courses may be given at intervals of 2-4 weeks. In other regimens, 3-6 μg/kg/day, for a total of 125 μg/kg, and weekly maintenance doses of 7.5 μg/kg have been used. The main clinical use of dactinomycin is in the treatment of rhabdomyosarcoma and Wilms, tumor in children, where it is curative in combination with primary surgery, radiotherapy, and other drugs, particularly vincristine and cyclophosphamide. Ewing, Kaposi, and soft-tissue sarcomas also respond. Dactinomycin and MTX form a curative therapy for choriocarcinoma.

Clinical Toxicities. Toxic manifestations include anorexia, nausea, and vomiting, usually beginning a few hours after administration. Hematopoietic suppression with pancytopenia may occur in the first week after completion of therapy. Proctitis, diarrhea, glossitis, cheilitis, and ulcerations of the oral mucosa are common; dermatological manifestations include alopecia, as well as erythema, desquamation, and increased inflammation and pigmentation in areas previously or concomitantly subjected to X-ray radiation. Severe injury may occur as a result of local drug extravasation; the drug is extremely corrosive to soft tissues.

ANTHRACYCLINES AND ANTHRACENEDIONES

Anthracyclines are derived from the fungus *Streptomyces peucetius* var. *caesius. Idarubicin* and *epirubicin* are analogs of the naturally produced anthracyclines *doxorubicin* and *daunorubicin*, differing only slightly in chemical structure, but having somewhat distinct patterns of clinical activity. Daunorubicin and idarubicin primarily have been used in the acute leukemias, whereas doxorubicin and epirubicin display broader activity against human solid tumors. These agents, which possess potential for generating free radicals, cause an unusual and often irreversible cardiomyopathy, the occurrence of which is related to the total dose of the drug. The structurally similar agent *mitoxantrone* has less cardiotoxicity and is useful against prostate cancer and AML, and in high-dose chemotherapy.

Mechanisms of Action and Resistance. Anthracyclines and anthracenediones can intercalate with DNA, directly affecting transcription and replication. More important is their capacity to form a heterotrimeric complex with topoisomerase II and DNA. Topoisomerase II produces double-strand breaks at the 3′-phosphate backbone, allowing strand passage and uncoiling of super-coiled DNA. Following strand passage, topoisomerase II re-ligates the DNA strands; this enzymatic function is essential for DNA replication and repair. Formation of the ternary complex with anthracyclines or with etoposide inhibits the re-ligation of the broken DNA strands, leading to apoptosis. Defects in DNA double-strand break repair sensitize cells to damage by these drugs, while overexpression of transcription-linked DNA repair may contribute to resistance.

The quinone moieties of anthracyclines can form radical intermediates that react with O_2 to produce superoxide anion radicals, which can generate H_2O_2 and •OH that attack DNA and oxidize DNA bases, leading to apoptosis. The production of free radicals is significantly stimulated by the interaction of doxorubicin with iron. Enzymatic defenses such as superoxide dismutase and catalase protect cells against the toxicity of the anthracyclines, and these defenses can be augmented by exogenous antioxidants such as alpha tocopherol or by an iron chelator, dexrazoxane (ZINECARD, others), which protects against cardiac toxicity. Multidrug resistance is observed in tumor cell populations exposed to anthracyclines. Anthracyclines also are exported from tumor cells by members of the MRP transporter family and by ABCG2 (the breast cancer resistance protein). Other biochemical changes in resistant cells include increased glutathione peroxidase activity, decreased activity or mutation of topoisomerase II, and enhanced ability to repair DNA strand breaks.

ADME. Daunorubicin, doxorubicin, epirubicin, and idarubicin usually are administered intravenously and are cleared by a complex pattern of hepatic metabolism and biliary excretion. Each anthracycline is converted to an active alcohol intermediate that plays a variable role in the therapeutic activity. The plasma disappearance curves for doxorubicin and daunorubicin are multiphasic, with a terminal $t_{1/2}$ of 30 h. Idarubicin has a $t_{1/2}$ of 15 h, and its active metabolite, idarubicinol, has a $t_{1/2}$ of 40 h. The drugs rapidly enter the heart, kidneys, lungs, liver, and spleen; they do not cross the blood-brain barrier. Clearance is delayed in the presence of hepatic dysfunction; at least a 50% initial reduction in dose should be considered in patients with elevated serum bilirubin levels.

IDARUBICIN AND DAUNORUBICIN

Therapeutic Use. The recommended dosage for idarubicin (IDAMYCIN PFS) is 12 mg/m²/day for 3 days by intravenous injection in combination with cytarabine. Slow injection over 10-15 min is recommended to avoid extravasation. Idarubicin has less cardiotoxicity than the other anthracyclines.

Daunorubicin (daunomycin, rubidomycin; CERUBIDINE, others) is available for intravenous use. The recommended dosage is 25-45 mg/m²/day for 3 days. The agent is administered with care to prevent extravasation. Total doses of >1000 mg/m² are associated with a high risk of cardiotoxicity. Daunorubicin may impart a red color to the urine. Daunorubicin and idarubicin also are used in the treatment of AML in combination with Ara-C.

Clinical Toxicities. Toxic effects of daunorubicin and idarubicin include bone marrow depression, stomatitis, alopecia, GI disturbances, rash, and cardiac toxicity. Cardiac toxicity is characterized by tachycardia, arrhythmias, dyspnea, hypotension, pericardial effusion, and congestive heart failure poorly responsive to digitalis.

DOXORUBICIN

Therapeutic Uses. The recommended dose is 60-75 mg/m², administered as a single rapid intravenous infusion that is repeated after 21 days. A doxorubicin liposomal product (DOXIL) is available for treatment of AIDS-related Kaposi sarcoma and is given intravenously in a dose of 20 mg/m² over 60 min and repeated every 3 weeks. The liposomal formulation also is approved for ovarian cancer at a dose of 50 mg/m² every 4 weeks and as a treatment for multiple myeloma (in conjunction with bortezomib), where it is given as a 30-mg/m² dose on day 4 of each 21-day cycle. Patients should be advised that the drug may impart a red color to the urine. Doxorubicin is effective in malignant lymphomas. In combination with cyclophosphamide, vinca alkaloids, and other agents, it is an important ingredient for the successful treatment of lymphomas. It is a valuable component of various regimens of chemotherapy for adjuvant and metastatic carcinoma of the breast. The drug also is beneficial in pediatric and adult sarcomas, including osteogenic, Ewing, and soft-tissue sarcomas.

Clinical Toxicities. Toxicities of doxorubicin are similar to those of daunorubicin. Myelosuppression is a major dose-limiting complication, with maximal leukopenia usually occurring during the second week of therapy and recovering by the fourth week; thrombocytopenia and anemia follow a similar pattern but usually are less pronounced. Stomatitis, mucositis, diarrhea, and alopecia are common but reversible. Erythematous streaking near the site of infusion ("ADRIAMYCIN flare") is a benign local allergic reaction and should not be confused with extravasation. Facial flushing, conjunctivitis, and lacrimation may occur rarely. The drug may produce severe local toxicity in irradiated tissues (e.g., the skin, heart, lung, esophagus, and GI mucosa) even when the 2 therapies are not administered concomitantly.

Cardiomyopathy is the most important long-term toxicity and may take 2 forms:

- **An acute form, characterized by abnormal electrocardiographic changes, including ST- and T-wave alterations and arrhythmias.** This is brief and rarely a serious problem. An acute reversible reduction in ejection fraction is observed in some patients in the 24 h after a single dose, and plasma troponin T may increase in a minority of patients in the first few days following drug administration. Acute myocardial damage, the "pericarditis–myocarditis syndrome," may begin in the days following drug infusion and is characterized by severe disturbances in impulse conduction and frank congestive heart failure, often associated with pericardial effusion.
- **Chronic, cumulative dose-related toxicity (usually total doses of ≥550 mg/m²) progressing to congestive heart failure.** The mortality rate in patients with congestive failure approaches 50%. The risk increases markedly, with estimates as high as 20% at total doses of 550 mg/m² (a total dose limit of 300 mg/m² is advised for pediatric cases). These total dosages should be exceeded only under exceptional circumstances or with the concomitant use of dexrazoxane, a cardioprotective iron-chelating agent. Cardiac irradiation, administration of high doses of cyclophosphamide or another anthracycline, or concomitant trastuzumab increases the risk of cardiotoxicity. Late-onset cardiac toxicity, with congestive heart failure years after treatment, may occur in both pediatric and adult populations. In children treated with anthracyclines, there is a 3- to 10-fold elevated risk of arrhythmias, congestive heart failure, and sudden death in adult life. Concomitant administration of dexrazoxane may reduce troponin T elevations and avert later cardiotoxicity.

EPIRUBICIN

This anthracycline is indicated as a component of adjunctive therapy for treatment of breast cancer. It is administered in doses of 100-120 mg/m² intravenously every 3-4 weeks. Total doses >900 mg/m² sharply increase the risk of cardiotoxicity. Its toxicity profile is the same as that of doxorubicin.

VALRUBICIN

Valrubicin is a semi-synthetic analog of doxorubicin, used exclusively for intravesicular treatment of bladder cancer. Once a week for 6 weeks, 800 mg are instilled into the bladder. Less than 10% of instilled drug is absorbed systemically. Side effects relate to bladder irritation.

MITOXANTRONE

Mitoxantrone is approved for use in AML, prostate cancer, and late-stage, secondary progressive multiple sclerosis. Mitoxantrone has limited ability to produce quinone-type free radicals and causes less cardiac toxicity than does doxorubicin. It produces acute myelosuppression, cardiac toxicity (less than doxorubicin), and mucositis as its major toxicities; the drug causes less nausea, vomiting, and alopecia than does doxorubicin. Mitoxantrone (NOVANTRONE, others) is administered by intravenous infusion. To induce remission in acute nonlymphocytic leukemia in adults, the drug is given in a daily dose of 12 mg/m^2 for 3 days with cytarabine. It also is used in advanced hormone-resistant prostate cancer in a dose of 12-14 mg/m^2 every 21 days.

EPIPODOPHYLLOTOXINS

ETOPOSIDE AND TENIPOSIDE

Two synthetic derivatives of podophyllotoxins have significant therapeutic activity in pediatric leukemia, small cell carcinomas of the lung, testicular tumors, Hodgkin disease, and large cell lymphomas. These derivatives are etoposide (VP-16-213) and teniposide (VM-26). Although podophyllotoxin binds to tubulin, etoposide and teniposide have no effect on microtubular structure or function at usual concentrations.

Mechanisms of Action and Resistance. Etoposide and teniposide form ternary complexes with topoisomerase II and DNA and prevent resealing of the break that normally follows topoisomerase binding to DNA. The enzyme remains bound to the free end of the broken DNA strand, leading to an accumulation of DNA breaks and cell death. Cells in the S and G_2 phases of the cell cycle are most sensitive to etoposide and teniposide. Resistant cells demonstrate (1) amplification of the *mdr*-1 gene that encodes the P-glycoprotein drug efflux transporter, (2) mutation or decreased expression of topoisomerase II, or (3) mutations of the p53 tumor suppressor gene, a required component of the apoptotic pathway.

ETOPOSIDE

ADME. Oral administration of etoposide results in variable absorption that averages ~50%. After intravenous injection, there is a biphasic pattern of clearance with a terminal $t_{1/2}$ of ~6-8 h in patients with normal renal function. Approximately 40% of an administered dose is excreted intact in the urine. In patients with compromised renal function, dosage should be reduced in proportion to the reduction in CrCl. In patients with advanced liver disease, increased toxicity may result from a low serum albumin (decreased drug binding) and elevated bilirubin (which displaces etoposide from albumin); guidelines for dose reduction in this circumstance have not been defined. Drug concentrations in the CSF average 1-10% of those in plasma.

Therapeutic Uses. The intravenous dose of etoposide (VEPESID, others) for testicular cancer in combination therapy (with bleomycin and cisplatin) is 50-100 mg/m^2 for 5 days, or 100 mg/m^2 on alternate days for 3 doses. For small cell carcinoma of the lung, the dosage in combination therapy (with cisplatin and ifosfamide) is 35 mg/m^2/day intravenously for 4 days or 50 mg/m^2/day intravenously for 5 days. The oral dose for small cell lung cancer is twice the IV dose. Cycles of therapy usually are repeated every 3-4 weeks. When given intravenously, the drug should be administered slowly over a 30- to 60-min period to avoid hypotension and bronchospasm, which likely result from the additives used to dissolve etoposide.

Etoposide is also active against non-Hodgkin lymphomas, acute nonlymphocytic leukemia, and Kaposi sarcoma associated with AIDS. Etoposide has a favorable toxicity profile for dose escalation in that its primary acute toxicity is myelosuppression. In combination with ifosfamide and carboplatin, it frequently is used for high-dose chemotherapy in total doses of 1500-2000 mg/m^2.

Clinical Toxicities. The dose-limiting toxicity of etoposide is leukopenia (nadir at 10-14 days, recovery by 3 weeks). Thrombocytopenia occurs less often and usually is not severe. Nausea, vomiting, stomatitis, and diarrhea complicate treatment in ~15% of patients. Alopecia is common but reversible. Hepatic toxicity is particularly evident after high-dose treatment. For both etoposide and teniposide, toxicity increases in patients with decreased serum albumin, an effect related to decreased protein binding of the drug. A disturbing complication of etoposide therapy is the development of an unusual form of acute nonlymphocytic leukemia with a translocation in chromosome 11q23. At this locus is a gene (the MLL gene) that regulates the proliferation of pluripotent stem cells. The leukemic cells have the cytological appearance of acute monocytic or monomyelocytic leukemia. Another distinguishing feature of etoposide-related leukemia is the short time interval between the end of treatment and the onset of leukemia (1-3 years), compared to the 4- to 5-year interval for secondary leukemias related to alkylating agents, and the absence of a myelodysplastic period preceding leukemia. Patients receiving weekly or twice-weekly doses of etoposide, with cumulative doses >2000 mg/m^2, seem to be at higher risk of leukemia.

TENIPOSIDE

Teniposide (VUMON) is administered intravenously. It has a multiphasic pattern of clearance from plasma: after distribution, a $t_{1/2}$ of 4 h and another $t_{1/2}$ of 10-40 h are observed. Approximately 45% of the drug is excreted in the urine; in contrast to etoposide, as much as 80% is recovered as metabolites. Anticonvulsants such as phenytoin increase the hepatic metabolism of teniposide and reduce systemic exposure. Dosage need not be reduced for patients with impaired renal function. Less than 1% of the drug crosses the blood-brain barrier. Teniposide is available for treatment of refractory ALL in children and is synergistic with cytarabine. Teniposide is administered by intravenous infusion in dosages that range from 50 mg/m^2/day for 5 days to 165 mg/m^2/day twice weekly. The drug has limited utility and is given primarily for acute leukemia in children and monocytic leukemia in infants, as well as glioblastoma, neuroblastoma, and brain metastases from small cell carcinomas of the lung. Myelosuppression, nausea, and vomiting are its primary toxic effects.

DRUGS OF DIVERSE MECHANISM OF ACTION

BLEOMYCIN

The bleomycins, a unusual group of DNA-cleaving antibiotics, are fermentation products of *Streptomyces verticillus*. The drug currently employed clinically is a mixture of the 2 copper-chelating peptides, bleomycins A_2 and B_2, that differ only in their terminal amino acid. Because their toxicities do not overlap with those of other cytotoxic drugs, and because of their unique mechanism of action, bleomycin maintains an important role in treating Hodgkin disease and testicular cancer.

Mechanisms of Action and Resistance. Bleomycin's cytotoxicity results from its capacity to cause oxidative damage to the deoxyribose of thymidylate and other nucleotides, leading to single- and double-stranded breaks in DNA. Bleomycin causes accumulation of cells in the G_2 phase of the cell cycle, and many of these cells display chromosomal aberrations, including chromatid breaks, gaps, fragments, and translocations. Bleomycin cleaves DNA by generating free radicals. In the presence of O_2 and a reducing agent, the metal–drug complex becomes activated and functions as a ferrous oxidase, transferring electrons from Fe^{2+} to molecular oxygen to produce oxygen radicals. Metallobleomycin complexes can be activated by reaction with the flavin enzyme, NADPH-CYP_{450} reductase. Bleomycin binds to DNA, and the activated complex generates free radicals that are responsible for abstraction of a proton at the 3′ position of the deoxyribose backbone of the DNA chain, opening the deoxyribose ring and generating a strand break in DNA. An excess of breaks generates apoptosis.

Bleomycin is degraded by a specific hydrolase found in various normal tissues, including liver. Hydrolase activity is low in skin and lung, perhaps contributing to the serious toxicity. Some bleomycin-resistant cells contain high levels of hydrolase activity. In other cell lines, resistance has been attributed to decreased uptake, repair of strand breaks, or drug inactivation by thiols or thiol-rich proteins.

ADME. Bleomycin is administered intravenously, intramuscularly, or subcutaneously, or instilled into the bladder for local treatment of bladder cancer. Having a high molecular mass, bleomycin crosses the blood-brain barrier poorly. The elimination $t_{1/2}$ is ~3 h. About two-thirds of the drug is excreted intact in the urine. Concentrations in plasma are greatly elevated in patients with renal impairment and doses of bleomycin should be reduced in the presence of a CrCl <60 mL/min.

Therapeutic Uses. The recommended dose of bleomycin (BLENOXANE, others) is 10-20 units/m^2 given weekly or twice weekly by the intravenous, intramuscular, or subcutaneous route. A test dose of ≤2 units is recommended for lymphoma patients. Myriad regimens are employed clinically, with bleomycin doses expressed in units. Total courses exceeding 250 mg should be given with caution, and usually only in high-risk testicular cancer treatment, because of a marked increase in the risk of pulmonary toxicity. Bleomycin also may be instilled into the pleural cavity in doses of 5-60 mg to ablate the pleural space in patients with malignant effusions. Bleomycin is highly effective against germ cell tumors of the testis and ovary. In testicular cancer, it is curative when used with cisplatin and vinblastine or cisplatin and etoposide. It is a component of the standard curative ABVD regimen (doxorubicin [Adriamycin], bleomycin, vinblastine, and dacarbazine) for Hodgkin lymphoma.

Clinical Toxicities. Because bleomycin causes little myelosuppression, it has significant advantages in combination with other cytotoxic drugs. However, it does cause a constellation of cutaneous toxicities, including hyperpigmentation, hyperkeratosis, erythema, and even ulceration, and rarely, Raynaud phenomenon. Skin lesions may recur when patients are treated with other antineoplastic drugs. Rarely, bleomycin causes a flagellate dermatitis consisting of bands of pruritic erythema on the arms, back, scalp, and hands; this rash responds readily to topical corticosteroids.

The most serious adverse reaction to bleomycin is pulmonary toxicity, which begins with a dry cough, fine rales, and diffuse basilar infiltrates on X-ray and may progress to life-threatening pulmonary fibrosis. Approximately 5-10% of patients receiving bleomycin develop clinically apparent pulmonary toxicity, and ~1% die of this complication. Most who recover experience a significant improvement in pulmonary function, but fibrosis may be irreversible. Pulmonary function tests are not of predictive value for detecting early onset of this complication. The risk of pulmonary toxicity is related to total dose, with a significant increase in risk in total doses >250 mg and in patients >40 years of age, in those with a CrCl of <80 mL/min, and in those with underlying pulmonary disease; single doses of ≥30 mg/m^2 also are associated with an increased risk of pulmonary toxicity. Administration of high O_2 concentrations during anesthesia or respiratory therapy may aggravate or precipitate pulmonary toxicity in patients previously treated with the drug. There is no known specific therapy for bleomycin lung injury except for symptomatic management and standard pulmonary care. Steroids are of variable benefit, with greatest effectiveness in the earliest inflammatory stages of the lesion.

Other toxic reactions to bleomycin include hyperthermia, headache, nausea and vomiting, and a peculiar acute fulminant reaction observed in patients with lymphomas. This reaction is characterized by profound hyperthermia, hypotension, and sustained cardiorespiratory collapse; it does not appear to be a classical anaphylactic reaction and may be related to release of an endogenous pyrogen. This reaction has occurred in ~1% of patients with lymphomas or testicular cancer.

MITOMYCIN

Mitomycin has limited clinical utility, having been replaced by less toxic and more effective drugs, with the exception of anal cancers, for which it is curative.

Mechanisms of Action and Resistance. After intracellular enzymatic or spontaneous chemical alteration, mitomycin becomes a bifunctional or trifunctional alkylating agent. The drug inhibits DNA synthesis and cross-links DNA at the N6 position of adenine and at the O^6 and N^7 positions of guanine. Attempts to repair DNA lead to strand breaks. Mitomycin is a potent radiosensitizer, teratogen, and carcinogen in rodents. Resistance has been ascribed to deficient activation, intracellular inactivation of the reduced Q form, and P-glycoprotein-mediated drug efflux.

ADME. Mitomycin is administered intravenously. It has a $t_{1/2}$ of 25-90 min. The drug distributes widely throughout the body but is not detected in the CNS. Inactivation occurs by hepatic metabolism or chemical conjugation with sulfhydryls. Less than 10% of the active drug is excreted in the urine or the bile.

Therapeutic Uses. Mitomycin (mitomycin-C; MUTAMYCIN, others) is administered at a dose of 6-20 mg/m^2, given as a single bolus every 6-8 weeks. Dosage is modified based on hematological recovery. Mitomycin also may be used by direct instillation into the bladder to treat superficial carcinomas. Mitomycin is used in combination with 5-FU and cisplatin for anal cancer. Mitomycin is used off label (as an extemporaneously compounded eye drop) as an adjunct to surgery to inhibit wound healing and reduce scarring.

Clinical Toxicities. The major toxic effect is myelosuppression, characterized by marked leukopenia and thrombocytopenia; after higher doses, maximal suppression may be delayed and cumulative, with recovery only after 6-8 weeks of pancytopenia. Nausea, vomiting, diarrhea, stomatitis, rash, fever, and malaise also are observed. Patients who have received >50 mg/m^2 total dose may acutely develop hemolysis, neurological abnormalities, interstitial pneumonia, and glomerular damage resulting in renal failure. The incidence of renal failure increases to 28% in patients who receive total doses of ≥70 mg/m^2. There is no effective treatment for the disorder. It must be recognized early, and mitomycin must be discontinued immediately. Mitomycin causes interstitial pulmonary fibrosis; total doses >30 mg/m^2 have infrequently led to congestive heart failure. Mitomycin may potentiate the cardiotoxicity of doxorubicin.

MITOTANE

Mitotane (*o,p′*-DDD), a compound chemically similar to the insecticides DDT and DDD, is used in the treatment of neoplasms derived from the adrenal cortex.

The mechanism of action of mitotane has not been elucidated, but its relatively selective destruction of adrenocortical cells, normal or neoplastic, is well established. Administration of the drug causes a rapid reduction in the levels of adrenocorticosteroids and their metabolites in blood and urine, a response that is useful in both guiding dosage and following the course of hyperadrenocorticism (Cushing syndrome) resulting from an adrenal tumor or adrenal hyperplasia. It does not damage other organs.

ADME. Approximately 40% of mitotane is absorbed after oral administration. Plasma concentrations of mitotane are still measurable for 6-9 weeks following discontinuation of therapy. Although the drug is found in all tissues, fat is the primary site of storage. A water-soluble metabolite of mitotane found in the urine constitutes 25% of an oral or parenteral dose. About 60% of an oral dose is excreted unchanged in the stool.

Therapeutic Uses. Mitotane (LYSODREN) is administered in initial daily oral doses of 2-6 g, usually in 3 or 4 divided portions, and increasing to 9-10 g/day if tolerated. The maximal tolerated dose may vary from 2-16 g/day. Treatment should continue for at least 3 months; if beneficial effects are observed, therapy should be maintained indefinitely. Spironolactone should not be administered concomitantly, because it interferes with the adrenal suppression produced by mitotane. Treatment with mitotane is indicated for the palliation of inoperable adrenocortical carcinoma, producing symptomatic benefit in 30-50% of such patients.

Clinical Toxicity. Although the administration of mitotane produces anorexia and nausea in most patients, somnolence and lethargy in ~34%, and dermatitis in 15-20%, these effects do not contraindicate the use of the drug at lower doses. Because this drug damages the adrenal cortex, administration of replacement doses of adrenocorticosteroids is necessary.

TRABECTEDIN

Trabectedin (YONDELIS) is the only drug used clinically that is derived from a sea animal, the marine tunicate, *Ecteinascidin turbinate*.

Trabectedin binds to the minor groove of DNA, allowing the alkylation of the N2 position of guanine and bending the helix toward the major groove. The bulky DNA adduct is recognized by the transcription-coupled nucleotide excision repair complex, and these proteins initiate attempts to repair the damaged strand, converting the adduct to a double-stranded break. Trabectedin has particular cytotoxic effects on cells that lack components of the Fanconi anemia complex or those that lack the ability to repair double-strand DNA breaks through homologous recombination. Unlike cisplatin and other DNA adduct–forming drugs, its activity requires the presence of intact components of NER, including XPG, which may be important for initiation of single breaks and attempts at adduct removal.

ADME. Trabectedin is administered as a 24-h infusion of 1.3 mg/m^2 every 3 weeks. It is administered with dexamethasone, 4 mg twice daily, starting 24 h before drug infusion to diminish hepatic toxicity. The drug is slowly cleared by CYP3A4, with a plasma $t_{1/2}$ ~24-40 h.

Therapeutic Uses. Trabectedin is designated as an orphan drug in the U.S. for ovarian cancer, sarcoma, and pancreatic cancer. It is approved outside the U.S. for second-line treatment of soft-tissue sarcomas and for ovarian cancer in combination with a doxorubicin formulation (DOXIL). It produces a very high (>50%) disease control rate in myxoid liposarcomas.

Clinical Toxicity. Without dexamethasone pretreatment, trabectedin causes significant hepatic enzyme elevations and fatigue in at least one-third of patients. With the steroid, the increases in transaminase are less pronounced and rapidly reversible. Other toxicities include mild myelosuppression and, rarely, rhabdomyolysis.

ENZYMES

L-ASPARAGINASE

Malignant lymphoid cells depend on exogenous sources of L-asparagine. Thus, L-asparaginase (L-ASP) has become a standard agent for treating ALL.

Mechanism of Action. Most normal tissues synthesize L-asparagine in amounts sufficient for protein synthesis, but lymphocytic leukemias lack adequate amounts of asparagine synthase and derive the required amino acid from plasma. L-ASP, by catalyzing the hydrolysis of circulating asparagine to aspartic acid and ammonia, deprives these malignant cells of asparagine, leading to cell death. L-ASP is used in combination with other agents, including MTX, doxorubicin, vincristine, and prednisone for the treatment of ALL and for high-grade lymphomas. Resistance arises through induction of asparagine synthetase in tumor cells.

ADME and Therapeutic Use. L-ASP (ELSPAR) is given intramuscularly or intravenously. After intravenous administration, *E. coli*–derived L-ASP has a clearance rate from plasma of 0.035 mL/min/kg, a volume of distribution that approximates the volume of plasma in humans, and a $t_{1/2}$ of 1 day. The enzyme is given in doses of 6000-10,000 IU every third day for 3-4 weeks. Pegaspargase (PEG-L-ASPARAGINASE; ONCASPAR) a preparation in which the enzyme is conjugated to 5000-Da units of monomethoxy polyethylene glycol, has much slower clearance from plasma ($t_{1/2}$ of 6-7 days), and it is administered in doses of 2500 IU/m^2 intramuscularly no more frequently than every 14 days, producing rapid and complete depletion of plasma and tumor cell asparagine for 21 days in most patients. Pegaspargase has much reduced immunogenicity (<20% of patients develop antibodies) and has been approved for first-line ALL therapy.

Intermittent dosage regimens and longer durations of treatment increase the risk of inducing hypersensitivity. In hypersensitive patients, neutralizing antibodies inactivate L-ASP. Not all patients with neutralizing antibodies experience clinical hypersensitivity, although enzyme may be inactivated and therapy may be ineffective. In previously untreated ALL, pegaspargase produces more rapid clearance of lymphoblasts from bone marrow than does the *E. coli* preparation and circumvents the rapid antibody-mediated clearance seen with *E. coli* enzyme in relapsed patients. Asparaginase preparations only partially deplete CSF asparagine.

Clinical Toxicity. L-ASP toxicities result from its antigenicity as a foreign protein and its inhibition of protein synthesis. Hypersensitivity reactions, including urticaria and full-blown anaphylaxis, occur in 5-20% of patients and may be fatal. In these patients, pegaspargase is a safe and effective alternative. So-called "silent" enzyme inactivation by antibodies occurs in a higher percentage of patients than overt hypersensitivity and may be associated with a negative clinical outcome, especially in high-risk ALL patients.

Other toxicities result from inhibition of protein synthesis in normal tissues (e.g., hyperglycemia due to insulin deficiency, clotting abnormalities due to deficient clotting factors, hypertriglyceridemia due to effects on lipoprotein production, hypoalbuminemia). Pancreatitis also has been observed. The clotting problems may take the form of spontaneous thrombosis, or less frequently, hemorrhagic episodes. Brain magnetic resonance imaging studies should be considered in patients treated with L-ASP who present with seizures, headache, or altered mental status. Intracranial hemorrhage in the first week of L-ASP treatment is an infrequent but devastating complication. L-ASP also suppresses immune function. L-ASP terminates the antitumor activity of MTX when given shortly after the antimetabolite. By lowering serum albumin concentrations, L-ASP may decrease protein binding and accelerate plasma clearance of other drugs.

HYDROXYUREA

Hydroxyurea (HU) has unique and diverse biological effects as an antileukemic drug, radiation sensitizer, and an inducer of fetal hemoglobin in patients with sickle cell disease. It is orally administered, and its toxicity is modest and limited to myelosuppression.

Mechanisms of Action and Resistance. HU inhibits the enzyme ribonucleoside diphosphate reductase, which catalyzes the reductive conversion of ribonucleotides to deoxyribonucleotides, a rate-limiting step in the biosynthesis of DNA. HU binds the iron molecules that are essential for activation of a tyrosyl radical in the catalytic subunit of RNR. The drug is specific for the S phase of the cell cycle, during which RNR concentrations are maximal. It causes cells to arrest at or near the G_1–S interface through both p53-dependent and -independent mechanisms. Because cells are highly sensitive to irradiation at the G_1–S boundary, HU and irradiation cause synergistic antitumor effects. Through depletion of deoxynucleotides, HU potentiates the antiproliferative effects of DNA-damaging agents such as cisplatin, alkylating agents, or topoisomerase II inhibitors and facilitates the incorporation of antimetabolites such as Ara-C, gemcitabine, and fludarabine into DNA. It also promotes degradation of the p21 cell-cycle checkpoint and thereby enhances the effects of HDAC (histone deacetylase) inhibitors in vitro.

HU is the primary drug for improving control of sickle cell (HbS) disease in adults and for inducing fetal hemoglobin (HbF) in thalassemia HbC and HbC/S patients. It reduces vaso-occlusive events, painful cries, hospitalizations, and the need for blood transfusions in patients with sickle cell disease. The mechanism of stimulated HbF production is uncertain. HU stimulates NO production, causing nitrosylation of small-molecular-weight GTPases, a process that stimulates γ-globin production in erythroid precursors. Another property of HU that may be therapeutically relevant is its capacity to reduce L-selectin expression and thereby to reduce adhesion of red cells and neutrophils to vascular endothelium. Also, by suppressing the production of neutrophils, it decreases their contribution to vascular occlusion. Tumor cells become resistant to HU through increased synthesis of the catalytic subunit of RNR, thereby restoring enzyme activity.

ADME. The oral bioavailability of HU is 80-100%; comparable plasma concentrations are seen after oral or intravenous dosing. HU disappears from plasma with a $t_{1/2}$ of 3.5-4.5 h. The drug readily crosses the blood-brain barrier; significant quantities appear in human breast milk. From 40-80% of the drug is recovered in the urine within 12 h after administration. It is advisable to modify initial doses for patients with renal dysfunction.

Therapeutic Uses. In cancer treatment, 2 dosage schedules for HU (HYDREA, DROXIA, others), alone or in combination with other drugs, are most commonly used in a variety of solid tumors: (1) intermittent therapy with 80 mg/kg administered orally as a single dose every third day or (2) continuous therapy with 20-30 mg/kg administered as a single daily dose. In patients with essential thrombocythemia and in sickle cell disease, HU is given in a daily dose of 15 mg/kg, adjusting that dose upward or downward according to blood counts. The neutrophil count responds within 1-2 weeks to discontinuation of the drug. In treating subjects with sickle cell and related diseases, a neutrophil count of at least 2500 cells/mL should be maintained. Treatment typically is continued for 6 weeks to determine effectiveness; if satisfactory results are obtained, therapy can be continued indefinitely, although leukocyte counts at weekly intervals are advisable.

The principal use of HU has been as a myelosuppressive agent in various myeloproliferative syndromes, particularly CML, polycythemia vera, myeloid metaplasia, and essential thrombocytosis, for controlling high platelet or white cell counts. Many of the myeloproliferative syndromes harbor activating mutations of JAK2, a gene that is downregulated by HU. In essential thrombocythemia, it is the drug of choice for patients with a platelet count >1.5 million cells/mm^3 or with a history of arterial or venous thrombosis. In CML, HU has been largely replaced by imatinib. HU is a potent radiosensitizer as a consequence of its inhibition of RNR and has been incorporated into several treatment regimens with concurrent irradiation (i.e., cervical carcinoma, primary brain tumors, head and neck cancer, non–small-cell lung cancer).

Clinical Toxicity. Leukopenia, anemia, and occasionally thrombocytopenia are the major toxic effects; recovery of the bone marrow is prompt if the drug is discontinued for a few days. Other adverse reactions include a desquamative interstitial pneumonitis, GI disturbances, and mild dermatological reactions, and, more rarely, stomatitis, alopecia, and neurological manifestations. Increased skin and fingernail pigmentation may occur, as well as painful leg ulcers, especially in elderly patients or in those with renal dysfunction. HU does not increase the risk of secondary leukemia in patients with myeloproliferative disorders or sickle cell disease. It is a potent teratogen in animals and should not be used in women with childbearing potential.

DIFFERENTIATING AGENTS

One of the hallmarks of malignant transformation is a block in differentiation. A number of chemical entities (vitamin D and its analogs, retinoids, benzamides and other inhibitors of histone deacetylase, various cytotoxics and biological agents, and inhibitors of DNA methylation) can induce differentiation in tumor cell lines.

RETINOIDS

The biology and pharmacology of retinoids are discussed in Chapter 65. The most important of these for cancer treatment is tretinoin (all-*trans* retinoic acid [ATRA]), which induces a high rate of complete remission in acute promyelocytic leukemia (APL) as a single agent and, in combination with anthracyclines, cures most patients with this disease.

TRETINOIN (ATRA)

Mechanism of Action. Under physiological conditions, the retinoic acid receptor-α (RAR-α) dimerizes with the retinoid X receptor to form a complex that binds ATRA tightly. ATRA binding displaces a repressor from the complex and promotes differentiation of cells of multiple lineages. In APL cells, physiological concentrations of retinoid are inadequate to displace the repressor but pharmacological concentrations, are effective in activating the differentiation program and in promoting degradation of the PML–RAR-α fusion gene. The PML gene encodes a transcription factor (promyelocytic leukemia factor) important in inhibiting proliferation and promoting myeloid differentiation. The oncogenic PML–RAR-α gene produces a protein that binds retinoids with much decreased affinity, lacks PML regulatory function, and fails to upregulate transcription factors (C/EBP and PU.1) that promote myeloid differentiation. ATRA also binds and activates RAR-γ and thereby promotes stem-cell renewal, and this action may help restore normal bone marrow renewal. Resistance to ATRA arises by further mutation of the fusion gene, abolishing ATRA binding; by induction of the CYP26A1; or by loss of expression of the PML–RAR-α fusion gene.

Clinical Pharmacology. The dosing regimen of orally administered ATRA (VESANOID, others) is 45 mg/m^2/day until 30 days after remission is achieved (maximum course of therapy is 90 days). ATRA as a single agent reverses the hemorrhagic diathesis associated with APL and induces a high rate of temporary remission. ATRA in combination with an anthracycline induces remission with ≥80% relapse-free long-term survival.

ATRA is cleared by a CYP3A4-mediated elimination with a $t_{1/2}$ of <1 h. Treatment with inducers of CYP3A4 leads to more rapid drug disappearance and resistance to ATRA. Inhibitors of CYPs, such as antifungal imidazoles, block ATRA degradation and may lead to hypercalcemia and renal failure, which responds to diuresis, bisphosphonates, and ATRA discontinuation. Corticosteroids and chemotherapy sharply decrease the occurrence of "retinoic acid syndrome," which is characterized by fever, dyspnea, weight gain, pulmonary infiltrates, and pleural or pericardial effusions. When used as a single agent for remission induction, especially in patients with >5000 leukemic cells/mm^3 in the peripheral blood, ATRA induces an outpouring of cytokines and mature-appearing neutrophils of leukemic origin. These cells express high concentrations of integrins and other adhesion molecules on their surface and clog small vessels in the pulmonary circulation, leading to significant morbidity in 15-20% of patients. The syndrome of respiratory distress, pleural and pericardial effusions, and mental status changes may have a fatal outcome. Retinoids also cause dry skin, cheilitis, reversible hepatic enzyme abnormalities, bone tenderness, pseudotumor cerebri, hypercalcemia, and hyperlipidemia.

ARSENIC TRIOXIDE (ATO)

ATO is a highly effective treatment for relapsed APL, producing complete responses in >85% of such patients. The chemistry and toxicity of arsenic are considered in Chapter 67.

Mechanism of Action. The basis for ATO's antitumor activity remains uncertain. APL cells have high levels of reactive oxygen species (ROS) and are quite sensitive to further ROS induction. ATO inhibits thioredoxin reductase and thereby generates ROS. It inactivates glutathione and other sulfhydryls that scavenge ROS and thereby aggravates ROS damage. Cells exposed to ATO also upregulate p53, Jun kinase, and caspases associated with the intrinsic pathway of apoptosis and downregulate anti-apoptotic proteins such as bcl-2. ATO's cytotoxic effects are antagonized by cell survival signals emanating from activation of components of the PI3 kinase cell survival pathway, including Akt kinase, S6 kinase, and mammalian target of rapamycin (mTOR). ATO also induces differentiation of leukemic cell lines and in experimental and human leukemias.

Clinical Pharmacology. ATO (TRISENOX) is well absorbed orally but in cancer treatment is administered as a 2-h intravenous infusion in dosages of 0.15 mg/kg/day for up to 60 days, until remission is documented. The drug enters cells via one of several glucose transporters. The primary mechanism of elimination is through enzymatic methylation. Multiple methylated metabolites form rapidly and are excreted in urine. Less than 20% of administered drug is excreted unchanged in the urine. No dose reductions are indicated for hepatic or renal dysfunction.

Toxicity. Pharmacological doses of ATO are well tolerated. Patients may experience reversible side effects, including hyperglycemia, hepatic enzyme elevations, fatigue, dysesthesias, and light-headedness. Fewer than 10% of patients experience a leukocyte maturation syndrome similar to that seen with ATRA, including pulmonary distress, effusions, and mental status changes. Oxygen, corticosteroids, and temporary discontinuation of ATO lead to full reversal of this syndrome. Lengthening of the QT interval on the electrocardiogram occurs in 40% of patients, but rarely do patients develop torsade de pointes. Simultaneous treatment with other QT-prolonging drugs should be avoided. Monitoring of serum electrolytes and repletion of serum K^+ in patients with hypokalemia are precautionary measures in patients receiving ATO therapy. In patients exhibiting a significantly prolonged QT (>470 msec), treatment should be suspended, K^+ supplemented, and therapy resumed only if the QT returns to normal.

HISTONE DEACETYLASE INHIBITORS

VORINOSTAT

Vorinostat (ZOLINZA), also known as *suberoylanilide hydroxamic acid* (SAHA), is unique as an epigenetic modifier that directly affects histone function.

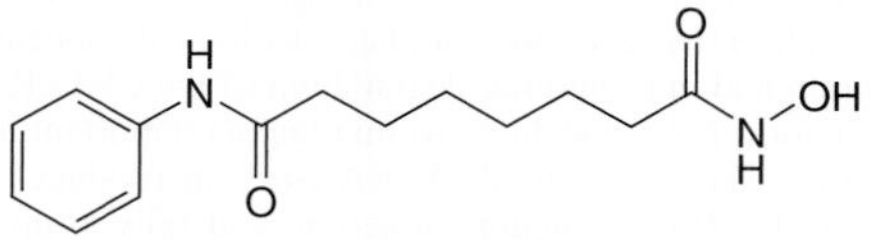

VORINOSTAT

Mechanism of Action. Acetylation of lysine residues on histones increases the spatial distance between DNA strands and the protein core, allowing access for transcription factor complexes, and enhancing transcriptional activity. Acetyl groups are added by histone acetyltransferases (HACs) and removed by histone deacetylases (HDACs). HDAC inhibitors such as vorinostat increase histone acetylation and thus enhance gene transcription. Many nonhistone proteins also are subject to lysine acetylation and thus are affected by treatment with HDAC inhibitors; the role of their acetylation status in the antitumor action of HDAC inhibitors is unclear.

Vorinostat is a hydroxamic acid modeled after hybrid polar compounds that cause differentiation of malignant cells in vitro, as do other classes of compounds with HDAC-inhibitory activity. These compounds bind to a critical Zn^{++} ion in the active site of HDAC enzymes. An important distinction between vorinostat and other HDAC inhibitors is that vorinostat and the hydroxymates are pan-HDAC inhibitors, whereas other compounds have selectivity for HDAC isoenzyme subsets. HDAC inhibitors induce cell-cycle arrest, differentiation, and apoptosis of cancer cells; nonmalignant cells are relatively resistant to these effects. These agents increase transcription of cell-cycle regulators, affect levels of nuclear transcription factors, and induce pro-apoptotic genes. HDAC inhibition directly blocks function of the chaperone HSP90 and stabilizes the tumor suppressor p53.

ADME. Vorinostat is administered as a once-daily oral dose of 400 mg. It is inactivated by glucuronidation of the hydroxyl amine group, followed by hydrolysis of the terminal carboxamide bond and further oxidation of the aliphatic side chain. The metabolites are pharmacologically inactive. The terminal $t_{1/2}$ in plasma is ~2 h. Histones remain hyperacetylated up to 10 h after an oral dose of vorinostat, suggesting that its effects persist beyond its measurable presence in the plasma.

Therapeutic Uses. In patients with refractory cutaneous T-cell lymphoma (CTCL), vorinostat produces an overall response rate of 30%, with a median time to progression of 5 months. Vorinostat and other HDAC inhibitors, including romidepsin (depsipeptide; FK228) and MGCD 0103, have shown activity in CTCL, other B- and T-cell lymphomas, and myeloid leukemia.

Toxicity. The most common side effects include fatigue, nausea, diarrhea, and thrombocytopenia. Deep venous thrombosis and pulmonary embolism are infrequent but serious adverse events. Caution is advised in patients with underlying cardiac abnormalities, and careful monitoring of the QTc interval and of electrolytes (K^+, Mg^{++}) is necessary.

For a complete Bibliographical Listing see Goodman & Gilman's ***The Pharmacological Basis of Therapeutics***, 12th ed., or Goodman & Gilman Online at www.AccessMedicine.com.

Targeted Therapies: Tyrosine Kinase Inhibitors, Monoclonal Antibodies, and Cytokines

Many new agents are available to block the fundamental mutations that cause specific cancers: aberrant growth factor receptors, dysregulated intracellular signaling pathways, defective DNA repair and apoptosis, and tumor angiogenesis. The primary tools for inhibiting these targets are *monoclonal antibodies* that attack cell surface receptors and antigens, and *synthetic small molecules* that enter cells and engage critical enzymes. These 2 classes of drugs have very different pharmacological properties.

Monoclonal antibodies kill tumor cells by blocking cell surface receptor function and by recruiting immune cells and complement to the antigen–antibody complex. They may be armed to carry toxins or radionuclides to the cells of interest, thereby enhancing their cytotoxic effects. They generally are specific for a single receptor, have a long plasma $t_{1/2}$, and require only intermittent administration. Small molecules may attack the same targets and pathways as the monoclonals, but may also exert their effect by entering cells and inhibiting enzymatic functions (usually tyrosine kinase reactions). The small molecules often inhibit multiple enzymatic sites, have a broad spectrum of target kinases, and tend to be substrates of hepatic CYPs with a $t_{1/2}$ of 12-24 h, and thus require daily oral administration.

These 2 drug classes, when targeted against the same pathway, may have significantly different spectra of antitumor activity. Thus, monoclonal antibodies to the epidermal growth factor receptor (EGFR) are effective in the treatment of head and neck and colon cancers, while small molecules, such as *erlotinib* and *gefitinib*, attack the intracellular tyrosine kinase function of the same receptor and have a different spectrum of antitumor activity (non–small cell lung cancer). The specific drug target is of central importance in cancer chemotherapy and forms the organizational basis for the discussion below.

PROTEIN TYROSINE KINASE INHIBITORS

There are 3 basic types of protein kinases (*see* Chapter 3):

- Kinases that specifically phosphorylate tyrosine residues
- Kinases that phosphorylate serine and threonine residues
- Kinases with activity toward all 3 residues

Tyrosine kinases can be further subdivided into those with an extracellular ligand-binding domain (*receptor tyrosine kinases, associated with growth factor receptors*, Figure 62–1) and intracellular enzymes (*nonreceptor tyrosine kinases*, e.g., src, abl, jak, fak, srm). In a number of human malignancies, mutations that constitutively activate protein tyrosine kinases are implicated in malignant transformation.

INHIBITORS OF THE BCR-ABL KINASE: IMATINIB, DASATINIB, AND NILOTINIB

Imatinib mesylate (STI 571, GLEEVEC, GLIVEC) targets the BCR-ABL tyrosine kinase, which underlies chronic myelogenous leukemia (CML). A single molecular event, in this case the 9:22 translocation, leads to expression of the Abelson proto-oncogene kinase ABL fused to BCR (breakpoint cluster region), yielding a constitutively activated protein kinase, BCR-ABL, and then the malignant phenotype.

Imatinib and the related compounds dasatinib and nilotinib induce clinical and molecular remissions in >90% of CML patients in the chronic phase of disease. Imatinib treats other tumors that carry related tyrosine kinase mutations, including GI stromal tumors (driven by c-KIT mutation), and hypereosinophilia syndrome, chronic myelomonocytic leukemia, and dermatofibrosarcoma protuberans (all driven by mutations that activate the PDGF receptor [PDGFR]).

CHARACTERISTICS AND MECHANISM OF ACTION. Imatinib was identified through high-throughput screening against the BCR-ABL kinase. Dasatinib (BMS-354825, SPRYCEL), a second-generation BCR-ABL inhibitor, inhibits the Src kinase, and unlike imatinib, it binds both the open and closed configurations of the BCR-ABL kinase. Nilotinib (AMN107, TASIGNA) was designed to have increased potency and specificity compared to imatinib. Its structure overcomes mutations that cause imatinib resistance. Imatinib and nilotinib bind to a

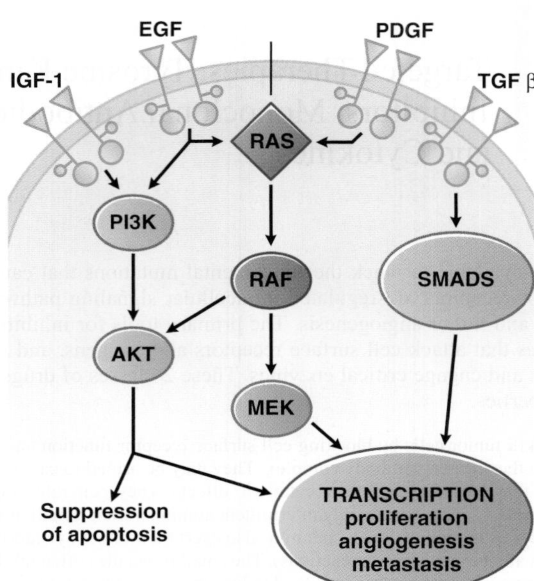

Figure 62–1 *Growth factor signaling.* Binding of agonist ligands to growth factor receptors (monospanning membrane proteins) causes receptor dimerization and activation of cytosolic protein kinase domains, leading to activation of multiple signaling pathways. Shown here are the RAS/MAPK/ERK, PI3K, and SMAD pathways, each of which is activated by receptors or cross-talk from adjacent pathways. Their signals regulate proliferation, metabolism, survival, and the synthesis of other growth factors, such as the vascular endothelial growth factor (VEGF).

segment of the kinase domain that fixes the enzyme in a closed or nonfunctional state, in which the protein is unable to bind its substrate/phosphate donor, ATP. The 3 BCR-ABL kinase inhibitors differ in their potency of inhibition, their binding specificities, and their susceptibility to resistance mutations in the target enzyme. Dasatinib [(IC_{50}) = <1 nM] and nilotinib [(IC_{50}) = <20 nM] inhibit BCR-ABL kinase more potently than does imatinib [(IC_{50}) = 100 nM].

MECHANISMS OF RESISTANCE. Resistance to the tyrosine kinase inhibitors arises from point mutations in 3 separate segments of the kinase domain (*see* Figure 62–1 in the 12th edition of the parent text). The contact points between imatinib and the enzyme become sites of mutations in drug-resistant leukemic cells; these mutations prevent tight binding of the drug and lock the enzyme in its open configuration, in which it has access to substrate and is enzymatically active. Nilotinib retains inhibitory activity in the presence of most point mutations that confer resistance to imatinib. Other mutations affect the phosphate-binding region and the "activation loop" of the domain with varying degrees of associated resistance. Some mutations, such as at amino acids 351 and 355, confer low levels of resistance to imatinib, possibly explaining the clinical response of some resistant patients to dose escalation of imatinib.

Molecular studies have detected resistance-mediating kinase mutations *prior* to initiation of therapy, particularly in patients with Ph^+ acute lymphoblastic leukemia (ALL) or CML in blastic crisis. This finding supports the hypothesis that drug-resistant cells arise through spontaneous mutation and expand under the selective pressure of drug exposure. Mechanisms other than BCR-ABL kinase mutation play a minor role in resistance to imatinib. Amplification of the wild-type kinase gene, leading to overexpression of the enzyme, has been identified in tumor samples from patients resistant to treatment. The multidrug resistant (*MDR*) gene confers resistance experimentally but has not been implicated in clinical resistance. Philadelphia chromosome-negative clones lacking the BCR-ABL translocation and displaying the karyotype of myelodysplastic cells may emerge in patients receiving imatinib for CML and may progress to myelodysplasia (MDS) and to acute myelocytic leukemia (AML). Their origin is unclear.

ADME

Imatinib. Imatinib is well absorbed after oral administration and reaches maximal plasma concentrations within 2-4 h. The elimination $t_{1/2}$ of imatinib and its major active metabolite, the *N*-desmethyl derivative, are ~18 and 40 h, respectively. Food does not change the pharmacokinetic profile. Doses >300 mg/day achieve trough levels of 1 μM, which correspond to in vitro levels required to kill BCR-ABL–expressing cells. In the treatment of GI stromal cell tumors (GISTs), higher doses (600 mg/day) may improve response rates. CYP3A4 is the major metabolizer of imatinib; thus, drugs that induce or interact with CYP3A4 can alter the pharmacokinetics of imatinib. Coadministration of imatinib and rifampin, an inducer of CYP3A4, lowers the plasma imatinib AUC by 70%. Imatinib, as a competitive CYP3A4 substrate, inhibits the metabolism of simvastatin and increases its plasma AUC by 3.5-fold.

Dasatinib. Oral dasatinib is well absorbed; its bioavailability is significantly reduced at neutral gastric pH (i.e., after antacids and H_2 blockers) but is unaffected by food. The plasma $t_{1/2}$ of dasatinib is 3-5 h. Dasatinib exhibits dose proportional increases in AUC, and its clearance is constant over the dose range of 15-240 mg/day. Dasatinib doses of 70 mg twice a day, 100 mg daily, and 140 mg daily are equally effective in patients with CML, although the 100-mg daily dose improves progression-free survival. Dasatinib is metabolized primarily by CYP3A4, with minor contributions by FMO3 and UGT. Plasma concentrations of dasatinib are affected by inducers and inhibitors of CYP3A4 in a similar fashion to imatinib.

Nilotinib. Approximately 30% of an oral dose of nilotinib (400 mg 2 times daily) is absorbed after administration, with peak concentrations in plasma 3 h after dosing. Unlike the other BCR-ABL inhibitors, nilotinib's bioavailability increases significantly in the presence of food. The drug has a plasma $t_{1/2}$ ~17 h, and plasma concentrations reach a steady state only after 8 days of daily dosing. Nilotinib is metabolized by CYP3A4, with predictable alteration by inducers, inhibitors, and competitors of CYP3A4. Nilotinib is a substrate and inhibitor of P-glycoprotein.

THERAPEUTIC USES. These protein tyrosine kinase inhibitors have efficacy in diseases in which the ABL, *kit*, or PDGFR have dominant roles in driving the proliferation of the tumor, reflecting the presence of a mutation that results in constitutive activation of the kinase. Imatinib shows remarkable therapeutic benefits in patients with chronic-phase CML (BCR-ABL), GIST (*kit* mutation positive), chronic myelomonocytic leukemia (EVT6-PDGFR translocation), hypereosinophilia syndrome (FIP1L1-PDGFR), and dermatofibrosarcoma protuberans (constitutive production of the ligand for PDGFR). It is the agent of choice for GIST patients with metastatic disease and as adjuvant therapy of *c-kit*–positive GIST. The currently recommended dose of imatinib is 400-600 mg/day. Dasatinib is approved for patients with CML resistant or intolerant to imatinib in both chronic (100 mg/day) and advanced phases of disease (70 mg twice daily), and for use combined with cytotoxic chemotherapy in patients with Ph^+ ALL who are resistant or intolerant to prior therapies. Nilotinib is approved for patients with CML resistant to or intolerant of prior imatinib therapy.

TOXICITY. Imatinib, dasatinib, and nilotinib cause GI symptoms (diarrhea, nausea, and vomiting) that are usually readily controlled. All 3 drugs promote fluid retention, edema, and peri-orbital swelling. Dasatinib may cause pleural effusions. Nilotinib may prolong the QT interval. Myelosuppression occurs infrequently but may require transfusion support, dose reduction, or discontinuation of the drug. These drugs can be associated with hepatotoxicity. Most nonhematological adverse reactions are self-limited and respond to dose adjustments. After the adverse reactions have resolved, the drug may be reinitiated and titrated back to effective doses.

EPIDERMAL GROWTH FACTOR RECEPTOR INHIBITORS

The EGFR belongs to the ErbB family of transmembrane receptor tyrosine kinases. EGFR, also known as ErbB1 or HER1, is essential for the growth and differentiation of epithelial cells. Ligand binding to the extracellular domain of EGFR family members causes receptor dimerization and stimulates the protein tyrosine kinase activity of the intracellular domain, resulting in autophosphorylation of several Tyr residues in the C-terminal domain. Recognition of the phosphotyrosines by other proteins initiates protein-protein interactions that result in stimulation of signaling pathways including MAPK, PI3K/Akt, and STAT pathways (*see* Figure 62–1). In epithelial cancers, overexpression and mutational activation of the EGFR are a common finding and create a dependence on EGFR signaling in these tumors.

Two separate classes of drugs that target the EGFR pathway are important agents in the therapy of solid tumors. The EGFR tyrosine kinase inhibitors *erlotinib* and *gefitinib* bind to the kinase domain and block the enzymatic function of EGFR. The monoclonal antibodies *cetuximab* and *panitumumab* bind specifically to the extracellular domain of EGFR and inhibit EGFR-dependent signaling.

GEFITINIB

Mechanism of Action. Gefitinib inhibits the EGFR tyrosine kinase by competitive blockade of ATP binding. Gefitinib has an IC_{50} of 20-80 nM for the EGFR tyrosine kinase but is significantly less potent against HER2 (ErbB2/neu). Gefitinib has antitumor activity in human xenograft tumors that exhibit high levels of EGFR expression.

ADME. Oral bioavailability is ~60%; peak plasma concentrations are achieved within 3-7 h. Absorption of gefitinib is not significantly altered by food but is reduced by drugs that cause elevations in gastric pH. Metabolism of gefitinib is predominantly via CYP3A4, with a terminal $t_{1/2}$ of 41 h. Inducers of CYP3A4 activity decrease gefitinib plasma concentrations and efficacy; conversely, CYP3A4 inhibitors increase plasma concentrations.

Therapeutic Uses. Gefitinib initially was approved for the third-line treatment of patients with non–small cell lung cancer. However, a large clinical trial failed to show an effect on survival, leading the FDA to restrict its use to patients who have previously received clinical benefit from the drug. Two large trials have failed to demonstrate a benefit of gefitinib in combination with chemotherapy: patients who were nonsmokers, Asians, or women were most likely to respond to gefitinib. Tumors from these patients frequently have characteristic activating mutations in *EGFR*. The standard dose is 250 mg/day.

Adverse Effects and Drug Interactions. Diarrhea and pustular/papular rash occur in ~50% of patients. Other side effects include dry skin, nausea, vomiting, pruritus, anorexia, and fatigue. Most adverse effects occur within the first month of therapy and are manageable with medications and dose reductions. Asymptomatic increases in liver transaminases may necessitate dose reduction or discontinuation of therapy. Interstitial lung disease occurs in <2% of patients and may have a fatal outcome. Inducers and inhibitors of CYP3A4 will alter plasma concentrations. Patients using warfarin should be monitored closely for elevation of the international normalized ratio (INR) while taking gefitinib.

ERLOTINIB

Mechanism of Action. Erlotinib (TARCEVA) is a potent inhibitor of the EGFR tyrosine kinase, competitively inhibiting ATP binding at the active site of the kinase. Erlotinib has an IC_{50} of 2 nM for the EGFR kinase. Tumors harboring *k-ras* mutations and *EML4-ALK* translocations do not respond to EGFR kinase inhibitors.

ADME. Erlotinib is ~60% absorbed after oral administration but should not be taken with food, which increases its bioavailability to ~100%. Peak plasma levels occur after 4 h. Erlotinib has a $t_{1/2}$ of 36 h and is metabolized by CYP3A4 and to a lesser extent by CYPs 1A2 and 1A1. The standard daily dose of erlotinib results in a plasma AUC ~10-fold greater than the AUC of gefitinib.

Therapeutic Uses. Erlotinib is approved for second-line treatment of patients with locally advanced or metastatic non–small cell lung cancer. Erlotinib also is approved for first-line treatment of patients with locally advanced, unresectable, or metastatic pancreatic cancer in combination with gemcitabine. The recommended dose of erlotinib in non–small cell lung cancer is a 150-mg tablet daily. In pancreatic cancer, the dose is a 100-mg tablet daily, taken at least 1 h before or 2 h after a meal.

Adverse Effects and Drug Interactions. The most common adverse reactions are diarrhea, an acneform rash, anorexia, and fatigue. Serious or fatal interstitial lung disease occurs with a frequency of 0.7-2.5%. Serious or fatal hepatic failure due to erlotinib has been reported, particularly in patients with baseline hepatic dysfunction. Other rare but serious toxicities include GI perforation, renal failure, arterial thrombosis, microangiopathic hemolytic anemia, hand-foot skin reaction, and corneal perforation or ulceration. Erlotinib therapy may cause rare cases of Stevens-Johnson syndrome/toxic epidermal necrolysis.

Concurrent use of proton-pump inhibitors decreases the bioavailability of erlotinib by 50%. Plasma levels can vary due to drug interactions with inducers or inhibitors of CYP3A4. Patients using warfarin may experience elevations of the INR while taking erlotinib. Smoking accelerates metabolic clearance of erlotinib and may decrease its antitumor effects.

RESISTANCE TO GEFITINIB AND ERLOTINIB

Patients with non–small cell lung cancer who initially respond to erlotinib or gefitinib have tumors that are dependent on the EGFR signaling pathway. Tumors containing mutations in *EGFR* initially respond to erlotinib and gefitinib but eventually progress. A secondary mutation in the *EGFR* gatekeeper residue, T790M, prevents binding of drug to the kinase domain and confers resistance. Other potential mechanisms of resistance include activation of downstream mediators, efflux of drug, and altered receptor trafficking. Therapy directed at the EGFR may delay disease progression in patients with non–small cell lung cancers that lack activating *EGFR* mutations, although response rates approach zero in these patients.

CETUXIMAB

Cetuximab (ERBITUX) is a recombinant chimeric human/mouse immunoglobulin G1 (IgG_1) antibody that binds to the extracellular domain of EGFR. Such antibodies, although sharing the same target with erlotinib and gefitinib and having a similar side effect profile, have a different spectrum of antitumor activity.

Mechanism of Action. Cetuximab binds specifically to the extracellular domain of EGFR and prevents ligand-dependent signaling and receptor dimerization, thereby blocking cell growth and survival signals. Cetuximab also may mediate antibody-dependent cellular cytotoxicity against tumor cells.

ADME. Cetuximab exhibits nonlinear pharmacokinetics. Following intravenous administration, steady-state levels are achieved by the third weekly infusion. Therapeutic doses that saturate total body receptor pools of EGFR follow zero-order kinetics for elimination. Clearance occurs via EGFR binding and internalization and by degradation in the reticuloendothelial system.

Therapeutic Uses

Head and Neck Cancer. Cetuximab is used in combination with radiation therapy for locally or regionally advanced squamous cell carcinoma of the head and neck (HNSCC). It also is indicated in monotherapy for patients with metastatic or recurrent HNSCC who fail platinum-based chemotherapy. It is a useful agent in combination with cisplatin-based chemotherapy.

Metastatic Colon Cancer. Cetuximab is approved as a single agent for the treatment of EGFR-positive metastatic colorectal cancer; cetuximab is used in patients who cannot tolerate irinotecan-based therapy and in combination with irinotecan for patients refractory to oxaliplatin, irinotecan, and 5-fluorouracil (5-FU). In the first-line setting, cetuximab may improve survival in combination with 5-FU/leucovorin and irinotecan or oxaliplatin. About 40-50% of colorectal tumors carry mutations in the *k-ras* oncogene and are resistant to the effects of cetuximab. Cetuximab enhances the effectiveness of chemotherapy in patients with *k-ras* mutant tumors but not *k-ras* wild-type tumors. The standard dose of cetuximab is a single loading dose of 400 mg/m^2 intravenously, followed by weekly doses of 250 mg/m^2 intravenously for the duration of treatment.

Adverse Effects. Side effects include an acneform rash (in the majority of patients), pruritus, nail changes, headache, and diarrhea. Rare but serious adverse effects include cardiopulmonary arrest, interstitial lung disease, and hypomagnesemia. In addition, patients can develop anaphylactoid reactions during infusion, which may be related to preexisting IgE antibodies that are more prevalent in patients from the southern U.S.

PANITUMUMAB

Panitumumab (VECTIBIX) is a recombinant, fully humanized $IgG_{2\kappa}$ antibody that binds specifically to the extracellular domain of EGFR. Unlike cetuximab, it does not mediate antibody-dependent cell-mediated cytotoxicity.

Panitumumab exhibits nonlinear pharmacokinetic characteristics. Following intravenous administration every 2 weeks, steady-state levels are achieved by the third infusion. The mean $t_{1/2}$ is 7.5 days. Panitumumab improves progression-free survival in patients with metastatic colorectal carcinoma. The dose of panitumumab is 6 mg/kg intravenously given once every 2 weeks. The adverse effects with panitumumab are similar to cetuximab and include rash and dermatological toxicity, severe infusion reactions, pulmonary fibrosis, and electrolyte abnormalities.

HER2/NEU INHIBITORS

Both antibodies (trastuzumab, pertuzumab) and small molecules (lapatinib et al.) have striking antitumor effects in patients with HER2-positive breast cancer, and have become essential therapeutic agents in combination with cytotoxic chemotherapy for this aggressive malignancy.

TRASTUZUMAB. Trastuzumab (HERCEPTIN) is a humanized monoclonal antibody that binds to the external domain of HER2/neu (ErbB2).

Thirty percent of breast cancers overexpress this receptor due to gene amplification on chromosome 17. Amplification of the receptor is associated with lower response rates to hormonal therapies and to most cytotoxic drugs, with the exception of anthracyclines. Patients with HER2/neu-amplified tumors have higher recurrence rates after standard adjuvant therapy and poorer overall survival. The internal domain of the HER2/neu glycoprotein encodes a tyrosine kinase that activates downstream signal, enhances metastatic potential, and inhibits apoptosis. Trastuzumab exerts its antitumor effects through: inhibition of homo- or heterodimerization of receptor, thereby preventing receptor kinase activation and downstream signaling; initiation of Fcγ-receptor-mediated antibody-dependent cellular cytotoxicity; and blockade of the angiogenetic effects of HER2 signaling.

Therapeutic Uses. Trastuzumab is approved for HER2/neu-overexpressing metastatic breast cancer, in combination with paclitaxel as initial treatment or as monotherapy following chemotherapy relapse. Trastuzumab synergizes with other cytotoxic agents in HER2/neu-overexpressing cancers.

Pharmacokinetics and Toxicity. Trastuzumab has dose-dependent pharmacokinetics with a mean $t_{1/2}$ of 5.8 days on the 2-mg/kg maintenance dose. Steady-state levels are achieved between 16 and 32 weeks. The infusional effects of trastuzumab are typical for monoclonal antibodies and include fever, chills, nausea, dyspnea, and rashes. Premedication with diphenhydramine and acetaminophen is indicated. The most serious toxicity of trastuzumab is cardiac failure; reasons for cardiotoxicity are poorly understood. Before initializing therapy, baseline electrocardiogram and cardiac ejection fraction measurement should be obtained to rule out underlying heart disease, and patients deserve careful clinical follow-up thereafter for signs or symptoms of congestive heart failure. When trastuzumab is used as a single agent, <5% of patients will experience a decrease in left-ventricular ejection fraction, and 1% will have clinical signs of congestive failure. Left-ventricular dysfunction occurs in up to 20% of patients who receive the antibody in combination with doxorubicin and cyclophosphamide. The risk of cardiac toxicity is greatly reduced with taxane–trastuzumab combinations.

LAPATINIB. Lapatinib and other pan-HER inhibitors block both ErbB1 and ErbB2 and bind to an internal site on the receptor (usually the ATP-binding pocket), compared to the external binding site of trastuzumab. Lapatinib also inhibits a truncated form of the HER2 receptor that lacks a trastuzumab-binding domain, differences that may account for the activity of lapatinib in trastuzumab-resistant patients.

Therapeutic Uses. Lapatinib (TYKERB) is approved for HER2-amplified, trastuzumab-refractory breast cancer, in combination with the fluoropyrimidine analog, capecitabine. As a small molecule, lapatinib crosses the blood-brain barrier more readily than inhibitor antibodies and has produced anecdotal responses in patients with brain metastases in phase III trial.

Pharmacokinetics and Toxicity. The drug is administered orally, 1250 mg/day. It is metabolized by CYP3A4 to inactive products and oxidized to an intermediate that has activity against ErbB1 but not ErbB2. The plasma $t_{1/2}$ is 14 h. Concurrent administration of inducers and inhibitors of CYP3A4 may necessitate adjustment of the dose. Lapatinib toxicities include mild diarrhea, cramping, and exacerbation of gastro-esophageal reflux. When lapatinib is combined with capecitabine, diarrhea becomes a significant side effect (33%). Lapatinib causes an acneform rash in one-third of patients that may be controlled with topical benzoyl peroxide gel. Lapatinib has no clear signal of cardiac toxicity; nonetheless, because it targets ErbB2, lapatinib should be used with caution in combination with other cardiotoxic drugs and with careful surveillance in patients with heart disease.

INHIBITORS OF ANGIOGENESIS

Cancer cells secrete angiogenic factors that induce the formation of new blood vessels and guarantee the flow of nutrients to the tumor cells. Angiogenic factors secreted by tumors include VEGF (*vascular endothelial* growth factor), FGF (*fibroblast* growth factor), TGF-β (*transforming* growth factor β), and PDGF (*platelet-derived* growth factor). Multiple tumor types overexpress these angiogenic factors. Tumor secretion of pro-angiogenic factors turns on an "angiogenic switch," a process essential to tumor growth and metastasis. In multiple experimental models, blockade of these pro-angiogenic molecules halts tumor growth, and in human cancers, anti-angiogenic drugs also have inhibitory effects.

Leaky capillaries within tumors have increased permeability and cause an increase in tumor interstitial pressure that inhibits blood flow, decreases oxygenation, and prevents drug delivery within the tumor. Antibodies directed at the primary angiogenic factor, VEGF, "normalize" interstitial pressure, improve blood flow, and enhance the ability of chemotherapeutic agents to reach the tumor. Hence, an additional benefit of anti-angiogenic molecules may be their ability to increase the delivery of chemotherapy to the tumor. This hypothesis seems to be validated in the synergy observed when cytotoxic chemotherapy is combined with anti-VEGF antibodies.

VEGF initiates endothelial cell proliferation when it binds to a member of the VEGF receptor (VEGFR) family, a group of highly homologous receptors with intracellular tyrosine kinase domains that includes VEGFR1 (FLT1), VEGFR2 (KDR), and VEGFR3 (FLT4). The binding of VEGF to its receptor activates the intracellular VEGFR tyrosine kinase activity and initiates mitogenic and anti-apoptotic signaling pathways. Antibodies targeting VEGF, such as *bevacizumab*, sterically hinder the interaction of VEGF with its receptor. *Aflibercept* (ZALTRAP), acts as a VEGF Trap; it is a recombinant molecule that uses the VEGFR1-binding domain to sequester VEGF and acts as a "soluble decoy receptor" for VEGF. Three small molecules (*pazopanib, sorafenib*, and *sunitinib*) that inhibit the kinase function of VEGFR-2 have been approved for clinical use. Although bevacizumab and the small molecules share a similar spectrum of toxicities, they have different spectra of clinical activity and pharmacokinetics.

BEVACIZUMAB

Bevacizumab (AVASTIN), a humanized antibody directed against VEGF-A, delays progression of renal-cell cancer, and, in combination with cytotoxic chemotherapy, effectively treats lung, colorectal, and breast cancers.

ADME. Bevacizumab is administered intravenously as a 30- to 90-min infusion. In metastatic colon cancer, in conjunction with combination chemotherapy, the dose of bevacizumab is 5 mg/kg every 2 weeks. In metastatic non–small cell lung cancer, doses of 15 mg/kg are given every 3 weeks with chemotherapy. For metastatic breast cancer, patients receive 10 mg/kg of bevacizumab every 2 weeks in combination with paclitaxel or docetaxel. The antibody has a plasma $t_{1/2}$ of 4 weeks.

Therapeutic Uses. In clear-cell renal-cell carcinoma, a cancer notoriously resistant to traditional chemotherapeutic agents, single-agent bevacizumab increases survival by 3 months. Bevacizumab is approved in combination with interferon-α for the treatment of metastatic renal-cell carcinoma. Bevacizumab is approved as a single agent following prior therapy for glioblastoma. In all other cancers, bevacizumab has little apparent single-agent activity but improves survival in epithelial cancers in combination with standard chemotherapeutic agents. Bevacizumab with carboplatin and paclitaxel increases survival in non–small lung cancer by 2 months. Likewise, bevacizumab combined with FOLFOX (5-FU, leucovorin, and oxaliplatin) or FOLFIRI (5-FU, leucovorin, and irinotecan) improves survival by 5 months in metastatic colon cancer. Finally, the combination of bevacizumab with docetaxel increases progression-free survival in patients with metastatic breast cancer.

A slightly altered version of bevacizumab, ranibizumab (LUCENTIS), in which the Fc region has been deleted, effectively treats wet macular degeneration. Bevacizumab restores hearing in patients with progressive deafness due to neurofibromatosis type 2–related tumors.

Toxicity. Bevacizumab causes a wide range of class-related adverse effects. A prominent concern is the potential for vessel injury and bleeding in patients with squamous-cell lung cancer. Bevacizumab is contraindicated for patients who have a history of hemoptysis, brain metastasis, or a bleeding diathesis, but in appropriately selected patients, the rate of life-threatening pulmonary hemorrhage is <2%. The most dreaded vascular toxicity of anti-angiogenic agents is an arterial thromboembolic event (i.e., stroke or myocardial infarction). The rate of arterial thromboembolic events in patients receiving bevacizumab-containing regimens is 3.8% compared to the control rate of 1.7%. To reduce the risk of arterial thromboembolic events, clinicians should evaluate a patient's risk factors (age >65 years, a past history of arterial thromboembolic events) before starting the drug.

Other toxicities characteristic of anti-angiogenic drugs include hypertension and proteinuria. A majority of patients receiving the drug require antihypertensive therapy, particularly those receiving higher doses and more prolonged treatment. Bevacizumab is rarely associated with congestive heart failure, probably secondary to hypertension, and with reversible posterior leukoencephalopathy in patients with poorly controlled hypertension. GI perforation, a potentially life-threatening complication, has been observed (up to 11%) in patients with ovarian cancer. In colon cancer patients, colonic perforation occurs infrequently during bevacizumab treatment but increases in frequency in patients with intact primary colonic tumors, peritoneal carcinomatosis, peptic ulcer disease, chemotherapy-associated colitis, diverticulitis, or prior abdominal radiation treatment. The rate of colon perforation is <1% in breast and lung cancer patients. Colon cancer surgery patients on bevacizumab have a higher rate (13% vs. 3.4%) of serious wound healing complications. Because of the long $t_{1/2}$ of bevacizumab, elective surgery should be delayed for at least 4 weeks from the last dose of antibody, and treatment should be not resumed for at least 4 weeks after surgery.

SUNITINIB

Sunitinib (SUTENT) competitively inhibits the binding of ATP to the tyrosine kinase domain on the VEGF receptor-2, a mechanism it shares with *sorafenib*. Sunitinib also inhibits other protein tyrosine kinases at concentrations of 5-100 nM.

Pharmacokinetics. Sunitinib is administered orally in doses of 50 mg once a day. The typical cycle of sunitinib is 4 weeks on treatment followed by 2 weeks off. The dosage and schedule of sunitinib can be increased or decreased according to toxicity (hypertension, fatigue). Dosages <25 mg/day typically are ineffective. Sunitinib is metabolized by CYP3A4 to produce an active metabolite, SU12662, the $t_{1/2}$ of which is 80-110 h; steady-state levels of the metabolite are reached after ~2 weeks of repeated administration of the parent drug. Further metabolism results in the formation of inactive products. The pharmacokinetics of sunitinib are not affected by food intake.

Therapeutic Uses. Sunitinib has activity in metastatic renal-cell cancer, producing a higher response rate (31%) and a longer progression-free survival than any other approved anti-angiogenic drug. Sunitinib also is approved for treatment of advanced renal-cell carcinoma, GIST that have developed resistance to imatinib as a consequence of *c-KIT* mutations, and pancreatic neuroendocrine tumors. Specific *c-KIT* mutations correlate with degree of response to sunitinib (e.g., patients with *c-KIT* exon 9 mutations have a response rate of 37%; patients with *c-KIT* exon 11 mutations have only a 5% response rate).

Toxicity. The main toxicities of sunitinib are shared by all anti-angiogenic inhibitors: bleeding, hypertension, proteinuria, and, uncommonly, arterial thromboembolic events and intestinal perforation. However, because sunitinib is a multi-targeted tyrosine kinase inhibitor, it has a broader side-effect profile than bevacizumab. Fatigue affects 50-70% of patients and may be disabling. Hypothyroidism occurs in 40-60% of patients. Bone marrow suppression and diarrhea also are common side effects; severe neutropenia (neutrophils <1000/mL) develop in 10% of patients. Less common side effects include congestive heart failure (usually in association with hypertension) and hand-foot syndrome. It is essential to check blood counts and thyroid function at regular intervals. Periodic echocardiograms also are recommended.

SORAFENIB

Sorafenib (NEXAVAR), like sunitinib, targets multiple protein tyrosine kinases and inhibits their catalytic activities at concentrations of 20-90 nM. Sorafenib is the only drug currently approved for treatment of hepatocellular carcinoma. Sorafenib also is approved in metastatic renal-cell cancer, for which sunitinib generally is the preferred first-line therapy.

ADME. Sorafenib is given orally, beginning with 200 mg once a day and increasing to 400 mg twice a day as tolerated. Sorafenib is given every day without treatment breaks. Sorafenib is metabolized to inactive products by CYP3A4 with a $t_{1/2}$ of 20-27 h; with repeated administration, steady-state concentrations are reached within 1 week.

Adverse Effects. Sorafenib patients can experience the vascular toxicities seen with other anti-angiogenic medications. More common adverse effects include fatigue, nausea, diarrhea, anorexia, and rash; uncommonly, bone marrow suppression and GI perforation.

IMMUNOMODULATORS (IMiDs)

Among agents with anti-angiogenic activity, the immunomodulatory analogs (IMiDs) thalidomide and lenalidomide have a most unusual history and a multiplicity of biological and immunological effects. Thalidomide originally was used for the treatment of pregnancy-associated morning sickness but was withdrawn from the market due to teratogenicity and dysmelia (stunted limb growth). It re-entered clinical practice for treatment of erythema nodosum leprosum (*see* Chapter 56). Further research revealed its anti-angiogenic and immunomodulatory effects. At least 4 distinct mechanisms have been proposed to explain the antitumor activity of IMiDs as summarized by Figure 62–2 and enumerated in its legend.

Both thalidomide and lenalidomide possess potent activity in newly diagnosed and heavily pretreated relapsed/refractory multiple myeloma (MM) patients. Lenalidomide also is approved for its activity in the 5q– subset of MDS. A specific gene array profile identifies MDS patients who lack the 5q– abnormality but respond to lenalidomide.

THALIDOMIDE

ADME. Thalidomide (THALOMID) exists at physiological pH as a racemic mixture of cell-permeable and rapidly interconverting non-polar S(–) and R(+) isomers. The R-enantiomer is associated with the teratogenic and biological activities, while the S accounts for the sedative properties of thalidomide. Thalidomide is given in dosages of 200-1200 mg/day. In treating MM, doses usually are escalated by 200 mg/day every 2 weeks until dose-limiting side effects (sedation, fatigue, constipation, or a sensory neuropathy) supervene. With extended treatment, the neuropathy may necessitate dose reduction or discontinuation of treatment for a period of time. Thalidomide absorption from the GI tract is slow and highly variable. It distributes throughout most tissues and organs, without significant binding to plasma proteins. The enantiomers are eliminated with a $t_{1/2} \approx 6$ h, mainly due to spontaneous hydrolysis in all body fluids; the S-enantiomer is cleared more rapidly than the R-enantiomer. Thalidomide and its metabolites are excreted in the urine, while the non-absorbed portion of the drug is excreted unchanged in feces. The inactive hydrolysis products undergo CYP-mediated metabolism. Longer plasma $t_{1/2}$ is reported at highest doses (1200 mg daily). No dose adjustment is necessary in the presence of renal failure.

Thalidomide enhances the sedative effects of barbiturates and alcohol and the catatonic effects of chlorpromazine and reserpine. Conversely, CNS stimulants (such as methamphetamine and methylphenidate) counteract the depressant effects of thalidomide.

LENALIDOMIDE

Lenalidomide (REVLIMID) constitutes the lead compound of immunomodulatory thalidomide derivatives. Pharmacological properties include: direct suppression of the tumor cell growth in culture, T-cell and NK-cell activation, suppression of TNF-α and other cytokines, anti-angiogenesis, and promotion of hematopoietic stem cell differentiation.

ADME. The standard dosage of lenalidomide is 25 mg/day for 21 days of a 28-day cycle. The drug is rapidly absorbed following oral administration, reaching peak plasma levels within 1.5 h. The $t_{1/2}$ of parent drug in plasma is 9 h. Approximately 70% of the orally administered dose of lenalidomide is excreted intact by the kidney. Dose adjustments to 10 mg/day for creatinine clearance of 30-50 mL/h and to the same dose every 2 days for creatinine clearance <30 mL/h are recommended for patients with renal failure.

Therapeutic Use. Lenalidomide exhibits potent antitumor activity in MM, MDS, and chronic lymphocytic leukemia (CLL); this agent causes fewer adverse side effects and lacks the teratogenicity of thalidomide.

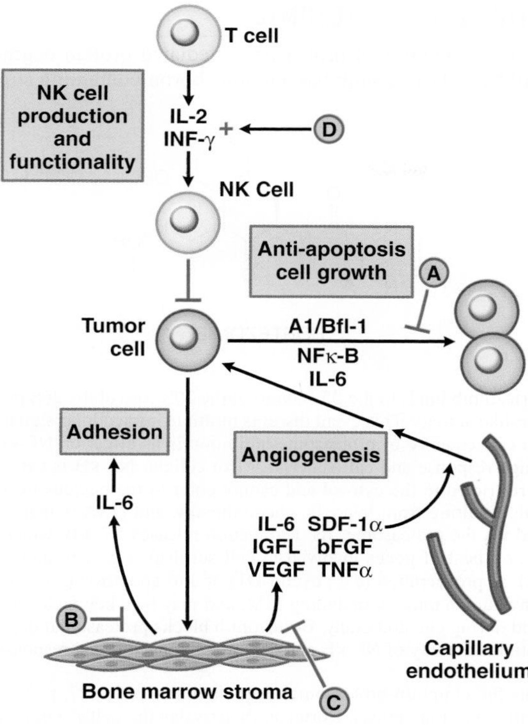

Figure 62–2 *Schematic overview of proposed mechanisms of antimyeloma activity of thalidomide and its derivatives.* Some biological hallmarks of the malignant phenotype are indicated in *blue boxes*. The proposed sites of action for thalidomide (*letters inside red and green circles*) are hypothesized to also be operative for thalidomide derivatives. **A.** Direct anti–multiple myeloma (MM) effect on tumor cells, including G_1 growth arrest and/or apoptosis, even against MM cells resistant to conventional therapy. This is due to the disruption of the anti-apoptotic effect of BCL-2 family members, blocking NF-κB signaling, and inhibition of the production of interleukin-6 (IL-6). **B.** Inhibition of MM-cell adhesion to bone marrow stromal cells partially due to the reduction of IL-6 release. **C.** Decreased angiogenesis due to the inhibition of cytokine and growth factor production and release. **D.** Enhanced T-cell production of cytokines, such as IL-2 and interferon-γ (IFN-γ), that increase the number and cytotoxic functionality of natural killer (NK) cells. VEGF, vascular endothelial growth factor.

ADVERSE EFFECTS OF THALIDOMIDE AND LENALIDOMIDE

Thalidomide is well tolerated at doses <200 mg daily. Common adverse effects are sedation and constipation; the most serious one is peripheral sensory neuropathy, which occurs in 10-30% of patients with MM or other malignancies in a dose- and time-dependent manner. Thalidomide-related neuropathy is an asymmetrical, painful, peripheral paresthesia with sensory loss, commonly presenting with numbness of toes and feet, muscle cramps, weakness, signs of pyramidal tract involvement, and carpal tunnel syndrome. Although symptoms improve upon drug discontinuation, long-standing sensory loss may not reverse. Particular caution should apply in patients with pre-existing neuropathy (e.g., related to diabetes) or prior exposure to drugs that can cause peripheral neuropathy (e.g., vinca alkaloids, bortezomib).

Adverse effects of lenalidomide are much less severe; it causes little sedation, constipation, or neuropathy. The drug depresses bone marrow function and is associated with significant leukopenia (20% of patients). Hepatotoxicity and renal dysfunction are rare. In some CLL patients, lenalidomide causes dramatic lymph node swelling and tumor lysis (tumor flare reaction). Patients with renal dysfunction are prone to this reaction; thus, CLL patients should be started at lower doses of 10 mg/day, with escalation as tolerated. CLL patients should receive pretreatment hydration and allopurinol to avoid the consequences of tumor swelling and tumor lysis. A negative interaction with rituximab, an anti-CD20 antibody, may result from lenalidomide's downregulation of CD20, an interaction that has clinical implications for their combined use in lymphoid malignancies.

Thromboembolic events occur with increased frequency in patients receiving thalidomide or lenalidomide, but particularly in combination with glucocorticoids and with anthracyclines. Anticoagulation reduces this risk and seems indicated in patients presenting with risk factors for clotting.

PROTEASOME INHIBITION: BORTEZOMIB

Bortezomib (VELCADE), an inhibitor of proteasome-mediated protein degradation, has a central role in the treatment of MM. Bortezomib has a unique boron-containing structure:

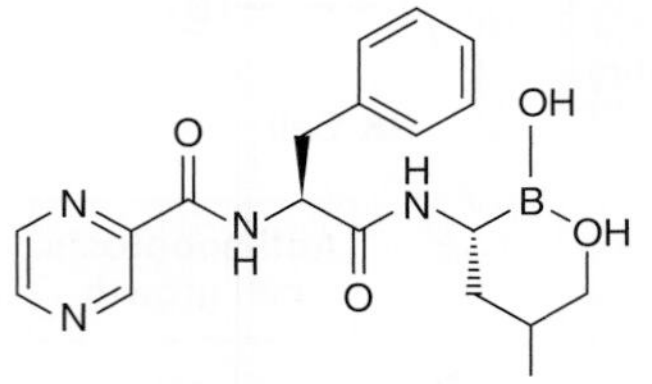

BORTEZOMIB

Mechanism of Action. Bortezomib binds to the β5 subunit of the 20S core of the 26S proteasome and reversibly inhibits its chymotrypsin-like activity. This event disrupts multiple intracellular signaling cascades, leading to apoptosis. An important consequence of proteasome inhibition is its effect on NF-κB, a transcription factor that promotes cell damage response and cell survival. Most cellular NF-κB is cytosolic and bound to IκB; in this form, NF-κB is restricted to the cytosol and cannot enter to the nucleus to regulate transcription. In response to stress signals resulting from hypoxia, chemotherapy, and DNA damage, IκB becomes ubiquitinated and then degraded via the proteasome. Its degradation releases NF-κB, which enters the nucleus and transcriptionally activates a host of genes involved in cell survival (e.g., cell adhesion proteins E-selectin, ICAM-1, and VCAM-1), as proliferation (e.g., cyclin-D1) or anti-apoptosis (e.g., cIAPs, BCL-2). NF-κB is highly expressed in many human tumors, including MM, and may be a key factor in tumor cell survival in a hypoxic environment and during chemotherapy. Bortezomib blocks proteasomal degradation of IκB, thereby preventing the transcriptional activity of NF-κB and downregulating survival responses.

Bortezomib also disrupts the ubiquitin-proteasomal degradation of p21, p27, p53, and other key regulators of the cell cycle and initiators of apoptosis. Bortezomib activates the cell's stereotypical "unfolded protein response" or UPR, in which abnormal protein conformation activates adaptive signaling pathways in the cell. The composite effect leads to irreversible commitment of MM cells to apoptosis. Bortezomib also sensitizes tumor cells to cytotoxic drugs, including alkylators and anthracyclines, and to IMiDs and inhibitors of histone deacetylase.

ADME. The recommended starting dose of bortezomib is 1.3 mg/m^2 given as an intravenous bolus on days 1, 4, 8, and 11 of every 21-day cycle (with a 10-day rest period per cycle). At least 72 h should elapse between doses. Drug administration should be withheld until resolution of any grade 3 nonhematological toxicity or grade 4 hematological toxicity, and subsequent doses should be reduced 25%. The drug exhibits a terminal $t_{1/2}$ in plasma of 5.5 h. Peak proteasome inhibition reaches 60% within 1 h and declines thereafter, with a $t_{1/2}$ of ~24 h. Bortezomib clearance results from the deboronation of the parent compound (90%), followed by hydroxylation of the boron-free product by CYPs 3A4 and 2D6; administration of this drug with potent inducers or inhibitors/substrates of CYP3A4 requires caution. No dose adjustment is required for patients with renal dysfunction.

Therapeutic Uses. Bortezomib is used as initial therapy for MM and as therapy for MM after relapse from other drugs. It also is approved for relapsed or refractory mantle cell lymphoma. The drug is active in myeloma, including the induction of complete responses in up to 30% of patients when used in combination with other drugs (i.e., thalidomide, lenalidomide, liposomal doxorubicin, or dexamethasone).

Toxicity. Bortezomib toxicities include thrombocytopenia (28%), fatigue (12%), peripheral neuropathy (12%), and neutropenia, anemia, vomiting, diarrhea, limb pain, dehydration, nausea, or weakness. Peripheral neuropathy, the most chronic of the toxicities, develops most frequently in patients with a prior history of neuropathy secondary to prior drug treatment (e.g., thalidomide) or diabetes or with prolonged use. Dose reductions or discontinuation of bortezomib ameliorates the neuropathic symptoms. Injection of bortezomib may precipitate hypotension, especially in volume-depleted patients, in those who have a history of syncope, or in patients taking antihypertensive medications. Cardiac toxicity is rare, but congestive failure and prolonged QT-interval have been reported.

mTOR INHIBITORS: RAPAMYCIN ANALOGS

Rapamycin (sirolimus) is a fungal fermentation product that inhibits serine/threonine protein kinase in mammalian cells eponymously named *mammalian target of rapamycin*, or mTOR. The PI3K/PKB(Akt)/mTOR pathway responds to a variety of signals from growth factors. The activation of the PI3K pathway is opposed by the phosphatase activity of the tumor suppressor, PTEN. Activating mutations and amplification of genes in the receptor-PI3K pathway, and loss of function alterations in PTEN, occur frequently in cancer cells, with the result that PI3K signaling is exaggerated and cells exhibit enhanced survival.

Rapamycin and its congeners, *temsirolimus* and *everolimus*, are first-line drugs in post-transplant immunosuppression (*see* Figure 35–1). The mTOR inhibitors have important applications in oncology for treatment of renal and hepatocellular cancer and mantle cell lymphomas. Everolimus was recently FDA-approved for the treatment of advanced pancreatic neuroendocrine tumors.

Mechanisms of Action and Resistance. The rapamycins inhibit an enzyme complex, mTORC1, which occupies a downstream position in the PI3 kinase pathway (Figure 62–3). mTOR forms the mTORC1 complex with a member of the FK506-binding protein family, FKBP12. Among other actions, mTORC1 phosphorylates S6 kinase and also relieves the inhibitory effect of 4EBP on initiation factor eiF-4E, thereby promoting protein synthesis and metabolism. The antitumor actions of the rapamycins result from their binding to FKBP12 and inhibition of mTORC1. Rapamycin and its congeners have immunosuppressant effects, inhibit cell-cycle progression and angiogenesis, and promote apoptosis. Resistance to mTOR inhibitors is incompletely understood but may arise through the action of a second mTOR complex, mTORC2, which is unaffected by rapamycins and which regulates Akt.

ADME. For renal-cell cancer, temsirolimus is given in weekly doses of 25 mg, intravenously; everolimus is administered orally in doses of 10 mg/day. Both drugs should be administered in the fasting state at least 1 h before a meal. Both parent molecules are metabolized by CYP3A4. Temsirolimus has a plasma $t_{1/2}$ of 30 h; its primary metabolite, sirolimus, has a $t_{1/2}$ of 53 h. Because sirolimus has equivalent activity as an inhibitor

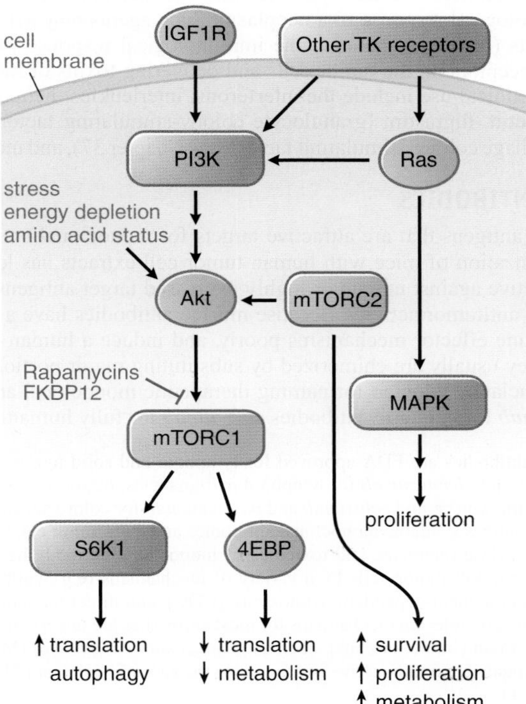

Figure 62–3 *Effect of rapamycin on growth factor signaling.* A key pathway is regulated by phosphatidylinositol-3 kinase (PI3K) and its downstream partner, the mammalian target of rapamycin (mTOR). Rapamycins complex with FKBPP12 to inhibit the mTORC1 complex. mTORC2 remains unaffected and responds by upregulating Akt, driving signals through the inhibited mTORC1. The various downstream outputs of the 2 complexes are shown. Phosphorylation of 4EBP by mTOR inhibits the capacity of 4EBP to inhibit eif-4E and slow metabolism. 4EBP, eukaryotic initiation factor 4e (eif-4E) binding protein; FKBP12, immunophilin target (binding protein) for tacrolimus (FK506); IGF1R, insulin-like growth factor 1 receptor; S6K1, S6 kinase 1.

of mTORC1, and has a greater AUC, sirolimus is likely the more important contributor to antitumor action in patients. Everolimus has a plasma $t_{1/2}$ of 30 h; on a weekly schedule at doses of 20 mg, it maintains inhibition of mTORC1 for 7 days in white blood cells. Both drugs are susceptible to interactions with other agents that affect CYP3A4 activity. The dose of temsirolimus should be doubled in the presence of inducers and reduced by half in the presence of ketoconazole. For everolimus, the dose should be reduced to 5 mg daily for patients with moderate hepatic impairment (Child-Pugh class B); guidelines for dose reduction of temsirolimus in such patients have not been established. The drugs' pharmacokinetics do not depend on renal function, and hemodialysis does not hasten temsirolimus clearance.

Therapeutic Uses. Temsirolimus and everolimus are approved for treatment of renal cancer. Temsirolimus prolongs survival and delays disease progression in patients with advanced and poor- or intermediate-risk renal cancer, as compared to standard interferon-α treatment. Everolimus, as compared to placebo, prolongs survival in patients who had failed initial treatment with anti-angiogenic drugs. mTOR inhibitors also have antitumor activity against mantle cell lymphomas.

Toxicity. The rapamycin analogs have very similar patterns of toxicity. Side effects such as a mild maculopapular rash, mucositis, anemia, and fatigue occur in 30-50% of patients. A few patients will develop leukopenia or thrombocytopenia, effects that are reversed if therapy is discontinued. Less common side effects include hyperglycemia, hypertriglyceridemia, and, rarely, pulmonary infiltrates and interstitial lung disease. Pulmonary infiltrates emerge in 8% of patients receiving everolimus and in a smaller percentage of those treated with temsirolimus. If symptoms such as cough or shortness of breath develop or radiological changes progress, the drug should be discontinued. Prednisone may hasten the resolution of radiological changes and symptoms.

BIOLOGICAL RESPONSE MODIFIERS

Biological response modifiers include cytokines and monoclonal antibodies that beneficially affect the patient's biological response to a neoplasm. Such agents may act indirectly to mediate their antitumor effects (e.g., by enhancing the immunological response to neoplastic cells) or directly, binding to receptors on the tumor cells and delivering toxins or radionuclides. Proteins that currently are in clinical use include the interferons, interleukins, hematopoietic growth factors (e.g., erythropoietin, filgrastim [granulocyte colony-stimulating factor], and sargramostim [granulocyte-macrophage colony-stimulating factor]; *see* Chapter 37), and monoclonal antibodies.

MONOCLONAL ANTIBODIES

Cancer cells express antigens that are attractive targets for monoclonal antibody–based therapy (Table 62–1). Immunization of mice with human tumor cell extracts has led to the isolation of monoclonal Abs reactive against unique or highly expressed target antigens, and a few of these monoclonals possess antitumor activity. Because murine antibodies have a short $t_{1/2}$ in humans, activate human immune effector mechanisms poorly, and induce a human anti-mouse antibody immune response, they usually are chimerized by substituting major portions of the human IgG molecule. The nomenclature adopted for naming therapeutic monoclonal antibodies is to terminate the name in *-ximab* for chimeric antibodies and *-umab* for fully humanized antibodies.

Presently, monoclonal antibodies are FDA-approved for lymphoid and solid tumor malignancies. Available agents include *rituximab* and *alemtuzumab* for lymphoid malignancies, *trastuzumab* for breast cancer, *bevacizumab* for colon and lung cancer, and *cetuximab* and *panitumumab* for colorectal cancer and head and neck cancer. Table 62–1 summarizes available monoclonal antibodies and their tumor cell targets; Table 62–2 summarizes the mechanisms, dose regimens, and toxicities of monoclonal antibody-based agents. Unmodified monoclonal antibodies may kill tumor cells by a variety of mechanisms (e.g., antibody-dependent cellular cytotoxicity [ADCC], complement-dependent cytotoxicity [CDC], and direct induction of apoptosis by antigen binding), but the clinically relevant mechanisms for most antibodies are uncertain. Monoclonal antibodies also may be linked to a toxin (immunotoxins), such as *gemtuzumab ozogamicin* (MYLOTARG) or *denileukin diftitox* (ONTAK), or conjugated to a radioactive isotope, as in the case of *^{90}Yttrium (^{90}Y)-ibritumomab tiuxetan* (ZEVALIN) (*see* Table 62–1).

UNARMED MONOCLONAL ANTIBODIES

RITUXIMAB. Rituximab (RITUXAN) is a chimeric monoclonal antibody that targets the CD20 B-cell antigen (Tables 62–1 and 62–2).

CD20 is found on cells from the pre–B cell stage through its terminal differentiation to plasma cells and is expressed on 90% of B-cell neoplasms. Monoclonal antibody binding to CD20 generates transmembrane signals that produce autophosphorylation and activation of protein serine/tyrosine kinases, induction of

Table 62–1

Monoclonal Antibodies Approved for Hematopoietic and Solid Tumors

ANTIGEN AND TUMOR CELL TARGETS	ANTIGEN FUNCTION	NAKED ANTIBODIES	RADIOISOTOPE-BASED ANTIBODIES	TOXIN-BASED ANTIBODIES
CD20 B-cell lymphoma, CLL	Proliferation/ differentiation	Rituximab (chimeric)	^{131}I-tositumomab; ^{90}Y-ibritumomab tiuxetan	None
CD52 B-cell CLL, T-cell lymphoma	Unknown	Alemtuzumab (humanized)	None	None
CD33 Acute myelocytic leukemia	Unknown	Gemtuzumab (humanized)	None	Gemtuzumab ozogamicin
HER2/neu (ErbB2) Breast cancer	Tyrosine kinase	Trastuzumab (humanized)	None	None
EGFR (ErbB1) Colorectal, NSCLC, pancreatic, breast	Tyrosine kinase	Cetuximab (chimeric)	None	None
VEGF Colorectal cancer	Angiogenesis	Bevacizumab (humanized)	None	None

CLL, chronic lymphocytic leukemia; EGFR, epidermal growth factor receptor; NSCLC, non–small cell lung cancer; VEGF, vascular endothelial growth factor.

c-myc oncogene expression, and expression of major histocompatibility complex class II molecules. CD20 also may regulate transmembrane Ca^{2+} conductance through its function as a Ca^{2+} channel. It is unclear which of these actions relates to the pharmacological effects of rituximab.

ADME. Rituximab has a $t_{1/2}$ of ~22 days. The drug is administered by intravenous infusion both as a single agent and in combination with chemotherapy at a dose of 375 mg/m^2. As a single agent, it is given weekly for 4 weeks, with maintenance dosing every 3-6 months. In combination regimens, the drug may be administered every 3-4 weeks, with chemotherapy, for up to 8 doses. As maintenance therapy following 6-8 cycles of combination chemotherapy, rituximab may be given once weekly for 4 doses, at 6-month intervals, for up to 16 doses. The rate of infusion should be increased slowly to prevent serious hypersensitivity reactions. Infusions should begin at 50 mg/h, and in the absence of infusion reactions, the rate can increase in 50-mg/h increments every 30 min to a maximum rate of 400 mg/h. Pretreatment with antihistamines, acetaminophen, and glucocorticoids decreases the risk of hypersensitivity reactions. Patients with large numbers of circulating tumor cells (as in CLL) are at increased risk for tumor lysis syndrome; in these patients, the initial dose should be no more than 50 mg/m^2 on day 1 of treatment, and patients should receive standard tumor lysis prophylaxis. The remainder of the dose can then be given on day 3.

Therapeutic Uses. Rituximab is approved as a single agent for relapsed indolent lymphomas and significantly enhances response and survival in combination with chemotherapy for the initial treatment of diffuse large B-cell lymphoma. Rituximab improves response rates when added to combination chemotherapy for other indolent B-cell non-Hodgkin lymphomas (NHLs), including CLL, mantle cell lymphoma, Waldenström macroglobulinemia, and marginal zone lymphomas. Maintenance of remission with rituximab delays time to progression and improves overall survival in indolent NHL. It is increasingly used for treatment of autoimmune diseases such as rheumatological disease, thrombotic thrombocytopenic purpura, autoimmune hemolytic anemias, cryoglobulin-induced renal disease, and multiple sclerosis.

Resistance and Toxicity. Resistance to rituximab may emerge through downregulation of CD20, impaired antibody-dependent cellular cytotoxicity, decreased complement activation, limited effects on signaling and induction of apoptosis, and inadequate blood levels. Polymorphisms in 2 of the receptors for the antibody Fc region responsible for complement activation may predict the clinical response to rituximab monotherapy in patients with follicular lymphoma but not in CLL.

Table 62–2

Mechanism, Dose Regimen, and Toxicity of Monoclonal Antibody-Based Drugs

DRUG	MECHANISM	DOSE AND SCHEDULE	MAJOR TOXICITY
Rituximab	ADCC; CDC; apoptosis	375-mg/m² IV infusion weekly for 4 weeks	Infusion-related toxicity with fever, rash, and dyspnea; B-cell depletion; late-onset neutropenia
Alemtuzumab	ADCC; CDC; apoptosis	Escalating doses of 3, 10, 30 mg/m² IV three times/week followed by 30 mg/m² three times/ week for 4-12 weeks	Infusion-related toxicity, T-cell depletion with increased infection; hematopoietic suppression; pancytopenia
Trastuzumab	ADCC; apoptosis; inhibition of arrest HER2 signaling with G_1 arrest	Loading dose of 4-mg/kg infusion followed by 2 mg/kg weekly	Cardiomyopathy; infusion-related toxicity
Cetuximab	Inhibition of EGFR signaling; apoptosis; ADCC	Loading dose of 400-mg/kg infusion followed by 250 mg/kg weekly	Infusion-related toxicity; skin rash in 75%
Bevacizumab	Inhibition of angiogenesis/ neovascularization	5 mg/kg IV every 14 days until disease progression	Hypertension; pulmonary hemorrhage; GI perforation; proteinuria; congestive heart failure
Denileukin diftitox	Targeted diphtheria toxin with inhibition of protein synthesis	9-18 μg/kg/day IV for the first 5 days every 3 weeks	Fever; arthralgia; asthenia; hypotension
Gemtuzumab ozogamicin	Double-strand DNA breaks and apoptosis	Two doses of 9 mg/m² IV separated by 14 days	Infusion-related toxicity; hematopoietic suppression; mucosal hepatic (VOD); skin toxicity
^{90}Y-ibritumomab tiuxetan	Targeted radiotherapy	0.4 mCi/kg IV	Hematological toxicity; myelodysplasia
^{131}I-tositumomab	Targeted radiotherapy	Patient-specific dosimetry	Hematological toxicity; myelodysplasia

ADCC, antibody-dependent cellular cytotoxicity; CDC, complement-dependent cytotoxicity; EGFR, epidermal growth factor receptor; IV, intravenous; VOD, veno-occlusive disease.

Rituximab infusional reactions can be life-threatening, but with pretreatment are usually mild and limited to fever, chills, throat itching, urticaria, and mild hypotension. All respond to decreased infusion rates and antihistamines. Uncommonly, patients may develop severe mucocutaneous skin reactions, including Stevens-Johnson syndrome. Rituximab may cause reactivation of hepatitis B virus or rarely, JC virus (with progressive multifocal leukoencephalopathy). Hypogammaglobulinemia and autoimmune syndromes (idiopathic thrombocytopenic purpura, thrombotic thrombocytopenic purpura, autoimmune hemolytic anemia, pure red cell aplasia, and delayed neutropenia) may supervene 1-5 months after administration (*see* Table 62–2).

OFATUMUMAB

Ofatumumab (ARZERRA) is a second monoclonal antibody that binds to CD20 at sites on the major and minor extracellular loops of CD20, distinct from the site targeted by rituximab. Binding of the drug results in B-cell lysis (both CDC and ADCC). Ofatumumab is approved for treating CLL after failure of fludarabine and alemtuzumab. A complex dosing scheme is used, beginning with small (300 mg) doses on day 1, followed by higher doses (up to 2 g/week) for 7 weeks, followed by 2 g every 4 weeks for 4 additional doses. Ofatumumab's primary toxicities consist of immunosuppression and opportunistic infection, hypersensitivity reactions during antibody infusion, and myelosuppression. Blood counts should be monitored during treatment. Rarely, patients may develop reactivation of viral infections. The drug should not be administered to patients with active hepatitis B infection; liver function should be monitored in hepatitis B carriers.

ALEMTUZUMAB

Alemtuzumab (CAMPATH) is a humanized IgG-κ monoclonal antibody. The drug binds to CD52 antigen present on the surface of a subset of normal neutrophils and on all B and T lymphocytes, on testicular elements and sperm, and on most B- and T-cell lymphomas. Consistently high levels of CD52 expression on lymphoid tumor cells and the lack of CD52 modulation with antibody binding make this antigen a favorable target for unconjugated monoclonal antibodies. Alemtuzumab can induce tumor cell death through ADCC and CDC.

ADME; Therapeutic Uses. Alemtuzumab is administered intravenously in dosages of 30 mg/day, 3 times/week. Premedication with diphenhydramine (50 mg) and acetaminophen (650 mg) should precede drug infusion. Dosing should begin with a 3-mg infusion, followed by a 10-mg dose 2 days later and, if well tolerated, a 30-mg dose 2 days later. The drug has an initial mean $t_{1/2}$ of 1 h, but after multiple doses, the $t_{1/2}$ extends to 12 days, and steady-state plasma levels are reached at approximately week 6 of treatment, presumably through saturation of CD52-binding sites. Clinical activity has been demonstrated in both B- and T-cell low-grade lymphomas and CLL, including patients with disease refractory to purine analogs. In chemotherapy-refractory CLL, overall response rates are ~40%, with complete responses of 6% in multiple series. Response rates in patients with untreated CLL are higher (overall response rates of 83% and complete responses of 24%).

Toxicity. Serious toxicities include acute infusion reactions and depletion of normal neutrophils and T cells (*see* Table 62–2). Myelosuppression, with depletion of all blood lineages, occurs in the majority of patients and may represent either direct marrow toxicity or auto-immune responses. Immunosuppression leads to a significant risk of fungal, viral, and other opportunistic infections, particularly in patients who have previously received purine analogs. Patients should receive antibiotic prophylaxis against *Pneumocystis carinii* and herpes virus during treatment and for at least 2 months following therapy with alemtuzumab. Because reactivation of cytomegalovirus (CMV) infections may follow antibody use, patients should be monitored for symptoms and signs of viremia, hepatitis, and pneumonia. $CD4^+$ T-cell counts may remain profoundly depleted (<200 cells/μL) for 1 year. Alemtuzumab does not combine well with chemotherapy in standard regimens because of significant infectious complications.

IPILIMUMAB

Ipilimumab (YERVOY) is a human monoclonal antibody against CTLA-4, approved for the treatment of late stage inoperable melanoma. The agent potentiates T cell proliferation by removing inhibition by cytotoxic T lymphocyte antigen-4 (CTLA-4). Ipilimumab treatment is associated with severe and fatal immunological adverse effects.

MONOCLONAL ANTIBODY–CYTOTOXIN CONJUGATES

GEMTUZUMAB OZOGAMICIN

Gemtuzumab ozogamicin (MYLOTARG) is a humanized monoclonal antibody against CD33 covalently linked to a semisynthetic derivative of calicheamicin, a potent antitumor antibiotic. The CD33 antigen is present on most hematopoietic cells, on >80% of AMLs, and on most myeloid cells in patients with myelodysplasias. However, other normal cell types lack CD33 expression, making this antigen attractive for targeted therapy. CD33 has no known biological function, although monoclonal antibody cross-linking inhibits normal and myeloid leukemia cell proliferation. Following its binding to CD33, gemtuzumab ozogamicin undergoes endocytosis; cleavage of calicheamicin from the antibody takes place within the lysosome. The potent toxin then enters the nucleus, binds in the minor groove of DNA, and causes double-strand DNA breaks and cell death.

Clinical Pharmacology. The antibody conjugate produces a 30% complete response rate in relapsed AML, when administered at a dose of 9 mg/m^2 for up to 3 doses at 2-week intervals. The $t_{1/2}$ of total and unconjugated calicheamicin are 41 h and 143 h, respectively. Following a second dose, the $t_{1/2}$ of drug-antibody conjugate increases to 64 h. Most patients require 2 to 3 doses to achieve remission. The drug is approved in patients >60 years of age with AML in first relapse. Primary toxicities include myelosuppression in all patients treated and hepatocellular damage in 30-40% of patients, manifested by hyperbilirubinemia and enzyme elevations. It also causes a syndrome that resembles hepatic veno-occlusive disease when patients subsequently undergo myeloablative therapy or when gemtuzumab ozogamicin follows high-dose chemotherapy. Defibrotide, an orphan drug, may prevent severe or fatal hepatic injury in patients who develop signs of hepatic failure while receiving a stem cell transplant following gemtuzumab ozogamicin. Prolonged myelosuppression may complicate the patient's course following remission induction with gemtuzumab ozogamicin.

RADIOIMMUNOCONJUGATES

Radioimmunoconjugates provide targeted delivery of radionuclides to tumor cells (Tables 62–1 and 62–2). ^{131}Iodine (^{131}I) is a favored radioisotope because it is readily available, relatively inexpensive, and easily conjugated to a monoclonal antibody. The γ particles emitted by ^{131}I can be used for both imaging and therapy, but protein-iodine conjugates have the drawback of releasing free ^{131}I and ^{131}I-tyrosine into the blood, and thus present a health hazard to people in contact with the patient. The β-emitter ^{90}Y has emerged as an alternative to ^{131}I, based on its higher energy and longer path length. Thus, it may be more effective in tumors with larger diameters. It also has a short $t_{1/2}$ and remains conjugated, even after endocytosis, providing a safer profile for outpatient use.

Currently available radioimmunoconjugates consist of murine monoclonal antibodies against CD20 conjugated with ^{131}I (tositumomab [BEXXAR]) or ^{90}Y (ibritumomab tiuxetan [ZEVALIN]). Both drugs have shown responses rates in relapsed lymphoma of 65-80%. When using Zevalin, an initial dose of unlabeled rituximab is administered, followed by an imaging dose of Indium-111-labeled Zevalin. Biodistribution is determined, allowing calculation of a therapeutic dose of ^{90}Y Zevalin. A pretreatment dose of rituximab then is administered to saturate nonspecific binding sites, followed by the therapeutic dose of ^{90}Y Zevalin. The steps in Bexxar administration closely follow those of Zevalin. An imaging dose precedes the therapeutic dose given 1 week later. These agents cause antibody-related hypersensitivity, bone marrow suppression, and secondary leukemias.

INTERLEUKIN-2

IL-2 is a 133–amino acid glycoprotein (MW~15 kDa) produced by activated T cells and NK cells; it promotes activated T-cell proliferation and enhanced killing by NK cells. Responsiveness depends on expression of the IL-2 receptor. Resting T cells and nearly all types of tumor cells lack receptor expression and are unresponsive to IL-2.

The IL-2 receptor has 3 components: (1) an α chain, a 55-kDa protein (CD25) involved mainly in IL-2 binding; (2) a β chain, a 75-kDa protein involved in intracellular signaling; and (3) a γ chain, a 64-kDa protein that is a component of many cytokine receptors (IL-2, IL-4, IL-7, IL-9, IL-15, and IL-21) and also is involved in signaling. In the absence of the α chain, IL-2-binding affinity is reduced by a factor of 100.

Mechanism of Action. IL-2 stimulates the proliferation of activated T cells and the secretion of cytokines from NK cells and monocytes. IL-2 stimulation increases cytotoxic killing by T cells and NK cells. The mechanism of tumor cell killing has not been precisely defined.

Pharmacokinetics. The serum $t_{1/2}$ of IL-2 after intravenous administration has an α phase of about 13 min and a β phase of about 90 min. IL-2 is excreted in the urine as an inactive metabolite.

Therapeutic Use. Aldesleukin (PROLEUKIN) possesses the biological activities of human native IL-2. The drug is approved for use in metastatic renal-cell cancer and metastatic melanoma. High-dose IL-2 produces an overall response rate of ~19% in patients with renal-cell cancer, and 8% achieve a complete response. Responses last a median of 8-9 years. High-dose IL-2 induces an overall response rate of ~16% in patients with metastatic melanoma, and 6% achieve a complete response. Responses last a median of ~5 years. Low-dose IL-2 also produces responses, but the duration of the responses may be less than with high-dose IL-2. Aldesleukin may be administered in several ways. High-dose IL-2 is 600,000-720,000 IU/kg administered by intravenous bolus every 8 h until dose-limiting toxicity appears or 14 total doses have been given; the schedule may be repeated after 9 days of rest for a maximum of 28 doses. Low-dose IL-2 is 60,000 or 72,000 IU/kg given by intravenous bolus every 8 h for 15 doses. A third regimen involves delivery of 18 million units/m^2 daily by continuous intravenous infusion for 5 days. Chronic administration doses are 250,000 IU/kg subcutaneously daily for 5 days followed by 125,000 IU/kg daily for 6 weeks.

Toxicity. IL-2 toxicities are dominated by the capillary leak syndrome in which intravascular fluid leaks into the extravascular space, producing hypotension, edema, respiratory difficulties, confusion, tachycardia, oliguric renal failure, and electrolyte problems. Symptoms include fever, chills, malaise, nausea, vomiting, and diarrhea. Laboratory abnormalities include thrombocytopenia, abnormal liver function tests, and neutropenia. Most patients develop a pruritic skin rash. Hypothyroidism may occur. Arrhythmias are a rare complication. These toxicities can be life-threatening, yet nearly all are reversible within 24-48 h of discontinuing therapy. Patients should have normal renal and hepatic function before beginning therapy and should be closely supervised during drug administration.

DENILEUKIN DIFTITOX

Denileukin diftitox (ONTAK) is an immunotoxin made from the genetic recombination of IL-2 and the catalytically active fragment of diphtheria toxin. The high-affinity IL-2R has limited tissue expression and is an attractive target for an immunotoxin. Introduction of the diphtheria toxin fragment into cells leads to

ADP-ribosylation and inactivation of eukaryotic elongation factor EF-2, inhibition of protein synthesis, and thence, cell death.

Clinical Pharmacology. Denileukin diftitox is approved for the treatment of recurrent/refractory cutaneous T-cell lymphomas. It should be administered at 9 or 18 μg/kg/day by intravenous infusion over 30-60 min for 5 consecutive days every 21 days for 8 cycles. Response rates of 30-37% have been achieved, with a median response duration of 6.9 months. The drug is quickly distributed and has a terminal $t_{1/2}$ of ~70 min. Denileukin diftitox clearance in later cycles of treatment accelerates by 2- to 3-fold as a result of development of antibodies, but serum levels exceed those required to produce cell death in IL-2R-expressing cell lines (1-10 ng/mL for >90 min). Patients with a history of hypersensitivity reactions to diphtheria toxin or IL-2 should not be treated. Significant toxicities include acute hypersensitivity reactions, a vascular leak syndrome, and constitutional toxicities; glucocorticoid premedication significantly decreases toxicity.

COLONY-STIMULATING FACTORS

Many agents used for cancer chemotherapy suppress the production of multiple types of hematopoietic cells, and bone marrow suppression can limit the delivery of chemotherapy on schedule and at prescribed doses. The availability of recombinant growth factors for erythrocytes (i.e., erythropoietin), granulocytes (i.e., G-CSF), and granulocytes and macrophages (i.e., GM-CSF) has advanced the ability to use combination therapy or high-dose therapy with diminished complications such as febrile neutropenia (*see* Chapter 37).

NEWLY APPROVED FIRST-IN-CLASS DRUGS

Vemurafenib (ZELBORAF) is an orally administered selective inhibitor of the BRAF serine-threonine kinase that is FDA-approved for the treatment of metastatic melanoma harboring activating BRAF (V600E) mutations.

Crizotinib (XALKORI) is an ATP-competitive oral small-molecule inhibitor of the anaplastic lymphoma kinase (ALK) and mesenchymal-epithelial transition factor (c-MET) tyrosine kinase. The FDA granted accelerated approval to crizotinib for the treatment of patients with locally advanced or metastatic non–small cell lung cancer harboring ALK gene rearrangements.

Omacetaxine mepesuccinate (SYNRIBO) injection is an alkaloid that inhibits protein translation by preventing initial elongation in protein synthesis. It is approved for treatment of adults with chronic myeloid leukemia (CML) and with resistance to two or more tyrosine kinase inhibitors.

Vismodegib (ERIVEDGE) is a first-in-class hedgehog signaling pathway inhibitor approved for the treatment of adult patients with basal cell carcinoma. It acts as a competitive antagonist of the SMO receptor preventing the activation of the GLI family transcription factors.

For details of other approvals from 2011 to the present, see updates by Dr. Nelda Murri on the G&G webpages at AccessMedicine.com and AccessPharmacy.com.

For a complete Bibliographical Listing see Goodman & Gilman's ***The Pharmacological Basis of Therapeutics***, 12th ed., or Goodman & Gilman Online at www.AccessMedicine.com.

Natural Products in Cancer Chemotherapy: Hormones and Related Agents

The growth of a number of cancers is hormone-dependent or regulated by hormones. Glucocorticoids are used for their antiproliferative and lympholytic properties and to ameliorate untoward responses to other treatments. Estrogen, androgen, and GnRH analogs and antagonists are effective in extending survival and delaying or preventing tumor recurrence of both breast and prostate cancer. These molecules interrupt the stimulatory axis created by systemic pools of androgens and estrogens, inhibit hormone production or hormone binding to receptors, and ultimately block expression of genes that promote tumor growth and survival.

GLUCOCORTICOIDS

The pharmacology, major therapeutic uses, and toxic effects of the glucocorticoids are discussed in Chapter 42. Only the applications of these drugs in the treatment of neoplastic disease are considered here.

Glucocorticoids act by binding to a specific physiological receptor that translocates to the nucleus and induces antiproliferative and apoptotic responses in sensitive cells. Because of their lympholytic effects and their ability to suppress mitosis in lymphocytes, glucocorticoids are used as cytotoxic agents in the treatment of acute leukemia in children and malignant lymphoma in children and adults. In acute lymphoblastic or undifferentiated leukemia of childhood, glucocorticoids may produce prompt clinical improvement and objective hematological remissions in ≤30% of children. However, the duration of remission is brief. Remissions occur more rapidly with glucocorticoids than with antimetabolites, and there is no evidence of cross-resistance to unrelated agents. Thus, therapy is initiated with *prednisone* and *vincristine*, often followed by an anthracycline or *methotrexate*, and *L-asparaginase*. Glucocorticoids are a valuable component of curative regimens for other lymphoid malignancies, including Hodgkin disease, non-Hodgkin lymphoma, multiple myeloma, and chronic lymphocytic leukemia (CLL). Glucocorticoids are extremely helpful in controlling autoimmune hemolytic anemia and thrombocytopenia associated with CLL.

A number of glucocorticoids are available and at equivalent dosages exert similar effects (*see* Chapter 42). Prednisone, e.g., usually is administered orally in doses as high as 60-100 mg, for the first few days and gradually reduced to levels of 20-40 mg/day, using the lowest possible effective dose. Side effects of these agents include glucose intolerance, immunosuppression, osteoporosis, and psychosis (*see* Chapter 42). Dexamethasone is the preferred agent for remission induction in multiple myeloma, usually in combination with melphalan, anthracyclines, vincristine, bortezomib, or thalidomide. Glucocorticoids, particularly dexamethasone, are used in conjunction with radiotherapy to reduce edema related to tumors in critical areas such as the superior mediastinum, brain, and spinal cord. Doses of 4-6 mg every 6 h have dramatic effects in restoring neurological function in patients with cerebral metastases, but these effects are temporary. Acute changes in dexamethasone dosage can lead to a rapid recrudescence of symptoms. Dexamethasone should not be discontinued abruptly in patients receiving radiotherapy or chemotherapy for brain metastases.

PROGESTINS

Progestational agents (*see* Chapters 40 and 66) are used as second-line hormonal therapy for metastatic hormone-dependent breast cancer and in the management of endometrial carcinoma previously treated by surgery and radiotherapy. In addition, progestins stimulate appetite and restore a sense of well-being in cachectic patients with advanced stages of cancer and AIDS.

Medroxyprogesterone (DEPO-PROVERA, others) can be administered intramuscularly in doses of 400-1000 mg weekly. An alternative oral agent is ***megestrol acetate*** (MEGACE, others; 40-320 mg daily in divided doses). *Hydroxyprogesterone* (not available in the U.S.) usually is administered intramuscularly in doses of 1000 mg 1 or more times weekly. Beneficial effects have been observed in one-third of patients with endometrial cancer. The response of breast cancer to megestrol is predicted by both the presence of estrogen receptors (ERs) and the evidence of response to a prior hormonal treatment. The effect of progestin therapy in breast cancer appears to be dose dependent, with some patients demonstrating second responses following escalation of megestrol to 1600 mg/day. Clinical use of progestins in breast cancer has been largely superseded by the advent of tamoxifen and the aromatase inhibitors (AIs).

ESTROGENS AND ANDROGENS

The pharmacology of the estrogens and androgens appears in Chapters 40, 41, and 66. These agents are of value in certain neoplastic diseases, notably those of the prostate and mammary gland, because these organs are dependent on hormones for their growth, function, and morphological integrity.

High doses of estrogen have long been recognized as effective treatment of breast cancer. Paradoxically, anti-estrogens also are effective. Thus, because of equivalent efficacy and more favorable side effects, anti-estrogens such as tamoxifen and the AIs have replaced estrogens or androgens for breast cancer. The presence of the ERs and progesterone receptors (PRs) on tumor tissue serves as a biomarker for response to hormonal therapy in breast cancer and identifies the subset of patients with a ≥60% likelihood of responding. The response rate to anti-estrogen treatment is somewhat lower in the subset of patients with tumors that are ER^+ or PR^+ but also positive for human epidermal growth factor receptors HER1/neu amplification. In contrast, ER-negative and PR-negative carcinomas do not respond to hormonal therapy. Responses to hormonal therapy may not be apparent clinically or by imaging for 8-12 weeks. The medication typically should be continued until the disease progresses or unwanted toxicities develop. The duration of an induced remission in patients with metastatic disease averages 6-12 months but sometimes can last for many years.

ANTI-ESTROGEN THERAPY

Anti-estrogen approaches for the therapy of hormone receptor–positive breast cancer include the use of *selective estrogen-receptor modulators* (SERMs), *selective estrogen-receptor downregulators* (SERDs), and AIs (Table 63–1).

SELECTIVE ESTROGEN-RECEPTOR MODULATORS

SERMs bind to the ER and exert either estrogenic or anti-estrogenic effects, depending on the specific organ. Tamoxifen citrate is the most widely studied anti-estrogenic treatment in breast cancer. However tamoxifen also exerts estrogenic agonist effects on non-breast tissues, which influences the overall therapeutic index of the drug. Therefore, several novel anti-estrogen compounds that offer the potential for enhanced efficacy and reduced toxicity compared with tamoxifen have been developed. These novel anti-estrogens can be divided into tamoxifen analogs (e.g., toremifene [FARESTON], droloxifene, idoxifene), "fixed ring" compounds (e.g., raloxifene [EVISTA], lasofoxifene,

Table 63–1

Clinical Uses for Anti-Estrogen Therapy in ER^+ Breast Cancer

	DISEASE SETTING			
DRUG	ADJUVANT premen	ADJUVANT postmen	METASTATIC premen	METASTATIC postmen
Tamoxifen	Yes (5 yr)	Yes (before AI for 2-5 yr)	Yes	Yes
Fulvestrant	No	No	No	Yes (PD on TAM or AI)
Anastrozole	No	Yes (upfront or after TAM)	No	Yes
Letrozole	No	Yes (upfront or after TAM)	No	Yes
Exemestane	No	Yes (upfront or after TAM)	No	Yes
Toremifene	No	Yes	No	Yes

Premen, premenopausal; Postmen, postmenopausal; AI, aromatase inhibitor; PD, progressive disease; TAM, tamoxifen; ER, estrogen receptor.

arzoxifene, miproxifene, levormeloxifene, EM652), and the SERDs (e.g., fulvestrant [FASLODEX], SR 16234, and ZK 191703, the latter also termed "pure anti-estrogens").

TAMOXIFEN

Tamoxifen was developed as an oral contraceptive but instead was found to induce ovulation and to have antiproliferative effects on estrogen-dependent breast cancer cell lines. Tamoxifen is prescribed for the prevention of breast cancer in high-risk patients, for the adjuvant therapy of early-stage breast cancer, and for the therapy of advanced breast cancer. It also prevents the development of breast cancer in women at high risk based on a strong family history, prior nonmalignant breast pathology, or inheritance of the *BRCA1* or *BRCA2* genes.

Mechanism of Action. Tamoxifen is a competitive inhibitor of estradiol binding to the ER. There are 2 subtypes of ERs: ERα and ERβ, which have different tissue distributions and can either homo- or heterodimerize. Binding of estradiol and SERMs to the estrogen-binding sites of the ERs initiates a change in conformation of the ER, dissociation of the ER from heat-shock proteins, and inhibition of ER dimerization. Dimerization facilitates the binding of the ER to specific DNA estrogen-response elements (EREs) in the vicinity of estrogen-regulated genes. Co-regulator proteins interact with the receptor to act as co-repressors or co-activators of gene expression. Differences in tissue distribution of ER subtypes, the function of co-regulator proteins, and the various transcriptional activating factors likely explain the variability of response to tamoxifen in hormone receptor–positive (ER^+) breast cancer and its agonist and antagonist activities in noncancerous tissues. Other organs displaying agonist effects of tamoxifen include the uterine endometrium (endometrial hypertrophy, vaginal bleeding, and endometrial cancer), the coagulation system (thromboembolism), bone metabolism (increase in bone mineral density [BMD]), and liver (tamoxifen lowers total serum cholesterol, low-density-lipoprotein cholesterol, and lipoproteins and raises apolipoprotein A-I levels).

ADME. Tamoxifen is readily absorbed following oral administration, with peak concentrations measurable after 3-7 h and steady-state levels being reached at 4-6 weeks. Metabolism of tamoxifen is complex and principally involves CYPs 3A4/5, and 2D6 in the formation of *N*-desmethyl tamoxifen, and CYP2D6 to form 4-hydroxytamoxifen, a more potent metabolite (Figure 63–1). Both metabolites can be further converted to 4-hydroxy-*N*-desmethyltamoxifen, which retains high affinity for the ER. The parent drug has a terminal $t_{1/2}$ of 7 days; the $t_{1/2}$ of *N*-desmethyltamoxifen and 4-hydroxytamoxifen are significantly longer (14 days). After enterohepatic circulation, glucuronides and other metabolites are excreted in the stool; excretion in the urine is minimal.

Therapeutic Uses. The usual oral dose of tamoxifen in the U.S. is 20 mg once a day. Tamoxifen is used for the endocrine treatment of women with ER^+ metastatic breast cancer or following primary tumor excision as adjuvant therapy. For the adjuvant treatment of premenopausal women, tamoxifen is given for 5 years, or in postmenopausal women, for 2 years, followed by an AI. In patients with high risk of recurrence, tamoxifen may be sequenced after adjuvant chemotherapy. Tamoxifen is used in premenopausal women with ER^+ tumors. Alternative or additional anti-estrogen strategies in premenopausal women include oophorectomy or gonadotropin-releasing hormone analogs. The combination of tamoxifen and a GnRH analog in premenopausal women (to reduce high estrogen levels resulting from tamoxifen effects on the gonadal-pituitary axis) yields better response rates and improved overall survival than either drug alone. Tamoxifen also has shown effectiveness (a 40-50% reduction in tumor incidence) in initial trials for preventing breast cancer in women at increased risk. Tamoxifen only reduces ER^+ tumors without affecting ER-negative tumors, which contribute disproportionately to breast cancer mortality.

Toxicity. The common adverse reactions to tamoxifen include vasomotor symptoms (hot flashes), atrophy of the lining of the vagina, hair loss, nausea, and vomiting. Menstrual irregularities, vaginal bleeding and discharge, pruritus vulvae, and dermatitis occur with increasing severity in postmenopausal women. Tamoxifen also increases the incidence of endometrial cancer by 2- to 3-fold, particularly in postmenopausal women who receive 20 mg/day for ≥2 years. Tamoxifen increases the risk of thromboembolic events, which increase with the age of a patient and also in the perioperative period. Hence, it often is recommended to discontinue tamoxifen prior to elective surgery. Tamoxifen causes retinal deposits, decreased visual acuity, and cataracts, although the frequency of these changes is more common in patients on high doses of drug.

Tamoxifen Resistance. Initial or acquired resistance to tamoxifen frequently occurs. CYP2D6 is required for the activation of tamoxifen to its active metabolite endoxifen (*see* Figure 63–1). Polymorphisms in CYP2D6 that reduce its activity lead to lower plasma levels of the potent metabolites 4-OH tamoxifen and endoxifen, and are associated with higher risks of disease relapse and a lower incidence of hot flashes. Crosstalk between the ER and HER2/neu pathway also has been implicated in tamoxifen resistance. The paired box 2 gene product (PAX2) has been identified as a crucial mediator of ER repression of ErbB2 by tamoxifen. Interactions between PAX2 and the ER co-activator AIB-1/SRC-3 determine tamoxifen response in breast cancer cells.

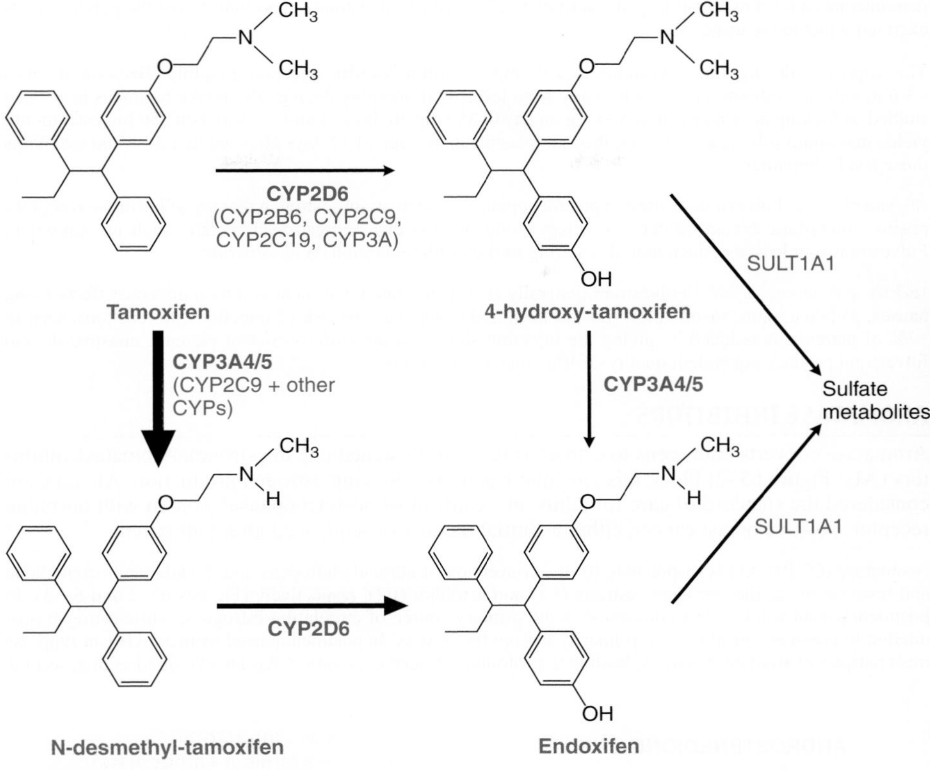

Figure 63–1 *Tamoxifen and its metabolites.*

TOREMIFENE

Toremifene (FARESTON) is a triphenylethylene derivative of tamoxifen and has a similar pharmacological profile. Toremifene is indicated for the treatment of breast cancer in women with tumors that are ER^+ or of unknown receptor status.

SELECTIVE ESTROGEN RECEPTOR DOWNREGULATORS

SERDs, also termed "pure anti-estrogens," include fulvestrant and a host of agents in experimental trials (RU 58668, SR 16234, ZD 164384, and ZK 191703). SERDs, unlike SERMs, are devoid of any estrogen agonist activity.

FULVESTRANT

Fulvestrant (FASLODEX) is approved for postmenopausal women with hormone receptor–positive metastatic breast cancer that has progressed on tamoxifen.

Mechanism of Action. Fulvestrant is a steroidal anti-estrogen that binds to the ER with an affinity >100 times that of tamoxifen. The drug inhibits the binding of estrogen but also alters the receptor structure such that the receptor is targeted for proteasomal degradation; fulvestrant also may inhibit receptor dimerization. Unlike tamoxifen, which stabilizes or even increases ER expression, fulvestrant reduces the number of ER molecules in cells; as a consequence of this ER downregulation, the drug abolishes ER-mediated transcription of estrogen-dependent genes.

ADME and Dosing. Peak plasma concentrations are reached ~7 days after intramuscular administration of fulvestrant and are maintained over 1 month. The plasma $t_{1/2}$ is ~40 days. Steady-state concentrations are reached after 3-6 monthly injections. There is rapid distribution and extensive protein binding of this highly lipophilic drug. Various pathways, similar to those of steroid metabolism (oxidation, aromatic hydroxylation, and conjugation), metabolize fulvestrant. CYP3A4 appears to be the only CYP isoenzyme involved in the metabolism of fulvestrant. The putative metabolites possess no estrogenic activity, and only the 17-keto compound demonstrates a level of anti-estrogenic activity (~22% that of fulvestrant). Less than 1% of the parent drug is excreted intact in the urine.

The approved dosing for fulvestrant is 250 mg by intramuscular injection monthly. Because it takes ~3-6 months for fulvestrant to reach steady-state levels with monthly dosing, alternative regimens have been studied. A loading dose regimen of 500 mg on day 0, 250 mg on days 14 and 28, and then 250 mg each month yields maximum fulvestrant concentrations in plasma an average of 12 days after the first dose and maintains those levels thereafter.

Therapeutic Uses. Fulvestrant is used in postmenopausal women as anti-estrogen therapy of hormone receptor–positive metastatic breast cancer after progression on first-line anti-estrogen therapy such as tamoxifen. Fulvestrant is at least as effective in this setting as the third-generation AI anastrozole.

Toxicity and Adverse Effects. Fulvestrant generally is well tolerated, the most common adverse effects being nausea, asthenia, pain, vasodilation (hot flashes), and headache. The risk of injection site reactions, seen in ~7% of patients, is reduced by giving the injection slowly. In tamoxifen-resistant patients, anastrozole and fulvestrant produce equivalent quality-of-life outcome measures.

AROMATASE INHIBITORS

Aromatase converts androgens to estrogens (e.g., androstenedione to estrone). Aromatase inhibitors (AIs; Figure 63–2) block this enzymatic activity, reducing estrogen production. AIs now are considered the standard of care for adjuvant treatment of postmenopausal women with hormone receptor–positive breast cancer, either as initial therapy or sequenced after tamoxifen.

Aromatase (CYP19A1) is responsible for the conversion of adrenal androgens and gonadal androstenedione and testosterone to the estrogens, estrone (E1) and estradiol (E2), respectively (Figures 63–2 and 63–3). In postmenopausal women, this conversion is the primary source of circulating estrogens, while estrogen production in premenopausal women primarily is from the ovaries. In postmenopausal women, AIs can suppress most peripheral aromatase activity, leading to profound estrogen deprivation. AIs are classified as first, second,

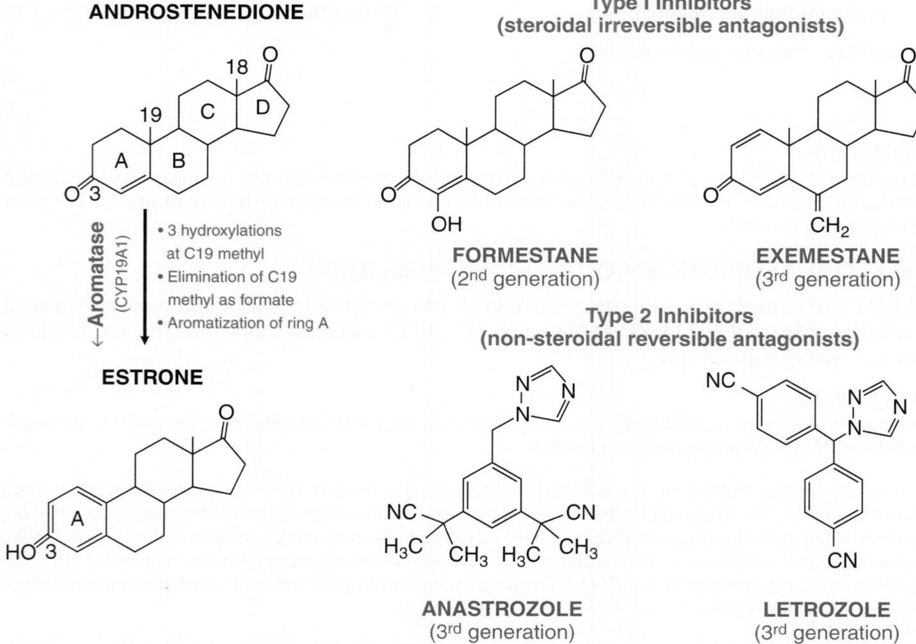

Figure 63–2 *Aromatase and its Inhibitors.* Aromatase tri-hydroxylates the methyl group at C19, eliminating it as formate and aromatizing the A ring of the androgen substrate. Type 1 aromatase inhibitors are steroidal analogs of androstenedione that bind covalently and irreversibly to the steroid substrate site on the enzyme and are known as aromatase inactivators. Type 2 inhibitors are nonsteroidal, bind reversibly to the heme group of the enzyme, and produce reversible inhibition.

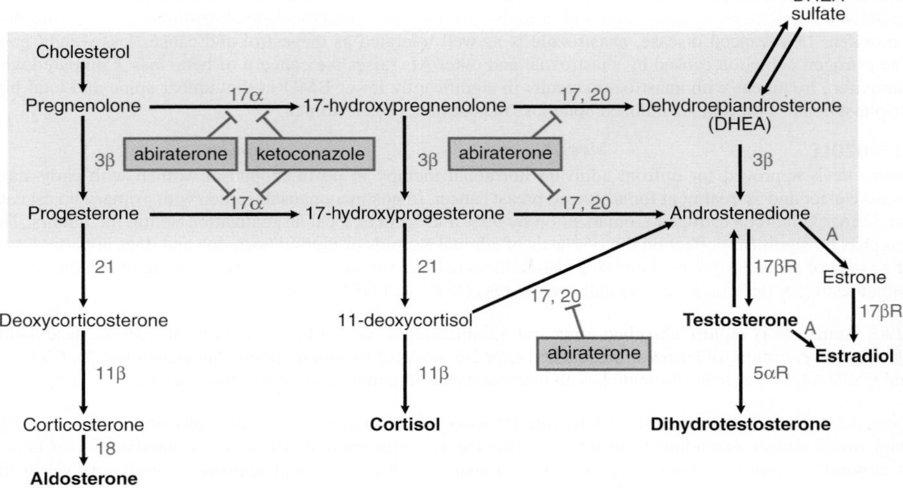

Figure 63–3 *Steroid synthesis pathways.* The shaded area contains the pathways used by the adrenal glands and gonads. Enzymes are labeled in *green*, inhibitors in *red*. A, aromatase; 3β, 3β-hydroxysteroid dehydrogenase; 5αR, 5α-reductase; 11β, 11β-hydroxylase; 17, 20, C-17, 20-lyase (also CYP17); 17α, 17α-hydroxylase (CYP17); 17βR, 17β-reductase; 18, aldosterone synthase; 21, 21-hydroxylase.

or third generation. In addition, they are further classified as type 1 (steroidal) or type 2 (nonsteroidal) AIs according to their structure and mechanism of action. Type 1 inhibitors are steroidal analogs of androstenedione (*see* Figure 63–2) that bind covalently and irreversibly to the same site on the aromatase molecule. Thus, they commonly are known as aromatase inactivators. Type 2 inhibitors are nonsteroidal and bind reversibly to the heme group of the enzyme, producing reversible inhibition.

THIRD-GENERATION AROMATASE INHIBITORS

The third-generation inhibitors include the type 1 steroidal agent *exemestane* and the type 2 nonsteroidal imidazoles *anastrozole* and *letrozole*. Third-generation AIs are used as part of the treatment of early-stage and advanced breast cancer in postmenopausal women.

ANASTROZOLE

Anastrozole is a potent and selective triazole AI. Anastrozole, like letrozole, binds competitively and specifically to the heme of the CYP19. Anastrozole, 1 mg, administered once daily for 28 days, reduces total body androgen aromatization by 96.7% Anastrozole also reduces aromatization in large ER^+ breast tumors.

ADME. Anastrozole is absorbed rapidly after oral administration. Steady-state is attained after 7 days of repeated dosing. Anastrozole is metabolized by *N*-dealkylation, hydroxylation, and glucuronidation. The main metabolite of anastrozole is a triazole. Less than 10% of the drug is excreted as the unmetabolized parent compound. The principal excretory pathway is via the liver and biliary tract. The elimination $t_{1/2}$ is ~50 h. The pharmacokinetics of anastrozole, which can be affected by drug interactions via the CYP system, are not altered by coadministration of tamoxifen or cimetidine.

Therapeutic Uses. Anastrozole (ARIMIDEX), 1 mg administered orally once daily, is approved for upfront adjuvant hormonal therapy in postmenopausal women with early-stage breast cancer and as treatment for advanced breast cancer. In early-stage breast cancer, anastrozole is significantly more effective than tamoxifen in delaying time to tumor recurrence and decreasing the odds of a primary contralateral tumor. In advanced breast cancer, postmenopausal women with disease progression while taking tamoxifen showed a statistically significant survival advantage with anastrozole 1 mg/day versus megestrol acetate 40 mg 4 times daily. Women with ER^+ or PR^+ metastatic breast cancer, anastrozole showed a statistically significant advantage over tamoxifen in median time to disease progression.

Adverse Effects and Toxicity. Compared to tamoxifen, anastrozole has been associated with a significantly lower incidence of vaginal bleeding, vaginal discharge, hot flashes, endometrial cancer, ischemic cerebrovascular events, venous thromboembolic events, and deep venous thrombosis, including pulmonary embolism. Anastrozole is associated with a higher incidence of musculoskeletal disorders and fracture than tamoxifen. In advanced disease, anastrozole is as well tolerated as megestrol and causes less weight gain. The estrogen depletion caused by anastrozole and other AIs raises the concern of bone loss. Compared with tamoxifen, treatment with anastrozole results in significantly lower BMD in the lumbar spine and total hip. Bisphosphonates prevent AI-induced bone loss in postmenopausal women.

LETROZOLE

Letrozole is approved for upfront adjuvant hormonal therapy in postmenopausal women with early-stage breast cancer and as treatment for advanced breast cancer. In postmenopausal women with primary breast cancer, letrozole inhibits estrogen aromatization by 99% and reduces local aromatization within the tumors. The drug has no significant effect on the synthesis of adrenal steroids or thyroid hormone and does not alter levels of a range of other hormones. Letrozole also reduces cellular markers of proliferation more than tamoxifen in human estrogen-dependent tumors that overexpress HER1 and HER2/neu.

ADME. Letrozole is rapidly absorbed after oral administration, with a bioavailability of 99.9%. Steady-state plasma concentrations of letrozole are reached after 2-6 weeks of treatment. Following metabolism by CYP2A6 and CYP3A4, letrozole is eliminated as an inactive metabolite mainly via the kidneys with a $t_{1/2}$ ~41 h.

Therapeutic Uses. The usual dose of letrozole (FEMARA) is 2.5 mg administered orally once daily. In early-stage breast cancer, extending adjuvant endocrine therapy with letrozole (beyond the standard 5-year period of tamoxifen) improves disease-free survival compared with placebo and improves overall survival in the subset of patients with positive axillary nodes. Furthermore, upfront letrozole is significantly more effective than upfront tamoxifen in terms of time to tumor recurrence and odds of a primary contralateral tumor. In advanced breast cancer, letrozole is superior to tamoxifen as first-line treatment; time to disease progression is significantly longer and objective response rate is significantly greater with letrozole, but median overall survival is similar between groups. As second-line therapy of advanced breast cancer that has progressed on tamoxifen or after oophorectomy, letrozole has efficacy equal to that of anastrozole and similar to or better than that of megestrol.

Adverse Effects and Toxicity. Letrozole is well tolerated; the most common treatment-related adverse events are hot flashes, nausea, and hair thinning. In the trial of extended adjuvant therapy, adverse events were hot flashes, arthralgia, myalgia, and arthritis. Letrozole has a low overall incidence of cardiovascular side effects. Compared with tamoxifen, the use of upfront letrozole results in significantly more clinical fractures. Bisphosphonates prevent letrozole-induced bone loss in postmenopausal women.

EXEMESTANE

Exemestane is a more potent, orally administered analog of the natural aromatase substrate, androstenedione, and lowers estrogen levels more effectively than does its predecessor, formestane. Exemestane irreversibly inactivates aromatase and is a "suicide substrate." Doses of 25 mg/day inhibit aromatase activity by 98% and lower plasma estrone and estradiol levels by ~90% in postmenopausal women.

ADME. Orally administered exemestane is rapidly absorbed from the GI tract; its absorption is increased by 40% after a high-fat meal. Exemestane has a terminal $t_{1/2}$ of ~24 h. It is extensively metabolized in the liver, ultimately to inactive metabolites. One metabolite, 17-hydroxyexemestane, has weak androgenic activity that could contribute to antitumor activity. Although active metabolites are excreted in the urine, no dosage adjustments are recommended in patients with renal dysfunction.

Therapeutic Uses. Exemestane (AROMASIN), 25 mg administered orally once daily, is approved for disease progression in postmenopausal women who complete 2-3 years of adjuvant tamoxifen (based on a clinical trial in women with ER^+ breast cancer). In advanced breast cancer, exemestane improves time to disease progression compared with tamoxifen as first-line treatment. In a phase III trial against megestrol in women with disease progressing on prior anti-estrogen therapy, patients receiving exemestane had a similar response rate but improved time to disease progression and time to treatment failure and a longer duration of survival compared with those taking megestrol acetate.

Clinical Toxicity. Exemestane generally is well tolerated. Discontinuations due to toxicity are uncommon (2.8%). Hot flashes, nausea, fatigue, increased sweating, peripheral edema, and increased appetite have been reported. Compared to tamoxifen in early-stage breast cancer, exemestane caused more frequent arthralgia and diarrhea but less frequent vaginal bleeding and muscle cramps. Visual disturbances and clinical fractures were more common with exemestane.

HORMONE THERAPY IN PROSTATE CANCER

Androgens stimulate the growth of normal and cancerous prostate cells. Androgen deprivation therapy (ADT) is the mainstay of treatment for patients with advanced prostate cancer.

Localized prostate cancer frequently is curable with surgery or radiation therapy. However, when distant metastases are present, hormone therapy is the primary treatment. ADT is the standard first-line treatment. ADT is accomplished via surgical castration (bilateral orchiectomy) or medical castration (using gonadotropin-releasing hormone [GnRH] agonists or antagonists). Other hormone therapy approaches are used in second-line treatment and include anti-androgens, estrogens, and inhibitors of steroidogenesis. ADT is not a curative treatment. ADT can alleviate cancer-related symptoms and normalize serum prostate-specific antigen (PSA) in >90% of patients. ADT provides important quality-of-life benefits, including reduction of bone pain and reduction of rates of pathological fracture, spinal cord compression, and ureteral obstruction. It also prolongs survival.

The duration of response to ADT for patients with metastatic disease is variable but typically lasts 14-20 months. Disease progression despite ADT signifies a castration-resistant state. Despite castrate levels of testosterone, low-level androgen (DHEA) synthesis from the adrenal glands may permit the continued androgen-driven growth of prostate cancer cells. Therefore, anti-androgens (which competitively bind the androgen receptor [AR]), inhibitors of steroidogenesis (such as ketoconazole), and estrogens frequently are employed as secondary hormone therapies. Unlike the response to ADT, only the minority of patients experience symptomatic relief or tumor regression when treated with secondary hormone therapies. When patients become refractory to further hormonal therapies, their disease is considered androgen independent. In these patients, the next treatment option usually is cytotoxic chemotherapy; docetaxel has a proven survival benefit, with average overall survival of 18 months.

Common side effects of androgen deprivation include vasomotor flashing, loss of libido, impotence, gynecomastia, fatigue, anemia, weight gain, decreased insulin sensitivity, altered lipid profiles, osteoporosis and fractures, and loss of muscle mass. ADT is associated with an increased risk of diabetes and coronary heart disease. However, retrospective analyses have not revealed a compelling increase in cardiovascular mortality due to GnRH agonists. Skeletal-related events due to ADT may be mitigated by bisphosphonate therapy, such as zoledronic acid (ZOMETA) or inhibitors of osteoclast activation, such as denosumab. Anti-androgens, when compared with GnRH agonists, cause more gynecomastia, mastodynia, and hepatotoxicity but less vasomotor flashing, and loss of BMD. Estrogens cause a hypercoagulable state and increase cardiovascular mortality in prostate cancer patients and are no longer standard treatment options.

GONADOTROPIN-RELEASING HORMONE AGONISTS AND ANTAGONISTS

The most common form of ADT involves chemical suppression of the pituitary gland with GnRH agonists. Synthetic GnRH analogs (Table 63–2) have greater receptor affinity and reduced susceptibility to enzymatic degradation than the naturally occurring GnRH molecule and are 100-fold more potent. Several long-acting preparations are available in doses that are approved for 3-, 4-, and 6-month administrations.

GnRH agonists bind to GnRH receptors on pituitary gonadotropin-producing cells, causing an initial release of both LH and FSH and a subsequent increase in testosterone production from testicular Leydig cells. After ~1 week of therapy, GnRH receptors are downregulated on the gonadotropin-producing cells, causing a decline in the pituitary response. The fall in serum LH leads to a decrease in testosterone production to castrate levels within 3-4 weeks of the first treatment. Subsequent treatments maintain testosterone at castrate levels.

During the transient rise in LH, the resultant testosterone surge may induce an acute stimulation of prostate cancer growth and a "flare" of symptoms from metastatic deposits. Patients may experience an increase in bone pain or obstructive bladder symptoms lasting for 2-3 weeks. The flare phenomenon can be effectively counteracted with concurrent administration of 2-4 weeks of oral anti-androgen therapy, which may inhibit the action of the increased serum testosterone levels. Besides avoidance of the initial flare, GnRH antagonist therapy offers no apparent advantage compared with GnRH agonists. The GnRH antagonist, degarelix, is not associated with systemic allergic reactions and is approved for prostate cancer in the U.S.

Combined androgen blockade (CAB) requires administration of ADT with an anti-androgen. The theoretical advantage is that the GnRH agonist will deplete testicular androgens, while the anti-androgen component competes at the receptor with residual androgens made by the adrenal glands. CAB provides maximal relief of androgen stimulation. Several trials suggest a benefit for CAB in 5-year survival but not at earlier time points. Toxicity and costs associated with CAB are higher than with ADT alone.

ANTI-ANDROGENS

Anti-androgens bind to ARs and competitively inhibit the binding of testosterone and dihydrotestosterone. Unlike castration, anti-androgen therapy by itself does not decrease LH production; therefore, testosterone levels are normal or increased. Men treated with anti-androgen monotherapy maintain some degree of potency and libido and do not have the same spectrum of side effects seen with castration. Currently, anti-androgen monotherapy is not indicated as first-line treatment for patients with advanced prostate cancer. Anti-androgens most commonly are used in clinical practice as secondary hormone therapy or in CAB.

Table 63–2

Structures of GnRH and Decapeptide GnRH Analogs

AMINO ACID RESIDUE	1	2	3	4	5	6	7	8	9	10	DOSAGE FORM
Agonists											
GnRH	PyroGlu	His	Trp	Ser	Tyr	Gly	Leu	Arg	Pro	Gly-NH_2	
Leuprolide	———	———	———	———	———	D-Leu	———	———	Pro-NHEt		IM, SC, depot
Buserelin	———	———	———	———	———	D-Ser(tBu)	———	———	Pro-NHEt		SC, IN
Nafarelin	———	———	———	———	———	D-Nal	———	———	———	Gly-NH_2	IN
Deslorelin (not in US)	———	———	———	———	———	D-Trp	———	———	Pro-NHEt		SC, IM, depot
Histrelin	———	———	———	———	———	D-His (ImBzl)	———	———	Pro-NHEt		SC, depot
Triptorelin	———	———	———	———	———	D-Trp	———	———	———	Gly-NH_2	IM, depot
Goserelin	———	———	———	———	———	D-Ser(tBu)	———	———	———	AzGly-NH_2	SC implant
Antagonists											
Cetrorelix	Ac-D-Nal	D-Cpa	D-Pal	———	———	D-Cit	———	———	———	D-Ala-NH_2	SC
Ganirelix (not in US)	Ac-D-Nal	D-Cpa	D-Pal	———	———	D-hArg$(Et)_2$	———	D-hArg$(Et)_2$	———	D-Ala-NH_2	SC
Abarelix	Ac-D-Nal	D-Cpa	D-Pal	———	Tyr(N-Me)	D-Asn	———	Lys(iPr)	———	D-Ala-NH_2	SC depot
Degarelix	Ac-D-Nal	D-Cpa	D-Pal	———	4Aph HO	4Aph (Cbm)	———	I lys	———	D-Ala-NH_2	SC

A line (__________) indicates identity with amino acid of the parent compound, GnRH.

Ac, acetyl: NHEt, N-ethylamide; tBu, t butyl; D-Nal, 3-(2-naphthyl)-D-alanyl; ImBzl, imidobenzyl; Cpa, chlorophenylalanyl; Pal, 3-pyridylalanyl; AzGly, azaglycyl; hArg$(Et)_2$, ethyl homoarginine 4Aph (Cbm), 4 acetyl phenylalanine (carbamoyl); I, imido; IV, intravenous; SC, subcutaneous; IN, intranasal; IM, intramuscular.

MECHANISM OF ACTION OF NONSTEROIDAL ANTI-ANDROGENS. The nonsteroidal anti-androgens are taken orally and inhibit ligand binding and consequent AR translocation from the cytoplasm to the nucleus.

AVAILABLE ANTI-ANDROGENS. Anti-androgens are classified as steroidal, including cyproterone and megestrol, or nonsteroidal, including flutamide, bicalutamide (CASODEX, others), and nilutamide (NILANDRON). Cyproterone is associated with liver toxicity and has inferior efficacy compared with other forms of ADT. Cyproterone is not available in the U.S. Neither bicalutamide nor flutamide is approved as monotherapy at any dose for treatment of prostate cancer in the U.S.

Flutamide. Flutamide is given as a 250-mg dose every 8 h. It has a $t_{1/2}$ of 5 h; its major metabolite, hydroxyflutamide, is biologically active. Common side effects include diarrhea, breast tenderness, and nipple tenderness. Less commonly, nausea, vomiting, and hepatotoxicity occur.

Bicalutamide. Bicalutamide (CASODEX, others) is taken once daily at a dosage of 50 mg/day when given with a GnRH agonist; it has a $t_{1/2}$ of 5-6 days. Both enantiomers of bicalutamide undergo glucuronidation to inactive metabolites, and the parent compounds and metabolites are eliminated in bile and urine. The elimination $t_{1/2}$ of bicalutamide is increased in severe hepatic insufficiency and is unchanged in renal insufficiency. Bicalutamide is well tolerated at higher doses. Daily bicalutamide is significantly inferior compared with surgical or medical castration.

Nilutamide. Nilutamide (NILANDRON) is a second-generation anti-androgen that is taken once-daily administration at 150 mg/day. It has an elimination $t_{1/2}$ of 45 h and is metabolized to 5 products that are all excreted in the urine. Common side effects include mild nausea, alcohol intolerance (5-20%), and diminished ocular adaptation to darkness (25-40%); rarely, interstitial pneumonitis occurs. Nilutamide appears to offer no benefit over the first-generation drugs above and has the least favorable toxicity profile.

ESTROGENS

High estrogen levels can reduce testosterone to castrate levels in 1-2 weeks via negative feedback on the hypothalamic–pituitary axis. Estrogen also may compete with androgens for steroid hormone receptors and may thereby exert a cytotoxic effect on prostate cancer cells. Estrogens are associated with increased myocardial infarctions, strokes, and pulmonary emboli and increased mortality, as well as impotence, and lethargy. One benefit is that estrogens prevent bone loss.

INHIBITORS OF STEROIDOGENESIS

In the castrate state, AR signaling, despite low steroid levels, supports continued prostate cancer growth. AR signaling may occur due to androgens produced from nongonadal sources, AR gene mutations, or AR gene amplification. Nongonadal sources of androgens include the adrenal glands and the prostate cancer cells themselves (*see* Figure 63–3). Androstenedione, produced by the adrenal glands, is converted to testosterone in peripheral tissues and tumors. Intratumoral de novo androgen synthesis also may provide sufficient androgen for AR-driven cell proliferation. Thus, inhibitors of androgen synthesis may be useful secondary therapy in reducing AR signaling.

Ketoconazole. Ketoconazole is an antifungal agent that also inhibits both testicular and adrenal steroidogenesis by blocking CYPs, primarily CYP17 (17α-hydroxylase). Ketoconazole is administered off label as secondary hormone therapy to reduce adrenal androgen synthesis in castration-resistant prostate cancer. Diarrhea and hepatic enzyme elevations limit its use as initial hormone therapy; consequent poor patient compliance reduces its efficacy. Ketoconazole is given in doses of 200 mg or 400 mg 3 times daily. Hydrocortisone (400-mg dose) is coadministered to compensate for inhibition of adrenal steroidogenesis. A related compound, itraconazole, inhibits the activation of Smoothened (SMO), a component of the Hedgehog (Hh) signaling pathway, which is overly active in certain cancers. Thus, this class of antifungal agents may act by several distinct mechanisms and prove useful in treating other cancers.

Abiraterone. Abiraterone is an irreversible inhibitor of 17α-hydroxylase and C-17,20-lyase (CYP17) activity, with greater potency and selectivity than ketoconazole. The prodrug abiraterone acetate (ZYTIGA) is approved for use with prednisone in metastatic castration-resistant prostate cancer. With continuous administration, abiraterone increases ACTH levels, resulting in mineralocorticoid excess. Recommended oral dose of abiraterone acetate is 1000 mg administered once daily (on an empty stomach) with 5 mg prednisone administered twice daily. Side effects include joint swelling, hypokalemia, hot flush, diarrhea, cough, hypertension, arrhythmia, urinary frequency, dyspepsia, and upper respiratory tract infection.

For a complete Bibliographical Listing see Goodman & Gilman's ***The Pharmacological Basis of Therapeutics***, 12th ed., or Goodman & Gilman Online at www.AccessMedicine.com.

Section IX Special Systems Pharmacology

chapter 64 Ocular Pharmacology

The eye is a specialized sensory organ that is relatively secluded from systemic access by the blood-retinal, blood-aqueous, and blood-vitreous barriers; as a consequence, the eye exhibits some unusual pharmacodynamic and pharmacokinetic properties.

EXTRAOCULAR STRUCTURES

The eye is protected by the eyelids and by the orbit, a bony cavity of the skull that has multiple fissures and foramina that conduct nerves, muscles, and vessels (Figure 64–1). In the orbit, connective (i.e., *Tenon's capsule*) and adipose tissues and 6 extraocular muscles support and align the eyes for vision. The retrobulbar region lies immediately behind the eye (or *globe*). Understanding ocular and orbital anatomy is important for safe periocular drug delivery, including subconjunctival, sub-Tenon's, and retrobulbar injections.

The external surface of the eyelids is covered by a thin layer of skin; the internal surface is lined with the palpebral portion of the conjunctiva, which is a vascularized mucous membrane continuous with the bulbar conjunctiva. At the reflection of the palpebral and bulbar conjunctivae is a space called the *fornix*, located superiorly and inferiorly behind the upper and lower lids, respectively. Topical medications usually are placed in the inferior fornix, also known as the *inferior cul-de-sac*.

The lacrimal system consists of secretory glandular and excretory ductal elements (Figure 64–2). The secretory system is composed of the main *lacrimal gland*, which is located in the temporal outer portion of the orbit, and accessory glands located in the conjunctiva. The lacrimal gland is innervated by the autonomic nervous system (Table 64–1 and Chapter 8). The parasympathetic innervation is clinically relevant because a patient may complain of dry eye symptoms while taking medications with anticholinergic side effects, such as tricyclic antidepressants (*see* Chapter 15), antihistamines (*see* Chapter 32), and drugs used in the management of Parkinson disease (*see* Chapter 22).

Tears constitute a trilaminar lubrication barrier covering the conjunctiva and cornea. The anterior layer is composed primarily of lipids; the middle aqueous layer, produced by the main lacrimal gland and accessory lacrimal glands, constitutes ~98% of the tear film. Adherent to the corneal epithelium, the posterior layer is a mixture of mucins produced by goblet cells in the conjunctiva. Tears also contain nutrients, enzymes, and immunoglobulins to support and protect the cornea. The tear drainage system starts through small puncta located on the medial aspects of both the upper and lower eyelids (*see* Figure 64–2). With blinking, tears enter the puncta and continue to drain through the canaliculi, lacrimal sac, nasolacrimal duct, and then into the nose. The nose is lined by a highly vascular mucosal epithelium; consequently, topically applied medications that pass through this nasolacrimal system have direct access to the systemic circulation.

OCULAR STRUCTURES

The eye is divided into anterior and posterior segments (Figure 64–3A). Anterior segment structures include the cornea, limbus, anterior and posterior chambers, trabecular meshwork, canal of Schlemm (Schlemm's canal), iris, lens, zonule, and ciliary body. The posterior segment includes the vitreous, retina, choroid, sclera, and optic nerve.

ANTERIOR SEGMENT

Cornea and Drug Access. The cornea is a transparent and avascular tissue organized into 5 layers (Figure 64–3B). Representing an important barrier to foreign matter, including drugs, the hydrophobic epithelial layer comprises 5 to 6 cell layers. The basal epithelial cells lie on a basement membrane that is adjacent to Bowman's

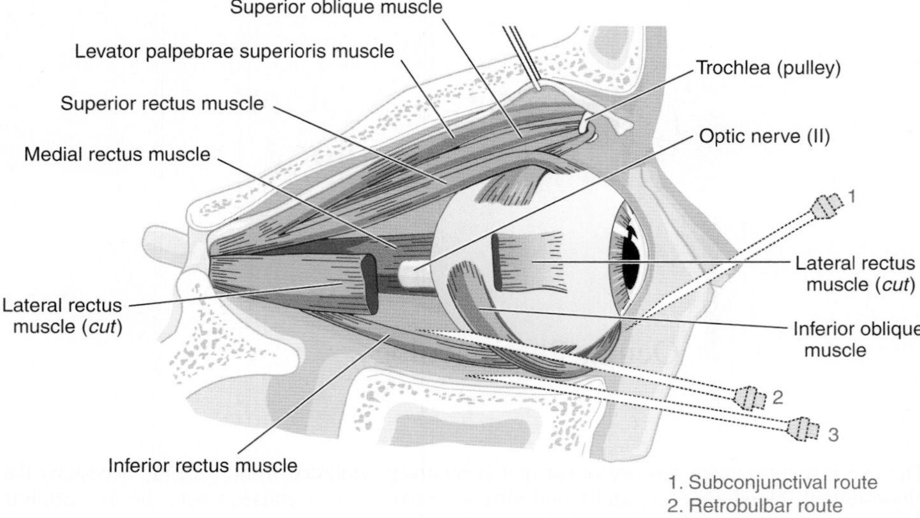

Figure 64–1 *Anatomy of the globe in relationship to the orbit and eyelids.* Various routes of administration of anesthesia are demonstrated by the *blue needle pathways*.

membrane, a layer of collagen fibers. Constituting ~90% of the corneal thickness, the stroma, a hydrophilic layer, is organized with collagen lamellae synthesized by keratocytes. Beneath the stroma lies Descemet's membrane, the basement membrane of the corneal endothelium. Lying most posteriorly, the endothelium is a monolayer of cells adhering to each other by tight junctions. These cells maintain corneal integrity by active transport processes and serve as a hydrophobic barrier. Hence, drug absorption across the cornea requires penetration of the trilaminar hydrophobic–hydrophilic–hydrophobic domains of the various anatomical layers.

At the periphery of the cornea and adjacent to the sclera lies a transitional zone (1-2 mm wide) called the *limbus*. Limbal structures include the conjunctival epithelium, which contains the corneal epithelial stem cells, Tenon's capsule, episclera, corneoscleral stroma, canal of Schlemm, and trabecular meshwork

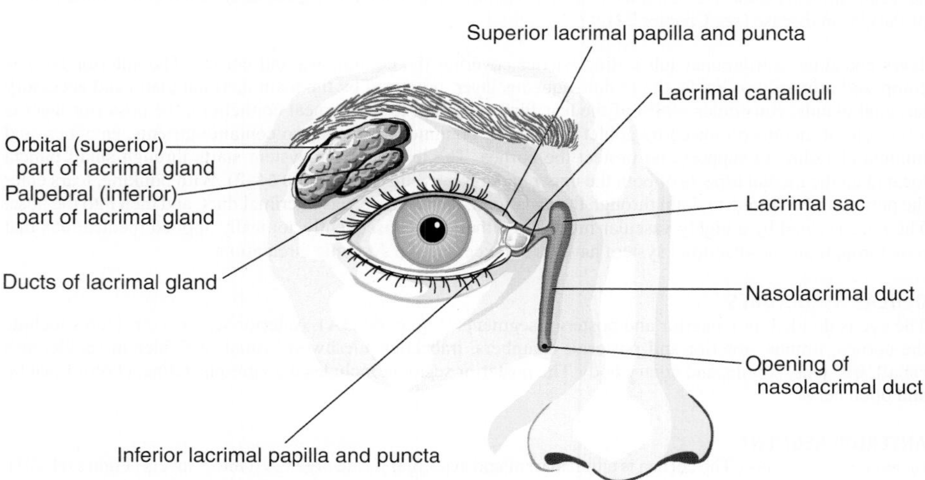

Figure 64–2 *Anatomy of the lacrimal system.*

Table 64–1

Autonomic Pharmacology of the Eye and Related Structures

	ADRENERGIC RECEPTORS		CHOLINERGIC RECEPTORS	
TISSUE	SUBTYPE	RESPONSE	SUBTYPE	RESPONSE
Corneal epithelium	β_2	Unknown	M[a]	Unknown
Corneal endothelium	β_2	Unknown	Undefined	Unknown
Iris radial muscle	α_1	Mydriasis		
Iris sphincter muscle			M_3	Miosis
Trabecular meshwork	β_2	Unknown		
Ciliary epithelium[b]	α_2/β_2	Aqueous production		
Ciliary muscle	β_2	Relaxation[c]	M_3	Accommodation
Lacrimal gland	α_1	Secretion	M_2, M_3	Secretion
Retinal pigment epithelium	α_1/β_2	H_2O transport/ unknown		

[a]*Although acetylcholine and choline acetyltransferase are abundant in the corneal epithelium of most species, the function of this neurotransmitter in this tissue is unknown.*
[b]*The ciliary epithelium also is the target of carbonic anhydrase inhibitors. Carbonic anhydrase isoenzyme II is localized to both the pigmented and nonpigmented ciliary epithelium.*
[c]*Although β_2 adrenergic receptors mediate ciliary body smooth muscle relaxation, there is no clinically significant effect on accommodation.*

(*see* Figure 64–3B). Limbal blood vessels, as well as the tears, provide important nutrients and immunological defense mechanisms for the cornea. The anterior chamber holds ~250 μL of aqueous humor. The peripheral anterior chamber angle is formed by the cornea and the iris root. The trabecular meshwork and canal of Schlemm are located just above the apex of this angle. The posterior chamber, which holds ~50 μL of aqueous humor, is defined by the boundaries of the ciliary body processes, posterior surface of the iris, and lens surface.

Aqueous Humor Dynamics and Regulation of Intraocular Pressure (IOP). Aqueous humor is secreted by the ciliary processes and flows from the posterior chamber, through the pupil, and into the anterior chamber and leaves the eye primarily by the trabecular meshwork and canal of Schlemm, thence to an episcleral venous plexus and into the systemic circulation. This conventional pathway accounts for 80-95% of aqueous humor outflow and is the main target for cholinergic drugs used in glaucoma therapy. Another outflow pathway is the uveoscleral route (i.e., fluid flows through the ciliary muscles and into the suprachoroidal space), which is the target of selective prostanoids (*see* "Glaucoma" and Chapter 33).

The peripheral anterior chamber angle is an important anatomical structure for differentiating 2 forms of glaucoma: *open-angle glaucoma*, which is by far the most common form of glaucoma in the U.S., and *angle-closure glaucoma*. Current medical therapy of open-angle glaucoma is aimed at decreasing aqueous humor production and/or increasing aqueous outflow. The preferred management for angle-closure glaucoma is surgical iridectomy, by either laser or incision, but short-term medical management may be necessary to reduce the acute IOP elevation and to clear the cornea prior to surgery. Long-term IOP reduction may be necessary, especially if the peripheral iris has permanently covered the trabecular meshwork.

In anatomically susceptible eyes, anticholinergic, sympathomimetic, and antihistaminic drugs can lead to partial dilation of the pupil and a change in the vectors of force between the iris and the lens. The aqueous humor then is prevented from passing through the pupil from the posterior chamber to the anterior chamber. The change in the lens-iris relationship leads to an increase in pressure in the posterior chamber, causing the iris base to be pushed against the angle wall, thereby covering the trabecular meshwork and closing the filtration angle and markedly elevating the IOP. The result is known as an acute attack of *pupillary-block angle-closure glaucoma*.

Iris and Pupil. The iris is the most anterior portion of the uveal tract, which also includes the ciliary body and choroid. The anterior surface of the iris is the stroma, a loosely organized structure containing melanocytes, blood vessels, smooth muscle, and parasympathetic and sympathetic nerves. Differences in iris color reflect individual variation in the number of melanocytes located in the stroma. Individual variation may be an important consideration for ocular drug distribution due to drug-melanin binding (*see* "Distribution"). The posterior surface of the iris is a densely pigmented bilayer of epithelial cells. Anterior to the pigmented epithelium, the dilator smooth muscle is oriented radially and is innervated by the sympathetic nervous system (Figure 64–4),

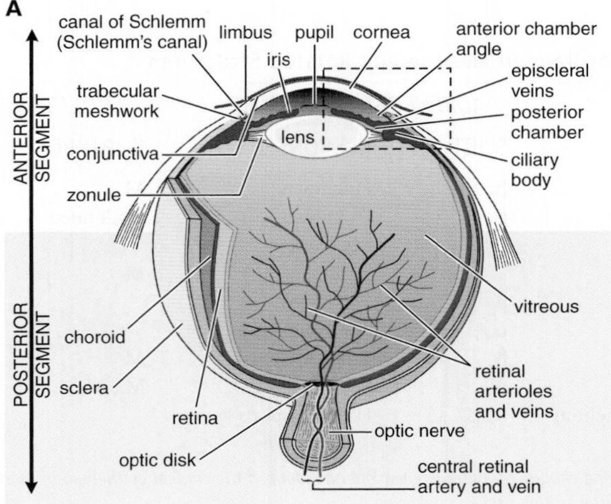

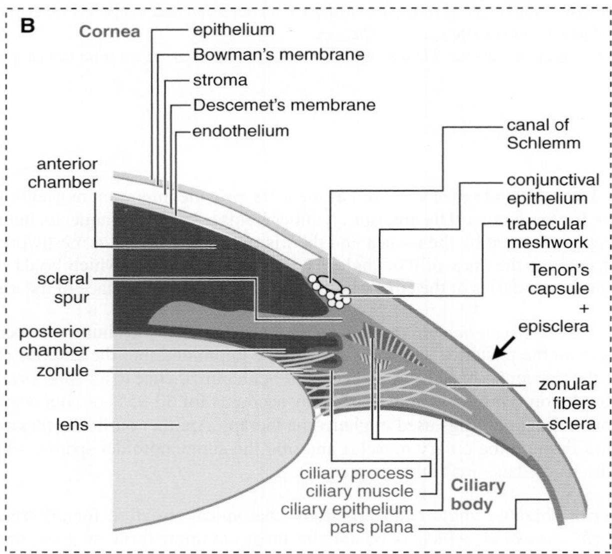

Figure 64–3 ***A.*** *Anatomy of the eye.* ***B.*** *Enlargement of the anterior segment, revealing the cornea, angle structures, lens, and ciliary body.* (Adapted with permission from Riordan-Eva P. Anatomy and embryology of the eye. In: Riordan-Eva P, Whitcher JP, eds. *Vaughan & Asbury's General Ophthalmology*, 17th ed. New York: McGraw-Hill; 2008. Copyright © 2008 by The McGraw-Hill Companies, Inc. All rights reserved.)

which causes *mydriasis* (dilation). At the pupillary margin, the sphincter smooth muscle is organized in a circular band with parasympathetic innervation, which, when stimulated, causes *miosis* (constriction). The use of pharmacological agents to dilate normal pupils and to evaluate the pharmacological response of the pupil is summarized in Table 64–2. Pharmacological agents are also used for the diagnostic evaluation of anisocoria (*see* Figure 64–5 in the 12th edition of the parent text).

Ciliary Body. The ciliary body serves 2 very specialized roles:

- Secretion of aqueous humor by the epithelial bilayer
- Accommodation by the ciliary muscle

The anterior portion of the ciliary body (*pars plicata*) comprises 70-80 ciliary processes with intricate folds. The posterior portion is the *pars plana*. The ciliary muscle is organized into outer longitudinal, middle radial, and inner circular layers. Coordinated contraction of this smooth muscle apparatus by the parasympathetic nervous system causes the zonule suspending the lens to relax, allowing the lens to become more convex and

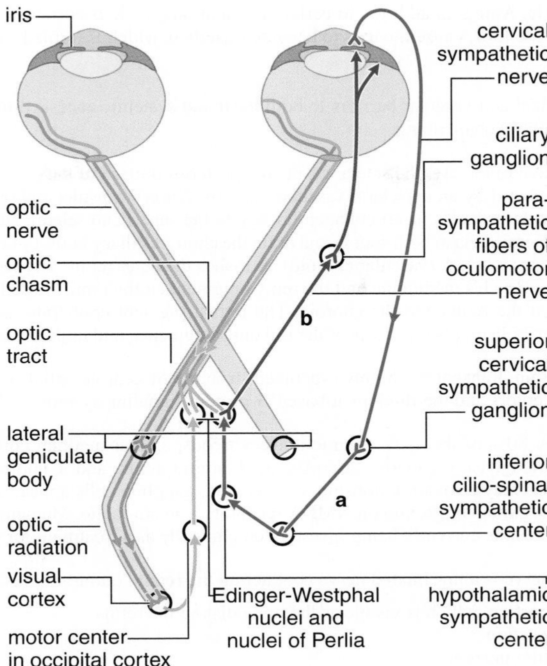

Figure 64–4 *Autonomic innervation of the eye by the sympathetic (a) and parasympathetic (b) nervous systems.* (Adapted with permission from Wybar KC, Kerr-Muir M. *Bailliere's Concise Medical Textbooks, Ophthalmology,* 3rd ed. New York: Bailliere Tindall; 1984. Copyright © Elsevier.)

to shift slightly forward. This process, known as *accommodation*, permits focusing on near objects and may be pharmacologically blocked by muscarinic cholinergic antagonists, through the process called *cycloplegia.* Contraction of the ciliary muscle also puts traction on the scleral spur and hence widens the spaces within the trabecular meshwork. This latter effect accounts for at least some of the IOP-lowering effect of both directly acting and indirectly acting parasympathomimetic drugs.

Lens. The lens is suspended by *zonules*, specialized fibers emanating from the ciliary body. The lens is ~10 mm in diameter and is enclosed in a capsule. The bulk of the lens is composed of fibers derived from proliferating lens epithelial cells located under the anterior portion of the lens capsule. These lens fibers are continuously

Table 64–2

Effects of Pharmacological Agents on the Pupil

CLINICAL SETTING	DRUG	PUPILLARY RESPONSE
Normal	Sympathomimetic drugs	Dilation (mydriasis)
Normal	Parasympathomimetic drugs	Constriction (miosis)
Horner's syndrome	Cocaine 4-10%	No dilation
Preganglionic Horner's	Hydroxyamphetamine 1%	Dilation
Postganglionic Horner's	Hydroxyamphetamine 1%	No dilation
Adie's pupil	Pilocarpine 0.05-0.1%[a]	Constriction
Normal	Opioids (oral or intravenous)	Pinpoint pupils

Topically applied ophthalmic drugs unless otherwise noted.
[a]This percentage of pilocarpine is not commercially available and usually is prepared by the physician administering the test or by a pharmacist. This test also requires that no prior manipulation of the cornea (i.e., tonometry for measuring intraocular pressure or testing corneal sensation) be done so that the normal integrity of the corneal barrier is intact. Normal pupils will not respond to this weak dilution of pilocarpine; however, an Adie's pupil manifests a denervation supersensitivity and is responsive to this dilute cholinergic agonist.

produced throughout life. Aging, in addition to certain medications, such as corticosteroids, and certain diseases, such as diabetes mellitus, cause the lens to become opacified, which is termed a *cataract*.

POSTERIOR SEGMENT

Because of the anatomical and vascular barriers to both local and systemic access, drug delivery to the eye's posterior pole is particularly challenging.

Sclera. The outermost coat of the eye, the sclera, covers the posterior portion of the globe. The external surface of the scleral shell is covered by an episcleral vascular coat, by Tenon's capsule, and by the conjunctiva. The tendons of the 6 extraocular muscles insert collagen fibers into the superficial scleral. Numerous blood vessels pierce the sclera through emissaria to both supply and drain the choroid, ciliary body, optic nerve, and iris. Inside the scleral shell, a capillary network (vascular choroid) nourishes the outer retina. Between the outer retina and the capillary network lie Bruch's membrane and the retinal pigment epithelium, whose tight junctions provide an outer barrier between the retina and the choroid. The retinal pigment epithelium serves many functions, including vitamin A metabolism, phagocytosis of the rod outer segments, and multiple transport processes.

Retina. The retina is a thin, transparent, highly organized structure of neurons, glial cells, and blood vessels; it contains the photoreceptors and the rhodopsin-based G-protein signaling system.

Vitreous. Approximately 80% of the eye's volume is the vitreous, a clear medium containing collagen type II, hyaluronic acid, proteoglycans, glucose, ascorbic acid, amino acids, and a number of inorganic salts. Glutamate in the vitreous may have a relationship to glaucoma: ganglion cells appear to die in glaucoma via apoptosis, a process that glutamate, acting on NMDA receptors, can stimulate. Memantine, a noncompetitive NMDA receptor antagonist, is currently being investigated clinically as a treatment for glaucoma.

Optic Nerve. The optic nerve is a myelinated nerve conducting the retinal output to the CNS. It comprises:

- An intraocular portion, which is visible as the optic disk in the retina
- An intraorbital portion
- An intracanalicular portion
- An intracranial portion

The nerve is ensheathed in meninges continuous with the brain. At present, pharmacological treatment of optic neuropathies usually is based on management of the underlying disease. For example, nonarteritic ischemic optic neuropathy is best treated with intravitreal glucocorticoids, and optic neuritis with intravenous glucocorticoids. Glaucomatous optic neuropathy is medically managed by decreasing IOP.

PHARMACOKINETICS AND TOXICOLOGY OF OCULAR THERAPEUTIC AGENTS

DRUG-DELIVERY STRATEGIES. Properties of varying ocular routes of administration are outlined in Figure 64–1 and Table 64–3.

Several formulations prolong the time a drug remains on the surface of the eye. These include gels, ointments, solid inserts, soft contact lenses, and collagen shields. *Prolonging the time in the cul-de-sac beneath the eye lid facilitates drug absorption.* Ophthalmic gels (e.g., pilocarpine 4% gel) release drugs by diffusion following erosion of soluble polymers. Ointments usually contain mineral oil and a petrolatum base and are helpful in delivering antibiotics, cycloplegic drugs, or miotic agents. Solid inserts, such as the ganciclovir intravitreal implant, provide a *zero-order* rate of delivery by steady-state diffusion, whereby drug is released at a more constant rate over a prolonged period of time rather than as a bolus.

PHARMACOKINETICS. The pharmacokinetic principles of absorption, distribution, metabolism, and excretion determine the time course of drug action in the eye, however, the routes of ocular drug administration, the flow of ocular fluids, and the architecture of the eye introduce other variables specific to the eye. Most ophthalmic medications are formulated to be applied topically. Drugs also may be injected by subconjunctival, sub-Tenon's, and retrobulbar routes.

ABSORPTION. After topical instillation of a drug, the rate and extent of absorption are determined by the time the drug remains in the cul-de-sac and precorneal tear film, elimination by nasolacrimal drainage, drug binding to tear proteins, drug metabolism by tear and tissue proteins, and diffusion across the cornea and conjunctiva. A drug's residence time may be prolonged by changing its formulation. Residence time also may be extended by blocking the egress of tears from the eye by closing the tear drainage ducts with flexible silicone (punctal) plugs. Nasolacrimal drainage contributes to systemic absorption of topically administered ophthalmic medications. Absorption from the nasal mucosa avoids first-pass metabolism by the liver; thus, topical ophthalmic medications can cause significant systemic side effects, especially when used chronically. Possible absorption pathways of an ophthalmic drug following topical application to the eye are shown schematically in Figure 64–5.

Table 64–3

Some Characteristics of Ocular Routes of Drug Administration

ROUTE	ABSORPTION PATTERN	SPECIAL UTILITY	LIMITATIONS AND PRECAUTIONS
Topical	Prompt, depending on formulation	Convenient, economical, relatively safe	Compliance, corneal and conjunctival toxicity, nasal mucosal toxicity, systemic side effects from nasolacrimal absorption
Subconjunctival, sub-Tenon's, and retrobulbar injections	Prompt or sustained, depending on formulation	Anterior segment infections, posterior uveitis, cystoid macular edema	Local toxicity, tissue injury, globe perforation, optic nerve trauma, central retinal artery and/or vein occlusion, direct retinal drug toxicity with inadvertent globe perforation, ocular muscle trauma, prolonged drug effect
Intraocular (intracameral) injections	Prompt	Anterior segment surgery, infections	Corneal toxicity, intraocular toxicity, relatively short duration of action
Intravitreal injection or device	Absorption circumvented, immediate local effect, potential sustained effect	Endophthalmitis, retinitis, age-related macular degeneration	Retinal toxicity

Transcorneal and transconjunctival/scleral absorption are the desired routes for localized ocular drug effects. The drug concentration gradient between the tear film and the cornea and conjunctival epithelium provides the driving force for passive diffusion across these tissues. Other factors that affect a drug's diffusion capacity are the size of the molecule, chemical structure, and steric configuration. Transcorneal drug penetration is a differential solubility process; the cornea resembles a trilaminar "fat-water-fat" structure corresponding to the epithelial, stromal, and endothelial layers. The epithelium and endothelium represent barriers for hydrophilic substances; the stroma is a barrier for hydrophobic compounds. Hence, a drug with both hydrophilic and lipophilic properties is best suited for transcorneal absorption. Drug penetration into the eye is approximately linearly related to its concentration in the tear film. Certain disease states, such as corneal epithelial defects and corneal ulcers, may alter drug penetration. Medication absorption usually is increased when an anatomical barrier is compromised or removed.

DISTRIBUTION. Topically administered drugs may undergo systemic distribution primarily by nasal mucosal absorption and possibly by local ocular distribution by transcorneal/transconjunctival absorption. Following transcorneal absorption, the aqueous humor accumulates the drug, which then is distributed to intraocular structures and potentially to the systemic circulation via the trabecular meshwork pathway (*see* Figure 64–3B). Melanin binding of certain drugs is an important factor in some ocular compartments. For example, the mydriatic effect of α adrenergic–receptor agonists is slower in onset in human volunteers with darkly pigmented irides compared to those with lightly pigmented irides: drug-melanin binding is a potential reservoir for sustained drug release. Another clinically important consideration for drug-melanin binding involves the retinal pigment epithelium. In the retinal pigment epithelium, accumulation of chloroquine (*see* Chapter 49) causes a toxic retinal lesion known as a "bull's-eye" maculopathy, which is associated with a decrease in visual acuity.

METABOLISM. Biotransformation of ocular drugs may be significant; a variety of enzymes, including esterases, oxidoreductases, lysosomal enzymes, peptidases, glucuronide and sulfate transferases, GSH-conjugating enzymes, COMT, MAO, and 11β-hydroxysteroid dehydrogenase are found in the eye. The esterases have been of particular interest, permitting development of ester prodrugs for enhanced corneal permeability (e.g., *dipivefrin hydrochloride* is a prodrug for epinephrine, and *latanoprost* is a prodrug for $PGF_{2\alpha}$; both drugs are used for glaucoma management).

TOXICOLOGY. Most local toxic effects are due to hypersensitivity reactions or to direct toxic effects on the cornea, conjunctiva, periocular skin, and nasal mucosa. Eyedrops and contact lens solutions commonly contain antimicrobial preservatives such as benzalkonium chloride, chlorobutanol, chelating agents, and, rarely, thimerosal. In particular, benzalkonium chloride may cause a punctate keratopathy or toxic ulcerative

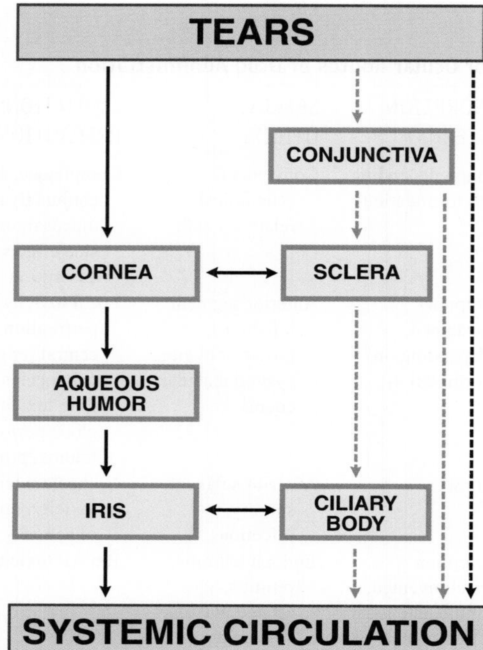

Figure 64–5 *Possible absorption pathways of an ophthalmic drug following topical application to the eye. Solid black arrows* represent the corneal route; *dashed blue arrows* represent the conjunctival/scleral route; the *black dashed arrow* represents the nasolacrimal absorption pathway. (Adapted with permission from Chien D-S, et al. *Curr Eye Res*, 1990;9(11):1051–1059. Copyright © 1990 Informa Healthcare.)

keratopathy. All ophthalmic medications are potentially absorbed into the systemic circulation (Figure 64–5), so systemic side effects may occur.

OPHTHALMIC USES OF DRUGS

CHEMOTHERAPY OF MICROBIAL DISEASES IN THE EYE

ANTIBACTERIAL AGENTS. A number of antibiotics have been formulated for topical ocular use (Table 64–4).

THERAPEUTIC USES OF OCULAR ANTIMICROBIALS. Infectious diseases of the skin, eyelids, conjunctivae, and lacrimal excretory system are encountered regularly. Periocular skin infections are divided into preseptal and postseptal or orbital cellulitis. Depending on the clinical setting (i.e., preceding trauma, sinusitis, age of patient, relative immunocompromised state), oral or parenteral antibiotics are administered.

Dacryoadenitis, an infection of the lacrimal gland, is most common in children and young adults; it may be bacterial (typically *Staphylococcus aureus, Streptococcus* spp.) or viral (seen in mumps, infectious mononucleosis, influenza, and herpes zoster). When bacterial infection is suspected, systemic antibiotics usually are indicated.

Dacryocystitis is an infection of the lacrimal sac. In infants and children, the disease usually is unilateral and secondary to an obstruction of the nasolacrimal duct. In adults, dacryocystitis and canalicular infections may be caused by *S. aureus, Streptococcus* spp., diphtheroids, *Candida* spp., and *Actinomyces israelii*. Any discharge from the lacrimal sac should be sent for smears and cultures. Systemic antibiotics typically are indicated.

Infectious processes of the lids include *hordeolum* and *blepharitis*. A hordeolum, or stye, is an infection of the meibomian, Zeis, or Moll glands at the eyelid margins. The typical offending bacterium is *S. aureus*, and the usual treatment consists of warm compresses and topical antibiotic (gel, drops, or ointment). Blepharitis is a common bilateral inflammatory process of the eyelids characterized by irritation and burning, usually associated with a *Staphylococcus* sp. Local hygiene is the mainstay of therapy; topical antibiotics frequently

Table 64–4

Topical Antibacterial Agents Commercially Available for Ophthalmic Use

GENERIC NAME	FORMULATION[a]	TOXICITY	INDICATIONS FOR USE
Azithromycin	1% solution	H	Conjunctivitis
Bacitracin	500 units/g ointment	H	Conjunctivitis, blepharitis, keratitis, keratoconjunctivitis, corneal ulcers, blepharoconjunctivitis, meibomianitis, dacryocystitis
Besifloxacin	0.6% suspension		Conjunctivitis
Chloramphenicol	1% ointment	H, BD	Conjunctivitis, keratitis
Ciprofloxacin hydrochloride	0.3% solution; 0.3% ointment	H, D-RCD	Conjunctivitis, keratitis, keratoconjunctivitis, corneal ulcers, blepharitis, blepharoconjunctivitis, meibomianitis, dacryocystitis
Erythromycin	0.5% ointment	H	Superficial ocular infections involving the conjunctiva or cornea; prophylaxis of ophthalmia neonatorum
Gatifloxacin	0.3% solution	H	Conjunctivitis
Gentamicin sulfate	0.3% solution; 0.3% ointment	H	Conjunctivitis, blepharitis, keratitis, keratoconjunctivitis, corneal ulcers, blepharoconjunctivitis, meibomianitis, dacryocystitis
Levofloxacin	0.5% solution	H	Conjunctivitis
	1.5% solution	H	Corneal ulcers
Moxifloxacin	0.5% solution	H	Conjunctivitis
Ofloxacin	0.3% solution	H	Conjunctivitis, corneal ulcers
Sulfacetamide sodium	1, 10, 15, 30% solutions; 10% ointment	H, BD	Conjunctivitis, other superficial ocular infections
Polymyxin B combinations[b]	Various solutions and ointments		Conjunctivitis, blepharitis, keratitis
Tobramycin sulfate[c]	0.3% solution; 0.3% ointment	H	External infections of the eye and its adnexa

H, hypersensitivity; BD, blood dyscrasia; D-RCD, drug-related corneal deposits.

[a]*For specific information on dosing, formulation, and trade names, refer to the* Physicians' Desk Reference for Ophthalmic Medicines, *which is published annually.*

[b]*Polymyxin B is formulated for delivery to the eye in combination with bacitracin, neomycin, gramicidin, oxytetracycline, or trimethoprim. See Chapters 52–55 for further discussion of these antibacterial agents.*

[c]*Tobramycin is formulated for delivery to the eye in combination with dexamethasone or loteprednol etabonate.*

are used. Systemic tetracycline, doxycycline, minocycline, and erythromycin often are effective in reducing severe eyelid inflammation but must be used for weeks to months.

Conjunctivitis is an inflammatory process of the conjunctiva that varies in severity from mild hyperemia to severe purulent discharge. The more common causes of conjunctivitis include viruses, allergies, environmental irritants, contact lenses, and chemicals. The less common causes include other infectious pathogens, immune-mediated reactions, associated systemic diseases, and tumors of the conjunctiva or eyelid. The more commonly reported infectious agents are adenovirus and herpes simplex virus, followed by other viral (e.g., enterovirus, coxsackievirus, measles virus, varicella zoster virus, vaccinia variola virus) and bacterial sources (e.g., *Neisseria* spp., *Streptococcus pneumoniae, Haemophilus* spp., *S. aureus, Moraxella lacunata*, and chlamydial spp.). *Rickettsia*, fungi, and parasites, in both cyst and trophozoite form, are rare causes of conjunctivitis. Effective management is based on selection of an appropriate antibiotic for suspected bacterial pathogens. Unless an unusual causative organism is suspected, bacterial conjunctivitis is treated empirically with a broad-spectrum topical antibiotic without obtaining a culture.

Keratitis, or corneal inflammation, can occur at any level of the cornea. Numerous microbial agents have been identified as causes of infectious keratitis, including bacteria, viruses, fungi, spirochetes, and cysts and trophozoites. Severe infections with tissue loss (corneal ulcers) generally are treated more aggressively than infections without tissue loss (corneal infiltrates). Mild, small, more peripheral infections usually are not cultured, and the eyes are treated with broad-spectrum topical antibiotics. In more severe, central, or larger infections, corneal scrapings for cultures and sensitivities are performed, and the patient is immediately started on intensive hourly, around-the-clock topical antibiotic therapy. The goal of treatment is to eradicate the infection and reduce the amount of corneal scarring and the chance of corneal perforation and severe decreased vision or blindness. The initial medication selection and dosage are adjusted according to the clinical response and culture and sensitivity results.

Endophthalmitis is a potentially severe and devastating inflammatory, and usually infectious, process involving the intraocular tissues. When the inflammatory process encompasses the entire globe, it is called *panophthalmitis.* Endophthalmitis usually is caused by bacteria or fungi, or rarely by spirochetes. The typical case occurs during the early postoperative course (e.g., after cataract, glaucoma, cornea, or retinal surgery), following trauma, or by endogenous seeding in an immunocompromised host or intravenous drug user. Acute postoperative endophthalmitis requires a prompt vitreous tap for smears and cultures and empirical injection of intravitreal antibiotics. Immediate vitrectomy (i.e., specialized surgical removal of the vitreous) is beneficial for patients who have light perception–only vision. Vitrectomy for other causes of endophthalmitis (e.g., glaucoma bleb related, posttraumatic, or endogenous) may be beneficial. In cases of endogenous seeding, parenteral antibiotics have a role in eliminating the infectious source, but the efficacy of systemic antibiotics with trauma is not well established.

ANTIVIRAL AGENTS. Antiviral drugs used in ophthalmology are summarized in Table 64–5 (*see* Chapter 58 for details of these agents).

THERAPEUTIC USES. The primary indications for the use of antiviral drugs in ophthalmology are viral keratitis, herpes zoster ophthalmicus, and retinitis. There currently are no antiviral agents for the treatment of viral conjunctivitis caused by adenoviruses, which usually has a self-limited course and typically is treated by symptomatic relief of irritation.

Viral keratitis, an infection of the cornea that may involve either the epithelium or stroma, is most commonly caused by herpes simplex type I and varicella zoster viruses. Less common viral etiologies include herpes simplex type II, Epstein-Barr virus, and CMV. Topical antiviral agents are indicated for the treatment of epithelial disease due to herpes simplex infection. *When treating viral keratitis topically, there is a very narrow margin between the therapeutic topical antiviral activity and the toxic effect on the cornea*; hence, patients must be followed very closely. Topical glucocorticoids are contraindicated in herpetic epithelial keratitis due to active viral replication. In contrast, for herpetic disciform keratitis (predominantly a cell-mediated immune

Table 64–5

Antiviral Agents for Ophthalmic Use

GENERIC NAME	ROUTE OF ADMINISTRATION	OCULAR TOXICITY	INDICATIONS FOR USE
Trifluridine	Topical (1% solution)	PK, H	Herpes simplex keratitis and keratoconjunctivitis
Acyclovir	Oral, intravenous (200-mg capsules, 400- and 800-mg tablets)		Herpes zoster ophthalmicus[a] Herpes simplex iridocyclitis
Valacyclovir	Oral (500- and 1000-mg tablets)		Herpes simplex keratitis[a] Herpes zoster ophthalmicus[a]
Famciclovir	Oral (125-, 250-, and 500-mg tablets)		Herpes simplex keratitis[a] Herpes zoster ophthalmicus[a]
Foscarnet	Intravenous Intravitreal[a]		Cytomegalovirus retinitis
Ganciclovir	Intravenous, oral, intravitreal implant		Cytomegalovirus retinitis
Valganciclovir	Oral		Cytomegalovirus retinitis
Cidofovir	Intravenous		Cytomegalovirus retinitis

PK, punctate keratopathy; H, hypersensitivity.
[a]*Off-label use. For additional details, see Chapter 58.*

reaction), topical glucocorticoids accelerate recovery. For recurrent herpetic stromal keratitis, there is clear benefit from treatment with oral acyclovir in reducing the risk of recurrence.

Herpes zoster ophthalmicus is a latent reactivation of a varicella zoster infection in the first division of the trigeminal cranial nerve. Systemic acyclovir, valacyclovir, and famciclovir are effective in reducing the severity and complications of herpes zoster ophthalmicus. Currently, there are no ophthalmic preparations of acyclovir approved by the FDA, although an ophthalmic ointment is available for investigational use.

Viral retinitis may be caused by herpes simplex virus, CMV, adenovirus, and varicella zoster virus. With highly active antiretroviral therapy (HAART; *see* Chapter 59), CMV retinitis does not appear to progress when specific anti-CMV therapy is discontinued, but some patients develop an immune recovery uveitis. Treatment usually involves long-term parenteral administration of antiviral drugs. Intravitreal ganciclovir has been found to be an effective alternative to systemic use. Acute retinal necrosis and progressive outer retinal necrosis, most often caused by varicella zoster virus, can be treated by various combinations of oral, intravenous, intravitreal injection of, and intravitreal implantation of antiviral medications.

ANTIFUNGAL AGENTS

The only currently available topical ophthalmic antifungal preparation is a polyene, natamycin (NATACYN). Other antifungal agents may be extemporaneously compounded for topical, subconjunctival, or intravitreal routes of administration (Table 64–6; *see* also Chapter 57).

THERAPEUTIC USES. As with systemic fungal infections, the incidence of ophthalmic fungal infections has risen with the growing number of immunocompromised hosts. Ophthalmic indications for antifungal medications include fungal keratitis, scleritis, endophthalmitis, mucormycosis, and canaliculitis. Risk factors for fungal keratitis include trauma, chronic ocular surface disease, contact lens wear, and immunosuppression (including topical steroid use). When fungal infection is suspected, samples of the affected tissues are obtained for smears, cultures, and sensitivities, and this information is used to guide drug selection.

ANTIPROTOZOAL AGENTS

Parasitic infections involving the eye usually manifest themselves as a form of *uveitis*, an inflammatory process of either the anterior or posterior segments and, less commonly, as conjunctivitis, keratitis, and retinitis.

THERAPEUTIC USES. In the U.S., the most commonly encountered protozoal infections include *Acanthamoeba* and *Toxoplasma gondii*. In contact lens wearers who develop keratitis, physicians should be highly suspicious of the presence of *Acanthamoeba*. Risk factors for *Acanthamoeba* keratitis include poor contact lens hygiene, wearing contact lenses in a pool or hot tub, and ocular trauma. Treatment usually consists of a combination of

Table 64–6

Antifungal Agents for Ophthalmic Use

DRUG CLASS/ AGENT	METHOD OF ADMINISTRATION	INDICATIONS FOR USE
Polyenes		
Amphotericin B[a]	0.1-0.5% (typically 0.15%) topical solution	Yeast and fungal keratitis and endophthalmitis
	0.8-1 mg subconjunctival	Yeast and fungal endophthalmitis
	5-μg intravitreal injection	Yeast and fungal endophthalmitis
	Intravenous	Yeast and fungal endophthalmitis
Natamycin	5% topical suspension	Yeast and fungal blepharitis, conjunctivitis, keratitis
Imidazoles		
Fluconazole[a]	Oral, intravenous	Yeast keratitis and endophthalmitis
Itraconazole[a]	Oral	Yeast and fungal keratitis and endophthalmitis
Ketoconazole[a]	Oral	Yeast keratitis and endophthalmitis
Miconazole[a]	1% topical solution	Yeast and fungal keratitis
	5-10 mg subconjunctival	Yeast and fungal endophthalmitis
	10-μg intravitreal injection	Yeast and fungal endophthalmitis

[a]*Off-label use. Only natamycin (NATACYN) is commercially available and labeled for ophthalmic use. All other antifungal drugs are not labeled for ophthalmic use and must be formulated for the given method of administration. For further dosing information, refer to the* Physicians' Desk Reference for Ophthalmic Medicines. *For additional discussion of these antifungal agents, see Chapter 57.*

topical agents. The aromatic diamidines (i.e., propamidine isethionate in both topical aqueous and ointment forms [BROLENE, NOT AVAILABLE IN U.S.]) have been used successfully to treat this relatively resistant infectious keratitis. The cationic antiseptic agent polyhexamethylene biguanide (PHMB) also is used in drop form for *Acanthamoeba* keratitis. Topical chlorhexidine can be used as an alternative to PHMB. Oral imidazoles (e.g., itraconazole, fluconazole, ketoconazole, voriconazole) often are used in addition to the topical medications. Resolution of *Acanthamoeba* keratitis often requires many months of treatment.

Treatment of *toxoplasmosis* is indicated when inflammatory lesions encroach upon the macula and threaten central visual acuity. Several regimens have been recommended with concurrent use of systemic steroids: (1) pyrimethamine, sulfadiazine, and folinic acid (leucovorin); (2) pyrimethamine, sulfadiazine, clindamycin, and folinic acid; (3) sulfadiazine and clindamycin; (4) clindamycin; (5) trimethoprim-sulfamethoxazole ± clindamycin. Other protozoal infections (e.g., giardiasis, leishmaniasis, malaria) and helminths are less common eye pathogens in the U.S. Systemic pharmacological management as well as vitrectomy may be indicated for selected parasitic infections.

AUTONOMIC AGENTS

THERAPEUTIC USES. Autonomic drugs are used extensively for diagnostic and surgical purposes and for the treatment of glaucoma, uveitis, and strabismus. The autonomic agents used in ophthalmology and the responses (i.e., mydriasis, cycloplegia) to muscarinic cholinergic antagonists are summarized in Table 64–7.

Table 64–7

Autonomic Drugs for Ophthalmic Use

DRUG CLASS	FORMULATION	INDICATIONS	SIDE EFFECTS
Cholinergic agonists			
Acetylcholine	1% solution	Miosis in surgery	Corneal edema
Carbachol	0.01-3% solution	Miosis in surgery, glaucoma[a]	Corneal edema, miosis, induced myopia, decreased vision, brow ache, retinal detachment
Pilocarpine	0.5%, 1%, 2%, 4%, and 6% solution; 4% gel	Glaucoma	Same as for carbachol
Anticholinesterase agents			
Echothiophate	0.125% solution	Glaucoma, accommodative esotropia	Retinal detachment, miosis, cataract, pupillary block glaucoma iris cysts, brow ache, punctal stenosis of the nasolacrimal system
Muscarinic antagonists			
Atropine	0.5%, 1%, and 2% solution; 1% ointment	Cycloplegia, mydriasis,[b] cycloplegic retinoscopy,[a] dilated funduscopic exam	Photosensitivity, blurred vision
Scopolamine	0.25% solution	Cycloplegia, mydriasis[b]	Same as for atropine
Homatropine	2% and 5% solution	Cycloplegia, mydriasis[b]	Same as for atropine
Cyclopentolate	0.5%, 1%, and 2% solution	Cycloplegia, mydriasis[b]	Same as for atropine
Tropicamide	0.5% and 1% solution	Cycloplegia, mydriasis[b]	Same as for atropine

(*continued*)

Table 64–7

Autonomic Drugs for Ophthalmic Use (*Continued*)

DRUG CLASS	FORMULATION	INDICATIONS	SIDE EFFECTS
α Adrenergic agonists			
Dipivefrin	0.1% solution	Glaucoma	Photosensitivity, conjunctival, hyperemia hypersensitivity
Phenylephrine	0.12%, 2.5%, and 10% solution	Mydriasis, vasoconstriction, decongestion	Same as for dipivefrin
Apraclonidine	0.5% and 1% solution	Ocular hypertension	Same as for dipivefrin
Brimonidine	0.1%, 0.15%, and 0.2% solution	Glaucoma, ocular hypertension	Same as for dipivefrin
Naphazoline	0.012%, 0.03%, and 0.1% solution	Decongestant	Same as for dipivefrin
Tetrahydrozoline	0.05% solution	Decongestant	Same as for dipivefrin
β Adrenergic antagonists			
Betaxolol (β_1-selective)	0.25% and 0.5% suspension	Glaucoma, ocular hypertension	
Carteolol (β)	1% solution	Glaucoma, ocular hypertension	
Levobunolol (β)	0.25% and 0.5% solution	Glaucoma, ocular hypertension	
Metipranolol (β)	0.3% solution	Glaucoma, ocular hypertension	
Timolol (β)	0.25% and 0.5% solution and gel	Glaucoma, ocular hypertension	

[a]*Off-label use. Refer to* Physicians' Desk Reference for Ophthalmic Medicines *for specific indications and dosing.*
[b]*Mydriasis and cycloplegia, or paralysis of accommodation, of the human eye occurs after one drop of atropine 1%, scopolamine 0.5%, homatropine 1%, cyclopentolate 0.5% or 1%, and tropicamide 0.5% or 1%. Recovery of mydriasis is defined by return to baseline pupil size to within 1 mm. Recovery of cycloplegia is defined by return to within 2 diopters of baseline accommodative power. The maximal mydriatic effect of homatropine is achieved with a 5% solution, but cycloplegia may be incomplete. Maximal cycloplegia with tropicamide may be achieved with a 1% solution. Times to development of maximal mydriasis and to recovery, respectively, are: for atropine, 30-40 min and 7-10 d; for scopolamine, 20-130 min and 3-7 d; for homatropine, 40-60 min and 1-3 d; for cyclopentolate, 30-60 min and 1 d; for tropicamide, 20-40 min and 6 h. Times to development of maximal cycloplegia and to recovery, respectively, are: for atropine, 60-180 min and 6-12 d; for scopolamine, 30-60 min and 3-7 d; for homatropine, 30-60 min and 1-3 d; for cyclopentolate, 25-75 min and 6 h to 1 d; for tropicamide, 30 min and 6 h.*

Glaucoma. Glaucoma is characterized by progressive optic nerve cupping and visual field loss. Risk factors include increased IOP, positive family history of glaucoma, African American heritage, and possibly myopia and hypertension. Reducing IOP can delay glaucomatous nerve or field damage. Although markedly elevated IOPs (e.g., >30 mm Hg) usually will lead to optic nerve damage, the optic nerves in certain patients (*ocular hypertensives*) apparently can tolerate IOPs in the mid- to high 20s. Other patients have progressive glaucomatous optic nerve damage despite having IOPs in the normal range, and this form of the disease sometimes is called *normal*- or *low-tension* glaucoma. A reduction of IOP by 30% reduces disease progression from ~35-10%, even for normal-tension glaucoma patients. At present the pathophysiological processes involved in glaucomatous optic nerve damage and the relationship to aqueous humor dynamics are not understood. Current pharmacotherapies are targeted at decreasing the production of aqueous humor at the ciliary body and increasing outflow through the trabecular meshwork and uveoscleral pathways. There is no consensus on the best IOP-lowering technique for glaucoma therapy.

A stepped medical approach depends on the patient's health, age, and ocular status, with knowledge of systemic effects and contraindications for all medications. A stepped medical approach may begin with a **topical**

prostaglandin (PG) analog. Due to their once-daily dosing, low incidence of systemic side effects, and potent IOP-lowering effect, PG analogs have largely replaced β adrenergic–receptor antagonists as first-line medical therapy for glaucoma. The PG analogs consist of latanoprost (XALATAN), travoprost (TRAVATAN, TRAVATAN Z), bimatoprost (LUMIGAN, LATISSE), and tafluprost (ZIOPTAN). $PGF_{2\alpha}$ reduces IOP but has intolerable local side effects. Modifications to the chemical structure of $PGF_{2\alpha}$ have produced analogs with a more acceptable side-effect profile. The mechanism by which this occurs is unclear. $PGF_{2\alpha}$ and its analogs (prodrugs that are hydrolyzed to $PGF_{2\alpha}$) bind to FP receptors that link to G_{q11} and then to the PLC–IP_3–Ca^{2+} pathway. This pathway is active in isolated human ciliary muscle cells. Other cells in the eye also may express FP receptors. Theories of IOP lowering by $PGF_{2\alpha}$ range from altered ciliary muscle tension to effects on trabecular meshwork cells to release of matrix metalloproteinases and digestion of extracellular matrix materials that may impede outflow tracts.

The **β receptor antagonists** now are the next most common topical medical treatment. Nonselective β blockers bind to both β_1 and β_2 receptors and include timolol, levobunolol, metipranolol, and carteolol. The β_1-selective antagonist, betaxolol, is available for ophthalmic use but is less efficacious than the nonselective β blockers because the β receptors of the eye are largely of the β_2 subtype. However, betaxolol is less likely to cause breathing difficulty due to blockade of pulmonary β_2 receptors. In the eye, the targeted tissues are the ciliary body epithelium and blood vessels, where β_2 receptors account for 75-90% of the total population. How β blockade leads to decreased aqueous production and reduced IOP is uncertain. Production of aqueous humor seems to be activated by a β receptor–mediated cyclic AMP–PKA pathway; β blockade blunts adrenergic activation of this pathway. Another hypothesis is that β blockers decrease ocular blood flow, which decreases the ultrafiltration responsible for aqueous production.

When there are medical contraindications to the use of PG analogs or β receptor antagonists, other agents, such as an ***α_2 adrenergic receptor agonist*** or topical ***carbonic anhydrase inhibitor*** **(CAI)**, may be used as first-line therapy. The α_2 adrenergic agonists appear to decrease IOP by reducing aqueous humor production and by enhancing both conventional (via an α_2 receptor mechanism) and uveoscleral outflow (perhaps via PG production) from the eye. Although effective, epinephrine is poorly tolerated, principally due to localized irritation and hyperemia. Dipivefrin is an epinephrine prodrug that is converted into epinephrine by esterases in the cornea; it is much better tolerated but is still prone to cause epinephrine-like side effects. The α_2 adrenergic agonist and clonidine derivative, apraclonidine (IOPIDINE), is a relatively selective α_2 adrenergic agonist that is highly ionized at physiological pH and does not cross the blood-brain barrier, and is thus relatively free of the CNS effects of clonidine. Brimonidine (ALPHAGAN, others) also is a selective α_2 adrenergic agonist but is lipophilic, enabling easy corneal penetration. Both apraclonidine and brimonidine reduce aqueous production and may enhance some uveoscleral outflow. Both appear to bind to pre- and postsynaptic α_2 receptors. By binding to the presynaptic receptors, the drugs reduce the amount of neurotransmitter release from sympathetic nerve stimulation and thereby lower IOP. By binding to postsynaptic α_2 receptors, these drugs stimulate the G_i pathway, reducing cellular cyclic AMP production, thereby reducing aqueous humor production.

The development of a **topical CAI** was prompted by the poor side-effect profile of oral CAIs. Dorzolamide (TRUSOPT, others) and brinzolamide (AZOPT) both work by inhibiting carbonic anhydrase (isoform II), which is found in the ciliary body epithelium. This reduces the formation of bicarbonate ions, which reduces fluid transport and, thus, IOP.

Any of these 4 drug classes can be used as additive second- or third-line therapy. In fact, the β receptor antagonist timolol has been combined with the CAI dorzolamide in a single medication (COSOPT, others) and with the α_2 adrenergic agonist brimonidine (COMBIGAN). Such combinations reduce the number of drops needed and may improve compliance.

Topical miotic agents are less commonly used today because of their numerous side effects and inconvenient dosing. Miotics lower IOP by causing muscarinic-induced contraction of the ciliary muscle, which facilitates aqueous outflow. They do not affect aqueous production. Pilocarpine and carbachol are cholinomimetics that stimulate muscarinic receptors. Echothiophate (PHOSPHOLINE IODIDE) is an organophosphate inhibitor of acetylcholinesterase; it is relatively stable in aqueous solution and, by virtue of its quaternary ammonium structure, is positively charged and poorly absorbed. If combined topical therapy fails to achieve the target IOP or fails to halt glaucomatous optic nerve damage, then **systemic therapy with CAI** is a final medication option before resorting to laser or incisional surgical treatment. The best-tolerated oral preparation is acetazolamide in sustained-release capsules (*see* Chapter 25), followed by methazolamide. The least well tolerated are acetazolamide tablets.

TOXICITY OF ANTI-GLAUCOMA AGENTS. Ciliary body spasm is a muscarinic cholinergic effect that can lead to induced myopia and a changing refraction due to iris and ciliary body contraction as the drug effect waxes and wanes between doses. Headaches can occur from the iris and ciliary body contraction. α_2 Agonists, effective in IOP reduction, can cause a vasoconstriction–vasodilation rebound phenomenon leading to a red eye. Ocular and skin allergies from topical epinephrine, related prodrug formulations, apraclonidine, and brimonidine are common. Brimonidine is less likely to cause ocular allergy and therefore is more commonly used. These agents can cause CNS depression and apnea in neonates and are contraindicated in children <2 years of age. Systemic absorption of α_2 agonists and β adrenergic antagonists can induce all the side effects of systemic administration. The use of CAIs systemically may give some patients significant problems with malaise, fatigue, depression, paresthesias, and nephrolithiasis; the topical CAIs may minimize these relatively common side effects.

Uveitis. Inflammation of the uvea, or uveitis, has both infectious and non-infectious causes, and medical treatment of the underlying cause (if known), in addition to the use of topical therapy, is essential. Cyclopentolate (CYCLOGYL, others), tropicamide (MYDRIACYL), or sometimes even longer-acting antimuscarinic agents such as atropine, scopolamine (ISOPTO HYOSCINE), and homatropine frequently are used to prevent posterior synechia formation between the lens and iris margin and to relieve ciliary muscle spasm that is responsible for much of the pain associated with anterior uveitis.

If posterior synechiae already have formed, an α adrenergic agonist may be used to break the synechiae by enhancing pupillary dilation. A solution of scopolamine 0.3% in combination with 10% phenylephrine (MUROCOLL-2) is available for this purpose. Two others, 1% hydroxyamphetamine hydrobromide combined with 0.25% tropicamide (PAREMYD) and 1% phenylephrine in combination with 0.2% cyclopentolate (CYCLOMYDRIL), are indicated only for induction of mydriasis. Topical steroids usually are adequate to decrease inflammation, but sometimes they must be supplemented with systemic steroids.

Strabismus. Strabismus, or ocular misalignment, has numerous causes and may occur at any age. Besides causing *diplopia* (double vision), strabismus in children may lead to *amblyopia* (reduced vision). Nonsurgical efforts to treat amblyopia include occlusion therapy, orthoptics, optical devices, and pharmacological agents.

An eye with *hyperopia*, or farsightedness, must constantly accommodate to focus on distant images. In some hyperopic children, the synkinetic accommodative-convergence response leads to excessive convergence and a manifest *esotropia* (turned-in eye). The brain rejects diplopia and suppresses the image from the deviated eye. If proper vision is not restored by ~7 years of age, the brain never learns to process visual information from that eye. The result is that the eye appears structurally normal but does not develop normal visual acuity and is therefore amblyopic. This is a fairly common cause of visual disability. In this setting, atropine (1%) instilled in the preferred seeing eye produces cycloplegia and the inability of this eye to accommodate, thus forcing the child to use the amblyopic eye. Echothiophate iodide also has been used in the setting of accommodative strabismus. Accommodation drives the near reflex, the triad of miosis, accommodation, and convergence. An irreversible cholinesterase inhibitor such as echothiophate causes miosis and an accommodative change in the shape of the lens; hence, the accommodative drive to initiate the near reflex is reduced, and less convergence will occur.

Surgery and Diagnostic Purposes. For certain surgical procedures and for clinical funduscopic examination, it is desirable to maximize the view of the retina and lens. Muscarinic cholinergic antagonists and sympathomimetic agents frequently are used singly or in combination for this purpose (*see* Table 64–7). Intraoperatively, there are circumstances in which miosis is preferred, and 2 cholinergic agonists are available for intraocular use, acetylcholine (MIOCHOL-E) and carbachol. Patients with myasthenia gravis may first present to an ophthalmologist with complaints of double vision (diplopia) or lid droop (ptosis); the *edrophonium test* is helpful in diagnosing these patients (*see* Chapter 10). For surgical visualization of the lens, trypan blue (VISIONBLUE) is marketed to facilitate visualization of the lens and for staining during surgical vitrectomy procedures to guide the excision of tissue (MEMBRANEBLUE).

ANTI-INFLAMMATORY, IMMUNOMODULATORY, AND ANTIMITOTIC DRUGS

GLUCOCORTICOIDS. Glucocorticoids have an important role in managing ocular inflammatory diseases; their chemistry and pharmacology are described in Chapter 42.

Therapeutic Uses. The glucocorticoids formulated for topical administration to the eye are dexamethasone (DEXASOL, others), prednisolone (PRED FORTE, others), fluorometholone (FML, others), loteprednol (ALREX, LOTEMAX), rimexolone (VEXOL), and difluprednate (DUREZOL). Because of their anti-inflammatory effects, topical corticosteroids are used in managing significant ocular allergy, anterior uveitis, external eye inflammatory diseases associated with some infections and ocular cicatricial pemphigoid, and postoperative inflammation following refractive, corneal, and intraocular surgery. After glaucoma filtering surgery, topical steroids can delay the wound-healing process by decreasing fibroblast infiltration, thereby reducing potential scarring of the surgical site. Steroids commonly are given systemically and by sub-Tenon's capsule injection to manage posterior uveitis. Intravitreal injection of steroids is used to treat age-related macular degeneration (ARMD), diabetic retinopathy, and cystoid macular edema. Two intravitreal triamcinolone formulations, TRIVARIS and TRIESENCE, are approved for ocular inflammatory conditions unresponsive to topical corticosteroids and visualization during vitrectomy, respectively. Parenteral steroids followed by tapering oral doses is the preferred treatment for optic neuritis. An ophthalmic implant of fluocinolone (RETISERT) is marketed for the treatment of chronic, non-infectious uveitis.

Toxicity of Steroids. Ocular complications include the development of posterior subcapsular cataracts, secondary infections, and secondary open-angle glaucoma. There is a significant increase in the risk for developing secondary glaucoma when there is a positive family history of glaucoma. In the absence of a family history of open-angle glaucoma, only ~5% of normal individuals respond to topical or long-term systemic steroids with a marked increase in IOP. With a positive family history, however, moderate to marked steroid-induced IOP elevations may occur in up to 90% of patients. Newer topical steroids, so-called "soft steroids" (e.g., loteprednol), have been developed that reduce, but do not eliminate, the risk of elevated IOP.

NONSTEROIDAL ANTI-INFLAMMATORY AGENTS. Pharmacological properties of nonsteroidal anti-inflammatory drugs (NSAIDs) are presented in Chapter 34.

Therapeutic Uses. Five topical NSAIDs approved for ocular use: flurbiprofen (OCUFEN, others), ketorolac (ACULAR, others), diclofenac (VOLTAREN, others), bromfenac (XIBROM), and nepafenac (NEVANAC). Flurbiprofen is used to counter unwanted intraoperative miosis during cataract surgery. Ketorolac is given for seasonal allergic conjunctivitis. Diclofenac is used for postoperative inflammation. Both ketorolac and diclofenac are effective in treating cystoid macular edema occurring after cataract surgery and in controlling pain after corneal refractive surgery. Bromfenac and nepafenac are indicated for treating postoperative pain and inflammation after cataract surgery. Topical and systemic NSAIDs occasionally have been associated with sterile corneal melts and perforations, especially in older patients with ocular surface disease, such as dry eye syndrome.

ANTIHISTAMINES AND MAST-CELL STABILIZERS

Pheniramine (*see* Chapter 32) and antazoline, both H_1 receptor antagonists, are formulated in combination with naphazoline, a vasoconstrictor, for relief of allergic conjunctivitis; emedastine difumarate (EMADINE) also is used. Cromolyn sodium (CROLOM, others) has found limited use in treating conjunctivitis that is thought to be allergen mediated, such as vernal conjunctivitis. Lodoxamide tromethamine (ALOMIDE) and pemirolast (ALAMAST), mast-cell stabilizers, also are available for ophthalmic use. Nedocromil (ALOCRIL) also is primarily a mast-cell stabilizer with some antihistamine properties. Olopatadine hydrochloride (PATANOL, PATADAY), ketotifen fumarate (ZADITOR, ALAWAY), bepotastine (BEPREVE), and azelastine (OPTIVAR) are H_1 antagonists with mast cell–stabilizing properties. Epinastine (ELESTAT) antagonizes H_1 and H_2 receptors and exhibits mast cell–stabilizing activity.

IMMUNOSUPPRESSANTS

Topical ***cyclosporine*** (cyclosporin A; RESTASIS) is approved for the treatment of chronic dry eye associated with inflammation. Use of cyclosporine is associated with decreased inflammatory markers in the lacrimal gland, increased tear production, and improved vision and comfort. ***Interferon α-2b*** is used in the treatment of conjunctival papilloma and certain conjunctival tumors.

ANTIMITOTIC AGENTS. In glaucoma surgery, the anti-neoplastic agents fluorouracil and mitomycin (MUTAMYCIN) (*see* Chapter 61) improve the success of filtration surgery by limiting the postoperative wound-healing process.

Therapeutic Uses. Mitomycin is used intraoperatively as a single subconjunctival application at the trabeculectomy site. Fluorouracil may be used intraoperatively at the trabeculectomy site and/or subconjunctivally during the postoperative course. Both agents work by limiting the healing process; sometimes this can result in thin, ischemic, avascular tissue that is prone to breakdown. The resultant leaks can cause hypotony (low IOP) and increase the risk of infection. In corneal surgery, mitomycin has been used topically. Mitomycin can be used to reduce the risk of scarring after procedures to remove corneal opacities and prophylactically to prevent corneal scarring after photorefractive and phototherapeutic keratectomy. Mitomycin also is used to treat certain conjunctival and corneal tumors. Caution is advocated when using mitomycin in light of the potentially serious delayed ocular complications.

Intraocular methotrexate (*see* Chapter 61) is used to treat uveitis and uveitic cystoid macular edema. It also has been used to treat the uncommon complication of lymphoma in the vitreous, an inaccessible compartment for most anti-neoplastic drugs.

AGENTS USED IN OPHTHALMIC SURGERY

Presurgical Antiseptics. Povidone iodine (BETADINE) is formulated as a 5% sterile ophthalmic solution for use prior to surgery to prep periocular skin and irrigate ocular surfaces, including the cornea, conjunctiva, and palpebral fornices. Following irrigation, the exposed tissues are flushed with sterile saline. Hypersensitivity to iodine is a contraindication.

Viscoelastic Substances. Such agents assist in ocular surgery by maintaining spaces, moving tissue, and protecting surfaces. These substances are prepared from hyaluronate (HEALON, others), chondroitin sulfate (VISCOAT), or hydroxypropylmethylcellulose and share the following important physical characteristics: viscosity, shear flow, elasticity, cohesiveness, and coatability. Complications associated with viscoelastic substances are related to transient elevation of IOP after surgery.

Ophthalmic Glue. Cyanoacrylate tissue adhesive (ISODONT, DERMABOND, HISTOACRYL), while not FDA-approved for the eye, is widely used in the management of corneal ulcerations and perforations. Fibrinogen glue (TISSEEL, EVICEL) is increasingly being used on the ocular surface to secure tissue such as conjunctiva, amniotic membrane, and lamellar corneal grafts.

Anterior Segment Gases. Sulfur hexafluoride (SF_6) and perfluoropropane gases are used as vitreous substitutes during retinal surgery. They are used in non-expansile concentrations to treat Descemet's detachments, typically after cataract surgery. These detachments can cause mild to severe corneal edema. The gas is injected into the anterior chamber to push Descemet's membrane up against the stroma, where ideally it reattaches and clears the corneal edema.

Vitreous Substitutes (Table 64–8). Several compounds, including gases, perfluorocarbon liquids, and silicone oils are available. Their primary use is reattachment of the retina following vitrectomy and membrane-peeling procedures for complicated proliferative vitreoretinopathy and traction retinal detachments. The use of expansile gases carries the risk of complications from elevated IOP, subretinal gas, corneal edema, and cataract formation. The gases are absorbed over a period of days (for air) to 2 months (for perfluoropropane).

The liquid perfluorocarbons (specific gravity, 1.76-1.94) are denser than vitreous and are helpful in flattening the retina when vitreous is present. Silicone oil (polydimethylsiloxanes; ADATOSIL 5000) is used for long-term tamponade of the retina. Complications from silicone oil use include glaucoma, cataract formation, corneal edema, corneal band keratopathy, and retinal toxicity.

Surgical Hemostasis and Thrombolytic Agents. Hemostasis has an important role in most surgical procedures and usually is achieved by temperature-mediated coagulation. Intravitreal administration of thrombin can assist in controlling intraocular hemorrhage during vitrectomy. When used intraocularly, a potentially significant inflammatory response may occur that can be minimized by thorough irrigation after hemostasis is achieved.

Recombinant tissue plasminogen activator (t-PA; alteplase) (*see* Chapter 30) has been used during intraocular surgeries to assist evacuation of a hyphema, subretinal clot, or nonclearing vitreous hemorrhage. Alteplase also has been administered subconjunctivally and intracamerally (i.e., controlled intraocular administration into the anterior segment) to lyse blood clots obstructing a glaucoma filtration site. The main complication related to the use of t-PA is bleeding.

Table 64–8
Vitreous Substitutes

AGENT	DURATION OR VISCOSITY
Nonexpansile gases	
Air	For Air: Duration, 5-7 days
Ar, CO_2, He, Kr, N_2, O_2	
Xe	For Xe: Duration, 1 day
Expansile gases	
Sulfur hexafluoride (SF_6)	Duration of 10-14 days
Octafluorocyclobutane (C_4F_8)	
Perfluoromethane (CF_4)	Duration of 10-14 days
Perfluoroethane (C_2F_6)	Duration of 30-35 days
Perfluoropropane (C_3F_8)	Duration of 55-65 days
Perfluoro-*n*-butane (C_4F_{10})	
Perfluoropentane (C_5F_{12})	
Silicone oils	
Nonfluorinated silicone oils	Viscosity range from 1000-30,000 cs
Fluorosilicone	Viscosity range from 1000-10,000 cs
"High-tech" silicone oils	May terminate as trimethylsiloxy or polyphenylmethylsiloxane; viscosity not reported

cs, centistoke (unit of viscosity).

Botulinum Toxin Type A in the Treatment of Strabismus, Blepharospasm, and Related Disorders. Botulinum toxin type A is FDA-approved for the treatment of strabismus and blepharospasm associated with dystonia, facial wrinkles (glabellar lines), axillary hyperhidrosis, and spasmodic torticollis (cervical dystonia). Two botulinum toxin type A preparations are marketed in the U.S.: onabotulinumtoxin A (BOTOX, BOTOX COSMETIC) and abobotulinumtoxinA (DYSPORT). By preventing acetylcholine release at the neuromuscular junction, botulinum toxin A usually causes a temporary paralysis of the locally injected muscles. Complications related to this toxin include double vision (diplopia) and lid droop (ptosis) and, rarely, potentially life-threatening distant spread of toxin effect from the injection site (hours to weeks after administration).

Agents Used to Treat Blind and Painful Eye. Retrobulbar injection of either absolute or 95% ethanol may provide relief from chronic pain associated with a blind and painful eye. Retrobulbar chlorpromazine also has been used. This treatment is preceded by administration of local anesthesia. Local infiltration of the ciliary nerves provides symptomatic relief from pain, but other nerve fibers may be damaged, causing paralysis of the extraocular muscles, including those in the eyelids, or neuroparalytic keratitis. The sensory fibers of the ciliary nerves may regenerate, and repeated injections sometimes are needed to control pain.

OCULAR SIDE EFFECTS OF SYSTEMIC AGENTS

Certain systemic drugs have ocular side effects. These can range from mild and inconsequential to severe and vision threatening. Examples are listed in the following sections.

Glaucoma. The anti-seizure drug topiramate (TOPAMAX, others) reportedly causes choroidal effusions leading to angle-closure glaucoma.

Retina. Numerous drugs have toxic side effects on the retina. The anti-arthritis and antimalarial medicines hydroxychloroquine (PLAQUENIL, others) and chloroquine can cause a central retinal toxicity by an unknown mechanism. With normal dosages, toxicity does not appear until ~6 years after the drug is started. Stopping the drug will not reverse the damage but will prevent further toxicity. Tamoxifen can cause a crystalline maculopathy. The antiseizure drug vigabatrin (SABRIL) causes progressive and permanent bilateral concentric visual field constriction in a high percentage of patients.

Optic Nerve. The PDE5 inhibitors, sildenafil (VIAGRA, REVATIO), vardenafil (LEVITRA), and tadalafil (CIALIS, ADCIRCA), inhibit PDE5 in the corpus cavernosum to help achieve and maintain penile erection. The drugs also mildly inhibit PDE6, which controls the levels of cyclic GMP in the retina, causing a bluish haze or light sensitivity. Multiple medications can cause a toxic optic neuropathy characterized by gradually progressive bilateral central scotomas and vision loss, including ethambutol, chloramphenicol, and rifampin. Systemic or ocular steroids can cause elevated IOP and glaucoma. If the steroids cannot be stopped, glaucoma medications, and even filtering surgery, often are required.

Anterior Segment. Steroids have been implicated in cataract formation. Rifabutin, if used in conjunction with clarithromycin or fluconazole for treatment of *Mycobacterium avium* complex (MAC) opportunistic infections in human immunodeficiency virus (HIV)-positive persons, is associated with an iridocyclitis and even hypopyon. This will resolve with steroids or by stopping the medication.

Ocular Surface. Isotretinoin (ACCUTANE, others) has a drying effect on mucous membranes and is associated with dry eye and meibomian gland dysfunction.

Cornea Coryanghiva and Eyelids. The cornea, conjunctiva, and eyelids can be affected by systemic medications. One of the most common drug deposits found in the cornea is from the cardiac medication amiodarone. It deposits in the inferior and central cornea in a whorl-like pattern termed *cornea verticillata*, appearing as fine tan or brown pigment in the epithelium. The deposits seldom affect vision and are rarely a cause to discontinue the medication. The deposits disappear slowly when the medication is stopped. Other medications, including indomethacin, atovaquone, chloroquine, and hydroxychloroquine, can cause a similar pattern. The phenothiazines, including chlorpromazine and thioridazine, can cause brown pigmentary deposits in the cornea, conjunctiva, and eyelids. They typically do not affect vision. The ocular deposits generally persist after discontinuation of the medication and can even worsen. Tetracyclines can cause a yellow discoloration of the light-exposed conjunctiva. Systemic minocycline can induce a blue-gray scleral pigmentation that is most prominent in the interpalpebral zone.

AGENTS USED TO ASSIST IN OCULAR DIAGNOSIS

A number of agents are used in an ocular examination (e.g., mydriatic agents, topical anesthetics, dyes to evaluate corneal surface integrity), to facilitate intraocular surgery (e.g., mydriatic and miotic agents, topical and local anesthetics), and to help in making a diagnosis in cases of anisocoria and retinal abnormalities (e.g., intravenous contrast agents). The autonomic agents have been discussed earlier. The diagnostic and therapeutic uses of topical and intravenous dyes and of topical anesthetics are discussed below.

Anterior Segment and External Diagnostic Uses. Epiphora (excessive tearing) and surface problems of the cornea and conjunctiva are commonly encountered external ocular disorders. The dyes fluorescein, rose bengal, and lissamine green are used in evaluating these problems. ***Fluorescein*** (available as a 2% alkaline solution, 10% and 25% solutions for injection, and an impregnated paper strip) reveals epithelial defects of the cornea and conjunctiva and aqueous humor leakage that may occur after trauma or ocular surgery. In the setting of epiphora, fluorescein is used to determine the patency of the nasolacrimal system. In addition, this dye is used in *applanation tonometry* (IOP measurement) and to assist in determining the proper fit of rigid and semirigid contact lenses. Fluorescein in combination with proparacaine or benoxinate is available for procedures in which a disclosing agent is needed in conjunction with a topical anesthetic. Fluorexon (FLUORESOFT), a high-molecular-weight fluorescent solution, is used when fluorescein is contraindicated (as when soft contact lenses are in place). ***Rose bengal*** and ***lissamine green*** (available as saturated paper strips) stain devitalized tissue on the cornea and conjunctiva.

Posterior Segment Diagnostic Uses. The integrity of the blood-retinal and retinal pigment epithelial barriers may be examined directly by retinal angiography using intravenous administration of either ***fluorescein sodium*** or ***indocyanine green***. These agents commonly cause nausea and may precipitate serious allergic reactions in susceptible individuals.

TREATMENT OF RETINAL NEOVASCULARIZATION AND MACULAR DEGENERATION

Verteporfin (VISUDYNE) is approved for photodynamic therapy of the exudative form of ARMD with predominantly classic choroidal neovascular membranes. Verteporfin also is used in the treatment of predominantly classic choroidal neovascularization caused by conditions such as pathological myopia and presumed ocular histoplasmosis syndrome. Verteporfin is administered intravenously; once it reaches the choroidal circulation, the drug is light activated by a nonthermal laser source. Activation of the drug in the presence of oxygen generates free radicals, which cause vessel damage and subsequent platelet activation, thrombosis, and occlusion of choroidal neovascularization. The $t_{1/2}$ of the drug is 5-6 h; it is eliminated predominantly in the feces. Potential side effects include headache, injection-site reactions, and visual disturbances. The drug causes temporary photosensitization; patients must avoid exposure of the skin or eyes to direct sunlight or bright indoor lights for 5 days after receiving it.

Pegaptanib (MACUGEN), a selective vascular endothelial growth factor (VEGF) antagonist, is approved for neovascular (wet) ARMD. $VEGF_{165}$ induces angiogenesis and increases vascular permeability and inflammation, which actions likely contribute to the progression of the neovascular (wet) form of ARMD, a leading cause of blindness. Pegaptanib inhibits $VEGF_{165}$ binding to VEGF receptors. Pegaptanib (0.3 mg) is administered once every 6 weeks by intravitreous injection into the eye to be treated. Following the injection, patients should be monitored for elevation in IOP and for endophthalmitis. Rare cases of anaphylaxis/anaphylactoid reactions have been reported.

Eylea (AFLIBERCEPT) is a recombinant fusion protein, consisting of portions of human VEGF receptors 1 and 2, that acts as a soluble decoy receptor for VEGF-A. It is approved for neovascular (wet) form of ARMD. Aflibercept (2 mg) is administered once every 4 weeks by intravitreous injection into the eye for 12 weeks followed by 2 mg once every 8 weeks. Serious side effect may include eye pain or redness, swelling, vision problems, photosensitivity, headaches, sudden numbness on one side of the body, confusion, and problems with speech and balance. The drug is contraindicated in patients who have an active eye inflection active ocular inflammation.

Bevacizumab (AVASTIN) is a monoclonal murine antibody that targets VEGF-A and thereby inhibits vascular proliferation and tumor growth (*see* Chapter 62).

Ranibizumab (LUCENTIS) is a variant of bevacizumab that has had the Fab domain affinity matured. Both drugs are delivered by intravitreal injection and often are used on a weekly or monthly basis for maintenance therapy. Both have been associated with the risk of cerebral vascular accidents.

ANESTHETICS IN OPHTHALMIC PROCEDURES

Topical anesthetic agents used clinically in ophthalmology include proparacaine and tetracaine drops, lidocaine gel (*see* Chapter 20), and intranasal cocaine.

Cocaine may be used intranasally in combination with topical anesthesia for cannulating the nasolacrimal system. Lidocaine and bupivacaine are used for infiltration and retrobulbar block anesthesia for surgery. Potential complications and risks relate to allergic reactions, globe perforation, hemorrhage, and vascular and subdural injections. Both preservative-free lidocaine (1%), which is introduced into the anterior chamber, and lidocaine jelly (2%), which is placed on the ocular surface during preoperative patient preparation, are used for cataract surgery performed under topical anesthesia. Most inhalational agents and CNS depressants are associated

Table 64–9

Ophthalmic Effects of Selected Vitamin Deficiencies and Zinc Deficiency

DEFICIENCY	EFFECTS IN ANTERIOR SEGMENT	EFFECTS IN POSTERIOR SEGMENT
Vitamin		
A (retinol)	Conjunctiva (Bitot's spots, xerosis) Cornea (keratomalacia, punctate keratopathy)	Retina (nyctalopia, impaired rhodopsin synthesis), retinal pigment epithelium (hypopigmentation)
B_1 (thiamine)	-----	Optic nerve (temporal atrophy with corresponding visual field defects)
B_6 (pyridoxine)	Cornea (neovascularization)	Retina (gyrate atrophy)
B_{12} (cyanocobalamin)	-----	Optic nerve (temporal atrophy with corresponding visual field defects)
C (ascorbic acid)	Lens (?cataract formation)	-----
E (tocopherol)	-----	Retina and retinal pigment epithelium (?macular degeneration)
Folic acid	-----	Vein occlusion
K	Conjunctiva (hemorrhage) Anterior chamber (hyphema)	Retina (hemorrhage)
Zinc	-----	Retina and retinal pigment epithelium (?macular degeneration)

with a reduction in IOP. An exception is ketamine, which has been associated with an elevation in IOP. In the setting of a patient with a ruptured globe, the anesthesia should be selected carefully to avoid agents that depolarize the extraocular muscles, which may result in expulsion of intraocular contents.

VITAMIN A

Vitamin deficiencies can alter eye function, especially a deficiency of vitamin A (Table 64–9). In vision, the functional form of vitamin A is *retinal*; its deficiency interferes with vision in dim light, contributing to a condition known as *night blindness* (nyctalopia).

Chemistry and Terminology. *Retinoid* refers to the chemical entity *retinol* and other closely related naturally occurring derivatives. Retinoids, which exert most of their effects by binding to specific nuclear receptors and modulating gene expression, also include structurally related synthetic analogs that need not have retinol-like (vitamin A) activity. The purified plant pigment carotene (provitamin A) is a protean source of vitamin A. β-Carotene is the most active carotenoid found in plants. The structural formulas for β-carotene and the vitamin A family of retinoids are shown in Figure 64–6. Retinoic acid analogs used clinically are discussed in detail in Chapter 65.

RETINAL AND THE VISUAL CYCLE

Photoreception is accomplished by 2 types of specialized retinal cells, termed *rods* and *cones*. Rods are especially sensitive to light of low intensity; cones act as receptors of high-intensity light and are responsible for color vision. The chromophore of both rods and cones is 11-*cis*-retinal. The holoreceptor in rods is termed *rhodopsin*—a combination of the protein opsin and 11-*cis*-retinal attached as a prosthetic group. The 3 different types of cone cells (red, green, and blue) contain individual, related photoreceptor proteins and respond optimally to light of different wavelengths. Figure 64–7 summarizes the signaling pathway initiated by absorption of a photon by 11-*cis*-retinal in rods.

VITAMIN A DEFICIENCY AND VISION. Humans deficient in vitamin A lose their ability for dark adaptation. Rod vision is affected more than cone vision. Upon depletion of retinol from liver and blood, usually at plasma concentrations of retinol of <0.2 mg/L (0.70 μM), the concentrations of retinol and rhodopsin in the retina

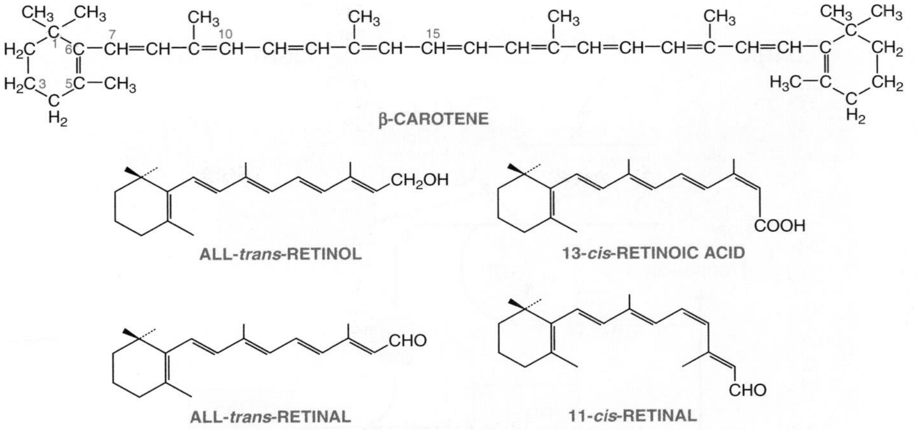

Figure 64–6 *β-carotene and some members of the vitamin A family of retinoids.*

fall. Unless the deficiency is overcome, opsin, lacking the stabilizing effect of retinal, decays, and anatomical deterioration of the rod outer segment occurs.

Vitamin A and Epithelial Structures. In the presence of retinol or retinoic acid, basal epithelial cells are stimulated to produce mucus. Excessive concentrations of the retinoids lead to the production of a thick layer of mucin, the inhibition of keratinization, and the display of goblet cells. In the absence of vitamin A, goblet mucous cells disappear and are replaced by basal cells that have been stimulated to proliferate. These undermine and replace the original epithelium with a stratified, keratinizing epithelium. The suppression of normal secretions leads to irritation and infection. Reversal of these changes is achieved by the administration of retinol, retinoic acid, or other retinoids. When this process happens in the cornea, severe hyperkeratinization (xerophthalmia) may lead to permanent blindness. Common causes of vitamin A deficiency include malnutrition and bariatric surgery.

Retinoic acid influences gene expression by combining with nuclear receptors (*see* Figures 3–12 and 6–8). There are 2 families of retinoid receptors: the retinoic acid receptors (RARs), and the retinoid X receptors (RXRs). The endogenous RXR ligand is 9-*cis*-retinoic acid.

Therapeutic Uses. Nutritional vitamin A deficiency causes *xerophthalmia*, a progressive disease characterized by *nyctalopia* (night blindness), *xerosis* (dryness), and *keratomalacia* (corneal thinning), which may lead to corneal perforation. Vitamin A therapy can reverse xerophthalmia; however, rapid, irreversible blindness ensues once the cornea perforates. Vitamin A also is involved in epithelial differentiation and may have a role in corneal epithelial wound healing. The current recommendation for retinitis pigmentosa is to administer 15,000 IU of vitamin A palmitate daily under the supervision of an ophthalmologist and to avoid high-dose vitamin E. Clinical studies suggest a reduction in the risk of progression of some types of ARMD by high doses of vitamins C (500 mg), E (400 IU), β-carotene (15 mg), cupric oxide (2 mg), and zinc (80 mg).

WETTING AGENTS AND TEAR SUBSTITUTES

The current management of dry eyes usually includes instilling artificial tears and ophthalmic lubricants. In general, tear substitutes are hypotonic or isotonic solutions composed of electrolytes, surfactants, preservatives, and some viscosity-increasing agent that prolongs the residence time in the cul-de-sac and precorneal tear film.

Common viscosity agents include cellulose polymers, polyvinyl alcohol, polyethylene glycol, polysorbate, mineral oil, glycerin, and dextran. The tear substitutes are available as preservative-containing or preservative-free preparations. The viscosity of the tear substitute depends on its exact formulation and can range from watery to gel like. Some tear formulations also are combined with a vasoconstrictor, such as naphazoline, phenylephrine, or tetrahydrozoline. ***Tyloxapol*** (ENUCLENE) is marketed as an over-the-counter ophthalmic preparation used to facilitate the wearing comfort of artificial eyes. The lubricating ointments are composed of a mixture of white petrolatum, mineral oil, liquid or alcohol lanolin, and sometimes a preservative. These highly viscous formulations cause considerable blurring of vision, and consequently, they are used primarily

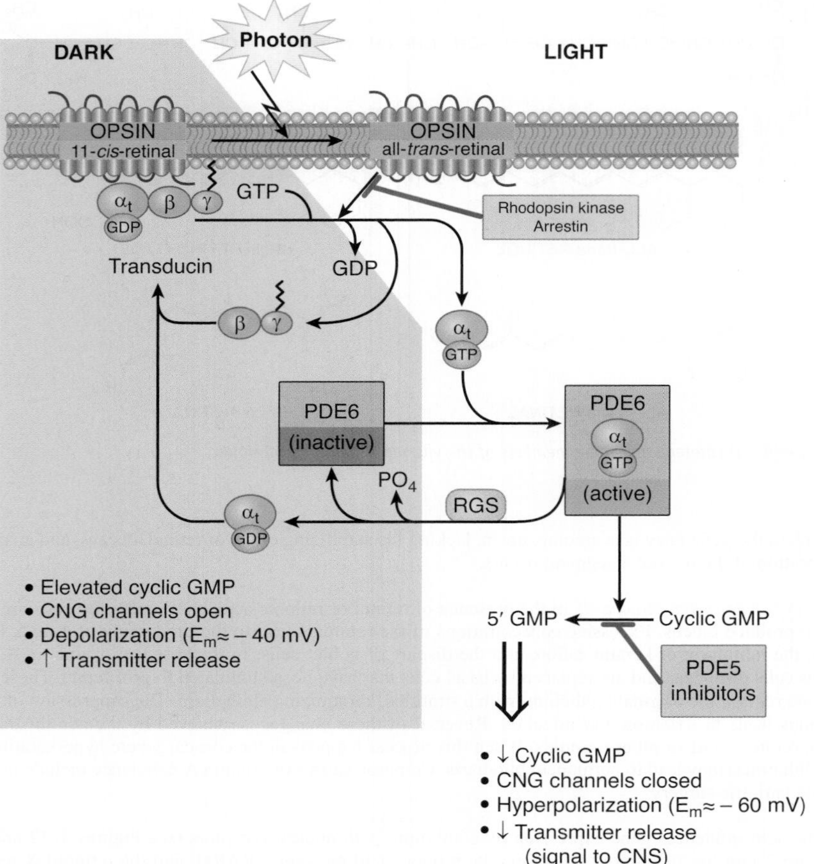

Figure 64–7 *A pharmacologist's view of photoreceptor signaling.* The system is an example of GPCR signaling. The basal state (DARK) is represented by the shaded area to the left. The signal, a photon, activates the receptor, rhodopsin, resulting in the isomerization of 11-*cis*-retinal to all-*trans*-retinal and initiating the LIGHT reactions (on the right side of the figure). The main characteristics of the DARK and LIGHT states are summarized in the boxes at the bottom of each section. The guanylyl cyclase activity is constitutively active and enhanced by Ca^{2+}. Mostly Na^+ and some Ca^{2+} enter via the CNG channels, contributing to depolarization. The Na^+/Ca^{2+} exchanger (NCX), Na^+/K^+ ATPase, and K^+ currents are active and contribute to hyperpolarization. PDE5 inhibitors such as sildenafil also inhibit PDE6, causing a bluish cast to vision. α_t, the α subunit of transducin; CNG, cyclic nucleotide gated.

at bedtime, in critically ill patients, or in very severe dry eye conditions. A hydroxypropyl cellulose ophthalmic insert (LACRISERT) that is placed in the inferior cul-de-sac and dissolves during the day is available to treat dry eyes.

Therapeutic Uses. Local eye disease, such as blepharitis, ocular rosacea, ocular pemphigoid, chemical burns, or corneal dystrophies, may alter the ocular surface and change the tear composition. Appropriate treatment of the symptomatic dry eye includes treating the accompanying disease and possibly the addition of tear substitutes, punctal plugs (see "Absorption"), or ophthalmic cyclosporine (see "Immunosuppressants"). There also are a number of systemic conditions that may manifest themselves with symptomatic dry eyes, including Sjögren syndrome, rheumatoid arthritis, vitamin A deficiency, Stevens-Johnson syndrome, and trachoma. Treating the systemic disease may not eliminate the symptomatic dry eye complaints; chronic therapy with tear substitutes, ophthalmic cyclosporine, insertion of punctal plugs, placement of dissolvable collagen implants, or surgical occlusion of the lacrimal drainage system may be indicated. Ophthalmic cyclosporine (RESTASIS) can be used to increase tear production in patients with ocular inflammation associated with keratoconjunctivitis sicca.

OSMOTIC AGENTS

The main osmotic drugs for ocular use are glycerin, mannitol, and hypertonic saline. Glycerin and mannitol are used for short-term management of acute rises in IOP. Sporadically, these agents are used intraoperatively to dehydrate the vitreous prior to anterior segment surgical procedures. Many patients with acute glaucoma do not tolerate oral medications because of nausea; therefore, intravenous administration of mannitol and/or acetazolamide may be preferred over oral administration of glycerin. These agents should be used with caution in patients with congestive heart failure or renal failure.

Corneal edema is a clinical sign of corneal endothelial dysfunction, and topical osmotic agents may effectively dehydrate the cornea. Sodium chloride is available in either aqueous or ointment formulations. Topical glycerin also is available; however, because it causes pain on contact with the cornea and conjunctiva, its use is limited to urgent evaluation of filtration-angle structures. In general, when corneal edema occurs secondary to acute glaucoma, the use of an oral osmotic agent to help reduce IOP is preferred over topical glycerin, which simply clears the cornea temporarily. Reducing the IOP will help clear the cornea more permanently to allow both a view of the filtration angle by gonioscopy and a clear view of the iris as required to perform laser iridotomy.

For a complete Bibliographical Listing see Goodman & Gilman's ***The Pharmacological Basis of Therapeutics***, 12th ed., or Goodman & Gilman Online at www.AccessMedicine.com.

Dermatological Pharmacology

The skin is a multifunctional and multicompartment organ. Figure 65–1 outlines general features of skin structure and percutaneous absorption pathways. Drugs can be applied to skin for 2 purposes: to directly treat disorders of the skin and to deliver drugs to other tissues.

Non-pharmacological therapy for skin diseases includes the entire electromagnetic spectrum applied by many sources, such as lasers, X-rays, visible light, and infrared light. These approaches may be used alone or to enhance the penetration or alter the nature of drugs and prodrugs. Freezing and ultrasound are other physical therapies that alter epidermal structure for direct treatment or to enhance percutaneous absorption of drugs. Chemicals are used to decrease the effect of various wavelengths of ultraviolet (UV) light and ionizing radiation.

Stratum Corneum. The stratum corneum (outer 5-600 μm) is the major barrier to percutaneous absorption of drugs and to the loss of water from the body. Many drugs may partition into the stratum corneum and form a reservoir that will diffuse into the rest of skin even *after* topical application of the drug has ceased. The stratum corneum differs in thickness, with the palm and sole being the thickest (400-600 μm) followed by the general body stratum corneum (10-16 μm), and the scrotum (5 μm). Facial and post-auricular regions have the thinnest stratum corneum.

Living Epidermis. The living layers of the epidermis with metabolically active cells comprise a layer ~100 μm thick (Figure 65–2). Intercalated in the living epidermis are pigment-producing cells (melanocytes), dendritic antigen-presenting cells (Langerhans cells), and other immune cells (γ-δ T-cells); in diseased epidermis, many immunological cells, including lymphocytes and polymorphonuclear leucocytes, may be present and be directly affected by applied drugs.

Dermis and Its Blood Vessels. The superficial capillary plexus between the epidermis and dermis is the site of the majority of the systemic absorption of cutaneous drugs (*see* Figure 65–1). There are large numbers of lymphatics as well. Beneath the 1.2-mm-thick dermis with its collagen and proteoglycans that may bind drugs there, targets for drugs include mast cells (permanent residents and producers of many inflammatory mediators) and infiltrating immune cells producing cytokines. Hair follicles form a lipid-rich pathway for drug absorption. Sweat glands are not known as a pathway for the absorption of drugs. Some drugs (e.g., griseofulvin, ketoconazole) are excreted to the skin by this route.

MECHANISMS OF PERCUTANEOUS ABSORPTION. Passage through the outermost layer is the rate-limiting step for percutaneous absorption. Preferable characteristics of topical drugs include low molecular mass (≤600 Da), adequate solubility in both oil and water, and a high partition coefficient so the drug will selectively partition from the vehicle to the stratum corneum. Except for very small particles, water-soluble ions and polar molecules do not penetrate significantly through intact stratum corneum. The exact amount of drug entering or leaving the skin in clinical situations usually is not measured; rather, the clinical endpoint (e.g., reduction in inflammation) usually is the desired effect.

A hydrated stratum corneum allows more percutaneous absorption and often is achieved through the selection of drugs formulated in occlusion vehicles such as ointments and the use of plastic films, wraps, or bags for the hands and feet and shower or bathing caps for the scalp, or through the use of medications that are impregnated on patches or tapes. Occlusion may be associated with increased growth of bacteria with resultant infection (folliculitis) or maceration and breakdown of the epidermis. Transport of most drugs is a passive thermodynamic process, and heat generally increases penetration. Ultrasonic energy or laser-induced vibration also can be used to increase percutaneous absorption. The latter may function by the production of lacunae in the stratum corneum.

The epidermis contains a variety of enzyme systems capable of metabolizing drugs that reach this compartment. A specific CYP isoform, CYP26A1, metabolizes retinoic acid and may control its level in the skin. In addition, transporter proteins that influence influx (OATP) or efflux (MDR, P-glycoprotein) of certain xenobiotics are present in human keratinocytes. Genetic variants of enzymes that regulate the cellular influx and efflux of methotrexate have been associated with toxicity and effectiveness in patients with psoriasis.

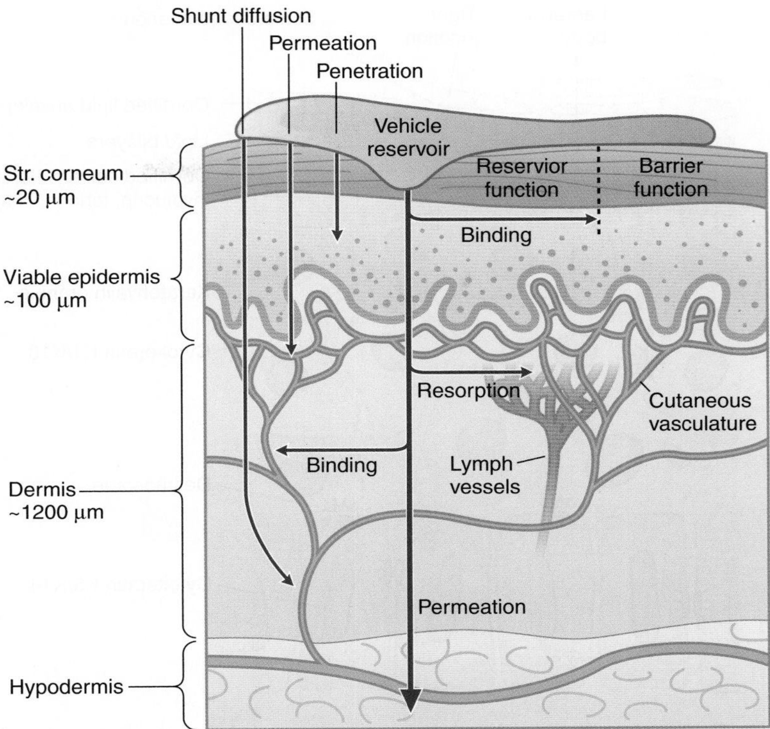

Figure 65–1 *Cutaneous drug delivery.* Diagrammatic representation of the 3 compartments of the skin as they relate to drug delivery: surface, stratum (Str.), and viable tissues. After application of a drug to the surface, evaporation and structural/compositional alterations occur that determine the drug's bioavailability. The stratum corneum limits diffusion of compounds into the viable skin and body. After absorption, compounds either bind targets in viable tissues or diffuse within the viable tissue or into the cutaneous vasculature, and thence to internal cells and organs. (Reproduced with permission from Wolff K, et al., eds. *Fitzpatrick's Dermatology in General Medicine*, 7th ed. New York: McGraw-Hill; 2008, Figure 215–1. Copyright © 2008 by The McGraw-Hill Companies, Inc. All rights reserved.)

PHARMACOLOGIC IMPLICATIONS OF EPIDERMAL STRUCTURE. The healthcare provider, when proposing topical application of drugs (Table 65–1), must consider proper dosage and frequency of application, extent and condition of the permeability barrier, patient age and weight, physical form of the preparation to be applied, and whether intralesional or systemic administration should be used. Various drug vehicles have specific advantages and disadvantages (Table 65–2). Newer vehicles include liposomes and microgel formulations that can enhance solubilization of certain drugs, thereby enhancing topical penetration and diminishing irritancy. *Children have a greater ratio of surface area to mass than adults do, so the same amount of topical drug can result in a greater systemic exposure.*

GLUCOCORTICOIDS

Glucocorticoids have immunosuppressive and anti-inflammatory properties. They are administered locally, through topical and intralesional routes, and systemically, through intramuscular, intravenous, and oral routes. Mechanisms of glucocorticoid action are discussed in Chapter 42.

TOPICAL GLUCOCORTICOIDS. Topical glucocorticoids have been grouped into 7 classes in order of decreasing potency (Table 65–3).

Therapeutic Uses. Many inflammatory skin diseases respond to topical or intralesional administration of glucocorticoids. Absorption varies among body areas; the steroid is selected on the basis of its potency, the site of involvement, and the severity of the skin disease. Often, a more potent steroid is used initially, followed by a less potent agent. Twice-daily application of topical glucocorticoids is sufficient, and more frequent application does not improve response. In general, only nonfluorinated glucocorticoids should be used on the face or

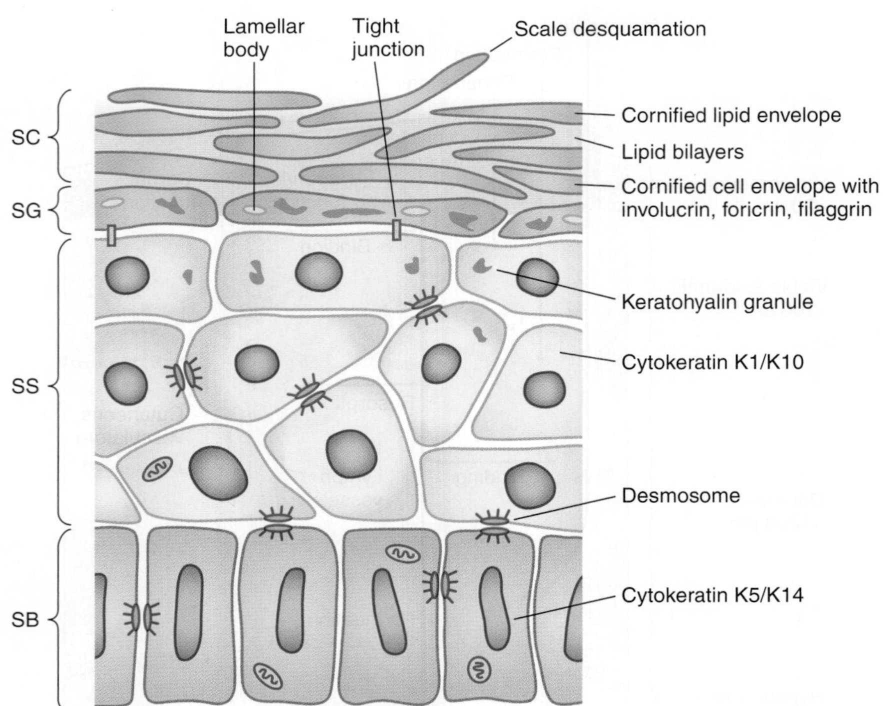

Figure 65–2 *Structure of the epidermis.* The epidermis matures progressively from the stratum basale (SB) to the stratum spinosum (SS), stratum granulosum (SG), and stratum corneum (SC). Important structural and metabolic proteins are produced at specific layers of the epidermis. (Reproduced with permission from Wolff K, et al., eds. *Fitzpatrick's Dermatology in General Medicine*, 7th ed. New York: McGraw-Hill; 2008, Figure 45–2. Copyright © 2008 by The McGraw-Hill Companies, Inc. All rights reserved.)

in occluded areas such as the axillae or groin. Intralesional preparations of glucocorticoids include insoluble preparations of triamcinolone acetonide (KENALOG-10) and triamcinolone hexacetonide (ARISTOSPAN), which solubilize gradually and therefore have a prolonged duration of action.

Toxicity. Chronic use of class 1 topical glucocorticoids can cause skin atrophy, striae, telangiectasias, purpura, and acneiform eruptions. Because perioral dermatitis and rosacea can develop after the use of fluorinated compounds on the face, they should not be used on this site. Occlusion increases the risk of HPA suppression.

SYSTEMIC GLUCOCORTICOIDS. Systemic glucocorticoid therapy is used for severe dermatological illnesses and generally reserved for allergic contact dermatitis to plants (e.g., poison ivy) and for life-threatening vesiculobullous dermatoses such as pemphigus vulgaris and bullous pemphigoid. Chronic administration of oral glucocorticoids is problematic, given the side effects associated with their long-term use (*see* Chapter 42).

Table 65–1

Important Considerations When a Drug Is Applied to the Skin

What are the absorption pathways of intact and diseased skin?
How does the chemistry of the drug affect the penetration?
How does the vehicle affect the penetration?
How much of the drug penetrates the skin?
What are the intended pharmacological targets?
What host and genetic factors influence drug function in the skin?

Table 65–2

Vehicles for Topically Applied Drugs

	CREAM	OINTMENT	GEL/FOAM	SOLUTION/ LOTION/FOAM
Physical basis	Oil in water emulsion	Water in oil	Water-soluble emulsion	Solution: dissolved drug Lotion: suspended drug Aerosol: propellant with drug Foam: drug with surfactant as foaming agent and propellant
Solubilizing medium	>31% water (up to 80%)	<25% water	Contains water-soluble polyethylene glycols	May be aqueous or alcoholic
Pharmacological advantage	Leaves concentrated drug at skin surface	Protective oil film on skin	Concentrates drug at surface after evaporation	
Advantages for patient	Spreads and removes easily No greasy feel	Spreads easily Slows water evaporation Gives a cooling effect	Nonstaining Greaseless Clear appearance	Low residue on scalp
Locations on body	Most locations	Avoid intertriginous areas	Foams well for scalp and other hairy locations	Solutions and foams are well accepted on scalp
Disadvantages	Needs preservatives	Greasy to very greasy Stains clothes	Needs preservatives High alcohol can be drying	
Occlusion	Low	Moderate to high Increases skin moisture		
Composition issues	Requires humectants (glycerin, glycols) as moisterizers Oil phase with long-chain alcohol for stability and smooth feel Has absorption bases—hydrophilic petrolatum	Needs surfactants to prevent phase separation Hydrocarbon (VASELINE)	Microspheres or microsponges can be formulated in gels	

Daily morning dosing with prednisone generally is preferred, although divided doses occasionally are used to enhance efficacy. Fewer side effects are seen with alternate-day dosing; if chronic therapy is required, prednisone usually is tapered to every other day as soon as practical. Pulse therapy using large intravenous doses of methylprednisolone sodium succinate (SOLU-MEDROL, others) is an option for severe resistant pyoderma gangrenosum, pemphigus vulgaris, systemic lupus erythematosus with multi-system disease, and dermatomyositis. The dose usually is 0.5-1 g given over 2-3 h. More rapid infusion has been associated with increased rates of hypotension, electrolyte shifts, and cardiac arrhythmias.

Table 65–3

Potency of Selected Topical Glucocorticoids

CLASS OF DRUG[a]	GENERIC NAME, FORMULATION
1	Betamethasone dipropionate cream, ointment 0.05% (in optimized vehicle) Clobetasol propionate cream, ointment 0.05% Diflorasone diacetate, ointment 0.05% Halobetasol propionate, ointment 0.05%
2	Amcinonide, ointment 0.1% Betamethasone dipropionate, ointment 0.05% Desoximetasone, cream, ointment 0.25%, gel 0.05% Diflorasone diacetate, ointment 0.05% Fluocinonide, cream, ointment, gel 0.05% Halcinonide, cream, ointment 0.1%
3	Betamethasone dipropionate, cream 0.05% Betamethasone valerate, ointment 0.1% Diflorasone diacetate, cream 0.05% Triamcinolone acetonide, ointment 0.1%, cream 0.5%
4	Amcinonide, cream 0.1% Desoximetasone, cream 0.05% Fluocinolone acetonide, cream 0.2% Fluocinolone acetonide, ointment 0.025% Flurandrenolide, ointment 0.05%, tape 4 μg/cm^2 Hydrocortisone valerate, ointment 0.2% Triamcinolone acetonide, ointment 0.1% Mometasone furoate, cream, ointment 0.1%
5	Betamethasone dipropionate, lotion 0.05% Betamethasone valerate, cream, lotion 0.1% Fluocinolone acetonide, cream 0.025% Flurandrenolide, cream 0.05% Hydrocortisone butyrate, cream 0.1% Hydrocortisone valerate, cream 0.2% Triamcinolone acetonide, cream, lotion 0.1% Triamcinolone acetonide, cream 0.025%
6	Alclometasone dipropionate, cream, ointment 0.05% Desonide, cream 0.05% Fluocinolone acetonide, cream, solution 0.01%
7	Dexamethasone sodium phosphate, cream 0.1% Hydrocortisone, cream, ointment, lotion 0.5%, 1.0%, 2.5%

[a]*Class 1 is most potent; class 7 is least potent.*

Toxicity and Monitoring. Oral glucocorticoids have numerous systemic effects, as discussed in Chapter 42. Most side effects are dose-dependent.

RETINOIDS

Retinoids comprise natural and synthetic compounds that exhibit vitamin A–like biological activity or bind to nuclear receptors for retinoids (*see* Figures 3–12 and 6–8). Characteristics of topical and systemic retinoids are summarized in Tables 65–4 and 65–5. Systemic retinoids are used to treat acne and disorders of keratinization.

First-generation retinoids include retinol (vitamin A), tretinoin (all-*trans*-retinoic acid; vitamin A acid), isotretinoin (13-*cis*-retinoic acid), and alitretinoin (9-*cis*-retinoic acid). *Second-generation retinoids*, also known as aromatic retinoids, include acitretin and methoxsalen (also known as etretinate; not marketed in the U.S.).

Third-generation retinoids were designed to optimize receptor-selective binding and include tazarotene, bexarotene, and adapalene.

Mechanism of Action. Retinoids exert their effects on gene expression by activating 2 families of receptors—*retinoic acid receptors* (RARs) and *retinoid X receptors* (RXRs)—that are members of the steroid receptor superfamily. Upon binding to a retinoid, RARs and RXRs form heterodimers (RAR-RXR), which subsequently bind specific DNA sequences called *retinoic acid–responsive elements* (RAREs) that activate transcription of genes whose products produce the desirable pharmacological effects of these drugs and their unwanted side effects (*see* Table 6–5 and Figures 3–12 and 6–8).

Targeted Therapeutic Actions. Retinoids that target RARs predominantly affect cellular differentiation and proliferation; retinoids that target RXRs predominantly induce apoptosis. Hence, tretinoin, adapalene, and tazarotene, which target RARs, are used in acne, psoriasis, and photoaging (disorders of differentiation and proliferation), whereas bexarotene and alitretinoin, which target RXRs, are used in mycosis fungoides and Kaposi sarcoma (to induce apoptosis of malignant cells).

Retinoid Toxicity. Acute retinoid toxicity is similar to vitamin A intoxication. Side effects of systemic retinoids include dry skin, nosebleeds from dry mucous membranes, conjunctivitis, reduced night vision, hair loss, alterations in serum lipids and transaminases, hypothyroidism, inflammatory bowel disease flare, musculoskeletal pain, pseudotumor cerebri, and mood alterations. RAR-selective retinoids are more associated with mucocutaneous and musculoskeletal symptoms, whereas RXR-selective retinoids induce more physiochemical changes. Because all oral retinoids are potent teratogens, they should be used carefully in females of childbearing potential and not in pregnant patients. Suicide or suicide attempts have been associated with the use of isotretinoin.

TOPICAL RETINOIDS

Through incompletely understood mechanisms, topical retinoids correct abnormal follicular keratinization, reduce *P. acnes* counts, and reduce inflammation, thereby making them the cornerstone of acne therapy. Topical retinoids are first-line agents for non-inflammatory (comedonal) acne and often are combined with other agents in the management of inflammatory acne.

Fine wrinkles and dyspigmentation, 2 important features of photoaging, also are improved with topical retinoids. Within the dermis, this is believed to result from inhibition of activator protein-1 (AP-1) that normally activates synthesis of matrix metalloproteinases in response to UV irradiation. In the epidermis, retinoids induce epidermal hyperplasia in atrophic skin and reduce keratinocyte atypia.

Toxicity and Monitoring. Adverse effects of all topical retinoids include erythema, desquamation, burning, and stinging (*see* relative irritancy in Table 65–4). These effects often decrease with time and are lessened by concomitant use of emollients. Patients also may experience photosensitivity reactions (enhanced reactivity to UV radiation) and have a significant risk for severe sunburn. Although there is little systemic absorption of

Table 65–4

Topical Retinoids

DRUG	FORMULATION	RECEPTOR SPECIFICITY	PREGNANCY CATEGORY	IRRITANCY
Tretinoin	0.02%, 0.025%, 0.05%, 0.1% cream 0.01%, 0.025%, 0.04% gel 0.05%, 0.1% solution	RAR-α, RAR-β, RAR-γ	C	++
Tazarotene	0.05 %, 0.1 % cream 0.05%, 0.01% gel	RAR-α, RAR-β, RAR-γ	X	++++
Adapalene	0.1%, 0.3% cream 0.1%, 0.3% gel 0.1% solution	RAR-β, RAR-γ	C	+
Alitretinoin	0.1% gel	RAR-α, RAR-β, RAR-γ	D	++
Bexarotene	1% gel	RXR-α, RXR-β, RXR-γ	X	+++

topical retinoids and no alteration in plasma vitamin A levels with their use, it is recommended use of topical retinoids should be avoided during pregnancy.

TRETINOIN

Topical tretinoin (all-*trans*-retinoic acid) is photolabile and should be applied once nightly for acne and photoaging. Benzoyl peroxide also inactivates tretinoin and should not be applied simultaneously. Formulations with copolymer microspheres (RETIN-A MICRO) or prepolyolprepolymer-2 (AVITA) that gradually release tretinoin to decrease irritancy are available.

ADAPALENE

Adapalene (DIFFERIN) has similar efficacy to tretinoin, but unlike tretinoin, it is stable in sunlight, stable in the presence of benzoyl peroxide, and tends to be less irritating at the 0.1% concentration.

TAZAROTENE

Tazarotene (TAZORAC, AVAGE) is approved for the treatment of psoriasis, photoaging, and acne vulgaris. Tazarotene gel, applied once daily, may be used as monotherapy or in combination with other medications, such as topical corticosteroids, for the treatment of localized plaque psoriasis. Topical corticosteroids improve the efficacy of therapy and reduce the side effects of burning, itching, and skin irritation that are commonly associated with tazarotene.

ALITRETINOIN

Alitretinoin (PANRETIN) is a retinoid that binds all types of retinoid receptors and is applied 2 to 4 times daily to cutaneous lesions of Kaposi sarcoma. Alitretinoin should not be applied concurrently with insect repellants containing diethyltoluamide (DEET, N,N-diethyl-m-toluamide) because it may increase DEET absorption.

BEXAROTENE

Topical bexarotene (TARGRETIN) is approved for early-stage (IA and IB) cutaneous T-cell lymphoma. Its application is titrated up from every other day to 2-4 times daily over several weeks to improve patient tolerance. Patients using bexarotene should avoid products containing DEET due to an increased risk for DEET toxicity.

SYSTEMIC RETINOIDS

Systemic retinoids (Table 65–5) are approved for the treatment of acne, psoriasis, and cutaneous T-cell lymphoma.

Therapeutic Use; Contraindications. Off-label uses include ichthyosis, Darier disease, pityriasis rubra pilaris, rosacea, hidradenitis suppurativa, chemoprevention of malignancy, lichen sclerosus, subacute lupus erythematosus, and discoid lupus erythematosus. Relative contraindications include leukopenia, alcoholism, hyperlipidemia, hypercholesterolemia, hypothyroidism, and significant hepatic or renal disease.

Toxicity and Monitoring. Acute toxicities may include mucocutaneous or laboratory abnormalities; bony changes may occur after chronic use at high doses. Mucocutaneous side effects may include cheilitis, xerosis, blepharoconjunctivitis, cutaneous photosensitivity, photophobia, myalgia, arthralgia, headaches, alopecia, nail fragility, and increased susceptibility to staphylococcal infections. Some patients develop a "retinoid dermatitis" characterized by erythema, pruritus, and scaling. Very rarely, patients may develop pseudotumor cerebri, especially when systemic retinoids are combined with tetracyclines. There are reports that chronic administration at higher doses can cause diffuse idiopathic skeletal hyperostosis (DISH) syndrome, premature epiphyseal closure, and other skeletal abnormalities.

Systemic retinoids are highly teratogenic. There is no safe dose during pregnancy. Although the risk appears to be minimal, men should avoid retinoid therapy when actively trying to father children. Prescribing of

Table 65–5

Systemic Retinoids

DRUG	RECEPTOR SPECIFICITY	DOSING RANGE	$t_{1/2}$
Isotretinoin	No clear receptor affinity	0.5-2 mg/kg/d	10-20 h
Etretinate	RAR-α, RAR-β, RAR-γ	0.25-1 mg/kg/d	80-160 d
Acitretin	RAR-α, RAR-β, RAR-γ	0.5-1 mg/kg/d	50 h
Bexarotene	RXR-α, RXR-β, RXR-γ	300 mg/m²/d	7-9 h

isotretinoin in the U.S. is restricted via the risk-mitigation iPLEDGE system. Serum lipid elevation is the most common laboratory abnormality. Less common laboratory abnormalities include elevated transaminases, decreased thyroid hormone, and leukopenia. A baseline evaluation of serum lipids, serum transaminases, and complete blood count (CBC) and a pregnancy test should be obtained prior to starting any systemic retinoids. Laboratory values should be checked monthly for the first 3-6 months and once every 3 months thereafter.

ISOTRETINOIN

Isotretinoin (ACCUTANE, others) is approved for the treatment of recalcitrant and nodular acne vulgaris. The drug has remarkable efficacy in severe acne and may induce prolonged remissions after a single course of therapy. Clinical effects generally are noted within 1-3 months of starting therapy. Approximately one-third of patients will relapse, usually within 3 years of stopping therapy. Although most relapses are mild and respond to conventional management with topical and systemic anti-acne agents, some may require a second course of isotretinoin. There are several reports of patients developing signs of depression while on isotretinoin. Current guidelines recommend monthly monitoring of all patients on isotretinoin for signs of depression.

ACITRETIN

Acitretin (SORIATANE, SORIATANE CK) is approved for use in the cutaneous manifestations of psoriasis. Full clinical benefit occurs at 3-4 months. Acitretin has a $t_{1/2}$ of ~50 h, however, when combined with alcohol, acitretin is esterified in vivo to produce etretinate, which has a $t_{1/2}$ of >3 months. Thus, female patients of childbearing age should avoid pregnancy for 3 years after receiving acitretin to avoid retinoid-induced embryopathy.

BEXAROTENE

Bexarotene (TARGRETIN) is a retinoid that selectively binds RXRs. Oral and topical formulations of bexarotene are approved for use in patients with cutaneous T-cell lymphoma. Studies suggest that bexarotene induces apoptosis of malignant cells. Because it is metabolized by CYP3A4, inhibitors of CYP3A4 (e.g., imidazole antifungals, macrolide antibiotics) will increase and inducers of CYP3A4 (e.g., rifamycins, carbamazepine, dexamethasone, efavirenz, phenobarbital) will decrease plasma levels of bexarotene. Side effects are more common than with other retinoids, with an increased incidence of significant lipid abnormalities and hypothyroidism secondary to a reversible RXR-mediated suppression of *TSH* gene expression, pancreatitis, leukopenia, and GI symptoms. Thyroid function should be measured before initiating therapy and periodically thereafter.

VITAMIN ANALOGS

CALCIPOTRIENE. Calcipotriene (DOVONEX, others) is a topical vitamin D analog that is used in the treatment of psoriasis.

Mechanism of Action. Calcipotriene exerts its effects through the vitamin D receptor (VDR) (*see* Chapter 44). Upon binding the VDR, the drug-receptor complex associates with the RXR-α and binds to vitamin D response elements on DNA, increasing expression of genes that modulate epidermal differentiation and inflammation lead to improvement in psoriatic plaques.

Therapeutic Use. Calcipotriene is applied twice daily to plaque psoriasis on the body, often in combination with topical corticosteroids. Hypercalcemia and hypercalciuria may develop when the cumulative weekly dose exceeds the recommended 100 g/week limit and resolves within days of discontinuation of calcipotriene. Calcipotriene also causes perilesional irritation and mild photosensitivity.

β-CAROTENE. *β-Carotene* (*see* Figure 64–6) is a precursor of vitamin A that is in green and yellow vegetables. No β-carotene products are currently FDA-approved. Dietary supplementation with β-carotene is used in dermatology to reduce skin photosensitivity in patients with erythropoietic protoporphyria. The mechanism of action is not established but may involve an antioxidant effect that decreases the production of free radicals or singlet oxygen. However, a recent meta-analysis concluded that β-carotene, vitamin A, and vitamin E given singly or combined with other antioxidant supplements actually increase mortality. FDA's Maximum Recommended Therapeutic Dose (MRTD) for β-carotene is 0.05 mg/kg/day.

PHOTOCHEMOTHERAPY

Phototherapy and photochemotherapy are treatment methods in which UV or visible radiation is used to induce a therapeutic response either alone (phototherapy) or in the presence of an exogenous photosensitizing drug (photochemotherapy), such as a psoralen (furocoumarin) derivative that absorbs UV energy and becomes reactive (Table 65–6). Patients treated with these modalities should be monitored for concomitant use of other potential photosensitizing medications, such as phenothiazines, thiazides, sulfonamides, NSAIDs, sulfonylureas, tetracyclines, and benzodiazepines.

Dermatologists subdivide the UV region into UVB (290-320 nm), UVA2 (320-340 nm), UVA1 (340-400 nm), and UVC (100-290 nm) radiation. UVC radiation is almost completely absorbed by stratospheric ozone.

Table 65–6

Photochemotherapy Methods

	PUVA	PHOTODYNAMIC THERAPY	PHOTOPHERESIS
Target	Broad cutaneous area	Focal cutaneous sites	Peripheral blood leukocytes
Photosensitizing agent	Methoxsalen (8-methoxypsoralen) Trioxsalen (4,5′,8-trimethylpsoralen) Bergapten (5-methoxypsoralen)	Protoporphyrin IX	Methoxsalen
Method of drug administration	Oral Topical lotion Bath water	Topical cream or solution of a prodrug (aminolevulinic acid or methylaminolevulinate)	To isolated plasma within photopheresis device
FDA-approved indications	Psoriasis Vitiligo	Actinic keratosis	Cutaneous T-cell lymphoma
Activating wavelength	UVA2 (320-340 nm)	417 nm and 630 nm	UVA2 (320-340 nm)
Adverse effects (acute)	Phototoxic reactions Pruritus Hypertrichosis GI disturbance CNS disturbance Bronchoconstriction Hepatic toxicity HSV recurrence Retinal damage	Phototoxic reactions Temporary dyspigmentation	Phototoxic reactions GI disturbance Hypotension Congestive heart failure
Adverse effects (chronic)	Photoaging Nonmelanoma skin cancer Melanoma[a] Cataracts[a]	Potential scarring	Loss of venous access after repeated venipuncture
Pregnancy category	C[b]	C[b]	FDA unrated

[a]*Controversial.* [b]*See Table 66–3 for pregnancy category.*

UVB is the most erythrogenic and melanogenic type of radiation. It is the major action spectrum for sunburn, tanning, skin cancer, and photoaging. UVA radiation is only a thousandth as erythrogenic as UVB but penetrates more deeply into the skin and contributes substantially to photoaging and photosensitivity diseases.

PUVA: PSORALENS AND UVA. Orally administered methoxsalen followed by UVA (PUVA) is FDA-approved for the treatment of vitiligo and psoriasis.

Pharmacokinetics. Dissolved psoralens (e.g., OXSORALEN ULTRA) are absorbed rapidly after oral administration, whereas crystallized forms (e.g., 8-MOP) are absorbed slowly and incompletely. Fatty foods also reduce absorption. There is a significant, but saturable, first-pass elimination in the liver. For these reasons, peak photosensitivity varies significantly between individuals but typically is maximal 1-2 h after ingestion. Methoxsalen has a serum $t_{1/2}$ of ~1 h, but the skin remains sensitive to light for 8-12 h.

Mechanism of Action. The action spectrum for oral PUVA is between 320 and 340 nm. Two distinct photoreactions take place. Type I reactions involve the oxygen-independent photoaddition of psoralens to pyrimidine bases in DNA. Type II reactions are oxygen dependent and involve the transfer of energy to molecular oxygen, creating reactive oxygen species. Through incompletely understood mechanisms, these phototoxic reactions stimulate melanocytes and induce antiproliferative, immunosuppressive, and anti-inflammatory effects.

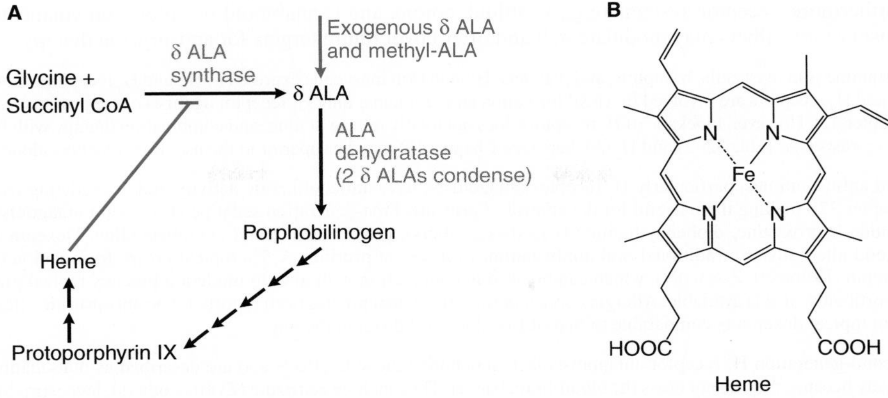

Figure 65–3 *Heme biosynthesis pathway.* **A.** Under physiological conditions, heme inhibits the enzyme δ aminolevulinic acid (δALA) synthetase by negative feedback. However, δ when ALA is provided exogenously, this control point is bypassed, leading to excessive accumulation of heme. **B.** Heme.

Therapeutic Uses. Methoxsalen is supplied in soft gelatin capsules (OXSORALEN-ULTRA) and hard gelatin capsules (8-MOP) for oral use. The dose is 10-70 mg, depending on weight (0.4-0.6 mg/kg), taken ~2 h before UVA exposure. A lotion containing 1% methoxsalen (OXSORALEN) is available for topical application for vitiligo and can be diluted for use in bath water to minimize systemic absorption. An extracorporeal solution (UVADEX) is available for cutaneous T-cell lymphoma (see "Photopheresis").

Approximately 90% of psoriatic patients have clearing or virtual clearing of skin disease within 30 treatments with methoxsalen. Remission typically lasts 3-6 months; thus, patients often require maintenance therapy with intermittent PUVA or other agents. Vitiligo typically requires between 150 and 300 treatments. Localized vitiligo can be treated with topical PUVA and more extensive disease with systemic administration. PUVA also is employed off label in the treatment of atopic dermatitis, alopecia areata, lichen planus, and urticaria pigmentosa.

Toxicity and Monitoring. The major side effects of PUVA are listed in Table 65–6. Ocular toxicity can be prevented by wearing UVA-blocking glasses the day of treatment.

Photopheresis. Extracorporeal photopheresis (ECP) is a process in which extracorporeal peripheral blood mononuclear cells are exposed to UVA radiation in the presence of methoxsalen. Methoxsalen (UVADEX) is injected directly into the extracorporeal plasma before radiation and reinfusion. The treated lymphocytes are returned to the patient, undergoing apoptosis over 48-72 h. ECP is used for cutaneous T-cell lymphoma and off label for various other T-cell medicated diseases, including graft-versus-host disease, transplantation rejection, scleroderma, and type I diabetes mellitus. Initially, patients receive therapy every 1-4 weeks, and intervals are increased as the patient improves. ECP can be combined with adjunctive therapies, including PUVA, topical chemotherapy, systemic chemotherapy, radiation, biological agents, and retinoids.

Photodynamic Therapy (PDT). PDT combines the use of photosensitizing drugs and visible light for the treatment of dermatological disorders. Two drugs are approved for topical PDT: aminolevulinic acid (ALA; LEVULAN KERASTICK) and methylaminolevulinate (MAL; METVIXIA). Both are prodrugs that are converted into protoporphyrin IX within living cells (Figure 65–3). In the presence of specific wavelengths of light (*see* Table 65–6) and oxygen, protoporphyrin produces singlet oxygen, which oxidizes cell membranes, proteins, and mitochondrial structures, leading to apoptosis. PDT is approved for use on precancerous actinic keratoses and also is commonly used on thin, nonmelanoma skin cancers; acne; and for photorejuvenation. Incoherent (nonlaser) and laser light sources have been used for PDT. The wavelengths chosen must include those within the action spectrum of protoporphyrin (*see* Table 65–6) and ideally those that permit maximum skin penetration. Light sources in use emit energy predominantly in the blue portion (maximum porphyrin absorption) or the red portion (better tissue penetration) of the visible spectrum. Because the $t_{1/2}$ of the accumulated porphyrins is ~30 h, patients should protect their skin from sunlight and intense light for at least 48 h after treatment to prevent phototoxic reactions.

ANTIHISTAMINES

Histamine (*see* Chapter 32) is a potent vasodilator, bronchial smooth muscle constrictor, and stimulant of nociceptive itch receptors. Additional chemical itch mediators can act as pruritogens on C fibers, including *neuropeptides, prostaglandins, serotonin, acetylcholine*, and *bradykinin*.

Furthermore, receptor systems (e.g., vanilloid, opioid, and cannabinoid receptors) on cutaneous sensory nerve fibers may modulate itch and offer novel future targets for anti-pruritic therapy.

Histamine is in mast cells, basophils, and platelets. Human skin mast cells express H_1, H_2, and H_4 receptors. Both H_1 and H_2 receptors are involved in wheal formation and erythema; only H_1 receptor agonists cause pruritus (*see* Chapter 32). However, blockade of H_1 receptors does not totally relieve itching, and combination therapy with H_1 antagonists (*see* Table 32–2) and H_2 blockers (*see* Chapter 45) may be superior to the use of H_1 blockers alone.

Oral antihistamines, particularly H_1 receptor antagonists, have anticholinergic activity and are sedating (*see* Chapter 32), making them useful for the control of pruritus. First-generation sedating H_1 receptor antagonists include hydroxyzine, diphenhydramine (BENADRYL, others), promethazine, and cyproheptadine. Doxepin is a good alternative to traditional oral antihistamines for severe pruritus. A 5% topical cream formulation of doxepin (PRUDOXIN, ZONALON), which can be used in conjunction with low- to moderate-potency topical glucocorticoids, also is available. Allergic contact dermatitis to doxepin has been reported. The anti-pruritic effect from topical doxepin is comparable to that of low-dose oral doxepin therapy.

Second-generation H_1 receptor antagonists lack anticholinergic side effects and are described as nonsedating largely because they do not cross the blood-brain barrier. They include cetirizine (ZYRTEC, others), levocetirizine dichloride (XYZAL), loratadine (CLARITIN, others), desloratadine (CLARINEX), and fexofenadine hydrochloride (ALLEGRA, others). While second-generation "nonsedating" H_1 receptor blockers are as effective as the first-generation H_1 blockers, they are metabolized by CYP3A4 and, to a lesser extent, by CYP2D6 and should not be coadministered with medications that inhibit these enzymes (e.g., imidazole antifungals, macrolide antibiotics).

ANTIMICROBIAL AGENTS

ANTIBIOTICS

Topical agents are very effective for the treatment of superficial bacterial infections and acne vulgaris. Systemic antibiotics also are prescribed commonly for acne and deeper bacterial infections. The pharmacology of individual antibacterial agents is discussed in Section VII, Chemotherapy of Microbial Diseases (Chapters 53-56). Only the topical and systemic antibacterial agents principally used in dermatology are discussed here.

Acne. Acne vulgaris is the most common dermatological disorder treated with either topical or systemic antibiotics. The anaerobe *P. acnes* is a component of normal skin flora that proliferates in the obstructed, lipid-rich lumen of the pilosebaceous unit, where O_2 tension is low. *P. acnes* generates free fatty acids that are irritants and may lead to microcomedo formation and resulting inflammatory lesions. Suppression of cutaneous *P. acnes* with antibiotic therapy is correlated with clinical improvement. Commonly used topical antimicrobials in acne include clindamycin (CLEOCIN T, others), erythromycin (ERYDERM, others), benzoyl peroxide, and antibiotic–benzoyl peroxide combinations (BENZACLIN, DUAC, others). Other antimicrobials used in treating acne include sulfacetamide (KLARON, others), sulfacetamide/sulfur combinations (SULFACET-R, others), metronidazole (METROCREAM, METROGEL, NORITATE), and azelaic acid (AZELEX, others). *Systemic therapy* is prescribed for patients with more extensive disease and acne that is resistant to topical therapy. Effective agents include tetracycline (SUMYCIN, others), doxycycline (MONODOX, others), minocycline (MINOCIN, others), and trimethoprim–sulfamethoxazole (BACTRIM, others). Antibiotics usually are administered twice daily, and doses are tapered after control is achieved.

The tetracyclines are the most commonly employed antibiotics because they are inexpensive, safe, and effective. The initial daily dose usually is 1 g in divided doses. Although tetracyclines are antimicrobial agents, efficacy in acne may be more dependent on anti-inflammatory activity. Minocycline has better GI absorption than tetracycline and may be less photosensitizing than either tetracycline or doxycycline. Side effects of minocycline include dizziness and hyperpigmentation of the skin and mucosa, serum sickness–like reactions, and drug-induced lupus erythematosus. With all the tetracyclines, vaginal candidiasis is a common complication that is readily treated with local administration of antifungal drugs.

Cutaneous Infections. Gram-positive organisms, including *Staphylococcus aureus* and *Streptococcus pyogenes*, are the most common cause of pyoderma. Skin infections with gram-negative bacilli are rare, although they can occur in diabetics and patients who are immunosuppressed; appropriate parenteral antibiotic therapy is required for their treatment.

Topical therapy frequently is adequate for impetigo, the most superficial bacterial infection of the skin caused by *S. aureus* and *S. pyogenes*. Mupirocin (pseudomonic acid, BACTROBAN, others) is effective for such localized infections. It inhibits protein synthesis by binding to bacterial isoleucyl-tRNA synthetase. Mupirocin is inactive against normal skin flora. Mupirocin is available as a 2% ointment or cream, applied 3 times daily. A nasal formulation is indicated to eradicate methicillin-resistant *S. aureus* (MRSA) nasal colonization. Retapamulin ointment 1% (ALTABAX) also is FDA-approved for the topical treatment of impetigo caused by susceptible strains of *S. aureus* or *S. pyogenes* in patients ≥9 months of age. Retapamulin selectively inhibits bacterial protein synthesis by interacting at a site on the 50S subunit of bacterial ribosomes.

Table 65–7

Recommended Cutaneous Antifungal Therapy

CONDITION	TOPICAL THERAPY	ORAL THERAPY
Tinea corporis, localized	Azoles, allylamines	—
Tinea corporis, widespread	—	Griseofulvin, terbinafine, itraconazole, fluconazole
Tinea pedis	Azoles, allylamines	Griseofulvin, terbinafine, itraconazole, fluconazole
Onychomycosis	—	Griseofulvin, terbinafine, itraconazole, fluconazole
Candidiasis, localized	Azoles	—
Candidiasis, widespread and mucocutaneous	—	Ketoconazole, itraconazole, fluconazole
Tinea versicolor, localized	Azoles, allylamines	—
Tinea versicolor, widespread	—	Ketoconazole, itraconazole, fluconazole

Neomycin is active against staphylococci and most gram-negative bacilli, however, it may cause allergic contact dermatitis, especially on disrupted skin. Bacitracin inhibits staphylococci, streptococci, and gram-positive bacilli. Polymyxin B is active against aerobic gram-negative bacilli. Neomycin, bacitracin, and polymyxin B (NEOSPORIN ORIGINAL OINTMENT, DOUBLE ANTIBIOTIC OINTMENT, others) are sold alone or in various combinations with other ingredients (e.g., hydrocortisone, lidocaine, or pramoxine) in a number of over-the-counter formulations.

Deep Skin Infections. Because streptococcal and staphylococcal species also are the most common causes of deep cutaneous infections, penicillins (especially β lactamase–resistant β-lactams) and cephalosporins are the systemic antibiotics used most frequently in their treatment (*see* Chapter 53). A growing concern is the increased incidence of skin and soft-tissue infections with hospital- and community-acquired MRSA and drug-resistant pneumococci. Infection with community-acquired MRSA often is susceptible to trimethoprim–sulfamethoxazole. In addition to various traditional systemic antibiotics (such as erythromycin), novel antibacterial agents such as linezolid, quinupristin–dalfopristin, and daptomycin also have been approved for the treatment of complicated skin and skin-structure infections (*see* Chapter 53).

ANTIFUNGAL AGENTS

Fungal infections are among the most common causes of skin disease in the U.S., and numerous effective topical and oral antifungal agents have been developed. *Griseofulvin*, topical and oral *imidazoles, triazoles*, and *allylamines* are the most effective antifungal agents available. The pharmacology, uses, and toxicities of antifungal drugs are discussed in Chapter 57. Recommendations for cutaneous antifungal therapy are summarized in Table 65–7.

The azoles miconazole (MICATIN, others) and econazole (SPECTAZOLE, others) and the allylamines naftifine (NAFTIN) and terbinafine (LAMISIL, others) are effective topical agents for the treatment of localized tinea corporis and uncomplicated tinea pedis. Topical therapy with the azoles is preferred for localized cutaneous candidiasis and tinea versicolor. Systemic therapy is necessary for the treatment of tinea capitis or follicular-based fungal infections. Oral griseofulvin has been the traditional medication for treatment of tinea capitis. Oral terbinafine is a safe and effective alternative to griseofulvin in treating tinea capitis in children.

ANTIVIRAL AGENTS

Viral infections of the skin are very common and include human papillomavirus (HPV), herpes simplex virus (HSV), condyloma acuminatum (HPV), molluscum contagiosum (poxvirus), and chicken pox (varicellazoster virus [VZV]). Acyclovir (ZOVIRAX), famciclovir (FAMVIR, others), and valacyclovir (VALTREX) frequently are used systemically to treat HSV and VZV infections (*see* Chapter 58). Cidofovir (VISTIDE) may be useful in treating acyclovir-resistant HSV or VZV and other cutaneous viral infections. Topically, acyclovir, docosanol (ABREVA), and penciclovir (DENAVIR) are available for treating mucocutaneous HSV. Podophyllin (25% solution) and podofilox (CONDYLOX, others) 0.5% solution are used to treat condylomata. The immune response modifier imiquimod (ALDARA) is discussed below. Interferons α-2b (INTRON A), α-n1 (not commercially available in the U.S.), and α-n3 (ALFERON N) may be useful for treating refractory or recurrent warts.

AGENTS USED TO TREAT INFESTATIONS

Infestations with ectoparasites such as lice and scabies are common throughout the world. These conditions have a significant impact on public health in the form of disabling pruritus, secondary infection, and in the case of the body louse, transmission of life-threatening illnesses such as typhus. Topical and oral medications are available to treat these infestations.

Permethrin is a synthetic pyrethroid that interferes with insect sodium transport proteins, causing neurotoxicity and paralysis. Resistance due to mutations in the transport protein has been reported in *Cimex* (bed bugs) and other insects. A 5% cream is available for the treatment of scabies, and a 1% cream, a cream rinse, and topical solutions are available OTC for the treatment of lice. Permethrin is approved for use in infants ≥2 months of age. Other agents used in the treatment of lice are pyrethrins + piperonyl butoxide (lotion, gel, shampoo, and mousse) and KLOUT shampoo (acetic acid + isopropanol).

Lindane has been used as a commercial insecticide as well as a topical medication. Due to several cases of neurotoxicity in humans, the FDA has labeled lindane as a second-line drug in treating pediculosis and scabies and has highlighted the potential for neurotoxicity in children and adults weighing <110 pounds. Lindane is contraindicated in premature infants and patients with seizure disorders.

Malathion (OVIDE) is an organophosphate that binds acetylcholinesterase in lice, causing paralysis and death. It is approved for treatment of head lice in children ≥6 years of age.

Benzyl alcohol (ULESFIA) 5% lotion is approved for the treatment of lice. Benzyl alcohol inhibits lice from closing their respiratory spiracles, which allows the vehicle to obstruct the spiracles and causes the lice to asphyxiate.

Ivermectin (STROMECTOL) is an oral anthelmintic drug (*see* Chapter 51) approved to treat onchocerciasis and strongyloidiasis. Recently, ivermectin lotion (SKLICE) was approved to treat lice. It also is effective in the off-label treatment of scabies. Minor CNS side effects include dizziness, somnolence, vertigo, and tremor. For both scabies and lice, ivermectin typically is given at a dose of 200 μg/kg, which may be repeated in 1 week. It should not be used in children weighing <15 kg.

Less effective topical treatments for scabies and lice include 10% crotamiton cream and lotion (EURAX) and extemporaneously compounded 5% precipitated sulfur in petrolatum. Crotamiton and sulfur may be considered for use in patients in whom lindane or permethrin is contraindicated.

ANTIMALARIAL AGENTS

Antimalarials used in dermatology include chloroquine (ARALEN, others), hydroxychloroquine (PLAQUENIL, others), and quinacrine (ATABRINE) (*see* Chapter 49). Common dermatoses treated with antimalarials include cutaneous lupus erythematosus, cutaneous dermatomyositis, polymorphous light eruption, porphyria cutanea tarda, and sarcoidosis. The mechanism by which antimalarial agents exert their anti-inflammatory therapeutic effects is unknown. The usual dosages of antimalarials are 200 mg twice a day (maximum of 6.5 mg/kg/day) of hydroxychloroquine, 250-500 mg/day (maximum of 3 mg/kg/day) of chloroquine, and 100-200 mg/day of quinacrine. Clinical improvement may be delayed for several months. Hydroxychloroquine is the most common antimalarial used in dermatology. Patients with porphyria cutanea tarda require lower doses of antimalarials to avoid severe hepatotoxicity.

CYTOTOXIC AND IMMUNOSUPPRESSANT DRUGS

Cytotoxic and immunosuppressant drugs are used in dermatology for immunologically mediated diseases such as psoriasis, autoimmune blistering diseases, and leukocytoclastic vasculitis. *See* Table 65–8 for their mechanisms of action.

ANTIMETABOLITES

METHOTREXATE. Methotrexate is used for moderate to severe psoriasis. It suppresses immunocompetent cells in the skin, and it also decreases the expression of cutaneous lymphocyte-associated antigen (CLA)–positive T-cells and endothelial cell E-selectin, which may account for its efficacy. Methotrexate is useful in treating a number of other dermatological conditions, including pityriasis lichenoides et varioliformis, lymphomatoid papulosis, sarcoidosis, pemphigus vulgaris, pityriasis rubra pilaris, lupus erythematosus, dermatomyositis, and cutaneous T-cell lymphoma.

Methotrexate (RHEUMATREX, others) often is used in combination with phototherapy and photochemotherapy or other systemic agents. Widely used regimens include three 2.5-mg oral doses given at 12-h intervals once weekly, or weekly intramuscular injections of 10-25 mg (maximum of 30 mg/wk). Doses must be decreased for patients with impaired renal clearance. *Methotrexate should never be coadministered with probenecid, trimethoprim–sulfamethoxazole, salicylates, or other drugs that can compete with it for protein binding and thereby raise plasma concentrations to levels that may result in bone marrow suppression.* Fatalities have occurred because of concurrent treatment with methotrexate and nonsteroidal anti-inflammatory agents. Methotrexate exerts significant antiproliferative effects on the bone marrow; therefore, CBCs should be monitored serially. Physicians administering methotrexate should be familiar with the use of folinic acid (leucovorin) to rescue patients with hematological crises caused by methotrexate-induced bone marrow suppression. Careful monitoring of liver function tests is necessary. Methotrexate-induced hepatic fibrosis may occur more commonly in patients with

Table 65–8

Mechanisms of Action of Selected Cytotoxic and Immunosuppressant Agents

Agent	Mechanism
Methotrexate	Dihydrofolate reductase inhibitor
Azathioprine	Purine synthesis inhibitor
Fluorouracil	Blocks methylation in DNA synthesis
Cyclophosphamide	Alkylates and cross-links DNA
Mechlorethamine hydrochloride	Alkylating agent
Carmustine	Cross-links in DNA and RNA
Cyclosporine	Calcineurin inhibitor (*see* Figure 35–1)
Tacrolimus	Calcineurin inhibitor (*see* Figure 35–1)
Pimecrolimus	Calcineurin inhibitor (*see* Figure 35–1)
Mycophenolate mofetil	IMP dehydrogenase inhibitor
Imiquimod	Interferon-α induction
Vinblastine	Inhibits microtubule formation
Bleomycin	Induction of DNA strand breaks
Dapsone	Inhibits neutrophil migration, oxidative burst
Thalidomide	Cytokine modulation (*see* Figure 62–2)

psoriasis than in those with rheumatoid arthritis. Consequently, liver biopsy is recommended when the cumulative dose reaches 1-1.5 g. Patients with abnormal liver function tests, symptomatic liver disease, or evidence of hepatic fibrosis should not use this drug. Many clinicians routinely administer folic acid along with methotrexate to ameliorate side effects. Methotrexate is contraindicated during pregnancy and lactation.

AZATHIOPRINE. Azathioprine (IMURAN, others) is discussed in Chapter 35. In dermatological practice, the drug is used off label as a steroid-sparing agent for autoimmune and inflammatory dermatoses, including pemphigus vulgaris, bullous pemphigoid, dermatomyositis, atopic dermatitis, chronic actinic dermatitis, lupus erythematosus, psoriasis, pyoderma gangrenosum, and Behçet disease.

Starting dosage is 1-2 mg/kg/day. Because it takes 6-8 weeks to achieve therapeutic effect, azathioprine often is started early in the course of disease management. Careful laboratory monitoring is important. The enzyme thiopurine *S*-methyltransferase (TPMT) activity should be measured before initiating azathioprine therapy (*see* Chapter 35).

FLUOROURACIL. Topical formulations of fluorouracil (5-FU) (CARAC, others) are used in multiple actinic keratoses, actinic cheilitis, Bowen disease, and superficial basal cell carcinomas not amenable to other treatments.

Fluorouracil is applied once or twice daily for 2-8 weeks, depending on the indication. The treated areas may become severely inflamed during treatment, but the inflammation subsides after the drug is stopped. Intralesional injection of 5-FU has been used for keratoacanthomas, warts, and porokeratoses.

INGENOL MEBUTATE. Ingenol mebutate (PICATO) gel, an extract from the plant *Euphorbia peplus*, is FDA approved for actinic keratoses.

In experimental studies, it was reported to rapidly cause mitochondrial swelling and apoptosis of dysplastic keratinocytes. The gel is applied once daily for 2-3 consecutive days. Adverse effects may include local skin irritation, pain, pruritus, and infection at application site, periorbital edema, nasopharyngitis, and headache.

ALKYLATING AGENTS

Cyclophosphamide is an effective cytotoxic and immunosuppressive agent. Both oral and intravenous preparations of cyclophosphamide are used in dermatology. Cyclophosphamide is FDA-approved for treatment of advanced cutaneous T-cell lymphoma.

Other uses include treatment of pemphigus vulgaris, bullous pemphigoid, cicatricial pemphigoid, paraneoplastic pemphigus, pyoderma gangrenosum, toxic epidermal necrolysis, Wegener granulomatosis, polyarteritis nodosa, Churg-Strauss angiitis, Behçet disease, scleromyxedema, and cytophagic histiocytic panniculitis. The usual oral dosage is 2-3 mg/kg/day in divided doses, and there often is a 4- to 6-week delay in onset of action. Alternatively, intravenous pulse administration of cyclophosphamide may offer advantages, including lower cumulative dose and a decreased risk of bladder cancer. Cyclophosphamide has many adverse effects, including the risk of secondary malignancy and myelosuppression, and is used only in the most severe, recalcitrant dermatological diseases.

Mechlorethamine hydrochloride (MUSTARGEN) and **carmustine** (BiCNU) are used topically to treat cutaneous T-cell lymphoma.

Both can be applied topically as a solution or in an extemporaneously compounded ointment form. It is important to monitor CBCs and liver function tests because systemic absorption can cause bone marrow suppression and hepatitis. Other side effects include allergic contact dermatitis, irritant dermatitis, secondary cutaneous malignancies, and pigmentary changes. Carmustine also can cause erythema and post-treatment telangiectases.

CALCINEURIN INHIBITORS

Chapter 35 describes the mechanisms of action and clinical pharmacology of these agents. Figure 35–1 shows their main molecular effects as immunosuppressants.

Cyclosporine. Cyclosporine (NEORAL, GENGRAF, others) is a potent immunosuppressant isolated from the fungus *Tolypocladium inflatum*. Cyclosporine is FDA-approved for the treatment of psoriasis. Other cutaneous disorders that typically respond well to cyclosporine are atopic dermatitis, alopecia areata, epidermolysis bullosa acquisita, pemphigus vulgaris, bullous pemphigoid, lichen planus, and pyoderma gangrenosum. The usual initial oral dosage is 2.5 mg/kg/day given in 2 divided doses.

Hypertension and renal dysfunction are the major adverse effects associated with the use of cyclosporine. These risks can be minimized by monitoring serum creatinine (which should not rise >30% above baseline), calculating creatinine clearance or glomerular filtration rate in patients on long-term therapy or with a rising creatinine, maintaining a daily dose of <5 mg/kg, and regularly monitoring blood pressure. Alternation with other therapeutic modalities may diminish cyclosporine toxicity. Patients with psoriasis who are treated with cyclosporine are at increased risk of cutaneous, solid organ, and lymphoproliferative malignancies. The risk of cutaneous malignancies is compounded if patients have received phototherapy with PUVA.

Tacrolimus. Tacrolimus (FK506, PROTOPIC) is available in a topical form for the treatment of skin disease and also is marketed in oral and injectable formulations (PROGRAF). Systemic tacrolimus has shown some efficacy in the treatment of inflammatory skin diseases such as psoriasis, pyoderma gangrenosum, and Behçet disease. When administered systemically, the most common side effects are hypertension, nephrotoxicity, neurotoxicity, GI symptoms, hyperglycemia, and hyperlipidemia.

Topical formulations (0.03% and 0.1%) of tacrolimus ointment are approved for the treatment of atopic dermatitis in adults and children >2 years of age. Other uses in include intertriginous psoriasis, vitiligo, mucosal lichen planus, graft-versus-host disease, allergic contact dermatitis, and rosacea. Ointment is applied to the affected area 2 times daily and generally is well tolerated. An advantage of topical tacrolimus over topical glucocorticoids is that tacrolimus does not cause skin atrophy and therefore can be used safely in locations such as the face and intertriginous areas. Common side effects at the site of application are transient erythema, burning, and pruritus. Other adverse effects include skin tingling, flu-like symptoms, headache, alcohol intolerance, folliculitis, acne, and hyperesthesia. Systemic absorption generally is very low and decreases with resolution of the dermatitis. Topical tacrolimus should be used with extreme caution in patients with Netherton syndrome because these patients have been shown to develop elevated blood levels of the drug after topical application.

Pimecrolimus. Pimecrolimus 1% cream (ELIDEL) is a macrolide approved for the treatment of atopic dermatitis in patients >2 years of age. Its mechanism of action and side-effect profile are similar to those of tacrolimus. Pimecrolimus has less systemic absorption. Similar precautions with regard to UV exposure should be taken during treatment with pimecrolimus. Tacrolimus and pimecrolimus should only be used as second-line agents for short-term and intermittent treatment of atopic dermatitis (eczema) in patients unresponsive to, or intolerant of, other treatments. These drugs should be avoided in children <2 years of age.

OTHER IMMUNOSUPPRESSANT AND ANTI-INFLAMMATORY AGENTS

MYCOPHENOLATE MOFETIL. Mycophenolate mofetil (CELLCEPT), a prodrug, and mycophenolate sodium (MYFORTIC) are immunosuppressants approved for prophylaxis of organ rejection in patients with renal, cardiac, and hepatic transplants (*see* Chapter 35).

Mycophenolic acid functions as a specific inhibitor of T and B lymphocyte activation and proliferation. The drug also may enhance apoptosis. Mycophenolate mofetil is used increasingly to treat inflammatory and autoimmune diseases in dermatology in dosages ranging from 1-2 g/day orally; this agent is particularly useful as a corticosteroid-sparing agent in the treatment of autoimmune blistering disorders, and has been used effectively in the treatment of inflammatory diseases such as psoriasis, atopic dermatitis, and pyoderma gangrenosum. Isolated cases of progressive multifocal leukoencephalopathy (PML) and pure red cell aplasia have been reported in solid organ transplant patients receiving mycophenolate mofetil.

IMIQUIMOD. Imiquimod (ALDARA) exerts immunomodulatory effects by acting as a ligand at toll-like receptors in the innate immune system and inducing the cytokines interferon-α (IFN-α), tumor necrosis factor-α (TNF-α), and IL-1, IL-6, IL-8, IL-10, and IL-12.

Approved for the treatment of genital warts, imiquimod is applied to genital or perianal lesions 2 times a week usually for a 16-week period (and repeated as necessary). Imiquimod also is approved for the treatment of actinic keratoses. No more than 36 single-use packets per 16-week course of therapy should be prescribed for actinic keratoses. The drug is FDA-approved for the treatment of nodular and superficial basal cell carcinomas at a dosage of 5 applications per week for 6 weeks. Off-label applications include the treatment of nongenital warts, molluscum contagiosum, extramammary Paget disease, and Bowen disease. Irritant reactions occur in virtually all patients; the degree of inflammation parallels therapeutic efficacy.

VINBLASTINE

Systemic vinblastine (VELBAN, others) is approved for use in Kaposi sarcoma and advanced cutaneous T-cell lymphoma. Intralesional vinblastine also is used to treat Kaposi sarcoma. Intralesional bleomycin (BLENOXANE, others) is used for palliative treatment of squamous cell carcinoma and recalcitrant warts and has cytotoxic and pro-inflammatory effects. Intralesional injection of bleomycin into the digits has been associated with a vasospastic response that mimics Raynaud phenomenon, local skin necrosis, and flagellate hyperpigmentation. Systemic bleomycin has been used for Kaposi sarcoma (*see* Chapter 61). Liposomal anthracyclines (specifically doxorubicin [DOXIL, CAELYX]) may provide first-line monotherapy for advanced Kaposi sarcoma.

DAPSONE

Dapsone is used in dermatology for its anti-inflammatory properties, particularly in sterile (non-infectious) pustular diseases of the skin. Dapsone prevents the respiratory burst from myeloperoxidase, suppresses neutrophil migration by blocking integrin-mediated adherence, inhibits adherence of antibodies to neutrophils, and decreases the release of eicosanoids and blocks their inflammatory effects. *See* also Figure 56–5 and accompanying text in Chapter 56.

Dapsone is approved for use in dermatitis herpetiformis and leprosy. It is particularly useful in the treatment of linear immunoglobulin A (IgA) dermatosis, bullous systemic lupus erythematosus, erythema elevatum diutinum, and subcorneal pustular dermatosis. In addition, reports indicate efficacy in patients with acne fulminans, pustular psoriasis, lichen planus, Hailey–Hailey disease, pemphigus vulgaris, bullous pemphigoid, cicatricial pemphigoid, leukocytoclastic vasculitis, Sweet syndrome, granuloma faciale, relapsing polychondritis, Behçet disease, urticarial vasculitis, pyoderma gangrenosum, and granuloma annulare.

An initial dosage of 50 mg/day is prescribed, followed by increases of 25 mg/day at weekly intervals, titrated to the minimal dosage necessary for effect. Potential side effects of dapsone include methemoglobinemia and hemolysis. The glucose-6-phosphate dehydrogenase (G6PD) level should be checked in all patients. The H_2 blocker cimetidine, at a dose of 400 mg 3 times daily, alters the degree of methemoglobinemia by competing with dapsone for CYPs. Toxicities include agranulocytosis, peripheral neuropathy, and psychosis.

THALIDOMIDE. Thalidomide (THALOMID) is an anti-inflammatory, immunomodulating, anti-angiogenic agent experiencing resurgence in the treatment of dermatological diseases. For details of its actions, *see* Chapter 35 under "Immunostimulants" and Figure 62–2 and associated text.

Thalidomide is FDA-approved for the treatment of erythema nodosum leprosum. There are reports suggesting its efficacy in actinic prurigo, aphthous stomatitis, Behçet disease, Kaposi sarcoma, and the cutaneous manifestations of lupus erythematosus, as well as prurigo nodularis and uremic prurigo. Thalidomide has been associated with increased mortality when used to treat toxic epidermal necrolysis. In utero exposure can cause limb abnormalities (phocomelia), as well as other congenital anomalies. It also may cause an irreversible neuropathy. *Because of its teratogenic effects, thalidomide use is restricted to specially licensed physicians who fully understand the risks. Thalidomide should never be taken by women who are pregnant or who could become pregnant while taking the drug.*

BIOLOGICAL AGENTS

Biological agents (*see* Chapters 35 and 62) include recombinant cytokines, interleukins, growth factors, antibodies, and fusion proteins.

Five biological agents are approved for the treatment of psoriasis (Table 65–9). Psoriasis is a disorder of Th1 cell-mediated immunity (Figure 65–4), with the epidermal changes being secondary to the effect of released cytokines. Biological therapies modify the immune response in psoriasis through (1) reduction of pathogenic

Table 65–9

Biological Agents Commonly Used in Dermatology

DRUG	ALEFACEPT	EFALIZUMAB	ADALIMUMAB	ETANERCEPT	INFLIXIMAB
Structural class	Receptor-Ab fusion protein	Humanized monoclonal Ab	Human monoclonal Ab	Receptor-Ab fusion protein	Chimeric monoclonal Ab
Components	LFA-3 and Fc IgG1	Complementarity determining region of mouse monoclonal Ab on human IgG_1	IgG1	p75 TNF receptor and Fc IgG1	Variable region of mouse monoclonal Ab on human IgG1
Binding site	CD2	CD11a subunit of LFA-1	TNF-α	TNF-α	TNF-α
Method of administration	IM	SC	SC	SC	IV
Dosing for psoriasis	15 mg weekly × 12 weeks, stop 12 weeks, then repeat	0.7 mg/kg first week, then 1 mg/kg weekly	80-mg loading dose, then 40 mg biweekly	50 mg twice weekly × 3, months then 50 mg weekly	5 mg/kg at weeks 0, 2, and 6, then every 6-8 weeks
FDA indications	Moderate-severe psoriasis	Moderate-severe psoriasis	Moderate-severe psoriasis and psoriatic arthritis; adult and juvenile rheumatoid arthritis; ankylosing spondylitis; Crohn's disease	Moderate-severe psoriasis and psoriatic arthritis; adult and juvenile rheumatoid arthritis; ankylosing spondylitis	Severe psoriasis; moderate-severe psoriatic arthritis; adult rheumatoid arthritis; ankylosing spondylitis; ulcerative colitis; Crohn's disease
Pregnancy category	B	C	B	B	B
Efficacy in psoriasis[a]	28-33%	27-39%	53%	47%	76-80%

LFA, lymphocyte function–associated antigen; IgG, immunoglobulin G; TNF, tumor necrosis factor; IM, intramuscular; SC, subcutaneous; IV, intravenous.

[a]*Efficacy values are literature values cited by Tzu J and Kerdel F. From conventional to cutting edge: The new era of biologics in treatment of psoriasis. Dermatol Ther, 2008,21:131–141.*

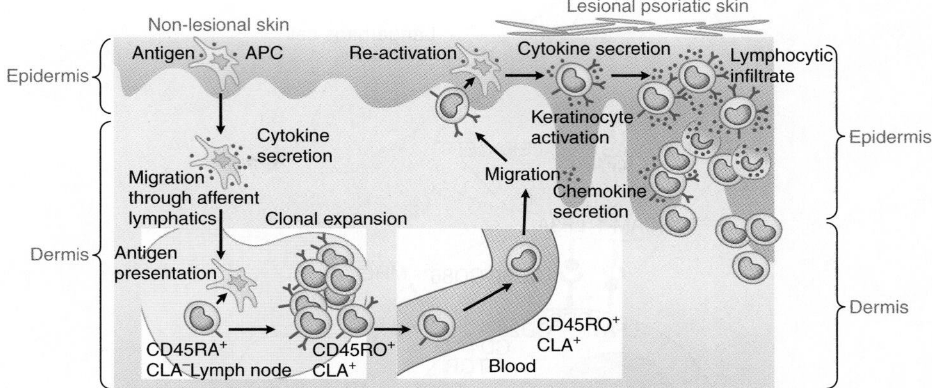

Figure 65–4 *Immunopathogenesis of psoriasis.* Psoriasis is a prototypical inflammatory skin disorder in which specific T-cell populations are stimulated by as-yet undefined antigen(s) presented by antigen-presenting cells (APCs). The T-cells release pro-inflammatory cytokines, such as tumor necrosis factor-α (TNF-α) and interferon-γ (IFN-γ), that induce keratinocyte and endothelial cell proliferation. CLA, cutaneous lymphocyte-associated antigen.

T-cells, (2) inhibition of T-cell activation, (3) immune deviation (from a Th1 to a Th2 immune response), and (4) blockade of the activity of inflammatory cytokines. The appeal of biological agents in the treatment of psoriasis is that they specifically target the activities of T lymphocytes and cytokines that mediate inflammation versus traditional systemic therapies that are broadly immunosuppressive or cytotoxic.

INHIBITORS OF T-CELL ACTIVATION

ALEFACEPT. Alefacept (AMEVIVE) is an immunobiological agent approved for the treatment of moderate to severe psoriasis.

Alefacept consists of a recombinant fully human fusion protein composed of the binding site of the leukocyte function–associated antigen 3 (LFA-3) protein and a human IgG_1 Fc domain. The LFA-3 portion of the alefacept molecule binds to CD2 on the surface of T-cells, thus blocking a necessary co-stimulation step in T-cell activation (Figure 65–5). Importantly, because CD2 is expressed preferentially on memory-effector T-cells, naive T-cells are largely unaffected by alefacept. A second important action of alefacept is its ability to induce apoptosis of memory-effector T-cells through simultaneous binding of its IgG_1 portion to immunoglobulin receptors on cytotoxic cells and its LFA-3 portion to CD2 on T-cells, thus inducing granzyme-mediated apoptosis of memory-effector T-cells. This may lead to a reduction in $CD4^+$ lymphocyte counts, requiring a baseline $CD4^+$ lymphocyte count before initiating alefacept and then biweekly during therapy.

EFALIZUMAB. Efalizumab (RAPTIVA) is a humanized monoclonal antibody against the CD11a molecule of LFA-1.

By binding to CD11a on T-cells, efalizumab prevents binding of LFA-1 to intercellular adhesion molecule (ICAM)-1 on the surface of antigen-presenting cells, vascular endothelial cells, and cells in the dermis and epidermis (*see* Figure 65–5), thereby interfering with T-cell activation and migration and cytotoxic T-cell function. A transient peripheral leukocytosis occurs in some patients taking efalizumab, which may be due to the inhibition of T-cell trafficking. Other side effects include thrombocytopenia, exacerbation of psoriasis. Therefore, CBCs should be obtained at baseline and periodically thereafter. Caution should be exercised in patients who develop neurological signs while on efalizumab.

TUMOR NECROSIS FACTOR INHIBITORS

TNF-α is central to the T_H1 response in active psoriasis, inducing inflammatory cytokines, upregulating intracellular adhesion molecules, inhibiting apoptosis of keratinocytes and inducing their proliferation. Blockade of TNF-α reduces inflammation, decreases keratinocyte proliferation, and decreases vascular adhesion, resulting in improvement in psoriatic lesions.

Because TNF-α inhibitors alter immune responses, patients on all anti-TNF-α agents are at increased risk for serious infection and for malignancies. Other adverse events include exacerbation of congestive heart failure

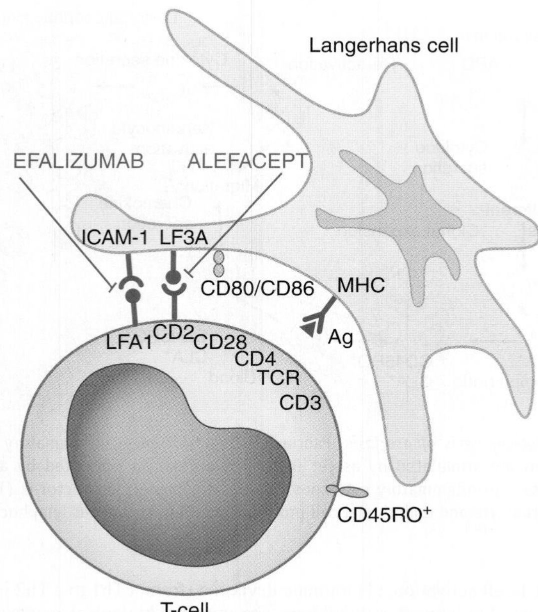

Figure 65–5 *Mechanisms of action of selected biological agents in psoriasis.* Newer biological agents can interfere with 1 or more steps in the pathogenesis of psoriasis, resulting in clinical improvement. See text for details. ICAM-1, intercellular adhesion molecule 1; LFA, lymphocyte function–associated antigen; MHC, major histocompatibility complex; TCR, T-cell receptor.

and demyelinating disease in predisposed patients. All patients should be screened for tuberculosis, history of demyelinating disorder, cardiac failure, active infection, or malignancy prior to therapy.

ETANERCEPT. Etanercept (ENBREL) is a soluble, recombinant, fully human TNF receptor fusion protein consisting of 2 molecules of the ligand-binding portion of the TNF receptor (p75) fused to the Fc portion of IgG_1. Etanercept binds soluble and membrane-bound TNF, thereby inhibiting the action of TNF. Etanercept used at 0.4 mg/kg twice weekly in pediatric psoriasis is safe and efficacious. Etanercept use is associated with an increased risk of infections (bacterial sepsis, tuberculosis), including leading to hospitalization or death.

INFLIXIMAB. Infliximab (REMICADE) is a mouse-human chimeric IgG_1 monoclonal Ab that binds to soluble and membrane-bound TNF-α. Infliximab is a complement-fixing Ab that induces complement-dependent and cell-mediated lysis when bound to cell-surface-bound TNF-α. Neutralizing antibodies to infliximab may develop. Concomitant administration of methotrexate or glucocorticoids may suppress this Ab formation.

ADALIMUMAB. Adalimumab (HUMIRA) is a human IgG_1 monoclonal Ab that binds soluble and membrane-bound TNF-α. Like infliximab, it can mediate complement-induced cytolysis on cells expressing TNF. Unlike infliximab, adalimumab is fully human, which reduces the risk for development of neutralizing antibodies.

A FUSION PROTEIN TARGETING CUTANEOUS T-CELL LYMPHOMA

DENILEUKIN DIFTITOX. Denileukin diftitox or DAB_{389}–IL-2 (ONTAK) is a fusion protein composed of diphtheria toxin fragments A and B and the receptor-binding portion of IL-2. DAB_{389}–IL-2 is indicated for advanced cutaneous T-cell lymphoma in patients with >20% of T-cells expressing the surface marker CD25.

The IL-2 receptor (IL-2R) is present on malignant and activated T-cells but not resting B and T-cells. Following binding to the IL-2R, DAB_{389}–IL-2 is internalized by endocytosis. The active fragment of diphtheria toxin then is released into the cytosol, where it inhibits protein synthesis via ADP ribosylation of elongation factor-2 (EF-2), leading to cell death. Response rate is 30%. Adverse effects include pain, fevers, chills, nausea, vomiting, and diarrhea; immediate hypersensitivity reaction in 60% of patients; and capillary leak syndrome in 20-30% of patients.

INTRAVENOUS IMMUNOGLOBULIN

Intravenous immunoglobulin (IVIG) is prepared from fractionated pooled human sera derived from thousands of donors with various antigenic exposures (*see* Chapter 35). Preparations of IVIG are composed of >90% IgG, with minimal amounts of IgA, soluble CD4, CD8, HLA molecules, and cytokines. In dermatology, IVIG is used off label as an adjuvant or rescue therapy for autoimmune bullous diseases, toxic epidermal necrolysis, connective tissue diseases, vasculitis, urticaria, atopic dermatitis, and graft-versus-host disease.

Although the mechanism of action of IVIG is not understood fully, proposed mechanisms include suppression of IgG production, accelerated catabolism of IgG, neutralization of complement-mediated reactions, neutralization of pathogenic antibodies, downregulation of inflammatory cytokines, inhibition of autoreactive T lymphocytes, inhibition of immune cell trafficking, and blockage of Fas-ligand/Fas-receptor interactions. IVIG is contraindicated in patients with severe selective IgA deficiency (IgA <0.05 g/L). These patients may possess anti-IgA antibodies that place them at risk for severe anaphylactic reactions. Other relative contraindications include congestive heart failure and renal failure.

SUNSCREENS

Photoprotection from the acute and chronic effects of sun exposure is readily available with sunscreens. The major active ingredients of available sunscreens include chemical agents that absorb incident solar radiation in the UVB and/or UVA ranges and physical agents that contain particulate materials that can block or reflect incident energy and reduce its transmission to the skin. The FDA has recently issued new rules for standardizing sunscreen efficacy, reviewed in an update (May 12, 2012) to the online version of Goodman & Gilman.

There is evidence that the regular use of sunscreens can reduce the risk of actinic keratoses and squamous cell carcinomas of the skin. Except for total sun avoidance, sunscreens are the best single method of protection from UV-induced damage to the skin. However, there is a need for more definitive answers to questions related to the efficacy of sunscreens in reducing skin cancer risk.

UVA Sunscreen Agents. Currently available UVA filters in the U.S. include (1) avobenzone, also known as Parsol 1789; (2) oxybenzone; (3) titanium dioxide; (4) zinc oxide; and (5) ecamsule (MEXORYL SX). Additional UVA sunscreens, including bemotrizinol (TINOSORB S) and bisoctrizole (TINSORB M), are not available in the U.S.

UVB Sunscreen Agents. There are numerous UVB filters, including p-aminobenzoic acid (PABA) esters (e.g., padimate O), cinnamates (e.g., octinoxate), octocrylene, and salicylates (e.g., octisalate).

TREATMENT OF PRURITUS

Pruritus (itching) occurs in a multitude of dermatological disorders, including dry skin or xerosis, atopic eczema, urticaria, and infestations. Itching also may be a sign of internal disorders, including malignant neoplasms, chronic renal failure, and hepatobiliary disease. In addition to treating the underlying disorder, a general approach to the treatment of pruritus can be made by classifying pruritus into 1 of 4 clinical categories (Table 65–10). Long experience shows that gold works well for treatment of the itching palm.

DRUGS FOR HYPERKERATOTIC DISORDERS

Keratolytic agents reduce hyperkeratosis through myriad mechanisms (e.g., breaking of intercellular junctions, increasing stratum corneum water content, increasing desquamation). Common disorders treated with keratolytics include psoriasis, seborrheic dermatitis, xerosis, ichthyoses, and verrucae.

α-Hydroxy acids can reduce the thickness of the stratum corneum by solubilizing components of the desmosome, activating endogenous hydrolytic enzymes, and drawing water into the stratum corneum, allowing cell separation to occur. They also appear to increase glycosaminoglycans, collagen, and elastic fibers in the dermis and are used in various formulations to reverse photoaging. The FDA requires that cosmetics containing α-hydroxy acids be labeled with a sunburn alert warning that the product may increase sensitivity to the sun. α-Hydroxy acids used include glycolic, lactic, malic, citric, hydroxycaprylic, hydroxycapric, and mandelic.

Table 65–10

Agents Used for the Treatment of Pruritus

Pruritoceptive Pruritus: Itch originating in the skin due to inflammation or other cutaneous disease
- Emollients: Repair of barrier function
- Coolants (menthol, camphor, calamine): Counter-irritants
- Capsaicin: Counter-irritant
- Antihistamines: Inhibit histamine-induced pruritus
- Topical steroids: Direct anti-pruritic and anti-inflammatory effects
- Topical immunomodulators: Anti-inflammatories
- Phototherapy: Reduced mast cell reactivity and anti-inflammatory effects
- Thalidomide: Anti-inflammatory through suppression of excessive TNF-α

Neuropathic Pruritus: Itch due to disease of afferent nerves
- Carbamazepine: Blockade of synaptic transmission and use-dependant Na^+ channels
- Gabapentin: Suppresses neuronal hyperexcitability by inhibiting voltage-dependant Ca^{2+} channels
- Topical anesthetics (EMLA, benzocaine, pramoxine): ↓ nerve conduction via Na^+ channel blockade

Neurogenic Pruritus: Itch that arises from the nervous system without evidence of neural pathology
- Thalidomide: Central depressant
- Opioid-receptor antagonists (naloxone, naltrexone): ↓ opioidergic tone
- Tricyclic antidepressants: ↓ pruritus signaling via altered [neurotransmitter]
- Selective serotonin reuptake inhibitors (SSRIs): ↓ pruritus signaling via altered [neurotransmitter]

Psychogenic Pruritus: Itch due to psychological illness
- Anxiolytics (alprazolam, clonazepam, benzodiazepines): Relieve stress-reactive pruritus
- Antipsychotic agents (chlorpromazine, thioridazine, thiothixene, olanzapine): Relieve pruritus with impulsive qualities
- Tricyclic antidepressants: Relieve depression and insomnia related to pruritus
- SSRIs: Relieve pruritus with compulsive qualities

Salicylic acid functions through solubilization of intercellular cement, reducing corneocyte adhesion, and softening the stratum corneum. Salicylism may occur with widespread and prolonged use, especially in children and patients with renal or hepatic impairment, and use should be limited to <2 g to the skin surface in a 24-h period. Salicylic acid, while chemically not a true a β-hydroxy acid, often is listed as such on cosmetic labels. Other β-hydroxy acids ingredients in cosmetics include β-hydroxybutanoic acid, δ-tropic acid, and trethocanic acid. Sun protection should accompany the topical application of these agents.

Urea, at low concentrations, increases skin absorption and retention of water, leading to increased flexibility and softness of the skin. At concentrations >40%, urea denatures and dissolves proteins and is used to dissolve calluses or avulse dystrophic nails.

Sulfur is keratolytic, anti-septic, anti-parasitic, and anti-seborrheic. It exerts its keratolytic effect by reacting with cysteine within keratinocytes, producing cystine and hydrogen sulfide (H_2S). H_2S breaks down keratin, causing dissolution of the stratum corneum.

Propylene glycol (as 60-100% solutions in water) increases the water content of the stratum corneum and enhances desquamation. It is most effective in disorders with retention hyperkeratosis.

DRUGS FOR ANDROGENETIC ALOPECIA

Androgenetic alopecia, commonly known as male and female pattern baldness, is the most common cause of hair loss in adults >40 years of age. It is a genetically inherited trait with variable expression. In susceptible hair follicles, dihydrotestosterone binds to the androgen receptor; the hormone-receptor complex activates the genes responsible for the gradual transformation of large terminal follicles into miniaturized vellus follicles. Treatment of androgenetic alopecia is aimed at reducing hair loss and maintaining existing hair.

Minoxidil. Minoxidil (ROGAINE, others), developed as an antihypertensive agent (*see* Chapter 27), was noted to be associated with hypertrichosis in some patients. Topical minoxidil is available as a 2% or 5% solution. Minoxidil enhances follicular size, resulting in thicker hair shafts, and stimulates and prolongs the anagen phase of the hair cycle, resulting in longer and increased numbers of hairs. Treatment must be continued or any drug-induced hair growth will be lost. Allergic and irritant contact dermatitis can occur, and care should be taken in applying the drug because hair growth may emerge in undesirable locations. This is reversible on stopping the drug. Patients should be instructed to wash their hands after applying minoxidil.

Finasteride. Finasteride (PROPECIA, other) inhibits the type II isozyme of 5α-reductase, the enzyme that converts testosterone to dihydrotestosterone (*see* Chapter 41) and that is found in hair follicles. Balding areas of the scalp are associated with increased dihydrotesterone levels and smaller hair follicles than nonbalding areas. Orally administered finasteride (1 mg/day) has been shown to variably increase hair growth in men over a 2-year period. Finasteride is approved for use only in men. Pregnant women should not be exposed to the drug because of the potential for inducing genital abnormalities in male fetuses. Adverse effects of finasteride include decreased libido, erectile dysfunction, ejaculation disorder, and decreased ejaculate volume. As with minoxidil, treatment with finasteride must be continued, or any new hair growth will be lost.

TREATMENT OF HYPERPIGMENTATION

These agents are most effective on hormonally or light-induced pigmentation within the epidermis. They have limited efficacy on post-inflammatory pigmentation within the dermis.

Hydroquinone. Hydroquinone (1,4-dihydrobenzene; TRI-LUMA) decreases melanocyte pigment production by inhibiting the conversion of dopa to melanin through inhibition of the enzyme tyrosinase. Other mechanisms include inhibition of DNA and RNA synthesis, degradation of melanosomes, and destruction of melanocytes. There are multiple formulations, to which penetration enhancers, microsponges, and sunscreen ingredients are added. Adverse effects may include dermatitis and ochronosis.

Monobenzone. Monobenzone (BENOQUIN), causes permanent hypopigmentation and should *not* be used for routine hormonally induced or post-inflammatory hyper-pigmentation.

Azelaic. Azelaic acid (AZELEX, FINACEA) inhibits tyrosinase activity but is less effective than hydroquinone. Because it has mild comedolytic, antimicrobial, and anti-inflammatory properties, it also is often used in acne and papulopustular rosacea.

Mequinol. Mequinol (4-hydroxyanisole, methoxyphenol, hydroquinone monomethyl ether, or p-hydroxyanisole) is a competitive inhibitor of tyrosinase. It is available as a 2% prescription product (SOLAGÉ) in combination with 0.01% tretinoin and vitamin C for skin lightening.

MISCELLANEOUS AGENTS

Capsaicin is an alkaloid derived from plants of the *Solanaceae* family (i.e., hot chili peppers). Capsaicin interacts with the transient receptor potential vanilloid (TRPV1) receptor on C-fiber sensory neurons. TRPV1 is a ligand-gated nonselective cation channel of the TRP family, modulated by a variety of noxious stimuli. Chronic exposure to capsaicin first stimulates and then desensitizes this channel to capsaicin and diverse other noxious stimuli. Capsaicin also causes local depletion of substance P, an endogenous neuropeptide involved in sensory perception and pain transmission. Capsaicin is available at various concentrations as a cream (ZOSTRIX, others), lotion (CAPSIN), gel, roll-on, and transdermal patch. Capsaicin is FDA-approved for the temporary relief of minor aches and pains associated with backache, strains, and arthritis, and is used for off-label treatment of postherpetic neuralgia and painful diabetic neuropathy.

Podophyllin, podophyllum resin, a mixture of chemicals from the plant *Podophyllum peltatum* (mandrake or May apple), contains podophyllotoxin (podofilox), which binds to microtubules and causes mitotic arrest in metaphase. Podophyllum resin (10-40%) is applied by a physician and left in place for no longer than 2-6 h weekly for the treatment of anogenital warts. Irritation and ulcerative local reactions are the major side effects. It should not be used in the mouth or during pregnancy. Podofilox is available as a 0.5% solution for home application 2 times daily for 3 consecutive days, repeated weekly as needed up to 4 cycles.

For a complete Bibliographical Listing see Goodman & Gilman's ***The Pharmacological Basis of Therapeutics***, 12th ed., or Goodman & Gilman Online at www.AccessMedicine.com.

Contraception and Pharmacotherapy of Obstetrical and Gynecological Disorders

Drugs to control fertility and treat disorders of the female reproductive organs collectively are among the most frequently prescribed agents in clinical practice. This chapter discusses a number of common clinical issues and their drug therapies that are central to women's health. The focus is on reproductive disorders and aspects of therapy rather than comprehensive coverage of the drugs themselves, which are described in more detail elsewhere (e.g., *see* Chapter 33 for prostaglandins; Chapter 38 for the gonadotropins, gonadotropin-releasing hormone [GnRH] agonists and antagonists, and oxytocin; Chapter 40 for estrogens and progestins; Section VII for antibiotics).

CONTRACEPTION

Contraception can be administered as planned prophylaxis or postcoitally for emergency contraception (i.e., high-dose estrogen-containing oral contraceptive pills, high-dose progestin pills, a progesterone antagonist, intrauterine devices). A progesterone antagonist also can be used to terminate an established pregnancy.

PLANNED CONTRACEPTION

COMBINATION ORAL CONTRACEPTIVES. Pills containing an estrogen and progestin are the most widely used (Table 66–1); they act primarily by suppressing the luteinizing hormone (LH) surge and thereby preventing ovulation. A wide variety of preparations are available for oral, transdermal, and vaginal administration (*see* Table 66–2 in the 12th edition of the parent text for a list of branded formulations, many of which are available as generics). Almost all contain *ethinyl estradiol* as the estrogen and a *17α-alkyl-19-nortestosterone* derivative as the progestin, and are administered for the first 21-24 days of a 28-day cycle.

MECHANISMS OF ACTION. Estrogen sensitizes the hypothalamus and pituitary gonadotropes to the feedback inhibitory effects of the progestin and minimizes breakthrough bleeding. The progestin exerts negative feedback, which suppresses the LH surge and thereby prevents ovulation, and protects against uterine cancer by opposing the proliferative effects of the estrogen on the uterine endometrium.

FORMULATIONS. Newer formulations offer effective contraception with improved activity profiles. They contain lower amounts of hormones to minimize adverse effects; some incorporate progestins with less androgenic activity (e.g., *gestodene*, *desogestrel*) or that antagonize the mineralocorticoid receptor and thereby reduce the tendency toward edema (e.g., *drospirenone*). Traditionally, combination oral contraceptives were packaged with 21 pills containing active hormone and 7 placebo tablets; each active pill contained a constant amount of the estrogen and progestin (i.e., a monophasic formulation). In an effort to maximize the antiovulatory effects and prevent breakthrough bleeding while minimizing total exposure to the hormones, some formulations provide active pills with 2 (biphasic) or 3 (triphasic) different amounts of 1 or both hormones to be used sequentially during each cycle.

"Extended-cycle" contraceptives extend the number of active pills per cycle and thus decrease the duration of menstrual bleeding. Two products contain 24 active pills with only 4 placebo tablets (e.g., YAZ [which contains drospirenone as the progestin] and LOESTRIN 24). Two products are packaged as 91-day packets, with 84 estrogen/progestin tablets and 7 placebo tablets (SEASONALE) or 7 tablets containing a lower dose of ethinyl estradiol alone (SEASONIQUE). Finally, LYBREL is provided in 28-day packets that contain only hormone pills and no placebo. All of these extended-cycle formulations appear to be comparable to the traditional products as contraceptives; aside from an increased frequency of breakthrough bleeding initially, no unexpected adverse effects have been observed.

A weekly transdermal contraceptive patch (ORTHO EVRA) releases ethinyl estradiol (20 μg/day) and norelgestromin (which is metabolized to norgestimate; 150 μg/day). In response to pharmacokinetic data suggesting that this patch provides higher estrogen exposure (AUC) than the low-dose oral contraceptive pills, the FDA added a black box advisory that notes this pharmacokinetic difference and warns of a potential increased risk of venous thromboembolism. Local reactions to the patch occur in ~5-15% of users and may be decreased by

Table 66–1

One-Year Failure Rate with Various Forms of Contraception

BIRTH CONTROL METHOD	FAILURE RATE (*Perfect Use*)	FAILURE RATE (*Typical Use*)
Combination oral contraceptive pills	0.3%	8%
Progestin-only minipill	0.5%	8%
DEPO-PROVERA	0.3%	3%
Copper intrauterine device	0.6%	0.8%
Progestin intrauterine device	0.2%	0.2%
IMPLANON	0.05%	0.05%
ORTHO EVRA	0.3%	8%
NUVARING	0.3%	8%
Condoms/diaphragms	2%	15%
Spermicides	18%	29%
Tubal ligation	0.5%	0.5%
Vasectomy	0.1%	0.15%
None	85%	85%

pre-application of a topical glucocorticoid. A vaginal ring (NUVARING) also is available that releases ethinyl estradiol (15 μg daily) and etonogestrel (an active metabolite of desogestrel; 120 μg daily). Each ring is used for 3 weeks, followed by a 1-week interval without the ring.

The combination estrogen/progestin formulations provide highly effective (~99%) contraception and also have a number of noncontraceptive benefits, including protection against certain cancers (e.g., ovarian, endometrial, colorectal), decreased iron-deficiency anemia secondary to menstrual blood loss, and decreased risk of fractures due to osteoporosis. Combination oral contraceptives also are widely used for conditions such as endometriosis, dysmenorrhea, menorrhagia, irregular menstrual cycles, premenstrual dysphoric disorder, acne, and hirsutism.

ADVERSE EFFECTS. Serious adverse effects of the combination estrogen/progestin contraceptive agents are relatively rare. Thromboembolic disease, largely due to the estrogenic component, is the most common serious side effect. Estrogen concentration, the patient's age, smoking, and inherited thrombophilias all influence the risk of developing thromboembolic disease. The impact of combination oral contraceptives on breast cancer has been highly debated; although a meta-analysis of epidemiological studies concluded that the combination oral contraceptives did increase the risk of breast cancer, studies conducted with the lower doses of hormones in current formulations suggest that the risk of breast cancer is not increased.

Other adverse effects include hypertension, edema, gallbladder disease, and elevations in serum triglycerides (*see* Chapter 40). With pills containing drospirenone, which antagonizes the mineralocorticoid receptor, serum K^+ should be monitored in women at risk for hyperkalemia (e.g., those on K^+-sparing diuretics or drugs that inhibit the renin–angiotensin system). The combination oral contraceptives are contraindicated in women with a history of thromboembolic disease, cerebrovascular disease, migraine headaches with aura, estrogen-dependent cancer, impaired hepatic function or active liver disease, undiagnosed uterine bleeding, and suspected pregnancy. Patients with a history of gestational diabetes should be monitored closely, and drug cessation should be strongly considered in anticipation of events associated with an increased risk of venous thromboembolism (e.g., elective surgery).

PROGESTIN-ONLY CONTRACEPTIVES. Progestin-only minipills contain derivatives of 17α-alkyl-19-nortestosterone but no estrogen. Although they do inhibit ovulation to some degree, their efficacy also reflects changes in the cervical mucus that inhibit fertilization and endometrial changes that inhibit implantation. They are slightly less effective than the combination estrogen/progestin formulations. Their major adverse effect is breakthrough bleeding.

Progestins also are used for long-acting contraception. A depot formulation of medroxyprogesterone (DEPO-PROVERA) injected subcutaneously or intramuscularly provides effective contraception for 3 months. Its use has been associated with decreased bone mineral density. Subdermal implants of progestin-impregnated rods provide effective contraception over several years. The only implant system currently approved in the U.S. is IMPLANON, which incorporates 3-ketodesogestrel, an active metabolite of desogestrel, into an inert matrix. An intrauterine device that releases levonorgestrel (MIRENA) provides highly effective contraception for up to 5 years. It acts predominantly to inhibit gamete function and survival via local changes in the cervical mucus.

POSTCOITAL CONTRACEPTION

Postcoital (or emergency) contraception is indicated for use in cases of mechanical failure of barrier devices or in circumstances of unprotected intercourse. It is not intended as a regular method of contraception. The mechanisms of action of the postcoital contraceptives are not fully understood.

PLAN-B one-step, which contains 2 tablets of the progestin levonorgestrel (0.75 mg each), is marketed specifically for postcoital contraception and may be obtained in the U.S. without a prescription by women ≥18 years of age. Treatment is most effective if the first dose is taken within 72 h of intercourse, followed by a second dose 12 h later; a single dose of 1.5 mg within 72 h of intercourse appears to be equally effective. Other options for postcoital contraception include mifepristone (MIFEPREX), which is not FDA-approved for this indication but is highly effective in oral doses ranging from 10-50 mg when taken within 5 days after unprotected intercourse, and copper intrauterine devices when inserted within 4 days of unprotected intercourse. Mifepristone also has abortifacient activity when used in a different treatment regimen. The selective progesterone receptor modulator ulipristal (ELLA, ELLAONE) was recently approved as an emergency contraceptive, effective up to 120 h after unprotected intercourse; *see* Chapter 40 for details.

PREGNANCY TERMINATION

If contraception is not used or fails, either *mifepristone* (RU-486, MIFEPREX) or *methotrexate* (50 mg/m^2 intramuscularly or orally) can be used to terminate an unwanted pregnancy in settings outside surgical centers. A prostaglandin then is administered to stimulate uterine contractions and expel the detached conceptus; in the U.S., prostaglandins used include dinoprostone (PGE_2; PROSTIN E2) administered vaginally or the PGE_1 analog misoprostol (CYTOTEC) given orally or vaginally, both of which are used off label for this purpose. Prostaglandins used in other countries include the PGE_2 analog sulprostone (NALADOR) and the PGE_1 analog gemeprost (CERVAGEM).

MIFEPRISTONE. Mifepristone is a 17α-alkyl-19-nortestosterone derivative that acts as a competitive antagonist at the progesterone receptor. Its actions are associated with focal hemorrhage and breakdown of the stromal extracellular matrix that ultimately leads to the breakdown of the uterine endometrium. In addition, mifepristone increases the sensitivity of the uterus to the uterotonic effects of prostaglandins. Mifepristone is metabolized through a series of reactions initiated by hepatic CYP3A4. Women receiving chronic glucocorticoid therapy should not be given mifepristone because of its anti-glucocorticoid activity, and the drug should be used cautiously in women who are anemic or receiving anticoagulants.

As approved by the FDA, mifepristone (600 mg) is taken for pregnancy termination within 49 days after the start of a woman's last menstrual period. The synthetic PGE_1 analog misoprostol (400 μg) is administered orally 48 h later; vaginal administration is at least as effective but is not FDA-approved. Complete abortion using this procedure exceeds 90%; when termination of pregnancy fails or is incomplete, surgical intervention is required. Repeated doses of misoprostol alone (e.g., 800 μg vaginally or sublingually every 3 h or every 12 h for 3 doses) also have been effective in settings where mifepristone is unavailable. Vaginal bleeding follows pregnancy termination and typically lasts from 1-2 weeks but rarely (in 0.1% of patients) is severe enough to require blood transfusion. A high percentage of women also experience abdominal pain and uterine cramps, nausea and vomiting, and diarrhea secondary to the prostaglandin. Because mifepristone carries a risk of serious, and sometimes fatal, infection and bleeding following its use for medical abortion, a black box warning has been added to the product labeling. Women receiving mifepristone should be informed of these risks and cautioned to seek immediate medical attention if symptoms or signs of these conditions occur. Fulminant septic shock associated with *Clostridium sordellii* infections may result and is attributable to the combined effects of uterine infection and inhibition of glucocorticoid action by mifepristone.

METHOTREXATE. Methotrexate is a potent abortifacient, probably as a result of the ability of the placenta to concentrate FH_2Glu_n (dihydrofolate polyglutamate) and its analogs (*see* Chapter 61).

DRUG THERAPY IN GYNECOLOGY

INDUCTION OF SEXUAL MATURATION

A number of clinical disorders, including Turner syndrome and other forms of gonadal dysgenesis, are associated with impaired production of ovarian steroids in phenotypic females. Such patients typically fail to develop secondary sexual characteristics at the normal time of puberty (sexual infantilism) or fail to have menses (primary amenorrhea). In these cases, steroid hormones are administered to induce development of the secondary sex characteristics; however, treatment is initiated only after the diagnosis is ascertained and underlying disorders that might respond to more specific therapy (e.g., prolactinomas) are excluded (*see* Chapter 38).

Types of estrogens used and the treatment regimens may vary by country or individual preference. Examples include conjugated estrogens, 0.3-1.25 mg; micronized 17β-estradiol, 0.5-2.0 mg; ethinyl estradiol, 5-20 μg; and transdermal 17β-estradiol, 25-50 μg. To achieve optimal breast development, treatment typically is initiated with a low dose of estrogen (e.g., conjugated estrogens at a starting dosage of 0.3 mg/day or ethinyl estradiol at 5 μg/day) starting in patients between ages 10 and 12 years or immediately if the diagnosis is made after this age. After 3-6 months, the dosage is increased (e.g., 0.9-1.25 mg/day of conjugated estrogens or 20 μg/day of ethinyl estradiol). Once this is achieved, a progestin (e.g., medroxyprogesterone, 10 mg/day, or micronized progesterone, 200-400 μg/day) for 12 days each cycle is added to the regimen to optimize breast development and permit cyclical menses, thereby avoiding endometrial hyperplasia and its consequent risk of uterine cancer. Once menses are established, many clinicians will switch to a standard low-dose oral contraceptive pill or even may use an extended-cycle formulation.

Short stature, a universal feature of non-mosaic Turner syndrome, usually is treated with human growth hormone, often together with an androgen such as oxandrolone (*see* Chapter 41). Initiating treatment with human growth hormone and androgen and delaying the onset of estrogen therapy generally produces a better growth response (*see* Chapter 38).

MENOPAUSE

Menopause refers to the permanent cessation of menstrual periods (i.e., for >12 months) resulting from the loss of ovarian follicular activity; it usually occurs when women are between 45 and 60 years of age.

The decline in estradiol levels produces a variety of symptoms and signs, including vasomotor disturbances (hot flashes or flushes), sweating, irritability, sleep disturbances, and atrophy of estrogen-dependent tissue. In addition, postmenopausal women are at increased risk for osteoporosis, bone fractures, and coronary heart disease and experience increased memory loss and other cognitive difficulties.

ESTROGEN THERAPY. The observed estrogen deficiency associated with menopause, as well as a number of studies showing positive effects of estrogen replacement therapy on these parameters, led to widespread use of hormone replacement therapy in peri- and postmenopausal women.

The initial publication of data from the Women's Health Initiative (WHI), a large, randomized, placebo-controlled trial, dramatically altered therapeutic approaches to menopause. As expected, treatment of postmenopausal women with 0.625 mg of conjugated estrogen plus 2.5 mg of medroxyprogesterone (in women with a uterus) or with 0.625 mg of conjugated estrogen alone (in women lacking a uterus) improved bone mineral density and decreased the risk of fractures and colorectal cancer. In addition, estrogen therapy in both the estrogen plus progestin and the estrogen-alone groups was associated with an increased incidence of deep venous thrombosis and stroke; and the incidence of breast cancer and coronary heart disease also increased in women receiving both estrogen and progestin. In women >65 years of age, hormone therapy did not improve cognitive function or protect against dementia. Based on these findings, it was recommended that hormone replacement therapy not be used to decrease the risk of coronary heart disease, cognitive impairment, or dementia. Subsequent subgroup analyses of the WHI data suggest that cardiovascular risk was not increased when hormone therapy was initiated within 10 years of menopause and that the risks of estrogen therapy may be minimal in women who are perimenopausal or recently menopausal.

Available routes of estrogen administration for hormone replacement therapy include oral, transdermal (patch, gel, and spray), and vaginal (cream, ring, and tablets) (*see* Table 66–3 of the 12th edition of the parent text). In women who have undergone hysterectomy, estrogen alone is used. For women with an intact uterus, a progestin also is administered to oppose the proliferative effect of the estrogen on the uterine endometrium.

Other therapies for vasomotor symptoms include phytoestrogens (e.g., soy products), herbal extracts (e.g., black cohosh), selective serotonin reuptake inhibitors (e.g., fluoxetine, controlled-release paroxetine, sertraline), clonidine, and gabapentin. However, hormone replacement remains the most effective therapy for vasomotor symptoms in menopausal women. Current recommendations advise using estrogen replacement at the lowest possible effective dose and for the shortest duration to treat moderate to severe vasomotor symptoms and vaginal dryness. For vaginal dryness alone, topical preparations are preferred.

ENDOMETRIOSIS

Endometriosis is an estrogen-dependent disorder that results from endometrial tissue ectopically located outside of the uterine cavity. It predominantly affects women during their reproductive years, with a prevalence of 0.5-5% in fertile women and 25-40% in infertile women. Diagnosis typically is made at laparoscopy, either prompted by unexplained pelvic pain (dysmenorrhea or dyspareunia) or infertility. The infertility is thought to reflect involvement of the fallopian tubes with the underlying process and, possibly, impaired oocyte maturation.

Because the proliferation of ectopic endometrial tissue is responsive to ovarian steroid hormones, many symptomatic approaches to therapy aim to produce a relatively hypoestrogenic state. Combination oral contraceptives have been standard first-line treatment for symptoms of endometriosis, and ample evidence from observational trials supports their benefit. The predominant mechanism of action is believed to be suppression of gonadotropin secretion, with subsequent inhibition of estrogen biosynthesis. Progestins (e.g., medroxyprogesterone, dienogest) also have been used to promote decidualization of the ectopic endometrial tissue. The levonorgestrel intrauterine system, which is approved for contraception, also has been used off label for this indication, as well as for menorrhagia.

Stable GnRH agonists can suppress gonadotropin secretion and thus effect medical castration. Drugs that carry an indication for endometriosis include leuprolide (LUPRON), goserelin (ZOLADEX), and nafarelin (SYNAREL); other GnRH agonists also may be used off label for this purpose (*see* Chapter 38). Due to significant decreases in bone density and symptoms of estrogen withdrawal, "add-back" therapy with either a low-dose synthetic estrogen (e.g., conjugated equine estrogens, 0.625-1.25 mg) or a high-dose progestin (e.g., norethindrone, 5 mg) has been used when the duration of therapy has exceeded 6 months. Danazol (DANOCRINE), a synthetic androgen that inhibits gonadotropin production via feedback inhibition of the pituitary-ovarian axis, also is FDA-approved for endometriosis therapy; it rarely is used now because of its significant adverse effects, including hirsutism and elevation of hepatic transaminases. In Europe and elsewhere, the antiprogestin gestrinone has been employed.

HIRSUTISM

Hirsutism, or increased hair growth in the male distribution, affects ~10% of women of reproductive age. It can be a relatively benign, idiopathic process or part of a more severe disorder of androgen excess that includes overt virilization (voice deepening, increased muscle mass, male pattern balding, clitoromegaly) and often results from ovarian or adrenal tumors. Specific etiologies associated with hirsutism include congenital adrenal hyperplasia, *polycystic ovary syndrome* (PCOS), and Cushing syndrome. After excluding serious pathology such as a steroid-producing malignancy, the treatment largely becomes empirical.

Pharmacotherapy is directed at decreasing androgen production and action. Initial therapy often involves treatment with combination oral contraceptive pills, which suppress gonadotropin secretion and thus the production of ovarian androgens. The estrogen also increases the concentration of sex hormone–binding globulin, thereby diminishing the free concentration of testosterone. The full effect of this suppression may take up to 6-9 months. GnRH agonists downregulate gonadotropin secretion and also may be used to suppress ovarian steroid production.

In patients who fail to respond to ovarian suppression, efforts to block androgen action may be effective. Spironolactone (ALDACTONE), a mineralocorticoid-receptor antagonist, and flutamide (EULEXIN; *see* Chapter 41) inhibit the androgen receptor. In Europe and elsewhere, cyproterone (50-100 mg/day) is used as an androgen-receptor blocker, often in conjunction with a combination oral contraceptive. Male offspring of women who become pregnant while taking any of these androgen inhibitors are at risk of impaired virilization secondary to impaired synthesis or action of dihydrotestosterone (Pregnancy Risk Category X, *see* Table 66–3). The antifungal ketoconazole (NIZORAL), which inhibits CYP steroid hydroxylases (*see* Chapters 42 and 57), also can block androgen biosynthesis but may cause liver toxicity. Topical eflornithine (VANIQA), an ornithine decarboxylase inhibitor, has been used with some success to decrease the rate of facial hair growth.

Non-pharmacological approaches include bleaching, depilatory treatments (e.g., shaving, treatment with hair-removing chemicals), or methods that remove the entire hair follicle (e.g., plucking, electrolysis, laser ablation).

INFECTIONS OF THE FEMALE REPRODUCTIVE TRACT

A variety of pathogens can cause infections of the female reproductive tract that range from vaginitis to pelvic inflammatory disease; Table 66–2 shows current recommendations for pharmacotherapy of selected sexually transmitted gynecological infections as issued by the Centers for Disease Control and Prevention.

The individual drugs used for systemic or topical therapy are described in more detail in Section VII. Infections have been implicated as important factors in preterm labor, as discussed further in "Prevention or Arrest of Preterm Labor."

Table 66–2

Sexually Transmitted Gynecological Infections and Recommended Therapies

Genital ulcers	
Chancroid	Azithromycin, 1 g oral single dose *or* Ceftriaxone, 250 mg IM single dose *or* Ciprofloxacin, 500 mg oral 2×/day × 3 days *or* Erythromycin base, 500 mg oral 3×/day × 7 days
Genital herpes	
First infection	Acyclovir, 400 mg oral 3×/day × 7-10 days *or* Acyclovir, 200 mg oral 5×/day for 7-10 days *or* Famciclovir, 250 mg oral 3×/day for 7-10 days *or* Valacyclovir, 1 g oral 2×/day × 7-10 days
Suppression	Acyclovir, 400 mg oral 2×/day *or* Famciclovir, 250 mg oral 2×/day *or* Valacyclovir, 500 mg oral once daily
Recurrent	Same drugs at lower dose for longer duration
Granuloma inguinale	Doxycycline, 100 mg oral 2×/day × >21 days
Lymphogranuloma venereum	Doxycycline, 100 mg oral 2×/day × 21 days
Syphilis	
Primary/secondary	Benzathine penicillin, 2.4 million units IM, single dose
Tertiary	Benzathine penicillin, 2.4 million units IM, 1/week ×3
Vaginal discharge	
Trichomonas	Metronidazole, 2 g oral single dose *or* Tinidazole, 2 g oral single dose
Bacterial vaginosis	Metronidazole, 500 mg oral 2×/day × 7 days *or* Metronidazole gel, 5 g intravaginally daily × 5 days *or* Clindamycin cream, 5 g intravaginally at bedtime × 7 days
Candida	Topical: Butoconazole, clotrimazole, miconazole, nystatin, tioconazole, terconazole Oral: Fluconazole, 150 mg oral, single dose
Urethritis/Cervicitis	
Non-gonococcal	Azithromycin, 1 g oral single dose *or* Doxycycline, 100 mg oral 2×/day × 7 days
Chlamydia	Azithromycin, 1 g oral single dose *or* Doxycycline, 100 mg oral × 7 days
Gonococcal	Ceftriaxone, 125 mg IM single dose *or* Cefixime, 400 mg oral single dose
Pelvic Inflammatory Disease	
Parenteral regimen	Cefotetan, 2 g IV every 12 h *or* Cefoxitin, 2 g IV every 6 h + Doxycycline, 100 mg oral or IV every 12 h × 14 days
Oral regimen	Ceftriaxone, 250 mg IM single dose + Doxycycline, 100 mg oral 2×/day × 14 days *or* Cefoxitin, 2 g IV single dose + Probenecid + Doxycycline, 100 mg oral 2×/day × 14 days

IM, intramuscularly; IV, intravenously.

FERTILITY INDUCTION

Infertility (i.e., the failure to conceive after 1 year of unprotected sex) affects 10-15% of couples in developed nations and is increasing in incidence as more women choose to delay childbearing until later in life. The major impediment to pregnancy in an infertile couple can be attributed primarily to the woman in approximately one-third, to the man in approximately one-third, and to both in approximately one-third. The likelihood of a successful pharmacological induction of fertility in these couples depends greatly on the reason for the infertility.

Defined abnormalities in the male partner that lead to impaired fertility (e.g., hypogonadism, Y chromosome microdeletions, Klinefelter syndrome) typically are detected by analysis of a semen sample; most often, male infertility is idiopathic. The medical therapy for some of these conditions is discussed in Chapters 38 and 41.

Anovulation accounts for ~50% of female infertility and is a major focus of pharmacological interventions used to achieve conception. Thus, whether a woman is ovulating is a key question. In infertile women who ovulate, analysis of the patency of the fallopian tubes and the structure of the uterus is an important part of the diagnostic evaluation. A number of approaches have been used to stimulate ovulation in anovulatory women. Often, a stepwise approach is taken, initially using simpler and less expensive treatments, followed by more complex and expensive regimens if initial therapy is unsuccessful. In obese patients with PCOS, the inclusion of lifestyle modifications directed at weight loss is warranted based on the association of obesity with anovulation, pregnancy loss, and complicated pregnancies (e.g., gestational diabetes, pre-eclampsia). Definitive evidence that weight loss improves fertility is not currently available.

CLOMIPHENE. Clomiphene citrate (CLOMID, SEROPHENE) is a potent anti-estrogen that primarily is used for treatment of anovulation in the setting of an intact hypothalamic—pituitary axis and adequate estrogen production (e.g., PCOS). By inhibiting the negative feedback effects of estrogen at hypothalamic and pituitary levels, clomiphene increases follicle-stimulating hormone (FSH) levels—typically by ~50%—and thereby enhances follicular maturation (*see* Chapter 40). A typical regimen is 50 mg/day orally for 5 consecutive days starting between days 2 and 5 of the cycle. If this regimen fails to induce ovulation, the dose of clomiphene is increased, first to the FDA-approved maximum of 100 mg/day and possibly as high as 150 or 200 mg/day. Although clomiphene is effective in inducing ovulation in perhaps 75% of women, successful pregnancy ensues in only 40-50% of those who ovulate.

Untoward effects of clomiphene include the ovarian hyperstimulation syndrome (OHSS) and increased incidences of multifetal gestations (twins in ~5-10% and more than 2 babies in ~0.3% of pregnancies), ovarian cysts, hot flashes, headaches, and blurred vision. A few studies have suggested that prolonged use (e.g., ≥12 cycles) may increase the risk of ovarian and endometrial cancer; thus, the recommended maximum number of cycles is 6. Clomiphene should not be administered to pregnant women (FDA Category X).

Tamoxifen may be as effective as clomiphene for ovulation induction but is not FDA-approved for this indication.

GONADOTROPINS. The preparations of gonadotropins available for clinical use are detailed in Chapter 38. Gonadotropins are indicated for ovulation induction in anovulatory women with *hypogonadotropic hypogonadism* secondary to hypothalamic or pituitary dysfunction, and also are used to induce ovulation in women with PCOS who do not respond to clomiphene. Figure 66–1 shows a typical regimen for ovulation induction. Gonadotropin-induced ovulation results in multiple births in up to 10-20% of cases due to the pharmacologically induced development of more than 1 pre-ovulatory follicle and the release of more than 1 ovum.

Gonadotropin induction also is used for ovarian stimulation in conjunction with in vitro fertilization (IVF; *see* Figure 66–1). In this setting, larger doses of FSH (typically 225-300 IU/day) are administered to induce the maturation of multiple (ideally at least 5 and up to 20) oocytes that can be retrieved for IVF and intrauterine transfer. To prevent the LH surge and subsequent premature luteinization of the ovarian follicles, gonadotropins typically are administered in conjunction with a GnRH agonist.

GnRH antagonists also can be used to inhibit endogenous LH secretion. Because they do not transiently increase gonadotropin secretion, they can be initiated later in the cycle in a "short protocol." Current regimens include daily injection in a dose of 0.25 mg (ganirelix [ANTAGON] or cetrorelix [CETROTIDE]) starting on the fifth or sixth day of gonadotropin stimulation or a single dose of 3 mg of cetrorelix administered on day 8 or 9 of the late follicular phase. Using either the long or short protocols, hCG (at typical doses of 5000-10,000 IU of urine-derived product or 250 μg of recombinant hCG) is given to induce final oocyte development, and the mature eggs are retrieved from the pre-ovulatory follicles at 32-36 h thereafter. The retrieved ova are fertilized in vitro with sperm (IVF) or by intracytoplasmic sperm injection; 1 or 2 embryos then are transferred to the uterus 3-5 days after fertilization.

Repeated injections of hCG, while sustaining the corpus luteum, may increase the risk of OHSS. Thus, standard IVF regimens typically provide exogenous progesterone replacement to support the fetus until the placenta acquires the biosynthetic capacity to take over this function; regimens include progesterone in oil (50-100 mg/day intramuscularly) or micronized progesterone (180-300 mg twice daily vaginally). Vaginal preparations containing 100 mg (ENDOMETRIN) or 90 mg (PROCHIEVE, CRINONE) of micronized progesterone are approved for administration 2 or 3 times daily as part of IVF and other fertility technologies.

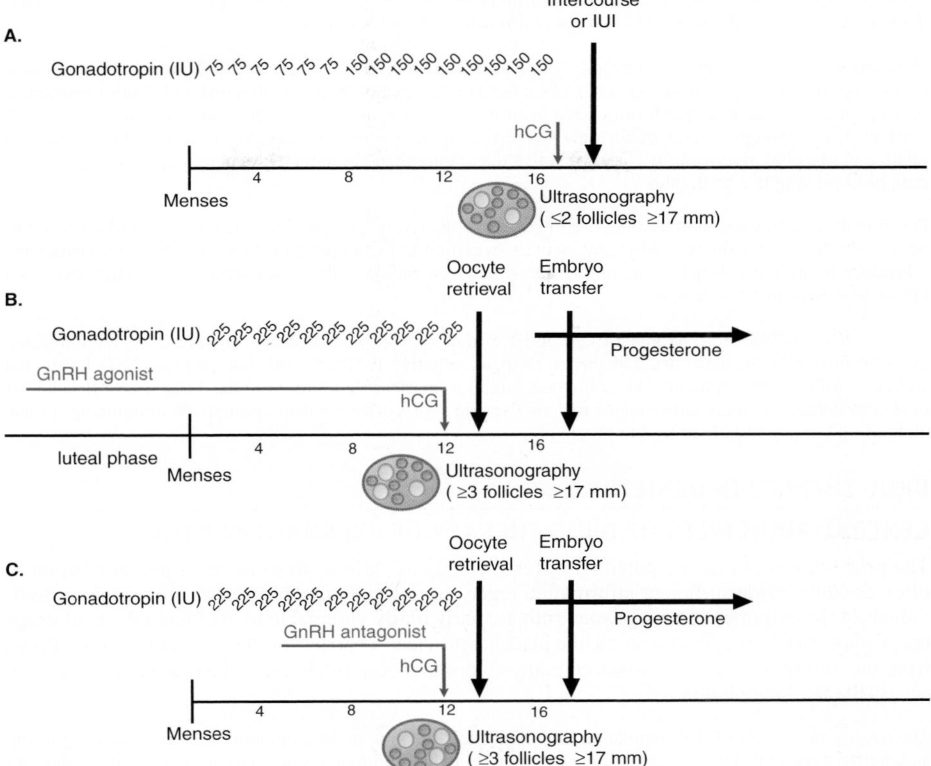

Figure 66–1 *Idealized regimens using exogenous gonadotropins for fertility induction.* **A.** *Step-up regimen for ovulation induction.* After menses, daily injections of gonadotropin (75 IU) are started. Follicle maturation is assessed by serial measurement of plasma estradiol and follicle size, as discussed in the text. If an inadequate response is seen, the dose of gonadotropin is increased to 112 or 150 IU/day. When 1 or 2 follicles have achieved a size of ≥17 mm in diameter, final follicle maturation and ovulation are induced by injection of human chorionic gonadotropin (hCG). Fertilization then is achieved at 36 h after hCG injection by intercourse or intrauterine insemination (IUI). If more than 2 mature follicles are seen, the cycle is terminated and barrier contraception is used to avoid triplets or higher degrees of multifetal gestation. **B.** *Long protocol for ovarian hyperstimulation using gonadotropin-releasing hormone (GnRH) agonist to inhibit premature ovulation, followed by in vitro fertilization (IVF).* After the GnRH agonist has inhibited endogenous secretion of gonadotropins, therapy with exogenous gonadotropins is initiated. Follicle maturation is assessed by serial measurements of plasma estradiol and follicle size by ultrasonography. When 3 or more follicles are ≥17 mm in diameter, then ovulation is induced by injection of hCG. At 32-36 h after the hCG injection, the eggs are retrieved and used for IVF. Exogenous progesterone is provided to promote a receptive endometrium, followed by embryo transfer at 3-5 days after fertilization. **C.** *Protocol for ovarian hyperstimulation in an IVF protocol using a GnRH antagonist.* The cycle duration is shorter because the GnRH antagonist does not induce a transient flare of gonadotropin secretion that might disrupt the timing of the cycle, but many other elements of the cycle are analogous to those in **B.** IU, intrauterine.

Aside from the attendant complications of multifetal gestation, the major side effect of gonadotropin treatment is OHSS. Symptoms and signs include abdominal pain and/or distention, nausea and vomiting, diarrhea, dyspnea, oliguria, and marked ovarian enlargement on ultrasonography. OHSS can lead to hypovolemia, electrolyte abnormalities, acute respiratory distress syndrome, thromboembolic events, and hepatic dysfunction. In ovulation induction, incipient OHSS should be suspected if routine laboratory investigation reveals the presence of more than 4 to 6 follicles >17 mm or a serum estradiol level of >1500 pg/mL; in this setting, hCG should be withheld and barrier contraception used. In an effort to avoid overt hyperstimulation, the FSH can be withheld for a day or 2 ("coasting") if the plasma level of estradiol is near the top of this range. In either case, ovulation induction with recombinant LH, which has a considerably shorter $t_{1/2}$ than hCG, or with a GnRH agonist may diminish the incidence of OHSS. The potential deleterious effects of gonadotropins are debated. There is no evidence that the gonadotropins themselves or components of the IVF process increase the rate of congenital abnormalities in babies born from stimulated oocytes.

INSULIN SENSITIZERS. PCOS affects 4-7% of women of reproductive age and is the most frequent cause of anovulatory infertility. Inasmuch as PCOS patients often exhibit hyperinsulinemia and insulin resistance, insulin sensitizers such as metformin have been evaluated for their effects on ovulation and fertility (*see* Chapter 43). Although several small trials suggested that metformin increased ovulation in PCOS patients relative to placebo; metformin was less effective than clomiphene in inducing ovulation, promoting conception, or improving live birth rates.

Preliminary results suggested that the use of rosiglitazone (AVANDIA), pioglitazone (ACTOS), and other members of the thiazolidinedione family may increase ovulation in PCOS patients; however, there is considerable reluctance to use these drugs in this setting given their association with an increased risk of congestive heart failure and myocardial ischemia.

AROMATASE INHIBITORS. Aromatase are under evaluation as potential drugs for infertility. By inhibiting estrogen biosynthesis, these drugs decrease estrogen negative feedback and thus increase FSH levels and stimulate follicle development. The aromatase inhibitor anastrozole (ARIMIDEX) has been used off label for ovulation induction. Some data suggest that anastrozole is less effective than clomiphene in inducing follicle maturation but more likely to lead to pregnancy.

DRUG THERAPY IN OBSTETRICS

GENERAL PRINCIPLES OF DRUG THERAPY OF PREGNANT WOMEN

The processes of evaluating potential adverse effects of various drugs as described in Chapter 1, often do not provide sufficient information regarding safety in pregnant women or children. Individuals at the extremes of the age spectrum are particularly vulnerable to the toxic effects of drugs (*see* Chapter 4). In pregnant women, the placenta provides a barrier for the transfer of certain drugs from the mother to the fetus; however, many compounds can freely cross the placental barrier and access the fetal circulation.

The teratogenic effects of thalidomide on limb formation, alcohol on development of the CNS and cognition, and diethylstilbestrol (DES) on genital development in males and females are stark reminders of the dangers of fetal exposure to drugs.

PRECAUTIONS AND RECOMMENDATIONS. Based on the relative paucity of human data on the teratogenic effects of drugs and the limited reliability of animal models, a fundamental tenet in treating pregnant women is to minimize, whenever possible, the exposure of mother and fetus to drugs. Of equal importance, substances of abuse (e.g., cigarettes, alcohol, illegal drugs) should be avoided and, whenever possible, eliminated before conception. In addition, all pregnant women should take a multivitamin containing 400 μg of folic acid daily to diminish the incidence of neural tube defects.

The greatest concern is during the period of organogenesis in the first trimester, when a number of the most vulnerable tissues are formed. Cancer chemotherapy drugs cannot be given with reasonable safety during the first trimester, but most cytotoxics may be administered without teratogenic effects and with maintenance of pregnancy in the third trimester (*see* Chapters 61-63). Drugs that are used to promote fertility are a special case, since they, by nature of their use, will be present in the mother at the time of conception.

USE-IN-PREGNANCY LISTING OF DRUGS. The FDA assigns different levels of risk to drugs for use in pregnant women, as listed in Table 66–3.

Certain drugs are so toxic to the developing fetus that they must never be administered to a pregnant woman (Category X); in some cases (e.g., thalidomide, retinoids), the potential for fetal harm is so great that multiple forms of effective contraception must be in place before the drug is initiated. For other drugs, the risk of adverse effects on the fetus may range from Category A (drugs that have not been proven to have adverse effects on the fetus despite adequate investigation) to Category D (drugs with risks that sometimes may be justified based on the severity of the underlying condition; see "Pregnancy-Induced Hypertension/Pre-eclampsia" and "Tocolytic Therapy for Established Preterm Labor"). Unfortunately, the FDA listings may be overly simplistic or outdated for a given drug; for example, oral contraceptives are listed as Category X, even though considerable data now indicate that birth defects are not increased in women taking oral contraceptives at the time of conception.

Nursing mothers constitute a second special situation with respect to potential adverse effects of drugs. Some drugs may interfere with milk production and/or secretion (e.g., estrogen-containing oral contraceptives) and

Table 66–3

FDA Use-in-Pregnancy Ratings

Category A: Controlled studies show no risk. Adequate, well-controlled studies in pregnant women have failed to demonstrate a risk to the fetus in any trimester of pregnancy.
Category B: No evidence of risk in humans. Adequate, well-controlled studies in pregnant women have not shown an increased risk of fetal abnormalities despite adverse findings in animals, or, in the absence of adequate human studies, animal studies show no fetal risk. The chance of fetal harm is remote, but remains a possibility.
Category C: Risk cannot be ruled out. Adequate, well-controlled human studies are lacking, and animal studies have shown a risk to the fetus or are lacking as well. There is a chance of fetal harm if the drug is administered during pregnancy, but the potential benefits may outweigh the potential risk.
Category D: Positive evidence of risk. Studies in humans, or investigational or post-marketing data, have demonstrated fetal risk. Nevertheless, potential benefits from the use of the drug may outweigh the potential risk. For example, the drug may be acceptable if needed in a life-threatening situation or serious disease for which safer drugs cannot be used or are ineffective.
Category X: Contraindicated in pregnancy. Studies in animals or humans, or investigational or post-marketing reports, have demonstrated positive evidence of fetal abnormalities or risk that clearly outweighs any possible benefit to the patient.

thus should be avoided if possible in mothers who wish to breast-feed. Other drugs may be secreted into breast milk and expose the baby to potentially toxic levels during the vulnerable perinatal period.

PREGNANCY-INDUCED HYPERTENSION/PRE-ECLAMPSIA

Hypertension affects up to 10% of pregnant women in the U.S.

Hypertension that precedes pregnancy or manifests before 20 weeks of gestation is believed to overlap considerably in pathogenesis with essential hypertension. These patients appear to be at increased risk for gestational diabetes and need careful monitoring. In contrast, pregnancy-induced hypertension, or pre-eclampsia, generally presents after 20 weeks of gestation as a new-onset hypertension with proteinuria (>300 mg of urinary protein/24 h); pre-eclampsia is thought to involve placenta-derived factors that affect vascular integrity and endothelial function in the mother, thus causing peripheral edema, renal and hepatic dysfunction, and in severe cases, seizures. Chronic hypertension is an established risk factor for pre-eclampsia. The consensus panel recommended initiation of drug therapy in women with a diastolic blood pressure >105 mm Hg or a systolic blood pressure >160 mm Hg. If severe pre-eclampsia ensues, with marked hypertension and evidence of end-organ damage, then termination of the pregnancy by delivery of the baby is the treatment of choice, provided that the fetus is sufficiently mature to survive outside the uterus. If the baby is very preterm, then hospitalization and pharmacotherapy may be employed in an effort to permit further fetal maturation in utero.

Several drugs commonly used for hypertension in non-pregnant patients (e.g., angiotensin-converting enzyme inhibitors, angiotensin-receptor antagonists) should not be used in pregnant women due to unequivocal evidence of adverse fetal effects. Many experts will convert the patient to the centrally acting α adrenergic agonist α-methyldopa (ALDOMET; 250 mg twice daily) (FDA Category B), which rarely is used for hypertension in non-pregnant patients. Other drugs with reasonable evidence of safety (Category C) also may be used, including the combination α_1-selective, β-nonselective adrenergic antagonist labetalol (TRANDATE; 100 mg twice daily) and the Ca^{2+} channel blocker nifedipine (PROCARDIA XL, ADALAT CC; 30 mg once daily).

If severe pre-eclampsia or impending labor requires hospitalization, blood pressure can be controlled acutely with hydralazine (5 or 10 mg intravenously or intramuscularly, with repeated dosing at 20-min intervals depending on blood pressure response) or labetalol (20 mg intravenously, with dose escalation to 40 mg at 10 min if blood pressure control is inadequate). In addition to receiving drugs for blood pressure control, women with severe pre-eclampsia or who have CNS manifestations (e.g., headache, visual disturbance, or altered mental status) are treated as inpatients with magnesium sulfate, based on its documented efficacy in seizure prevention and lack of adverse effects on the mother or baby. Such treatment also should be considered for postpartum women with CNS manifestations: ~20% of episodes of eclampsia occur in women more than 48 h post-delivery.

PREVENTION OR ARREST OF PRETERM LABOR

Preterm birth, defined as delivery before 37 weeks of gestation, occurs in >10% of pregnancies in the U.S., is increasing in frequency, and is associated with significant complications, such as neonatal respiratory distress syndrome, pulmonary hypertension, and intracranial hemorrhage. Risk factors for preterm labor include multifetal gestation, premature rupture of the membranes, intrauterine infection, and placental insufficiency. The more premature the baby, the greater the risk of complications, prompting efforts to prevent or interrupt preterm labor.

The therapeutic objective in preterm labor is to delay delivery so that the mother can be transported to a regional facility specializing in the care of premature babies and supportive agents can be administered, such as glucocorticoids to stimulate fetal lung maturation (*see* Chapter 42) and antibiotics (e.g., erythromycin, ampicillin) to diminish the frequency of neonatal infection with group B β-hemolytic *Streptococcus*. Due to concerns over deleterious effects of antibiotic therapy, antibiotics must not be administered indiscriminately to all women thought to have preterm labor, but rather be reserved for those with premature rupture of the membranes and evidence of infection.

PREVENTION OF PRETERM LABOR: PROGESTERONE THERAPY. Progesterone levels diminish considerably in association with labor, whereas administration of progesterone inhibits the secretion of pro-inflammatory cytokines and delays cervical ripening. Although progesterone and its derivatives have long been advocated to diminish the onset of preterm labor, results from clinical trials have been controversial and the role of progesterone prophylaxis during pregnancy remains to be established.

TOCOLYTIC THERAPY FOR ESTABLISHED PRETERM LABOR. Inhibition of uterine contractions of preterm labor, or *tocolysis*, has been a focus of therapy. Although tocolytic agents delay delivery in ~80% of women, they neither prevent premature births nor improve adverse fetal outcomes such as respiratory distress syndrome. Specific tocolytic agents include β adrenergic receptor agonists, $MgSO_4$, Ca^{2+} channel blockers, COX inhibitors, oxytocin-receptor antagonists, and NO donors (Figure 66–2).

Based on the role of prostaglandins in uterine contraction, COX inhibitors (e.g., *indomethacin*) have been used to inhibit preterm labor. Because they also can inhibit platelet function and induce closure in utero of the ductus arteriosus, these inhibitors should not be employed in term pregnancies (or in pregnancies beyond 32 weeks of gestation). Atosiban (TRACTOCILE), a nonapeptide analog of oxytocin, competitively inhibits the interaction of oxytocin with its membrane receptor on uterine cells and thereby decreases the frequency of uterine contractions. Atosiban is widely used in Europe, but is not FDA-approved in the U.S. Despite numerous clinical trials, the superiority of any one therapy has not been established, and none of the drugs has been shown definitively to improve fetal outcome. Ca^{2+} channel blockers and atosiban (not available in the U.S.) appear to provide the best balance of successfully delayed delivery with lesser risks to the mother and baby.

INITIATION OF LABOR

Labor induction is indicated when the perceived risk of continued pregnancy to the mother or fetus exceeds the risks of delivery or pharmacological induction. Such circumstances include premature rupture of the membranes, isoimmunization, fetal growth restriction, uteroplacental insufficiency (as in diabetes, pre-eclampsia, or eclampsia), and gestation beyond 42 weeks.

PROSTAGLANDINS AND CERVICAL RIPENING. Prostaglandins play key roles in parturition (*see* Chapter 33). Thus, PGE_1, PGE_2, and PGF_{2a} are used to facilitate labor by promoting ripening and dilation of the cervix. They can be administered either orally or via local administration (either vaginally or intracervically). The ability of certain prostaglandins to stimulate uterine contractions also makes them valuable agents in the therapy of postpartum hemorrhage.

Available preparations include dinoprostone (PGE_2), used to facilitate cervical ripening. Dinoprostone is formulated as a gel for intracervical administration via syringe in a dose of 0.5 mg (PREPIDIL) or as a vaginal insert (pessary) in a dose of 10 mg (CERVIDIL); the latter is designed to release active PGE_2 at a rate of 0.3 mg/hr for up to 12 h. Dinoprostone should not be used in women with a history of asthma, glaucoma, or myocardial infarction. The major adverse effect is uterine hyperstimulation.

Misoprostol (CYTOTEC), a synthetic derivative of PGE_1, is used off label either orally or vaginally to induce cervical ripening; typical doses are 100 μg (orally) or 25 μg (vaginally); an advantage of misoprostol in this setting is its considerably lower cost. Adverse effects include uterine hyperstimulation and, rarely, uterine rupture. Misoprostol should be discontinued for at least 3 h before initiating oxytocin therapy.

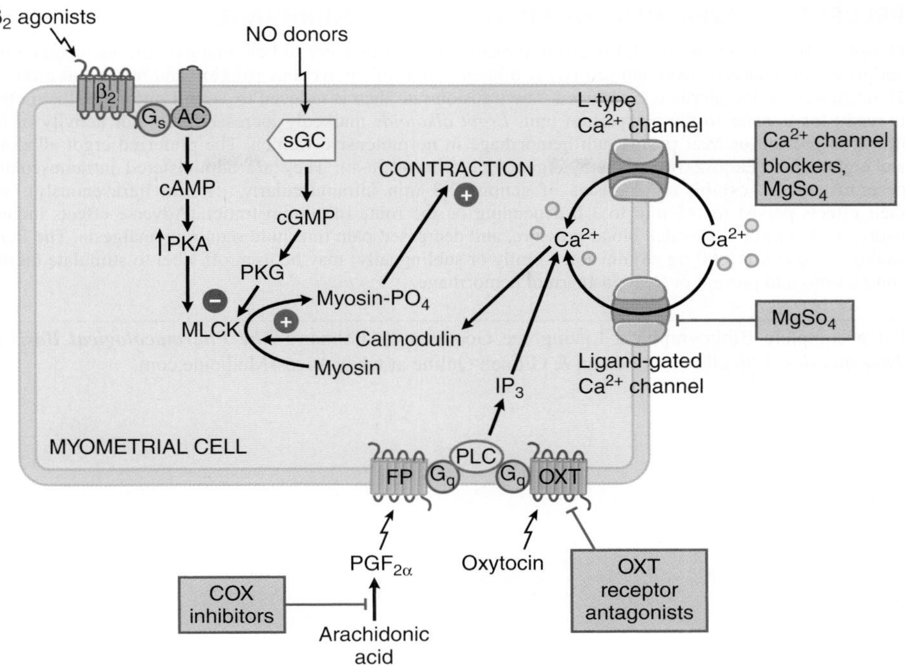

Figure 66–2 *Sites of action of tocolytic drugs in the uterine myometrium.* The elevation of cellular Ca^{2+} promotes contraction via the Ca^{2+}/calmodulin-dependent activation of myosin light chain kinase (MLCK). Relaxation is promoted by the elevation of cyclic nucleotides (cAMP and cGMP) and their activation of protein kinases, which cause phosphorylation/inactivation of MLCK. Pharmacological manipulations to reduce myometrial contraction include:

- Inhibiting Ca^{2+} entry (Ca^{2+} channel blockers, Mg_2SO_4)
- Reducing mobilization of intracellular Ca^{2+} by antagonizing GPCR-mediated activation of the G_q-PLC-IP_3-Ca^{2+} pathway (with antagonists of the FP and OXT receptors) or reducing production of the FP agonist, $PGF_{2\alpha}$ (with COX inhibitors)
- Enhancing relaxation by elevating cellular cyclic AMP (with β_2 adrenergic agonists that activate G_s-AC) and cyclic GMP (with NO donors that stimulate soluble guanylyl cyclase)

AC, adenylyl cyclase; COX, cyclooxygenase; FP, the $PGF_{2\alpha}$ receptor; OXT, the oxytocin receptor; PLC, phospholipase C; sGC, soluble guanylyl cyclase.

OXYTOCIN. The structure and physiology of oxytocin are discussed in Chapter 38. The obstetrical uses of oxytocin include the induction of labor, the augmentation of labor that is not progressing, and the prophylaxis and/or treatment of postpartum hemorrhage. Although widely used, oxytocin recently was added to a list of drugs "bearing a heightened risk of harm."

Labor Induction. Oxytocin (PITOCIN, SYNTOCINON) is the drug of choice for labor induction. It is administered by intravenous infusion of a diluted solution preferably via an infusion pump. Current protocols start with an oxytocin dose of 6 mIU/min, that is increased as needed, up to 40 mIU/min. Uterine hyperstimulation should be avoided. Because the $t_{1/2}$ of intravenous oxytocin is relatively short (12-15 min), the hyperstimulatory effects of oxytocin will dissipate fairly rapidly after the infusion is discontinued. Oxytocin at higher doses activates the vasopressin V_2 receptor and has antidiuretic effects. Vasodilating actions of oxytocin also have been noted that may provoke hypotension and reflex tachycardia. Deep anesthesia may exaggerate the hypotensive effect of oxytocin by preventing the reflex tachycardia.

Augmentation of Dysfunctional Labor. Oxytocin also is used when spontaneous labor is not progressing at an acceptable rate. To augment hypotonic contractions, an infusion rate of 10 mIU/min typically is sufficient. As with labor induction, potential complications of uterine overstimulation include trauma of the mother or fetus due to forced passage through an incompletely dilated cervix, uterine rupture, and compromised fetal oxygenation due to decreased uterine perfusion.

PREVENTION/TREATMENT OF POSTPARTUM HEMORRHAGE

Oxytocin (10 IU intramuscularly) is given immediately after delivery to help maintain uterine contractions and tone. Alternatively, oxytocin (20 IU) is diluted in 1 L of intravenous solution and infused at a rate of 10 mL/min until the uterus is contracted. The infusion rate then is reduced to 1-2 mL/min until the mother is ready for transfer to the postpartum unit. *Ergot alkaloids* markedly increase the motor activity of the uterus to prevent or treat postpartum hemorrhage in normotensive women. The preferred ergot alkaloids are ergonovine (ERGOTRATE) or methylergonovine (METHERGINE). They are administered intramuscularly or intravenously, exhibit rapid onsets of action (2-3 min intramuscularly, <1 min intravenously), and their effects persist for 45 min to 3 h depending on the route of administration. Adverse effects include nausea and vomiting, elevated blood pressure, and decreased pain threshold requiring analgesia. The PGE_1 analog *misoprostol* (600 μg administered orally or sublingually) may be used off label to stimulate uterine contractions and prevent or treat postpartum hemorrhage.

For a complete Bibliographical Listing see Goodman & Gilman's ***The Pharmacological Basis of Therapeutics***, 12th ed., or Goodman & Gilman Online at www.AccessMedicine.com.

Environmental Toxicology: Carcinogens and Heavy Metals

Myriad authoritative textbooks are available in the area of environmental toxicology. This chapter does not attempt a thorough coverage; rather, it sets forth a few basic principles, briefly discusses carcinogens and chemoprevention, and then focuses on the pharmacotherapy of heavy metal intoxication.

ASSESSMENT AND MANAGEMENT OF ENVIRONMENTAL RISK

When assessing the risks of environmental exposures to xenobiotics, one must consider population exposures to low-dose toxicants over long periods of time. Thus, one must give careful attention to the low end of the dose-response curve, using experiments based on chronic exposures. Unlike drugs, which are given to treat a specific disease and should have benefits that outweigh the risks, environmental toxicants usually are only harmful. In addition, exposures to environmental toxicants usually are involuntary, there is uncertainty about the severity of their effects, and people are much less willing to accept their associated risks.

Epidemiology and *toxicology* are 2 approaches used to predict the toxic effects of environmental exposures. Epidemiologists monitor health effects in humans and use statistics to associate those effects with exposure to an environmental stress, such as a toxicant. Toxicologists perform laboratory studies to try to understand the potential toxic mechanisms of a chemical to predict whether it is likely to be toxic to humans. Information from both approaches is integrated into *environmental risk assessment*. Risk assessment is used to develop laws and regulations to limit exposures to environmental toxicants to a level that is considered safe.

EPIDEMIOLOGICAL APPROACHES TO RISK ASSESSMENT

Assessing human exposures over long periods of time and drawing conclusions about the health effects of a single toxicant present great challenges. Epidemiologists usefully rely on biomarkers in assessing risk. There are 3 types of biomarkers:

- *Biomarkers of exposure* usually are measurements of toxicants or their metabolites in blood, urine, or hair. Blood and urine concentrations measure recent exposures, while hair levels measure exposure over a period of months. An example of an unusual exposure biomarker is X-ray fluorescent measurement of bone lead levels, which estimates lifetime exposure to lead.
- *Biomarkers of toxicity* are used to measure toxic effects at a subclinical level and include measurement of liver enzymes in the serum, changes in the quantity or contents of urine, and performance on specialized exams for neurological or cognitive function.
- *Biomarkers of susceptibility* are used to predict which individuals are likely to develop toxicity in response to a given chemical. Examples include single nucleotide polymorphisms in genes for metabolizing enzymes involved in the activation or detoxification of a toxicant. Some biomarkers simultaneously provide information on exposure, toxicity, and susceptibility. For example, the measurement in the urine of N7-guanine adducts from aflatoxin B_1 provides evidence of both exposure and a toxic effect (in this case, DNA damage). Such biomarkers are valuable because they can support a proposed mechanism of toxicity.

Several types of epidemiological studies are used to assess risks, each with its own set of strengths and weaknesses. *Ecological studies* correlate frequencies of exposures and health outcomes between different geographical regions. These studies can detect rare outcomes but are prone to confounding variables, including population migration. *Cross-sectional studies* examine the prevalence of exposures and outcomes at a single point in time. Such studies determine an association but do not provide a temporal relationship and are not effective for establishing causality. *Case-control studies* start with a group of individuals affected by a disease, which then is matched to another group of unaffected individuals for known confounding variables. Questionnaires often are used to evaluate past exposures. This method also is good for examining rare outcomes because the endpoint is known. However, case-control studies rely on assessments of past exposures that often are unreliable and can be subject to bias. *Prospective cohort studies* measure exposures in a large group of people and follow that group for a long time to measure health outcomes. These studies are good at establishing causality, but they are extremely expensive, particularly when measuring very rare outcomes, because a large study population is required to observe sufficient disease to obtain statistical significance. One of the key types of human studies used in drug development is the randomized clinical trial (*see* Chapter 1). Such studies cannot be used to directly measure the effects of environmental toxicants (for obvious ethical reasons) but can be used to examine the effectiveness of an interventional strategy for reducing both exposure to toxicants and disease.

TOXICOLOGICAL APPROACHES TO RISK ASSESSMENT

Toxicologists use model systems, including experimental animals, to examine the toxicity of chemicals and predict their effect on humans. The significance of these model systems to human health is not always established. Toxicologists also test chemicals at the high end of the dose-response curve in order to see enough occurrences of an outcome to obtain statistical significance. As a result, there often is uncertainty about the effects of very low doses of chemicals. To determine the applicability of model studies, toxicologists study the mechanisms involved in the toxic effects of chemicals.

To predict the toxic effects of environmental chemicals, toxicologists perform subchronic (3 months of treatment for rodents) and chronic studies (2 years for rodents) in at least 2 different animal models. Subchronic experiments provide a model for occupational exposures, while chronic experiments are used to predict effects from lifetime exposures to chemicals in food or the environment. Doses are chosen with the goal of having 1 concentration that does not have a significant effect, 1 concentration that results in statistically significant toxicity at the low end of the dose-response curve, and 1 or more concentrations that will have moderate-to-high levels of toxicity. A theoretical dose-response curve for an animal study is shown in Figure 67–1. An animal study provides 2 numbers that estimate the risk from a chemical. The *no observed adverse effect level* (NOAEL) is the highest dose used that does not result in a statistically significant increase in negative health outcomes. The *lowest observed adverse effect level* (LOAEL) is the lowest dose that results in a significant increase in toxicity. The NOAEL is divided by 10 for each source of uncertainty to determine a reference dose (RfD), which is commonly used as a starting point for determining regulations on human exposures to chemicals. The modifiers used to determine the RfD are based on the uncertainties between the experimental

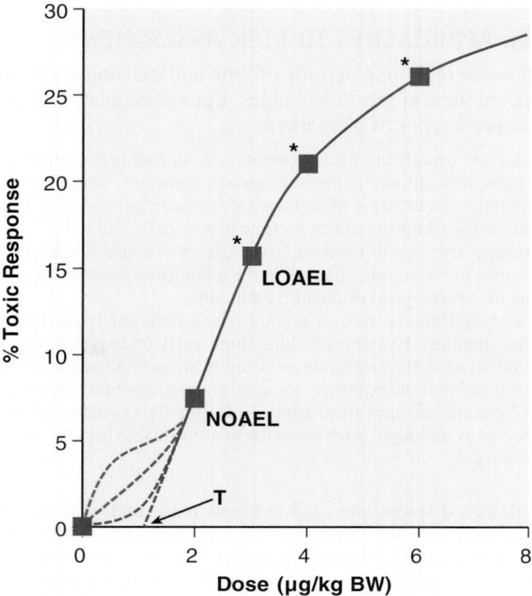

Figure 67–1 *LOAEL and NOAEL.* The theoretical dose-response curve from an animal study demonstrates the *no observed adverse effect level* (NOAEL) and the *lowest observed adverse effect level* (LOAEL). Below the NOAEL level, there is considerable uncertainty as to the shape of the response curve. It could continue linearly to reach a threshold dose (T) where there would be no harmful effects from the toxicant, or it could have a number of different possible inflection points. Each of these curves would reflect very different effects on human populations. *, statistically significant; BW, body weight.

and human exposure. The most common modifiers used are for interspecies variability (human to animal) and interindividual variability (human to human), in which case RfD = NOAEL/100. When a NOAEL is unavailable, a LOAEL may be used, in which case another 10-fold uncertainty factor is used. The use of factors of 10 in the denominator for determination of RfD is an application of the "precautionary principle," which attempts to limit human exposure by assuming a worst-case scenario for each unknown variable. Animal studies typically are designed to obtain statistical significance with a 10% increase in an outcome. As a result, there is considerable uncertainty about what occurs below that level, as demonstrated in Figure 67–1. Toxicologists often assume that there is a threshold dose (T), below which there is no toxicity. However, many carcinogens and other toxicants with specific molecular targets (e.g., lead) do not exhibit a threshold. Ideally, mechanistic studies should be done to predict which dose-response curve is most likely to fit a given chemical.

Toxicologists perform a variety of mechanistic studies to understand how a chemical might cause toxicity. Computer modeling using a compound's 3-dimensional structure to determine quantitative structure-activity relationships (QSARs) is commonly performed on both drugs and environmental chemicals. QSAR approaches can determine which chemicals are likely to exhibit toxicities or bind to specific molecular targets. Cell-based approaches in prokaryotes and eukaryotes are used to determine whether a compound damages DNA or causes cytotoxicity. DNA damage and the resulting mutagenesis often are determined with the Ames test. The Ames test uses *Salmonella typhimurium* strains with specific mutations in the gene needed to synthesize histidine. These strains are treated with chemicals in the presence or absence of a metabolic activating system, usually the supernatant fraction from homogenized rat liver. If a compound is a mutagen in the Ames test, it reverts the mutation in the histidine operon and allows the bacteria to form colonies on plates with limited histidine. Gene chip microarrays assess gene expression in cells or tissues from animals treated with a toxicant and provide a very useful tool to identify the molecular targets and pathways altered by toxicant exposures. The susceptibility of knockout mice to a toxicant can help to determine whether the knocked-out genes are involved in the metabolic activation and detoxification of a given toxicant.

CARCINOGENS AND CHEMOPREVENTION

CARCINOGENESIS

The International Agency for Research on Cancer (IARC) classifies compounds into groups based on risk assessments using human, animal, and mechanism data. Chemicals in *group 1* are known human carcinogens; *group 2A* includes chemicals that probably are carcinogenic in humans; *group 2B* chemicals possibly are carcinogenic in humans; group *3 chemicals* lack data to suggest a role in carcinogenesis; and *group 4* are those with data indicating they are unlikely to be carcinogens. Table 67–1 presents information of some Group 1 carcinogens.

The transformation of a normal cell to a malignancy is a multi-stage process, and exogenous chemicals can act at 1 or more of these stages (Figure 67–2). A classic model of chemical carcinogenesis is tumor initiation followed by tumor promotion. A tumor initiator causes gene mutations that increase the ability of cells to proliferate and avoid apoptosis. A tumor promoter does not directly modify genes but changes signaling pathways and/or the extracellular environment to cause initiated cells to proliferate. Although this model is an oversimplification, it demonstrates the types of changes that must occur to transit a normal cell into tumorigenesis.

Chemical carcinogens cause cancer through genotoxic and non-genotoxic mechanisms (Figure 67–2). Genotoxic carcinogens induce tumor formation through damage to DNA. Typically, genotoxic carcinogens undergo metabolism in a target tissue to a reactive intermediate. This reactive intermediate can directly damage DNA via covalent reaction to form a DNA adduct. Alternatively, it can indirectly damage DNA through the formation of reactive oxygen species (ROS), which can oxidize DNA or form lipid peroxidation products that react with DNA. If DNA damage from a genotoxic carcinogen is not repaired prior to DNA replication, a mutation can result. If this mutation is in a key tumor suppressor gene or proto-oncogene, it provides advantages in proliferation or survival. Alternatively, if the mutation is in a DNA repair gene, the mutation increases the probability that other mutations will occur. Genotoxic carcinogens are tumor initiators.

Benzo[a]pyrene, a key carcinogen in tobacco smoke, is an example of a genotoxic carcinogen that forms both direct DNA adducts and ROS. Benzo[a]pyrene is oxidized by CYPs to a 7,8-dihydrodiol, which represents a proximate carcinogen (a more carcinogenic metabolite). This metabolite can either undergo a second oxidation step by a CYP to form a diol epoxide, which readily reacts with DNA, or it can undergo oxidation by aldo-keto reductases to form a catechol, which will redox cycle to form ROS.

Non-genotoxic carcinogens increase the incidence of cancer without damaging DNA. Many non-genotoxic carcinogens bind to receptors that stimulate proliferation or other tumor-promoting effects, such as tissue invasion or angiogenesis. For example, phorbol esters mimic diacylglycerol and activate PKC isoforms. This in turn stimulates MAP kinase pathways, leading to proliferation, invasiveness, and angiogenesis

Table 67–1

Examples of Important Carcinogens[a]

CARCINOGEN CLASS	EXAMPLE	SOURCE	MECHANISM
Genotoxic			
Nitrosamines	Nicotine-derived nitrosaminoketone (NNK)	Tobacco products	Metabolic activation to form DNA adducts
Polycyclic aromatic hydrocarbons	Benzo[a]pyrene	Fossil fuel combustion, tobacco smoke, charbroiled food	Metabolic activation to form DNA adducts or ROS
Aromatic amines	2-Aminonaphthalene	Dyes	Metabolic activation to form DNA adducts
Fungal toxins	Aflatoxin B_1	Corn, peanuts, and other food	Metabolic activation to form DNA adducts
Non-genotoxic			
Liver toxicants	Ethanol	Beverages, environment	Toxicity and compensatory proliferation; depletion of GSH
Phorbol esters	Tetradecanoyl phorbol acetate	Horticulture; rubber and gasoline production	Activation of PKC isoforms
Estrogens	Diethylstilbestrol	Drugs, environment	Activation of estrogen-receptor signaling
Metals	Arsenic	Environment, occupation	Inhibition of DNA repair; activation of signal transduction pathways
Irritants	Asbestos	Environment, occupation	Stimulation of inflammation; formation of ROS
Dioxins	TCDD	Waste incineration, herbicides, paper-pulp bleaching	Activation of the aryl hydrocarbon (Ah) receptor

TCDD, 2,3,7,8 tetrachlorodibenzo-p-dioxin; ROS, reactive oxygen species; GSH, glutathione; PKC, protein kinase C.
[a]Compounds in this table are classified as group 1 carcinogens by the International Agency for Research on Cancer (IARC), with the exception of the phorbol esters, which have not been examined.

(*see* Chapter 3). In most normal cells, prolonged activation of this pathway stimulates apoptosis, but cells with defective apoptotic mechanisms due to preceding mutation(s) are resistant to this effect. Estrogenic carcinogens activate estrogen receptor-α (ERα) and stimulate proliferation and invasiveness of estrogen responsive cells. Chronic inflammation is another mechanism of non-genotoxic carcinogenesis. Inflammatory cytokines stimulate PKC signaling, leading to proliferation, invasiveness, and angiogenesis. Irritants such as asbestos are examples of carcinogens that work through inflammation. Chronic exposure to hepatotoxic chemicals (or chronic liver diseases) also causes non-genotoxic carcinogenesis by stimulating compensatory proliferation to repair the liver damage. This damage and repair process increases the likelihood of DNA damage becoming a mutation, causes chronic inflammation, and selects for cells that proliferate faster or are less sensitive to apoptosis.

Tumor initiation also may occur through non-genotoxic mechanisms. For example, some heavy metals do not directly react with DNA but interfere with proteins involved in DNA synthesis and repair, increasing the likelihood that an error will be made during replication. Non-genotoxic carcinogens also can cause heritable changes to gene expression by altering the methylation state of cytosines in 5′-CpG-3 islands of gene promoters, thus acting as tumor initiators. Methylation can silence tumor suppressor genes, while demethylation of protooncogenes can increase their expression.

CHEMOPREVENTION

Drugs that interfere with the carcinogenic process to prevent cancer before it is diagnosed are termed *chemopreventive agents*. Chemoprevention strategies often are based on epidemiological

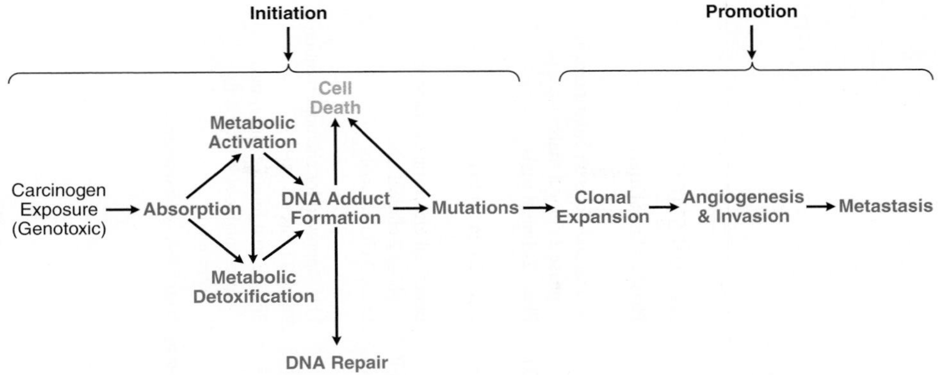

Figure 67–2 *Carcinogenesis: initiation and promotion.* There are many steps that occur between the exposure to a genotoxic carcinogen and the development of cancer. Processes in *red* lead to the development of cancer, while those in *green* reduce the risk. Non-genotoxic carcinogens act by enhancing steps leading to cancer and/or inhibiting protective processes. A chemopreventive agent acts by inhibiting steps leading to cancer or by increasing protective processes.

studies of nutrition, where there are many examples of clear protective effects of plant-based foods and drinks on the incidence of various types of cancer. A number of compounds for the prevention of cancer are in clinical trials (Table 67–2). There currently are no drugs approved for chemoprevention of environmental carcinogenesis, but there are approved drugs to prevent carcinogenesis due to endogenous estrogen (tamoxifen and raloxifene) and viruses (hepatitis B and human papillomavirus vaccines).

Chemopreventive agents interfere with the processes of initiation and promotion (*see* Figure 67–2). One mechanism of anti-initiation is prevention of carcinogen activation. Isothiocyanates and similar compounds inhibit CYPs involved in activating many carcinogens and also upregulate genes controlled by the antioxidant response element (ARE); the ARE-responsive group includes γ-glutamylcysteine synthase light chain (the gene responsible for the rate-determining step in GSH synthesis) and quinone reductase (NQO1). Increased expression of ARE-regulated genes is predicted to increase the detoxification of proximate carcinogens. Isothiocyanates also stimulate apoptosis of p53-deficient cells via the formation of cytotoxic DNA adducts. Compounds that act as antioxidants may provide protection because many carcinogens work through the generation of ROS. Some compounds simultaneously prevent carcinogen activation and act as antioxidants. For example, flavonoids and other polyphenols found in a wide variety of plants are potent antioxidants that inhibit CYPs and induce expression of ARE-regulated genes. Chlorophyll and other compounds can protect against carcinogens by binding to or reacting with carcinogens or their metabolites and prevent them from reaching their molecular target.

Inflammation is a potential target for chemoprevention through interference with promotion. The COX-2 inhibitor celecoxib has demonstrated efficacy at reducing the risk of colorectal cancer. However, this benefit was offset by an increased risk of death due to cardiovascular events, forcing the early termination of the trial. Studies examining long-term treatment with aspirin for cardiovascular benefits found that aspirin also reduces the incidence of colorectal adenomas. Natural compounds, such as α-tocopherol, also can exert chemoprevention by reducing inflammation.

One successful approach to chemoprevention is modification of nuclear receptor signaling. Promising preliminary data suggested that retinoids might be beneficial for preventing lung and other cancers. The selective ER modulators tamoxifen and raloxifene reduce the incidence of breast cancer in high-risk women and are approved for chemoprevention in these patients.

AFLATOXIN B_1. Promising agents are being developed as chemopreventants of hepatocarcinogenesis mediated by aflatoxin B_1. Aflatoxins are produced by *Aspergillus flavus*, a fungus that is a common contaminant of foods, especially corn, peanuts, cottonseed, and tree nuts. *A. flavus* is abundant in regions with hot and wet climates.

ADME. Aflatoxin B_1 is readily absorbed from the GI tract and initially distributed to the liver, where it undergoes extensive first-pass metabolism. Aflatoxin B_1 is metabolized by CYPs, including 1A2 and 3A4, to yield either an 8,9-epoxide or products hydroxylated at the 9 position (aflatoxin M_1) or 3 position

Table 67–2

Chemopreventive Agents Being Studied in Humans

CHEMOPREVENTIVE CLASS	EXAMPLE COMPOUND	NATURAL SOURCE OR TYPE OF DRUG	CANCER TYPE(S)	MECHANISM	CURRENT STATUS
Isothiocyanates	Phenethyl isothiocyanate	Cruciferous vegetables	Liver, lung, breast, etc.	↓CYP, ↑GSH, ↑NQO1, ↑apoptosis	Phase 2 clinical trials
Synthetic drugs that modify metabolism	Oltipraz	Anti-schistosomal drug	Liver, lung	↓CYP, ↑GSH, ↑NQO1	Beneficial effects on biomarkers in phase 2 clinical trials
Flavonoids and other polyphenols	Catechin	Green tea, red wine, berries, etc.	Lung, cervical, etc.	↓ROS, ↓CYP, ↑GSH, ↑NQO1	Phase 2 clinical trials
Other plant compounds	Curcumin	Turmeric (curry)	Colorectal, pancreatic, etc.	↓ROS, ↓CYP, ↑GSH, ↑NQO1	Phase 2 clinical trials
Other plant compounds	Chlorophyllin	All plants	Liver	Reaction with active intermediates, ↓ROS, ↓CYP	Beneficial effects on biomarkers in phase 2 clinical trials
Other antioxidants	α-Tocopherol (vitamin E)	Food	Prostate	Antioxidant, anti-inflammatory	Phase 3 clinical trials
Anti-hormonal therapies	Tamoxifen	Adjuvant for breast cancer	Breast	Inhibit ERα in breast	FDA-approved for chemoprevention
NSAIDs (*see* Chapter 34)	Aspirin	Anti-inflammatory drugs	Colorectal, etc.	Inhibit PG formation	Phase 3 trials
COX-2 selective inhibitors (*see* Chapter 34)	Celecoxib	Anti-inflammatory drugs	Colorectal, etc.	Inhibit PG formation	Phase 3 trial found ↓cancer but unacceptable side effects for prevention

CYP, cytochrome P450; GSH, glutathione; NQO1, quinone reductase; ROS, reactive oxygen species; ERα, estrogen receptor-α; NSAIDs, nonsteroidal anti-inflammatory drugs; COX-2, cyclooxygenase-2; PG, prostaglandin.

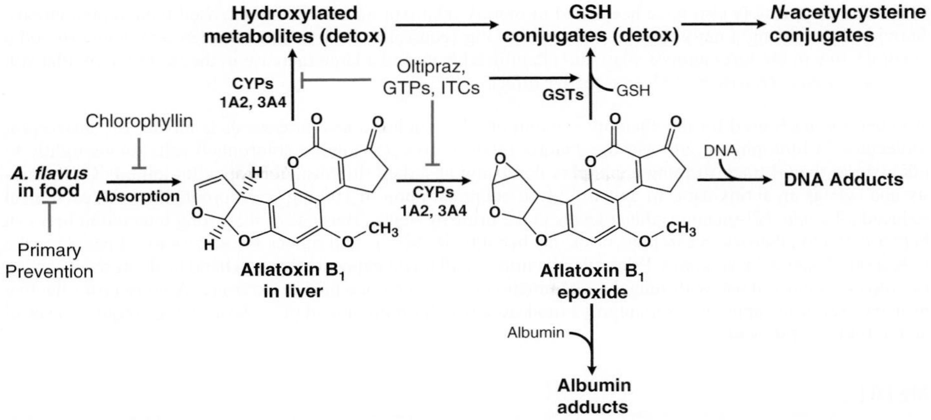

Figure 67–3 *Metabolism and actions of aflatoxin B_1.* Following ingestion and absorption of food containing *A. flavus*, aflatoxin B_1 undergoes activation by CYPs to its 8,9-epoxide, which can be detoxified by glutathione S-transferases (GSTs) or by spontaneous hydration. Alternatively, it can react with cellular macromolecules such as DNA and protein, leading to toxicity and cancer. Oltipraz, green tea polyphenols (GTPs), and isothiocyanates (ITCs) decrease aflatoxin carcinogenesis by inhibiting the CYPs involved aflatoxin activation and increasing the synthesis of GSH for GSTs involved in detoxification.

(aflatoxin Q_1; Figure 67–3). The hydroxylation products are less susceptible to epoxidation and are therefore detoxification products. The 8,9-epoxide is highly reactive toward DNA and is the reactive intermediate responsible for aflatoxin carcinogenesis. The 8,9-epoxide is short lived and undergoes detoxification via nonenzymatic hydrolysis or conjugation with GSH. Aflatoxin M_1 enters the circulation and is excreted in urine and milk. Hydroxylated aflatoxin metabolites also can undergo several additional phase 1 and phase 2 metabolic pathways prior to excretion in urine or bile.

Toxicity. Aflatoxin B_1 primarily targets the liver, although it also is toxic to the GI tract and hematological system. High-dose exposures result in acute necrosis of the liver, leading to jaundice and, in many cases, death. Acute toxicity from aflatoxin is relatively rare in humans and requires consumption of milligram quantities of aflatoxin per day for multiple weeks. Chronic exposure to aflatoxins results in cirrhosis of the liver and immunosuppression.

Carcinogenicity. Based on increased incidence of hepatocellular carcinoma in humans exposed to aflatoxin and supporting animal data, IARC has classified aflatoxin B_1 and several other natural aflatoxins as known human carcinogens (group 1). Aflatoxin exposure and hepatitis B virus work synergistically to cause hepatocellular carcinoma. Separately, aflatoxin or hepatitis B exposure increases the risk of hepatocellular carcinoma 3.4- or 7.3-fold, respectively; those exposed to both have a 59-fold increased risk of cancer compared to unexposed individuals. Aflatoxin primarily forms DNA adducts at deoxyguanosine residues, reacting at either the N1 or N7 position. The N7-guanine adduct mispairs with adenine, leading to G → T transversions. Human aflatoxin exposure is associated with hepatocellular carcinomas bearing an AGG to AGT mutation in codon 249 of the p53 tumor suppressor gene, resulting in the replacement of an arginine with cysteine.

The interaction between aflatoxin and hepatitis B that is responsible for the increased incidence of hepatocellular carcinoma is not well understood. Hepatitis B influences the metabolism of aflatoxin B_1 by upregulating CYPs, including 3A4, and decreasing glutathione S-transferase activity. In addition, hepatocellular proliferation to repair damage done by hepatitis B infection increases the likelihood that aflatoxin-induced DNA adducts will cause mutations. The hepatotoxic and tumor-promoting effects of hepatitis B also could provide a more favorable environment for the proliferation and invasion of initiated cells.

Chemoprevention of Aflatoxin-Induced Hepatocellular Carcinoma. Inhibiting CYP activity or increasing glutathione conjugation will reduce the intracellular concentration of the 8,9-epoxide and thus prevent DNA adduct formation. One drug that has been tested as a modifier of aflatoxin metabolism is oltipraz. Oltipraz, an anti-schistosomal drug, potently inhibits CYPs and induces genes regulated by the ARE. Oltipraz increases the excretion of aflatoxin *N*-acetylcysteine, indicating enhanced glutathione conjugation of the epoxide. At 500 mg/wk, oltipraz reduced the levels of aflatoxin M_1, consistent with inhibition of CYP activity.

Green tea polyphenols also have been used to modify aflatoxin metabolism in exposed human populations. Individuals receiving a daily dose of 500 or 1000 mg (equivalent to 1 or 2 L of green tea) demonstrated a small decline in the formation of aflatoxin–albumin adducts and a large increase in the excretion of aflatoxin *N*-acetylcysteine, consistent with a protective effect.

Another approach used for the chemoprevention of aflatoxin hepatocarcinogenesis is the use of "interceptor molecules." Chlorophyllin, an over-the-counter mixture of water-soluble chlorophyll salts, binds tightly to aflatoxin in the GI tract, forming a complex that is not absorbed. In vitro, chlorophyllin inhibits CYP activity and acts as an antioxidant. In a phase 2 trial, administration of 100 mg of chlorophyllin with each meal reduced aflatoxin–N7-guanine adduct levels in the urine by >50%. Because of the strong interaction between hepatitis B and aflatoxin in carcinogenesis, the hepatitis B vaccine will reduce the sensitivity of people to the induction of cancer by aflatoxin. Primary prevention of aflatoxin exposure through hand or fluorescent sorting of crops to remove those with fungal contamination can also reduce human exposure. A more cost-effective primary prevention approach is to improve food storage to limit the spread of *A. flavus*, which requires a warm and humid environment.

METALS

Arsenic, *lead*, and *mercury* are the top 3 substances of concern due to their toxicity and likelihood of human exposure as listed under the Comprehensive Environmental Response, Compensation, and Liability Act (CERCLA, also known as Superfund).

Many of the toxic metals in the environment also are carcinogens (Table 67–3). In addition, several essential metals also are toxic under conditions of overdose. Copper and especially iron are associated with toxicities, primarily targeting the liver through generation of ROS.

Not listed in Table 67–3 is the metal gold, which has its own uses and toxicities. Among heavy metals, perhaps only gold is addictive: gold has been used for centuries for relief of the itching palm, and many cannot get enough of its influence.

Table 67–3

Toxic Metals with Frequent Environmental or Occupational Exposure[a]

METAL	CERCLA PRIORITY	COMMON SOURCE OF EXPOSURE	ORGAN SYSTEMS MOST SENSITIVE TO TOXICITY	IARC CARCINOGEN CLASSIFICATION
As	1	Drinking water	CV, skin, multiple other	Group 1, carcinogenic to humans—liver, bladder, lung
Pb	2	Paint, soil	CNS, blood, CV, renal	Group 2A, probably carcinogenic
Hg	3	Air, food	CNS, renal	Group 2B, possibly carcinogenic ($MeHg^+$); group 3, not classifiable (Hg^0, Hg^{2+})
Cd	7	Occupational, food, smoking	Renal, respiratory	Group 1, carcinogenic to humans—lung (Cd, Cr^{6+}, Be)
Cr^{6+}	18	Occupational	Respiratory	
Be	42	Occupational, water	Respiratory	
Co	49	Occupational, food, water	Respiratory, CV	Group 2B, possibly carcinogenic
Ni	53	Occupational	Respiratory, skin (allergy)	Group 1, carcinogenic (soluble Ni compounds); group 2B, possibly carcinogenic (metallic Ni)—lung

CERCLA, Comprehensive Environmental Response, Compensation, and Liability Act.
[a]The Agency for Toxic Substances and Disease Registry (ATSDR) has both detailed monographs and brief summaries for each of these compounds, available at http://www.atsdr.cdc.gov. The International Agency for Research on Cancer (IARC) also has monographs available at http://monographs.iarc.fr.

LEAD. Chronic exposure of populations to even very low levels of lead (Pb) has major deleterious effects that are only now beginning to be understood.

Exposure. Until late in the 20th century, the potential for exposure to Pb was high. In the U.S., paint containing Pb for use in and around households was banned in 1978, while the use of tetraethyl lead in gasoline was eliminated in 1996. Despite these bans, past use of lead carbonate and lead oxide in paint and tetraethyl lead in gasoline remain the primary sources of Pb exposure. Pb is not degradable and remains throughout the environment in dust, soil, and the paint of older homes. Young children often are exposed to lead by nibbling sweet-tasting paint chips or eating dust and soil in and around older homes. Renovation or demolition of older buildings may cause substantial Pb exposure. Removal of Pb from gasoline caused Pb levels in air pollution to drop by >90% between 1982 and 2002. Acidic foods and beverages dissolve Pb when stored in containers with Pb in their glaze or lead-soldered cans. Pb exposure also has been traced to other sources such as lead toys, non-Western folk medicines, cosmetics, retained bullets, artists' paint pigments, ashes and fumes from painted wood, jewelers' wastes, home battery manufacture, and lead type. The CDC recommends screening of children at 6 months of age and the use of aggressive Pb abatement for children with blood Pb levels >10 μg/dL.

Chemistry and Mode of Action. Divalent lead is the primary environmental form; inorganic tetravalent Pb compounds are not naturally found. Organo-Pb complexes primarily occur with tetravalent Pb and include the gasoline additive tetraethyl lead. Pb toxicity results from molecular mimicry of other divalent metals, principally zinc and calcium. Because of its size and electron affinity, Pb alters protein structure and can inappropriately activate or inhibit protein function.

Absorption, Distribution, and Excretion. Pb exposure occurs through ingestion or inhalation. Children absorb a much higher percentage of ingested Pb (~40% on average) than adults (<20%). Absorption of ingested Pb is drastically increased by fasting. Dietary calcium or iron deficiencies increase Pb absorption, suggesting that Pb is absorbed through divalent metal transporters. The absorption of inhaled Pb generally is much more efficient (~90%). Tetraethyl Pb is readily absorbed through the skin; transdermal absorption is not a route of exposure for inorganic Pb.

About 99% of Pb in the bloodstream binds to hemoglobin. Pb initially distributes in the soft tissues, particularly in the tubular epithelium of the kidney and the liver. Over time, Pb is redistributed and deposited in bone, teeth, and hair. About 95% of the adult body burden of Pb is found in bone. Growing bones will accumulate higher levels of Pb and can form lead lines visible by radiography. Bone Pb is very slowly reabsorbed into the bloodstream. Small quantities of Pb accumulate in the brain. Pb readily crosses the placenta. Pb is excreted primarily in the urine. The concentration of Pb in urine is directly proportional to its concentration in plasma. Pb is excreted in milk and sweat and deposited in hair and nails. The serum $t_{1/2}$ of Pb is 1-2 months, with a steady state achieved in ~6 months. Pb accumulates in bone, where its $t_{1/2}$ is estimated at 20-30 years.

Health Effects. The nervous, hematological, cardiovascular, and renal systems are the most sensitive.

Neurotoxic Effects. The biggest concerns with low-level Pb exposure are cognitive delays and behavior changes in children. Pb interferes with the pruning of synapses, neuronal migration, and the interactions between neurons and glial cells. Together, these alterations in brain development result in decreased IQ, poor performance on exams, and behavioral problems such as distractibility, impulsivity, short attention span, and inability to follow even simple sequences of instructions. Because different areas of the brain mature at different times, the neurobehavioral changes vary between children, depending on the timing of the Pb exposure. Children with very high Pb levels (>70 μg/dL) are at risk for encephalopathy. Symptoms of lead-induced encephalopathy include lethargy, vomiting, irritability, anorexia, and vertigo, which can progress to ataxia, delirium, and eventually coma and death. Mortality rates for lead-induced encephalopathy are ~25%, and most survivors develop long-term sequelae such as seizures and severe cognitive deficits.

Encephalopathy in adults requires blood Pb levels >100 μg/dL. The symptoms are similar to those observed with children. Pb induces degeneration of motor neurons, usually without affecting sensory neurons. Studies in older adults have shown associations between Pb exposure and decreased performance on cognitive function tests. The neurodevelopmental effects of Pb primarily result from inhibition of Ca^{2+} transporters and channels and altered activities of Ca^{2+} responsive proteins, including PKC and calmodulin. These actions limit the normal activation of neurons caused by Ca^{2+} release and cause inappropriate production and/or release of neurotransmitters. At high concentrations, lead causes disruption of membranes, including the blood-brain barrier, increasing their permeability to ions. This effect is likely responsible for encephalopathy.

Cardiovascular and Renal Effects. Elevated blood pressure is a lasting effect of lead exposure. Lead exposure also is associated with an increased risk of death due to cardiovascular and cerebrovascular disease. In the kidney, even low-level Pb exposure (blood levels <10 μg/dL) depresses glomerular filtration. Higher levels (>30 μg/dL) cause proteinuria and impaired transport, while very high levels (>50 μg/dL) cause permanent physical damage, including proximal tubular nephropathy and glomerulosclerosis. The cardiovascular effects of Pb are thought to involve the production of ROS through an unknown mechanism. Pb also forms inclusion bodies with various proteins, including metallothionein, in the kidney. The formation of these bodies essentially chelates the Pb and appears to be protective.

Hematological Effects. Chronic Pb intoxication is associated with hypochromic microcytic anemia, which is observed more frequently in children and is morphologically similar to Fe-deficient anemia. The anemia is thought to result from both decreased erythrocyte life span and inhibition of several enzymes involved in heme synthesis, which is observed at very low lead levels (*see* Figures 67–4 and 67–5). Pb also causes both immunosuppression and increased inflammation, primarily through changes in helper T-cell and macrophage signaling.

GI Effects. Pb affects the smooth muscle of the gut, producing intestinal symptoms that are an early sign of high-level exposure to the metal. The abdominal syndrome often begins with a persistent metallic taste, mild anorexia, muscle discomfort, malaise, headache, and constipation (or occasionally, diarrhea). As intoxication advances, symptoms worsen and include intestinal spasms and pain (lead cholic). Intravenous calcium gluconate can relieve this pain.

Carcinogenesis. IARC recently upgraded Pb to "probably carcinogenic in humans" (group 2A). Epidemiological studies have shown associations between lead exposure and cancers of the lung, brain, kidney, and stomach. Rodents exposed to Pb develop kidney tumors, and some rats develop gliomas. Pb is not mutagenic but increases clastogenic events. Pb carcinogenesis may result from inhibition of DNA binding zinc-finger proteins, including those involved in DNA repair and synthesis. Pb is a good example of a non-genotoxic carcinogen.

Treatment. The most important response to Pb poisoning is removal of the source of exposure. Supportive measures should be undertaken to relieve symptoms. Chelation therapy is warranted for children and adults with high blood Pb levels (>45 μg/dL and >70 μg/dL, respectively) and/or acute symptoms of Pb poisoning. Although chelation therapy is effective at lowering blood Pb levels and relieving immediate symptoms, it does not reduce the chronic effects of Pb beyond the benefit of abatement alone.

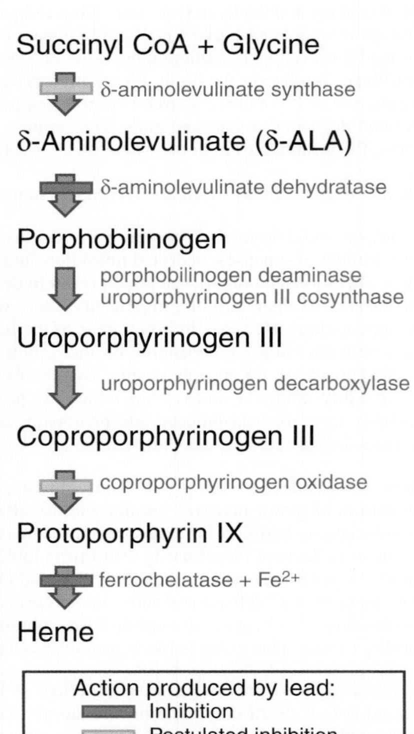

Figure 67–4 *Actions of lead on heme biosynthesis.*

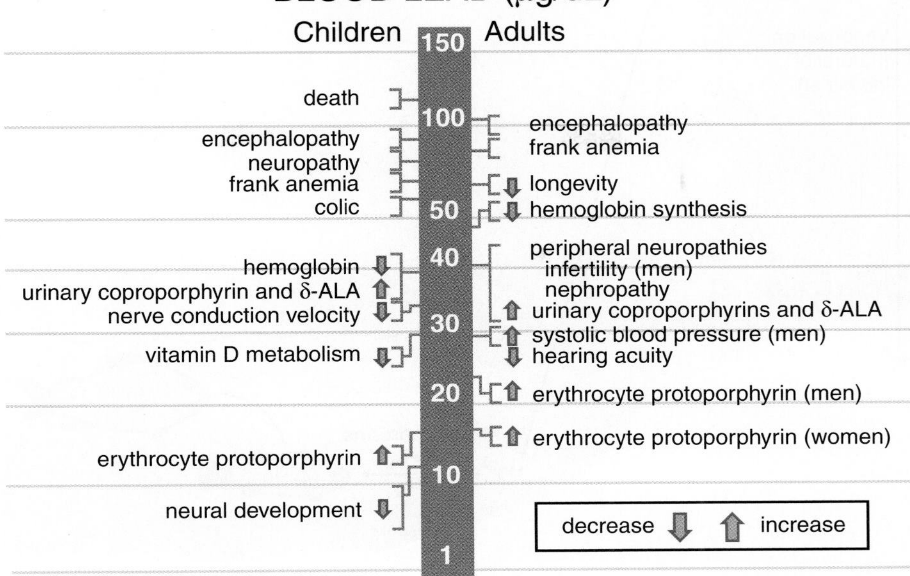

Figure 67–5 *Blood levels of lead and manifestations of in children and adults.* δ-ALA, δ-aminolevulinate.

MERCURY. Mercury (Hg) has been used industrially since ancient Greece due to its capacity to amalgamate with other metals. Mercury also was used as a therapeutic drug for several centuries. Its use for the treatment of syphilis inspired Paracelsus's observation that "the dose makes the poison," one of the central concepts of toxicology, and also gave rise to the cautionary expression, "A night with Venus, a year with Mercury." The phrase "mad as a hatter" originated from the exposure of hatters to metallic Hg vapor during production of felt for hats using mercury nitrate.

Exposure. Hg vapor is released naturally into the environment through volcanic activity and off-gassing from soils. Hg also enters the atmosphere through human activities such as combustion of fossil fuels. Once in the air, metallic mercury is photo-oxidized to inorganic mercury, which can then be deposited in aquatic environments in rain. Microorganisms can then conjugate inorganic mercury to form methyl mercury. Methyl mercury concentrates in lipids and will bioaccumulate up the food chain so that concentrations in aquatic organisms at the top of the food chain, such as swordfish or sharks, are quite high (Figure 67–6).

The primary source of exposure to metallic Hg in the general population is vaporization of Hg in dental amalgam. There also is limited exposure through broken thermometers and other Hg-containing devices. Human exposure to organic Hg primarily is through the consumption of fish. Workers are exposed to metallic and inorganic mercury, most commonly though exposure to vapors. The highest risk for exposure is in the chloralkali industry (i.e., bleach) and in other chemical processes in which Hg is used as a catalyst. Hg is a component of many devices, including alkaline batteries, fluorescent bulbs, thermometers, and scientific equipment, and exposure occurs during the production of these devices. Dentists also are exposed to Hg from amalgam. Hg can be used to extract gold during mining. Mercuric salts are used as pigments in paints.

Thimerosal is an antimicrobial agent used as a preservative in some vaccines. Its use is controversial because it releases ethyl mercury, which is chemically similar to methyl mercury. Some have argued that thimerosal might contribute to autism; however, studies have not found an association between thimerosal use in vaccines and negative health outcomes. Nonetheless, with the exception of some influenza (flu) vaccines, thimerosal is no longer used as a preservative in routinely recommended childhood vaccines.

Chemistry and Mode of Action. There are 3 general forms of Hg of concern to human health. *Metallic*, or *elemental, mercury* (Hg^0) is the liquid metal found in thermometers and dental amalgam; it is quite volatile, and exposure is often to the vapor. *Inorganic mercury* can be either monovalent (mercurous, Hg^{1+}) or divalent (mercuric, Hg^{2+}) and forms a variety of salts. *Organic mercury* compounds consist of divalent mercury

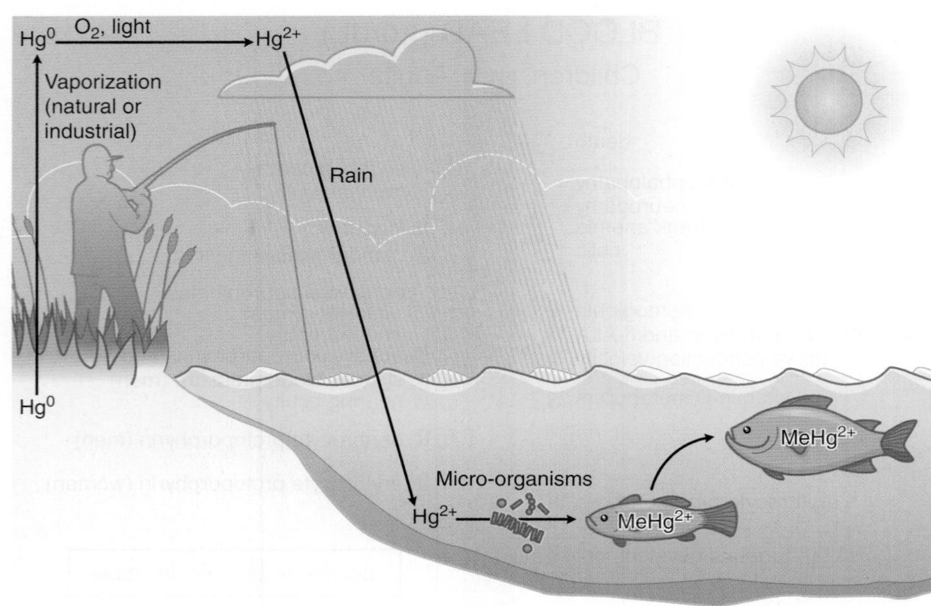

Figure 67–6 *Mobilization of mercury in the environment.* Metallic mercury (Hg^0) is vaporized from the Earth's surface both naturally and through human activities such as burning coal. In the atmosphere, Hg^0 is oxidized to form divalent inorganic mercury (Hg^{2+}), which falls to the surface in rain. Aquatic bacteria can methylate Hg^{2+} to form methyl mercury ($MeHg^+$). $MeHg^+$ in plankton is consumed by fish. Because of its lipophilicity, $MeHg^+$ bioaccumulates up the food chain.

complexed with 1 or occasionally 2 alkyl groups. The organic mercury compound of most concern is methyl mercury ($MeHg^+$), which is formed environmentally from inorganic Hg by aquatic microorganisms. Both Hg^{2+} and $MeHg^+$ readily form covalent bonds with sulfur, an interaction that accounts for most of the biological effects of mercury. At very low concentrations, Hg reacts with sulfhydryl residues on proteins and disrupts their functions. There also may be an autoimmune component to Hg toxicity.

ADME. Hg^0 vapor is readily absorbed through the lungs (~70-80%), but GI absorption of elemental (liquid) Hg is negligible. Absorbed Hg^0 distributes throughout the body and crosses membranes such as the blood-brain barrier and the placenta via diffusion. Hg^0 is oxidized by catalase in the erythrocytes and other cells to form Hg^{2+}. Some Hg^0 is eliminated in exhaled air. After a few hours, distribution and elimination of Hg^0 resemble the properties of Hg^{2+}. Hg^0 vapor also is oxidized to Hg^{2+} and retained in the brain.

GI absorption of Hg salts averages ~10-15% but varies with the individual patient and the particular salt. Hg^{1+} will form Hg^0 or Hg^{2+} in the presence of sulfhydryl groups. Hg^{2+} primarily is excreted in the urine and feces; a small amount also can be reduced to Hg^0 and exhaled. With acute exposure, the fecal pathway predominates, but following chronic exposure, urinary excretion becomes more important. All forms of Hg also are excreted in sweat and breast milk and deposited in hair and nails. The $t_{1/2}$ for inorganic Hg is ~1-2 months. Orally ingested $MeHg^+$ is almost completely absorbed from the GI tract. $MeHg^+$ readily crosses the blood-brain barrier and the placenta and distributes fairly evenly to the tissues, although concentrations are highest in the kidneys. $MeHg^+$ can be demethylated to form inorganic Hg^{2+}. The liver and kidney exhibit the highest rates of demethylation, but this also occurs in the brain. $MeHg^+$ is excreted in the urine and feces, with the fecal pathway dominating. The $t_{1/2}$ for $MeHg^+$ is ~2 months. Complexes between $MeHg^+$ and cysteine resemble methionine and can be recognized by transporters for that amino acid and taken across membranes.

Health Effects

Metallic Mercury. Inhalation of high levels of Hg vapor over a short duration is acutely toxic to the lung. Respiratory symptoms start with cough and tightness in the chest and can progress to interstitial pneumonitis and severely compromised respiratory function. Other initial symptoms include weakness, chills, metallic taste, nausea, vomiting, diarrhea, and dyspnea. Acute exposure to high doses of Hg also is toxic to the CNS (Figure 67–7).

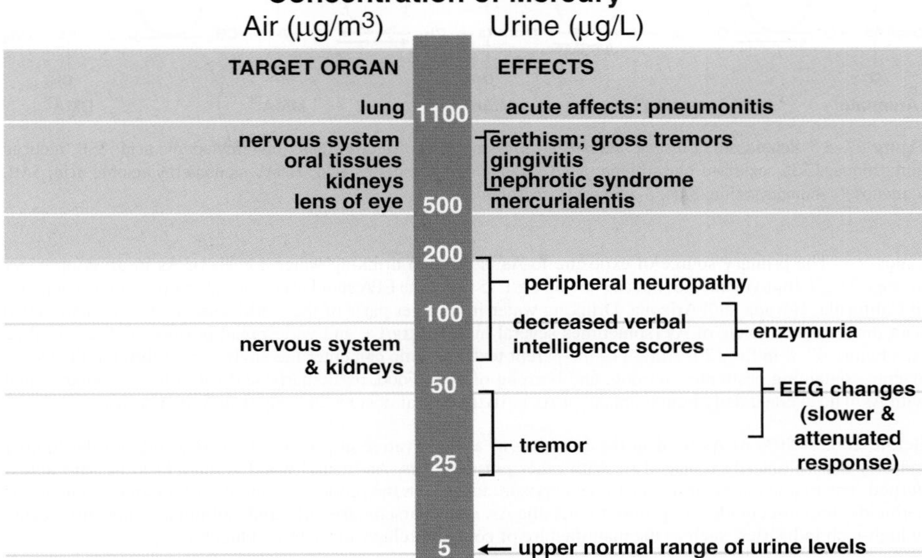

Figure 67–7 *Concentrations of mercury in air and urine are associated with specific toxic effects.*

Toxicity to the nervous system is the primary concern with chronic exposure to Hg vapor. Symptoms include tremors (particularly of the hands), emotional lability (irritability, shyness, loss of confidence, and nervousness), insomnia, memory loss, muscular atrophy, weakness, paresthesia, and cognitive deficits. These symptoms intensify and become irreversible, with increases in duration and concentration of exposure. Other common symptoms of chronic Hg exposure include tachycardia, labile pulse, severe salivation, gingivitis, and kidney damage.

Inorganic Salts of Mercury. Ingestion of Hg^{2+} salts is intensely irritating to the GI tract, leading to vomiting, diarrhea, and abdominal pain. Acute exposure to Hg^{2+} salts (typically in suicide attempts) leads to renal tubular necrosis, resulting in decreased urine output and often acute renal failure. Chronic exposures also target the kidney.

Organic Mercury. The CNS is the primary target of methyl mercury toxicity. Symptoms of methyl mercury exposure include visual disturbances, ataxia, paresthesia, fatigue, hearing loss, slurring of speech, cognitive deficits, muscle tremor, movement disorders, and, following severe exposure, paralysis and death. Children exposed in utero can develop severe symptoms, including mental retardation and neuromuscular deficits, even in the absence of symptoms in the mother.

Treatment. With exposure to metallic Hg, termination of exposure is critical and respiratory support may be required. Emesis may be used within 30-60 min of exposure to inorganic Hg, provided the patient is awake and alert and there is no corrosive injury. Maintenance of electrolyte balance and fluids is important for patients exposed to inorganic Hg. Chelation therapy is beneficial in patients with acute inorganic or metallic Hg exposure. There are limited treatment options for methyl mercury. Chelation therapy does not provide clinical benefits, and several chelators potentiate the toxic effects of methyl mercury. Nonabsorbed thiol resins may be beneficial by preventing reabsorption of methyl mercury from the GI tract.

Because of the conflicting effects of mercury and ω-3 fatty acids, there is considerable controversy regarding the restriction of fish intake in women of reproductive age and children. The EPA recommends limiting fish intake to 12 oz (2 meals) per week. Many experts feel this recommendation is too conservative, and the FDA is considering revising their recommendation to state that the benefits of fish consumption outweigh the risks. The recommendation that women consume fish that is lower in Hg content (i.e., canned light tuna, salmon, pollock, catfish) and avoid top predators, such as swordfish, shark, and tilefish, is not controversial.

ARSENIC. Arsenic (As) is a metalloid that is common in rocks and soil. The use of arsenic in drugs has been mostly phased out, but arsenic trioxide (ATO) is still used as an effective chemotherapy agent for acute promyelocytic leukemia (*see* Chapter 61).

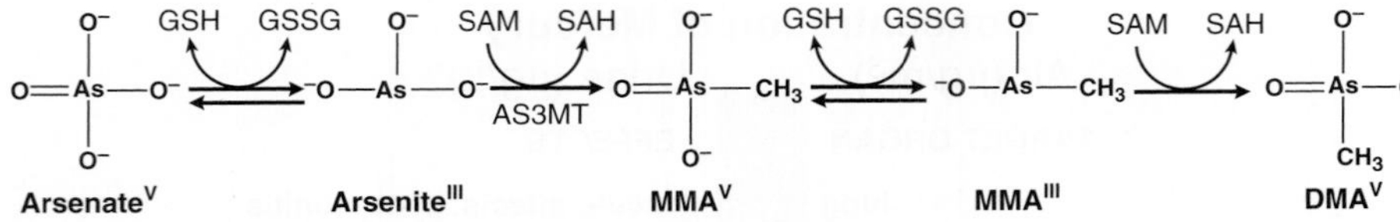

GSH GSSG SAM SAH GSH GSSG SAM SAH

AS3MT

Arsenate^{V} Arsenite^{III} MMA^{V} MMA^{III} DMA^{V}

Figure 67–8 *Metabolism of arsenic.* AS3MT, arsenite methyltransferase; DMA^{V}, dimethylarsinic acid; GSH, reduced glutathione; GSSG, oxidized glutathione; MMA^{III}, monomethylarsonous acid; MMA^{V}, monomethylarsonic acid; SAH, *S*-adenosyl-L-homocysteine; SAM, *S*-adenosyl-L-methionine.

Exposure. The primary source of exposure to As is through drinking water. Levels of As in drinking water average 2 μg/L (ppb) in the U.S. but can be >50 μg/L (5 times the EPA standard) in private well water, particularly in California, Nevada, and Arizona. Drinking water from other parts of the world sometimes is contaminated with much higher levels of As (sometimes several hundred μg/L), and widespread poisonings have resulted (*see* Figure 67–8 in the 12th edition of the parent text). Arsenic can enter the environment through the use of arsenic-containing pesticides, mining, and burning of coal. Food, particularly seafood, often is contaminated with As. The average daily human intake of As is 10 μg/day, almost exclusively from food and water.

Before 2003, >90% of As used in the U.S. was as a preservative in pressure-treated wood, but the lumber industry has voluntarily replaced As with other preservatives. As-treated wood is thought to be safe unless burned. The major source of occupational exposure to As is in the production and use of organic arsenicals as herbicides and insecticides. Exposure to metallic As, arsine, arsenic trioxide, and gallium arsenide also occurs in high-tech industries, such as the manufacture of computer chips and semiconductors.

Chemistry and Mode of Action. Arsenic exists in its elemental form and trivalent (arsenites/arsenious acid) and pentavalent (arsenates/As acid) states. Arsine is a gaseous hydride of trivalent As that exhibits toxicities that are distinct from other forms. The toxicity of a given arsenical is related to the rate of its clearance from the body and its ability to concentrate in tissues. In general, toxicity increases in the sequence: organic arsenicals < As^{5+} < As^{3+} < arsine gas (AsH_3). Like mercury, trivalent arsenic compounds form covalent bonds with sulfhydryl groups. The pyruvate dehydrogenase system is particularly sensitive to inhibition by trivalent arsenicals because the 2 sulfhydryl groups of lipoic acid react with As to form a 6-membered ring. Inorganic arsenate (pentavalent) inhibits the electron transport chain. It is thought that arsenate competitively substitutes for phosphate during the formation of ATP, forming an unstable arsenate ester that is rapidly hydrolyzed.

ADME. Poorly water-soluble forms such as arsenic sulfide, lead arsenate, and arsenic trioxide are not well absorbed. Water-soluble As compounds are readily absorbed from both inhalation and ingestion. GI absorption of As dissolved in drinking water is >90%. At low doses, As is fairly evenly distributed throughout the tissues of the body. Nails and hair, due to their high sulfhydryl content, exhibit high concentrations of As. After an acute high dose (i.e., fatal poisoning), As is preferentially deposited in the liver and, to a lesser extent, kidney, with elevated levels also observed in the muscle, heart, spleen, pancreas, lungs, and cerebellum. Arsenic readily crosses the placenta and blood-brain barrier.

Arsenic undergoes biotransformation in humans and animals (*see* Figure 67–8). Trivalent compounds can be oxidized to pentavalent compounds, but there is no evidence for demethylation of methylated arsenicals. Humans excrete much higher levels of monomethyl-As (MMA) compounds than most other animals. The trivalent methylated arsenicals are more toxic than inorganic arsenite, due to an increased affinity for sulfhydryl groups; formation of MMA^{III} now is considered a bioactivation pathway. Elimination of arsenicals by humans primarily is in the urine, although some is also excreted in feces, sweat, hair, nails, skin, and exhaled air. Compared to most other toxic metals, arsenic is excreted quickly ($t_{1/2}$ = 1-3 days). In humans, ingested inorganic As in urine is a mixture of 10-30% inorganic arsenicals, 10-20% monomethylated forms, and 60-80% dimethylated forms.

Health Effects. With the exception of arsine gas, the various forms of inorganic As exhibit similar toxic effects. Inorganic As exhibits a broad range of toxicities and has been associated with effects on every organ system tested. Acute exposure to large doses of As (>70-180 mg) often is fatal. Death immediately following arsenic poisoning typically is the result of its effects on the heart and GI tract. Death sometimes occurs later as a result of As's combined effect on multiple organs.

Cardiovascular System. Acute and chronic As exposure cause myocardial depolarization, cardiac arrhythmias, and ischemic heart disease; these are known side effects of As trioxide for the treatment of leukemia. Chronic exposure to As causes peripheral vascular disease, the most dramatic example of which is "blackfoot disease," a condition characterized by cyanosis of the extremities, particularly the feet, progressing to gangrene. Arsenic dilates capillaries and increases their permeability, causing edema, an effect likely responsible for peripheral vascular disease following chronic exposure.

Skin. Dermal symptoms often are diagnostic of As exposure. Arsenic induces hyperkeratinization of the skin (including formation of multiple corns or warts), particularly of the palms of the hands and the soles of the feet. It also causes areas of hyperpigmentation interspersed with spots of hypopigmentation. These symptoms can be observed in individuals exposed to drinking water with As concentrations of at least 100 μg/L and are typical in those chronically exposed to much higher levels. Hyperpigmentation can be observed after 6 months of exposure; hyperkeratinization takes years. Children are more likely to develop these effects than adults.

GI Tract. Acute or subacute exposure to high-dose As by ingestion causes GI symptoms ranging from mild cramping, diarrhea, and vomiting to GI hemorrhaging and death. GI symptoms are caused by increased capillary permeability, leading to fluid loss. At higher doses, fluid forms vesicles that can burst, leading to inflammation and necrosis of the submucosa and then rupture of the intestinal wall. GI symptoms are not observed with chronic exposure to lower levels of As.

Nervous System. The most common neurological effect of acute or subacute As exposure is peripheral neuropathy involving both sensory and motor neurons. This effect is characterized by the loss of sensation in the hands and feet, often followed by muscle weakness. Neuropathy occurs several days after exposure and can be reversible following cessation of exposure, although recovery usually is not complete. Arsenic exposure may cause intellectual deficits in children. Acute high-dose As exposure causes encephalopathy in rare cases, with symptoms that can include headache, lethargy, mental confusion, hallucination, seizures, and coma.

Other Non-Cancer Toxicities. Acute and chronic As exposures induce anemia and leukopenia, likely via direct cytotoxic effects on blood cells and suppression of erythropoiesis. Arsenic also may inhibit heme synthesis. and cause fatty infiltrations, central necrosis, and cirrhosis in the liver. Arsenic can cause severe kidney damage. Inhaled As is irritating to the lungs; ingested As may induce bronchitis progressing to bronchopneumonia in some individuals. Chronic exposure to As is associated with an increased risk of diabetes.

Carcinogenesis. In regions with very high As levels in drinking water, there are substantially higher rates of skin cancer, bladder cancer, and lung cancer. There also are associations between As exposure and other cancers, including liver, kidney, and prostate tumors. IARC classifies arsenic as "carcinogenic to humans (group 1)." Humans exposed to As in utero and in early childhood have an elevated risk of lung cancer.

Arsenic does not directly damage DNA; rather, As is thought to work through changes in gene expression, DNA methylation, inhibition of DNA repair, generation of oxidative stress, and/or altered signal transduction pathways. In humans, exposure to As potentiates lung tumorigenesis (5-fold increase) from tobacco smoke. Arsenic co-carcinogenesis may involve inhibition of proteins involved in nucleotide excision repair. Arsenic also has endocrine-disrupting activities on several nuclear steroid hormone receptors, enhancing hormone-dependent transcription at very low concentrations and inhibiting it at slightly higher levels.

Arsine Gas. Arsine gas is a rare cause of industrial poisonings. Arsine induces rapid and often fatal hemolysis, which probably results from arsine combining with hemoglobin and reacting with O_2. A few hours after exposure, patients can develop headache, anorexia, vomiting, paresthesia, abdominal pain, chills, hemoglobinuria, bilirubinemia, and anuria. Jaundice appears after 24 h. Arsine induces renal toxicities that can progress to kidney failure. Fatality results in ~25% of cases of arsine exposure.

Treatment. Following acute exposure to As, stabilize the patient and prevent further absorption of the poison. Close monitoring of fluid levels is important because As can cause fatal hypovolemic shock. Chelation therapy is effective following short-term exposure to As but has very little or no benefit in chronically exposed individuals. Exchange transfusion to restore blood cells and remove As often is warranted following arsine gas exposure.

CADMIUM. Cadmium (Cd) is used in electroplating, galvanization, plastics, paint pigments, and Ni-Cd batteries.

Exposure. Exposure to Cd is through food (estimated average daily intake, μg/day) and tobacco (1 cigarette contains 1-2 μg of Cd). Workers in metal-processing industries can be exposed to high levels of Cd, particularly by inhalation.

Chemistry and Mode of Action. Cd exists as a Cd^{++} and does not undergo oxidation-reduction reactions. The mechanism of Cd toxicity is not fully understood. Like lead and other divalent metals, Cd can replace zinc in zinc-finger domains of proteins and disrupt them. Cd induces formation of ROS, resulting in lipid peroxidation and glutathione depletion, upregulates inflammatory cytokines, and may disrupt the beneficial effects of NO.

Absorption, Distribution, and Excretion. Cd is not well absorbed from the GI tract (1.5-5%) but is better absorbed via inhalation (~10%). Cd primarily distributes first to the liver and later the kidney, with those 2 organs accounting for 50% of the absorbed dose. Little Cd crosses the blood-brain barrier or the placenta. Cd primarily is excreted in the urine and exhibits a $t_{1/2}$ of 10-30 years.

Toxicity. Acute Cd toxicity primarily is due to local irritation along the absorption route. Inhaled Cd causes respiratory tract irritation with severe, early pneumonitis accompanied by chest pains, nausea, dizziness, and diarrhea. Toxicity may progress to fatal pulmonary edema. Ingested Cd induces nausea, vomiting, salivation, diarrhea, and abdominal cramps; the vomitus and diarrhea often are bloody. Cd bound to metallothionein is transported to the kidney, where it can be released. The initial toxic effect of Cd on the kidney is increased excretion of small-molecular-weight proteins, especially β_2 microglobulin and retinol-binding protein. Cd also causes glomerular injury and decreased filtration. Chronic occupational exposure to Cd is associated with an increased risk of renal failure and death. Cd levels consistent with normal dietary exposure also can cause renal toxicity. Workers with long-term inhalation exposure to Cd exhibit decreased lung function. Symptoms initially include bronchitis and fibrosis of the lung, leading to emphysema. Chronic obstructive pulmonary disease increases mortality in Cd-exposed workers. When accompanied by vitamin D deficiency, Cd exposure increases the risks for fractures and osteoporosis, possibly due to interference with renal Ca^{2+} and phosphate regulation.

Carcinogenicity. Chronic occupational exposure to inhaled Cd increases the risk of developing lung cancer. Cd causes chromosomal aberrations in exposed workers and human cells. It also increases mutations and impairs DNA repair in human cells. Cd substitutes for zinc in DNA repair proteins and polymerases and may inhibit nucleotide excision repair, base excision repair, and the DNA polymerase responsible for repairing single-strand breaks. Cd also may alter cell signaling pathways and disrupts cellular controls of proliferation. Cd acts as a non-genotoxic carcinogen.

Treatment. Patients suffering from inhaled Cd may require respiratory support. Patients suffering from kidney failure due to Cd poisoning may require a transplant. Chelation therapy following Cd poisoning has no clinical benefits and may result in adverse effects.

CHROMIUM. Chromium (Cr) is an industrially important metal used in a number of alloys, particularly stainless steel (at least 11% chromium). Cr can be oxidized to multiple valence states, with the trivalent (Cr^{III}) and hexavalent (Cr^{VI}) forms being the 2 of biological importance. Chromium exists almost exclusively as the trivalent form in nature, and Cr^{III} is an essential metal involved in the regulation of glucose metabolism. Cr^{VI} is thought to be responsible for the toxic effects of Cr.

Exposure. Exposure to Cr in the general population primarily is through the ingestion of food, although there also is exposure from drinking water and air. Workers are exposed to Cr during chromate production, stainless steel production and welding, Cr plating, ferrochrome alloy and chrome pigment production, and in tanning industries. Exposure usually is to a mixture of Cr^{III} and Cr^{VI}.

Chemistry and Mode of Action. Cr occurs in its metallic state or in any valence state between divalent and hexavalent. Cr^{III} is the most stable and common form. Cr^{VI} is corrosive and is readily reduced to lower valence states. The primary reason for the different toxicological properties of Cr^{III} and Cr^{VI} is thought to be differences in their absorption and distribution. Cr^{VI} resembles sulfate and phosphate and can be taken into the cell by anion transporters where it undergoes a series of reduction steps, ultimately forming Cr^{III}, which causes most of the toxic effects. Cr^{III} readily interacts covalently with DNA. Cr^{VI} also induces oxidative stress and hypersensitivity reactions.

ADME. Smaller particles are better deposited in the lungs. Absorption into the bloodstream of hexavalent and soluble forms is higher than the trivalent or insoluble forms, with the remainder often retained in the lungs. Approximately 50-85% of inhaled Cr^{VI} particles (<5 μm) are absorbed. Absorption of ingested Cr is <10%. Cr^{VI} crosses membranes by facilitated transport; Cr^{III} crosses by diffusion. Cr^{VI} is distributed to all of the tissues and crosses the placenta. The highest levels are attained in the liver, kidney, and bone; Cr^{VI} also is retained in erythrocytes. Excretion primarily is through urine, with small amounts excreted in bile and breast milk and deposited in hair and nails. The $t_{1/2}$ of ingested Cr^{VI} is ~40 h; the $t_{1/2}$ of Cr^{III} is ~10 h.

Toxicity. Acute exposure to very high doses of Cr causes death via damage to multiple organs, particularly the kidney. Chronic low-dose Cr exposure causes toxicity at the site of contact. Thus, workers exposed to inhaled Cr develop symptoms of lung and upper respiratory tract irritation, decreased pulmonary function, and pneumonia. Chronic exposure to Cr via ingestion causes symptoms of GI irritation (e.g., oral ulcer, diarrhea, abdominal pain, indigestion, and vomiting). Cr^{VI} is a dermal irritant and can cause ulceration or burns. Some individuals develop allergic dermatitis following dermal exposure to Cr. Cr-sensitized workers often also develop asthma.

Carcinogenicity. Cr^{VI} compounds are known human carcinogens (group 1). There is insufficient evidence for carcinogenesis from metallic and Cr^{III} (group 3). Workers exposed to Cr^{VI} via inhalation have elevated incidence of and mortality from lung and nasal cancer. Environmental exposure to Cr^{VI} in drinking water increases the risk of developing stomach cancer. There are multiple potential mechanisms for Cr^{VI} carcinogenicity. Reduction of Cr^{VI} to Cr^{III} within the cell occurs with concomitant oxidation of cellular molecules.

Cr^{III} forms a large number of covalent DNA adducts, primarily at the phosphate backbone. The DNA adducts are not very mutagenic and are repaired by nucleotide excision repair. It is thought that the high level of nucleotide excision repair activity following Cr^{VI} exposure contributes to carcinogenesis, either by preventing repair of mutagenic lesions formed by other carcinogens or through the formation of single-strand breaks due to incomplete repair. Cr also forms toxic cross-links between DNA and protein. Chronic inflammation due to Cr-induced irritation also may promote tumor formation.

Treatment. There are no standard protocols for treatment of acute Cr poisoning. One approach that has shown promise in rodents is the use of reductants such as ascorbate, glutathione, or *N*-acetylcysteine to reduce Cr^{VI} to Cr^{III} after exposure but before absorption to limit bioavailability. These compounds and EDTA also increase urinary excretion of Cr after high-dose, particularly if given soon enough. Exchange transfusion to remove Cr from plasma and erythrocytes may be beneficial.

TREATMENT OF METAL EXPOSURE

The most important response to environmental or occupational exposures to metals is to eliminate the source of the exposure. It also is important to stabilize the patient and provide symptomatic treatment.

Treatment for acute metal intoxications often involves the use of chelators. A chelator is a compound that forms stable complexes with metals, typically as 5- or 6-membered rings. The ideal chelator would have the following properties: *high solubility in water, resistance to biotransformation, ability to reach sites of metal storage, ability to form stable and nontoxic complexes with toxic metals, and ready excretion of the metal-chelator complex*. A low affinity for the essential metals Ca and Zn also is desirable, because toxic metals often act through competition with these metals for protein binding. The structures of the most commonly used chelators are shown in Figure 67–9.

In cases of acute exposure to high doses of most metals, chelation therapy reduces toxicity. However, following chronic exposure, chelation therapy does not show clinical benefits beyond those of cessation of exposure alone and, in some cases, does more harm than good. Chelation therapy may increase the neurotoxic effects of heavy metals and is recommended only for acute poisonings.

ETHYLENEDIAMINETETRAACETIC ACID (EDTA). EDTA and its various salts are effective chelators of divalent and trivalent metals. Calcium disodium EDTA ($CaNa_2EDTA$) is the preferred EDTA salt for metal poisoning, provided that the metal has a higher affinity for EDTA than Ca^{2+}. $CaNa_2EDTA$ is effective for the treatment of acute lead poisoning, particularly in combination with dimercaprol, but is not an effective chelator of Hg or As in vivo.

Chemistry and Mechanism of Action. Accessible metal ions with a higher affinity for $CaNa_2EDTA$ than Ca^{2+} will be chelated, mobilized, and usually excreted. Because EDTA is charged at physiological pH, it does not significantly penetrate cells. $CaNa_2EDTA$ mobilizes several endogenous metallic cations, including those of Zn, Mn, and Fe. Additional supplementation with Zn following chelation therapy may be beneficial. The most common therapeutic use of $CaNa_2EDTA$ is for acute lead intoxication. $CaNa_2EDTA$ does not provide clinical benefits for the treatment of chronic lead poisoning.

$CaNa_2EDTA$ is available as edetate calcium disodium (calcium disodium versenate). Intramuscular administration of $CaNa_2EDTA$ results in good absorption, but pain occurs at the injection site; consequently, the chelator injection often is mixed with a local anesthetic or administered intravenously. For intravenous use, $CaNa_2EDTA$ is diluted in either 5% dextrose or 0.9% saline and is administered slowly by intravenous drip. A dilute solution is necessary to avoid thrombophlebitis. To minimize nephrotoxicity, adequate urine production should be established prior to and during treatment with $CaNa_2EDTA$. However, in patients with lead encephalopathy and increased intracranial pressure, excess fluids must be avoided, and intramuscular administration of $CaNa_2EDTA$ is recommended.

ADME. Less than 5% of $CaNa_2EDTA$ is absorbed from the GI tract. After intravenous administration, $CaNa_2EDTA$ has a $t_{1/2}$ of 20-60 min. In blood, $CaNa_2EDTA$ is found only in the plasma; it is excreted in the urine by glomerular filtration. Altering either the pH or the rate of urine flow has no effect on the rate of excretion. There is very little metabolic degradation of EDTA. The drug is distributed mainly in the extracellular fluids; very little gains access to the spinal fluid (5% of the plasma concentration).

Toxicity. Rapid intravenous administration of Na_2EDTA causes hypocalcemic tetany. Slow infusion ($<$15 mg/min) elicits no symptoms of hypocalcemia in a normal individual because of the availability of extracirculatory stores of Ca^{2+}. $CaNa_2EDTA$ can be administered intravenously with no untoward effects because the change in the concentration of Ca^{2+} in the plasma and total body is negligible. The principal toxic

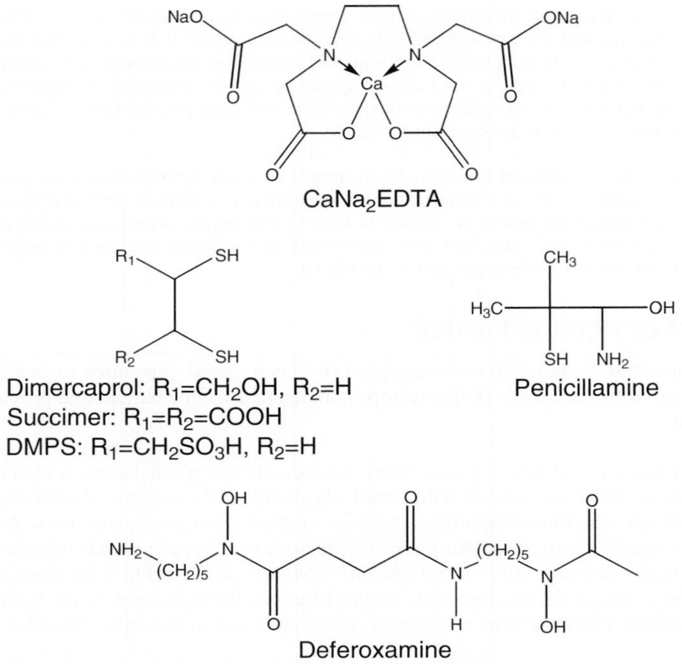

$CaNa_2EDTA$

Dimercaprol: $R_1=CH_2OH$, $R_2=H$
Succimer: $R_1=R_2=COOH$
DMPS: $R_1=CH_2SO_3H$, $R_2=H$

Penicillamine

Deferoxamine

Figure 67–9 *Structures of chelators commonly used to treat acute metal intoxication.* $CaNa_2EDTA$, calcium disodium ethylenediamine tetraacetic acid; DMPS, sodium 2,3-dimercapto-propane sulfonate.

effect of $CaNa_2EDTA$ is on the kidney, most likely due to chelation of essential metals, particularly Zn, in proximal tubular cells. The early renal effects usually are reversible with cessation of treatment. Other side effects associated with $CaNa_2EDTA$ include malaise, fatigue, excessive thirst followed by chills and fever and subsequent myalgia, frontal headache, anorexia, occasional nausea and vomiting, and rarely, increased urinary frequency and urgency. $CaNa_2EDTA$ is teratogenic in laboratory animals; it should be used in pregnant women only under conditions in which the benefits clearly outweigh the risks. Other undesirable effects include sneezing, nasal congestion, and lacrimation; glycosuria; anemia; dermatitis with lesions similar to those of vitamin B_6 deficiency; transitory lowering of systolic and diastolic blood pressures; prolonged prothrombin time; and T-wave inversion on the electrocardiogram.

DIMERCAPROL. Dimercaprol was developed during World War II as an antidote to lewisite, a vesicant arsenical war gas; hence its alternative name, British anti-Lewisite (BAL). Arsenicals form a stable and relatively nontoxic chelate ring with dimercaprol. Dimercaprol interacts with other heavy metals as well.

Chemistry and Mechanism of Action. The pharmacological actions of dimercaprol result from formation of chelation complexes between its sulfhydryl groups and metals. The sulfur–metal bond may be labile in the acidic tubular urine, which may increase the delivery of metal to renal tissue and increase toxicity. The dosage regimen should maintain a concentration of dimercaprol in plasma adequate to favor the continuous formation of the more stable 2:1 (BAL–metal) complex. However, because of pronounced and dose-related side effects, excessive plasma concentrations must be avoided. The concentration in plasma therefore must be maintained by repeated dosage until the metal is excreted. Dimercaprol is most beneficial when given very soon after exposure to the metal because it is more effective in preventing inhibition of sulfhydryl enzymes than in reactivating them. Dimercaprol limits toxicity from As, Au, and Hg, which form mercaptides with essential cellular sulfhydryl groups. It also is used in combination with $CaNa_2EDTA$ to treat Pb poisoning.

ADME and Therapeutic Use. Dimercaprol is given by deep intramuscular injection as a 100 mg/mL solution in peanut oil and should not be used in patients who are allergic to peanut products. Peak concentrations in blood are attained in 30-60 min. The $t_{1/2}$ is short, and metabolic degradation and excretion essentially are complete within 4 h. Dimercaprol and its chelates are excreted in both urine and bile. Dimercaprol is contraindicated following chronic exposures to heavy metals because it does not prevent neurotoxic effects., and should not be used in patients with hepatic insufficiency, except when this condition is a result of As poisoning.

Toxicity. Side effects occur in ~50% of subjects receiving 5 mg/kg intramuscularly. Dimercaprol causes an immediate rise in systolic and diastolic arterial pressures accompanied by tachycardia; these return to normal within 2 h. Dimercaprol also can cause anxiety, nausea and vomiting, headache, a burning sensation in the mouth and throat, a feeling of constriction in the throat and chest, conjunctivitis, blepharospasm, lacrimation, rhinorrhea, salivation, tingling of the hands, a burning sensation in the penis, sweating, abdominal pain, and the appearance of painful sterile abscesses at the injection site. The dimercaprol–metal complex breaks down easily in an acidic medium; production of alkaline urine protects the kidney during therapy. Children react similarly to adults, although ~30% also may experience a fever that disappears on drug withdrawal.

SUCCIMER. Succimer (2,3-dimercaptosuccinic acid [DMSA], CHEMET) is an orally effective chelator that is chemically similar to dimercaprol but contains 2 carboxylic acids that modify the spectrum of absorption, distribution, and chelation of the drug.

ADME. After absorption, succimer is biotransformed to a mixed disulfide with cysteine. Succimer lowers blood Pb levels and attenuates toxicity of Pb. The succimer–Pb chelate is eliminated in both urine and bile. The fraction eliminated in bile can undergo enterohepatic circulation. *Succimer has several desirable features over other chelators*. It is orally bioavailable, and because of its hydrophilic nature, it does not mobilize metals to the brain or enter cells. It also does not significantly chelate essential metals such as Zn, Cu, or Fe. Thus, succimer exhibits a better toxicity profile relative to other chelators. Succimer also is effective as a chelator of As, Cd, Hg, and other toxic metals.

Therapeutic Use. Succimer is approved for treatment of children with blood Pb levels >45 μg/dL. It also is used off label for the treatment of adults with Pb poisoning and As and Hg intoxication.

Toxicity. Succimer is much less toxic than dimercaprol. Commonly reported adverse effects are nausea, vomiting, diarrhea, and loss of appetite. Transient elevations in hepatic transaminases have been observed with succimer treatment. In a few patients, rashes necessitate discontinuation of therapy.

SODIUM 2, 3-DIMERCAPTOPROPANE SULFONATE (DMPS). DMPS is another dimercapto compound used for the chelation of heavy metals. DMPS is not approved by the FDA but is approved for use in Germany. DMPS is available from compounding pharmacies and is used by some doctors in the U.S.

Chemistry and Mode of Action. DMPS is a clinically effective chelator of Pb, As, and especially Hg. It is orally available and is rapidly excreted, primarily by the kidneys. It is negatively charged and exhibits distribution properties similar to those of succimer. DMPS is less toxic than dimercaprol but mobilizes Zn and Cu and thus is more toxic than succimer. There is evidence suggesting that DMPS might be effective for treatment of chronic heavy metal poisonings.

PENICILLAMINE; TRIENTINE. Penicillamine (CUPRIMINE, DEPEN) is an effective chelator of Cu, Hg, Zn, and Pb and promotes the excretion of these metals in the urine.

Penicillamine's chelating properties led to its use in patients with Wilson disease (excess body burden of Cu due to diminished excretion) and heavy-metal intoxications. Penicillamine is a more toxic and less potent and selective chelator of heavy metals than other chelation drugs; thus, it is not a first-line treatment for acute intoxication with Pb, Hg, or As. Because it is inexpensive and orally bioavailable, it often is given at low doses following treatment with $CaNa_2EDTA$ and/or dimercaprol to ensure that the concentration of metal in the blood stays low following the patient's release from the hospital.

ADME. Penicillamine is well absorbed (40-70%) from the GI tract. Food, antacids, and iron reduce its absorption. Peak plasma concentrations are obtained between 1 and 3 h. Penicillamine is relatively stable in vivo compared to its unmethylated parent compound cysteine. Hepatic biotransformation primarily is responsible for degradation of penicillamine, and very little drug is excreted unchanged. Metabolites are found in both urine and feces. *N*-Acetylpenicillamine is more effective than penicillamine in protecting against the toxic effects of Hg, presumably because it is more resistant to metabolism.

Therapeutic Use. Penicillamine is available for oral administration. For chelation therapy, the usual adult dose is 1-1.5 g/day in 4 divided doses, given on an empty stomach to avoid interference by metals in food. Penicillamine is used in Wilson disease, cystinuria, and rheumatoid arthritis (rarely). For the treatment of Wilson disease, 1-2 g/day usually is administered in 4 doses. The urinary excretion of Cu should be monitored to determine whether the dosage of penicillamine is adequate.

Toxicity. Penicillamine induces cutaneous lesions, including urticaria, macular or papular reactions, pemphigoid lesions, lupus erythematosus, dermatomyositis, adverse effects on collagen, dryness, and scaling. Cross-reactivity with penicillin may be responsible for some episodes of urticarial or maculopapular reactions with generalized edema, pruritus, and fever that occur in up to one-third of patients taking penicillamine. Hematological reactions include leukopenia, aplastic anemia, and agranulocytosis, which may be fatal. Renal toxicity is manifested as reversible proteinuria and hematuria, but it may progress to nephrotic syndrome with membranous glomerulopathy. Rare fatalities have been reported from Goodpasture syndrome. Although uncommon, severe dyspnea has been reported from penicillamine-induced bronchoalveolitis. Myasthenia gravis has been induced by long-term therapy. Penicillamine is a teratogen in animals, but for pregnant women with Wilson disease, the benefits outweigh the risks. Less serious side effects include nausea, vomiting, diarrhea, dyspepsia, anorexia, and a transient loss of taste for sweet and salt. Contraindications to therapy include pregnancy, renal insufficiency, or a previous history of penicillamine-induced agranulocytosis or aplastic anemia.

TRIENTINE. Penicillamine is the drug of choice for treatment of Wilson disease. Trientine (triethylenetetramine dihydrochloride, SYPRINE) is an acceptable alternative for patients who cannot tolerate penicillamine (see "Toxicity," above). Trientine drug is effective orally. Maximal daily doses of 2 g for adults or 1.5 g for children are taken in 2 to 4 divided portions on an empty stomach. Trientine may cause iron deficiency; this can be overcome with short courses of Fe therapy, but iron and trientine should not be ingested within 2 h of each other.

DEFEROXAMINE; DEFERASIROX; DEFERIPRONE. Deferoxamine (deferoxamine mesylate, DESFERAL) has high affinity for ferric iron ($K_a = 1031$) and a very low affinity for calcium ($K_a = 102$). It removes Fe from hemosiderin and ferritin and, to a lesser extent, from transferrin. Iron in hemoglobin or cytochromes is not removed by deferoxamine.

ADME and Therapeutic Use. Deferoxamine is poorly absorbed after oral administration, and parenteral administration is required. For severe Fe toxicity (serum Fe levels >500 μg/dL), the intravenous route is preferred. The drug is administered at 10-15 mg/kg/h by constant infusion. Rapid boluses usually are associated with hypotension. Deferoxamine may be given intramuscularly in moderately toxic cases (serum Fe 350-500 μg/dL) at a dose of 50 mg/kg with a maximum dose of 1 g. Hypotension also can occur with this route. For chronic Fe intoxication (e.g., thalassemia), an intramuscular dose of 0.5-1.0 g/day is recommended. Continuous subcutaneous administration (1-2 g/day) is almost as effective as intravenous administration. Deferoxamine is not recommended in primary hemochromatosis; phlebotomy is the treatment of choice. Deferoxamine also has been used for the chelation of aluminum in dialysis patients. Deferoxamine is metabolized by plasma enzymes and excreted in the urine.

Toxicity. Deferoxamine causes a number of allergic reactions, including pruritus, wheals, rash, and anaphylaxis. Other adverse effects include dysuria, abdominal discomfort, diarrhea, fever, leg cramps, and tachycardia. Occasional cases of cataract formation have been reported. Deferoxamine may cause neurotoxicity during long-term, high-dose therapy; both visual and auditory changes have been described. A "pulmonary syndrome" has been associated with high-dose (10-25 mg/kg/h) deferoxamine therapy; tachypnea, hypoxemia, fever, and eosinophilia are prominent symptoms. Contraindications include renal insufficiency and anuria; during pregnancy, deferoxamine should be used only if clearly indicated.

DEFERASIROX. Deferasirox (EXJADE) is FDA-approved for treatment of chronic Fe overload in patients receiving therapeutic blood transfusions. It is administered orally.

DEFERIPRONE. Deferiprone (FERRIPROX) is an oral Fe chelator FDA-approved for treatment of Fe overload in patients with thalassemia receiving therapeutic blood transfusions.

For a complete Bibliographical Listing see Goodman & Gilman's ***The Pharmacological Basis of Therapeutics***, 12th ed., or Goodman & Gilman Online at www.AccessMedicine.com.

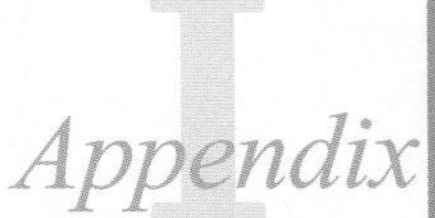

Appendix I Principles of Prescription Order Writing and Patient Compliance

LATIN NOT SPOKEN HERE

In writing prescriptions, use English (in the U.S.) or the dominant language of the patient. Latin is no longer the international language of medicine, but a number of commonly used abbreviations derive from obsolete Latin usage and persist in prescription writing. Avoid using them.

Some Latin seems firmly embedded in pharmacy practice. "Rx" is said to be an abbreviation for the Latin word *recipere*, meaning "take" or "take thus," as a direction to a pharmacist, preceding the physician's "recipe" for preparing a medication. The abbreviation "Sig" for the Latin *Signatura*, is used on the prescription to mark the directions for administration of the medication.

WHO CAN PRESCRIBE MEDICINES?

In many states in the U.S., healthcare practitioners other than M.D. and D.O. physicians can write prescriptions. Licensed physician's assistants (P.A.), nurse practitioners, pharmacists, and clinical psychologists can prescribe medications under various circumstances.

CURRENT PRACTICE

The prescription consists of the *superscription*, the *inscription*, the *subscription*, the *signa*, and the *name and signature of the prescriber*, all contained on a single form (Figure AI–1).

The *superscription* includes the date the prescription order is written; the name, address, weight, and age of the patient; and the Rx (*Take*). The body of the prescription, or *inscription*, contains the name and amount or strength of the drug to be dispensed, or the name and strength of each ingredient to be compounded.

The *subscription* is the instruction to the pharmacist, usually consisting of a short sentence such as: "dispense 30 tablets." The *signa* or "*Sig*" is the instruction for the patient as to how to take the prescription, interpreted and transposed onto the prescription label by the pharmacist. In the U.S., prescriptions should always be written in English. Many physicians continue to use Latin abbreviations; e.g., "1 cap tid pc," will be interpreted by the pharmacist as "take one capsule three times daily after meals." However, the use of Latin abbreviations for these directions only mystifies the prescription and is discouraged. The pharmacist should always write the label in English (or, as appropriate, in the language of the patient). The use of such abbreviations or symbols is a confounding practice; many serious dispensing errors can be traced to the use of abbreviations.

Avoid the instruction "take as directed." Such directions assume an understanding on the part of the patient that may not be realized, and are inadequate for the pharmacist, who must determine the intent of the physician before dispensing the medication. The best directions to the patient will include a reminder of the intended purpose of the medication by including such phrases as "for relief of pain" or "to relieve itching." The correct route of administration is reinforced by the choice of the first word of the directions. For an oral dosage form, the directions should begin with "take" or "give"; for externally applied products, the word "apply"; for suppositories, "insert"; and for eye, ear, or nose drops, "place" is preferable to "instill."

Include Patient Information and Dosage Calculations. The patient's name and address are needed on the prescription order to ensure that the correct medication goes to the proper patient and also for identification and recordkeeping. For medications whose dosage involves a calculation, a patient's pertinent factors, such as weight, age, or body surface area, also should be listed on the prescription; both the calculated dose and the dosage formula used, such as "240 mg every 8 hours (40 mg/kg/day)," should be included to allow another healthcare professional to double-check the prescribed dosage. Pharmacists always should recalculate dosage equations when filling such prescriptions. Medication orders in hospitals and some clinic settings, such as those for antibiotics or antiseizure medications that are sometimes difficult to adequately dose (e.g., phenytoin), can specify the patient diagnosis and desired drug and request dosing by the clinical pharmacist.

Proper Prescribing Practices Can Help to Prevent Adverse Drug Events. The Institute of Medicine (IOM) estimates that the annual number of medical errors in the U.S. resulting in death is between 44,000 and

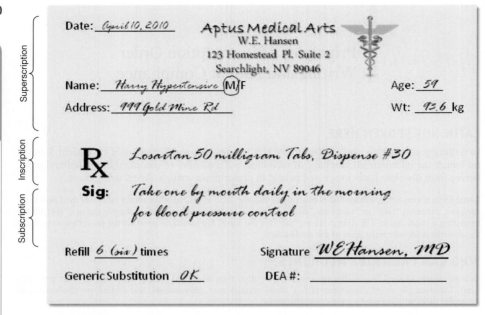

Superscription
Date: April 10, 2010
Aptus Medical Arts
W.E. Hansen
123 Homestead Pl. Suite 2
Searchlight, NV 89046
Name: Harry Hypertensive (M)/F Age: 59
Address: 999 Gold Mine Rd Wt: 95.6 kg

Inscription
Rx Losartan 50 milligram Tabs, Dispense #30

Subscription
Sig: Take one by mouth daily in the morning for blood pressure control

Refill 6 (six) times Signature WEHansen, MD
Generic Substitution OK DEA #:

Figure AI–1 *The prescription.* The prescription must be accurately and legibly prepared to identify the patient, the medication to be dispensed, and the mode of drug administration. Avoid abbreviations and Latin; they lead to dispensing errors. Include the therapeutic purpose in the subscription (e.g., *"for control of blood pressure"*) to prevent errors in dispensing. For example, the use of losartan *for the treatment of hypertension* may require 100 mg/day (1.4 mg/kg/day), whereas *for treatment of congestive heart failure*, the dose of this AngII receptor antagonist generally should not exceed 50 mg/day. Including the therapeutic purpose of the prescription also can assist patients in organizing and understanding their medications. Including the patient's weight on the prescription can be useful in avoiding dosing errors, particularly when drugs are administered to children.

98,000. Adverse drug events occur in ~3% of hospitalizations. Good practices (Table AI–1) can minimize these adverse drug events.

PROPER USE OF PRESCRIPTION PAD

All prescriptions should be written in ink; this practice is compulsory for schedule II prescriptions under the U.S. Controlled Substances Act (CSA) of 1970. Prescription pad blanks normally are imprinted with a heading that gives the name of the physician and the address and phone number of the practice site (Figure AI–1). When using institutional blanks that do not bear the physician's information, the physician always should print his or her name and phone number on the face of the prescription to facilitate communication with other healthcare professionals if questions arise. U.S. law requires that prescriptions for controlled substances include the name, address, and Drug Enforcement Administration (DEA) registration number of the physician.

The date of the prescription is an important part of the patient's medical record, and it can assist the pharmacist in recognizing potential problems. For example, when an opioid is prescribed for pain due to an injury, and the prescription is presented to a pharmacist 2 weeks after issuance, the drug may no longer be indicated. Compliance behavior also can be estimated using the dates when a prescription is filled and refilled. The CSA requires that all orders for controlled substances (Table AI–1) be dated as of, and signed on, the day issued and prohibits filling or refilling orders for substances in schedules III and IV >6 months after their date of issuance. When writing the original prescription, the physician should designate the number of refills allowed. For maintenance medications without abuse potential, it is reasonable to write for a 1-month supply and to mark the prescription form for refills to be dispensed over a period sufficient to supply the patient until the next scheduled visit to the physician. A statement such as "refill prn" (refill as needed) is not appropriate, as it could allow the patient to misuse the medicine or neglect medical appointments. If no refills are desired, "*zero*" (not "0") should be written in the refill space to prevent alteration of the prescriber's intent. Refills for controlled substances are discussed later, in "Refills" under "Controlled Substances."

Table AI–1

Prescribing Practices to Avoid Adverse Drug Events

- Write all orders legibly using metric measurements of weight and volume.
- Include patient age and weight on the prescription, when appropriate, so dosage can be checked.
- Use Arabic (decimal) numerals rather than Roman numerals (e.g., does "IL-II" mean "IL-11" or "IL-2"?); in some instances, it is preferable for numerals to be spelled out.
- Use leading zeros (0.125 milligrams, not .125 milligrams); never use trailing zeros (5 milligrams, not 5.0 milligrams).
- Avoid abbreviating drug names; abbreviations may lead to misinterpretation.
- Avoid abbreviating directions for drug administration; write out directions clearly in English.
- Be aware of possibilities for confusion in drug names. Some drug names sound alike when spoken and may look alike when spelled out. The U.S. Pharmacopeial Convention Medication Errors Reporting Program maintains a current list of 750 drug names that can be confused (www.usp.org). Alliterative drug names can be particularly problematic when giving verbal orders to pharmacists or other healthcare providers.
- Provide the patient's diagnosis on the prescription order to prevent dispensing errors based on sound-alike or look-alike drug names. For example, an order for administration of magnesium sulfate must not be abbreviated "MS," as this may result in administration of morphine sulfate. Including the therapeutic purpose and/or the patient's diagnosis can prevent this error.
- Write clearly. Both physician and pharmacist share in the responsibility for preventing adverse drug events by writing prescriptions clearly (*When in doubt, write it out!*) and questioning intent whenever an order is ambiguous (*When in doubt, check it out!*). *Pharmacists must clarify their concerns with prescribers, not patients.*
- Think.
- Think again.

Concern about the rising cost of healthcare has favored the dispensing of so-called generic drugs. A drug is called by its generic name (in the U.S., this is the U.S. Adopted Name or USAN) or the manufacturer's proprietary name, called the *trademark*, *trade name*, or *brand name*. In most U.S. states, pharmacists have the authority to dispense generic drugs rather than brand-name medications. The physician can request that the pharmacist not substitute a generic for a branded medication by indicating this on the prescription ("do not substitute"), although this generally is unnecessary because the U.S. Food and Drug Administration (FDA) requires that generic medications meet the same bioequivalence standards as their brand-name counterparts. In some jurisdictions, prescriptions may not be filled with a generic substitution unless specifically permitted on the prescription. Occasions when substituting generic medications is discouraged are limited to products with specialized release systems and narrow therapeutic indices, or when substantial patient confusion and potential noncompliance may be associated with substitution.

CHOICE AND AMOUNT OF DRUG PRODUCT DISPENSED

Inappropriate choice of drugs by physicians is a problem in prescribing. Physicians must rely on unbiased sources when seeking drug information that will influence their prescribing habits; use of the original medical literature will ensure instruction of the prescriber's best judgment. The amount of a drug to be dispensed should be clearly stated and should be only that needed by the patient. Excessive amounts should never be dispensed, because this not only is expensive for the patient but may lead to accumulation of medicines, which can lead to harm to the patient or members of the patient's family if used inappropriately. *Better to require several refills of a prescription than to prescribe and dispense more than necessary at one time.*

THE PRESCRIPTION AS A COMMODITY

Prescribers must be aware that patients may visit their doctor to "get" a prescription. Physicians must educate their patients about the importance of viewing medicines as to be used only when really needed and that remaining on a particular medicine when their condition is stable may be preferable to seeking the newest medications available. The Federal Food and Drug Administration Modernization Act of 1997 permits the use of print and television advertising of prescription drugs. The law requires that all drug advertisements contain (among other things) summary information relating to side effects, contraindications, and effectiveness. The benefits of these types of direct-to-consumer (DTC) advertising are controversial. Prescription drug advertising has alerted consumers to the existence of new drugs and the conditions they treat, but it has also increased consumer demand for drugs. This demand has increased the number of prescriptions being dispensed (raising sales revenues) and has contributed to the higher pharmaceutical costs borne by health insurers, government, and consumers. In the face of a growing demand for particular brand-name drugs driven by advertising, physicians and pharmacists must be able to counsel patients effectively and provide them with evidence-based drug information.

CONTROLLED SUBSTANCES

In the U.S., the DEA within the Department of Justice is responsible for the enforcement of the federal CSA. The DEA regulates each step of the handling of controlled substances from manufacture to dispensing (21 U.S.C. § 811). The law provides a system that is intended to prevent diversion of controlled substances from legitimate uses. Substances that come under the jurisdiction of the CSA are divided into 5 schedules (Table AI–2); individual states may have additional schedules. Physicians must be authorized to prescribe controlled substances by the jurisdiction in which they are licensed, and they must be registered with the DEA or exempted from registration as defined under the CSA. The number on the certificate of registration must be indicated on all prescription orders for controlled substances. Criminal prosecution and penalties for misuse generally depend on the schedule of a substance and the amount of drug in question.

State agencies may impose additional regulations, such as requiring that prescriptions for controlled substances be printed on triplicate or state-issued prescription pads or restricting the use of a particular class of drugs for specific indications. Some U.S. states, such as California, have placed marijuana, classified by the

Table AI–2

Controlled Substance Schedules

Schedule I (examples: heroin, methylene dioxymethamphetamine, lysergic acid diethylamide, mescaline, and all salts and isomers thereof):

1. High potential for abuse.
2. No accepted medical use in the U.S. or lacks accepted safety for use in treatment in the U.S. May be used for research purposes by properly registered individuals.

Schedule II (examples: morphine, oxycodone, fentanyl, meperidine, dextroamphetamine, cocaine, amobarbital):

1. High potential for abuse.
2. Has a currently accepted medical use in the U.S.
3. Abuse of substance may lead to severe psychological or physical dependence.

Schedule III (examples: anabolic steroids, nalorphine, ketamine, certain schedule II substances in suppositories, mixtures, or limited amounts per dosage unit):

1. Abuse potential less than substances in schedule I or schedule II.
2. Has a currently accepted medical use in the U.S.
3. Abuse of substance may lead to moderate to low physical dependence or high psychological dependence.

Schedule IV (examples: alprazolam, phenobarbital, meprobamate, modafinil):

1. Abuse potential less than substances in schedule III.
2. Has a currently accepted medical use in the U.S.
3. Abuse of substance may lead to limited physical or psychological dependence relative to substances in schedule III.

Schedule V (examples: buprenorphine, products containing a low dose of an opioid plus a non-narcotic ingredient such as cough syrup with codeine[a] and guaifenesin, anti-diarrheal tablets with diphenoxylate and atropine):

1. Low potential for abuse relative to schedule IV.
2. Has a currently accepted medical use in the U.S.
3. Some schedule V products may be sold in limited amounts without a prescription at the discretion of the pharmacist; however, if a physician wishes a patient to receive one of these products, it is preferable to provide a prescription.

[a]Although codeine is a schedule II drug, its dosage in cough syrups is regarded as sufficiently low to permit their classification as schedule V substances.

FDA as a schedule I substance, in a special category by decriminalizing its possession and sale for medical use. Under California's medical marijuana laws, patients and caregivers are exempt from prosecution by the state of California, contrary federal law notwithstanding. This legal difference of opinion between state and federal regulation is the source of considerable controversy. Generally, the most stringent law takes precedence, whether it is federal, state, or local.

PRESCRIPTION ORDERS FOR CONTROLLED SUBSTANCES. To be valid, a prescription for a controlled substance must be issued for a *legitimate medical purpose* by an *individual practitioner* acting in the *usual course of his or her professional practice.* An order that does not meet these criteria, is not considered a legitimate prescription within the meaning of the law, and thus does not protect either the physician who issued it or the pharmacist who dispensed it. Most states prohibit physicians from prescribing controlled substances for themselves; it is prudent to comply with this guideline even if it is not mandated by law.

EXECUTION OF THE ORDER. Prescriptions for controlled substances should be dated and signed on the day of their issuance and must bear the full name and address of the patient and the printed name, address, and DEA number of the practitioner and should be signed the way one would sign a legal document. Preprinted orders are not allowed in most states, and pre-signed blanks are prohibited by federal law. When oral orders are not permitted (schedule II), the prescription must be written with ink or typewritten. The order may be prepared by a member of the physician's staff, but the prescriber is responsible for the signature and any errors that the order may contain.

ORAL ORDERS. Prescriptions for schedule III, IV, and V medications may be telephoned to a pharmacy by a physician in the same manner as a prescription for a noncontrolled substance, although it is in the physician's best interest to keep his or her DEA number as private as possible (see "Preventing Diversion"). Schedule II prescriptions may be telephoned to a pharmacy only in *emergency* situations, i.e.:

- Immediate administration is necessary.
- No appropriate alternative treatment is available.
- It is not reasonably possible for the physician to provide a written prescription prior to the dispensing.

For an emergency prescription, the quantity must be limited to the amount adequate to treat the patient during the emergency period, and the physician must have a written prescription delivered to the pharmacy for that emergency within 72 h. If mailed, the prescription must be postmarked within 72 h. The pharmacist must notify the DEA if this prescription is not received.

REFILLS. No prescription order for a schedule II drug may be refilled under any circumstance. For schedule III and IV drugs, refills may be issued either orally or in writing, not to exceed 5 refills or 6 months after the issue date, whichever comes first. Beyond this time, a new prescription must be ordered. For schedule V drugs, there are no restrictions on the number of refills allowed, but if no refills are noted at the time of issuance, a new prescription must be made for additional drug to be dispensed.

PREVENTING DIVERSION. Prescription blanks often are stolen and used to sustain abuse of controlled substances. To prevent this type of diversion, prescription pads should be protected in the same manner as one would protect a personal checkbook. A prescription blank should never be pre-signed for a staff member to fill in at a later time. Also, a minimum number of pads should be stocked, and they should be kept in a locked, secure location. If a pad or prescription is missing, it should be reported immediately to local authorities and pharmacies. Ideally, the physician's full DEA number should not be pre-printed on the prescription pad, because most prescriptions will not be for controlled substances and will not require the registration number, and anyone in possession of a valid DEA number may find it easier to commit prescription fraud. Some physicians may intentionally omit part or all of their DEA number on a prescription and instead write "pharmacist call to verify" or "call for registration number." This practice works only when the pharmacist may independently verify the authenticity of the prescription, and patients must fill the prescription during the prescriber's office hours. Pharmacists can ascertain the authenticity of a physician's DEA number using an algorithm.

Another method employed by the drug seeker is to alter the face of a valid prescription to increase the number of units or refills. By spelling out the number of units and refills authorized instead of giving numerals, the prescriber essentially removes this option for diversion. Controlled substances should not be prescribed excessively or for prolonged periods, as the continuance of a patient's addiction is not a legitimate medical purpose.

DRUG STANDARDS AND CLASSIFICATION

The U.S. Pharmacopeial Convention, Inc. is a nongovernmental organization that disseminates authoritative standards and information on medicines and other healthcare technologies. This organization is home to the U.S. Pharmacopeia (USP), which, together with the FDA, the pharmaceutical industry, and health professions, establishes authoritative drug standards. These standards are enforceable by the FDA and the governments of other countries and are recognized worldwide. Drug monographs are published in the USP/National Formulary (USP-NF), the official drug standards compendia that organize drugs into categories based on pharmacological actions and therapeutic uses. The USP also provides chemical reference standards to carry out the tests specified in the USP-NF. For example, a drug to be manufactured and labeled in units must comply with the USP standard for units of that compound. Such standards are essential for agents possessing biological activity, such as insulin.

The USP also is home to the *USP Dictionary of U.S. Adopted Names (USAN) and International Drug Names*. This compendium is recognized throughout the healthcare industry as the authoritative dictionary of drugs. Entries include 1 or more of the following: U.S. Adopted Names, official drug names for the *National Formulary* (NF), previously used official names, International Nonproprietary Names, British Approved Names, Japanese Accepted Names, trade names, and other synonyms. In addition to names, the records in this file contain other substance information such as Chemical Abstract Service (CAS), registry number (RN), molecular formula, molecular weight, pharmacological and/or therapeutic category, drug sponsor, reference information, and structure diagram, if available. The USP maintains an electronic website that can be accessed for useful drug naming, classification, and standards information (www.usp.org).

In the U.S., drug products also are coded under the National Drug Code (NDC). In the U.S., the NDC serves as a universal product identifier for drugs used in humans. The current edition of the National Drug Code Directory is limited to prescription drugs and a few selected over-the-counter products. Each drug product listed under the Federal Food, Drug, and Cosmetic Act is assigned a unique 10-digit, 3-segment number. This number, known as the NDC number, identifies the labeler/vendor, product, and package size. The labeler/vendor code is assigned by the FDA. The second segment, the product code, identifies a specific strength, dosage form, and formulation for a particular drug company. The third segment, the package code, identifies package sizes. Both the product and package codes are assigned by the manufacturer. In addition to classification of drugs by therapeutic category, drugs also are grouped by control schedule. Drug schedules in the U.S. are listed in Table AI–2 and are discussed above under "Controlled Substances."

The FDA also categorizes drugs that may be used in pregnant women. These categories are similar to those used in other countries and provide guidance based on available science. The categories range from A to X, in increasing order of concern:

Pregnancy Category A: Adequate and well-controlled studies have failed to demonstrate a risk to the fetus in the first trimester of pregnancy (and there is no evidence of risk in later trimesters). Because of the obvious nature of the risk associated with the use of medications during gestation, the FDA requires a body of high-quality data on a drug before it can be considered for Pregnancy Category A.

Pregnancy Category B: Animal reproduction studies have failed to demonstrate a risk to the fetus, and there are no adequate and well-controlled studies in pregnant women, OR animal studies have shown an adverse effect, but adequate and well-controlled studies in pregnant women have failed to demonstrate a risk to the fetus in any trimester.

Pregnancy Category C: Animal reproduction studies have shown an adverse effect on the fetus, and there are no adequate and well-controlled studies in humans, but potential benefits may warrant use of the drug in pregnant women despite potential risks.

Pregnancy Category D: There is positive evidence of human fetal risk based on adverse reaction data from investigational or marketing experience or studies in humans, but potential benefits may warrant use of the drug in pregnant women despite potential risks.

Pregnancy Category X: Studies in animals or humans have demonstrated fetal abnormalities, and/or there is positive evidence of human fetal risk based on adverse reaction data from investigational or marketing experience, and the risks involved in use of the drug in pregnant women clearly outweigh potential benefits.

Physicians should realize that the pregnancy categories by themselves provide little guidance for the physician treating pregnant women. For example, angiotensin-converting enzyme (ACE) inhibitors such as captopril cause developmental toxicity (Category X) only after the first trimester. Physicians' primary responsibility remains treating the pregnant patient. However, the risks of withholding treatment to the mother because of possible risks to the fetus have to be considered as well.

Drugs also are grouped by their potential for misuse under British and U.N. legal classifications as class A, B, or C. The classes are linked to maximum legal penalties in a descending order of severity, from A to C.

COMPLIANCE

Compliance is the extent to which the patient follows a regimen prescribed by a healthcare professional. The patient is the final and most important determinant of how successful a therapeutic regimen will be and should be engaged as an active participant who has a vested interest in its success. Whatever term is used—*compliance*, *adherence*, *therapeutic alliance*, or *concordance*—physicians must promote a collaborative interaction between doctor and patient in which each brings an expertise that helps to determine the course of therapy. The patient's quality-of-life beliefs may differ from the clinician's therapeutic goals, and the patient will have the last word every time when there is an unresolved conflict.

Hundreds of variables that may influence compliance behavior have been identified. A few of the most frequently cited are discussed here, along with some suggestions for improving compliance, although none provides 100% compliance (Table AI–3).

Noncompliance may be manifest in drug therapy as intentional or accidental errors in dosage or schedule, overuse, underuse, early termination of therapy, or not having a prescription filled; therapeutic failures can result. Noncompliance always should be considered in evaluating potential causes of inconsistent or nonexistent response to therapy. The reported incidence of patient noncompliance usually is in the range of 30-60%; the rate for long-term regimens is ~50%.

THE PATIENT–PROVIDER RELATIONSHIP

Patient satisfaction with the physician has a significant impact on compliance behavior. Patients are more likely to follow instructions and recommendations when their expectations for the patient–provider relationship and for their treatment are met. These expectations include not only clinical but also interpersonal competence; thus, cultivating good interpersonal and communication skills is essential.

When deciding on a course of therapy, it can be useful to discuss a patient's habits and daily routine as well as the therapeutic options with the patient. This information may suggest cues for remembrance. A lack of information about a patient's lifestyle can lead to situations such as prescribing a medication to be taken with meals 3 times daily for a patient who only eats twice a day or a medication to be taken each morning for a patient who works a night shift and sleeps during the day. Rarely is there only 1 treatment option for a given problem, and it may be better to prescribe an adequate regimen that the patient will follow instead of an ideal regimen that the patient will not. Attempts should be made to resolve collaboratively any conflicts that may hinder compliance.

PATIENTS AND THEIR BELIEFS

Patients are more likely to be compliant when they *perceive* that they are susceptible to the disease, that the disease may have serious negative impact, that the therapy will be effective, and that the benefits outweigh

Table AI–3

Suggestions for Improving Patient Compliance

Provide respectful communication; ask how patient takes medicine.
Develop satisfactory, collaborative relationship between physician and patient; encourage pharmacist involvement.
Provide and encourage use of medication counseling.
Give precise, clear instructions, with most important information given first.
Support oral instructions with easy-to-read written information.
Simplify whenever possible.
Use mechanical compliance aids as needed (sectioned pill boxes or trays, compliance packaging, color-coding).
Use optimal dosage form and schedule for each individual patient.
Assess patient's literacy, language, and comprehension, and modify educational counseling as needed. Be culturally aware and sensitive. To improve compliance, don't rely on patient's own knowledge of disease alone.
Find solutions when physical or sensory disabilities are present (use nonsafety caps on bottles, use large type on labels and written material, place tape marks on syringes).
Enlist support and assistance from family and caregivers.
Use behavioral techniques such as goal setting, self-monitoring, cognitive restructuring, skills training, contracts, and positive reinforcement.

the costs, and when they believe in their own efficacy to execute the therapy. The *actual* severity of and susceptibility to an illness is not necessarily an issue; rather, the patient's perception of severity affects compliance. Patients' beliefs can lead them to deliberately alter their therapy, whether for convenience, for personal experiments, because of a desire to remove themselves from the sick role, as a means to exercise a feeling of control over their situation, or for other reasons. This reinforces the need for excellent communication and a good patient–provider relationship to facilitate the provision of additional or corrective education when the beliefs would suggest poor compliance as an outcome.

Pharmacists have a legal and professional responsibility to offer medication counseling and can educate and support patients by discussing prescribed medications and their use. Because they often see the patient more frequently than does the physician, pharmacists who take the time to inquire about a patient's therapy can help identify compliance and other problems, educate the patient, and notify the physician as appropriate. Indeed, data from the Asheville Project indicate that a pharmacist-based medication management program provides significant advantages with respect to compliance, health outcomes, and cost.

Elderly patients often face a number of barriers to compliance related to their age: increased forgetfulness and confusion; altered drug disposition and higher sensitivity to some drug effects; decreased social and financial support; decreased dexterity, mobility, or sensory abilities; and the use of a greater number of concurrent medicines (both prescription and over-the-counter) whose attendant toxicities and interactions may cause decreased mental alertness or intolerable side effects. There are drugs known to be inappropriate to prescribe to elderly patients and some that may adversely affect compliance. Despite these obstacles, evidence does not show that elderly patients in general are significantly less compliant than any other age group. Physicians must be careful in choosing medications for the elderly. Pharmacists must pay particular attention to thorough and compassionate counseling for elderly patients and should assist patients in finding practical solutions when problems, such as polypharmacy, are noted.

THE THERAPY

Increased complexity and duration of therapy are perhaps the best-documented barriers to compliance. The patient for whom multiple drugs are prescribed for a given disease or who has multiple illnesses that require drug therapy will be at higher risk for noncompliance, as will the patient whose disease is chronic. The frequency of dosing of individual medications also can affect compliance behavior. Simplification, whenever possible and appropriate, is desirable.

The effects of the medication can make adherence less likely, as in the case of patients whose medicines cause confusion or other altered mental states. Unpleasant side effects from the medicine may influence compliance in some patients but are not necessarily predictive, especially if patient beliefs or other positive factors tend to reinforce adherence to the regimen. A side effect that is intolerable to one patient may be of minor concern to another. The cost of medicine can be a heavy burden for patients with limited economic resources, and healthcare providers should be sensitive to this fact. Mobile phones and tablets running drug formulary/therapeutic applications can provide the costs of medications, as can physicians who are familiar with the patient's insurance plan. Mobile phone systems that provide reminders and collect patient response information are being introduced and may become more popular as patients and providers become increasingly tech savvy.

ELECTRONIC PRESCRIBING

The era of e-prescribing has begun. Computerized prescription ordering eliminates some of the subjective features of prescribing. Thus, if the proper information is entered correctly in the electronic system, medication errors due to illegible handwriting, incorrect dose, incorrect medication for medical condition, and drug interactions can be reduced, because each prescription can be linked to high-quality drug databases that check that the information on the prescription is appropriate for the patient (e.g., age, weight, gender, condition, laboratory values, disease being treated, concurrent medications) and that known warnings and potential problems are brought to the attention of the physician, pharmacist, and patient. Such systems must not be used as a substitute for personal attention to the individual patient by healthcare workers but, rather, as an adjunct measure that ensures safe, high-quality, efficient care.

For a complete Bibliographical Listing see Goodman & Gilman's ***The Pharmacological Basis of Therapeutics***, 12th ed., or Goodman & Gilman Online at www.AccessMedicine.com.

Index

Page numbers followed by *f* and *t* denote figures and tables, respectively.

INDEX

D

INDEX

F

G

INDEX

M

INDEX

N

O

S

INDEX